RADIATION ONCOLOGY
IMAGING AND TREATMENT

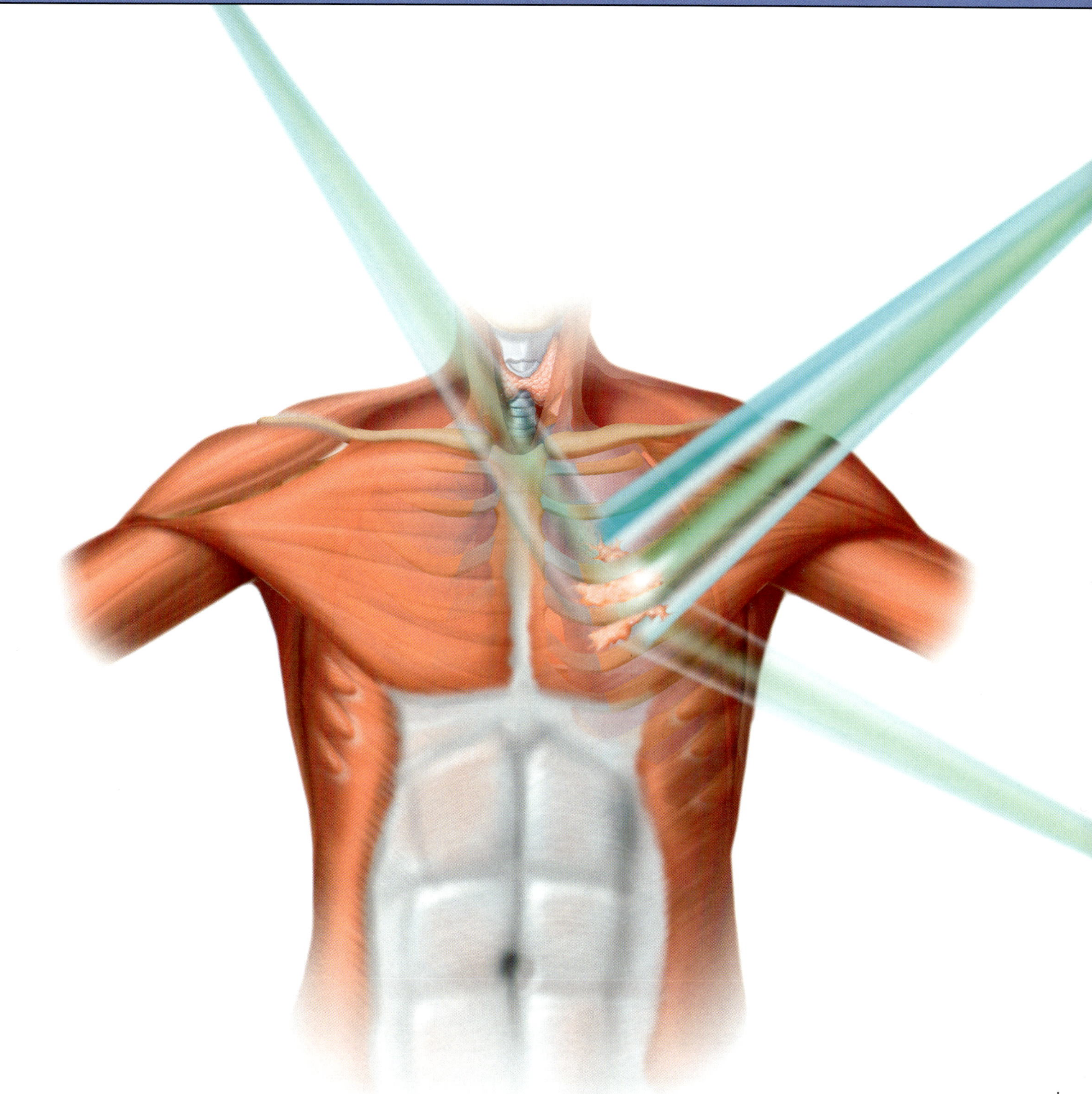

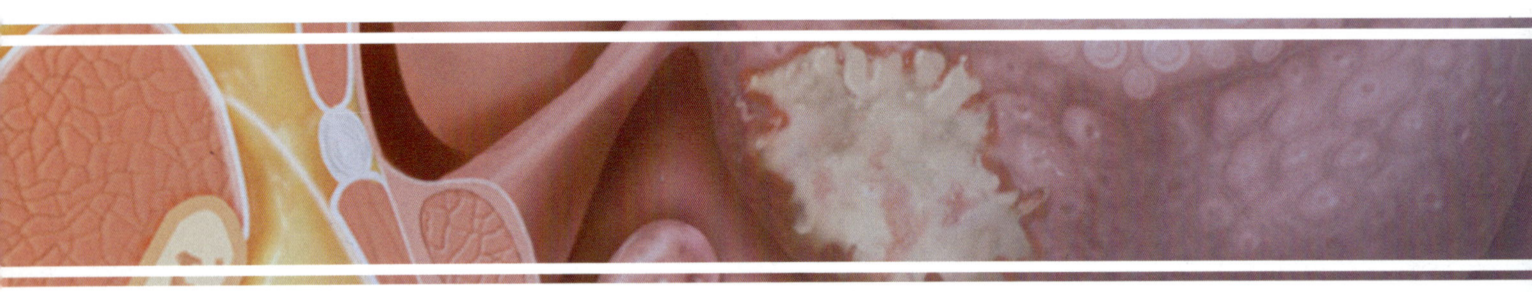

RADIATION ONCOLOGY
IMAGING AND TREATMENT

David K. Gaffney, MD, PhD
Professor of Radiation Oncology
Vice-Chair and Medical Director
Huntsman Cancer Hospital
University of Utah School of Medicine
Salt Lake City, Utah

Dennis Shrieve, MD, PhD
Professor of Radiation Oncology
Chair of the Department of Radiation Oncology
Huntsman Cancer Hospital
University of Utah School of Medicine
Salt Lake City, Utah

Feng-Ming (Spring) Kong, MD, PhD, MPH
Associate Professor of Radiation Oncology
Department of Radiation Oncology
University of Michigan and Veteran Affairs Hospital
Ann Arbor, Michigan

Christopher J. Anker, MD, PhD
Assistant Professor of Radiation Oncology
Huntsman Cancer Hospital
University of Utah School of Medicine
Salt Lake City, Utah

Ying J. Hitchcock, MD
Associate Professor of Radiation Oncology
Department of Radiation Oncology
Huntsman Cancer Hospital
University of Utah School of Medicine
Salt Lake City, Utah

Mark K. Buyyounouski, MD, MS
Associate Professor of Radiation Oncology
Director of Clinical Research
Fox Chase Cancer Center
Philadelphia, Pennsylvania

Jonathan D. Tward, MD, PhD
Assistant Professor of Radiation Oncology
Department of Radiation Oncology
Huntsman Cancer Hospital
University of Utah School of Medicine
Salt Lake City, Utah

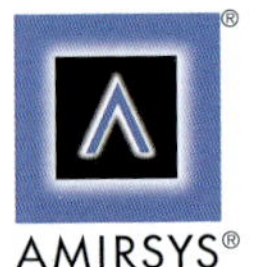

AMIRSYS®
Names you know. Content you trust.®

First Edition

Printed in Canada by Friesens, Altona, Manitoba, Canada

ISBN: 978-1-931884-70-9

Notice and Disclaimer

Library of Congress Cataloging-in-Publication Data

Gaffney, David K.
Radiation oncology : imaging and treatment / David K. Gaffney. -- 1st ed.
p. ; cm.
Includes bibliographical references and index.
ISBN 978-1-931884-70-9
I. Title.
[DNLM: 1. Neoplasms--diagnosis. 2. Diagnostic Imaging. 3. Neoplasms--radiotherapy. 4. Radiation Oncology--methods. QZ 241]

616.99'40757--dc23

2012037063

I am grateful to all medical professionals who share their knowledge and participate in multidisciplinary care of the cancer patient. Working together, I believe we achieve powerful results.

And to the three brightest stars in the sky: My wife, Lorrie, and our girls, Samantha and Jessica.

DKG

CONTRIBUTORS

Aaron E. Wagner, MD
Resident
Department of Radiation Oncology
Huntsman Cancer Hospital
University of Utah School of Medicine
Salt Lake City, Utah

Robert Amdur, MD
Professor of Radiation Oncology
Department of Radiation Oncology
University of Florida College of Medicine
Gainesville, Florida

Beth M. Beadle, MD, PhD
Assistant Professor of Radiation Oncology
Department of Radiation Oncology
University of Texas MD Anderson Cancer Center
Houston, Texas

Andrea A. Bezjak, MSc, MDCM, FRCPC
Professor of Radiation Oncology
Department of Radiation Oncology
Princess Margaret Hospital/University Health Network
Radiation Medicine Program, University of Toronto
Toronto, Canada

Anthony Brade, MDCM, PhD, FRCPC
Assistant Professor of Radiation Oncology
Department of Radiation Oncology
Princess Margaret Hospital/University Health Network
Radiation Medicine Program, University of Toronto
Toronto, Canada

L. Andy Chen, MD, PhD
Resident
Department of Radiation Oncology
Huntsman Cancer Hospital
University of Utah School of Medicine
Salt Lake City, Utah

B. C. John Cho, MD, PhD
Assistant Professor
Department of Radiation Oncology
Princess Margaret Hospital/University Health Network
Radiation Medicine Program, University of Toronto
Toronto, Canada

Mehee Choi, MD
Resident
Department of Radiation Oncology
Northwestern University Feinberg School of Medicine
Chicago, Illinois

Prajnan (Proggan) Das, MD, MS, MPH
Associate Professor and Quality Officer
Department of Radiation Oncology
University of Texas MD Anderson Cancer Center
Houston, Texas

Gerald B. Fogarty, MBBS, FRANZCR
Director
Mater Sydney Radiation Oncology
Genesis Cancer Care
Melanoma Institute of Australia
Sydney, Australia

Thomas J. Galloway, MD
Assistant Professor of Radiation Oncology
Fox Chase Cancer Center
Philadelphia, Pennsylvania

G. Brandon Gunn, MD
Assistant Professor
Department of Radiation Oncology
Division of Radiation Oncology
University of Texas MD Anderson Cancer Center
Houston, Texas

Mark A. Hallman, MD, PhD
Resident
Department of Radiation Oncology
Fox Chase Cancer Center
Philadelphia, Pennsylvania

Y. Jessica Huang, PhD, DABR

Assistant Professor of Radiation Oncology
Division of Medical Physics
Huntsman Cancer Hospital
University of Utah School of Medicine
Salt Lake City, Utah

Anuja Jhingran, MD

Professor of Radiation Oncology
Department of Radiation Oncology
University of Texas MD Anderson Cancer Center
Houston, Texas

Candice A. Johnstone, MD, MPH

Assistant Professor of Radiation Oncology
Medical Director, Froedtert and the Medical College of Wisconsin Cancer Network
Medical Director, Radiation Oncology, Kraemer Cancer Center
St. Joseph's West Bend
Milwaukee, Wisconsin

Bronwyn King, MBBS, FRANZCR

Radiation Oncologist
Department of Radiation Oncology
Cancer Imaging Peter MacCallum Cancer Centre
Melbourne, Australia

Ryan O'Hara, MD

Assistant Professor of Radiology
Chief of Department of Interventional Radiology
Director of Interventional Oncology
Huntsman Cancer Hospital
University of Utah School of Medicine
Salt Lake City, Utah

Brandi R. Page, MD

Resident
Department of Radiation Oncology
Huntsman Cancer Hospital
University of Utah School of Medicine
Salt Lake City, Utah

Jack Phan, MD, PhD

Assistant Professor
Department of Radiation Oncology
Division of Radiation Oncology
University of Texas MD Anderson Cancer Center
Houston, Texas

Matthew M. Poppe, MD

Assistant Professor of Radiation Oncology
Department of Radiation Oncology
Huntsman Cancer Hospital
University of Utah School of Medicine
Salt Lake City, Utah

Lorraine Portelance, MD

Associate Professor
Department of Radiation Oncology
Sylvester Comprehensive Cancer Center
Miller School of Medicine, University of Miami
Miami, Florida

William Small Jr., MD, FACRO, FACR, FASTRO

Professor and Vice Chairman
Department of Radiation Oncology
Associate Medical Director
Robert H. Lurie Comprehensive Cancer Center
Northwestern University Feinberg School of Medicine
Chicago, Illinois

Jeffrey M. Vainshtein, MD

Resident
Department of Radiation Oncology
University of Michigan and Veteran Affairs Hospital
Ann Arbor, Michigan

Akila N. Viswanathan, MD, MPH

Associate Professor of Radiation Oncology
Director of Gynecologic Radiation
Department of Radiation Oncology
Brigham and Women's Hospital/Dana-Farber Cancer Center
Harvard Medical School
Boston, Massachusetts

Dian Wang, MD, PhD

Professor of Radiation Oncology
Medical College of Wisconsin
Milwaukee, Wisconsin

Jessica Zhou, MD

Resident
Department of Radiation Oncology
University of Michigan and Veteran Affairs Hospital
Ann Arbor, Michigan

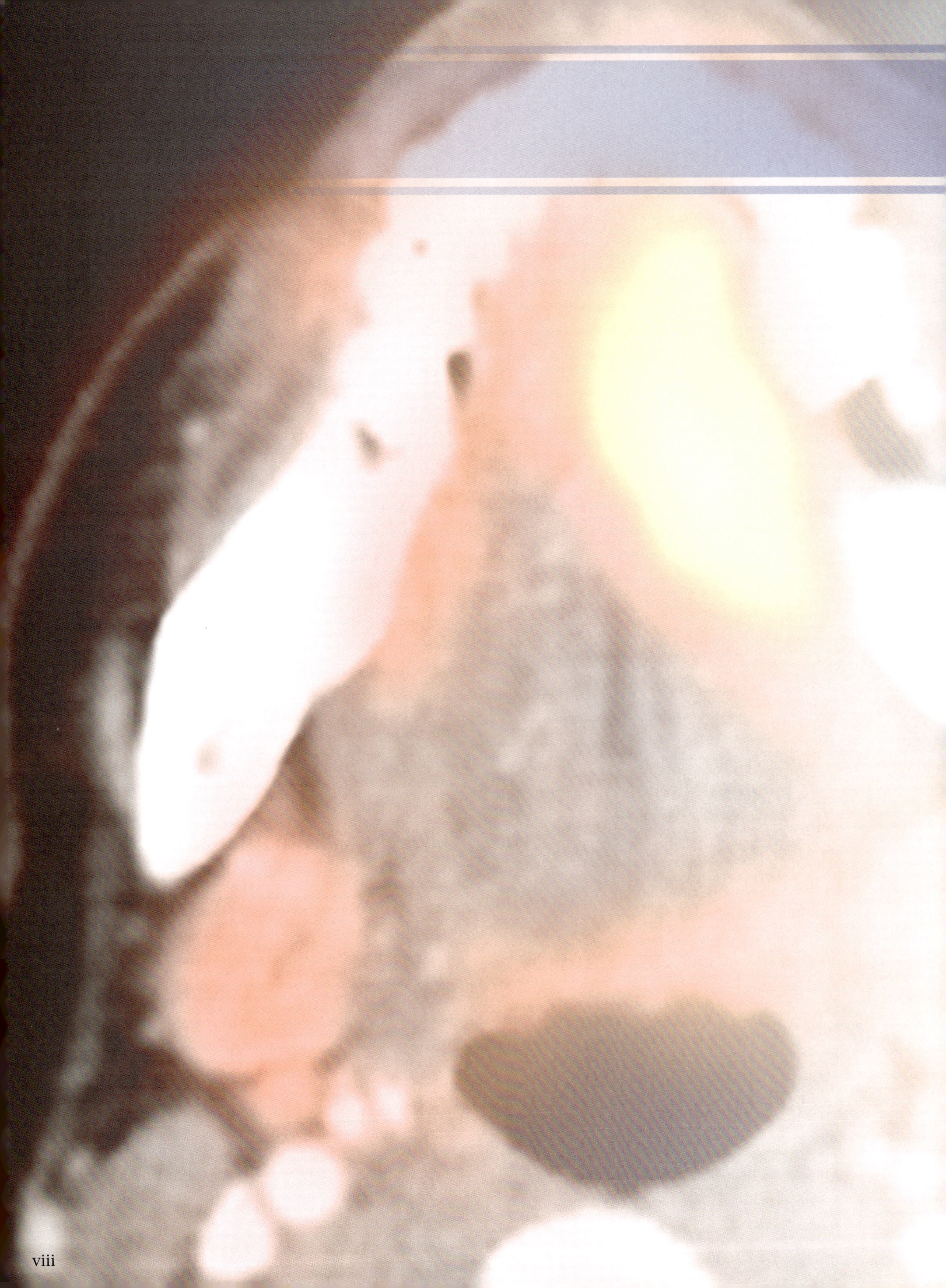

PREFACE

We are pleased to present *Radiation Oncology: Imaging and Treatment*, the most up-to-date collection of staging, imaging, and radiotherapy planning information for cancers of the entire body. This text unites the sister disciplines of diagnostic radiology and radiation oncology.

Each lavishly illustrated chapter highlights critical aspects of a particular cancer. Bulleted text distills pertinent information to the essentials. Reference tables provide quick access to definitions for TNM staging and AJCC prognostic groups. Rich drawings illuminate these categories. High-quality images demonstrate the clinical appearance of and treatment approach for practically every stage of every tumor. All of these vivid images—more than 2,500 in the volume—are fully annotated to maximize their illustrative potential. Whether you are looking for routes of spread, imaging techniques for local staging, treatment options, or effects of treatment, you will find it quickly in this easy-to-use yet comprehensive reference.

Radiation Oncology: Imaging and Treatment was designed with you, the reader, in mind. We think you'll find this new volume a handy and wonderfully rich resource that will enhance your practice and find a welcome place on your bookshelf.

David K. Gaffney, MD, PhD
Professor of Radiation Oncology
Vice-Chair and Medical Director
Huntsman Cancer Hospital
University of Utah School of Medicine
Salt Lake City, Utah

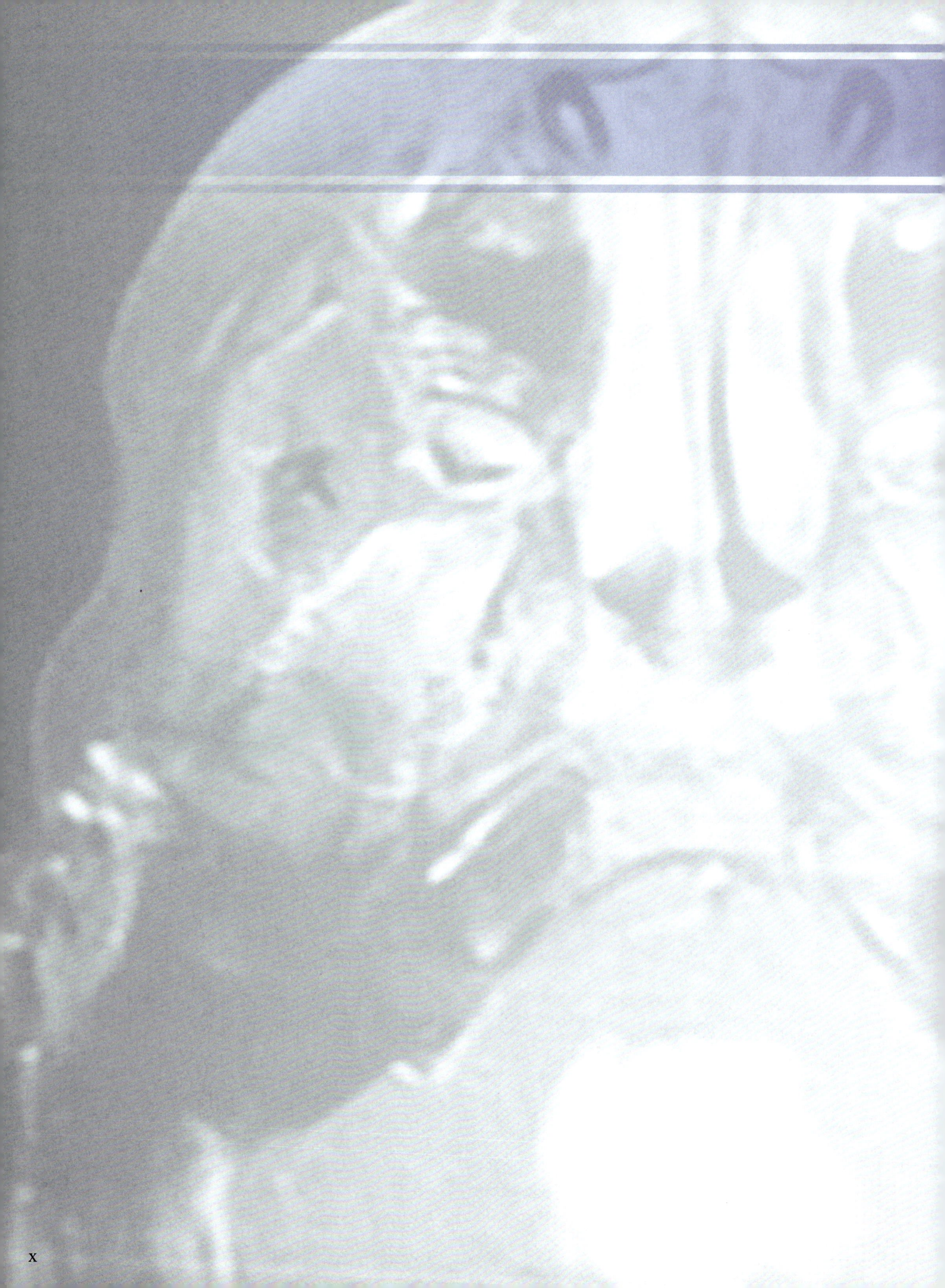

ACKNOWLEDGMENTS

Text Editing
Dave L. Chance, MA
Arthur G. Gelsinger, MA
Lorna Kennington, MS
Rebecca L. Hutchinson, BA
Angela M. Green, BA
Kalina K. Lowery, MS

Image Editing
Jeffrey J. Marmorstone, BS
Lisa A. M. Steadman, BS

Medical Editing
Aaron P. Brown, MD

Illustrations
Laura C. Sesto, MA
Lane R. Bennion, MS
Richard Coombs, MS

Art Direction and Design
Laura C. Sesto, MA
Lisa A. M. Steadman, BS

Publishing Lead
Katherine L. Riser, MA

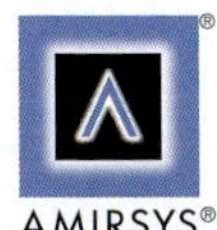

AMIRSYS®
Names you know. Content you trust.®

Table of Contents

SECTION 6
Genitourinary System

SECTION 7
Gynecology

SECTION 8
Mesenchymal Tumors

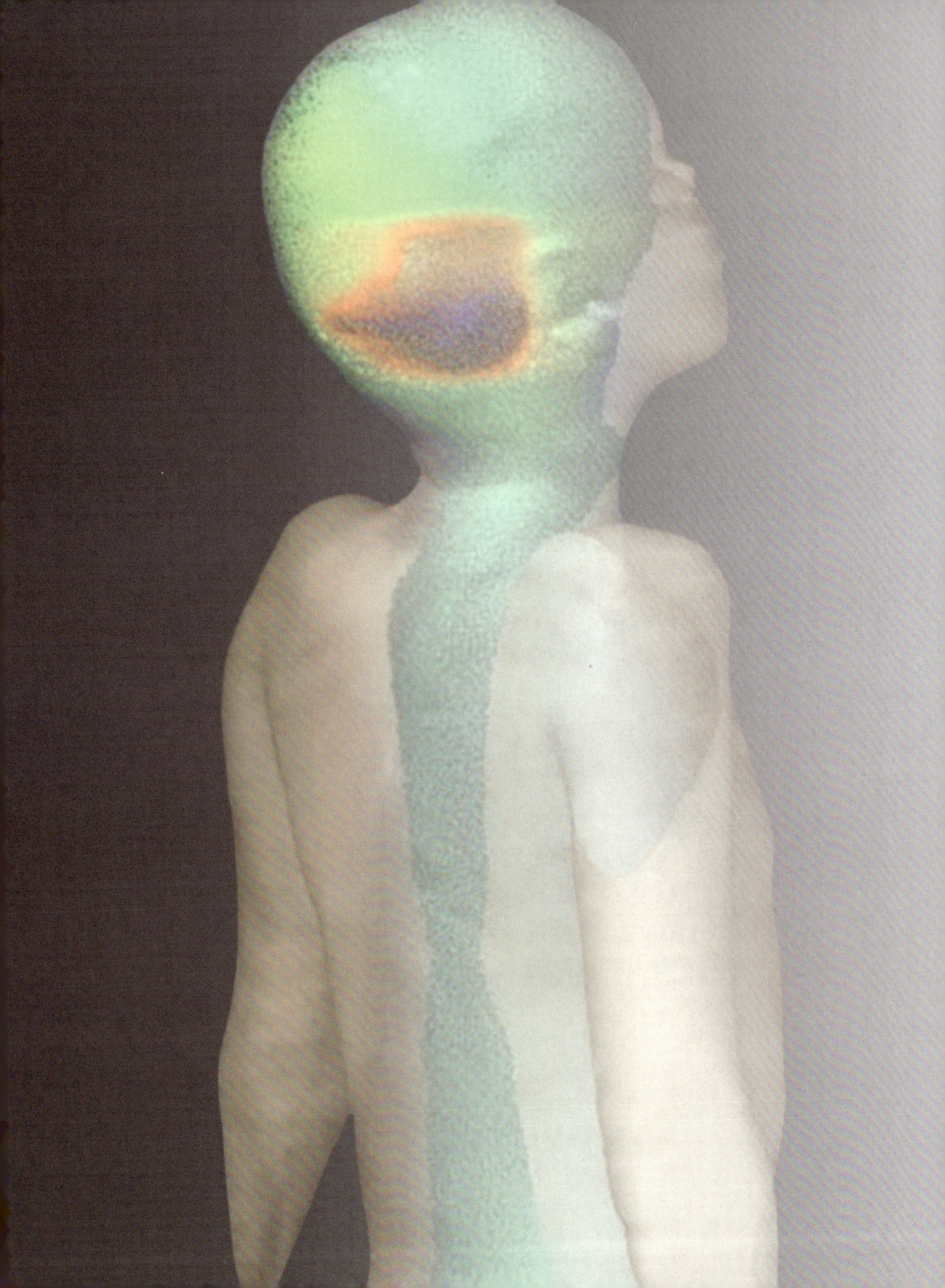

SECTION 1
Central Nervous System

GLIOMAS

RPA Classification

Stage	*Characteristics*	*Median Survival (Months)*	*2-year OS (%)*
High-Grade Tumors Without Temozolomide			
I	Age < 50, normal MS	59	76
II	Age ≥ 50, KPS ≥ 70, symptoms > 3 months	37	68
III	Age < 50, abnormal MS	18	35
	GBM: Age < 50, KPS > 90		
IV	Age ≥ 50, KPS ≥ 70, symptoms ≤ 3 months	11	15
	Age < 50, KPS < 90; or GBM S/P resection able to work		
V	Age ≥ 50, KPS < 70 and normal MS	9	6
	Age ≥ 50, KPS ≥ 70, and S/P surgery not able to work, or S/P biopsy receiving at least 54.4 Gy; or age ≥ 50, KPS < 70 with normal mental status		
VI	Age ≥ 50, KPS < 70, abnormal MS; or S/P biopsy receiving ≤ 54.4 Gy	5	4
Update for GBM With Temozolomide			
III	Age < 50, WHO PS 0	21	43
IV	Age < 50, WHO PS 1-2; age ≥ 50, S/P surgery, MMSE ≥ 27	16	28
V	Age ≥ 50, S/P surgery with MMSE < 27 or biopsy only	10	17

Low-Grade Glioma: EORTC Risk Group Stratification

Risk Group	*Score*	*Median OS (Years)*
Low	0-2	7.8
High	3-5	3.7

**Risk factors: Age ≥ 40, astrocytoma histology, tumor size ≥ 6 cm, tumor crosses midline, neurologic deficit.*

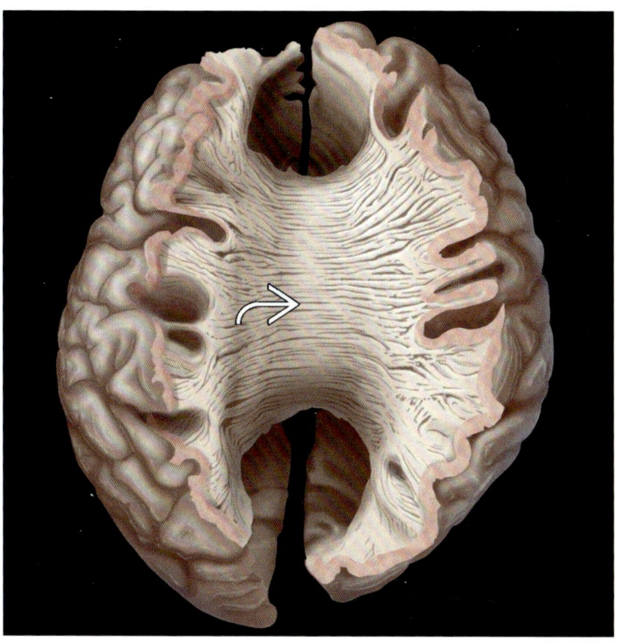

This graphic demonstrates white matter tracts within the brain. In particular, the corpus callosum ➔ can be seen yielding a connection between the right and left hemispheres. A glioma's primary route of spread is along white matter tracts.

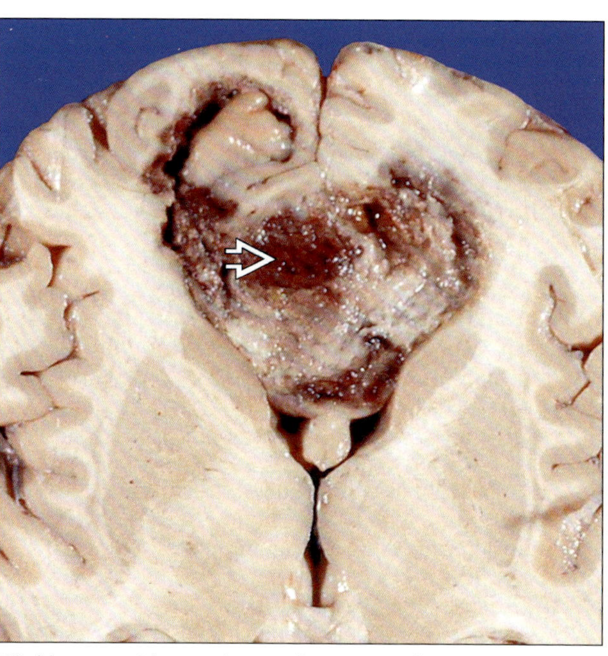

Glioblastoma with spread across the corpus callosum gives a "butterfly" appearance. Central necrosis can also be seen ➔. (Courtesy R. McComb, MD, P. Burger, MD.)

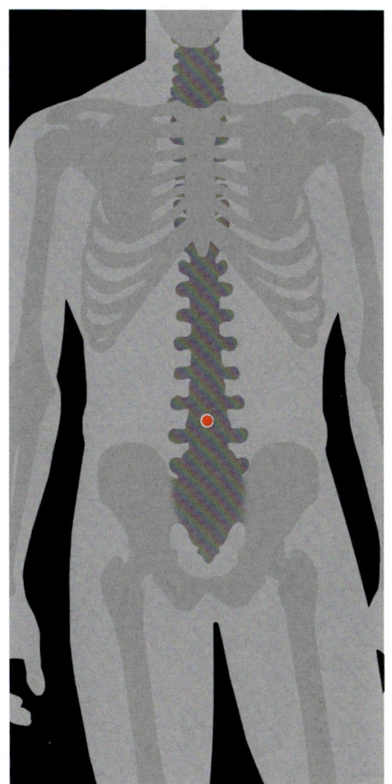

INITIAL SITE OF RECURRENCE

Spinal Drop Metastases 1.1 % (3/267)

Stark AM et al: Glioblastoma multiforme-report of 267 cases treated at a single institution. Surg Neurol. 63(2):162-9; discussion 169, 2005

GLIOMAS

OVERVIEW

General Comments

- Tumors arising from glial cells within the CNS parenchyma
  - Main histologic subtypes
    - Astrocytomas
    - Oligodendrogliomas
  - Divided into low- and high-grade tumors due to dichotomous behavior and treatment approaches

Classification

- WHO classification divides tumors into grades I-IV
- WHO grade relies on 4 factors: Nuclear atypia, mitoses, microvascular/endothelial proliferation, and necrosis
  - Grade I: Pilocytic astrocytoma, subependymal giant cell astrocytoma
  - Grade II: Cellular atypia
  - Grade III: Atypia, mitoses
  - Grade IV: Atypia, mitoses, microvascular proliferation, or necrosis
  - Grade determines treatment approach
- RPA classification
  - Used to predict overall prognosis
  - Update of table was performed for GBM patients receiving temozolomide

NATURAL HISTORY

General Features

- Comments
  - GBM most common primary malignant CNS tumor in adults
- Location
  - Most commonly in the supratentorial white matter
    - Cerebral hemispheres > brainstem > cerebellum
    - Frontal, temporal, parietal > occipital lobes

Etiology

- Risk factors
  - Prior cranial ionizing radiation
  - Hereditary
    - NF 1-2, tuberous sclerosis; Li-Fraumeni and Turcot syndromes

Epidemiology & Cancer Incidence

- Number of cases in USA per year
  - Low grade: 2,000-4,000 per year
  - Grade III: 1,000-2,500 per year
  - Grade IV (GBM): 8,000-10,000 per year
- Sex predilection
  - Low grade: Slight male predominance but varies with histology
  - High grade: M > F (1.5:1)
- Age of onset
  - Low grade: Varies with histology; generally occurs at younger ages than high grade
    - Juvenile pilocytic astrocytoma (JPA): 1st-2nd decades
    - Subependymal giant cell tumors: 1st-3rd decades
  - High grade: 5th-6th decades

Genetics

- Common alterations
  - *MGMT* methylation: DNA alkylation repair gene; promoter methylation inactivates gene; imparts positive prognosis regardless of treatment
  - 1p19q loss of heterozygosity: Improved prognosis and chemosensitivity; most common in oligodendrogliomas
  - Isocitrate dehydrogenase-1 (IDH-1) mutation: Can be present in all gliomas; positive prognostic effect

Gross Pathology & Surgical Features

- Low grade
  - Diffuse slowly growing tumors involving white matter tracts
  - Exhibit intrinsic mass effect on surrounding anatomy
  - Demonstrate more well-demarcated borders than higher grade
- High grade
  - Poorly delineated heterogeneous tumors involving white matter tracts
  - Demonstrate intrinsic mass effect with blurring of anatomical boundaries and indistinct margins (oligodendrogliomas demonstrate clearer borders)
  - Classical hallmarks
    - GBM: Hemorrhage, rim of tissue with central necrosis
    - Oligos: Calcifications

Microscopic Pathology

- H&E
  - Low grade
    - Mixed glial cells with fibrillary matrix
    - Mild: Moderate cellular atypia, low mitotic counts
    - Low-grade oligos generally demonstrate perinuclear halos with "chicken wire" vascular network
  - High grade
    - Increased cellularity with cellular pleomorphism, atypia, and mitoses
      - GBM: Necrosis, microvascularity, pseudopalisading appearance
      - Anaplastic astro: High cellularity with nuclear atypia, no necrosis or microvascular proliferation
      - Anaplastic oligo: Perinuclear halos, "chicken wire" capillary network, microcalcifications
- Special stains
  - Glial fibrillary acidic protein (GFAP)
    - Generally positive in astrocytomas, rare in oligos
  - MIB-1
    - Antibody against Ki-67, expressed in proliferating cells
    - Used as a marker for cell proliferation

Routes of Spread

- Local spread
  - Generally follow white matter tracts
    - Higher grade tumors can demonstrate subependymal spread and dissemination

IMAGING

Low Grade

- CT
  - Nonenhanced CT
    - Iso-hypodense mass

- Enhanced CT
  - Nonenhancing
  - Enhancement raises suspicion of transformation to high grade
- Exceptions
  - JPA: Cystic cerebellar mass, frequently with enhancing mural nodule and compressing 4th ventricle
  - Subependymal giant cell astrocytoma: Foramen of Monro solid mass, which is strongly enhancing

- MR
  - T1WI
    - Hypo-isointense mass compared to gray matter
  - T2WI
    - Hyperintense mass compared to gray matter
  - T2 FLAIR
    - Hyperintense mass compared to gray matter
  - T1 post contrast
    - Generally nonenhancing; enhancement concerning for progression to high grade
  - Exceptions
    - JPA: Cerebellar cystic mass; frequently compresses 4th ventricle; cystic fluid can be hyperintense to CSF on T1, T2, and T2 FLAIR; mural nodule can demonstrate enhancement
    - Subependymal giant cell astrocytoma: Solid mass located close to foramen of Monro, demonstrates enhancement

High Grade

- CT
  - Nonenhanced CT
    - Low to hypodense ill-defined mass
    - May see hemorrhage in GBM or oligo, and Ca++ in oligo
  - Enhanced CT
    - Rim enhancement seen in GBM
    - May see patchy enhancement in anaplastic oligo (AO), less often in anaplastic astro (AA)
- AO
  - T1WI
    - Heterogeneous hypointense infiltrative mass centered in white matter
    - Can appear circumscribed
    - Ca++, necrosis and blood products may be seen
  - T2WI
    - Heterogeneous hyperintense infiltrative mass
      - Heterogeneity related to hemorrhage, Ca++, and cystic changes
    - Necrosis and hemorrhage can be seen
  - T2 FLAIR
    - Heterogeneous hyperintense infiltrative mass
  - T1 post contrast
    - Variable enhancement, present ≈ 50% of the time
- AA
  - T1WI
    - Iso-hypointense white matter mass
    - Ca++, hemorrhage, cysts rare in contrast to oligos
  - T2WI
    - Heterogeneously hyperintense
    - Frequently invades adjacent brain, even with discrete appearance
    - Ca++, hemorrhage, cysts rare
  - T2 FLAIR
    - Heterogeneously hyperintense
  - T1 post contrast
    - Generally nonenhancing
    - Occasional focal areas of enhancement seen
- GBM
  - T1WI
    - Iso-hypointense white matter mass
    - Necrosis, cysts, and hemorrhage frequently seen
    - Thickened margin common
  - T2WI
    - Heterogeneous, hyperintense mass
    - Adjacent infiltration/vasogenic edema usually seen
    - Flow voids (neovascularity) may be seen
    - Tumor usually infiltrates beyond visualized signal changes
  - T2 FLAIR
    - Heterogeneous, hyperintense mass with adjacent tumor infiltration/vasogenic edema
  - T1 post contrast
    - Classically, area of central necrosis surrounded by irregular rind of enhancement
    - Enhancement pattern can vary: Patchy, focal, ring-like

CLINICAL PRESENTATION & WORK-UP

Presentation

- Headaches, altered mental status, seizures, neurologic deficits
- Onset may be insidious

Prognosis

- Low grade
  - Relatively good compared to high grade
  - MS ranges from 6-10 years
  - Eventual transformation to high grade 70-80%
- Grade III
  - Heterogeneous group based off of histology, genetics, age, and KPS
  - In general, oligos have better prognosis than astros
  - Good prognostic indicators: *MGMT* methylation, LOH 1p19q, mutated *IDH1*
  - MS ranges from 1.7 years (AA, *IDH1* wild type) to 7.5 years (AO, LOH 1p19q)
- Grade IV (GBM)
  - Unrelenting progression
  - MS 8-14 months
  - Survival varies with RPA class

Work-Up

- Clinical
  - Complete H&P
    - Include comprehensive neurological exam

Radiographic

- CT brain frequently obtained at presentation secondary to symptoms
- MR brain ± contrast

TREATMENT

Treatment Options by Stage

- Low grade

GLIOMAS

- ○ Maximal surgical resection
- ○ Adjuvant treatment controversial
  - ■ NCCN acceptable options
    - Observation (with RT or chemo salvage): Age < 40 or low risk
    - RT
    - Chemotherapy: TMZ, PCV, or nitrosourea
- ○ Special cases
  - ■ JPA/subependymal giant cell astrocytoma: Surgical resection with observation (regardless of resection)
    - RT if unresectable and causing symptoms in adults
- Grade III
  - ○ Maximal surgical resection
  - ○ Adjuvant treatment controversial
    - ■ NCCN acceptable options
      - RT (with chemo salvage)
      - Chemotherapy: TMZ (preferred) or PCV, with RT salvage
      - ChemoRT
    - ■ No current change in therapy based on molecular prognostic indices, but investigational
- Grade IV (GBM)
  - ○ Surgery followed by radiation with concurrent/adjuvant TMZ
- Surgical note
  - ○ Complete resections not always possible based upon tumor location, patient age, and performance status; biopsy at minimum for pathologic confirmation
  - ○ Notably in high grade, prognosis improves with increasing resection

Dose Response

- Low grade
  - ○ No proven dose response above 45 Gy
- High grade
  - ○ Dose response up to 60 Gy with standard fractionation
  - ○ No benefit to dose escalation higher than 60 Gy, either with conventional or stereotactic boost

Standard Doses

- Low grade
  - ○ 45-54 Gy in 1.8-2 Gy fractions
- High grade
  - ○ 59.4-60 Gy in 1.8-2 Gy fractions
  - ○ Elderly patients or poor performance status
    - ■ Hypofx RT acceptable
    - ■ 40-50 Gy in 15-20 fx

Organs at Risk Parameters

- Optic nerves/chiasm: < 54 Gy (< 1% optic neuropathy, QUANTEC)
- Retina: 45 Gy (< 5% retinopathy, Emami)
- Lens: 10 Gy (< 5% cataract [probably higher], Emami)
- Cochlea: Mean dose 35-45 Gy (minimize risk, QUANTEC)
- Brainstem: < 54 Gy (< 5% necrosis/neuropathy, QUANTEC)

Common Techniques

- Contouring
  - ○ Low grade
    - ■ GTV: T2 FLAIR with T1 enhancement (if present)
    - ■ CTV: GTV + 1-2 cm
    - ■ PTV: CTV + 3-5 mm
  - ○ High grade
    - ■ EORTC (Stupp) approach
      - GTV: Resection cavity + residual T1 enhancement
      - CTV: GTV + 2-3 cm (typically 2.5)
      - Can constrain off of regular anatomical boundaries (i.e., skull, tentorium, etc.)
      - Expand to include any T2 FLAIR signal outside of contour
      - PTV: CTV + 3-5 mm
    - ■ RTOG approach
      - GTV1: T1 enhancement + T2 FLAIR; GTV2: T1 enhancement
      - CTV1: GTV1 + 2 cm; CTV2: GTV2 + 2 cm
      - PTV: CTV + 3-5 mm
      - PTV1: Treated to 45-46 Gy; PTV2: Treated to 59.4-60 Gy
- Planning
  - ○ 3D conformal plan using 3-5 beams; arrangement varies by location
  - ○ IMRT can be used if in close proximity to OARs
    - ■ Will create hotspots; verify hotspots outside of OARs

Landmark Trials

- Low grade
  - ○ "Nonbelievers trial" EORTC 22845: Early vs. delayed RT
    - ■ No OS benefit to early RT, but improves PFS and reduces frequency of seizures
  - ○ "Believers trial" EORTC 22844: Low dose (45 Gy) vs. high dose (59.4 Gy) RT
    - ■ No dose response above 45 Gy
- Grade III
  - ○ RTOG 9402: Sequential PCV followed by RT vs. RT alone
    - ■ Showed no OS benefit
    - ■ PFS benefit (2.6 vs. 1.7 years) but with increased toxicity
  - ○ EORTC 26951: RT ± adjuvant PCV
    - ■ PFS benefit but no OS benefit
  - ○ NOA-4: RT vs. PCV vs. TMZ with alternate modality salvage
    - ■ No survival difference or time to failure difference
- Grade IV (GBM)
  - ○ Stupp trial: RT ± concurrent/adjuvant temozolomide
    - ■ Survival benefit with addition of TMZ (5-year OS 9.8% vs. 1.9%)

RECOMMENDED FOLLOW-UP

Clinical

- 2-6 weeks after completion of RT
- Every 2-4 months for 2-3 years
- Can then widen follow-up (commonly every 6 months until 5 years out, then annually)

Radiographic

- Serial MRs with above clinical schedule
  - ○ 1st MR should be at least 4 weeks out, 8 weeks is common
- Recurrence interval
  - ○ Low grade: On average, 5-6 years for recurrence, 9-11 years for progression to higher grade

- ○ Grade III: On average, 1-2 years to recurrence or progression to higher grade
  - ▪ Recurrence may be later depending upon favorable histology and molecular markers
- ○ Grade IV (GBM): 6-8 months
- "Pseudo-progression" treatment effect vs. tumor progression difficult to distinguish
  - ○ Specialty imaging
    - ▪ Perfusion MR
      - Tumor: Elevated relative cerebral blood volume (rCBV): > 2.6
      - Pseudo-progression: Decreased rCBV: < 0.6
    - ▪ MR spectroscopy
      - Tumor: Elevated Cho, Cho:NAA ratio
      - Pseudo-progression: Decreased Cho, Cr, NAA
      - Increased lipid or lactate can be seen in either case
    - ▪ PET
      - Tumor: FDG avid
      - Pseudo-progression: Can also be FDG avid, especially within 8 weeks of treatment
      - Necrosis: Not usually hypermetabolic unless mixed with post-treatment inflammation
      - Note: Low-grade tumors frequently show avidity similar to white matter, not usually hypermetabolic

Laboratory

- Obtain CBC with platelets during TMZ therapy

SELECTED REFERENCES

1. Wick W et al: NOA-04 randomized phase III trial of sequential radiochemotherapy of anaplastic glioma with procarbazine, lomustine, and vincristine or temozolomide. J Clin Oncol. 28(4):708, 2010
2. Stupp R et al: Effects of radiotherapy with concomitant and adjuvant temozolomide versus radiotherapy alone on survival in glioblastoma in a randomised phase III study: 5-year analysis of the EORTC-NCIC trial. Lancet Oncol. 10(5):459-66, 2009
3. Intergroup Radiation Therapy Oncology Group Trial 9402 et al: Phase III trial of chemotherapy plus radiotherapy compared with radiotherapy alone for pure and mixed anaplastic oligodendroglioma: Intergroup Radiation Therapy Oncology Group Trial 9402. J Clin Oncol. 24(18):2707-14, 2006
4. Mirimanoff RO et al: Radiotherapy and temozolomide for newly diagnosed glioblastoma: recursive partitioning analysis of the EORTC 26981/22981-NCIC CE3 phase III randomized trial. J Clin Oncol. 24(16):2563-9, 2006
5. van den Bent MJ et al: Adjuvant procarbazine, lomustine, and vincristine improves progression-free survival but not overall survival in newly diagnosed anaplastic oligodendrogliomas and oligoastrocytomas: a randomized European Organisation for Research and Treatment of Cancer phase III trial. J Clin Oncol. 24(18):2715-22, 2006
6. van den Bent MJ et al: Long-term efficacy of early versus delayed radiotherapy for low-grade astrocytoma and oligodendroglioma in adults: the EORTC 22845 randomised trial. Lancet. 2005 Sep 17-23;366(9490):985-90. Erratum in: Lancet. 367(9525):1818, 2006
7. Pignatti F et al: Prognostic factors for survival in adult patients with cerebral low-grade glioma. J Clin Oncol. 20(8):2076-84, 2002
8. Karim AB et al: A randomized trial on dose-response in radiation therapy of low-grade cerebral glioma: European Organization for Research and Treatment of Cancer (EORTC) Study 22844. Int J Radiat Oncol Biol Phys. 36(3):549-56, 1996
9. Curran WJ Jr et al: Recursive partitioning analysis of prognostic factors in three Radiation Therapy Oncology Group malignant glioma trials. J Natl Cancer Inst. 85(9):704-10, 1993
10. CBTRUS. "CBTRUS Statistical Report: Primary Brain and Central Nervous System Tumors Diagnosed in the United States in 2004-2006." Central Brain Tumor Registry of the United States. www.cbtrus.org (2010)

WHO II Low-Grade Diffuse Astrocytoma

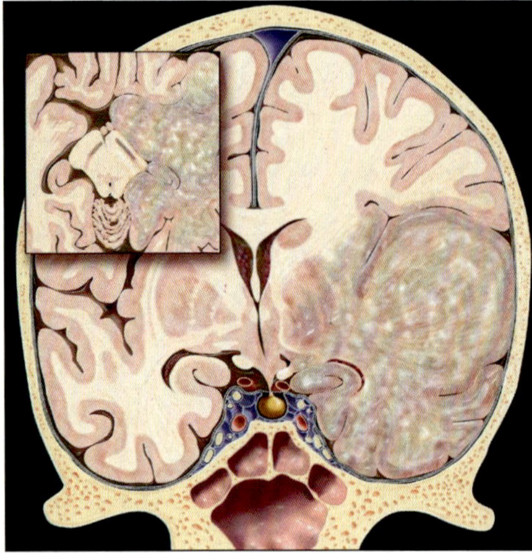

WHO II Low-Grade Diffuse Astrocytoma

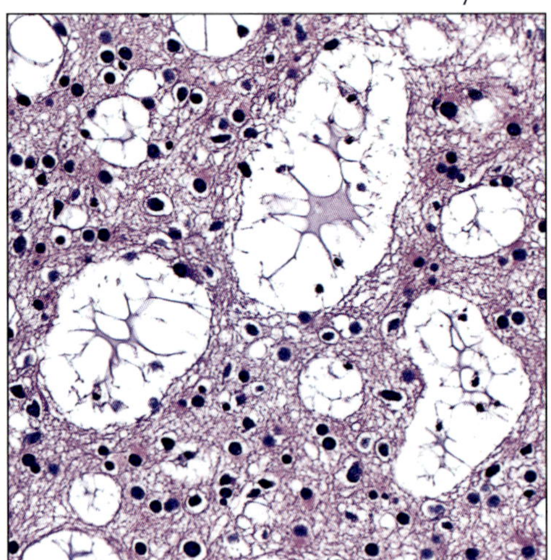

(Left) *Coronal graphic shows an infiltrative mass within the left temporal lobe. Axial inset shows mild mass effect upon the midbrain. Low-grade astrocytomas typically affect young adults.* ***(Right)*** *H&E of grade II diffuse astrocytoma shows hypercellularity, pleomorphism, and microcysts. (Courtesy P. Burger, MD.)*

WHO II Low-Grade Diffuse Astrocytoma

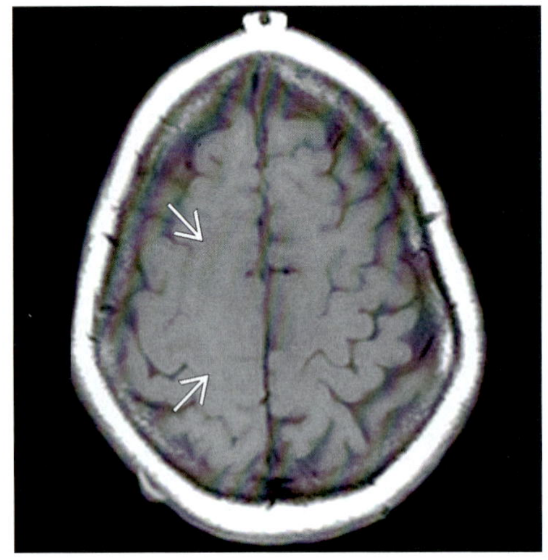

WHO II Low-Grade Diffuse Astrocytoma

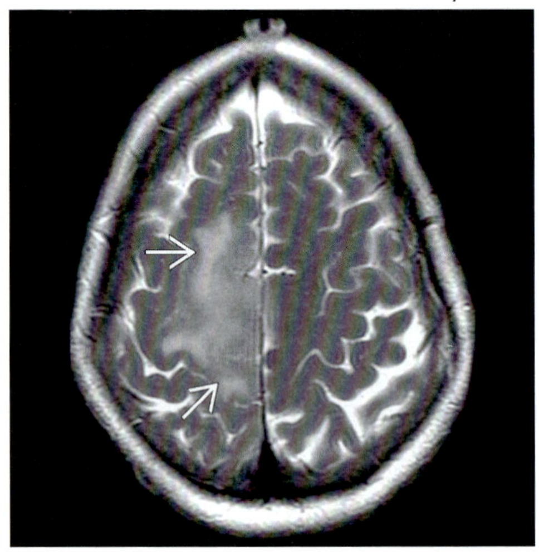

(Left) *This is an axial T1 image with iso-hypointense signal involving the right superior frontal and precentral gyri ➔. There is adjacent sulcal effacement.* ***(Right)*** *Axial T2 MR in the same patient shows an infiltrative hyperintense mass ➔.*

WHO II Low-Grade Diffuse Astrocytoma

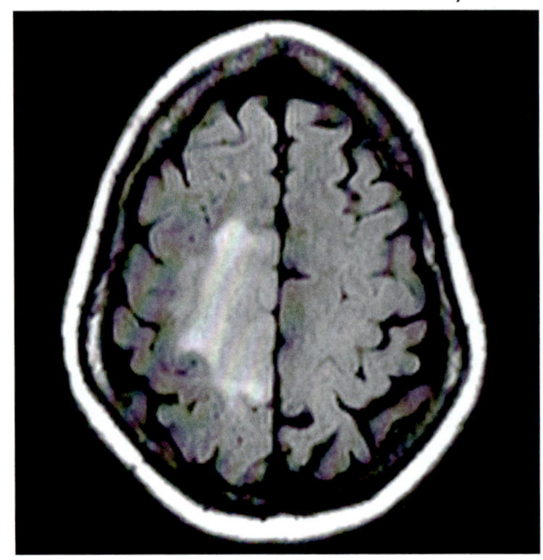

WHO II Low-Grade Diffuse Astrocytoma

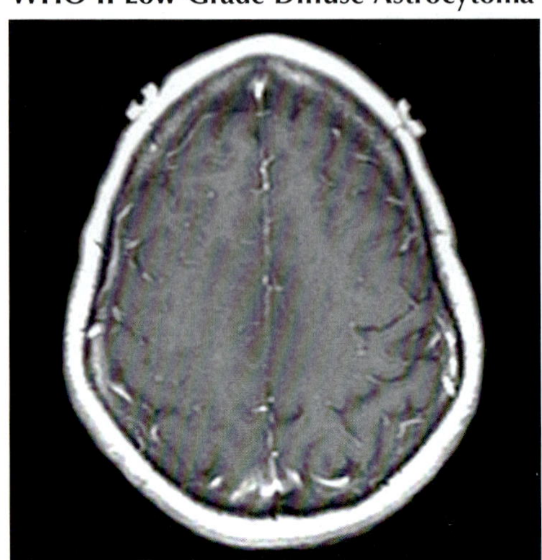

(Left) *Axial FLAIR MR in the same patient shows an infiltrative hyperintense mass similar to T2WI.* ***(Right)*** *This is an axial post-contrast T1 image in the same patient without demonstration of any enhancement. The absence of enhancement is characteristic of low-grade gliomas.*

WHO Grade II Oligodendroglioma

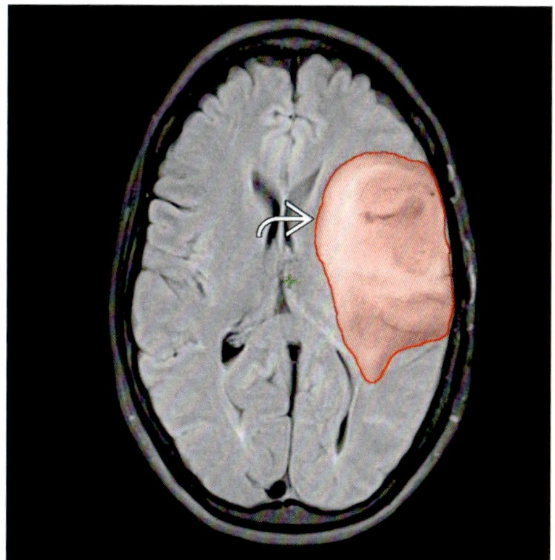

WHO Grade II Oligodendroglioma

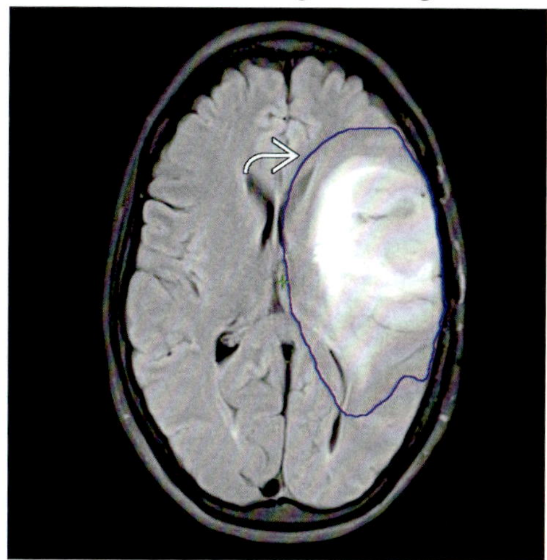

(Left) *This is an axial FLAIR MR with the GTV ➡ highlighting the edema. Note there is no contrast enhancement in typical low-grade gliomas.* ***(Right)*** *Axial FLAIR MR in the same patient shows CTV ➡ as a 1 cm expansion on the GTV and constrained by anatomical boundaries.*

WHO Grade II Oligodendroglioma

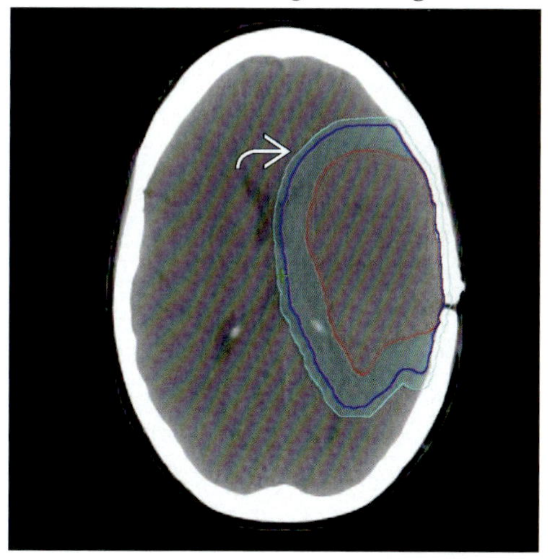

WHO Grade II Oligodendroglioma

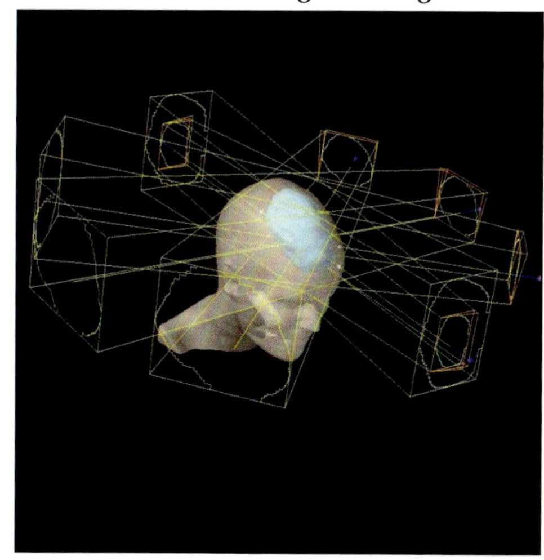

(Left) *Planning CT in the same patient shows GTV, CTV, and PTV ➡. PTV in this case is a 3 mm expansion from the CTV.* ***(Right)*** *This beam arrangement was used to deliver 54 Gy in the same patient. In this case, a 5-field 3D conformal plan was implemented.*

WHO Grade II Oligodendroglioma

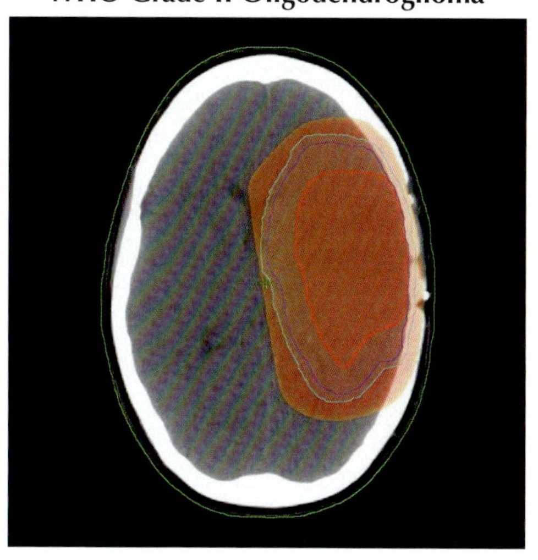

WHO Grade II Oligodendroglioma

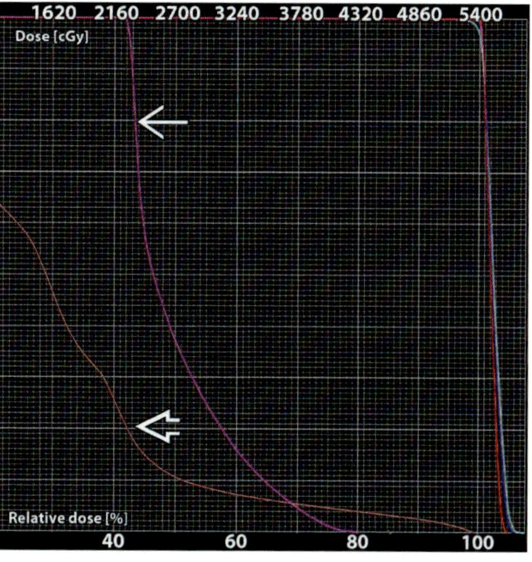

(Left) *A 95% dose colorwash is illustrated showing the target coverage in the same patient.* ***(Right)*** *DVH in the same patient depicts the coverage of the target. 54 Gy was the prescription for this low-grade glioma. Note that the optic chiasm ➡ and brainstem ➡ are well below tolerance.*

WHO Grade III Anaplastic Oligodendroglioma

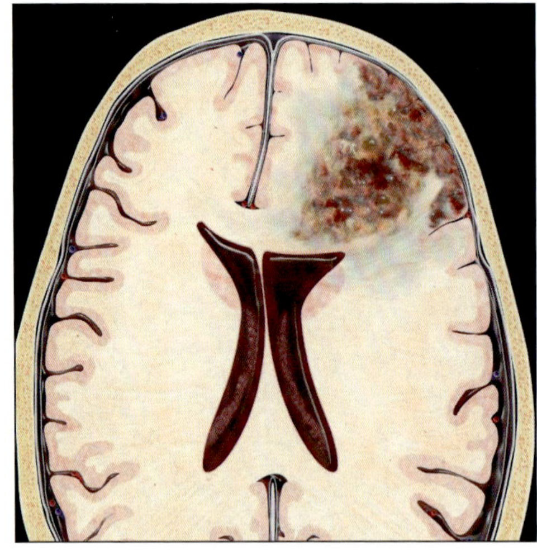

WHO Grade III Anaplastic Oligodendroglioma

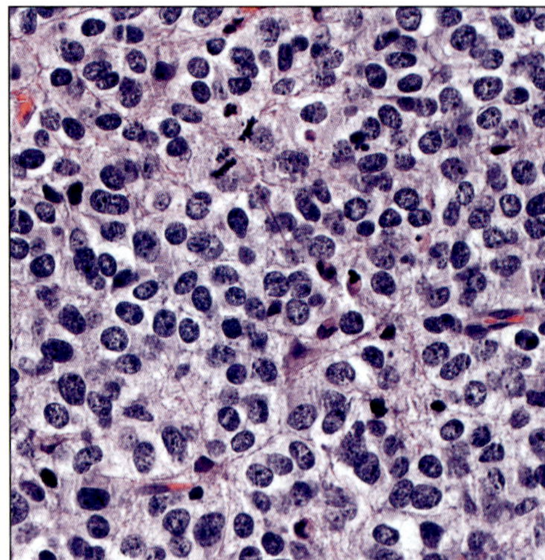

*(**Left**) Axial graphic shows a heterogeneous frontal mass with areas of necrosis and hemorrhage. Mass effect and infiltrative margins can be seen, typical of anaplastic grade III oligodendroglioma. (**Right**) H&E stain shows a highly cellular and mitotically active anaplastic oligodendroglioma. (Courtesy P. Burger, MD.)*

WHO Grade III Anaplastic Oligodendroglioma

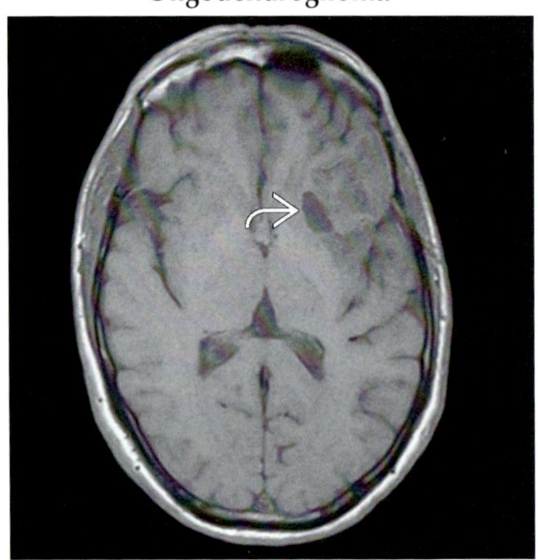

WHO Grade III Anaplastic Oligodendroglioma

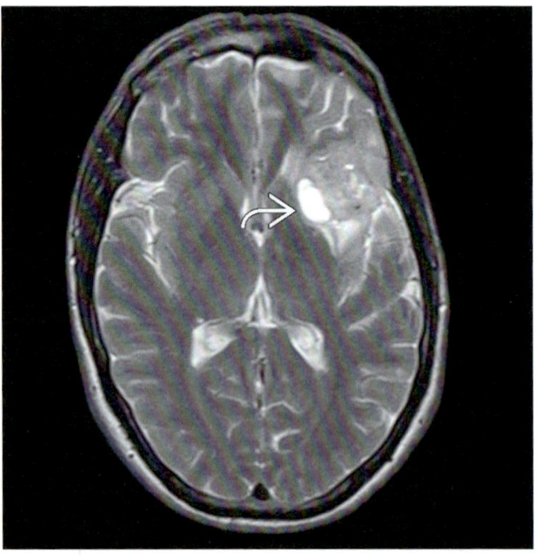

*(**Left**) Axial T1 MR shows iso-hypointense mass and cystic changes ➔ within the left frontal lobe. (**Right**) Axial T2 MR in the same patient shows cystic changes ➔ with surrounding hyperintensity within the left frontal lobe.*

WHO Grade III Anaplastic Oligodendroglioma

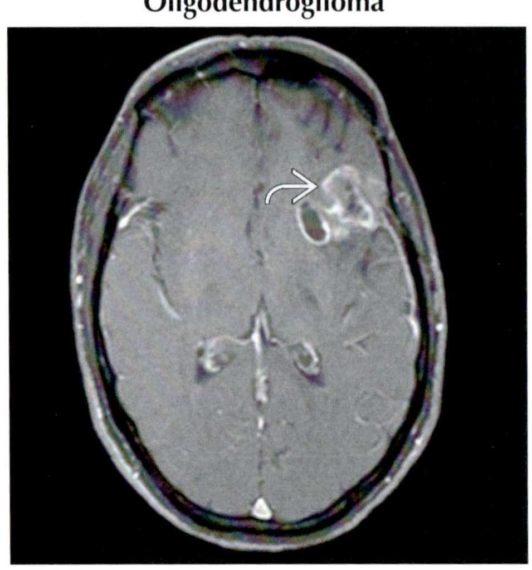

WHO Grade III Anaplastic Oligodendroglioma

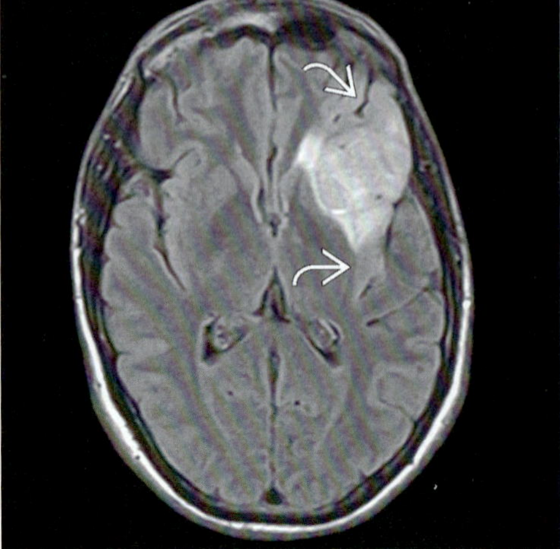

*(**Left**) Axial T1 post-contrast MR in the same patient shows nodular enhancement ➔ within the left frontal lobe. (**Right**) Axial FLAIR MR in the same patient shows hyperintense nodular mass with surrounding edema ➔.*

Grade III Anaplastic Oligodendroglioma

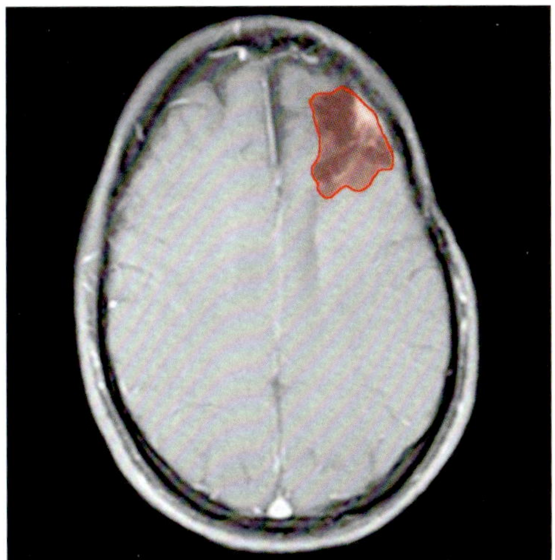

Grade III Anaplastic Oligodendroglioma

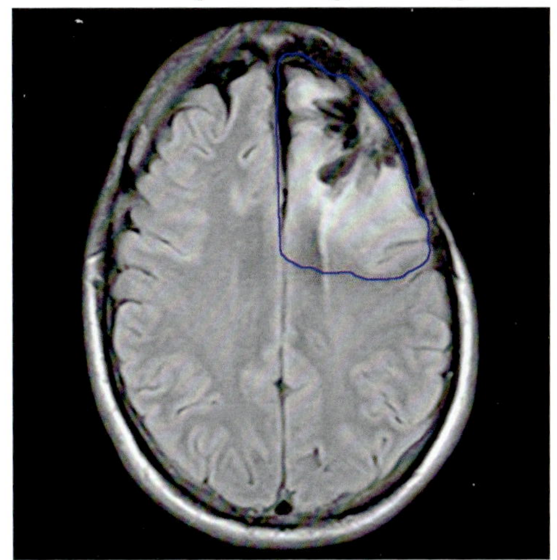

(Left) *Axial T1 contrast-enhanced MR shows the GTV outlining the resection cavity as well as the residual enhancement.* ***(Right)*** *Axial FLAIR MR in the same patient shows the CTV as a 2.5 cm expansion from the GTV, constrained by the skull as well as the tentorium cerebri, and including all FLAIR signals.*

Grade III Anaplastic Oligodendroglioma

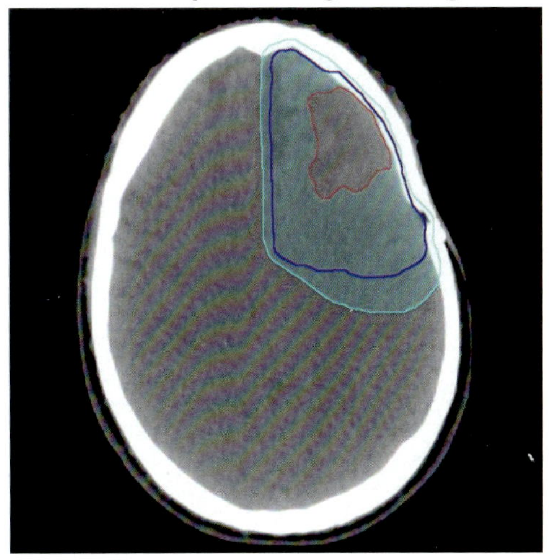

Grade III Anaplastic Oligodendroglioma

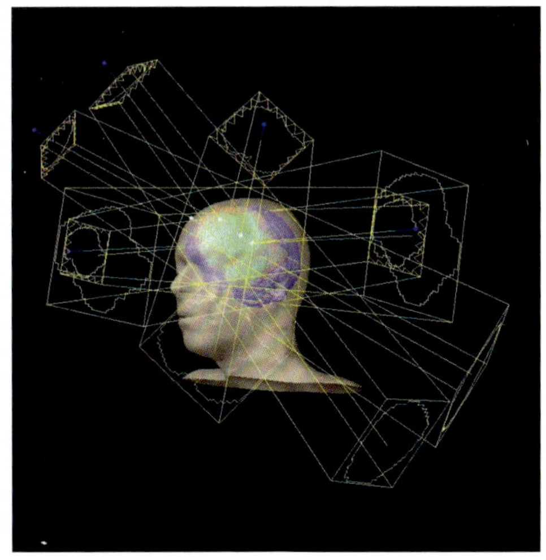

(Left) *Planning CT in the same patient shows GTV, CTV, and PTV. The PTV is a 3 mm expansion from the CTV.* ***(Right)*** *Beam arrangement of the 5-field IMRT plan in the same patient is shown. IMRT permitted reduction in dose to the cochleae, optic chiasm, and brainstem in this case.*

Grade III Anaplastic Oligodendroglioma

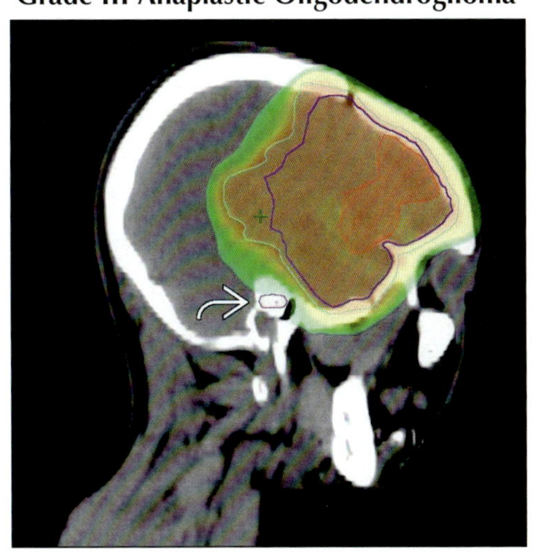

Grade III Anaplastic Oligodendroglioma

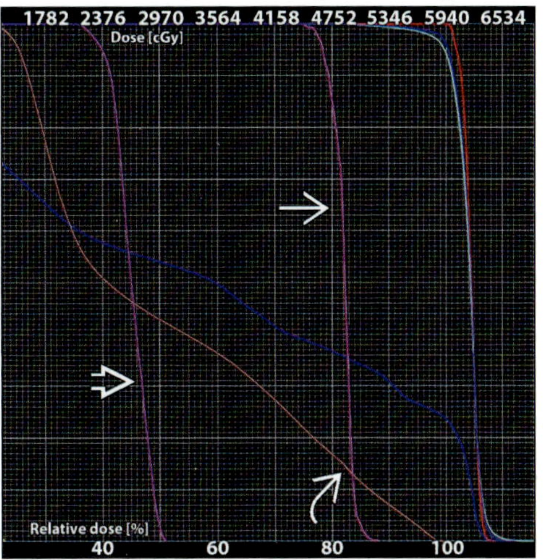

(Left) *The dose colorwash is shown set at a 30 Gy minimum in the same patient. Note the dose wrapping around the cochlea ➚.* ***(Right)*** *DVH shows target coverage in the same patient. The optic chiasm was limited to 54 Gy ➔, the brainstem < 60 Gy with only a small peripheral volume > 54 Gy ➚, and the cochleae < 30 Gy ➩.*

GLIOMAS

(**Left**) Axial graphic shows an infiltrative white matter mass with focal hemorrhage ➔ and local mass effect. In addition, extension along the corpus callosum can be seen; white matter extension is typical of anaplastic astrocytoma. (**Right**) H&E shows pleomorphism and mitoses ➔ indicative of a grade III anaplastic astrocytoma. (Courtesy P. Burger, MD.)

WHO Grade III Anaplastic Astrocytoma

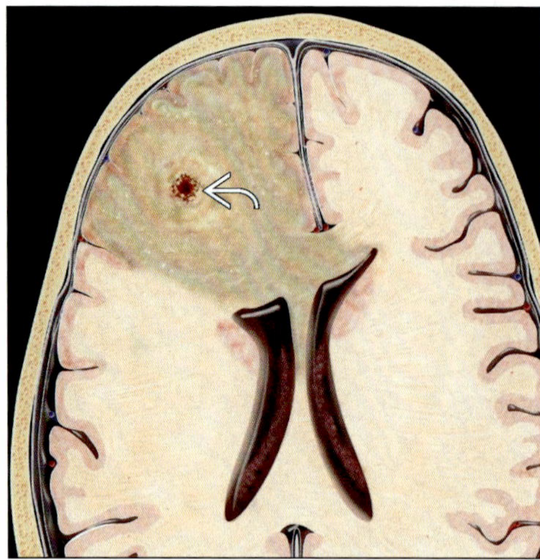

WHO Grade III Anaplastic Astrocytoma

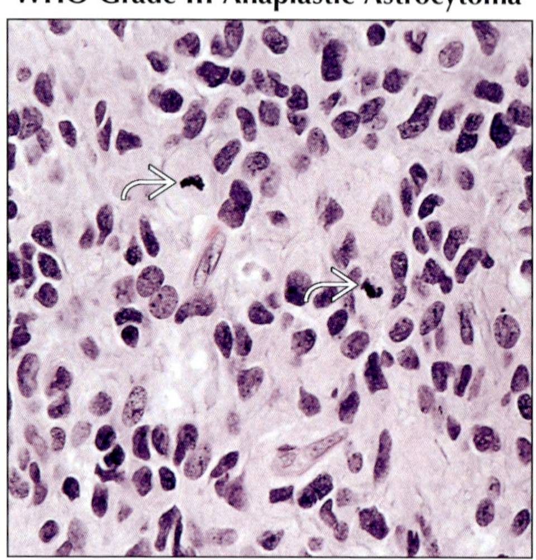

(**Left**) Axial T1 MR shows a hypointense infiltrative mass in the left temporal region. Mild mass effect can be seen. (**Right**) Axial T2 MR image in the same patient shows a hyperintense temporal mass centered in the white matter.

WHO Grade III Anaplastic Astrocytoma

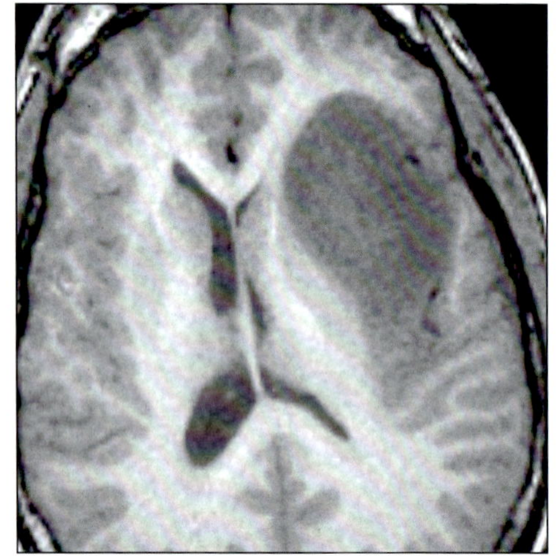

WHO Grade III Anaplastic Astrocytoma

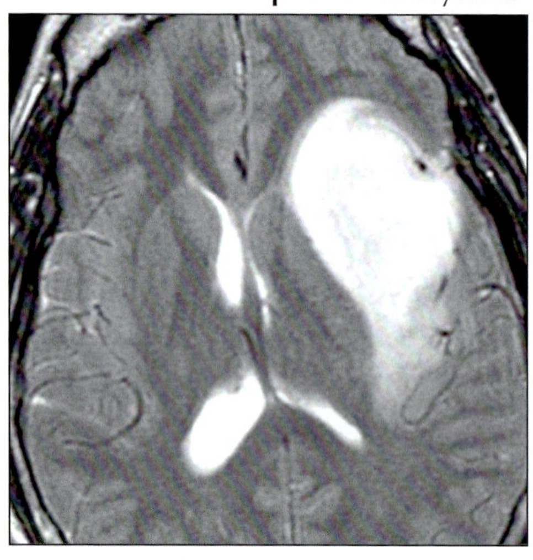

(**Left**) Axial T1 post-contrast MR in the same patient reveals no enhancement. This is typical for anaplastic astrocytomas. (**Right**) Axial FLAIR MR image in the same patient shows a similar hyperintense temporal mass as seen on T2WI. While the borders appear to be discrete, high-grade tumors typically demonstrate microscopic infiltration beyond the radiographic signal abnormalities.

WHO Grade III Anaplastic Astrocytoma

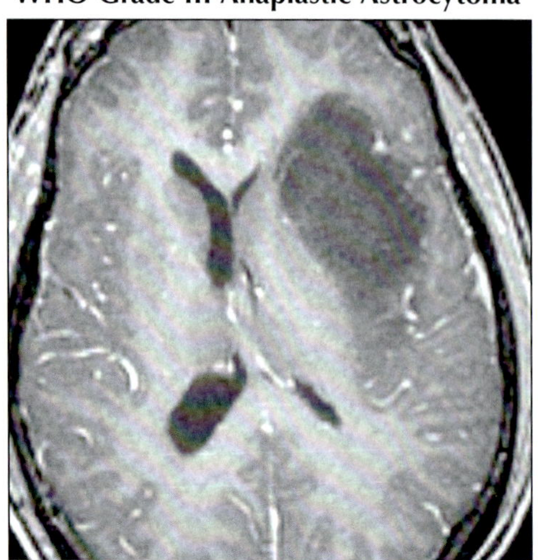

WHO Grade III Anaplastic Astrocytoma

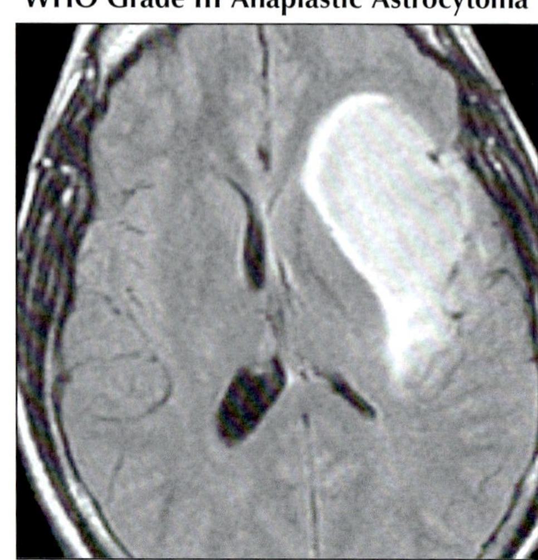

WHO Grade III Anaplastic Astrocytoma

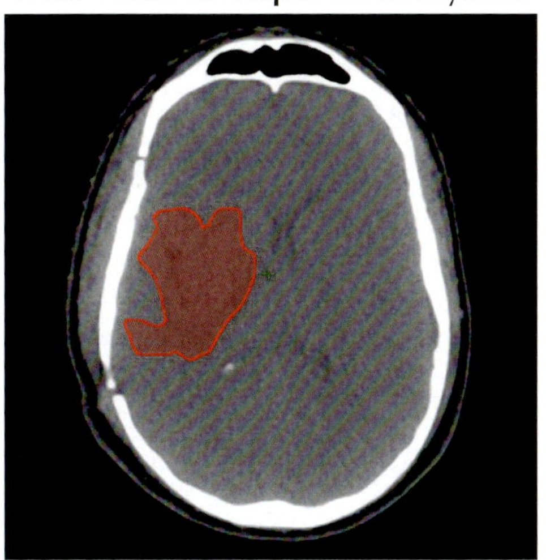

WHO Grade III Anaplastic Astrocytoma

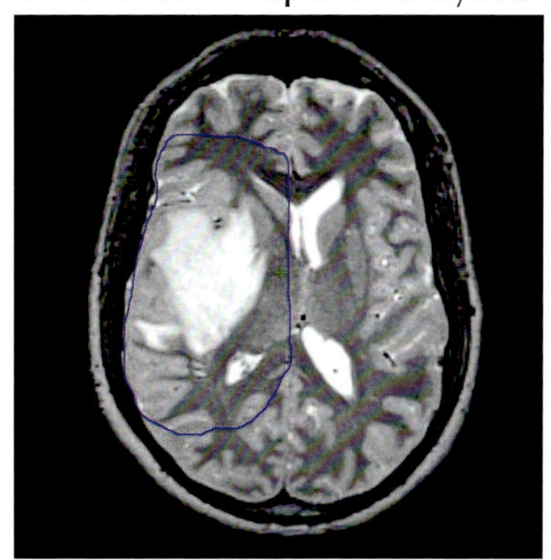

(Left) *Planning CT from a different case shows the GTV outlining the resection cavity and the residual tumor.* ***(Right)*** *Fused T2 MR in the same patient shows CTV as a 2 cm expansion, and including all edema. CTV was subtracted from the calvarium and the falx.*

WHO Grade III Anaplastic Astrocytoma

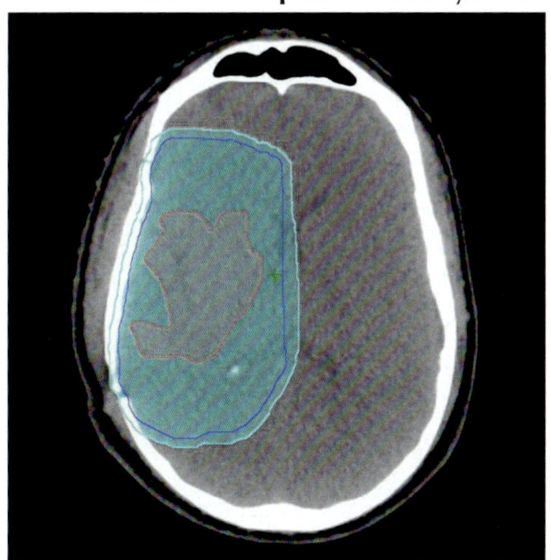

WHO Grade III Anaplastic Astrocytoma

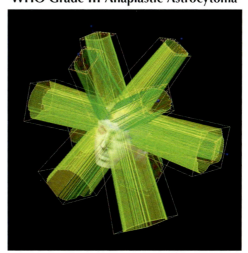

(Left) *Planning CT in the same patient demonstrates GTV, CTV, and PTV. PTV is a 3 mm expansion from the CTV.* ***(Right)*** *Six-field IMRT was used to deliver 59.4 Gy in 33 fx in the same patient. IMRT was used to reduce dose to critical structures.*

WHO Grade III Anaplastic Astrocytoma

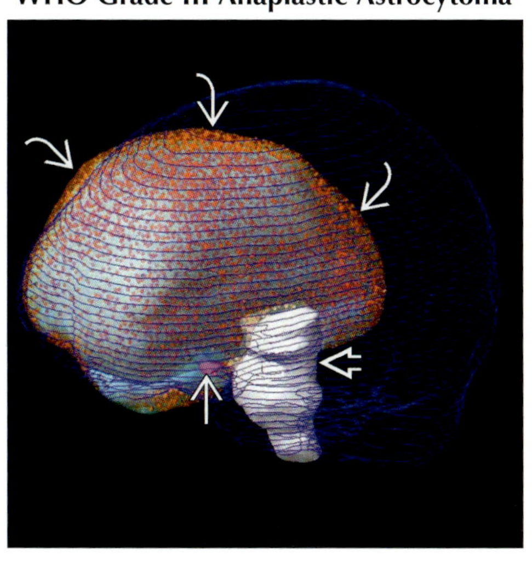

WHO Grade III Anaplastic Astrocytoma

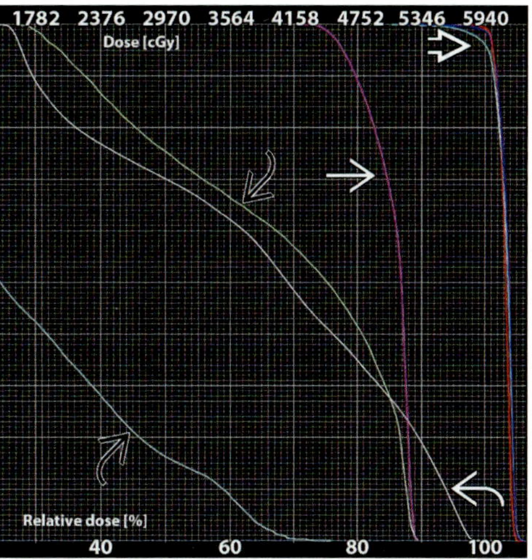

(Left) *3D representation in the same patient shows 54 Gy dose cloud. Note the shaping of the dose around the brainstem and chiasm.* ***(Right)*** *DVH in the same patient shows target coverage. Note the optic chiasm and optic nerves are limited to 54 Gy. The brainstem was limited to < 60 Gy, with only a small portion of the periphery with > 54 Gy.*

*(**Left**) Axial graphic shows an infiltrating mass within the left frontal lobe. Central necrosis can be seen, as well as extension across the corpus callosum. These findings are characteristic of a GBM. (**Right**) H&E shows glioblastoma multiforme with classic hallmarks of neovascularity ➡ and necrosis ⇨.*

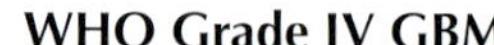

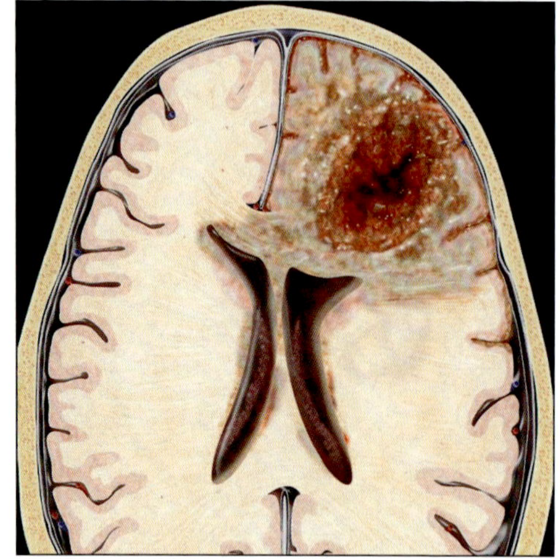

WHO Grade IV GBM

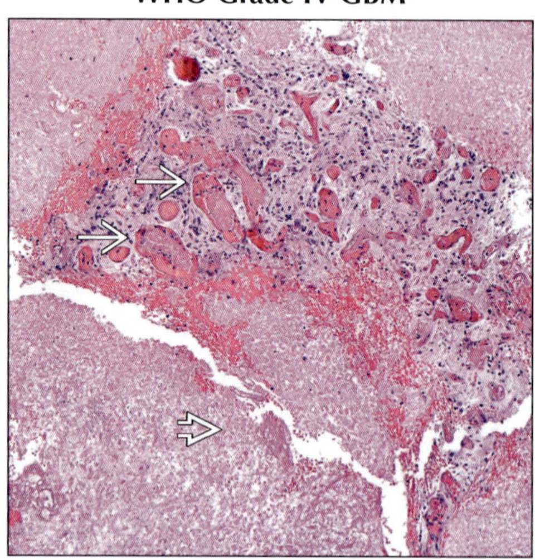

*(**Left**) Axial T1WI in a different case shows a heterogeneous mass. Surrounding edema can be seen, as well as focal areas of subacute hemorrhage ➡. (**Right**) Axial T2WI in the same patient shows mixed hyper-hypointense regions within the mass →. Significant edema can be seen throughout the temporal lobe.*

WHO Grade IV GBM

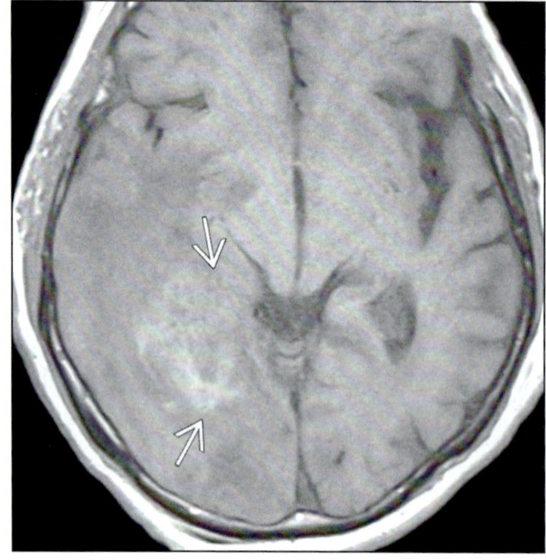

WHO Grade IV GBM

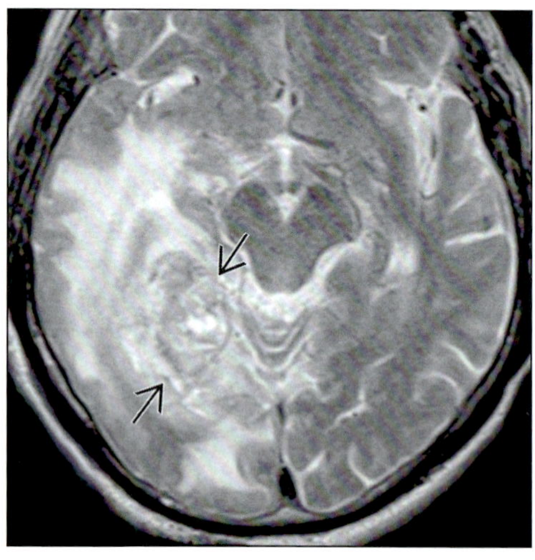

*(**Left**) Axial T1 contrast-enhanced MR in the same patient shows an irregular area of enhancement surrounding a central area of necrosis. (**Right**) Axial FLAIR MR in the same patient shows edema as visualized on the T2WI.*

WHO Grade IV GBM

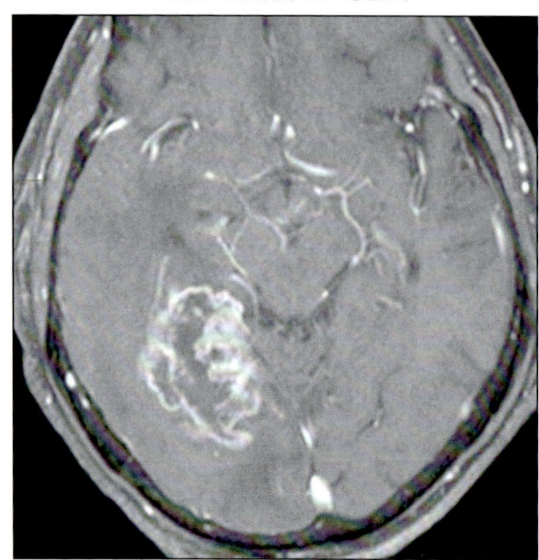

WHO Grade IV GBM

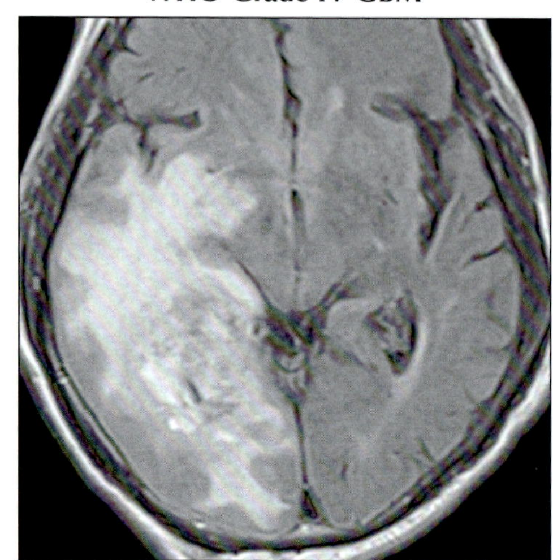

WHO Grade IV GBM

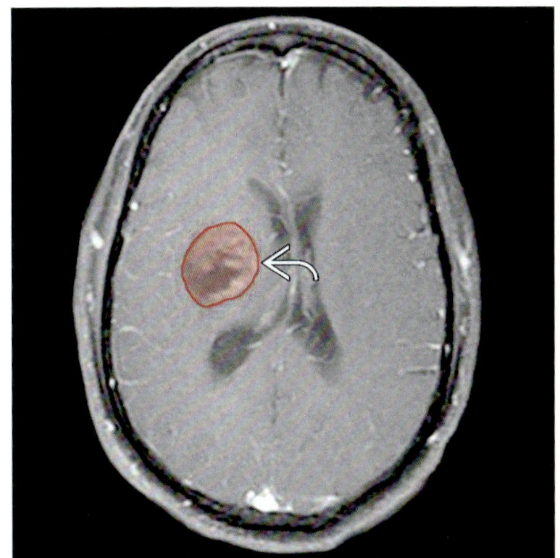

WHO Grade IV GBM

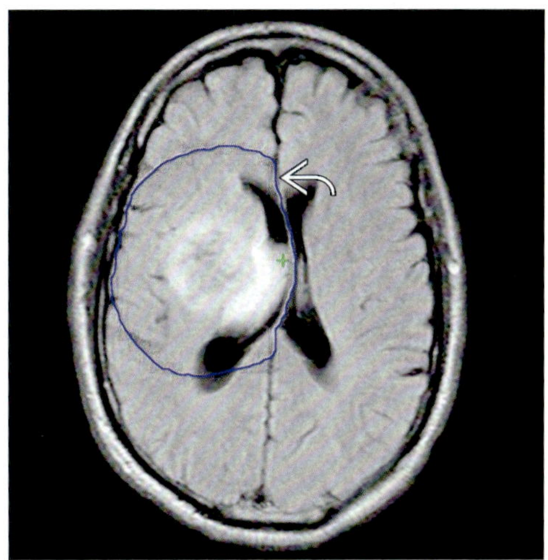

*(**Left**) Axial T1 post-contrast MR delineating the GTV is shown. Note the GTV ➔ encompasses the entire contrast enhancement. (**Right**) Axial FLAIR MR in the same patient was used to delineate CTV. CTV ➔ is a 2.5 cm expansion of GTV. Note that it encompasses the entire FLAIR signal and is constrained by natural anatomic boundaries.*

WHO Grade IV GBM

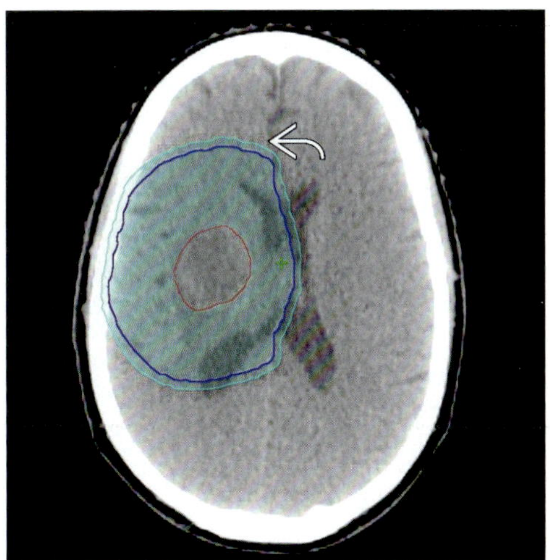

WHO Grade IV GBM

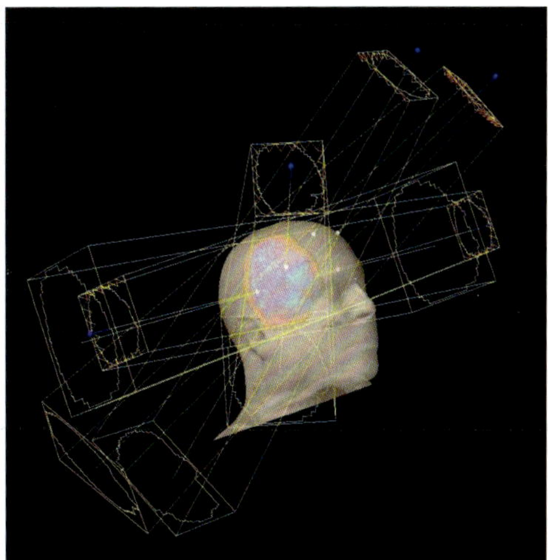

*(**Left**) Planning CT in the same patient demonstrates GTV, CTV, and PTV. PTV ➔ is a 0.3 mm margin expanded from the CTV. (**Right**) Beam arrangement in the same patient shows a 5-field IMRT plan. IMRT was used to reduce dose to the chiasm and brainstem in this case.*

WHO Grade IV GBM

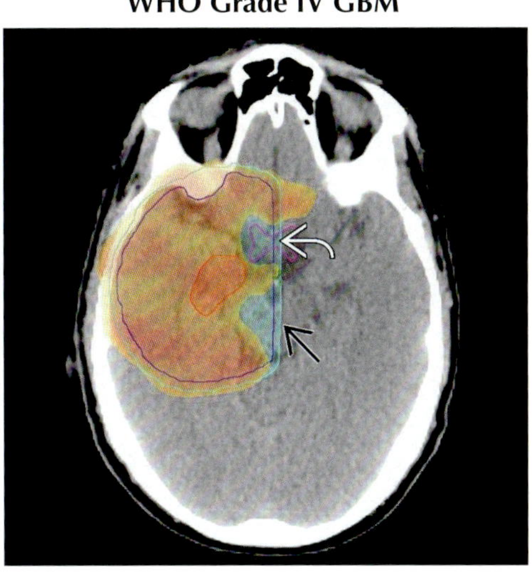

WHO Grade IV GBM

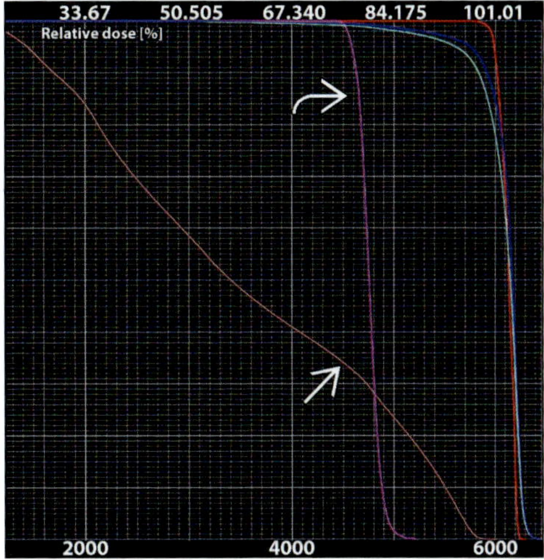

*(**Left**) Axial CT in the same patient shows the dose colorwash with the minimum dose set at 54 Gy. Note the optic chiasm ➔ and brainstem exclusion accomplished with IMRT ➔. (**Right**) DVH in the same patient shows target coverage and OARs. Note the chiasm is kept below 54 Gy ➔ and the brainstem volume is limited to < 60 Gy with limited volumes (peripheral, not central) above 54 Gy ➔.*

GLIOMAS

(**Left**) Axial T2WI in a patient with left hemispheric lesion shows no contrast enhancement of the lesion. The overlayed MRS shows a high choline (Cho) peak and a low NAA peak. This spectrum is nonspecific but is suggestive of low-grade malignancy. (**Right**) Single voxel MRS in the same patient shows an elevated choline peak relative to NAA. Note the absence of a lactate peak, which would be concerning for high-grade malignancy.

WHO Grade II (MRS)

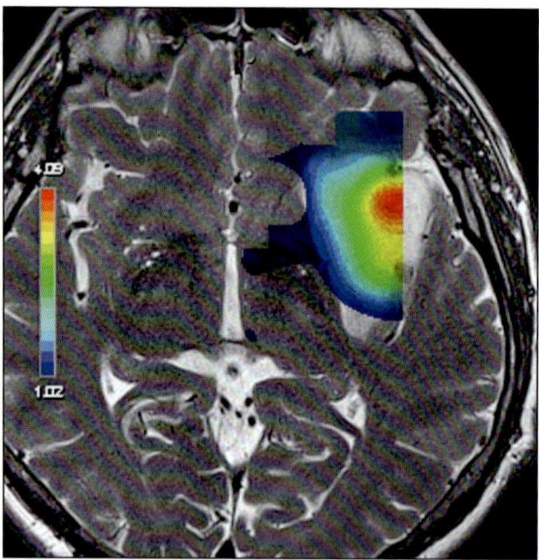

WHO Grade II (MRS)

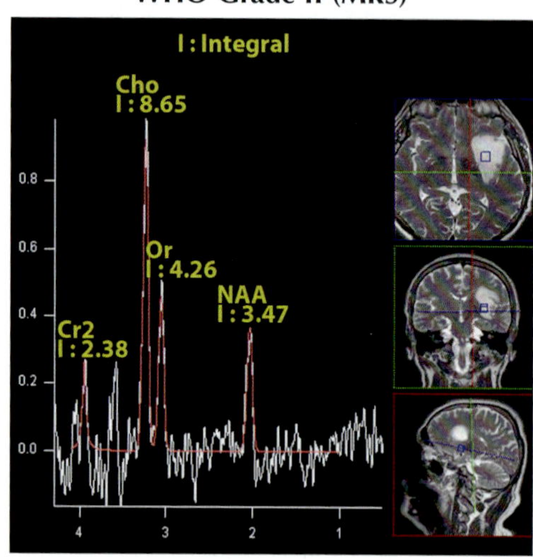

(**Left**) Axial MR perfusion shows relatively low cerebral blood volume (CBV) ➔ in the frontotemporal mass, suggesting a low-grade tumor. (**Right**) Multivoxel MRS in the same patient shows abnormal spectra. These findings are consistent with a tumor, i.e., marked elevation of Cho and decreased NAA ➔ in the area of signal abnormality seen on the underlying MR.

WHO Grade II Oligo (Perfusion)

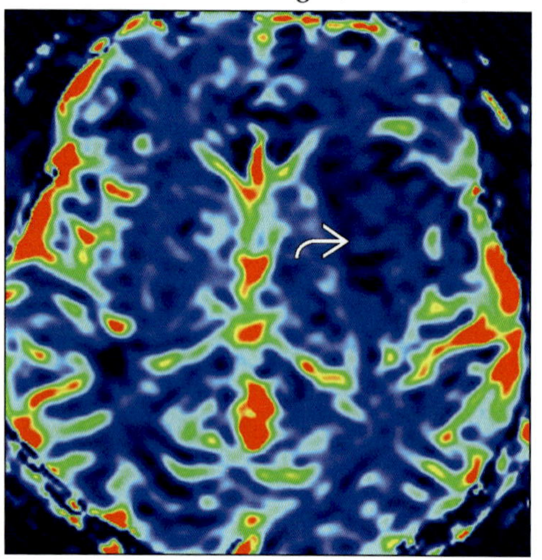

WHO Grade II Oligo (MRS)

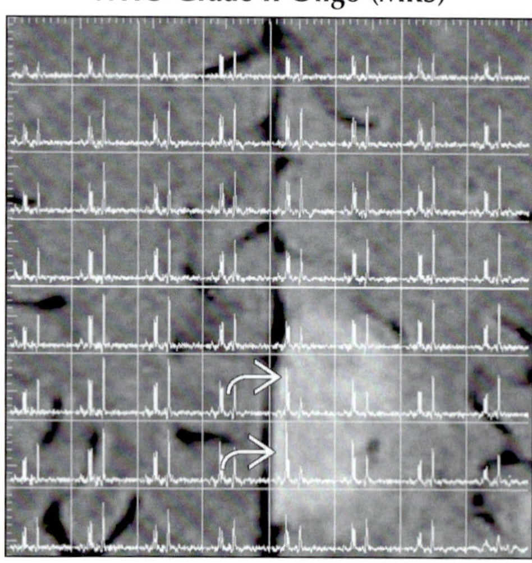

(**Left**) Axial T1 contrast-enhanced MR shows a right hemispheric GBM. (**Right**) Perfusion scan in the same patient shows increased CBV in solid portions of the tumor ➔ and decreased CBV in the necrotic center ➔.

WHO Grade IV (Perfusion)

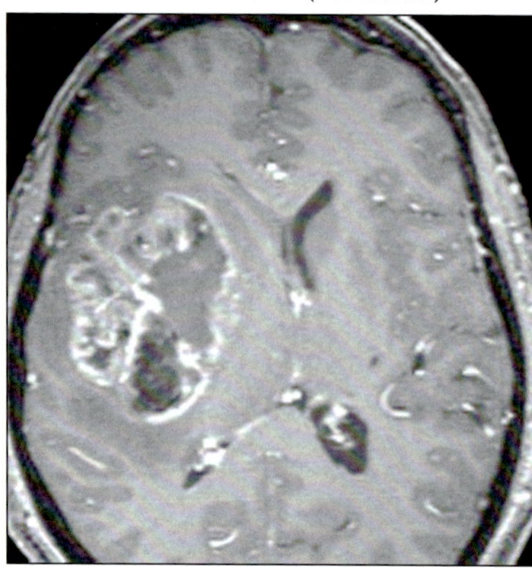

WHO Grade IV (Perfusion)

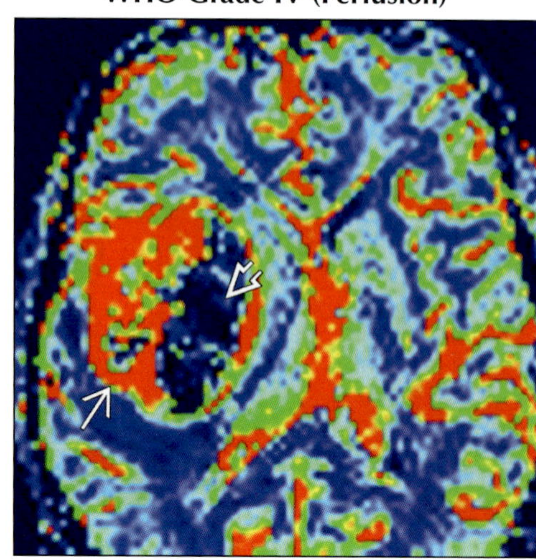

GBM After Radiation

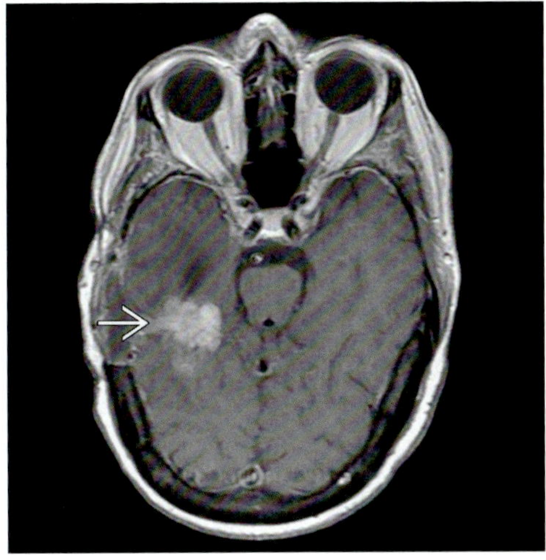

GBM After Radiation

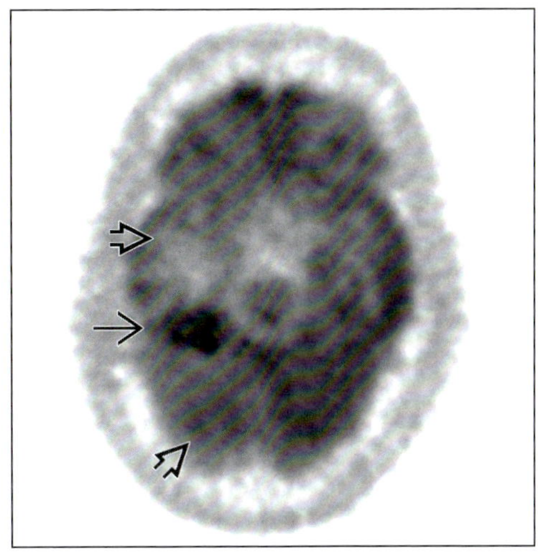

(Left) *GBM of the right temporal lobe is shown 4-6 months after RT. Axial T1 post-contrast MR shows an abnormal enhancing lesion in the medial right temporal lobe ➔, concerning for tumor recurrence. Radiation necrosis may appear similar.* ***(Right)*** *Axial FDG PET in the same patient shows the medial right temporal lobe lesion to be FDG avid ➔, consistent with recurrence. The surrounding parenchyma demonstrates mildly decreased activity ⇨, consistent with edema.*

Treatment Effect vs. Recurrence/Progression

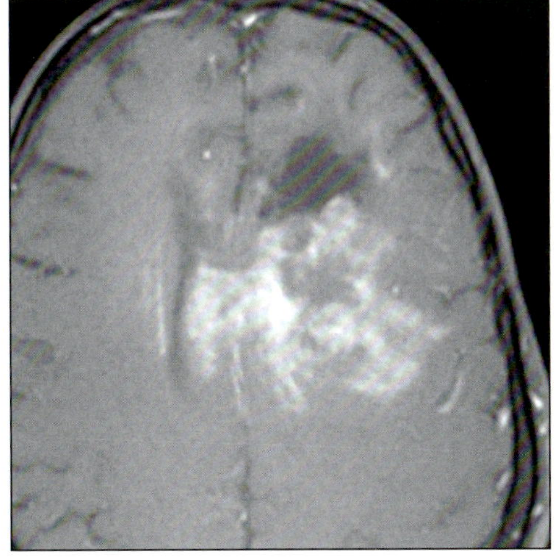

Treatment Effect vs. Recurrence/Progression

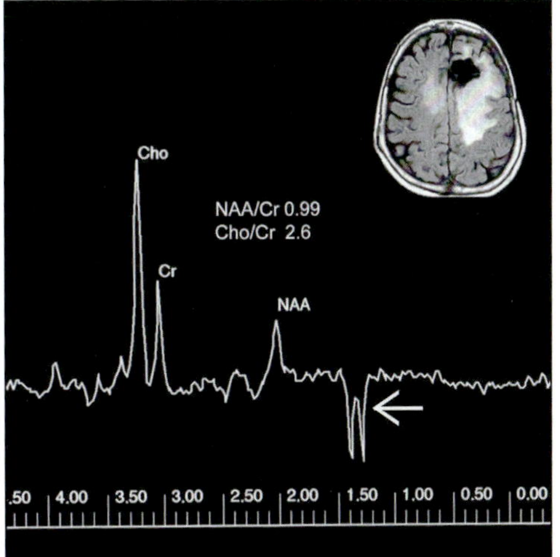

(Left) *Axial T1 contrast-enhanced MR shows previously treated anaplastic astrocytoma, now with significant heterogeneous enhancement. This is concerning for recurrence &/or progression.* ***(Right)*** *Single voxel MRS in the same patient with inlay image shows findings consistent with a high-grade tumor recurrence, with elevated choline, decreased NAA, and a lactate doublet ➔.*

Treatment Effect vs. Recurrence/Progression

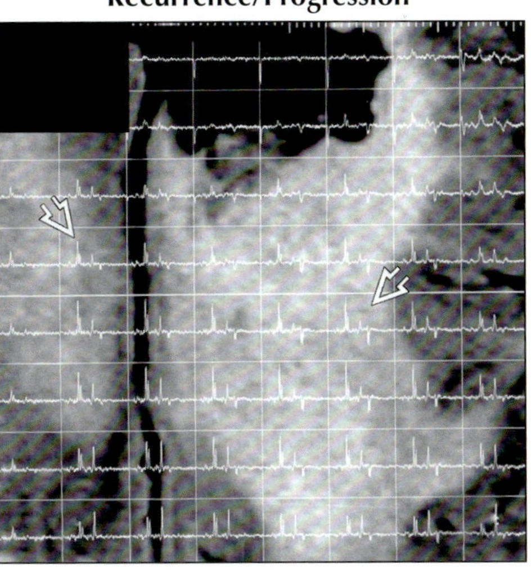

Treatment Effect vs. Recurrence/Progression

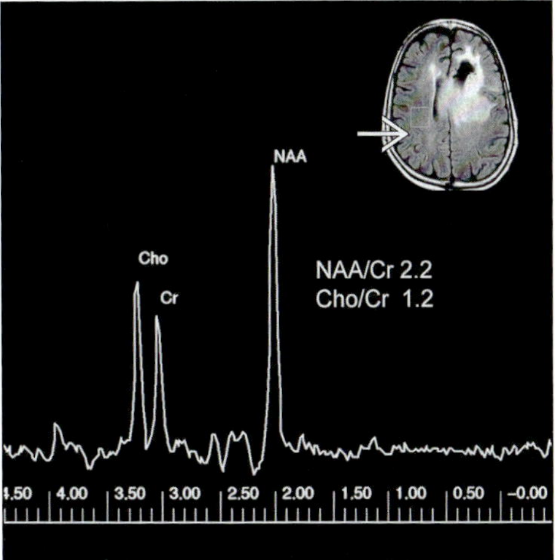

(Left) *Multivoxel MRS in the same patient shows abnormal tumor spectra ⇨ (high Cho:NAA) within the area of abnormal signal in the underlying MR.* ***(Right)*** *MRS of the contralateral normal brain (see voxel selection ➔) shows a normal white matter spectrum.*

*(**Left**) Axial T1 post-contrast MR shows an area of enhancement within the left occipital lobe. (**Right**) Axial FLAIR MR in the same patient shows diffuse edema within the left occipital lobe, surrounding the area of enhancement.*

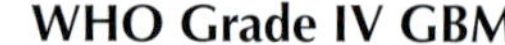

WHO Grade IV GBM

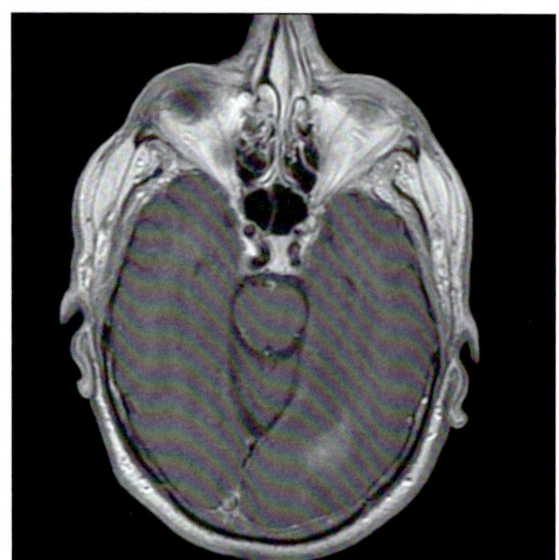

WHO Grade IV GBM

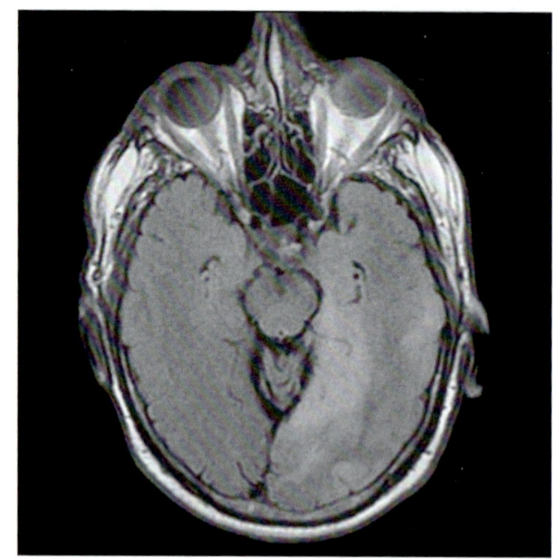

*(**Left**) Axial T1 post-contrast MR demonstrates the previously seen lesion status post resection. The area of enhancement in the cavity was also hyperintense on T1 imaging without contrast, indicating blood products rather than residual tumor. (**Right**) Axial FLAIR MR in the same patient shows the resection cavity with surrounding edema.*

WHO Grade IV GBM

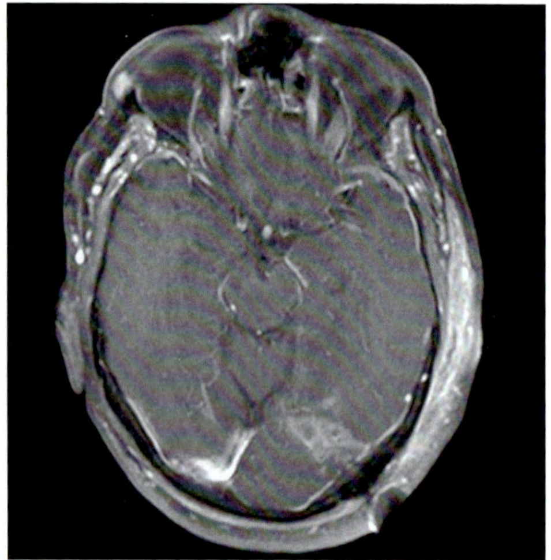

WHO Grade IV GBM

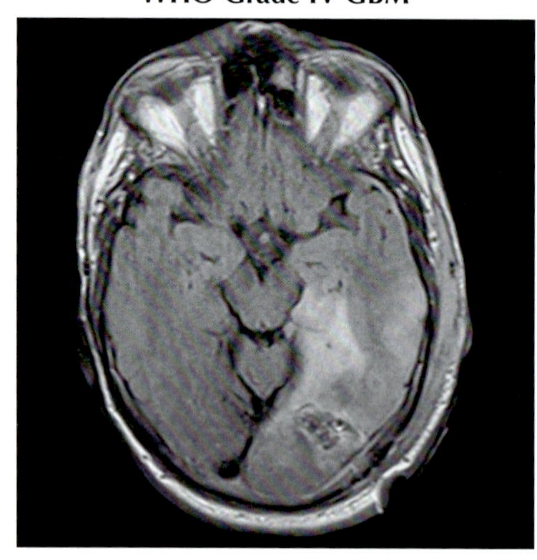

*(**Left**) Axial T1 post-contrast MR in the same patient illustrates the GTV ➔ outlining the resection cavity. (**Right**) Axial FLAIR MR in the same patient shows the CTV ➔. The CTV is a 2.5 cm expansion from the GTV, which was further expanded anteriorly to include the areas of edema.*

WHO Grade IV GBM

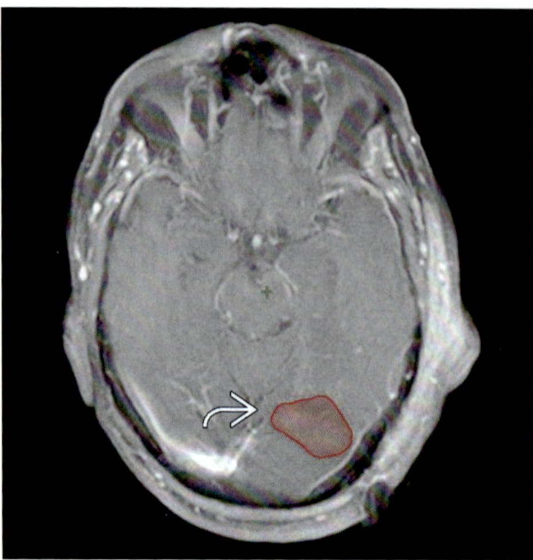

WHO Grade IV GBM

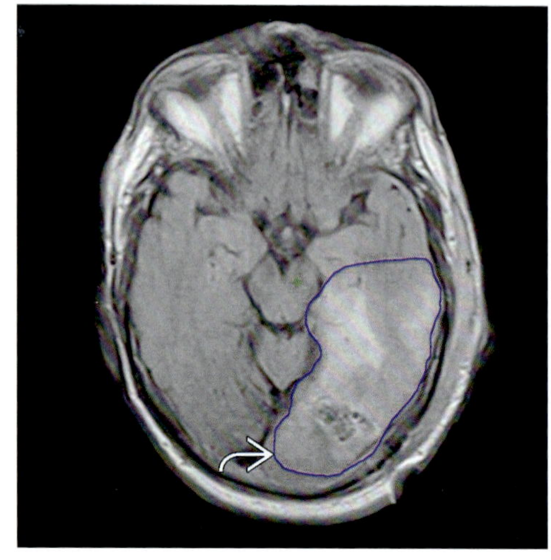

WHO Grade IV GBM

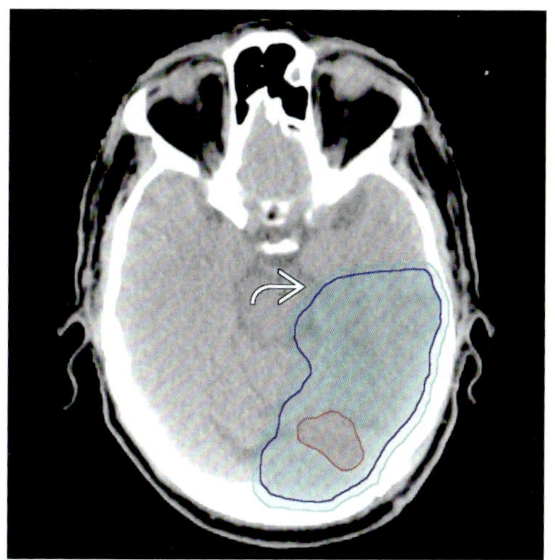

WHO Grade IV GBM

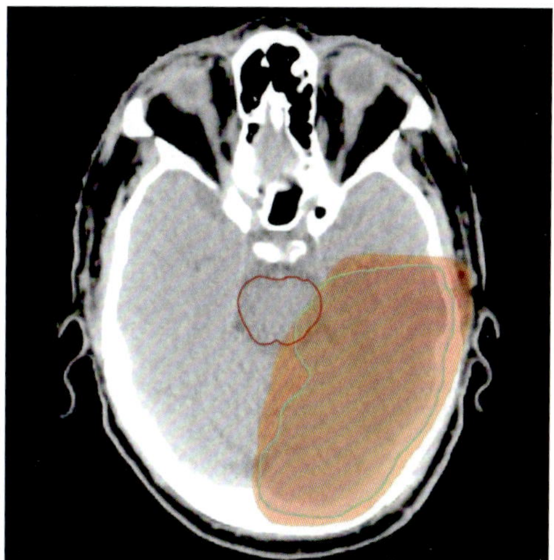

(Left) *Planning CT shows the GTV, CTV, and PTV. The PTV is a 3 mm expansion on the CTV.* ***(Right)*** *Dose colorwash in the same patient shows 95% coverage of the PTV.*

WHO Grade IV GBM

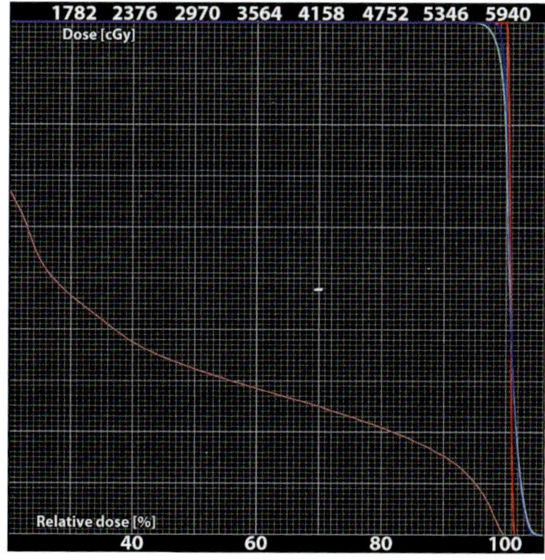

WHO Grade IV GBM

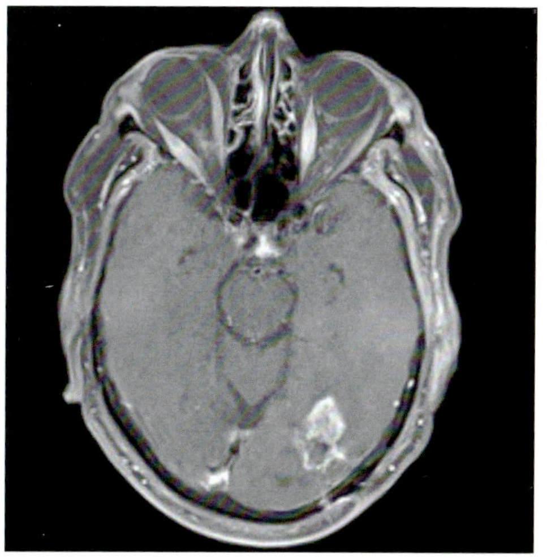

(Left) *DVH in the same patient shows 95% of the volume covered by 98% of the dose.* ***(Right)*** *Axial T1 post-contrast MR in the same patient was taken 3 months after completing RT. Note the nodular area of enhancement anterior to the resection cavity, concerning for treatment effect vs. recurrence.*

WHO Grade IV GBM

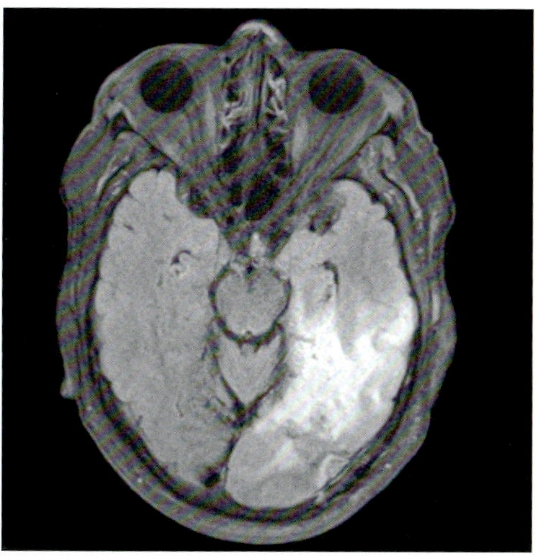

WHO Grade IV GBM

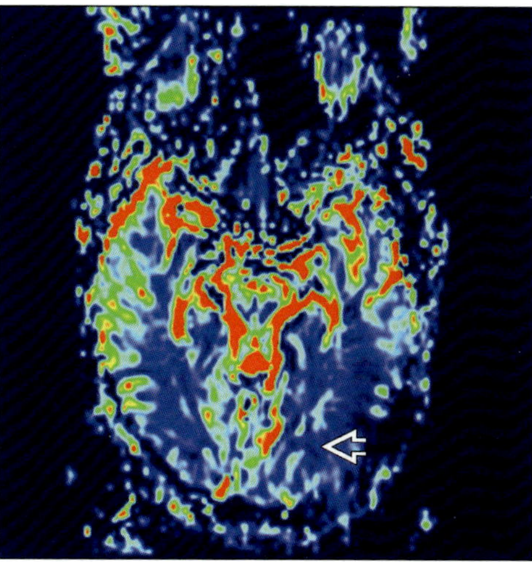

(Left) *Axial FLAIR MR in the same patient shows edema surrounding the resection cavity. This could be due to recurrent tumor or treatment effect.* ***(Right)*** *Shown is an axial perfusion MR in the same patient performed 3 months after completing RT. Note the absence of increased blood flow in the area of nodular enhancement seen on the contrast-enhanced MR. This was classified as treatment effect, with a plan for repeat imaging in 3 months.*

EPENDYMOMA

OVERVIEW

General Comments
- Tumors arising from ependymal cells lining the ventricular system

Classification
- WHO classifies tumors into grades I-III

NATURAL HISTORY

General Features
- Location
  - While mostly intracranial, can occur anywhere within ventricular system and spinal canal
    - Pediatric: 80-90% intracranial, mostly posterior fossa
    - Adult: 60-70% spinal cord, more supratentorial lesions than children

Epidemiology & Cancer Incidence
- Represents 8-10% of pediatric CNS tumors; < 4% of adult CNS tumors

Genetics
- Links with *NF2* and *MEN1*
- Chromosomal aberrations common, i.e., LOH 22q

Gross Pathology & Surgical Features
- Tumors are usually well-delineated, lobular masses

Microscopic Pathology
- Both glial and epithelial features common
- Perivascular pseudorosettes are a hallmark
- Considered anaplastic (grade III) when abundant mitosis, necrosis, or endothelial proliferation

IMAGING

CT
- Hypo-hyperdense: Varies with cystic/solid components
- Calcifications common

MR
- T1WI: Heterogeneously iso- to hypointense
- T2WI: Usually hyperintense, but varies with cystic and solid content
- T1 post contrast: Solid portions generally enhance (i.e., mural nodules/ring enhancement around cysts)

CLINICAL PRESENTATION & WORK-UP

Presentation
- Frequently signs of elevated intracranial pressure (ICP)
  - Headaches, N/V, ataxia, vertigo, papilledema
- Focal neurologic deficits depending on location

Prognosis
- 5-year PFS 50-95%
  - Pediatric patients with intracranial low-grade lesions have control rates > 80%
- ~ 90% of recurrences local, surgery most important prognostic factor

Work-Up
- H&P with neurologic exam
- Brain and spinal MR, ± contrast
- CSF evaluation, if postop delay 2-3 weeks (to prevent false positives)

TREATMENT

Overview
- Maximal resection, then focal RT
  - Complete resection most important prognostic factor
- Craniospinal irradiation (CSI) after resection if positive CSF or spinal MR
- Observation for low-grade supratentorial lesions controversial
  - Pediatric patients currently being observed in this category

Standard Doses
- Intracranial: 54-59.4 Gy in 1.8-2.0 Gy fractions
  - Pediatric: 59.4 Gy unless < 18 months, then 54 Gy
- CSI: 36 Gy in 1.8 Gy fractions
  - Spinal lesions boosted to 45 Gy

Common Techniques
- Intracranial: 3D conformal, IMRT, or arc therapy depending on location
- CSI: Process described for medulloblastoma
- Contouring
  - GTV: Resection cavity + residual tumor or enhancement
    - Utilize preop imaging to include all areas contacted by tumor
    - Cysts will be markedly decompressed after surgery
  - CTV: GTV + 1-2 cm
    - GTV + 0.5-1 cm for pediatric patients
    - Constrain for natural anatomic boundaries (i.e., calvarium, falx, tentorium)
  - PTV: CTV + 3-5 mm

Landmark Trials
- Rogers: Addition of RT after GTR improves LC and trends toward improved overall survival (OS)
- HIT-SKK87/HIT-SKK92: Omission or delay of RT in pediatric patients jeopardized survival

RECOMMENDED FOLLOW-UP

Routine
- Follow up every 3-4 months with repeat MR imaging for 1st year
  - 4-6 months during year 2
  - 6 months to annually from year 3 onward

Suspected Recurrence
- Repeat staging with suspected recurrence, including brain/spine MR and CSF evaluation

Posterior Fossa Ependymoma

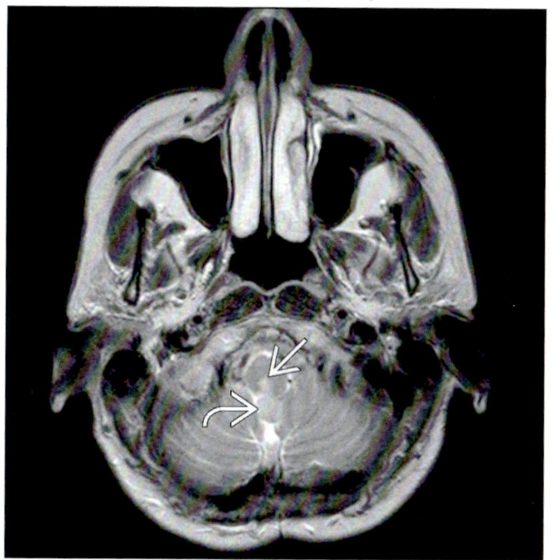

Posterior Fossa Ependymoma

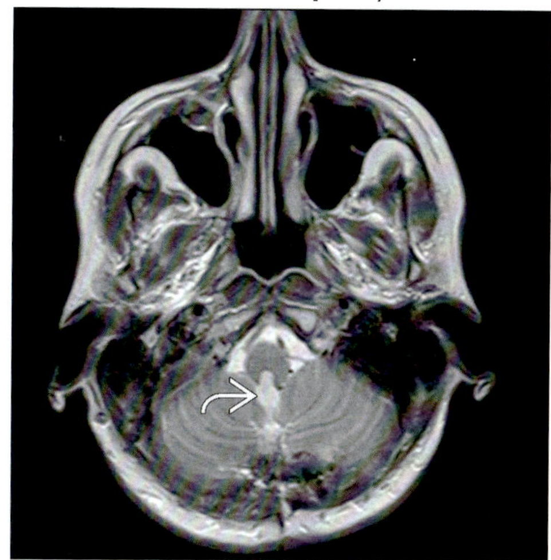

(Left) *Axial T2WI shows a mass ➔ centered in the 4th ventricle with extension ➔ into the brainstem.* ***(Right)*** *Axial T2WI postoperatively shows resection cavity ➔ of the 4th ventricular mass. No residual mass was seen. Spinal imaging (not shown) and CSF evaluation were negative, and CSI was not required.*

Posterior Fossa Ependymoma

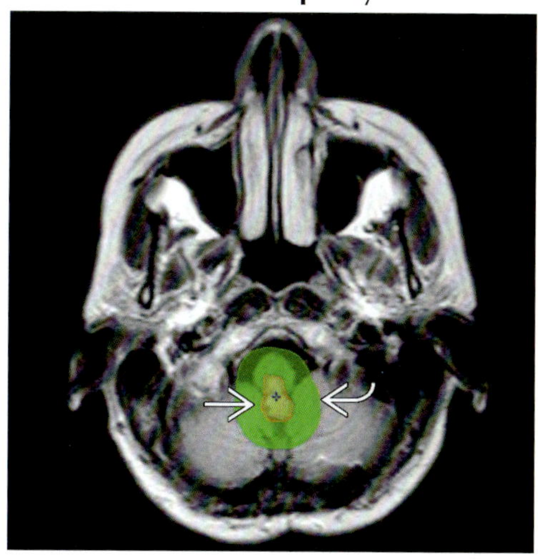

Posterior Fossa Ependymoma

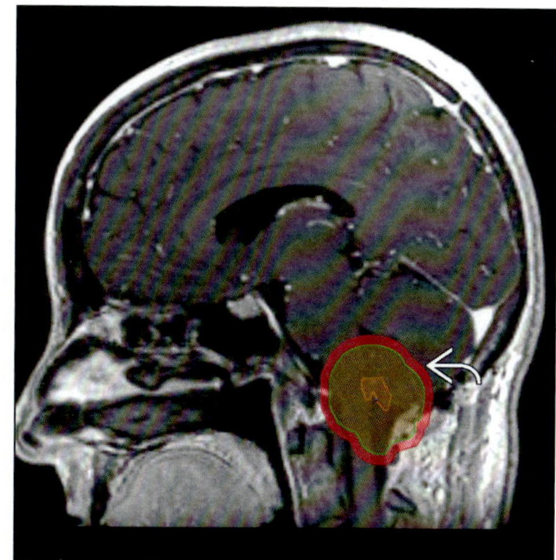

(Left) *Fused postop and preop planning FLAIR MR shows the resection cavity outlined as the GTV ➔, with the CTV ➔ added as a 1 cm expansion.* ***(Right)*** *Sagittal fused SPGR MR shows GTV, CTV, and PTV ➔. PTV was a 3 mm expansion in this case.*

Posterior Fossa Ependymoma

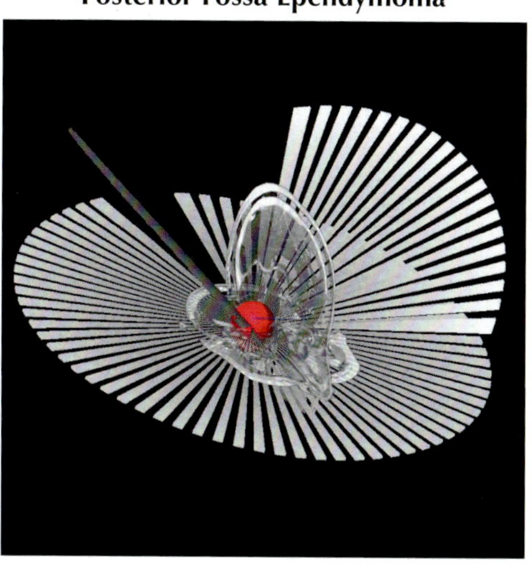

Posterior Fossa Ependymoma

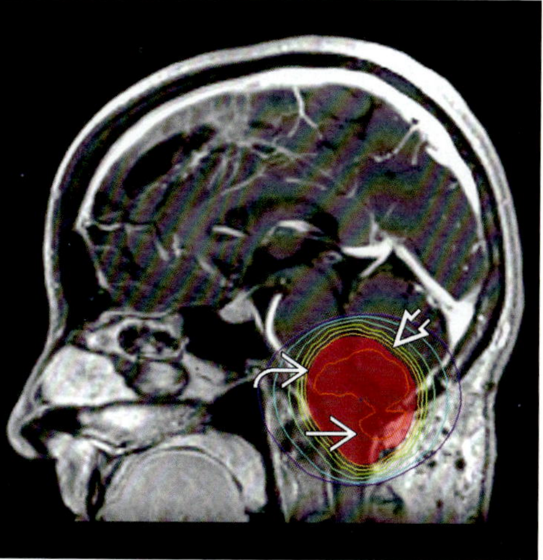

(Left) *Three dynamic conformal arcs were used to deliver 54 Gy in 30 fx with a Novalis Brainlab treatment platform.* ***(Right)*** *Treatment plan shows dose coverage of the PTV ➔. Note the brainstem was allowed to go to 54 Gy, with hotspots excluded. The orange isodose line ➔ represents 100% and the yellow isodose line ➔ represents 95% coverage.*

CRANIOPHARYNGIOMA

OVERVIEW

General Comments
- Suprasellar benign tumor arising from Rathke pouch ectodermal remnant

Classification
- Adamantinomatous and papillary subtypes

NATURAL HISTORY

General Features
- Comments
  - Benign tumor with solid and cystic components

Epidemiology & Cancer Incidence
- Most common non-glial CNS tumor in pediatrics (~ 350 cases/year in USA)
- Bimodal distribution: 5-14 years old; 50-75 years old

Gross Pathology & Surgical Features
- Mixed solid/cystic lesion

Microscopic Pathology
- Squamous cells in columnar layers (adamantinomatous) or papillary architecture
- "Crankcase oil" appearance of cystic fluid is result of high lipid/cholesterol crystal content

IMAGING

CT
- Mixed cystic/solid (hypodense/isodense) mass in suprasellar region
- Can see local mass effect &/or surrounding invasion
- Calcifications frequently present

MR
- T1WI: Hyperintense (cyst) to isointense (solid)
- T2WI: Hyperintense cysts with iso-/hyperintense solid portions
- T2 FLAIR: Hyperintensity seen in cystic portions
- T1 post contrast: Enhancement in solid portions and cyst walls

CLINICAL PRESENTATION & WORK-UP

Presentation
- Visual disturbances 2° to compression of optic chiasm
  - Classically bitemporal hemianopsia
- Pituitary dysfunction/growth failure

Prognosis
- Benign tumor but locally aggressive
- Recurrence rates increase with tumor size
- 10-year disease-free survival: 70-100%
  - Aggressive surgery may lead to high morbidity

Work-Up
- H&P with complete neurologic exam and visual testing

Radiographic
- CT and MR brain

Laboratory
- Endocrine evaluation: TSH, T4, FSH, LH, IGF-1 (insulin-like growth factor-1), AM cortisol, ACTH

TREATMENT

Overview
- Surgical resection > postop RT if STR
  - Achieving GTR can have high morbidity
    - GTR morbidity frequently higher than STR + RT
    - STR + RT ~ equal to GTR in disease control

Standard Doses
- 50-60 Gy in 1.8 Gy/fx
  - 54 Gy most common

Organs at Risk Parameters
- Optic nerves/chiasm: < 54 Gy (< 1% optic neuropathy, QUANTEC)
- Retina: 45 Gy (< 5% retinopathy, Emami)
- Lens: 10 Gy (< 5% cataract, Emami)
- Cochlea: Mean dose 35-45 Gy (minimize risk, QUANTEC)
- Brainstem: < 54 Gy (< 5% necrosis, neuropathy, QUANTEC)

Common Techniques
- 3D conformal, intensity-modulated radiation therapy (IMRT), dynamic conformal arcs, or proton beam

Contouring
- GTV: Resection cavity + residual tumor seen on MR or CT
- CTV: 0.5-1.5 cm expansion of GTV
  - May constrain to natural anatomic boundaries
  - Consider accounting for cystic expansion during treatment; alternatively, may account for this in PTV
- PTV: 3-5 mm expansion from CTV

RECOMMENDED FOLLOW-UP

Follow-Up Based on Symptomatology
- Generally annual follow-up with MR, visual field testing, and endocrine testing (if needed)

CRANIOPHARYNGIOMA

Craniopharyngioma

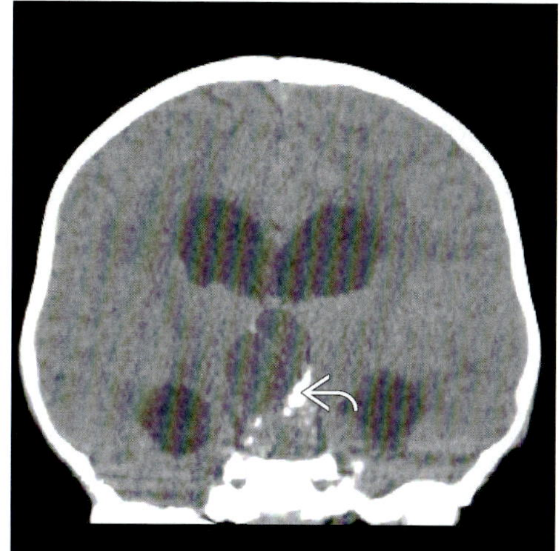

Craniopharyngioma

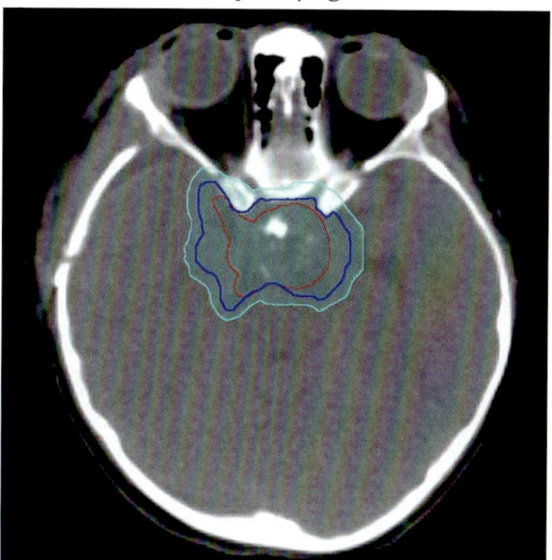

(Left) *Coronal CT of a 7-year-old girl shows a mixed cystic/solid mass with calcifications in the sellar/suprasellar region. The patient underwent subtotal resection with a plan for postop RT. Note that complete resection in this location would cause significant morbidity.* ***(Right)*** *Axial planning CT in the same patient shows target. GTV is the residual tumor/resection cavity. CTV is a 0.5 cm expansion constrained from natural boundaries and the PTV is a 3 mm expansion of CTV.*

Craniopharyngioma

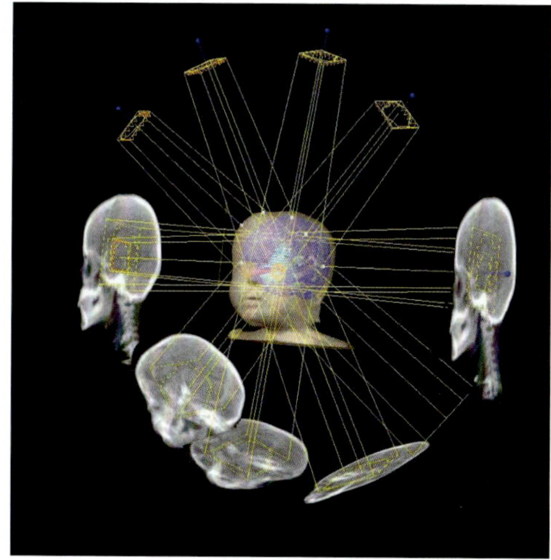

Craniopharyngioma

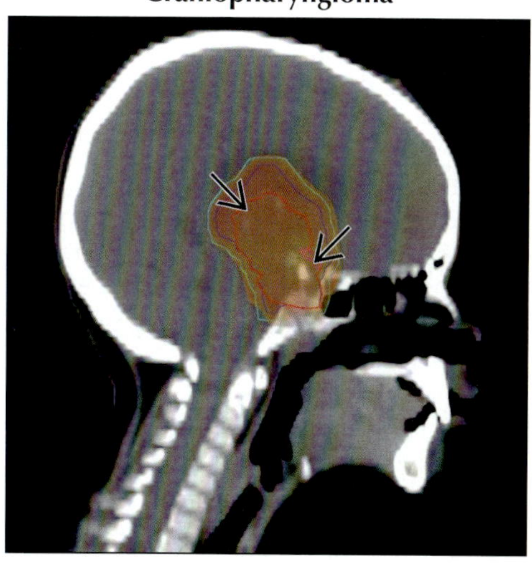

(Left) *Beam orientation was used in the same patient to deliver 54 Gy. A 5-field IMRT plan was required to increase conformality in this pediatric patient and to maintain OAR tolerances.* ***(Right)*** *Dose colorwash in the same patient on a sagittal CT shows 95% dose coverage of the target. Note the calcifications and cephalad extension of the cystic mass.*

Craniopharyngioma

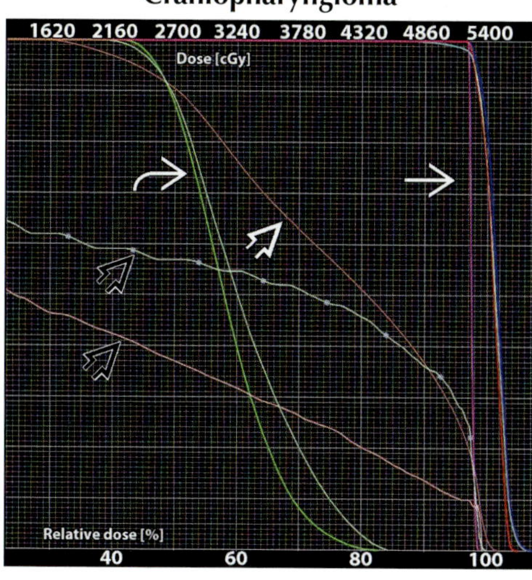

Craniopharyngioma

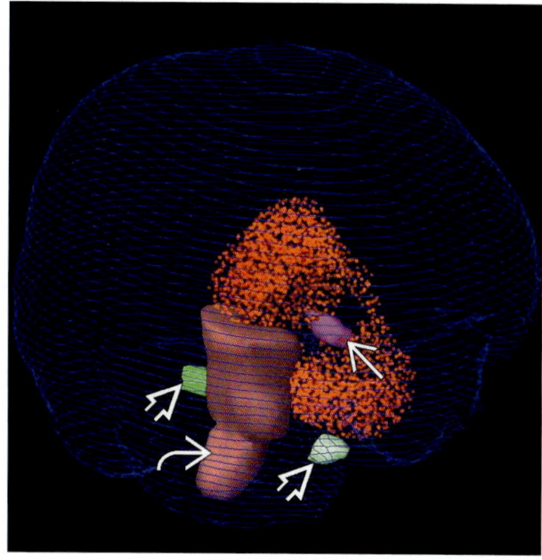

(Left) *DVH in the same patient shows adequate target coverage. A sharp drop-off of dose occurs at 54 Gy to conform to OAR tolerances: Chiasm, optic nerves, brainstem, and cochleae.* ***(Right)*** *3D illustration in the same patient shows a dose cloud > 54 Gy. Note how dose avoids the brainstem, chiasm, and cochleae so as not to exceed tolerances.*

MEDULLOBLASTOMA

OVERVIEW

General Comments

- Malignancy of posterior fossa seen primarily in children

Classification

- Standard risk: Age > 3 years, postsurgical residual < 1.5 cm^2, M0
- High risk: Age < 3 years, postsurgical residual > 1.5 cm^2, M+
  - Anaplastic histology considered high risk
- M staging
  - M0: No subarachnoid or hematogenous mets
  - M1: Microscopic tumor cells in CSF
  - M2: Gross nodular seeding intracranially distant from primary site
  - M3a: Gross nodular seeding in spinal subarachnoid space w/o intracranial seeding
  - M3b: Gross nodular seeding in spinal subarachnoid space and intracranial seeding
  - M4: Mets outside cerebrospinal axis

NATURAL HISTORY

General Features

- Comments
  - Generally arise from roof of 4th ventricle, within cerebellar vermis
  - High propensity to spread along CSF tracts
    - CSF seeding present in up to 35% at diagnosis

Etiology

- Previously classified as a primitive neuroectodermal tumor (PNET) of posterior fossa
  - Distinct molecular profile, now classified separately
- Derived from granule cells within cerebellum
- Exact cause unknown
- Several subtypes seen
  - Classic
  - Desmoplastic
  - Extensive nodular
  - Large cell

Epidemiology & Cancer Incidence

- Primarily found in children
  - 70% found at ages < 20 years old
- Most common malignant brain tumor of childhood
- Incidence: ~ 500 cases/year in USA

Genetics

- Associated genetic abnormalities
  - Gorlin syndrome
  - Turcot syndrome
- Frequently demonstrates loss of information on distal chromosome 17

Gross Pathology & Surgical Features

- Soft, fleshy, midline tumors frequently found in cerebellar vermis
  - Hemorrhage and necrosis can be seen
- May demonstrate frank invasion of surrounding structures
- May demonstrate meningeal or subarachnoid spread

Microscopic Pathology

- Small blue cell tumor: Highly cellular, hyperchromatic nuclei, scant cytoplasm
- Homer Wright rosettes seen in up to 40%

IMAGING

CT

- Solid hyperdense mass in 4th ventricle
- > 90% enhance, usually homogeneously
- Calcifications can be present
- Hydrocephalus can be seen

MR

- T1WI: Hypointense mass in posterior fossa
- T2WI: Iso-/hyperintense to gray matter
- FLAIR: Hyperintense mass
  - Helps distinguish from CSF
- T1 post contrast: Heterogeneous enhancement
  - Contrast needed to help evaluate for CSF dissemination

Special Imaging

- MR spine with contrast to evaluate for leptomeningeal disease

CLINICAL PRESENTATION & WORK-UP

Presentation

- Signs of increased intracranial pressure (ICP): Headaches, N/V, AMS, ataxia
- Pediatric patients can demonstrate macrocephaly with open sutures
- Can demonstrate cranial nerve deficits from direct involvement or indirectly from elevated ICP

Prognosis

- Historic risk stratification: Standard and high risk (see classification)
- Tumors can be very responsive to treatment secondary to height mitotic rate
- Heterogeneous prognosis
  - Standard risk: 5-year DFS 60-90%
  - High risk: 5-year DFS 30-60%
- Multiple molecular and histologic markers identified with prognosis
  - Wnt and hedgehog pathway activation associated with good prognosis

Work-Up

- H&P
- MR brain: ± contrast, preop and postop within 48 hours
- MR spine: ± contrast
- CSF cytology
- Bone scan if clinically indicated
  - One of few CNS tumors that can demonstrate bone involvement (rare)
- Baseline endocrine, growth, IQ, and audiometric evaluations

TREATMENT

Overview

- Max surgical resection > craniospinal RT and posterior fossa boost + concurrent vincristine > adjuvant PCV chemo
- Current investigations
  - Ages 3-7 years
    - Reduced craniospinal dose
    - Focal boost instead of entire posterior fossa
  - Children < 3 years
    - Chemo only; RT reserved for salvage

Standard Doses

- Standard risk
  - Craniospinal irradiation (CSI): 23.4 Gy in 1.8 Gy/fx
    - 18 Gy being investigated
  - Posterior fossa: Boost to 54 Gy in 1.8 Gy/fx
    - Limited volume being investigated
- High risk
  - CSI: 36 Gy in 1.8 Gy/fx
    - Diffuse spine involvement (M3); CSI goes to 39 Gy
    - Focal deposits get boosted to 45 Gy or 50.4 Gy (cauda equina)
  - Posterior fossa: 55.8 Gy in 1.8 Gy/fx

Organs at Risk Parameters

- Brainstem: < 54 Gy (< 5% necrosis/neuropathy, QUANTEC)
- Cochlea: Mean dose 35-45 Gy (minimize risk, QUANTEC)
- Retina: 45 Gy (< 5% retinopathy, Emami)
- Lens: 10 Gy (< 5% cataract, Emami)
- Optic nerves/chiasm: < 54 Gy (< 1% optic neuropathy, QUANTEC)

Common Techniques

- CSI
  - Whole brain + spinal fields
  - Simulate with neck extended and thermoplastic mask
  - Spine fields to include entire thecal sac
    - Superior: Matched to whole brain field
    - Inferior: 2 cm below termination of subdural space (usually S2-3)
- Posterior fossa
  - Include entire contents of posterior fossa
    - C1 inferiorly to tentorium superiorly
    - Bony confines laterally and posteriorly
    - Brainstem/midbrain anteriorly
- Limited volume posterior fossa (if used)
  - GTV: Residual tumor + resection cavity, include preop tumor imaging for target delineation
  - CTV: GTV + 1.5 cm (constrain to posterior fossa contents)
  - PTV: CTV + 3-5 mm
- CSI field adjustments: Requires collimator rotation of whole brain field, couch kick, and gap for spinal field (if numerous fields used)
  - Collimator angle = arctangent (upper spine field length x 1/2/SSD)
  - Couch angle = atan ([1/2 cranial field length]/SAD)
  - Skin gap = (1st field length/2) x (d/SSD1) + (2nd field length/2) x (depth/SSD2)
  - Field junctions frequently feathered (5 mm to 1 cm) weekly to mitigate hot/cold spots

Landmark Trials

- SIOP I: CSI ± adjuvant chemo
  - Full dose CSI; no benefit to adjuvant chemo except in advanced disease
- French SFOP M4: RT to spine and posterior fossa ± supratentorium
  - Supratentorium cannot be spared
- POG 8631/CCG 923: CSI 23.4 Gy vs. 36 Gy
  - Reduced dose CSI not adequate with RT alone
- SIOP II: ± pre-RT chemo, CSI 25 Gy vs. 36 Gy
  - No benefit to pre-RT chemo, low-dose chemo and RT did especially poorly
- CCG 9892: Reduced dose RT with concurrent and adjuvant chemo
  - Reduced dose CSI (23.4 Gy) acceptable with concurrent and adjuvant chemo
- Baby POG 1: Children < 3 years old, chemo upfront to delay RT
  - Similar outcomes to older patients with RT upfront, chemo to delay RT acceptable approach
- Baby brain French SIOP: Children < 5 years old, postop chemo only
  - Acceptable if GTR achieved, not adequate for M+ or STR

RECOMMENDED FOLLOW-UP

Clinical

- H&P and physical exam every 3 months for 1st year, then 6 months until year 3, then annually

Radiographic

- MR brain and spine with time intervals corresponding to clinical appointments

Laboratory

- Endocrine evaluation at 6 months, then annually
- CSF evaluation if suspect recurrence

MEDULLOBLASTOMA

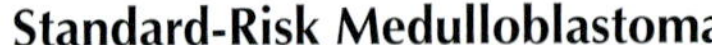

Standard-Risk Medulloblastoma

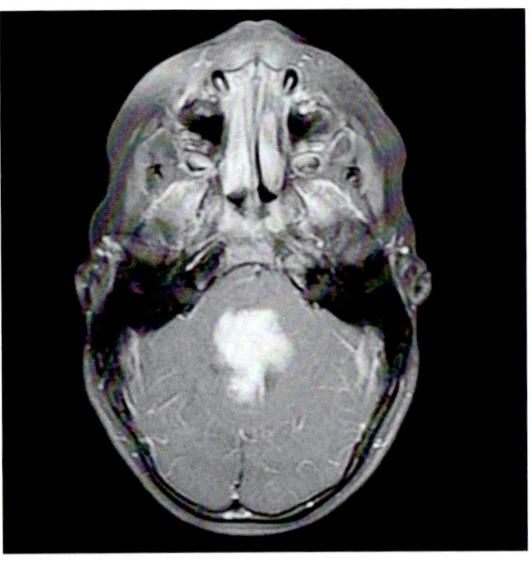

Standard-Risk Medulloblastoma

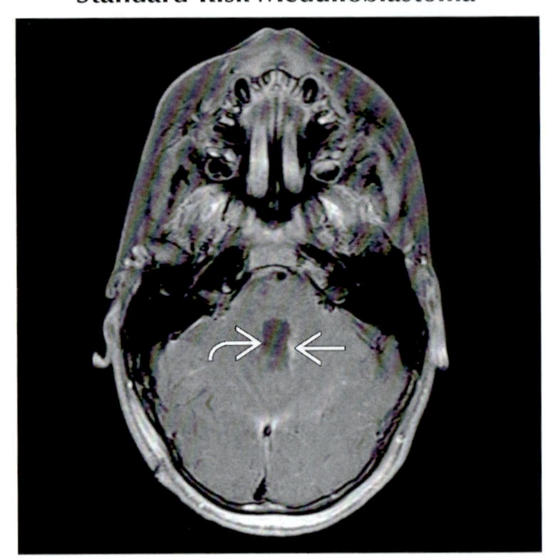

(Left) *Preop T1WI C+ MR shows an enhancing posterior fossa mass in a 7-year-old boy presenting with headaches.* ***(Right)*** *Axial T1WI C+ MR in the same patient (after resection) shows a cavity ↪ with no residual disease. The slight area of enhancement → was also bright on T1, indicating that it is the result of blood products. Spinal MR (not shown) and CSF evaluation were negative, making this case a standard-risk medulloblastoma.*

Standard-Risk Medulloblastoma

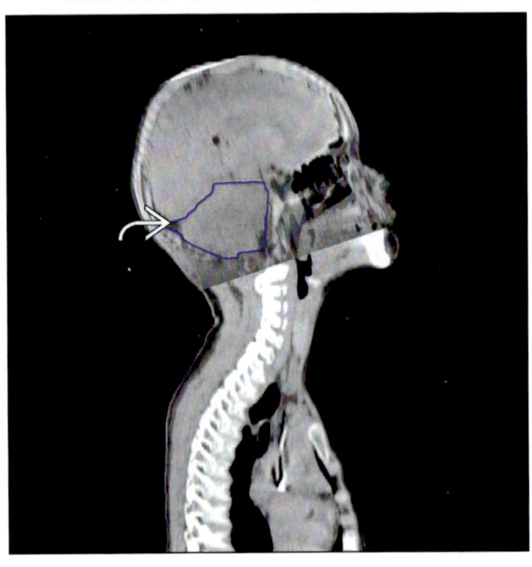

Standard-Risk Medulloblastoma

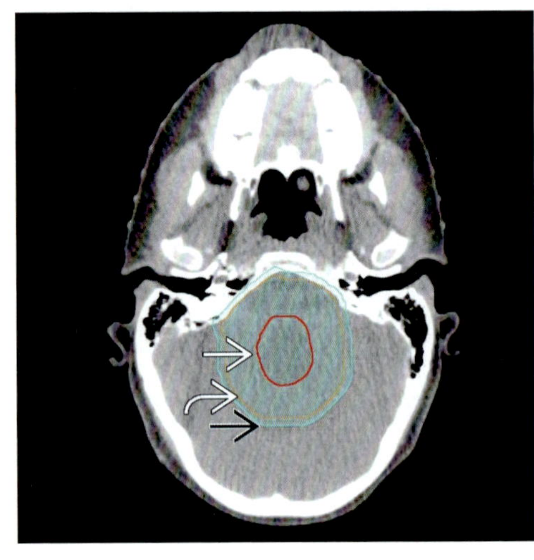

(Left) *Planning CT with fused MR in the same patient shows the outline of the posterior fossa ↪. Traditionally, the entire posterior fossa serves as the boost volume.* ***(Right)*** *Planning CT in the same patient shows volumes if treating to a limited boost volume. The GTV → includes the resection cavity and any residual disease (preop MR helpful in verifying volumes). The CTV ↪ is a 1.5 cm expansion of the GTV, and the PTV → is a 3 mm expansion.*

Standard-Risk Medulloblastoma

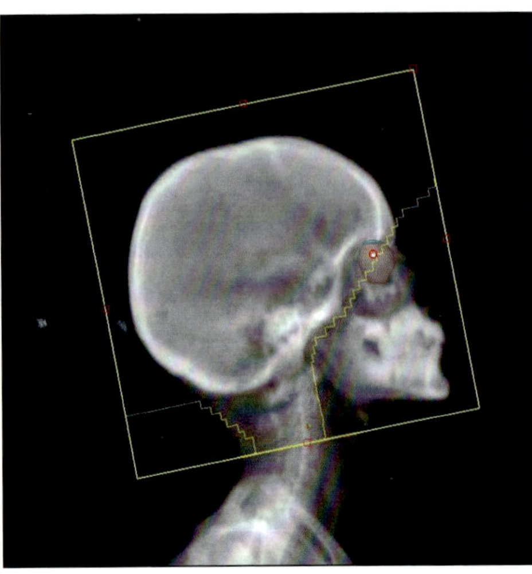

Standard-Risk Medulloblastoma

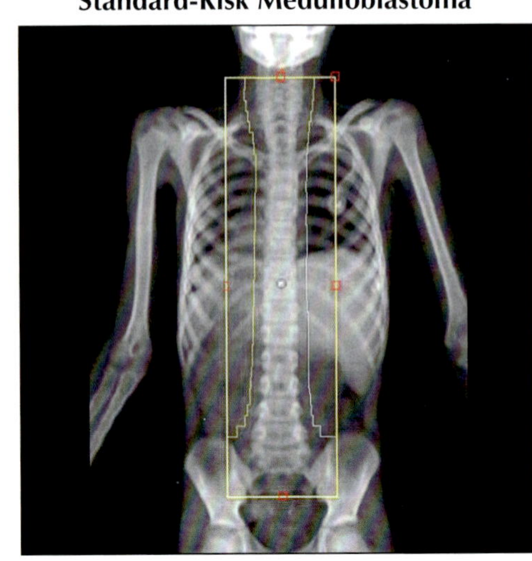

(Left) *DRR representation in the same patient shows the whole brain field outline.* ***(Right)*** *DRR in the same patient shows outline of spinal field. The inferior border was set at 2 cm below the thecal sac, with a lateral border of 1.5 cm from the vertebral bodies. Sagittal MR is useful in identifying the distal aspect of the thecal sac.*

Standard-Risk Medulloblastoma

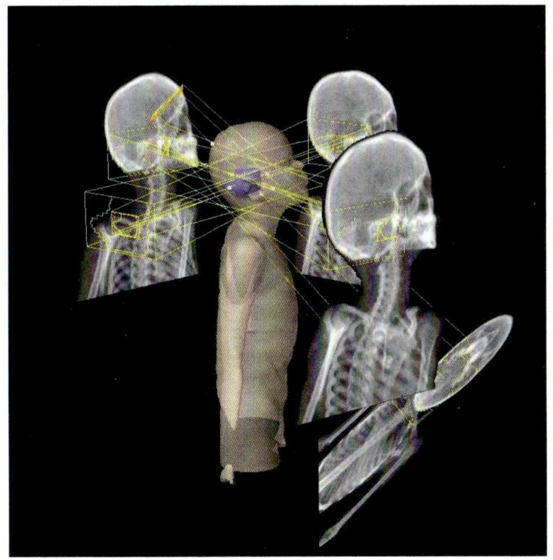

Standard-Risk Medulloblastoma

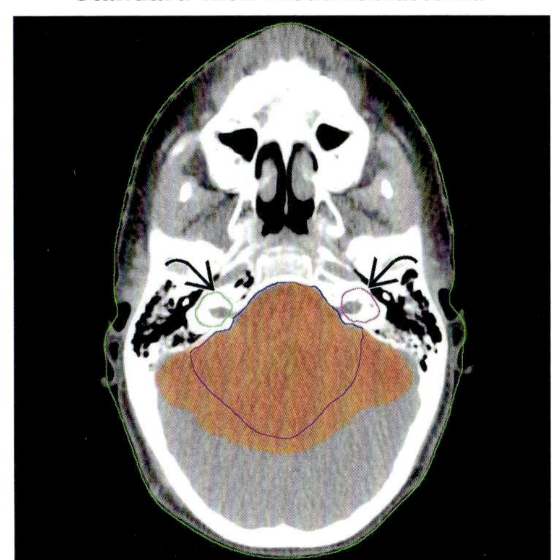

*(**Left**) 3D representation shows the fields used for the posterior fossa boost. In this case, a 5-field IMRT plan was used. (**Right**) Dose colorwash shows 95% coverage of the boost volume (the entire posterior fossa in this case). IMRT was utilized to reduce the dose to the cochleae ➩.*

Cranial Spinal Irradiation

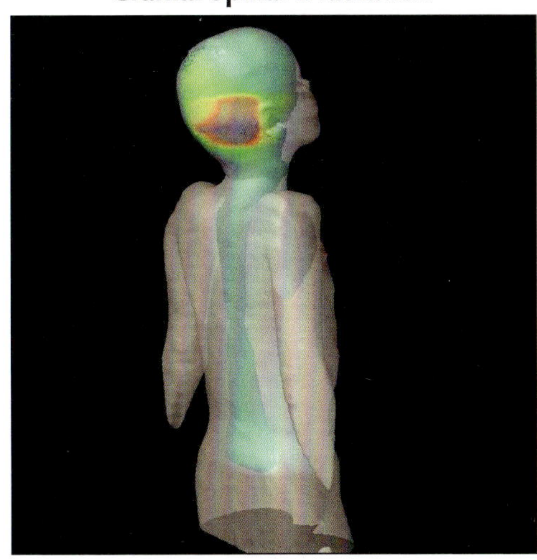

Cranial Spinal Irradiation

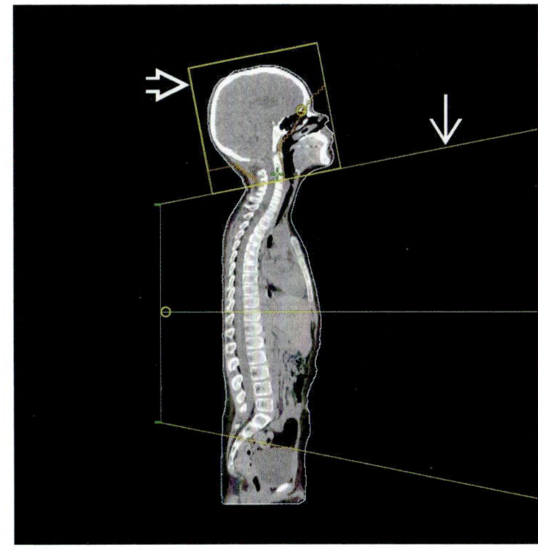

*(**Left**) 3D representation with dose colorwash indicates the CSI dose of 23.4 Gy and the posterior fossa boost of 54 Gy. Note that this was a standard-risk medulloblastoma; a high-risk patient would have received CSI to 36 Gy and a boost to 55.8 Gy. (**Right**) Beam arrangement for initial CSI shows the collimator rotation of the whole brain field ➩ to match the divergence of the spinal field ➔.*

Cranial Spinal Irradiation

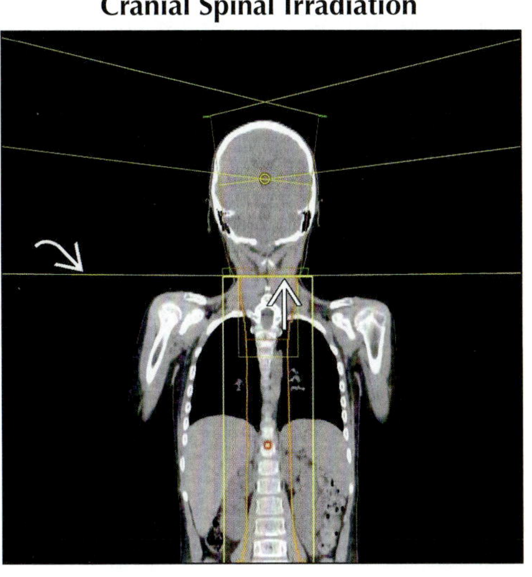

Cranial Spinal Irradiation

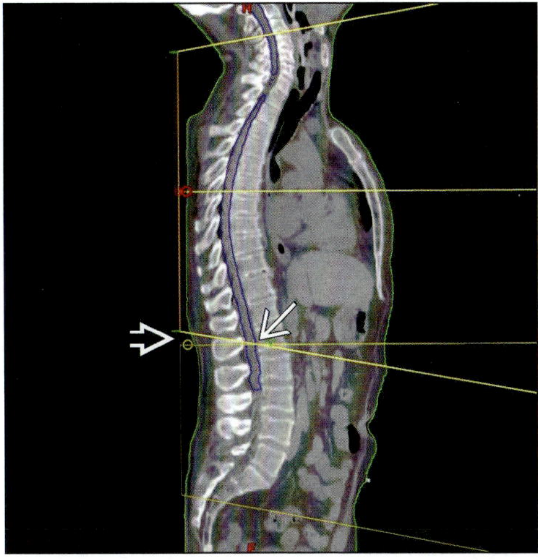

*(**Left**) Beam arrangement of CSI is shown. Note that a couch kick is used for the upper border of the spinal field ➔ to match the divergence of the whole brain field ➩ (if required). (**Right**) Beam arrangement for an adult patient demonstrates a skin gap ➩ between the 2 spinal fields. Note the point of field overlap ➔, which in this case has been placed anterior to the spinal cord to minimize the cord dose.*

GERMINOMA

OVERVIEW

General Comments

- Midline tumors arising from ectopic germ cell rests during development

Classification

- CNS germ cell tumors: WHO classification
  - Germinomas: 50-60%
  - Nongerminomatous germ cell tumors (NGGCT)
    - Embryonal, yolk sac tumor, choriocarcinoma, teratomas, mixed germ cell tumor
- Metastatic classification
  - M0: Localized lesion
  - M+: Synchronous lesions
    - Synchronous pineal and suprasellar lesions M+ in US, considered M0 in Europe

NATURAL HISTORY

General Features

- Midline tumors closely associated with 3rd ventricle
  - Pineal (45%) > suprasellar (35%) > both > other

Etiology

- Thought to arise from primordial germ cells, which fail normal migration during development

Epidemiology & Cancer Incidence

- Peak onset 2nd decade; adult presentation rare
  - 1-3% of pediatric brain tumors (up to 11% in Asia)

Associated Diseases, Abnormalities

- Klinefelter syndrome (47XXY), NF1, Down syndrome

Gross Pathology & Surgical Features

- Well circumscribed with soft/solid components
  - Cysts can be present, necrosis usually absent

Microscopic Pathology

- Polyhedral large cells in sheets
  - Fibrous septa between lobules with lymphocytic infiltrations

IMAGING

CT

- Circumscribed hyperdense mass
- Strong uniform enhancement with contrast

MR

- T1WI
  - Iso- to hyperintense to gray matter
- T2WI
  - Iso- to hyperintense, cysts common
- T2 FLAIR
  - Mildly hyperintense
- T1 post contrast
  - Strong homogeneous enhancement
    - Evaluate for CSF seeding/ventricular wall infiltration

CLINICAL PRESENTATION & WORK-UP

Presentation

- Varies with location
  - Pineal
    - Obstructive hydrocephalus: Elevated ICP
    - Parinaud syndrome: Upgaze paralysis, loss of light perception/accommodation, nystagmus
  - Suprasellar
    - Hypothalamic/pituitary dysfunction: DI classic
    - Visual disturbances, bitemporal hemianopsia

Prognosis

- Long-term PFS > 90%

Work-Up

- H&P + neuro exam, MR brain/spine w/wo contrast, CSF evaluation
- Tumor markers: Both serum and CSF (more sensitive)
  - Germinoma: Absent AFP, b-HCG < 50 IU/L
  - NGGCT: AFP > 10 micrograms/L, b-HCG > 50 IU/L
- Tissue sample encouraged
  - Biopsies/tumor markers can be discordant, treat by worse histology

TREATMENT

Overview

- Traditionally RT alone (CSI with focal boost)
  - Local control > 95%, tx evolving to limit side effects
- Current accepted options
  - M0
    - IFRT to reduced dose with neoadjuvant chemo
    - Whole ventricular RT with focal boost or WBRT
    - CSI with focal boost
  - M+
    - CSI with focal boost
- Reduced doses and volumes for focal disease being investigated

Standard Doses

- IFRT: 30.6-50.4 Gy depending on chemo response
- Focal boost: 40-50.4 Gy in 1.5-2 Gy/fx
- CSI or whole brain/ventricular RT
  - 23.4-30.6 Gy in 1.5-2 Gy/fx

Common Techniques

- Intracranial: 3D conformal, IMRT, or arc therapy
- CSI: Procedure described for medulloblastoma
- Contouring
  - GTV: Entire tumor volume
    - Pre-chemo volume if neoadjuvant chemo utilized
  - CTV: GTV + 1-2 cm
  - PTV: CTV + 0.3-0.5 cm

RECOMMENDED FOLLOW-UP

Routine

- Follow-up every 3-6 months initially, with MR brain/spine ± contrast and tumor markers
- Can increase interval if disease free

Germinoma

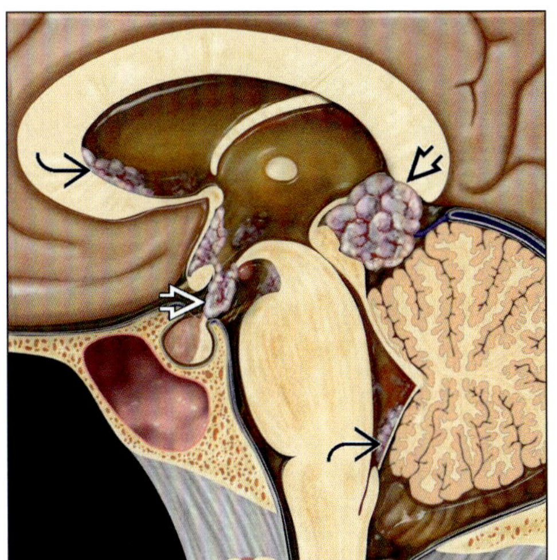

Germinoma (M0)

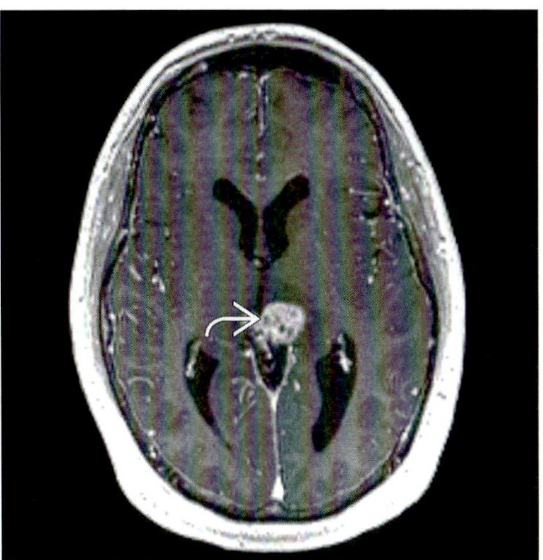

(Left) *Graphic shows common locations for germinoma in midline structures: Pineal gland ⇨, suprasellar ➡, and ventricular seeding ↷.* ***(Right)*** *A 28-year-old man presented with the development of sensory deficits. A T1 post-contrast MR shows an enhancing lesion ➡ in the region of the pineal gland with extension to midbrain and bilateral thalami. A biopsy proved the mass to be a germinoma, and further staging indicated that the patient was M0.*

Germinoma (M0)

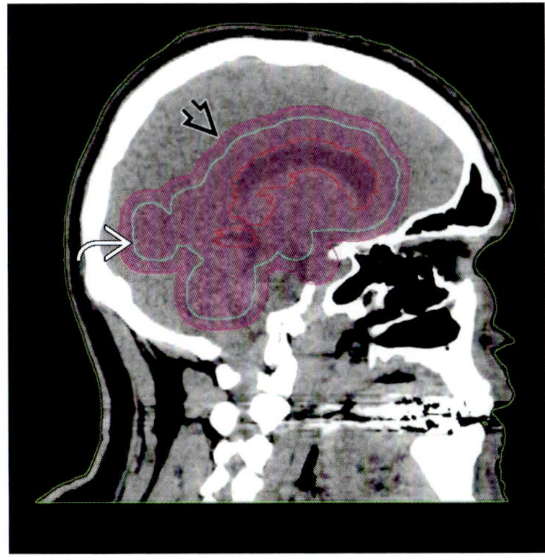

Germinoma (M0)

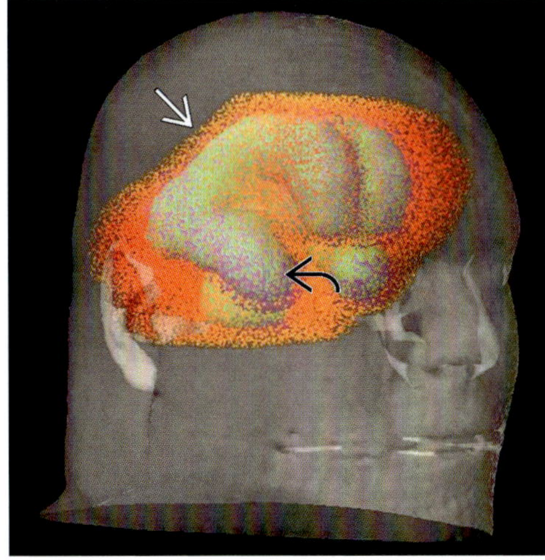

(Left) *In the same patient, whole ventricular radiation was planned, with a focal boost. This is shown on the planning CT depicting the ventricles with a 1 cm expansion as a CTV ➡ and 3 mm expansion as a PTV ⇨.* ***(Right)*** *3D representation in the same patient shows the 24 Gy colorwash ➡ surrounding the ventricular PTV ↷. This patient received 24 Gy whole ventricular radiation, with a 16 Gy focal boost.*

Germinoma (M0)

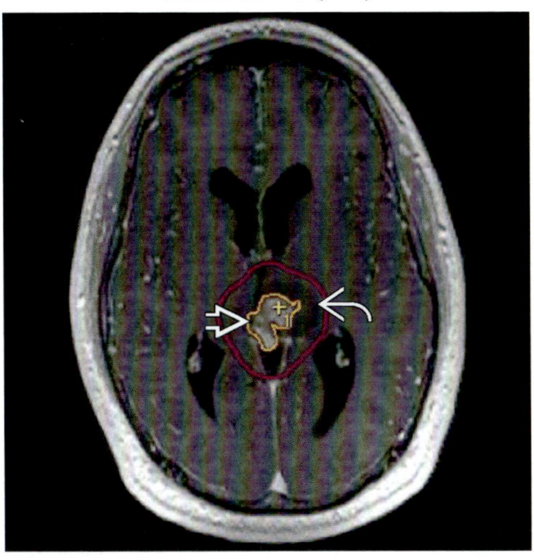

Germinoma (M0)

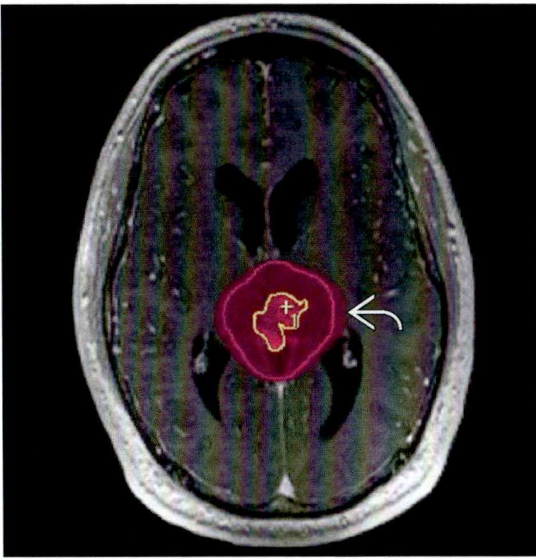

(Left) *T1 post-contrast fused MR in the same patient showing the focal boost GTV ➡ and a 1 cm CTV ↷ expansion.* ***(Right)*** *Ninety-five percent dose colorwash ↷ for the same patient shows coverage of the boost volume. A 16 Gy boost was given for a total of 40 Gy.*

MENINGIOMA

OVERVIEW

General Comments

- Dural-based extraaxial lesions arising from cellular components of leptomeninges

Classification

- WHO classification
  - Grade I: Benign meningioma (90-95%)
  - Grade II: Atypical meningioma (5-7%)
  - Grade III: Anaplastic/malignant meningioma (1-2%)
- Simpson grade: I-IV based on extent of resection
  - Prognostic for local recurrence

NATURAL HISTORY

General Features

- Comments
  - Arise from arachnoid cap cells within arachnoid granulations
- Location
  - Supratentorial (90%) > infratentorial (< 10%) > extracranial (rare)
  - Convexity/parasagittal > sphenoid ridge > other

Etiology

- Risk factors
  - Neurofibromatosis type 2
  - Hormone replacement therapy in women
  - Prior cranial RT: Therapeutic or incidental
    - Latency of ~ 20 years

Epidemiology & Cancer Incidence

- 20-30% of primary CNS tumors
  - Most common benign CNS tumor
- Usually presents in 4th-6th decades
- Present in 1-2% of general population on autopsy

Gross Pathology & Surgical Features

- Dural based with invagination (not invasion) into brain
  - Can be well demarcated and globular, or sheet-like along dura

Microscopic Pathology

- Multiple pathologic subtypes within each WHO grade
  - Microscopic appearance varies with subtype
  - Variety of IHC markers and surface receptors seen

IMAGING

CT

- Well-circumscribed, hyperdense, extraaxial mass abutting dura
  - Calcifications often indicate more benign course
  - Bone hyperostosis/irregularity common
- Usually homogeneously enhancing

MR

- T1: Iso- to hypointense mass with broad-based dural attachment
- T1: Post contrast; homogeneous enhancement (> 95%); dural "tail" is classic, but nonspecific
- T2: Varies, usually iso- to hyperintense

CLINICAL PRESENTATION & WORK-UP

Presentation

- Frequently asymptomatic and found incidentally
- Seizures/focal neurologic deficits possible, deficits vary by location

Prognosis

- Usually excellent, but varies with histology and tx
  - 5-year OS: WHO grade I > 90%, grade III 40-60%
  - LC > 95% for typical benign meningioma

Work-Up

- H&P with neurologic exam
- MR brain ± contrast
- Biopsy/resection if radiographic diagnosis in doubt

TREATMENT

Overview

- Observation for small asymptomatic lesions
- Definitive tx with either surgery or RT if lesions are large or symptomatic
  - Surgery preferred for easily accessible lesions
    - Subtotal resection (STR) with adjuvant RT equivalent to gross total resection (GTR) in long-term survival
- Adjuvant RT: WHO grade III, STR grade II, and consider for STR grade I

Standard Doses

- Conventional RT
  - Benign: 45-54 Gy in 1.8-2 Gy/fx
  - Malignant: 54-60 Gy in 1.8-2 Gy/fx
    - 54 Gy standard with 60 Gy for known malignant tumors
- SRS
  - 12-15 Gy, varies by location and adjacent OAR

Common Techniques

- 3D conformal, IMRT, arc therapy, or SRS as indicated
- Contouring
  - Conventional fx
    - GTV: Enhancing tumor + tumor bed (if resected)
      - Inclusion of dural tail controversial (not included on latest RTOG protocol)
    - CTV (on latest protocol if postop, controversial): GTV + 1-2 cm
      - 0.5 cm against natural boundary, such as bone
    - PTV: CTV + 3-5 mm
  - SRS
    - Enhancing tumor
      - Dural "tail" controversial, but frequently included

RECOMMENDED FOLLOW-UP

Routine

- Follow-up with neuro exam and MR brain ± contrast
  - 3, 6, 12 months, then q. 6-12 months for 5 years, and q. 1-3 years thereafter

Planum Sphenoidale Meningioma

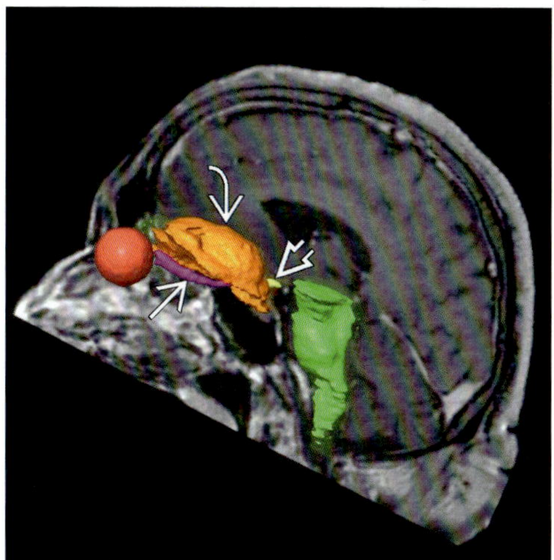

Planum Sphenoidale Meningioma

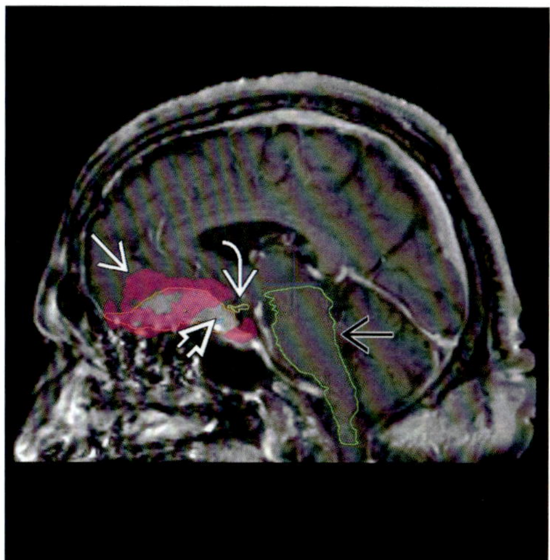

(Left) *Fused MR shows the meningioma with the tumor volume ➔ encompassing the optic nerves ➔ and chiasm ➔. Definitive RT was used to deliver 54 Gy/30 fx with a 7-field IMRT plan.* ***(Right)*** *T1 post-contrast MR of the same patient shows dose > 54 Gy ➔. Note the optic nerves ➔ and chiasm ➔ being obscured by the tumor, as well as the proximity to the brainstem ➔. Due to a tolerance of 54 Gy, hotspots were omitted from the optic nerves, chiasm, and brainstem.*

Grade II Meningioma, Postop SRS

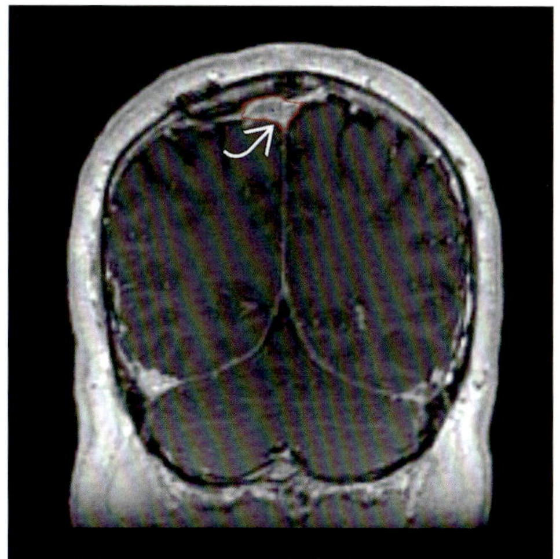

Grade II Meningioma, Postop SRS

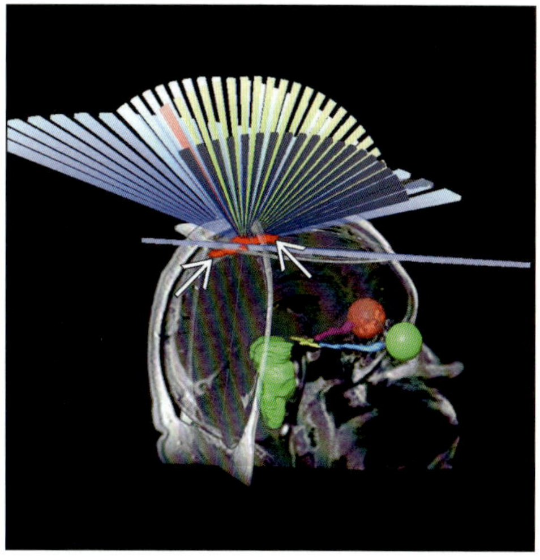

(Left) *Fused T1 post-contrast MR shows residual tumor ➔ involving the right superior sagittal sinus.* ***(Right)*** *Beam arrangement for the same patient shows radiosurgical delivery of 15 Gy to the 85% isodose line using 5 dynamic conformal arcs. Note the tumor spreading sheet-like along the sagittal sinus ➔, which can lead to difficulty in conformality during radiosurgical planning.*

Grade II Meningioma, Postop

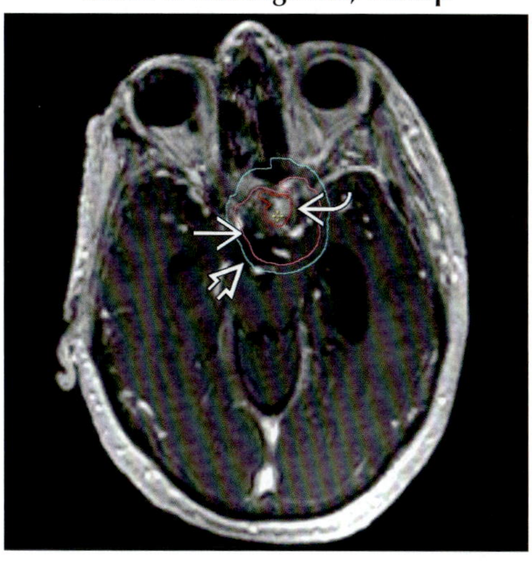

Grade II Meningioma, Postop

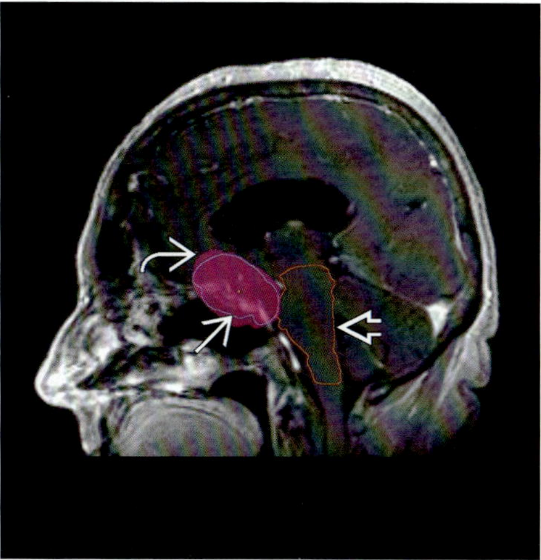

(Left) *Axial T1 post-contrast MR shows GTV ➔, with CTV ➔ as a 1 cm expansion (reduced to 0.5 cm for bone) and PTV ➔ as a 3 mm expansion.* ***(Right)*** *Sagittal fused T1 post-contrast MR for the same patient shows 54 Gy colorwash ➔ covering the PTV ➔ and being excluded from the brainstem ➔. This was delivered in 30 fx with a 6-field IMRT plan.*

PITUITARY ADENOMA

OVERVIEW

General Comments
- Benign tumor within pituitary gland

Classification
- Size: Micro < 1.0 cm, macro ≥ 1.0 cm
- Secretion
  - Nonfunctional: 25%
  - Functional: 75%
    - Prolactin (50%), GH (20-25%), ACTH (20%), TSH (1-2%)

NATURAL HISTORY

General Features
- Location
  - Arises from anterior pituitary
  - Confined by bony sella, generally expands upward
    - Can compress pituitary stalk and optic chiasm
    - Can expand laterally into cavernous sinus

Epidemiology & Cancer Incidence
- 10-15% of intracranial tumors
- Median age varies, usually presents 20-50 years

Associated Diseases, Abnormalities
- Increased incidence in *MEN1*

Gross Pathology & Surgical Features
- Reddish-brown, well-circumscribed mass

Microscopic Pathology
- Monomorphic cells with granular cytoplasm and sheet-like growth

IMAGING

MR
- T1: Frequently isointense
  - Mass can be seen bulging upward if large
- T1 post contrast: Pituitary normally enhances
  - Micro: Enhancement, but hypointense relative to pituitary
  - Macro: Heterogeneous enhancement
- T2: Frequently isointense
- FLAIR: Can appear hyperintense

CLINICAL PRESENTATION & WORK-UP

Presentation
- Microadenomas: Frequently found incidentally
- Macroadenomas: Compressive symptoms, headaches
  - Optic chiasm: Bitemporal hemianopsia
  - Cavernous sinus: CN palsies
- Functional tumors can present with endocrine abnormalities
  - Prolactin: Galactorrhea, amenorrhea, infertility
  - ACTH: Cushing disease, Nelson syndrome
  - Growth hormone: Acromegaly
  - TSH: Hyperthyroidism

Work-Up
- H&P with neurologic exam
- MR brain ± contrast (thin cut/fat saturated)
- Endocrine evaluation
  - Serum prolactin, IGF-1, TSH, free T4, 24-hr urine cortisol, ACTH, LH, FSH
    - Further hormone testing may be required

TREATMENT

Overview
- Treatment options
  - Observation/medical management
    - Up-front therapy for adenomas when no neurologic symptoms
  - Surgery
    - Indications
      - Neurologic symptoms, failed medical therapy, rapid growth/large tumors
      - Cushing/acromegaly often surgery up front
    - Trans-sphenoidal microsurgery standard approach
    - Tumor control 80-90% for microadenomas, 50-80% overall
  - RT
    - Indications
      - Medically inoperable, incomplete resection, surgical failure of endocrine control, recurrence
    - Tumor control 80-90%, endocrine control (GH 80%, ACTH 50-80%, prolactin 25-50%)
    - ↑ endocrine control with long-term F/U > 10 years

Standard Doses
- Fractionated RT
  - 45-54 Gy in 1.8-2Gy/fx
    - Functional tumors generally 50.4-54 Gy
- SRS
  - Functional: 15-30 Gy
  - Nonfunctioning: 12-20 Gy

Common Techniques
- SRS or fx RT (stereotactic techniques encouraged)
- Contouring
  - GTV: Tumor volume, residual tumor if postop
  - CTV: Not usually required
  - PTV (if fx): GTV + 3-5 mm

Organs at Risk Parameters
- Optic chiasm/nerves
  - Fx: < 54 Gy
  - SRS: 8 Gy; if prior RT 4 Gy

RECOMMENDED FOLLOW-UP

Routine
- Follow-up with MR brain ± contrast
  - Every 6 months x 1 year, then annually
- Annual visual field testing
- Endocrine evaluation
  - Radiosensitivity GH > FSH/LH > ACTH > TSH
  - Prolactin levels difficult to predict
    - Loss of inhibitory effect from hypothalamus may lead to paradoxical increase

Pituitary Macroadenoma

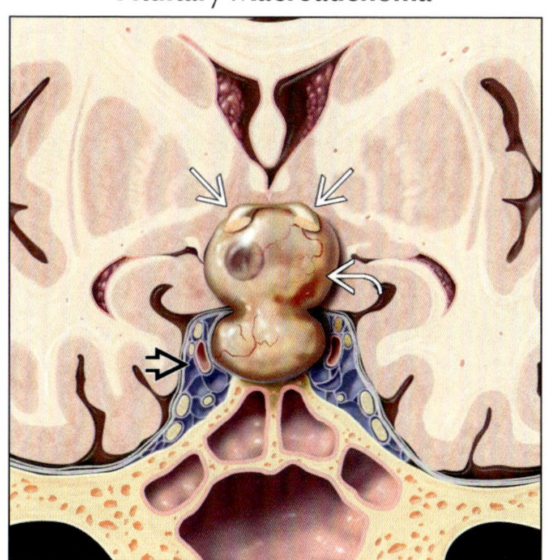

Pituitary Macroadenoma

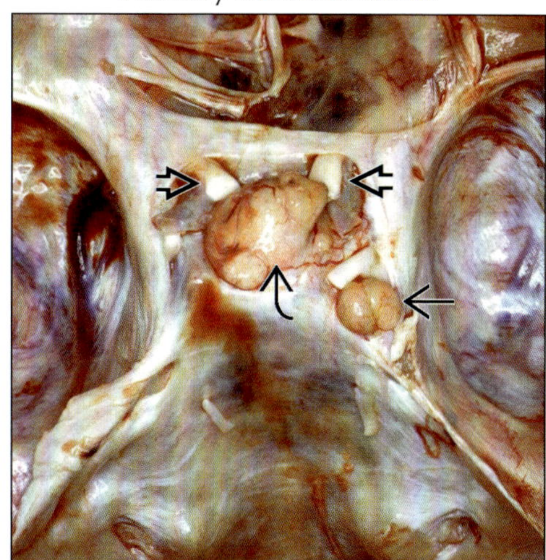

(Left) *Graphic shows a pituitary macroadenoma ➡ with extension upward through the diaphragma sellae displacing the optic nerves ➡. When locally invasive, invasion into the cavernous sinus ➡ can be seen.* ***(Right)*** *Gross pathology shows a pituitary macroadenoma ➡ with extension superiorly through the diaphragma sellae, as well as laterally into the cavernous sinus ➡. Note the proximity of the optic nerves ➡. (Courtesy R. Hewlett, MD.)*

Nonfunctional Pituitary Macroadenoma

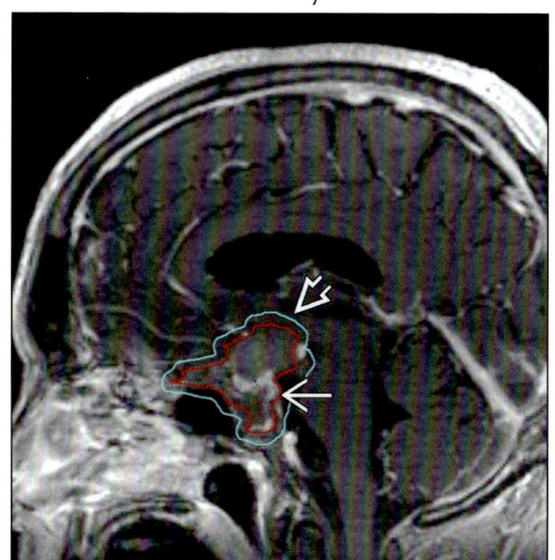

Nonfunctional Pituitary Macroadenoma

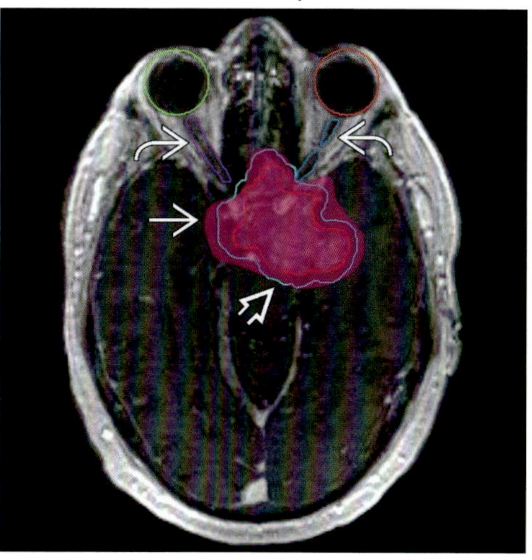

(Left) *Fused T1 C + SPGR MR in a 54-year-old man shows a nonsecreting macroadenoma with lateral cavernous sinus extension. The GTV is shown ➡ with a 3 mm PTV expansion ➡.* ***(Right)*** *Fused MR in the same patient shows the 95% dose colorwash ➡ covering the PTV. An IMRT plan was utilized to deliver 50.4 Gy. Note the dose conforming to the optic nerves ➡ and brainstem ➡ (with IMRT, ensure no hotspots occur on critical structures).*

Nonfunctional Pituitary Macroadenoma, Postop

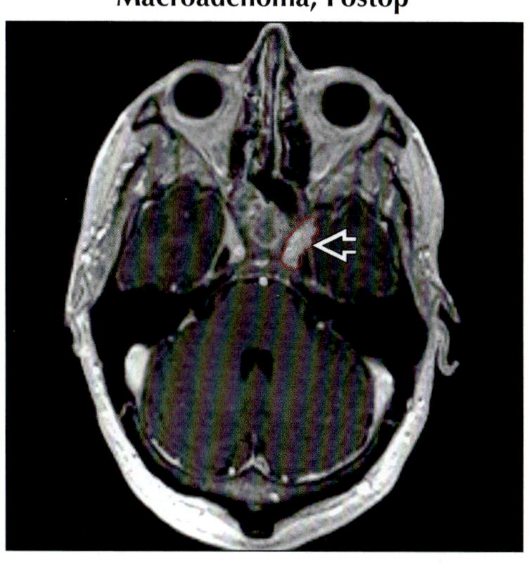

Nonfunctional Pituitary Macroadenoma, Postop

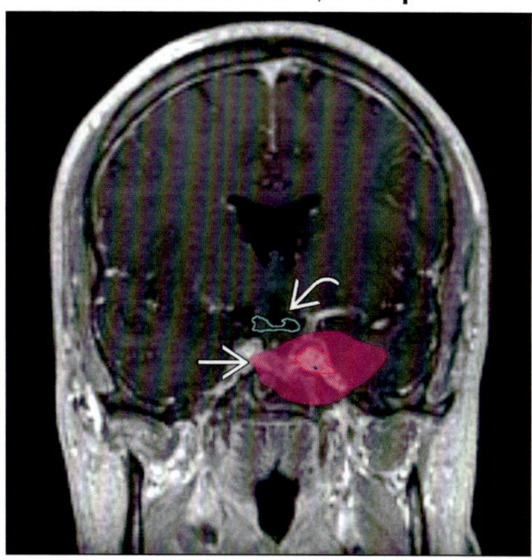

(Left) *Shown is a T1 C+ SPGR MR in a 41-year-old man with a nonfunctional pituitary macroadenoma, with residual right-sided cavernous sinus disease postoperatively. The residual cavernous sinus disease is shown ➡.* ***(Right)*** *In the same patient, a 9-field IMRT plan was used to radiosurgically deliver 15 Gy to the tumor bed. The optic nerves and chiasm ➡ were limited to 8 Gy, as is shown with the 8 Gy dose colorwash ➡.*

ACOUSTIC NEUROMA

OVERVIEW

General Comments

- Tumor arising from Schwann cells along vestibulocochlear nerve

NATURAL HISTORY

General Features

- Comments
  - Arise at transition zone between central oligodendrocytes and peripheral Schwann cells
- Location
  - Occur along superior/inferior branches of vestibular nerve, usually within internal auditory canal (IAC)
    - Rarely occurs along cochlear portion of nerve
  - > 90% unilateral
    - Bilateral generally → neurofibromatosis type 2
  - Can cause local mass effect on CNs V/VII

Etiology

- Risk factors
  - Neurofibromatosis type 2: Bilateral lesions classic
  - Other associated risks
    - Chronic loud noise exposure, parathyroid adenomas, childhood low-dose RT exposure

Epidemiology & Cancer Incidence

- 6-8% of intracranial primary neoplasms
  - 80-90% of cerebellar pontine (CP) angle tumors
- Arises 3rd-7th decades
  - Median age of onset: 5th decade

Gross Pathology & Surgical Features

- Encapsulated globular tumors surrounding nerve

Microscopic Pathology

- Composed entirely of Schwann cells
  - Alternating zones of Antoni A (dense cellularity) and B (sparse cellularity)
- Stain positive for S100 protein on IHC

IMAGING

CT

- Enhancing, well-demarcated mass in IAC/CPA cistern
  - Calcifications absent, can help differentiate from meningioma

MR

- T1: Iso- to hypointense, similar to normal brain
- T1 post contrast: Strongly enhancing mass within IAC/CPA cistern
- T2: Heterogeneously hyperintense
- CISS/FIESTA: Tumor outlined by CSF signal, helpful in delineating nerves

CLINICAL PRESENTATION & WORK-UP

Presentation

- Usually present with slowly progressive CN symptoms
  - CN VIII cochlear (95%), CN VIII vestibular (60%), CN V (15-20%), CN VII (< 10%)
    - Hearing loss present > 95%, patients symptomatic in ~ 2/3

Prognosis

- Slow-growing tumors
  - 40-60% of tumors will show no significant growth
  - 20% of patients who undergo observation will eventually require tx

Work-Up

- H&P with neurologic exam
  - Evaluate for unilateral sensorineural hearing loss
- Audiometry evaluation
- MR ± contrast: High resolution through IAC/CPA region
  - CISS/FIESTA sequences helpful to evaluate nerves

TREATMENT

Overview

- Observation: Older patients with small tumors and minimal symptoms
- Surgery
  - 3 different surgical approaches, morbidity varies with each approach
  - Hearing preservation (30-60%), CN VII disturbance (5-40%), CN V disturbance (20-30%)
- Radiation
  - Hearing preservation (60-80%), CN V and VII preservation (> 90%)
  - SRS and fractionated RT roughly equal in tumor control and side effects
    - Increased concern for side effects with SRS for tumors > 3 cm

Standard Doses

- Fractionated: 50-54 Gy in 1.8-2 Gy/fx
  - 20-25 Gy in 4-5 Gy/fx also been shown to have good results
- SRS: 12-13 Gy marginal dose
  - Doses > 14 Gy have shown increasing toxicity

Common Techniques

- Fractionated: IMRT or arc therapy usually required
  - Tx with stereotactic techniques/mask strongly encouraged
- SRS: Gamma knife or linac-based radiosurgery
- Contouring
  - GTV: Tumor volume
  - PTV: GTV + 0-3 mm (no margin for SRS)
- Organs at risk
  - Cochlea and brainstem not specifically avoided (but limit hot spots with IMRT)
  - Toxicity is as detailed above

RECOMMENDED FOLLOW-UP

Routine

- Yearly follow-up with neurologic exam, audiometric evaluation, and MR (contrast-enhanced or high-resolution CISS/FIESTA)
  - Audiometry only required if hearing preserved

Internal Auditory Canal

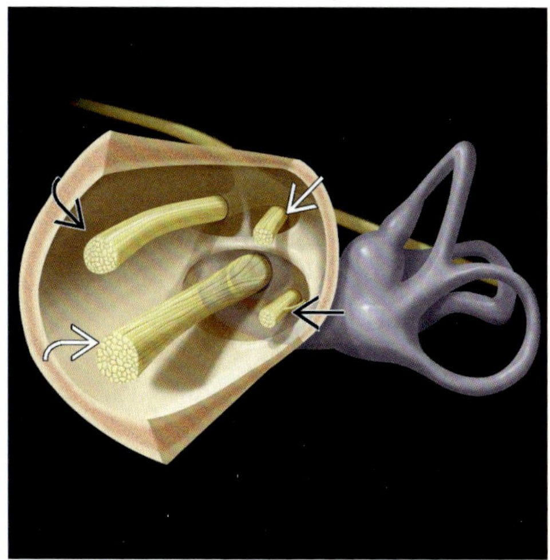

Acoustic Neuroma

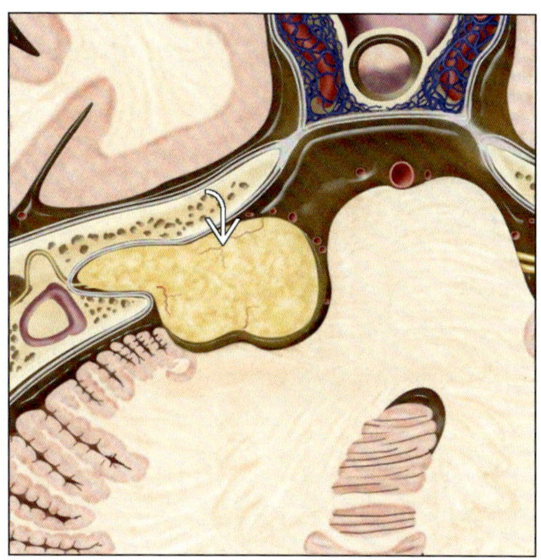

(Left) Graphic demonstrates the anatomy of the IAC. Note the relationship of the CN VII ⇗ to the the cochlear ⇗ and vestibular portions of the CN VIII. The superior ➡ and inferior ⇒ portions of the vestibular nerve are the most common locations for acoustic neuromas. ***(Right)*** Graphic depicts an acoustic neuroma involving the right IAC ⇗, with extension into the CPA cistern. Note the mass effect on the brainstem.

Acoustic Neuroma

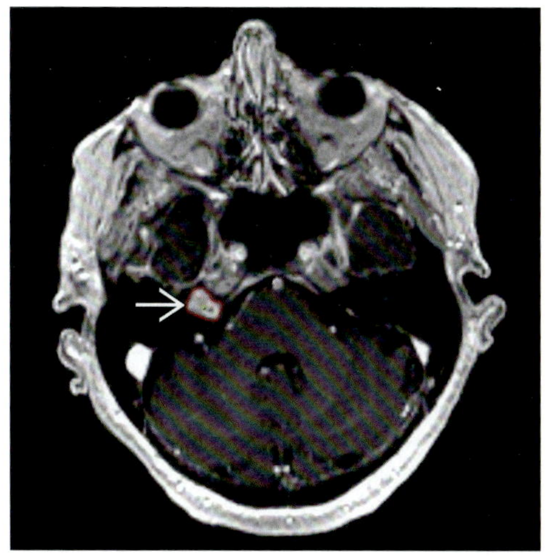

Acoustic Neuroma

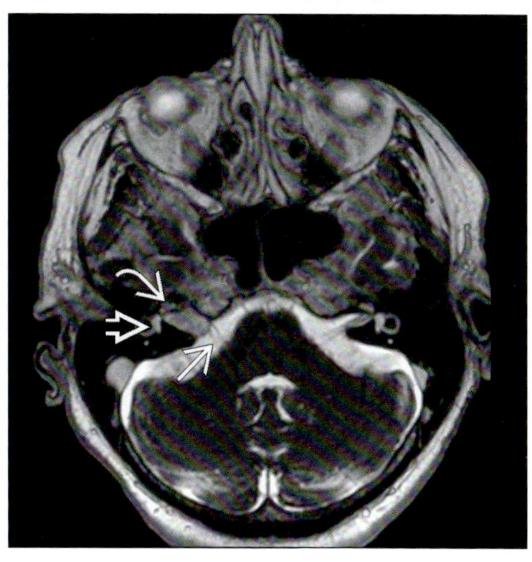

(Left) Axial T1 post-contrast SPGR MR in a 76-year-old woman with hearing loss showing an enhancing mass within the right IAC ➡. High-resolution contrast-enhanced sequences remain the gold standard for tumor characterization. ***(Right)*** Axial CISS sequence MR in the same patient shows the relationship of the mass to vestibulocochlear nerve ➡. This sequence can be helpful in visualizing the cranial nerves as well as the cochlea ⇗ and semicircular canals ⇨.

Acoustic Neuroma

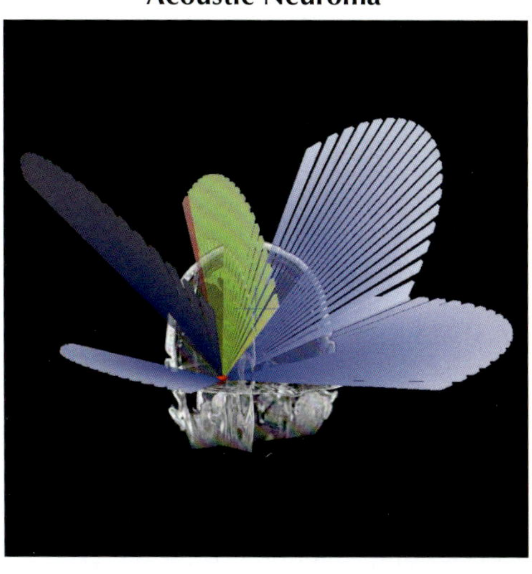

Acoustic Neuroma

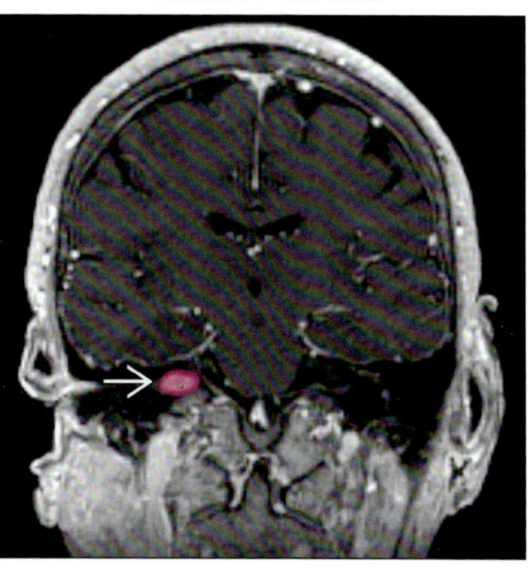

(Left) Beam arrangement for the same patient shows planned delivery of 12 Gy to the 80% isodose line using 5 dynamic conformal arcs. ***(Right)*** Dose colorwash for the same patient ➡ shows the prescription of 12 Gy covering the tumor.

ARTERIOVENOUS MALFORMATION

OVERVIEW

General Comments
- Abnormal arterial-venous communication resulting in tangle of fragile blood vessels

Classification
- Spetzler-Martin grading
  - Size
    - I: < 3 cm; II: 3-6 cm; III: > 6 cm
  - Eloquence of adjacent brain
    - 0: Non-eloquent; I: Eloquent
  - Venous drainage pattern
    - 0: Superficial only; I: Deep
  - Grade = number of points (I-V, VI is inoperable)

NATURAL HISTORY

General Features
- Comments
  - Direct arterial to venous communication → shunting without intervening capillary structure
    - High pressure in venous system → dilation and increased risk of rupture
    - Surrounding hypoxia → increased angiogenic factors → vascular proliferation
  - Thought to arise from embryologic malformations, with manifestations later in life

Epidemiology & Cancer Incidence
- Occurs in 0.1% of population
  - Incidence increased with imaging advancements
- Usually presents at ages 20-40 years

Associated Diseases, Abnormalities
- Higher incidence with Osler-Weber-Rendu and Sturge-Weber syndromes

Gross Pathology & Surgical Features
- Tangle of blood vessels with dilated venous drainage system
  - Nidus is point of abnormal AV communication

IMAGING

CT
- Tortuous iso- to hyperdense vessels ± calcifications
  - May appear normal if small nidus
  - Strongly enhance with contrast
  - ± surrounding hemorrhage

CTA
- Enhancing nidus position with feeding arteries and draining veins visualized

MR
- T1/T2: Tangle of flow voids frequently seen
- T1 post contrast: Enhancement of nidus and draining veins
  - Flow may be so rapid that only flow voids seen

Angiogram
- Best delineates vascular structure
- 3 phases seen: Feeding arteries, nidus, draining veins

CLINICAL PRESENTATION & WORK-UP

Presentation
- Hemorrhage (~ 50%), seizures, headaches, focal neurologic deficits

Prognosis
- Risk of hemorrhage: 1-4%/year
  - Incidentally found deep lesions closer to 1%/year
  - Fatality with hemorrhage: 10-25%

Work-Up
- H&P with neurologic exam
- CT/MR ± angiography: Frequently performed at presentation
- Angiography: Gold standard for evaluation
  - CTA/MRA required for radiation tx planning

TREATMENT

Overview
- Tx recommended for Spetzler-Martin grade I-III
  - Surgery or SRS
    - SRS used if high surgical risk
  - Endovascular embolization frequently performed neoadjuvantly for grade III lesions
    - Not usually curative unless lesions < 1 cm
    - Clipping of arterial aneurysms > 7 mm performed prior to further tx
      - ↑ pressure after SRS ↑ risk of aneurysm bleed
- Grade IV-VI lesions controversial
  - Balance between morbidity and hemorrhage risk
  - Observation vs. tx varies with case
- Stereotactic radiosurgery
  - Latency period 1-3 years for obliteration
    - Risk of hemorrhage during latency ↓ by ~ 50%
  - Complete obliteration 80-90% for lesions < 3 cm
    - ↓ for larger lesions

Common Techniques
- Gamma knife (GK) or linear accelerator-based radiosurgery
  - Poor results with fractionated RT
- Contouring: Fuse CTA or MRA (± digital subtraction)
  - Target volume: Nidus on angiography
- Doses: 15-25 Gy to periphery
  - Varies with tumor size and location
  - Increased neurologic sequelae for location/volume > 12 Gy
- Staged procedures (separated by ~ 6 months) can be performed for lesions > 15 mL
  - Goal to increase efficacy and decrease side effects

RECOMMENDED FOLLOW-UP

Routine
- Follow-up with neurologic exam with imaging
  - MR/MRA/CTA at 6 and 12 months, then annually until obliteration
    - Confirm obliteration at 3 years
      - Not obliterated → further therapy

Spetzler-Martin Grade III AVM

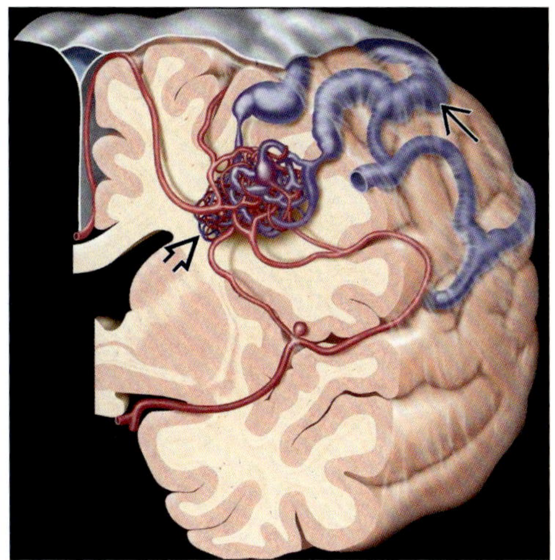

Spetzler-Martin Grade III AVM

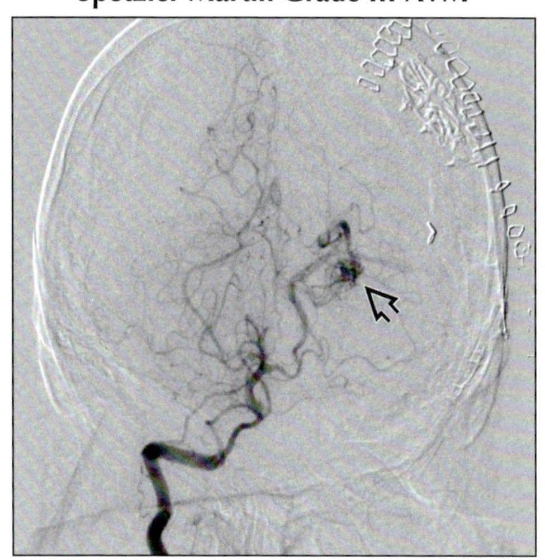

(Left) Graphic shows classic AVM nidus ⇨. Note the abnormally dilated draining veins → secondary to elevated pressure within the venous system. **(Right)** Shown is an angiogram for a 57-year-old woman with left temporal lobe AVM found secondary to visual symptoms. She underwent partial resection, but postoperatively was found to have persistent AVM ⇨.

Spetzler-Martin Grade III AVM

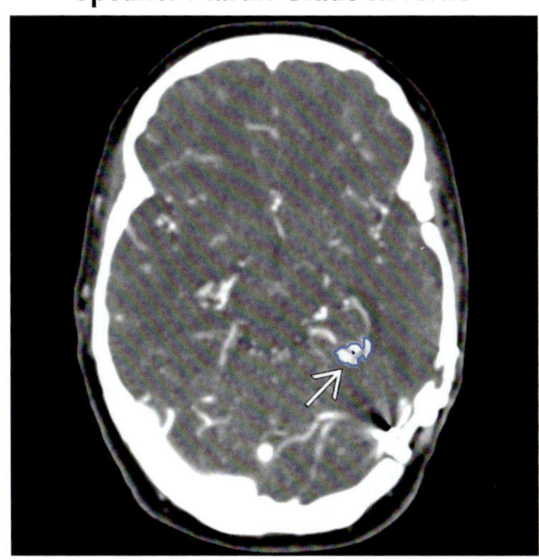

Spetzler-Martin Grade III AVM

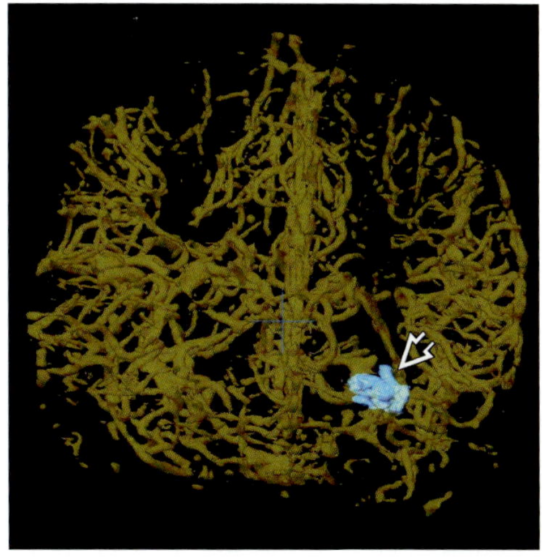

(Left) CT angiogram of the same patient was fused to the planning CT, and the persisting nidus → is shown. Note that digital subtraction CTA/MRAs can be used to help delineate the extent of the nidus. **(Right)** 3D representation of internal vasculature shows the AVM contour ⇨ in the same patient. The predominant vascular supply was from the left posterior cerebral artery.

Spetzler-Martin Grade III AVM

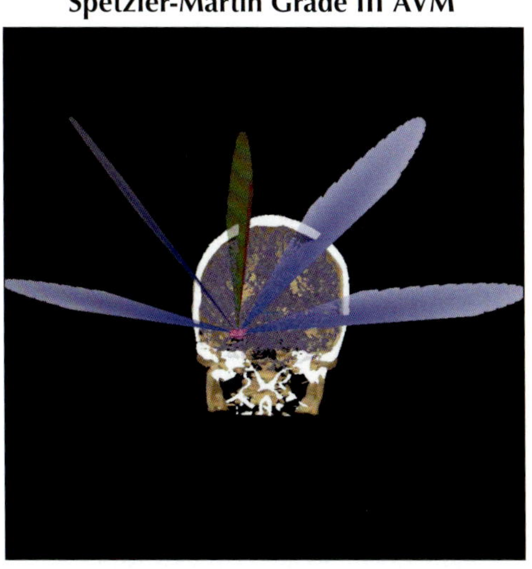

Spetzler-Martin Grade III AVM

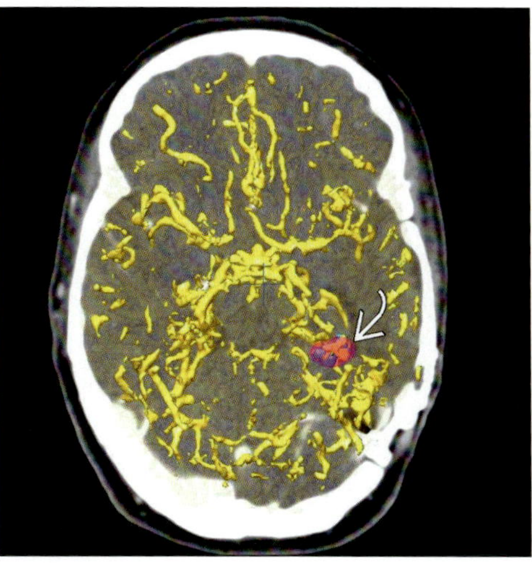

(Left) Five dynamic conformal arcs were used for the same patient to deliver 20 Gy to the 82% isodose line using a Brainlab treatment planning platform. **(Right)** Planning CT in the same patient shows the 20 Gy dose colorwash ↷ covering the residual AVM.

TRIGEMINAL NEURALGIA

OVERVIEW

General Comments
- Stereotypical pain in the distribution of CN V

Classification
- International Headache Society classification
  - Classic: Idiopathic with stereotypical presentation
    - Majority thought to be secondary to vascular compression
  - Secondary: Same as classic but attributed to structural lesion (i.e., neuroma, meningioma, etc.)
- Diagnostic criteria
  - Paroxysmal pain lasting up to 2 minutes involving ≥ 1 division of trigeminal nerve
  - Pain characteristics (at least 1)
    - Intense, superficial, stabbing
    - Precipitated from trigger areas or by trigger factors
  - Stereotyped attacks
  - No neurologic deficit
  - Not attributable to other disorders

NATURAL HISTORY

General Features
- Comments
  - Stereotyped attacks of pain involving trigeminal nerve distribution
    - Typically unilateral involving V2/3
    - V1 < 5% (V1 common with postherpetic neuralgia)

Etiology
- Most cases secondary to compression of trigeminal nerve root at root entry zone
  - Root entry zone: Cisternal portion of trigeminal nerve as it enters the pons
    - Transition point of oligodendrocytic and Schwann cells
      - Hypothesized as more radiosensitive
  - Aberrant vessel causing compression thought to be causative agent in 80-90% of cases

Epidemiology & Cancer Incidence
- ~ 15,000 cases per year in USA
- Usually arises after age 50

IMAGING

MR
- T1/T2: Trigeminal nerve exits from lateral pons
  - Courses anterosuperiorly through prepontine cistern
  - Enters Meckel cave, becomes trigeminal ganglion
- Thin cut or CISS/FIESTA helpful to delineate nerves

CLINICAL PRESENTATION & WORK-UP

Work-Up
- H&P with complete neuro exam
  - Diagnosis is based on history and exam
- Imaging
  - May be helpful in identifying structural causes
    - Consider for patients with trigeminal sensory loss, bilateral symptoms, young age (< 40 years)
    - High-resolution MR/MRA controversial for identifying neurovascular compression
    - Thin cut MR necessary for radiosurgical planning
- Electrophysiologic testing also not routinely required
  - Trigeminal reflex and masseter reflex recordings should be normal in patients with classic vs. secondary TN

TREATMENT

Overview
- Medical management: First-line treatment
  - Anticonvulsant therapy, typically carbamazepine
- Surgery: Utilized when patients medically refractory
  - Microvascular decompression
    - Craniotomy with separation/removal of vascular structures from the trigeminal nerve
  - Percutaneous procedures
    - Gasserian ganglion accessed, usually via foramen ovale, followed by intervention
      - Balloon compression: Compresses ganglion
      - Glycerol rhizotomy: Glycerol injected into cistern
      - Radiofrequency rhizotomy: Destruction secondary to heat
- Radiosurgery: Utilized for patients who are not operative candidates, or as alternative therapy
  - Response rates: Partial response 70-90%, complete response 40-60%
  - Side effects: Facial dysesthesia 5-30% (usually mild)

Standard Doses
- 70-90 Gy

Common Techniques
- SRS: Gamma knife or LINAC based
  - Typically a 4-5 mm cone (LINAC) or 4 mm shot (gamma knife) utilized
    - Beam channel plugging can be utilized on gamma knife to help avoid brainstem
  - Isocenter is placed at trigeminal root entry zone
    - Location chosen so that brainstem surface limited to 30-50%
    - Tx with multiple isocenters (longer section of nerve) is controversial
  - Immobilization important with long tx time
    - Caution advised when considering frameless immobilization devices
  - Gamma knife and LINAC-based tx demonstrate similar dose fall-off characteristics
    - Utilize > 7 arcs and high MU/min on LINAC-based systems

RECOMMENDED FOLLOW-UP

Routine
- Follow-up with neuro exam in 6 months to assess toxicity, then yearly

Trigeminal Nerve

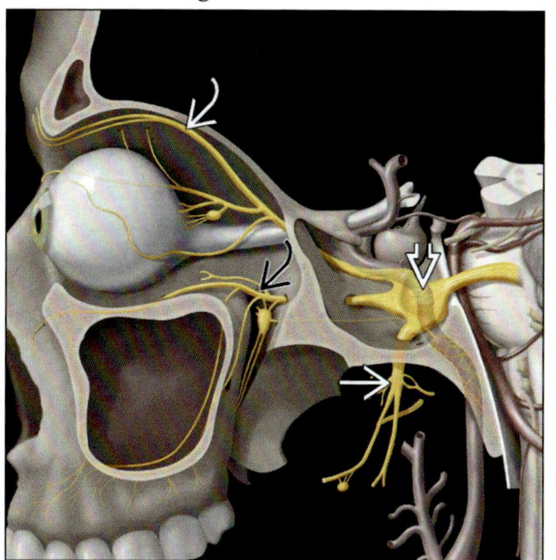

Trigeminal Nerve

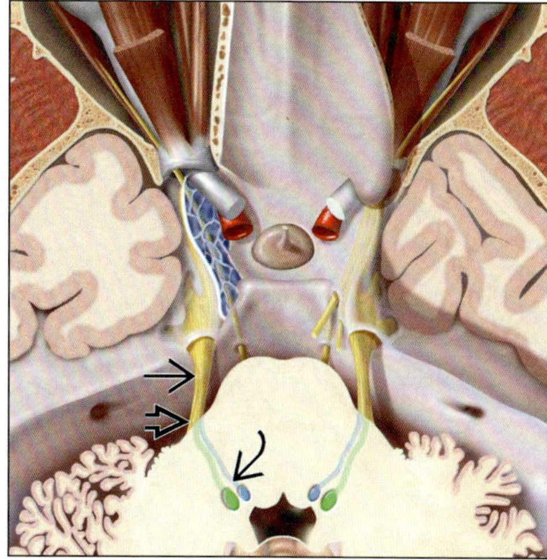

(Left) *Graphic depicts the trigeminal nerve exiting from the lateral pons, entering Meckel cave to form the trigeminal ganglion ➡ before splitting into V1 ➡, V2 ➡, and V3 ➡.* ***(Right)*** *Axial graphic shows the preganglionic portion of the trigeminal nerve ➡ originating from the main motor and sensory nuclei ➡ within the pons and exiting from the root entry zone ➡. The preganglionic portion is the radiosurgical target.*

Trigeminal Neuralgia

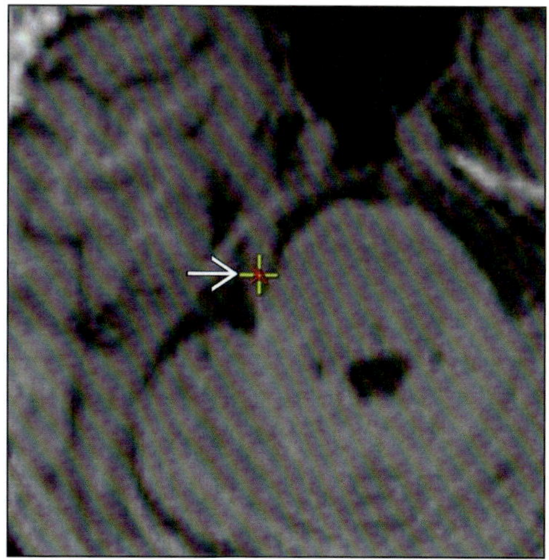

Trigeminal Neuralgia

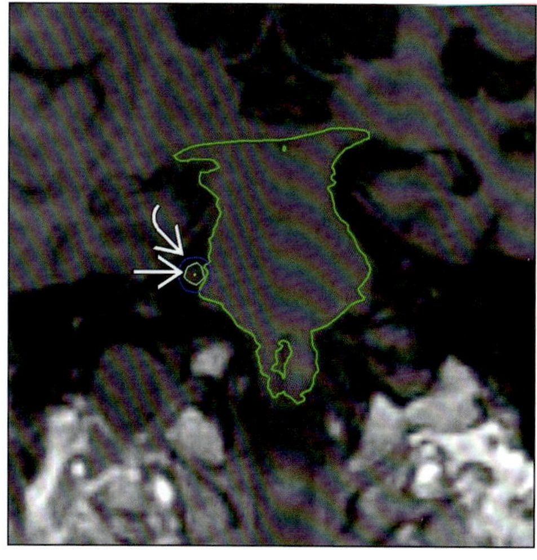

(Left) *Fused T1 SPGR MR shows the placement of the isocenter ➡ on the preganglionic portion of the trigeminal nerve.* ***(Right)*** *Fused MR in the same patient shows the 30% ➡ and 50% ➡ isodose lines after radiosurgical planning. The isocenter was moved along the nerve until the 50% isodose line was excluded from the brainstem, and the 30% tangentially involved the surface.*

Trigeminal Neuralgia

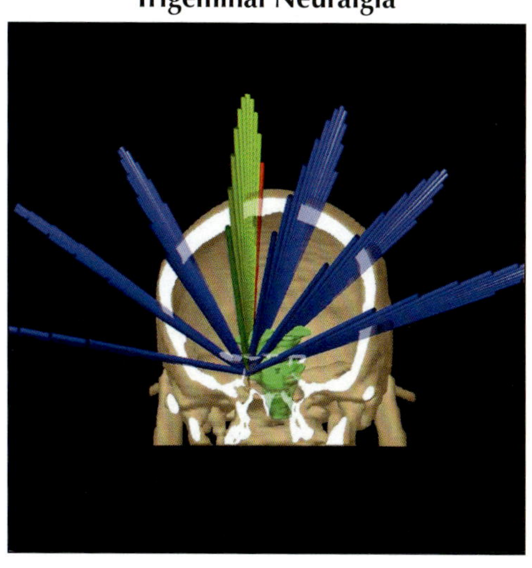

Trigeminal Neuralgia

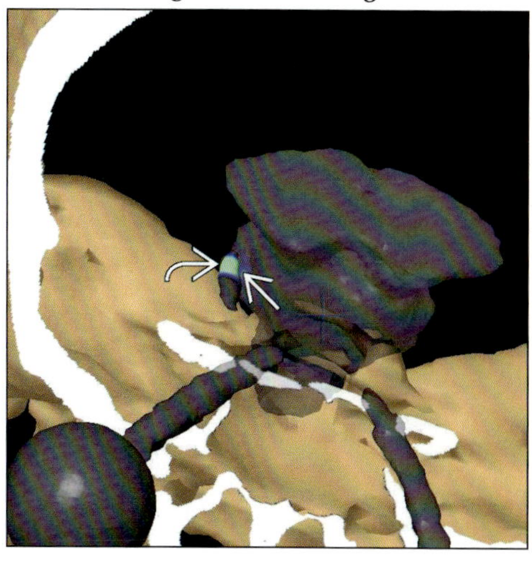

(Left) *LINAC-based radiosurgery was used to deliver 90 Gy to the isocenter using 7 arcs with a 4 mm collimator. Note that at least 7 arcs should be utilized for LINAC-based systems to achieve adequately sharp dose fall-off.* ***(Right)*** *3D representation in the same patient shows the dose colorwash of 30% and 50% along the nerve ➡. Note that the 30% dose contacts the brainstem surface but the 50% is excluded ➡.*

UVEAL MELANOMA

OVERVIEW

General Comments
- Melanoma arising within uvea of eye

Classification
- Collaborative Ocular Melanoma Study (COMS) classification
  - Small: Height = 1-3 mm, diameter = 5-16 mm
  - Medium: Height = 2.5-10 mm, diameter = 5-16 mm
    - Overlap in classification from height of 2.5-3 mm
  - Large: Height > 10 mm, diameter > 16 mm
- AJCC staging classification also exists

NATURAL HISTORY

General Features
- Comments
  - Arise from uveal melanocytes
    - Can develop from transition of pigmented nevi within uvea
- Location
  - Located within uvea of eye
    - Can be located in iris, ciliary body, or choroid

Etiology
- Risk factors
  - Fair skin, light eyes, prone to sunburn, cutaneous and ocular nevi, UV exposure

Epidemiology & Cancer Incidence
- Most common intraocular malignancy
  - ~ 1,500 cases each year
- Median age range: 50-60 years

Gross Pathology & Surgical Features
- Frequently dome-shaped, variably pigmented mass

Microscopic Pathology
- 3 major cell types
  - Spindle cell (type A and B), mixed cell, and epithelioid cell (worst prognosis)
    - Classification based upon cell type and histologic characteristics

IMAGING

Ultrasound
- A and B scans performed
  - Usual characteristics: Dome/mushroom shape, low to medium internal reflectivity, and internal vascularity

CLINICAL PRESENTATION & WORK-UP

Presentation
- Frequently asymptomatic > incidental discovery
- Visual disturbances include blurred vision, scotomas, visual field loss

Prognosis
- 5-year OS: Small (~ 95%), medium (80-88%), large (55-65%)

Work-Up
- H&P
  - Ophthalmologic examination with tumor characterization
    - Classic findings: Thickness > 2 mm, subretinal fluid, symptomatic, orange pigment, and margin near optic disc
  - Ocular ultrasound with A/B modes
- CBC, CMP with LFTs, LDH
  - Liver imaging if liver enzymes abnormal
- Chest x-ray

TREATMENT

Overview
- Small: May be observed until growth
  - ~ 1/4 to 1/3 will grow within 5 years
  - Transpupillary thermotherapy, photodynamic therapy, and other interventions also being used
- Medium: RT with plaque brachytherapy (most common); proton/heavy ion therapy and SRS also being investigated
  - Surgery may also be employed, but no difference in mortality with increased morbidity
- Large: Enucleation

Plaque Brachytherapy
- American Brachytherapy Society recommendations
  - If I-125, 85 Gy to apex delivered at dose rate of 0.6-1.05 Gy/hr (3-7 days)
  - Pd-103, Ru-106, Co-60, Ir-192 also used
  - Standard circular, notched, or custom plaques may be used
    - Plaques usually designed with 2-3 mm free margin around tumor (less if unrimmed)
    - Plaques may be loaded uniformly or nonuniformly
  - AAPM TG-43 utilized for dose calculation
  - Cases not suitable for plaque brachytherapy
    - Gross extrascleral extension
    - Ring melanoma
    - > 1/2 ciliary body involvement

RECOMMENDED FOLLOW-UP

Routine
- F/U primarily with ophthalmologist to monitor for complications
  - q. 3-6 months for 1 year, then q. 6 months to yearly
  - Ocular ultrasound performed at least yearly
  - Hepatic labs yearly with imaging if indicated

Plaque Brachytherapy Complications
- Visual acuity preserved > 20/200: ~ 50-60% of patients
- Other: Radiation retinopathy, cataracts, glaucoma, dry eyes
  - Rates vary widely based on tumor location
    - Retinopathy: 10-63%
    - Cataracts: 10-69%

UVEAL MELANOMA

Globe

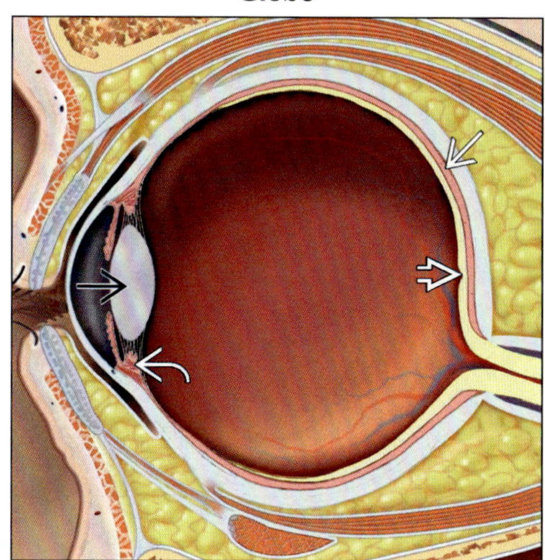

Funduscopy, COMS Medium Tumor

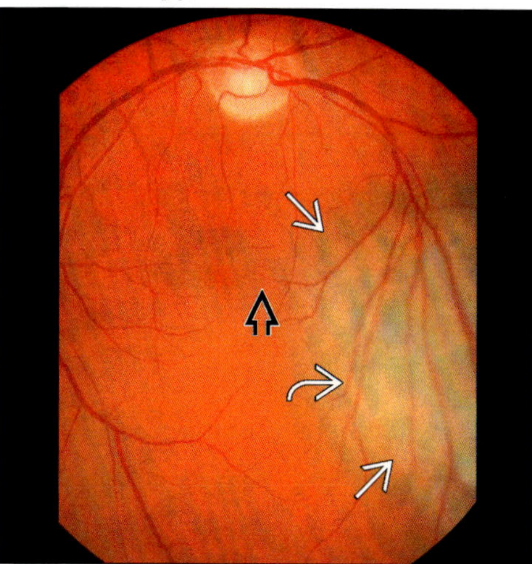

(Left) *Graphic depicts the normal globe, with the lens → separating the anterior and posterior chambers. Uveal melanomas can arise anywhere within the posterior choroid → or ciliary body →, classically causing retinal → elevation.* ***(Right)*** *Funduscopic photograph shows a choroidal tumor → of the left eye, with elevation of the choroid. The elevation continues up to the edge → of the macula. Classic orange pigmentation → can be seen. (Courtesy K. E. Winward, MD.)*

COMS Medium Tumor

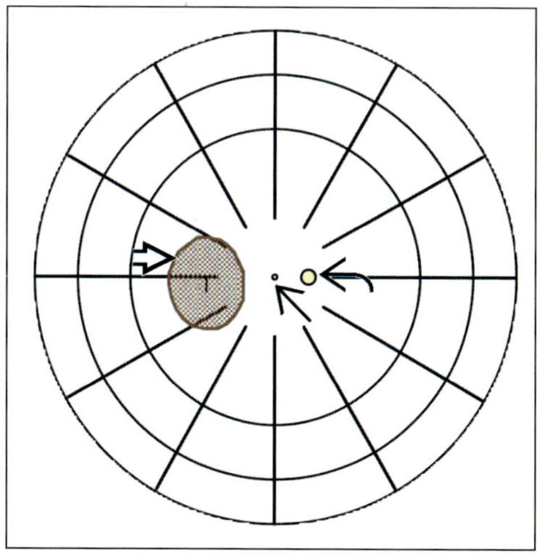

COMS Medium Tumor

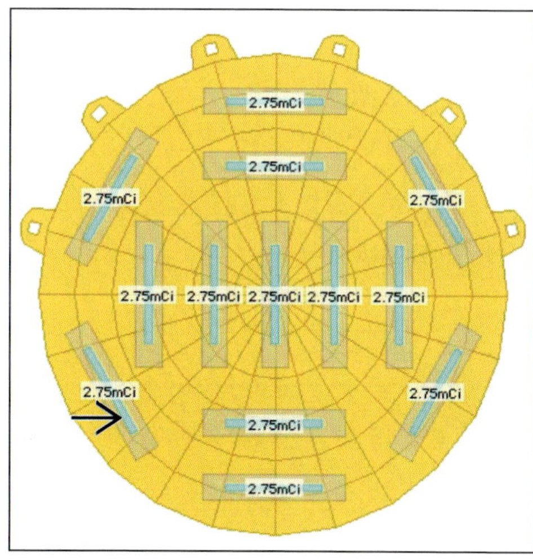

(Left) *Ocular schematic in a 55-year-old female with COMS medium melanoma → shows the right eye located lateral to macula → and optic nerve →. She was recommended to undergo plaque brachytherapy.* ***(Right)*** *Loading diagram for the plaque utilized in the same patient shows uniform seed loading with 13 I-125 seeds → placed.*

COMS Medium Tumor

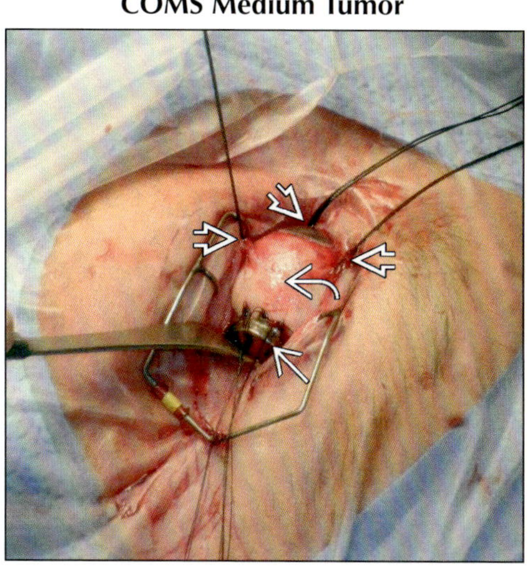

COMS Medium Tumor

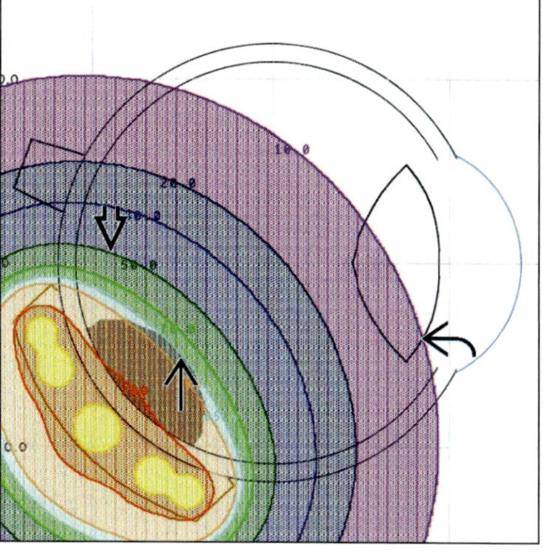

(Left) *Intraoperative photograph of the same patient shows plaque placement →. Note the isolation of the rectus musculature → to allow for globe manipulation. The lateral rectus muscle has been detached →. (Courtesy K. E. Winward, MD.)* ***(Right)*** *Dose distribution for the same patient shows the 85 Gy prescription covering the tumor apex →. While the dose fall-off is rapid (note the 50 Gy dose line →), the lens still partially receives 10 Gy →.*

GRAVES OPHTHALMOPATHY

OVERVIEW

General Comments

- Autoimmune disease of retroorbital tissues associated with Graves hyperthyroidism

NATURAL HISTORY

Etiology

- Risk factors
  - Family autoimmune Hx, females, smoking (odds ratio 7.7)
- Pathogenesis: Not completely understood
  - Antibodies to TSH receptor in Graves disease
  - Higher concentration of TSH receptors in retroorbital fibroblasts and adipocytes
  - T-cell activation → inflammation → glycosaminoglycan (GAG) deposition
  - ↑ osmotic pressure → retroorbital swelling → proptosis

Epidemiology & Cancer Incidence

- Clinically present in ~ 1/3 of patients with Graves
  - Higher nonclinical incidence rates

Gross Pathology & Surgical Features

- Infiltration/enlargement of extraocular muscles (EOM) and fat

Microscopic Pathology

- Lymphocytic and inflammatory infiltration of retroorbital tissues
  - Collagen and GAG deposition

IMAGING

CT

- NECT: Isodense EOM enlargement
- Proptosis can be seen relative to lateral orbital rim

MR

- T1WI: Isointense EOM enlargement
  - Increased retroorbital fat
- T2WI FS: Can demonstrate increased signal in EOM
  - Secondary to ↑ fluid accumulation
  - Not seen in chronic disease with ↑ fibrosis
- T1 post-contrast FS: Muscle enhancement, but less than normal EOM muscles 2° ↓ perfusion

CLINICAL PRESENTATION & WORK-UP

Presentation

- Orbital symptoms
  - ↑ lid retraction and lid lag with downward gaze
  - Can also demonstrate conjunctival irritation, retroorbital pain, diplopia, visual loss
- Symptoms usually concurrent (~ 40%) with hyperthyroidism presentation
  - May occur prior or post diagnosis of Graves disease

Work-Up

- H&P
  - Conjunctival/EOM/visual field/visual acuity evaluation
    - Lid lag can be seen with downward gaze
  - Exophthalmometer to evaluate proptosis
    - Borders: Lateral bony orbit to anterior cornea
      - 20-22 mm upper limit of normal
- Ophthalmology evaluation if abnormal visual fields/ acuity/corneal ulceration
- Endocrine evaluation to confirm Graves disease if not already performed
  - TSH, free T4, T3
- Imaging with CT/MR if evaluating for RT

TREATMENT

Overview

- Mild symptoms
  - Symptomatic management
  - Selenium
- Progressive or severe symptoms
  - Medical: Primary treatment with glucocorticoid therapy (prednisone)
    - Rituximab being investigated with good responses
  - RT: Medically refractory, cannot tolerate medications, alternative therapy
    - RT most effective for diplopia and ocular motility
      - Response rate 50-80%
      - Not been shown to prevent progression
    - Caution in diabetic patients secondary to concerns for retinopathy
    - Steroids helpful early during treatment to avoid worsening symptoms from edema
  - Orbital decompressive surgery: Refractory to other therapies, threatened visual loss, cosmetic reconstruction

Standard Doses

- 20 Gy in 2 Gy/fx

Common Techniques

- Classic fields
  - Opposed laterals, anterior block 5-6 mm behind iris
    - Anterior border can be decreased with stereotactic techniques to ensure complete coverage
    - Blocks to create D-shaped field to include bony confines of retroorbital compartment
  - Half beam block &/or posterior angulation (3-10°) to help spare anterior globe and lens
- IMRT and other advanced techniques investigational

RECOMMENDED FOLLOW-UP

Routine

- Follow-up with physical examination every 3-6 months for 1 year, then annually
- Ophthalmologist evaluation to evaluate for retinopathy, visual complications, and cataracts
  - Retinopathy 0-15%
    - Varies with other risk factors, such as diabetes
  - Cataracts 10-30%

Graves Ophthalmopathy

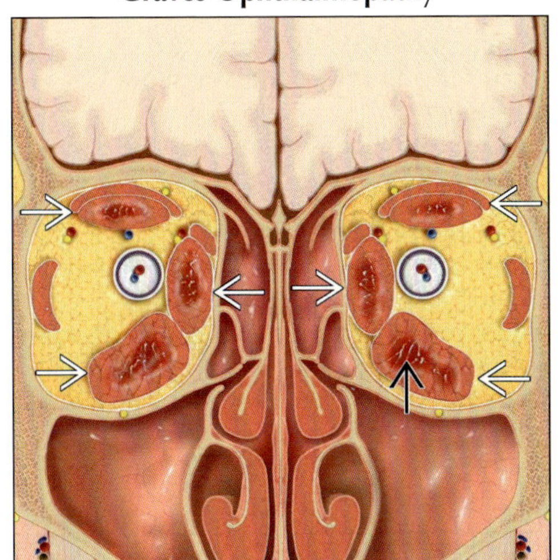

Graves Ophthalmopathy

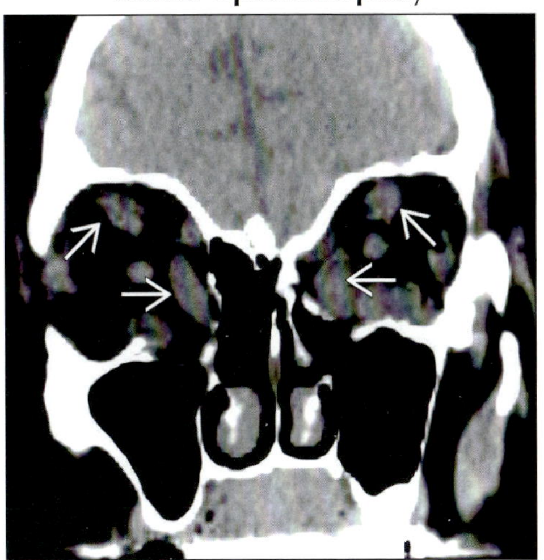

(Left) Graphic depicts bilateral enlarged extraocular muscles ➔. Note the mucopolysaccharide deposition within the musculature ➔. (Right) Shown is a planning CT for a 72-year-old woman with symptomatic Graves ophthalmopathy, with progressive disease on corticosteroids. Note the enlargement of the bilateral rectus muscles ➔.

Graves Ophthalmopathy

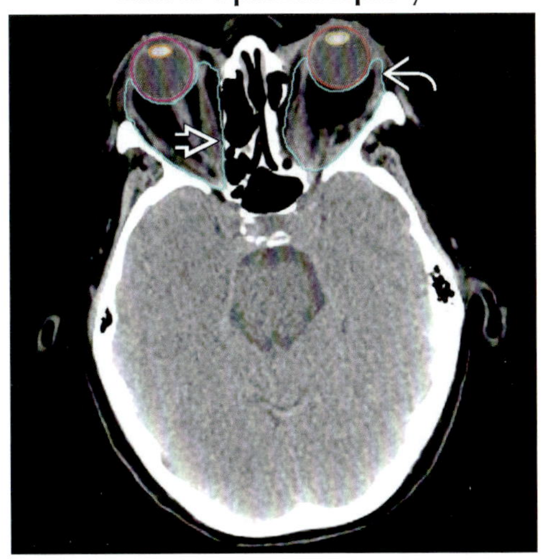

Graves Ophthalmopathy

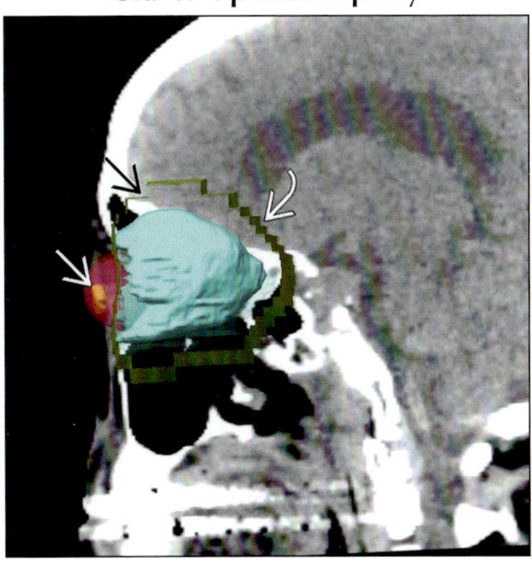

(Left) Planning CT in the same patient shows the retroorbital contents contoured as the target volume ➔. Note the inclusion of the muscular attachments ➔. (Right) Planning CT in the same patient shows a traditional D-shaped treatment field ➔. The anterior border was placed 3 mm behind the lens ➔ (stereotactic treatment techniques were utilized), and the remaining field shaped 7 mm from the treatment volume to allow for beam penumbra ➔.

Graves Ophthalmopathy

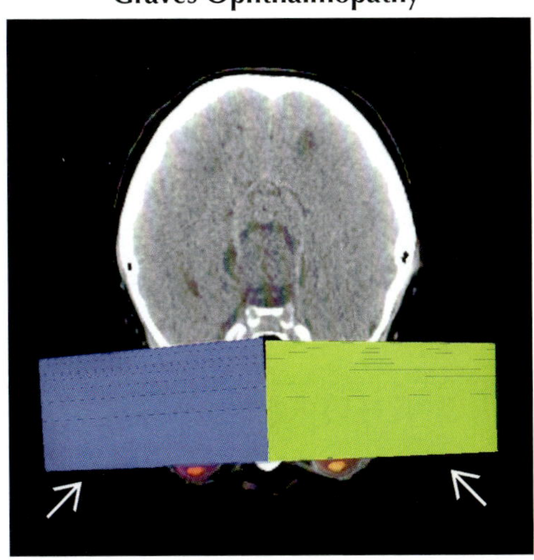

Graves Ophthalmopathy

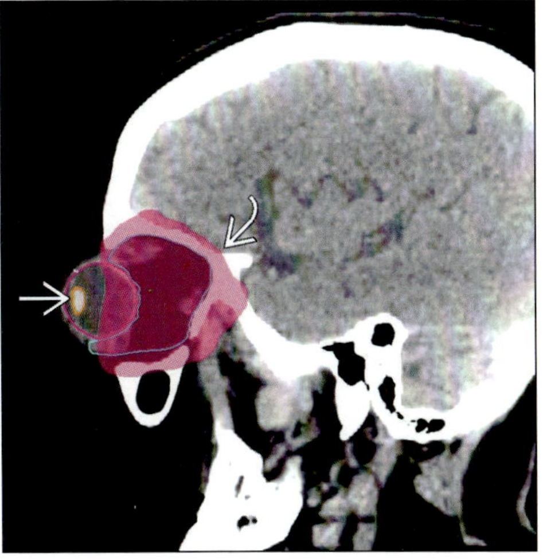

(Left) Axial images in the same patient show an opposed lateral beam arrangement ➔ utilized to deliver 20 Gy in 10 fractions. Posterior angulation of 6 degrees was used to avoid the contralateral structures. (Right) The 95% dose colorwash is shown for the same patient demonstrating target volume coverage ➔. Note the avoidance of the anterior chamber and lens ➔.

OPTIC GLIOMA

OVERVIEW

General Comments
- Neuroglial tumor arising along optic nerves, chiasm, or optic tracts

Classification
- Dodge classification
  - Stage 1: Optic nerve involvement only
  - Stage 2: Optic chiasm ± optic nerve involvement
  - Stage 3: Hypothalamic or adjacent structures

NATURAL HISTORY

General Features
- Comments
  - Majority of lesions occur in children and are low grade (WHO grade 1 pilocytic astrocytomas)
  - When occurs in adults, typically more aggressive and can be higher grade

Etiology
- Risk factors
  - NF 1: Most common CNS tumor with NF 1 (~ 15%)
    - 10-70% of optic gliomas associated with NF 1

Epidemiology & Cancer Incidence
- 2% of CNS gliomas
  - 5% of pediatric brain tumors
- Age of onset
  - 90% at age < 20 years (usually at age < 10 years)

Microscopic Pathology
- Varies with histology
  - Most appear as WHO grade 1 pilocytic astrocytomas

IMAGING

CT
- Isodense fusiform enlargement of optic nerves
- Calcifications rare (help differentiate from optic nerve meningioma)

MR
- T1WI: Iso- to hypointense enlargement of optic nerve
- T2WI: Variable, but typically hyperintense
- T1 post contrast: Varies, slight to hyperintense enhancement
  - NF 1 typically with slight enhancement

CLINICAL PRESENTATION & WORK-UP

Presentation
- Varies with location
  - Anterior: Proptosis, gaze abnormalities, visual disturbances
  - Posterior: Visual disturbances, obstructive hydrocephalus, endocrine abnormalities (hypothalamic involvement)

Prognosis
- Varies, more indolent course with NF 1, spontaneous regression can be seen
- In children, median survival > 15 years
  - Worse prognosis in adults secondary to more malignant histology
- Anterior tumors more favorable than posterior

Work-Up
- H&P with retinal and neurologic exam
- Imaging: MR with or without contrast, ± CT for bony abnormalities
- Endocrine evaluation may be required depending upon location and symptoms
- Biopsy may be required for posterior tumors to establish diagnosis
  - Differential large for suprasellar lesions

TREATMENT

Overview
- Pediatric
  - Treatment controversial
    - Observation encouraged initially
    - Chemotherapy for progression or significant symptoms
    - RT
      - Usually deferred until progression on chemo
      - May be utilized sooner when patients > 10 yo
    - Surgery
      - If clinically necessary or to help defer RT
      - May be utilized if complete visual loss present or for cosmetic concerns
- Adults
  - Treatment controversial
    - Surgery if resectable without significant morbidity
    - Chemo, RT, chemoRT may all be utilized
    - Treat more aggressively than pediatric patients, or as dictated by pathology

Standard Doses
- 45-54 Gy in 1.8 Gy/fx

Techniques
- 3D conformal, IMRT, or arc therapy as indicated
  - Stereotactic techniques encouraged
- Contouring
  - GTV: Gross tumor as visualized on MR
    - Includes enhancing volume (if present) and T1 or T2 abnormality
  - CTV: Controversial, GTV + 5 mm on latest pediatric protocols
  - PTV: CTV + 3-5 mm

RECOMMENDED FOLLOW-UP

Routine
- Follow-up with MR every 3 months for 2 years, then every 6 months for 2 years, then annually
  - Endocrine evaluation for pediatric patients or as indicated
    - Serum prolactin, IGF-1, TSH, free T4, AM cortisol, ACTH, LH/FSH

Visual Pathways

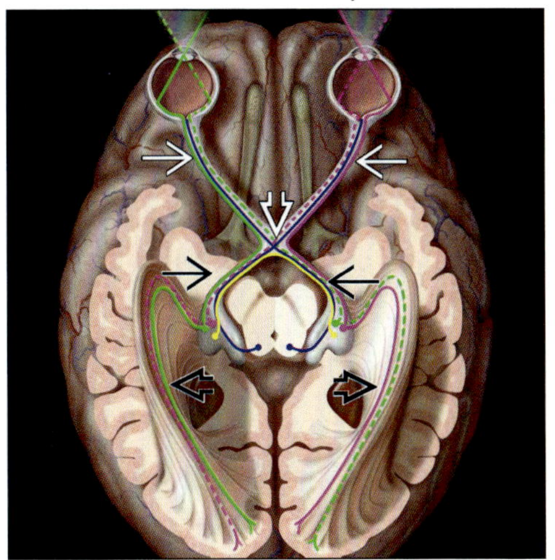

Optic Glioma

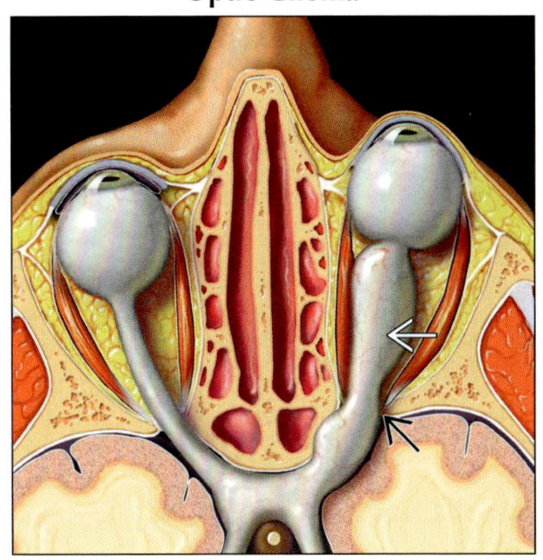

(Left) *Axial graphic demonstrates the visual pathway. The left and right optic nerves ➡ can be seen, with the medial nerve fibers crossing at the optic chiasm ➡. The optic tracts course posteriorly ➡ before becoming the optic radiations ➡.* ***(Right)*** *Axial graphic shows fusiform enlargement of the left optic nerve ➡ extending through the optic canal ➡. Proptosis of the left eye secondary to the enlargement can also be seen.*

Optic Tract/Hypothalamic Glioma

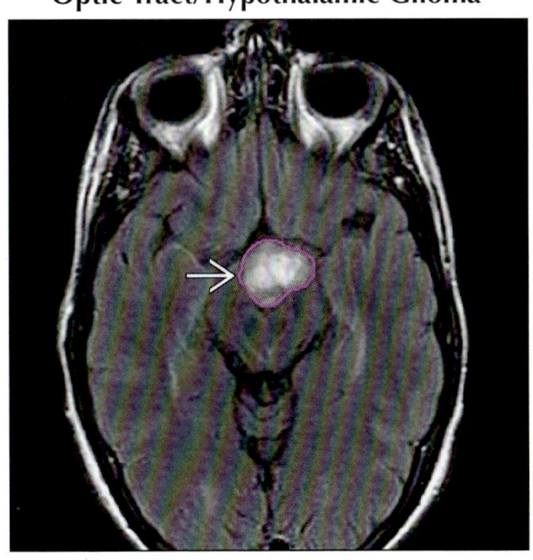

Optic Tract/Hypothalamic Glioma

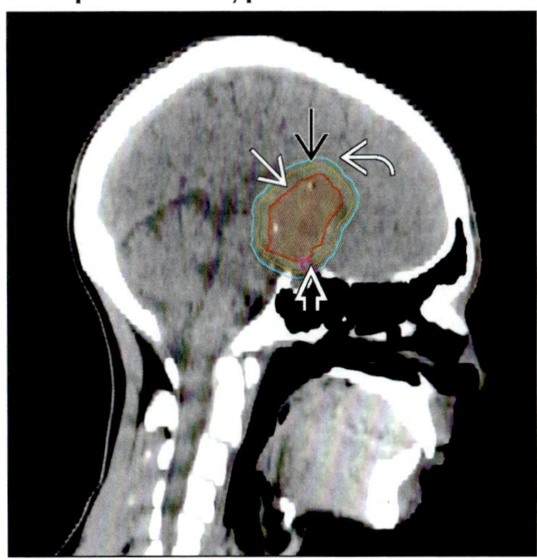

(Left) *Fused T2 FLAIR MR in an 18-year-old man shows a WHO grade I pilocytic astrocytoma demonstrating involvement of the optic tracts and hypothalamus. He demonstrated progression after chemotherapy with symptoms of headaches and visual disturbances. Radiation was recommended, and the GTV is shown ➡.* ***(Right)*** *Planning CT in the same patient shows the GTV ➡, CTV ➡ (GTV + 5 mm), and PTV ➡ (CTV + 3 mm). Note the location of the optic chiasm ➡.*

Optic Tract/Hypothalamic Glioma

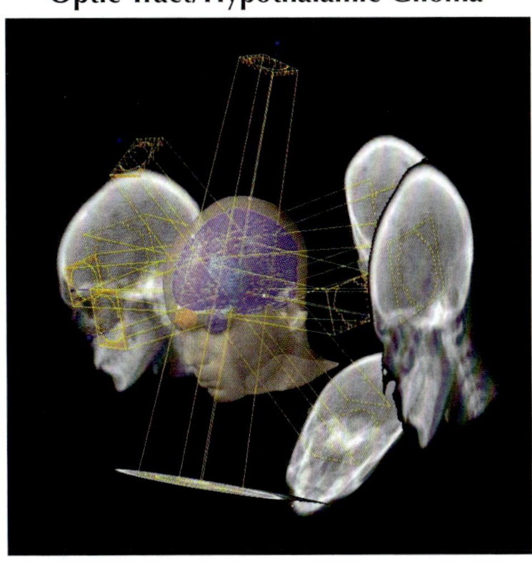

Optic Tract/Hypothalamic Glioma

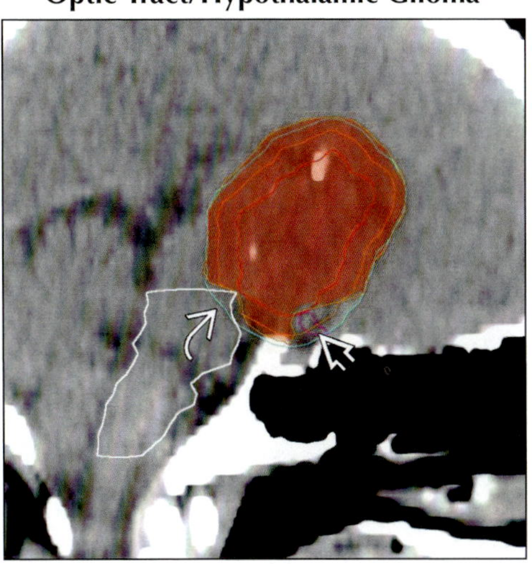

(Left) *Beam arrangement in the same patient shows a 5-field IMRT plan used to deliver 54 Gy in 30 fractions.* ***(Right)*** *Planning CT in the same patient shows the 54 Gy dose colorwash. Note the exclusion of dose > 54 Gy from the brainstem ➡ and optic chiasm ➡.*

CNS LYMPHOMA

OVERVIEW

General Comments
- Variant of non-Hodgkin lymphoma localized to brain, leptomeninges, eyes, or spinal cord

NATURAL HISTORY

General Features
- Location
  - Most periventricular in deep white matter
  - ~ 90% supratentorial
  - Solitary mass in 75%, multifocal in 25%

Etiology
- Risk factors
  - Immunodeficiency
    - 5-10% of AIDS patients develop CNS lymphoma
- Etiology unclear
  - CNS normally does not contain lymphatic tissue
  - Causal link with Epstein-Barr virus (EBV) in some cases

Epidemiology & Cancer Incidence
- Median age: 5th decade
  - Younger in AIDS patients
- ~ 4% of CNS tumors
- Rise in incidence since 1970s, now stabilizing
  - Attributable in part to HIV

Gross Pathology & Surgical Features
- Grayish brown tumors
- Infiltrative with poorly defined borders

Microscopic Pathology
- Histology consistent with NHL
  - 95% B-cell histology
    - DLBCL most common
- Hallmark is angiocentric infiltration with perivascular cell cuffs

IMAGING

CT
- Iso-/hyperdense mass
- Most uniformly enhance

MR
- T1: Iso-/hypointense to gray matter
- T1 post contrast: Strong homogeneous enhancement
  - Can appear infectious with peripheral ring enhancement
  - Well-demarcated appearance in contrast to histologically infiltrative borders
- T2: Iso-/hypointense

CLINICAL PRESENTATION & WORK-UP

Presentation
- Varies with location
  - Neurologic deficits, psychiatric disturbances, signs of elevated ICP

Prognosis
- No tx: Median survival (MS) = 1.5 months
- Whole brain radiotherapy (WBRT): MS 10-18 months
- Chemo ± WBRT: MS 44 months

Work-Up
- Clinical
  - H&P with neuro exam
    - Ophthalmologist slit lamp evaluation
      - Evaluate for ocular lymphoma
    - CSF evaluation
      - Contraindicated if signs of elevated ICP
    - Bone marrow biopsy
    - Systemic evaluation for extracranial lymphoma
    - HIV evaluation
  - MR neuroaxis ± contrast
  - Stereotactic needle biopsy
    - May be able to avoid if confirmation by CSF

TREATMENT

Overview
- Tx controversial
  - WBRT used historically
    - Very radiosensitive, but local recurrence inevitable
      - Dose escalation → ↑ toxicity, no survival benefit
    - Addition of chemo ± WBRT consolidation improves survival
      - ↑ toxicity with WBRT, especially for age > 60 y
- NCCN accepted options
  - Initiate steroids once diagnosis confirmed
    - Avoid steroids before diagnosis established
  - KPS ≥ 40
    - High-dose methotrexate-based chemotherapy
    - ± WBRT
      - Utilized more often for younger patients with good performance status
  - KPS < 40
    - WBRT or chemotherapy if able to tolerate

Standard Doses
- WBRT: 24-36 Gy in 1.8-2 Gy/fx
- Focal boost if < CR to chemo
  - Boost gross disease to 45 Gy

Common Techniques
- WBRT: Opposed lateral fields most common
  - WBRT techniques described elsewhere
- Focal boost: 3D conformal, IMRT, or arc therapy
  - GTV: Gross tumor (contrast-enhancing volume)
  - CTV: GTV + 1-2 cm
  - PTV: CTV + 3-5 mm

RECOMMENDED FOLLOW-UP

Routine
- F/U with H&P and neuro exam q. 3 months for 1st 2 yrs, q. 6 months for the following 3 yrs, then annually
  - CSF and ocular examination depending upon initial presentation

Primary CNS Lymphoma

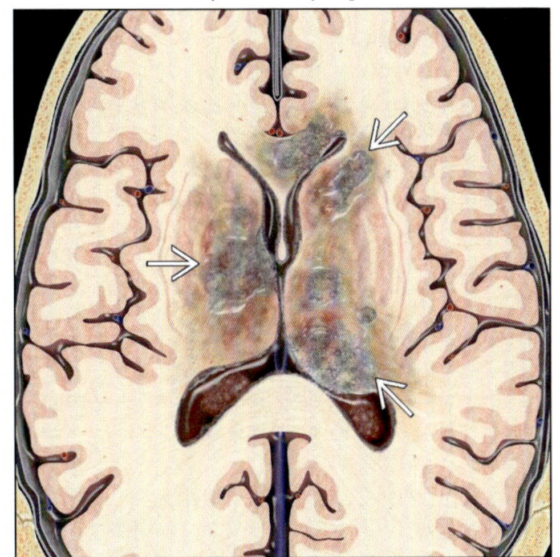

Primary CNS Lymphoma

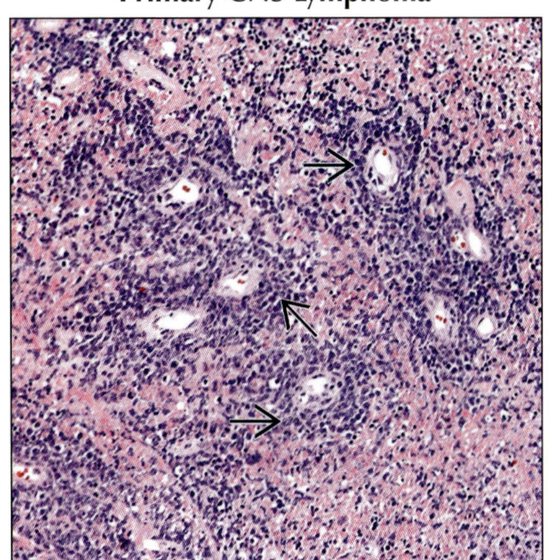

(Left) *Graphic illustrates a primary CNS lymphoma with multifocal periventricular involvement ➡. Multifocal disease is more often seen in immunocompromised patients, but diffuse infiltration is usually present despite the discrete appearance often seen on imaging.* ***(Right)*** *Classic appearance of CNS lymphoma is shown, with angiocentric perivascular cuffs ➡. (Courtesy T. Tihan, MD, PhD.)*

Primary CNS Lymphoma

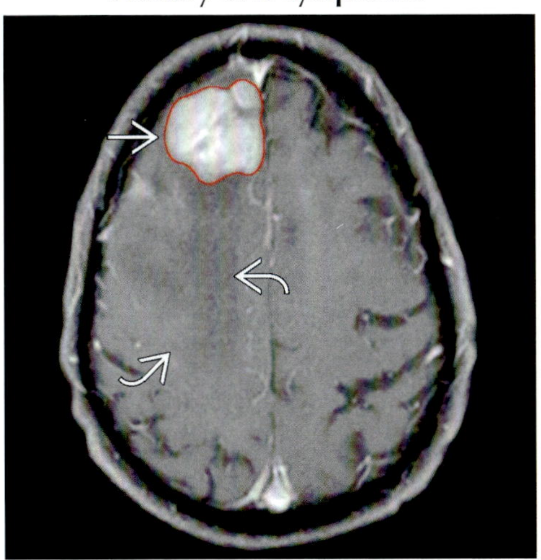

Primary CNS Lymphoma

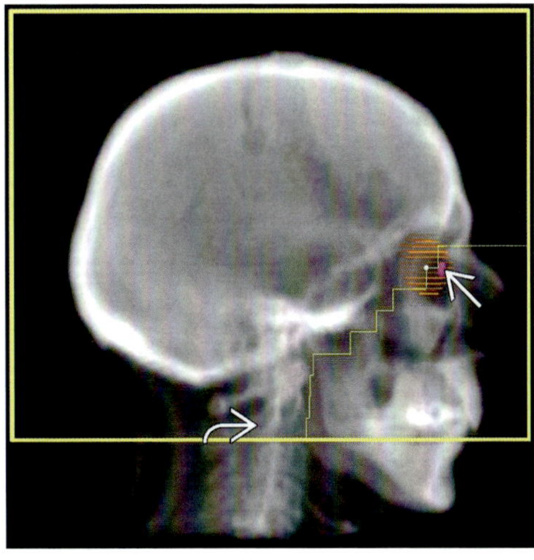

(Left) *T1 post-contrast MR of an 80 year old with biopsy-confirmed primary CNS lymphoma shows the GTV outlining the enhancement ➡. Multifocal involvement was present in other portions of the scan. Note the surrounding edema ➡.* ***(Right)*** *DRR shows that the whole brain blocks in the same patient. Due to age and comorbidities, chemotherapy was not an option, and RT was recommended. Note the exclusion of the lens ➡ and the inclusion of C1-C2 ➡.*

Primary CNS Lymphoma

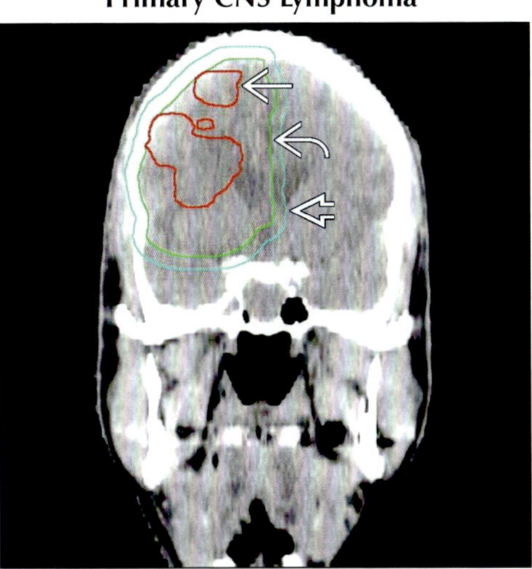

Primary CNS Lymphoma

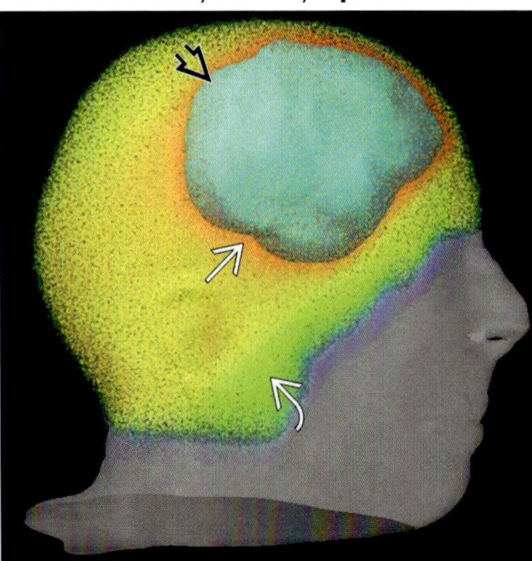

(Left) *Planning CT in the same patient shows the GTV ➡ with a 2 cm margin as the CTV ➡, and a 3 mm PTV margin ➡. The CTV was constrained from the midline as a natural anatomic boundary. Note the multifocal involvement.* ***(Right)*** *Dose colorwash in the same patient demonstrates the initial WBRT dose of 36 Gy ➡, followed by a conformal boost to the PTV ➡ to a total dose of 45 Gy ➡.*

CNS METASTASES

OVERVIEW

General Comments
- Metastases from tumors originating outside the CNS

Classification
- RPA class
  - I: Age < 65 years, KPS ≥ 70, primary controlled, brain-only metastases
  - II: All others
  - III: KPS < 70
- Graded prognostic assessment (GPA) classification
  - Total score predicts survival
    - Age: 0 (≥ 60), 0.5 (50-59), 1 (< 50)
    - KPS: 0 (< 70), 0.5 (70-80), 1 (90-100)
    - Number of cranial metastases: 0 (> 3), 0.5 (2-3), 1 (1)
    - Number of extracranial metastases: 0 (present), 1 (absent)
  - Update of GPA classification allows for site-specific prognosis

NATURAL HISTORY

General Features
- Location
  - Most are found at gray matter-white matter (GM-WM) junction
    - Hematogenous spread is most common mechanism of spread to CNS
    - Blood vessel diameter decreases at GM-WM junction: Leads to trapping of tumor cells
  - Cerebral hemispheres (80%) > cerebellum (15%) > brainstem (5%)

Epidemiology & Cancer Incidence
- 20-40% of cancer patients develop brain metastases
  - Incidence varies with histology
    - Most common histologies include lung, breast, renal, colorectal, and melanoma
  - Incidence increasing in many histologies
    - Imaging advances and increased screening → increased detection rates
    - Improved survival with newer systemic therapies → higher prevalence
- Metastases:primary brain malignancies = 10:1

Gross Pathology & Surgical Features
- Classically well-demarcated round lesions
  - Calcifications are not usually seen
  - Hemorrhage can be seen
    - More common in melanoma, renal cell, choriocarcinoma
  - Vasogenic edema common in surrounding parenchyma

IMAGING

CT
- NECT: Hypo-/isodense masses, usually seen at GM-WM interface
  - Edema commonly present
  - Hemorrhage may be present
- CECT
  - Strongly enhancing, well-demarcated mass

MR
- T1WI: Iso-/hypointense mass
  - Hemorrhage may be seen as hyperintensity
    - T1 can help distinguish blood products from contrast enhancement
- T2WI: Iso-hyperintense mass, varies
  - Surrounding edema frequently seen
- T1 FLAIR: Commonly hyperintense
  - Peritumoral edema often striking in appearance
- T1 post contrast: Almost all mets strongly enhance
  - Variable patterns of enhancement
- DWI: Most with no diffusion restriction
  - Can help differentiate between abscesses and tumor
- Dynamic susceptibility contrast-enhanced MR: Measure of rCBV
  - May be elevated in metastases and gliomas
  - Peritumoral region usually shows higher rCBV in gliomas than metastases

CLINICAL PRESENTATION & WORK-UP

Presentation
- Variable
  - Headaches: Most common
    - Early morning headaches classic
  - Focal neurologic deficits: 20-40%
  - Cognitive dysfunction: 30-35%
  - Seizures/strokes: 5-20%

Prognosis
- By classification
  - RPA class
    - I: 7.1 months median survival (MS)
    - II: 4.2 months MS
    - III: 2.3 months MS
  - GPA classification
    - 0-1: 2.6 months MS
    - 1.5-2.5: 3.8 months MS
    - 3.0: 6.9 months MS
    - 3.5-4: 11 months MS
    - GPA update allows for site-specific prognosis
- Varies with primary site histology
  - Long survival with good histologies
    - Breast: 11.9 months MS (6.1-18.7 months [GPA scores 0-4])
    - Renal cell: 9.6 months MS (3.3-14.8)
  - Poor histologies
    - GI malignancies: 5.4 months MS (3.1-13.5)
    - Small cell lung: 4.9 months MS (2.8-17.0)
- No treatment or steroids alone: Survival 1-3 months

Work-Up
- Clinical
  - H&P with neurologic exam
  - Stereotactic/open biopsy: Needed in specific cases
    - Diagnosis in doubt
    - Unknown primary on work-up
  - If no known primary
    - Chest x-ray or CT
    - CT abdomen/pelvis

- PET can be considered if > 1 lesion
- Systemic work-up as indicated

TREATMENT

Overview

- Historically WBRT standard tx
  - Surgery for severely symptomatic lesions
- Tx controversial with advent of SRS
  - Variation in prioritization of WBRT vs. SRS
  - Addition of WBRT to SRS being investigated in clinical trials

NCCN Accepted Options

- 1-3 lesions
  - Limited/stable systemic disease with good systemic treatment options
    - Resectable
      - Surgery + WBRT/SRS
      - SRS + WBRT
      - SRS
    - Unresectable
      - SRS + WBRT
      - SRS
  - Extensive systemic disease + poor treatment options
    - WBRT
- > 3 lesions
  - WBRT
  - SRS considered for select patients
- Surgery considered for symptom relief in all cases

Standard Doses

- WBRT
  - 20-40 Gy in 5-20 fx
    - 30 Gy in 10 fx: Common regimen
    - 37.5 Gy in 15 fx: Preferred if life expectancy > 6 months
      - Increased concern for neurocognitive dysfunction with fx size ≥ 3 Gy
    - 20 Gy in 5 fx for patients with limited life expectancy
- SRS
  - Lesion size
    - ≤ 2 cm: 24 Gy
    - 2-3 cm: 18 Gy
    - 3-4 cm: 15 Gy
    - Close proximity to optic structures
      - 25 Gy in 5 fx well tolerated
    - Brainstem lesions: Dose varies
      - 15 Gy well tolerated
      - Doses up to 19 Gy have been used and tolerated

Organs at Risk Parameters

- SRS
  - Optic nerves: ≤ 8-10 Gy
  - Optic chiasm: ≤ 8-10 Gy
  - Pituitary: Mean ≤ 15 Gy
  - Brainstem: ≤ 16 Gy
    - Small volumes to 20 Gy have been tolerated

Common Techniques

- WBRT
  - Typically opposed lateral fields with blocks inferior to base of skull
    - Superior/anterior/posterior: 2 cm margin from bony skull
      - Typically open field
    - Inferiorly: Inferior border is C1/C2 and 1-2 cm from base of skull
      - Adjust blocks to exclude bilateral lens as able
      - Margin for block should account for motion movement (frequently 3 mm with mask) and dose buildup (typically 7 mm)
      - In patients with leukemia requiring WBRT, coverage should include the posterior globe, a sanctuary site for leukemic cells
- SRS
  - LINAC based or gamma knife
    - Gamma knife: Multiple shots placed to cover tumor volume
      - Shot size selected for maximal conformality
      - Typically, dose prescribed to 50% isodose line
    - LINAC based: Can utilize dynamic conformal arcs, cone-based arc therapy, or IMRT
      - Improved conformality with micro-multileaf collimator advent, dynamic conformal arcs (DCAs) common implementation
      - Dose typically prescribed to 70-90% isodose line
      - Conformity index varies with prescription isodose level
      - Standardized approach: Prescribe to isodose line covering 95% of volume; ensure that 95% of this dose covers 99% of volume
    - Conformity index
      - (PIV/PVTV)/(PVTV/TV)
      - PIV = prescription isodose volume, TV = tumor volume, PVTV = tumor volume (TV) encompassed by prescription isodose
      - Ideally < 2.0
  - Contouring
    - Target: Gross tumor or resection cavity if postop
    - Use of additional margin is controversial
      - Autopsy series indicates that 1-2 mm margins should be used to cover tumor infiltration
      - Clinical series have not shown benefit but have shown increased toxicity
      - Generally, no margin used

Landmark Trials

- Patchell: Surgery prior to WBRT with single brain metastasis improved intracranial recurrence, neurologic death, median survival, and QOL
- Patchell: Addition of WBRT after surgical resection of single brain metastasis decreased intracranial recurrence and death secondary to neurologic causes
- RTOG 9508 (Andrews): Addition of radiosurgical boost after WBRT improved survival for patients with single brain met and improved or stabilized KPS
- RTOG 9005 (Shaw): Dose escalation of SRS for brain metastases; doses of 24, 18, and 15 Gy for lesions < 2, 2-3, and 3-4 cm, respectively

RECOMMENDED FOLLOW-UP

Routine

- Follow-up with MR w/wo contrast q. 3 months for 1 year, then as clinically indicated

CNS METASTASES

(**Left**) *Graphic depicting CNS metastases shows the discrete, round appearance with surrounding edema characteristic of metastases. The location at the GM-WM junction is typical.* (**Right**) *Shown is a 3D planning reconstruction of a 58-year-old woman with metastatic lung adenocarcinoma with multiple intracranial metastases. WBRT was recommended, and classic opposed lateral fields were used.*

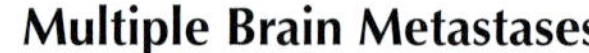

Multiple Brain Metastases

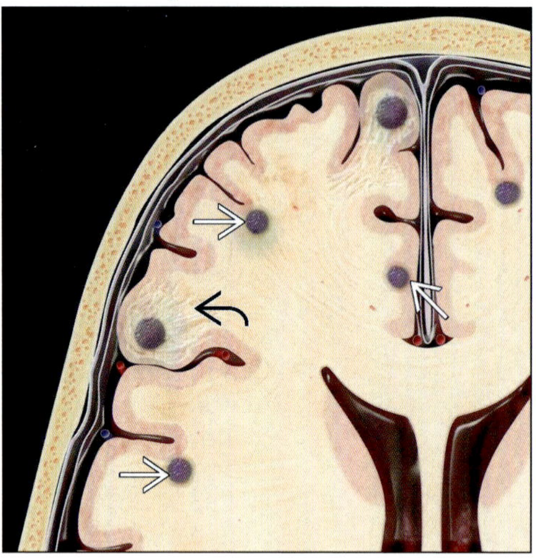

Multiple Brain Metastases

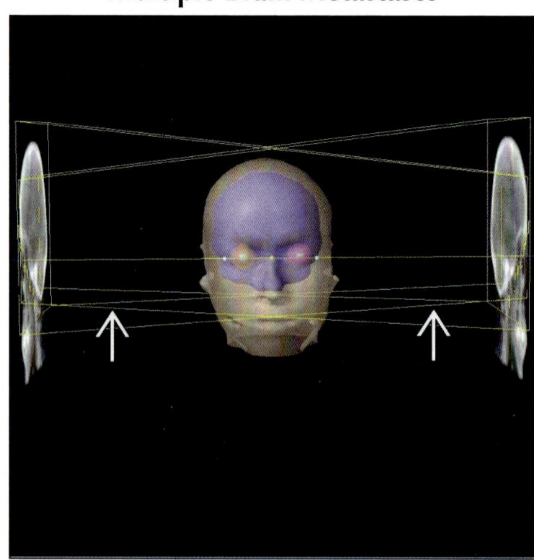

(**Left**) *Planning CT in the same patient shows the isocenter placement in the midline behind the lenses. Note the resulting absence of divergence anteriorly compared to posteriorly, which would otherwise result in dose to the opposite lens.* (**Right**) *DRR in the same patient shows MLC shaping. The inferior border was C1 or 1 cm from the contoured brain. Leaves were adjusted to block out the lenses, but note that care must be taken to include the cribriform plate.*

Multiple Brain Metastases

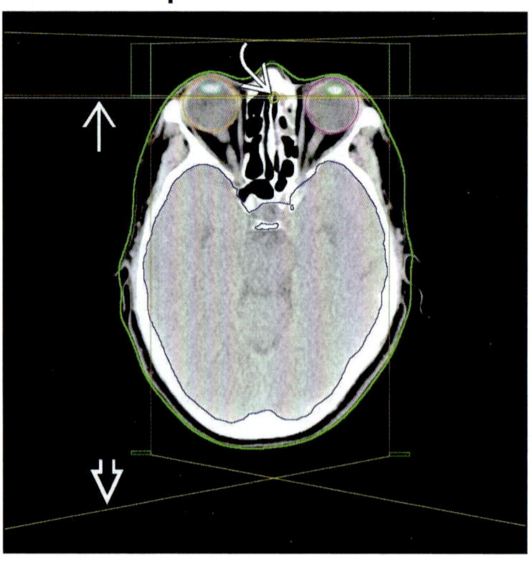

Multiple Brain Metastases

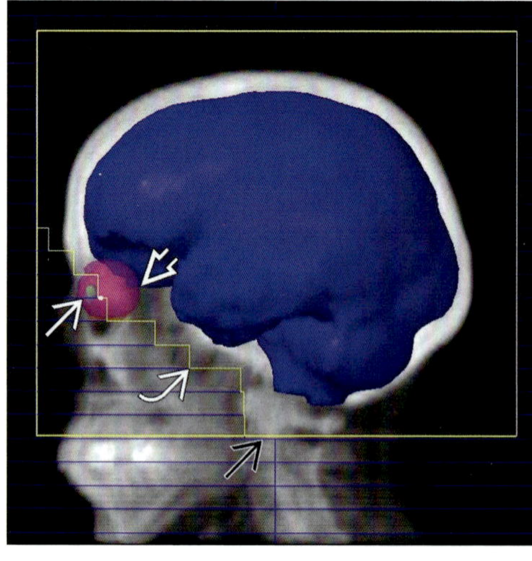

(**Left**) *Dose colorwash in the same patient shows the 95% dose coverage. Note the buildup distance required from the leaves to achieve full dose. The 7 mm buildup region (typical) and a 3 mm PTV results in the minimum required 1 cm MLC shaping distance.* (**Right**) *3D representation in the same patient shows typical midline vertex hotspot, as illustrated by the 105% dose colorwash. This can be minimized with the use of field-in-field blocking if desired.*

Multiple Brain Metastases

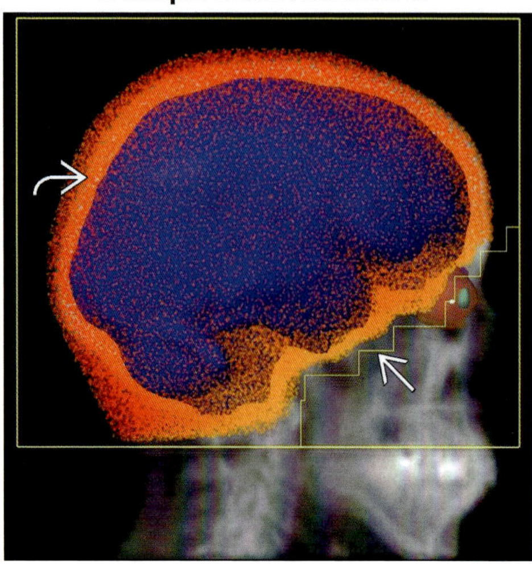

Multiple Brain Metastases

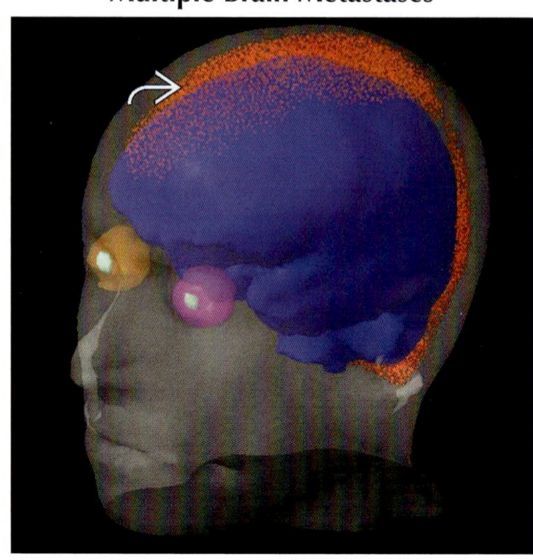

CNS Metastases, SRS of 2 Lesions

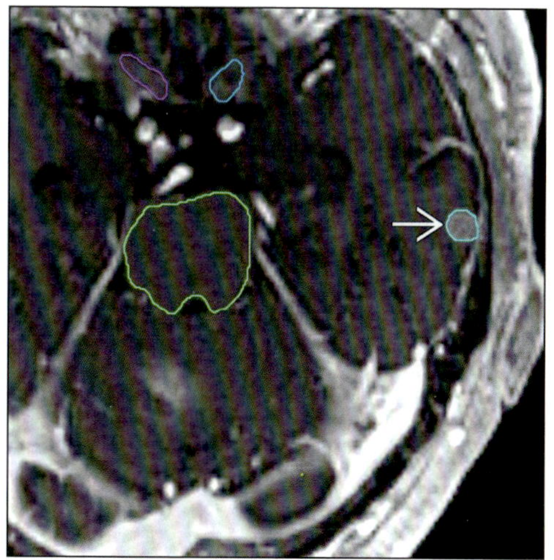

CNS Metastases, SRS of 2 Lesions

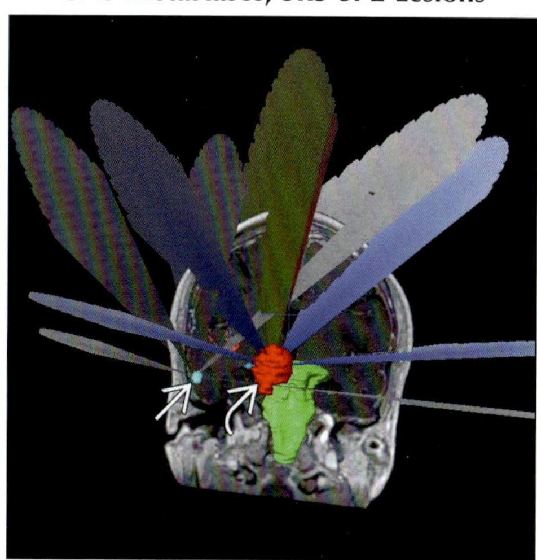

(Left) *Fused SPGR MR of a 54-year-old man shows metastatic esophageal adenocarcinoma with left temporal and left occipital metastases. Radiosurgery was recommended. The left temporal lesion is shown here outlined as the target ➡.* ***(Right)*** *LINAC-based SRS was used in the same patient to deliver 24 Gy to the temporal lesion (0.7 cm) ➡ and 18 Gy to the occipital lesion (2.7 cm) ➡, prescribed to the 86% and 66% isodose lines, respectively, with 5 DCAs used for each lesion.*

CNS Metastases, SRS of 2 Lesions

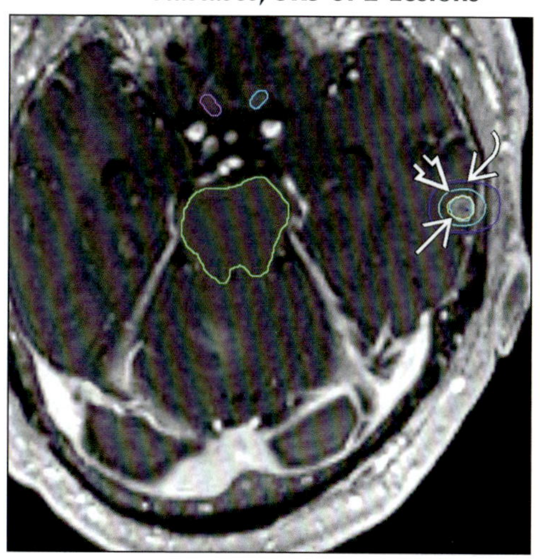

CNS Metastases, Postop SRS

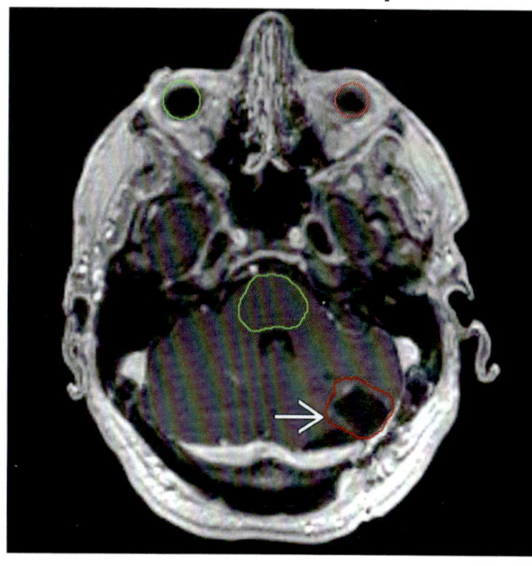

(Left) *The left temporal isodose lines are shown in the same patient. Note the rapid dose fall-off from the prescription isodose ➡ for the 50% ➡ and 30% ➡ isodose lines. The conformity index was 1.5 (ideally < 2).* ***(Right)*** *Fused SPGR MR in a 35-year-old man with metastatic thyroid carcinoma S/P resection of a solitary left cerebellar metastasis. 18 Gy was prescribed to the 85% isodose line. The resection bed (2.6 cm) ➡ is shown.*

CNS Metastases, Fractionated SRS

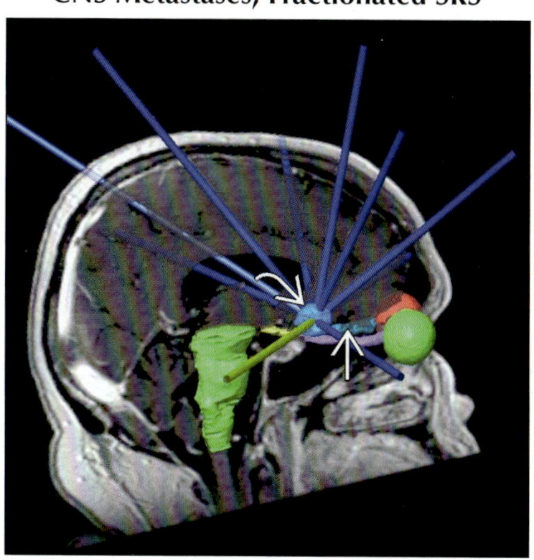

CNS Metastases, Brainstem Lesion

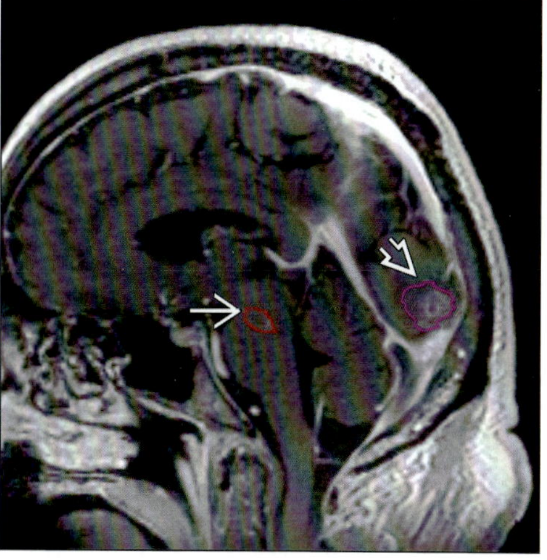

(Left) *Fused SPGR MR in a 43-year-old woman with metastatic melanoma shows a single lesion ➡ that can be seen superior to right optic nerve ➡. Due to proximity, 25 Gy/5 fx was prescribed using a 9-field IMRT plan.* ***(Right)*** *Fused SPGR MR in a 71-year-old man with metastatic melanoma shows brainstem and right occipital lesion. 15 Gy was delivered to brainstem (1.3 cm) ➡ and 24 Gy to occipital lesion (1.7 cm) ➡, prescribed to global 50% and 80% isodose lines, respectively.*

CNS TUMORS: RELATED REFERENCES

RELATED REFERENCES

1. Kano H et al: Stereotactic radiosurgery for arteriovenous malformations, part 6: multistaged volumetric management of large arteriovenous malformations. J Neurosurg. 116(1):54-65, 2012
2. Marchetti M et al: Multisession radiosurgery for optic nerve sheath meningiomas-an effective option: preliminary results of a single-center experience. Neurosurgery. 69(5):1116-22; discussion 1122-3, 2011
3. Linskey ME et al: The role of stereotactic radiosurgery in the management of patients with newly diagnosed brain metastases: a systematic review and evidence-based clinical practice guideline. J Neurooncol. 2010 Jan;96(1):45-68. Epub 2009 Dec 4. Review. Erratum in: J Neurooncol. 96(1):69-70, 2010
4. Schalin-Jäntti C et al: Outcome of fractionated stereotactic radiotherapy in patients with pituitary adenomas resistant to conventional treatments: a 5.25-year follow-up study. Clin Endocrinol (Oxf). 73(1):72-7, 2010
5. Sperduto PW et al: Diagnosis-specific prognostic factors, indexes, and treatment outcomes for patients with newly diagnosed brain metastases: a multi-institutional analysis of 4,259 patients. Int J Radiat Oncol Biol Phys. 77(3):655-61, 2010
6. Thiel E et al: High-dose methotrexate with or without whole brain radiotherapy for primary CNS lymphoma (G-PCNSL-SG-1): a phase 3, randomised, non-inferiority trial. Lancet Oncol. 11(11):1036-47, 2010
7. Hazard LJ et al: Conformity of LINAC-based stereotactic radiosurgery using dynamic conformal arcs and micro-multileaf collimator. Int J Radiat Oncol Biol Phys. 73(2):562-70, 2009
8. Kobayashi T: Long-term results of stereotactic gamma knife radiosurgery for pituitary adenomas. Specific strategies for different types of adenoma. Prog Neurol Surg. 22:77-95, 2009
9. Merchant TE et al: Conformal radiotherapy after surgery for paediatric ependymoma: a prospective study. Lancet Oncol. 10(3):258-66, 2009
10. Wen JC et al: Ocular complications following I-125 brachytherapy for choroidal melanoma. Eye (Lond). 23(6):1254-68, 2009
11. Brada M et al: Radiotherapy for pituitary adenomas. Endocrinol Metab Clin North Am. 37(1):263-75, xi, 2008
12. Eom KY et al: Upfront chemotherapy and involved-field radiotherapy results in more relapses than extended radiotherapy for intracranial germinomas: modification in radiotherapy volume might be needed. Int J Radiat Oncol Biol Phys. 71(3):667-71, 2008
13. Lunsford LD et al: Arteriovenous malformation radiosurgery: a twenty year perspective. Clin Neurosurg. 55:108-19, 2008
14. Nataf F et al: Radiosurgery with or without a 2-mm margin for 93 single brain metastases. Int J Radiat Oncol Biol Phys. 70(3):766-72, 2008
15. Chopra R et al: Long-term follow-up of acoustic schwannoma radiosurgery with marginal tumor doses of 12 to 13 Gy. Int J Radiat Oncol Biol Phys. 68(3):845-51, 2007
16. Koh ES et al: Fractionated stereotactic radiotherapy for acoustic neuroma: single-institution experience at The Princess Margaret Hospital. Cancer. 109(6):1203-10, 2007
17. Kollová A et al: Gamma Knife surgery for benign meningioma. J Neurosurg. 107(2):325-36, 2007
18. Kretschmar C et al: Pre-radiation chemotherapy with response-based radiation therapy in children with central nervous system germ cell tumors: a report from the Children's Oncology Group. Pediatr Blood Cancer. 48(3):285-91, 2007
19. Pollock BE: Radiosurgery for pituitary adenomas. Prog Neurol Surg. 20:164-71, 2007
20. van den Bergh AC et al: Immediate postoperative radiotherapy in residual nonfunctioning pituitary adenoma: beneficial effect on local control without additional negative impact on pituitary function and life expectancy. Int J Radiat Oncol Biol Phys. 67(3):863-9, 2007
21. Baumert BG et al: A pathology-based substrate for target definition in radiosurgery of brain metastases. Int J Radiat Oncol Biol Phys. 66(1):187-94, 2006
22. Bhatnagar AK et al: Stereotactic radiosurgery for four or more intracranial metastases. Int J Radiat Oncol Biol Phys. 64(3):898-903, 2006
23. Collaborative Ocular Melanoma Study Group: The COMS randomized trial of iodine 125 brachytherapy for choroidal melanoma: V. Twelve-year mortality rates and prognostic factors: COMS report No. 28. Arch Ophthalmol. 124(12):1684-93, 2006
24. Fuentes S et al: Brainstem metastases: management using gamma knife radiosurgery. Neurosurgery. 58(1):37-42; discussion 37-42, 2006
25. Gavrilovic IT et al: Long-term follow-up of high-dose methotrexate-based therapy with and without whole brain irradiation for newly diagnosed primary CNS lymphoma. J Clin Oncol. 24(28):4570-4, 2006
26. Jahraus CD et al: Optic pathway gliomas. Pediatr Blood Cancer. 46(5):586-96, 2006
27. Régis J et al: Prospective controlled trial of gamma knife surgery for essential trigeminal neuralgia. J Neurosurg. 104(6):913-24, 2006
28. Sharif S et al: Second primary tumors in neurofibromatosis 1 patients treated for optic glioma: substantial risks after radiotherapy. J Clin Oncol. 24(16):2570-5, 2006
29. Chan AW et al: Stereotactic radiotherapy for vestibular schwannomas: favorable outcome with minimal toxicity. Neurosurgery. 57(1):60-70; discussion 60-70, 2005
30. Combs SE et al: Fractionated stereotactic radiotherapy of optic pathway gliomas: tolerance and long-term outcome. Int J Radiat Oncol Biol Phys. 62(3):814-9, 2005
31. Grill J et al: Treatment of medulloblastoma with postoperative chemotherapy alone: an SFOP prospective trial in young children. Lancet Oncol. 6(8):573-80, 2005
32. Jensen AW et al: Radiation complications and tumor control after 125I plaque brachytherapy for ocular melanoma. Int J Radiat Oncol Biol Phys. 63(1):101-8, 2005
33. Ma L et al: Comparative analyses of linac and Gamma Knife radiosurgery for trigeminal neuralgia treatments. Phys Med Biol. 50(22):5217-27, 2005
34. Marcus KJ et al: Stereotactic radiotherapy for localized low-grade gliomas in children: final results of a prospective trial. Int J Radiat Oncol Biol Phys. 61(2):374-9, 2005
35. Maruyama K et al: The risk of hemorrhage after radiosurgery for cerebral arteriovenous malformations. N Engl J Med. 352(2):146-53, 2005
36. Richards GM et al: Linear accelerator radiosurgery for trigeminal neuralgia. Neurosurgery. 57(6):1193-200; discussion 1193-200, 2005
37. Rogers L et al: Is gross-total resection sufficient treatment for posterior fossa ependymomas? J Neurosurg. 102(4):629-36, 2005
38. Rogers SJ et al: Radiotherapy of localised intracranial germinoma: time to sever historical ties? Lancet Oncol. 6(7):509-19, 2005
39. Sheehan JP et al: Stereotactic radiosurgery for pituitary adenomas: an intermediate review of its safety, efficacy, and role in the neurosurgical treatment armamentarium. J Neurosurg. 102(4):678-91, 2005
40. Andrews DW et al: Whole brain radiation therapy with or without stereotactic radiosurgery boost for patients with one to three brain metastases: phase III results of the RTOG 9508 randomised trial. Lancet. 363(9422):1665-72, 2004
41. Merchant TE et al: Preliminary results from a phase II trial of conformal radiation therapy and evaluation of radiation-

related CNS effects for pediatric patients with localized ependymoma. J Clin Oncol. 22(15):3156-62, 2004
42. Prummel MF et al: A randomized controlled trial of orbital radiotherapy versus sham irradiation in patients with mild Graves' ophthalmopathy. J Clin Endocrinol Metab. 89(1):15-20, 2004
43. Taylor RE: Review of radiotherapy dose and volume for intracranial ependymoma. Pediatr Blood Cancer. 42(5):457-60, 2004
44. Wakelkamp IM et al: Orbital irradiation for Graves' ophthalmopathy: Is it safe? A long-term follow-up study. Ophthalmology. 111(8):1557-62, 2004
45. Choi JY et al: Radiological and hormonal responses of functioning pituitary adenomas after gamma knife radiosurgery. Yonsei Med J. 44(4):602-7, 2003
46. Goss BW et al: Linear accelerator radiosurgery using 90 gray for essential trigeminal neuralgia: results and dose volume histogram analysis. Neurosurgery. 53(4):823-8; discussion 828-30, 2003
47. Meijer OW et al: Single-fraction vs. fractionated linac-based stereotactic radiosurgery for vestibular schwannoma: a single-institution study. Int J Radiat Oncol Biol Phys. 56(5):1390-6, 2003
48. Nag S et al: The American Brachytherapy Society recommendations for brachytherapy of uveal melanomas. Int J Radiat Oncol Biol Phys. 56(2):544-55, 2003
49. Pollock BE et al: Stereotactic radiosurgery provides equivalent tumor control to Simpson Grade 1 resection for patients with small- to medium-size meningiomas. Int J Radiat Oncol Biol Phys. 55(4):1000-5, 2003
50. DeAngelis LM et al: Combination chemotherapy and radiotherapy for primary central nervous system lymphoma: Radiation Therapy Oncology Group Study 93-10. J Clin Oncol. 20(24):4643-8, 2002
51. Flickinger JC et al: An analysis of the dose-response for arteriovenous malformation radiosurgery and other factors affecting obliteration. Radiother Oncol. 63(3):347-54, 2002
52. Lee JY et al: Stereotactic radiosurgery providing long-term tumor control of cavernous sinus meningiomas. J Neurosurg. 97(1):65-72, 2002
53. Mehta VK et al: Image guided stereotactic radiosurgery for lesions in proximity to the anterior visual pathways: a preliminary report. Technol Cancer Res Treat. 1(3):173-80, 2002
54. Merchant TE et al: Craniopharyngioma: the St. Jude Children's Research Hospital experience 1984-2001. Int J Radiat Oncol Biol Phys. 53(3):533-42, 2002
55. Merchant TE et al: Preliminary results from a Phase II trail of conformal radiation therapy for pediatric patients with localised low-grade astrocytoma and ependymoma. Int J Radiat Oncol Biol Phys. 52(2):325-32, 2002
56. Flickinger JC et al: Does increased nerve length within the treatment volume improve trigeminal neuralgia radiosurgery? A prospective double-blind, randomized study. Int J Radiat Oncol Biol Phys. 51(2):449-54, 2001
57. Goyal LK et al: Local control and overall survival in atypical meningioma: a retrospective study. Int J Radiat Oncol Biol Phys. 46(1):57-61, 2000
58. Kahaly GJ et al: Low- versus high-dose radiotherapy for Graves' ophthalmopathy: a randomized, single blind trial. J Clin Endocrinol Metab. 85(1):102-8, 2000
59. Shaw E et al: Single dose radiosurgical treatment of recurrent previously irradiated primary brain tumors and brain metastases: final report of RTOG protocol 90-05. Int J Radiat Oncol Biol Phys. 47(2):291-8, 2000
60. Shields CL et al: Plaque radiotherapy for uveal melanoma: long-term visual outcome in 1106 consecutive patients. Arch Ophthalmol. 118(9):1219-28, 2000
61. Thomas PR et al: Low-stage medulloblastoma: final analysis of trial comparing standard-dose with reduced-dose neuraxis irradiation. J Clin Oncol. 18(16):3004-11, 2000
62. Bamberg M et al: Radiation therapy for intracranial germinoma: results of the German cooperative prospective trials MAKEI 83/86/89. J Clin Oncol. 17(8):2585-92, 1999
63. Duffner PK et al: The treatment of malignant brain tumors in infants and very young children: an update of the Pediatric Oncology Group experience. Neuro Oncol. 1(2):152-61, 1999
64. Kondziolka D et al: Long-term outcomes after meningioma radiosurgery: physician and patient perspectives. J Neurosurg. 91(1):44-50, 1999
65. Kondziolka D et al: Stereotactic radiosurgery plus whole brain radiotherapy versus radiotherapy alone for patients with multiple brain metastases. Int J Radiat Oncol Biol Phys. 45(2):427-34, 1999
66. Packer RJ et al: Treatment of children with medulloblastomas with reduced-dose craniospinal radiation therapy and adjuvant chemotherapy: A Children's Cancer Group Study. J Clin Oncol. 17(7):2127-36, 1999
67. Flickinger JC et al: Analysis of neurological sequelae from radiosurgery of arteriovenous malformations: how location affects outcome. Int J Radiat Oncol Biol Phys. 40(2):273-8, 1998
68. Hukin J et al: Treatment of intracranial ependymoma by surgery alone. Pediatr Neurosurg. 29(1):40-5, 1998
69. Patchell RA et al: Postoperative radiotherapy in the treatment of single metastases to the brain: a randomized trial. JAMA. 280(17):1485-9, 1998
70. Huh SJ et al: Radiotherapy of intracranial germinomas. Radiother Oncol. 38(1):19-23, 1996
71. Milosevic MF et al: Radiotherapy for atypical or malignant intracranial meningioma. Int J Radiat Oncol Biol Phys. 34(4):817-22, 1996
72. Bailey CC et al: Prospective randomised trial of chemotherapy given before radiotherapy in childhood medulloblastoma. International Society of Paediatric Oncology (SIOP) and the (German) Society of Paediatric Oncology (GPO): SIOP II. Med Pediatr Oncol. 25(3):166-78, 1995
73. Goldsmith BJ et al: Postoperative irradiation for subtotally resected meningiomas. A retrospective analysis of 140 patients treated from 1967 to 1990. J Neurosurg. 80(2):195-201, 1994
74. Hetelekidis S et al: 20-year experience in childhood craniopharyngioma. Int J Radiat Oncol Biol Phys. 27(2):189-95, 1993
75. Bouffet E et al: M4 protocol for cerebellar medulloblastoma: supratentorial radiotherapy may not be avoided. Int J Radiat Oncol Biol Phys. 24(1):79-85, 1992
76. Nelson DF et al: Non-Hodgkin's lymphoma of the brain: can high dose, large volume radiation therapy improve survival? Report on a prospective trial by the Radiation Therapy Oncology Group (RTOG): RTOG 8315. Int J Radiat Oncol Biol Phys. 23(1):9-17, 1992
77. Regine WF et al: Pediatric craniopharyngiomas: long term results of combined treatment with surgery and radiation. Int J Radiat Oncol Biol Phys. 24(4):611-7, 1992
78. Healey EA et al: The prognostic significance of postoperative residual tumor in ependymoma. Neurosurgery. 28(5):666-71; discussion 671-2, 1991
79. Patchell RA et al: A randomized trial of surgery in the treatment of single metastases to the brain. N Engl J Med. 322(8):494-500, 1990
80. Tait DM et al: Adjuvant chemotherapy for medulloblastoma: the first multi-centre control trial of the International Society of Paediatric Oncology (SIOP I). Eur J Cancer. 26(4):464-9, 1990
81. Spetzler RF et al: A proposed grading system for arteriovenous malformations. J Neurosurg. 65(4):476-83, 1986

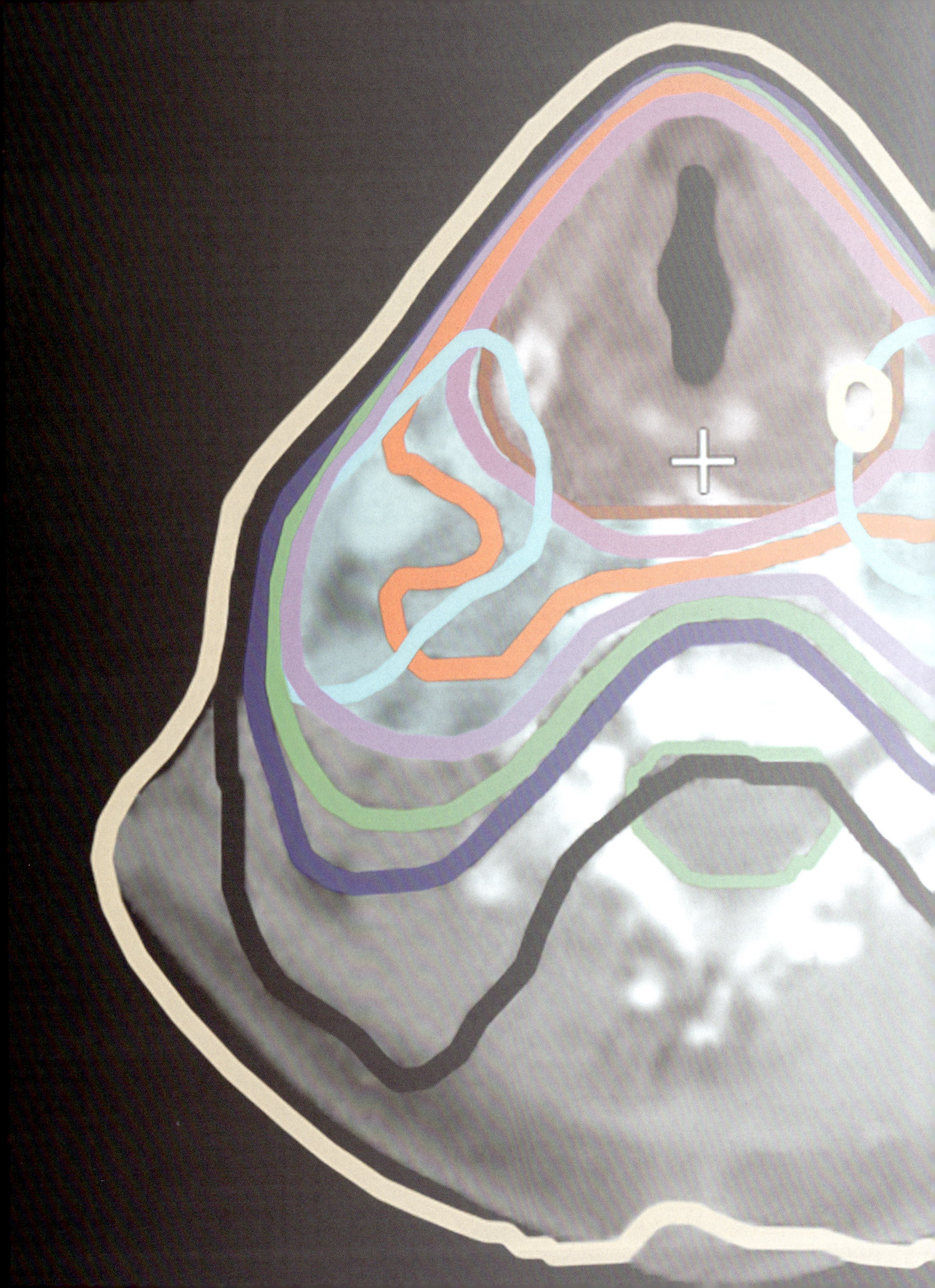

SECTION 2
Head and Neck

ORAL CAVITY

(T) Primary Tumor

Adapted from 7th edition AJCC Staging Forms.

TNM	*Definitions*
TX	Primary tumor cannot be assessed
T0	No evidence of primary tumor
Tis	Carcinoma in situ
T1	Tumor ≤ 2 cm in greatest dimension
T2	Tumor > 2 cm but ≤ 4 cm in greatest dimension
T3	Tumor > 4 cm in greatest dimension
T4a	Moderately advanced local disease*
Lip	Tumor invades through cortical bone, inferior alveolar nerve, floor of mouth, or skin of face, that is, chin or nose
Oral cavity	Tumor invades adjacent structures only (e.g., through cortical bone [mandible or maxilla] into deep [extrinsic] muscle of tongue [genioglossus, hyoglossus, palatoglossus, and styloglossus], maxillary sinus, skin of face)
T4b	Very advanced local disease: Tumor invades masticator space, pterygoid plates, or skull base &/or encases internal carotid artery

(N) Regional Lymph Nodes

NX	Regional lymph nodes cannot be assessed
N0	No regional lymph node metastasis
N1	Metastasis in a single ipsilateral lymph node, ≤ 3 cm in greatest dimension
N2	Metastasis in a single ipsilateral lymph node, > 3 cm but ≤ 6 cm in greatest dimension; or in multiple ipsilateral lymph nodes, none > 6 cm in greatest dimension; or in bilateral or contralateral lymph nodes, none > 6 cm in greatest dimension
N2a	Metastasis in single ipsilateral lymph node > 3 cm but ≤ 6 cm in greatest dimension
N2b	Metastasis in multiple ipsilateral lymph nodes, none > 6 cm in greatest dimension
N2c	Metastasis in bilateral or contralateral lymph nodes, none > 6 cm in greatest dimension
N3	Metastasis in a lymph node > 6 cm in greatest dimension

(M) Distant Metastasis

M0	No distant metastasis
M1	Distant metastasis

(G) Histologic Grade

GX	Grade cannot be assessed
G1	Well differentiated
G2	Moderately differentiated
G3	Poorly differentiated
G4	Undifferentiated

**Superficial erosion alone of bone/tooth socket by gingival primary is not sufficient to classify a tumor as T4.*

AJCC Stages/Prognostic Groups

Adapted from 7th edition AJCC Staging Forms.

Stage	*T*	*N*	*M*
0	Tis	N0	M0
I	T1	N0	M0
II	T2	N0	M0
III	T3	N0	M0
	T1	N1	M0
	T2	N1	M0
	T3	N1	M0
IVA	T4a	N0	M0
	T4a	N1	M0
	T1	N2	M0
	T2	N2	M0
	T3	N2	M0
	T4a	N2	M0
IVB	Any T	N3	M0
	T4b	Any N	M0
IVC	Any T	Any N	M1

Boundaries of the Neck Levels and Sub-Levels, Sites of Origin

Boundary Level	*Superior*	*Inferior*	*Anterior (Medial)*	*Posterior (Lateral)*	*Sites of Origin*
IA	Symphysis of mandible	Body of hyoid	Anterior belly of contralateral digastric muscle	Anterior belly of ipsilateral digastric muscle	Floor of mouth, anterior tongue, anterior mandible, lower lip
IB	Body of mandible	Posterior belly of digastric muscle	Anterior belly of digastric muscle	Stylohyoid muscle	Oral cavity, anterior nasal cavity, submandibular gland
IIA	Skull base	Horizontal plane defined by the inferior border of the hyoid bone	The stylohyoid muscle	Vertical plane defined by the spinal accessory nerve	Oral cavity, nasal cavity, nasopharynx, oropharynx, hypopharynx, parotid gland, larynx
IIB	Skull base	Horizontal plane defined by the inferior body of the hyoid bone	Vertical plane defined by the spinal accessory nerve	Lateral border of the SCM muscle	Oral cavity, nasal cavity, nasopharynx, oropharynx, hypopharynx, parotid gland, larynx
III	Horizontal plane defined by the inferior body of hyoid	Horizontal plane defined by the inferior border of the cricoid cartilage	Lateral border of the sternohyoid muscle	Lateral border of the SCM muscle or sensory branches of cervical plexus	Oral cavity, nasopharynx, oropharynx, hypopharynx, larynx
IV	Horizontal plane defined by the inferior border of the cricoid cartilage	Clavicle	Lateral border of the sternohyoid muscle	Lateral border of the SCM or sensory branches of cervical plexus	Hypopharynx, thyroid, esophagus, larynx
VA	Apex of the convergence of the SCM and trapezius muscles	Horizontal plane defined by the lower border of the cricoid cartilage	Posterior border of the SCM muscle or sensory branches of cervical plexus	Anterior border of the trapezius muscle	Nasopharynx, oropharynx, skin of posterior scalp and neck
VB	Horizontal plane defined by the lower border of the cricoid cartilage	Clavicle	Posterior border of the SCM muscle	Anterior border of the trapezius muscle	Nasopharynx, oropharynx, skin of posterior scalp and neck
VI	Hyoid bone	Suprasternal notch	Common carotid artery	Common carotid artery	Thyroid, larynx, apex of piriform sinus, esophagus
VII	Suprasternal notch	Innominate artery	Sternum	Trachea, esophagus, and prevertebral fascia	Thyroid, esophagus

Lymph Node Levels

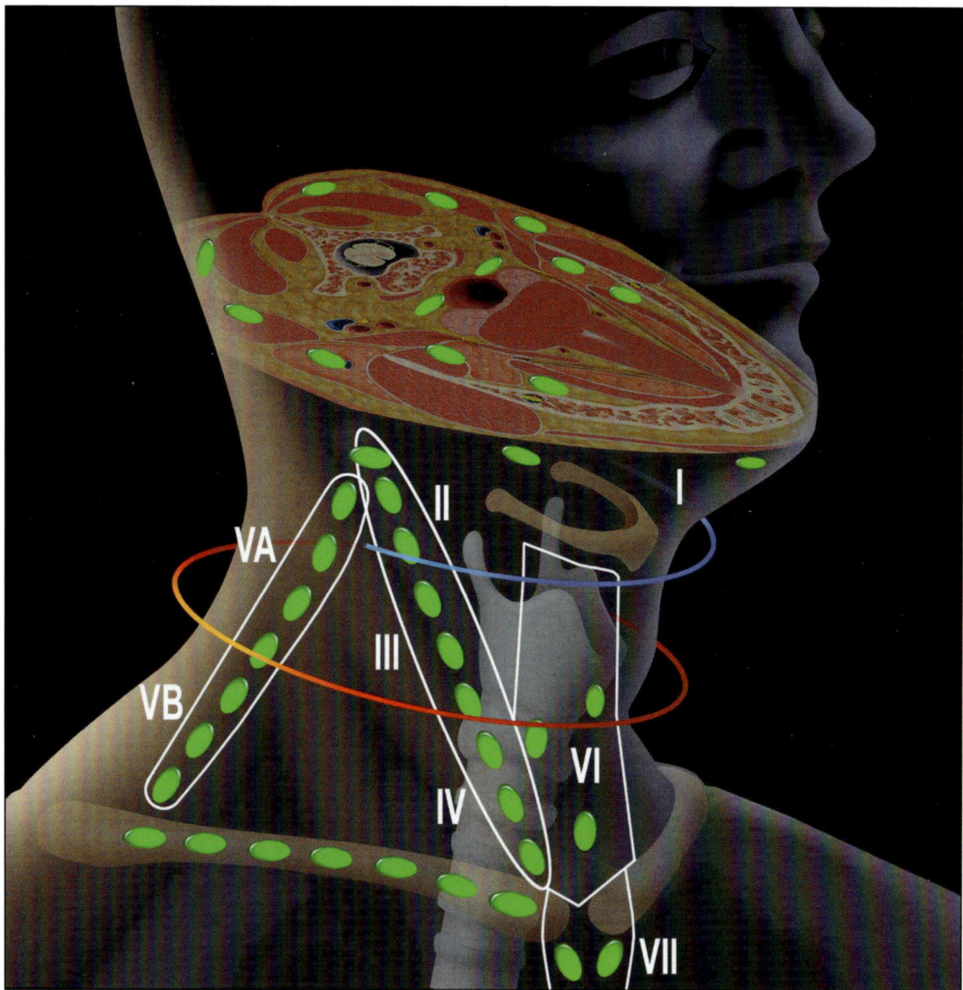

Schematic indicates the location of the lymph node levels in the neck. Lymph node levels II and III are separated by a horizontal plane defined by the inferior border of the hyoid bone. Lymph node levels III and IV are separated by a horizontal plane defined by the inferior border of the cricoid cartilage. Lymph node levels VA and VB are located posterior to the sternocleidomastoid muscle.

ORAL CAVITY

T1

Graphic illustrates T1 disease of the oral tongue and lip as tumor → that is ≤ 2 cm. Although the AJCC classification of oral cavity tumor includes all of the freely mobile portions of the tongue, the WHO considers the undersurface of the tongue to be a separate category.

T2

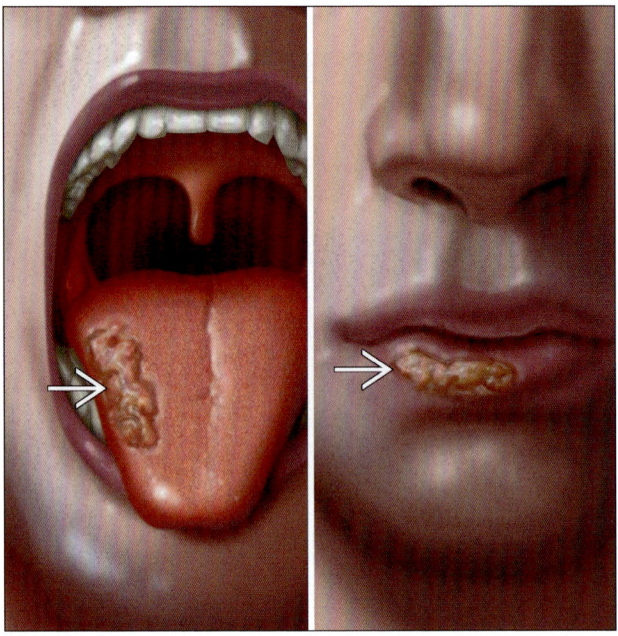

Graphic illustrates T2 disease of the oral tongue and lip as a tumor → that is > 2 cm but ≤ 4 cm in greatest dimension. Assessment of lip and oral cavity tumors is primarily performed by visual inspection and palpation; small lesions may not require imaging.

T3

Graphic illustrates T3 disease of the oral tongue and lip as tumor → that is > 4 cm in greatest dimension. Imaging is generally more helpful in patients with larger lesions for evaluating the thickness of the lesion and possible invasion of underlying structures.

T4a: Lip

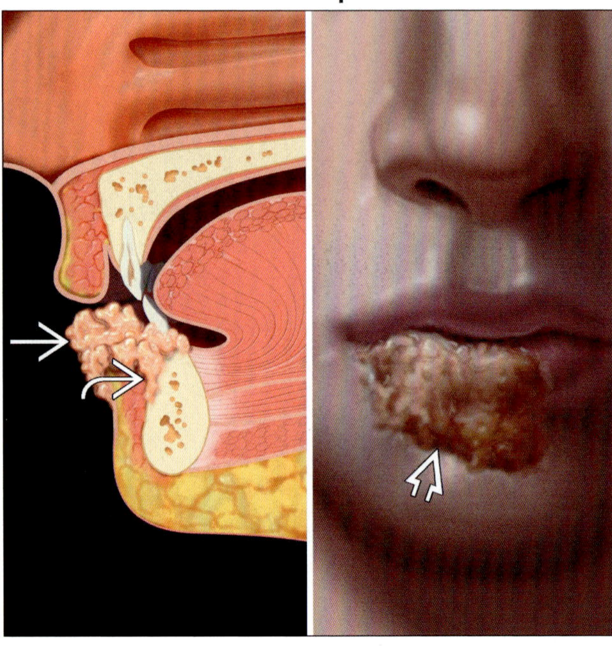

Sagittal graphic illustrates tumor → invading through the cortex of the mandible ↪. Frontal drawing shows tumor invading the skin ⇨ of the face. Both of these are sufficient to classify a carcinoma of the lip as T4a. Invasion into the floor of the mouth or inferior alveolar nerve also warrants such classification.

T4a: Oral Cavity

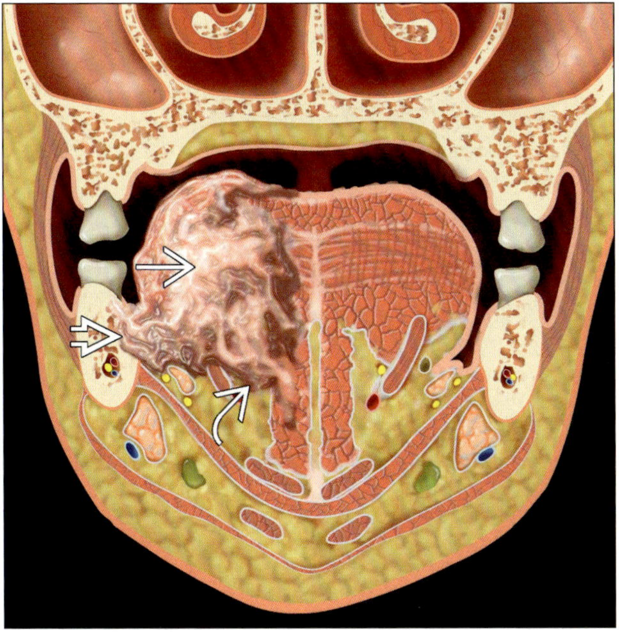

Axial graphic illustrates moderately advanced local disease, with an oral cavity tumor invading adjacent structures. Any oral cavity tumor invading through the cortical bone into the deep muscle of the tongue, the maxillary sinus, or the skin of the face is staged as T4a.

T4b

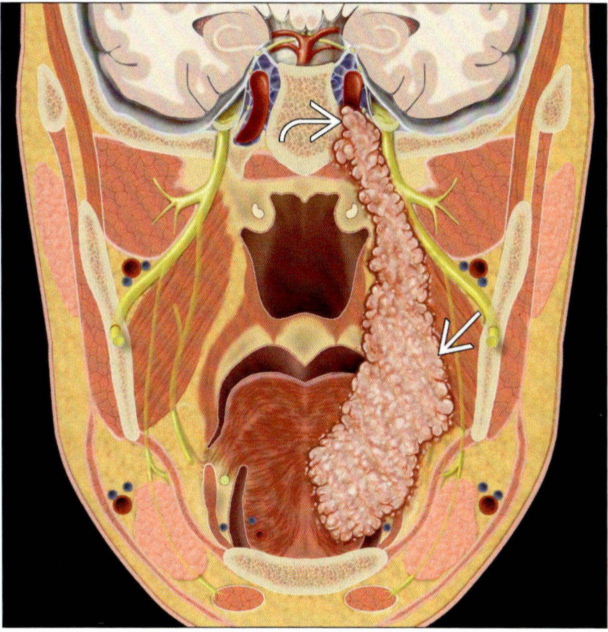

Coronal graphic illustrates very advanced local disease, with the tumor invading the masticator space, pterygoid plates, and skull base. T4b tumors may also encase the internal carotid artery.

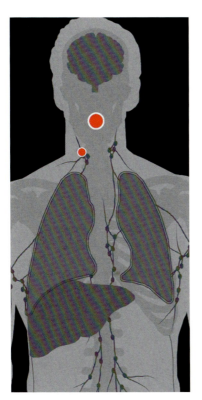

INITIAL SITE OF RECURRENCE

Local	23.2%
Neck Failure	10.5%

Distant metastases at diagnosis are extremely low. Metastasis depends on extent of TNM stage and extent of local regional recurrence. Lymph node involvement occurs in 5-10% of patients at initial diagnosis. Million RR et al: Management of Head and Neck Cancer, a multidisciplinary approach. Philadelphia, JB Lippincott. 208-234, 322, 1994; Decroix Y et al: Experience of Curie Institute in treatment of cancer of the mobile tongue, treatment policies and results. Cancer. 47; 47-500, 1981.

ORAL CAVITY

OVERVIEW

General Comments

- Squamous cell carcinoma (SCC) represents 90-95% of oral cavity malignancies
- Subsites of the oral cavity
  - Mucosal lip
  - Buccal mucosa
  - Floor of mouth
  - Lower and upper alveolar ridge
  - Retromolar trigone
  - Hard palate
  - Anterior 2/3 of tongue

Classification

- Histology
  - Premalignant erythroplakia or leukoplakia may precede carcinoma on mucosal surfaces
  - Malignant epithelial tumors
    - Squamous cell carcinomas
      - Verrucous cell carcinoma
      - Basaloid squamous cell carcinoma
      - Papillary squamous cell carcinoma
      - Spindle cell carcinoma
      - Acantholytic squamous cell carcinoma
      - Adenosquamous cell carcinoma
      - Carcinoma cuniculatum
    - Lymphoepithelial carcinoma
    - Most squamous cell carcinomas of oral cavity have mutations in *p53* gene
    - Minor salivary gland tumors
    - Adenoid cystic carcinomas
  - **Soft tissue tumors**
    - Kaposi sarcoma
    - Lymphangioma
    - Ectomesenchymal chondromyxoid tumor
    - Focal oral mucinosis
    - Congenital granular cell epulis
  - **Hematolymphoid tumors**
    - Diffuse large B-cell lymphoma
    - Mantle cell lymphoma
    - Follicular lymphoma
    - Extranodal marginal zone B-cell lymphoma of MALT type
    - Burkitt lymphoma
    - T-cell lymphoma
    - Extramedullary plasmacytoma
    - Langerhans cell histiocytosis
    - Extramedullary myeloid sarcoma (chloroma)
    - Follicular dendritic cell sarcoma/tumor
  - **Mucosal malignant melanoma**
  - Secondary tumor

NATURAL HISTORY

General Features

- Comments
  - Oral cavity cancers mostly develop from premalignant lesions resulting in both clinical and histological changes to mucosa

Etiology

- Risk factors
  - Tobacco smoking
  - Extensive alcohol use
  - Prolonged sun exposure (lip carcinoma)
  - Human papillomavirus (HPV) infection
  - Poor oral hygiene
  - Betel-containing substances
- Genetics
  - Oral cavity cancer shows relatively small effect of genetic and familial predisposition
  - Most squamous cell carcinomas of oral cavity have mutations in *p53* gene

Epidemiology & Cancer Incidence

- Number of cases in USA per year
  - 26,740 estimated new cases in USA in 2012
    - 9,380 estimated deaths in USA in 2012
    - More prevalent in parts of Asia (various forms of tobacco use and consumption of betel-containing substances)
    - Overall decrease in incidence from 1970s in USA
      - Largely attributed to decreases in smoking
- Sex predilection
  - Males > females
    - Incidence in females rising secondary to tobacco use and HPV
- Age of onset
  - Oral cavity carcinoma is more prevalent in elderly; mean age: 60 years

Associated Diseases, Abnormalities

- HPV infection
  - Approximately 70% of oral cavity SCC are HPV(+)
    - 44% are high-risk HPV(+)
      - High-risk HPV subtypes: 16, 18, 31, 33, 35, 39, 45, 51, 52, 53, 56, 58, 59, and 66
    - 26% are low-risk HPV(+)
      - Low-risk HPV subtypes: 6, 11, 40, 42, 43, 44, 54, 61, 72, 73, and 81
  - HPV(+) tumors ↑ overall survival (OS) than HPV(-) in oropharyngeal cancers; effect of HPV on oral cavity cancers is unknown

Routes of Spread

- Local spread
  - Direct extension
- Lymphatic extension
  - Cancer of lip
    - Low potential for metastases
    - Submental (level IA) and submandibular (level IB)
  - Cancer of alveolar ridge and hard palate
    - Low potential for metastases
    - Buccinator
    - Submandibular (level IB)
    - Jugular (level II-IV)
    - Retropharyngeal (less common)
      - Level IB and IIA
      - III and IV (rare)
  - Cancer of oral tongue
    - Submental (level IA) or submandibular (level IB) depending on primary tumor location
    - Level II
  - Primary site closer to midline increases risk of bilateral nodal spread
  - Risk factors for nodal metastases
    - Poorly differentiated histology

- Large lesions
- Tumor thickness (particularly in oral tongue)
- Invasion of muscle

- Metastatic sites
  - Lung/pleura: 60-80%
  - Bone: 20-25%
  - Liver: 10-13%
  - Dermis: 2-5%
  - Brain: 1-5%
  - Other: 1-5%

IMAGING

Detection

- Clinical examination is more accurate than imaging for mucosal lesions stages T1-T3
- Imaging important for deep extent and lymph nodes
- **Assessing imaging for malignant vs. benign tumors**
  - Benign
    - Well-defined morphology
    - Normal or displaced surrounding tissue
    - Bones are unaffected or regressively remodeled
    - Nerves are unaffected or only have focal lesion present
    - Calcification may or may not be present
  - Malignant
    - Poorly defined or ulcerated morphology
    - Invasion of surrounding tissue
    - Invasion or destruction of cortical bone
    - Perineural invasion present with either diffuse involvement or skip lesions
- **CECT soft tissues and neck**
  - Primary tumor
    - Poorly marginated oral mass
    - Invasion often follows muscle planes (lingual tumors)
    - Diagnostic coronal and sagittal reformatted images helpful
  - Large metastatic nodes show necrosis with rim enhancement; necrosis is heterogeneously enhancing
    - Metastatic lymph nodes appear round with loss of fatty hilum on CT
    - > 1.5 cm in jugulodigastric region and > 1 cm in other locations
  - Extracapsular nodal spread is more common in larger nodes but possible in smaller nodes as well
  - Larger lymph nodes may become cystic; wall of node may be thin
  - Valuable in evaluating cortical bone invasion
- **MR**
  - Advantages
    - Multiplanar capabilities, better soft tissue contrast
    - Dental amalgam artifact less severe than CT
    - Evaluation of perineural invasion
    - Evaluation of retropharyngeal lymph nodes, hard palate tumor, and tumor's skull base extension
  - Disadvantages
    - Nondiagnostic if bulky tumors cause pooling of secretion and constant swallowing
    - Long acquisition time requiring patient compliance (at least 30 minutes)
- **PET/CT**
  - Helpful to find primary lesion and diagnosis in cases of unknown primary
    - Perform before directed biopsies
    - Submucosal tumors may be located via PET/CT when searching for unknown primaries
    - Excellent for detecting unsuspected tumor foci in distant or nonenlarged nodes
    - Limitation: FDG activity may be underestimated in nodes < 1 cm; PET/CT cannot detect micrometastatic disease
    - Cystic lymph node metastases may have less FDG uptake or more peripheral uptake of FDG
  - Several normal structures in neck may take up FDG physiologically
    - Muscle, brown fat, lymphoid tissues, mucosa
    - Infection and surgical sites may also take up FDG

Staging

- General nodal spread
  - 1st-order nodal spread from most oral cavity cancers is submandibular nodes (level IB), then to jugulodigastric nodes (level IIA), to top of internal jugular chain
  - May spread directly to level III or IV
  - Extracapsular extension is more common in larger nodes but possible in smaller nodes
    - Associated with poorer prognosis and higher rate of regional recurrence
- Radiographic characteristics of nodal disease
  - Size criteria: > 1.5 cm in jugulodigastric region or > 1 cm in other locations
  - Lymph node rim enhancement
  - Nodal central necrosis
  - Heterogeneous enhancement
  - Loss of nodal fat plane
  - May have focal metastases or necrosis in "normal-sized" nodes

CLINICAL PRESENTATION & WORK-UP

Presentation

- General symptoms may include
  - Nonhealing ulcers of oral cavity
  - Dysphagia
  - Odynophagia
  - Bleeding
  - Weight loss
  - Referral otalgia
- Lip cancer
  - Exophytic or ulcerative mass
  - Bleeding or pain
  - Chin numbness resulting from mental nerve involvement
- Oral tongue cancer
  - Exophytic or infiltrative growth pattern
  - Possible history of leukoplakia

Prognosis

- Observed 5-year survival by stage for SCC of lip
  - **Stage I**: 89.6%
  - **Stage II**: 83.5%
  - **Stage III**: 54.6%

- Stage IV: 47.2%
- Observed 5-year survival by stage for SCC of oral cavity
  - **Stage I**: 71.5%
  - **Stage II**: 57.9%
  - **Stage III**: 44.5%
  - **Stage IV**: 31.9%

Work-Up

- Clinical
  - History and physical with complete head and neck exam
    - Fiberoptic examination
    - Biopsy
    - Examination under anesthesia with endoscopy, if indicated
    - Dental evaluation prior to radiotherapy; dental repairs made before radiotherapy
    - Nutrition, speech, and swallowing evaluation
    - Hearing evaluation if concurrent cisplatin is planned
- Radiographic
  - CT with contrast of neck/soft tissue
  - MR with gadolinium for lesions involving oral tongue, base of tongue, or base of skull
  - Consider PET/CT for local regional advanced disease
- Laboratory
  - CBC, metabolic panel, B-hCG in females of childbearing age

TREATMENT

Major Treatment Alternatives

- Surgery is primary treatment for most oral cavity cancers
- Radiotherapy (RT) ± chemo for early-stage primary tumor
- Adjuvant RT ± chemo
- Definitive RT ± chemo for very advanced or unresectable disease
- **Surgery**
  - Depends on medical and technical operability
    - Types of resection
      - Lip: Mohs microscopic surgery for superficial lip skin lesion, V or W excision with primary closure or reconstruction
      - Oral tongue: Partial or total glossectomy with or without free-flap reconstruction
      - Carcinomas involving bone: Marginal or segmental mandibulectomy with reconstruction, maxillectomy with prosthetic reconstruction
      - ± selective or modified neck dissection
  - Resectable disease if primary tumor extends to
    - Mandible
    - Maxillary sinus
    - Floor of mouth
    - Skin
  - Unresectable disease if it has involved
    - Masticator space
    - Pterygoid plates
    - Skull base
    - Encasement of internal carotid artery
- **Chemotherapy**
  - Cisplatin
    - Adverse side effects: Nausea, nephrotoxicity, neurotoxicity, hearing impairment
  - Carboplatin
    - More myelosuppressive than cisplatin but less neurotoxicity, nephrotoxicity, nausea, and vomiting
    - Option for patients with renal disease, poorer performance status, or difficulty tolerating fluid volume associated with bolus cisplatin
  - Cetuximab
    - Monoclonal antibody inhibits EGFR receptor activity
    - Most common side effect: Acne-like skin rash
- **Radiotherapy** and general guidelines
  - **External beam radiotherapy (EBRT)**
    - Alone or with concomitant chemotherapy dependent on stage or pathologic risk features
    - 3D conformal radiotherapy
      - Can mix photons/electrons
    - **IMRT (intensity-modulated radiation therapy)**
      - Inversely planned with respect to organ dose constraints
  - **Interstitial brachytherapy**
    - Considered in selected cases
    - High dose rate (HDR) brachytherapy
      - Consider HDR boost 21 Gy at 3 Gy/fraction if combined with 40-50 Gy EBRT; or 45-60 Gy at 3-6 Gy/fraction if HDR as sole therapy
    - Low dose rate (LDR) brachytherapy
      - Consider LDR boost 20-35 Gy if combined with 50 Gy EBRT, or 60-70 Gy over several days if LDR as sole therapy
  - Indications for postoperative RT
    - T4 or selected T3
    - Close surgical margins
    - Multiple N(+) nodes
    - PNI
    - LVSI
    - Level IV or V N(+)
  - Indications for postop-chemoradiation therapy (CRT)
    - Microscopic positive margin
    - ECE(+)
- **3D conformal RT dosage**
  - Postoperative radiotherapy
    - Primary tumor and positive nodal sites: 50 Gy
      - Additional 10-16 Gy boost to high-risk sites: Close or positive surgical margins, ECE(+), PNI, LVSI(+), positive node(s)
  - Uninvolved, elective neck: 44-54 Gy
  - Primary radiotherapy
    - Conventional RT 50-54 Gy followed by 16-20 Gy boost to gross tumor volume 70 Gy total or concomitant boost RT to total dose of 72 Gy
- IMRT dosage
  - Postoperative RT
    - PTV1 (high-risk sites): 60-66 Gy at 2.0 Gy per fraction
      - Reconstructed preoperative primary tumor and high-risk nodal sites plus 1.0-1.5 cm margins
    - PTV2 (intermediate-risk sites): 56-60 Gy at 1.7-1.8 Gy per fraction
      - Surgical bed &/or areas having risk of harboring microscopic tumor cells

- PTV3 (elective nodal sites): 52-56 Gy at 1.6-1.7 Gy per fraction
  - Elective nodal sites, such as uninvolved contralateral neck &/or bilateral lower neck and supraclavicular fossa

- **Radiation dose constraints on critical structures**
  - Brachial plexus: 66 Gy max dose
  - Brainstem: 54 Gy max dose
  - Cervical esophagus: 30 Gy mean dose
  - Glottic larynx: 20 Gy mean dose, or max dose 45 Gy
  - Lips: < 20 Gy mean dose
  - Mandible/TM joint: 66 Gy max dose
  - Oral cavity (non-involved): 30 Gy mean dose, 60 Gy max dose
  - Parotid glands: < 26 Gy mean for 1 gland, < 20 Gy for 20 mL combined
  - Posterior wall of pharynx: 45 Gy mean dose, 33% to < 50 Gy, 15% to < 60 Gy
  - Spinal cord: ≤ 45 Gy or 48 Gy point dose (≤ 0.03 mL)
  - Submandibular gland: < 39 Gy mean dose
- **Most common side effects of radiotherapy**
  - Related to target location
    - **Acute side effects**
      - Skin erythema, dry or moist desquamation
      - Mucositis (worse with concurrent chemotherapy)
      - Xerostomia
      - Dysgeusia
      - Esophagitis
      - Dehydration
      - Malnutrition
    - **Intermediate term risks**
      - Spinal cord: Lhermitte syndrome
      - Lungs: Radiation pneumonitis
    - **Late effects**
      - Skin hyperpigmentation, fibrosis, telangiectasias
      - Soft tissue fibrosis, or soft tissue necrosis
      - Hypothyroidism
      - Speech and swallowing deficits
      - Cervical esophageal stricture
      - Trismus
      - Osteoradionecrosis

Treatment Options by Stage

- **Lip**
  - Early stage
    - May be cured equally well with surgery or local RT
      - Surgical resection with satisfactory cosmetic outcome for tumor < 2 cm that do not involve the commissure
      - V- or W-shaped excision with primary closure if lesion < 1.5 cm
    - Consider RT alone by EBRT or interstitial brachytherapy
  - Local regional advanced
    - Primary tumor resection with reconstruction if surgical removal causes poorly cosmetic defect or functional impairment
    - Selective neck dissection for clinical N0 or modified radical neck dissection for N(+)
  - Postoperative RT for pathological features of close margins, PNI, positive nodes, or consider CRT for microscopic positive margins or ECE(+)
  - EBRT dose: 60-66 Gy
- **Buccal mucosa**
  - T1-2 N0-1, primary surgery or definitive RT or chemoradiation; RT fields cover primary tumor and ipsilateral neck
  - T3-4 N0-3, surgical resection is preferred, adjuvant RT or CRT dependent on postoperative pathologic features
  - Postoperative RT for pathological features
    - Adjuvant RT: Close margins, PNI, positive nodes, T4 or selected T3
    - Adjuvant CRT for microscopic positive margins &/ or ECE(+)
    - EBRT dose: 60-66 Gy
- **Floor of mouth**
  - Surgical resection is preferred for early and locally advanced disease
  - Selected neck dissection for clinical N0; modified or comprehensive neck dissection for N(+) neck
  - Postoperative RT or CRT dependent on postoperative pathologic features
    - Adjuvant RT: T4 or selected T3, close margins, PNI, positive nodes
    - Adjuvant CRT for microscopic positive margins &/ or ECE(+)
    - EBRT dose: 60-66 Gy
- **Retromolar trigone**
  - Surgical resection is preferred
  - Postoperative RT or CRT dependent on postoperative pathologic features
    - Adjuvant RT: Close margins, PNI, positive nodes, selected T3, T4 disease, particularly when tumor involves pterygoid muscles, pterygoid plates, parapharyngeal space, or retropharyngeal nodes
    - Adjuvant CRT for microscopic positive margins &/ or ECE(+)
- **Oral tongue**
  - T1-2 N0, primary surgery with selected neck dissection
    - Consider selected neck dissection depending on primary tumor size and depth
  - T3-4 or N1-3, glossectomy with free flap reconstructed, neck dissection
  - Postoperative RT or CRT dependent on postoperative pathologic features
    - Adjuvant RT: T3 or T4, close margins, PNI, positive nodes
    - Adjuvant CRT for microscopic positive margins &/ or ECE(+)
    - EBRT dose: 60-66 Gy or consider interstitial brachytherapy as sole therapy or as a boost combination with EBRT

Dose Response

- 50 Gy controls subclinical disease > 97% of the time
- 50 Gy controls a 2 cm tumor 50% of the time
- 65 Gy controls a 2 cm 90% of the time
- Postoperatively, subclinical disease needs slightly higher doses
  - Surgical interruption of normal vasculature and tumor bed scarring can cause hypoxia
  - Density of infiltration of tissues by tumor cells potentially greater in postoperative setting

Landmark Trials

- **Mishra**: Postop RT in carcinoma of buccal mucosa

- Randomized stage III and IV SCC of buccal mucosa to surgery alone vs. surgery then postoperative RT (PORT)
- Disease-free survival (DFS) for surgery alone: 38%; PORT: 68%
- Disease-free survival improved with PORT

- **Fu (RTOG 90-03):** Accelerated hyperfractionation vs. standard fractionation radiotherapy
  - Randomized, 4 arms; stages III-IV (oral cavity, oropharynx, or supraglottic larynx) or stages II-IV (base of tongue, hypopharynx)
    - Arm 1: Standard fractionation 70 Gy in 35 fractions (2 Gy/fraction)
      - 2-year LRC 46%
    - Arm 2: Hyperfractionated 81.6 Gy in 68 fractions (1.2 Gy b.i.d.)
      - 2-year LRC 54% (SS), increased acute effects but no increase in late effects
    - Arm 3: Split course accelerated fractionation 67.2 in 42 fractions (1.6 Gy b.i.d.) with 2-week break after 38.4 Gy
      - 2-year LRC 47%
    - Arm 4: Concomitant boost 72 Gy given as 54 Gy in 30 fractions (1.8 Gy/fraction) + 18 Gy/12 fractions (1.5 Gy concurrent b.i.d. boost)
      - 2-year LRC 54% (SS), increased acute effects but no increase in late effects
  - Conclusion: Hyperfractionated or concomitant boost RT improves LRC compared to standard fractionation, no impact on DFS and OS
- **Bernier (EORTC 22931):** Postop RT ± chemo for locally advanced head and neck cancer
- Randomized; locally advanced oral cavity, oropharynx, hypopharynx, or larynx
  - T3-4 any N with negative margins; T1-2 N2-3; T1-2 N0-1 with high-risk features (ECE, SM[+], PNI, LVI); or oral cavity/oropharynx with LN(+) at levels IV or V
  - Arm 1: RT alone to 54 Gy/27 fractions + boost to 66 Gy to high-risk areas
    - 5-year PFS: 36%, OS: 40%, LRC: 69%
  - Arm 2: Same RT + concurrent cisplatin 100 mg/m2 every 21 days
    - 5-year PFS: 47% (SS), OS: 53% (SS), LRC: 82% (SS)
  - High-risk groups: 56% with 2+ LN, 26% with positive margins, 53% with extracapsular extension
  - No difference in distant metastasis rate or toxicity
  - Conclusion: Postop CRT is more effective in locally advanced H&N, with no difference in complication rate

RECOMMENDED FOLLOW-UP

Clinical

- History and physical
  - Every 1-3 months for year 1
  - Every 2-4 months for year 2
  - Every 6 months for years 3-5
  - Annually after year 5
  - If recurrence is suspected, rebiopsy; if negative, follow-up monthly until resolution

Radiographic

- Head and neck post-treatment baseline imaging is recommended within 3-6 months from end of therapy
- Chest CT as clinically indicated or chest x-ray annually

Laboratory

- TSH every 6-12 months if neck is irradiated

Others

- Speech, hearing, and swallowing evaluation if clinically indicated
- Smoking cessation and alcohol counseling if clinically indicated
- Dental evaluation

SELECTED REFERENCES

1. Duray A et al: Human papillomavirus DNA strongly correlates with a poorer prognosis in oral cavity carcinoma. Laryngoscope. 122(7):1558-65, 2012
2. Ang KK et al: Human papillomavirus and survival of patients with oropharyngeal cancer. N Engl J Med. 363(1):24-35, 2010
3. Bonner JA et al: Radiotherapy plus cetuximab for locoregionally advanced head and neck cancer: 5-year survival data from a phase 3 randomised trial, and relation between cetuximab-induced rash and survival. Lancet Oncol. 2010 Jan;11(1):21-8. Epub 2009 Nov 10. Erratum in: Lancet Oncol. 11(1):14, 2010
4. Gross ND et al: Nomogram for deciding adjuvant treatment after surgery for oral cavity squamous cell carcinoma. Head Neck. 30(10):1352-60, 2008
5. Mendenhall WM et al: Retromolar trigone squamous cell carcinoma treated with radiotherapy alone or combined with surgery. Cancer. 103(11):2320-5, 2005
6. Umeda M et al: A comparison of brachytherapy and surgery for the treatment of stage I-II squamous cell carcinoma of the tongue. Int J Oral Maxillofac Surg. 34(7):739-44, 2005
7. Bernier J et al: Postoperative irradiation with or without concomitant chemotherapy for locally advanced head and neck cancer. N Engl J Med. 350(19):1945-52, 2004
8. Cooper JS et al: Postoperative concurrent radiotherapy and chemotherapy for high-risk squamous-cell carcinoma of the head and neck. N Engl J Med. 350(19):1937-44, 2004
9. Fu KK et al: A Radiation Therapy Oncology Group (RTOG) phase III randomized study to compare hyperfractionation and two variants of accelerated fractionation to standard fractionation radiotherapy for head and neck squamous cell carcinomas: first report of RTOG 9003. Int J Radiat Oncol Biol Phys. 48(1):7-16, 2000
10. Mishra RC et al: Post-operative radiotherapy in carcinoma of buccal mucosa, a prospective randomized trial. Eur J Surg Oncol. 22(5):502-4, 1996
11. Rodgers LW Jr et al: Management of squamous cell carcinoma of the floor of mouth. Head Neck. 15(1):16-9, 1993
12. Tupchong L et al: Randomized study of preoperative versus postoperative radiation therapy in advanced head and neck carcinoma: long-term follow-up of RTOG study 73-03. Int J Radiat Oncol Biol Phys. 20(1):21-8, 1991
13. Fletcher GH: Irradiation of subclinical disease in the draining lymphatics. Int J Radiat Oncol Biol Phys. 10(6):939-42, 1984
14. Fletcher GH. Textbook of Radiotherapy. 3rd ed. Philadelphia: Lea & Febiger. 180-219, 1980

Epithelial Dysplasia

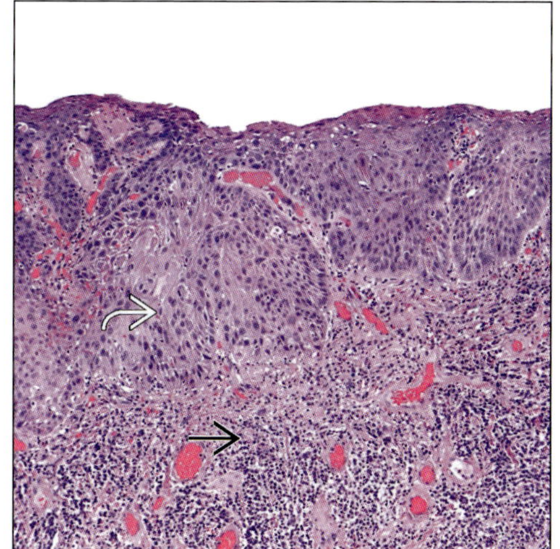

SCC in Setting of Dysplasia

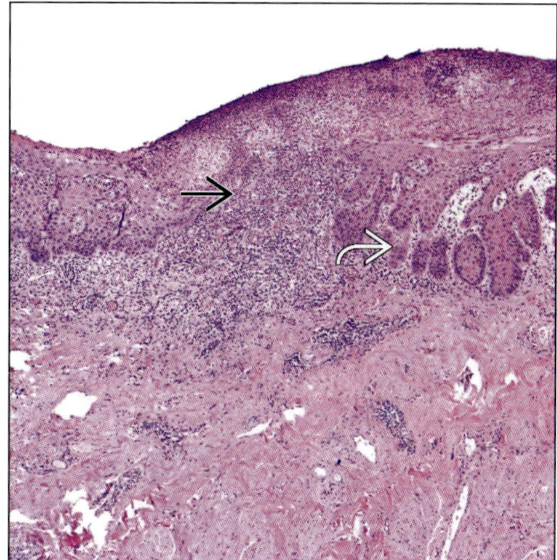

*(**Left**) On hematoxylin and eosin staining, inflamed submucosa is seen beneath development of epithelial dysplasia. (Courtesy G. Ellis, DDS.) (**Right**) This image shows epithelial dysplasia with squamous cell carcinoma, illustrating transformation. (Courtesy G. Ellis, DDS.)*

SCC

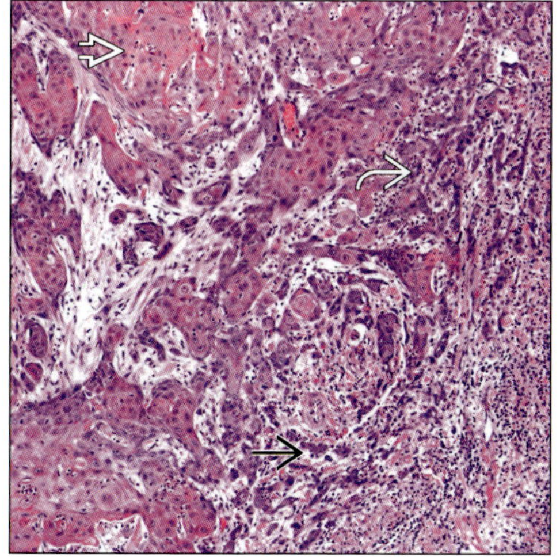

Verrucous Carcinoma

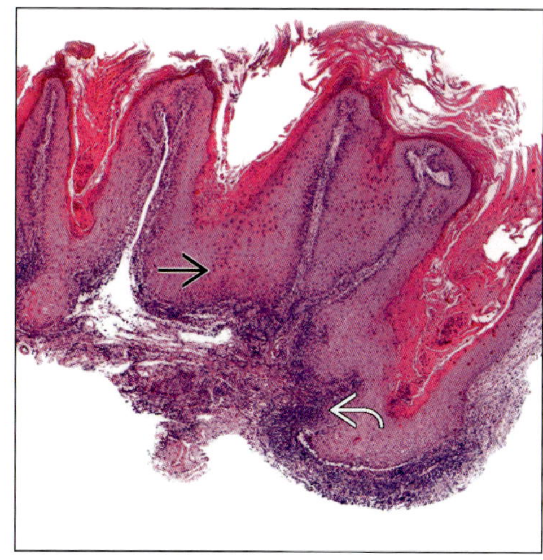

*(**Left**) The same patient developed overt SCC in the oral mucosa, exhibiting pleomorphic cell types of various sizes, infiltrating fingers of cells with islands of tumor, and inflammatory infiltrate. (Courtesy G. Ellis, DDS.) (**Right**) This specimen of verrucous carcinoma on the oral tongue is characterized by thickening of keratinocytes (acanthosis) and a "pushing border" with a thick band of chronic inflammation without infiltration. (Courtesy G. Ellis, DDS.)*

SCC of the Alveolar Ridge

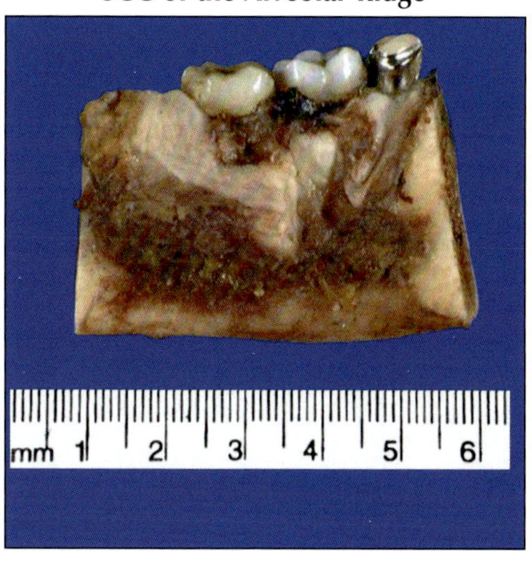

SCC of the Oral Tongue

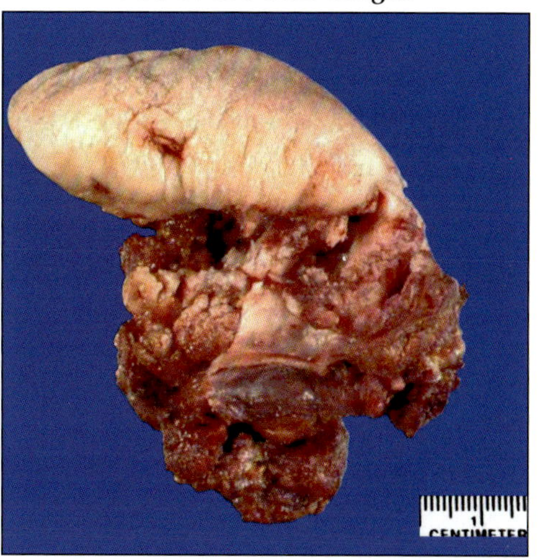

*(**Left**) This photograph shows the gross appearance of a squamous cell carcinoma of the alveolar ridge. (**Right**) This photograph shows a resected advanced squamous cell carcinoma involving the oral tongue and the floor of the mouth.*

Stage II (T2 N0 M0) Oral Tongue, 3D RT

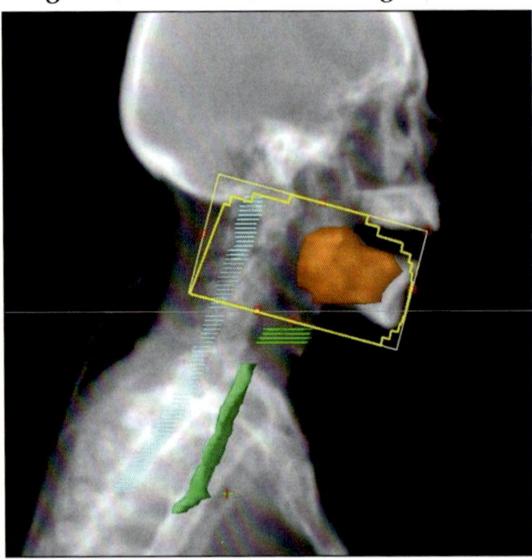

Stage II (T2 N0 M0) Oral Tongue, 3D RT

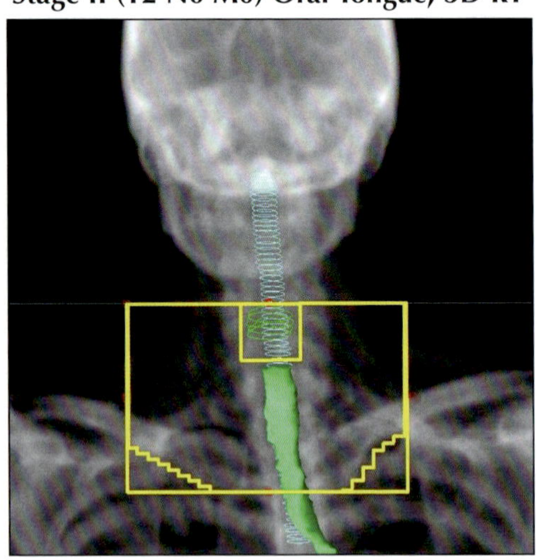

*(**Left**) DRR shows initial lateral field. Postoperative RT was indicated due to PNI and close margins after partial glossectomy. Initial treatment fields were taken to 42 Gy, off-cord laterals to 54 Gy, and then final boost to 60 Gy, all in 2 Gy fractions. (**Right**) DRR shows an AP field for elective lower neck irradiation to 50 Gy in 2 Gy fractions. Note the laryngeal and spinal cord block. Spinal cord is in blue, esophagus and larynx in light green.*

Stage II (T2 N0 M0) Oral Tongue, 3D RT

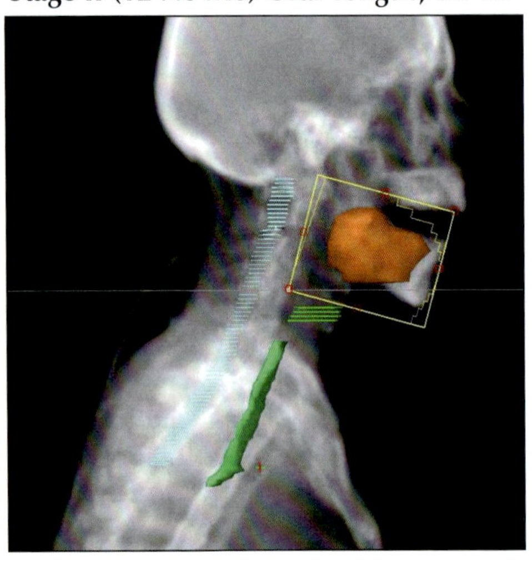

Stage II (T2 N0 M0) Oral Tongue, 3D RT

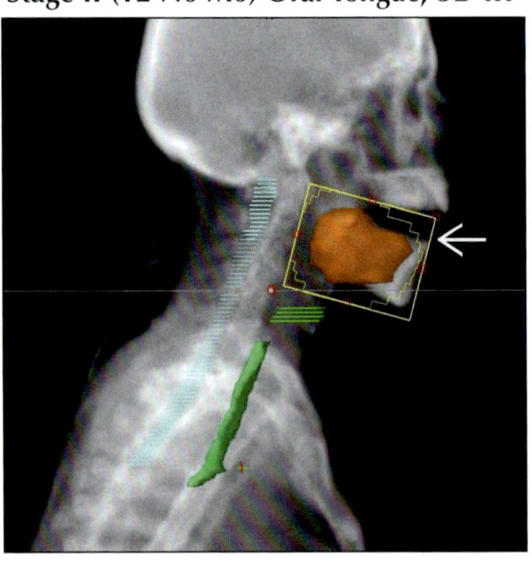

*(**Left**) DRR illustrates an upper neck off-cord field. The above field was treated to 54 Gy at 2 Gy per fraction. A high match (above the larynx) permits sparing the larynx in the lateral fields. (**Right**) The final boost field covering the entire remaining tongue and base of tongue was taken to 60 Gy. Field shaping should be performed to spare normal structures such as the lower lip ➔.*

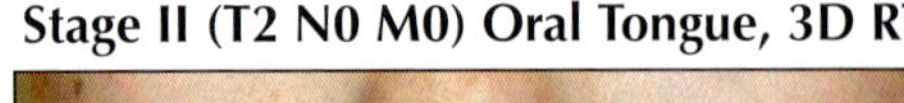

Stage II (T2 N0 M0) Oral Tongue, 3D RT

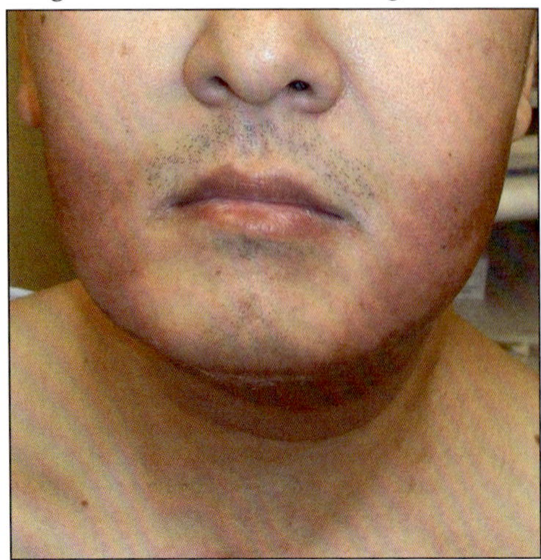

Stage II (T2 N0 M0) Oral Tongue, 3D RT

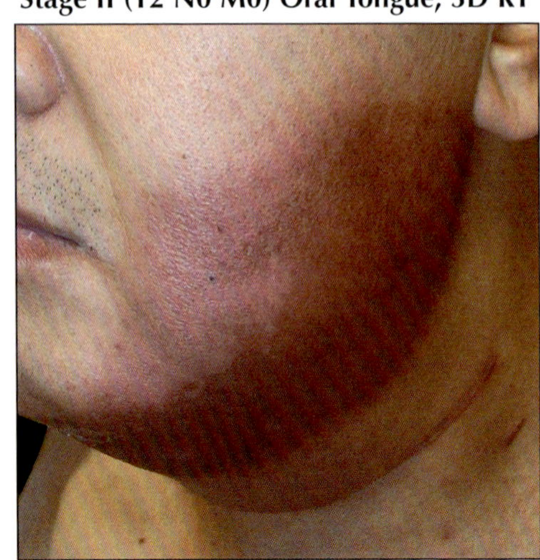

*(**Left**) Note erythematous skin reaction laterally, with anterior chin and lip being spared. Patient was treated with a 3-field technique, including opposed laterals to oral cavity and a matched anterior neck field, as illustrated. (**Right**) This photograph shows the erythematous skin reaction in the distribution of the opposed lateral fields at a dose level of 60 Gy.*

Stage I (T1 N0 M0)

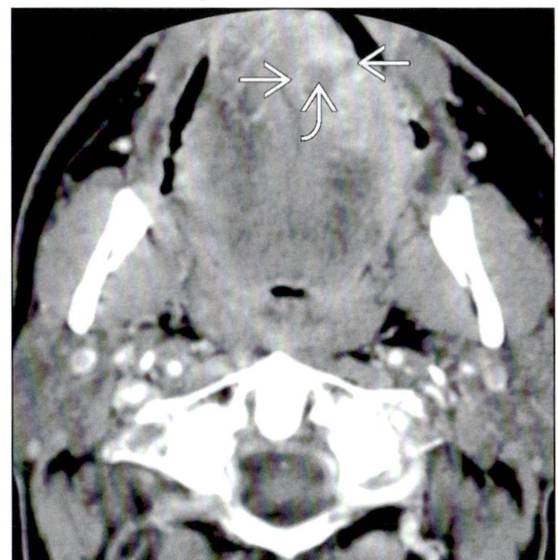

Stage II (T2 N0 M0)

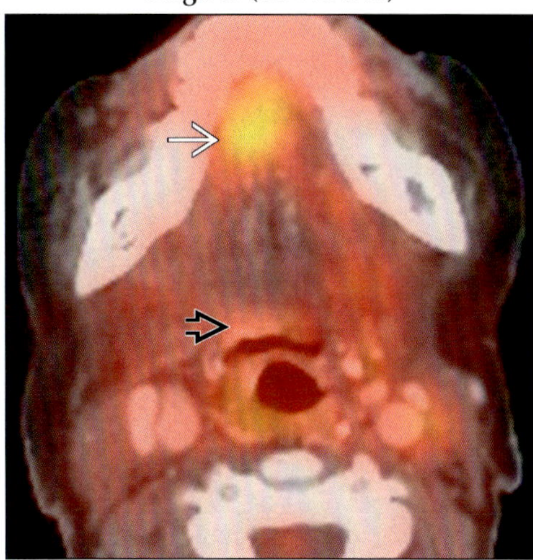

(Left) *Axial CECT shows a small enhancing 1.7 cm lesion at the anterior left oral tongue with some peripheral enhancement of the lesion with central necrosis.* ***(Right)*** *Axial fused PET/CT shows increased FDG activity compatible with a 3 cm vaguely enhancing mass on CECT. Symmetric metabolic activity in lymphoid tissue at the base of the tongue is normal.*

Stage III (T3 N0 M0)

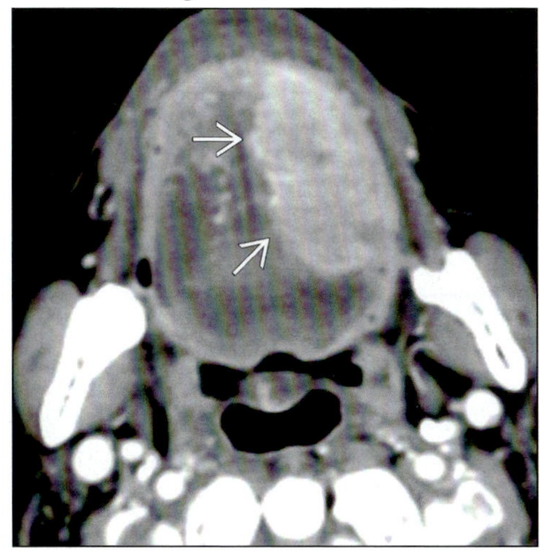

Stage III (T3 N0 M0)

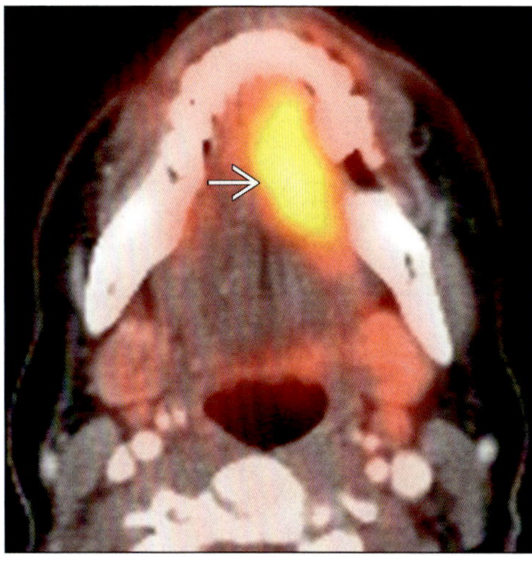

(Left) *Axial CECT of SCC of the tongue shows an irregularly shaped 5.6 cm enhancing lesion. The mass does not cross midline, which should allow the patient to have a hemiglossectomy.* ***(Right)*** *Axial fused PET/CT in a patient with a left lateral tongue mass shows intense FDG activity corresponding to an enhancing mass on CECT. The degree of increased metabolic activity in this case is characteristic of most squamous cell carcinomas.*

Stage IVA (T4a N2 M0)

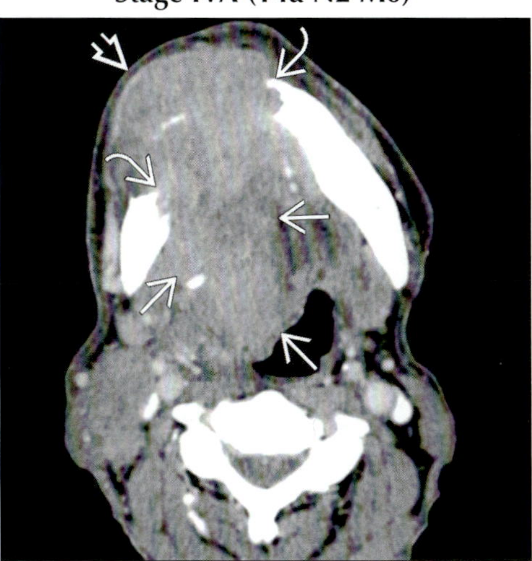

Stage IVA (T4a N2 M0)

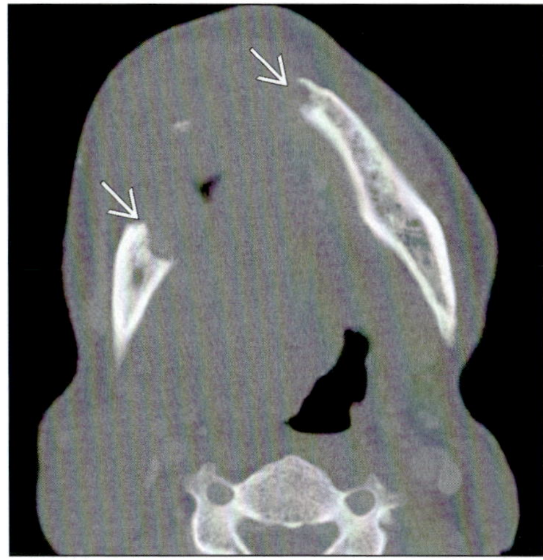

(Left) *Axial CECT shows a large enhancing mass centered in the anterior aspect of the tongue with complete erosion through the mandible and almost extending to the surface of the skin.* ***(Right)*** *Axial CECT with bone windows in the same patient shows destruction of a large portion of the mandible. Invasion into the mandible, deep muscles of the tongue, maxillary sinus, or skin of the face by an oral cavity tumor is considered T4a disease.*

ORAL CAVITY

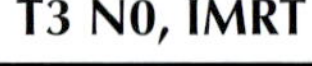

T3 N0, IMRT

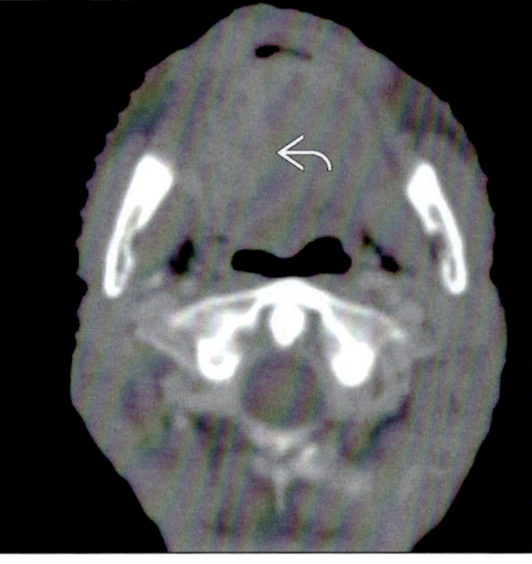

T3 N0, IMRT

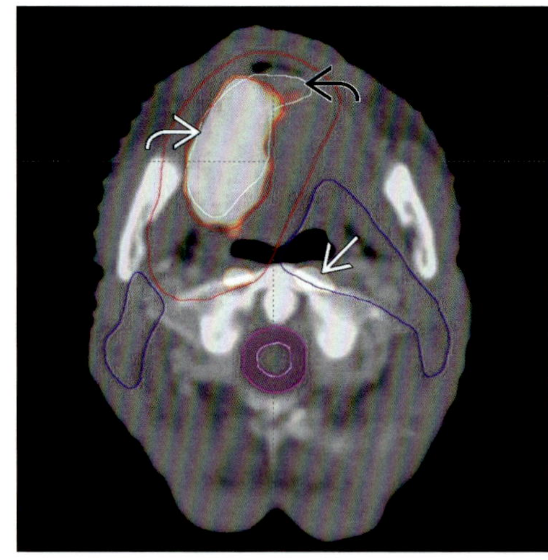

(Left) *Axial CECT shows a 4.5 cm tumor with floor of mouth extension in a 52 year old with biopsy-proven SCC of the oral tongue. He underwent definitive chemoradiation with PET/CT integrated into RT planning.* **(Right)** *Primary GTV in the same patient was contoured separately on PET/CT and planning simulation CT images, which were fused. PTV1 encompassed both GTVs. Posterior pharyngeal FDG uptake was from normal muscular activity.*

T3 N0, IMRT

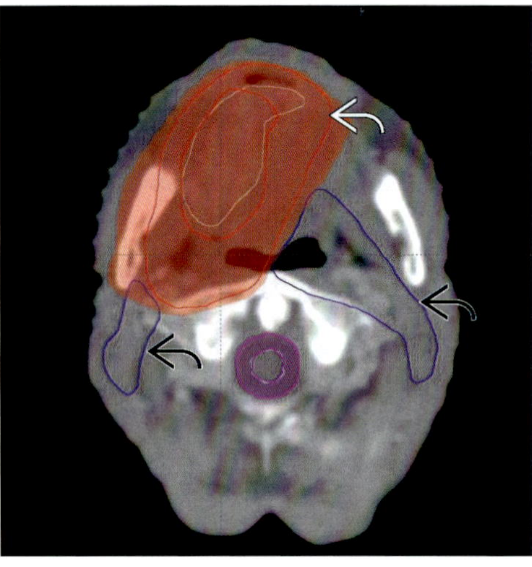

T3 N0, IMRT

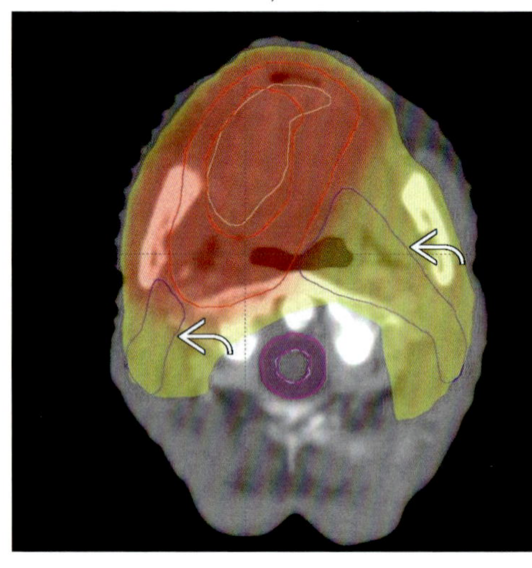

(Left) *PTV1 (combined GTV + margins) in the same patient is shown in colorwash, representing 95% of isodose coverage. PTV2 (intermediate nodal risk volumes) is outlined in blue and spinal canal in purple.* **(Right)** *PTV2 (intermediate nodal risk sites) in the same patient is shown in blue lines with dose covered in yellow colorwash. PTV1 was prescribed to 67.5 Gy and PTV2 to 54 Gy, both in 30 fractions.*

T3 N0, IMRT

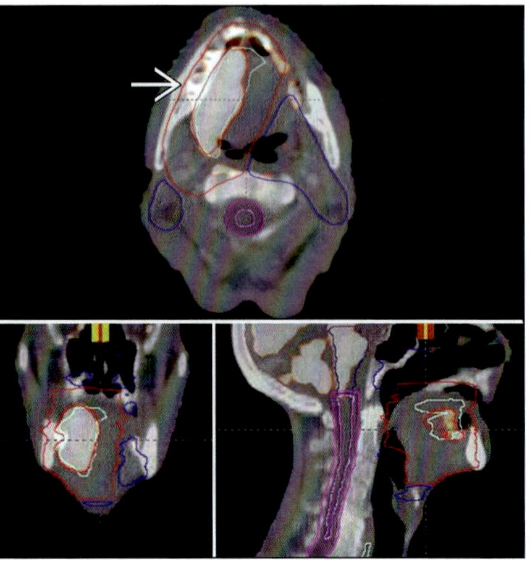

T3 N0, IMRT

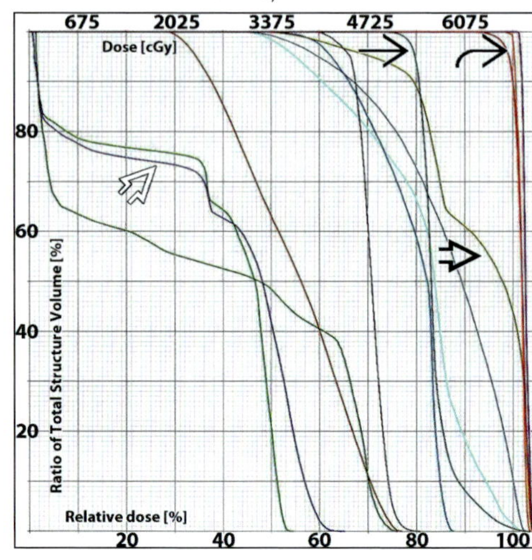

(Left) *This image set of the same patient shows integrated PET/CT and planning CT images. Metabolic activity on right molars was from recent tooth extraction.* **(Right)** *This image shows a DVH in the same patient. PTV1 (GTVs + margin) and PTV2 (intermediate nodal risk) are shown, respectively. Spinal cord and mandible are within acceptable limits. This patient is disease free 5 years post treatment and has hypothyroidism.*

Stage IVA (T3 N2b M0)

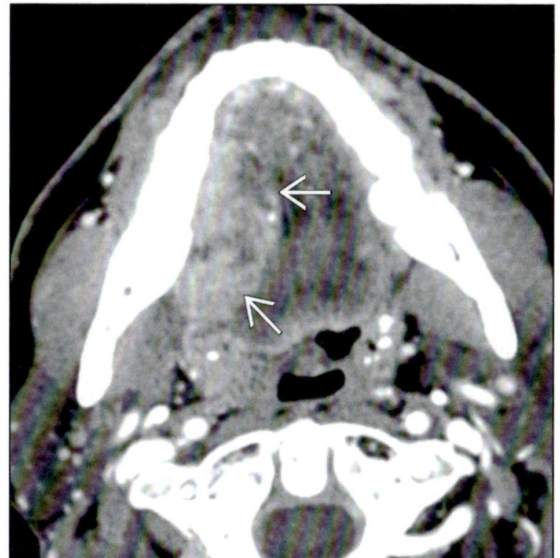

Stage IVA (T3 N2b M0)

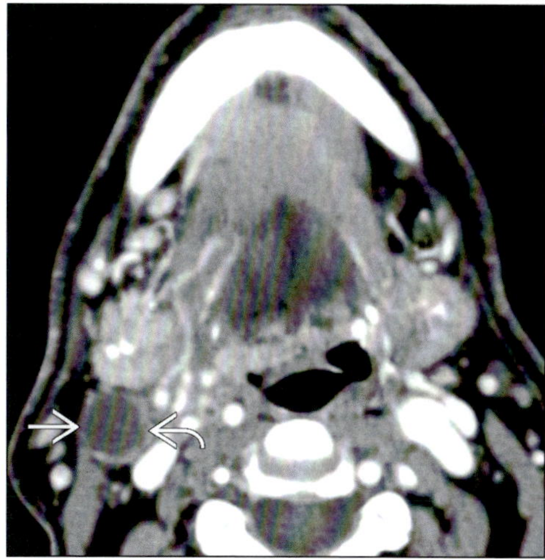

*(**Left**) Axial CECT shows an irregularly enhancing 4.3 cm mass ➡ along the right lateral aspect of the oral tongue, extending posteriorly into the posterior 1/3 of the tongue. This patient also has multiple right-sided lymph nodes < 6 cm. (**Right**) Axial CECT in the same patient shows a cystic level II lymph node ➡ in the right neck with a barely perceptible enhancing medial wall ↪.*

Cystic metastatic nodes are common in squamous cell carcinoma in the head and neck.

Stage III (T2 N1 M0)

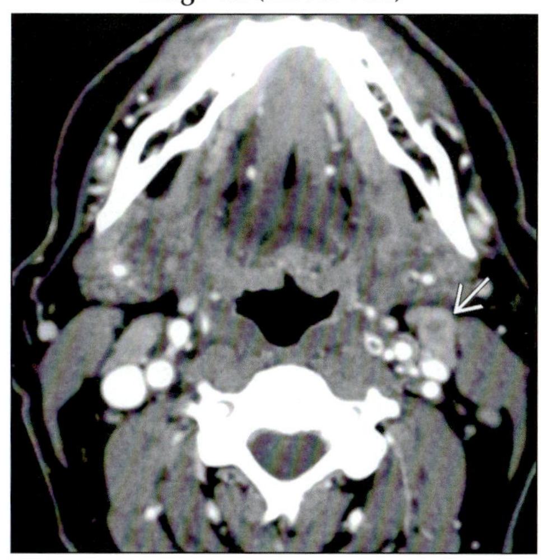

Stage IVA (T3 N2b M0)

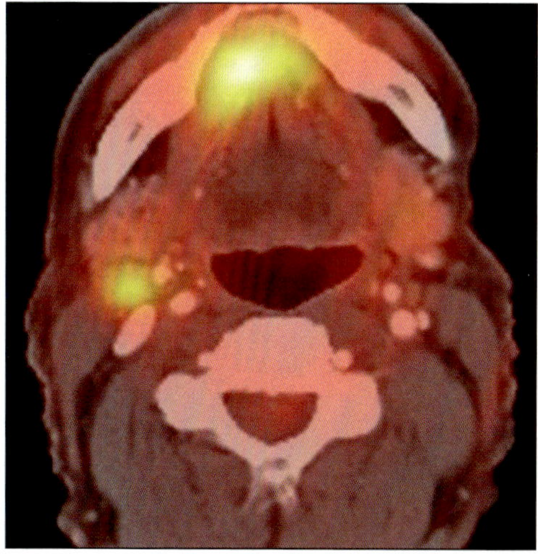

*(**Left**) Axial CECT shows an enlarged, suspicious left level II lymph node ➡. Metastatic lymph nodes may or may not be enlarged, but may have CECT evidence of extracapsular spread, central necrosis, or peripheral enhancement on CT. (**Right**) Axial FDG PET/CT shows hypermetabolic activity in a patient with a 4.5 cm oral tongue tumor and level II lymph node. This scan may be fused with the planning CT to help guide contouring high, intermediate, and lower risk target volumes.*

Stage IVC (T3 N2c M1)

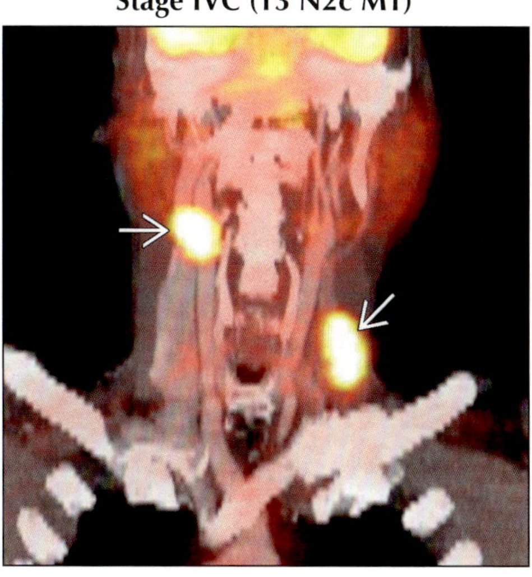

Stage IVB (T3 N3 M0)

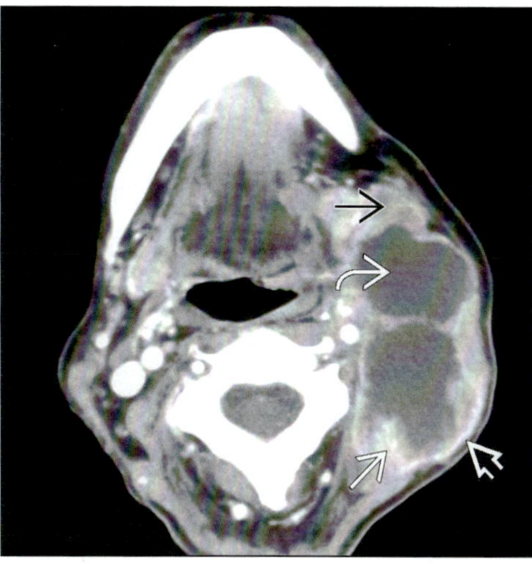

*(**Left**) Coronal fused PET/CT in a patient with bilateral neck metastases (all < 6 cm in size) shows bilateral hypermetabolic activity in the neck ➡. (**Right**) Axial CECT in a patient with metastatic lymph nodes measuring > 6 cm shows central necrosis ↪ with more solid components ➡ and an enhancing rim ➤. Extranodal extension and infiltration of the subcutaneous tissues are also noted ➡.*

ORAL CAVITY

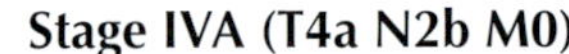

Stage IVA (T4a N2b M0)

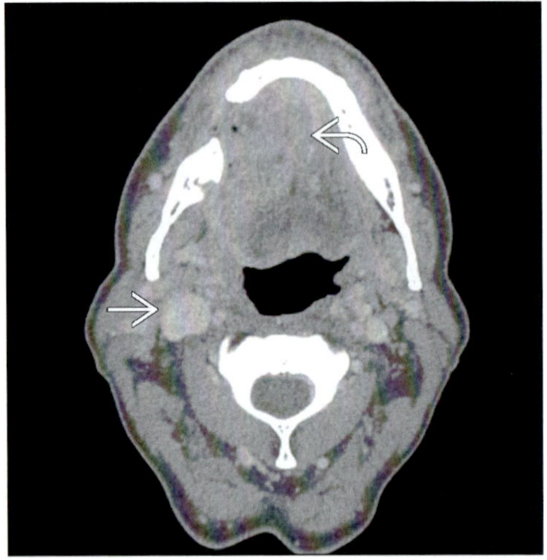

Stage IVA (T4a N2b M0)

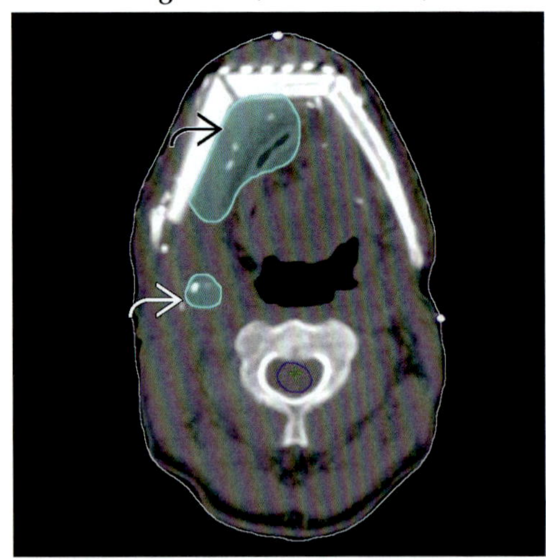

(Left) *Axial CECT shows a right-sided 5.2 cm oral tongue SCC extending to the floor of the mouth, extending past midline with loss of mandibular cortex, and enlarged lymph nodes.* ***(Right)*** *Axial CT shows the same patient after partial glossectomy, mandibulectomy, partial palatectomy, floor of mouth resection, bilateral dissections, and fibular free-flap reconstruction. The reconstructed primary tumor and involved node are shown.*

Stage IVA (T4a N2b M0)

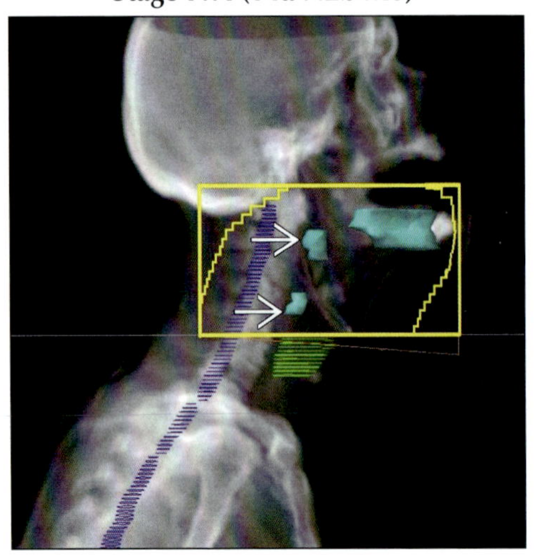

Stage IVA (T4a N2b M0)

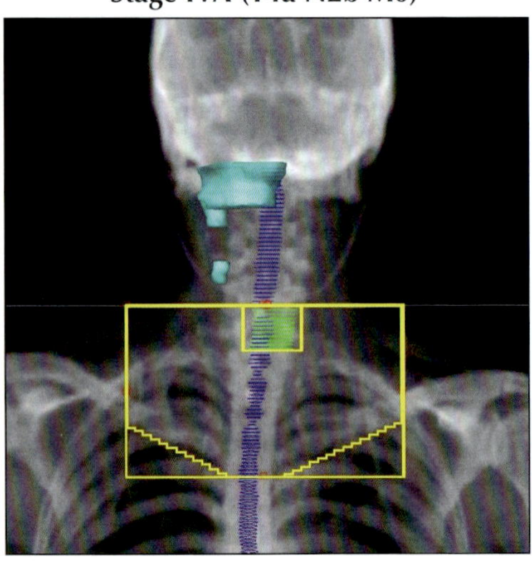

(Left) *DRR (same patient) shows initial bilateral upper neck fields, reconstructed primary tumor, and metastatic lymph nodes. Note larynx (light green) below upper neck fields. The mouth is open to prevent dose to the hard palate. The dose to this initial field was 42 Gy given in 21 fractions.* ***(Right)*** *AP field (same patient) shows bilateral lower neck and supraclavicular fossa for elective nodal irradiation. Note spinal cord and larynx are blocked at the match line.*

Stage IVA (T4a N2b M0)

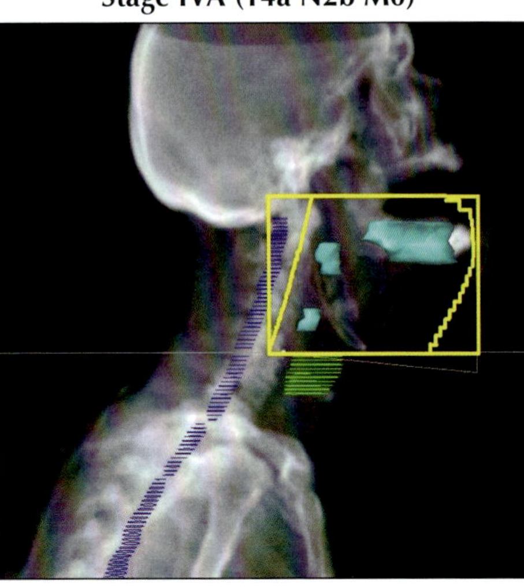

Stage IVA (T4a N2b M0)

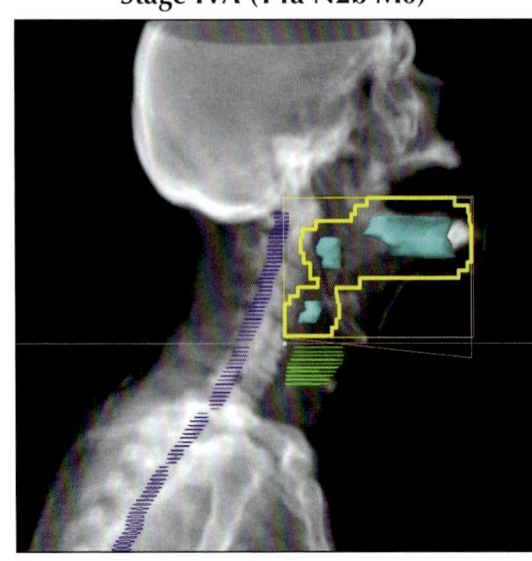

(Left) *This lateral DRR shows upper neck off-cord field in the same patient. The dose to this field was 54 Gy.* ***(Right)*** *This image shows the final boost volume in the same patient covering the preoperative primary and nodal sites. The final dose in this postop case was 60 Gy given with cisplatin chemotherapy. Patient is free of disease at 2 years.*

Stage II (T2 N0 M0) Interstitial Implant

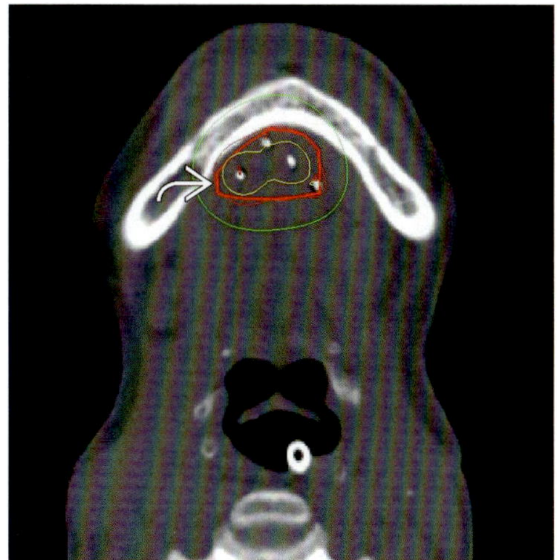

Stage II (T2 N0 M0) Interstitial Implant

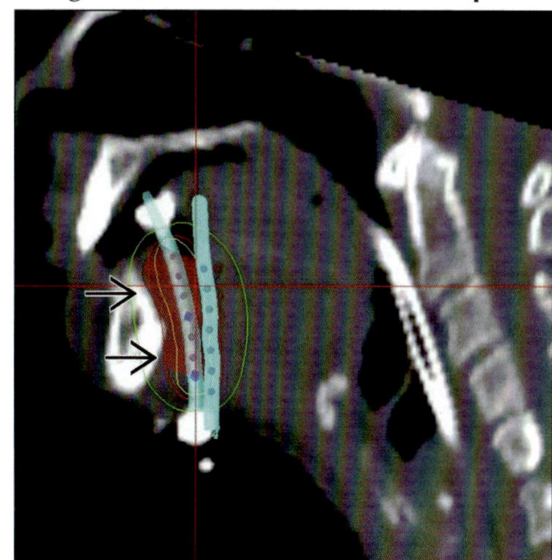

(Left) *This axial CT shows an interstitial implant for a 2.1 cm floor of mouth SCC, with positive margins and PNI. The patient received 39 Gy (3.25 Gy x 12 fractions b.i.d. > 6 hours between fractions). The CTV is shown in red* →*.* ***(Right)*** *The sagittal view illustrates placement of transoral catheters. Interstitial implants permit excellent conformality* → *and limit dose to OARs. The patient had no evidence of recurrence or mucosal abnormalities at 1.5 years post implant.*

Stage IVA (T4a N0 M0) Alveolar Ridge

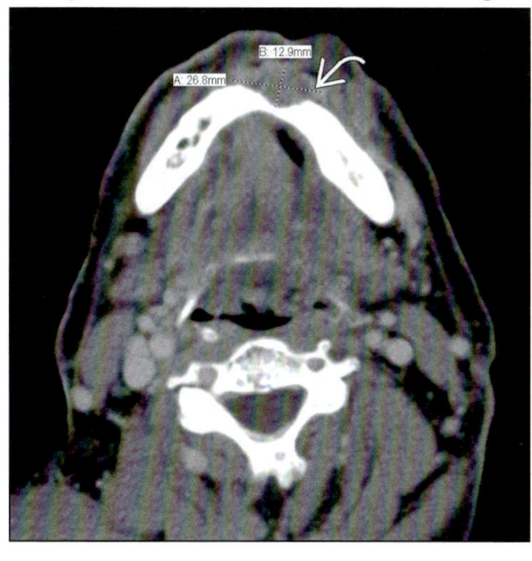

Stage IVA (T4a N0 M0) Alveolar Ridge

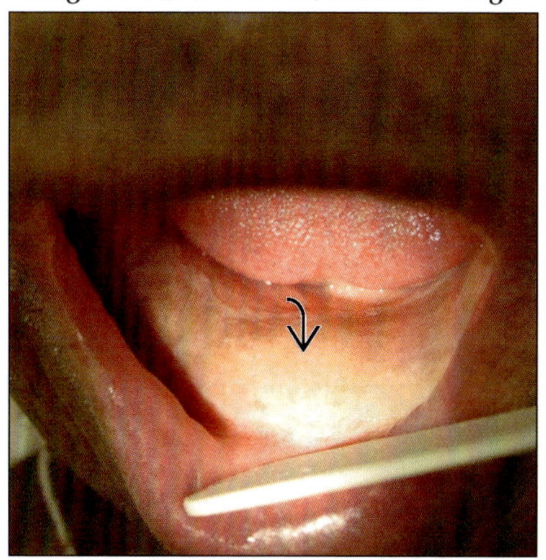

(Left) *This axial CECT in a 72-year-old man reveals a mandibular alveolar ridge tumor* →*. He underwent resection with reconstruction for a 2.6 cm lesion with a 0.2 cm close margin. He received a course of adjuvant 3D conformal radiotherapy, 60 Gy in 30 fractions.* ***(Right)*** *Six months post radiation follow-up shows a well-healed reconstructed osteocutaneous free flap* →*. There is no evidence of local or regional recurrence.*

Stage IVA (T4a N0 M0) Alveolar Ridge

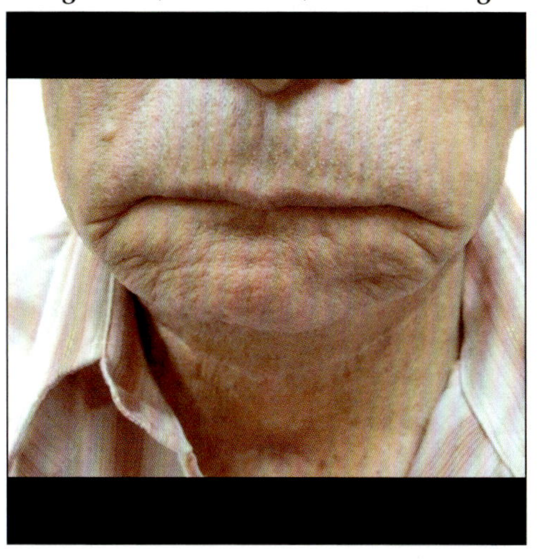

Stage IVA (T4a N0 M0) Alveolar Ridge

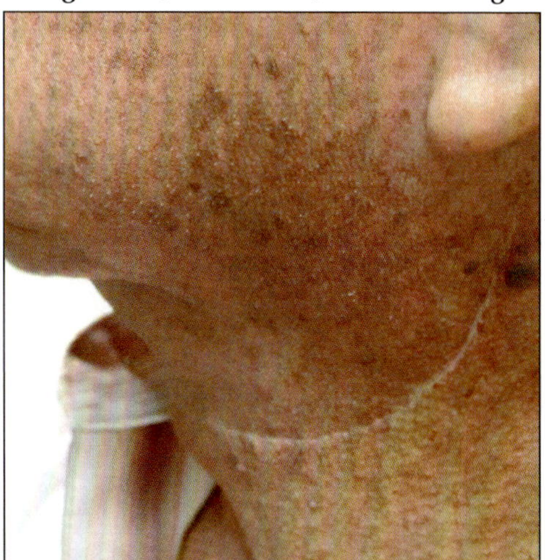

(Left) *This photo shows cosmetic changes following segmental anterior mandibular resection with fibular osteocutaneous free-flap reconstruction.* ***(Right)*** *The photo shows residual skin dryness and mild hyperpigmentation 3 months status post adjuvant RT.*

PHARYNX

(T) Primary Tumor

Adapted from 7th edition AJCC Staging Forms.

TNM	*Definitions*
TX	Primary tumor cannot be assessed
T0	No evidence of primary tumor
Tis	Carcinoma in situ
Oropharynx	
T1	Tumor ≤ 2 cm in greatest dimension
T2	Tumor > 2 cm but ≤ 4 cm in greatest dimension
T3	Tumor > 4 cm in greatest dimension or extension to lingual surface of epiglottis
T4a	Moderately advanced local disease: Tumor invades larynx, extrinsic muscle of tongue, medial pterygoid, hard palate, or mandible[1]
T4b	Very advanced local disease: Tumor invades lateral pterygoid muscle, pterygoid plates, lateral nasopharynx, or skull base or encases carotid artery
Hypopharynx	
T1	Tumor limited to 1 subsite of hypopharynx &/or ≤ 2 cm in greatest dimension
T2	Tumor invades > 1 subsite of hypopharynx or an adjacent site, or measures > 2 cm but ≤ 4 cm in greatest dimension without fixation of hemilarynx
T3	Tumor > 4 cm in greatest dimension or with fixation of hemilarynx or extension to esophagus
T4a	Moderately advanced local disease: Tumor invades thyroid/cricoid cartilage, hyoid bone, thyroid gland, or central compartment soft tissue[2]
T4b	Very advanced local disease: Tumor invades prevertebral fascia, encases carotid artery, or involves mediastinal structures

[1]*Mucosal extension to lingual surface of epiglottis from primary tumors of the base of the tongue and vallecula does not constitute invasion of larynx.*

[2]*Central compartment soft tissue includes prelaryngeal strap muscles and subcutaneous fat.*

(N) Regional Lymph Nodes for Oropharynx and Hypopharynx

Adapted from 7th edition AJCC Staging Forms.

TNM	*Definitions*
NX	Regional lymph nodes cannot be assessed
N0	No regional lymph node metastasis*
N1	Metastasis in a single ipsilateral lymph node, ≤ 3 cm in greatest dimension
N2	Metastasis in a single ipsilateral lymph node, > 3 cm but ≤ 6 cm in greatest dimension, or in bilateral or contralateral lymph nodes, none > 6 cm in greatest dimension
N2a	Metastasis in a single ipsilateral lymph node, > 3 cm but ≤ 6 cm in greatest dimension
N2b	Metastasis in multiple ipsilateral lymph nodes, none > 6 cm in greatest dimension
N2c	Metastasis in bilateral or contralateral lymph nodes, none > 6 cm in greatest dimension
N3	Metastasis in a lymph node, > 6 cm in greatest dimension

**Metastases at level VII are considered regional lymph node metastases.*

(M) Distant Metastasis

Adapted from 7th edition AJCC Staging Forms.

TNM	*Definitions*
M0	No distant metastasis
M1	Distant metastasis

AJCC Stages/Prognostic Groups

Adapted from 7th edition AJCC Staging Forms.

Stage	*T*	*N*	*M*
Oropharynx, Hypopharynx			
0	Tis	N0	M0
I	T1	N0	M0
II	T2	N0	M0
III	T3	N0	M0
	T1	N1	M0
	T2	N1	M0
	T3	N1	M0
IVA	T4a	N0	M0
	T4a	N1	M0
	T1	N2	M0
	T2	N2	M0
	T3	N2	M0
	T4a	N2	M0
IVB	T4b	Any N	M0
	Any T	N3	M0
IVC	Any T	Any N	M1

T1 and T2: Oropharynx

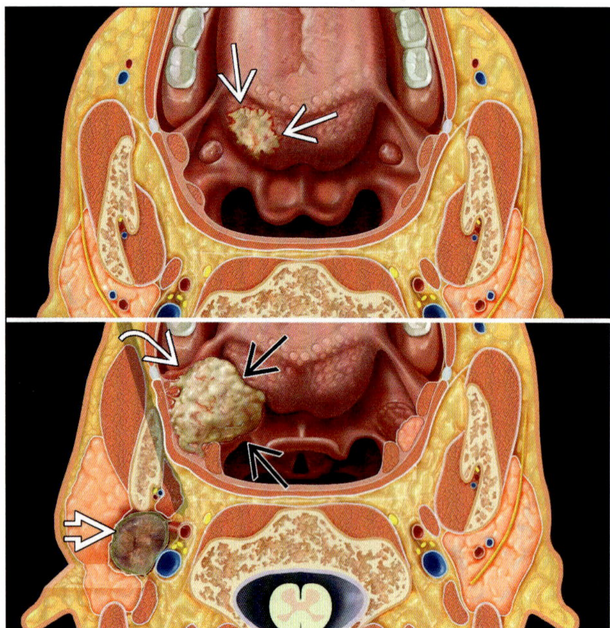

Top depicts a small, < 2 cm tumor confined to right lingual tonsil →, stage T1. Oropharyngeal tumors may arise from lingual tonsil, palatine tonsillar complex, posterior oropharyngeal wall, or soft palate. Bottom shows a larger tumor → involving the anterior tonsillar pillar →. A tumor > 2 cm but ≤ 4 cm is stage T2. Note ipsilateral level IIA node →, a frequently seen finding.

T3: Oropharynx

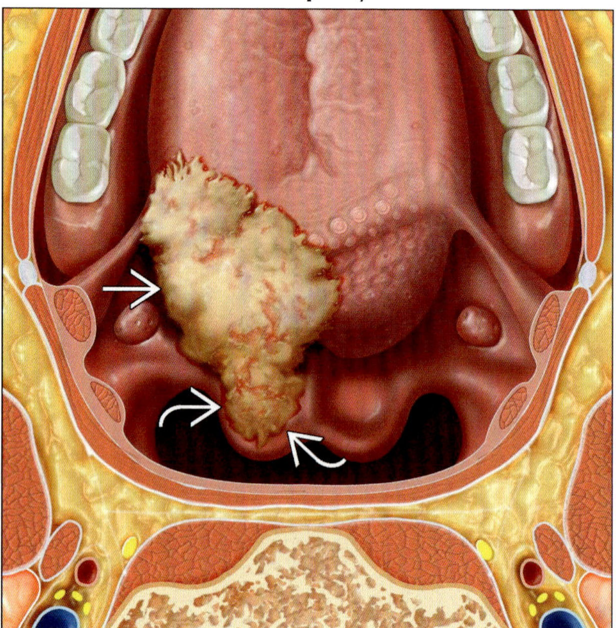

Graphic shows a tumor → that is > 4 cm in greatest dimension and extends to the lingual surface of the epiglottis →. Either condition would classify an oropharyngeal tumor as T3.

T4a: Oropharynx

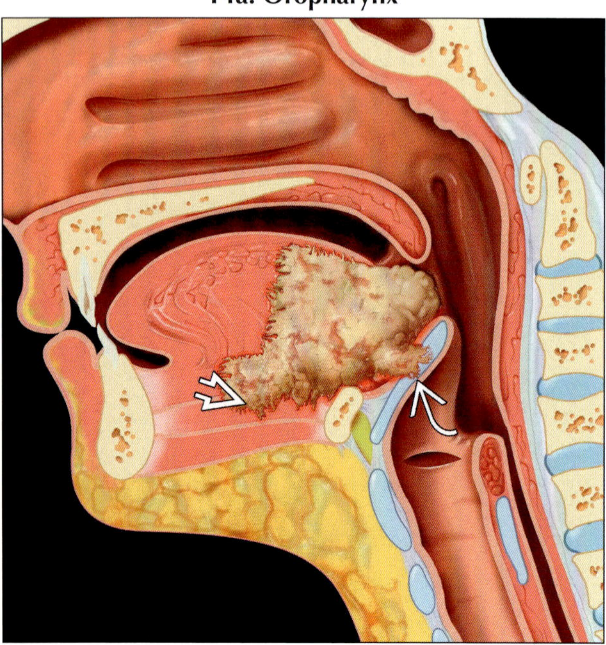

Graphic depicts an oropharyngeal tumor that invades the larynx → and extrinsic muscle of tongue →. Involvement of these areas, along with the medial pterygoid, hard palate, or mandible, is consistent with T4a disease. This is considered moderately advanced local disease.

T4a: Oropharynx

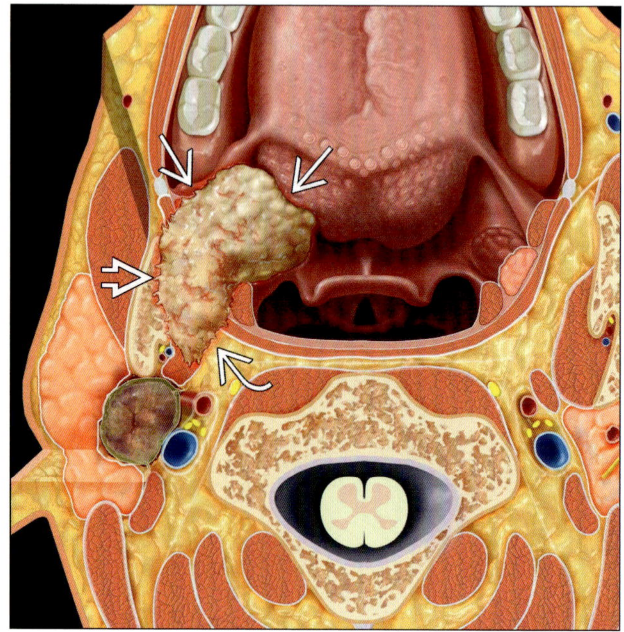

Graphic illustrates more extensive palatine tonsillar SCCa →, which infiltrates through the lateral oropharyngeal wall to invade both the medial pterygoid muscle → and mandible →. Either area of invasion stages this tumor as T4a or moderately advanced local disease.

T4b: Oropharynx

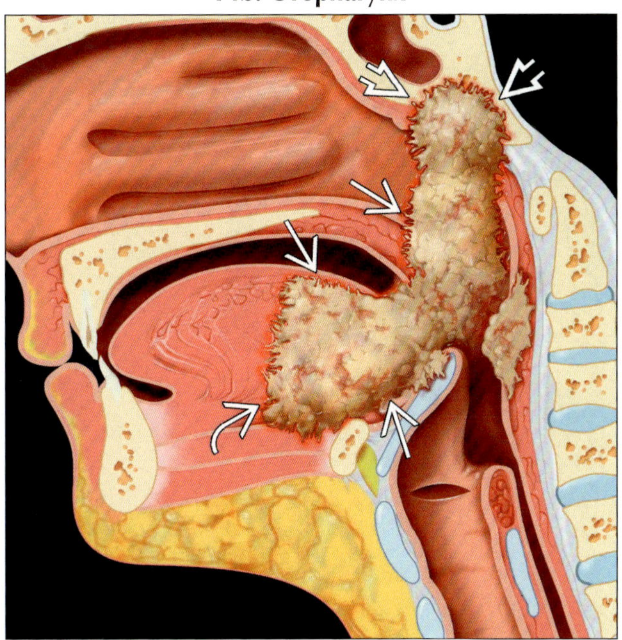

Graphic depicts advanced local disease with large SCCa involving tongue base and lateral pharyngeal wall and extending both anteriorly to oral tongue and genioglossus muscle and superiorly to skull base. Extrinsic tongue muscle involvement denotes T4a disease, but skull base invasion upstages this to T4b tumor.

T4b: Oropharynx

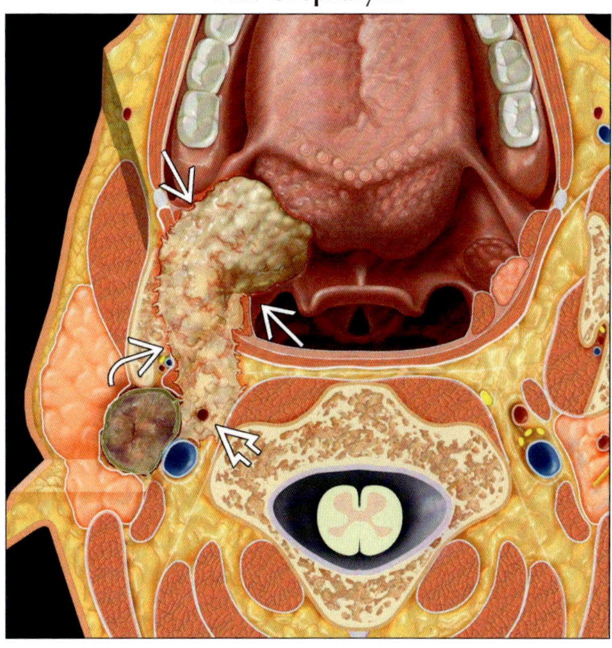

Graphic illustrates advanced tumor arising from right palatine tonsil and invading posteriorly through medial pterygoid muscle and mandible to encase internal carotid artery (ICA). T4b is determined by invasion of lateral pterygoid muscle, pterygoid plate, lateral nasopharynx, or skull base, or by encasement of the carotid.

T1 and T2: Hypopharynx

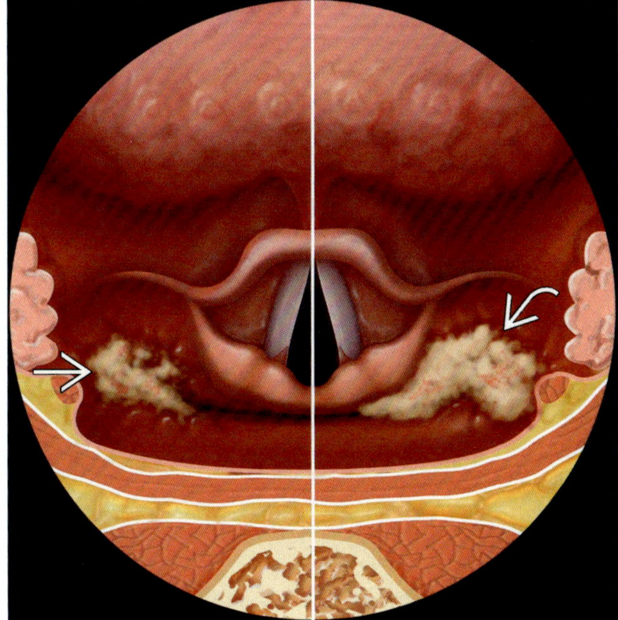

T1 and T2 hypopharyngeal tumors are defined by both size and subsite involvement (i.e., left and right pyriform sinuses, lateral and posterior hypopharyngeal walls, postcricoid region). T1 tumors are limited to 1 subsite and no more than 2 cm in size. T2 tumors invade > 1 subsite or measure 2-4 cm.

T3: Hypopharynx

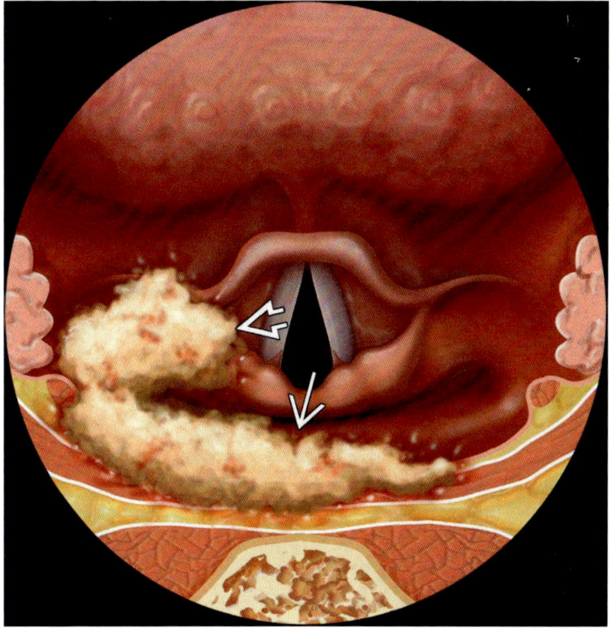

Graphic depicts a T3 tumor of the hypopharynx involving the pyriform sinus and posterior wall. Such tumors are > 4 cm in greatest dimension, create fixation of the hemilarynx, or extend to the esophagus.

T4a: Hypopharynx

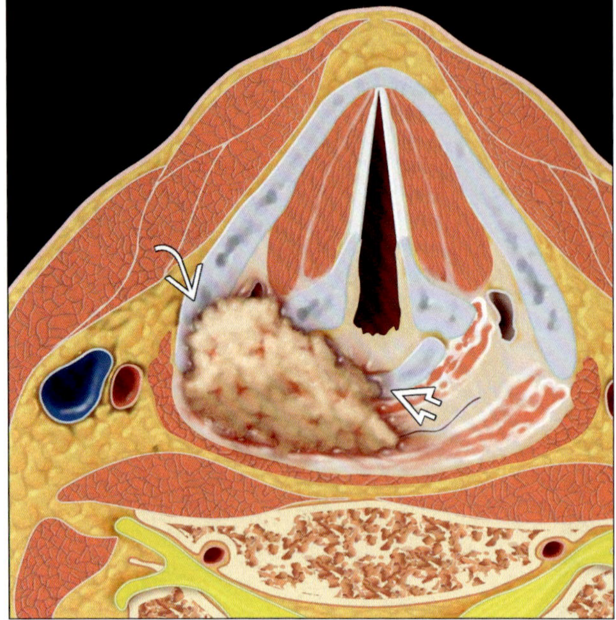

Graphic shows tumor that invades thyroid ➔ and cricoid ➔ cartilage. Invasion of these structures or involvement of the hyoid bone, thyroid gland, or central compartment soft tissues is consistent with T4a disease. This is considered moderately advanced local disease, a category introduced in 2010.

T4b: Hypopharynx

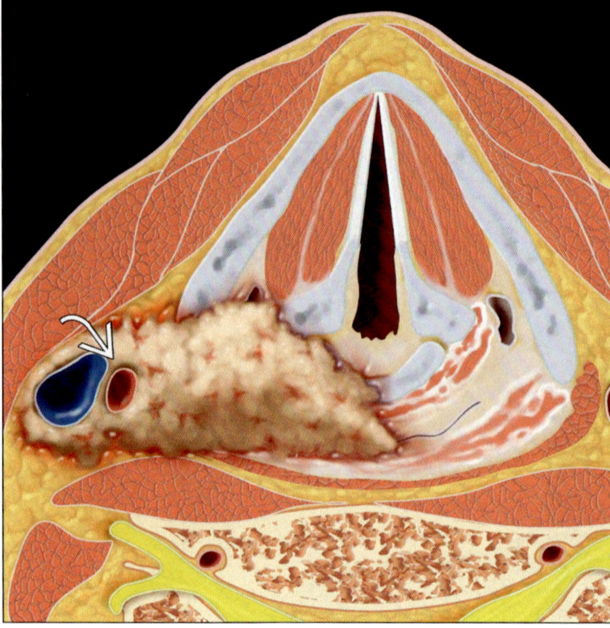

Graphic shows a T4b tumor of the hypopharynx that encases the carotid artery ➔. Such tumors are considered T4b, very advanced local disease, as are tumors that invade the prevertebral fascia or involve mediastinal structures.

T4a Post-Cricoid Region

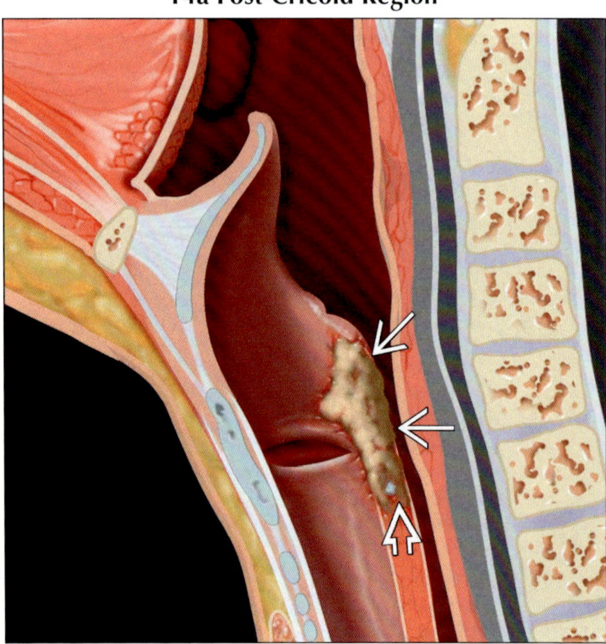

Graphic illustrates a moderately advanced hypopharyngeal tumor arising from post-cricoid mucosa ➔ and invading through the cricoid cartilage ➔.

T4b Posterior Hypopharyngeal Wall

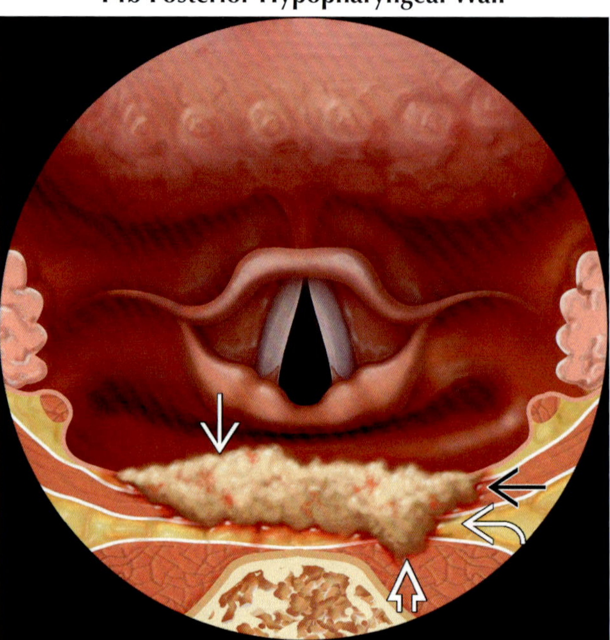

Graphic illustrates a sessile posterior hypopharyngeal wall SCCa ➔. This tumor has extended through the posterior pharyngeal wall →, then the prevertebral fascia ➔ and the left prevertebral muscle ➔. This is T4b disease.

T4 SCCa of Base of Tongue

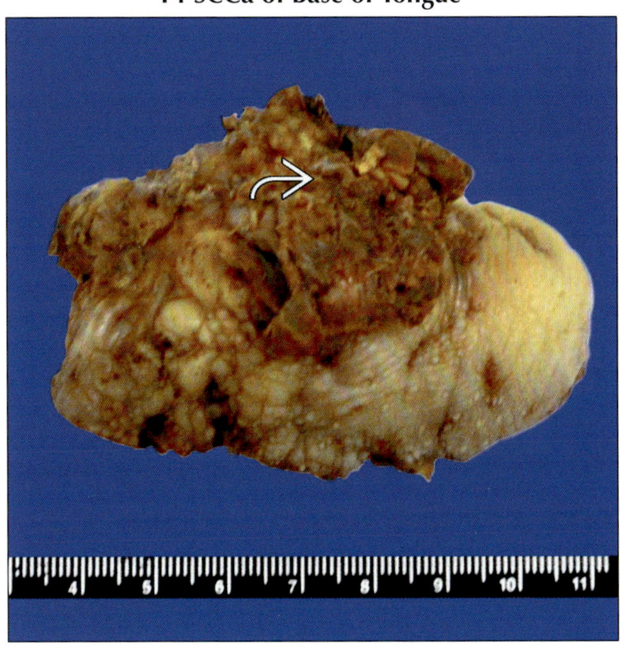

Gross specimen of SCCa of base of tongue ➦ shows an exophytic tumor involving the base of tongue. (Courtesy G. Ellis, DDS.)

T4 Squamous Cell Carcinoma of Pyriform Sinus

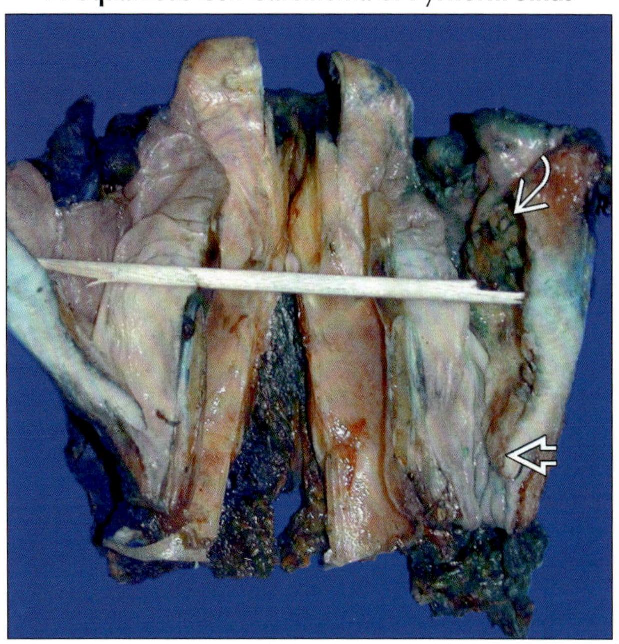

Gross specimen of SCCa of pyriform sinus shows an exophytic lesion ➦. The apex of the pyriform sinus is also involved ⇨. (Courtesy G. Ellis, DDS.)

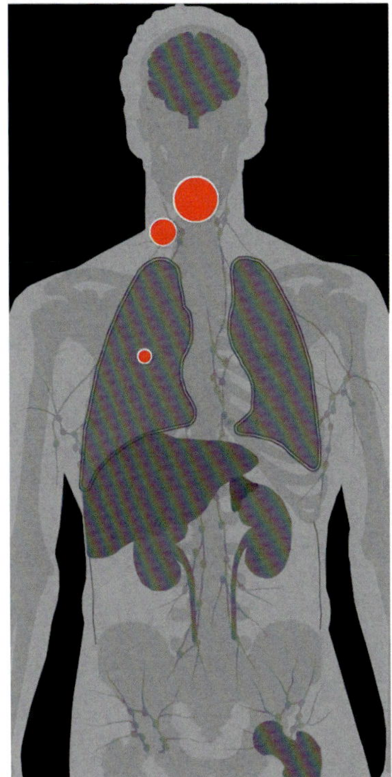

INITIAL SITE OF RECURRENCE

Local	41-58%
Regional	19-33%
Distant	18%

Data obtained from a randomized study of 226 stages III and IV patients with locoregional advanced squamous cell carcinoma of the oropharynx. Study compared RT alone vs. chemoradiation. Denis F et al: Final results of the 94-01 French Head and Neck Oncology and Radiotherapy Group randomized trial comparing radiotherapy alone with concomitant radiochemotherapy in advanced-stage oropharynx carcinoma. J Clin Oncol 2004. 22(1): 69-76, 2004.

PHARYNX

OVERVIEW

General Comments

- **Oropharyngeal carcinoma**
  - Squamous cell carcinoma (SCCa) accounts for 95% of oropharyngeal cancer
  - Lymphomas account for 5% of tonsillar and 1-2% of base of tongue cancers
  - Others: Minor salivary gland, plasmacytoma, etc.
  - Anatomic subsites of oropharynx
    - Base of tongue (lingual tonsil)
    - Tonsillar region (palatine/faucial tonsils): Most common site of oropharyngeal cancer
    - Soft palate
    - Pharyngeal walls (posterior and lateral)
- **Hypopharyngeal carcinoma**
  - Relatively uncommon malignancy
  - More advanced T stage and ↑ N stage at time of diagnosis
  - Majority are SCCa (> 95%)
  - Anatomic divisions of hypopharynx
    - Pyriform sinuses
    - Postcricoid area
    - Lateral and posterior pharyngeal walls
  - Primary site of malignancy
    - Pyriform sinuses: 65-85% (in USA and Canada)
    - Posterior pharyngeal wall: 10-20%
    - Postcricoid area: 5-15%

NATURAL HISTORY

Epidemiology & Cancer Incidence

- **Oropharyngeal carcinoma**
  - Worldwide
    - 123,000 new cases per year
    - 79,000 deaths per year
    - M:F = 3-5:1
  - In USA
    - 35,000 new cases per year
    - 7,590 deaths per year
  - Tobacco and alcohol exposure
  - High-risk HPV infection
    - Especially HPV-16
    - High-risk HPV positive commonly seen
      - Tend to be younger
      - No tobacco or alcohol use
      - History of multiple sex partners (particularly oral-genital sex)
      - Better prognosis
  - Diets with few fruits and vegetables
  - Certain stimulant beverages and preparations
- **Hypopharyngeal carcinoma**
  - Accounts for 7% of upper aerodigestive tract malignancies
  - In USA
    - 2,600 hypopharynx cases per year
  - Primary etiologies
    - Alcohol abuse
    - Tobacco use
  - Other etiologies
    - Nutritional deficiencies (e.g., iron and vitamin C suggested)
    - Plummer-Vinson syndrome also known as Paterson-Kelly syndrome in the UK
      - Triad of dysphagia from esophageal webs, glossitis, and iron deficiency anemia
      - Particularly associated with postcricoid carcinomas
  - Age
    - Incidence ↑ over age of 40
    - Uncommon under age of 30

Genetics

- **Oropharyngeal carcinoma**
  - Inactive mutant alleles of alcohol dehydrogenase-2
    - Cause impaired elimination of acetaldehyde, a carcinogen
    - Alcohol use results in increased susceptibility to oropharyngeal cancers (multiple metachronous)
    - Mainly seen in East Asian population
- **Hypopharyngeal carcinoma**
  - Suggested genetic associations include loss of chromosome 18

Gross Pathology & Surgical Features

- **Oropharyngeal carcinoma**
  - Tonsillar carcinoma
    - Ulcerated mass
      - Raised edges
    - Morphological findings
      - Firm
      - Gritty
      - Whitish color
      - Occasionally cystic degeneration or necrosis seen
- **Hypopharyngeal carcinoma**
  - May appear as flat plaque
    - Edges may be well defined and raised or appear polypoid and exophytic
  - Surface may appear ulcerated

Microscopic Pathology

- H&E
  - **Oropharyngeal carcinoma**
    - SCCa classification
      - May be noninvasive or invasive
      - Invasive SCCa may be undifferentiated or differentiated
  - **Hypopharyngeal carcinoma**
    - More than 95% of hypopharyngeal neoplasms are SCCa
      - 60% of carcinomas are keratinizing
      - 33% are nonkeratinizing
      - Generally poorly differentiated
    - Infiltrating margins are often present (80% of cases)
    - Multifocal disease or skip lesions may be seen
- Special stains
  - **Oropharyngeal carcinoma**
    - Immunohistochemistry
      - Expression of Ki-67 antigen by the MIB-1 biomarker may be complimentary to histologic grading
  - **Hypopharyngeal carcinoma**
    - Ki-67 expression
      - Lower proliferation index correlates with improved 5-year survival

Routes of Spread

- **Oropharyngeal carcinoma**
  - Direct extension
  - Lymphatic-rich lymphatic drainage present
    - Primarily to levels I-IV nodes
      - Level II: Most common node
    - Base of tongue carcinomas
      - 30% of patients have bilateral nodal metastasis
    - Soft palate carcinomas
      - Nodal metastasis particularly common
      - Nodal spread present in 60% of patients at time of diagnosis
  - Distant metastasis
    - Lung
    - Bone
- **Hypopharyngeal carcinoma**
  - Direct extension
    - Lesions arising on medial wall of pyriform sinuses often extend
      - Medially to aryepiglottic fold, arytenoid, and false vocal cord
      - Posteriorly to the postcricoid region
    - Potentially with further invasion into paraglottic space and larynx
    - Lesions arising on lateral wall tend to invade
      - Posterior thyroid cartilage
      - Thyroid gland
      - Posterior cricoid cartilage
      - Posterior pharyngeal wall
    - Cervical esophagus spread as a late event
    - Postcricoid region cancer tends to invade posterior pharyngeal wall or arytenoid area, depending on its origin
  - Lymphatic spread
    - Rich lymphatic drainage → frequent regional nodal metastasis
    - Asymptomatic neck mass is present in 20% of cases
      - Generally represents regional nodal metastasis
      - Most typically jugulodigastric or jugulo-omohyoid lymph node
    - Nodal involvement in pharyngeal wall carcinomas according to study of neck dissections
      - Level I: 0%
      - Level II: 67%
      - Level III: 33%
      - Level IV: 7%
    - Nodal involvement in pyriform sinus carcinomas according to study of neck dissections
      - Level I: 20%
      - Level II: 80%
      - Level III: 40%
      - Level IV: 40%
  - Distant metastasis
    - Lung
    - Bone

IMAGING

Detection

- **Oropharynx-lingual tonsil** (base of tongue [BOT])
  - CT
    - Invasive mass centered in lingual tonsil
      - BOT defined as Waldeyer lymphatic ring component posterior to circumvallate papilla, extending inferiorly to vallecula (posterior 1/3 of tongue)
    - Symptoms from BOT-SCCa occur late
      - Tumors often large (> 4 cm) at presentation
    - Mucosal lesion can be either invasive or exophytic, filling airway
    - Lingual tonsil SCCa spread patterns
      - Anterior: Sublingual space, tongue root, and floor of mouth
      - Inferior: Supraglottic larynx and preepiglottic space
      - Posterolateral: Anterior tonsillar pillar, faucial (palatine) tonsil
    - Small tumors appear as mucosal asymmetry
      - Tumor surrounded by enhancing lymphoid tissue
      - Normal lymphoid tissue variably enhances and may be asymmetric, further hindering CECT detection of small tumors
      - Imaging essential for deep extension and nodal stage
    - Moderate enhancement
    - Deep tumor invasion more easily appreciated than superficial spread
  - **MR**
    - T1WI
      - Isointense to tongue musculature
      - Extension into fat-filled sublingual space easily detected
      - Sagittal plane best shows invasion of preepiglottic space
      - Larynx involvement important in determining treatment course
      - If surgery is considered, will need to include supraglottic larynx in imaging field
    - T2WI
      - BOT-SCCa may be isointense or slightly hyperintense on T2 MR to muscle in tongue and floor of mouth
      - Sagittal & coronal planes helpful to assess spread into root of tongue (genioglossus and geniohyoid muscles)
    - T1WI C+
      - BOT-SCCa enhances
      - Especially helpful to appreciate interface between tumor and muscle
  - **PET/CT**
    - Normal lingual tissue at tongue base is FDG avid
    - Small lesions may be indistinguishable from normal physiologic uptake in tonsillar tissue
    - May detect primary tumor if lesion occult
    - Possible multifocal disease
      - 15% of patients have 2nd primary SCCa in neck and chest
- **Oropharynx-palatine tonsil**
  - CECT
    - Enhancing mass centered in faucial tonsil with invasive deep margins
    - Location: Tonsillar fossa > anterior tonsillar pillar > posterior tonsillar fossa
    - Small lesion may be difficult to differentiate from asymmetric faucial tonsil

- Tonsil may enhance like SCCa
- Larger lesions enhance moderately, invade locally
- Enlarged lymph nodes (LNs) ± central nodal necrosis ± extranodal tumor
  - Level II internal jugular chain most likely location
- PET/CT
  - Tonsillar tissue normally FDG avid
    - Therefore, symmetric uptake important
  - Tumor and metastatic nodes strongly FDG avid
  - Recommended in "occult primary" clinical setting
    - Presents as necrotic, almost cystic-appearing, level II node with no obvious primary on imaging or mucosal examination
    - Work-up includes direct laryngoscopy in operating room with random superficial & deep mucosal biopsies
    - May obviate need for random biopsies if primary detected in faucial tonsil or oropharynx
- **Hypopharynx**
  - **General**
    - Assessment of clinical tumor stage through endoscopy enables more focused imaging evaluation of deep tissue below lesions of mucosa
    - Pyriform sinuses are primary site of majority
  - **CECT**
    - Invasive mass with moderate enhancement
    - Pyriform sinus SCCa: Destruction of cartilage in posterior thyroid, neck invasion with carotid space involvement
    - Posterior hypopharyngeal wall SCCa: Invasion of prevertebral space and retropharyngeal nodes through deep layer of deep cervical fascia
    - Postcricoid SCCa: Endolarynx invasion and associated cartilage destruction of cricoid or thyroid
  - **MR**
    - T1WI
      - Mass with low to intermediate signal
    - T2WI
      - Mass with intermediate to high signal
    - STIR
      - Mass with intermediate to high signal
    - T1WI C+
      - Heterogeneously enhancing
  - **PET/CT**
    - Shown to add diagnostic value in staging of hypopharyngeal cancers
    - FDG avidity useful to
      - Detect occult primary site
      - Gauge response to treatment
      - Distinguish post-treatment changes from neoplastic tissue (e.g., scar tissue vs. early recurrence)

Staging

- N staging
  - Similar findings for all pharyngeal tumors with exception of nodes involved
  - **CT**
    - Metastatic lymph nodes appear round with loss of fatty hilum on CT
    - Extracapsular nodal spread is more common in larger nodes but possible in smaller nodes as well
    - Metastatic cervical adenopathy is commonly seen on contrast-enhanced CT
      - CT is preferred over MR for cervical metastatic disease, except retropharyngeal disease
      - Nodal metastasis is heterogeneously enhancing
      - Rim enhancement and central necrosis of lymph node are abnormal irrespective of size
  - **MR**
    - Superior at evaluating metastatic retropharyngeal lymph nodes
      - T1WI C+ or T2WI with fat saturation superior to CECT in visualization
    - Large tumors show necrosis with rim enhancement
      - Regions of necrosis often heterogeneously enhancing
  - **PET/CT**
    - Strong FDG avidity seen in primary and metastatic nodes
    - Excellent modality for detecting unsuspected tumor foci in distant or nonenlarged nodes
- M staging
  - **General**
    - Distant metastases are present < 10% of time at presentation
      - Lung > bone > liver
    - Node-positive patients with nasopharyngeal carcinoma are at high risk of developing metastases
  - **CT**
    - Moderately enhancing solid mass that shows aggressive destruction of bone
    - Parenchymal metastases may show hyperenhancement
    - Large metastatic foci may be nonenhancing
    - CT superior in evaluating cortical bone invasion
      - Thin slice (1-2 mm) helps assess bone invasion
      - Bone lesions may show enhancement
      - Erosion into skull base indicates poor prognosis
  - **MR**
    - Also best tool for evaluating intracranial extent via direct, perivascular, and perineural routes
    - May reveal subtle bony erosions of skull base
    - Limiting factors include long acquisition time (~ 30 minutes)
    - T1WI
      - Intermediate signal mass
      - Hypointense to isointense compared to muscle
      - Increased T1 signal may be seen in intratumoral hemorrhage areas
      - Replaced bone marrow is easier to appreciate on pre-contrast T1-weighted images than on other sequences
    - T2WI
      - Moderate hyperintensity to muscle
      - Mucosal extent of tumor difficult to determine on MR as normal mucosa and tumor nearly isointense
      - Cystic degeneration: Appears hyperintense
      - Foci of hemorrhage: Appear hypointense to hyperintense based on age of blood
    - T1WI C+
      - Post-contrast fat saturation for differentiation of tumor from adjacent muscle/fat
      - Enhancement typically mild to moderate, heterogeneous, and diffuse

- Necrotic areas do not enhance
- SCCa enhances less than adenocarcinoma
- PET/CT
  - Strong FDG avidity seen in distant metastasis
  - Sensitivity greatest in metastases with diameter > 1 cm
  - Submucosal tumors may be located via PET/CT
  - Careful attention to artifacts and patterns of physiologic uptake is essential to avoid inaccurate staging

Restaging

- CT
  - Widely used for regular monitoring of patients who have undergone surgical treatment of pharyngeal carcinoma
    - Useful for bone erosion/involvement
    - May show asymmetry of nasopharynx
  - Contrast-enhanced CT recommended to evaluate recurrent cervical lymphadenopathy
- MR
  - Trend toward higher accuracy than PET/CT in detecting residual &/or recurrent nasopharyngeal carcinoma
  - Restaging is more accurate when both MR and PET/CT are used than when either is used alone
  - Cannot reliably differentiate tumor from XRT changes, but T2 hypointensity and poor enhancement are often seen with fibrosis
- PET/CT
  - Superior to CT and MR in restaging and evaluating treatment effectiveness of nasopharyngeal carcinoma
  - Early restaging by single whole-body 18F FDG PET scan after 1st or 2nd course of induction chemotherapy
    - Useful in predicting response in patients with advanced nasopharyngeal carcinoma
  - MR and PET/CT are more accurate when combined

CLINICAL PRESENTATION & WORK-UP

Presentation

- **Oropharyngeal carcinoma**
  - BOT (lingual tonsil)
    - Insidious clinically
    - Base of tongue malignancies often symptomatic only after significant disease progression
      - Due to lack of pain fibers in base of tongue
    - Symptoms
      - Pain
      - Dysphagia
      - Loss of weight
      - Referred otalgia secondary to cranial nerve IX involvement
      - Trismus secondary manifestation of involvement of pterygoid muscle
      - Tongue fixation due to deep muscle infiltration
      - Neck mass
    - Lymph node metastasis is frequent
      - Base of tongue has rich lymphatic drainage
      - Common sites include ipsilateral cervical node (≥ 70% of cases) and bilateral cervical lymph node (≤ 30% of cases)
  - Tonsillar region
    - Most common location for primary tumor of oropharynx
    - Symptoms
      - Pain
      - Dysphagia
      - Loss of weight
      - Ipsilateral referred otalgia
      - Neck mass
    - Tonsillar fossa lesions
      - Exophytic or ulcerative morphology
      - More commonly presents as advanced disease relative to tonsillar pillar cancers
      - Approximately 75% of patients present with stage III or stage IV disease
      - Lymphatic drainage of this region is most frequently to lymph nodes located in posterior triangle
    - Anterior pillar of tonsil lesions
      - May present as superficial spreading lesions
      - Spread to buccal mucosa, base of tongue, and retromolar trigone area
      - Spread to level II nodes often prior to other levels
  - Soft palate tumors
    - Found mainly on anterior surface
    - Tumors may stay superficial and in earlier disease stage
    - Lymphatic drainage of these lesions is mainly to upper jugular lymph nodes superior to digastric muscle
  - Pharyngeal wall tumors
    - Symptoms
      - Pain
      - Bleeding
      - Loss of weight
      - Neck mass
    - Commonly, diagnosis is made at advanced stage of disease due to clinically silent location
- **Hypopharyngeal carcinoma**
  - Symptoms
    - Sore throat
      - Often unilateral and localized
    - Hoarseness
      - Indicates invasions of intrinsic muscles of larynx, cricoarytenoid joints, or, less commonly, recurrent laryngeal nerve involvement
    - Dysphagia
    - Otalgia
    - Hemoptysis
    - Halitosis
    - Stridor
    - Nodal metastases approximately 50% at initial presentation

Prognosis

- **Oropharyngeal carcinoma**
  - Prognostic factors
    - Overall patient health
      - Comorbidities can be classified by Karnofsky scale score
    - Continued carcinogen exposure
      - Tobacco

- Alcohol
- Prognosis: Relative survival rate for oropharyngeal squamous cell carcinomas
  - 5-year survival rate
    - Stage I: 80-90%
    - Stage II: 70-80%
    - Stage III: 60-70%
    - Stage IV: 30-50%
- Distant metastases
  - Associated risks
    - High N stage (N3)
    - Low neck involvement
    - Poor response to definitive chemoradiation therapy (CRT)
- Recurrence
  - 80-90% of local or regional recurrence occurs within the 1st 2-3 years

- **Hypopharyngeal carcinoma**
  - Factors associated with poor prognosis
    - Distant metastases
    - Lymph node metastases
    - Lymphatic invasion
    - Positive surgical margin
    - Comorbidities
      - Alcohol abuse
      - Tobacco use
  - Prognosis is related to specific location of primary site
    - Pyriform sinus location associated with poor prognosis and early metastasis
    - Postcricoid location associated with poor prognosis; tumors often present at advanced stage and are associated with paratracheal/mediastinal metastasis
    - Posterior wall of hypopharynx: Stage I and II cancers in this area are associated with generally good prognosis
  - Prognosis: Relative survival rate for hypopharyngeal squamous cell carcinomas
    - 5-year survival rate
      - Stage I: 70-80%
      - Stage II: 50-60%
      - Stage III: 40-50%
      - Stage IV: 10-30%
  - Distant metastases
    - High risk of distant metastases
      - Advanced T stage
      - High N stage, bilateral neck or N3 disease
      - Low neck involvement, level IV or level V
  - Recurrence
    - Majority locoregional recurrence occurs within 1st 2-3 years

Work-Up

- Clinical
  - History and physical examination
    - Include otalgia, dysphagia, odynophagia, weight loss, and trismus
  - Nasopharyngolaryngoscopy to evaluate tumor extension and vocal cord mobility
  - Bronchoscopy and esophagoscopy for locally advanced primary tumor or if clinically indicated
  - Pretreatment dental care
    - 10-14 days required for extraction wound healing before RT
  - Audiometry baseline before RT
  - Speech and swallow evaluation
- Radiographic
  - Contrast-enhancing CT of neck soft tissue
  - Chest imaging
  - PET with contrast-enhancing CT for stage III or IV disease
- Laboratory
  - CBC, CMP, baseline thyroid stimulating hormone (TSH)

TREATMENT

Major Treatment Alternatives

- **Oropharyngeal carcinoma**
  - Radiation therapy (RT)
    - May be used as definitive therapy in stages I and II cancers
      - Generally equally successful when compared to surgery
    - Concurrent RT and chemotherapy recommended for most stage III and IV tumors
    - Indication of adjuvant RT or CRT is based on pathological features for high risk of recurrences
  - Surgery
    - May be used in stages I and II cancers
    - Similar success as RT except in cases where there may be significant functional deficit
    - In cases of primary tumor disease involving thyroid cartilage or mandible
  - Chemotherapy
    - Concurrent with radiotherapy most often
    - Cisplatin is most common agent
- **Hypopharyngeal carcinoma**
  - Radiation therapy
    - Definitive RT alone for very selected stages I or II cancer
    - Radiotherapy concurrent with chemoradiation
      - Often used in local regional advanced tumors
      - Adjuvant chemoradiation for high-risk pathological features (microscopic positive margins, extracapsular extension, or selected T4 disease)
      - Cisplatin is most used agent
  - Surgery
    - Partial laryngopharyngectomy with laryngeal organ preservation for T1 or T2 pyriform sinus carcinoma
    - Total laryngopharyngectomy for advanced disease with total laryngectomy and pharyngeal wall resection
    - Approach and decision for surgery must be weighed against functional considerations and quality of life going forward
    - Advanced stage cancer often requires combined therapies as opposed to sole treatment with surgery
  - Induction chemotherapy
    - If complete response (CR), generally RT or CRT follows
    - CRT if partial response
    - CRT or radical surgery if disease progression
- Indication for adjuvant RT
  - Close margins (< 5 mm)

- T4 disease with primary tumor invasion of bone, soft tissue, or cartilage
    - LVSI
    - Perineural invasion
    - Nodal metastasis to 2 or more nodes
- Indication for adjuvant CRT
    - Extracapsular extension
    - Microscopic positive margins

Major Treatment Roadblocks/ Contraindications

- **Oropharyngeal carcinoma**
    - Adverse side effects associated with RT
        - Skin reaction
            - e.g., erythema, moist desquamation, ulceration, skin pigmentation
        - Mucositis
        - Dysphagia
        - Odynophagia
        - Xerostomia
        - Dysgeusia
- **Hypopharyngeal carcinoma**
    - Functional outcomes related to preservation of larynx must be considered
    - Complications of therapy, including surgery, can include difficulties in
        - Feeding
        - Speaking
        - Swallowing
        - Pharyngoesophageal stenosis/stricture
    - Treatment plan must be designed to avoid functional impairment as much as possible

Treatment Options by Stage

- **Oropharyngeal carcinoma**
    - Stages I and II
        - RT and surgery show equal success
        - In cases where functional deficit is significant, such as in BOT or tonsil, RT is preferred modality
        - In cases where functional deficit is relatively small, as in tonsil pillar, surgery is preferred modality
    - Stage III
        - Surgical treatment with either RT or CRT postoperatively in select high-risk patients
        - RT can be used in cases of tonsil cancer and combination CRT
    - Stage IV
        - Surgical treatment with both RT and CRT postoperatively in selected high-risk patients
        - CRT used most often
        - Generally, management of these patients is highly complex
        - Surgery is sole treatment in cases of stage IVA tonsillar cancer that has not deeply invaded base of tongue
- **Hypopharyngeal carcinoma**
    - Stage I
        - Radiotherapy alone
        - Surgery (laryngopharyngectomy and neck dissection) ± postoperative radiation
        - Partial laryngopharyngectomy may be considered if pyriform sinus malignancy arises from upper lateral wall
    - Stage II
        - Surgery (laryngopharyngectomy and neck dissection) ± postoperative RT
        - Partial laryngopharyngectomy may be considered if pyriform sinus malignancy arises from upper lateral wall
        - Neoadjuvant chemotherapy may be given to enhance treatment success with surgery or radiation
    - Stage III
        - Surgery
            - Often with postoperative radiation therapy
        - Neoadjuvant chemotherapy may be given to enhance treatment success with surgery or radiation
        - Combinations of adjuvant postoperative RT and CRT may be also given
    - Stage IVA: Resectable cancers
        - Surgery
            - Often with postoperative radiation therapy
        - Neoadjuvant chemotherapy may be given to enhance treatment success with surgery or radiation
        - Combinations of adjuvant postoperative radiotherapy and CRT
    - Stage IVB: Unresectable cancers
        - CRT

Dose Response

- Well-established radiation regimens, total dose and dose per fraction, similar to other sites of head and neck squamous cell carcinomas
- Accelerated fractionation and hyperfractionated RT ↑ local control compared to standard fractionation RT (RTOG 9003)
- Accelerated fractionation with chemotherapy has not shown any tumor control benefit compared to standard radiation fraction with concurrent chemotherapy
- Dose-painting IMRT technique and simultaneous in-field boost have been widely used

Standard Doses

- Definitive RT alone for stage I or stage II oropharyngeal carcinoma
    - Conventional RT
        - 70 Gy in 35 fractions at 2 Gy per fraction, 5 treatments per week
    - Accelerated fractionation with concomitant boost RT
        - 72 Gy in 40 fractions (54 Gy in 30 fractions over 6 weeks, 1.5 Gy as a daily boost during the last 2.5 weeks)
    - Hyperfractionated RT
        - 81.6 Gy at 1.2 Gy per fraction, 2x per day with at least 6 hours between 2 daily fractions
- IMRT
    - High-dose CTV
        - 70 Gy at 2 Gy per fraction to cover the GTVs + 1.0-1.5 cm margins
    - Intermediate-dose CTV
        - 56-63 Gy at 1.7-1.8 Gy per fraction encompasses the intermediate nodal risk sites
    - Elective-dose CTV
        - 56-59.5 Gy at 1.6-1.7 Gy encompasses the elective nodal risk sites
- Simultaneous in-field boost IMRT
    - High-dose CTV

- 66-67.5 Gy at 2.2-2.25 Gy per fraction to cover the GTVs + 1.0-1.5 cm margins
  - Intermediate-dose CTV
    - 60 Gy at 2.0 per fraction encompasses the intermediate nodal risk sites
  - Elective-dose CTV
    - 54 Gy at 1.8 encompasses the elective nodal risk sites
- Adjuvant radiotherapy
  - Indications for adjuvant RT
    - Close surgical margin, multiple nodal involvement, perineural invasion, T4 disease
  - Adjuvant CRT
    - Microscopic positive margins, extracapsular extension, selected T4 tumor
  - 60-66 Gy at 2 Gy per fraction

Organs at Risk Parameters

- Mean dose to bilateral parotid glands: < 26 Gy
- Spinal cord: < 45 Gy
- Brainstem: < 54 Gy
- Mandible: 70 Gy
- Retina: < 45 Gy

Common Techniques

- Thermoplastic mark for immobilization
- Mouth guard placement
- 2.5 mm per axis CT simulation and IV contrast are preferred to distinguish vessels and nodal disease
- PET/CT integrated into RT treatment planning with same setup position when PET/CT to neck area
- 3D conformal
- Whole-neck IMRT
- Upper-neck IMRT with AP to bilateral neck and supraclavicular fossa
  - Tumor located in tonsil or BOT with adequate margin to larynx
  - Larynx and entire cervical esophagus are well spared from high-dose radiation
- Ipsilateral neck irradiation is considered if primary tumor is well lateralized ± only minimal tongue base extension

Landmark Trials

- RTOG 90-03
  - N = 268 locally advanced head & neck cancer (4-arm study)
  - 70 Gy at 2 Gy/fx vs. 81.6 Gy at 1.2 Gy/fx, b.i.d. vs. 67.2 Gy at 1.6 Gy/fx with 2-week break vs. 72 Gy at 1.8 Gy/fx and 1.5 Gy/fx concomitant boost, b.i.d. for last 12 fractions
  - Hyperfractionation and accelerated fractionation with concomitant boost had better locoregional control (LRC); no difference in overall survival (OS)
- GORTEC 94-01
  - N = 226 stage III/IV oropharyngeal carcinoma, randomized RT 70 Gy/35 ± 3 cycles of carboplatin and 5-fluorouracil
  - For CRT and RT, 5-year OS, disease-free survival (DFS), and LRC rates were 22% vs. 16%, 27% vs. 15%, and 48% vs. 25%, respectively
  - Increased acute toxicity in CRT arm (P value not significant), not statistically different in late toxicity
- RTOG 95-10 and EORTC 22931
  - Both studies included local regional advanced head and neck SCCa with pathological high risk features, randomized postoperative RT (60-66 Gy at 2 Gy per fraction) ± concomitant cisplatin (cisplatin 100 mg/m2, days 1, 22, and 43)
    - RTOG 95-10: N = 459, risk factors: 2 or more involved LNs, ECE(+), and microscopic positive margins
      - 3-year DFS 36% → 47%; OS 47% → 56%; local or regional failure 33% → 22% favoring CRT
    - EORTC 22931: N = 334, risk factors: Levels IV or V nodes, PNI(+), ECE(+), positive margin, intravascular embolisms
      - 5-year PFS 36% → 47%; OS 40% → 53%; local or regional relapse 31% → 18% favoring CRT; grade 3 or higher toxicities more frequent in CRT arm
  - ECE &/or microscopically involved surgical margins were most important risk factors
- Head and neck cancer and high-risk HPV
  - Retrospective analysis of RTOG 0129 patients with stage III/IV oropharyngeal SCCa
  - Randomized accelerated RT vs. standard RT, each with concurrent cisplatin
  - N = 323, 64% had HPV-DNA(+) and 68% were p16(+), median follow-up 4.8 years
  - No differences of 3-year OS in groups between accelerated and standard RT arms, 70.3% vs. 64.3%, P = .18
  - HPV(+) patients had better 3-year OS, 82.4% vs. 57.1%, P < .001, and 58% reduction in risk of death

RECOMMENDED FOLLOW-UP

Clinical

- Exam: Every 2-3 months during years 1-2; every 4-6 months during years 2-5; every 12 months at > 5 years
- Speech, hearing, and swallowing evaluation and rehabilitation as indicated
- Smoking cessation and alcohol counseling as indicated
- Dental care with periodic teeth cleaning and fluoride supplement as indicated

Radiographic

- Post-treatment baseline imaging of primary and neck: 3 months
- Annual chest imaging or as clinically indicated

Laboratory

- TSH every 6-12 months if neck irradiated

SELECTED REFERENCES

1. American Joint Committee on Cancer: AJCC Cancer Staging Manual. 7th ed. New York: Springer. 41-56, 2010
2. Ang KK et al: Human papillomavirus and survival of patients with oropharyngeal cancer. N Engl J Med. 363(1):24-35, 2010
3. Guido A et al: Combined 18F-FDG-PET/CT imaging in radiotherapy target delineation for head-and-neck cancer. Int J Radiat Oncol Biol Phys. 73(3):759-63, 2009
4. Lee NY et al: Concurrent chemotherapy and intensity-modulated radiotherapy for locoregionally advanced laryngeal and hypopharyngeal cancers. Int J Radiat Oncol Biol Phys. 69(2):459-68, 2007

5. Bernier J et al: Defining risk levels in locally advanced head and neck cancers: a comparative analysis of concurrent postoperative radiation plus chemotherapy trials of the EORTC (#22931) and RTOG (# 9501). Head Neck. 27(10):843-50, 2005
6. Bernier J et al: Postoperative irradiation with or without concomitant chemotherapy for locally advanced head and neck cancer. N Engl J Med. 350(19):1945-52, 2004
7. Cooper JS et al: Postoperative concurrent radiotherapy and chemotherapy for high-risk squamous-cell carcinoma of the head and neck. N Engl J Med. 350(19):1937-44, 2004
8. O'Sullivan B et al: The benefits and pitfalls of ipsilateral radiotherapy in carcinoma of the tonsillar region. Int J Radiat Oncol Biol Phys. 51(2):332-43, 2001
9. Fu KK et al: A Radiation Therapy Oncology Group (RTOG) phase III randomized study to compare hyperfractionation and two variants of accelerated fractionation to standard fractionation radiotherapy for head and neck squamous cell carcinomas: first report of RTOG 9003. Int J Radiat Oncol Biol Phys. 48(1):7-16, 2000

(*Left*) *Axial PET/CECT of a 70-year-old man shows squamous cell carcinoma of the posterior wall. The large hypermetabolic lesion* ➔ *arising from the left-sided posterior pharyngeal wall extends across the midline.* (*Right*) *Axial PET/CECT of the same patient shows bilateral FDG uptake in level II lymph nodes* ➔. *The primary* ➔ *is still apparent on this axial image.*

T3 N2c M0 Posterior Pharyngeal Wall

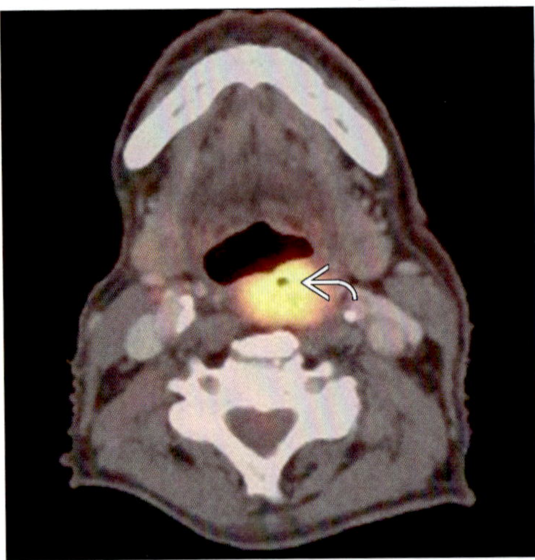

T3 N2c M0 Posterior Pharyngeal Wall

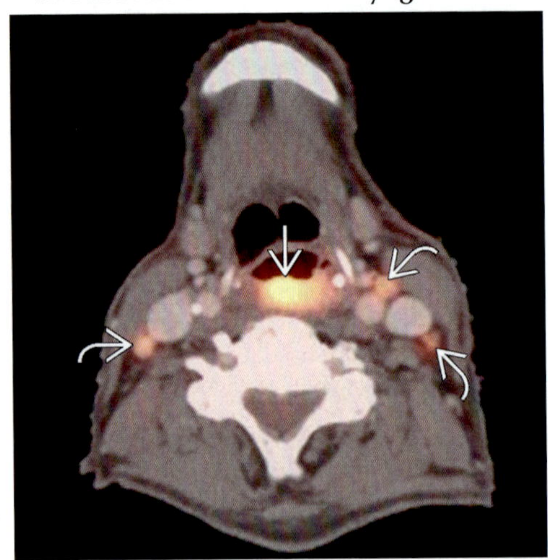

(*Left*) *Axial fused PET/CT in the same patient integrated into IMRT planning shows the PTV1* ➔ *receiving 70 Gy at 2 Gy per fraction, and PTV2* ➔ *covers the intermediate nodal risk sites (59.5 Gy at 1.7 Gy per fraction).* (*Right*) *Coronal image of the same patient with PET/CT integrated IMRT planning shows that PTV1* ➔ *encompasses the primary* ➔ *and bilateral nodal disease* ➔. *PTV2* ➔ *covers the intermediate nodal risk sites.*

T3 N2c M0 Posterior Pharyngeal Wall

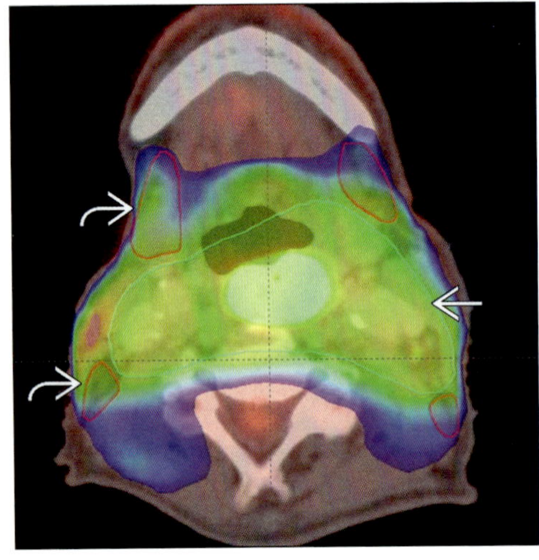

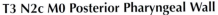

T3 N2c M0 Posterior Pharyngeal Wall

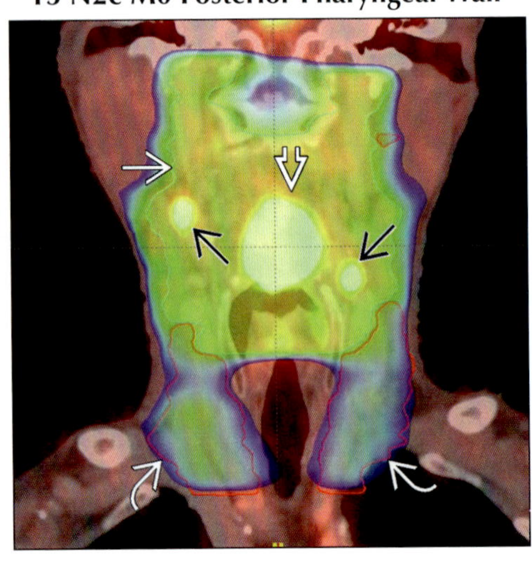

(*Left*) *Follow-up contrast-enhanced PET/CT in the same patient 3 months after definitive chemoradiation shows complete resolution in the posterior pharyngeal wall.* (*Right*) *Axial contrast-enhancing PET/CT image of the same patient demonstrates complete resolution of the bilateral lymphadenopathy. Ten months post CRT, the patient developed widely metastatic disease without locoregional recurrence and died a few months later.*

T3 N2c M0 3-Month Follow-Up

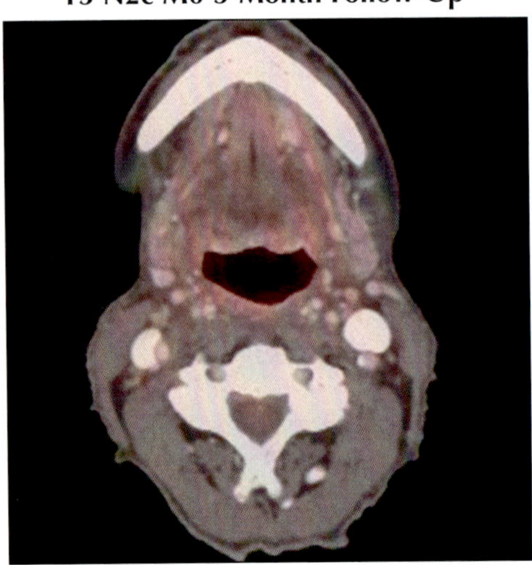

T3 N2c M0 3-Month Follow-Up

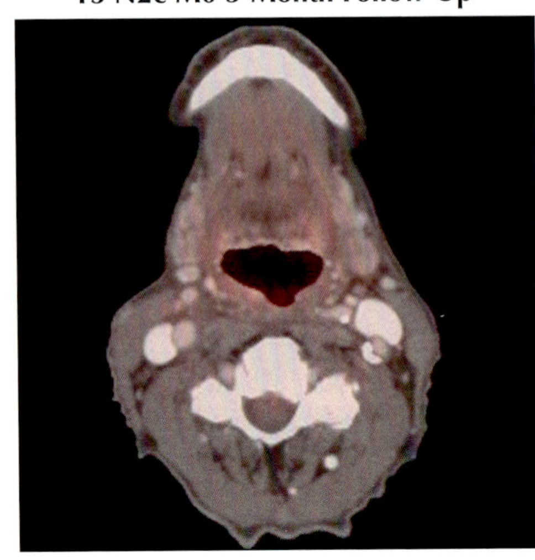

T3 N3 M0 Right Tonsil

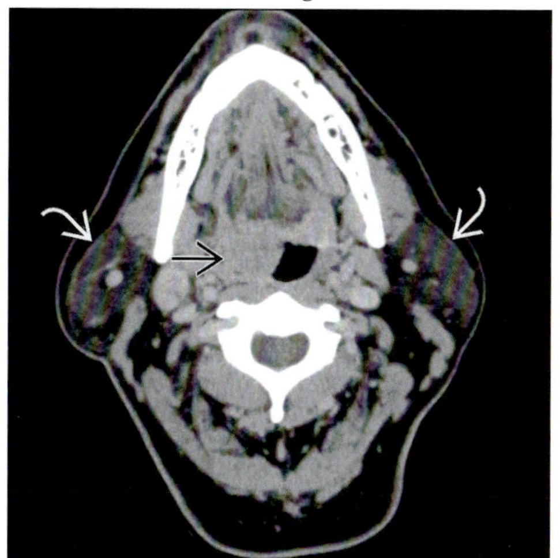

T3 N3 M0 Right Tonsil

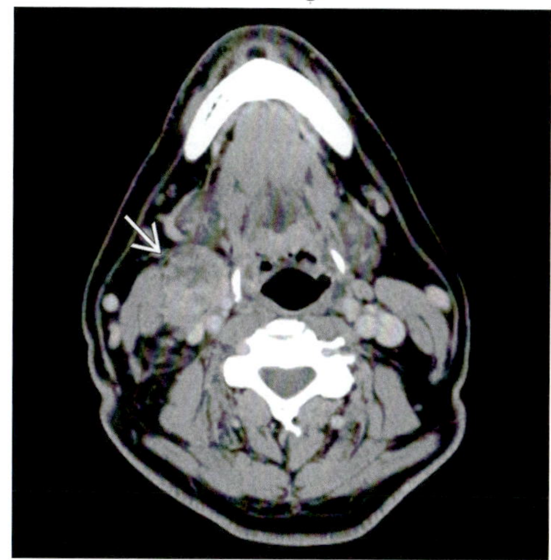

(Left) *Axial CECT shows a 4.5 cm SCCa of the right tonsil ➙ in 57-year-old man with T3 N3 M0, stage IVB disease. The > 4 cm tumor indicates stage T3. The parotid glands ➙ are easily seen bilaterally.* ***(Right)*** *Axial CECT shows a large necrotic lymph node ➙ with extracapsular involvement. The node measured 6.5 cm pathologically, hence, it was stage N3.*

T3 N3 M0 Right Tonsil: Robotic Surgery

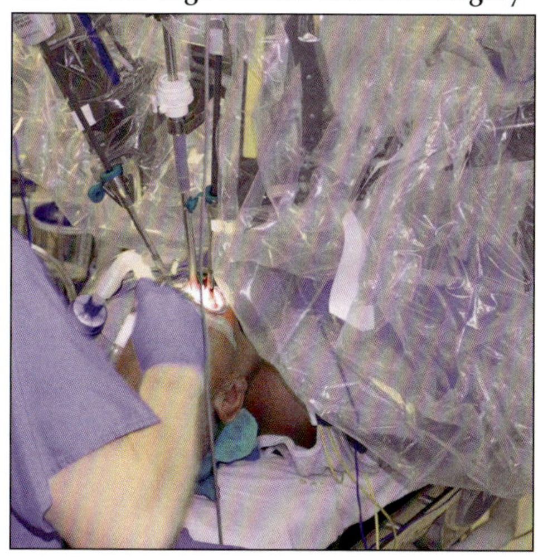

T3 N3 M0 Right Tonsil: Robotic Surgery

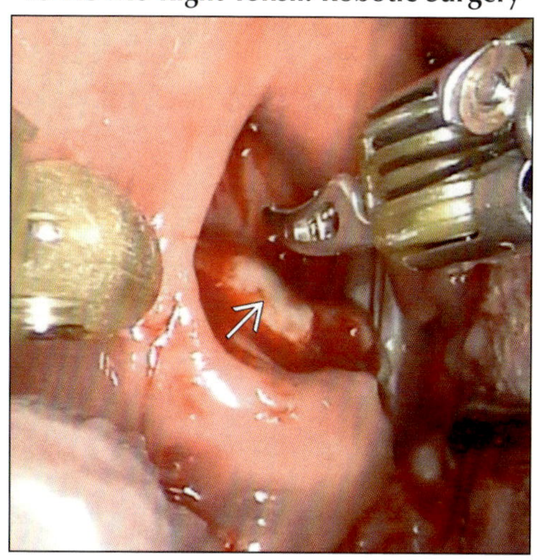

(Left) *Intraoperative photograph shows the transoral robotic surgery for right tonsillar tumor resection and a right-modified neck dissection. (Courtesy J. Hunt, MD.)* ***(Right)*** *Photograph shows the right tonsillar tumor ➙, which was resected via a transoral robotic surgery. Margins were pathologically involved. (Courtesy J. Hunt, MD.)*

T3 N3 M0 Right Tonsil: Postop CRT

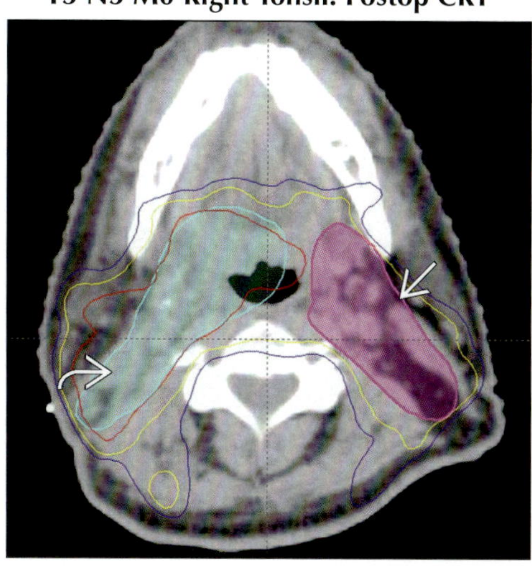

T3 N3 M0 Right Tonsil: Postop CRT

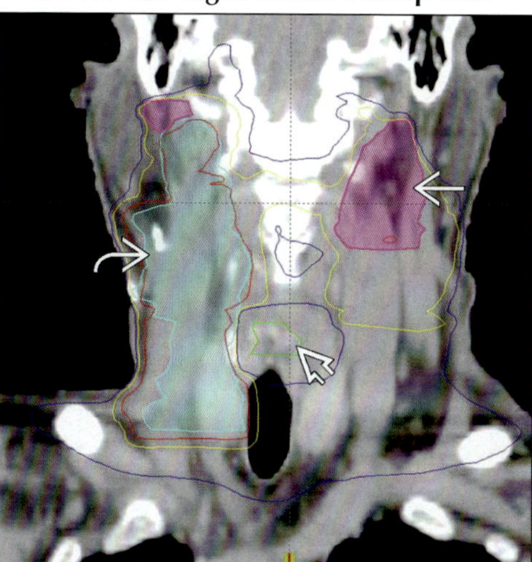

(Left) *Axial CT shows postop chemo IMRT. 66 Gy was delivered to PTV1 ➙ covering preop GTVs positive margins, and 56.1 Gy to PTV2 ➙ to elective nodal sites. Red, yellow, and blue lines indicate the 66 Gy, 56 Gy, and 50 Gy, respectively.* ***(Right)*** *Coronal CT of the same patient shows coverage of PTV1 ➙ and PTV2 ➙. With an AP field to the bilateral lower neck and supraclavicular fossa, the larynx ➙ and the entire esophagus were blocked.*

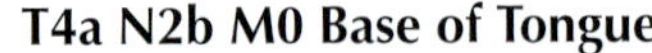
T4a N2b M0 Base of Tongue

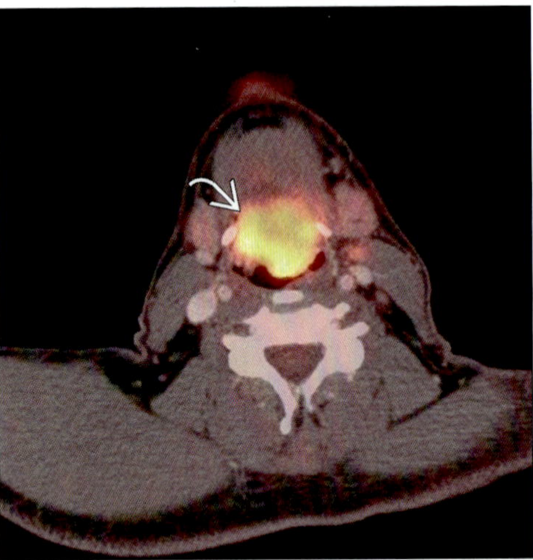

T4a N2b M0 Base of Tongue

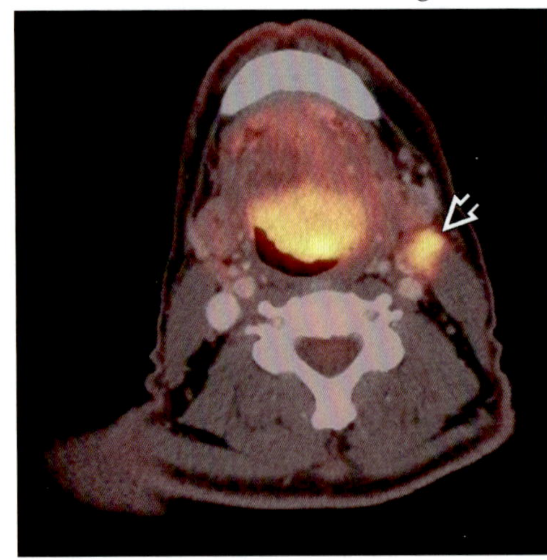

*(**Left**) Axial fused contrast-enhanced PET/CT in a 63-year-old man shows a SCCa involving extrinsic muscles of the tongue (T4a). (**Right**) Axial fused contrast-enhanced PET/CT of the same patient shows a hypermetabolic node in the left level II region with the primary readily evident. Multiple involved ipsilateral nodes with none > 6 cm indicates N2b.*

T4a N2b M0 Base of Tongue

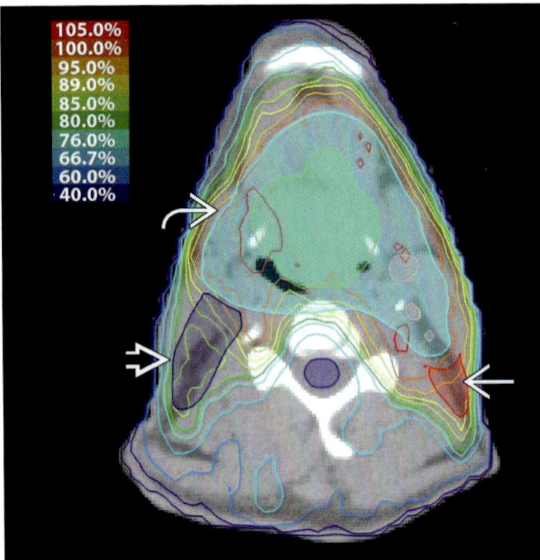

T4a N2b M0 Base of Tongue

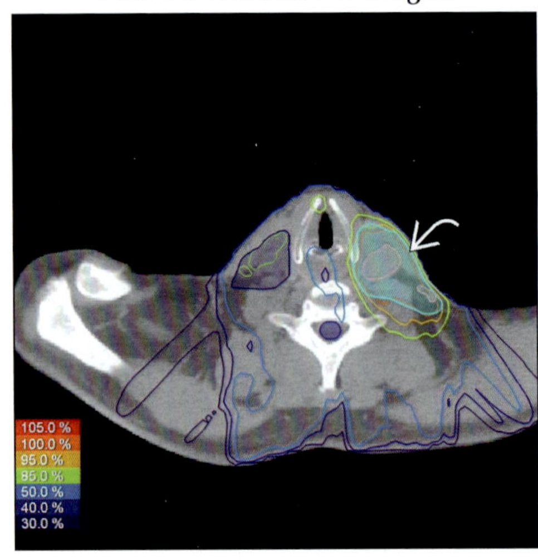

*(**Left**) Axial image in the same patient of IMRT plan: 67.5 Gy at 2.25 Gy/fx to PTV1, 60 Gy at 2.0 Gy/fx to PTV2, and 54 Gy at 1.8 Gy/fx to PTV3. (**Right**) Axial CT shows IMRT plan of the same patient with PTV1 getting 67.5 Gy in 30 fractions with simultaneous in-field boost technique to the left level III nodes. The larynx was covered by 50% isodose line with a small area of the anterior commissure receiving 85% of prescription dose.*

T4a N2b M0 Base of Tongue: 3 Months Post Treatment

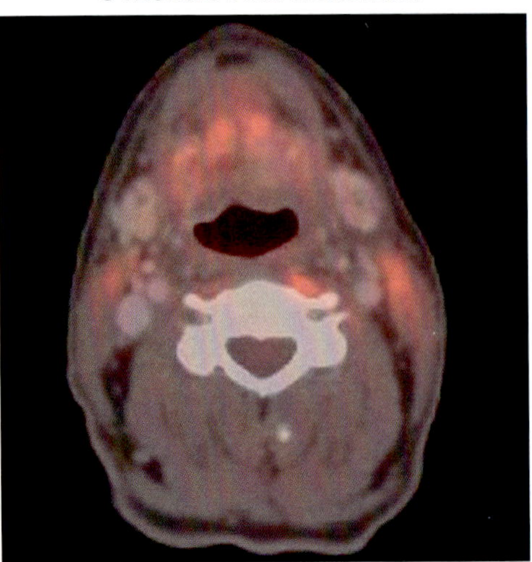

T4a N2b M0 Base of Tongue: 3 Months Post Treatment

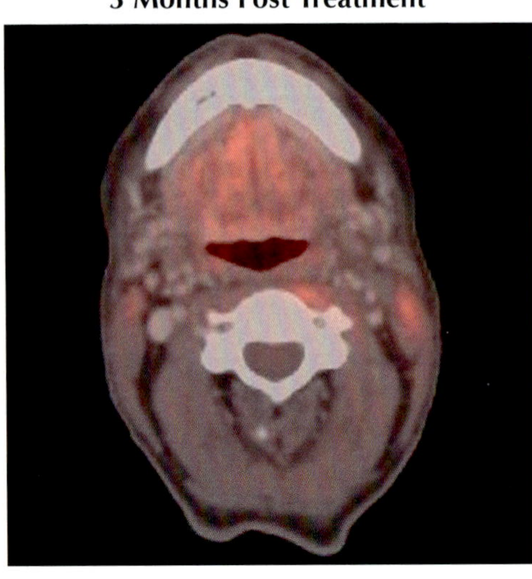

*(**Left**) Follow-up contrast-enhanced PET/CT in the same patient 3 months after completion of CRT shows complete resolution in the primary base of tongue. Note mildly avid FDG uptake in the normal muscular structures. (**Right**) Post-treatment PET/CT in the same patient demonstrated complete response in the nodal sites. There was no locoregional recurrence over 2 years of follow-up. There was also no evidence of laryngeal edema or soft tissue fibrosis.*

T4a N2c M0 Base of Tongue

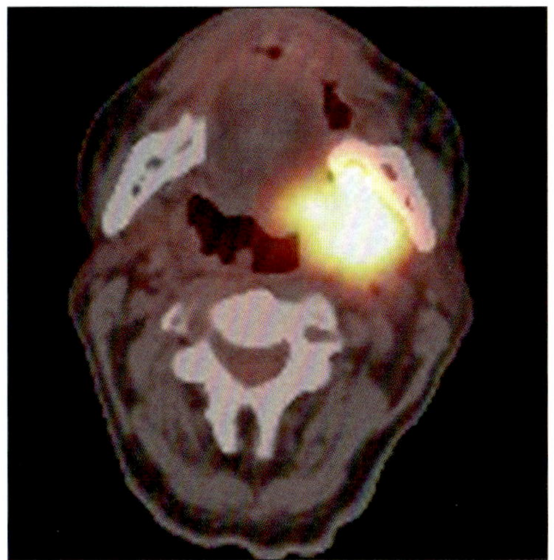

T4a N2c M0 Base of Tongue

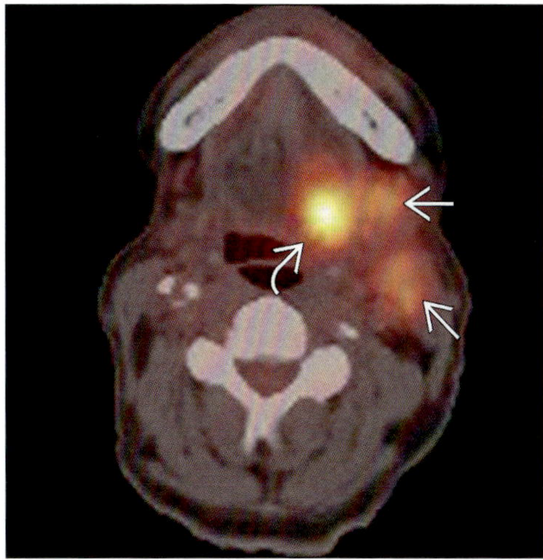

*(**Left**) Axial PET/CT demonstrates a large hypermetabolic soft tissue mass arising from the left-sided base of tongue with left parapharyngeal space extension in a 61-year-old woman with a diagnosis of T4a N2c M0, stage IVA SCCa. (**Right**) Axial PET/CT in the same patient shows the primary base of tongue tumor deeply involving the extrinsic muscles ➩, with 2 hypermetabolic lymph nodes ➔ in the left level II region.*

T4a N2c M0 Base of Tongue

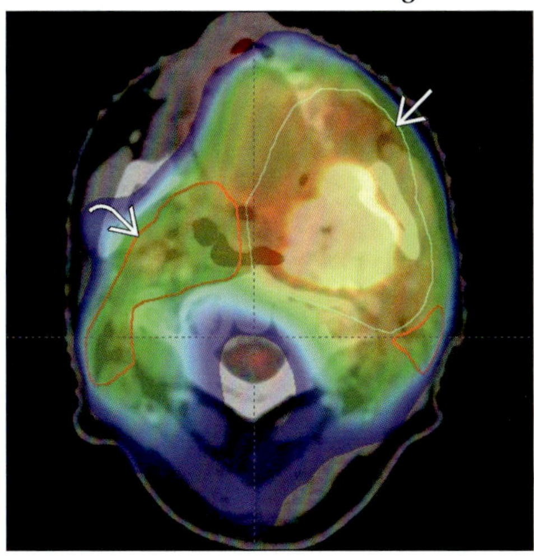

T4a N2c M0 Base of Tongue

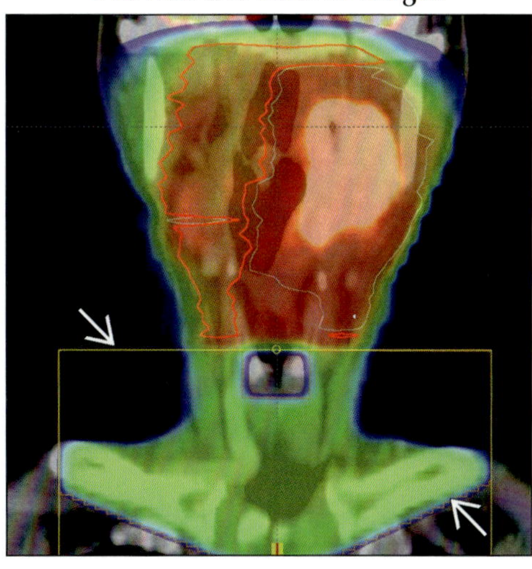

*(**Left**) PET/CT in the same patient integrated into IMRT planning with 70 Gy delivered at 2 Gy/fx to PTV1 ➔, 59.5 Gy at 1.7 Gy/fx to PTV2 ➩, and 56 Gy at 1.6 Gy/fx to PTV3 (not shown). Note avoidance of spinal cord with IMRT (blue = 45 Gy). (**Right**) Coronal PET/CT in the same patient shows IMRT to the upper neck matched to an AP field ➔ to the lower neck and supraclavicular fossa. A block was used to omit dose to the larynx.*

T4a N2c M0 Base of Tongue: 3 Months Post Treatment

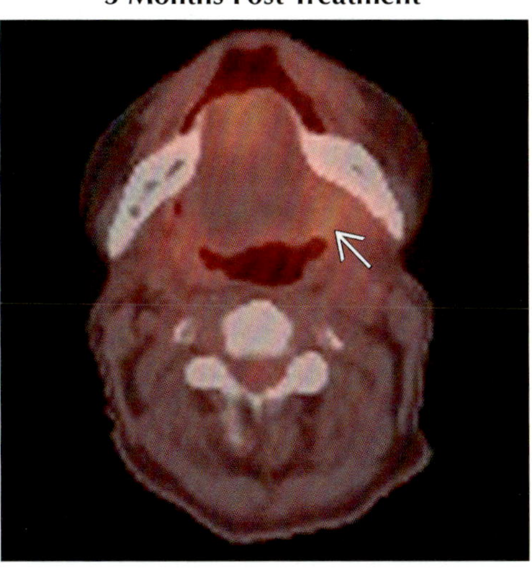

T4a N2c M0 Base of Tongue: 3 Months Post Treatment

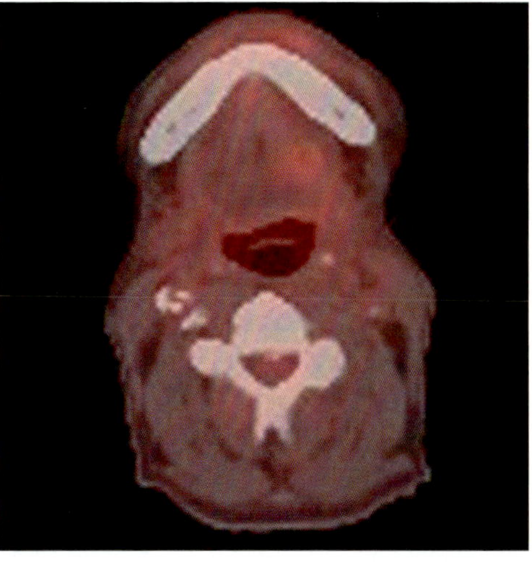

*(**Left**) Axial image in the same patient on a 3-month post-CRT PET/CT shows mild hypermetabolic uptake at the primary ➔. Biopsy of the area showed no evidence of residual disease, and there was no evidence of recurrence over 4 years of follow-up. (**Right**) Axial fused PET/CT documents complete resolution in the nodal sites and primary 3 months after definitive chemoradiation.*

T4a N3 M0 Pyriform Sinus

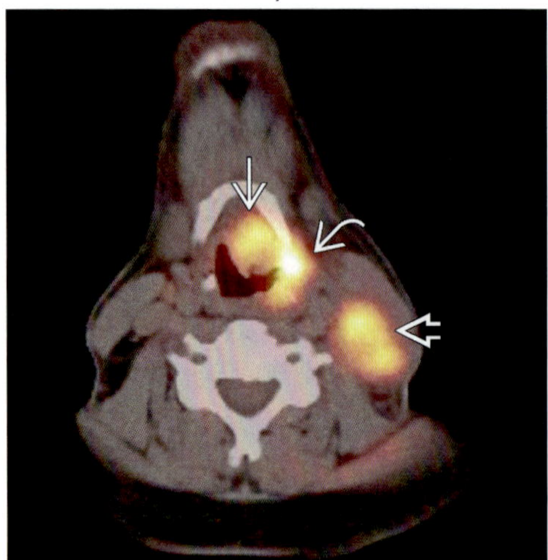

T4a N3 M0 Pyriform Sinus

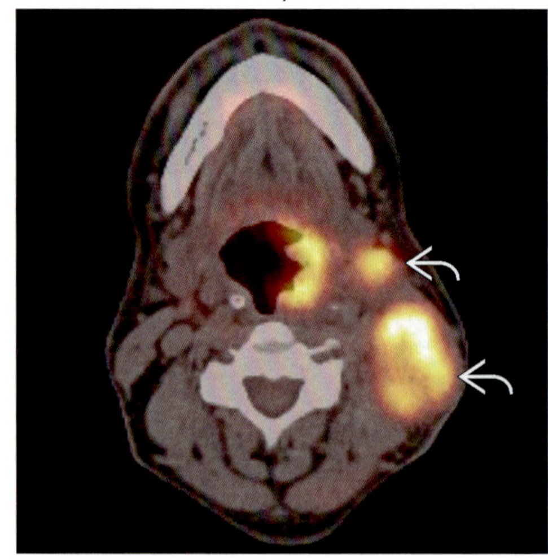

(Left) Axial fused PET/CT of a 61-year-old man demonstrates the pyriform sinus tumor extending into the preepiglottic space ➡ and left neck soft tissue ➡ with a hypermetabolic lymph node ➡. *(Right)* Axial PET/CT of the same patient shows hypermetabolic level II lymph nodes ➡.

T4a N3 M0 Pyriform Sinus

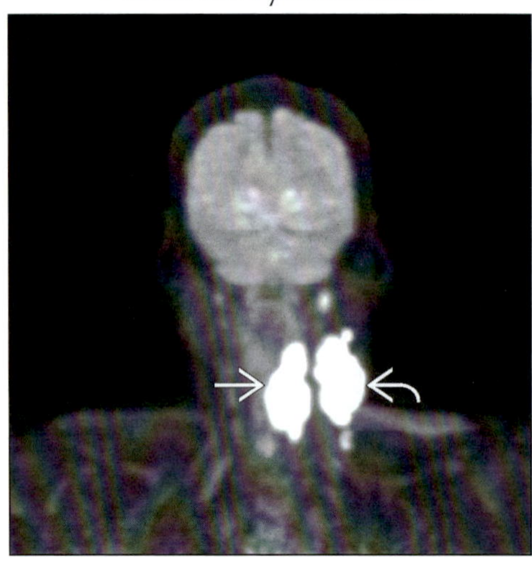

T4a N3 M0 Pyriform Sinus

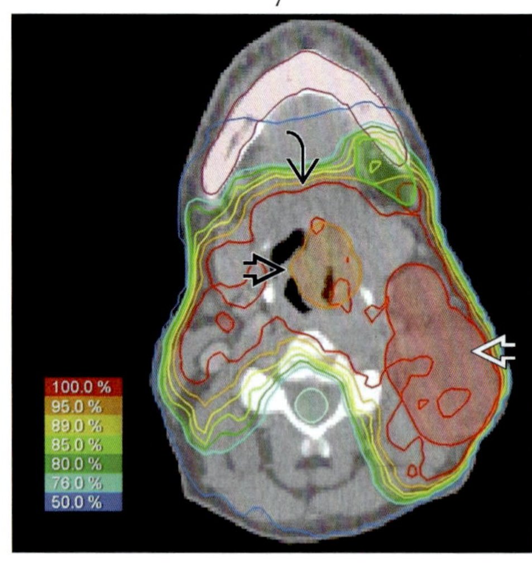

(Left) Coronal PET of the same patient shows hypermetabolic left pyriform sinus tumor ➡ and bulky left neck node ➡. *(Right)* IMRT plan in the same patient shows 100% isodose line ➡ covering the GTV ➡ and neck nodes ➡. Simultaneous in-field boost was used: 67.5 Gy at 2.25 Gy/fx to PTV1 (GTVs + margins), 60 Gy at 2 Gy/fx to PTV2 (intermediate risk sites), and 54 Gy at 1.8 Gy/fx to PTV3 (elective nodal sites).

T4a N3 M0 Pyriform Sinus

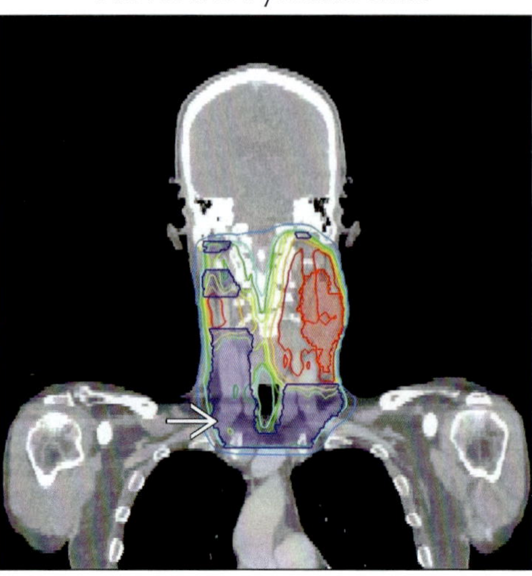

T4a N3 M0 Pyriform Sinus

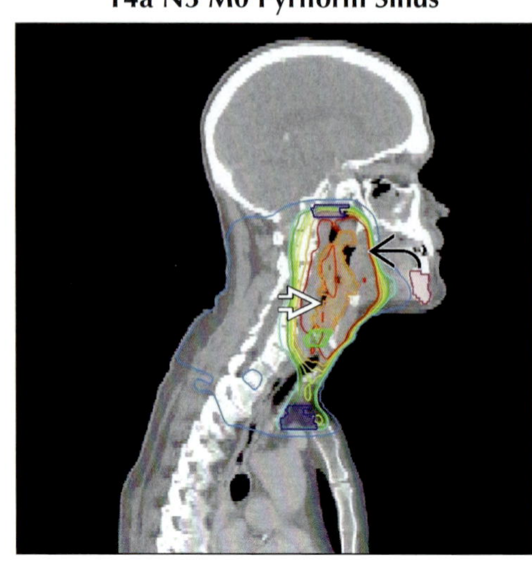

(Left) Coronal image of the same patient shows the volume of elective irradiation in blue ➡ to the bilateral lower neck and supraclavicular fossa. Uninvolved nodes were treated to 54 Gy at 1/8 Gy/fx. Concurrent chemo was used. *(Right)* Sagittal image of the same patient shows primary tumor extension ➡ in orange and 100% prescription dose coverage ➡ to the gross disease.

Acute Skin Reaction

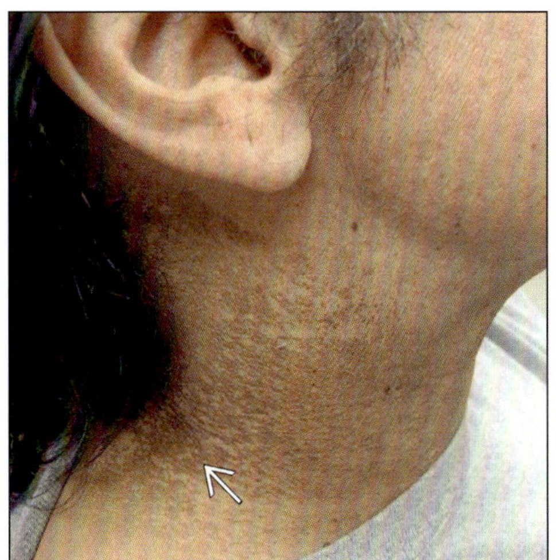

Fibrosis and Skin Telangiectasia

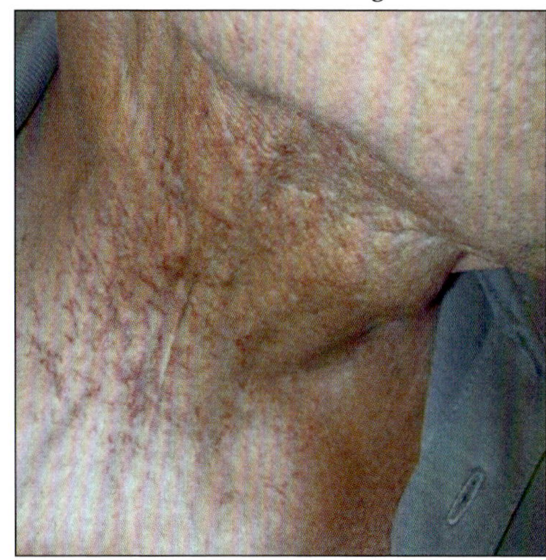

*(**Left**) Photo shows skin hyperpigmentation ➡ 1 month post definitive chemoradiation for SCCa of the base of tongue. The degree of hyperpigmentation is variable between patients. (**Right**) Photo shows a patient with T1 N2b SCCa of the tonsil, who received postoperative CRT 66 Gy with concomitant cisplatin 5 years previously. There was no evidence of recurrence, but soft tissue fibrosis and skin telangiectasias are evident.*

Soft Tissue Edema

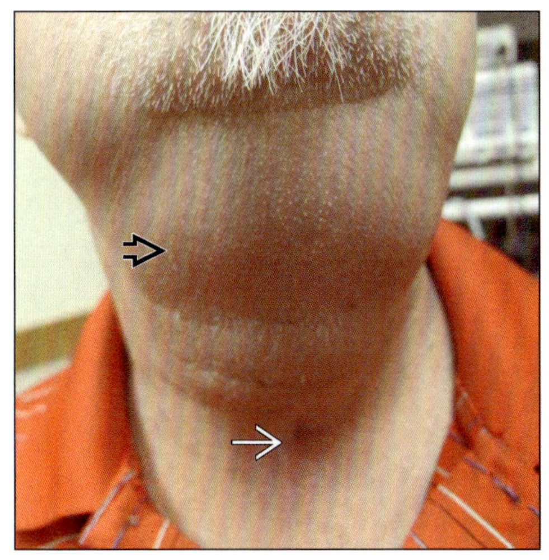

Soft Tissue Edema

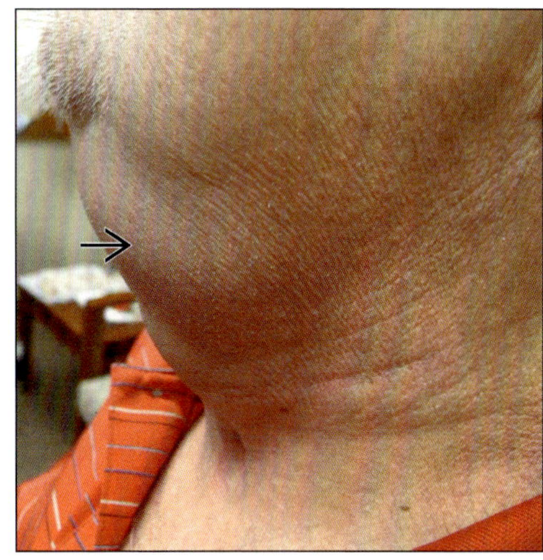

*(**Left**) Photo shows a patient with stage IVA (T4a N2c M0) SCCa of the base of tongue, status post tracheostomy prior to CRT for airway obstruction. Soft tissue edema ⇨ was seen at 3 months post-treatment with no evidence of residual disease at primary and nodal sites. The well-healed tracheostomy site ➡ is seen. (**Right**) Lateral photo in the same patient displays the soft tissue edema →.*

Brachial Plexus Injury

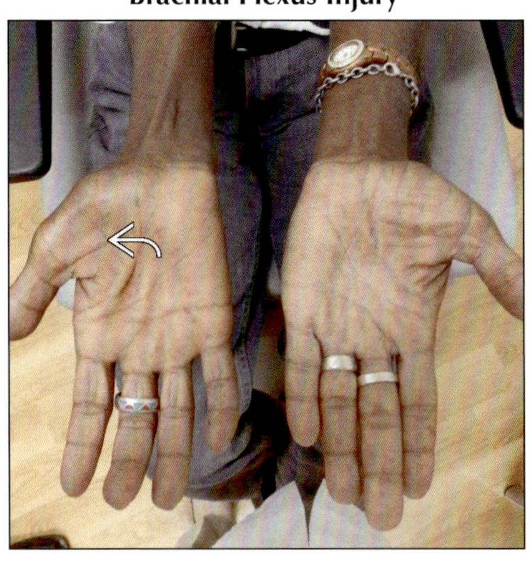

Brachial Plexus Injury

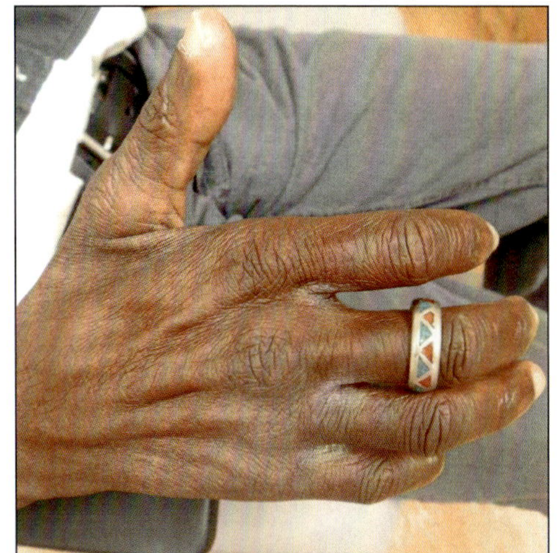

*(**Left**) Photo shows a patient with T4a N2c M0 SCCa of the base of tongue who received 70 Gy in 35 fractions concurrent with cisplatin. The right lower neck and supraclavicular fossa received 70 Gy for gross disease. A 9-month follow-up exam demonstrates lack of sensation, weakness, and muscular atrophy ➡ of the thenar eminence. (**Right**) Photo shows the same patient with a "claw hand" from brachial plexus injury.*

LARYNX

(T) Primary Tumor

Adapted from 7th edition AJCC Staging Forms.

TNM	*Definitions*
TX	Primary tumor cannot be assessed
T0	No evidence of primary tumor
Tis	Carcinoma in situ
Supraglottis	
T1	Tumor limited to 1 subsite of supraglottis with normal vocal cord mobility
T2	Tumor invades mucosa of > 1 adjacent subsite of supraglottis or glottis or region outside the supraglottis (e.g., mucosa of base of tongue, vallecula, medial wall of pyriform sinus) without fixation of the larynx
T3	Tumor limited to larynx with vocal cord fixation &/or invades any of the following: Postcricoid area, preepiglottic space, paraglottic space, &/or inner cortex of thyroid cartilage
T4a	Moderately advanced local disease: Tumor invades through the thyroid cartilage &/or invades tissues beyond the larynx (e.g., trachea, soft tissues of neck including deep extrinsic muscle of the tongue, strap muscles, thyroid, or esophagus)
T4b	Very advanced local disease: Tumor invades prevertebral space, encases carotid artery, or invades mediastinal structures
Glottis	
T1	Tumor limited to the vocal cord(s) (may involve anterior or posterior commissure) with normal mobility
T1a	Tumor limited to 1 vocal cord
T1b	Tumor involves both vocal cords
T2	Tumor extends to supraglottis &/or subglottis, &/or with impaired vocal cord mobility
T3	Tumor limited to the larynx with vocal cord fixation &/or invasion of paraglottic space, &/or inner cortex of the thyroid cartilage
T4a	Moderately advanced local disease: Tumor invades through the outer cortex of the thyroid cartilage &/or invades tissues beyond the larynx (e.g., trachea, soft tissues of neck including deep extrinsic muscle of the tongue, strap muscles, thyroid, or esophagus)
T4b	Very advanced local disease: Tumor invades prevertebral space, encases carotid artery, or invades mediastinal structures
Subglottis	
T1	Tumor limited to the subglottis
T2	Tumor extends to vocal cord(s) with normal or impaired mobility
T3	Tumor limited to larynx with vocal cord fixation
T4a	Moderately advanced local disease: Tumor invades cricoid or thyroid cartilage &/or invades tissues beyond the larynx (e.g., trachea, soft tissues of neck including deep extrinsic muscles of the tongue, strap muscles, thyroid, or esophagus)
T4b	Very advanced local disease: Tumor invades prevertebral space, encases carotid artery, or invades mediastinal structures

(N) Regional Lymph Nodes	*Adapted from 7th edition AJCC Staging Forms.*
NX	Regional lymph nodes cannot be assessed
N0	No regional lymph node metastasis*
N1	Metastasis in a single ipsilateral lymph node, ≤ 3 cm in greatest dimension
N2	Metastasis in a single ipsilateral lymph node, > 3 cm but ≤ 6 cm in greatest dimension, or in multiple ipsilateral lymph nodes, none > 6 cm in greatest dimension, or in bilateral or contralateral lymph nodes, none > 6 cm in greatest dimension
N2a	Metastasis in a single ipsilateral lymph node > 3 cm but ≤ 6 cm in greatest dimension
N2b	Metastasis in multiple ipsilateral lymph nodes, none > 6 cm in greatest dimension
N2c	Metastasis in bilateral or contralateral lymph nodes, none > 6 cm in greatest dimension
N3	Metastasis in a lymph node > 6 cm in greatest dimension

**Metastases at level VII are considered regional lymph node metastases.*

(M) Distant Metastasis	*Adapted from 7th edition AJCC Staging Forms.*
M0	No distant metastasis
M1	Distant metastasis

(G) Histologic Grade	*Adapted from 7th edition AJCC Staging Forms.*
GX	Grade cannot be assessed
G1	Well differentiated
G2	Moderately differentiated
G3	Poorly differentiated
G4	Undifferentiated

LARYNX

AJCC Stages/Prognostic Groups

Adapted from 7th edition AJCC Staging Forms.

Stage	*T*	*N*	*M*
0	Tis	N0	M0
I	T1	N0	M0
II	T2	N0	M0
III	T3	N0	M0
	T1	N1	M0
	T2	N1	M0
	T3	N1	M0
IVA	T4a	N0	M0
	T4a	N1	M0
	T1	N2	M0
	T2	N2	M0
	T3	N2	M0
	T4a	N2	M0
IVB	T4b	Any N	M0
	Any T	N3	M0
IVC	Any T	Any N	M1

T1a: Glottis

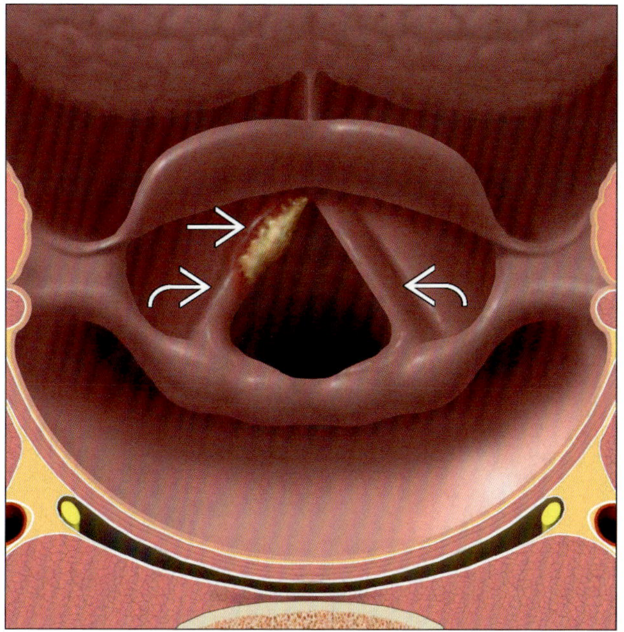

Graphic depicts the true vocal cords ➦, with tumor ➡ affecting 1 vocal cord. Cord mobility is normal in T1a glottic disease.

T1b: Glottis

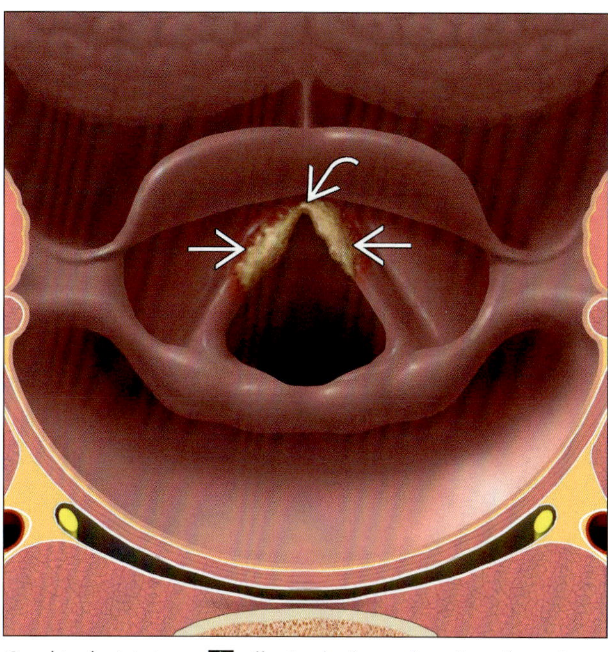

Graphic depicts tumor ➡ affecting both vocal cords and crossing along the anterior commissure ➦, consistent with T1b glottic disease. As with a T1a tumor, mobility is not impaired in T1b glottic disease.

T1: Supraglottis

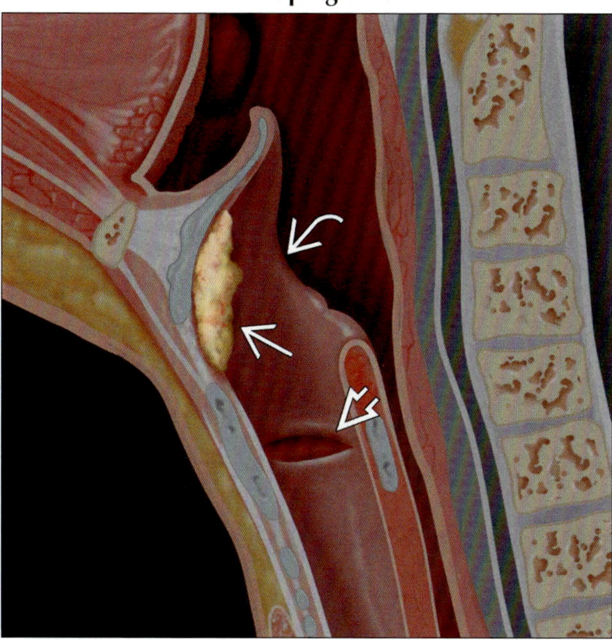

Graphic depicts a T1 supraglottic tumor ➡ involving the epiglottis. For purposes of staging, the AJCC divides the supraglottis into the supra- and infrahyoid epiglottis, the aryepiglottic folds ➦ (laryngeal aspect), arytenoids, and ventricular bands ⇨ (false cords). T1 tumors are those limited to 1 supraglottic subsite.

T1: Subglottis

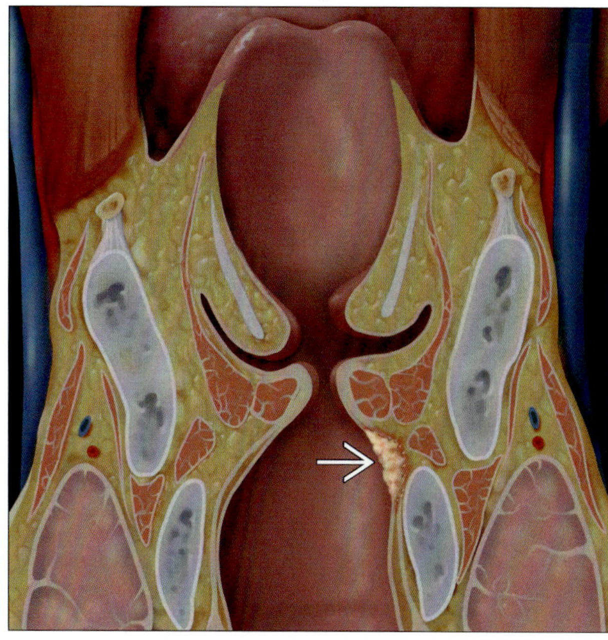

Graphic shows tumor ➡ limited to the subglottis, which includes mucosa of the undersurface of the true vocal cords, consistent with T1 disease. As with T1 tumors of the supraglottis and the glottis, T1 subglottic tumors do not affect normal vocal cord mobility.

T2: Glottis

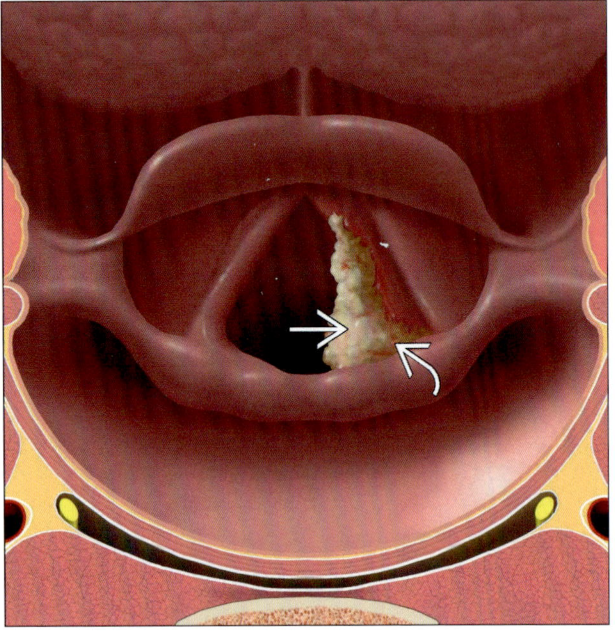

Graphic shows tumor ➡ with extension into the aryepiglottic fold ↪ with distortion of the vocal cord.

T2: Glottis

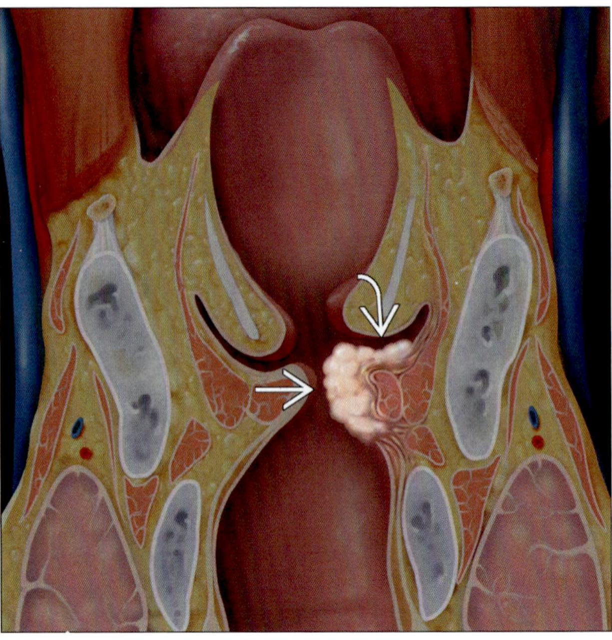

Coronal graphic shows tumor ➡ that extends from the glottis to the laryngeal ventricle ↪, part of the supraglottis. This is consistent with T2 disease.

T2: Supraglottis

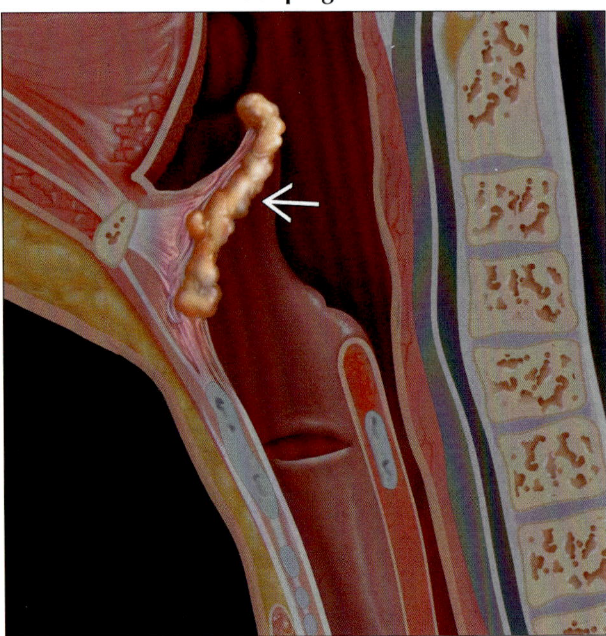

Sagittal graphic depicts a T2 supraglottic tumor ➡, which invades both suprahyoid and infrahyoid portions of the epiglottis. Involvement of more than 1 adjacent subsite of the supraglottis or glottis or region outside the supraglottis (e.g., mucosa of base of tongue) without fixation of the larynx is T2 disease.

T2: Subglottis

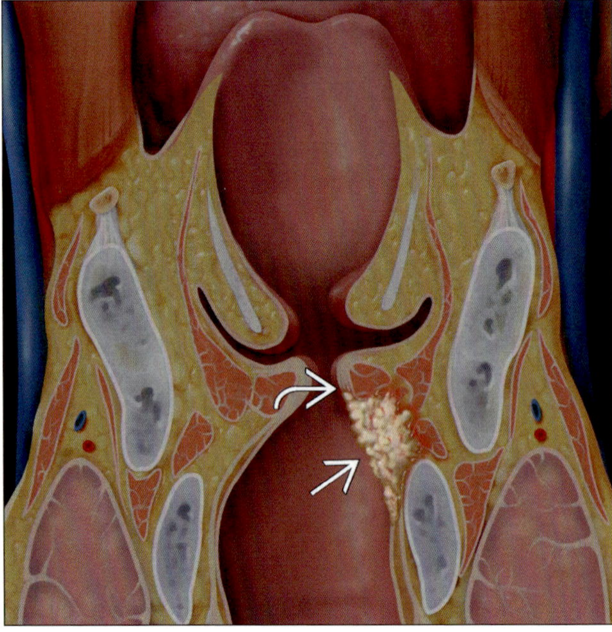

Graphic depicts tumor ➡ that extends from the subglottis to the true vocal cord ↪, consistent with T2 disease. Vocal cord mobility may be either normal or impaired, but the vocal cords are not fixed in T2 disease. Either 1 or both vocal cords may be affected.

T3: Glottis

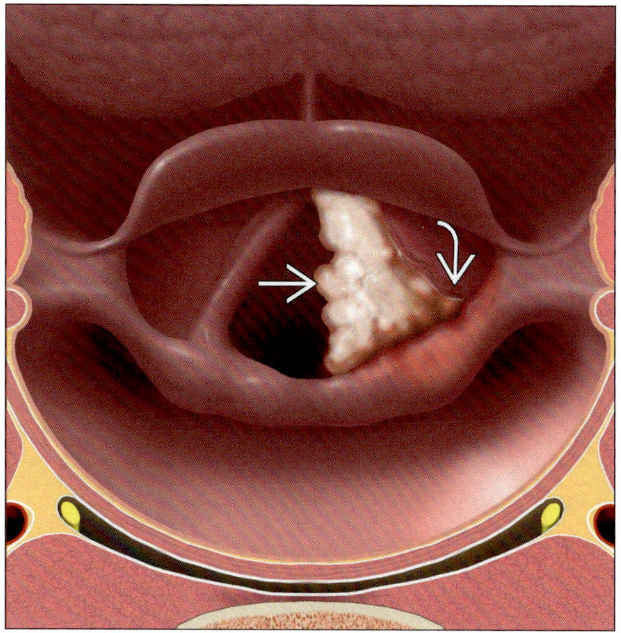

Graphic illustrates T3 glottic disease ➡, defined as tumor limited to the larynx with vocal cord fixation &/or invasion of paraglottic space ➡ &/or inner cortex of the thyroid cartilage.

T3: Glottis

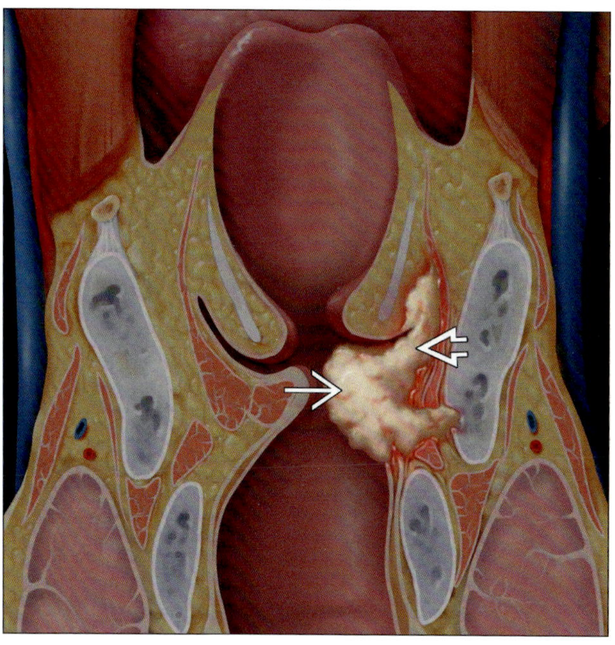

Coronal graphic depicts tumor ➡ involving the true vocal cords with extension into the laryngeal ventricle (supraglottis) and paraglottic space ➡. Tumor can extend to the inner cortex of the thyroid cartilage and still be considered a T3 tumor.

T3: Supraglottis

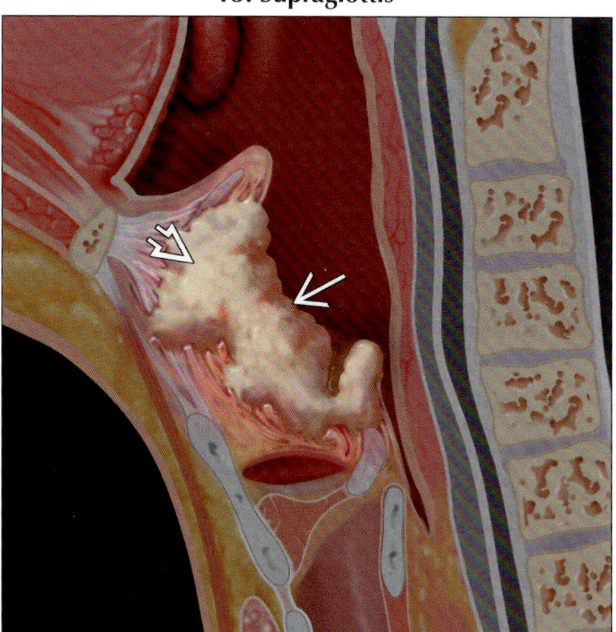

Graphic depicts tumor ➡ involving the epiglottis, false cords, and aryepiglottic folds with local invasion. If the postcricoid area, preepiglottic space ➡, paraglottic space, or inner cortex of the thyroid cartilage is affected by a supraglottic tumor (or if there is vocal cord fixation), the tumor is graded as T3.

T3: Subglottis

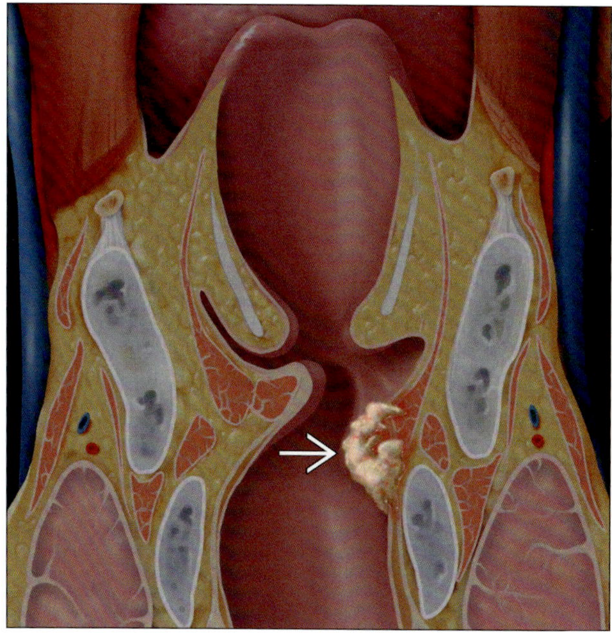

Graphic demonstrates a subglottic tumor ➡ with invasion of the true vocal cord. Clinically evident vocal cord fixation makes this T3 subglottic disease.

T4a: Glottis

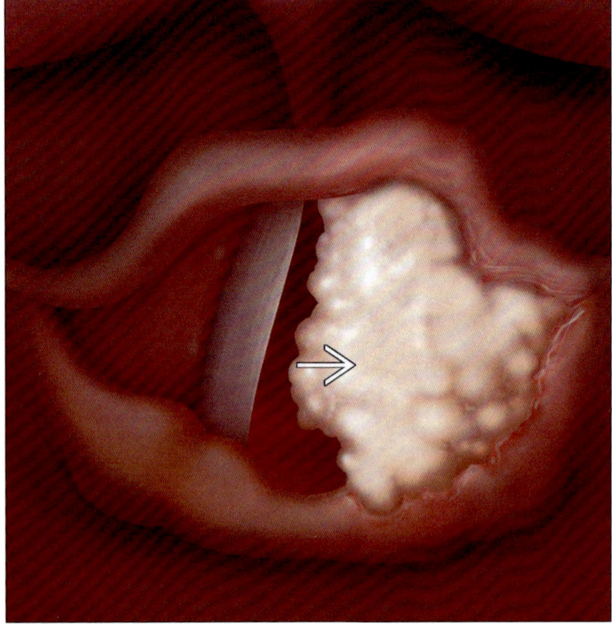

Graphic depicts a T4a glottic tumor ➔ with invasion of the paraglottic fat and adjacent structures, which is moderately advanced local disease. The distinction between "moderately" and "very" advanced local disease (T4a vs. T4b) for laryngeal tumors was introduced by the AJCC in 2010.

T4a: Glottis

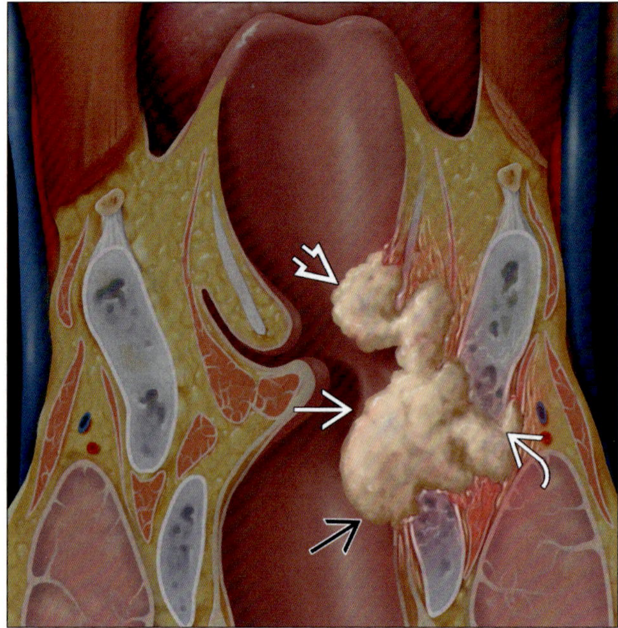

Graphic depicts a T4a transglottic tumor that involves the false vocal cord ➔, glottis ➔, and subglottis ➔, with invasion through the outer cortex of the thyroid cartilage ➔.

T4a: Supraglottis

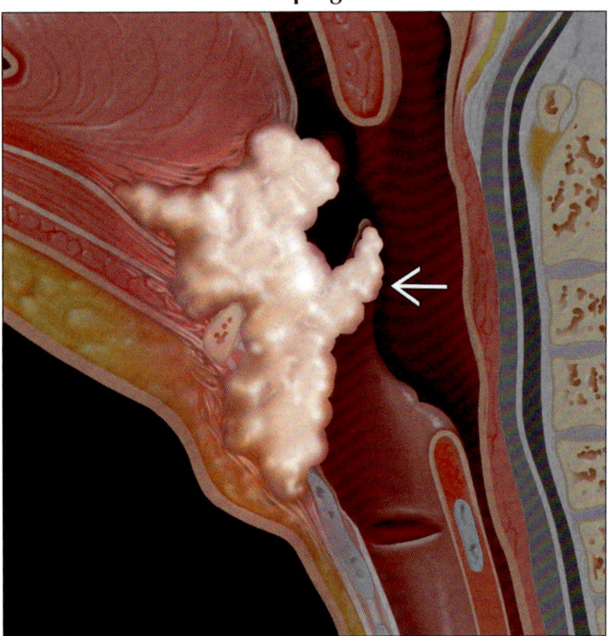

Graphic depicts a T4a supraglottic tumor ➔ involving the epiglottis with invasion of the tongue base and extrinsic tongue musculature, as well as the thyroid cartilage. The definitions of T4a for glottic, supraglottic, and subglottic tumors vary only in the precise type of cartilage that is most immediately vulnerable.

T4a: Subglottis

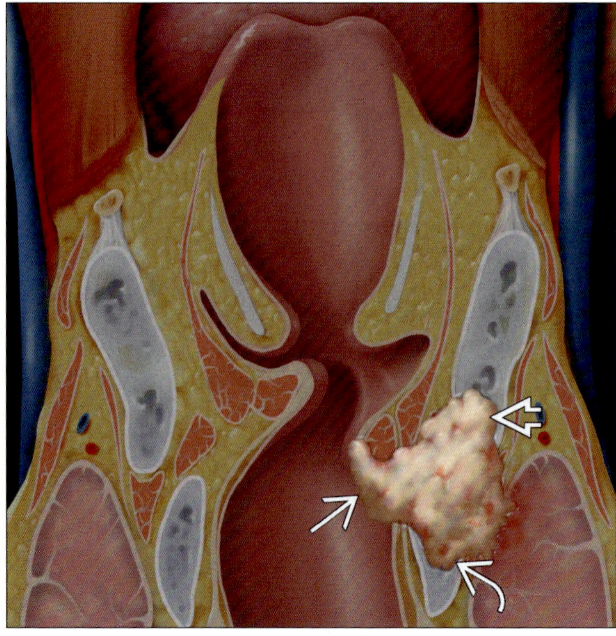

Graphic depicts a T4a subglottic tumor ➔ that invades the cricoid ➔ and thyroid cartilage ➔. T4a tumors also may invade tissues beyond the larynx (e.g., trachea, soft tissues of neck including deep extrinsic muscle of the tongue, strap muscles, thyroid, or esophagus).

T4b: All Laryngeal Sites

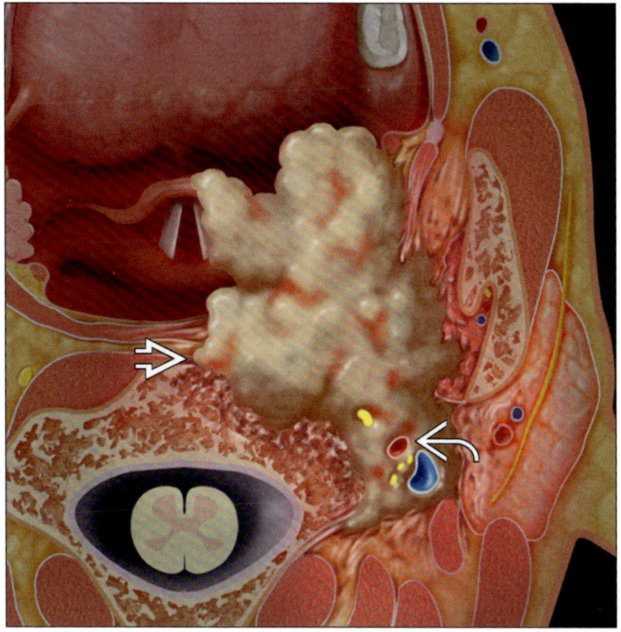

T4b tumors are characterized as very advanced local disease and the definition is the same for tumors of the supraglottis, glottis, and subglottis. T4b tumors may invade the prevertebral space, encase the carotid artery, or invade mediastinal structures.

T4b: All Laryngeal Sites

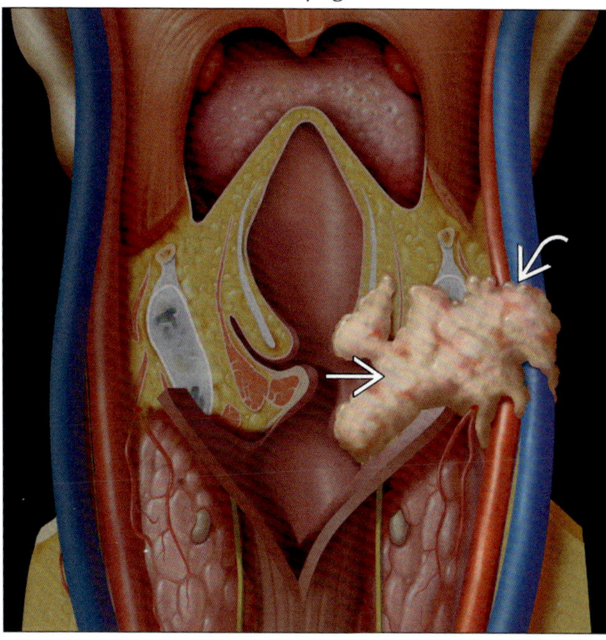

Coronal graphic depicts tumor that invades posterolaterally to encase the carotid artery. Tumor may also spread inferiorly into the mediastinum.

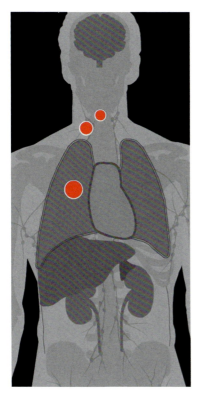

INITIAL SITE OF RECURRENCE

Distant	30.4%
Neck/Regional	21.1%
Local	14.4%
Second Primary	14.4%

Data obtained from larynx preservation in pyriform sinus cancer: Preliminary results of a EORTC Phase III trial. Trial evaluated 194 patients (T2-T4 and N0-N3) treated with surgery and postop RT vs. induction chemo + CRT for responders. Median follow-up: 51 months. Distant metastases were reduced in the induction chemo arm: 25% vs. 36%, P = 0.04. Lefebvre J et al: JNCI 88(13):890-9, 1996.

OVERVIEW

General Comments

- Squamous cell carcinoma (SCCa) is most common histology of laryngeal cancer (~ 95%)
- Laryngeal tumors originate from mucosal surface
- There are 3 anatomic subdivisions of the larynx; location of tumor affects treatment recommendations
  - **Supraglottic carcinoma**
    - 2nd most common location of laryngeal cancer (glottic cancer most common)
    - Represents 30% of all laryngeal squamous cell carcinomas
    - Supraglottis anatomically includes
      - False cords
      - Aryepiglottic (AE) folds
      - Suprahyoid epiglottis
      - Infrahyoid epiglottis
      - Arytenoids
      - Laryngeal ventricle
  - **Glottic carcinoma**
    - Most frequently involved site of laryngeal cancers (at least 60% of cases)
    - Glottis anatomically includes
      - True vocal cords
      - Anterior commissure
      - Posterior commissure
  - **Subglottic carcinoma**
    - Primary subglottic carcinoma is rare
    - Anatomically spans mucosa from inferior true vocal cords to lower edge of cricoid cartilage

Classification

- **WHO histological classification for tumors of larynx**
  - **Malignant epithelial tumors**
  - SCCa: Most commonly well to moderately differentiated (> 90%)
    - Verrucous carcinoma
      - 1-3% of all larynx cancers
      - Characterized by bulky exophytic lesion and papillomatous appearance
    - Basaloid squamous cell carcinoma
      - Uncommon variant, typically not HPV initiated
      - Characterized by aggressive spread pattern
    - Adenosquamous carcinoma
      - 2 distinct malignant components: Squamous and glandular
    - Spindle cell carcinoma
      - Consists of squamous cell carcinoma and sarcoma-like lesions composed of spindle cells
    - Papillary squamous cell carcinoma
      - Must be "predominantly" papillary to qualify
      - Associated with favorable prognosis
    - Acantholytic squamous cell carcinoma
  - Giant cell carcinoma
  - Lymphoepithelial carcinoma
  - **Neuroendocrine tumors**
    - Typical carcinoid
    - Atypical carcinoid tumor
    - Extrapulmonary small cell carcinoma
    - Paraganglioma
  - **Soft tissue tumors**
    - Malignant tumors
      - Fibrosarcoma
      - Malignant fibrous histiocytoma
      - Liposarcoma
      - Leiomyosarcoma
      - Rhabdomyosarcoma
      - Angiosarcoma
      - Kaposi sarcoma
      - Malignant peripheral nerve sheath tumor
      - Synovial sarcoma
    - Tumors with low malignant potential/borderline tumors
      - Inflammatory myofibroblastic tumor
  - **Hematolymphoid tumors**
  - **Tumors of bone and cartilage**
    - Chondrosarcoma
    - Osteosarcoma
    - Chondroma
    - Giant cell tumor
  - **Mucosal malignant melanoma**
  - **Secondary tumors**

NATURAL HISTORY

General Features

- Comments
  - **Supraglottic carcinoma**
    - Tumors often do not start near vocal cords
      - Both physical examination and imaging is necessary for accurate staging of advanced tumors
  - **Glottic carcinoma**
    - Most lesions arise from free margin and upper surface of true vocal cord
    - Lesions can be diagnosed early; even a small lesion can produce symptoms (dysphonia)
    - Both physical examination and imaging are necessary for accurate staging of advanced tumors
      - Impaired vocal cord mobility is T2
      - Paralyzed vocal cord is T3
  - **Subglottic carcinoma**
    - Rarely causes symptom until primary tumor is advanced

Etiology

- **Laryngeal cancers overall**
  - Among head and neck cancers, carcinogenic effects of tobacco appear to be most pronounced in larynx
    - Tobacco-related carcinogenesis appears to be p53 mediated
  - p53 loss of expression is associated with history of tobacco and alcohol
  - Environmental exposures
    - Nickel
    - Sulfuric acid mist
    - Asbestos
- **Supraglottic carcinoma**
  - Risk greater from black (air-cured) tobaccos compared to blonde (flue-cured) tobaccos
    - Characteristic not seen in glottic cancers

Epidemiology & Cancer Incidence

- Sex predilection
  - M:F = 5:1
- Age of onset

- Median age: 65 years old
- Estimated statistics of laryngeal cancer in United States for 2012
  - 12,360 new cases
  - 3,650 deaths
- Risk factors related to personal habits
  - Single most important risk is history of smoking
  - Heavy alcohol usage
  - History of both smoking with heavy alcohol usage results in profound increase in risk
    - 100x that of nonsmokers who do not drink
- Other risk factors
  - Age
  - Male gender
  - African-Americans are at increased risk compared to Caucasians

Genetics

- **Supraglottic carcinoma**
  - Loss of p23 region of chromosome 8 is independent predictor of poor prognosis
  - *HER-2/neu* (*c-erB-2*) oncogene expression
    - Association with distant metastasis
- **Glottic and subglottic carcinoma**
  - p53 overexpression
    - ~ 50-60% of patients
  - p16 absence
    - ~ 90% of patients
  - Loss of Rb protein expression
    - ~ 20% of patients
    - May play relatively minor role

Gross Pathology & Surgical Features

- **Supraglottic carcinoma**
  - Mucosal lesions display following pathological characteristics
    - Poorly marginated
    - Ulcerative
    - Indurated
- **Glottic carcinoma**
  - Small tumor
    - Irregular thickening of mucosa that is often not visible on imaging
  - Large tumor
    - Ulcerating, invasive, or exophytic lesion
- **Subglottic carcinoma**
  - Lesions display following pathological characteristics
    - Poorly marginated
    - Ulcerative
    - Indurated
    - May also manifest as large exophytic or fungating mass

Microscopic Pathology

- H&E
  - **Laryngeal cancers overall**
    - Squamous cell carcinomas represent great majority of laryngeal cancers
    - Squamous cell carcinoma in situ (CIS) is infrequently encountered (0.4 per 100,000 persons)
      - Approximately 25-30% of laryngeal CIS will proceed to invasive tumors; untreated cases transform at higher rates
    - Carcinomas that are not squamous cell are staged the same as squamous cell carcinomas
  - **Supraglottic carcinoma**
    - Nonkeratinizing
    - Moderate to poor differentiation
    - Squamous differentiation
      - Intracellular bridges or keratinization present
  - **Glottic carcinoma**
    - Typically keratinizing
    - Well to moderately differentiated
  - **Subglottic carcinoma**
    - Mainly squamous differentiation with intracellular bridges or keratinization (possibly keratin pearls as well)
    - Undifferentiated carcinomas are more likely in subglottic carcinomas
- Special stains
  - **Laryngeal cancers overall**
    - Keratin immunoreactivity
      - Types of keratin vary between tumors
    - Epidermal growth factor receptor expression present
      - May be prognostic factor for neck node relapse
  - **Supraglottic carcinoma**
    - Immune staining for expression of *HER-2/neu* (*c-erB-2*) oncogene

Routes of Spread

- Local spread
  - **Supraglottic carcinoma**
    - Tends to remain confined to organ or origin, although there is no barrier to extralaryngeal spread
    - Can invade deep laryngeal tissues, such as preepiglottic and paraglottic spaces
      - Invasion of either upstages to T3 disease
    - Can extend inferiorly toward glottis and subglottis
  - **Glottic carcinoma**
    - Typically spreads horizontally across free margin of vocal cord in direction of anterior commissure
    - Anatomic structures of glottis typically pose barrier to spread
    - Extension to contralateral vocal cord does not change AJCC stage (bilateral cord involvement is still stage I)
    - Cord fixation may result after eventual invasion of underlying thyroarytenoid muscle
    - Extension into subglottis may occur by invasion through conus elasticus
  - **Subglottic carcinoma**
    - Spreads anteriorly into thyroid gland through cricothyroid membrane
    - Spreads posteriorly to
      - Cricoid cartilage
      - Esophagus
    - Spreads cephalad to
      - True vocal cords
      - Supraglottis
    - Spreads inferiorly to
      - Tracheal lumen
      - Cartilaginous rings
- Lymphatic extension
  - Supraglottic carcinoma
    - Lymphatic metastases at diagnosis are common (> 50%)

LARYNX

- Midline structure with dense lymphatic drainage that can potentially drain to bilateral necks
- Level II is most commonly involved lymph node level
  - Glottic carcinoma
    - T1-2 N0 have relatively low rate of occult lymphatic spread (< 10%)
    - T3/T4 cancers have much higher rate of involved lymphatics (33-50%)
    - Level VI (anterior compartment) lymph nodes at high risk in certain situations
      - More than minimal subglottic extension
      - Emergent tracheotomy
  - Subglottic carcinoma
    - Incidence of positive lymph nodes at diagnosis is 10-20%
    - Primarily drains to paratracheal lymph nodes
- Hematogenous spread
  - Rare in N0 patients
- Metastatic sites
  - Common sites for laryngeal cancers overall include
    - Lung
    - Liver
    - Diaphragm/pleura

IMAGING

Detection

- **Supraglottic carcinoma**
  - **General**
    - Mass of epiglottis, aryepiglottic folds, and potentially false vocal cords
    - Mass appears moderately enhancing and infiltrating
    - Morphologic features
      - Invasion of deep laryngeal tissues including deep preepiglottic space and potentially paraglottic space (T3 disease)
      - Larger tumors may destroy laryngeal cartilage &/ or exhibit malignant spread to lymph nodes
  - **CT**
    - NECT
      - Asymmetric appearance of supraglottic soft tissue
      - Mass effect
      - Sclerosis of cartilage seen (low specificity)
    - CECT
      - Mass of epiglottis, aryepiglottic folds, ± false vocal cords with moderate enhancement
      - Epiglottic carcinoma: Symmetric epiglottic enlargement in side-to-side fashion may be seen, which leads to missed diagnoses if only looking for asymmetry
      - Important to note that preepiglottic space is blind spot clinically (upstages to T3)
      - Aryepiglottic fold carcinoma: Posterior extension to involve pyriform sinus/hypopharynx or anterior extension to involve false cord
      - False cord carcinoma: Deep invasion to paraglottic space should be looked for
  - **MR**
    - T1WI
      - Low to intermediate signal mass
    - T2WI
      - Intermediate to high signal mass
    - T1WI C+
      - Homogeneously or heterogeneously enhancing
  - **PET/CT**
    - Functional imaging can help determine the involvement of lymph nodes that are borderline by anatomic imaging criteria
    - Functional imaging can demonstrate submucosal tumor spread that is not evident on physical examination or anatomic imaging
- **Glottic carcinoma**
  - **General**
    - Enhancing and invasive mass located in true vocal cords
    - Variability in size of mass
      - Typically small at time of detection
      - Certain primaries will be too small to view on imaging
    - Often displays invasive or exophytic morphology
  - **CT**
    - NECT
      - May show asymmetric soft tissue located in true vocal cords
      - Thin slice (1-2 mm) helps assess bone invasion
    - CECT
      - May show enhancing infiltrative or exophytic mass in true vocal cords
      - If tumor is large, necrosis may be seen as nonenhancing
  - **MR**
    - T1WI
      - Low to intermediate signal true vocal cord mass
      - Increased T1 signal may be seen in intratumoral hemorrhage areas
    - T2WI
      - High to intermediate signal true vocal cord mass
    - T1WI C+
      - Homogeneous enhancement
      - Superior delineation of tumor from muscle (if patient holds still without swallowing or moving)
    - MR imaging may be nondiagnostic when bulky tumors cause pooling of secretion and constant swallowing
  - **PET/CT**
    - Displays increased glucose uptake of tumor
    - Appreciation of submucosal tumor spread may be enhanced by PET/CT
- **Subglottic carcinoma**
  - **General**
    - Enhancing and invasive mass centered inferior to glottis and superior to inferior margin of cricoid cartilage
  - **CT**
    - NECT
      - Prominent density of soft tissue at level of cricoid cartilage within airway
    - CECT
      - Enhancing mass centered inferior to true vocal cords (can be invasive or exophytic)
  - **MR**
    - T1WI
      - Low to intermediate signal mass

- T2WI
  - High to intermediate signal mass
- T1WI C+
  - Subglottic mass with heterogeneous or homogeneous enhancement
- PET/CT
  - Diagnostic value in post-laryngectomy patients if tumor recurrence is suspected based on CT or MR findings
  - FDG avidity in areas of malignancy
- **Imaging recommendations**
  - CECT is preferred modality due to laryngeal motion caused by breathing, coughing, and swallowing
  - MR can play adjunctive role in cases of suspected cartilage invasion
  - CECT protocol 2-pass method
    - 1st pass: 2-3 mm axial images from mandibular fillings to clavicles
      - During quiet respiration
      - Given with maximum intravascular contrast
      - Searches for nodes
    - 2nd pass: Axial image set from hyoid to 2nd tracheal ring
      - During breath-holding to allow imaging of true vocal cord mobility
      - Multiplanar reconstruction in coronal plane offers best estimate of craniocaudal extension
    - Multislice CT can reformat volumetric data sets in oblique planes
      - Enables reconstruction of single-stacked axial acquisition through cervical soft tissues in sagittal and coronal planes
      - Oblique reformations may be obtained around dental amalgam

Staging

- **General**
  - **CT**
    - Coronal imaging is helpful to determine involvement of laryngeal ventricle and transglottic spread
    - Cartilage sclerosis may be periostitis due to adjacent tumor or true cartilage invasion
    - Advanced lesions arising within anterior aspect of vocal cord or along posterior 1/3 of cord may
      - Extend posteriorly to involve cricoarytenoid joint and interarytenoid region
      - Extend inferiorly, either mucosally or submucosally, to involve subglottic region
    - Clinical blind spots for endoscopic examination include paraglottic space and cartilage invasion
  - **MR**
    - Invasion of cartilage may be detected with both CT and MR
      - MR is more sensitive, but less specific, than CT in demonstrating cartilage involvement
    - MR has adjunctive role in complex cases
      - In addition to cartilage invasion, direct coronal images show craniocaudal extent
    - Midsagittal images are helpful to demonstrate relationship between tumor and anterior commissure
  - **T1WI**
    - Fatty marrow in ossified cartilage has high signal
      - Tumor infiltration into cartilage results in decreased signal intensity of marrow
    - Focal sclerosis or low signal intensity on T1 is suggestive of cartilage involvement
  - **T2WI**
    - More helpful because tumor is usually hyperintense relative to nonossified cartilage
      - Unfortunately, edema may be mistaken for tumor invasion on T2WI
  - **T1WI C+**: Cartilage enhancement suggests invasion
- T staging
  - **Supraglottis**
    - > 50% have nodal metastases at presentation
      - Level II is 1st-order drainage
    - Moderately enhancing mass invades deep tissues of larynx, including preepiglottic space ± paraglottic space
    - Aryepiglottic fold SCCa may spread
      - Posteriorly to involve pyriform sinus (hypopharynx)
      - Anteriorly to involve false cord
    - False cord SCCa may invade deep into paraglottic space (T3)
    - Advanced lesions may extend
      - Superiorly to invade vallecula and base of tongue
      - Laterally to involve aryepiglottic folds, false vocal cord, and paralaryngeal space
    - Direct inferior extension to involve anterior commissure and subglottis is seen only in advanced lesions
  - **Glottis**
    - Glottic SCCa spread patterns
      - Anteromedial to anterior commissure
      - Posterior to arytenoids or cricoid cartilage
      - Superiorly into supraglottic paraglottic space
      - Inferiorly into subglottis
    - Cartilage invasion more common than in subglottic carcinomas
  - **Subglottis**
    - Inherent motion of larynx makes CECT better staging tool than MR for subglottic SCCa
    - CECT protocol: 2-pass method for subglottic SCCa
      - 1st pass: Quiet respiration 2-3 mm axial images from mandibular fillings to clavicles with maximum intravascular contrast (node search)
      - 2nd pass: Breath-holding axial image set from hyoid to 2nd tracheal ring
      - Multiplanar reconstruction in coronal plane gives best sense of craniocaudal extent of subglottic SCCa
    - Subglottic SCCa spread patterns
      - Anterior through cricothyroid membrane or lateral through cricoid cartilage into thyroid gland
      - Posterior into cricoid cartilage and esophagus
      - Cephalad to invade true vocal cords and supraglottis
      - Inferior into tracheal lumen and cartilaginous rings
- N staging
  - **CT**
    - Metastatic lymph nodes appear round with loss of fatty hilum on CT

- Extracapsular nodal spread is more common in larger nodes but possible in smaller nodes as well
- Small volume lymphatic disease detection is based on size and morphology
  - > 1.5 cm in jugulodigastric region and > 1 cm in other locations
- Contrast-enhanced CT is recommended to evaluate cervical lymphadenopathy
  - Lymph node rim enhancement and central necrosis are abnormal irrespective of size
- **MR**
  - T1WI: Low to intermediate intensity
  - T1WI C+: Homogeneous or heterogeneous enhancement
  - T2WI: High signal intensity
    - MR is superior at evaluating metastatic retropharyngeal lymph nodes
  - T1WI C+ or T2WI superior to CECT in visualization of retropharyngeal lymph nodes
  - Interest is growing in use of dextran-coated, ultrasmall, supramagnetic iron oxide (USPIO) to detect metastatic nodal disease
    - Reported sensitivity and specificity in detecting nodal metastases are 87% and 90%, respectively
- **PET/CT**
  - Strong FDG avidity seen in large, non-necrotic metastatic nodes
  - Necrotic lymph nodes may not have strong FDG avidity, despite involvement with metastatic cancer
- M staging
  - **General**
    - Use of preoperative CT or MR is important to determine extent of tumor
    - Coronal and sagittal reformatted images helpful
  - **CT**
    - CECT more sensitive for evaluation of organs and non-nodal soft tissue, such as muscle
      - Moderately enhancing solid mass
      - Parenchymal metastases may show hyperenhancement
      - If tumor is large, necrosis may be seen as nonenhancing
    - CT superior in evaluating cortical bone invasion
      - Bone lesions may show enhancement
  - **MR**
    - Superior delineation of tumor from muscle (if patient holds still without swallowing or moving)
      - MR imaging may become nondiagnostic when bulky tumors cause pooling of secretion and constant swallowing
    - Dental amalgam artifact less severe than with CT
    - T1WI
      - Isointense to muscle
      - Increased T1 signal may be seen in intratumoral hemorrhage areas
      - Replaced bone marrow is easier to appreciate on pre-contrast T1WI
    - T2WI
      - High-grade tumors tend to be lower in intensity
      - Moderate hyperintensity to muscle
      - High signal intensity best seen with fat saturation
    - T1WI C+
      - Variable enhancement
      - Necrotic areas do not enhance
      - Axial and coronal reconstruction superior for showing tumor interface with surrounding structures
  - **PET/CT**
    - Sensitivity greatest in metastases with diameter > 1 cm
    - Careful attention to artifacts and patterns of physiologic uptake is essential to avoid incorrect staging
      - Biopsy sites may show FDG uptake in short term

Restaging

- CT
  - Use of preoperative CT or MR is important to determine extent of tumor for more sensitive surveillance imaging
  - CT in particular is widely used for regular monitoring of patients who have undergone surgical treatment of laryngeal carcinoma
  - Stomal recurrences following total laryngectomy are most commonly level VI nodal recurrences
  - **Post-XRT changes**
    - Diffuse laryngeal/supraglottic edema without discrete mass in patients previously irradiated for head and neck cancer
    - Mild to moderate thickening of skin, platysma, false cords, epiglottis, & aryepiglottic folds
    - Increased "stranding" or "reticulation" in cervical fat due to lymphedema, perilymphatic fibrosis
    - Chondronecrosis (laryngeal cartilage sclerosis, fragmentation, gas) is a rare but serious late complication
    - Enlargement (acutely) or atrophy (chronically) and increased enhancement of salivary glands due to XRT-induced sialadenitis
    - Narrowing of hypopharyngeal, supraglottic, glottic airway
    - Dynamic CT perfusion studies may help differentiate tumor from XRT changes
- MR
  - **Post-XRT changes**
    - MR may help differentiate tumor from XRT changes; T2 hypointensity and poor enhancement are often seen with fibrosis
    - T1WI
      - Decreased signal in edematous mucosa
      - Reduction in T1 hyperintensity of fat
    - T2WI
      - Changes vary with time
      - T2 hyperintense edema subsides in many cases, but mucosal thickening may persist
      - Thickening of epiglottis, aryepiglottic folds
      - Retropharyngeal edema, thickening and edema of posterior pharyngeal wall
      - Subacute: Increased signal in edematous mucosa, edematous subcutaneous and deep fat planes, and salivary glands
      - Chronic: Salivary gland atrophy, decreased signal compared to early post-XRT findings
    - T1WI C+: Increased enhancement of mucosa, salivary glands, retropharyngeal space
- PET/CT

- Increased uptake of FDG with tumor helps differentiate from XRT-induced changes
- False-positives due to laryngeal muscle activation with contralateral vocal cord paralysis
- PET most useful in post-laryngectomy patient if CT or MR is suspicious but not definite for recurrent tumor

CLINICAL PRESENTATION & WORK-UP

Presentation

- **Supraglottic laryngeal cancer**
  - Common presenting symptoms
    - Odynophagia
    - Dysphagia
    - Painless neck mass
    - Otalgia (referred via superior laryngeal nerve to auricular nerve of Arnold)
    - Chronic cough
  - Less common symptoms suggestive of neglected, advanced local disease
    - Stridor
    - Hemoptysis
- **Glottic laryngeal cancer**
  - Common presenting symptoms
    - Hoarseness (dysphonia)
  - Uncommon presenting symptoms suggestive of neglected, advanced disease
    - Odynophagia
    - Dysphagia
    - Stridor
    - Hemoptysis
- **Subglottic laryngeal cancer**
  - Given the anatomic confines of the subglottis, presentation is most typically with advanced tumor
  - Common presenting symptoms
    - Stridor
    - Emergent tracheostomy
- Complete head and neck examination should be performed in patients who potentially have any laryngeal cancer, including
  - Laryngeal examination, often through use of following devices
    - Laryngeal mirror
    - Flexible endoscope
    - Rigid endoscope
  - Specific focuses of head and neck examination should include examinations of
    - Skin
    - Oral cavity
      - Check for 2nd primary tumors
      - Check adequacy of dentition
    - Neck
      - Palpation of lymphadenopathy
      - Laryngotracheal complex mobility
      - Direct extension of tumor
    - Larynx
      - Movement of cords
      - Involvement of different sites influences staging
      - Superficial tumor spread on visual inspection may not be adequately represented by imaging

Prognosis

- Glottic tumor may remain initially confined to larynx due to anatomical barriers
- Without treatment, invasion will continue and become transglottic in nature
- Prognosis: Relative survival rate
  - **Supraglottic carcinoma**
    - Supraglottic cancers (vs. glottic cancers)
      - Worse prognosis
      - Increased likelihood of being high-grade cancer
    - Due to often late presenting signs, supraglottic cancers are often diagnosed later than other laryngeal cancers
      - After lymph node spread has occurred
    - Most important negative prognostic indicators
      - Metastases to regional lymph nodes
      - Lymph node extracapsular spread
    - 5-year survival rate:
      - Stage I: 83.4%
      - Stage II: 69.5%
      - Stage III: 57.4%
      - Stage IV: 42.6%
  - **Glottic carcinoma 5-year survival rate**
    - Stage I: 65.1%
    - Stage II: 62.1%
    - Stage III: 54.7%
    - Stage IV: 36.8%
  - **Subglottic carcinoma 5-year survival rate**
    - Stage I: 54.1%
    - Stage II: 68.2%
    - Stage III: 53.2%
    - Stage IV: 36.0%
- Distant metastases
  - Risk of metastases mostly influenced by nodal status
    - Bulky (i.e., N3) nodal disease
    - Low neck (e.g., level IV or level V) nodes
- Recurrence
  - Greatest recurrence risk within 2-3 years, emphasizing importance of clinical follow-up
    - After organ preservation therapy, surgical salvage of larynx tumors has favorable success rates
  - After 5 years, risk is greatly reduced; new malignancies are likely primary in origin as opposed to recurrent
  - Subglottic stoma is common site for recurrence

TREATMENT

Major Treatment Alternatives

- **Supraglottic carcinoma**
  - Radiation therapy (RT)
    - Primary radiotherapy can be used as sole treatment in stages I-II tumors
      - Elective radiation to bilateral necks is indicated in all cases
    - Concurrent radiotherapy and chemotherapy recommended for most stages III-IV tumors
    - Adjuvant radiotherapy ± concurrent chemotherapy is recommended for patients managed initially with operation who are thought to have high recurrence risk
    - At simulation
      - Thermoplastic mask essential

- Use bolus for superficial tumors/nodes or if anterior commissure is involved
- Requires judicious placement of isocenter

- Chemotherapy
  - Most commonly delivered concurrently with radiotherapy
  - Most common agent is cisplatin
- Surgical treatment
  - Supraglottic laryngectomy is an option for T1-3 supraglottic tumors
    - Adjuvant radiation is often necessary secondary to close/involved margins or regional metastases
  - Laser microsurgery: Offers precise ablation of tissue, which is a surgical alternative to supraglottic laryngectomy in early stage diseases such as T1 or T2 lesions
  - Bilateral elective neck dissections or adjuvant radiotherapy is generally required
  - Total laryngectomy: Often for advanced stage cancers, generally in combination with adjuvant radiotherapy ± chemotherapy

- **Glottic carcinoma**
  - Radiation therapy
    - Main nonsurgical option in early stage glottic cancers (stages I-II tumors)
      - Treatment generally does not require elective nodal irradiation
    - Voice quality is generally better after treatment of early glottic cancers when compared to advanced cancer; useful voice remains in 80-95% of cured patients
    - Radiation therapy is associated with thickening of true vocal cords
    - Pattern of thickening is typically diffuse and symmetric and occurs in dose-dependent fashion
    - Used adjuvantly for patients thought to be at high risk for recurrence
  - Chemotherapy
    - Chemotherapy and radiotherapy may be administered in combination for stages III-IV tumors, offering improved disease control
  - Surgical treatment
    - Endoscopic surgery: Stage I carcinomas, some stage II glottic carcinomas, premalignant lesions
    - Vertical partial laryngectomy is open procedure that addresses tumors of true vocal cords that have limited extent of spread to anterior commissure; tracheotomy is required for variable time postoperatively
    - Supracricoid laryngectomy removes both vocal cords and requires reconstruction
      - Major disadvantage of the many open organ sparing surgeries is that they are appropriate for relatively small number of patients
    - Total laryngectomy: Advanced glottic cancers
  - Immunotherapy
    - Investigational
- **Subglottic carcinoma**
  - Radiation therapy
    - If used as primary treatment, may offer conservation of larynx
      - Tumor spread frequently inferior via trachea and is poorly imaged
      - Tumor volumes rely heavily on intraoperative examination to determine inferior extent of disease
    - Thickening of subglottic mucosa and submucosa can be seen following XRT
    - Used in combination with total laryngectomy for large tumors
  - Surgical therapy
    - Total laryngectomy with radiation therapy for large tumors
- Voice outcomes
  - Important consideration as both surgical and nonsurgical modalities offer similar rates of tumor control and long-term cure
  - Little prospective data to investigate which modality (primary radiation or primary surgery) is best
  - Patients with well-demarcated lesions amenable to laser surgery generally have good voice outcome with either modality
  - Patients with poorly demarcated &/or deep lesions generally do better with primary radiotherapy

Major Treatment Roadblocks/ Contraindications

- Adverse effects associated with radiotherapy
  - Adverse effects associated with both early and advanced glottic larynx cancer
    - Skin reaction
    - Dysphagia
    - Odynophagia
  - Adverse effects associated primarily with advanced glottic larynx cancer or supraglottic larynx cancer
    - Loss of taste (dysgeusia)
    - Mucositis
    - Xerostomia
    - Need for gastrotomy feeding tube
- Adverse effects of vertical partial laryngectomy
  - Wound infection
  - Formation of fistula
  - Glottic incompetence associated with aspiration
  - Granulation tissue that leads to inferior voice quality
  - Laryngeal stenosis
- Adverse effects of total laryngectomy
  - Loss of voice and airway protection
  - Early complications include
    - Wound dehiscence
    - Wound infection
    - Pharyngocutaneous fistula
    - Hematoma
  - Late complications also include
    - Hypothyroidism
    - Stomal stenosis
    - Pharyngoesophageal stenosis and stricture
- Adverse effects of neck dissection
  - Wound infection
  - Wound dehiscence
  - Hematoma
  - Chylous fistula
  - Dysphagia
  - Rupture of carotid artery represents most grave complication
- Endoscopic procedures are rarely associated with adverse effects
  - Aspiration is infrequent complication

Treatment Options by Stage

- **Supraglottic carcinoma**
  - Stages I and II
    - Sole treatment via external beam radiation therapy or laser surgery
    - Supraglottic laryngectomy vs. total laryngectomy
      - Decision based on anatomical location of lesion and patient's clinical status
      - Postoperative care important to maintain pulmonary and swallowing function
    - Radiation therapy may be preferred due to preservation of voice and potential to be salvaged
  - Stages III and IV
    - Surgical excision ± postop RT
    - RT with surgical excision: Definitive treatment in cases of salvage for failures in RT
    - Combination therapy of chemotherapy with RT, alternative to total laryngectomy
    - Laryngectomy may also be performed
- **Glottic carcinoma**
  - Stage I
    - RT or laser excision
    - Cordectomy in very specifically chosen patients (e.g., T1 cancers in which lesion is limited and superficial)
    - Vertical partial laryngectomy
  - Stage II
    - RT or laser excision
    - Partial or total laryngectomy based on anatomic nature of disease
  - Stage III
    - Organ preservation consisting of concurrent chemotherapy and RT
    - RT alone (for patient who cannot tolerate concurrent chemotherapy) provides similar survival rate as combined modality therapy with worse rate of locoregional control
    - Surgical excision ± adjuvant RT
    - Laryngectomy performed if response to chemotherapy < 50% or persistence of disease after RT
  - Stage IV
    - Total laryngectomy with postop RT
    - RT with surgical excision: Definitive treatment in cases of salvage for failures in RT
    - Combination therapy of chemotherapy with RT may be considered as alternative to total laryngectomy RT
    - Laryngectomy performed if response to chemotherapy < 50% tumor reduction
- **Subglottic carcinoma**
  - Stages I and II
    - RT: Offers good outcomes with voice preservation
    - Surgery if RT fails or not easy to treat with RT
  - Stage III
    - Surgical approach consisting of laryngectomy with isolated thyroidectomy, dissection of tracheoesophageal node; postop RT typically performed
    - RT: Sole treatment in nonsurgical candidates; patients need to be followed closely with potential alternative of surgical salvage
  - Stage IV
    - Surgical approach consisting of laryngectomy with total thyroidectomy, lymphadenectomy of nodes located in throat; adjuvant RT typically performed
    - RT as sole treatment

Dose Response

- Total dose to high-risk volume is similar to doses used to other sites in head and neck; higher total dose is required in setting of gross disease

Standard Doses

- Early glottic cancer: 63 Gy in 28 fractions (QD treatment)
  - T2 disease can be treated with 79.2 Gy in 66 fractions (b.i.d. treatment)
- Advanced larynx cancer: 70 Gy in 35 fractions (QD treatment)
- Adjuvant therapy of resected larynx cancer: 60 Gy in 30 fractions (QD treatment)

Organs at Risk Parameters

- Bilateral parotid glands: < 25 Gy can usually prevent severe xerostomia
- Spinal cord: 45 Gy
- Many other normal tissue structures have been proposed: Safety and efficacy is unclear

Common Techniques

- Early larynx cancer
  - Parallel opposed fields to larynx only
  - IMRT used for carotid sparing
- Supraglottic larynx and advanced larynx cancer
  - Parallel opposed fields with sequential reductions
  - IMRT

Landmark Trials

- Veterans Affairs (VA) Laryngeal Cancer Study Group larynx trial
  - Surgery + postoperative radiation vs. induction chemotherapy and chemoradiation (if PR/CR), n = 332, stage III/IV
  - Similar overall survival in both arms: 68%
  - Chemoradiation arm had decreased rate of distant metastases (11% vs. 17%, P = 0.001) and higher rate of local failure (12% vs. 2%, P = 0.001) than primary surgery arm
  - Larynx preservation: 64% at 2 years in chemoradiation arm
  - 56% of patients with T4 required laryngectomy
- RTOG 91-11
  - 3 arms: Radiation alone vs. induction chemotherapy followed radiation (sequential chemoradiation) vs. concurrent chemoradiation, n = 547, stage III/IV
  - Concurrent chemoradiation improved larynx preservation and locoregional control at 2 years
  - Both chemotherapy including regimens suppressed distant metastases when compared to radiation alone arm
  - No difference in overall survival was detected

RECOMMENDED FOLLOW-UP

Clinical

- Clinical examination every 6-8 weeks after organ preservation; interval can be lengthened at physician's discretion

Radiographic

- Follow-up imaging of early larynx cancer patient with normal physical examination is optional
- CECT at 4-6 weeks after completion of treatment to evaluate response of primary and nodes
- PET/CT after treatment appears to have quite good negative predictive value (NPV); ideal time to obtain scan is unclear
- Routine imaging in absence of symptoms is not recommended

SELECTED REFERENCES

1. Siegel R et al: Cancer statistics, 2012. CA Cancer J Clin. 62(1):10-29, 2012
2. American Joint Committee on Cancer: AJCC Cancer Staging Manual. 7th ed. New York: Springer. 57-67, 2010
3. Yao M et al: Clinical significance of postradiotherapy [18F]-fluorodeoxyglucose positron emission tomography imaging in management of head-and-neck cancer: a long-term outcome report. Int J Radiat Oncol Biol Phys. 74(1):9-14, 2009
4. Becker M et al: Imaging of the larynx and hypopharynx. Eur J Radiol. 66(3):460-79, 2008
5. Blitz AM et al: Radiologic evaluation of larynx cancer. Otolaryngol Clin North Am. 41(4):697-713, vi, 2008
6. Chong VF: Tumour volume measurement in head and neck cancer. Cancer Imaging. 7 Spec No A:S47-9, 2007
7. Connor S: Laryngeal cancer: how does the radiologist help? Cancer Imaging. 7:93-103, 2007
8. Mendenhall WM et al: Multidisciplinary management of laryngeal carcinoma. Int J Radiat Oncol Biol Phys. 69(2 Suppl):S12-4, 2007
9. Roh JL et al: 2-[18F]-Fluoro-2-deoxy-D-glucose positron emission tomography as guidance for primary treatment in patients with advanced-stage resectable squamous cell carcinoma of the larynx and hypopharynx. Eur J Surg Oncol. 33(6):790-5, 2007
10. Daisne JF et al: Tumor volume in pharyngolaryngeal squamous cell carcinoma: comparison at CT, MR imaging, and FDG PET and validation with surgical specimen. Radiology. 2004 Oct;233(1):93-100. Epub 2004 Aug 18. Erratum in: Radiology. 235(3):1086, 2005
11. Mendenhall WM et al: Management of T1-T2 glottic carcinomas. Cancer. 100(9):1786-92, 2004
12. Forastiere AA et al: Concurrent chemotherapy and radiotherapy for organ preservation in advanced laryngeal cancer. N Engl J Med. 349(22):2091-8, 2003
13. Wax MK et al: The role of positron emission tomography in the evaluation of the N-positive neck. Otolaryngol Head Neck Surg. 129(3):163-7, 2003
14. Zinreich SJ: Imaging in laryngeal cancer: computed tomography, magnetic resonance imaging, positron emission tomography. Otolaryngol Clin North Am. 35(5):971-91, Review, 2002
15. Induction chemotherapy plus radiation compared with surgery plus radiation in patients with advanced laryngeal cancer: The Department of Veterans Affairs Laryngeal Cancer Study Group. N Engl J Med. 324(24):1685-90, 1991

Well-Differentiated Keratinizing SCCa of the True Glottis

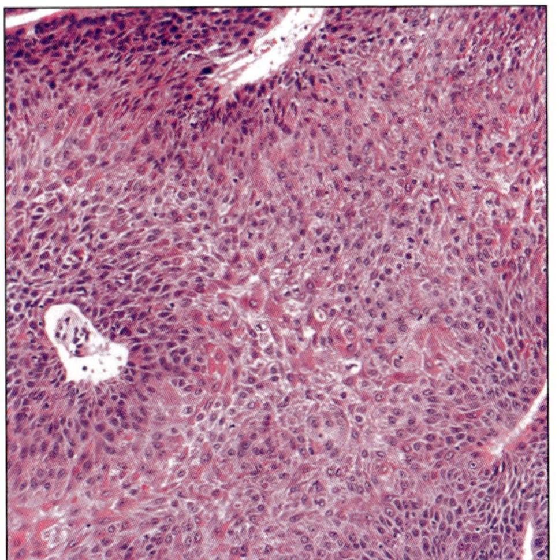

Poorly Differentiated Non-Keratinizing SCCa of the Supraglottis

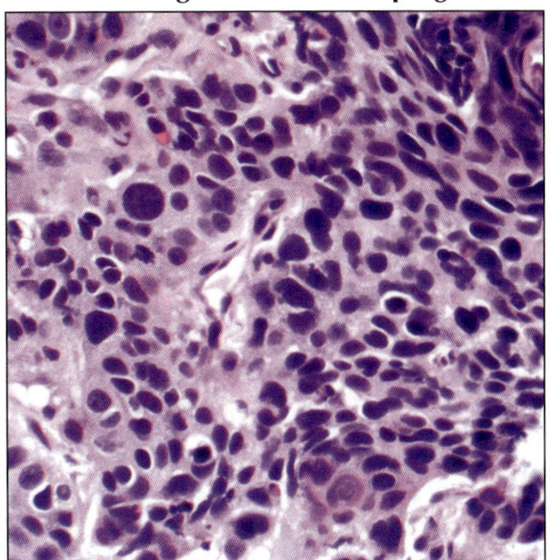

*(**Left**) This low-power image of an early larynx tumor demonstrates a well-differentiated, keratinizing tumor. Note the intensely pink (eosinophilic) cytoplasm, evidence of keratinization, and distinct cell borders. (**Right**) This high-power image demonstrates a supraglottic larynx tumor with little squamous differentiation. Hence, it is poorly differentiated. The cells are highly atypical, with bizarre nuclei and indistinct cell borders.*

Stage I (T1a N0 M0)

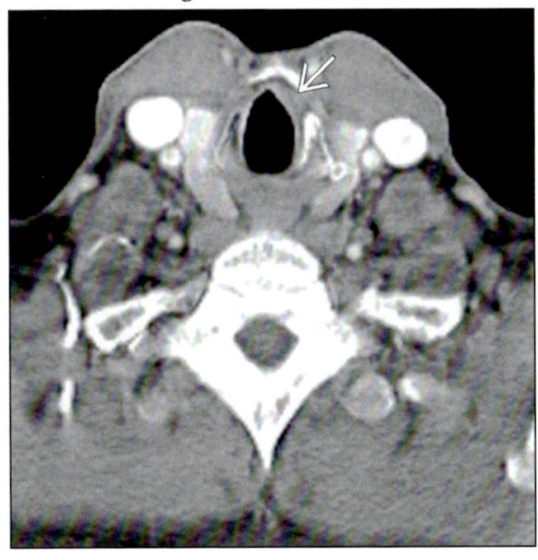

Stage I (T1a N0 M0)

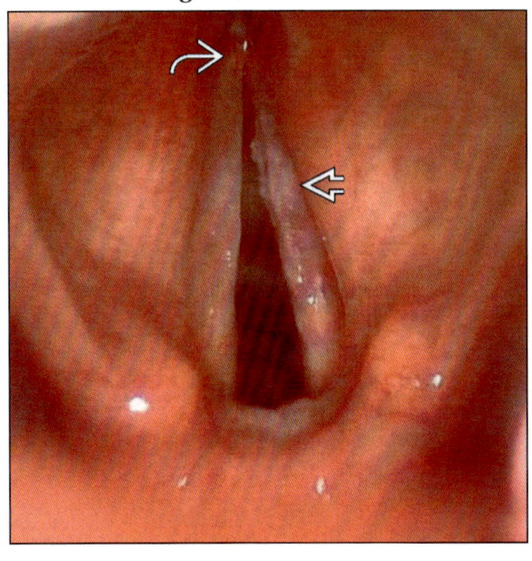

*(**Left**) Axial CECT shows a small left laryngeal mass ➡, which is almost invisible on CT, with the exception of slight asymmetry of the left inferior true vocal cord. (**Right**) Indirect laryngoscopy image demonstrates nodularity along the medial aspect of the right true vocal cord ➡. The anterior commissure ➡ is not involved with carcinoma. With phonation, cords were mobile and symmetric bilaterally.*

Stage I (T1 N0 M0)

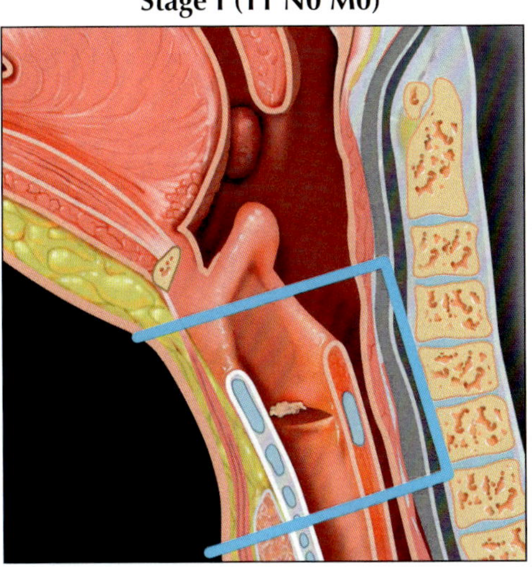

Vocal Cord Mobility

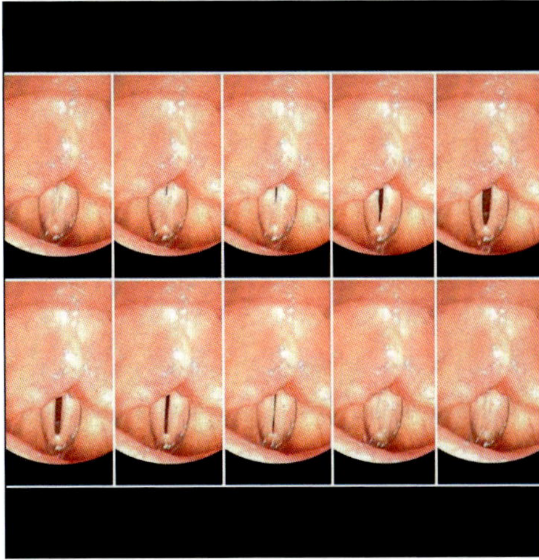

*(**Left**) Drawing demonstrates a typical treatment portal for early vocal cord carcinoma. The top border's relation to the thyroid notch is adjusted according to the lesion. Posterior border is at the posterior extent of the thyroid cartilage. Inferior border is placed at the bottom of the thyroid cartilage when there is no subglottic extension. (**Right**) Photograph of a stroboscopy demonstrates a normal cycle of phonation. Note that both vocal cords appear to be moving symmetrically.*

(Left) *Axial noncontrast treatment planning CT demonstrates typical homogeneous dose distribution for parallel opposed fields. Wedges (heel anterior) → accommodate for the changing thickness of the neck.* **(Right)** *Coronal noncontrast CT demonstrates isodose distribution for early larynx cancer treated without elective nodal irradiation. Note the distance of the treated volume to the oral cavity →, resulting in extremely low dose to the parotids and oral cavity.*

Stage I (T1 N0 M0)

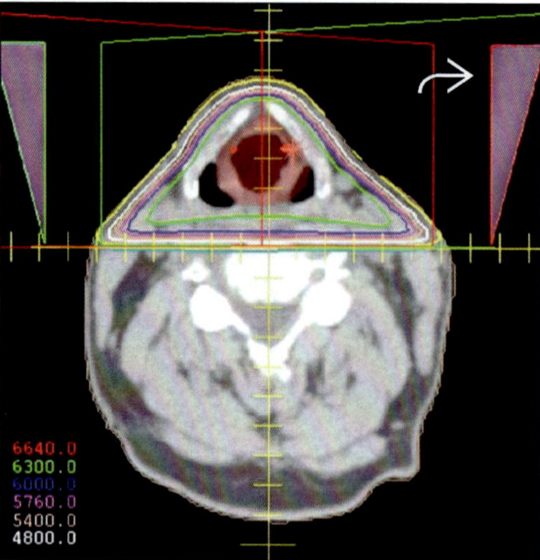

Stage I (T1 N0 M0)

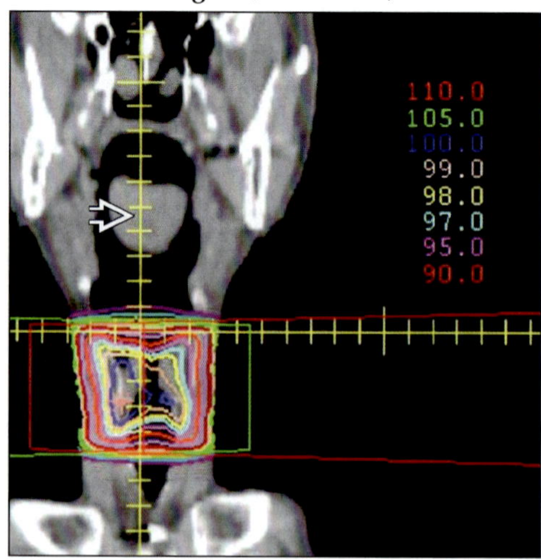

(Left) *Axial CECT shows a small, slightly enhancing mass in the anterior aspect of the left true vocal cord →. The lesion bulges minimally into the airway. There is thickening of the anterior commissure →.* **(Right)** *Indirect laryngoscopy demonstrates a bulky, exophytic mass on the left true vocal cord → that fills the ventricle and involves the false cord of the supraglottic larynx →.*

Stage II (T2 N0 M0)

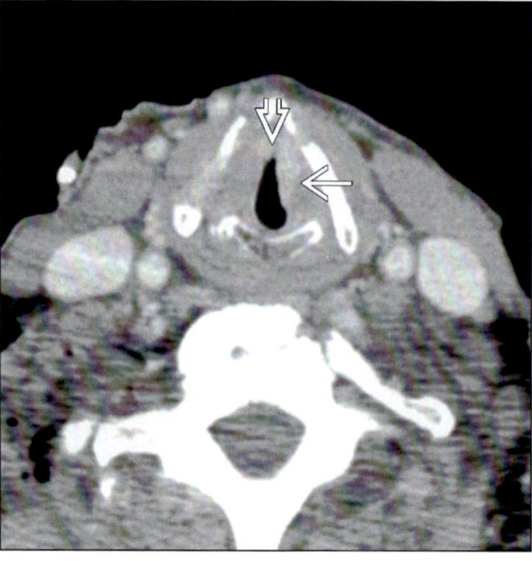

Stage II (T2 N0 M0)

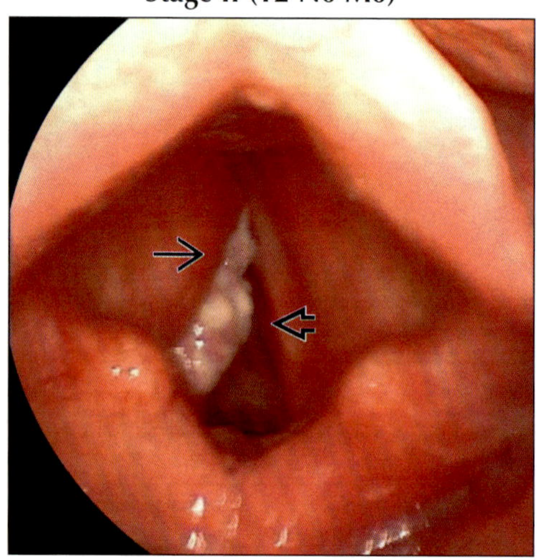

(Left) *This axial CECT demonstrates a bulky mass in the supraglottic larynx →, consistent with a T2 primary tumor.* **(Right)** *Indirect laryngoscopy image demonstrates a supraglottic squamous cell carcinoma that is centered on the left false vocal cord and involves the ipsilateral arytenoid cartilage → and a portion of the aryepiglottic fold →.*

Stage II (T2 N0 M0)

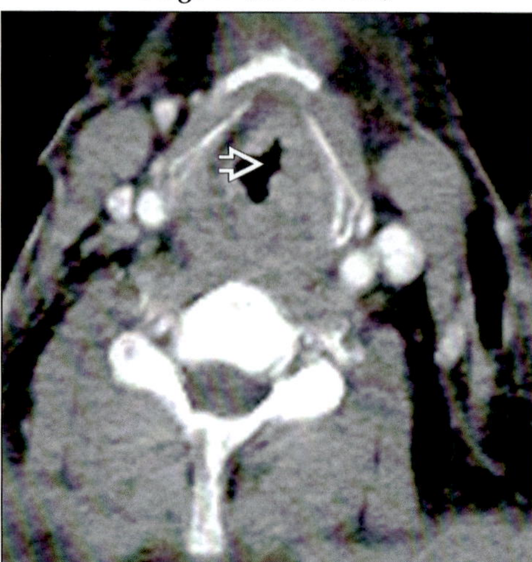

Stage II (T2 N0 M0)

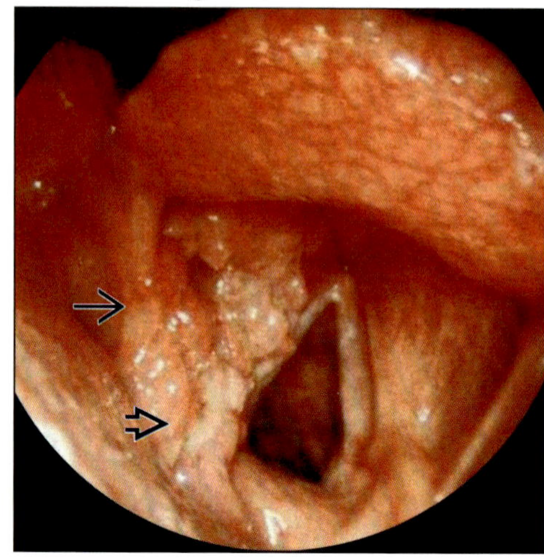

Stage II (T2 N0 M0)

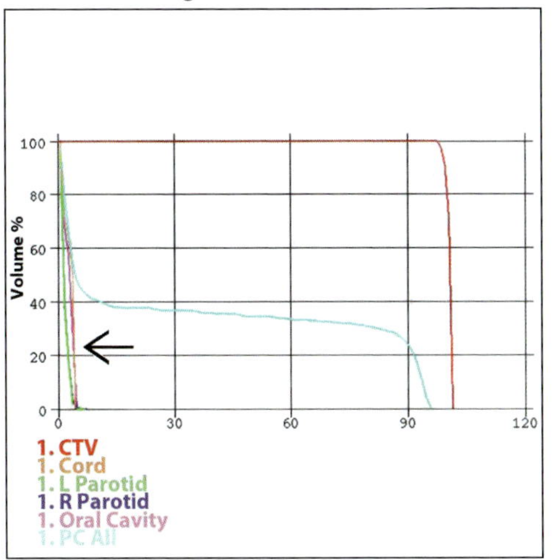

Stage II (T2 N0 M0) with Elective Nodal RT

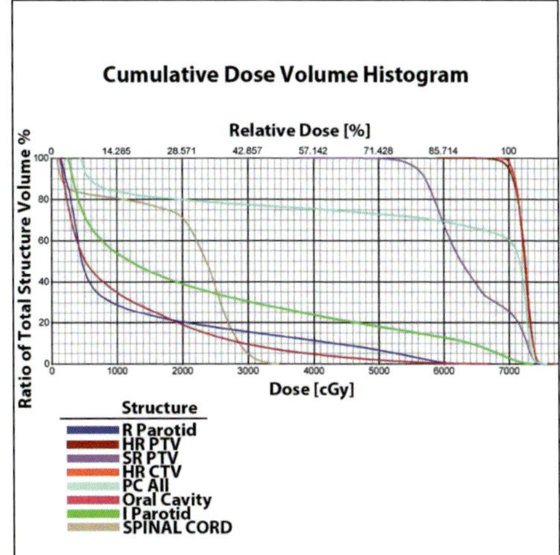

(Left) This is a representative DVH of a parallel opposed plan for a T2 N0 squamous cell carcinoma of the true vocal cord. Note that limiting the radiotherapy field to the larynx significantly limits dose to most avoidance structures ➔. *(Right)* This is a representative DVH of an IMRT plan for a T2 N0 squamous cell carcinoma of the supraglottic larynx. Note the increase in normal tissue dose as a consequence of elective nodal irradiation.

Stage III (T2 N1 M0)

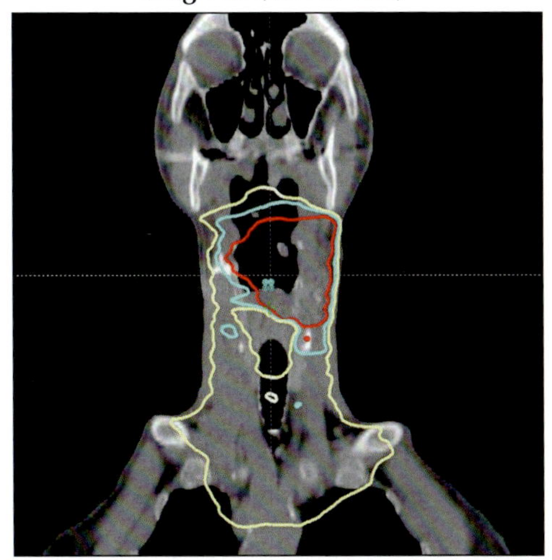

Stage III (T2 N1 M0)

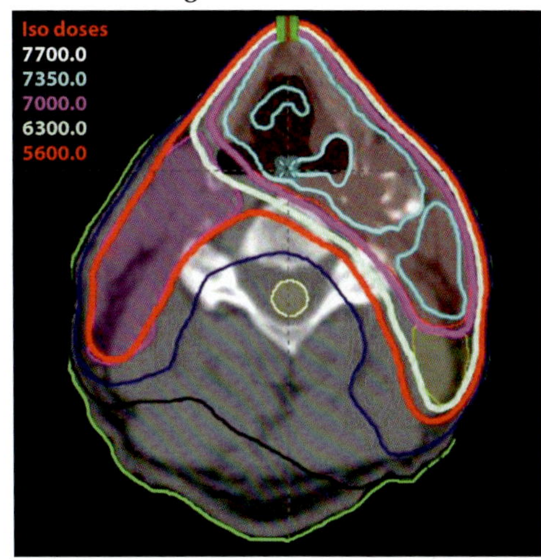

(Left) This is a coronal CECT demonstrating isodose distribution for a supraglottic tumor with a left-sided level III node. *(Right)* This is an axial image from a treatment planning CECT for a patient treated with IMRT for a lymph node positive supraglottic larynx cancer. Note that the IMRT treatment causes much of the PTV 70 Gy volume to receive 73.5 Gy, a dose escalation compared to parallel opposed fields.

Stage III (T2 N1 M0)

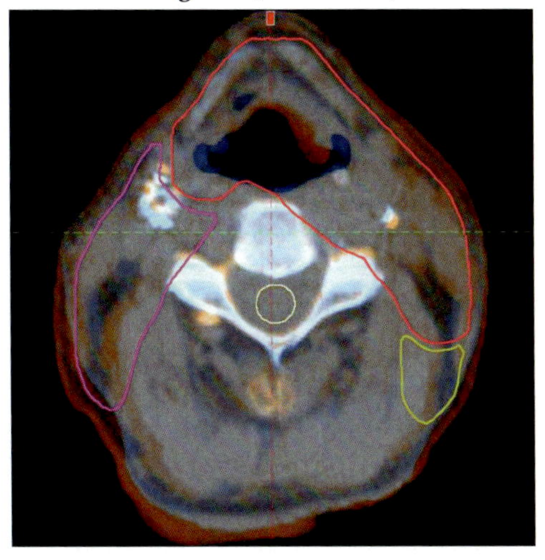

Stage III (T2 N1 M0)

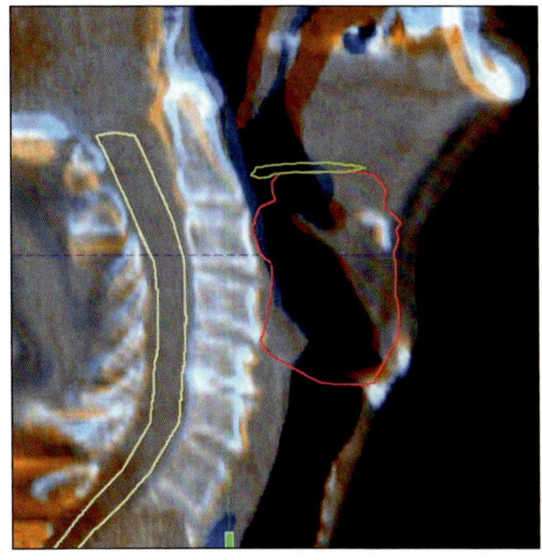

(Left) This is an axial CBCT demonstrating bony alignment at the level of the supraglottis. The blue image is obtained the day of treatment. The orange image is obtained at the day of simulation. *(Right)* This is a sagittal CBCT demonstrating bony alignment along the cervical spine. The blue image is obtained the day of treatment. The orange image is obtained the day of simulation. Image-guided radiotherapy can limit daily setup variability.

Stage III (T3 N0 M0)

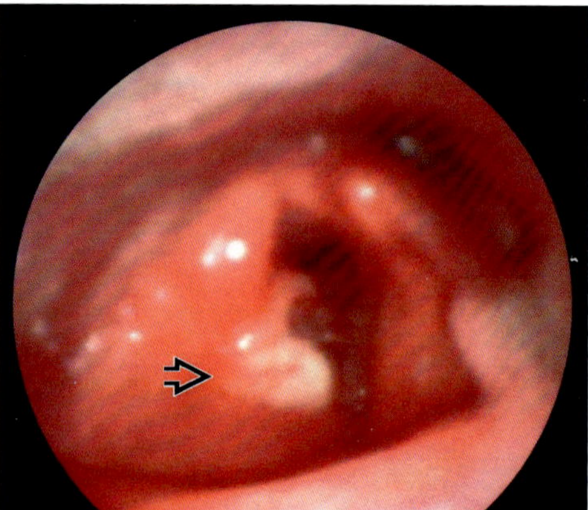

Stages III-IV (T3 or T4 N0 M0)

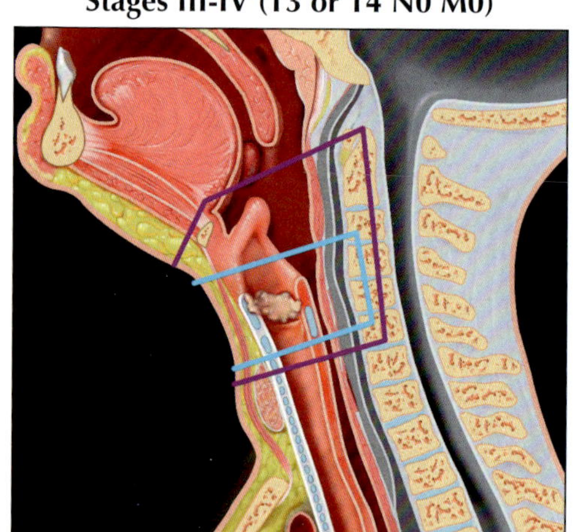

***(Left)** This is an indirect laryngoscopy image demonstrating a bulky tumor of the left true vocal cord. On phonation, the cord was immobile. **(Right)** This is a sagittal graphic demonstrating typical fields for node-negative advanced true glottis cancer or supraglottic cancer. The initial portal includes levels 2 and 3 lymph node stations bilaterally. The placement of the inferior border depends on the presence/absence and degree of subglottic extension.*

Stage III (T3 N0 M0)

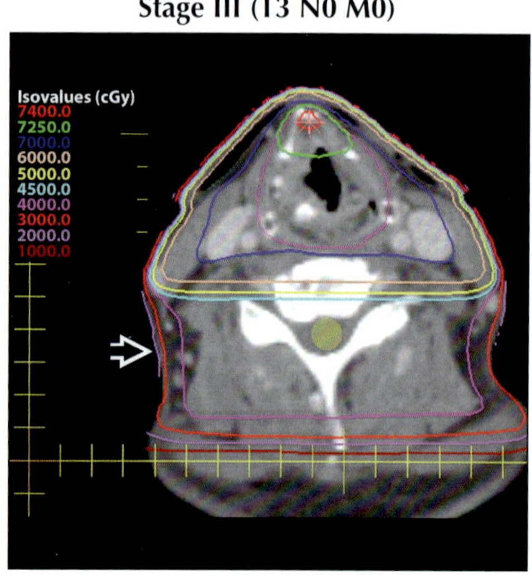

Stage III (T3 N0 M0)

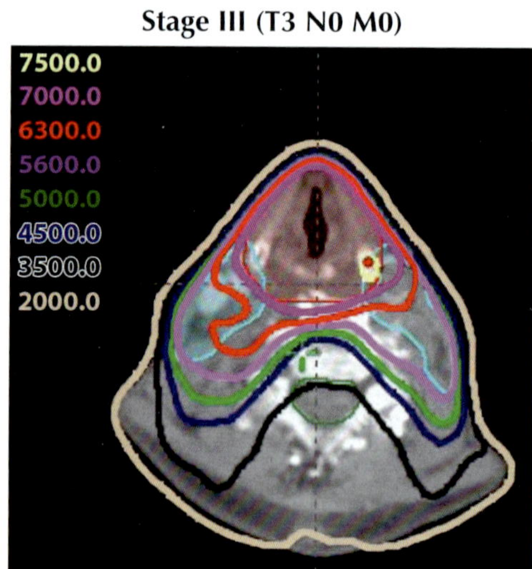

***(Left)** Axial CECT demonstrates a typical isodose distribution for an advanced larynx cancer treated with parallel opposed fields. Electron fields are added clinically to deliver 5,000 cGy to the posterior aspects of the field. **(Right)** This is an axial CECT demonstrating a typical isodose distribution for an advanced larynx cancer treated with a dose painting IMRT plan.*

Stage III (T3 N0)

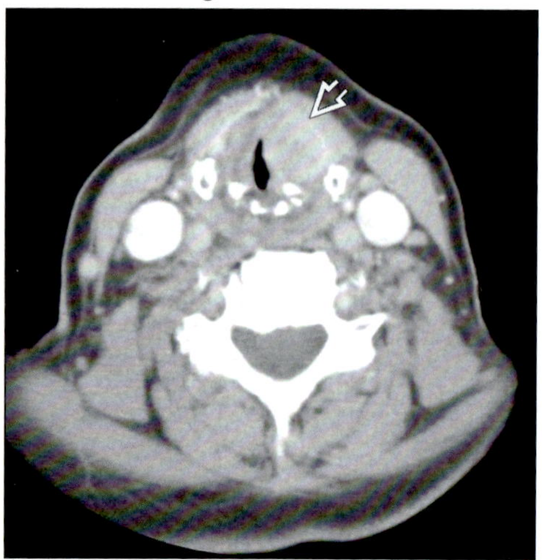

Stage III (T3 N1 M0)

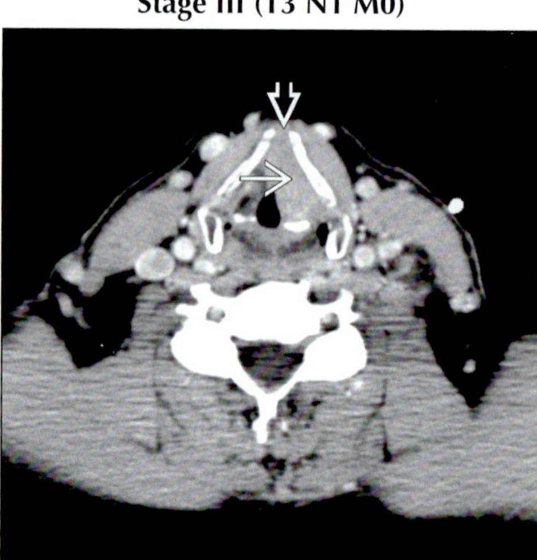

***(Left)** This is an axial CECT of a patient with a bulky transglottic tumor. On laryngoscopy, the left cord was noted to be paralyzed. **(Right)** This is an axial CECT of a patient with a T3 supraglottic of the left false vocal cord and by virtue of paraglottic fat space invasion. Note the extension anteriorly to the thyroid notch.*

Stage IVA (T3 N2b M0)

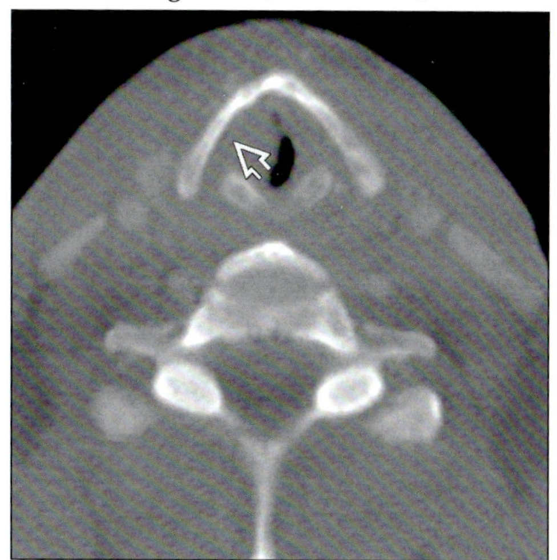

Stage IVA (T3 N2c M0)
Supraglottic Larynx

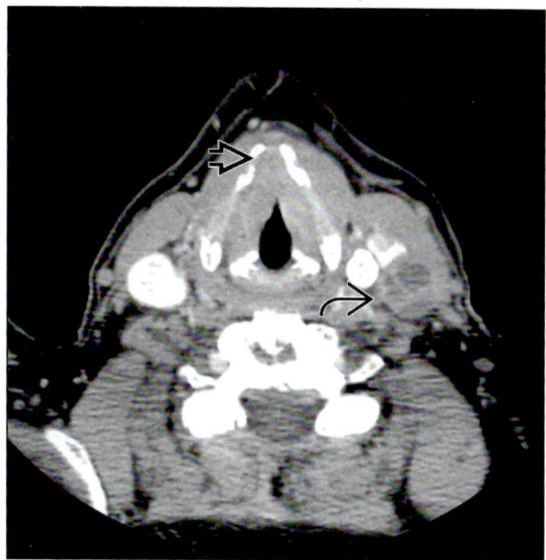

(Left) *This is an axial CT of a patient with T3 N2b carcinoma of the glottic larynx demonstrating subtle inner table thyroid cartilage invasion on the right .* ***(Right)*** *Axial CECT of a patient with a T3 N2c supraglottic squamous cell carcinoma demonstrates preepiglottic space invasion , making this a T3 primary tumor. There is also an enlarged, partially necrotic jugular chain lymph node .*

Stage IVA (T3 N2c M0)

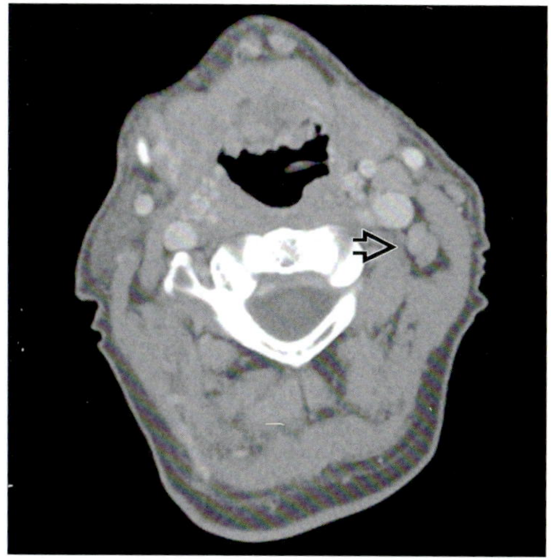

Stage IVA (T3 N2c M0)

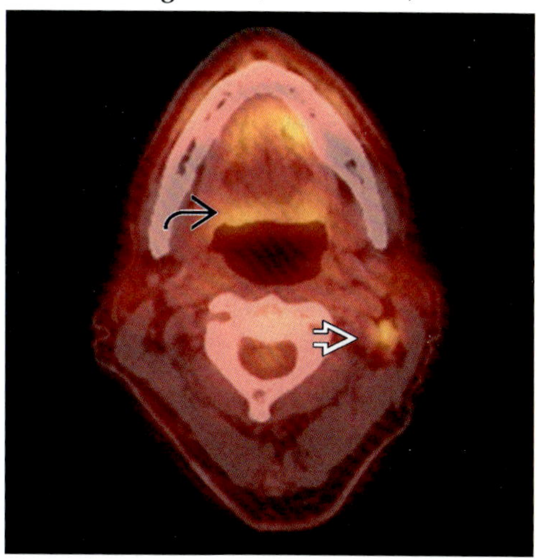

(Left) *Axial CECT of a patient with a supraglottic squamous cell carcinoma demonstrates a left level 2 node that is potentially involved with carcinoma.* ***(Right)*** *Subsequent axial PET/CT at the same level demonstrates that the lymph node has an SUV of 4.7 and is considered involved with carcinoma. Low-level uptake in the base of tongue in the absence of a soft tissue abnormality on the CT portion of the exam is within normal limits.*

Stage IVA (T4a N2b M0)

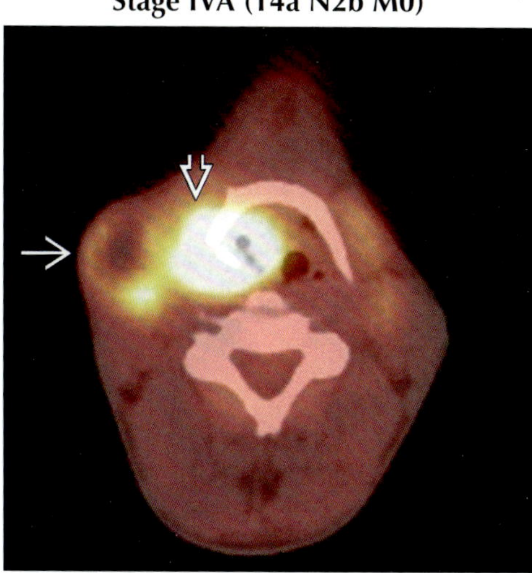

Stage IVB (T4b N2b M0)

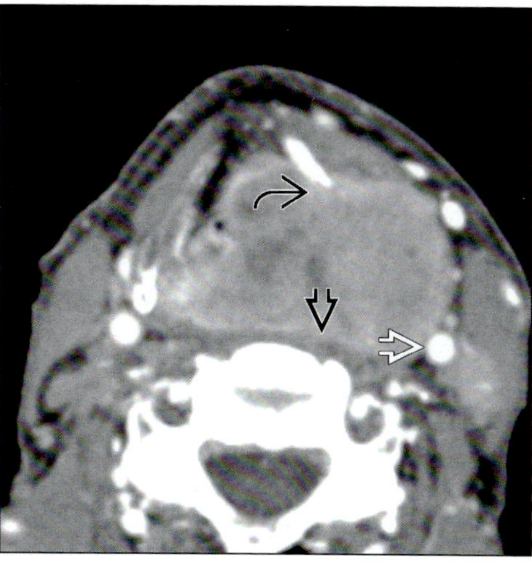

(Left) *This is an axial PET/CT of a patient with a T4a N2b carcinoma of the glottic larynx. Note the significant extralaryngeal spread into the soft tissues of the neck (classifying this as a T4a primary) and partially necrotic ipsilateral lymph node .* ***(Right)*** *Axial CECT demonstrates a large, enhancing mass that demonstrates spread through the thyroid cartilage and encroaches upon the prevertebral space and carotid artery .*

Stage IVA (T4a N0 M0)

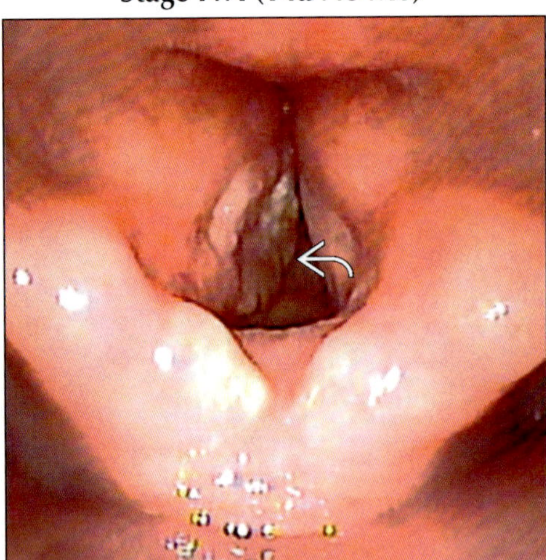

Stage IVA (T4a N0 M0)

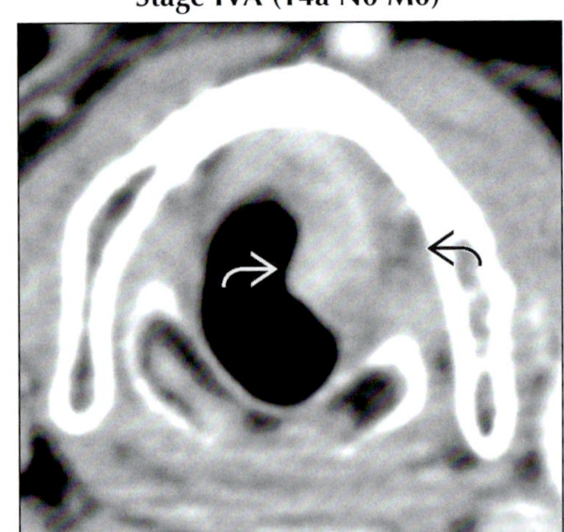

(Left) *This image demonstrates laryngoscopy at diagnosis. It demonstrates a primary tumor of the glottic larynx that is at least T2 by virtue of subglottic extension ➔.* ***(Right)*** *Axial CECT in the same patient at the level of the true glottis demonstrates an exophytic mass in the left true vocal cord ➔. The paraglottic space does not appear to be involved ➔.*

Stage IVA (T4a N0 M0)

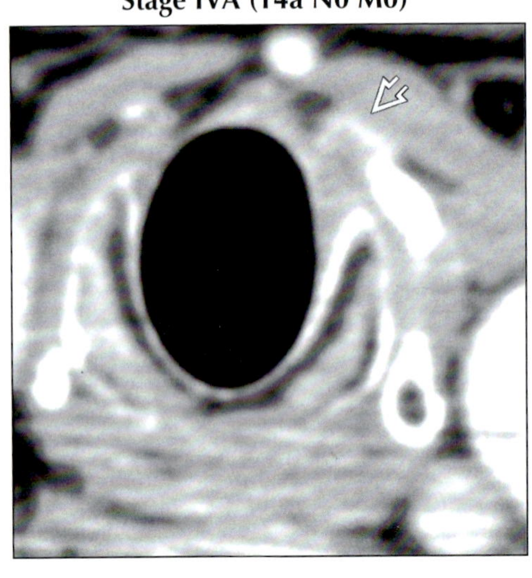

Stage IVA (T4a N0 M0)

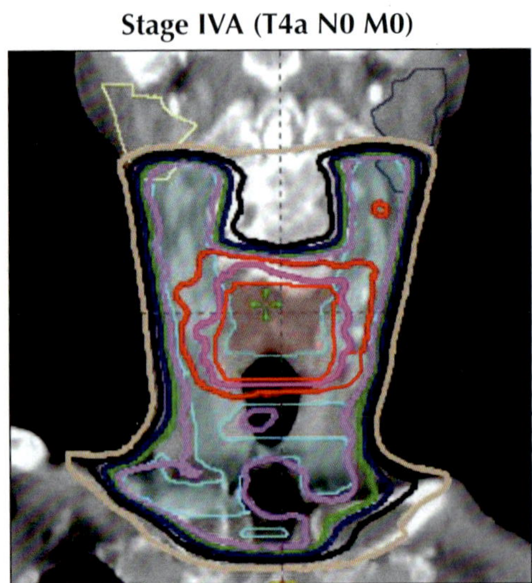

(Left) *Axial CECT in a more inferior cut in the same patient demonstrates invasion of the outer cortex of the thyroid cartilage ➔. Thus, this represents a T4a N0 M0 stage designation. Given the subtle imaging finding upstaging, the decision was made to proceed ahead with organ preservation.* ***(Right)*** *Coronal treatment planning CECT in the same patient demonstrates the volume treated in a dose painting technique.*

Stage IVA (T4a N0 M0)

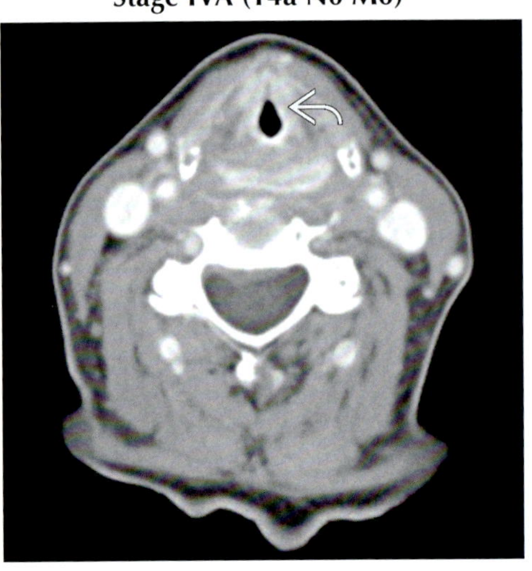

Stage IVA (T4a N0 M0)

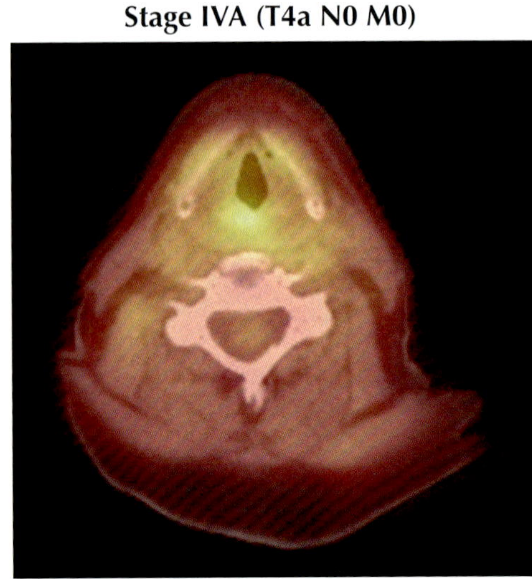

(Left) *Axial CECT in the same patient at 4 months post treatment demonstrates complete resolution of tumor, with nonspecific contrast uptake symmetrically in the larynx, likely representing post-treatment inflammation ➔.* ***(Right)*** *Axial PET/CT in the same patient 3 months after the completion of therapy demonstrates mild and diffuse uptake with no corresponding soft tissue abnormality. Physical examination demonstrated no persistence of disease.*

Esophageal Stricture

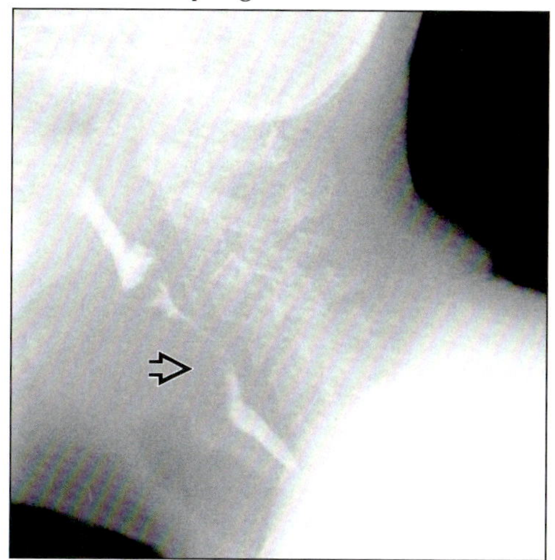

Paralyzed Cord

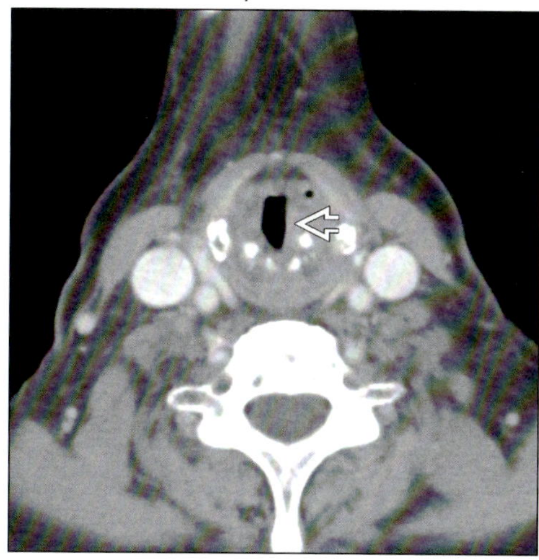

*(**Left**) Sagittal fluoroscopy obtained as a component of a modified barium swallow examination demonstrates a stricture ⇨ in the cervical esophagus 3 months post treatment for a supraglottic cancer with extensive pyriform sinus involvement. (**Right**) Axial CECT 6 months after completion of chemoradiation for advanced larynx cancer shows the vocal cord ➡ that was paralyzed on presentation continues to be paralyzed after eradication of tumor.*

Skin Reaction

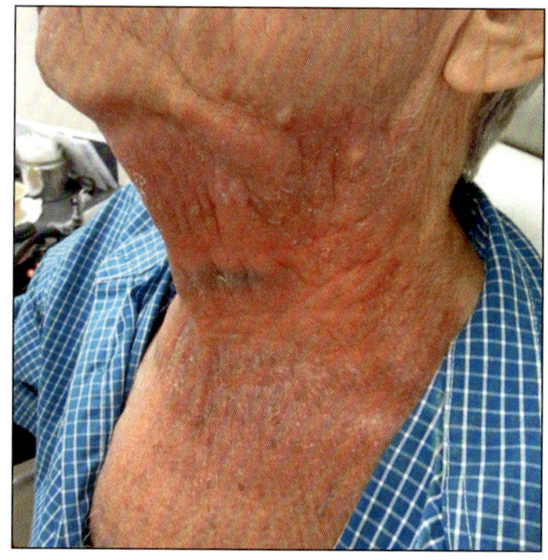

Treatment Response

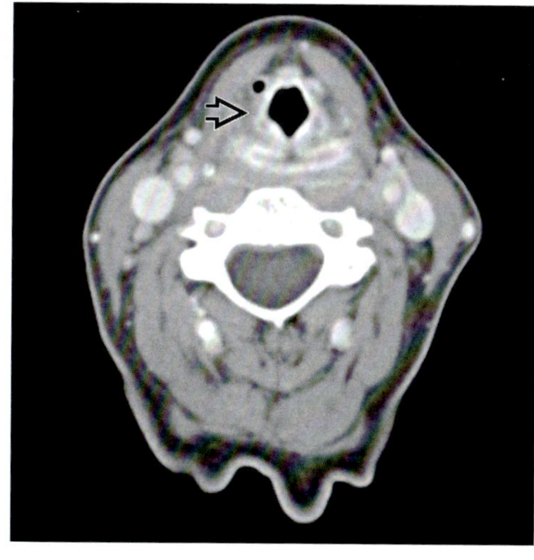

*(**Left**) Photograph of a patient 3 weeks after radiation demonstrates erythema in the treatment field likely secondary to exit dose from 6 MV beams, with a parallel opposed beam orientation. (**Right**) Axial CECT 4 weeks after the completion of chemoradiation for a T3 N0 larynx cancer demonstrates symmetric enhancement of the mucosa of the supraglottis ⇨ with no identifiable soft tissue mass, a finding consistent with disease control.*

Edema and Mucositis

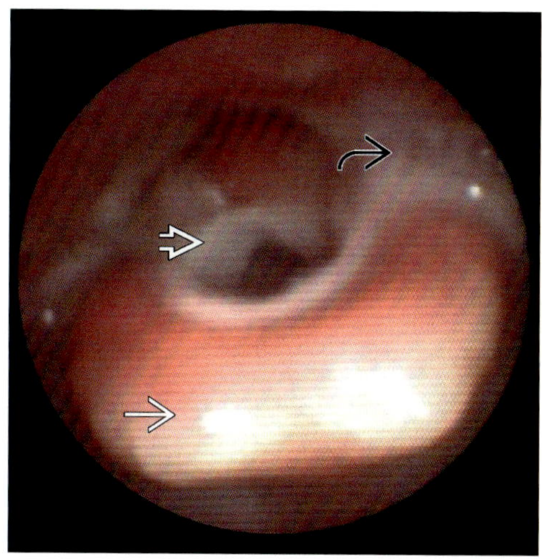

Edema

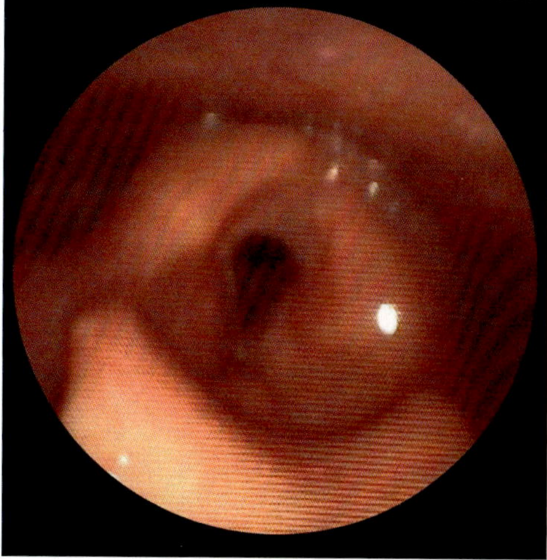

*(**Left**) Indirect laryngoscopy photograph of a larynx 4 weeks after completion of chemoradiation shows a swollen, blunted epiglottis ➡, persistent mucositis along the visualized aspects of the laryngeal epiglottis and false cords ➡, and pooling secretion ↗. (**Right**) Indirect laryngoscopy image demonstrates a symmetrically swollen larynx 2 months after radiotherapy with no evidence of persistent disease.*

NASAL CAVITY/PARANASAL SINUSES

(T) Primary Tumor

Adapted from 7th edition AJCC Staging Forms.

TNM	*Definitions*
TX	Primary tumor cannot be assessed
T0	No evidence of primary tumor
Tis	Carcinoma in situ
Maxillary Sinus	
T1	Tumor limited to maxillary sinus mucosa with no erosion or destruction of bone
T2	Tumor causing bone erosion or destruction including extension into hard palate &/or middle nasal meatus, except extension to posterior wall of maxillary sinus and pterygoid plates
T3	Tumor invades any of the following: Bone of posterior wall of maxillary sinus, subcutaneous tissues, floor or medial wall of orbit, pterygoid fossa, ethmoid sinuses
T4a	Moderately advanced local disease: Tumor invades anterior orbital contents, skin of cheek, pterygoid plates, infratemporal fossa, cribriform plate, sphenoid or frontal sinuses
T4b	Very advanced local disease: Tumor invades any of the following: Orbital apex, dura, brain, middle cranial fossa, cranial nerves other than maxillary division of trigeminal nerve (V2), nasopharynx, or clivus
Nasal Cavity and Ethmoid Sinus	
T1	Tumor restricted to any 1 subsite, ± bony invasion
T2	Tumor invading 2 subsites in a single region or extending to involve an adjacent region within nasoethmoidal complex, with or without bony invasion
T3	Tumor extends to invade medial wall or floor of orbit, maxillary sinus, palate, or cribriform plate
T4a	Moderately advanced local disease: Tumor invades any of the following: Anterior orbital contents, skin of nose or cheek, minimal extension to anterior cranial fossa, pterygoid plates, sphenoid or frontal sinuses
T4b	Very advanced local disease: Tumor invades any of the following: Orbital apex, dura, brain, middle cranial fossa, cranial nerves other than (V2), nasopharynx, or clivus

(N) Regional Lymph Nodes

NX	Regional lymph nodes cannot be assessed
N0	No regional lymph node metastasis
N1	Metastasis in a single ipsilateral lymph node, ≤ 3 cm in greatest dimension
N2	Metastasis in a single ipsilateral lymph node, > 3 cm but ≤ 6 cm in greatest dimension, or in multiple ipsilateral lymph nodes, none > 6 cm in greatest dimension, or in bilateral or contralateral lymph nodes, none > 6 cm in greatest dimension
N2a	Metastasis in a single ipsilateral lymph node, > 3 cm but ≤ 6 cm in greatest dimension
N2b	Metastasis in multiple ipsilateral lymph nodes, none > 6 cm in greatest dimension
N2c	Metastasis in bilateral or contralateral lymph nodes, none > 6 cm in greatest dimension
N3	Metastasis in a lymph node, > 6 cm in greatest dimension

(M) Distant Metastasis

M0	No distant metastasis
M1	Distant metastasis

(G) Histologic Grade

Adapted from 7th edition AJCC Staging Forms.

TNM	*Definitions*
GX	Grade cannot be assessed
G1	Well differentiated
G2	Moderately differentiated
G3	Poorly differentiated
G4	Undifferentiated

AJCC Stages/Prognostic Groups

Adapted from 7th edition AJCC Staging Forms.

Stage	*T*	*N*	*M*
0	Tis	N0	M0
I	T1	N0	M0
II	T2	N0	M0
III	T3	N0	M0
	T1	N1	M0
	T2	N1	M0
	T3	N1	M0
IVA	T4a	N0	M0
	T4a	N1	M0
	T1	N2	M0
	T2	N2	M0
	T3	N2	M0
	T4a	N2	M0
IVB	T4b	Any N	M0
	Any T	N3	M0
IVC	Any T	Any N	M1

Kadish Staging System for Esthesioneuroblastoma

Group A	Tumor localized to nasal cavity
Group B	Tumor localized to nasal cavity and sinuses
Group C	Tumor extends beyond nasal cavity and sinuses to skull base, anterior cranial fossa, orbit, or neck nodes, with or without distant metastases

Hyams Histologic Grading System for Esthesioneuroblastoma

Microscopic Features	*Grade 1*	*Grade 2*	*Grade 3*	*Grade 4*
Architecture	Lobular	Lobular	± lobular	± lobular
Pleomorphism	Absent to slight	Present	Prominent	Marked
Neurofibrillary matrix	Prominent	Present	May be present	Absent
Rosettes	Present[1]	Present[1]	May be present[2]	May be present[2]
Mitoses	Absent	Present	Prominent	Marked
Necrosis	Absent	Absent	Present	Prominent
Glands	May be present	May be present	May be present	May be present
Calcification	Variable	Variable	Absent	Absent

Adapted from Barnes L et al: World Health Organization Classification of Tumours: Pathology and Genetics of Head and Neck Tumours. Lyon: IARC Press, 2005.

[1]*Homer Wright rosettes (pseudorosettes).*

[2]*Flexner-Wintersteiner rosettes (true neural rosettes).*

T1/T2 Maxillary Sinus

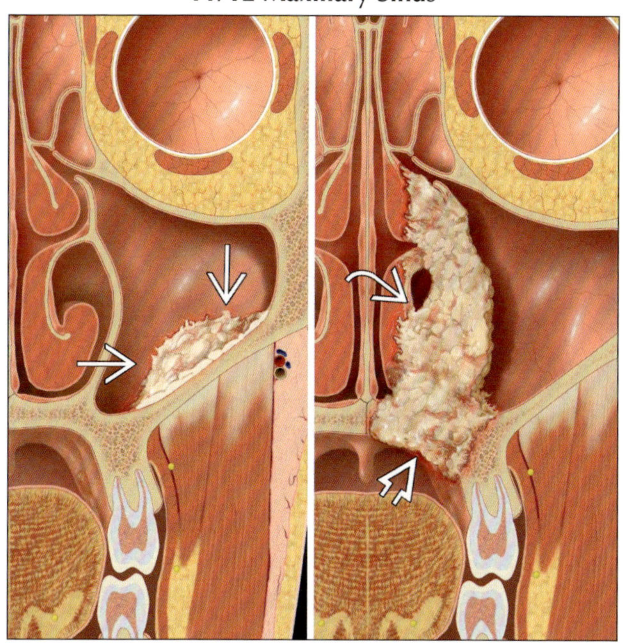

Coronal graphic shows a small T1 tumor ➔ confined to the maxillary mucosa without bone destruction. On the right, there is a larger tumor that destroys bone and also extends to the hard palate ➔ and middle meatus ➔. Any of these features designate this as a T2 tumor.

T3 Maxillary Sinus

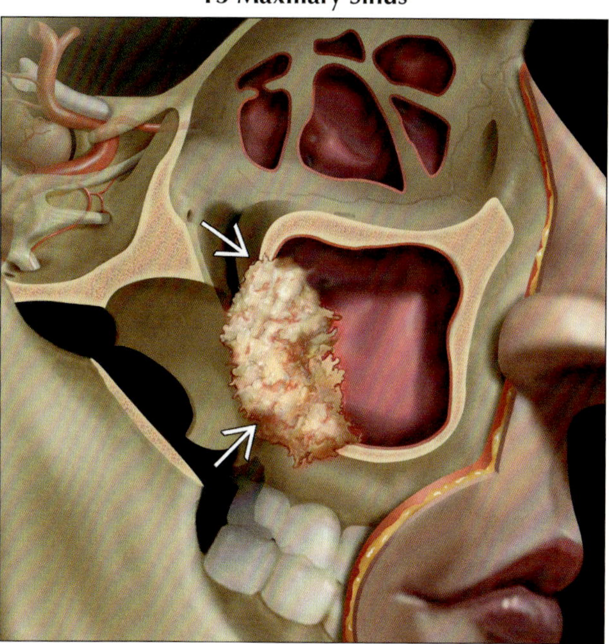

Graphic shows a T3 carcinoma invading the posterior bony wall of the maxillary sinus ➔. T3 disease is also determined by invasion of the floor or medial wall of the orbit &/or involvement of the ethmoid sinus, pterygoid fossa, or subcutaneous tissues.

T4a Maxillary Sinus

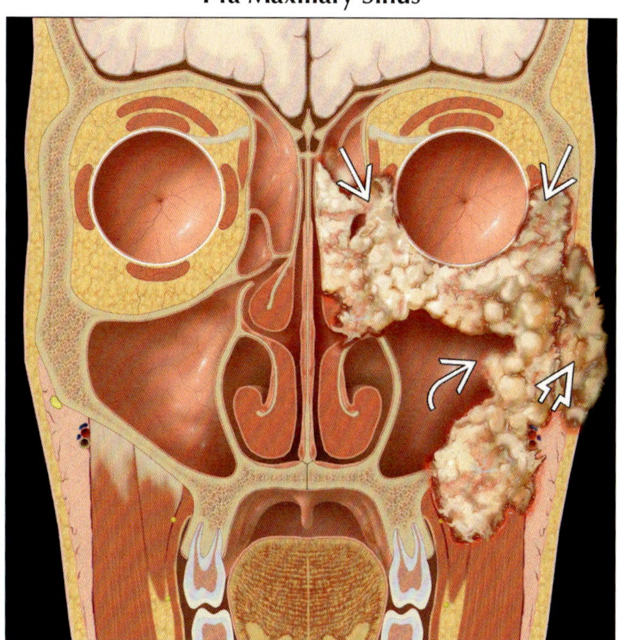

Coronal graphic shows a T4a maxillary sinus carcinoma ➔, which is invading the anterior orbit ➔ as well as extending out to the skin of the cheek ➔. T4a disease is also determined by invasion of pterygoid plates, infratemporal fossa, cribriform plate, and sphenoid or frontal sinuses.

T4b Maxillary Sinus

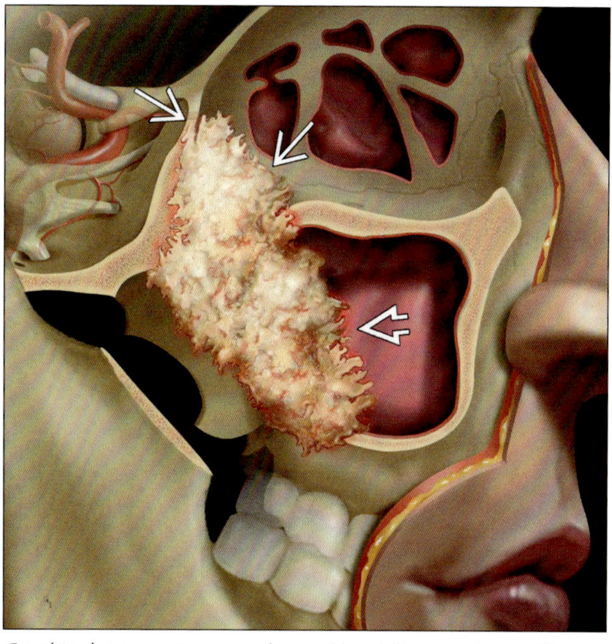

Graphic demonstrates very advanced local disease with maxillary sinus tumor ➔ invading posteriorly and superiorly to the orbital apex ➔. T4b disease is also designated when there is invasion of dura, brain, middle cranial fossa, nasopharynx, clivus, or cranial nerves other than maxillary division of trigeminal nerve.

T1 Ethmoid Sinus/T2 Nasal Cavity

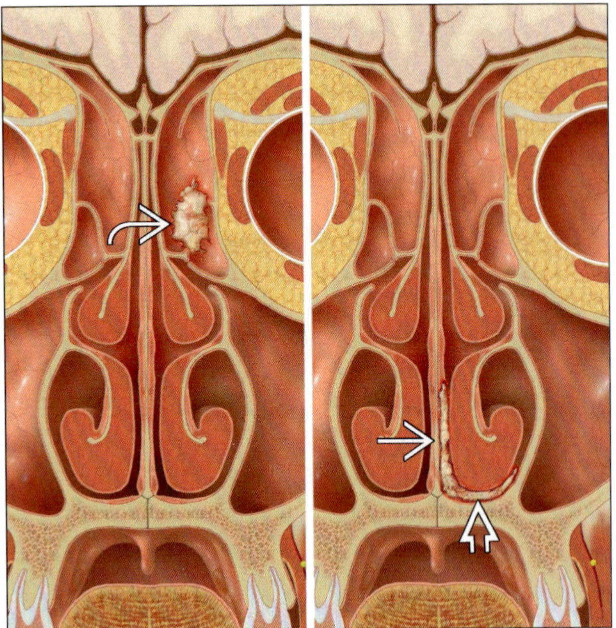

Coronal graphic (left) shows a small tumor confined to the left ethmoid air cells ➡, which is a T1 tumor. On the right, there is a small tumor involving the nasal septum ➡ and nasal floor ➡. Involvement of two subsites in the nasal cavity makes this a T2 tumor.

T3 Ethmoid Sinus/Nasal Cavity

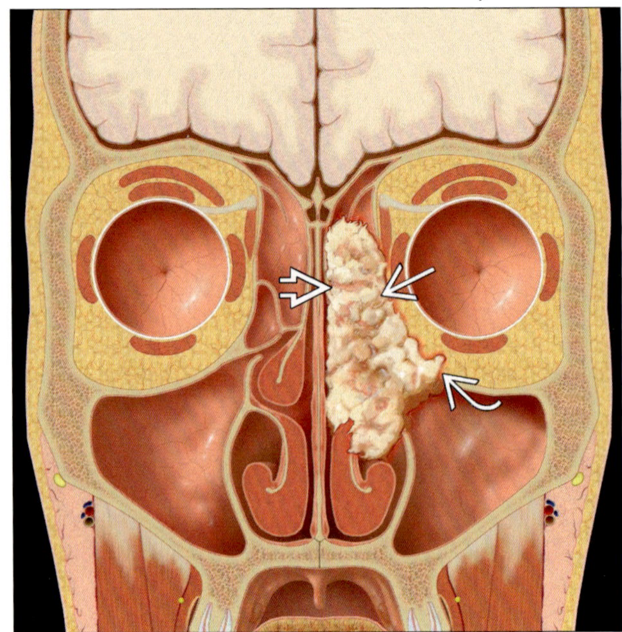

Coronal graphic shows an ethmoid tumor ➡, which extends to the medial orbital wall ➡ and orbital floor ➡. Maxillary sinus, palate, or cribriform plate invasion also constitute T3 disease.

T4a Ethmoid Sinus

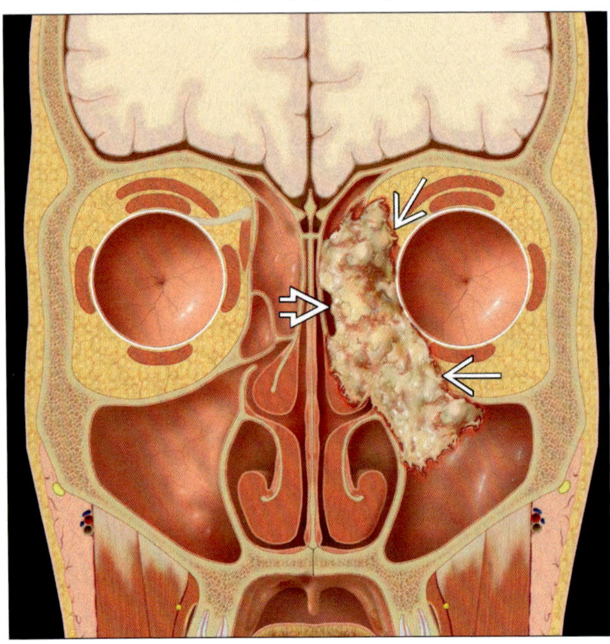

Coronal graphic illustrates a T4a ethmoid sinus carcinoma ➡ invading the anterior orbit ➡. T4a disease is also determined by invasion of the skin of the nose or cheek, minimal extension to the anterior cranial fossa, pterygoid plates, or sphenoid or frontal sinuses.

T4b Ethmoid Sinus

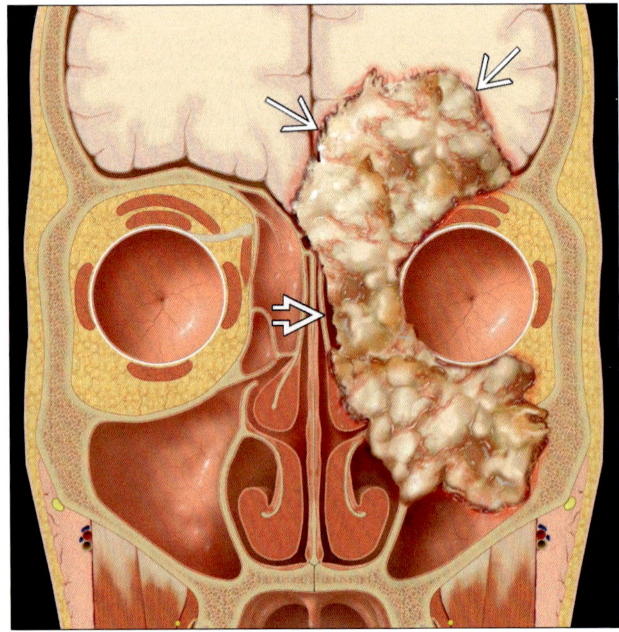

Coronal graphic shows a very advanced local ethmoid tumor ➡ with extensive intracranial invasion ➡ in addition to orbital and maxillary sinus invasion. T4b disease is also evident when there is orbital apex, middle cranial fossa, clivus, nasopharynx, or cranial nerve (other than CN V2) involvement.

Kadish A/Kadish B Esthesioneuroblastoma

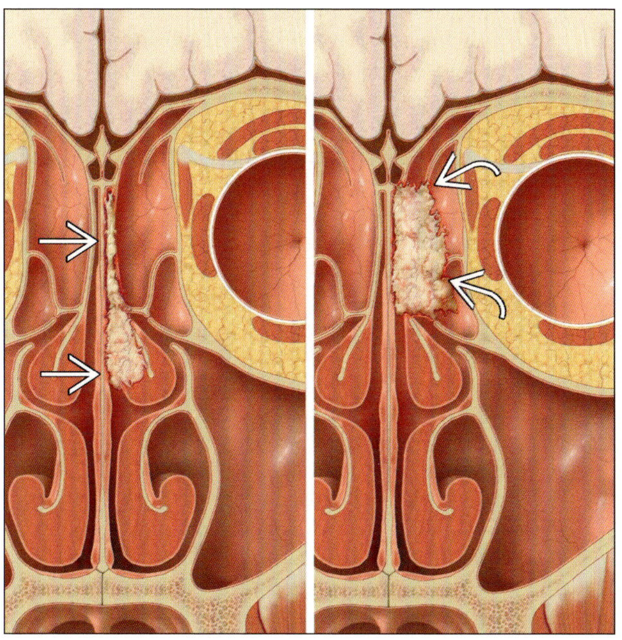

Coronal graphic (left) demonstrates a small tumor confined to the nasal cavity ➡, which is Kadish A and the least common form. On the right, there is extension of tumor from the nasal cavity to the paranasal sinuses ↪, which is Kadish B.

Kadish C Esthesioneuroblastoma

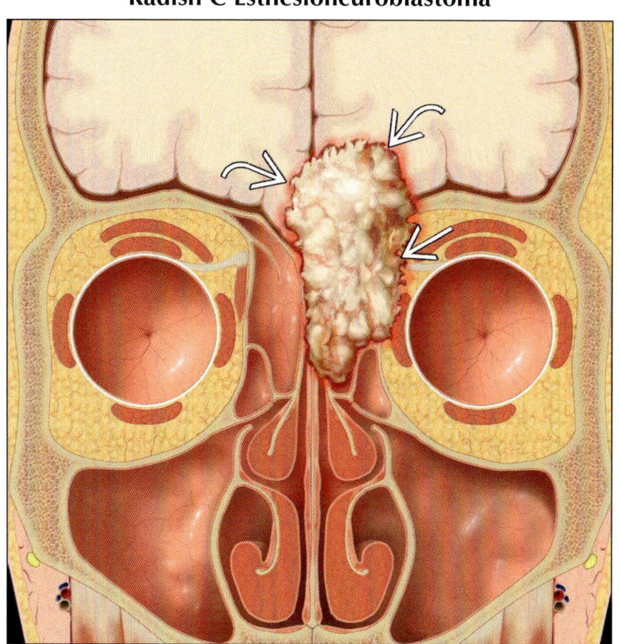

Coronal graphic illustrates a Kadish C tumor with extension beyond the nasal cavity and sinuses, into both the orbit ➡ and anterior cranial fossa ↪. Kadish D was not in the original staging system, but indicates nodal &/or distant metastases.

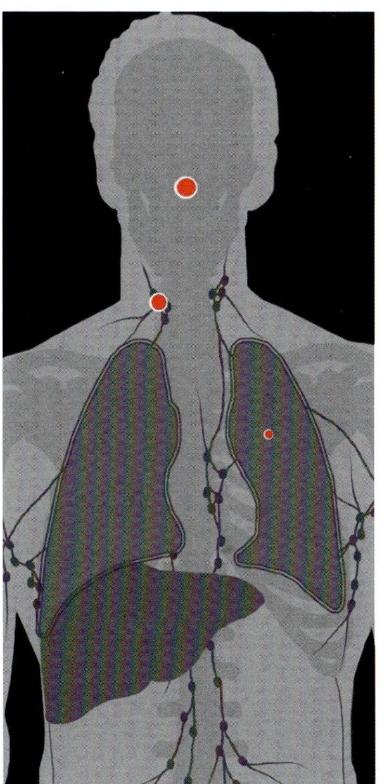

INITIAL SITE OF RECURRENCE

Local	10-30%
Regional	10-20%
Distant	0-20%

KK Ang et al: Radiotherapy for Head and Neck Cancers. 4th edition. 217-9, 2012.

NASAL CAVITY/PARANASAL SINUSES

OVERVIEW

General Comments

- Rare malignancies arising from nasal cavity and paranasal sinus
- Incidence of 1 per 100,000 or 3% of upper respiratory cancers
- Maxillary sinus is the most common site of sinonasal malignancies
- 60-80% of paranasal sinus tumors arise from maxillary antrum
- Squamous cell carcinoma is the most common histology
- Adenocarcinomas tend to occur in ethmoid sinuses or upper nasal cavity
- Esthesioneuroblastoma (ENB) originates from neuroectoderm; rare (2% of nasal malignancies)
  - Referred to as olfactory neuroblastoma
  - Arises from olfactory mucosa of superior 1/3 of nasal septum, cribriform plate, and superior turbinates
- Subsites anatomy
  - Nasal cavity
    - Nasal vestibule
    - Nasal fossa: Septum, floor, lateral wall
  - Paranasal sinuses
    - Maxillary sinuses
    - Ethmoid sinuses
    - Sphenoid sinuses
    - Frontal sinuses
- Late clinical presentation often results in advanced stage of disease
- Regional LN spread is relatively uncommon, can occur in advanced T stage tumors
  - Involvement of nodal sites: Buccinator, submandibular, upper jugular, and retropharyngeal nodes
  - Bilateral spread may occur when primary extends beyond midline

Classification

- **Primary malignant tumors (WHO classification)**
  - **Carcinomas**
    - Squamous cell carcinomas
      - Verrucous carcinoma
      - Papillary squamous cell carcinoma
      - Basaloid squamous cell carcinoma
      - Spindle cell carcinoma
      - Adenosquamous carcinoma
      - Acantholytic squamous cell carcinoma
    - Lymphoepithelial carcinoma
    - Sinonasal undifferentiated carcinoma
    - Adenocarcinoma
      - Intestinal-type adenocarcinoma
      - Non-intestinal-type adenocarcinoma
  - **Neuroendocrine tumors**
    - Typical carcinoid
    - Atypical carcinoid
    - Small cell carcinoma, neuroendocrine type
  - **Soft tissue tumors**
    - Malignant tumors
      - Fibrosarcoma
      - Malignant fibrous histiocytoma
      - Leiomyosarcoma
      - Rhabdomyosarcoma
      - Angiosarcoma
      - Malignant peripheral nerve sheath tumor
    - Tumors with low malignant potential/borderline tumors
      - Desmoid-type fibromatosis
      - Inflammatory myofibroblastic tumor
      - Glomangiopericytoma (sinonasal-type hemangiopericytoma)
      - Extrapleural solitary fibrous tumor
  - **Tumors of bone and cartilage (malignant subtype)**
    - Chondrosarcoma
    - Mesenchymal chondrosarcoma
    - Osteosarcoma
    - Chordoma
  - **Hematolymphoid tumors**
    - Extranodal NK-/T-cell lymphoma
    - Diffuse large B-cell lymphoma
    - Extramedullary plasmacytoma
    - Extramedullary myeloid sarcoma
    - Histiocytic sarcoma
    - Langerhans cell histiocytosis
  - **Neuroectodermal tumors**
    - Ewing sarcoma
    - Primitive neuroectodermal tumor
    - Olfactory neuroblastoma (ENB)
    - Melanotic neuroectodermal tumor of infancy
    - Mucosal malignant melanoma
  - **Germ cell tumors**
    - Immature teratoma
    - Teratoma with malignant transformation
    - Sinonasal yolk sac tumor (endodermal sinus tumor)
    - Sinonasal teratocarcinosarcoma
    - Mature teratoma
    - Dermoid cyst
  - **Mucosal melanoma**
  - **Secondary tumors**

NATURAL HISTORY

General Features

- Comments
  - Sinonasal carcinoma
    - Most patients older than 40 years of age
    - Minor salivary gland tumors and ENB tend to appear before age 20
    - Early symptoms are vague
      - Nasal cavity: Unilateral nasal obstruction, epistaxis
      - Maxillary sinus: Most often do not present early
    - Advanced stage
      - Aggressively spreads to adjacent structures, facial pain, intranasal/intraoral mass, ocular symptoms

Epidemiology & Cancer Incidence

- Sinonasal carcinoma
  - Generally a relatively rare cancer, although more prevalent in Japan, South Africa
  - Demographics
    - Age: 95% of patients > 45 years of age
    - Gender: M:F =2:1
  - Approximately 2,000 new cases per year in USA
  - Approximately 3% of head and neck cancers

- European data show incidence < 2 per 100,000 men and 1 per 100,000 women
- Risk factors
  - Tobacco use
  - Alcohol use
  - Viruses
    - Associations with HPV and EBV have been postulated
    - HPV is especially important in carcinomas arising from inverted papillomas
  - Occupational exposures (e.g., textile, leather, formaldehyde, and wood dust)
  - Age
- ENB
  - Age
    - Broad range: 3-88 years
    - Bimodal distribution centered in 2nd and 6th decades of life
  - Gender: Slightly more common in females

Genetics

- Sinonasal carcinoma
  - Possible link to abnormal expression of *p53*
- ENB
  - Cytogenetic abnormalities (e.g., translocations)

Gross Pathology & Surgical Features

- Sinonasal carcinoma
  - Polypoid morphology
  - Papillary or fungating growth
  - Tan-white or pinkish red color
- ENB
  - Broad-based, pedunculated, lobulated, soft, glistening mass covered in mucosa
  - Red-gray, red-brown color

Microscopic Pathology

- H&E
  - Squamous cell carcinoma
    - Keratinizing subtype (80%)
      - Papillary, exophytic, or inverted patterns in architecture
      - Surface and individual cell keratinization
      - Dyskeratosis
      - Poorly to well differentiated
    - Nonkeratinizing subtype (20%)
      - Papillary or exophytic growth pattern
      - Interconnecting bands of neoplastic epithelium
      - Hypercellular
      - Pleomorphic
      - Mitotic activity
  - Undifferentiated carcinoma
    - Lack of squamous or glandular differentiation
    - Cytokeratin/EMA positive
  - Adenocarcinoma
    - Papillary morphology
  - Squamous cell carcinoma variants include
    - Verrucous
      - Exophytic
      - Broad based
      - "Church spire" hyperkeratosis
      - Deep margin of bulbous processes
    - Papillary
      - Focal invasion at base
    - Basaloid
      - Palisaded basaloid cells
      - Hyalinized stroma
    - Spindle cell
      - Polypoid
      - Pleomorphic
      - Cytokeratin positive
    - Adenoid squamous
      - Acantholytic
    - Adenosquamous
      - Mixed differentiation squamous cell carcinoma and adenocarcinoma
      - Solid with cells positive for mucin or obvious glands
  - **ENB**
    - Grows in circumscribed lobules or nests
      - Separated by fibrous stroma rich in vasculature
    - Diffuse growth pattern may also be seen
      - Less common
    - Vast majority of ENBs have in situ component
    - Uniform, small, and round nuclei
      - Scant cytoplasm
      - Coarse to fine chromatin ("salt and pepper")
      - Inconspicuous nucleoli
    - Rosettes
      - Homer Wright (pseudorosettes) in up to 30%
      - Flexner-Wintersteiner (true neural rosettes) in < 30% of ENB
    - Criteria for Hyams system of histologic grading (grades 1-4)
      - Architecture
      - Pleomorphism
      - Neurofibrillary matrix
      - Rosette formation
      - Mitoses
      - Necrosis
      - Presence of gland formation
      - Presence of calcifications
- Special stains
  - Sinonasal carcinoma
    - Keratin profile correlates with microscopic subtype
  - ENB markers
    - Neuron-specific enolase (NSE)
      - Most consistently expressed marker
    - Other markers seen in majority of tumors
      - Synaptophysin
      - Neurofilament protein (NFP)
      - Class III β-tubulin
      - Microtubule-associated protein

Routes of Spread

- Nasal vestibule
  - Invade nasal skin, alar and septal cartilage, upper lip
  - Lymphatics
    - Ipsilateral facial nodes and level IB nodes
- Nasal cavity
  - Direct extension depending on primary tumor site
    - Tumor arising from olfactory bulb tends to invade ethmoid sinus, orbit, or cribriform plate
  - Lymphatics
    - Nasal cavity: Drain to lateral retropharyngeal nodes or level II nodes
- Sinonasal carcinoma
  - Direct extension (most common)
  - Lymphatic (lymphatic metastases to regional nodes are uncommon)

- Paranasal sinus: Rare nodal spread in T1-2 disease, about 15% in T3-4, drain to lateral levels IB and II
- ENB
  - Direct extension, submucosal extension, or along olfactory nerves with frontal lobe invasion
  - Metastases
    - 20-40% of ENBs metastasize to regional lymph nodes, lungs, bone
    - Most common sites of nodal spread are retropharyngeal nodes or parapharyngeal nodes
- Hematogenous
  - May involve bone, lung, liver, CNS
  - Organ metastases are uncommon

IMAGING

Detection

- **Sinonasal carcinoma**
  - Radiologist constructs presurgical map of tumor spread
    - Anterior
      - Subcutaneous cheek tissues
    - Posterior
      - Retroantral fat pad and pterygopalatine fossa
    - Cephalad
      - Pterygopalatine fossa to inferior orbital fissure to orbit
    - Lateral
      - Malar eminence and subcutaneous tissues
    - Superior
      - Into orbit proper through orbital floor
    - Inferior
      - Maxillary alveolar ridge, buccal space, and hard palate
    - Perineural spread
      - Inferior orbital nerve or pterygopalatine fossa to foramen rotundum (V2) to cavernous sinus
  - Majority of initial diagnoses made on NECT when evaluating "sinusitis type" symptoms
  - CT
    - NECT
      - Soft tissue density mass with irregular margins
      - Conspicuous destruction of bone
    - CECT
      - Moderately enhancing, heterogeneous, solid mass that shows aggressive destruction of bone
  - MR
    - T1WI
      - Intermediate-signal mass
      - Increased T1 signal may be seen in intratumoral hemorrhage areas
    - T2WI
      - Intermediate to high signal when compared against musculature, yet lower than majority of sinonasal malignancies
      - Lower signal is result of high cellularity and higher nuclear to cytoplasmic ratio
      - T2 differentiates tumor from high signal due to obstructed sinus secretions
    - T1WI C+
      - Enhancement typically mild to moderate, heterogeneous, and diffuse
      - Necrotic areas do not enhance
      - Squamous cell carcinoma enhances less than adenocarcinoma, ENB, and melanoma
      - T1WI C+ fat-saturated imaging is excellent for perineural tumor spread
- **ENB**
  - **General**
    - Key diagnostic findings
      - Classic finding: "Dumbbell" mass with superior part of tumor in intracranial fossa and inferior part of tumor in upper nasal cavity
      - Peripheral cysts of tumor located at intracranial tumor margin strongly suggestive of ENB
    - Anatomic location
      - Small ENB: Unilateral mass in nasal cavity with center of mass located at superior nasal wall
      - Larger ENB: Mass located in anterior cranial fossa and ethmoid and maxillary sinuses ipsilaterally (involvement of orbit occurs late)
    - Size
      - Nodule < 1 cm to occupying whole nasal cavity and inferior anterior cranial fossa
    - Morphological characteristics
      - If tumor size is small, it is a polypoid mass
      - If tumor size is large, it is dumbbell-shaped
  - CT
    - NECT
      - Remodeling of bone enlarges nasal cavity and causes destruction of bone (particularly in area of cribriform plate)
      - Speckled pattern of calcification in lesion is uncommon
    - CECT
      - Homogeneous enhancement
      - Necrosis (nonenhancing) may be seen in large tumors
  - **MR**
    - T1WI
      - Compared to brain, hypointense to intermediate intensity
      - Hemorrhage: May appear hyperintense
    - T2WI
      - Compared to brain, intermediate intensity to hyperintensity
      - Cystic degeneration: Hyperintense
      - Obstructed secretions of adjacent sinuses: Hyperintense
      - Foci of hemorrhage: Hypointense to hyperintense based on age of blood
    - T1WI C+
      - Avid homogeneous enhancement
      - Regions of necrosis: Heterogeneously enhancing
  - **PET/CT**
    - SUV measurements may correlate with tumor grade
  - **Imaging recommendations**
    - Map tumor for en bloc craniofacial surgery
      - Enhanced MR combined with CT (bone only)
    - Key diagnostic tool
      - Enhanced MR (axial and coronal) T2 sequences: Superior to distinguish tumor from sinus secretions
    - Bone-only CT
      - Offers precise assessment of bone destruction

- Can change extent of tissue removal in potential craniofacial resection
- If ENB is suspected, scan
  - Anterior cranial fossa
  - Sinonasal region
  - Cervical neck (20% of ENB patients have malignant lymph nodes at presentation)
- Surveillance
  - Follow-up over long term (5-10 years)

Staging

- **Sinonasal carcinoma**
  - **Nodal disease**
    - **General**
      - Regional lymph metastasis is indicator of poor prognosis, potentially signifying neoplastic spread beyond sinonasal cavity
      - Paranasal carcinomas primarily drain to lateral retropharyngeal nodes, which cannot be evaluated clinically; can result in underestimation of nodal metastasis
      - Other frequent sites of nodal metastasis include upper internal jugular (level II) and submandibular nodes (level IB)
      - Maxillary antrum: Most common primary site associated with cervical lymph node metastasis (seen in up to 15% of patients at time of presentation)
      - Ethmoid, sphenoid, and frontal sinus neoplasms: Less frequently associated with lymph node metastasis
    - **CT**
      - Commonly used modality for evaluation of neck nodes
      - Generally superior in detecting necrosis of neck nodes
      - Size evaluation criteria: > 1.5 cm in jugulodigastric region and > 1 cm in other nodes considered abnormal
      - Other pathologic characteristics to evaluate include extracapsular spread, carotid encasement, and fixation of lymph node(s), all of which are poor prognostic indicators
      - Findings worrisome for extracapsular spread include increased node size, poorly defined margins, stranding in soft tissue
    - **MR**
      - Superior soft tissue contrast
      - Offers ability to evaluate tissue characteristics with different sequences
    - **PET/CT**
      - Nodal FDG avidity more predictive of disease than size criteria alone, although FDG avidity can also represent inflammation
      - Can offer additional diagnostic value in addition to mainstay modalities of CT/MR
  - **Metastatic disease**
    - **CT**
      - Evaluates osseous involvement
      - CECT can be beneficial in detection of intracranial tumor spread, meningeal/ parenchymal involvement
      - Commonly used to evaluate extension to skull base
    - **MR**
      - Superior differentiation of malignancy from background inflammation, soft tissue, and sinus secretions
      - Precise assessment of borders of neoplasm if it extends to soft tissues outside sinuses
      - Complementary role to CT, superior in evaluating intracranial tumor spread
      - Contrast-enhanced MR: Preferred modality in evaluation of perineural spread, orbit extension, cavernous sinus spread, and intracranial compartment extension
      - Commonly used to evaluate extension to skull base
      - T1WI, before and after contrast, with fat suppression from sellar floor to hyoid bone: Used to map tumor spread and evaluate perineural spread
    - **PET/CT**
      - Can offer additional diagnostic value in addition to mainstay modalities of CT/MR
      - Can detect both regional and distant metastasis
      - Limited evaluation of perineural spread
- **ENB**
  - **Nodal disease**
    - **General**
      - Nodal metastasis to cervical nodes most commonly seen (20% at presentation)
    - **CT**
      - Evaluates size criteria: > 1.5 cm in jugulodigastric region and > 1 cm in other nodes considered abnormal
      - Given high rate of metastasis, CECT with IV contrast often routinely performed to detect occult metastasis
    - **MR**
      - Generally preferred modality for evaluation of retropharyngeal lymph nodes
      - Proposed criteria to assess lateral retropharyngeal adenopathy range from size > 10 mm considered abnormal to shortest axial diameter > 5 mm considered abnormal
      - Any visible node seen in median retropharyngeal area considered malignant
    - **PET/CT**
      - Can offer additional diagnostic value in addition to mainstay modalities of CT/MR
  - **Metastatic disease**
    - **General**
      - Common sites of metastasis: Lung, skin, parotid gland, bone, liver, eye, spinal cord/canal
    - **CT**
      - Beneficial in assessing extension to lamina papyracea, cribriform plate, and anterior cranial base (particularly coronal CT)
      - Chest and abdominal CT may be performed to rule out metastatic disease
    - **MR**
      - Superior assessment of precise margins of tumor extension to intracranial and intraorbital region
      - Offers differentiation between neoplasm and background inflammation

- Often used in Kadish stage C disease for further diagnostic assessment (often gadolinium-enhanced T1WI); especially important when erosion/thinning of bone walls
- PET/CT
  - Can offer additional diagnostic value in addition to mainstay modalities of CT/MR
  - Can detect both regional and distant metastasis
  - Limited evaluation of perineural spread

Restaging

- CT
  - Can evaluate change in post-treatment phase
  - Following treatment, can be difficult to differentiate neoplasm from scar tissue, as tissues have similar densities
- MR
  - Beneficial in distinguishing neoplastic tissue from scar tissue if interpretation on CT is difficult
  - Early scar tissue and granulation tissue
    - Often hyperintense with T2-weighted imaging, enhancing with contrast administration
  - Mature scar tissue
    - Little or no mass effect, hypointense on T2-weighted images due to fibrosis, lack of avid contrast enhancement
- PET/CT
  - Can be used if residual malignancy or recurrent malignancy cannot be ruled out
  - Less useful immediately following treatment given FDG-avid background inflammation

CLINICAL PRESENTATION & WORK-UP

Presentation

- **Nasal vestibule**
  - Slow-growing lesion with crusting, superficial bleeding
  - Upper lip or anterior hard palate involvement when tumor is advanced
- **Nasal cavity**
  - Nasal obstruction, discharge, intermittent bleeding
  - In advanced disease, tumor can invade skin, nasal septum, orbit, or other paranasal sinuses
- Maxillary sinus
  - Larger maxillary tumors present with
    - Unilateral nasal obstruction
    - Epistaxis
    - Nasal discharge
    - Numbness of cheek
  - Advanced local invasion may present with
    - Tooth pain or loosening
    - Proptosis
    - Diplopia
    - Trismus
    - Facial asymmetry
    - Nonhealing ulcer or sore
- **Ethmoid sinus**
  - Soft tissue mass in inner canthus or frontonasal region; nasal obstruction, intermittent bleeding; orbital extension with proptosis or diplopia
- **Sphenoid sinus**
  - Extremely rare; could present with headache, CNs III, IV, V1, V2, or VI symptoms if cavernous sinus invasion
- **ENB**
  - Nonspecificity of signs and symptoms typically results in late diagnosis
  - Signs and symptoms
    - Most common: Unilateral nasal obstruction or congestion
    - Others: Epistaxis, anosmia, rhinorrhea, headache, pain, ocular disturbances
  - Findings on rhinoscopy
    - Mass may not be distinguishable from other conditions (e.g., polyposis, chronic sinusitis, or other malignancies of nasal cavity)
  - Profuse bleeding of tumor may occur upon biopsy

Prognosis

- **Sinonasal carcinoma**
  - Poor prognostic factors
    - Primary tumor origins from structure above Ohngren line (line that connects medial canthus of eye to angle of mandible)
    - Locally advanced disease
    - Nodal metastases
    - Perineural invasion
    - Positive surgical margins
    - Multiple recurrences
  - Overall 5-year, disease-free survival rate: 50%
    - Squamous cell carcinoma (30-40%)
    - Adenocarcinoma (70-80%)
  - 5-year disease local control
    - T1: 90-100%
    - T2: 70-90%
    - T3: 30-50%
    - T4: 0-30%
  - 5-year regional control
    - With postop neck RT: 80-100%
    - No postop neck RT: 40-80%
  - 5-year overall survival
    - Stage I: 62.9%
    - Stage II: 60.6%
    - Stage III: 50.3%
    - Stage IV: 35.9%
  - Tumor T and N stages and postop RT are the most common prognostic factors affecting disease local or regional control and overall survival
- **ENB**
  - Kadish group C most common stage
  - Late nodal failure (2-3 years) or late distant failure (5-10 years) is not rare
  - Failure rates: Local up to 70% reported; nodal 15%; distant: 20-30%, usually bone and lung
  - Negative prognostic indicators
    - Tumor grade
    - Extensive disease or intracranial extension
    - Distant metastasis or cervical metastasis
    - Tumor recurrence
  - Tumor stage and grade are both significant prognostic indicators
    - Kadish stage A (tumor confined to nasal cavity)
      - > 90% 3-year survival rate
    - Kadish stage B (tumor in nasal cavity that extends to paranasal sinus)
      - > 80% 3-year survival rate

- Kadish stage C (tumor extends to orbit, skull base, or intracranial or cervical/distant metastases
  - < 30-50% 3-year survival rate
- Low-grade histology
  - 80% 5-year survival rate
- High-grade histology
  - 40% 5-year survival rate

Work-Up

- Clinical
  - H&P including complete head and neck exam, rhinoscopy or fiberoptic exam
  - Biopsy
  - Dental or prosthetic consult if indicated
    - Pretreatment dental care, 10-14 days required for extraction wound healing before RT
  - Audiometry baseline before RT
  - Speech and swallow evaluation if indicated
  - Ophthalmology consult if indicated
- Radiographic
  - Diagnostic sinonasal imaging: CECT and MR of maxillofacial images; CT neck soft tissue, or PET/CT for locally advanced disease; chest imaging
    - Differential diagnosis whether inflammation or malignancy
    - Extension of primary tumor or nodal metastases, including intracranial, intraorbital, infratemporal fossa, nasopharynx, subcutaneous fat, pharyngea or retropharyngeal space, perineural or neurovascular bundle invasion, etc.
- Laboratory
  - CBC, CMP

TREATMENT

Major Treatment Alternatives

- **Sinonasal carcinoma**
  - Surgery
    - Most nasal cavity or paranasal sinus cancers are treated with surgery
    - Neck dissection if clinical N(+)
    - Consider reexcision if feasible
  - Radiation therapy (RT)
    - RT is often used in postop setting
    - Adjuvant RT for pathologic adverse features: Close or microscopic positive margins, perineural invasion, any T3 or T4 disease, N(+) or ECE(+)
    - Adjuvant RT for most adenoid cystic carcinomas, especially if tumor arising from suprastructure
    - Consider preoperative RT or chemoradiation therapy (CRT) if tumor is marginally resectable
    - Consider definitive RT or CRT for locoregional advanced or unresectable tumor
  - Chemotherapy
    - Adjuvant CRT for postop adverse features: Microscopic margins, nodal ECE(+)
    - Definitive concurrent CRT for advanced or unresectable disease
    - Induction chemotherapy followed by CRT as indicated
    - Palliative chemotherapy may increase quality of life and length of survival
- **ENB**
  - Combination of radical craniofacial surgery (en bloc resection) and postop RT
  - Definitive CRT for unresectable disease
  - Preop RT or CRT for marginal resectable disease
  - Chemotherapy reserved for
    - Larger, higher grade tumors
    - Tumors that have disseminated

Major Treatment Roadblocks/ Contraindications

- **Sinonasal carcinoma**
  - Complex anatomy and critical local structures (e.g., brain, dura, cranial nerves, and orbits)
  - Relapse at primary site is more common than at primary lymph nodes
  - 90% of patients with tumor recurrences have < 1 year of survival
- **ENB**
  - Given its rare nature, little clear data or evidence regarding optimal treatment of ENB
- **Adverse side effects associated with RT or CRT**
  - Skin reaction: Erythema, moist desquamation, pigmentation, etc.
  - Alopecia
  - Mucositis
  - Xerostomia
  - Neurosensory injury, hearing impairment
  - Vision impairment possible from injury of cornea, lens, retina, optic nerve, or chiasm
  - Watery eye secondary tear duct stenosis
  - Pituitary hormone deficiencies
  - Osteomyelitis, aseptic brain necrosis, meningitis

Treatment Options by Stage

- **Sinonasal carcinoma**
  - Stage I
    - Surgical resection is preferred for early stage tumor
    - Postop RT for close or positive margins or perineural invasion (+)
    - Sometimes RT alone for early stage ethmoid sinus cancer
  - Stage II
    - Surgical resection
    - Postop RT should be given after incomplete resection or close or positive margins
    - Sometimes RT alone for T1-2 N0 ethmoid sinus tumor, and postop RT if indicated, such as close or positive margin, PNI(+)
  - Stage III
    - Surgical resection followed by postop RT if indicated: N(+), close margins, PNI(+)
    - Consider postop CRT if margins (+) &/or ECE(+)
    - Definitive RT or CRT
    - Cisplatin is the common chemo agent
  - Stage IV
    - Definitive CRT for local or regional advanced tumor
    - Prophylactic RT to ipsilateral or bilateral upper neck nodal sites for T3 or T4 disease
    - Induction chemotherapy followed by RT or CRT if initial RT ports have high risks to organs at risk (OARs)
    - Salvage chemotherapy or clinical trial for metastatic disease
- **ENB**

NASAL CAVITY/PARANASAL SINUSES

- Localized esthesioneuroblastoma
  - Anterior craniofacial resection with postop RT
- Advanced disease
  - Systemic chemo in treatment regimen likely consisting of multiple modalities
  - Definitive CRT
  - Induction chemotherapy followed by CRT or RT

Dose Response

- Well-established RT regimens, total dose and dose per fraction similar to other sites of head and neck SCCs
  - To minimize toxicity, recommend 1.8 Gy/fx if volumes are close to eye, optic nerve, and chiasm
- IMRT is strongly recommended if tumor volume adjacent to critical structures, such as eyes, optic pathways, brain
- Dose-painting IMRT technique has been widely used

Standard Doses

- Standard RT dose
  - Adjuvant RT or CRT: 60-66 Gy at 1.8-2.0 Gy/fx
  - Definitive RT or CRT: 70 Gy at 1.8-2.0 Gy/fx
  - Preop RT or CRT: 50 Gy at 1.8-2.0 Gy/fx

Organs at Risk Parameters

- Mean dose to bilateral parotid glands: 26 Gy
- Spinal cord: < 45 Gy
- Brainstem: < 54 Gy
- Mandible: < 70 Gy
- Retina: < 45 Gy
- Optic nerve: < 54 Gy
- Chiasm: < 54 Gy
- Lens: < 7 Gy

Common Techniques

- Mouth guard and bite block to protect teeth and separate hard palate from oral tongue, if indicated
  - Consider water balloon or stent to fill surgical defects
- Thermoplastic mask for immobilization
- 2.5 mm axial CT scan
- Diagnostic MR with T1 post-contrast images fusion if tumor is located near or invades base of skull or brain
- 3D conformal
- IMRT is recommended for tumor coverage and to minimize high dose to OARs
- Monoisocentric technique with IMRT to upper neck and AP field to lower neck and supraclavicular fossa
- For nasal vestibule primary tumor: "Fu Manchu mustache" area needs be treated if poorly differentiated tumor or well-differentiated tumor > 1.5 cm
  - "Fu Manchu mustache" covers bilateral facial lymphatics, levels IB and IIA nodes; levels III and IV should be treated if there is N(+) in upper neck

RECOMMENDED FOLLOW-UP

Clinical

- Exam: Every 2-3 months for years 1-2; every 4-6 months for years 2-5; every 12 months after 5 years
- Pre- and post-treatment ophthalmology or prosthodontics evaluation as indicated
- Speech, swallowing, and hearing assessment, and rehabilitation as indicated
- Endoscopic exam as indicated
- Post-RT dental care with periodic teeth cleaning and fluoride supplement as indicated
- Prosthetic organs (eye, nose, teeth, etc.) as indicated

Radiographic

- Baseline post-treatment CT &/or MR of maxillofacial images
- Follow-up imaging as indicated
- Annual chest imaging or as clinically indicated

Laboratory

- Thyroid-stimulating hormone (TSH) every 6-12 months if neck irradiated

SELECTED REFERENCES

1. American Joint Committee on Cancer: AJCC Cancer Staging Manual. 7th ed. New York: Springer. 69-78, 2010
2. Khademi B et al: Malignant neoplasms of the sinonasal tract: report of 71 patients and literature review and analysis. Oral Maxillofac Surg. 13(4):191-9, 2009
3. Gabriele AM et al: Stage III-IV sinonasal and nasal cavity carcinoma treated with three-dimensional conformal radiotherapy. Tumori. 94(3):320-6, 2008
4. Daly ME et al: Intensity-modulated radiation therapy for malignancies of the nasal cavity and paranasal sinuses. Int J Radiat Oncol Biol Phys. 67(1):151-7, 2007
5. Lee CH et al: Survival rates of sinonasal squamous cell carcinoma with the new AJCC staging system. Arch Otolaryngol Head Neck Surg. 133(2):131-4, 2007
6. Raghavan P et al: Magnetic resonance imaging of sinonasal malignancies. Top Magn Reson Imaging. 18(4):259-67, 2007
7. Mendenhall WM et al: Sinonasal undifferentiated carcinoma. Am J Clin Oncol. 29(1):27-31, 2006
8. Loevner LA et al: Imaging of neoplasms of the paranasal sinuses. Magn Reson Imaging Clin N Am. 10(3):467-93, 2002
9. Goffart Y et al: Minimally invasive endoscopic management of malignant sinonasal tumours. Acta Otorhinolaryngol Belg. 54(2):221-32, 2000
10. Le QT et al: Lymph node metastasis in maxillary sinus carcinoma. Int J Radiat Oncol Biol Phys. 46(3):541-9, 2000
11. Resto VA et al: Esthesioneuroblastoma: the Johns Hopkins experience. Head Neck. 22(6):550-8, 2000
12. Ng SH et al: Nasopharyngeal carcinoma: MRI and CT assessment. Neuroradiology. 39(10):741-6, 1997
13. Parsons JT et al: Response of the normal eye to high dose radiotherapy. Oncology (Williston Park). 10(6):837-47; discussion 847-8, 851-2, 1996
14. Jiang GL et al: Radiation-induced injury to the visual pathway. Radiother Oncol. 30(1):17-25, 1994

Malignant Transformation of Inverted Papilloma

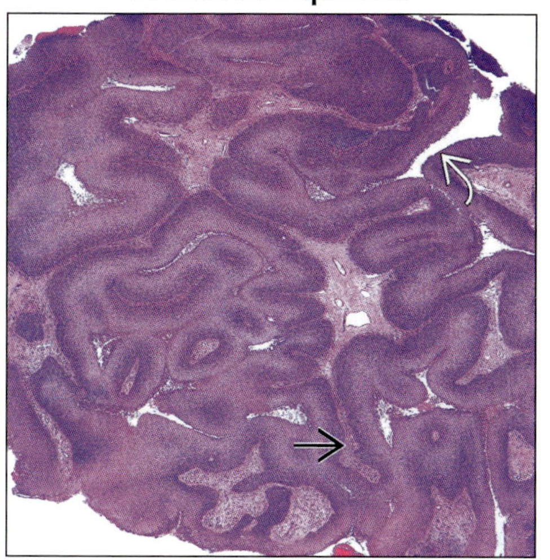

Squamous Cell Carcinoma

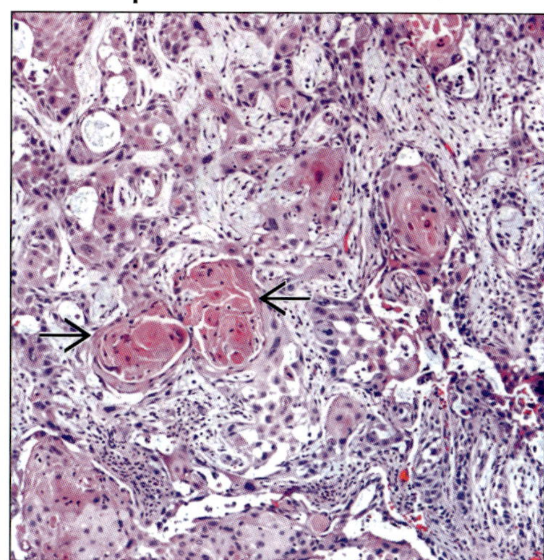

(Left) *An inverted papilloma specimen from the maxillary sinus and nasal cavity has prominent infolding ➔ of nonkeratinizing stratified squamous epithelium into the lamina propria as well as exophytic papillary protrusions ➔. (Courtesy G. Ellis, DDS.)* ***(Right)*** *Photo shows a moderately differentiated SCC of the maxilla. There are interconnecting cords of epithelial cells with nests of keratinization ➔. (Courtesy G. Ellis, DDS.)*

Olfactory Neuroblastoma

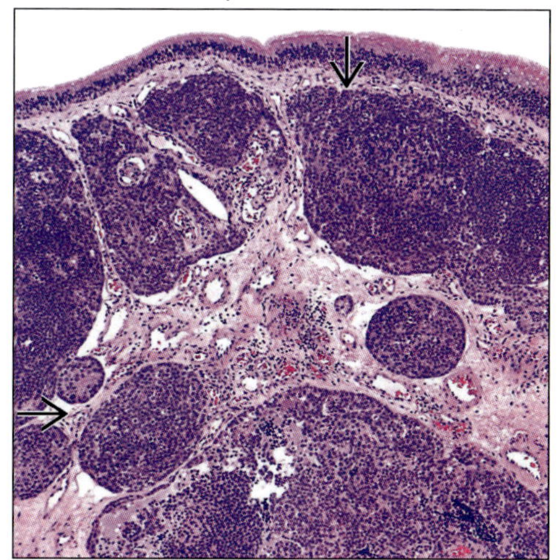

Olfactory Neuroblastoma

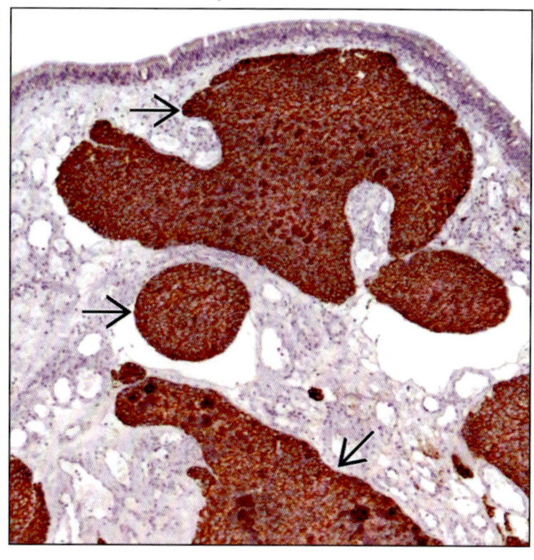

(Left) *This olfactory neuroblastoma in the lamina propria of the nasal cavity mucosa is composed of variably sized, well-demarcated nests of uniform small round cells with a high nuclear:cytoplasmic ratio ➔. (Courtesy G. Ellis, DDS.)* ***(Right)*** *An immunostain for synaptophysin, a neuroendocrine marker, is strongly reactive in nests of olfactory neuroblastoma ➔. Immunostains for cytokeratins (not shown) were unreactive in the tumor cells. (Courtesy G. Ellis, DDS.)*

Stage II (T2 N0 M0) of the Nasal Cavity

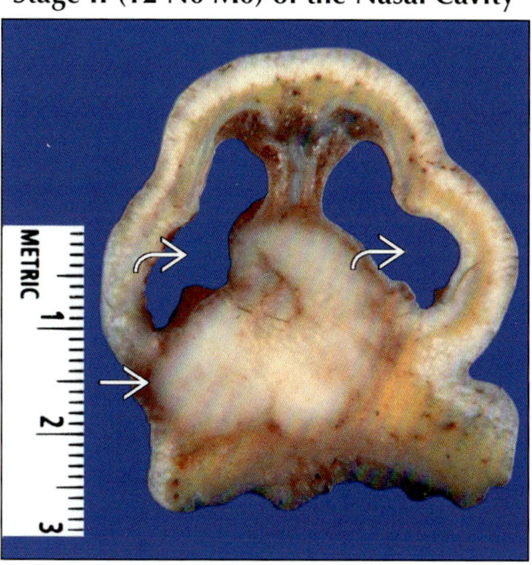

Stage III (T3 N0 M0) of the Nasal Cavity

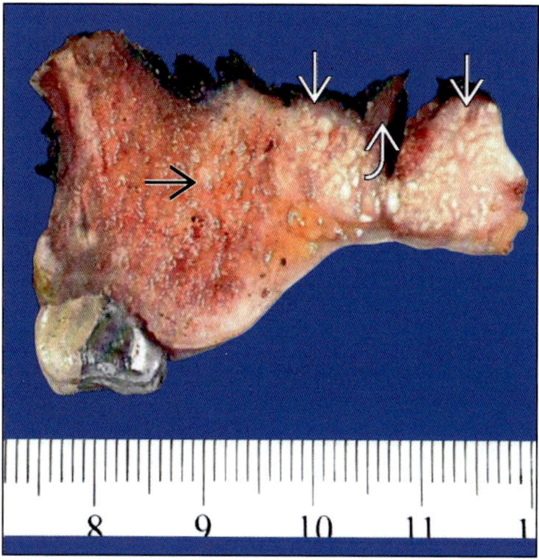

(Left) *Gross pathology shows a whitish-tan mass ➔ centered slightly to the right of midline, causing mild narrowing of the nasal cavities ➔. Since the tumor invades 2 subsites (septum and floor), it is classified as T2 disease.* ***(Right)*** *Gross specimen shows a coronal image of primary stage III (T3 N0 M0) SCCs of the nasal cavity ➔ with right maxillary sinus bony invasion ➔. The nasal septum is visible ➔.*

Stage I (T1 N0 M0)

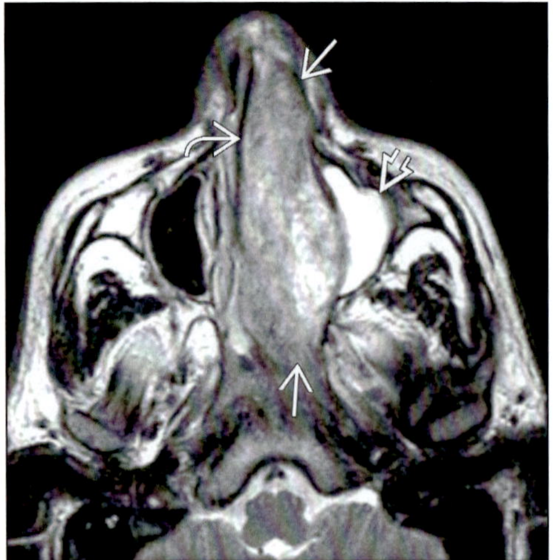

Stage I (T1 N0 M0)

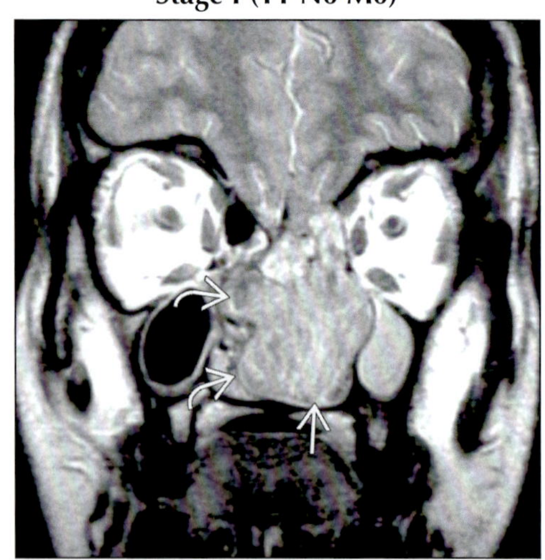

(Left) Axial T2WI MR shows a nasal cavity adenocarcinoma that has filled the left nasal cavity ➡, obstructed the ipsilateral maxillary sinus ➡, and pushed the nasal septum into the right nasal cavity ➡. (Right) Coronal T2WI MR in the same patient shows the heterogeneous tumor ➡ and rightward displacement of the nasal septum ➡. Tumor limited to the nasal cavity is T1.

Stage III (T3 N0 M0)

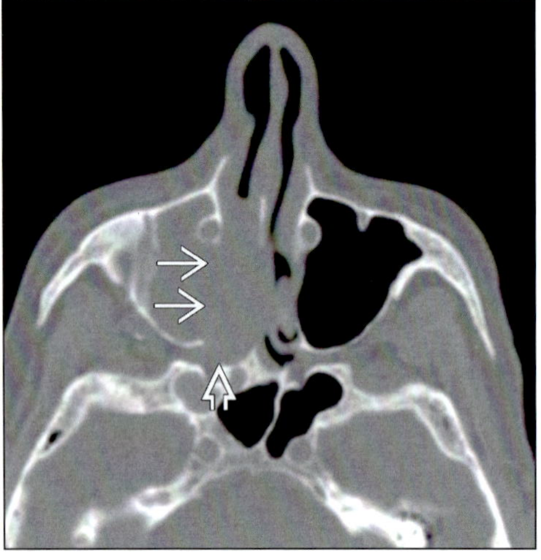

Stage III (T3 N0 M0)

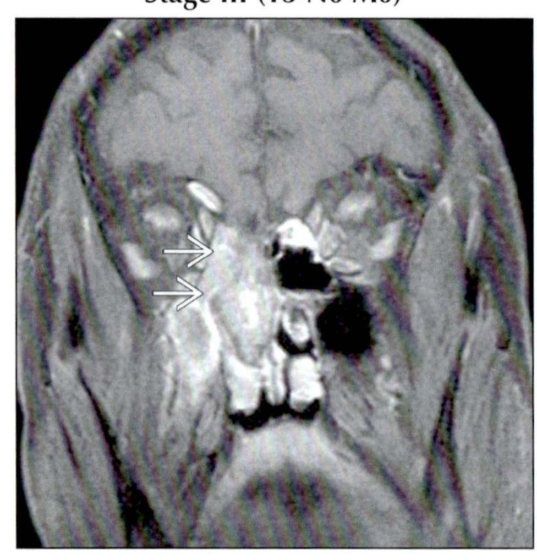

(Left) Axial bone CT in a patient with diagnosed nasal cavity carcinoma demonstrates a destructive lesion in the right sinonasal cavities with erosion of the medial antral wall ➡, extension into the maxillary sinus, and spread into the pterygopalatine fossa ➡. (Right) Coronal T1WI C+ FS MR in the same patient shows heterogeneous enhancement of the lesion ➡. Note the lack of extension to the anterior cranial fossa, which would, if present, upstage this tumor to T4a.

Stage IVB (T4b N0 M0)

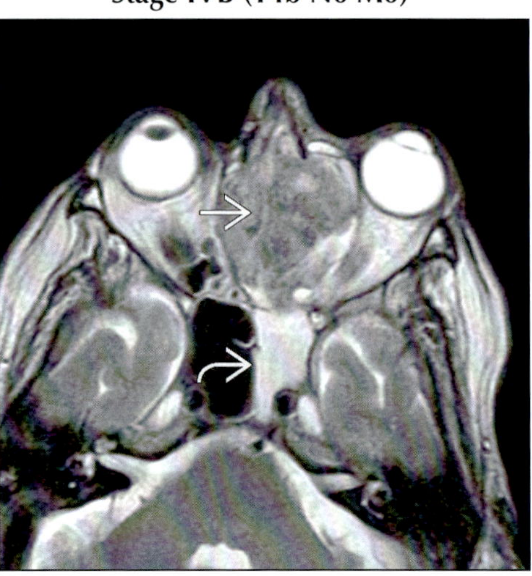

Stage IVB (T4b N0 M0)

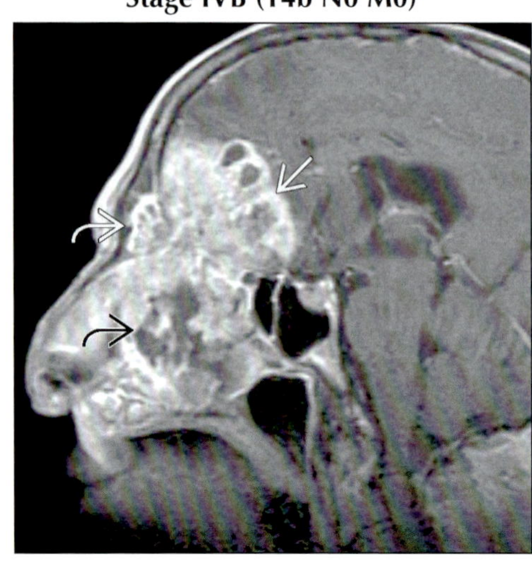

(Left) Axial T2WI MR shows the tumor to be largely low signal intensity ➡, a common finding in high-grade sinonasal neoplasia. The obstructive secretions in the sphenoid sinus ➡ are well contrasted. (Right) Sagittal T1WI C+ MR in the same patient shows heterogeneous enhancement of tumor ➡. There is significant invasion into the surrounding structures, with extension into the nasal vestibule, frontal sinus ➡, and inferior frontal lobes ➡.

Stage IVA (T4a N0 M0) Nasal Cavity

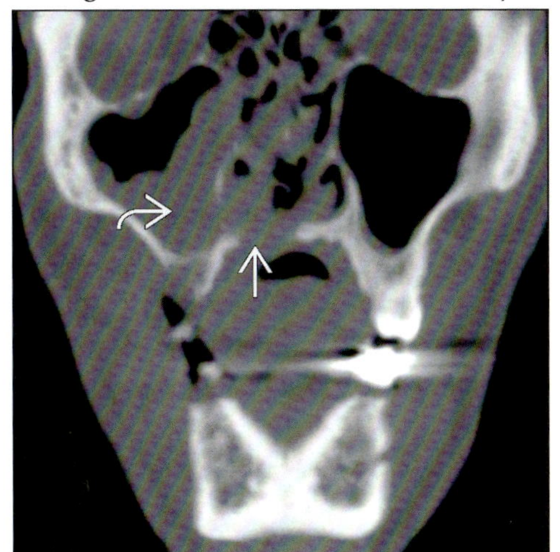

Stage IVA (T4a N0 M0) Nasal Cavity

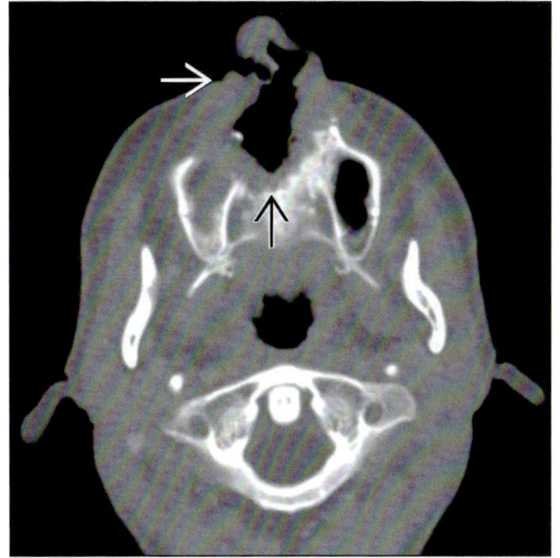

(Left) *Coronal NECT in a 54-year-old man with stage IVA (T4a N0 M0) SCC of the nasal cavity shows tumor involving the hard palate ➡ and extending into the right maxillary sinus ↪.* ***(Right)*** *In the same patient, tumor invaded the facial skin ➡, upper lip, and hard palate ➡. Surgical margins were microscopically positive. Skin involvement makes this T4a. Patient was treated with total rhinectomy and hard palate resection with reconstruction.*

Stage IVA (T4a N0 M0) Nasal Cavity

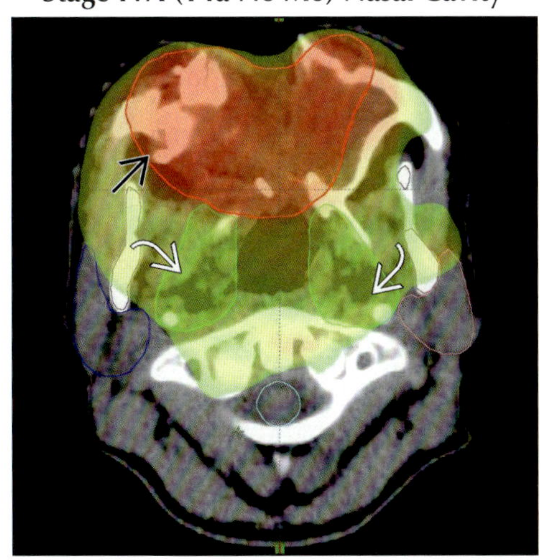

Stage IVA (T4a N0 M0) Nasal Cavity

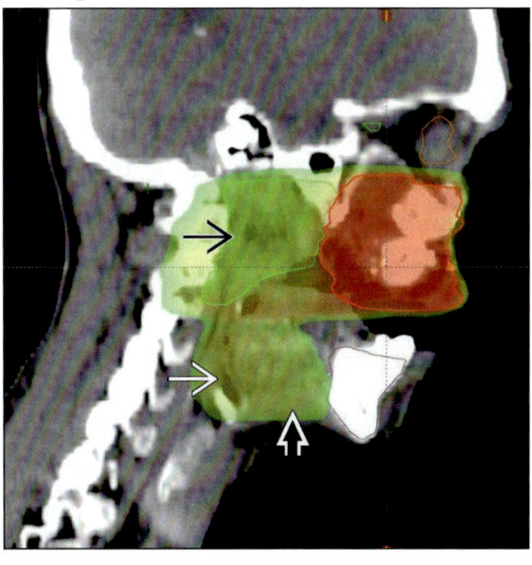

(Left) *Same patient received postop CRT with IMRT to upper neck, 66 Gy to PTV1 ➡, 54 Gy to PTV2 ↪, and 50 Gy to bilateral neck and supraclavicular fossa. Six weekly cycles of cisplatin were given concomitantly.* ***(Right)*** *Sagittal CT shows IMRT plan of the same patient. Bilateral parapharyngeal nodal sites ➡ and level IB ➡ and II areas ➡ were prophylactically treated. Bite block (not shown) was used to separate oral tongue from high-dose areas.*

Stage IVA (T4a N0 M0) Nasal Cavity

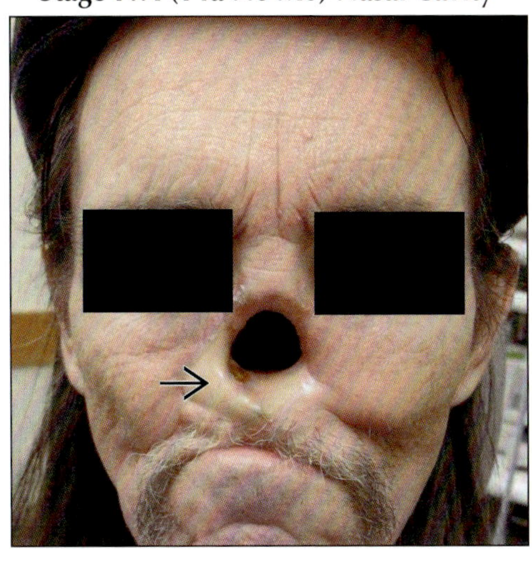

Stage IVA (T4a N0 M0) Nasal Cavity

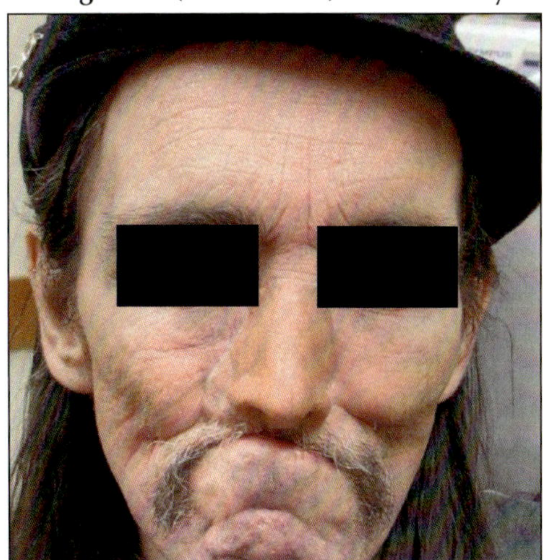

(Left) *Photo of the same patient 3 months after postop CRT shows a well-healed osteocutaneous flap ➡ with total rhinectomy defect.* ***(Right)*** *Photo shows the same patient with a prosthetic nose. There is no evidence of local or regional relapse at 2-year follow-up.*

Stage IVA (T4a N1 M0) SCC of the Maxillary Sinus

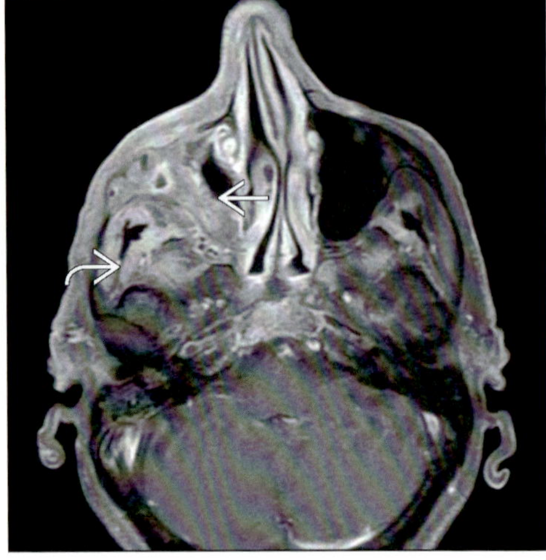

Stage IVA (T4a N1 M0) SCC of the Maxillary Sinus

*(**Left**) Axial T1 MR post gadolinium shows a right maxillary sinus tumor → with infratemporal extension →. (**Right**) Coronal MR image of the same patient shows tumor involving inferior and lateral orbital walls →, buccal mucosa →, and extension into the infratemporal fossa →.*

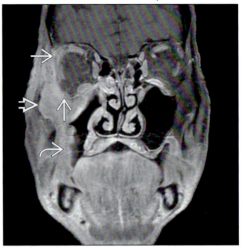

Stage IVA (T4a N1 M0) SCC of the Maxillary Sinus

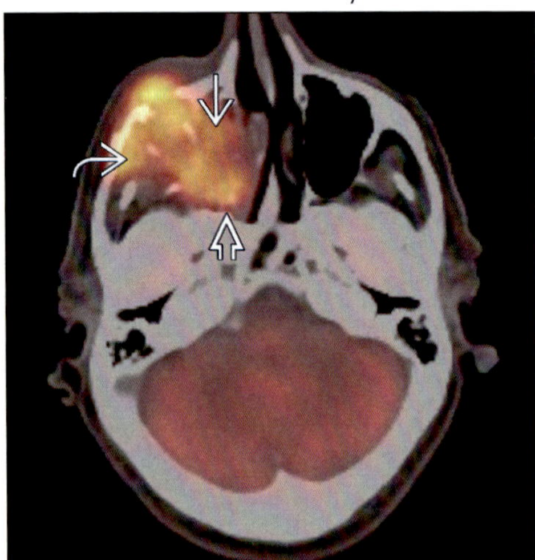

Stage IVA (T4a N1 M0) SCC of the Maxillary Sinus

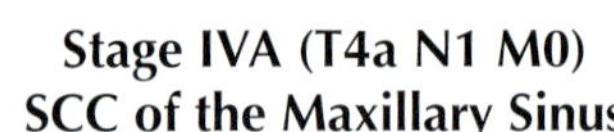

*(**Left**) Axial PET/CT demonstrates a large hypermetabolic soft tissue mass involving the right maxillary sinus →, infratemporal fossa →, and pterygoid fossa →. (**Right**) Axial PET/CT demonstrates lateral wall involvement of the orbit →. Involvement of orbital contents and infratemporal fossa makes this T4a.*

Stage IVA (T4a N1 M0) SCC of the Maxillary Sinus

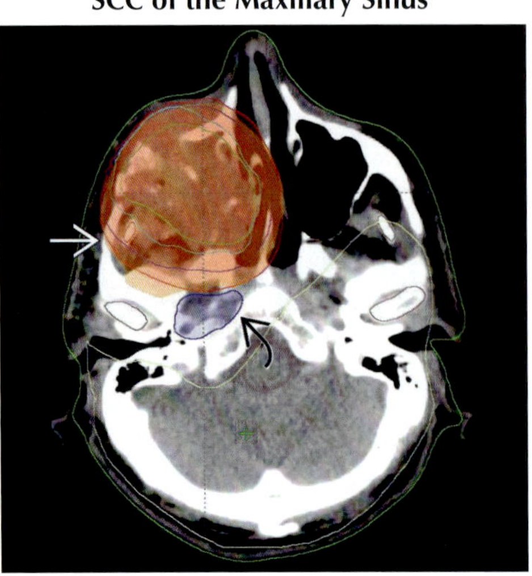

Stage IVA (T4a N1 M0) SCC of the Maxillary Sinus

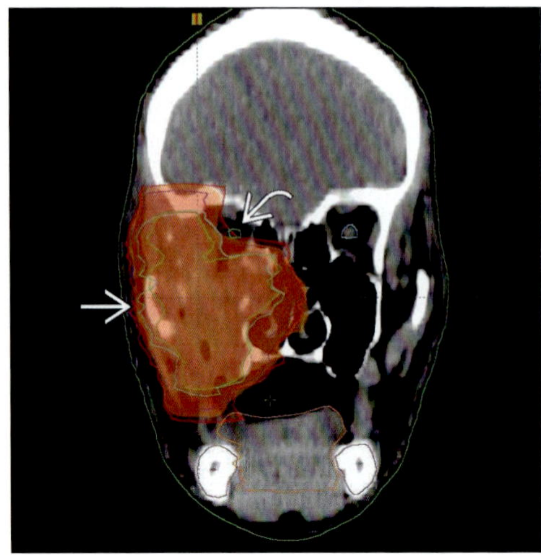

*(**Left**) The same patient received IMRT with initial 50.4 Gy at 1.8 Gy/fx to PTV1 (GTV[+] margins), and a rescan was performed to deliver a 19.8 Gy boost to residual tumor →. PTV2 → covers parapharyngeal/retropharyngeal nodal sites. A total dose of 70.2 Gy was delivered with 7 cycles of concurrent weekly cisplatin 40 mg/m2. (**Right**) Coronal image of IMRT shows > 95% PTV1 coverage → with superior/medial orbit sparing →. A CR was achieved and patient has functional vision.*

Kadish C Esthesioneuroblastoma

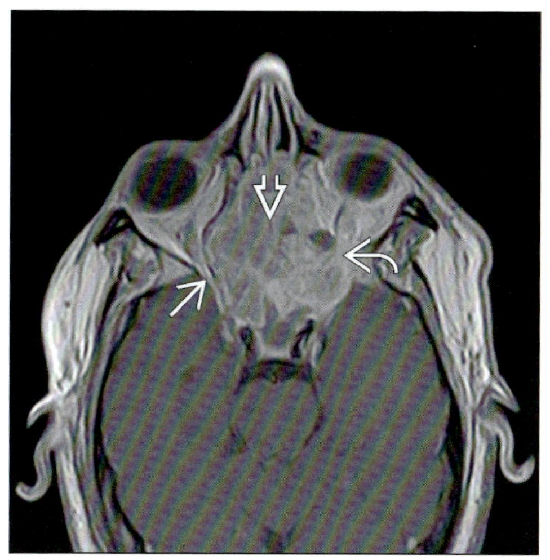

Kadish C Esthesioneuroblastoma

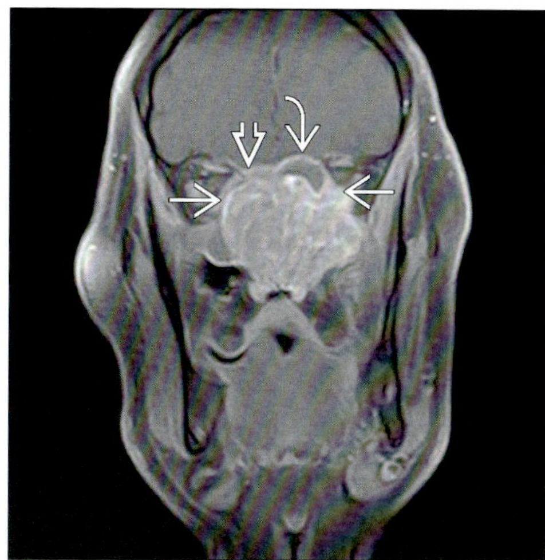

(Left) *Axial T1WI MR post gadolinium shows a large, multiloculated, heterogeneous enhancing mass centered in the nasal cavity vault ➡ with left optic nerve encased ➡ and right optic nerve impinged ➡ in a 41 year old with Kadish C esthesioneuroblastoma.* ***(Right)*** *Coronal image of the same patient shows tumor invading the left frontal sinus ➡, and brain ➡, through the lamina papyracea into extraconal orbital fat ➡.*

Kadish C Esthesioneuroblastoma

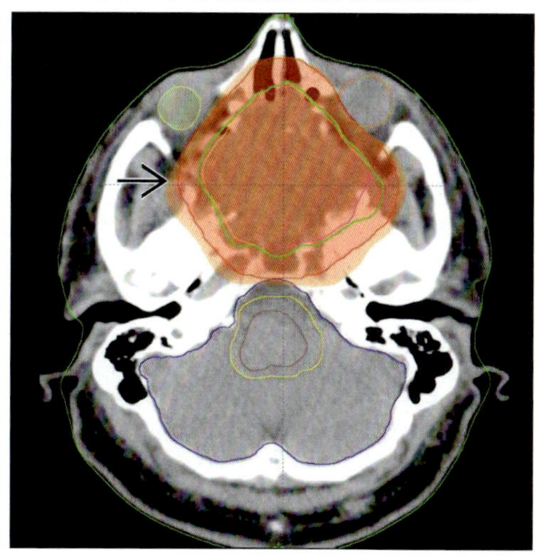

Kadish C Esthesioneuroblastoma

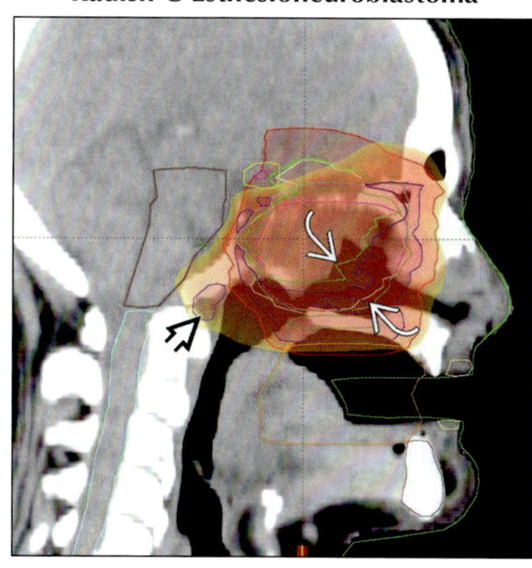

(Left) *The same patient received emergent RT, 3 Gy x 2, followed by 46.8 Gy at 1.8 Gy/fx. After 52.8 Gy, the patient was rescanned and an additional 19.8 Gy was delivered to boost residual disease to a total dose of 72.6 Gy ➡. Weekly cisplatin was given concurrently.* ***(Right)*** *Sagittal IMRT boost plan of the same patient shows tumor regression from pretreatment and boost planning ➡. Note coverage of the retropharyngeal area ➡.*

Kadish C Esthesioneuroblastoma

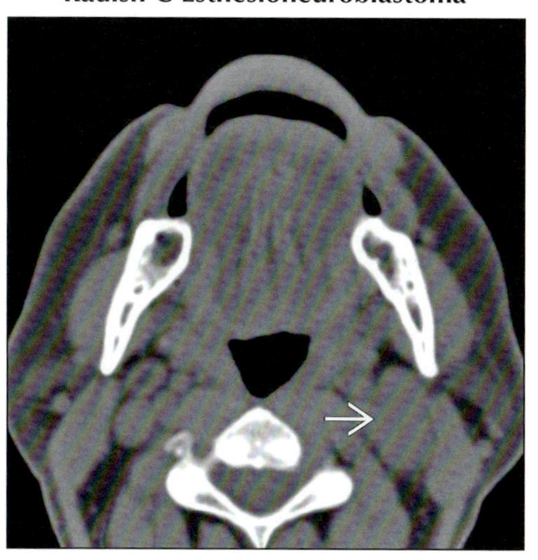

Kadish C Esthesioneuroblastoma

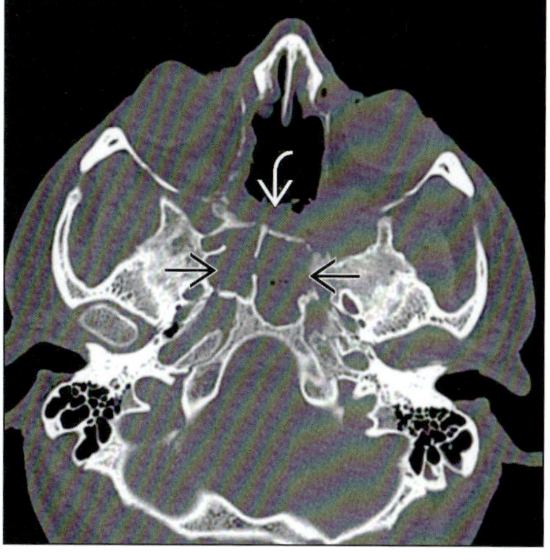

(Left) *Axial CT 12 months after CRT shows a left level II node ➡. Biopsy was positive for recurrent esthesioneuroblastoma. Pathology from left neck dissection demonstrated a 2.2 cm positive node with ECE(+).* ***(Right)*** *Axial CT of the same patient demonstrates soft tissue thickening ➡ and sphenoid sinus opacity ➡. Endoscopic surgery of nasal cavity and sinuses shows inflamed mucosa and fibrous tissue. Biopsy was negative for tumor cells, indicating local control.*

NASOPHARYNX

(T) Primary Tumor

Adapted from 7th edition AJCC Staging Forms.

TNM	*Definitions*
TX	Primary tumor cannot be assessed
T0	No evidence of primary tumor
Tis	Carcinoma in situ
T1	Tumor confined to nasopharynx or extends to oropharynx &/or nasal cavity without parapharyngeal extension
T2	Tumor with parapharyngeal extension
T3	Tumor involves bony structures of skull base &/or paranasal sinuses
T4	Tumor with intracranial extension &/or involvement of cranial nerves, hypopharynx, orbit, or with extension to infratemporal fossa/masticator space

(N) Regional Lymph Nodes

NX	Regional lymph nodes cannot be assessed
N0	No regional lymph node metastasis
N1	Unilateral metastasis in cervical lymph node(s), ≤ 6 cm in greatest dimension, above supraclavicular fossa, &/or unilateral or bilateral, retropharyngeal lymph nodes, ≤ 6 cm, in greatest dimension
N2	Bilateral metastasis in cervical lymph node(s), ≤ 6 cm in greatest dimension, above supraclavicular fossa
N3	Metastasis in lymph node(s) > 6 cm &/or to supraclavicular fossa
N3a	> 6 cm in dimension
N3b	Extension to supraclavicular fossa

(M) Distant Metastasis

M0	No distant metastasis
M1	Distant metastasis

AJCC Stages/Prognostic Groups

Adapted from 7th edition AJCC Staging Forms.

Stage	*T*	*N*	*M*
0	Tis	N0	M0
I	T1	N0	M0
II	T1	N1	M0
	T2	N0	M0
	T2	N1	M0
III	T1	N2	M0
	T2	N2	M0
	T3	N0	M0
	T3	N1	M0
	T3	N2	M0
IVA	T4	N0	M0
	T4	N1	M0
	T4	N2	M0
IVB	Any T	N3	M0
IVC	Any T	Any N	M1

T1: Nasopharynx

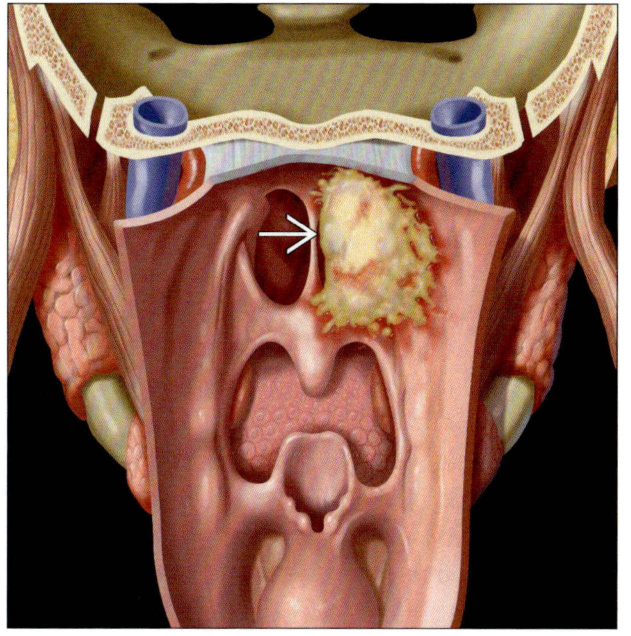

Graphic shows T1 nasopharyngeal tumor ➡, confined to the nasopharynx. Tumor that extends to the oropharynx &/or nasal cavity without parapharyngeal extension, although previously T2a, is considered T1 in the 2010 AJCC staging system.

T2: Nasopharynx

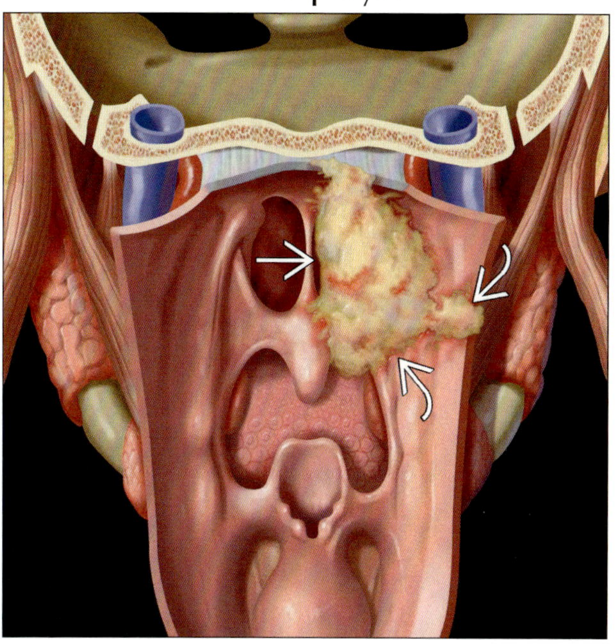

Graphic shows tumor ➡ that extends from the nasopharynx to affect the parapharyngeal space ➡. Although T2 was previously subdivided, in 2010 the AJCC consolidated the staging to reflect the prognostic importance of involvement of the parapharyngeal space.

T3: Nasopharynx

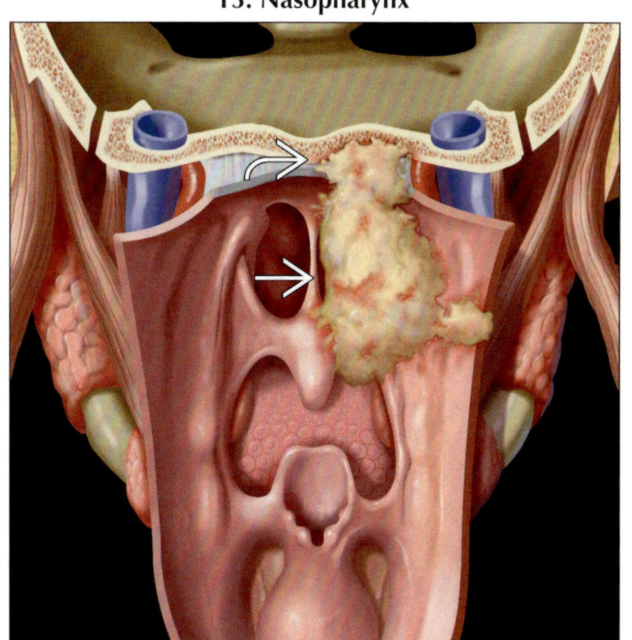

Graphic depicts tumor ➡ involving the bony structures of the skull base ➡, consistent with T3 disease. T3 nasopharyngeal disease may involve the skull base &/or the paranasal sinuses.

T4: Nasopharynx

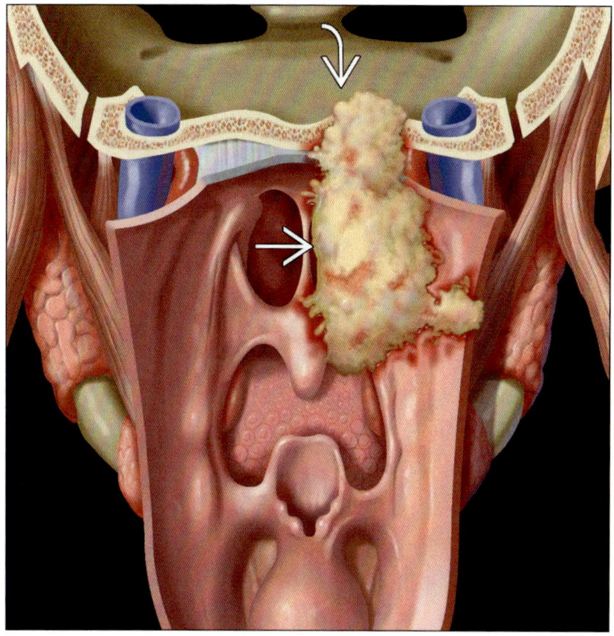

Graphic depicts tumor ➡ with intracranial extension ➡, consistent with T4 disease. Involvement of cranial nerves, hypopharynx, or orbit, or extension to the infratemporal fossa/masticator space, would also be T4. Unlike staging for other pharyngeal tumors, T4 staging for nasopharynx is not subdivided.

Normal Parapharyngeal Space

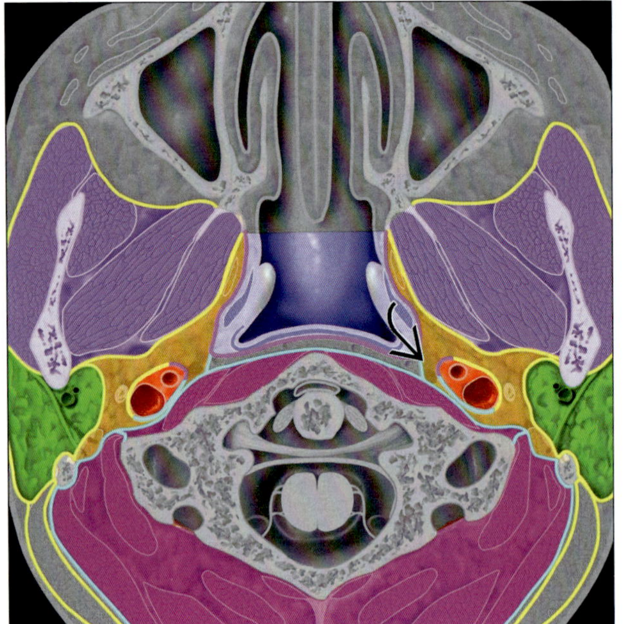

Axial graphic of the normal parapharyngeal space at the level of the nasopharynx demonstrates the complex fascial margins and the fat-only contents. Mass lesions originating in the surrounding pharyngeal mucosal can extend into the parapharyngeal space ⮫. Parapharyngeal space invasion is considered a T2 lesion.

Potential Routes of Spread

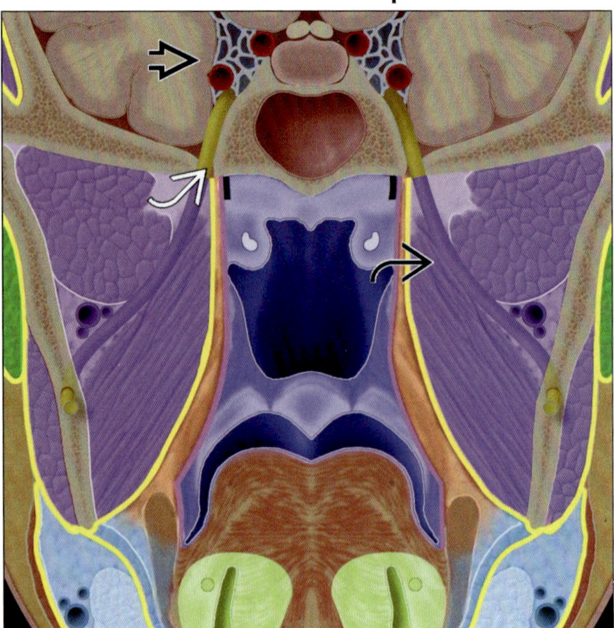

Coronal graphic depicts various potential routes of spread of NPC (parapharyngeal invasion ⮫ and intracranial spread through skull base foramina ➡). Further intracranial extension can lead to invasion of cavernous sinus ⇨.

Parapharyngeal Space on MR

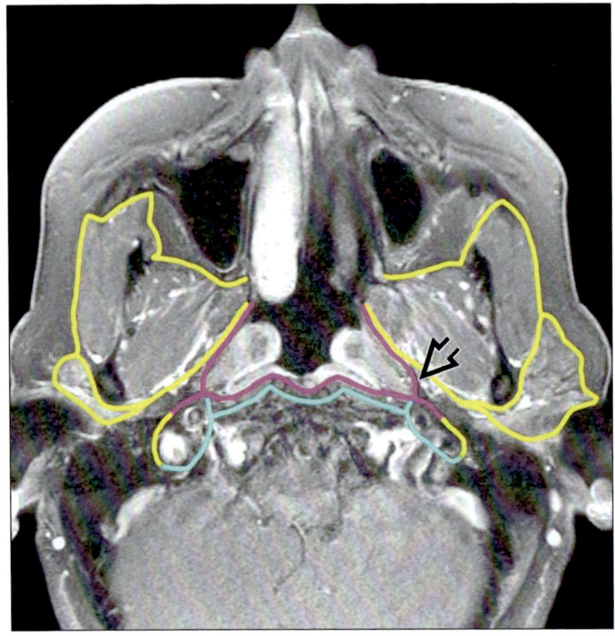

Axial T1WI MR shows relation of nasopharyngeal mucosa and access to parapharyngeal space and surrounding structures ⇨. Nearby structures include skull base foramina for intracranial access of tumor.

Roof of Nasopharynx

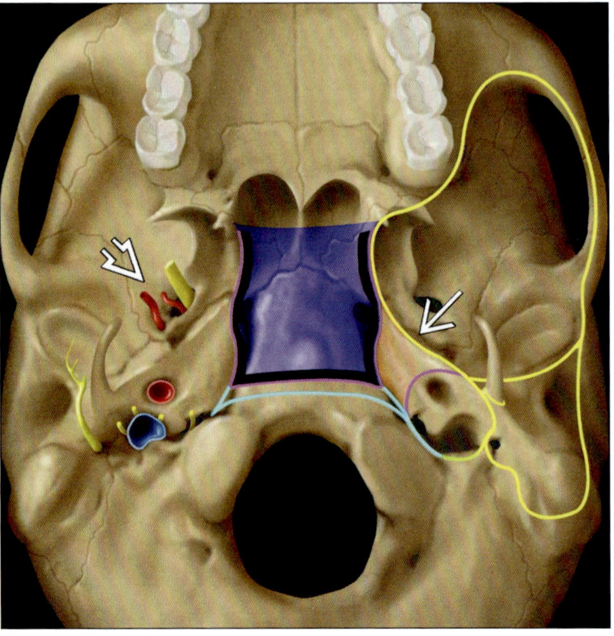

Axial graphic shows the roof of the nasopharynx, which is the floor of the sphenoid sinus (blue). The yellow outline depicts the parapharyngeal space ➡. Note the close proximity to cranial nerve foramina ➡. Cranial nerve(s) involvement is seen in 20% of NPC cases.

Stage IVC (T2 N3 M1)

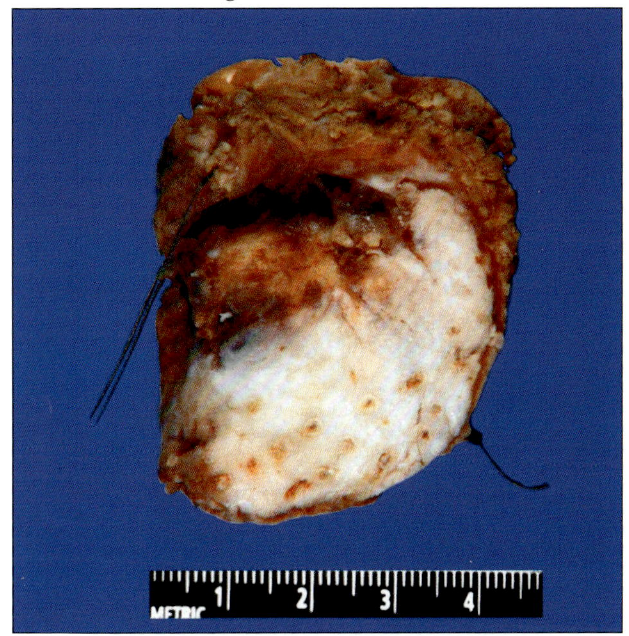

This primary nasopharyngeal carcinoma measures 4 cm x 7 cm. The tumor appears as a reddish-gray, vascular, polypoid mass.

Stage IVC (T2 N3 M1)

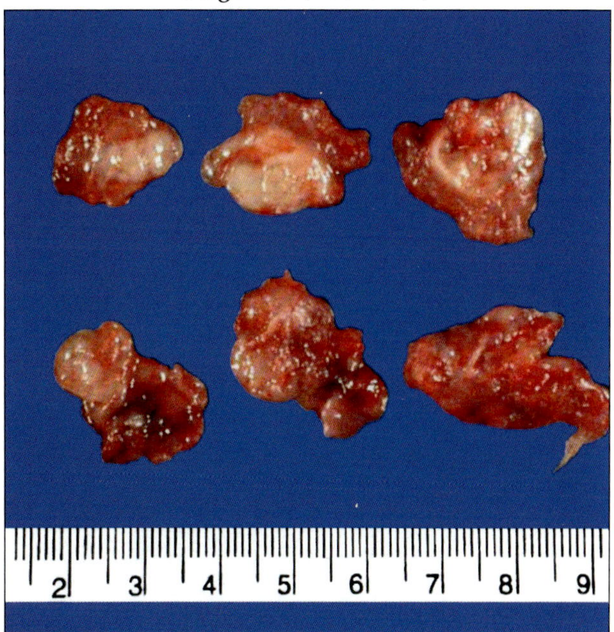

Enlarged lymph nodes were resected from the same patient with N3 disease. Final pathology was positive for WHO grade III carcinoma.

Stage IVC (T2 N3 M1)

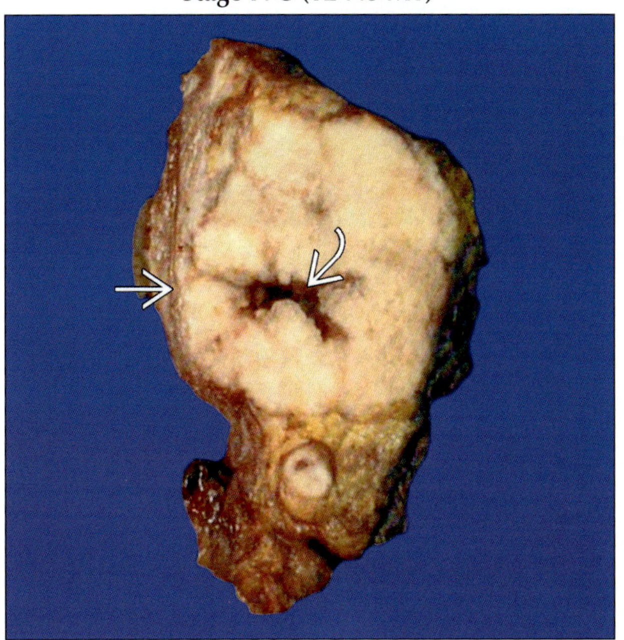

Gross pathologic specimen from the same patient shows a well-circumscribed whitish-tan mass ➡ corresponding to the large node with a central area of necrosis ↙.

Stage IVC (T2 N3 M1)

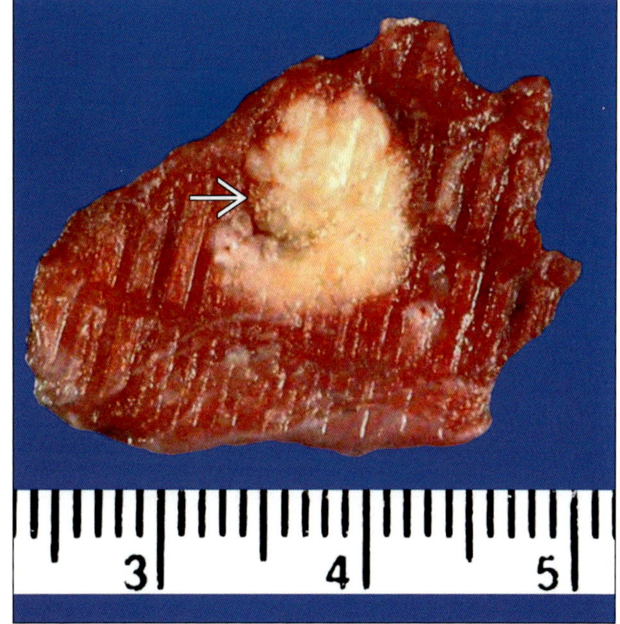

Gross pathologic specimen from the same patient (right lower lobe wedge resection) shows a tannish nodule ➡ measuring just over 1 cm and confirmed as a metastatic lesion. Overall stage is therefore IVC (T2 N3 M1).

Cervical Lymph Nodes

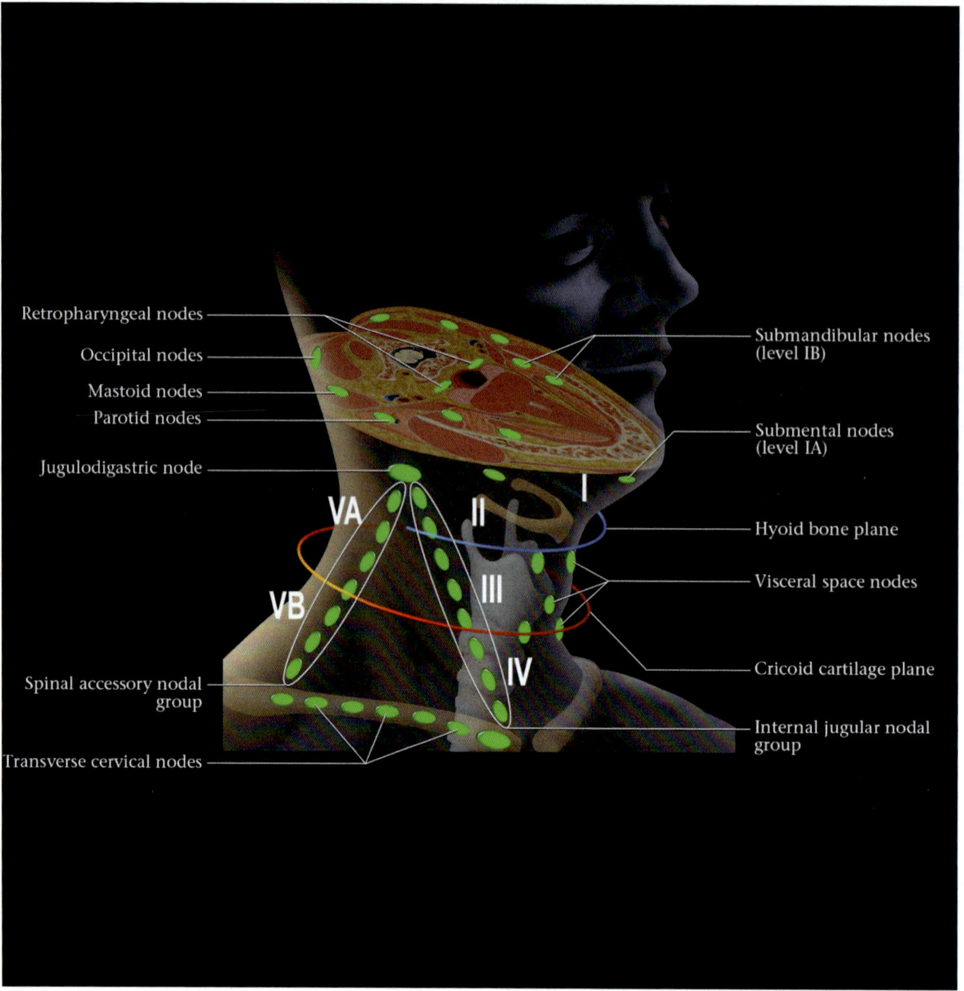

Lateral oblique graphic of cervical neck depicts an axial slice through the suprahyoid neck. The retropharyngeal nodes behind the pharynx are often clinically occult. The hyoid bone (blue arc) and cricoid cartilage (orange circle) planes are highlighted, as they serve to subdivide the internal jugular and spinal accessory nodal group levels.

Regional lymph nodes are staged the same way for almost all head and neck tumors, largely based on size, bilaterality, and number of nodes involved. N stages for tumors of the oropharynx and hypopharynx are determined by this generic head and neck nodal classification.

Tumors of the nasopharynx, however, have a unique N classification scheme. In particular, it considers whether metastasis occurs in the supraclavicular zone or fossa. This triangular region, originally described by Ho, is defined by 3 points, the sternal and lateral ends of the clavicle and the junction of neck and shoulder. This includes the caudal portions of levels IV and VB.

For nasopharyngeal tumors, N1 is applied to unilateral metastasis in cervical lymph node(s), 6 cm or less, above the supraclavicular fossa. Also classified as N1 are metastases smaller than 6 cm to retropharyngeal lymph nodes, whether unilateral or bilateral.

N2

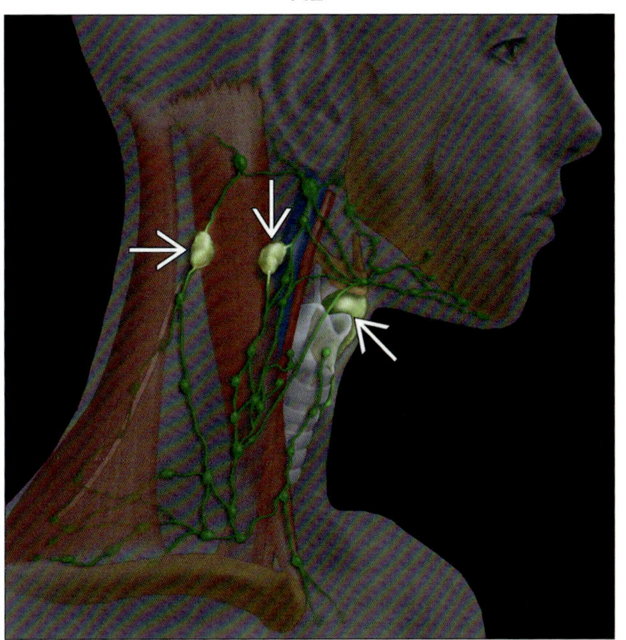

Graphic demonstrates the N2 staging for nasopharyngeal cancers. There are bilateral metastasis in cervical lymph nodes ➡, each 6 cm or less, all above the supraclavicular fossa, consistent with the N2 classification for nasopharyngeal tumors. This N staging is different from that used for other locations in the head and neck.

N3a and N3b

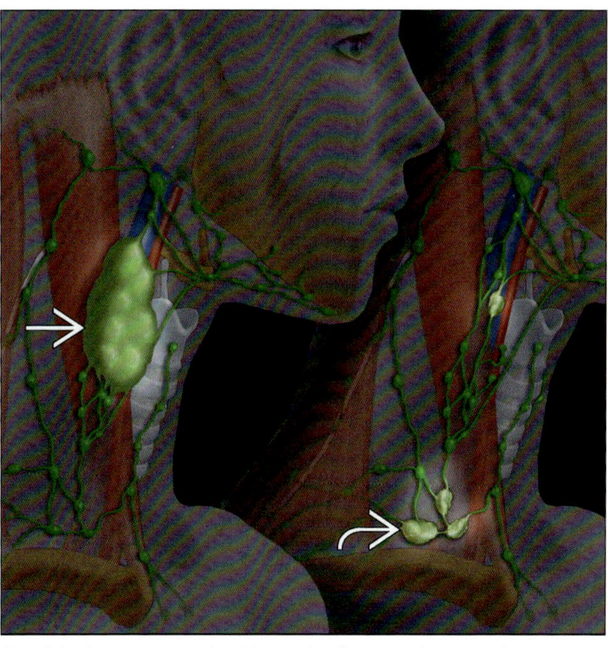

Graphic demonstrates the N3 staging for nasopharyngeal cancers. On the left, the nodes ➡ are larger than 6 cm, consistent with N3a disease. On the right, the metastasis extends to the supraclavicular fossa ↪, which is considered N3b regardless of size.

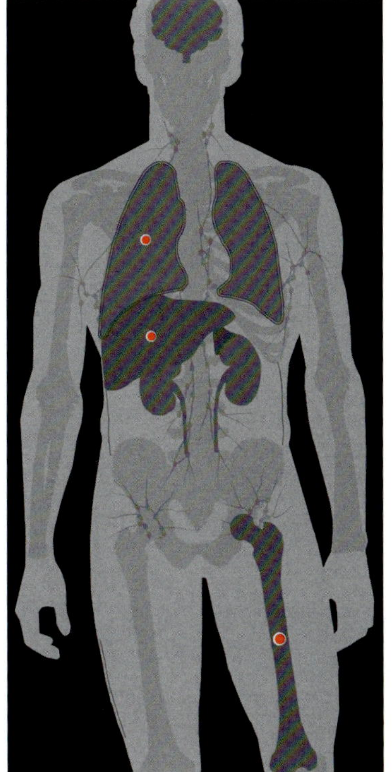

INITIAL SITE OF RECURRENCE	
Bone	15%
Lung	9%
Liver	8%
Multiple Organs	11%

In a review of 629 cases of NPC, distant metastasis occurred in 125 cases. Data refer to metastatic sites per total number of patients. Most distant relapses (95%) occurred within 3 years after completion of radiotherapy. Huang CJ et al: Patterns of metastasis nasopharyngeal cancer. Kaohsiung J Med Sci. 12(4): 229-34, 1996.

NASOPHARYNX

OVERVIEW

General Comments

- **Nasopharyngeal carcinoma (NPC)**
  - Malignancy of nasopharyngeal epithelium
  - NPC represents nearly all nasopharyngeal malignancies in adults
  - Uncommon in Western countries but endemic in Southeast Asia and those of Asian decent
    - Epstein-Barr virus (EBV) is strongly associated with NPC in endemic regions
  - Radiation is standard of care treatment
    - Radiotherapy alone can be given for small localized primary tumors
    - Addition of chemotherapy has been shown to improve disease control rates in locally advanced NPC

Classification

- **WHO classification for malignant nasopharyngeal tumors**
  - Keratinizing squamous cell carcinoma (type 1)
    - 20% prevalence in United States
    - Worse prognosis (35% 5-year survival)
    - Typically associated with smoking and alcohol use
  - Nonkeratinizing carcinoma (type 2)
    - 20% overall prevalence
  - Undifferentiated carcinoma (type 3)
    - 99% prevalence in endemic areas
    - More favorable prognosis (50% 5-year survival)

NATURAL HISTORY

General Features

- Location
  - Anatomic borders of the nasopharynx
    - Anterior border is posterior nasal cavity (choanae)
    - Posterior border is clivus and C1-C2 vertebrae
    - Superior border is floor of sphenoid (skull base)
    - Inferior border is soft palate (oropharynx)

Etiology

- Risk factors
  - Generally considered combination of genetic and environmental factors
    - Ethnicity/genetics: Chinese native > Chinese immigrant > North American native
    - Nitrosamines: Salted fish, preserved meats
    - Viral: EBV associated with nonkeratinizing type and Asian ancestry
    - Others: Polycyclic hydrocarbons, chronic nasal infection, poor hygiene, poor ventilation
    - Smoking and alcohol association with NPC is controversial

Epidemiology & Cancer Incidence

- Number of cases in USA per year
  - 0.3-0.8 cases per 100,000 in USA
  - 25-50 cases per 100,000 in China and Hong Kong
- Sex predilection
  - Male predominance (3:1)
- Age of onset
  - Bimodal peak incidence in age ranges from 30-40 and 50-60 years
    - Can be seen in all age groups

Associated Diseases, Abnormalities

- EBV
  - Evidence of EBV DNA has been found in tumor cells
  - Many NPC patients have anti-EBV antibodies
  - Most strongly associated with type III (nonkeratinizing undifferentiated) form

Gross Pathology & Surgical Features

- May be difficult to detect on gross pathology
- Most are exophytic
- Random biopsies from nasopharynx recommended when diagnosis suspected (neck mass from unknown primary)

Microscopic Pathology

- H&E
  - Crucial distinction is between keratinizing and nonkeratinizing carcinomas
    - Keratinizing
      - Show clear-cut evidence of keratinization
      - Lesser association with EBV than nonkeratinizing
    - Nonkeratinizing
      - Differentiated
      - Stratified or tiled arrangement
      - Well-defined cell margins
    - Undifferentiated
      - Indistinct cell margins
      - Some spindle-shaped tumor cells
      - High proportion accompanied by inflammatory infiltrate of lymphocytic cells
      - Nuclear chromatin is clear or vesicular, accentuating prominent nucleoli
      - High nuclear to cytoplasmic ratio with amphophilic cytoplasm
      - Syncytial appearance

Routes of Spread

- Local spread
  - Direct extension
    - Spreads along nasopharyngeal wall
    - Invasion into parapharyngeal space
    - Intracranial extension
  - Jacod syndrome
    - Direct tumor extension via foramen lacerum to cavernous sinus
    - Affects cranial nerves (CNs) VI, then III, V1, V2, and IV
    - Ptosis, ophthalmoplegia, neuralgia in supraorbital and maxillary distribution
  - Villaret syndrome
    - Tumor invasion into parapharyngeal space, then gains access to jugular foramen and hypoglossal canal
    - Dysphagia, taste change, numbness of soft palate, paralysis of vocal cords, trapezius muscle and sternocleidomastoid muscle, Horner syndrome (cervical sympathetics)
    - Affects cranial nerves IX, X, X, and XII
- Lymphatic extension
  - Lymphatic spread common
    - > 80% present with nodal involvement
    - Bilateral nodal presentation in ~ 50%
  - Nodal location

- Commonly involved nodal basins include levels II, III, IV, and V
  - Upper & mid jugulodigastric nodes (levels II-III)
  - Retropharyngeal (RP) nodes
  - Spinal accessory nodes (level V)
- RP nodes are more difficult to detect on CT (30-40% detection rate) than MR (70-80% detection rate)
  - Most RP nodes are located at C1 level and incidence decreases from C1 to C3
- Hematogenous spread
  - Distant metastases (DM) is less common at initial presentation but more common in recurrent disease
    - Rare at initial presentation (< 10%)
    - High metastatic potential
      - In recurrent disease, NPC has highest rates of DM among head and neck cancers
      - WHO type III has highest rate of DM among head and neck cancers
      - High rate of multiorgan involvement (57%)
    - DM rates correlate with nodal stage
      - N1: 10-20%
      - N2: 30-40%
      - N3: 40-70%
- Metastatic sites
  - Common metastatic sites include
    - Bones (70-80%)
    - Lungs (40-50%)
    - Liver (30-40%)
    - Brain

IMAGING

Detection

- Common radiologic presentations
  - Best diagnostic clue
    - Mass in lateral pharyngeal recess of nasopharynx with deep extension and cervical adenopathy
  - Non-contrast-enhanced CT
    - Bone CT
      - Destruction of clival cortex, pterygoid plates, or posterior skull base may be seen
  - Contrast-enhanced CT
    - Mildly enhancing mass
      - Most frequently located in lateral pharyngeal recess
    - Extension into surrounding spaces is common
      - Often enables differentiation between malignant and benign tumors; most benign lesions displace tissue rather than invade
      - Lateral extension to parapharyngeal space and masticator space (pterygoid muscles) commonly seen
      - Intracranial spread, commonly via posterior extension through cervical fascia and into carotid space
  - MR
    - Generally preferred imaging modality for nasopharyngeal carcinoma
      - Improved soft tissue contrast
      - Decreased amalgam/dental artifact
    - T1WI
      - Mass in lateral nasopharynx hypointense to isointense compared to muscle
      - Multiplanar images superior for seeing invasion of clivus, sphenoid bone, and sinus, C1 and C2 vertebral bodies
      - Perineural spread suggested by obliterated normal fat at foramina of skull base, particularly foramen ovale
    - T2WI
      - Nasopharyngeal mass moderate hyperintensity to muscle
      - Obstructed secretions of benign nature in mastoid, middle ear, or sinuses tend to be strongly hyperintense as opposed to mild hyperintensity of tumor
    - T1WI C+
      - Mild homogeneous enhancement
      - T1 C+ axial and coronal imaging superior to show tumor interface with surrounding structures
  - **PET/CT**
    - Strong FDG avidity seen in primary nasopharyngeal carcinoma
    - Useful in cases of unknown primaries to find primary lesion

Staging

- N staging
  - Similar findings for all pharyngeal tumors with exception of nodes involved
  - **CT**
    - Metastatic lymph nodes (LNs) appear round with loss of fatty hilum on CT
    - Extracapsular extension is more common in larger nodes but possible in smaller nodes as well
    - Metastatic cervical adenopathy is commonly seen on contrast-enhanced CT
      - CT is preferred over MR for cervical metastatic disease, except retropharyngeal disease
      - Nodal metastasis is heterogeneously enhancing
      - Rim enhancement and central necrosis of lymph node are abnormal irrespective of size
  - **MR**
    - Superior at evaluating metastatic retropharyngeal lymph nodes
      - T1WI C+ or T2WI with fat saturation superior to CECT in visualization
    - Large tumors show necrosis with rim enhancement
      - Regions of necrosis often heterogeneously enhancing
  - **PET/CT**
    - Strong FDG avidity seen in metastatic nodes
    - Excellent modality for detecting unsuspected tumor foci in distant or nonenlarged nodes
- M staging
  - **General**
    - Distant metastases are present < 10% of time at presentation
    - Node-positive patients with nasopharyngeal carcinoma are at high risk of developing metastases
  - **CT**
    - Moderately enhancing solid mass that shows aggressive destruction of bone
    - Parenchymal metastases may show hyperenhancement
    - Large metastatic foci may be nonenhancing
    - CT superior in evaluating cortical bone invasion

- Thin slice (1-2 mm) helps assess bone invasion
- Bone lesions may show enhancement
- Important to evaluate as erosion into skull base suggests poor prognosis and requires change in RT field

- MR
  - Enhanced MR imaging is recommended for staging known nasopharyngeal malignancies
  - Also best tool for evaluating intracranial extent via direct, perivascular, and perineural routes
  - May reveal subtle bony erosions of skull base
  - Limiting factors include long acquisition time (~ 30 minutes)
  - T1WI
    - Intermediate signal mass
    - Hypointense to isointense compared to muscle
    - Increased T1 signal may be seen in intratumoral hemorrhage areas
    - Replaced bone marrow is easier to appreciate on pre-contrast T1WI than on other sequences
  - T2WI
    - Moderate hyperintensity to muscle
    - Mucosal extent of tumor difficult to determine on MR as normal mucosa and tumor nearly isointense
    - Cystic degeneration: Appears hyperintense
    - Foci of hemorrhage: Appear hypointense to hyperintense based on age of blood
  - T1WI C+
    - Post-contrast fat saturation for differentiation of tumor from adjacent muscle/fat
    - Enhancement typically mild to moderate, heterogeneous, and diffuse
    - Necrotic areas do not enhance
    - Squamous cell carcinoma enhances less than adenocarcinoma
- PET/CT
  - Strong FDG avidity seen in distant metastasis
  - Sensitivity greatest in metastases with diameter > 1 cm
  - Submucosal tumors may be located via PET/CT
  - Careful attention to artifacts and patterns of physiologic uptake is essential to avoid inaccurate staging

Restaging

- CT
  - Use of preoperative CT scanning or MR is important for determining extent of tumor
  - CT widely used for regular monitoring
    - Useful for bone erosion/involvement
    - May show asymmetry of nasopharynx
  - Contrast-enhanced CT recommended to evaluate recurrent cervical lymphadenopathy
- MR
  - Has demonstrated trend toward higher accuracy than PET/CT in detecting residual &/or recurrent nasopharyngeal carcinoma
  - Restaging is more accurate when both MR and PET/CT are used than when either is used alone
  - Cannot reliably differentiate tumor from XRT changes, but T2 hypointensity and poor enhancement are often seen with fibrosis
- PET/CT
  - Superior to CT and MR in restaging in some studies
  - Early restaging by single whole-body 18F FDG PET scan after 1st or 2nd course of induction chemotherapy
    - Useful in predicting therapeutic response and outcome in patients with locoregionally advanced nasopharyngeal carcinoma
  - As above, MR and PET/CT are more accurate when combined than when used alone

CLINICAL PRESENTATION & WORK-UP

Presentation

- Often misdiagnosed early because of vague presenting symptoms and difficulty examining nasopharynx
  - Most cases are detected late in disease course
    - In endemic areas, patients are diagnosed earlier
  - #1 complaint is neck mass (66%)
- Most common finding
  - Clinical triad (neck, nose, ear)
    - Neck mass
    - Nasal obstruction with epistaxis
    - Otitis media
  - Unilateral hearing loss from middle ear effusion
- Nonspecific, early symptoms include
  - Nasal obstruction
  - Blood-tinged sputum
  - Nasal discharge
  - Tinnitus
  - Headache
  - Ear fullness
  - Unilateral conductive hearing loss, due to either
    - Serous otitis media
    - Recurrent acute otitis media
- Advanced disease may show invasion of base of skull and spread intracranially through foramina
  - Results in cranial nerve involvement (CNs III-VI)
    - Indicates cavernous sinus involvement
  - Clinical signs include
    - Diplopia
    - Facial numbness

Prognosis

- Smaller nasopharyngeal carcinomas
  - Radiation therapy (RT) cures 90%
- More advanced carcinomas without nodal disease
  - RT cures approximately 60%
- Prognostic factors
  - Advanced carcinomas with nodes and distant metastases are associated with poor prognosis
  - Overall patient health
    - Comorbidities can be classified by Karnofsky performance score or Kaplan-Feinstein index
- Prognosis: Relative 5-year survival rate for nasopharyngeal squamous cell carcinomas
  - Stage I: 71.5%
  - Stage II: 64.2%
  - Stage III: 62.2%
  - Stage IV: 38.4%

Work-Up

- Clinical
  - History and physical

- Examination under anesthesia (EUA) and endoscopy
- Biopsy
- Dental, speech, swallowing, and audiogram as indicated

- Radiographic
  - Thin slice CT &/or MR
    - MR useful for advanced lesions and evaluating retropharyngeal LN
  - Consider PET/CT
  - Chest imaging
- Laboratory
  - Consider EBV evaluation

TREATMENT

Major Treatment Alternatives

- Radiation therapy
  - Mainstay of treatment
  - Surgery plays minimal role due to anatomic location of NPC and high rate of nodal presentation
- Combined radiation and chemotherapy used for
  - Locally advanced nasopharyngeal carcinomas (stages II-IV)
  - Typically concurrent chemoradiation followed by adjuvant chemotherapy
- Neck dissection
  - Used for nodal disease unresponsive to radiation
  - Residual nodal disease often assessed 6-8 weeks after completion of RT

Major Treatment Roadblocks/ Contraindications

- Local radiation treatment failure can be further managed by re-irradiation or salvage nasopharyngectomy
  - Re-irradiation associated with high rate of complications
  - Consideration for stereotactic radiosurgery (i.e., gamma knife radiosurgery) for intracranial recurrences
- Distant metastases becoming major pattern of disease relapse as locoregional control (LRC) rates improve
  - Current treatment options ineffective in curing distant metastases
  - Chemotherapy is mainstay therapy for metastatic disease
  - Commonly used systemic agents include cisplatin, 5-fluorouracil, carboplatin, docetaxel, paclitaxel, gemcitabine
  - Trials currently underway comparing neoadjuvant chemotherapy + concurrent chemotherapy vs. concurrent chemotherapy alone in locally advanced NPC

Treatment Options by Stage

- Stages I and II
  - RT alone
    - 5-year overall survival (OS) 70-80%
  - Standard fractionation radiotherapy for T1 tumors
  - Altered fractionation for bulky T1 or T2 tumors
- Stages III and IV
  - Radiation alone outcomes poor in locally advanced stage NPC
    - 5-year OS only 10-40%
  - Concurrent chemoradiation therapy (CRT) mainstay for patients with advanced NPC
    - Level I evidence demonstrates that concurrent CRT is superior to RT alone
    - Chemo often consists of high-dose cisplatin with fluorouracil
    - Improvement in LRC and OS
    - Further adjuvant chemo often given
      - Benefit of additional adjuvant chemo after CRT is not clear
  - Use of neoadjuvant chemo remains controversial
    - Multiple randomized trials yield mixed results with no clear survival benefit
    - Meta-analysis indicates improved outcomes with concurrent CRT compared to neoadjuvant sequential CRT
    - Potential benefits of neoadjuvant therapy include better toleration of concurrent CRT course, which is considered the most important part
    - Consideration for induction chemo given for stage N2 patients followed by RT alone or concurrent CRT
- Radiation target
  - T1 lesions: Nasopharynx, clivus, floor of sphenoid sinus, pterygoid fossa, parapharyngeal space, retropharyngeal nodes, and bilateral cervical nodes (including level V)
  - T2 lesions: Extend target volume to include tumor extension into parapharyngeal space
  - T3-T4 lesions: Ensure generous coverage of skull base and known intracranial extension, respecting tolerance of nearby normal critical tissues (optic chiasm, brainstem, temporal lobe)

Standard Doses

- Clinical target volumes (CTV) and RT dose using intensity-modulated radiation therapy (IMRT)
  - 2 CTVs are generally delineated in treatment of NPC
    - High-dose CTV (HD-CTV): 66-70 Gy to gross disease plus margin (typically 0.5-1.0 cm)
    - Intermediate-dose CTV (ID-CTV): 57-60 Gy to subclinical disease
    - Narrow margins on GTV may be required for skull base and intracranial disease to protect critical neural structures
  - Fraction sizes range from 1.8 Gy (intermediate-dose CTV) to 2.12 Gy (high-dose CTV)
- Elective nodal irradiation
  - Elective nodal coverage includes uninvolved levels II-V and bilateral retropharyngeal nodes
  - Where IMRT is used to treat primary tumor and upper neck nodes, uninvolved low neck can be treated with matching anterior &/or posterior fields
    - Permits lower mean dose to larynx
    - Done using monoisocentric technique and placement of isocenter for matching fields 1.5 cm above arytenoids (typically at thyroid notch)
    - Comparison of mean larynx dose between whole-field IMRT to half-beam IMRT demonstrates lower larynx dose using monoisocentric technique

Organs at Risk Parameters

- Brainstem margin should be only a few millimeters to avoid delivering doses of > 60 Gy
- Avoid temporal lobe doses > 66 Gy

- Optic chiasm dose should be < 54 Gy

Common Techniques

- IMRT is ideal modality for treatment of NPC due to horseshoe shape and proximity to nearby critical structures
  - Steeper dose fall-off allows for more conformal plans
  - Higher conformality may increase normal tissue sparing and dose escalation for improved tumor control
    - Optic chiasm, brainstem, temporal lobe, spinal cord, cochlea, parotid glands
  - Incorporates accelerated fractionation and hyperfractionation
    - Higher biological dose can be given to tumor
    - Potential for improved local tumor control
  - Available data demonstrate that IMRT improves LRC and reduces toxicity such as xerostomia

Landmark Trials

- Intergroup 0099 study: Phase III randomized trial comparing concurrent CRT followed by adjuvant chemo vs. RT alone for locally advanced NPC
  - CRT improved PFS and OS compared to RT alone
  - Concurrent chemotherapy regimen
    - High-dose cisplatin 100 mg/m2 given weeks 1, 4, and 7 of radiotherapy
  - Adjuvant chemotherapy regimen
    - Cisplatin 80 mg/m2 on day 1 and fluorouracil on days 1-4
    - Regimen repeated every 3-4 weeks x 3 cycles
  - Radiotherapy
    - 70 Gy total dose to primary tumor and neck nodes > 2 cm
    - 66 Gy to gross neck nodes ≤ 2 cm
    - 50-54 Gy elective nodal RT to bilateral neck for N0 disease
    - 1.8-2.0 Gy fraction sizes

RECOMMENDED FOLLOW-UP

Clinical

- Exam every 1-3 months for year 1, every 2-6 months for year 2, every 4-8 months for years 2-5, then annually
- Speech, swallowing, hearing, and dental rehabilitation as indicated
- Smoking cessation and alcohol counseling as indicated

Radiographic

- Baseline imaging within 6 months
  - PET/CT may be preferred for monitoring distant sites
- Chest imaging as indicated

Laboratory

- Thyroid-stimulating hormone (TSH) monitoring every 6 months if RT used
- Consider EBV monitored

SELECTED REFERENCES

1. American Joint Committee on Cancer: AJCC Cancer Staging Manual. 7th ed. New York: Springer. 41-56, 2010
2. Bonner JA et al: Radiotherapy plus cetuximab for locoregionally advanced head and neck cancer: 5-year survival data from a phase 3 randomised trial, and relation between cetuximab-induced rash and survival. Lancet Oncol. 2010 Jan;11(1):21-8. Epub 2009 Nov 10. Erratum in: Lancet Oncol. 11(1):14, 2010
3. Guido A et al: Combined 18F-FDG-PET/CT imaging in radiotherapy target delineation for head-and-neck cancer. Int J Radiat Oncol Biol Phys. 73(3):759-63, 2009
4. Ng SH et al: Staging of untreated nasopharyngeal carcinoma with PET/CT: comparison with conventional imaging work-up. Eur J Nucl Med Mol Imaging. 2009 Jan;36(1):12-22. Epub 2008 Aug 15. Erratum in: Eur J Nucl Med Mol Imaging. 36(3):538, 2009
5. Pignon JP et al: Meta-analysis of chemotherapy in head and neck cancer (MACH-NC): an update on 93 randomised trials and 17,346 patients. Radiother Oncol. 92(1):4-14, 2009
6. Chong VF et al: Nasopharyngeal carcinoma. Eur J Radiol. 66(3):437-47, 2008
7. Chu ST et al: Primary tumor volume of nasopharyngeal carcinoma: significance for recurrence and survival. J Chin Med Assoc. 71(9):461-6, 2008
8. Comoretto M et al: Detection and restaging of residual and/or recurrent nasopharyngeal carcinoma after chemotherapy and radiation therapy: comparison of MR imaging and FDG PET/CT. Radiology. 249(1):203-11, 2008
9. Guigay J: Advances in nasopharyngeal carcinoma. Curr Opin Oncol. 20(3):264-9, 2008
10. Glastonbury CM: Nasopharyngeal carcinoma: the role of magnetic resonance imaging in diagnosis, staging, treatment, and follow-up. Top Magn Reson Imaging. 18(4):225-35, 2007
11. Lee AW et al: Preliminary results of a randomized study (NPC-9902 Trial) on therapeutic gain by concurrent chemotherapy and/or accelerated fractionation for locally advanced nasopharyngeal carcinoma. Int J Radiat Oncol Biol Phys. 66(1):142-51, 2006
12. Pow EH et al: Xerostomia and quality of life after intensity-modulated radiotherapy vs. conventional radiotherapy for early-stage nasopharyngeal carcinoma: initial report on a randomized controlled clinical trial. Int J Radiat Oncol Biol Phys. 66(4):981-91, 2006
13. Dabaja B et al: Intensity-modulated radiation therapy (IMRT) of cancers of the head and neck: comparison of split-field and whole-field techniques. Int J Radiat Oncol Biol Phys. 63(4):1000-5, 2005
14. Yen RF et al: Early restaging whole-body (18)F-FDG PET during induction chemotherapy predicts clinical outcome in patients with locoregionally advanced nasopharyngeal carcinoma. Eur J Nucl Med Mol Imaging. 32(10):1152-9, 2005
15. Lin JC et al: Quantification of plasma Epstein-Barr virus DNA in patients with advanced nasopharyngeal carcinoma. N Engl J Med. 350(24):2461-70, 2004
16. Lee N et al: Intensity-modulated radiation therapy for head-and-neck cancer: the UCSF experience focusing on target volume delineation. Int J Radiat Oncol Biol Phys. 57(1):49-60, 2003
17. Lee N et al: Intensity-modulated radiotherapy in the treatment of nasopharyngeal carcinoma: an update of the UCSF experience. Int J Radiat Oncol Biol Phys. 53(1):12-22, 2002
18. Al-Sarraf M et al: Chemoradiotherapy versus radiotherapy in patients with advanced nasopharyngeal cancer: phase III randomized Intergroup study 0099. J Clin Oncol. 16(4):1310-7, 1998

Stage II (T1 N1)

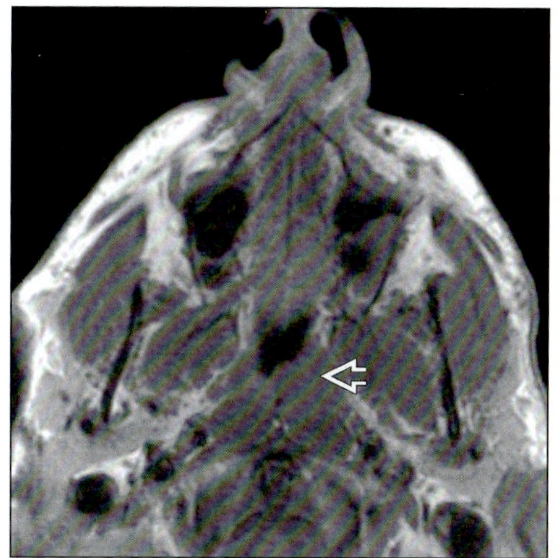

Stage II (T1 N1)

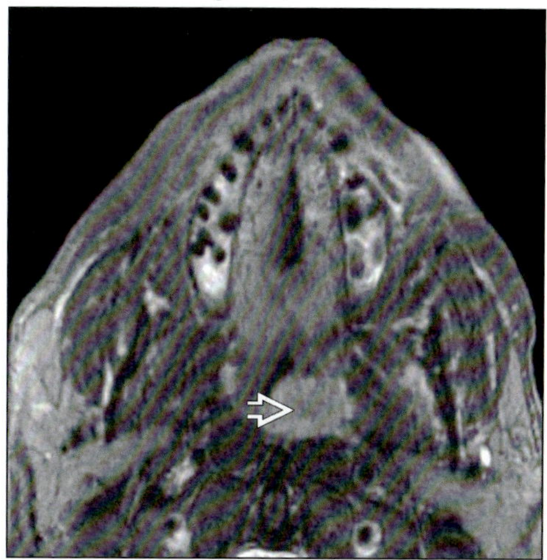

(Left) *Axial T1WI non-contrast MR in a 77-year-old man presenting with left neck mass shows nasopharyngeal tumor isointense to muscle. Mass emanates from left fossa of Rosenmuller ➡. Due to poor renal function, contrast was not administered.* ***(Right)*** *Axial T2WI MR in the same patient shows left nasopharyngeal mass ➡, which appears hyperintense to muscle. Biopsy revealed NPC, WHO type II. Tumor limited to nasopharynx is a T1 lesion.*

Stage II (T1 N1)

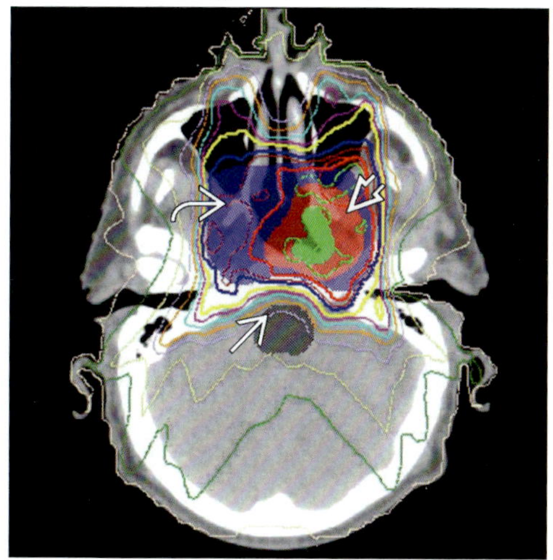

Stage II (T1 N1)

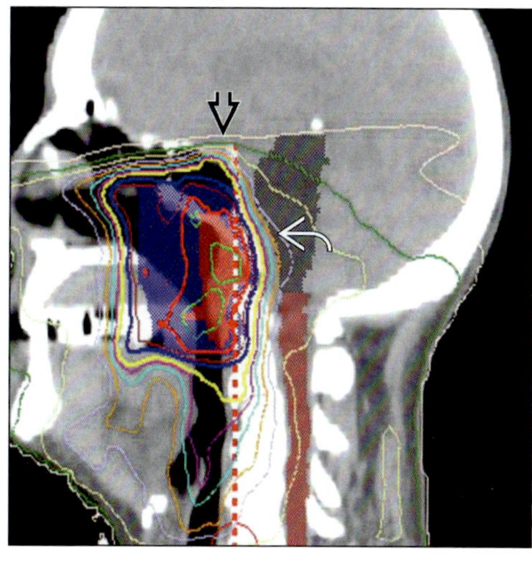

(Left) *High-dose CTV (red shading ➡) received 70 Gy and encompassed gross tumor with 0.5-1.0 cm margin. Intermediate-dose CTV (blue shading ➡) received 63 Gy and includes parapharyngeal space, clivus, retropharyngeal nodes, posterior nasal cavity, and maxillary and ethmoid sinuses. Brainstem ➡ sparing was achieved using IMRT.* ***(Right)*** *Sagittal view of same plan shows sparing of the brainstem ➡ and optic chiasm ➡ using IMRT.*

Stage II (T1 N1)

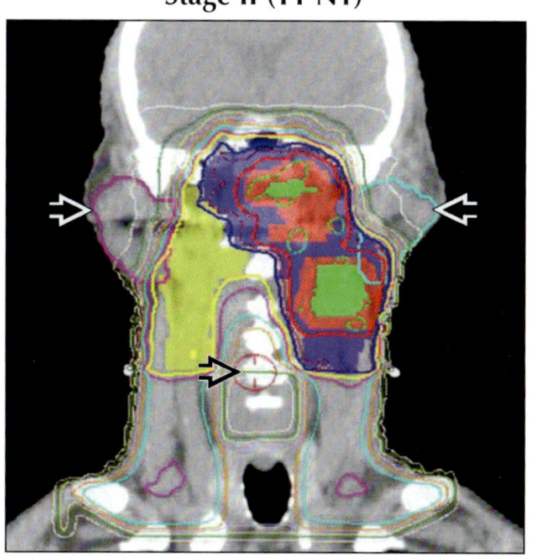

Stage II (T1 N1)

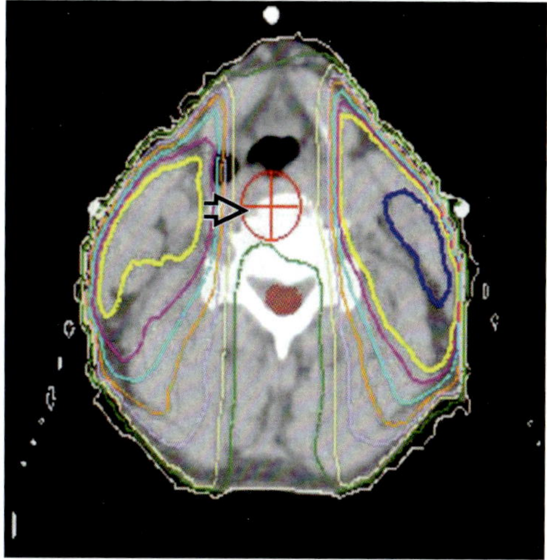

(Left) *Coronal view shows parotid sparing using IMRT ➡. Contralateral neck received subclinical dose of 57 Gy in 33 fractions (yellow). Low neck received 50 Gy in 25 fractions, which is below isocenter ➡.* ***(Right)*** *Axial CT shows isocenter placed above thyroid notch (about 1.5 cm above arytenoids) ➡. Anterior and posterior matching portals are used to treat the low neck using monoisocentric technique with half-beam blocking. This improves larynx sparing.*

(Left) Axial contrast-enhanced CT (CECT) shows left nasopharyngeal mass with extension across midline ➡. Parapharyngeal space invasion is seen here ↪. (Right) Axial fused PET/CT in the same patient shows intense FDG activity ➡ corresponding to the nasopharyngeal mass. Extension to the left parapharyngeal space is considered a T2 lesion.

Stage III (T2 N2 M0)

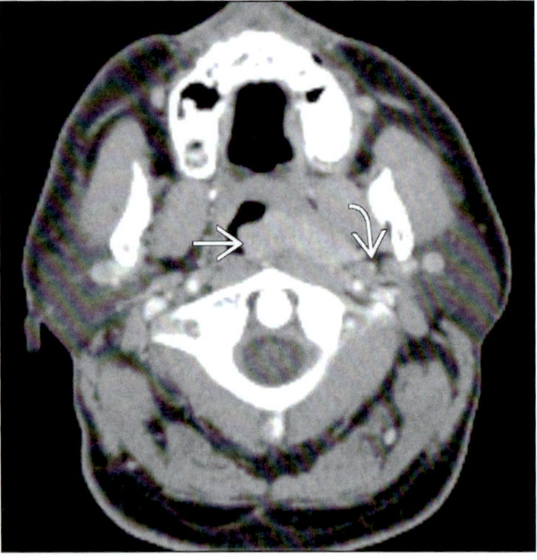

Stage III (T2 N2 M0)

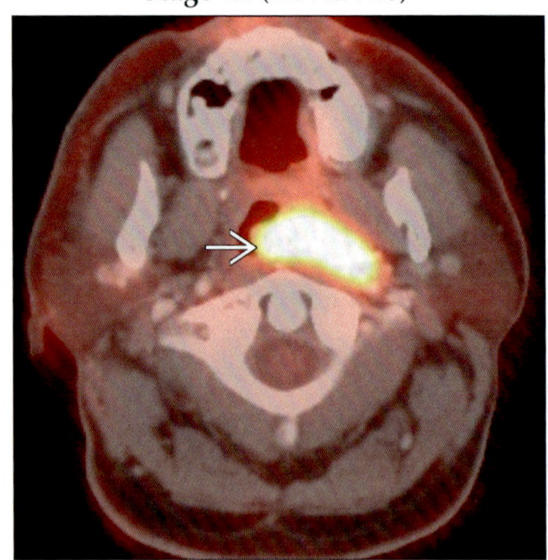

(Left) Axial T2WI MR in the same patient shows extent of local tumor extension. This tumor involves bilateral nasopharynx and invades into parapharyngeal space ➡. The retropharyngeal space behind the pharyngeal constrictor muscles does not appear involved ↪. (Right) Axial CECT in the same patient shows an enlarged right level IIA lymph node ➡ that is worrisome for metastatic disease. Additional smaller metastatic nodes were present bilaterally (not shown).

Stage III (T2 N2 M0)

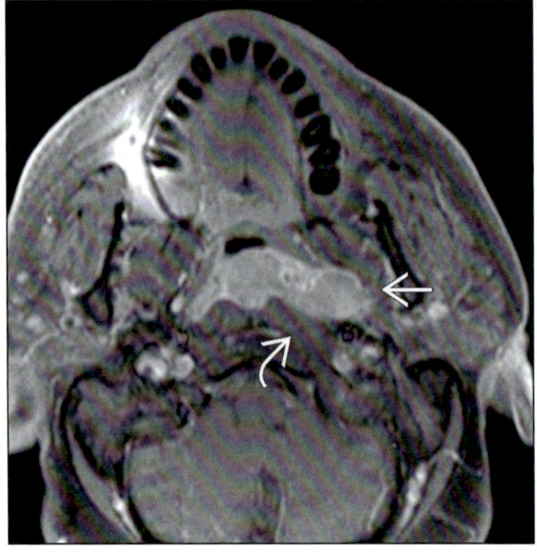

Stage III (T2 N2 M0)

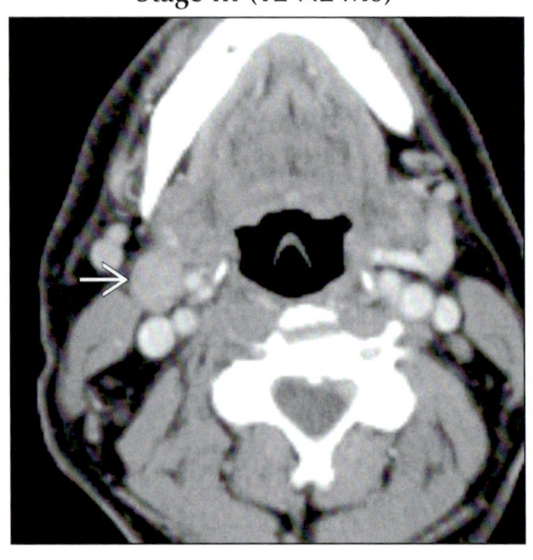

(Left) Axial fused PET/CT in the same patient shows an enlarged hypermetabolic contralateral metastatic lymph node ➡. (Right) Prominent contralateral nodes are seen ↪ in the same patient. These were biopsied positive for carcinoma. This is considered N2 disease due to the bilateral lymph node involvement.

Stage III (T2 N2 M0)

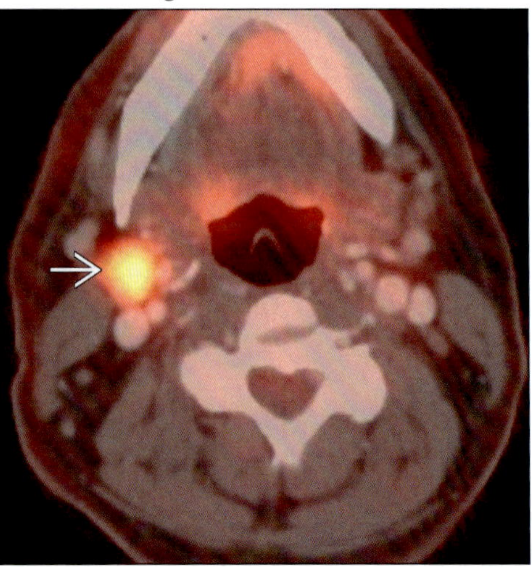

Stage III (T2 N2 M0)

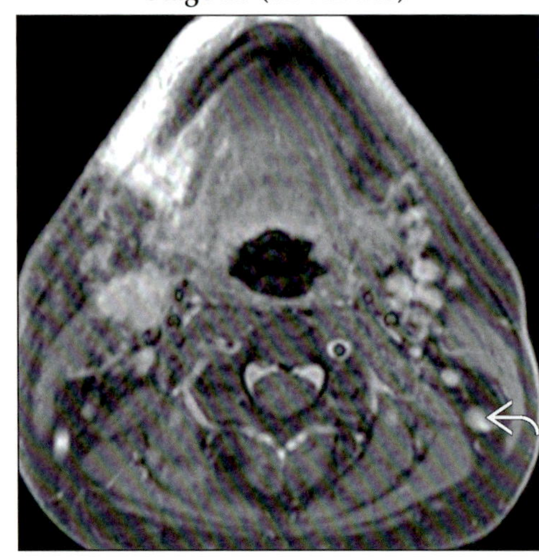

Stage II (T2 N1)

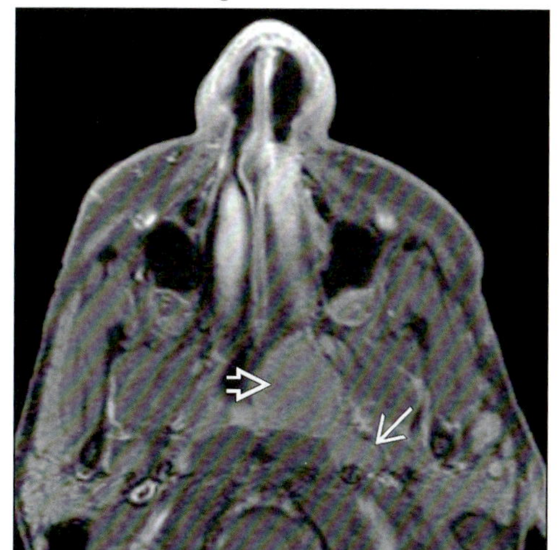

Stage II (T2 N1)

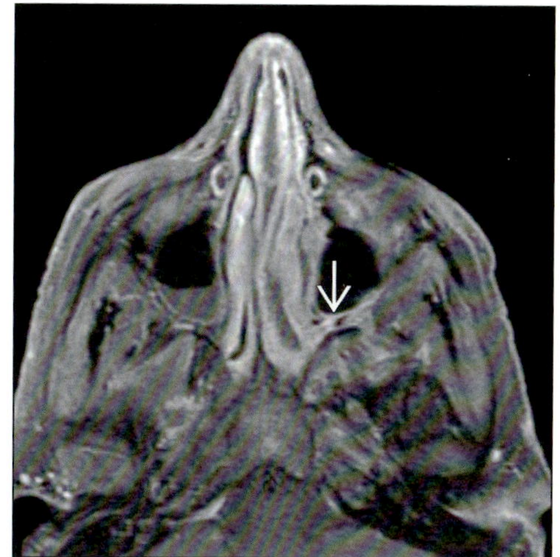

(Left) *T1WI C+ MR shows an exophytic left nasopharyngeal mass* ➔ *in a 17-year-old with a T2 N1, WHO type III nasopharyngeal carcinoma who presented with left-ear fullness. There is a prominent but not necrotic left retropharyngeal node* ➔ *(1.6 cm). Nodal enlargement is typical in this age group.* ***(Right)*** *Axial T1WI C+ MR in the same patient shows the mass extending through the sphenopalatine foramen into the pterygopalatine fossa* ➔*.*

Stage II (T2 N1)

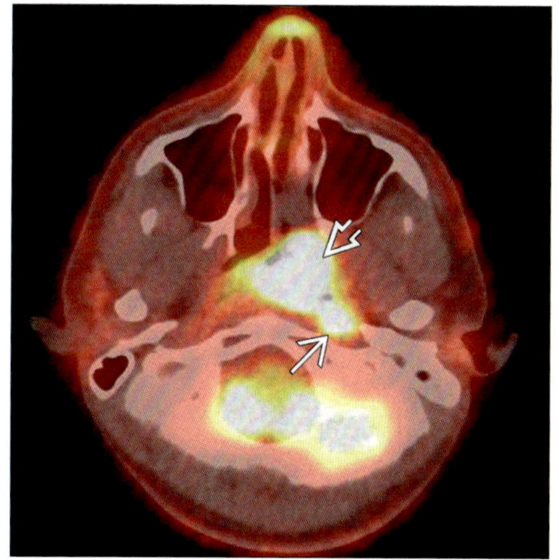

Stage II (T2 N1)

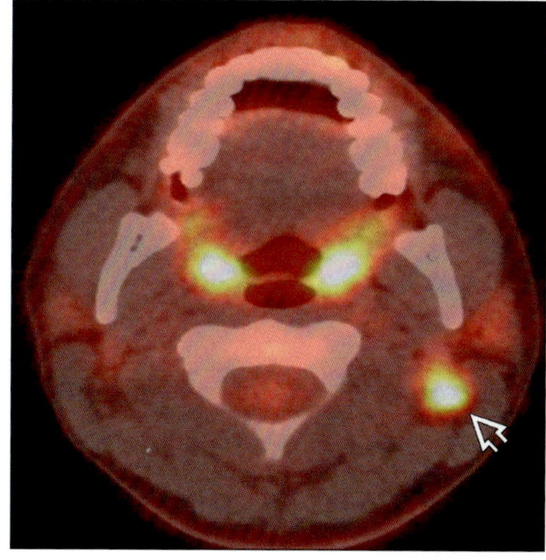

(Left) *Axial PET/CT in the same patient shows a hypermetabolic mass in the left nasopharynx* ➔ *(SUV 28.0), with a separate focus of activity posterior and lateral to this* ➔ *representing retropharyngeal nodal metastasis (SUV 14.7).* ***(Right)*** *In the same patient, a 2nd FDG-avid lymph node is demonstrated in the left cervical level II region* ➔*. This patient has ipsilateral cervical nodal metastases. His nodal staging is N1.*

Stage II (T2 N1)

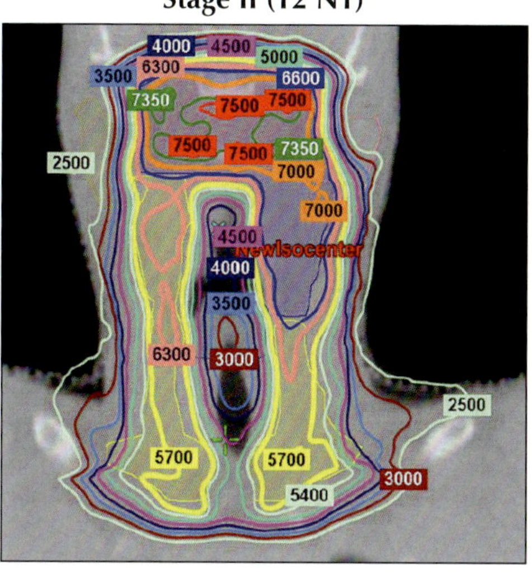

Stage II (T2 N1)

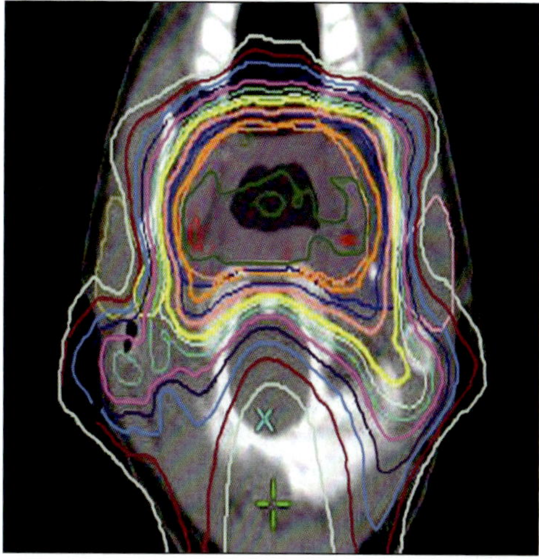

(Left) *The same patient was treated with concurrent CRT followed by chemo. He was treated to a total dose of 70 Gy in 33 fractions. Due to his young age and proximity of skull base, the patient was treated with intensity-modulated proton therapy (IMPT) to minimize dose to skull, brain, brainstem, spinal cord, parotids, and oral cavity.* ***(Right)*** *Oral cavity and parotid gland sparing with IMPT of the same patient is shown. He had grade 2 oral mucositis upon completion of RT.*

*(**Left**) Axial T1WI C+ MR in a 38 year old presenting with otalgia and headaches shows an extensive submucosal mass of right nasopharynx ➔. Biopsy showed adenoid cystic carcinoma. There is direct invasion of the right retropharyngeal space ➔. This patient did not have lymphadenopathy, a typical finding for adenoid cystic cancer. (**Right**) Axial T1WI C+ MR in the same patient shows tumor accessing the carotid canal ➔ to gain access to the cavernous sinus.*

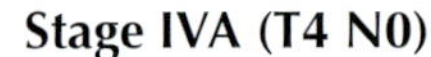

Stage IVA (T4 N0)

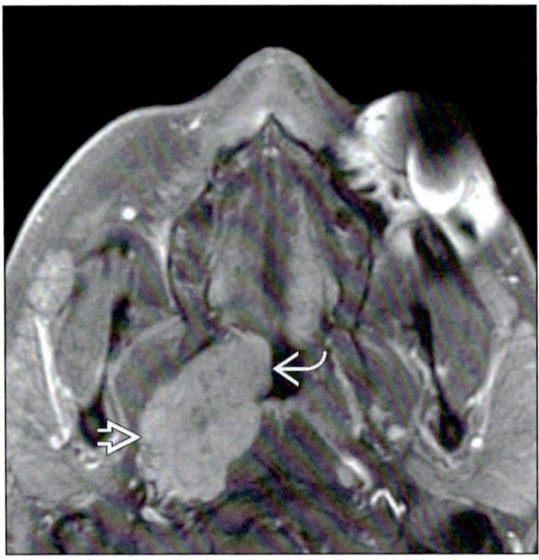

Stage IVA (T4 N0)

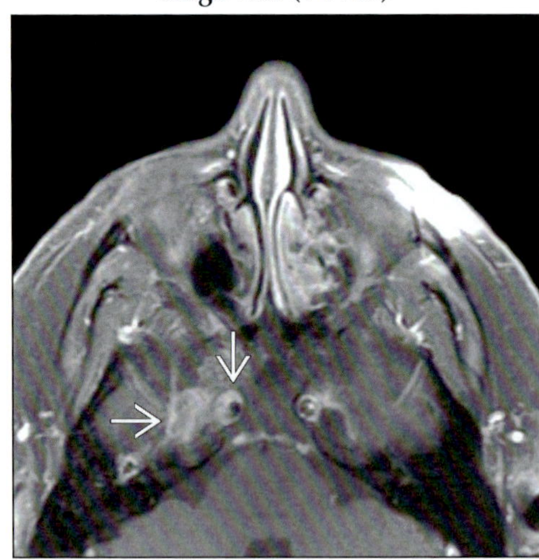

*(**Left**) Coronal T1WI C+ MR in the same patient shows the tumor is extending through right foramen ovale ➔ into the floor of the middle cranial fossa and inferior aspect of Meckel cave ➔. (**Right**) Sagittal T1WI C+ MR in the same patient shows intracranial tumor extension ➔ of bulky nasopharyngeal tumor ➔; hence the T4 designation.*

Stage IVA (T4 N0)

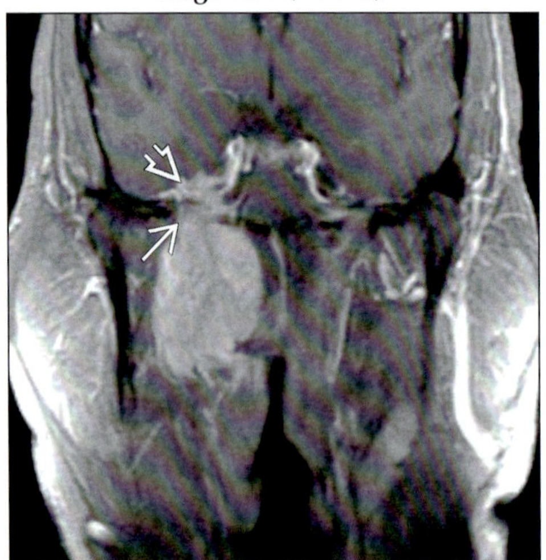

Stage IVA (T4 N0)

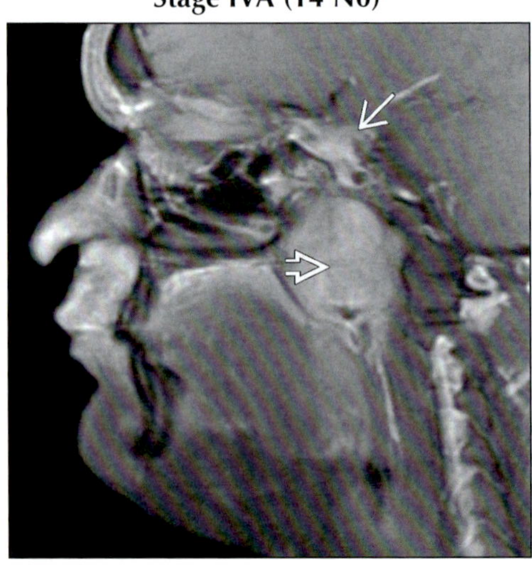

*(**Left**) Axial T1WI C+ MR in the same patient shows submucosal spread along several routes. Tumor invades right petroclival fissure ➔ and infiltrates pterygopalatine fossa, vidian canal ➔, and foramen lacerum ➔. (**Right**) In the same patient, HD-CTV includes gross disease (red) treated to 70 Gy. Subclinical disease received 57 Gy (yellow). Dose was limited to right temporal lobe (< 66 Gy), brainstem and optic chiasm (< 54 Gy), and spinal cord (< 45 Gy).*

Stage IVA (T4 N0)

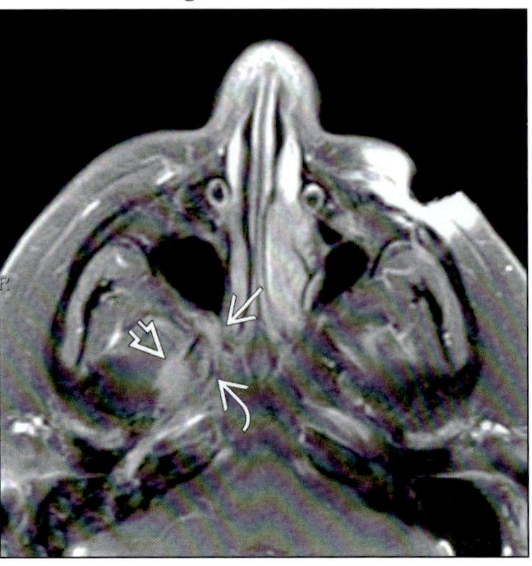

Stage IVA (T4 N0)

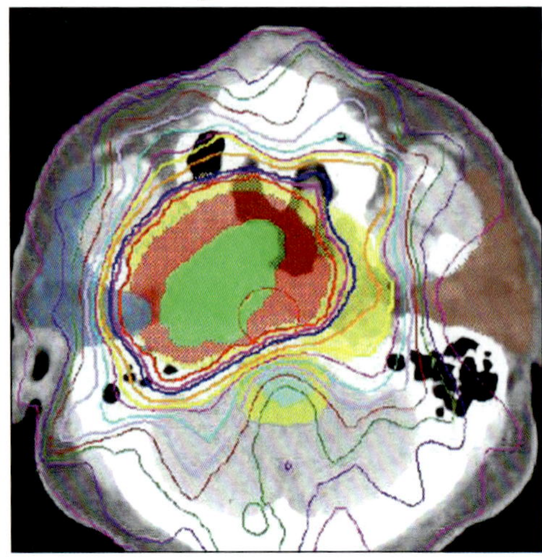

Stage IVA (T4 N2)

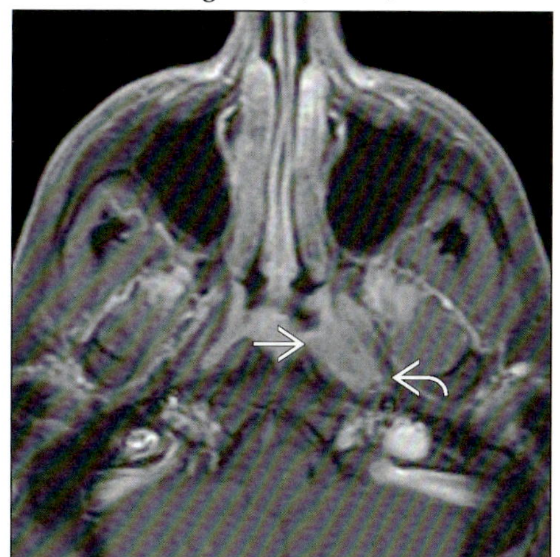

Stage IVA (T4 N2)

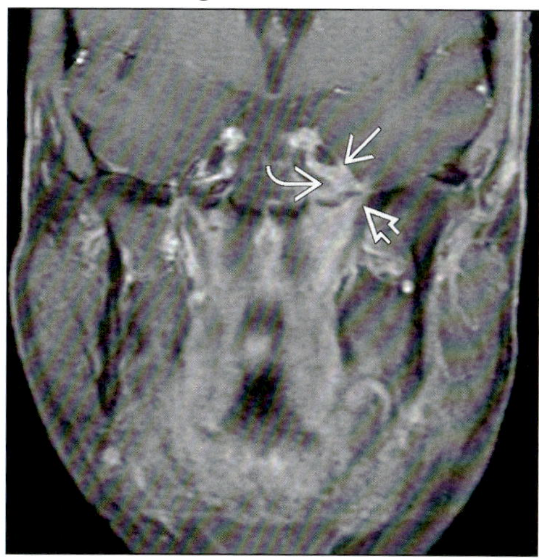

(Left) *48 year old with undifferentiated nasopharyngeal carcinoma (WHO type III) presented with left hearing loss and epistaxis. T1WI MR with contrast reveals nasopharyngeal mass → with parapharyngeal space invasion →.* ***(Right)*** *Coronal T1WI C+ MR in the same patient shows extension superiorly through foramen ovale → to the inferior aspect of Meckel cave →. There is soft tissue enhancement around the left internal carotid artery →.*

Stage IVA (T4 N2)

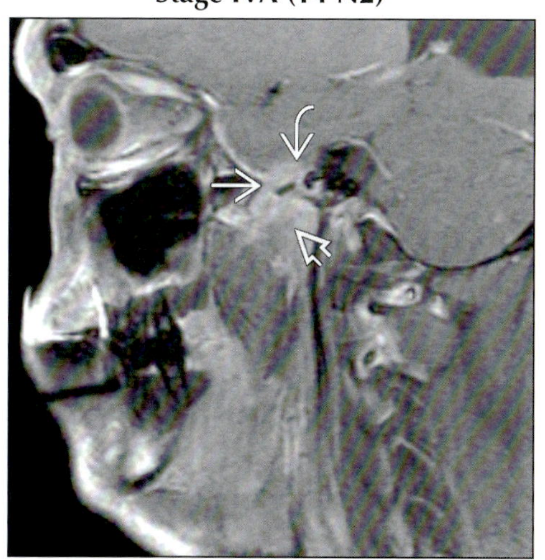

Stage IVA (T4 N2)

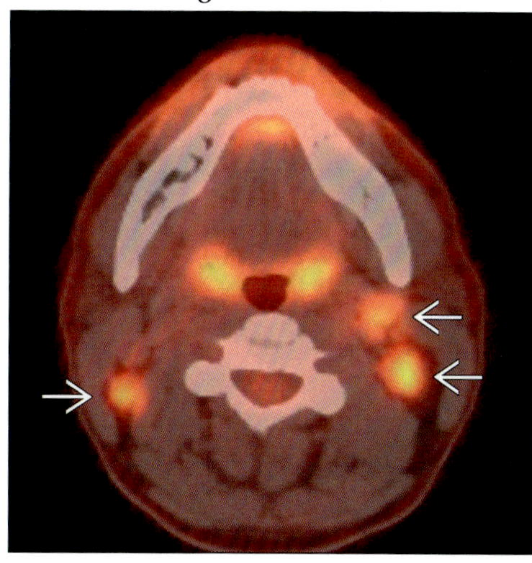

(Left) *Sagittal MR with contrast in the same patient demonstrates superior extension of tumor → through foramen ovale → into middle cranial fossa →, which makes this a T4 disease.* ***(Right)*** *Axial fused PET/CT in the same patient shows multiple FDG-avid lymph nodes bilaterally →. Ultrasound-guided biopsy confirmed metastatic carcinoma. Nodal staging for this patient is N2.*

Stage IVA (T4 N2)

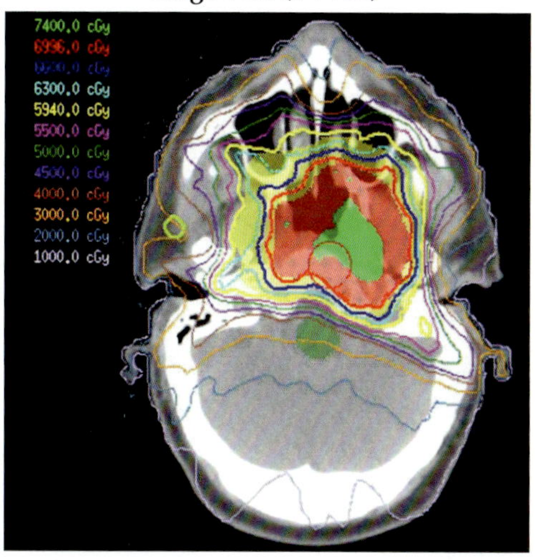

Stage IVA (T4 N2)

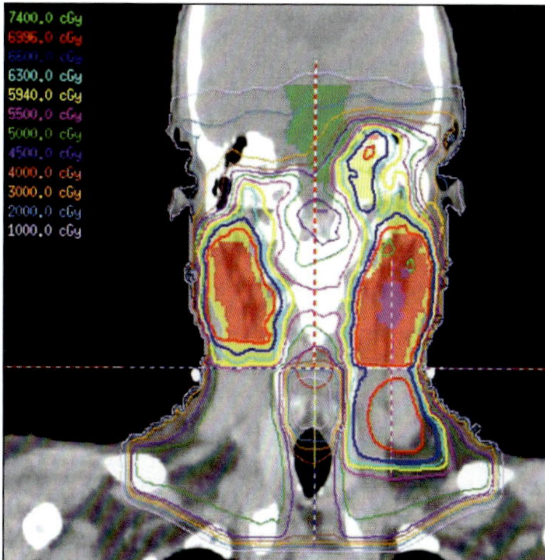

(Left) *Same patient was staged T4 N2c M0 and treated with IMRT with concurrent weekly cisplatin at 40 mg/m2. The tumor with margin (red) received 70 Gy in 33 fractions. At-risk structures, including pterygoid fossa (yellow), received 59.4 Gy in 33 fractions.* ***(Right)*** *Coronal imaging in the same patient shows IMRT field matched at isocenter to half-beam AP/PA fields below. Left mid-neck boost to 10 Gy using oblique PA beam was given to level IV nodal basin.*

SALIVARY GLAND

(T) Primary Tumor

Adapted from 7th edition AJCC Staging Forms.

TNM	*Definitions*
TX	Primary tumor cannot be assessed
T0	No evidence of primary tumor
T1	Tumor ≤ 2 cm in greatest dimension without extraparenchymal extension*
T2	Tumor > 2 cm but ≤ 4 cm in greatest dimension without extraparenchymal extension*
T3	Tumor > 4 cm &/or tumor having extraparenchymal extension*
T4a	Moderately advanced disease: Tumor invades skin, mandible, ear canal, &/or facial nerve
T4b	Very advanced disease: Tumor invades skull base &/or pterygoid plates &/or encases carotid artery

(N) Regional Lymph Nodes

NX	Regional lymph nodes cannot be assessed
N0	No regional lymph node metastasis
N1	Metastasis in a single ipsilateral lymph node, ≤ 3 cm in greatest dimension
N2	Metastasis in a single ipsilateral lymph node, > 3 cm but ≤ 6 cm in greatest dimension, or in multiple ipsilateral lymph nodes, none > 6 cm in greatest dimension, or in bilateral or contralateral lymph nodes, none > 6 cm in greatest dimension
N2a	Metastasis in a single ipsilateral lymph node, > 3 cm but ≤ 6 cm in greatest dimension
N2b	Metastasis in multiple ipsilateral lymph nodes, none > 6 cm in greatest dimension
N2c	Metastasis in bilateral or contralateral lymph nodes, none > 6 cm in greatest dimension
N3	Metastasis in a lymph node, > 6 cm in greatest dimension

(M) Distant Metastasis

M0	No distant metastasis
M1	Distant metastasis

**Extraparenchymal extension is clinical or macroscopic evidence of invasion of soft tissues. Microscopic evidence alone does not constitute extraparenchymal extension for classification purposes.*

AJCC Stages/Prognostic Groups

Adapted from 7th edition AJCC Staging Forms.

Stage	*T*	*N*	*M*
I	T1	N0	M0
II	T2	N0	M0
III	T3	N0	M0
	T1	N1	M0
	T2	N1	M0
	T3	N1	M0
IVA	T4a	N0	M0
	T4a	N1	M0
	T1	N2	M0
	T2	N2	M0
	T3	N2	M0
	T4a	N2	M0
IVB	T4b	Any N	M0
	Any T	N3	M0
IVC	Any T	Any N	M1

T1

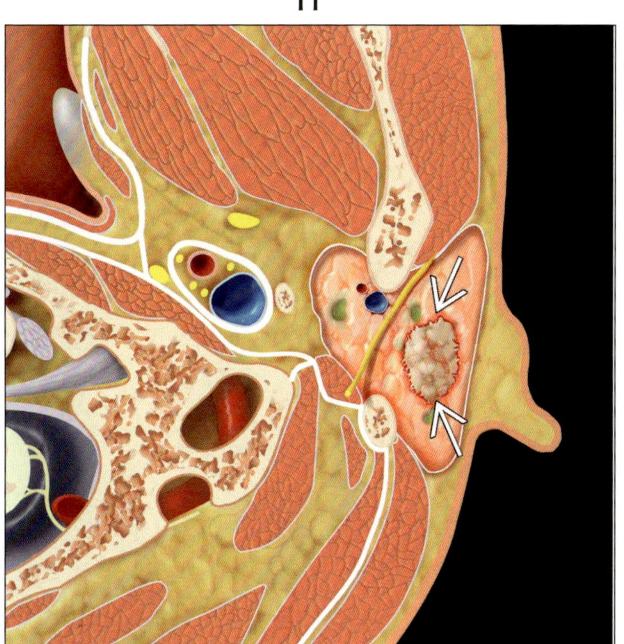

Axial graphic illustrates a tumor in the superficial parotid lobe. A T1 tumor is up to 2 cm in maximal size and does not macroscopically nor by clinical examination extend beyond the margins of the gland.

T2

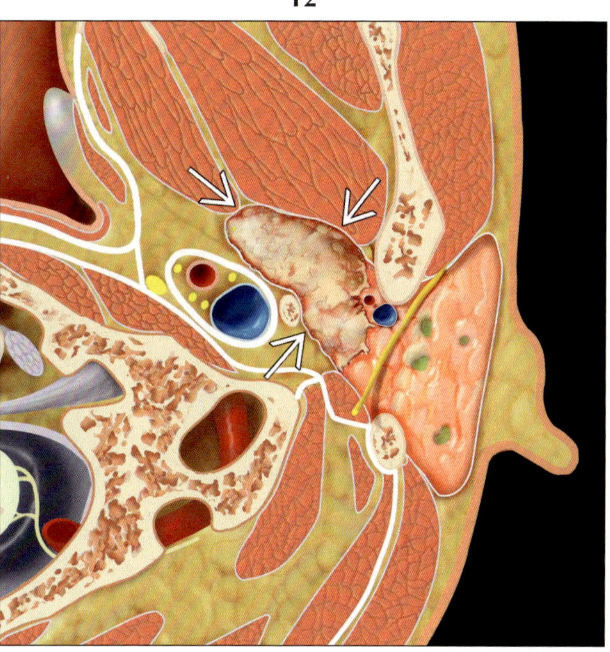

Axial graphic illustrates a larger tumor, this time arising within the deep lobe of parotid. T2 tumors are > 2 cm and up to 4 cm in size, without extension beyond the gland.

T3

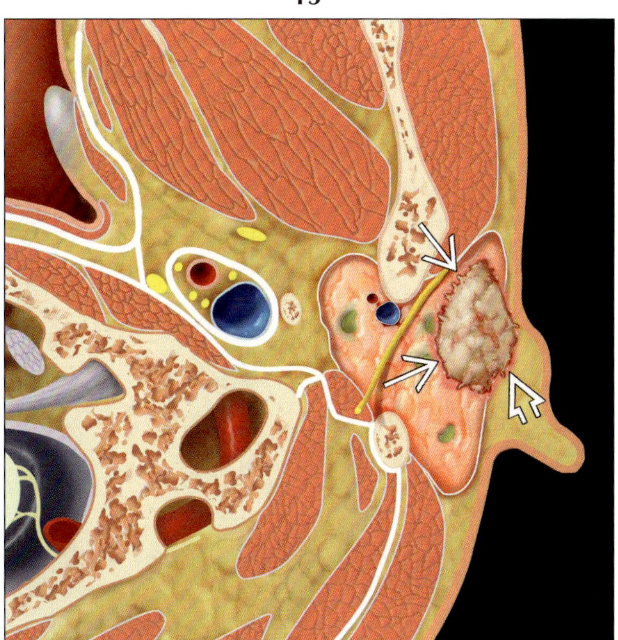

Axial graphic shows a tumor that extends beyond the gland to extraparenchymal tissue. T3 salivary tumors are > 4 cm in size or extend beyond the gland.

T3

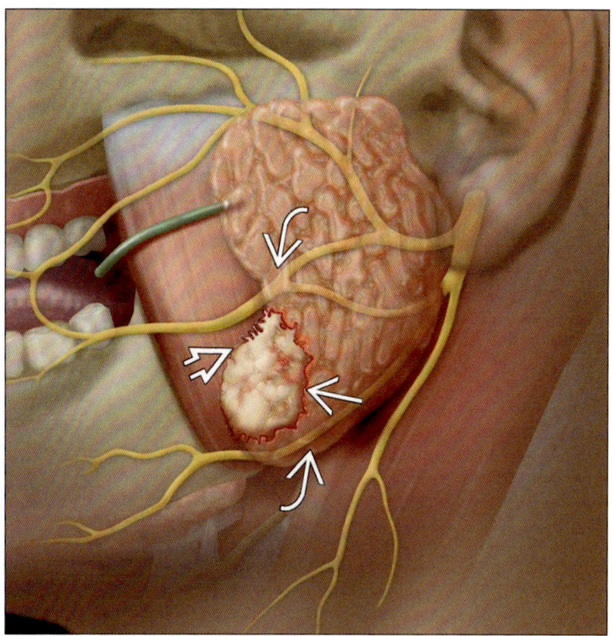

Graphic illustrates a small parotid tumor that is designated T3 since it extends from the gland to extraparenchymal tissue. There is, however, no involvement of facial nerve branches.

T4a

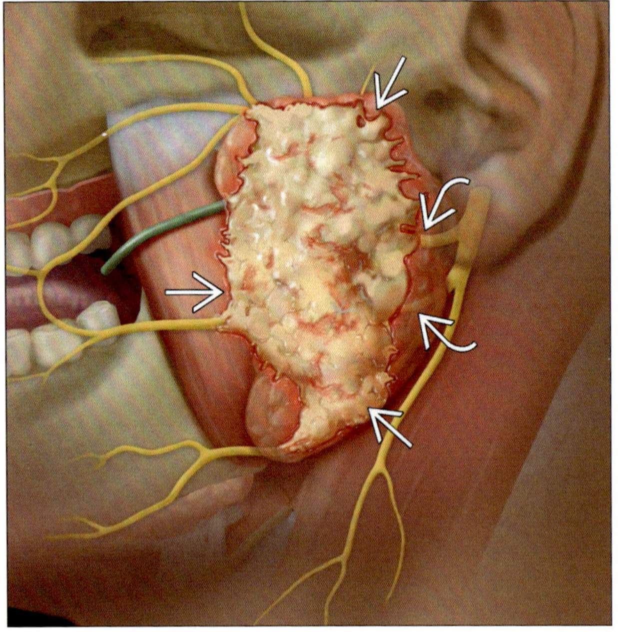

Graphic illustrates a large parotid tumor ➔ involving the superficial lobe. A lesion > 4 cm should be at least a T3 tumor. Involvement of facial nerve branches ➔, however, designates this a T4a moderately advanced tumor.

T4a

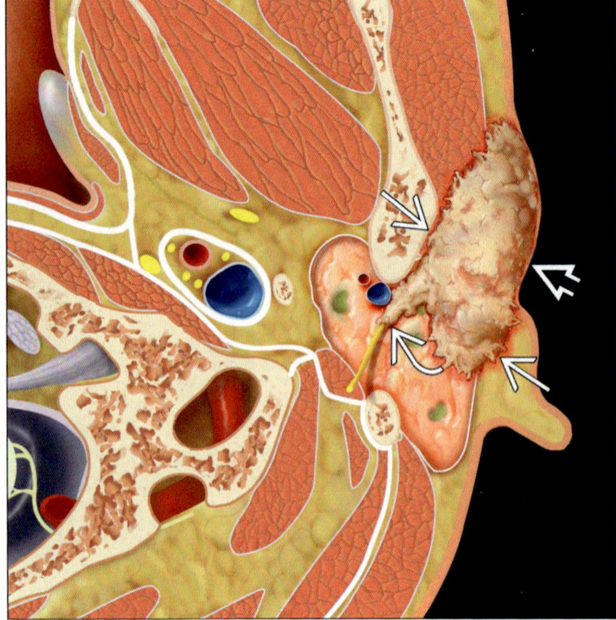

Axial graphic depicts a T4a superficial lobe parotid tumor ➔ with involvement of the facial nerve ➔ and extension to the skin ➔. T4a is determined by invasion of mandible, ear canal, skin, &/or facial nerve.

T4b

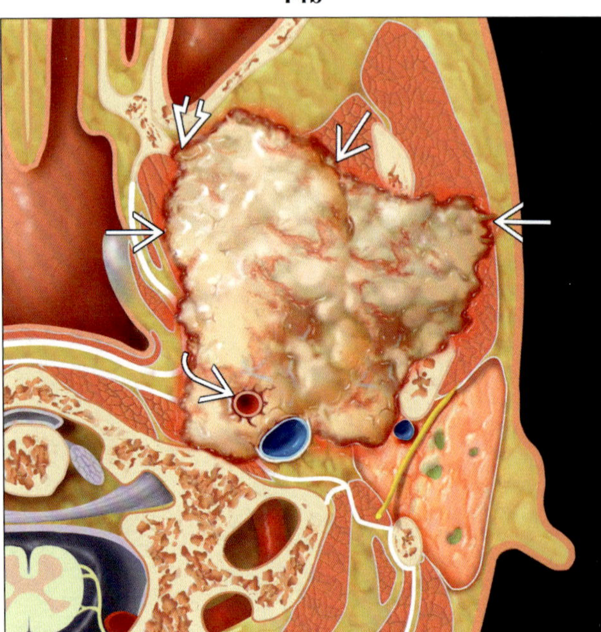

Axial graphic demonstrates very advanced disease with a T4b tumor arising from the deep parotid lobe and invading the masticator space ➔, mandible and pterygoid plates ➔ with encasement of the carotid ➔.

T4b

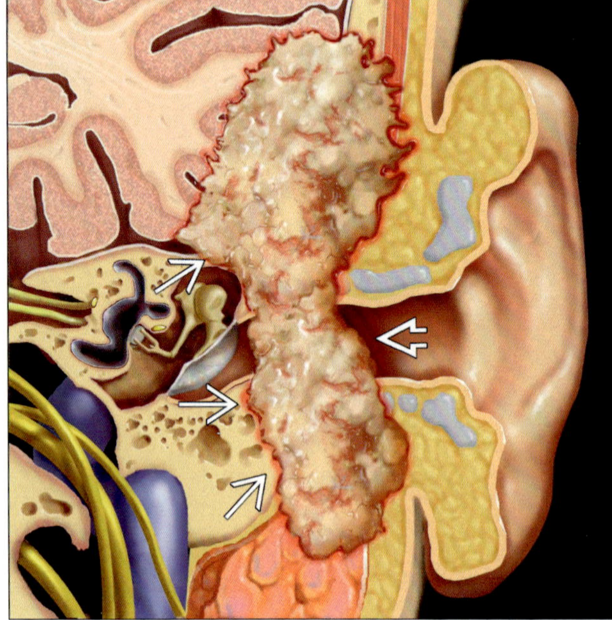

Coronal graphic illustrates another T4b tumor with extensive skull base ➔ and external auditory canal ➔ invasion. T4b is determined by invasion of skull base, pterygoid plates, &/or encasement of the carotid artery.

T2

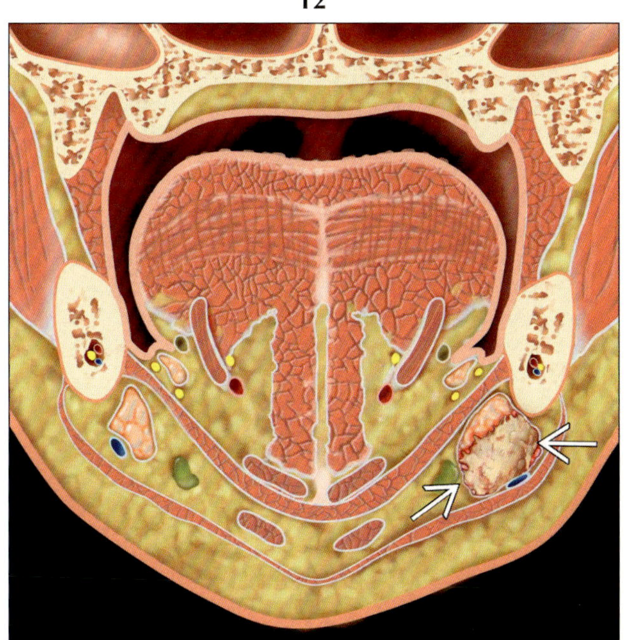

Coronal graphic illustrates submandibular gland carcinoma ➡. This T2 tumor expands the gland but is < 4 cm in greatest diameter and does not extend outside of the gland parenchyma.

T3

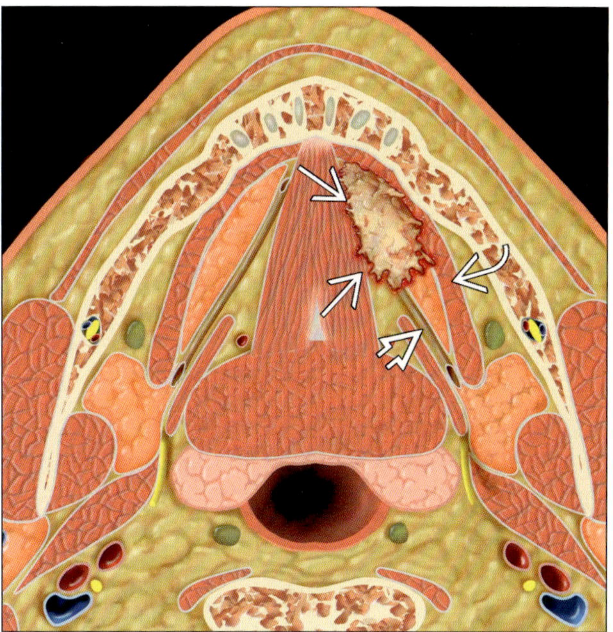

Axial graphic illustrates T3 sublingual gland carcinoma ➡. Although tumor is not > 4 cm in greatest diameter, there is extraparenchymal extension to mylohyoid muscle ↪. Such a tumor may also present with symptoms from obstruction of submandibular (Wharton) duct ⇨.

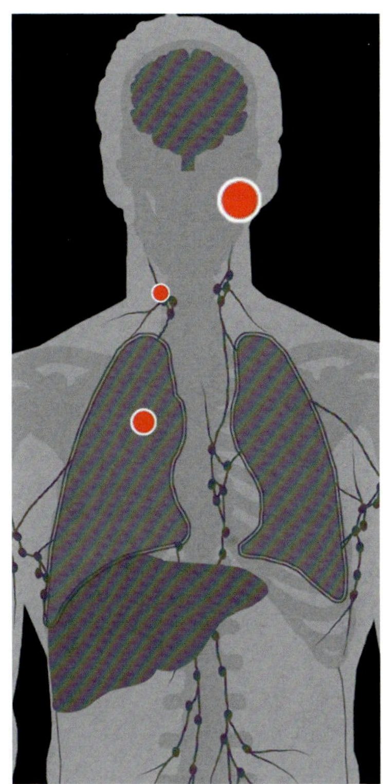

INITIAL SITE OF RECURRENCE

T1 (LF)	5%
T2 (LF)	9%
T3/T4 (LF)	16%
Incomplete Margins (LF)	18%
Bone Invasion (LF)	14%
Perineural Invasion (LF)	12%
Regional Failure (N0)	7%
Regional Failure (N+)	14%
Distant Failure	27%

Local and regional failure patterns were obtained from 386 patients treated with surgery and radiotherapy. LF indicates 10-year local failure rate. Terhaard CHJ et al: The Role of Radiotherapy in the Treatment of Malignant Salivary Gland Tumors. IJROBP 61(1):103-11, 2005. Distant failure rate obtained from Garden AS et al: Postoperative Radiotherapy for Malignant Tumors of the Minor Salivary Glands. Outcomes and Patterns of Failure. Cancer 73(10):2563-9, 1994.

SALIVARY GLAND

OVERVIEW

General Comments

- Rare; represent only 6% of head and neck neoplasms
  - Challenging to study given enormous heterogeneity in location, histology, and clinical behavior
  - Possible locations of salivary gland tumors and frequency of tumors arising in each
    - Parotid glands: 70%
      - Approximately 50% malignant
    - Submandibular glands: 10%
      - Approximately 50% malignant
    - Sublingual glands: < 1%
    - Minor salivary glands: 20%
      - Almost all malignant
      - Scattered throughout upper aerodigestive tract
  - Evaluation and treatment warranted for all neoplasms, benign and malignant
- Most common malignancies
  - Mucoepidermoid carcinoma
  - Adenoid cystic carcinoma
  - Polymorphous low-grade adenocarcinoma
  - Acinic cell carcinoma
  - Carcinoma ex-pleomorphic adenoma
  - Adenocarcinoma, not otherwise specified (NOS)
- Multidisciplinary evaluation crucial to adequate staging, treatment, and follow-up

Classification

- **World Health Organization (WHO) histological classification for tumors of salivary glands**
  - **Malignant epithelial tumors**
    - Acinic cell carcinoma (7%)
    - Mucoepidermoid carcinoma (34%)
      - Low-grade mucoepidermoid carcinoma
      - High-grade mucoepidermoid carcinoma
    - Adenoid cystic carcinoma (22%)
    - Polymorphous low-grade adenocarcinoma
    - Epithelial-myoepithelial carcinoma
    - Clear cell carcinoma, NOS
    - Basal cell adenocarcinoma
    - Sebaceous carcinoma
    - Sebaceous lymphadenocarcinoma
    - Cystadenocarcinoma
    - Low-grade cribriform cystadenocarcinoma
    - Mucinous adenocarcinoma
    - Oncocytic carcinoma
    - Salivary duct carcinoma
    - Adenocarcinoma, NOS
    - Myoepithelial carcinoma
    - Carcinoma ex-pleomorphic adenoma (9%)
    - Carcinosarcoma
    - Metastasizing pleomorphic adenoma
    - Squamous cell carcinoma
    - Small cell carcinoma
    - Large cell carcinoma
    - Lymphoepithelial carcinoma
    - Sialoblastoma
  - **Benign epithelial tumors**
    - Pleomorphic adenoma
    - Myoepithelioma
    - Basal cell adenoma
    - Warthin tumor
    - Oncocytoma
    - Canalicular adenoma
    - Sebaceous adenoma
    - Lymphadenoma
      - Sebaceous
      - Nonsebaceous
    - Ductal papillomas
      - Inverted ductal papilloma
      - Intraductal papilloma
      - Sialadenoma papilliferum
    - Cystadenoma
  - **Soft tissue tumors**
    - Hemangioma
  - **Hematologic tumors**
    - Hodgkin lymphoma
    - Diffuse large B-cell lymphoma
    - Extranodal marginal zone B-cell lymphoma
  - **Metastatic tumors**

NATURAL HISTORY

General Features

- Comments
  - Incredibly varied in clinical behavior
    - Differentiation based on location and histology determines optimal treatment regimen
- Location
  - Lesions from any of major or minor salivary glands
    - Histology and location identify salivary gland tumors as such

Etiology

- Risk factors
  - Low-dose radiation associated with salivary gland neoplasms 15-20 years later, including
    - Pleomorphic adenoma
    - Mucoepidermoid carcinoma
    - Squamous cell carcinoma
  - Silica dust and nitrosamines associated with salivary gland neoplasms in some reports
  - Unlike other head and neck cancers, no association between alcohol/tobacco and salivary gland malignant tumors
  - Tobacco exposure associated with development of Warthin tumors, which are benign

Epidemiology & Cancer Incidence

- Number of cases in USA per year
  - 1.5 cases diagnosed per 100,000 individuals
  - 700 deaths each year
- Sex predilection
  - Women more likely to develop benign neoplasms
  - Women and men equally likely to develop malignant neoplasms
- Age of onset
  - Malignant lesions typically present after age 60
  - Benign lesions typically present earlier, after age 40

Genetics

- Characteristic molecular and hormonal profiles
  - Serve as potential therapeutic targets
- Common molecular and hormonal markers in salivary gland cancers
  - C-kit overexpression
    - 80-90% adenoid cystic carcinoma

- Rarely in mucoepidermoid carcinoma, adenocarcinoma, salivary duct carcinoma
  - Epidermal growth factor receptor (EGFR) overexpression
    - 0-37% adenoid cystic carcinoma
    - 40% mucoepidermoid carcinoma
    - 30-40% adenocarcinoma and salivary duct carcinoma
  - HER2 expression
    - Rarely in adenoid cystic carcinoma
    - 25-35% mucoepidermoid carcinoma
    - 20-30% adenocarcinoma and salivary duct carcinoma
  - Vascular epidermal growth factor (VEGF) expression
    - 85% adenoid cystic carcinoma
    - 50% mucoepidermoid carcinoma
    - 65% adenocarcinoma and salivary duct carcinoma
  - Androgen receptor expression
    - 15-40% salivary duct carcinoma (marker for this histology)
    - Rarely in other types
- Chromosomal translocations identified in adenoid cystic carcinoma and mucoepidermoid carcinoma
  - t(6;9)(q22-23;p23-24) in adenoid cystic carcinoma
  - t(11;19) in mucoepidermoid carcinoma

Gross Pathology & Surgical Features

- Mucoepidermoid carcinoma
  - Low grade
    - Typically, well circumscribed with cystic areas containing mucin
  - High grade
    - Typically, solid with more infiltrative growth pattern
- Adenoid cystic carcinoma
  - Typically, solid masses with infiltrative growth pattern, especially along perineural routes
- Salivary gland carcinoma
  - Typically, locally infiltrative with multiple metastatic lymph nodes

Microscopic Pathology

- H&E
  - Heterogeneous array of histologies
    - Controversy in grading of salivary gland tumors
  - Grading of salivary gland tumors
    - Low grade
      - Acinic cell carcinoma
      - Basal cell adenocarcinoma
      - Clear cell carcinoma
      - Cystadenocarcinoma
      - Epithelial-myoepithelial carcinoma
      - Mucinous adenocarcinoma
      - Polymorphous low-grade adenocarcinoma
    - Low, intermediate, or high grade
      - Adenocarcinoma, NOS
      - Mucoepidermoid carcinoma
      - Squamous cell carcinoma
    - Intermediate or high grade
      - Myoepithelial carcinoma
    - High grade
      - Anaplastic small cell carcinoma
      - Carcinosarcoma
      - Large cell undifferentiated carcinoma
      - Small cell undifferentiated carcinoma
      - Salivary duct carcinoma
- Special stains
  - Mucoepidermoid carcinoma
    - Simple mucin-type carbohydrate antigens
      - T, Tn, syalosyl-Tn
    - Low-grade mucoepidermoid carcinoma associated with striated duct differentiation pattern
      - CK7
      - CK14
      - Mitochondrial antibodies
  - Adenoid cystic carcinoma
    - Malignant cells in ductal structures share similar phenotype with intercalated ducts
      - Keratin
      - CEA
      - Lysozyme
      - Lactoferrin
      - α-1-antichymotrypsin
      - S100 protein
      - CD117 (c-kit)
    - Phenotype of malignant cells around gland-like spaces suggestive for myoepithelial cell differentiation
      - S100 protein
      - Actin
    - Strong reactivity seen for components of basement membrane
      - Type IV collagen
      - Laminin
      - Integrin ligands
      - Heparan sulfate proteoglycan (perlecan)
      - α-1-antitrypsin

Routes of Spread

- Local spread
  - Can be locally invasive into soft tissue or surrounding areas, depending on subtype
    - Adenoid cystic carcinoma most commonly associated with perineural spread
- Lymphatic extension
  - Compared to squamous cell carcinomas of the head and neck, lymph node spread from salivary cancers relatively rare
  - Lymph node metastases related to size and histology of primary tumor
    - High-grade tumors more likely to spread to regional lymph nodes
    - Low-grade tumors rarely spread to regional lymph nodes
  - Typically, orderly spread of lymph node disease from site of primary tumor
    - Intraglandular lymph nodes
    - Periglandular lymph nodes
    - Upper neck lymph nodes
    - Lower neck lymph nodes
  - Typically, unilateral lymph node metastases (vs. bilateral)
- Metastatic sites
  - Distant metastasis related to histology of tumor
    - High-grade tumors, i.e., adenocarcinoma and salivary duct carcinoma, most commonly spread to distant sites
    - Adenoid cystic carcinomas with relatively high rates of bone and lung metastases
    - Low-grade tumors rarely metastasize

- Most common sites of metastases from salivary duct tumors
  - Lung
  - Brain
  - Bone
- Predictors of distant metastases
  - Tumor > 3 cm
  - Solid histologic pattern
  - Local recurrence
  - Nodal metastases

IMAGING

Detection

- **General**
  - 3D imaging crucial for evaluation of newly diagnosed salivary gland mass, including
    - Extent of tumor
    - Extraglandular extension
    - Involvement of critical adjacent structures, e.g., facial nerve, deep lobe of parotid, or bone
    - Involvement of regional lymph nodes
    - Concurrent tumors in other glands
  - Mucoepidermoid carcinoma
    - Most commonly located in superficial lobe of parotid gland (more so than deep lobe)
    - Typically 1-4 cm in size at presentation
  - Adenoid cystic carcinoma
    - Most commonly located in parotid gland
      - Followed by submandibular gland and hard palate
    - Size at presentation may vary; typically 1-3 cm
- **CT**
  - Standard imaging for evaluation of a newly diagnosed salivary gland mass and potentially involved lymph nodes
    - Important to determine size and location of lesion
    - Less helpful in predicting histologic diagnosis
  - Low-grade tumors
    - Often well-circumscribed masses with sharp margins on CT imaging
  - High-grade tumors
    - Often enhancing infiltrative masses with poorly defined margins on CT imaging
- **MR**
  - Excellent imaging for evaluation of salivary gland masses and preferred modality if cancer is suspected
    - Specifically important in evaluation of cranial nerve palsies and meningeal symptoms
    - Helpful in delineating perineural invasion and proximity to nerves prior to surgery
    - Less effective at imaging obstructive or inflammatory processes
  - T1 images ± contrast useful in delineating extent of tumor and pathways of spread
    - Perineural invasion
    - Bone invasion
    - Intracranial extension
  - T2 images relatively good predictors of type of neoplasm (benign vs. malignant)
    - Some subtypes hyperintense on T2 images, e.g., pleomorphic adenomas
    - High-grade tumors tend to be lower in signal intensity
  - Mucoepidermoid carcinoma
    - Low-grade tumors typically heterogeneous well-defined masses with predominantly low signal on T1 imaging and heterogeneous signal on T2 imaging
    - High-grade tumors typically solid masses with soft tissue signal on T1 imaging and intermediate signal on T2 imaging
  - Adenoid cystic carcinoma
    - Typically low to intermediate signal intensity on T1 imaging
    - Especially important to determine perineural invasion, which can be extensive
- **PET/CT**
  - Most commonly used to identify lymph node and distant metastases
    - Less commonly used for evaluation of primary tumors of salivary glands
  - False-positive rate for malignancy is 30%
    - Typically due to Warthin tumors
    - Pleomorphic adenomas may also have FDG avidity
  - High-grade salivary tumors generally FDG-avid
    - Typical SUVs above 5
    - Adenoid cystic carcinoma, however, is an exception, with typically low SUVs
  - Normal salivary glands with minimal to moderate uptake or diffuse asymmetric uptake
    - Mean SUV of normal parotid ~ 2
    - May be asymmetrical if gland inflammation
    - Symmetrical activity with no anatomic abnormality typically benign, regardless of SUV
- **Ultrasound**
  - Can be used to assess primary tumor and suspicious adenopathy
    - Can be coupled with fine-needle aspiration (FNA) for diagnosis or staging
  - Low-grade mucoepidermoid carcinoma
    - Well-defined, solid, hypoechoic, homogeneous/heterogeneous mass
  - High-grade mucoepidermoid carcinoma
    - Ill-defined, hypoechoic, heterogeneous mass ± infiltration into adjacent tissues and associated lymphadenopathy

Restaging

- Post-treatment imaging provides new baseline for comparison
- No data for routine imaging, but should be employed based on symptom development
  - Some centers routinely image for surveillance, especially in cases at high risk for perineural spread or distant disease

CLINICAL PRESENTATION & WORK-UP

Presentation

- 98% of parotid malignancies present with palpable, discrete, painless mass
- Parotid malignancies may also present with
  - Facial nerve dysfunction (24%)

- Lymphadenopathy (6%)

Prognosis

- Prognostic factors
  - Positive prognostic indicators
    - Tumor location in major salivary gland
      - Best prognosis associated with location in parotid gland
  - Negative prognostic indicators
    - Tumor location in
      - Sublingual glands
      - Minor salivary glands
    - Facial nerve invasion
    - Tumor fixed to skin or deep structures
- 5-year prognosis of parotid malignancies
  - Good
    - Acinic cell carcinoma
    - Adenoid cystic carcinoma
    - Low-grade mucoepidermoid carcinoma
  - Poor
    - High-grade mucoepidermoid carcinoma
    - Adenocarcinoma
    - Squamous cell carcinoma (often metastatic from skin primary)
    - Carcinoma ex-pleomorphic adenoma
    - Undifferentiated or poorly differentiated carcinoma
- Prognosis (relative survival rate of cancers of major salivary glands)
  - Stage I survival rate
    - 2-year: 92.5%
    - 5-year: 85.8%
  - Stage II survival rate
    - 2-year: 80.7%
    - 5-year: 66.2%
  - Stage III survival rate
    - 2-year: 71.2%
    - 5-year: 53.3%
  - Stage IV survival rate
    - 2-year: 48.5%
    - 5-year: 31.9%

Work-Up

- Clinical
  - Clinical history
  - Focused head and neck examination
  - Biopsy or FNA for diagnosis
  - Dental evaluation, if radiation planned
  - Supportive care with nutrition, speech/swallowing, as warranted
- Radiographic
  - Baseline 3D imaging
    - CT or MR
      - Favor MR for lesions with high risk of perineural spread, for instance adenoid cystic carcinoma
    - Ultrasound (with FNA as warranted)
  - CT of chest or chest x-ray
  - PET/CT if high risk for distant metastases

TREATMENT

Major Treatment Alternatives

- Surgery
  - Principal treatment modality if resectable
  - Goal of complete margin negative (R0) excision without undue morbidity
  - Extent of primary surgery and approach dependent on location of tumor, including
    - Superficial parotidectomy for lesions of superficial lobe
    - Total parotidectomy for lesions extending to or originating in deep lobe
      - Facial nerve dissected and preserved unless directly infiltrated or surrounded by tumor
      - Facial nerve monitoring to minimize injury
    - En bloc submandibular gland excision for lesions of submandibular gland
      - Lingual, hypoglossal, and marginal mandibular nerves should be preserved unless involved
    - Minor salivary gland tumor excision based on location and extent of disease
  - Neck dissection in selected patients
    - Ipsilateral neck dissection in patients with known neck disease or high-risk histology with N0 neck, including
      - Advanced primary disease
      - Undifferentiated carcinoma
      - High-grade mucoepidermoid carcinoma
      - Adenocarcinoma
      - Salivary duct carcinoma
    - Bilateral neck dissection rarely used; indicated for
      - Bilateral clinically positive neck disease
      - Minor salivary gland lesion that crosses midline (for instance, base of tongue)
  - Reconstruction used based on extent of resection required
    - Free flaps to reconstruct tissue deficits from extensive salivary gland resections
    - Nerve grafts as needed for reconstruction if surgery or tumor compromises function
- Radiation therapy
  - For low-grade lesions, surgical resection alone sufficient
  - For intermediate-grade lesions, postoperative therapy controversial
  - Postoperative radiation therapy indicated for
    - High-grade histologies
    - Locally advanced disease
    - Bone or nerve involvement
    - Perineural invasion
    - Lymphovascular space invasion
    - Close or positive margins
    - Lymph node positivity
    - Recurrent disease
  - For postoperative therapy, targets include
    - Tumor bed with margin (60 Gy in 30 fractions)
    - Dissected areas and margin around tumor bed (57 Gy in 30 fractions)
    - Low-risk areas and perineural tracts, if indicated (54 Gy in 30 fractions)
    - Consider boost to 66 Gy for positive margins
  - Definitive radiation therapy for unresectable disease
  - Techniques include
    - Intensity-modulated radiation therapy (IMRT): Considered standard of care
    - Electron beam therapy: For superficial treatments
    - Neutron beam therapy: Previously used, less common now due to normal tissue complications

- Proton and carbon ion therapy: Under investigation
  - Concurrent chemoradiation with cisplatin under investigation
- Systemic therapy
  - Typically used for advanced or incurable disease
  - Difficult to study due to heterogeneity of tumor types and locations
  - Most commonly cisplatin or cisplatin-containing regimens
  - Other agents under investigation
    - Paclitaxel
    - Gemcitabine
    - Imatinib (c-kit inhibitor) for adenoid cystic carcinoma
    - Lapatinib (oral tyrosine kinase inhibitor of EGFR and HER2)
    - Gefitinib and cetuximab (EGFR inhibitors)
    - Trastuzumab (anti-HER2 agent)
  - Concurrent chemoradiation with cisplatin being studied

Major Treatment Roadblocks/ Contraindications

- Morbidity of surgery often related to possible nerve complications
  - Facial nerve
  - Hypoglossal nerve
  - Lingual nerve

Treatment Options by Stage

- Stages I-III
  - Low-grade tumors
    - Surgery as sole treatment
    - If resection margins positive, consider reresection or postoperative radiation
  - High-grade tumors
    - Surgery with postoperative radiation therapy
- Stage IV
  - Systemic therapy for distant metastatic disease
  - Consider locoregional therapy (surgery &/or radiation) for palliation

Standard Doses

- Postoperative radiation with IMRT
  - 60 Gy to tumor bed with margin (primary and involved lymph nodes)
  - 57 Gy to high-risk areas and entire operative bed
  - 54 Gy to low-risk areas and undissected regions, including perineural tracts (if indicated)
  - Delivered in 30 fractions (Monday-Friday)
  - Consider boost to 66 Gy for positive margins
- Definitive radiation with IMRT for unresectable/gross residual disease
  - 70 Gy to tumor with margin
  - 63 Gy to high-risk areas
  - 57 Gy to low-risk areas, including perineural tracts, if indicated
  - Delivered in 33 fractions (Monday-Friday)

Organs at Risk Parameters

- Spinal cord < 45 Gy
- Brainstem < 54 Gy
- Mandible < 70 Gy
- Retina < 45 Gy

RECOMMENDED FOLLOW-UP

Clinical

- For the 1st year, clinical examination every 1-3 months
- For year 2, clinical examination every 2-6 months
- For years 3-5, clinical examination every 4-8 months
- For years 5 and more, clinical examination annually

Radiographic

- Post-treatment baseline imaging within 6 months following treatment completion
- Further imaging based on symptoms; no data on routine follow-up imaging

SELECTED REFERENCES

1. Adelstein DJ et al: Biology and management of salivary gland cancers. Semin Radiat Oncol. 22(3):245-53, 2012
2. Papaspyrou G et al: Chemotherapy and targeted therapy in adenoid cystic carcinoma of the head and neck: a review. Head Neck. 33(6):905-11, 2011
3. Shah K et al: Parotid cancer treatment with surgery followed by radiotherapy in Oxford over 15 years. Ann R Coll Surg Engl. 93(3):218-22, 2011
4. American Joint Committee on Cancer: AJCC Cancer Staging Manual. 7th ed. New York: Springer. 79-86, 2010
5. Guzzo M et al: Major and minor salivary gland tumors. Crit Rev Oncol Hematol. 74(2):134-48, 2010
6. Boukheris H et al: Incidence of carcinoma of the major salivary glands according to the WHO classification, 1992 to 2006: a population-based study in the United States. Cancer Epidemiol Biomarkers Prev. 18(11):2899-906, 2009
7. Nagliati M et al: Surgery and radiotherapy in the treatment of malignant parotid tumors: a retrospective multicenter study. Tumori. 95(4):442-8, 2009
8. Bell RB et al: Management and outcome of patients with malignant salivary gland tumors. J Oral Maxillofac Surg. 63(7):917-28, 2005
9. Fiorella R et al: Major salivary gland diseases. Multicentre study. Acta Otorhinolaryngol Ital. 2005 Jun;25(3):182-90. Erratum in: Acta Otorhinolaryngol Ital. 25(5):following 337, 2005
10. Witt RL: Major salivary gland cancer. Surg Oncol Clin N Am. 13(1):113-27, 2004
11. Garden AS et al: The influence of positive margins and nerve invasion in adenoid cystic carcinoma of the head and neck treated with surgery and radiation. Int J Radiat Oncol Biol Phys. 32(3):619-26, 1995
12. Armstrong JG et al: Malignant tumors of major salivary gland origin. A matched-pair analysis of the role of combined surgery and postoperative radiotherapy. Arch Otolaryngol Head Neck Surg. 116(3):290-3, 1990
13. Spiro RH: Salivary neoplasms: overview of a 35-year experience with 2,807 patients. Head Neck Surg. 8(3):177-84, 1986

T1 N0 M0

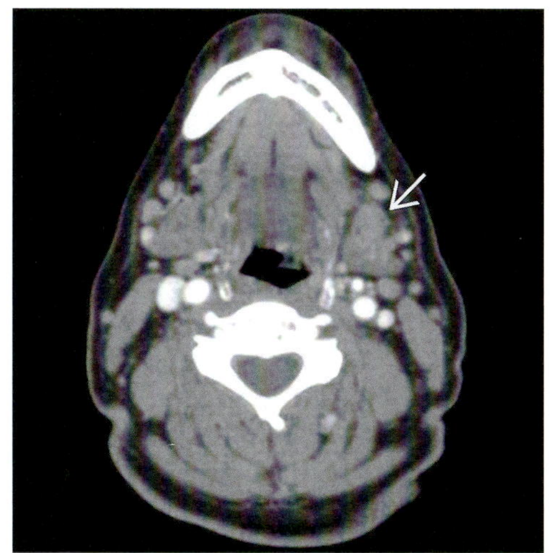

T1 N0 M0

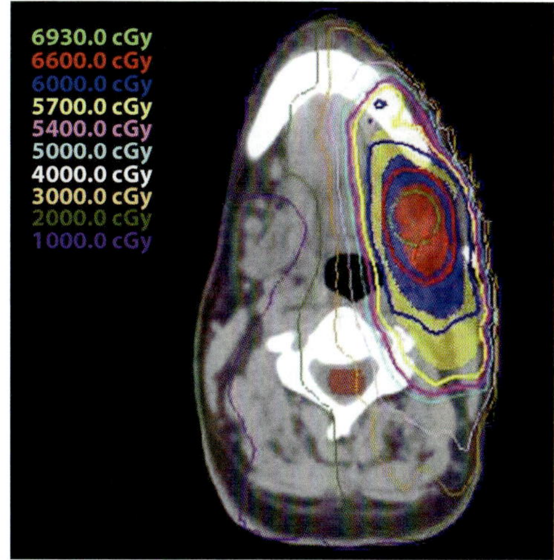

(Left) *Axial CECT shows a 63-year-old woman with a left submandibular mass ➡. Surgical pathology revealed a 1.4 cm adenoid cystic carcinoma with perineural invasion and close margins.* ***(Right)*** *Axial noncontrast simulation CT of the same patient shows the boost volume (66 Gy) in red, postoperative bed (60 Gy) in blue, and intermediate risk (57 Gy) in yellow in 30 fractions. Perineural tracts were covered; lymph nodes were not.*

T4 N0 M0

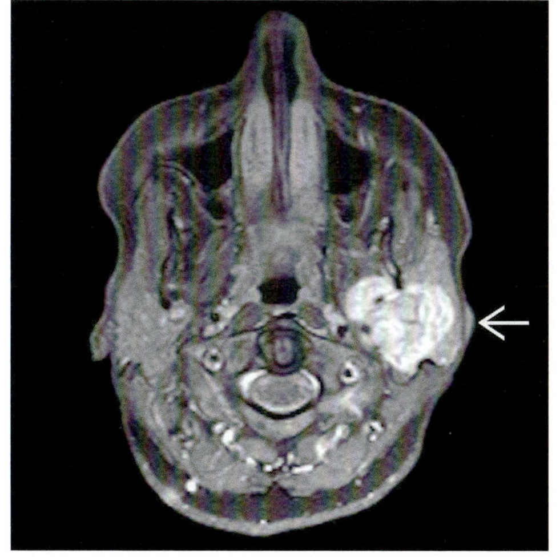

T4 N0 M0

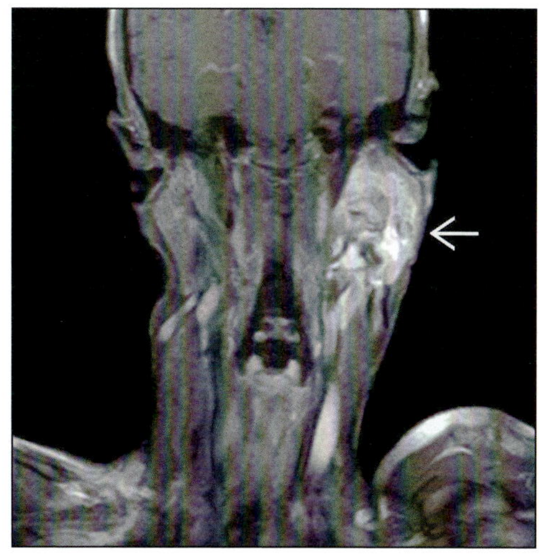

(Left) *Axial T1WI C+ MR revealed a parotid mass ➡ that was palpable in a 41-year-old woman with left facial paralysis. The lesion involved the superficial and deep lobes and parapharyngeal fat. Biopsy was positive for adenoid cystic carcinoma.* ***(Right)*** *Coronal T1WI C + MR of the same patient documents the extent of the left parotid lesion ➡. Facial asymmetry is seen from the bulky lesion.*

T4 N0 M0

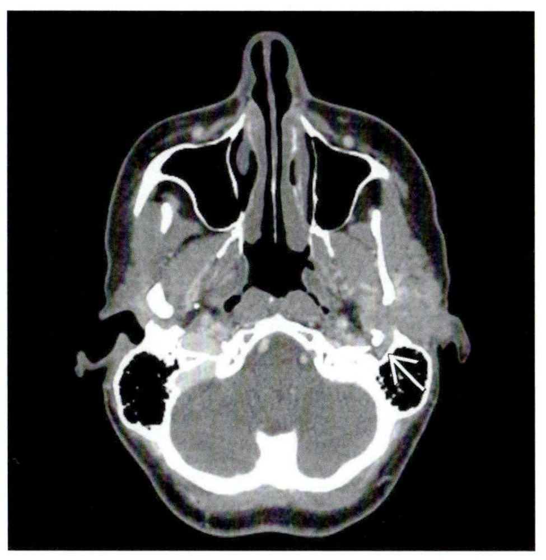

T4 N0 M0

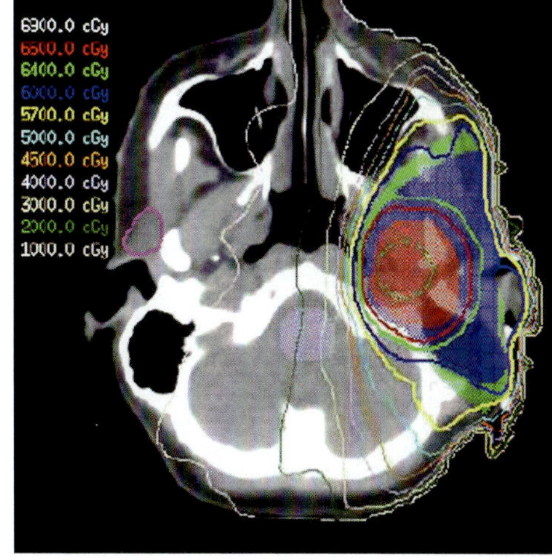

(Left) *Axial CECT of the same patient demonstrates the lesion and widening of the stylomastoid foramen ➡, consistent with facial nerve involvement. Surgical pathology revealed a 4.5 cm adenoid cystic carcinoma with positive margin at the stylomastoid foramen and facial nerve involvement.* ***(Right)*** *Axial noncontrast simulation CT of the same patient shows high-risk areas (66 Gy) in red, postoperative bed (60 Gy) in blue, and intermediate risk (57 Gy) in green.*

(Left) *Axial CECT of a 47-year-old woman shows a recurrent left parotid mass of the deep lobe ➡. Note the heterogeneous mass and asymmetry.* **(Right)** *Axial noncontrast CT-guided biopsy of the deep parotid lesion in the same patient shows the needle ➡. Pathology was positive for recurrent acinic cell carcinoma. She underwent parotidectomy and neck dissection; pathology revealed a 2.5 cm acinic cell carcinoma with no perineural invasion and no positive lymph nodes.*

Recurrent

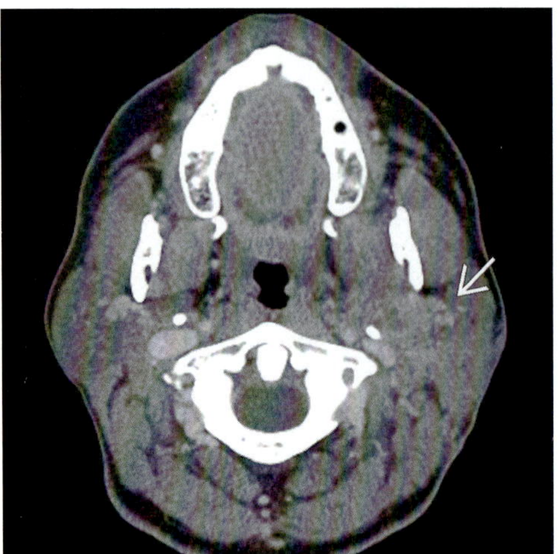

Recurrent

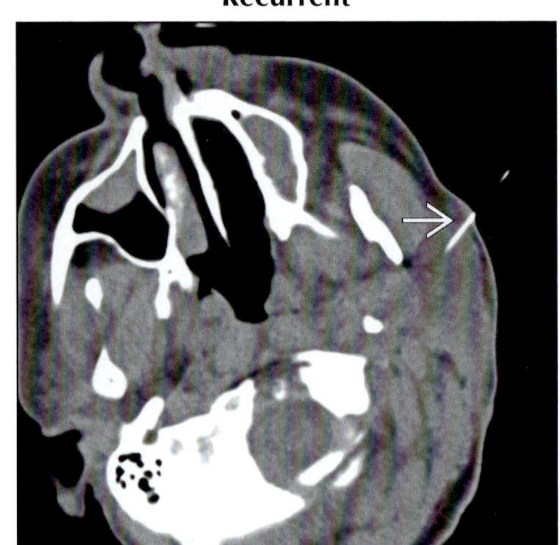

(Left) *Axial noncontrast simulation CT in the same patient shows high-risk areas (60 Gy) in red and intermediate (57 Gy) in blue. A tongue-lateralizing stent is used ➡. Radiation was used due to the recurrent nature.* **(Right)** *Coronal simulation CT of the same patient shows the high-risk areas (60 Gy) in red and intermediate (57 Gy) in blue. The surgical bed was targeted; uninvolved lymph nodes were not. Perineural tracts were not covered.*

Recurrent

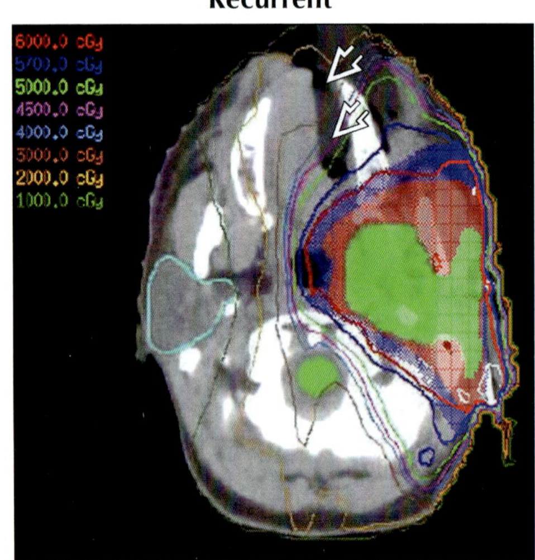

Recurrent

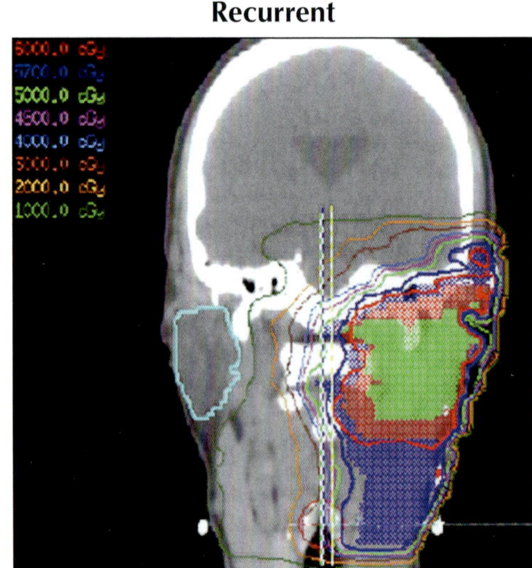

(Left) *Axial CECT of a 49-year-old man presenting with dysarthria shows a left base of tongue mass ➡ with multiple ipsilateral lymph nodes ➡. Biopsy was positive for adenoid cystic carcinoma (minor salivary gland).* **(Right)** *Axial T1WI C + FS MR of the same patient shows the hyperintense mass ➡. Subsequent resection with a total glossectomy, left neck dissection, and reconstruction revealed a 4.5 cm adenoid cystic carcinoma with 1 of 19 positive lymph nodes.*

T4 N1 M0

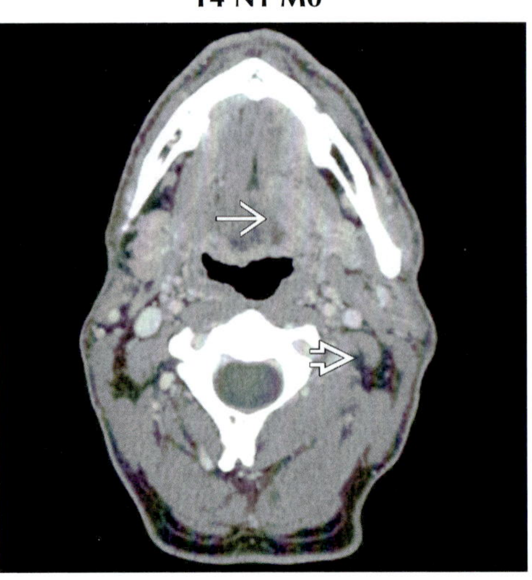

T4 N1 M0

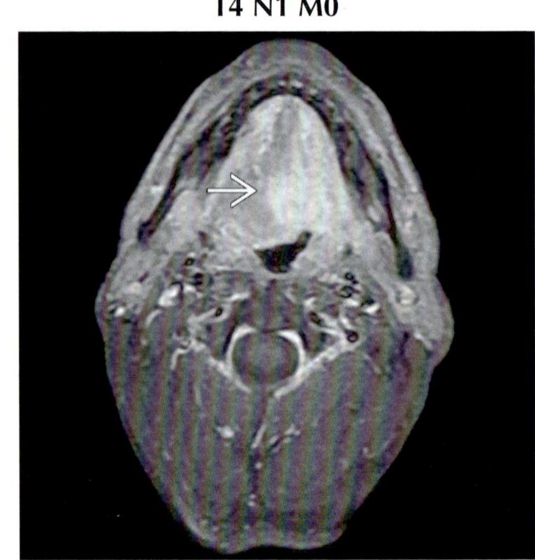

T4 N1 M0

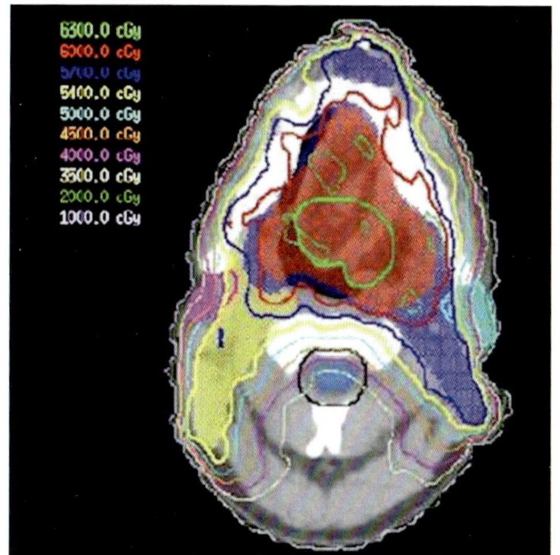

T4 N1 M0

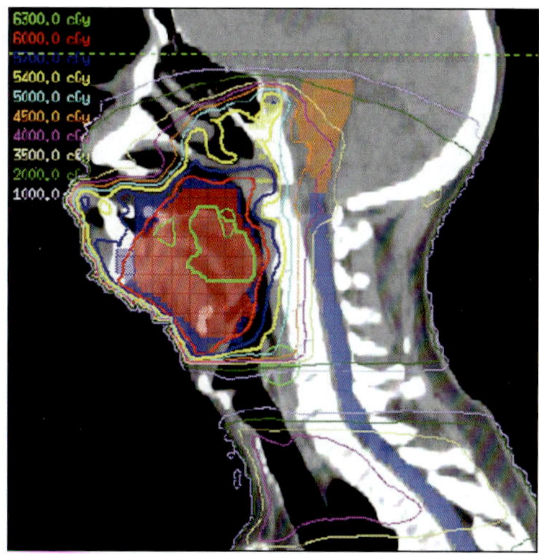

(Left) *Axial simulation CT of the same patient shows high-risk areas (60 Gy) in red, intermediate (57 Gy) in blue, and low (54 Gy) in yellow. The contralateral neck was treated due to the extension of the primary past midline. Perineural tracts were treated bilaterally due to adenoid cystic histology.* ***(Right)*** *Sagittal simulation CT of the same patient shows the high-risk areas (60 Gy) in red, intermediate (57 Gy) in blue, and low (54 Gy) in yellow.*

T4 N0 M0

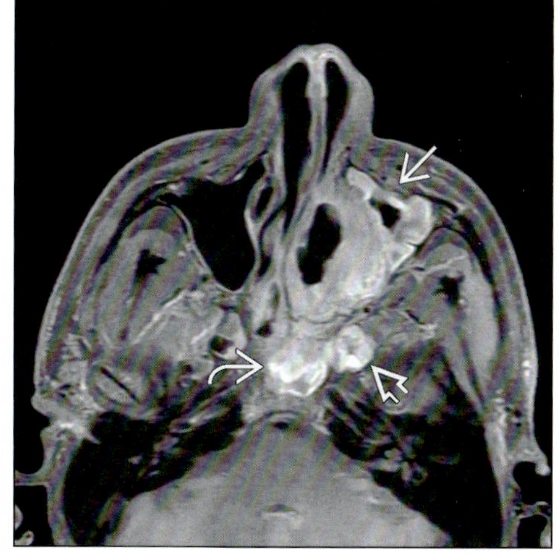

T4 N0 M0

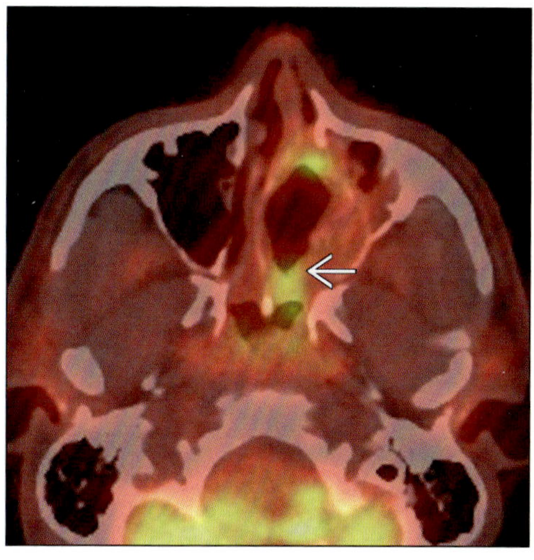

(Left) *Axial T1WI C+ MR in a 39-year-old man presenting with epistaxis shows a large left nasoethmoid mass* ➔ *with extension to the sphenoid sinus* ➔ *and left pterygopalatine fossa* ➔. *Biopsy was positive for adenoid cystic carcinoma.* ***(Right)*** *Axial fused PET/CT of the same patient shows the minor salivary gland mass (SUV 4.7)* ➔. *There were no distant metastases and no adenopathy. The patient underwent craniofacial resection of the tumor.*

T4 N0 M0

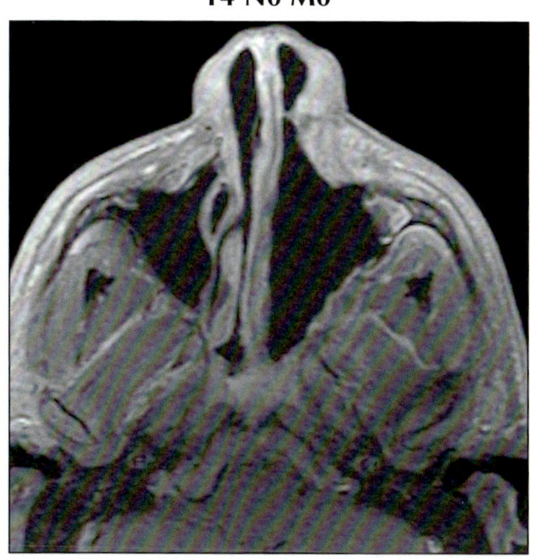

T4 N0 M0

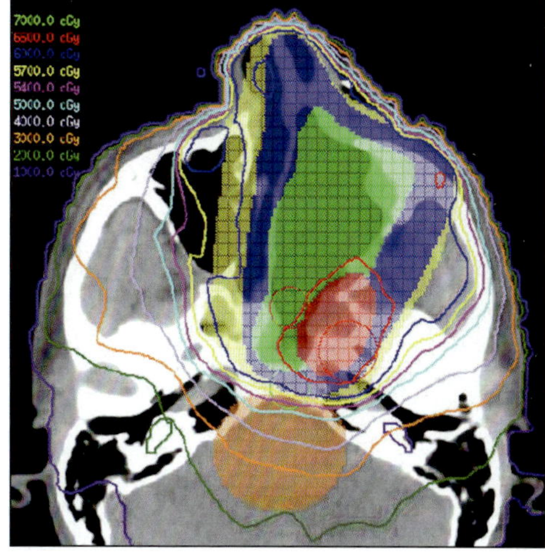

(Left) *Axial T1WI C+ MR of the same patient following gross total resection shows a 3.5 cm adenoid cystic carcinoma, cribriform type, with soft tissue extension in the pterygopalatine fossa.* ***(Right)*** *Axial noncontrast simulation CT in the same patient shows the boost volume in red (66 Gy) with the tumor bed in blue (60 Gy) and intermediate-risk areas in yellow (57 Gy) in 30 fractions. Perineural tracts were covered; lymph nodes were not.*

(Left) Axial T1WI C+ MR of a 62-year-old man presenting with left facial palsy shows a heterogeneous left parotid mass. **(Right)** Axial T1WI C+ MR of the same patient shows the perineural extension along the left auriculotemporal nerve.

T4 N2b M0

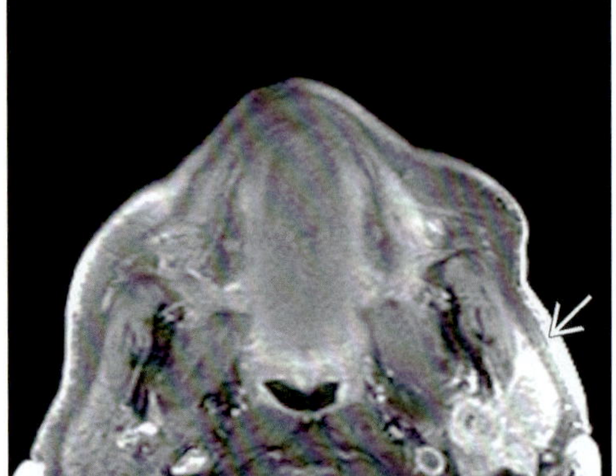

T4 N2b M0

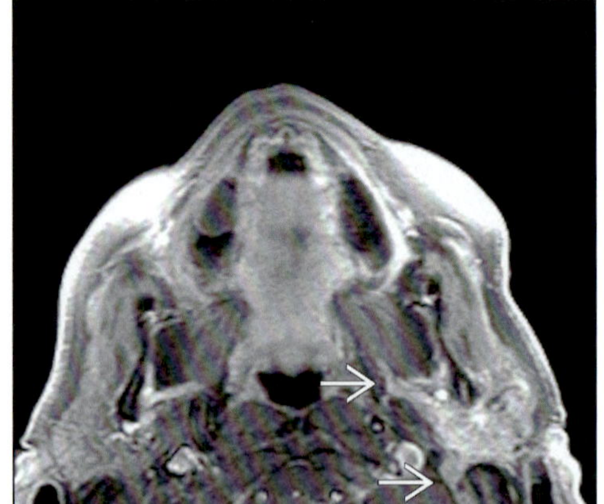

(Left) Axial T1WI C+ MR of the same patient shows the perineural invasion along the left facial nerve. **(Right)** Axial T1WI C+ MR of the same patient shows the ipsilateral suspicious lymph nodes. The patient was treated with surgical resection and reconstruction; pathology revealed a 1.7 cm high-grade salivary duct carcinoma with 57 out of 59 lymph nodes positive with extracapsular extension.

T4 N2b M0

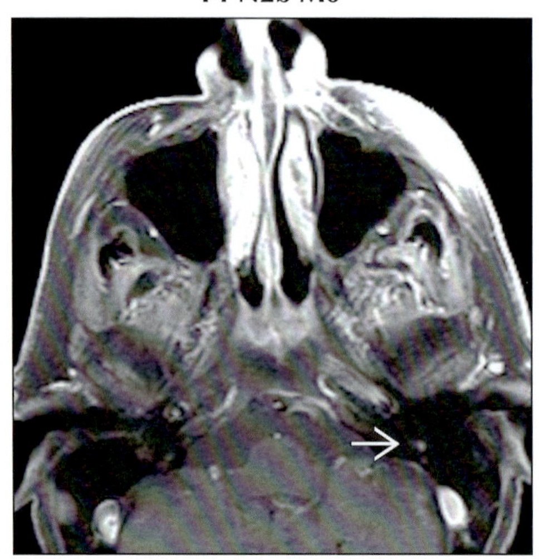

T4 N2b M0

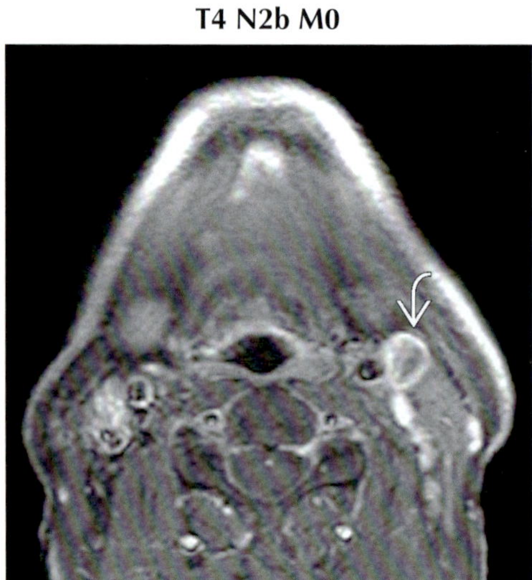

(Left) Axial noncontrast simulation CT of the same patient shows the high-risk areas (60 Gy) in red and intermediate (57 Gy) in blue. A tongue-deviating stent nicely displaces the tongue to minimize dose and prevent radiation injury. Note the avoidance of dose to the contralateral parotid gland. **(Right)** Coronal noncontrast simulation CT of the same patient shows high-risk areas (60 Gy) in red and intermediate-risk areas (57 Gy) in blue.

T4 N2b M0

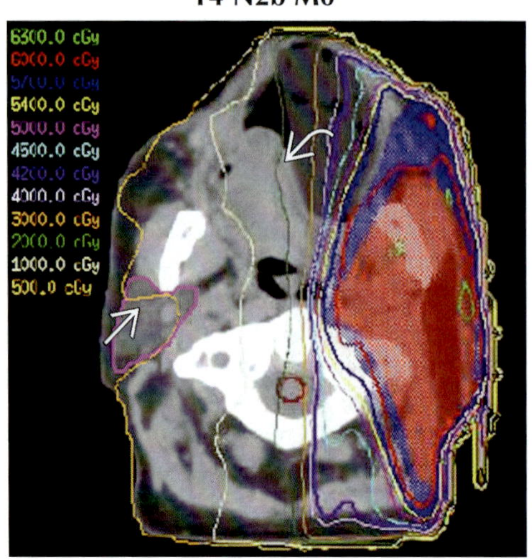

T4 N2b M0

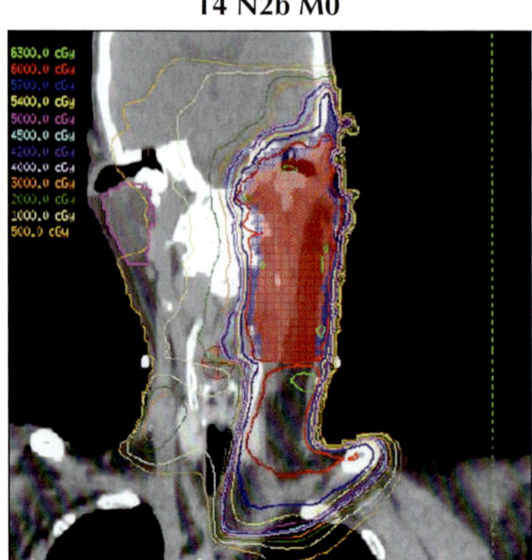

T2 N2b M0

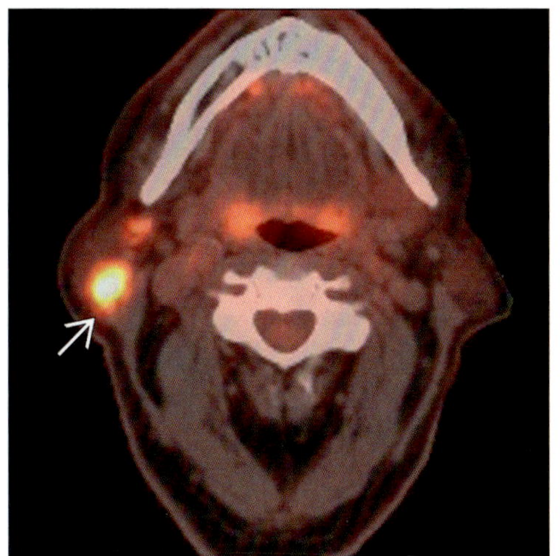

T2 N2b M0

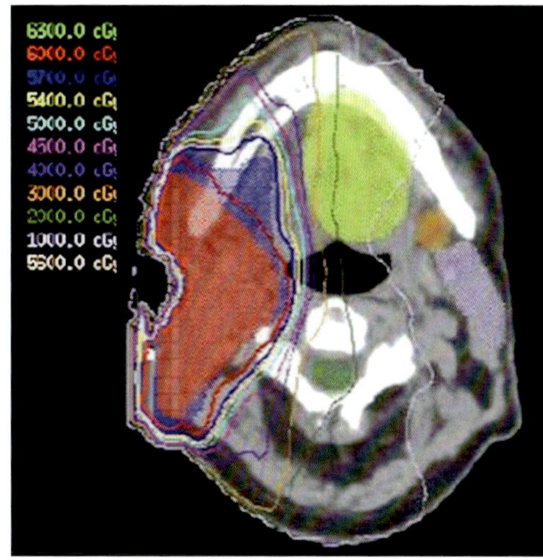

(Left) *Axial fused PET/CT in a 71-year-old man with prior right temple skin cancer with no regional or distant disease shows a right parotid mass ➔. Pathology confirmed a 2.2 cm poorly differentiated carcinoma and 2 positive lymph nodes with extracapsular extension.* ***(Right)*** *Axial noncontrast simulation CT of the same patient shows high-risk areas (60 Gy) in red and intermediate-risk areas (57 Gy) in blue. Concurrent chemotherapy was given due to extracapsular extension.*

T2 N2b M0

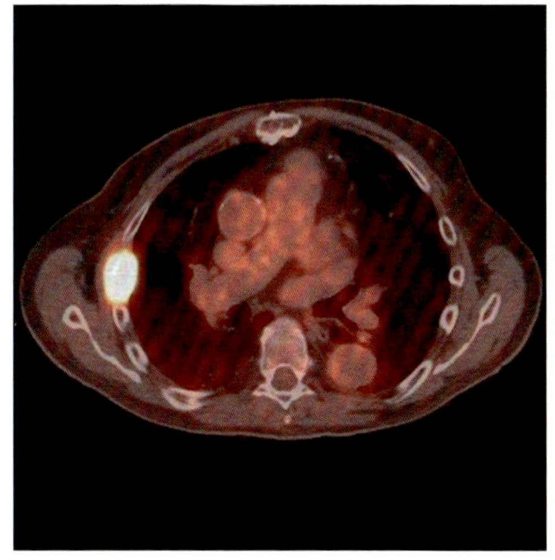

T2 N2b M0

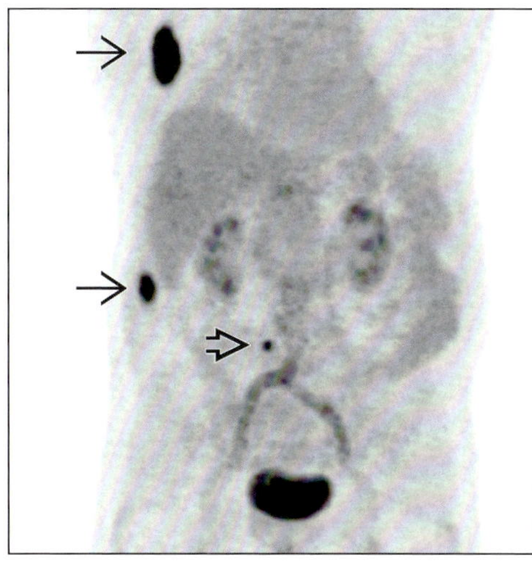

(Left) *Axial fused PET/CT shows the same patient presenting with right rib pain 6 weeks after finishing definitive treatment. Biopsy revealed metastatic disease.* ***(Right)*** *Coronal PET of the same patient reveals metastases in the ribs ➔ and superior facet ➔ of the L4 vertebral body. He received palliative radiation to the 3 sites, followed by systemic chemotherapy, but ultimately died of disease.*

T4b N3 M1

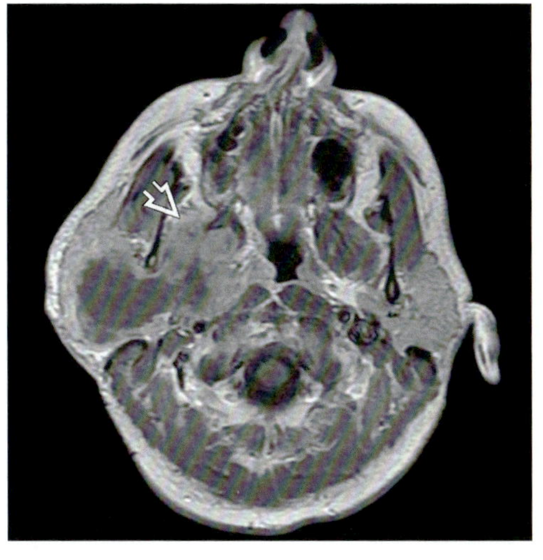

T4b N3 M1

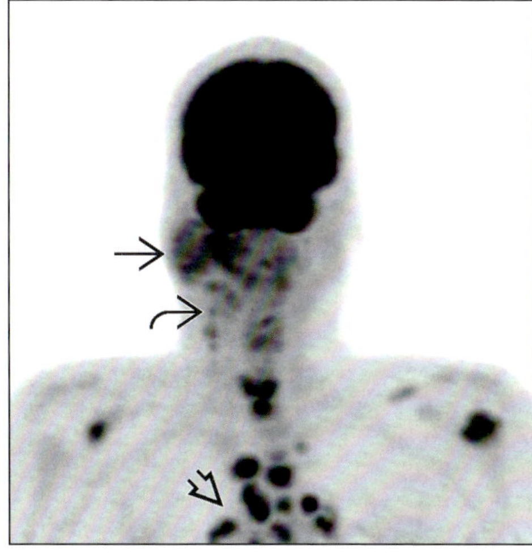

(Left) *Axial T1WI C+ MR shows a 36-year-old man presenting with a right facial mass and facial nerve palsy. There was a massive right parotid lesion with extension to the pterygoids ➔ and displacement of the tonsil. Biopsy was positive for salivary duct adenocarcinoma.* ***(Right)*** *Coronal PET of the same patient shows widespread local ➔, regional ➔, and distant ➔ metastases. He was treated with palliative radiation to the primary followed by chemotherapy.*

THYROID

Adapted from 7th edition AJCC Staging Forms.

(T) Primary Tumor

TNM	*Definitions*
TX	Primary tumor cannot be assessed
T0	No evidence of primary tumor
T1	Tumor ≤ 2 cm in greatest dimension, limited to thyroid
T1a	Tumor ≤ 1 cm in greatest dimension, limited to thyroid
T1b	Tumor > 1 cm but ≤ 2 cm in greatest dimension, limited to thyroid
T2	Tumor > 2 cm but ≤ 4 cm in greatest dimension, limited to thyroid
T3	Tumor > 4 cm in greatest dimension, limited to thyroid, or any tumor with minimal extrathyroid extension (e.g., extension to sternothyroid muscle or perithyroid soft tissues)
T4	
T4a	Moderately advanced disease: Tumor of any size extending beyond thyroid capsule to invade subcutaneous soft tissues, larynx, trachea, esophagus, or recurrent laryngeal nerve
T4b	Very advanced disease: Tumor invades prevertebral fascia or encases carotid artery or mediastinal vessels
	Anaplastic carcinoma with gross extrathyroid extension
Anaplastic Carcinoma[1]	
T4a	Intrathyroidal anaplastic carcinoma
T4b	Anaplastic carcinoma with gross extrathyroid extension

(N) Regional Lymph Nodes

NX	Regional lymph nodes cannot be assessed
N0	No regional lymph node metastasis[2]
N1	Regional lymph node metastasis[2]
N1a	Metastasis to level VI (pretracheal, paratracheal, and prelaryngeal/Delphian lymph nodes)
N1b	Metastasis to unilateral, bilateral, or contralateral cervical (levels I, II, III, IV, or V) or retropharyngeal or superior mediastinal lymph nodes (level VII)

(M) Distant Metastasis

M0	No distant metastasis
M1	Distant metastasis

All (T) categories may be subdivided into (s) solitary tumor and (m) multifocal tumor; the largest determines the classification.

[1]*All anaplastic carcinomas are considered T4 tumors.*

[2]*Regional lymph nodes are the central compartment, lateral cervical, and upper mediastinal lymph nodes.*

AJCC Stages/Prognostic Groups for Papillary or Follicular (Differentiated) Carcinoma

Adapted from 7th edition AJCC Staging Forms.

Stage	*T*	*N*	*M*
Under 45 Years			
I	Any T	Any N	M0
II	Any T	Any N	M1
45 Years and Older			
I	T1	N0	M0
II	T2	N0	M0
III	T3	N0	M0
	T1, T2, T3	N1a	M0
IVA	T4a	N0	M0
	T4a	N1a	M0
	T1, T2, T3, T4a	N1b	M0
IVB	T4b	Any N	M0
IVC	Any T	Any N	M1

AJCC Stages/Prognostic Groups for Medullary Carcinoma (All Ages)

Adapted from 7th edition AJCC Staging Forms.

Stage	*T*	*N*	*M*
I	T1	N0	M0
II	T2	N0	M0
	T3	N0	M0
III	T1, T2, T3	N1a	M0
IVA	T4a	N0	M0
	T4a	N1a	M0
	T1, T2, T3, T4a	N1b	M0
IVB	T4b	Any N	M0
IVC	Any T	Any N	M1

AJCC Stages/Prognostic Groups for Anaplastic Carcinoma

Adapted from 7th edition AJCC Staging Forms.

Stage	*T*	*N*	*M*
IVA	T4a	Any N	M0
IVB	T4b	Any N	M0
IVC	Any T	Any N	M1

All anaplastic carcinomas are considered stage IV tumors.

THYROID

T1

Coronal graphic shows T1 lesion ➔ that is < 2 cm and confined to the gland.

T1a/T1b

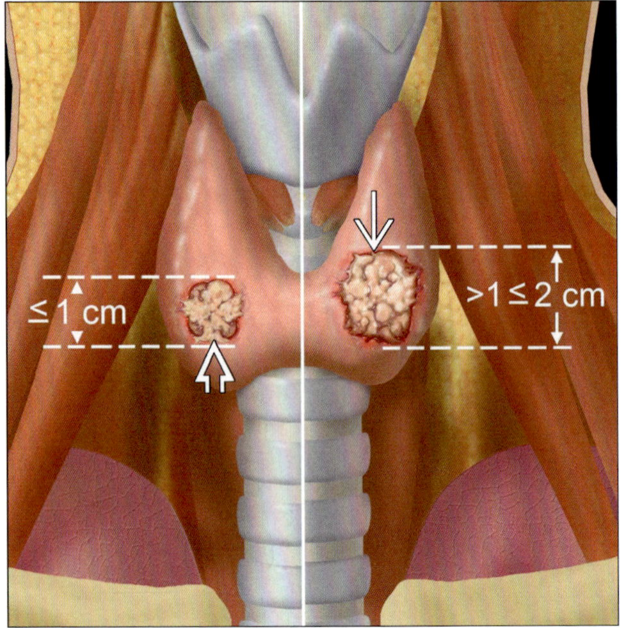

Coronal graphic illustrates the distinction between T1a ➔ and T1b ➔ tumors. If multifocal neoplasia is present, the T staging is determined by the largest tumor.

T2

Coronal graphic demonstrates a T2 primary thyroid carcinoma ➔, confined wholly to the thyroid gland and > 2 cm but ≤ 4 cm in size. All differentiated thyroid carcinomas and medullary thyroid carcinomas use the same T staging criteria.

T3

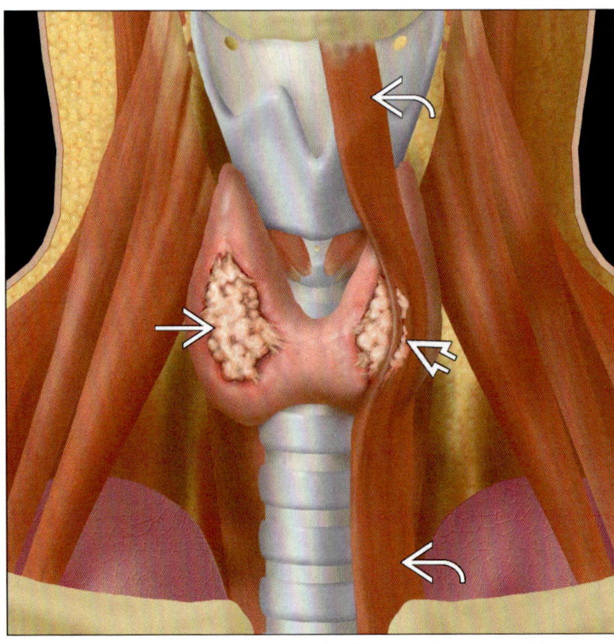

Graphic shows 2 tumors, both of which are T3 by virtue of being > 4 cm. The tumor in the right lobe ➔ is confined whereas the tumor in the left lobe ➔ has minimal extrathyroidal extension to sternohyoid muscle ➔ (still T3 disease).

T4a

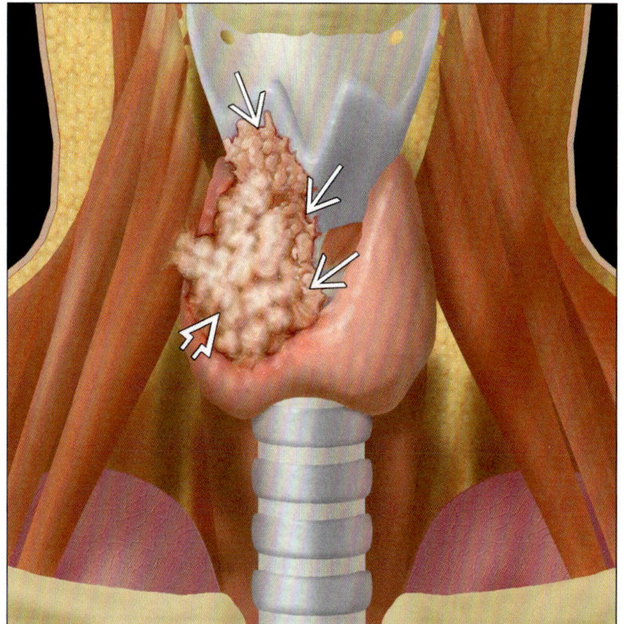

Graphic shows T4a medullary or DTC ⮚ with invasion of adjacent structures, particularly the larynx ➡. All anaplastic thyroid carcinomas are T4a when confined to the thyroid gland and T4b if there is gross extrathyroidal extension.

T4a

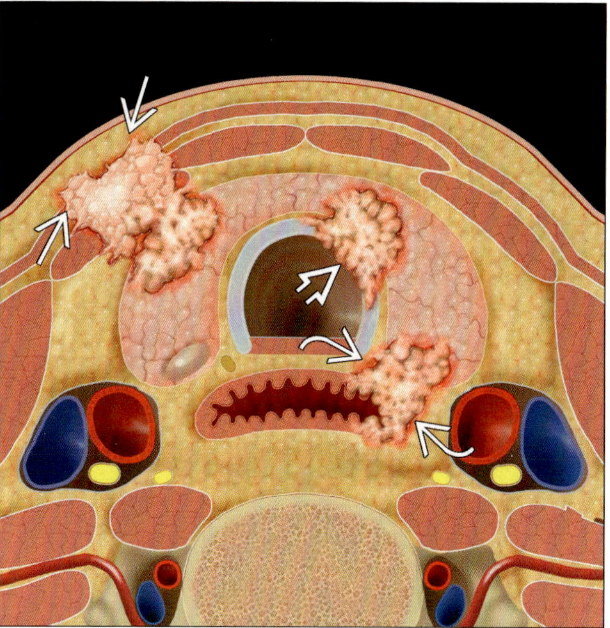

Graphic shows 3 different T4a tumors. One extends to subcutaneous tissues ➡ and another invades the trachea ⮚. The 3rd tumor invades the esophagus ↷ with likely involvement of the left recurrent laryngeal nerve, which lies in the TE groove.

T4b

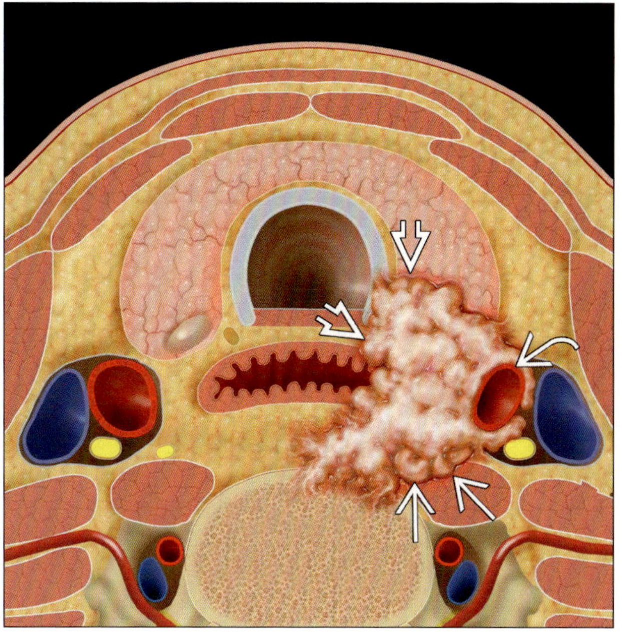

Graphic shows very advanced T4b thyroid carcinoma ⮚. This tumor extends beyond the gland, invades the prevertebral fascia ➡, and involves the prevertebral space and encasement of the carotid artery ↷.

Regional Lymph Nodes

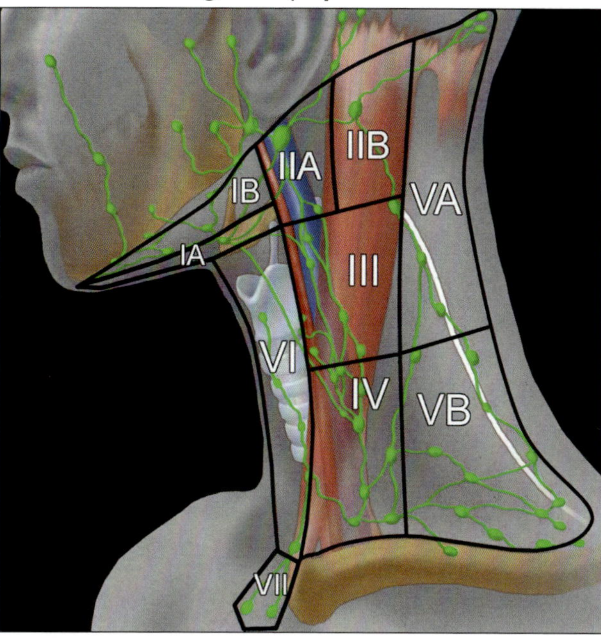

Graphic depicts regional cervical lymph node levels I-VII.

Regional Lymph Nodes

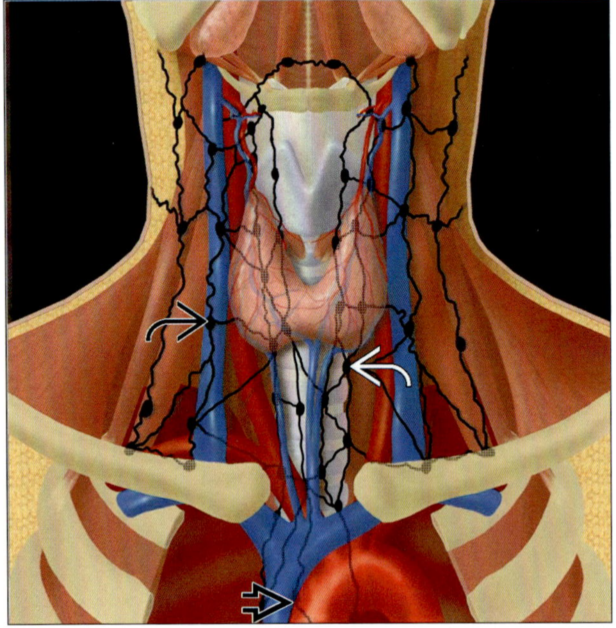

Regional paratracheal, cervical, and upper mediastinal lymph node stations are further illustrated.

T3 N1a

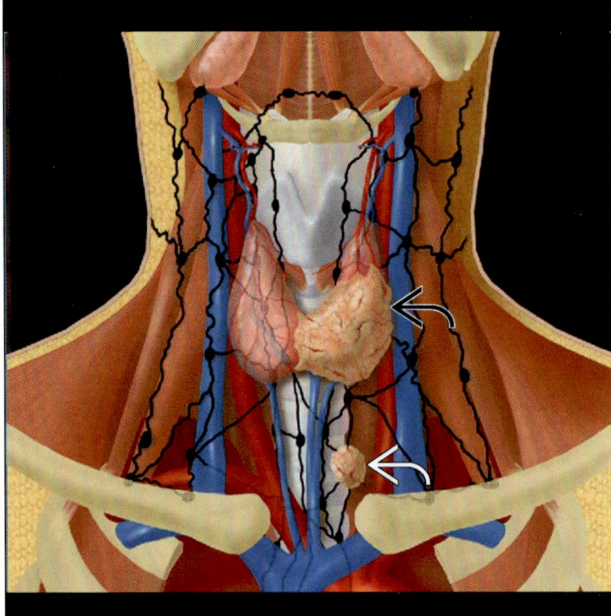

Paratracheal, pretracheal, and prelaryngeal (Delphian) lymph nodes are category N1a. This graphic shows a T3 tumor in the left side of the thyroid gland (> 4 cm) and a single left paratracheal lymph node.

T3 N1b

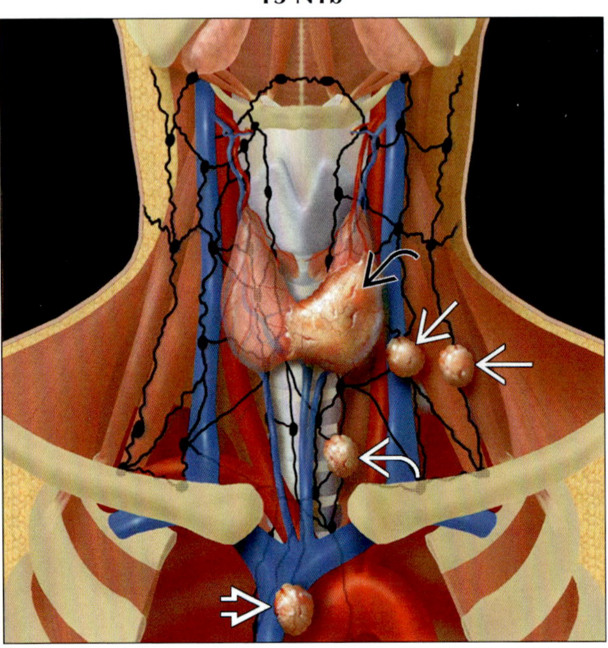

Lateral cervical, retropharyngeal, and upper mediastinal lymph nodes are category N1b. This graphic shows a T3 tumor in the left side of the thyroid gland (> 4 cm), a single left paratracheal lymph node, multiple left lateral cervical lymph nodes, and an upper mediastinal lymph node.

Node of Rouvière

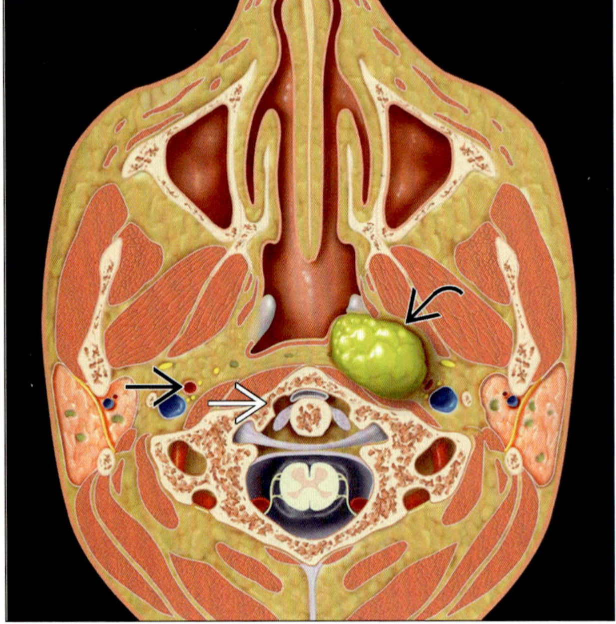

Retropharyngeal lymph nodes are category N1b. An enlarged left lateral retropharyngeal lymph node is shown. This lymph node group, which lies anterior to C1 and just medial to the carotid artery, was first described by Henri Rouvière in 1936 in Anatomie des Lymphatiques de l'Homme.

Papillary Thyroid Carcinoma H&E

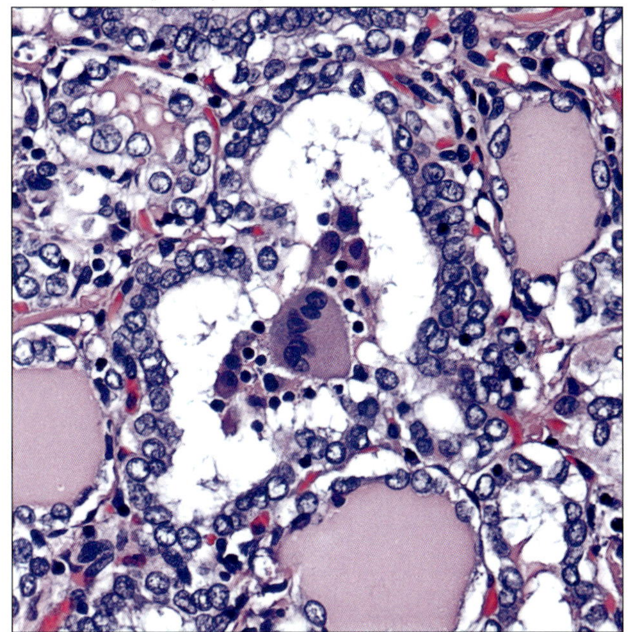

Classic cytomorphonuclear features are seen: Enlarged cells, high N:C ratio, irregular placement around follicles, nuclear grooves, nuclear contour irregularities, optical clearing, and giant cells within colloid. (Courtesy L. D. R. Thompson, MD.)

Anaplastic Thyroid Carcinoma H&E

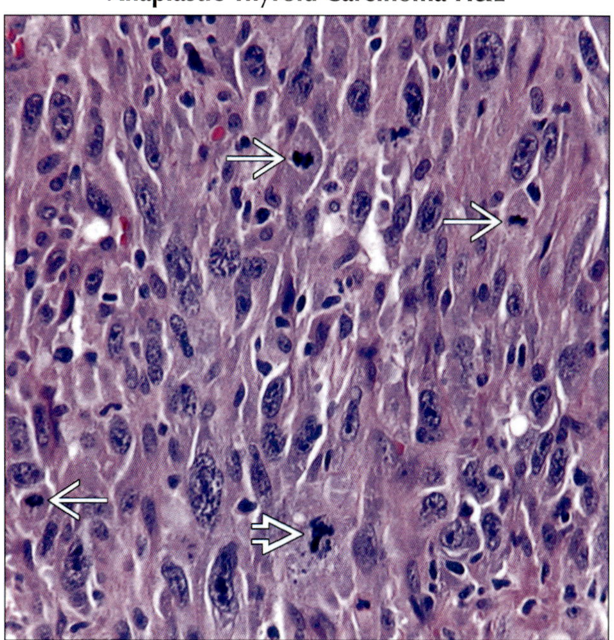

A fascicle composed of spindled cells is noted in this undifferentiated carcinoma. There is significant pleomorphism as well as numerous mitotic figures ➔, including atypical forms ➲. (Courtesy B. M. Wenig, MD.)

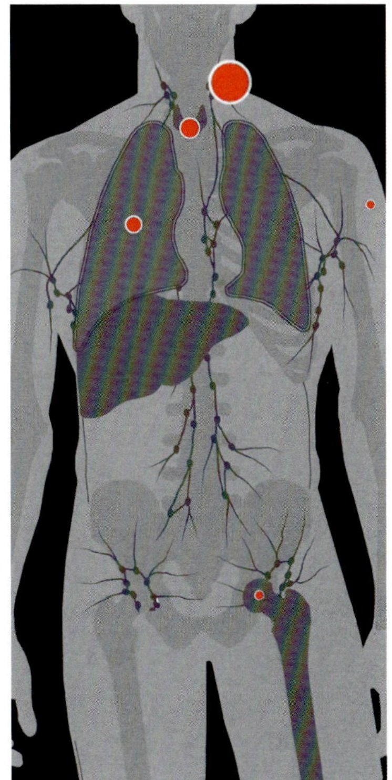

INITIAL SITE OF RECURRENCE

Neck Lymph Nodes	58%
Residual Thyroid	16%
Lungs Alone	13%
Trachea or Muscle	5%
Bone Alone	4%
Multiple Sites	4%

Overall recurrence rate was 21% in a study of over 1,300 patients with DTC in long-term follow-up after surgical and medical therapy. Mazzaferri EL et al: Long-term impact of initial surgical and medical therapy on papillary and follicular thyroid cancer. Am J Med. Nov; 97(5):418-28, 1994.

THYROID

OVERVIEW

General Comments

- **4 major histopathologic subtypes**
  - Papillary carcinoma
  - Follicular carcinoma
  - Medullary carcinoma
  - Anaplastic (undifferentiated) carcinoma
- Most common endocrine malignancy but still relatively rare
  - Represents about 1% of all cancers
- Differentiated thyroid carcinoma (DTC) includes
  - Papillary carcinoma
  - Follicular carcinoma

Classification

- **WHO histologic classification**
  - **Malignant tumors of follicular cells**
    - Papillary carcinoma (80%)
    - Follicular carcinoma (13%)
      - Hürthle cell carcinoma
    - Poorly differentiated carcinoma
    - Anaplastic (undifferentiated) carcinoma (1-2%)
  - **Malignant tumors of C cells**
    - Medullary carcinoma (3-4%)
  - **Malignant tumors of mixed follicular and C cells**
  - **Miscellaneous epithelial tumors**
    - Squamous cell carcinoma
    - Adenosquamous carcinoma
    - Mucin-producing carcinoma
    - Mucoepidermoid carcinoma
  - **Malignant nonepithelial tumors**
    - Lymphoma (5%)
    - Sarcoma
  - **Miscellaneous**
    - Fibrosarcoma
    - Malignant hemangioendothelioma
    - Metastasis to thyroid gland

NATURAL HISTORY

General Features

- Comments
  - **DTC**
    - Both papillary and follicular types arise from thyroid-stimulating hormone (TSH)-sensitive follicular cells
    - Generally takes up iodine and produces thyroglobulin in response to TSH stimulation

Etiology

- Risk factors
  - Majority of cases are sporadic with no known cause
  - Prior radiation to head and neck increases risk to 30%; age at exposure is important
  - Relatively low percentage of familial-associated malignancies
  - Impact of diet, smoking, alcohol, hormones not clear

Epidemiology & Cancer Incidence

- Number of cases in USA per year
  - 56,460 new cases with 1,780 deaths
  - Steady increase in incidence over the past 20 years, perhaps due to greater detection of early cancers
    - DTC accounts for approximately 94% of all thyroid malignancies
  - 1% of all malignant tumors overall, but 5% of malignant tumors in females
- Sex predilection
  - Women account for 77% of new cases but only 56% of deaths
    - Reflects female predominance of DTC
- Age of onset
  - Age at diagnosis is strong prognostic factor and considered in staging system and risk stratification algorithms

Genetics

- **Papillary carcinoma**
  - 5-10% of patients have positive family history for thyroid malignancy
- **Medullary carcinoma**
  - 20-30% familial
    - Isolated familial medullary thyroid carcinoma (MTC)
    - Part of MEN type 2 syndrome

Associated Diseases, Abnormalities

- Gardner syndrome
- Cowden syndrome: Increased risk of follicular cancer
- Hashimoto thyroiditis is associated with thyroid lymphoma
- Important gene mutations in thyroid cancers include mutations in *RET*, *BRAF*, *RAS*, *p53*
  - *PTC* with *BRAF* mutation demonstrate more aggressive behavior
  - *RET* mutation present in 100% of hereditary medullary cases

Microscopic Pathology

- H&E
  - **Papillary carcinoma**
    - Nuclear grooves
    - Empty "ground-glass" nuclei
    - Psammoma bodies
  - **Follicular carcinoma**
    - Solid
    - Follicular or trabeculated growth
    - Differentiated from benign follicular adenomas by tumor capsular invasion or vascular invasion
- Special stains
  - Positive IHC stain for thyroglobulin

Routes of Spread

- Local spread
  - Extrathyroidal extension via capsule breech
  - Can be invasive of central compartment structures
    - Trachea
    - Esophagus
    - Recurrent laryngeal nerve, which lies in tracheoesophageal (TE) groove
    - Vascular structures (carotid artery &/or internal jugular vein)
    - Neck musculature
    - Cricoid and larynx in advanced cases
- Lymphatic extension
  - Regional lymphatics: Paratracheal, prelaryngeal, cervical chains, retropharyngeal, and upper mediastinum
- Hematogenous spread

- Lung most common metastatic site
- Metastatic sites
  - Lung, bone, CNS, multisite involvement

IMAGING

Detection

- Common radiologic presentations
  - Incidental discovery on various imaging modalities
- **General**
  - Often indistinguishable from adenomas or other benign pathology on most imaging modalities unless invasive
  - US important in initial thyroid nodule evaluation, image-guided biopsy, and staging evaluation of thyroid, thyroid bed, paratracheal region, and lateral neck lymph node compartments
  - Cross-sectional and functional imaging (in select situations) key for local, regional, and distant staging, and surgical and RT planning

CLINICAL PRESENTATION & WORK-UP

Presentation

- **General symptoms**
  - Most often painless palpable neck nodule or incidentally discovered on imaging
  - Other symptoms
    - Hoarseness from vocal fold paralysis due to recurrent laryngeal nerve compression/invasion
    - Dysphagia
    - Bone pain
    - Cough
- **Papillary carcinoma**
  - Elevated thyroglobulin levels
- **Follicular carcinoma**
  - Asymptomatic neck mass
  - Rapid growth
  - Elevated thyroglobulin levels
  - 25% present with extrathyroidal invasion
  - 5-10% present with adenopathy
  - 10-20% will have distant metastases
- **Medullary carcinoma**
  - Painless palpable mass
  - Elevated serum calcitonin, important in diagnosis and post-treatment surveillance
  - Rarely paraneoplastic syndromes
  - ≤ 75% have lymphadenopathy at diagnosis
- **Anaplastic carcinoma**
  - Rapidly growing mass in older patient
  - Approximately 50% have symptoms related to local invasion of structures
    - Dyspnea from invasion of trachea
    - Hoarseness from invasion/compression of recurrent laryngeal nerve
    - Dysphagia from invasion/compression of esophagus
  - Often painful
  - Often adenopathy &/or distant spread at time of presentation, thus staging work-up is comprehensive, including brain imaging

Prognosis

- **DTC**
  - 5-year survival rate: ~ 100% for stages I and II
  - Papillary 10-year survival rate: 93%
  - Follicular 10-year survival rate: 85%
  - Best prognosis for young women
- **MTC**
  - 10-year survival rate: 75%
    - 90% when confined to gland
    - 70% when cervical lymph nodes
    - 20% when distant metastases
- **Anaplastic thyroid carcinoma**
  - Rapidly fatal, generally within 6-9 months
    - 5-year survival rate: ~ 5%
  - Patients often expire secondary to central airway compromise

TREATMENT

Major Treatment Alternatives

- **General treatment strategies**
  - Surgical resection is primary treatment, generally followed by adjuvant RAI for functioning (iodine-avid) DTC cancers
  - Extent of surgery and neck dissection often guided by histologic type, differentiation, extent of local invasion, and presence of regional lymph node involvement
  - RAI is given to ablate the thyroid remnant after thyroidectomy and for treatment of functioning DTC distant metastases
  - TSH suppression also important component of treatment
  - External beam radiation can be considered in postop setting in patients at high risk for local regional recurrence or in palliation of distant metastatic disease
  - Relative indications for postoperative radiation therapy (PORT)
    - DTC
      - Incomplete resection of nonfunctioning (non-iodine avid) cancers
      - Direct invasion of central structures, such as trachea, cricoid, esophagus, strap muscles, and other neck musculature
      - Extracapsular nodal extension
      - Recurrent disease
      - Mediastinal structure invasion or extensive mediastinal nodal disease
    - Medullary
      - In addition to indications for DTC, PORT also considered for persistently elevated calcitonin after complete surgery and no evident distant metastases
    - Poorly differentiated variants and frankly anaplastic cancers
      - Combination of surgery and PORT preferred, but anaplastic cancers rarely resectable
      - Concurrent chemotherapy considered
      - Treatment in clinical trial preferred for anaplastic cancers

- When conformal PORT is given for high-risk medullary or DTC, local regional control can reach 80-87%
  - Increased understanding of key molecular pathways and use of targeted therapy for refractory or incurable disease, particularly small molecule TKIs
    - Vandetanib recently FDA approved for use in patients with progressive, symptomatic, &/or unresectable medullary thyroid carcinoma
- **Anaplastic carcinoma**
  - Treatment often multimodal, with strong preference for treatment in clinical trial
    - RT is commonly the backbone of local-regional treatment since commonly unresectable at presentation
      - There is no standard combination of chemo and RT or RT fractionation schedule, but accelerated-hyperfractionated programs have been used
      - Even in setting of distant metastatic disease, local treatment often prioritized to stave off morbidity and mortality from uncontrolled central neck disease
    - Chemo can be given as concurrent radiosensitizer, in adjuvant setting, and for palliation
      - Targeted agents are being investigated in clinical trial
    - Surgery is considered in select cases but is often limited by invasion of critical structures; PORT considered in all cases
  - Palliative measures should be initiated early

Major Treatment Roadblocks/ Contraindications

- Maximum I-131 radioiodine dose limited by bone marrow and lung exposure

Treatment Options by Stage

- Surgical resection of isolated metastatic lesions or recurrence considered
- Can re-treat iodine-avid malignancies with I-131
- Stereotactic radiosurgery (SRS) considered for limited brain metastases

Dose Response

- Historically a radioresistant histology; standard of care is surgery when gross disease is present and resectable

Standard Doses

- When treating microscopic disease in postop setting, traditional doses are 50-66 Gy in 2 Gy fractions
  - High-risk target volume: Typically 60 Gy in 30 fractions
    - Includes areas of resected disease with margin: Primary tumor bed, involved lymph node bed, and often entirety of thyroid bed, central compartment, both TE groves, and tracheal and esophageal walls
    - Boost to areas of residual disease considered: 63-66 Gy
  - Intermediate-risk target volume: 57 Gy in 30 fractions
    - Includes uninvolved operative bed
  - Standard-risk target volume: 54 Gy in 30 fractions
    - Includes areas at risk beyond operative bed
- Higher doses to thyroid bed and lower neck problematic because of tolerance of subglottic region (stenosis), upper esophagus (stricture), and brachial plexus (neuropathy/plexopathy)

Organs at Risk Parameters

- Primary critical structures: Spinal cord < 45 Gy, brachial plexus < 60 Gy preferred
- Secondary organs at risk: Larynx, esophagus, submandibular glands, parotid glands, oral cavity, oropharynx, pharyngeal constrictors, mandible, lungs
  - Inferior aspect of larynx, cricoid, laryngeal inlet (as recurrent laryngeal nerves enter larynx), posterior cricoid region, and cervical esophagus are commonly part of clinical target volumes and receive prescription doses
- Dose to lungs must be considered and minimized, particularly when target includes mediastinum

Common Techniques

- IMRT technique favored due to difficulty delivering needed doses to low central neck because of complex and mostly concave shape of target and proximity to spinal cord and lungs
- Conventional radiation therapy techniques commonly used for palliation of metastases
- SRS considered for limited brain metastases
- SBRT considered for limited metastatic sites
- Traditional PORT beam arrangements are AP/PA followed by off-cord obliques to boost high-risk areas (or electron boost)
  - Initial field borders are guided by extent of nodal disease and operative bed
    - Superior border can be mastoid tip (when upper neck disease is present) or at hyoid level (when most superior radiation target is mid neck)
    - Inferior border typically at carina when upper mediastinal disease is present
    - Lateral borders set to encompass supraclavicular fossa

SELECTED REFERENCES

1. Siegel R et al: Cancer statistics, 2012. CA Cancer J Clin. 62(1):10-29, 2012
2. Ang KK et al: Radiotherapy for Head and Neck Cancer: Indications and Techniques. 4th ed. Philadelphia: Lippincott Williams & Wilkins, 2011
3. American Joint Committee on Cancer: AJCC Cancer Staging Manual. 7th ed. New York: Springer. 87-96, 2010
4. Bhatia A et al: Anaplastic thyroid cancer: Clinical outcomes with conformal radiotherapy. Head Neck. 32(7):829-36, 2010
5. Schwartz DL et al: Postoperative external beam radiotherapy for differentiated thyroid cancer: outcomes and morbidity with conformal treatment. Int J Radiat Oncol Biol Phys. 74(4):1083-91, 2009
6. Grubbs EG et al: Recent advances in thyroid cancer. Curr Probl Surg. 45(3):156-250, 2008
7. Schwartz DL et al: Postoperative radiotherapy for advanced medullary thyroid cancer--local disease control in the modern era. Head Neck. 30(7):883-8, 2008
8. Sherman SI: Thyroid carcinoma. Lancet. 361(9356):501-11, 2003

Follicular Thyroid Carcinoma, T2 N0 M0

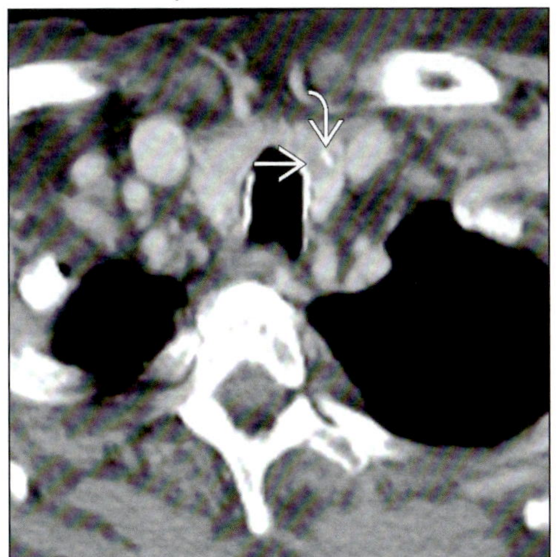

Follicular Thyroid Carcinoma, T2 N0 M0

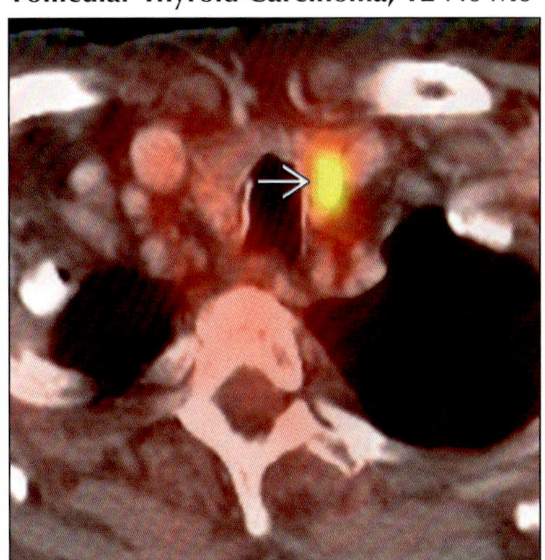

*(**Left**) Axial CECT shows a 2.2 cm, slightly low-attenuation left lobe lesion → with calcifications ↷. (**Right**) Axial PET/CT in the same patient shows intense asymmetric FDG activity → in the nodule in the left lobe. Appropriate evaluation of patient would be follow-up ultrasound and FNA. Subsequent biopsy showed follicular carcinoma.*

Papillary Thyroid Carcinoma, T3 N1b M0

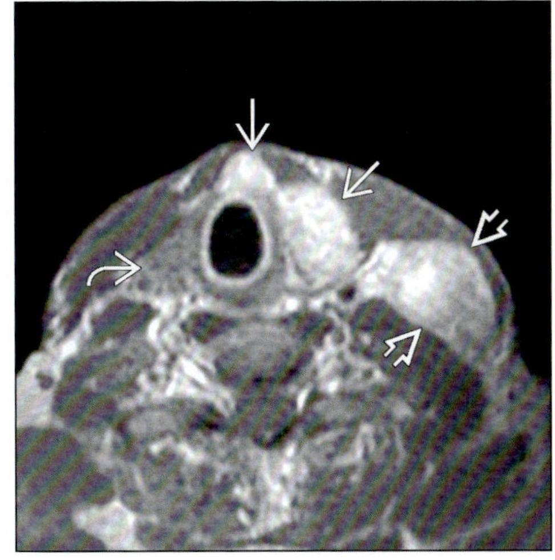

Papillary Thyroid Carcinoma, T3 N1b M0

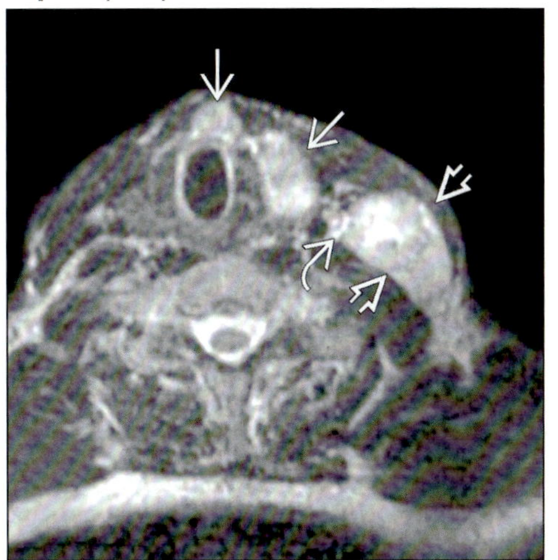

*(**Left**) Axial T1WI C+ MR shows several enhancing neck masses. The normal right thyroid gland ↷ is lateral to the trachea; the left thyroid lobe and the thyroid isthmus are replaced by enhancing lobular masses →. Also note a large enhancing level IV node ⇨. (**Right**) Axial T2WI fat-saturated MR in the same patient shows heterogeneous high signal intensity of the thyroid → and nodal ⇨ masses. High signal ↷ medial to the nodal mass represents thrombosed jugular vein.*

Recurrent Papillary Thyroid Carcinoma

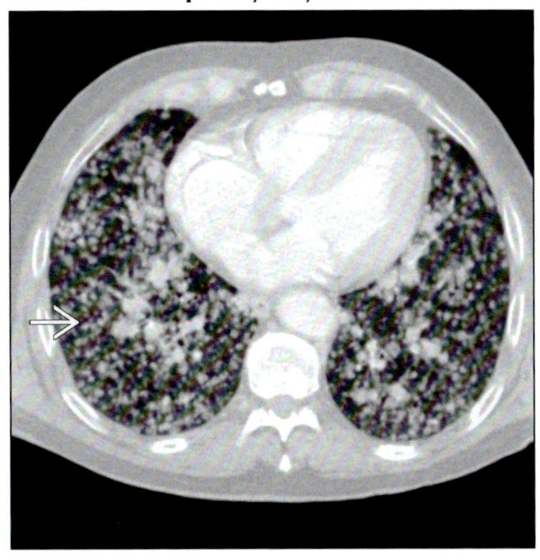

Recurrent Papillary Thyroid Carcinoma

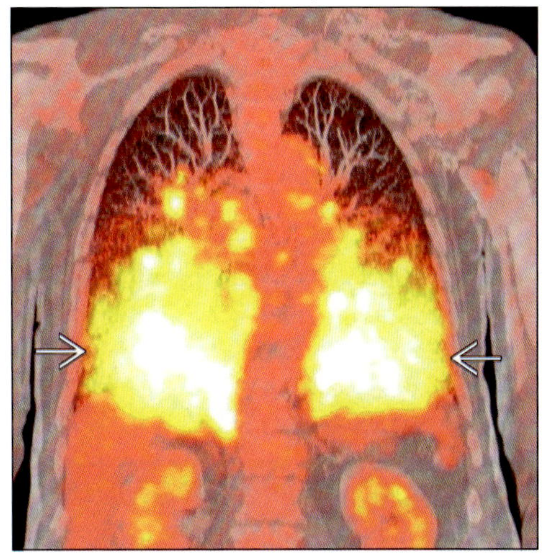

*(**Left**) Axial CECT shows innumerable well-circumscribed pulmonary nodules → in a "miliary" pattern, a finding that may be seen occasionally in patients with metastatic disease from thyroid cancer. (**Right**) Coronal fused PET/CT MIP in the same patient shows the lower lobe distribution → typical of vascular metastases. Many of the smaller nodules affecting the upper lobes are below the resolution of the PET camera and do not have appreciable increased FDG activity.*

THYROID

(Left) Coronal PET MIP image shows extensive FDG-avid multisite metastatic lesions, some of which are noted ➔. This patient had a history of papillary thyroid carcinoma, multiple recurrences, and RAI refractory. **(Right)** Axial NECT shows a large, cystic nodal metastasis ➔ involving a left level IV lymph node with punctate calcifications peripherally ➔.

Recurrent Papillary Thyroid Carcinoma

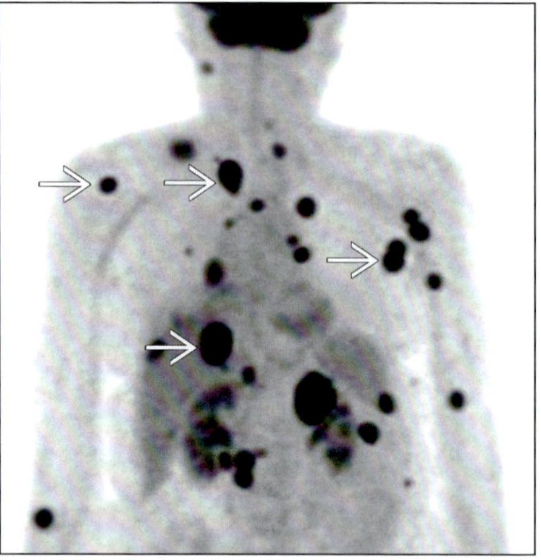

Recurrent Papillary Thyroid Carcinoma

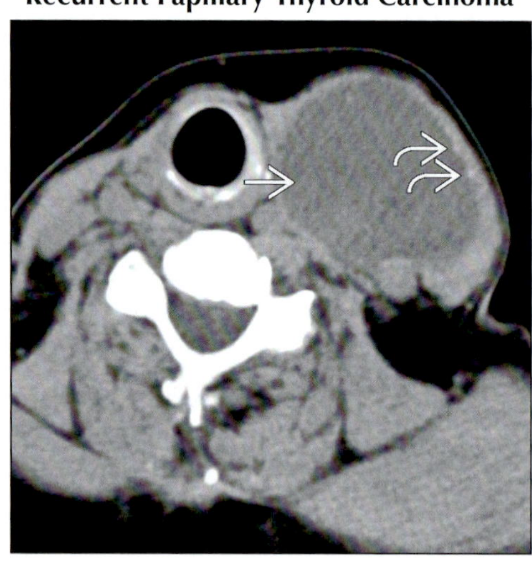

(Left) Color Doppler ultrasound shows a 4 cm (T2) hypoechogenic lesion in the thyroid ➔ with nonspecific increased vascularity ➔. **(Right)** This patient had a history of PTC requiring sacrifice of left recurrent laryngeal nerve. PET/CT demonstrates left vocal fold position, consistent with paralysis ➔ with asymmetric hypermetabolic activity of the larynx ➔ due to compensatory hypertrophy of the right vocal fold.

Papillary Thyroid Carcinoma, Stage II (T2 N0 M0)

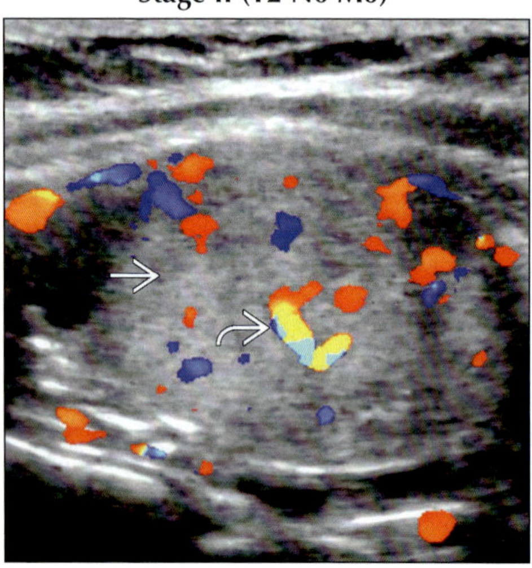

Vocal Fold Paralysis

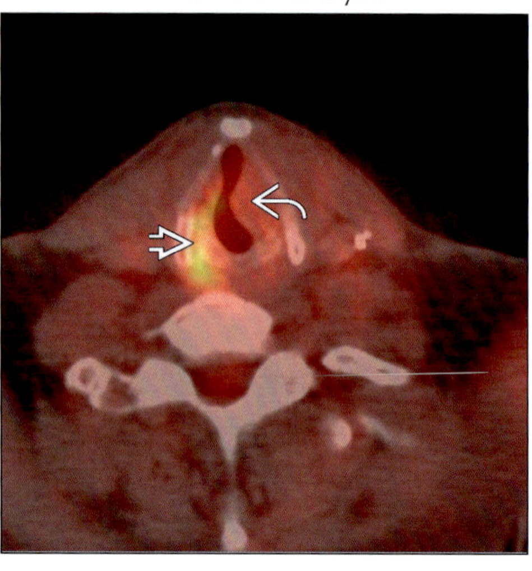

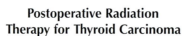

(Left) Traditional anterior radiation portal is shown with the inferior border at the level of carina ➔. The superior border on the right was extended up to the mastoid ➔ due to the presence of upper neck disease. **(Right)** Important anatomical landmarks help guide delineation of CTVs of the central compartment on CT.

Postoperative Radiation Therapy for Thyroid Carcinoma

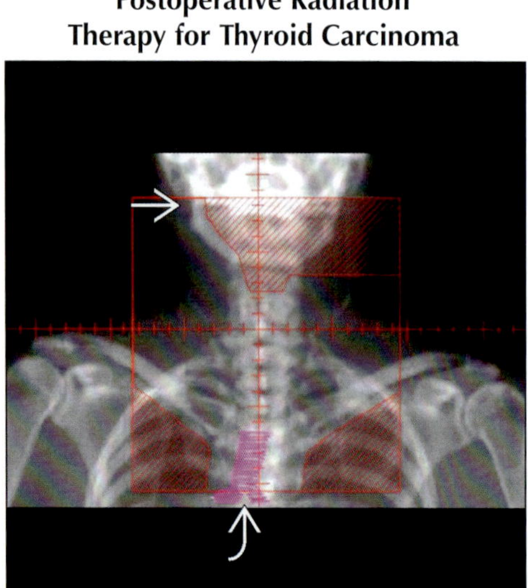

Normal Structures

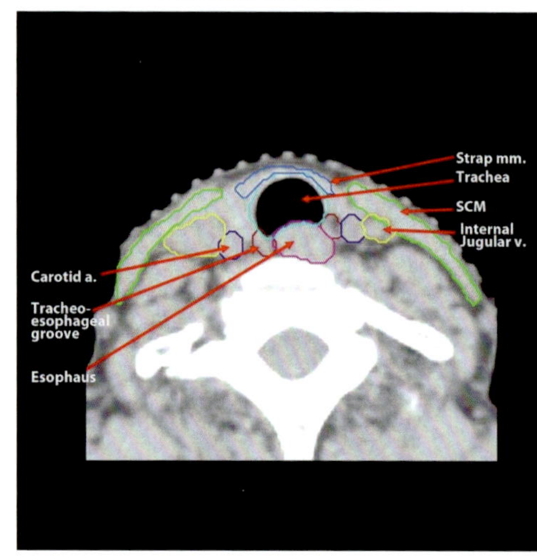

CT Simulation

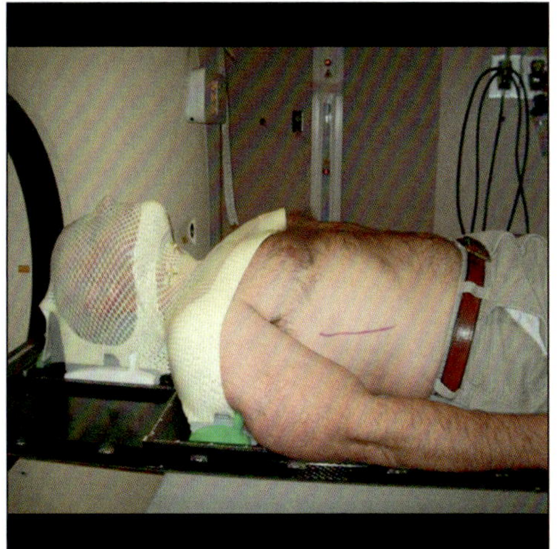

IMRT Clinical Target Volumes

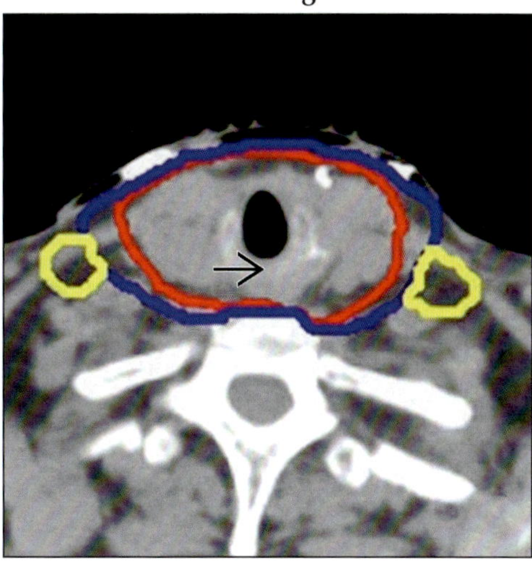

(Left) *This photograph shows patient setup at time of CT simulation with custom thermoplastic mask for head, neck, and shoulder immobilization.* ***(Right)*** *Representative CTVs are shown at caudal aspect of cricoid cartilage →. In this case, high-risk CTV (in red) is targeting thyroid bed, central compartment, and both TE grooves; intermediate-risk CTV (in blue) includes operative bed; and standard-risk CTV (in yellow) includes undissected cervical lymph nodes at risk.*

IMRT Clinical Target Volumes

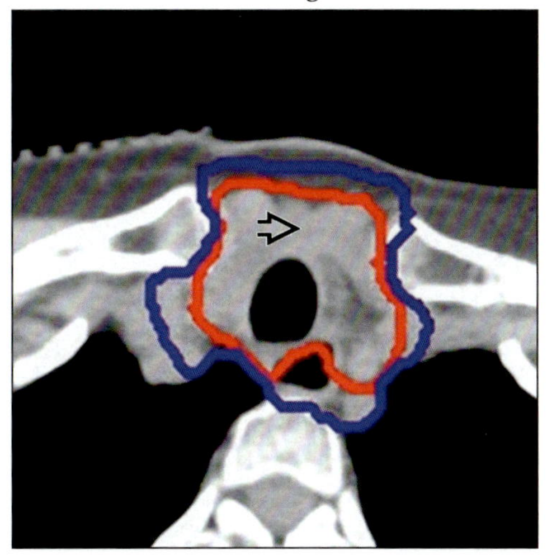

IMRT Clinical Target Volumes

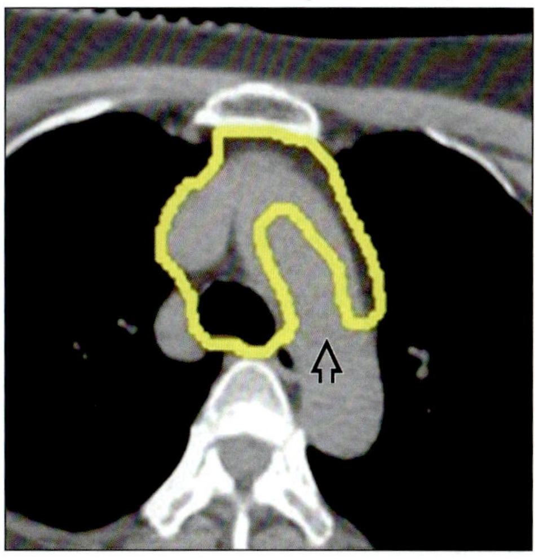

(Left) *Representative CTVs (high and intermediate risk) are shown in red and blue, respectively, at the level of the suprasternal notch ⇨.* ***(Right)*** *Representative standard-risk CTV is shown at the superior mediastinum at the level of the mid-aortic arch ⇨. Note the sparing of the mid aspect of the aortic arch.*

Intensity-Modulated Radiation Therapy

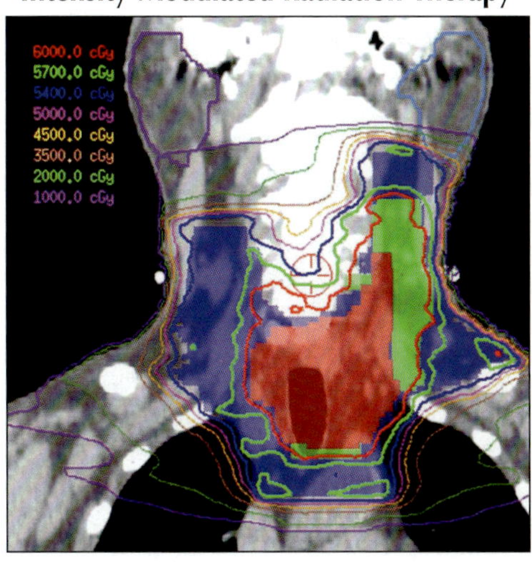

IMRT Dose Volume Histogram

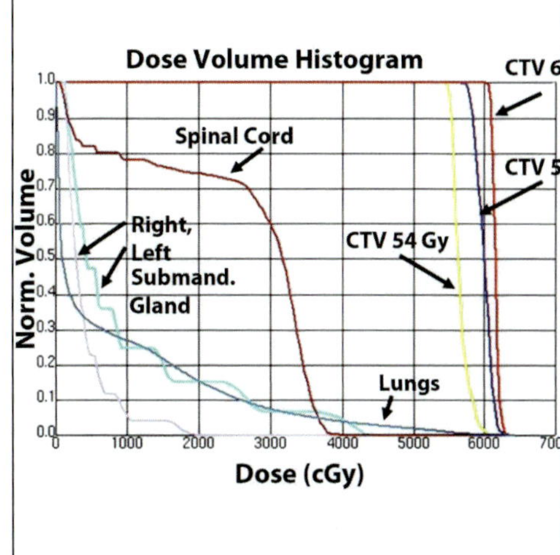

(Left) *Postoperative IMRT dose distributions are shown in coronal plane, demonstrating potential for differential targeting of cervical lymph node regions, treating upper mediastinum, bilateral levels III, IV, VI, and left levels II and V.* ***(Right)*** *Dose volume histogram demonstrates coverage of CTVs with relative sparing of selected avoidance structures.*

(Left) This photograph of a patient demonstrates acute radiation-associated dermatitis at end of treatment. **(Right)** This esophagram shows a post-RT cervical esophagus stricture ➔ resolved with dilatation.

Acute Effects of Radiation Therapy

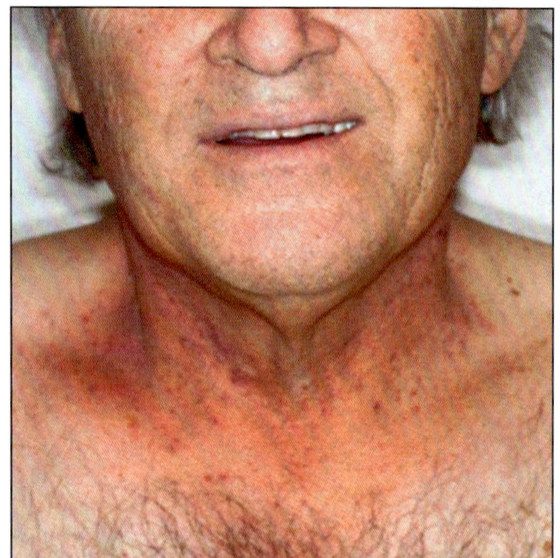

Late Effects of Radiation Therapy

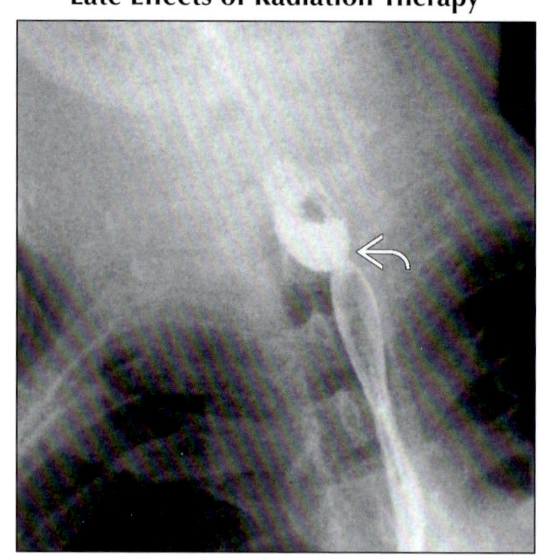

(Left) *A 57-year-old woman with history of papillary thyroid carcinoma presents with cough. This CECT demonstrates recurrence with tracheal compression and invasion ➔.* **(Right)** *Following surgery, including tracheal resection, the same patient received IMRT to 60, 57, and 54 Gy in 30 fx to the tumor bed, operative bed, and undissected neck at risk, respectively. CTVs in colorwash and corresponding isodoses are shown: Red = 60 Gy, sky blue = 57 Gy, and yellow = 54 Gy.*

Recurrent Papillary Thyroid Carcinoma

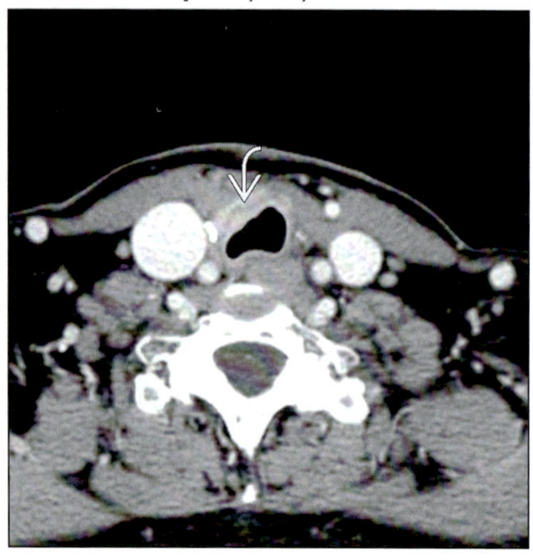

Recurrent Papillary Thyroid Carcinoma

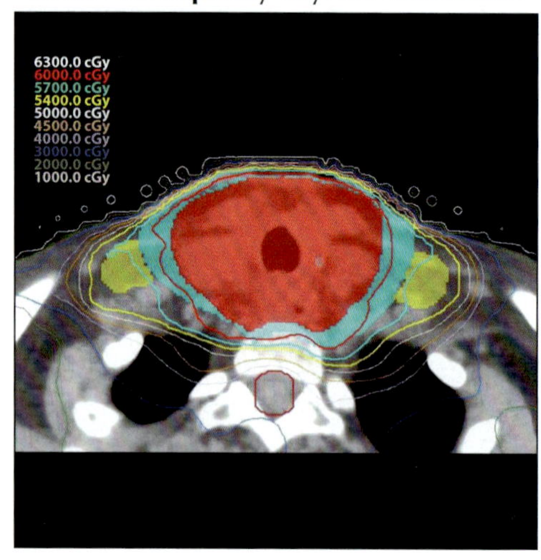

(Left) *This 62-year-old man with known metastatic non-iodine avid papillary thyroid cancer presented with left shoulder pain. PET/CT shows hypermetabolic metastasis of left clavicular head with extensive soft tissue involvement.* **(Right)** *The same patient was treated with palliative 3D conformal RT, wedge pair beam arrangement, and 50 Gy in 20 fx to the dominant metastasis with subsequent pain relief. Axial CT shows representative isodose distributions.*

Metastatic Papillary Thyroid Carcinoma

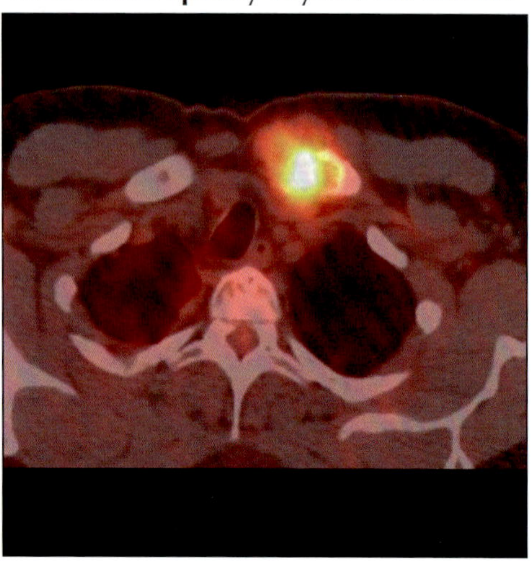

Metastatic Papillary Thyroid Carcinoma

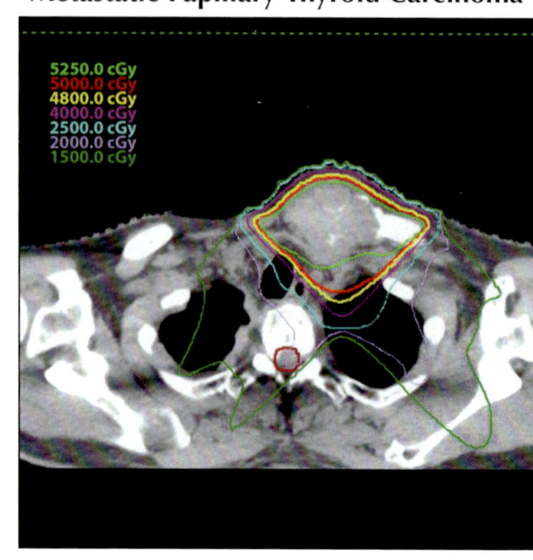

Anaplastic Thyroid Carcinoma, Stage IVB

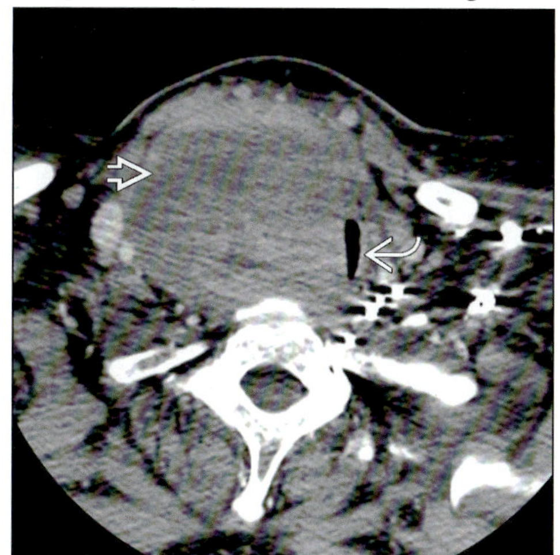

Anaplastic Thyroid Carcinoma, Stage IVB

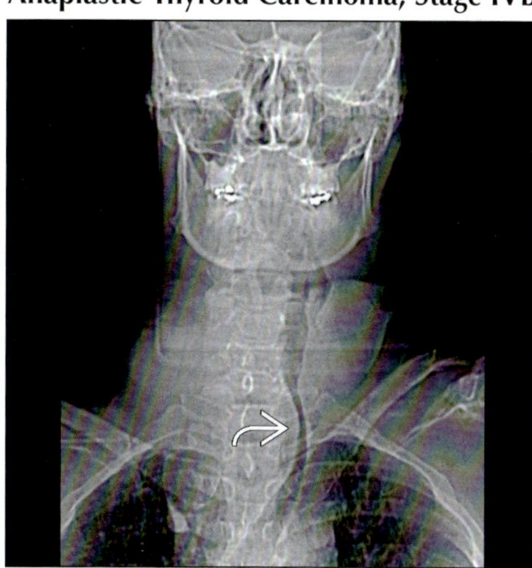

*(**Left**) A 58-year-old woman presented with shortness of breath and a rapidly enlarging low anterior neck mass. CECT demonstrates heterogeneous thyroid mass ➪ with extensive tracheal compression ↪. (**Right**) Radiograph of the same patient shows extensive tracheal compression and displacement of the upper airway ↪. Core biopsy showed anaplastic thyroid carcinoma.*

Anaplastic Thyroid Carcinoma, Stage IVB

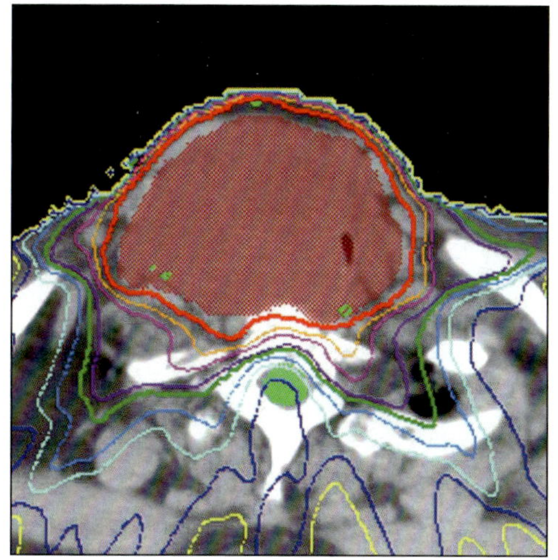

Anaplastic Thyroid Carcinoma, Stage IVB

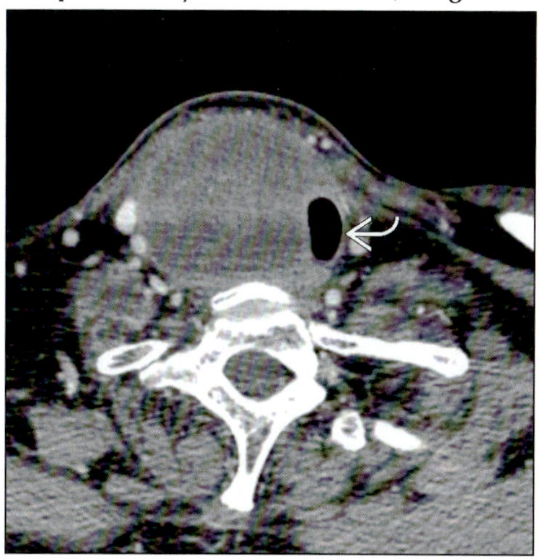

*(**Left**) The same patient was treated with concurrent chemo-IMRT to 66 Gy in 44 fx, 150 cGy 2x daily over 4.5 weeks. She received concurrent carboplatin and paclitaxel. Maximum spinal cord dose was 32 Gy. Red colorwash = CTV 66 Gy, red line = 66 Gy, and green colorwash = spinal cord. (**Right**) Post-treatment CECT of the same patient shows disease stabilization of dominant mass with improved tracheal narrowing ↪.*

Anaplastic Thyroid Carcinoma, Stage IVB

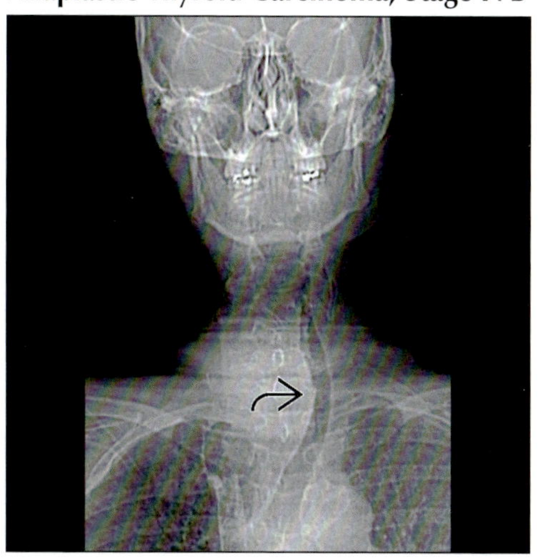

Anaplastic Thyroid Carcinoma, Stage IVB

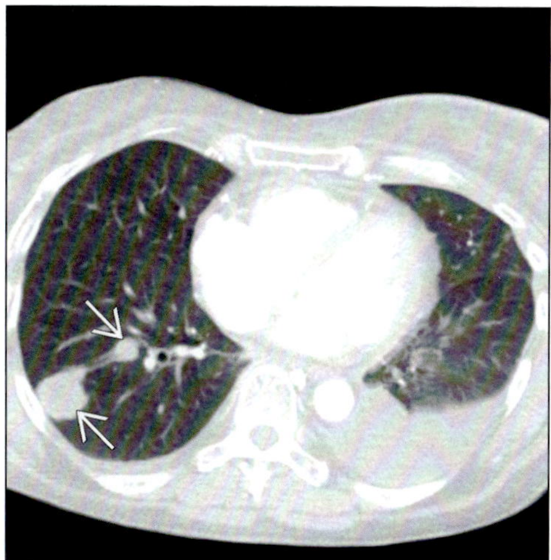

*(**Left**) This post-treatment radiograph of the same patient further demonstrates the improved tracheal compression and airway displacement ↪ compared to pre-treatment images. (**Right**) The same patient developed distant metastatic disease to lungs ➔ and died 10 months after completing radiation therapy, but durable central airway patency was maintained.*

(Left) 68-year-old woman with history of follicular carcinoma presented with dysphagia. CECT shows multicentric recurrence involving sternocleidomastoid ➡ and esophagus ➡. *(Right)* Post surgery, including partial esophagectomy, same patient received IMRT to 60, 57, and 54 Gy to central compartment, operative bed, and undissected neck at risk, respectively. CTVs in colorwash with corresponding isodoses are shown: Red = 60 Gy, blue = 57 Gy, yellow = 54 Gy.

Recurrent Follicular Thyroid Carcinoma

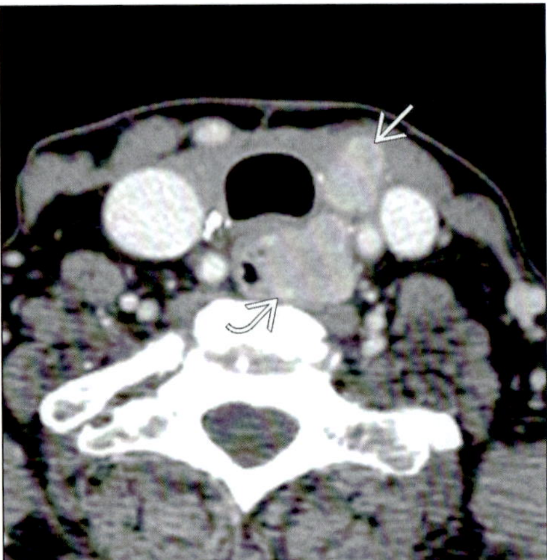

Recurrent Follicular Thyroid Carcinoma

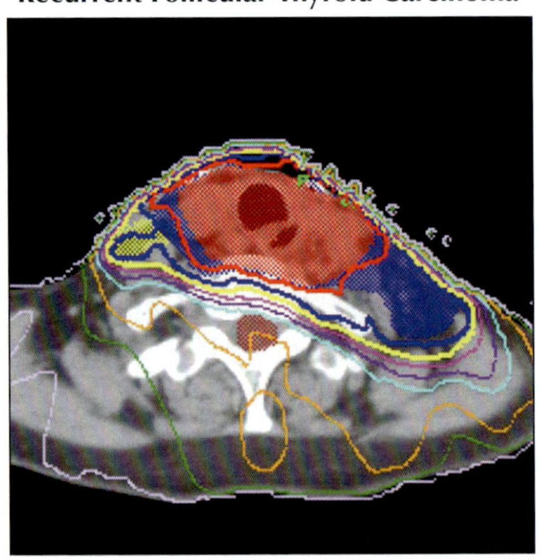

(Left) A 47-year-old woman with history of follicular thyroid cancer presented with mid back pain. T1-weighted nonenhanced MR shows metastasis ➡ to T6 with spinal cord compression ➡. *(Right)* CT myelogram of the same patient further characterizes the metastasis ➡ to T6 and spinal cord ➡. The tumor can be seen displacing the cord ➡.

Metastatic Follicular Thyroid Carcinoma

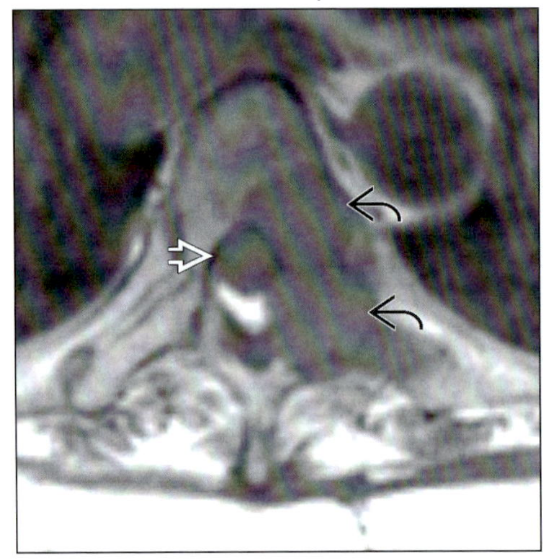

Metastatic Follicular Thyroid Carcinoma

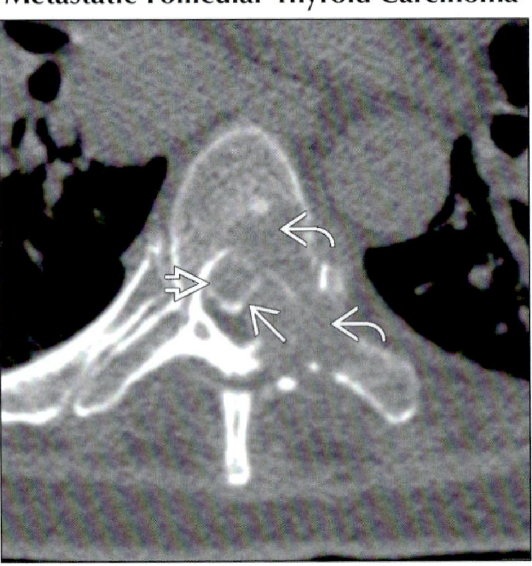

(Left) The same patient had previous spine surgery and palliative RT adjacent to this area, and additional surgery was not feasible. She was treated with palliative CT-guided intensity-modulated SBRT on protocol; 18 Gy in a single fraction was delivered to the tumor while strictly limiting maximum doses to the spinal cord, esophagus, aorta, and surface. *(Right)* Post-treatment CT of the same patient 1 year after SBRT shows disease stabilization.

Metastatic Follicular Thyroid Carcinoma

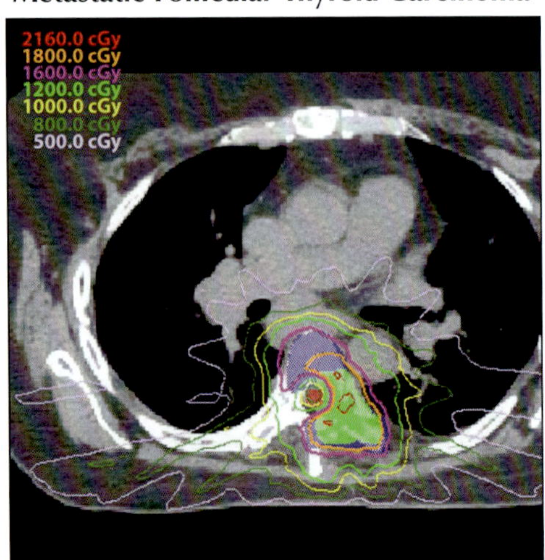

Metastatic Follicular Thyroid Carcinoma

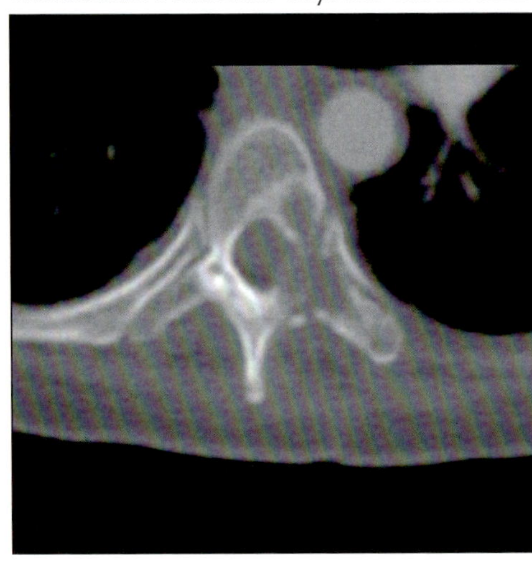

Metastatic Follicular Thyroid Carcinoma

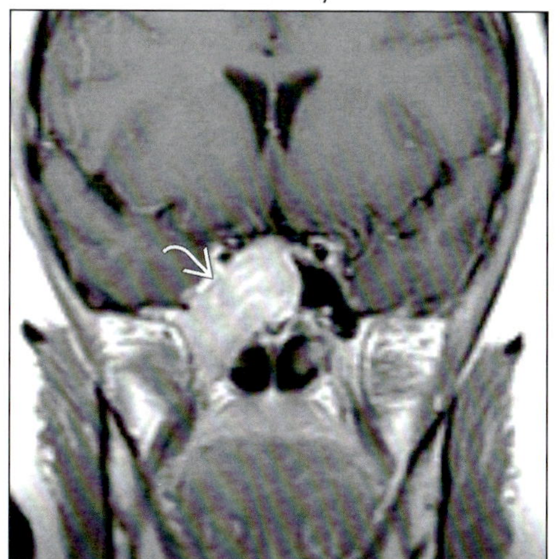

Metastatic Follicular Thyroid Carcinoma

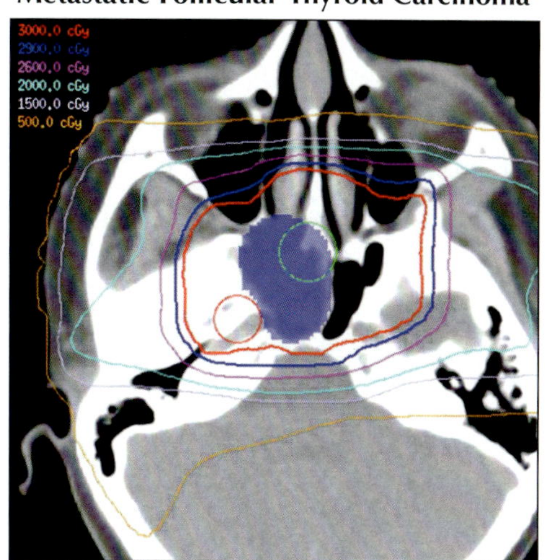

(Left) *A 48-year-old woman with recurrent metastatic follicular thyroid carcinoma presented with headache and right eye vision decrement. Coronal MR with gadolinium shows enhancing right skull base metastasis ➔ involving the right sphenoid sinus.* ***(Right)*** *The same patient was treated with emergent palliative radiation therapy, 30 Gy in 10 fractions with complete resolution of symptoms. Blue colorwash = GTV.*

Metastatic Follicular Thyroid Carcinoma

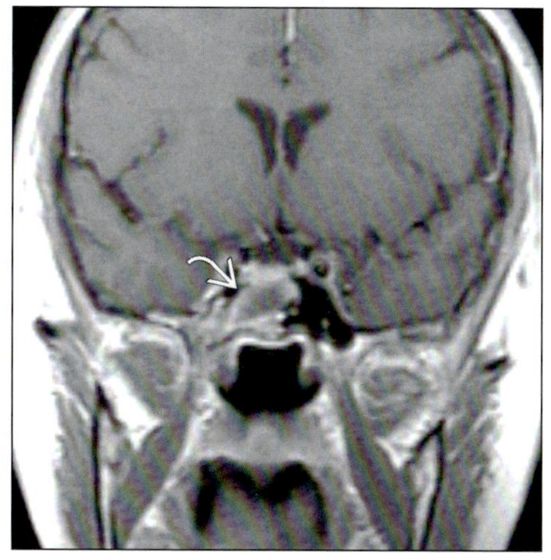

Poorly Differentiated Thyroid Carcinoma

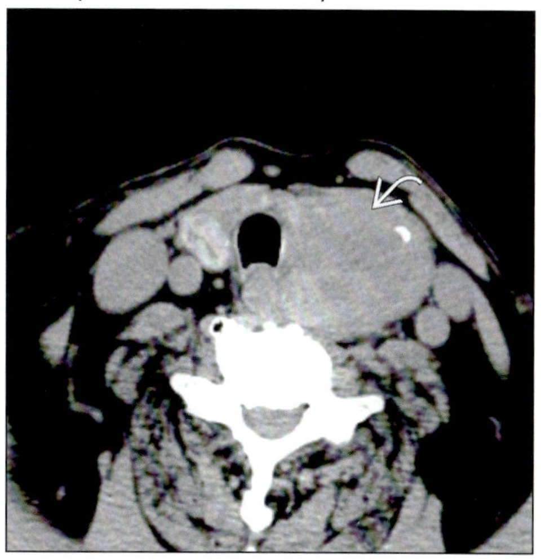

(Left) *Post-treatment MR of the same patient shows a nearly complete resolution of the mass ➔ 14 months after RT.* ***(Right)*** *This 75-year-old man presented with hoarseness. NECT shows heterogeneous thyroid mass ➔. The patient underwent total thyroidectomy; the mass was resected from the retroesophageal region. Pathology revealed papillary thyroid carcinoma, follicular variant, with areas of poor differentiation, extrathyroidal extension, and narrow resection margin.*

Poorly Differentiated Thyroid Carcinoma

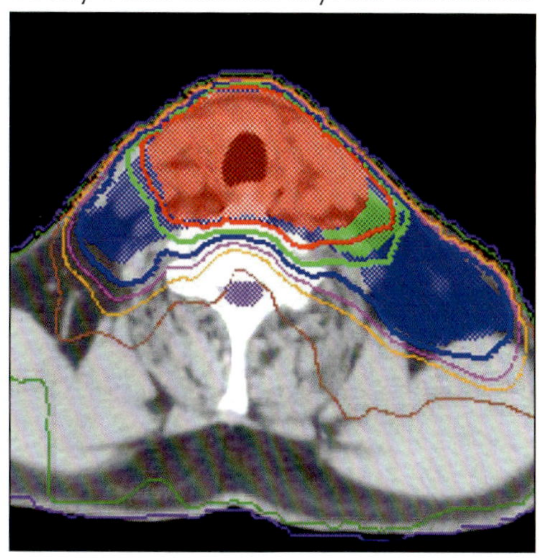

Poorly Differentiated Thyroid Carcinoma

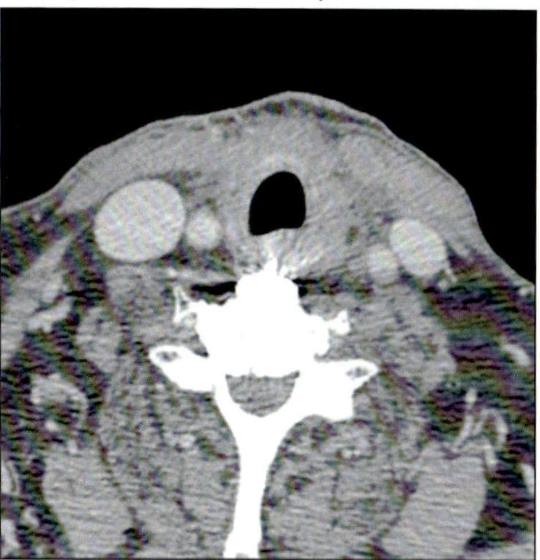

(Left) *The same patient was treated with postoperative RAI followed by IMRT to 60, 57, and 54 Gy in 30 daily fractions to the tumor bed/central compartment, operative bed, and bilateral undissected neck at risk, respectively. CTVs in colorwash with corresponding isodoses are shown: Red = 60 Gy, green = 57 Gy, and blue = 54 Gy.* ***(Right)*** *Post-treatment CECT of the same patient shows interval resection of the mass and post-therapy-related changes only.*

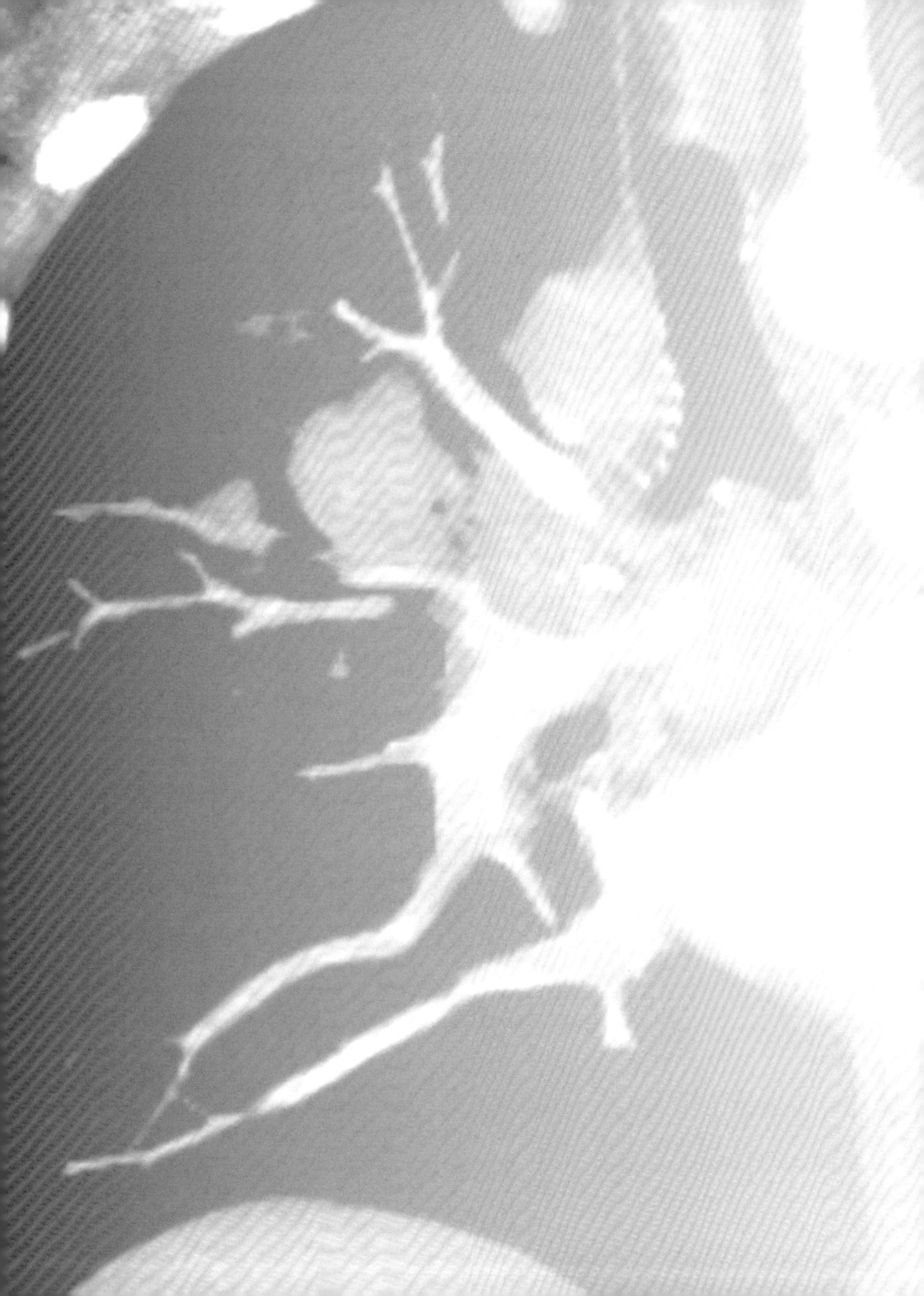

SECTION 3
Thorax

NON-SMALL CELL LUNG CANCER

(T) Primary Tumor

Adapted from 7th edition AJCC Staging Forms.

TNM	*Definitions*
TX	Primary tumor cannot be assessed **or** tumor proven by presence of malignant cells in sputum or bronchial washings but not visualized by imaging or bronchoscopy
T0	No evidence of primary tumor
Tis	Carcinoma in situ
T1	Tumor ≤ 3 cm in greatest dimension, surrounded by lung or visceral pleura, without bronchoscopic evidence of invasion more proximal than lobar bronchus (i.e., not in main bronchus)[1]
T1a	Tumor ≤ 2 cm in greatest dimension
T1b	Tumor > 2 cm but ≤ 3 cm in greatest dimension
T2	Tumor > 3 cm but ≤ 7 cm or tumor with any of the following features: Involves main bronchus, ≥ 2 cm distal to carina; invades visceral pleura (PL1 or PL2); associated with atelectasis or obstructive pneumonitis that extends to hilar region but does not involve entire lung
T2a	Tumor > 3 cm but ≤ 5 cm in greatest dimension
T2b	Tumor > 5 cm but ≤ 7 cm in greatest dimension
T3	Tumor > 7 cm or tumor that directly invades any of the following: Parietal pleural (PL3) chest wall (including superior sulcus tumors), diaphragm, phrenic nerve, mediastinal pleura, parietal pericardium; or tumor in main bronchus (≤ 2 cm distal to carina[1] but without involvement of carina); or associated atelectasis or obstructive pneumonitis of entire lung or separate tumor nodule(s) in same lobe
T4	Tumor of any size that invades any of the following: Mediastinum, heart, great vessels, trachea, recurrent laryngeal nerve, esophagus, vertebral body, carina, separate tumor nodule(s) in different ipsilateral lobe

(N) Regional Lymph Nodes

NX	Regional lymph nodes cannot be assessed
N0	No regional lymph node metastases
N1	Metastasis in ipsilateral peribronchial &/or ipsilateral hilar lymph nodes and intrapulmonary nodes, including involvement by direct extension
N2	Metastasis in ipsilateral mediastinal &/or subcarinal lymph node(s)
N3	Metastasis in contralateral mediastinal, contralateral hilar, ipsilateral or contralateral scalene, or supraclavicular lymph node(s)

(M) Distant Metastasis

M0	No distant metastasis
M1	Distant metastasis
M1a	Separate tumor nodule(s) in contralateral lobe tumor with pleural nodules or malignant pleural (or pericardial) effusion[2]
M1b	Distant metastasis

[1]*The uncommon superficial spreading tumor of any size with its invasive component limited to bronchial wall, which may extend proximally to the main bronchus, is also classified as T1a.*

[2]*Most pleural (and pericardial) effusions with lung cancer are due to tumor. In a few patients, however, multiple cytopathologic examinations of pleural (pericardial) fluid are negative for tumor, and the fluid is not bloody and is not an exudate. Where these elements and clinical judgment dictate that the effusion is not related to the tumor, the effusion should be excluded as a staging element and the patient's disease should be classified as M0.*

NON-SMALL CELL LUNG CANCER

AJCC Stages/Prognostic Groups

Adapted from 7th edition AJCC Staging Forms.

Stage	*T*	*N*	*M*
Occult carcinoma	TX	N0	M0
0	Tis	N0	M0
IA	T1a	N0	M0
	T1b	N0	M0
IB	T2a	N0	M0
IIA	T2b	N0	M0
	T1a	N1	M0
	T1b	N1	M0
	T2a	N1	M0
IIB	T2b	N1	M0
	T3	N0	M0
IIIA	T1a	N2	M0
	T1b	N2	M0
	T2a	N2	M0
	T2b	N2	M0
	T3	N1	M0
	T3	N2	M0
	T4	N0	M0
	T4	N1	M0
IIIB	T1a	N3	M0
	T1b	N3	M0
	T2a	N3	M0
	T2b	N3	M0
	T3	N3	M0
	T4	N2	M0
	T4	N3	M0
IV	Any T	Any N	M1a
	Any T	Any N	M1b

NON-SMALL CELL LUNG CANCER

T1

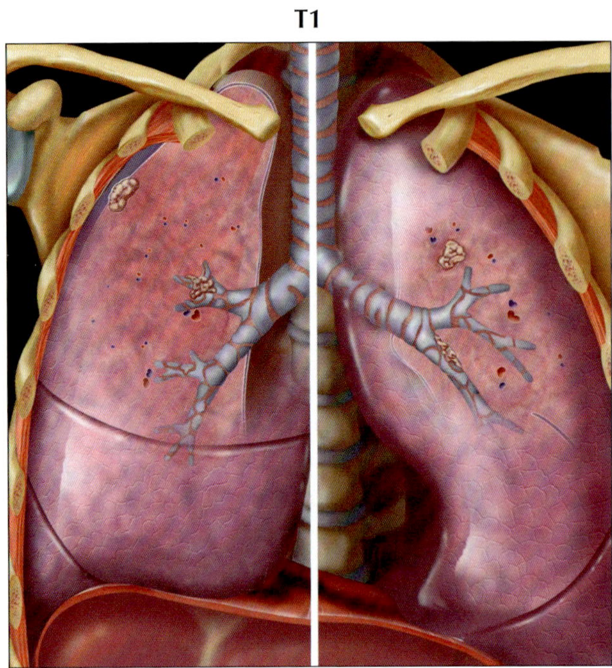

Graphic depicts T1 tumors, all < 3 cm, surrounded by lung/visceral pleura, with no invasion of the main bronchus. T1a (left) designates tumor ≤ 2 cm or superficial spreading tumor invading bronchial wall (may extend to main bronchus). T1b (right) indicates tumor > 2 cm but ≤ 3 cm.

T2

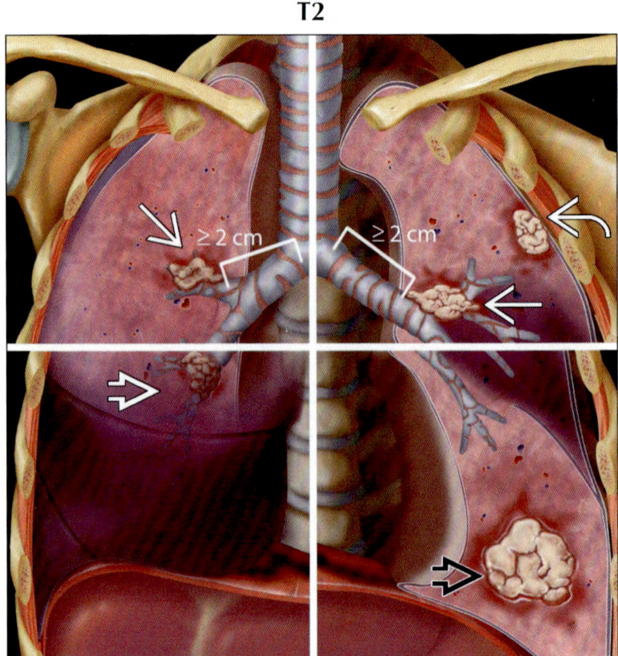

Graphic depicts T2 tumors involving main pulmonary bronchus, > 2 cm distal to carina, invading visceral pleura, and associated with atelectasis/pneumonitis of portion of lung. T2a applies to tumor > 3 cm but ≤ 5 cm, and T2b refers to tumor > 5 cm but ≤ 7 cm.

T3

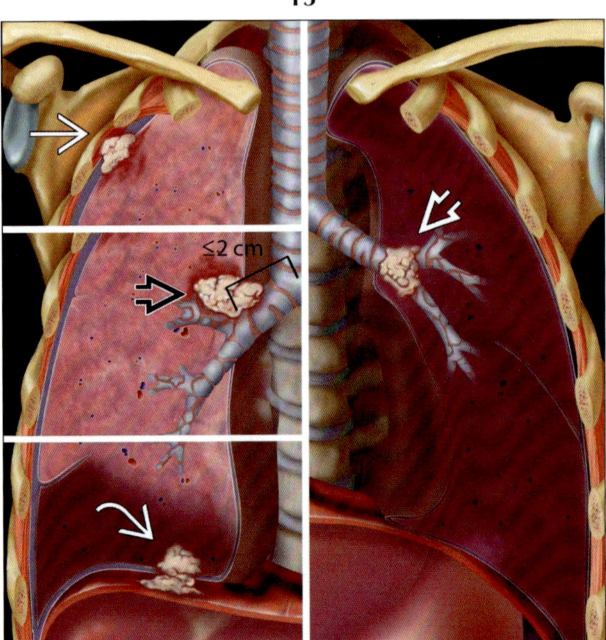

Graphic depicts T3 tumor invading the chest wall, tumor in main bronchus < 2 cm distal to carina, tumor invading the diaphragm, and tumor with associated atelectasis/pneumonitis of entire left lung. Any of these tumors alone would be considered T3 disease. Separate tumor nodules in the same lobe is also T3.

T4

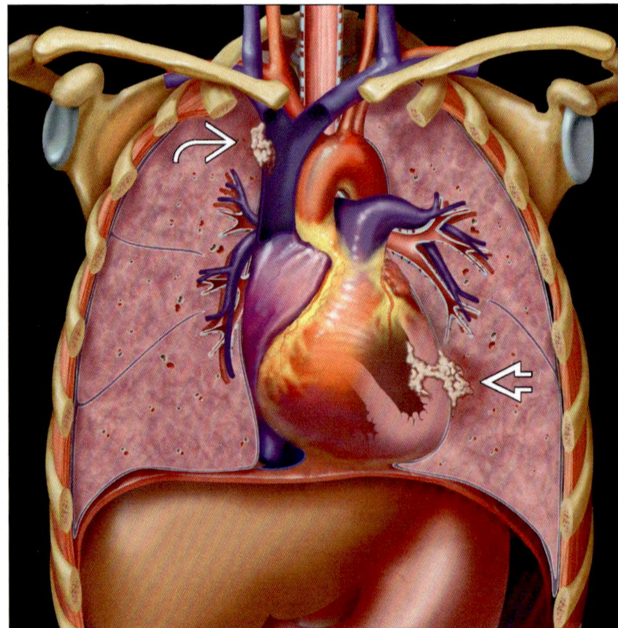

Graphic depicts 2 T4 tumors. One invades the superior vena cava; another invades the myocardium. Invasion of the mediastinum, heart, great vessels, trachea, recurrent laryngeal nerve, esophagus, vertebral body, carina, and separate tumor nodules in different ipsilateral lobe are all T4.

Adenocarcinoma

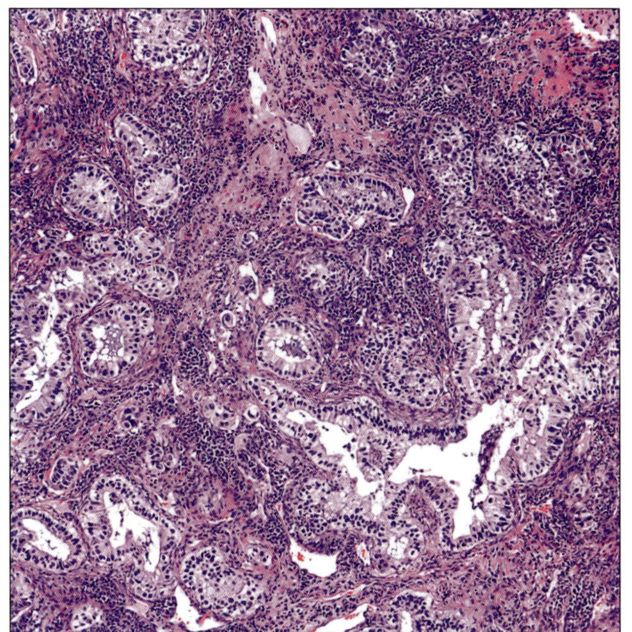

Moderately differentiated adenocarcinoma shows sparse gland formation. Malignant glandular proliferation is admixed with areas of fibrosis and inflammatory reaction. (Courtesy C. Moran, MD.)

Squamous Cell Carcinoma

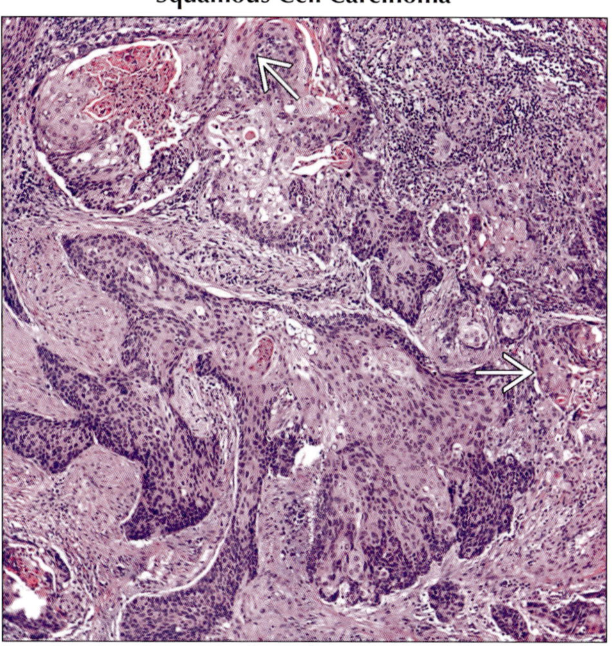

Keratinizing well-differentiated SCCa is shown. Note keratin formation ➔. (Courtesy C. Moran, MD.)

Large Cell Carcinoma

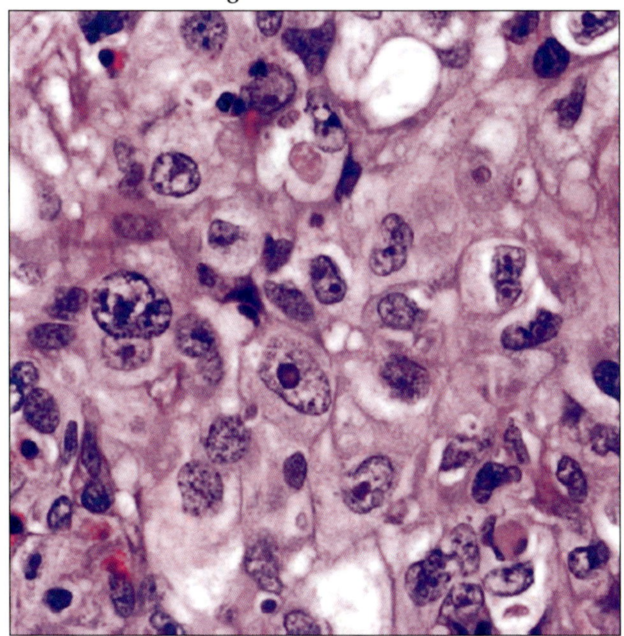

Large cell carcinoma is shown. Note sheets of large tumor cells without evidence of glandular or squamous differentiation. Cells are mostly ovoid in shape. (Courtesy S. Suster, MD.)

Bronchoalveolar Carcinoma

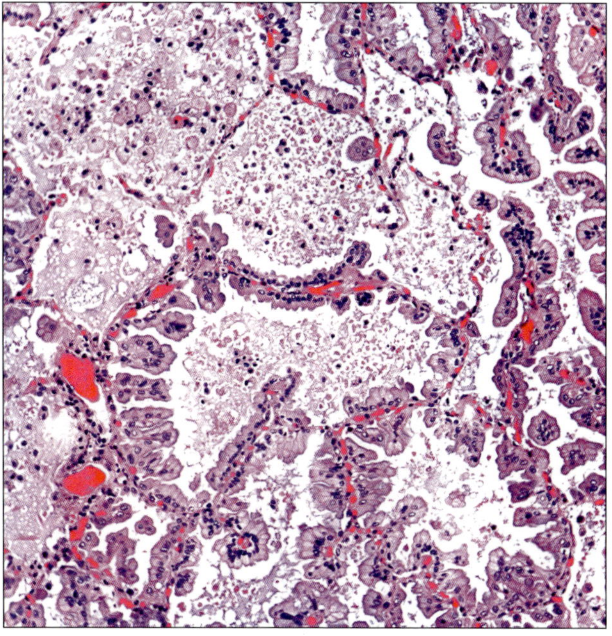

Bronchoalveolar carcinoma is shown. Note presence of tall columnar, peg-shaped neoplastic cells lining the alveolar wall in a "picket fence" fashion. (Courtesy S. Suster, MD.)

Lymph Node Map

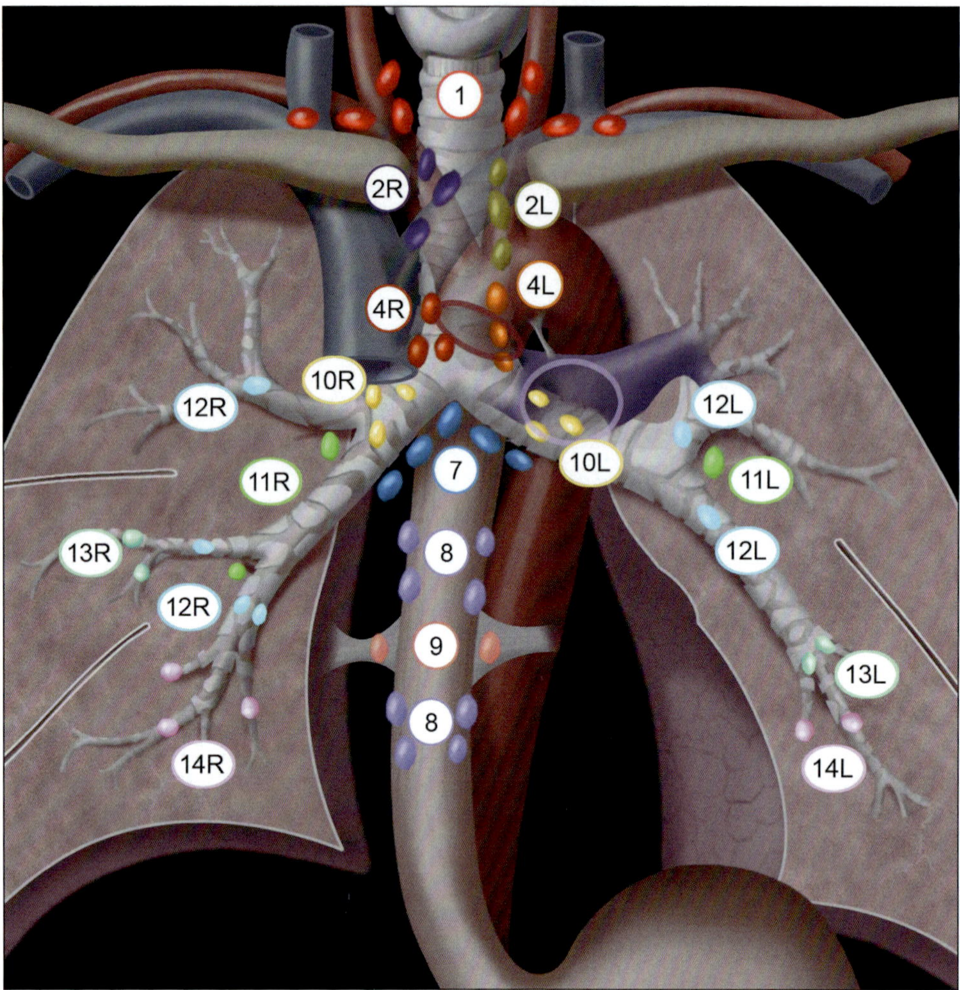

Graphic depicts the International Association for the Study of Lung Cancer (IASLC) lymph node map.

***Supraclavicular zone**: 1) Low cervical, supraclavicular, and sternal notch nodes.*

***Upper zone**: 2R) Upper paratracheal, right; 2L) upper paratracheal, left; 4R) lower paratracheal, right; 4L) lower paratracheal, left.*

***AP zone**: 7) Subcarinal nodes.*

***Lower zone**: 8) Paraesophageal (below carina); 9) pulmonary ligament.*

***Hilar/interlobar zone**: 10) Hilar, 11) interlobar.*

***Peripheral zone**: 12) Lobar, 13) segmental, 14) subsegmental.*

Other nodes are shown in the following graphics.

Prevascular and Retrotracheal Lymph Nodes

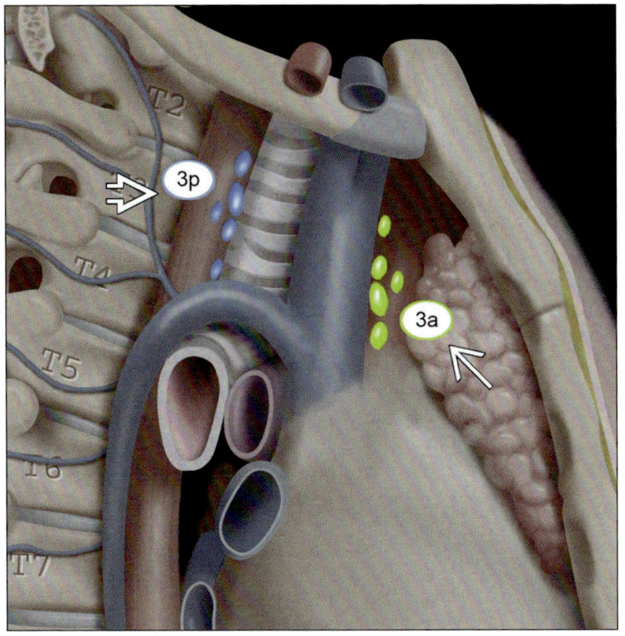

Graphic depicts 3a) prevascular ➡ and 3p) retrotracheal ➡ lymph nodes.

Subaortic and Paraaortic Lymph Nodes

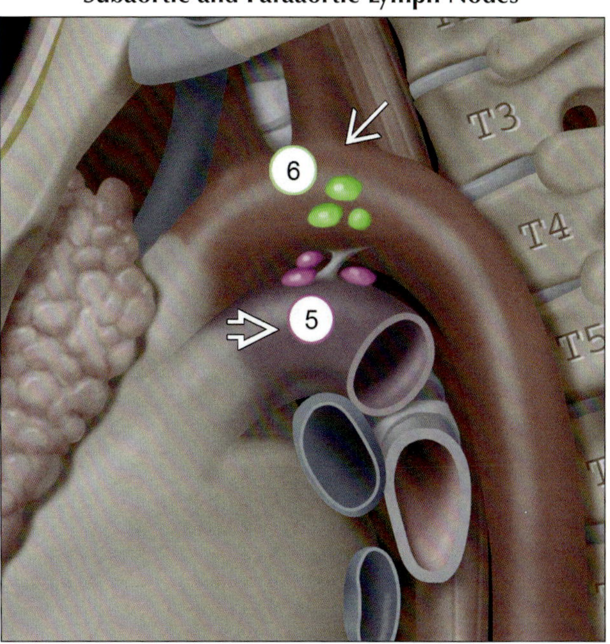

Graphic depicts AP zone lymph nodes: 5) Subaortic ➡ and 6) paraaortic (ascending aorta or phrenic) ➡.

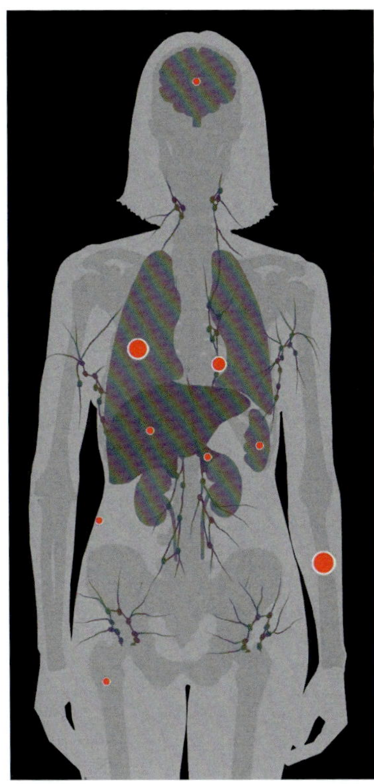

INITIAL SITE OF RECURRENCE	
Distant Metastases	47%
Primary Tumor	29%
Regional Nodes	16%
DISTANT SITES OF METASTASES	
Brain	47%
Bone	36%
Liver	22%
Adrenal Glands	15%
Body Wall	13%
Spleen	6%

The distribution of site of initial recurrence is from RTOG 9410, arm 2 concurrent chemoradiation for patients with stages II/III NSCLC. The distribution of sites of distant metastases is from a study of 72 patients with M1 disease, as diagnosed by CT.

NON-SMALL CELL LUNG CANCER

OVERVIEW

General Comments

- Non-small cell lung cancer (NSCLC) should be staged per 7th edition of AJCC system (2010)

Classification

- NSCLC
  - Adenocarcinoma, including bronchioloalveolar carcinoma (BAC)
  - Squamous cell carcinoma (SCCa)
  - Large cell carcinoma

NATURAL HISTORY

General Features

- Comments
  - Vast majority of NSCLC patients die from cancer
- Location
  - 53% upper lobe, 23% lower lobe, 3% middle lobe, 4.4% bronchus, 2% overlapping sites, and remaining unknown

Etiology

- Risk factors
  - Cigarette smoking (~ 90% of lung cancers in males, ~ 80% lung cancer in females)
    - Lung cancer development directly related to number of cigarettes smoked, length of smoking history, and tar and nicotine content of cigarettes
    - Smoking cessation reduces risk of cancer
  - Passive smoking (secondhand smoke)
    - Carcinogenic material can be inhaled passively by nonsmokers
    - Accounts for up to 25% of lung cancers in persons who do not smoke
  - Asbestos
    - Silicate type of asbestos fiber is important carcinogen
    - Exposure increases risk of developing lung cancer by as much as 5x
    - Tobacco smoke and asbestos exposure act synergistically
  - Radon
    - Inert gas produced from uranium decay
    - Accounts for 2-3% of lung cancers annually
    - Household exposure to radon has never been clearly shown to cause lung cancer
  - HIV
    - 6.5x ↑ in lung cancer in patients infected with HIV
  - Environmental agents
    - Exposure to beryllium, nickel, copper, chromium, and cadmium all linked to lung cancer risk

Epidemiology & Cancer Incidence

- Number of cases in USA per year
  - 226,160 estimated new lung cancer cases in 2012
  - 60,340 estimated deaths from lung cancer in 2012
  - Most common cause of cancer deaths in USA and worldwide
    - Surpassing breast, prostate, colon, and ovarian cancer combined
    - Accounts for approximately 12% of global cancer burden (2007)
- NSCLC accounts for 80-85% of lung cancer

Genetics

- Advanced molecular techniques have identified amplification of oncogenes and inactivation of tumor suppressor genes
  - *Ras* family of oncogene mutations
    - Occur almost exclusively in adenocarcinoma (30% of all cases)
    - Mutations not identified in adenocarcinomas that develop in persons who do not smoke
- Adverse biologic factors
  - *TTF1*, Cox2, *EGFR* overexpression, *Ras*, Ki-67, *HER2*, *VEGF*, microvascular density, *p53*, aneuploidy
- Favorable biologic factors
  - *BCL2*, *EGFR* mutation, *ALK* translocation

Associated Diseases, Abnormalities

- Paraneoplastic syndromes
  - Squamous cell carcinomas are more likely to be associated with hypercalcemia due to parathyroid-like hormone production
  - Ectopic adrenocorticotropic hormone (ACTH) production can result in Cushing syndrome
  - Adenocarcinomas
    - Digital clubbing
    - Hypertrophic pulmonary osteoarthropathy
    - Trousseau syndrome of hypercoagulability

Gross Pathology & Surgical Features

- Gross specimens from thoracotomy or thoracoscopy
- Core specimens from CT or bronchoscopy-guided procedures
- Pathologic assessment of lung cancers is based on
  - Histologic type
  - Tumor size and location
  - Involvement of visceral pleura
  - Extension to regional lymph nodes and adjacent organs
- Squamous cell carcinomas are often centrally located
  - Either in main bronchus or proximal portion of lobar bronchus
  - Can lead to partial or complete bronchial obstruction
  - Larger tumors demonstrate central cavitation as tumors outgrow their blood supply
- Adenocarcinomas are commonly peripheral in location
  - Solitary nodule or mass

Microscopic Pathology

- H&E
  - Adenocarcinoma
    - Gland formation (acinar, papillary, bronchoalveolar, mucus secreting)
    - Lepidic growth pattern
    - Mucinous or nonmucinous
  - Squamous cell carcinoma
    - Very high rates of cell division, necrosis
    - Keratin, intercellular desmosomes ("bridges")
  - Large cell carcinoma
    - Round or polygonal cells, prominent nucleoli, pale cytoplasm; none of these features is associated with other lung carcinomas
- Special stains
  - Periodic acid-Schiff (PAS) staining for non-small cell lung cancer
  - Intracytoplasmic mucin on PAS in cases of BAC

NON-SMALL CELL LUNG CANCER

Routes of Spread

- Local extension
  - Direct extension from tumor to surrounding tissues/ organs
  - Most commonly involves
    - Pleura
      - Most frequently results in pleural metastases in caudal and posterior parts of pleural cavities
    - Chest wall
    - Vertebral body
    - Esophagus
    - Great vessels
    - Thymus
    - Pericardium/heart
  - Spread into airways is rare
- Lymphatic spread
  - Through lymphatic system to neighboring or distant lymph nodes
  - Lymphangitic spread can be associated with hematogenous dissemination
    - Followed by invasion of adjacent interstitium and lymphatics
    - Subsequent tumor spread toward hila or lung periphery
  - Most commonly involve hilar, subcarinal, and pretracheal regions
- Distant metastases
  - Pulmonary veins are common route for metastases
    - Rich vascular supply draining directly into systemic venous system
  - Spread via bronchial arteries may be responsible for some endobronchial metastases

IMAGING

Detection

- **Chest x-ray**
  - Solitary pulmonary nodule
    - May be relatively well marginated, appears as rounded lung opacity
    - Diameter < 3 cm
    - Ill-defined or spiculated margin
    - Thick-walled cavity
    - All patterns of calcification, except eccentric or scattered punctate (stippled) calcification, are associated with benign lesion
  - Hilar mass
    - Central bronchogenic carcinomas manifest as added opacity in hilar region
    - Infiltration of lymphatics may be demonstrated as linear opacities radiating from hilar mass into lung periphery
  - Nonresolving pneumonia
    - Ill-defined homogeneous or patchy consolidation in segmental or nonsegmental distribution
    - Air bronchograms and air alveolograms can be seen with adenocarcinoma and bronchoalveolar carcinoma
  - Bronchial stenosis
    - Endobronchial lesion commonly leads to partial or complete lobar atelectasis
    - Common because most non-small cell carcinomas demonstrate intraluminal growth
    - Narrowing of main bronchi or complete cut-off can be identified
  - Regional hyperlucency
    - Hypoxic vasoconstriction reduces lung perfusion, and attenuation is seen as hyperlucency
    - Endobronchial lesion reduces ventilation despite normal or increased air volume
  - Mediastinal lymph node enlargement
    - Widened mediastinum
    - Right paratracheal stripe increase
    - Convex margin of mediastinum
    - Absence of concavity in aortopulmonary window
    - Splaying of carina
  - Used less often now due to use of CT scans
- CECT (contrast-enhanced CT)
  - Adenocarcinoma
    - Nodule (spiculated, lobulated), pleural tail
    - Peripheral nodule with ill-defined, irregular, and spiculated border is malignant in > 90% of patients
    - CT densitometry may help in differentiating between benign and malignant lesions
  - BAC
    - Ground-glass opacity (GGO); solid; mixed/ semisolid (solid and GGO); air bronchograms/ cystic or bubbly lucency
    - Features that favor malignancy
      - > 1 cm, increasing size, increase in solid component of mixed lesion
      - Development of solid component in prior GGO
      - Coarse spiculation
      - Round shape
  - SCCa
    - Nodule, characteristically cavitary (especially with wall thickness > 15 mm)
  - Large cell carcinoma
    - Large, peripheral mass with necrosis

Staging

- **CECT**: Thorax to adrenal glands with inclusion of liver
  - Evaluate extent of primary tumor
    - Size
    - Proximal extent of tumor (usually confirmed by bronchoscopy)
    - Invasion of main bronchus, visceral pleura, associated atelectasis/obstructive pneumonia (part of lung)
    - Invasion of chest wall, diaphragm, mediastinal pleura, parietal pericardium, extension into main bronchus < 2 cm distal to carina, associated atelectasis/pneumonitis (entire lung)
    - Findings favoring chest wall invasion on CT
      - > 3 cm of tumor-pleura contact
      - Obtuse angle of tumor-pleura interface
      - Thickened pleura
      - Hyperattenuation of extrapleural fat
      - Sensitivity and specificity of CT for chest wall invasion: 63-90% and 84-86%, respectively; similar to MR
    - Subtle mediastinal invasion suggested by
      - Tumor-mediastinal contact > 3 cm
      - Obliteration of fat plane between tumor and mediastinum
      - Tumor extending > 90° of aortic circumference

NON-SMALL CELL LUNG CANCER

- Sensitivity and specificity of CT for subtle mediastinal invasion: 56-89% and 50-93%, respectively; similar to MR
  - Invasion of heart, great vessels, trachea, esophagus, vertebral body, carina
  - Pleural/pericardial effusion
    - Malignancy should be confirmed with cytology
  - Presence of separate tumor nodules
- Nodal disease
  - Size criteria
    - Mediastinal lymph nodes (LNs) > 10 mm (> 13-15 mm subcarinal) more likely malignant
    - Retrocrural, paraaortic, pericardial LN > 8 mm more likely malignant
  - If meets size criteria, grade based on location
  - Sensitivity and specificity of CT in predicting mediastinal lymphadenopathy: 51% and 86%, respectively
- Distant metastases
  - Lung
    - Tumor in contralateral lung
    - Tumor with pleural nodules
    - Malignant pleural/pericardial effusion
  - Adrenal gland
    - Malignancy favored if > 3 cm, poorly defined margin, irregular rim enhancement, invasion of adjacent structures
    - Benign etiology favored if attenuation values are < 10 HU on CT (sensitivity 71%, specificity 98%)
  - Bone
    - Vertebral bodies, ribs, pelvis, proximal appendicular skeleton
    - Osteolytic lesions more common than osteoblastic
    - CT alone insufficient to exclude bone metastases

- **PET/CT**
  - In patients with biopsy-confirmed carcinoma, hypermetabolic activity highly specific for additional sites of malignant disease can improve staging accuracy by 20%
    - For mediastinal nodal staging, sensitivity is 0.84 and specificity is 0.89
  - Brain metastasis best evaluated with MR due to sensitivity/resolution limits of PET for small lesions
    - However, PET can detect unsuspected brain metastases, especially those ~ 1.5 cm or larger
  - Adrenals: Compare hypermetabolic activity to liver
    - If greater activity than liver, most likely metastasis
  - Note: BAC and carcinoid often show minimal activity on PET; staging/restaging with PET may be inaccurate
- **MR**
  - Chest
    - Helpful for determining chest wall and mediastinal invasion with sensitivity/specificity similar to CT
    - Useful to evaluate for cardiac invasion
    - Used to determine extent of involvement of brachial plexus, subclavian vessels, vertebral bodies
      - Subclavian vessel or carotid/vertebral artery invasion often precludes surgery
      - Absolute surgical contraindications: Invasion of brachial plexus roots/trunks above T1; invasion of > 50% vertebral body; invasion of esophagus/trachea
    - Not part of routine staging work-up of lung cancer
  - Brain
    - MR most sensitive to detect brain metastasis
  - Adrenals
    - Useful if CT or PET findings are equivocal
- **Radionuclide bone scan**
  - Provides images of extremities that may be missed on other imaging
  - Often used to evaluate new-onset bone pain in patient with cancer diagnosis but not necessary if PET already obtained
    - Can be associated with elevated laboratory values of serum calcium &/or alkaline phosphatase levels
- **Transthoracic percutaneous fine-needle aspiration**
  - Less invasive than bronchoscopy
  - Reserved for accessible tumors
    - Those tumors not accessible via bronchoscope
  - Via CT-fluoro guidance
- **Thoracentesis**
  - Presence of malignant pleural effusion upstages disease to M1a
    - For adequate staging, pleural effusions should be aspirated and examined for malignant cells if no other sites of distant spread are identified
  - Therapeutic thoracentesis provides symptomatic relief in patients with large pleural effusions

Restaging

- Monitoring tumor response to evaluate efficacy of chemo &/or radiation therapy (RT)
- CT represents primary imaging modality; however, PET more accurate in detecting residual and recurrent neoplasm
- Response evaluation criteria in solid tumors (RECIST)
  - Unidimensional measurements
  - Presence of at least 1 measurable lesion at baseline
  - For MDCT scanners, minimum size of lesion may be 10 mm, provided that 10 mm collimation is used and reconstructions are performed at 5 mm intervals
- World Health Organization (WHO)
  - Bidimensional measurements

CLINICAL PRESENTATION & WORK-UP

Presentation

- More common in men than in women
  - Increasing prevalence in women and younger patients
  - Risk of developing lung cancer remains higher among men over age 40
- Symptoms due to primary tumor
  - Central tumors are generally squamous cell carcinomas
    - Cough, dyspnea, wheezing, and hemoptysis
  - Most peripheral tumors are adenocarcinomas or large cell carcinomas
    - Cough and dyspnea
    - Can cause symptoms due to pleural effusion and severe pain as result of infiltration of parietal pleura and chest wall
- Usually advanced disease at presentation
  - Aggressive disease

- Low-dose CT screening can detect early cancers and reduce mortality
- Advanced intrathoracic disease, extrathoracic metastases

- Nonspecific or no symptoms until advanced disease
- Hoarseness due to recurrent laryngeal nerve involvement
- Superior vena cava syndrome
  - Obstruction of blood flow to heart from head and neck regions and upper extremities due to tumor compression of superior vena cava
    - Early physical findings: Facial edema, dusky skin coloration, and, possibly, conjunctival edema
    - Late physical findings: Upper extremity edema and prominent upper chest wall veins with retrograde flow
- Pancoast syndrome
  - Pain of shoulder and arm, atrophy of hand muscles, Horner syndrome
  - From tumor of superior pulmonary sulcus (uppermost extent of costovertebral recess)
    - Tumor centered on 2nd rib or lower is not Pancoast tumor
  - Superior rib tumor invasion
    - Causes shoulder pain
  - Compression of brachial plexus roots
    - Causes intense, radiating neuropathic arm pain and muscle atrophy in ipsilateral upper extremity
  - Horner syndrome
    - Ipsilateral ptosis, miosis, enophthalmos, and anhidrosis (i.e., lack of sweating)
    - Cause by tumor invasion of stellate ganglion
- Liver, lung, bone metastases with associated morbidity
- Hypercoagulable state
- Anemia, thrombocytosis, leukocytosis
- Sites of distant metastasis
  - Brain: 47%
  - Bone: 36%
  - Liver: 22%
  - Adrenal glands: 15%
  - Body wall: 13%
  - Lung: 11%
  - Spleen: 6%

Prognosis

- Overall 5-year survival by clinical stage grouping
  - Stage IA: 50%
  - Stage IB: 43%
  - Stage IIA: 36%
  - Stage IIB: 25%
  - Stage IIIA: 19%
  - Stage IIIB: 7%
  - Stage IV: 2%

Work-Up

- Clinical
  - Complete history and physical exam, including smoking history and assessment of performance status and weight loss
  - Bronchoscopy can visualize proximal tracheobronchial tree to subsegmental level
    - Endobronchial ultrasound with biopsy
  - Mediastinoscopy is used to detect N2 and N3 disease; nodal levels sampled are levels 2 (R and L) and 4 (R and L)
    - Video-assisted thoracoscopic surgery (VATS) or Chamberlain procedure (anterior mediastinotomy) can be used to sample levels 5 and 6
  - Preoperative evaluation of pulmonary function
    - Desirable parameters: Forced expiratory volume at 1 second (FEV1) > 1.5 L for lobectomy, > 2 L for pneumonectomy
    - For borderline cases: Quantitative ventilation and perfusion scans to calculate predicted postop FEV1 to > 1.0 L; maximum oxygen consumption > 15 mL/kg/min; assessment by board-certified thoracic surgeon
    - Medically inoperable for lobectomy: FEV1 < 60% or < 1.2 L; diffusion capacity of lung for carbon monoxide (DLCO) < 60%
- Radiographic
  - CECT chest and abdomen, PET for all patients, MR brain for stage II or higher diseases, bone scan is rarely needed now with wide use of PET
- Laboratory
  - Pathology: Bronchoscopy for central lesions, CT-guided biopsy for peripheral lesions
  - CBC, metabolic panel including BUN and Cr, LFTs, alkaline phosphatase, and LDH

TREATMENT

Major Treatment Alternatives

- Surgery
  - Typically reserved for patients with no evidence of mediastinal disease or invasion of local organs
    - Stages I and II non-small cell lung cancers only
    - Patients with completely resectable primary tumors (i.e., T1 N0) have much better prognosis
  - Lobectomy
    - Helps preserve pulmonary function while allowing good resection
    - Hilar and other proximal tumors may require more extensive surgery, including pneumonectomy
  - Wedge resection/segmentectomy
    - Used in patients with poor pulmonary reserve, high-risk population
  - VATS
    - Minimally invasive, shorter hospital stay
    - Used for both diagnostic and therapeutic lung cancer surgery
    - Similar recurrence rates, 5-year and long-term overall survival (OS) as compared to open thoracotomies
    - Low perioperative morbidity and mortality
    - Less chest pain compared with open thoracotomy
    - More intraoperative bleeding
    - Better tolerated in older populations
  - Complications (perioperative mortality rate)
    - Pneumonectomy (6%)
    - Lobectomy (3%)
    - Segmentectomy (1%)
  - RT
    - Mainstay local treatment for inoperable/unresectable diseases
    - Response rate 70-90%
- Combined chemoradiation therapy (CRT)

- Current standard of care for locally advanced unresectable (stage III) or inoperable stages II/III NSCLC is concurrent CRT for patients with a good performance status
- Sequential CRT for those who cannot tolerate concurrent regimen
- Concurrent CRT provides better survival than sequential

- Systemic therapy: Chemotherapy
  - Chemo alone has no role in potentially curative therapy for NSCLC
    - NSCLC is only moderately sensitive to chemo, response rate < 30%
  - Cisplatin is cornerstone of most combination regimens studied in advanced non-small cell lung cancer
- Systemic therapy: Targeted therapy
  - Recent research efforts have focused heavily on identifying molecular targets
  - Response rate reaches 70%
  - Approved agents include erlotinib (for EGFR mutants) and crizotinib for ALK rearrangement

Major Treatment Roadblocks/ Contraindications

- Poor performance, severe comorbid conditions

Treatment Options by Stage

- Stages I-II, operable patients
  - Surgical resection ± adjuvant chemo is current standard of care
  - Lobectomy is generally considered optimum procedure
  - Patients with limited pulmonary reserve: More limited resection with either segmental or wedge resection
  - Early lung study group reported higher risk of local recurrence with more limited resection
  - After surgery
    - If positive margins in stage IA disease, re-resection is preferred or, alternatively, adjuvant radiation
    - If negative margins in stage IB or IIA (N0) disease, observe or consider adjuvant chemo for high-risk patients (including poorly differentiated tumors, vascular invasion, wedge resection, tumors > 4 cm, visceral pleural involvement, or unknown nodal status)
    - If positive margins in stage IB or IIA (N0) disease, consider re-resection ± adjuvant chemotherapy, or adjuvant radiation ± chemotherapy (for IIA or high-risk IB patients)
- Stages I-II, medically inoperable
  - Stereotactic body radiation therapy (SBRT) is standard of care for nodal negative early stage diseases
  - Conventional fractionated or hypofractionated high dose RT when SBRT is not available
  - SBRT delivers focal high-dose radiation precisely targeted to tumor
  - Biologically effective dose (BED) ≥ 100 Gy provides 90% of local tumor control
  - High conformal plan is essential
  - Tumor motion management is mandated
  - Image guidance during treatment delivery is required
  - SBRT is generally used for lesions < 5 cm in size
  - Larger lesions can be treated if normal tissue dose constraints are met
  - Peripheral lesions can be safely treated with fewer fractions (3 or 1)
  - Central lesions are treated with smaller fraction sizes (total of 4 or more)
  - Tumors involving chest wall are better treated with 5 fractions to ↓ risk of chest pain
- Stage IIIA
  - Marginally operable
    - Concurrent CRT (45 Gy), if no progression then surgery; otherwise boost to 63 Gy
  - Inoperable and stage IIIB
    - Concurrent CRT
- Stage IV
  - Chemotherapy
  - RT for palliation

Dose Response

- Dose response exists in stages I/II NSCLC, particularly in SBRT series
- Controversial RT dose-response relationship in locally advanced NSCLC
  - 60 Gy is better than 50 or 40 Gy (RTOG 7301): 3-year OS is 15% for 60 Gy group vs. 10% for 50 Gy and 6% for 40 Gy groups
    - Established 60 Gy as standard dose
  - Single institution studies (e.g., University of Michigan) showed positive dose response
  - RTOG secondary analysis demonstrated positive dose response with concurrent CRT
  - RTOG 0617 preliminary results reported inferior 1-year survival with 74 Gy

Standard Doses

- Typical dose and fractionation is 1.8-2.0 Gy per day to a total dose of 60-70 Gy for definitive treatment
- 45-50 Gy for preoperative treatment
- 50-54 Gy ± boost for positive margins or extranodal extension for postoperative treatment
- Commonly used SBRT doses
  - 25-34 Gy in 1 fx
  - 45-60 Gy in 3 fx
  - 48-50 Gy in 4 fx
  - 50-60 Gy in 5 fx
  - 60-70 Gy in 8-10 fx

Organs at Risk Parameters

- Spinal cord: Maximum dose to ≤ 45 Gy, or 36 Gy if b.i.d. fractionation
- Lung: Mean lung dose ≤ 20 Gy; volume receiving ≥ 20 Gy (V20) ≤ 30-35%
- Esophagus: Mean dose ≤ 34 Gy
- Heart: Limit 1/3 to ≤ 65 Gy
- Brachial plexus: Maximum dose to < 66 Gy

Common Techniques

- Radiation simulation
  - Simulation CT scans obtained in RT treatment position
  - Immobilization devices typically used include head rest, thorax board (arms-up position), alpha cradle, or vacuum bag, and knee fix

- Tumor motion secondary to respiration assessed at time of simulation with 4D CT to aid in treatment planning and target decision
- Respiratory motion, especially for technique requiring highly precise treatment such as SBRT, can be limited with active breathing control (ABC), abdominal compression devices, beam gating with respiratory cycle, or dynamic tumor tracking

- Treatment planning
  - GTV: Gross primary and nodal disease including nodes 1 cm or greater, or hypermetabolic on PET scan or positive on biopsy
  - CTV: GTV + 0.5-0.8 cm margin
  - PTV: CTV + 0.5-1.0 cm margin to account for setup error and respiratory motion

Landmark Trials

- Lung cancer screening
  - National lung screening trial: 53,454 patients at high risk for lung cancer; 3 annual screenings with low-dose CT vs. single-view PA x-ray
    - ↓ lung cancer mortality with CT screening of 20% (P = 0.004)
- SBRT
  - RTOG 0236 phase II trial: 55 patients; T1-3 N0, inoperable; dose = 60 Gy in 3 fractions
    - Results: 3-year tumor control rate 97.6%, 3-year OS 55.8%
- CRT ± surgery
  - Intergroup 0139: 396 patients with stage T1-3 pN2 disease; CRT, then either surgery or more CRT
    - Median OS: 23.6 months with surgery vs. 22.2 months without surgery (P = .24)
    - For lobectomy patients, median OS is 33.6 months vs. 21.7 months for matched set of NS patients
    - For pneumonectomy patients, median OS is 18.9 months with surgery vs. 29.4 months with CRT alone (NS)
    - CRT + resection for patients with resectable stage IIIA (N2) disease without need of pneumonectomy
- Sequential CRT is better than RT alone
  - CALGB 8433: 155 patients with stage IIIA/B disease; chemo (cisplatin and vinblastine) followed by RT (60 Gy in 2 Gy per fx) vs. RT alone
    - Median OS: 13.7 months with CRT vs. 9.6 months with RT (P = 0.012)
  - RTOG 8808 (Sause et al, 2000): 458 patients with stage II, IIA/B disease; chemo followed by RT (60 Gy in 2 Gy per fx) vs. same RT alone vs. hyperfractionated RT alone
    - CRT superior to other 2 arms (P = 0.04)
- Concurrent CRT is better than sequential CRT
  - RTOG 9410: 577 patients with unresectable stages II and IIIA/B disease
    - Randomized to 1) concurrent chemo with RT (63 Gy), 2) sequential chemo followed by RT, or 3) concurrent oral chemo with hyperfractionated RT b.i.d.
    - Median OS: 17 months concurrent vs. 14.6 months sequential vs. 15.6 months hyperfractionated
  - Auperin meta-analysis: 6 randomized trials of 1,205 patients comparing concurrent to sequential CRT
  - Significant benefit in locoregional control favoring concurrent
  - Survival benefit: 5.7% at 3 years, 4.5% at 5 years
  - Grade 3-4 esophagitis increased from 4-18%
  - Pneumonitis no differences between 2 arms
- Lack of benefit of consolidation chemotherapy
  - Hoosier trial (Hanna et al): Randomized 203 patients with stage IIIA/B disease to consolidation chemo (docetaxel) x 3 cycles after CRT vs. CRT alone
    - Results showed no benefit with consolidation
- Lack of benefit of induction chemotherapy
  - CALGB 39801 trial: Randomized 366 patients with stage IIIA/B disease to induction chemo followed by CRT vs. CRT alone
    - Results showed no benefit to induction chemo
- Postoperative radiation
  - Adjuvant Navelbine International Trialists Association (ANITA) trial
    - 840 patients with completely resected stages IB-IIIA disease; adjuvant chemo (cisplatin and vinorelbine) vs. observation; postoperative radiation therapy (PORT) was recommended for N2 disease (45-50 Gy over 5 weeks) per treating physician
      - Chemo significantly ↑ OS; median: 65.7 months of chemotherapy vs. 43.7 months of no chemotherapy
      - PORT ↓ survival in N0/N1 disease
      - PORT improved survival in all N2 patients, ± chemotherapy
  - SEER analysis of PORT showed ↓ survival in N0/N1 but improved survival in N2 disease
  - PORT meta-analysis demonstrated detrimental effect for N0/N1 disease, borderline improvement in survival in N0 patients
- Clinical trials
  - RTOG 0617: 423 patients with stage IIIA/B disease; 60 Gy vs. 74 Gy, ± cetuximab to chemo
    - Trial closed prematurely for high dose arm due to inferior 1-year survival, mature results awaited
  - RTOG 1106: Phase II randomized study to assess benefit of individualized adaptive RT dose escalation

Radiation Complications

- Acute complications
  - Severe radiation pneumonitis can be lethal, thus dose limiting
    - Begins 1-3 months after completing treatment
    - Symptoms and signs
      - Nonproductive cough, dyspnea on exertion, low-grade fever, chest pain, malaise, weight loss
      - Physical exam may show crackles, pleural rub, or pleural effusions
      - On x-ray and CT, diffuse haziness with sharp edges that do not follow anatomic borders
      - Pulmonary function testing: Reduction in lung volumes, DLCO, and lung compliance
      - Diagnosis should exclude tumor progression, infection, or other known etiology
    - Lung dosimetric factors have been shown to be predictive factor in development of radiation pneumonitis; NCCN recommends V20 of ≤ 30%, mean lung dose ≤ 20 Gy
    - Treatment includes corticosteroids (i.e., prednisone) at least 60 mg/day for 2-4 weeks and tapered slowly over 3-12 weeks; pentoxifylline may be used

- Esophagitis: Acute RTOG grade 3+ esophagitis seen in ~ 15-20% of concurrent CRT patients and 5% of sequential CRT patients, according to randomized trials
- Pericarditis/pericardial effusion: More commonly seen in patients treated with concurrent chemo
- Fatigue: 80-90% patients
- Skin irritation: Less common now with use of megavoltage photons and 3D conformal technique

- Late complications
  - Radiation fibrosis can be seen 6-24 months after completing radiation; patients can present with fibrosis without pneumonitis
  - Radiographic fibrosis visible in majority of patients
  - Bronchial stenosis/collapsed lung occur in < 5% of patients
  - Esophageal constricture requires dilatation in < 1% of patients
  - Late heart toxicity from lung cancer radiation is poorly defined, probably underreported
  - Rib fracture related to local radiation dose; small risk overall (< 1% per year)
  - Development of secondary malignancy from radiation, usually > 10 years after treatment within treated field

RECOMMENDED FOLLOW-UP

Clinical

- H&P every 3-6 months for 2 years, then annually thereafter
- Smoking cessation advice, counseling, and pharmacotherapy as indicated

Radiographic

- Chest CT ± contrast every 3-6 months for 2 years, then chest NECT annually thereafter
- PET scan or brain MR not indicated for routine follow-up

Laboratory

- As clinically indicated

SELECTED REFERENCES

1. Curran WJ Jr et al: Sequential vs. concurrent chemoradiation for stage III non-small cell lung cancer: randomized phase III trial RTOG 9410. J Natl Cancer Inst. 2011 Oct 5;103(19):1452-60. Epub 2011 Sep 8. Erratum in: J Natl Cancer Inst. 104(1):79, 2012
2. Siegel R et al: Cancer statistics, 2012. CA Cancer J Clin. 62(1):10-29, 2012
3. Kong FM et al: Consideration of dose limits for organs at risk of thoracic radiotherapy: atlas for lung, proximal bronchial tree, esophagus, spinal cord, ribs, and brachial plexus. Int J Radiat Oncol Biol Phys. 81(5):1442-57, 2011
4. National Lung Screening Trial Research Team et al: Reduced lung-cancer mortality with low-dose computed tomographic screening. N Engl J Med. 365(5):395-409, 2011
5. Volterrani L et al: MSCT multi-criteria: a novel approach in assessment of mediastinal lymph node metastases in non-small cell lung cancer. Eur J Radiol. 79(3):459-66, 2011
6. Almeida FA et al: Initial evaluation of the nonsmall cell lung cancer patient: diagnosis and staging. Curr Opin Pulm Med. 16(4):307-14, 2010
7. American Joint Committee on Cancer: AJCC Cancer Staging Manual. 7th ed. New York: Springer. 253-70, 2010
8. Aupérin A et al: Meta-analysis of concomitant versus sequential radiochemotherapy in locally advanced non-small-cell lung cancer. J Clin Oncol. 28(13):2181-90, 2010
9. Grills IS et al: Outcomes after stereotactic lung radiotherapy or wedge resection for stage I non-small-cell lung cancer. J Clin Oncol. 28(6):928-35, 2010
10. Kligerman S et al: A radiologic review of the new TNM classification for lung cancer. AJR Am J Roentgenol. 2010 Mar;194(3):562-73. Review. Erratum in: AJR Am J Roentgenol. 194(5):1404, 2010
11. Timmerman R et al: Stereotactic body radiation therapy for inoperable early stage lung cancer. JAMA. 303(11):1070-6, 2010
12. Albain KS et al: Radiotherapy plus chemotherapy with or without surgical resection for stage III non-small-cell lung cancer: a phase III randomised controlled trial. Lancet. 374(9687):379-86, 2009
13. Hicks RJ: Role of 18F-FDG PET in assessment of response in non-small cell lung cancer. J Nucl Med. 50 Suppl 1:31S-42S, 2009
14. Hanna N et al: Phase III study of cisplatin, etoposide, and concurrent chest radiation with or without consolidation docetaxel in patients with inoperable stage III non-small-cell lung cancer: the Hoosier Oncology Group and U.S. Oncology. J Clin Oncol. 26(35):5755-60, 2008
15. Chapet O: [Acute and late toxicities in thoracic irradiation.] Cancer Radiother. 11(1-2):92-100, 2007
16. Gould MK et al: Evaluation of patients with pulmonary nodules: when is it lung cancer?: ACCP evidence-based clinical practice guidelines (2nd edition). Chest. 132(3 Suppl):108S-130S, 2007
17. Raz DJ et al: Natural history of stage I non-small cell lung cancer: implications for early detection. Chest. 132(1):193-9, 2007
18. Vokes EE et al: Induction chemotherapy followed by chemoradiotherapy compared with chemoradiotherapy alone for regionally advanced unresectable stage III Non-small-cell lung cancer: Cancer and Leukemia Group B. J Clin Oncol. 25(13):1698-704, 2007
19. Yuan S et al: A randomized study of involved-field irradiation versus elective nodal irradiation in combination with concurrent chemotherapy for inoperable stage III nonsmall cell lung cancer. Am J Clin Oncol. 30(3):239-44, 2007
20. Baumann P et al: Factors important for efficacy of stereotactic body radiotherapy of medically inoperable stage I lung cancer. A retrospective analysis of patients treated in the Nordic countries. Acta Oncol. 45(7):787-95, 2006
21. Douillard JY et al: Adjuvant vinorelbine plus cisplatin versus observation in patients with completely resected stage IB-IIIA non-small-cell lung cancer (Adjuvant Navelbine International Trialist Association [ANITA]): a randomised controlled trial. Lancet Oncol. 2006 Sep;7(9):719-27. Erratum in: Lancet Oncol. 7(10):797, 2006
22. Kong FM et al: Final toxicity results of a radiation-dose escalation study in patients with non-small-cell lung cancer (NSCLC): predictors for radiation pneumonitis and fibrosis. Int J Radiat Oncol Biol Phys. 65(4):1075-86, 2006
23. Vansteenkiste JF: FDG-PET for lymph node staging in NSCLC: a major step forward, but beware of the pitfalls. Lung Cancer. 47(2):151-3, 2005
24. Giraud P et al: Conformal radiotherapy for lung cancer: different delineation of the gross tumor volume (GTV) by radiologists and radiation oncologists. Radiother Oncol. 62(1):27-36, 2002
25. Postoperative radiotherapy in non-small-cell lung cancer: systematic review and meta-analysis of individual patient data from nine randomised controlled trials: PORT Meta-analysis Trialists Group. Lancet. 352(9124):257-63, 1998

Stage IA (T1a N0 M0)

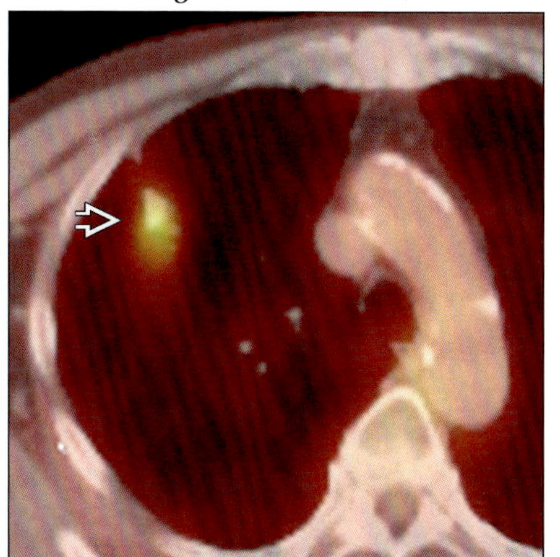

Stage IA (T1a N0 M0)

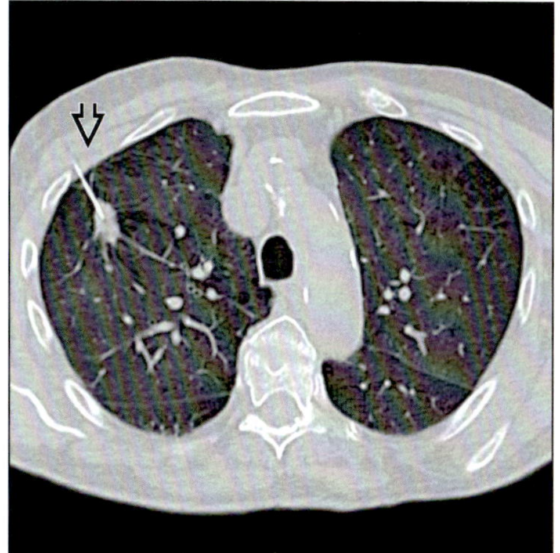

*(**Left**) Axial fused PET/CT shows increased FDG activity in anterior right upper lobe ➡, correlating with a primary lung tumor no larger than 2 cm. Given its size and lack of adenopathy, this lesion was staged as IA. PET is very useful in evaluating solitary pulmonary nodules. (**Right**) Axial CT in the same patient shows CT-guided biopsy of right upper lobe nodule ⇨. Non-small cell carcinoma was subsequently diagnosed.*

Stage IB (T2a N0 M0)

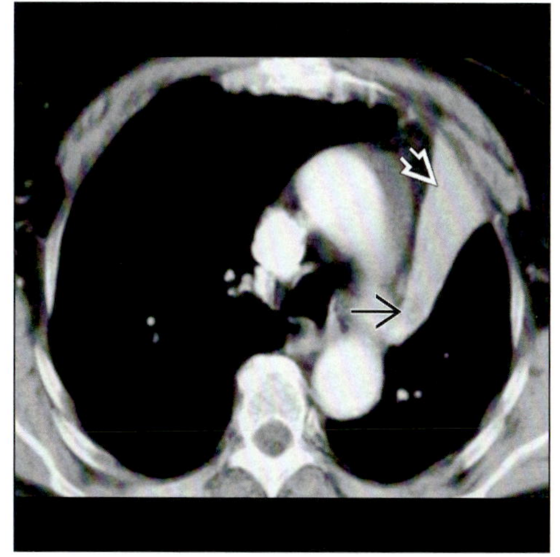

Stage IB (T2a N0 M0)

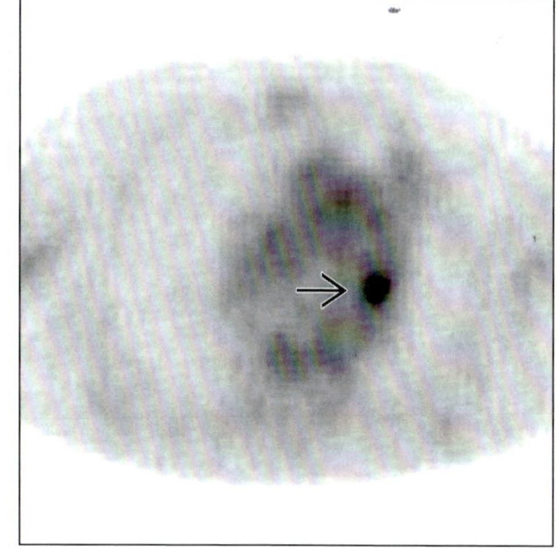

*(**Left**) Axial CECT shows a centrally located primary neoplasm →. Note extensive postobstructive pneumonitis ➡ that extends from the hilum, involving the majority of lingula. Since the lesion was > 3 cm, this is T2a N0, stage IB. (**Right**) Axial PET in the same patient shows rounded FDG activity in the left hilum →, corresponding with primary lung neoplasm. PET can aid in distinguishing tumor from atelectasis in some cases.*

Stage IB (T2a N0 M0)

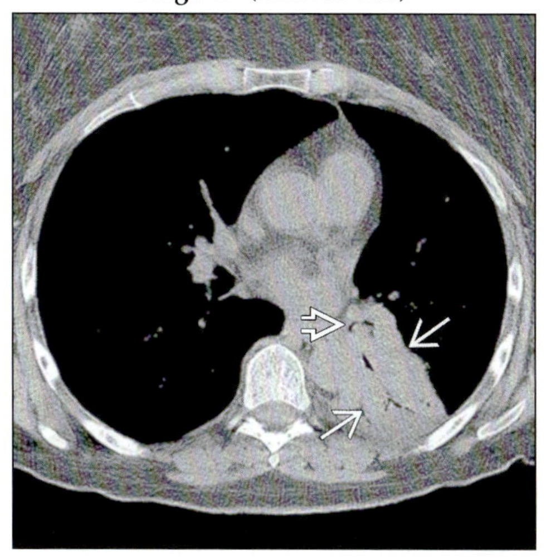

Stage IB (T2a N0 M0)

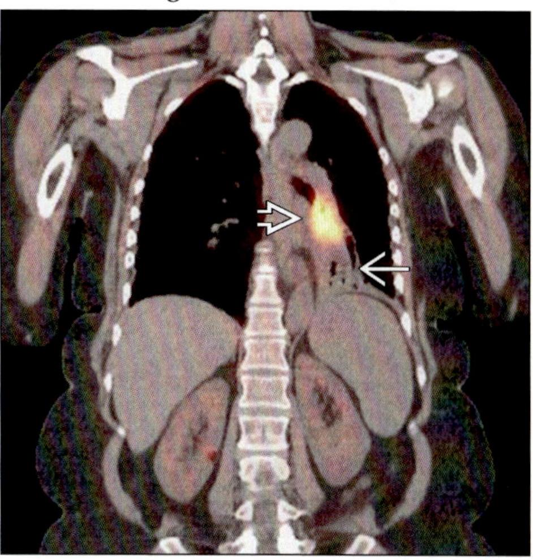

*(**Left**) Axial NECT from HRCT shows proximal left lower lobe endobronchial neoplasm ➡. Tumor causes complete left lower lobe collapse ➡. Findings correspond to stage IB primary lung cancer. (**Right**) Coronal fused PET/CT in the same patient shows focal increased FDG activity ➡ that correlates with endobronchial lesion discovered on prior image. Again, note left lower lobe collapse ➡ that is not FDG avid. Diagnosis was made via endobronchial biopsy.*

NON-SMALL CELL LUNG CANCER

(Left) Axial CECT shows mild enhancement of the centrally located, round nodule ➡ that proved to be endobronchial in origin. This is a typical CECT appearance of carcinoid. Diagnosis was made via endobronchial biopsy. Since it was < 2 cm, this was a T1a lesion. *(Right)* Typical simulation CT setup for lung treatment is shown, utilizing a thorax board with arms situated above the head. 4D scans are preferred in definitive cases.

Stage IA (T1a N0 M0)

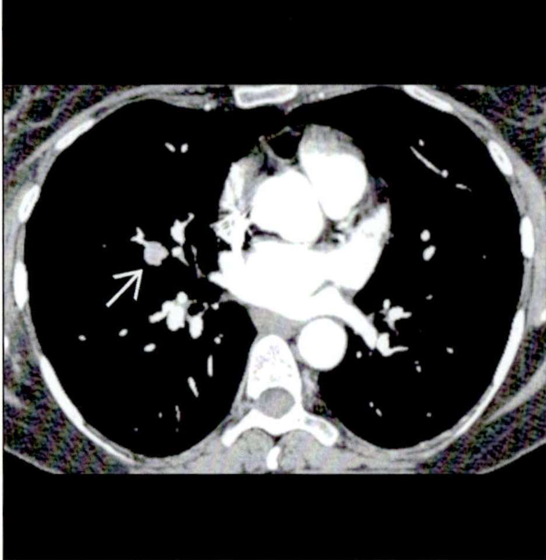

Simulation

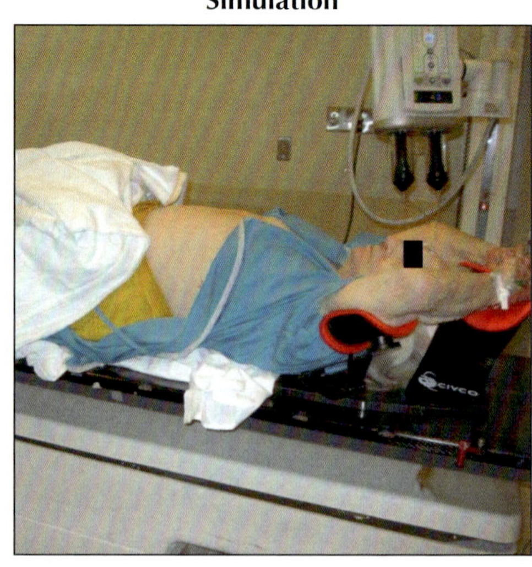

(Left) Contouring atlas for thoracic structures is shown in axial view. Representative GTVs = gross tumor/nodal volumes as defined by CT &/or PET. DA = descending aorta, AA = ascending aorta, PA = pulmonary artery, and SVC = superior vena cava. *(Right)* Contouring atlas for thoracic structures is shown in coronal view.

Contouring of Mediastinal Structures

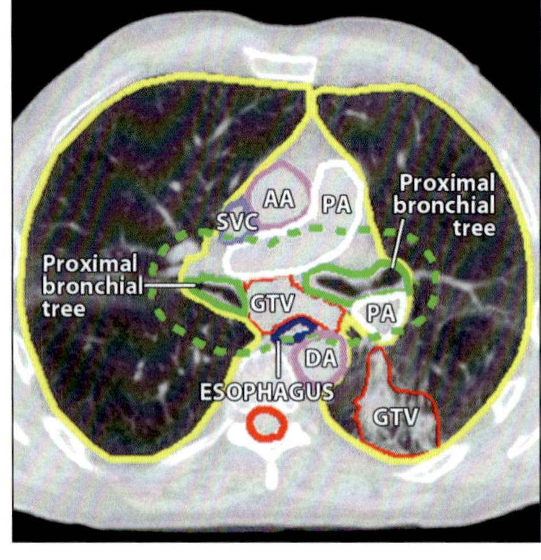

Contouring of Mediastinal Structures

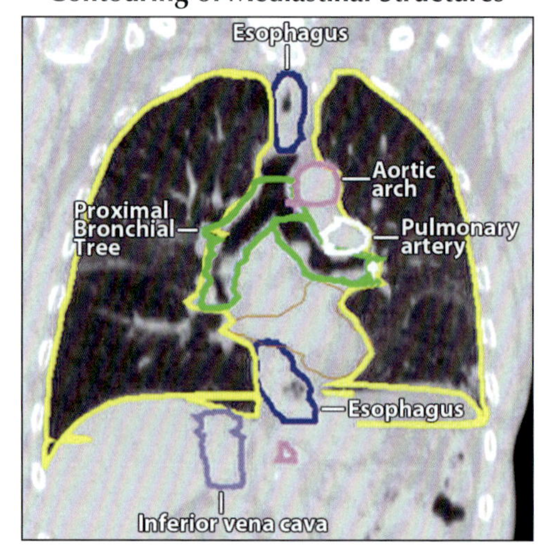

(Left) Multileaf collimators shape each beam, seen here as "beam's eye view" (each oriented perpendicular to the target). Non-coplanar fields can assist in reducing high-dose regions. *(Right)* CTV (yellow) and uniformly expanded PTV (pink) are shown for a resected T3 N0 adenocarcinoma of the right upper lung (RUL). There was a positive margin at the mediastinum (marked by surgical clips ➡).

3D Planning

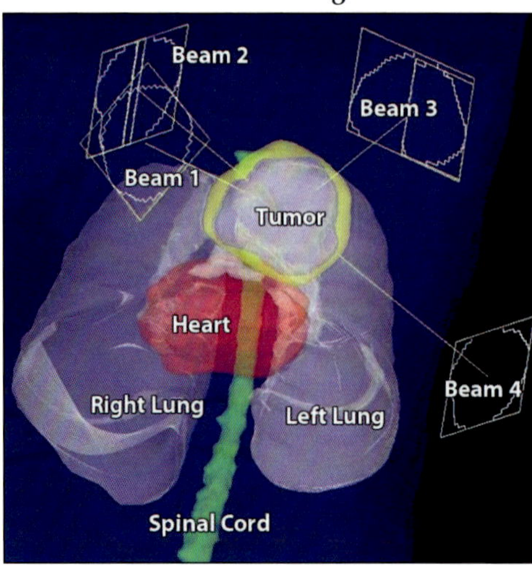

CTV Contouring

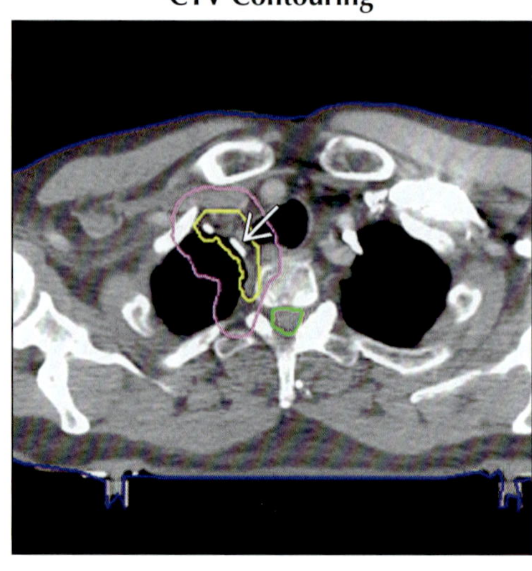

Stage IA (T1 N0) Adenocarcinoma

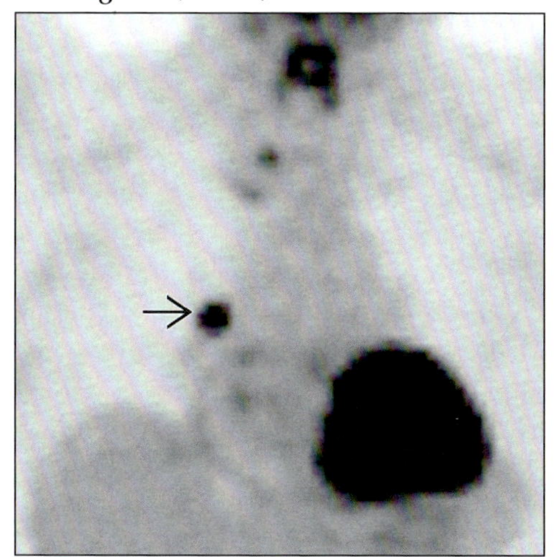

Stage IA (T1 N0) Adenocarcinoma

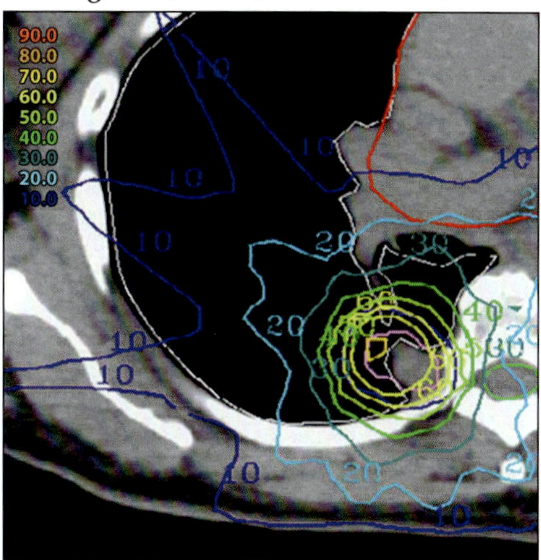

(Left) Patient with a T1 N0 right lower lobe adenocarcinoma ⇒ was an operative candidate but elected for RT instead. Pretreatment PET scan shows an intensely FDG-avid tumor. *(Right)* The same patient was treated with SBRT to a total dose of 55 Gy in 5 fractions. Treatment was prescribed to the 82% isodose line for the 1st 3 fractions and to the 80% isodose line for the last 2 fractions. Fourteen fields with 6 and 16 mV photons were used.

Stage IA (T1 N0) Adenocarcinoma

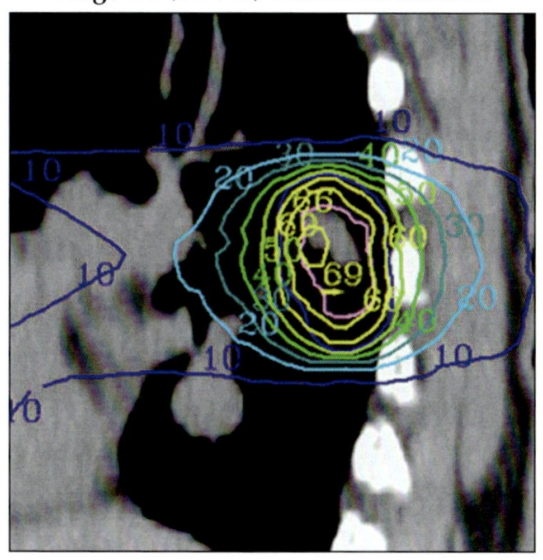

Stage IA (T1 N0) Adenocarcinoma

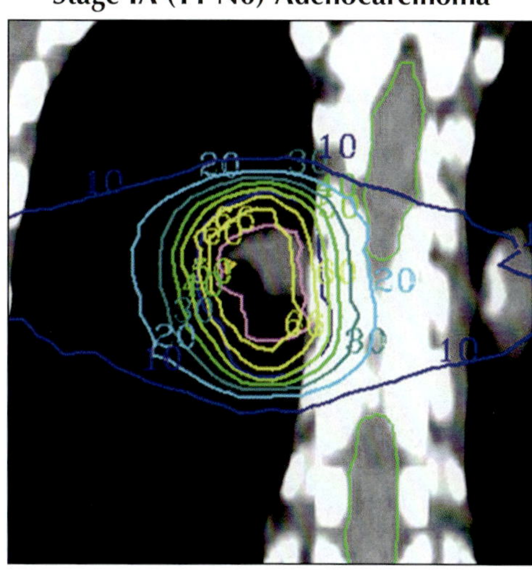

(Left) The same treatment plan is shown in sagittal view. Fourteen fields with 6 and 16 mV photons were used. 4D CT simulation and on-board cone beam were used for accurate tumor targeting. Representative isodose lines include inner yellow (66 Gy), outer yellow (60 Gy), light green (50 Gy), green (40 Gy), and light blue (20 Gy) lines. Due to proximity of chest wall, 5 fractions were used. *(Right)* The same treatment plan is shown in coronal view. 4D scan and ITV are essential in SBRT.

Stage IA (T1 N0) Adenocarcinoma

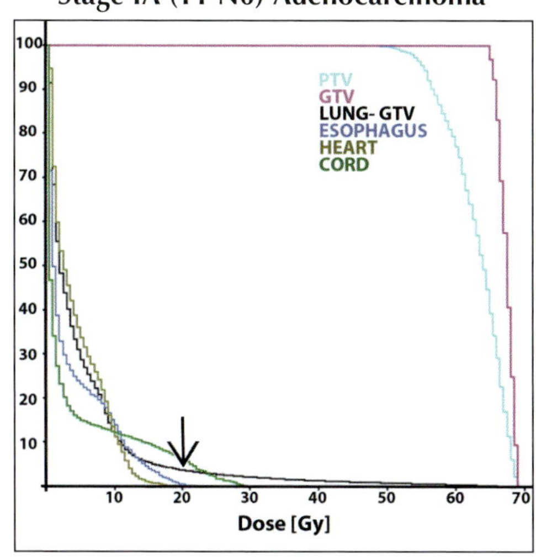

Stage IA (T1 N0) Adenocarcinoma

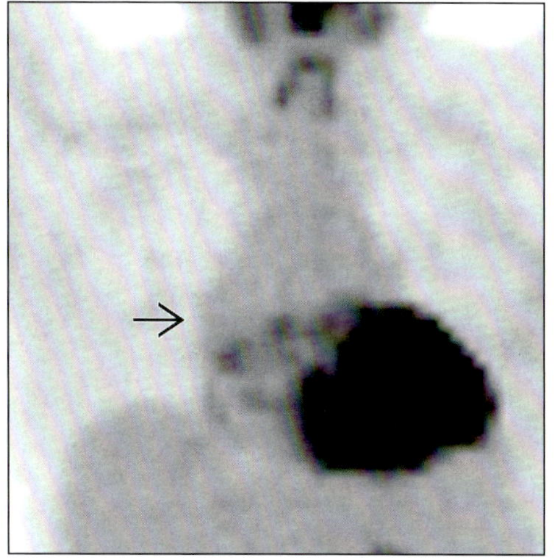

(Left) Dose volume histogram in the same patient shows that 3% of the total lung volume receives at least 20 Gy ⇒. Again, a significant hot spot (higher dose than prescribed) of radiation is seen in the center of PTV and GTV. *(Right)* Post-treatment PET scan in the same patient 8 months after treatment shows significantly decreased tumor activity ⇒. SBRT can provide local control in ~ 90% of lesions.

NON-SMALL CELL LUNG CANCER

*(**Left**) Pretreatment CT scan for another patient with an intensely FDG avid (not shown) shows a T1 N0 tumor in the right lower lobe ➔. Peripheral lesions like this are typically adenocarcinomas. (**Right**) The same patient received 60 Gy in 3 fractions using 6 and 16 mV photons with a 15-field arrangement. Axial view shows scattering of low-dose radiation through the thorax (dark blue regions at the periphery represent areas receiving approximately 6 Gy).*

Stage IA (T1 N0)

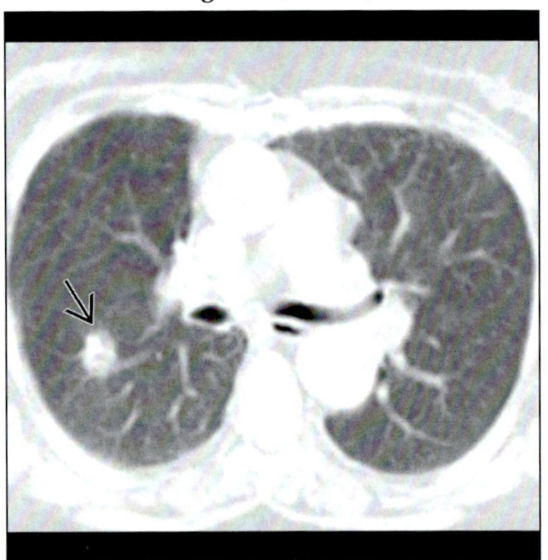

Stage IA (T1 N0)

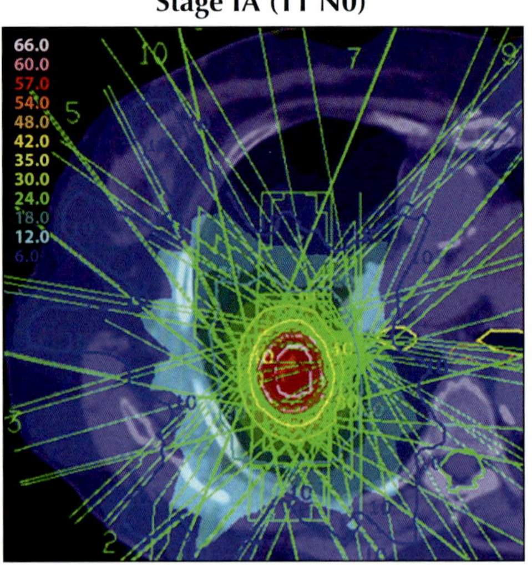

*(**Left**) Sagittal view of the same plan shows non-coplanar beams in a superior and inferior oblique arrangement. This aids in reducing high-dose regions. Three 20 Gy fractions were used since the lesion is not central and not near the chest wall. (**Right**) Dose volume histogram (DVH) in the same patient shows that 4% of the total lung volume receives at least 20 Gy ➔.*

Stage IA (T1 N0)

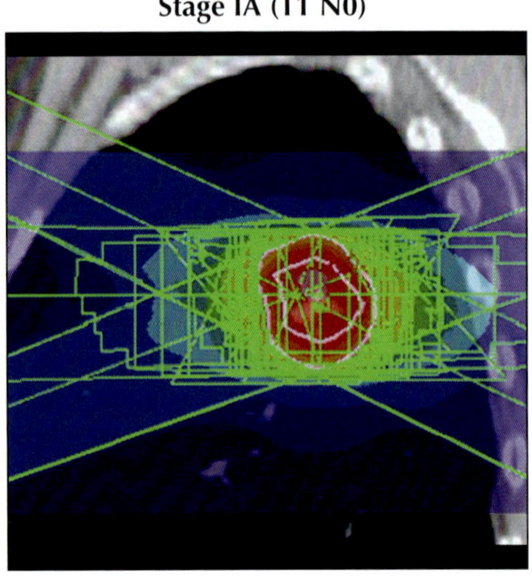

Stage IA (T1 N0)

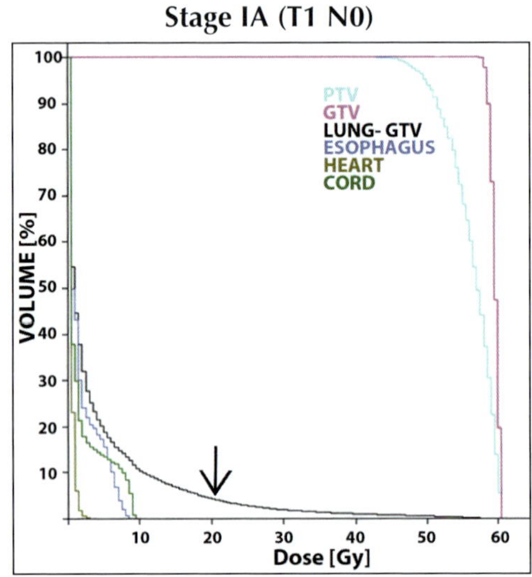

*(**Left**) Post-treatment CT scan in the same patient shows stability of the nodule ➔. The lesion was not avid on PET at this time (not shown). (**Right**) The same patient experienced no side effects until 1 year later when cough and shortness of breath developed. PFTs also showed significant reduction (DLCO 44%, initially 56%). The patient was started on prednisone with improvement of symptoms. On CT, an area of patchy airspace disease ➔ at the periphery of the right lung is seen.*

Stage IA (T1 N0)

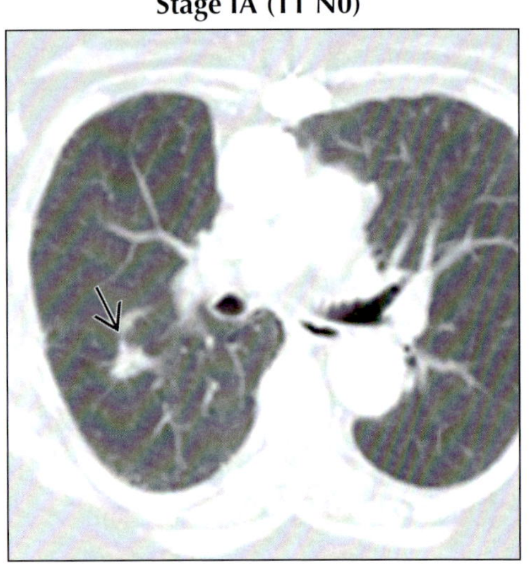

Stage IA (T1 N0)

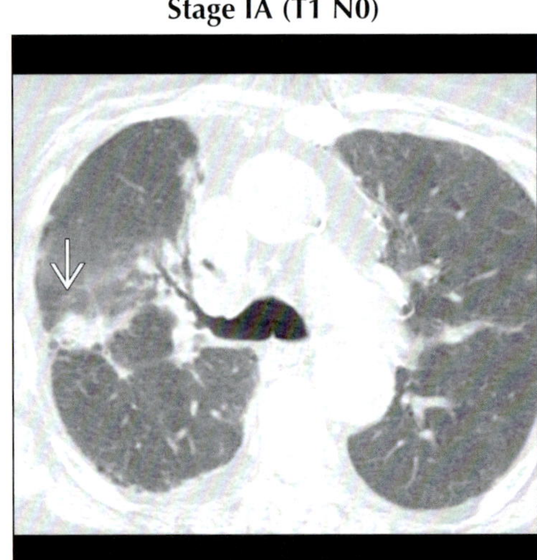

Stage IA (T1b N0) Adenocarcinoma

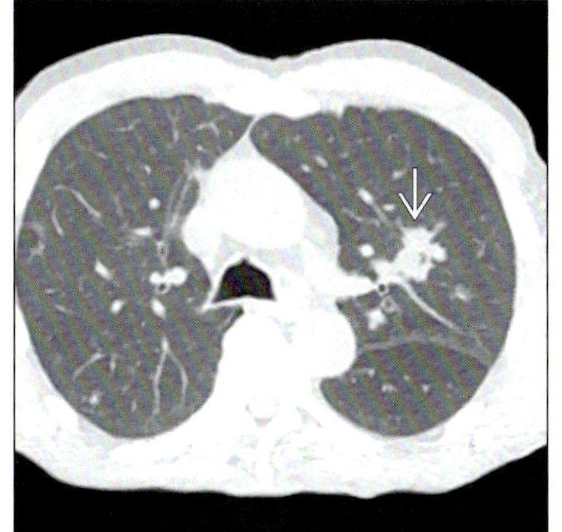

Stage IA (T1b N0) Adenocarcinoma

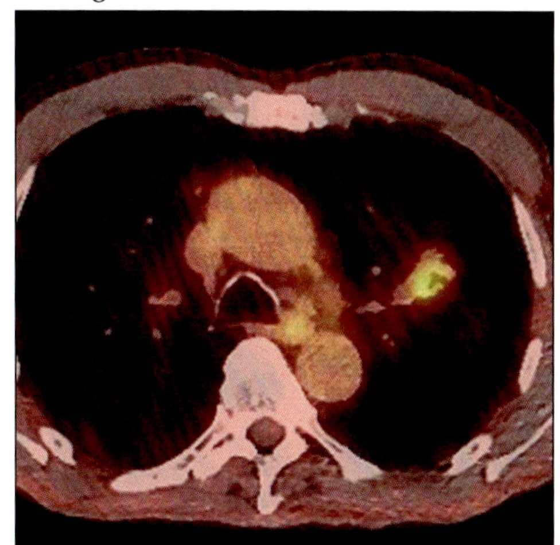

(Left) *Pretreatment CT shows a bilobed left upper lobe mass in a patient with an adenocarcinoma that is 2.7 cm in size ➔. Tumors > 2 cm but ≤ 3 cm are T1b.* ***(Right)*** *Corresponding fused pretreatment PET/CT in the same patient shows increased uptake in the mass with SUV of 2.6. PET scans are invaluable for ruling out distant disease. Staging accuracy increases by 20% with PET.*

Stage IA (T1b N0) Adenocarcinoma

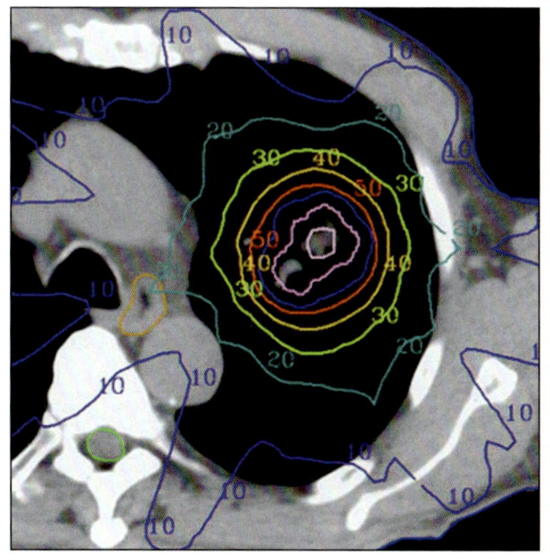

Stage IA (T1b N0) Adenocarcinoma

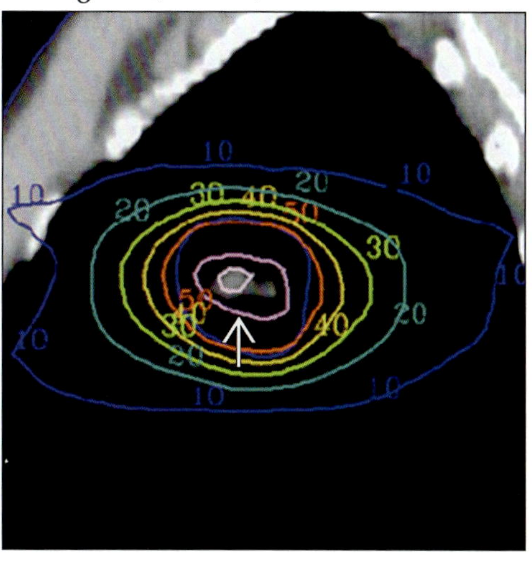

(Left) *In the same patient, SBRT treatment plan in axial view is shown. The plan was prescribed to a total dose of 54 Gy in 3 fractions to the 72% isodose line. Fourteen beams were used, achieving a conformality index of 1.072. Inner light pink is 60 Gy, dark pink is 54 Gy, red is 50 Gy, orange is 40 Gy, and green is 30 Gy.* ***(Right)*** *Sagittal view in the same patient shows the margin from the 60 Gy line (pink) ➔ to the GTV. Creation of an ITV by use of a 4D scan and image guidance ensures accuracy.*

Stage IA (T1b N0) Adenocarcinoma

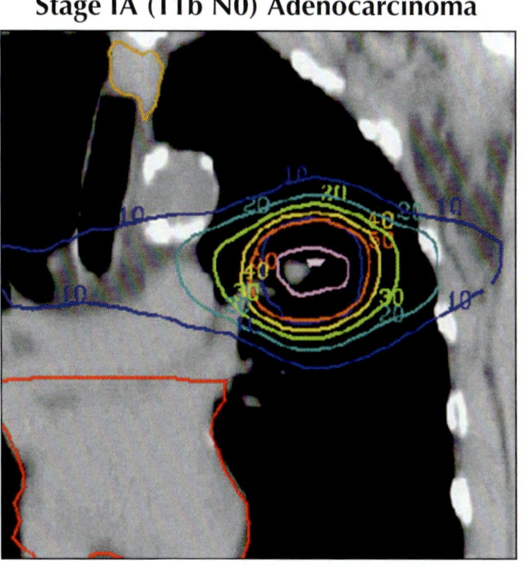

Stage IA (T1b N0) Adenocarcinoma

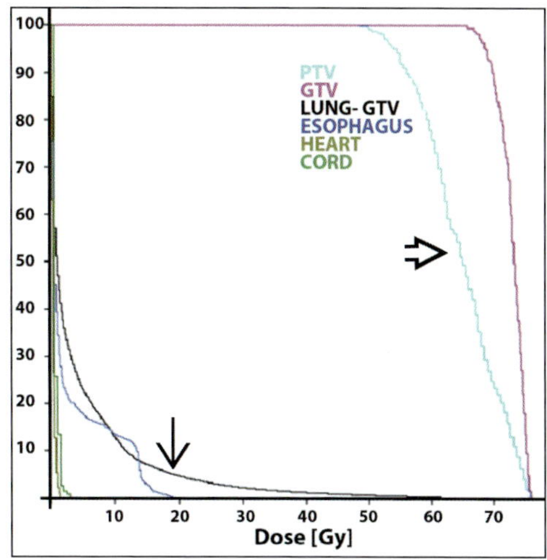

(Left) *Coronal view in the same patient demonstrates central left lung location; hence, 3 fractions were used.* ***(Right)*** *DVH in the same patient shows that 5% of the total lung volume receives 20 Gy (under the 10% limit for 3-fraction SBRT ➔). Also note that the PTV (light blue line ➩) is covered by a dose of 54 Gy, which is set as 72% of the maximum dose. The center of the PTV, especially the GTV, thus receives a very high dose of > 70 Gy.*

NON-SMALL CELL LUNG CANCER

*(**Left**) Coronal fused PET/CT shows a rounded mass ➔ invading the left chest wall and axilla. Central necrosis ➔ is seen. Central photopenia on PET is typical of necrosis. Chest wall involvement makes this T3. (**Right**) Axial NECT reveals left prevascular adenopathy ➔. A faint soft tissue nodule can also be seen in left upper lobe ➔. Despite small primary neoplasm, bulky ipsilateral mediastinal adenopathy (N2) indicates stage IIIA disease.*

Stage IIB (T3 N0 M0)

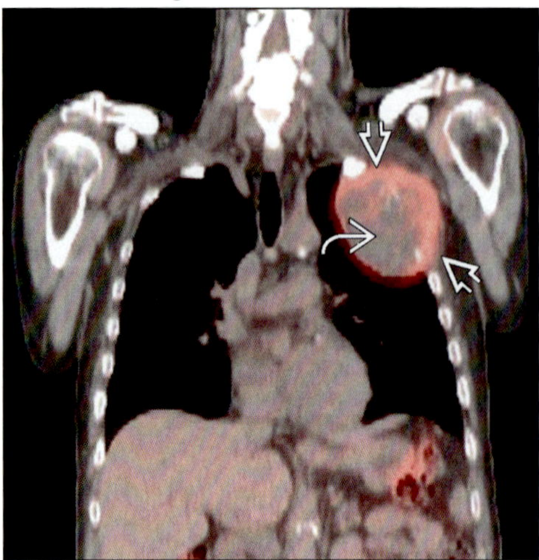

Stage IIIA (T1a N2 M0)

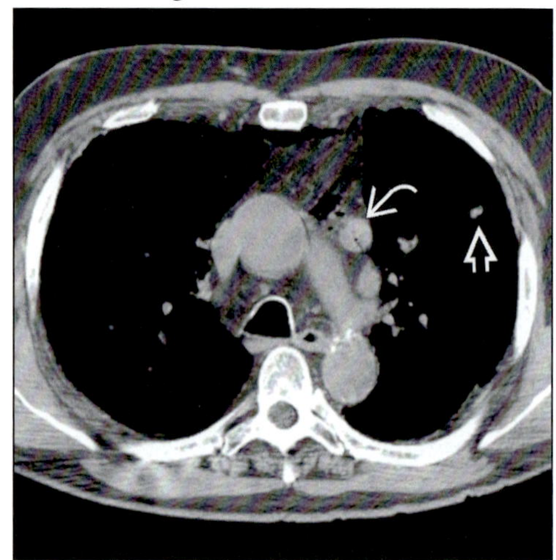

*(**Left**) Axial CECT shows an asymmetric soft tissue density in the right lung apex ➔. Superior sulcus tumor (Pancoast tumor) was subsequently diagnosed. (**Right**) Coronal T1WI MR in the same patient better delineates Pancoast tumor ➔. Also note degree of extension beyond chest wall ➔. Horner syndrome can result by involvement of the stellate ganglion causing meiosis, ptosis, anhydrosis, and enophthalmos.*

Stage IIIA (T3 N2 M0)

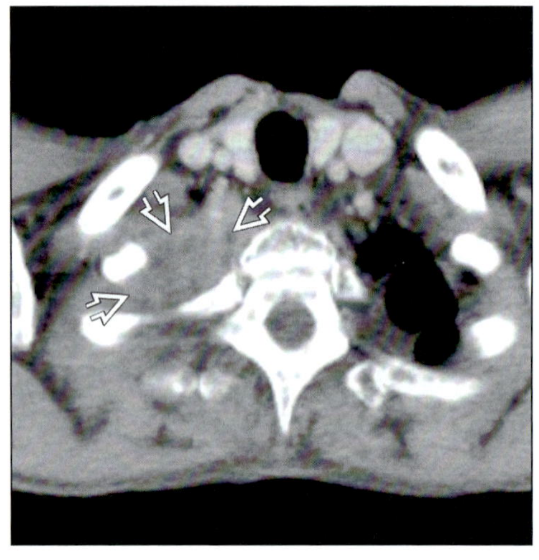

Stage IIIA (T3 N2 M0)

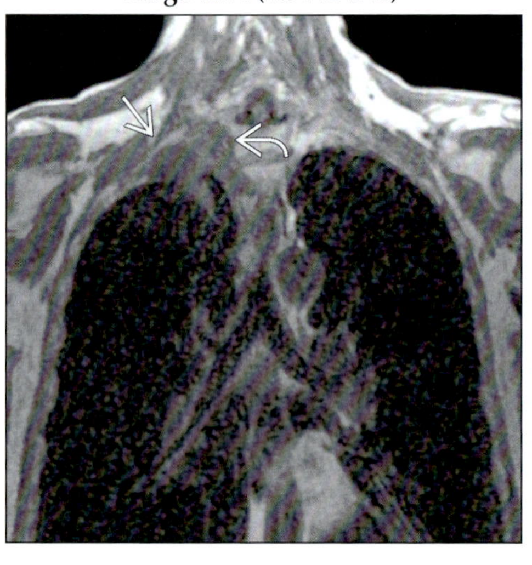

*(**Left**) Coronal PET maximum-intensity projection (MIP) shows primary tumor ➔ centered in left hilum. Note extent of tumor thrombus invading left atrium ➔. NSCLC was diagnosed via hilar biopsy. (**Right**) Maximum-intensity PET in another patient shows a T4 tumor ➔ invading the mediastinum. Multiple FDG-avid foci correspond to lymphadenopathy extending to contralateral mediastinum and supraclavicular nodes ➔. Contralateral adenopathy indicates N3 disease.*

Stage IIIA (T4 N0 M0)

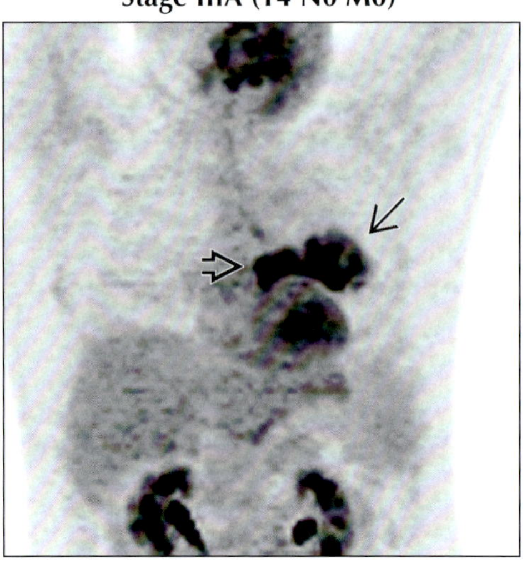

Stage IIIB (T4 N3 M0)

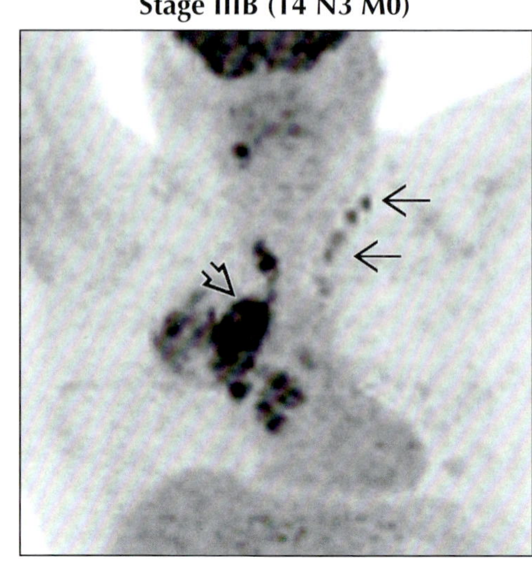

Stage IIB (T3 N0 M0)

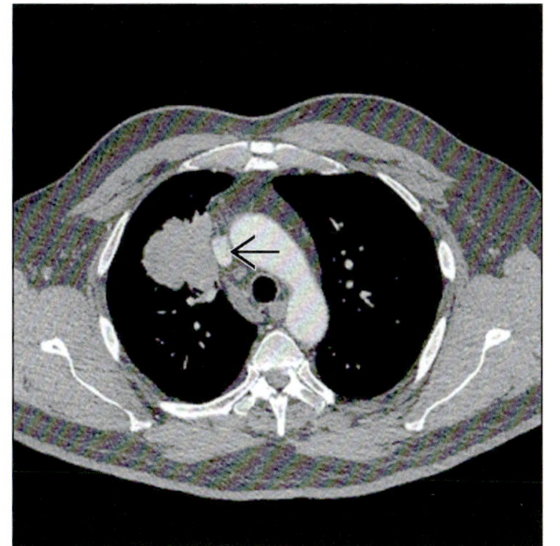

Stage IIB (T3 N0 M0)

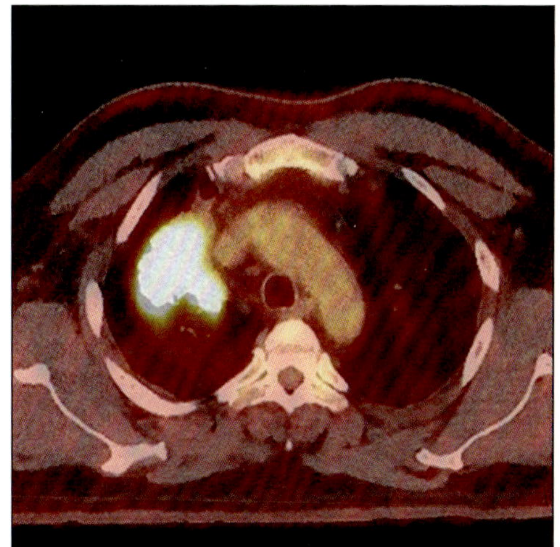

(Left) *This patient has an 8 cm, T3 N0 M0, stage IIB non-small cell carcinoma. Pretreatment CT chest shows a mass with broad surface of contact with the mediastinal pleura along the region of superior vena cava* ⇨ *without mediastinal invasion.* ***(Right)*** *Pretreatment fused PET/CT in the same patient shows intense avidity in the mass, with SUV of 13.3.*

Stage IIB (T3 N0 M0)

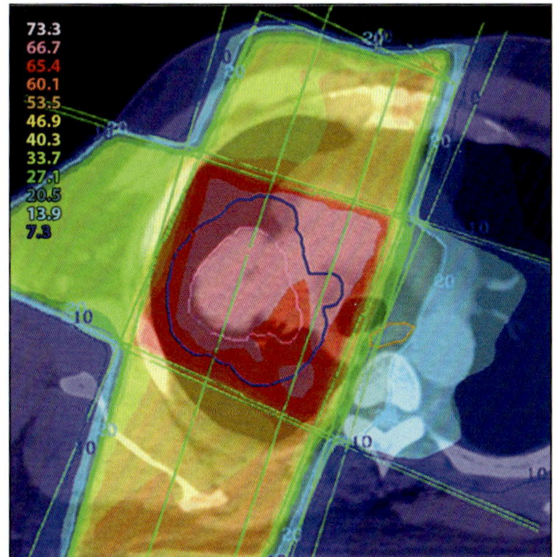

Stage IIB (T3 N0 M0)

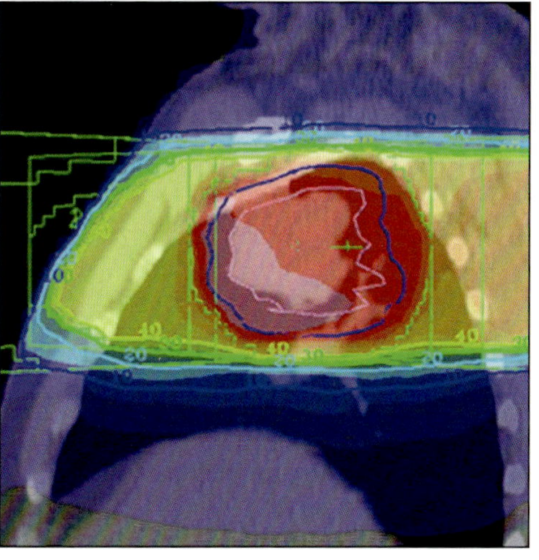

(Left) *The same patient was treated with a 3D conformal plan with 3 beams and 2 segments (partial beams) to a total dose of 66 Gy in 2 Gy per fraction prescribed to the 100% isodose line. Pink area is 67 Gy isodose line, red is 63 Gy, orange is 54 Gy, yellow is 40 Gy, green is 27 Gy, and light blue is 14 Gy.* ***(Right)*** *Sagittal view of the same plan demonstrates good coverage of the PTV.*

Stage IIB (T3 N0 M0)

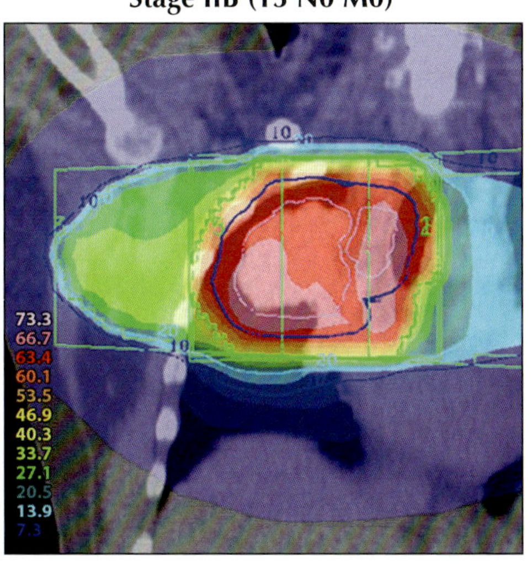

Stage IIB (T3 N0 M0)

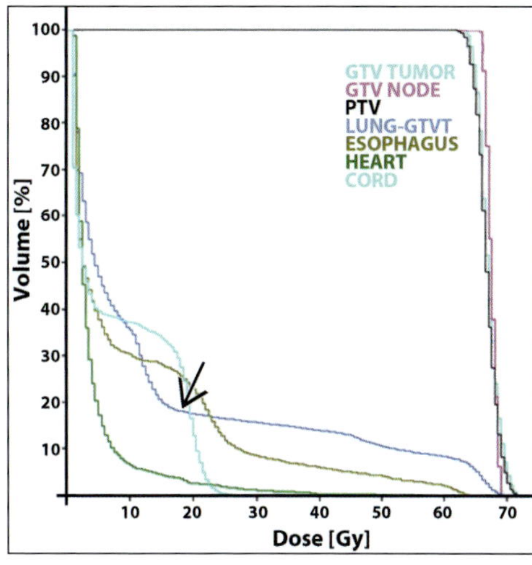

(Left) *Coronal view shows the same plan. Since this case was node negative, there was no planned coverage of elective nodes.* ***(Right)*** *DVH in the same patient shows that approximately 17% of the total lung volume (dark blue line) receives at least 20 Gy* ⇨*. The mean esophagus dose is < 10 Gy. The other OARs (heart and cord) also received a low dose.*

NON-SMALL CELL LUNG CANCER

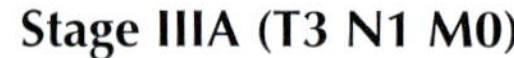

Stage IIIA (T3 N1 M0)

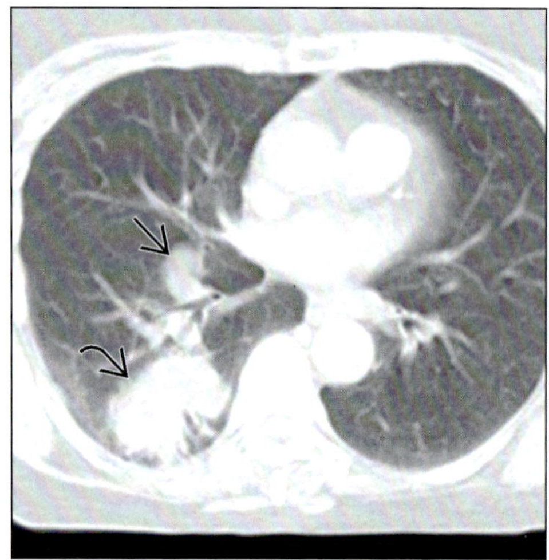

Stage IIIA (T3 N1 M0)

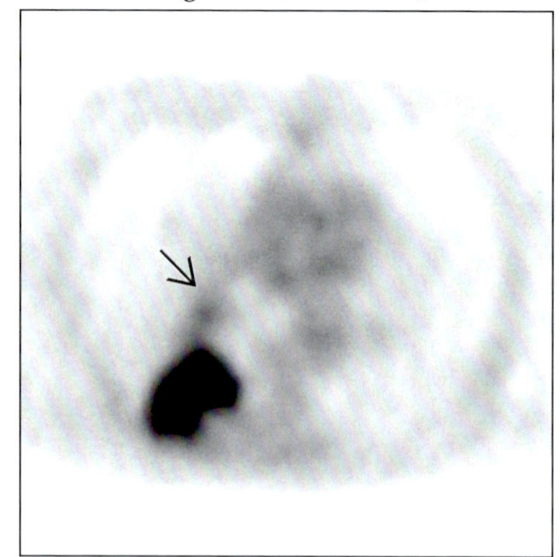

(Left) *This is a patient with a 9 cm mass with extension to posterior pleural surface and large right hilar nodes* →*, T3 N1 M0, stage IIIA disease. Pretreatment CT shows a large right lower lobe mass* ⇨*.* ***(Right)*** *Pretreatment PET in the same patient shows SUV max of 9.2 in the right lower lobe mass, also mild to moderate increased uptake in right hilar nodes* → *compared to the left.*

Stage IIIA (T3 N1 M0)

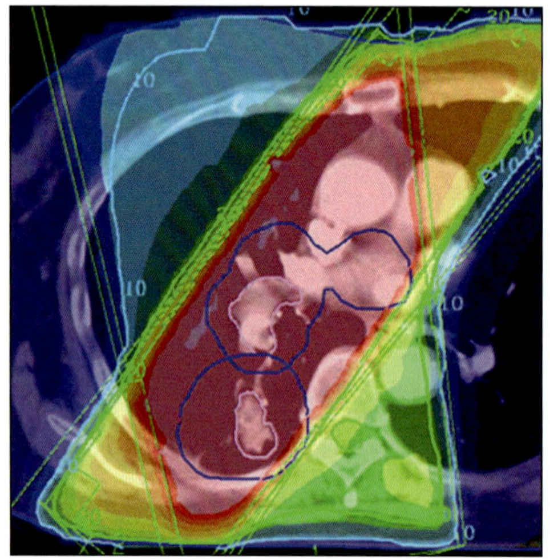

Stage IIIA (T3 N1 M0)

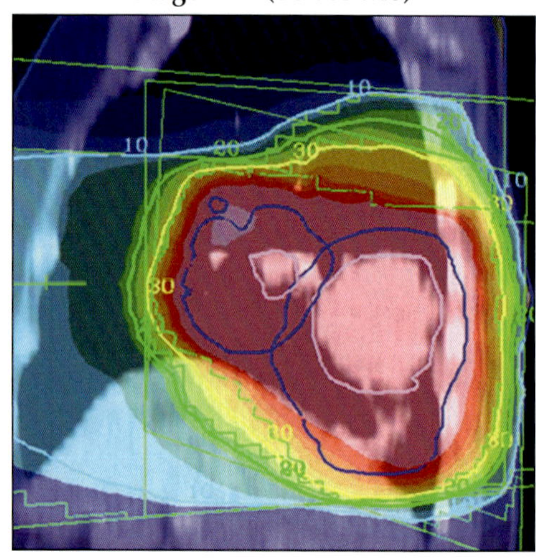

(Left) *The same patient received neoadjuvant radiation to a total of 45 Gy in 1.8 Gy fractions to the mass with a 3-field arrangement. Pink area is 45 Gy, red is 43 Gy, orange is 36 Gy, green is 18 Gy, and light blue is 10 Gy.* ***(Right)*** *Sagittal view in the same patient shows coverage of primary and N1 disease.*

Stage IIIA (T3 N1 M0)

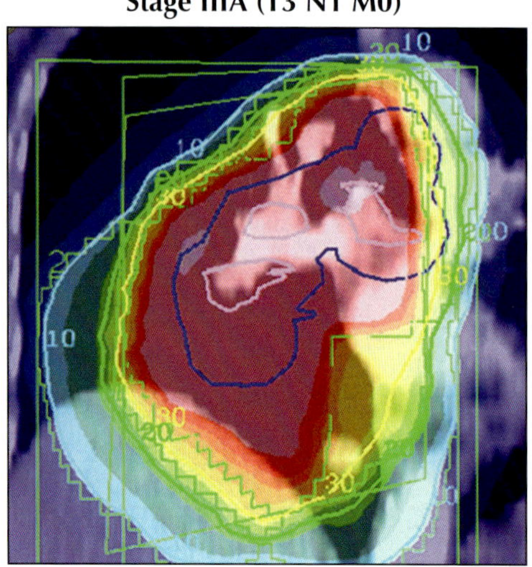

Stage IIIA (T3 N1 M0)

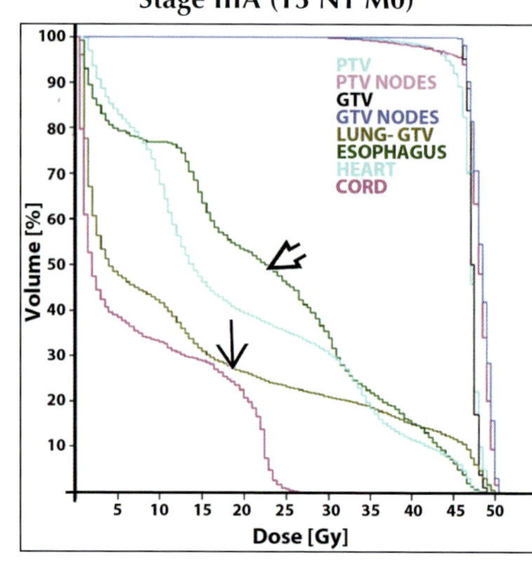

(Left) *The same patient subsequently underwent right lower lobectomy and mediastinal node dissection, followed by adjuvant chemotherapy. Pathology showed pT2 N0 disease with a positive visceral margin. She had no evidence of disease on CT more than 5 years later.* ***(Right)*** *DVH in the same patient shows 27% of the total lung volume receiving at least 20 Gy* →*. Esophagus mean dose is 22 Gy* ⇨*.*

Stage IV (T1 N0 M1a)

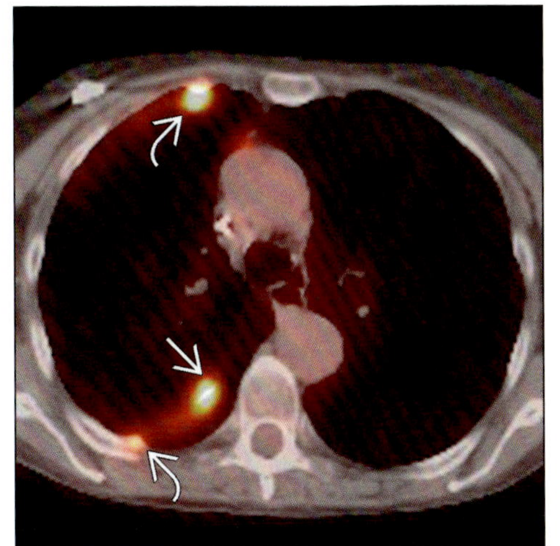

Stage IV (T2 N0 M1a)

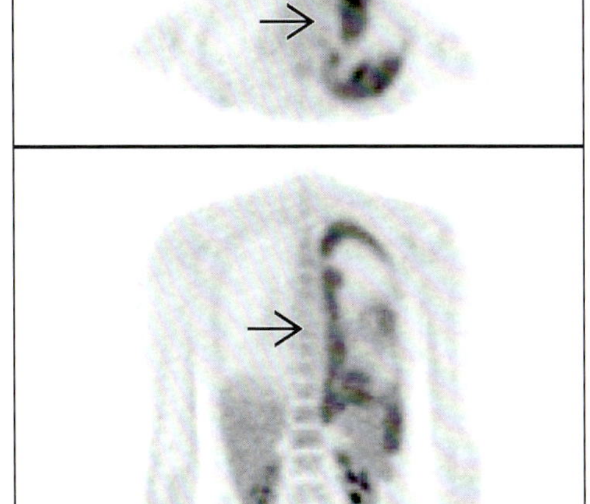

*(**Left**) Axial PET/CT shows primary lung neoplasm ➡ and ipsilateral pleural nodules ↪. Presence of pleural nodules is designated M1a disease. (**Right**) In a different patient with non-small cell lung carcinoma, axial and coronal PET images show malignant pleural effusion →, which requires M1a staging.*

Stage IV (T2b N1 M1a)

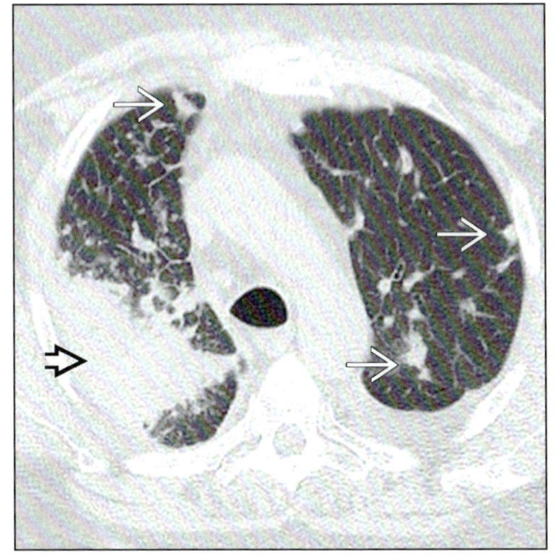

Stage IV (T2 N2 M1b)

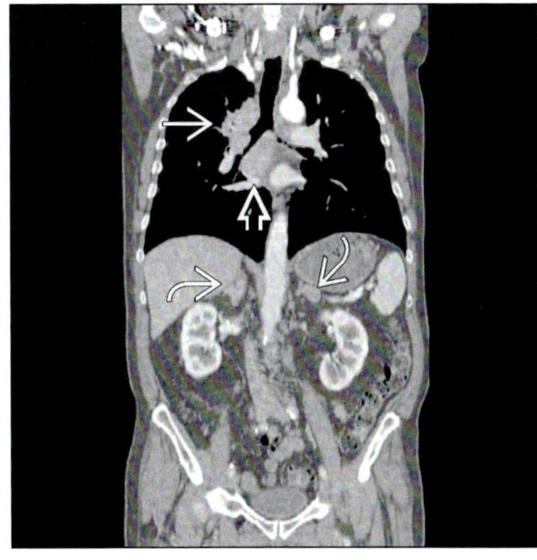

*(**Left**) Axial NECT shows a right upper lobe mass ⇨. Additionally, multiple bilateral pulmonary nodules are present ➡. Contralateral lung metastasis is consistent with M1a disease. (**Right**) Coronal CECT shows paramediastinal ➡ and subcarinal ⇨ lymphadenopathy from primary non-small cell lung carcinoma. Note bilateral adrenal metastases ↪, consistent with stage IV disease.*

Stage IV (T4 N2 M1b)

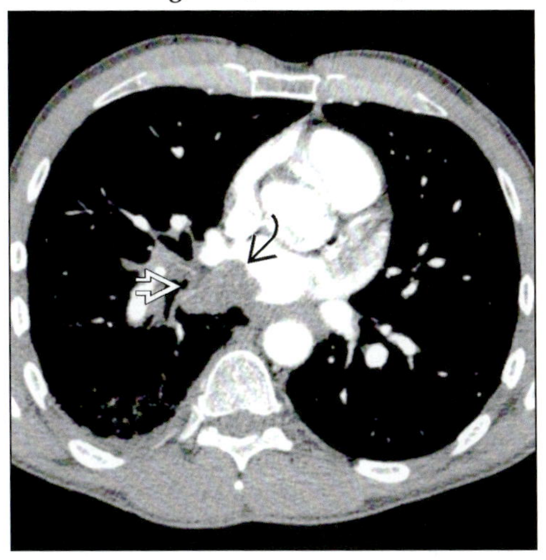

Stage IV (T4 N3 M1b)

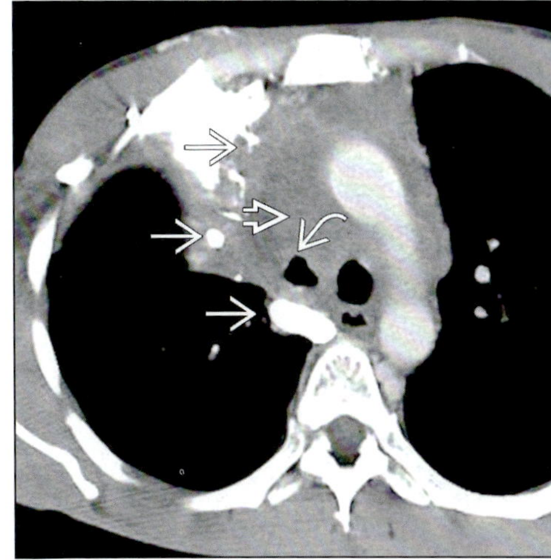

*(**Left**) Axial CECT depicts a lobular right perihilar soft tissue mass obliterating the right inferior pulmonary vein ⇨ and extending into the left atrium ↪. Invasion into the cardiac chambers can cause emboli. (**Right**) Axial CECT reveals a conglomerate, necrotic right paratracheal mass. The tumor has central low attenuation ⇨, representing necrosis. Central cavitation is also seen ↪. Note partial obstruction of superior vena cava and azygous veins ➡.*

SMALL CELL LUNG CANCER

(T) Primary Tumor

Adapted from 7th edition AJCC Staging Forms.

TNM	*Definitions*
TX	Primary tumor cannot be assessed or tumor proven by presence of malignant cells in sputum or bronchial washings but not visualized by imaging or bronchoscopy
T0	No evidence of primary tumor
Tis	Carcinoma in situ
T1	Tumor ≤ 3 cm in greatest dimension, surrounded by lung or visceral pleura, without bronchoscopic evidence of invasion more proximal than lobar bronchus (i.e., not in main bronchus)[1]
T1a	Tumor ≤ 2 cm in greatest dimension
T1b	Tumor > 2 cm but ≤ 3 cm in greatest dimension
T2	Tumor > 3 cm but ≤ 7 cm or tumor with any of the following features: Involves main bronchus, ≥ 2 cm distal to carina; invades visceral pleura (PL1 or PL2); associated with atelectasis or obstructive pneumonitis that extends to hilar region but does not involve entire lung
T2a	Tumor > 3 cm but ≤ 5 cm in greatest dimension
T2b	Tumor > 5 cm but ≤ 7 cm in greatest dimension
T3	Tumor > 7 cm or tumor that directly invades any of the following: Parietal pleural (PL3) chest wall (including superior sulcus tumors), diaphragm, phrenic nerve, mediastinal pleura, parietal pericardium; or tumor in main bronchus (≤ 2 cm distal to carina[1] but without involvement of the carina); or associated atelectasis or obstructive pneumonitis of entire lung or separate tumor nodule(s) in same lobe
T4	Tumor of any size that invades any of the following: Mediastinum, heart, great vessels, trachea, recurrent laryngeal nerve, esophagus, vertebral body, carina, separate tumor nodule(s) in a different ipsilateral lobe

(N) Regional Lymph Nodes

NX	Regional lymph nodes cannot be assessed
N0	No regional lymph node metastases
N1	Metastasis in ipsilateral peribronchial &/or ipsilateral hilar lymph nodes and intrapulmonary nodes, including involvement by direct extension
N2	Metastasis in ipsilateral mediastinal &/or subcarinal lymph node(s)
N3	Metastasis in contralateral mediastinal, contralateral hilar, ipsilateral or contralateral scalene, or supraclavicular lymph node(s)

(M) Distant Metastasis

M0	No distant metastasis
M1	Distant metastasis
M1a	Separate tumor nodule(s) in a contralateral lobe tumor with pleural nodules or malignant pleural (or pericardial) effusion[2]
M1b	Distant metastasis

[1]*The uncommon superficial spreading tumor of any size, with its invasive component limited to bronchial wall, which may extend proximally to the main bronchus, is also classified as T1a.*

[2]*Most pleural (and pericardial) effusions with lung cancer are due to tumor. In a few patients, however, multiple cytopathologic examinations of pleural (pericardial) fluid are negative for tumor, and the fluid is not bloody and is not an exudate. Where these elements and clinical judgment dictate that the effusion is not related to the tumor, the effusion should be excluded as a staging element and the patient's disease should be classified as M0.*

AJCC Stages/Prognostic Groups

Adapted from 7th edition AJCC Staging Forms.

Stage	*T*	*N*	*M*
Occult carcinoma	TX	N0	M0
0	Tis	N0	M0
IA	T1a	N0	M0
	T1b	N0	M0
IB	T2a	N0	M0
IIA	T2b	N0	M0
	T1a	N1	M0
	T1b	N1	M0
	T2a	N1	M0
IIB	T2b	N1	M0
	T3	N0	M0
IIIA	T1a	N2	M0
	T1b	N2	M0
	T2a	N2	M0
	T2b	N2	M0
	T3	N1	M0
	T3	N2	M0
	T4	N0	M0
	T4	N1	M0
IIIB	T1a	N3	M0
	T1b	N3	M0
	T2a	N3	M0
	T2b	N3	M0
	T3	N3	M0
	T4	N2	M0
	T4	N3	M0
IV	Any T	Any N	M1a
	Any T	Any N	M1b

SMALL CELL LUNG CANCER

The Veterans' Administration Lung Study Group (VALSG) Staging System

Limited stage	Disease extension confined to 1 hemithorax that could be encompassed within a "reasonable" radiation therapy field (i.e., ipsilateral lung & hilum, ipsilateral or contralateral mediastinum, ipsilateral supraclavicular fossa)
Extensive stage	Disease extension beyond limited stage (including contralateral lung nodules, malignant pleural effusion, and distant disease)

Limited and extensive stage is most commonly used to describe extent of disease for SCLC; however, the AJCC staging system for lung cancer can also be used.

Metastatic Sites of Involvement

Site	*At Presentation*	*At Autopsy*
Liver	21-27%	69%
Bone	27-41%	54%
Adrenal glands	5-31%	35-65%
Brain	10-14%	28-50%
Bone marrow	15-30%	N/A
Pleural effusion	16-20%	30%
Retroperitoneal lymph nodes	3-12%	29-52%
Soft tissues	5%	19%
Contralateral lung	1-12%	8-27%

Adapted from Argiris et al, 2004. N/A = not available.

Core Biopsy

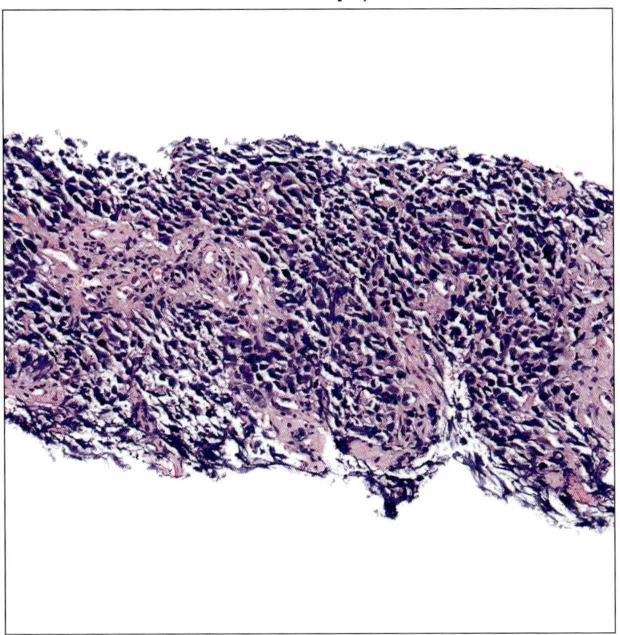

Core biopsy specimen shows small cell carcinoma. Often, core biopsy causes less crush artifact compared with transbronchial biopsy technique. Cells have classic oat-like appearance. Each cell is ~ 2x the size of a lymphocyte. Cells have lymphocyte-like appearance and high mitotic rate. (Courtesy C. Moran, MD.)

Central Tumors

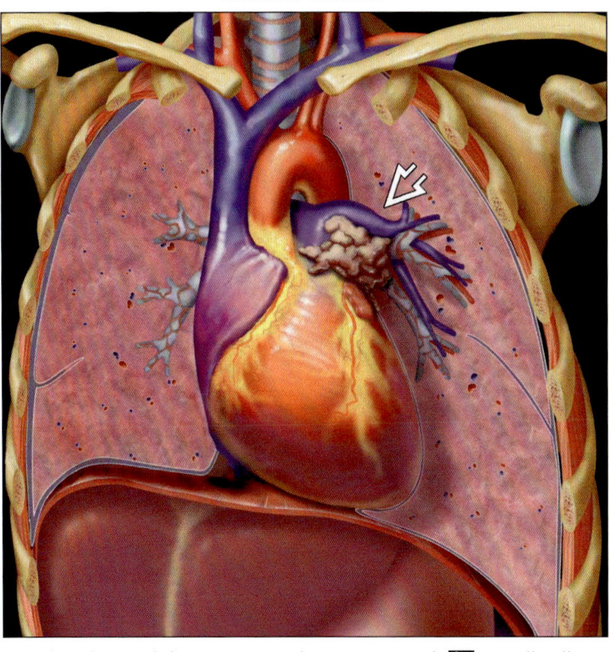

Graphic depicts hilar tumor invading great vessels ➨. Small cell lung cancer (SCLC) is typically a central mass and often invades mediastinum (T4). Limited stage includes disease that can be encompassed within a single RT port, and extensive stage includes contralateral lung nodules, malignant pleural effusion, and distant disease.

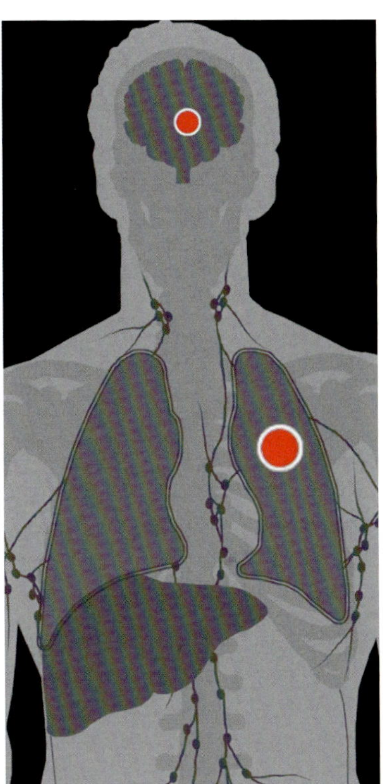

INITIAL SITE OF RECURRENCE

Thorax (i.e., locoregional failure)	16-52%
Brain	6%*-46%**
Liver	Not reported
Adrenal Gland	Not reported
Bone	Not reported

*Data represent initial sites of failure after concurrent CRT for limited-stage small cell lung carcinoma. *With and **without prophylactic cranial irradiation. Warde P et al, Turrisi AT 3rd et al, Guiliani ME et al, Coy P et al, Watkins JM et al, Murray N et al, Tai P et al, Arriagada R et al.*

SMALL CELL LUNG CANCER

OVERVIEW

Classification

- Uses same TNM staging system as non-small cell lung cancer (NSCLC), per AJCC 7th edition
- Veterans' Administration Lung Study Group (VALSG) staging system is still commonly used in practice, and classifies patients into
  - Limited stage (LS): Disease extension confined to 1 hemithorax that could be encompassed within "reasonable" radiation therapy field (i.e., ipsilateral lung & hilum, ipsilateral or contralateral mediastinum, ipsilateral supraclavicular fossa)
  - Extensive stage (ES): Disease extension beyond limited stage (including multiple/contralateral nodules and malignant pleural effusion)

NATURAL HISTORY

General Features

- Highly malignant neuroendocrine tumor of lung origin with predilection for early nodal and distant metastases
- SCLC has a shorter overall survival than NSCLC if left untreated
- Location
  - At diagnosis, 1/3 of patients are LS and 2/3 are ES
    - LS disease typically presents as large, locally invasive central lung mass with hilar and mediastinal lymphadenopathy
    - ES disease commonly involves distant metastatic spread to brain, adrenal glands, liver, and bone

Etiology

- Risk factors
  - Cigarette smoking (> 95% of cases)
    - Lung cancer development directly related to number of cigarettes smoked, length of smoking history, as well as tar and nicotine content of cigarettes
    - Smoking cessation reduces risk of developing SCLC
  - Passive smoking (secondhand smoke)
    - Carcinogens can be inhaled passively by nonsmokers
    - Accounts for up to 25% of lung cancers in persons who do not smoke
  - Asbestos
  - Radon

Epidemiology & Cancer Incidence

- Number of cases in USA per year
  - In 2010, estimated 33,380 new cases of SCLC and 23,600 deaths
- Sex predilection
  - Slightly over 50% of newly diagnosed patients are male, representative of growing proportion of newly diagnosed females over past 25 years
- Age of onset
  - Most patients are > 65 years old

Genetics

- Common genetic alterations
  - Deletion of chromosome 3p14-23 region (80%)
  - Retinoblastoma (*RB1*) gene inactivation on chromosome 13 (> 90%)
  - Mutation of *TP53* tumor suppressor gene on chromosome 17p (> 75%)
  - *BCL2* overexpression (95% of cases)
  - *MYC* family amplification or protein overexpression (i.e., c-myc, N-myc, L-myc)

Associated Diseases, Abnormalities

- Paraneoplastic syndromes
  - Ectopic antidiuretic hormone (ADH) production causing syndrome of inappropriate antidiuretic hormone secretion (SIADH)
  - Ectopic ACTH production causes Cushing syndrome
  - Atrial natriuretic peptide (ANP) syndrome causes hyponatremia, hypotension, and natriuresis
  - Cerebellar degeneration syndrome (due to autoimmune reaction targeted against Purkinje cells) causes ataxia
  - Lambert-Eaton syndrome causes muscle weakness, typically involving legs and arms, worse with repeated muscle use

Gross Pathology & Surgical Features

- Gross specimens from thoracotomy or thoracoscopy
- Core specimens from CT or bronchoscopy-guided biopsies
- Pathologic assessment of lung cancers is based on
  - Histologic type
  - Tumor size and location
  - Involvement of visceral pleura
  - Extension to regional and distant lymph nodes and organs

Microscopic Pathology

- H&E
  - Small cells with scant cytoplasm, ill-defined cell borders, finely granular nuclear chromatin, and absent or inconspicuous nucleoli
    - Prominent necrosis and high mitotic rate common
    - Thought to arise from Kulchitsky cells
  - Combined small cell carcinoma histological variant: SCLC with any NSCLC histological type (i.e., adenocarcinoma, squamous cell carcinoma)

Routes of Spread

- Local spread
  - Typically presents as large, bulky central mass invading or compressing central airways and mediastinum
    - Peripheral masses invading chest wall are uncommon
  - SCLC presenting as solitary pulmonary nodule is rare
- Lymphatic extension
  - Frequent hilar and mediastinal lymph node involvement
- Hematogenous spread
  - About 60% of patients present with stage IV disease from hematogenous spread
- Metastatic sites
  - Brain
    - Present at diagnosis in 10-20% of patients
    - Occur in 50-80% of patients at 2 years in absence of cranial irradiation
      - Presence at autopsy in 70-80% of patients
  - Bone, bone marrow, adrenal, and hepatic metastases all additional common sites of distant metastases

IMAGING

Detection

- Common radiologic presentations
  - Large central mass
    - Bronchial obstruction
      - Atelectasis present in 1/3 of patients (sublobar, lobar, or entire lung)
      - Postobstructive pneumonia
    - Mediastinal invasion
      - Encasement and compression of mediastinal structures (i.e., great vessels, heart, carina, trachea)
      - Superior vena cava compression or invasion common (10%)
  - Hilar &/or mediastinal lymphadenopathy
  - Elevated hemidiaphragm due to phrenic nerve involvement by central tumor
  - Solitary pulmonary nodule or peripheral mass are rare
  - Pleural effusion
  - Distant metastases to brain, bone, adrenal glands, and liver

Staging

- **Contrast-enhanced CT**: Thorax to adrenal glands
  - Evaluate extent of primary tumor
    - Size
    - Proximal extent of tumor (usually confirmed by bronchoscopy)
    - Invasion of main bronchus, visceral pleura, associated atelectasis/pneumonitis (part of lung)
    - Invasion of chest wall, diaphragm, mediastinal pleura, parietal pericardium, extension into main bronchus < 2 cm distal to carina, associated atelectasis/pneumonitis (entire lung)
    - Invasion of heart, great vessels, trachea, esophagus, vertebral body, carina
    - Pleural/pericardial effusion
      - Malignancy should be confirmed with cytology
    - Presence of separate tumor nodules
  - Nodal disease
    - Size criteria
      - Mediastinal lymph nodes (LN) > 10 mm (> 13-15 mm subcarinal) more likely malignant
      - Retrocrural, paraaortic, pericardial LN > 8 mm more likely malignant
    - Locations
      - Hilum, mediastinum, & supraclavicular fossa all common sites of lymph node involvement
  - Distant metastases
    - Lung
      - Tumor in contralateral lung
      - Malignant pleural/pericardial effusion
    - Adrenal gland
      - Malignancy favored if > 3 cm, poorly defined margin, irregular rim enhancement, invasion of adjacent structures
      - Benign etiology favored if attenuation values < 10 HU on CT (sensitivity 71%, specificity 98%)
    - Bone
      - Vertebral bodies, ribs, pelvis, proximal appendicular skeleton
      - Osteolytic lesions more common than osteoblastic
      - CT alone insufficient to exclude bone metastases
- **PET/CT**
  - Whole-body PET/CT is most accurate for staging intra- and extrathoracic disease in single study
  - In patient with biopsy-confirmed carcinoma, hypermetabolic activity highly specific for additional sites of malignant disease
  - Confirm highest stage lesion with biopsy, if possible, as false positives occur
  - Brain metastasis best evaluated with MR due to sensitivity/resolution limits of PET for small lesions
    - However, PET can detect unsuspected brain metastases, especially those ~ 1.5 cm or larger
  - Adrenals: Compare hypermetabolic activity to liver
    - If greater activity than liver, most likely metastasis
  - Note that BAC and carcinoid often show minimal activity on PET; staging/restaging with PET may be inaccurate
- **MR**
  - Chest
    - Rarely used for evaluation of intrathoracic disease
    - Not part of routine staging work-up of either SCLC or NSCLC
  - Brain
    - MR most sensitive to detect brain metastasis
    - Gadolinium-enhanced brain MR mandatory for staging of all limited-stage SCLC patients
  - Adrenals
    - Useful if CT or PET findings equivocal
- **Radionuclide bone scan**
  - Potentially useful for detection of skeletal metastases
    - Not typically indicated due to high sensitivity of PET/CT
- **Transthoracic percutaneous fine-needle aspiration**
  - Less invasive than bronchoscopy
  - Reserved for accessible tumors
    - Those tumors not accessible through bronchoscope
  - Via CT-fluoro guidance
- **Thoracentesis**
  - Presence of malignant pleural effusion or suspected malignant effusion (i.e., transudative or bloody effusion) upstages disease to stage IV (ES)
    - For adequate staging, pleural effusions should be aspirated and examined for malignant cells if no other sites of distant spread are identified
  - Therapeutic thoracentesis provides symptomatic relief in patients with large pleural effusions

Restaging

- Monitoring tumor response to evaluate efficacy of chemo &/or RT
  - Contrast-enhanced CT chest/abdomen represents primary imaging modality
  - Brain evaluation with MR (preferred) or CT with IV contrast for patients in whom prophylactic cranial irradiation (PCI) is considered
- Response evaluation criteria in solid tumors (RECIST)
  - Unidimensional measurements
  - Presence of at least 1 measurable lesion at baseline, maximum of 5 target lesions used

  - For MDCT scanners, minimum size of lesion may be 10 mm, provided that 10 mm collimation is used and reconstructions are performed at 5 mm intervals
- WHO (World Health Organization)
  - Bidimensional measurements

CLINICAL PRESENTATION & WORK-UP

Presentation

- Symptoms due to primary tumor extension
  - Cough
  - Dyspnea
  - Chest pain
  - Wheezing
  - Hemoptysis
  - Hoarseness (due to recurrent laryngeal nerve involvement)
  - Superior vena cava syndrome
    - Obstruction of blood flow to heart from head and neck regions and upper extremities due to tumor compression of superior vena cava
      - Early physical findings: Facial edema, dusky skin coloration, and, possibly, conjunctival edema
      - Late physical findings: Upper extremity edema and prominent upper chest wall veins with retrograde flow
- Paraneoplastic syndromes
- Constitutional symptoms associated with distant spread
  - Weight loss
  - Weakness
  - Anorexia
  - Fever
- Liver, brain, and bone metastases with associated site-specific symptomatology

Prognosis

- Prognosis remains poor; weight loss, performance status, and stage are most important prognostic factors
  - Male gender, continued tobacco use, and lactate dehydrogenase (LDH) elevation are additional adverse prognostic factors
- Median survival by clinical stage grouping
  - Stage IA: 30 months
  - Stage IB: 18 months
  - Stage IIA: 33 months
  - Stage IIB: 18 months
  - Stage IIIA: 14 months
  - Stage IIIB: 12 months
  - Stage IV: 7 months
  - Limited stage: 16-22 months
  - Extensive stage: 10 months

Work-Up

- Clinical
  - History and physical
  - Biopsy
  - Pulmonary function testing including diffusion capacity of lungs for carbon monoxide (DLCO)
- Radiographic
  - Contrast-enhanced CT chest/liver/adrenals
  - Brain MR (preferred) or brain CT with IV contrast
  - Whole-body PET/CT (for limited-stage disease)
    - Bone scan if PET/CT unable to be obtained
- Laboratory
  - Complete blood count
  - Comprehensive metabolic panel
  - LDH
  - Bone marrow biopsy (if suspicion of bone marrow involvement due to nucleated RBCs on peripheral smear, neutropenia, or thrombocytopenia)

TREATMENT

Major Treatment Alternatives

- Combined chemo and RT (CRT) is standard of care for SCLC
  - Current standard of care for LS disease (i.e., stages IA-IIIB)
    - Concurrent CRT improves overall survival (OS) compared with either chemo alone or sequential chemo followed by RT
    - Early initiation of thoracic RT concurrent with cycle 1 or 2 of platinum-based chemo associated with improved OS compared with late RT (i.e., with cycle 3 or later)
    - Optimal dose currently unknown
      - Current standard of care is 45 Gy RT delivered 2x daily (1.5 Gy per fx at least 6 hours apart), based on improvement in OS compared with 1x daily (1.8 Gy per fx) RT to 45 Gy, although at cost of increased acute esophageal toxicity
      - 45 Gy in 30 fx (1.5 Gy 2x daily) is currently being compared with 70 Gy in 2 Gy daily fx and 61.2 Gy in concomitant boost fractionation in CALGB 30610 phase III study
    - Etoposide & cisplatin (EP) for 4-6 cycles is considered standard first-line concurrent CRT regimen
      - Carboplatin may be safely substituted for cisplatin without apparent compromise of efficacy
- Surgery
  - Not routinely performed in standard management of SCLC due to high rate of mediastinal lymph node involvement and resultant low complete resection rates
  - Potential role in carefully selected patients with T1-2 N0 M0 SCLC, good performance status, and negative pathological mediastinal staging
    - Lobectomy with mediastinal lymph node dissection or sampling recommended
    - Adjuvant chemo recommended following complete resection for N0 patients
    - Adjuvant chemo and RT recommended following either incomplete resection or resection of node-positive disease
  - No benefit for surgical resection of residual disease after completion of chemo or CRT
- PCI
  - Improves OS and reduces rates of brain metastases in LS patients with complete response (CR) after CRT, and ES patients with at least partial response (PR) to chemotherapy

- 25 Gy in 10 fx is standard of care dose for PCI (due to failure of higher doses to improve outcomes)
- Consolidative thoracic radiotherapy
  - May be beneficial for ES patients who achieve an extrathoracic CR and at least intrathoracic PR to chemo
  - No optimal established dose
    - 45 Gy in 15 daily fx currently being studied in Radiation Therapy Oncology Group (RTOG) 0937 study
- Systemic therapy: Chemo alone
  - Standard of care for extensive stage (M1) disease
    - EP x 4-6 cycles considered first-line
      - Carboplatin may be potentially substituted for cisplatin
  - May be appropriate in limited-stage disease for poor PS patients

Major Treatment Roadblocks/ Contraindications

- Prior thoracic RT (potential contraindication to curative RT)
- Renal impairment (potential contraindication to platinum-based chemotherapy)
- Poor performance status (may reduce tolerability of all therapies)
- Prior CNS RT or dementia (contraindication to PCI)

Treatment Options by Stage

- Limited stage
  - T1-2 N0 M0
    - Concurrent CRT (preferred)
    - Surgery + adjuvant chemotherapy
    - Consolidative PCI recommended for patients with any response to therapy
  - T3-4 (any N stage) or N1-3 (any T stage) & M0
    - Concurrent chemoradiotherapy with early RT (with chemotherapy cycles #1 or 2)
    - Consolidative PCI recommended for patients with any response to therapy
- Extensive stage
  - M1 (any T or N stage)
    - Systemic chemo
    - Consolidative RT may be considered for patients with extrathoracic CR and intrathoracic CR or PR to chemotherapy
    - PCI recommended for patients with any response to chemotherapy

Dose Response

- Optimal dose remains unknown
  - 45 Gy in 30 fx (1.5 Gy/fx delivered 2x daily) showed improved OS and local control compared with 45 Gy in 25 daily fx
- Prophylactic cranial irradiation (for either LS or ES)
  - 25 Gy in 10 daily fx is current standard of care
    - No demonstrated benefit for higher dose PCI (survival decrement observed with 36 Gy in 18 daily fx or 24 b.i.d. fx)
- Consolidative thoracic RT (for ES)
  - Optimal dose and fractionation currently undetermined
  - RTOG phase III study to confirm the role of consolidation RT

Standard Doses

- Thoracic radiation therapy (TRT) with concurrent EP
  - 45 Gy in 30 fx of 1.5 Gy each b.i.d. (6 hours apart)
- PCI
  - 25 Gy in 10 daily fx
- Consolidative TRT (ES only)
  - 45 Gy in 15 daily fx (3 Gy per fx)
  - 30 Gy in 10 daily fx (3 Gy per fx)

Organs at Risk Parameters

- Spinal cord
  - Maximum dose < 50 Gy (if using 1.8-2 Gy daily fx)
  - Maximum dose < 36 Gy (if using 1.5 Gy fx b.i.d.)
- Lung (defined as lung minus gross tumor volume)
  - Volume receiving ≥ 20 Gy (V20) ≤ 35%
  - Mean lung dose (MLD) ≤ 20 Gy
- Esophagus (defined from bottom of cricoid to gastroesophageal junction [GEJ])
  - Mean dose ≤ 34 Gy
- Heart (defined from pulmonary artery trunk to apex)
  - Dose to 1/3 < 60 Gy
  - Dose to 2/3 < 45 Gy
  - Dose to entire organ < 40 Gy

Common Techniques

- Simulation
  - CT-based simulation considered standard of care
  - 4D CT or alternative form of breathing motion assessment or motion control preferred
    - Motion management mandatory if using intensity-modulated radiation therapy (IMRT)
      - If no motion management utilized, larger planning target volume (PTV) expansion is required
  - IV contrast whenever possible to aid in differentiation of central tumor from mediastinal vasculature
  - Reproducible immobilization essential
- Target volume delineation
  - PET/CT fusion with simulation CT may aid in gross tumor volume (GTV) delineation
  - For patients without PET/CT, GTV should include primary tumor and all LNs > 1 cm in short axis
  - Use of elective nodal irradiation (ENI) is controversial
    - Traditional ENI included ipsilateral hilum (level 10), bilateral mediastinal LNs from 3 cm below carina to level of aortic arch (levels 3, 4R, 4L, & 7), as well as AP window (level 6) and paraaortic LNs (level 5) for left-sided tumors
      - Inclusion of supraclavicular fossa in ENI is controversial
  - ACR and NCCN practice guidelines recommend omission of ENI
  - PET may have role in designing RT volumes; selective nodal RT on basis of FDG PET scans in LS-SCLC was also examined by prospective study
    - PET-based involved nodal RT resulted in low rate of isolated nodal failures (3%), with low percentage of acute esophagitis, while CT-based selective nodal RT resulted in unexpectedly high percentage of isolated nodal failures (11%)
- Treatment planning (per RTOG 0538/CALGB 30610)
  - GTV = summed from inhale and exhale CT scan or 4D CT scan where possible

- Clinical target volume (CTV) = GTV + margin for microscopic disease + elective nodal regions (if using ENI)
- PTV definitions
  - If using 4D CT or composite inhale/exhale scan: PTV = CTV + 1.0 cm circumferentially
  - If using free-breathing CT simulation: PTV = CTV + 1.5 cm (craniocaudally) + 1.0 cm (axially)
  - If using breath-hold technique: PTV = CTV + 1.0 cm (craniocaudally) + 0.5 cm (axially)
- 3D conformal RT technique is considered standard
  - IMRT may be considered in selected patients although careful motion management required

Landmark Trials

- Use of TRT for LS disease
  - Meta-analysis of 13 trials involving 2,140 patients randomized to either chemo alone or with concurrent CRT demonstrated that TRT improved OS with absolute benefit of 5.4% at 3 years
    - Local control was similarly improved from 23.3-48.0% (P < 0.001)
- Concurrent vs. sequential TRT for LS disease
  - Japanese Clinical Oncology Group phase III trial that randomized 231 patients to 4 cycles of PE with RT (45 Gy in 1.5 Gy fx 2x daily over 3 weeks) beginning either with cycle 1 (concurrent arm) or after cycle 4 (sequential arm)
    - Concurrent CRT showed trend toward superior OS, with median survival of 27.2 months vs. 19.7 months and 5-year OS of 23.7% vs. 18.3% (P = 0.097)
    - Concurrent CRT is associated with higher hematologic toxicity, with modest grade 3 or higher esophagitis rates in both arms (9% vs. 4%)
- Early vs. late TRT in LS disease
  - 8 randomized trials and 3 meta-analyses address this issue; early initiation of TRT (before chemotherapy cycle #3) is preferred, comparing to late (with or after cycle #3) initiation of TRT
    - National Cancer Institute of Canada phase III randomized controlled trial (RCT) in 308 patients compared RT (40 Gy in 15 daily fx) delivered during cycle 2 or cycle 6 chemo (CAV, EP alternating) concurrently with the 1st cycle of EP
      - 5-year survival rates showed significant benefit for early TRT compared to late TRT (22% vs. 13%, respectively)
      - Median progression-free survival (PFS) was 15.4 months in early TRT group vs. 11.8 months in late TRT group (P = 0.036)
      - Median OS times were 21.2 months and 16 months, respectively (P = 0.008)
    - Meta-analysis of RCTs published after 1985 showed relative risk (RR) of 1.17 (95% CI, 1.02-1.35) for OS at 2 years favoring early TRT
      - On subgroup analysis, survival benefit seen only for patients receiving hyperfractionated TRT (2-year OS RR 1.44, absolute benefit 17%) and for those receiving platinum-based chemo (2-year OS RR 1.30, absolute benefit 10%)
    - Meta-analysis by de Ruysscher et al similarly showed that time from start of any therapy to end of TRT was most important predictor of OS at 5 years, with absolute decrease in 5-year OS of 1.83% for every week extended
- Fractionation and dose of TRT in LS disease
  - Intergroup trial compared TRT dose of 45 Gy delivered via either accelerated hyperfractionation (30 fx of 1.5 Gy delivered 2x daily over 3 weeks) or conventional fractionation (25 fx of 1.8 Gy daily delivered over 5 weeks), both began day 1 of concurrent PE x 4 cycles
    - 2x-daily TRT improved median survival from 19 months to 23 months, and 5-year OS from 16% to 26% (P = 0.04); intrathoracic failures were decreased from 52-36% (P = 0.06)
    - Acute esophagitis (grade 3 or higher) rates were significantly increased in 2x daily arm (32% vs. 16%, P < 0.001)
    - Study criticized due to lack of biologically equivalent RT dose in daily TRT arm compared to 2x-daily TRT arm
  - CALGB phase II study of 63 patients utilized 70 Gy in daily 2 Gy fx with concurrent carboplatin and etoposide (after 2 cycles of paclitaxel and topotecan induction chemotherapy)
    - Median OS of 22.4 months compared favorably with intergroup 2x-daily TRT results
  - 3-arm phase III study currently being conducted by CALGB and RTOG to compare
    - 45 Gy in 1.5 Gy 2x-daily fx
    - 70 Gy in 2 Gy daily fx
    - 61.2 Gy with delayed accelerated hyperfractionation
- PCI
  - Meta-analysis of 987 patients in CR on 7 RCTs of PCI vs. no PCI demonstrated absolute 5.4% improvement in 3-year OS, and decrease in cumulative incidence of brain metastases for PCI patients
  - Phase III study conducted by EORTC randomized 286 patients with ES-SCLC who had response to 4-6 cycles of chemotherapy and no clinical evidence of brain metastases (brain imaging not required) to PCI or no PCI
    - PCI reduced risk of brain metastases at 1 year (14.6% vs. 40.4%, HR 0.27, P < 0.001) and improved OS (1-year OS 27.1% vs. 13.3%, HR 0.68, P = 0.003)
    - PCI was associated with significantly increased fatigue and trend toward worse cognitive functioning and global health status
  - International consortium study involving EORTC, RTOG, CALGB, and SWOG randomized 720 patients with LS-SCLC in CR after chemoradiotherapy to either
    - Standard-dose PCI (25 Gy in 10 daily fx) or
    - Higher dose PCI (36 Gy in either daily 2 Gy fx or 2x-daily 1.5 Gy fx)
    - OS at 2 years was superior in standard-dose PCI group (42% vs. 37%, HR 1.20, P = 0.05), and incidence of brain metastases at 2 years was not significantly different between standard- and higher dose PCI
- Consolidative TRT

- Addition of TRT significantly improved OS (median 17 vs. 11 months, 5-year OS 9.1% vs. 3.7%, P = 0.041)

RECOMMENDED FOLLOW-UP

Clinical

- Clinical follow-up visits every 3-4 months for years 1-2, every 6 months for years 3-5, then annually
- Smoking cessation intervention recommended

Radiographic

- Chest CECT recommended at each clinic follow-up visit
- PET/CT and brain imaging (MR or CT) are not recommended during routine follow-up

Laboratory

- CBC, comprehensive metabolic panel, & LDH with each clinical follow-up

SELECTED REFERENCES

1. Giuliani ME et al: Locoregional failures following thoracic irradiation in patients with limited-stage small cell lung carcinoma. Radiother Oncol. 102(2):263-7, 2012
2. Rossi A et al: Carboplatin- or cisplatin-based chemotherapy in first-line treatment of small-cell lung cancer: the COCIS meta-analysis of individual patient data. J Clin Oncol. 30(14):1692-8, 2012
3. Siegel R et al: Cancer statistics, 2012. CA Cancer J Clin. 62(1):10-29, 2012
4. Kalemkerian GP et al: Small cell lung cancer. J Natl Compr Canc Netw. 9(10):1086-113, 2011
5. Kong FM et al: Consideration of dose limits for organs at risk of thoracic radiotherapy: atlas for lung, proximal bronchial tree, esophagus, spinal cord, ribs, and brachial plexus. Int J Radiat Oncol Biol Phys. 81(5):1442-57, 2011
6. Terasaki H et al: Lung adenocarcinoma, mixed subtype: histopathologic basis for high-resolution computed tomography findings. J Thorac Imaging. 26(1):74-81, 2011
7. van Meerbeeck JP et al: Small-cell lung cancer. Lancet. 378(9804):1741-55, 2011
8. Volterrani L et al: MSCT multi-criteria: a novel approach in assessment of mediastinal lymph node metastases in non-small cell lung cancer. Eur J Radiol. 79(3):459-66, 2011
9. American Joint Committee on Cancer: AJCC Cancer Staging Manual. 7th ed. New York: Springer. 253-70, 2010
10. van Loon J et al: Selective nodal irradiation on basis of (18)FDG-PET scans in limited-disease small-cell lung cancer: a prospective study. Int J Radiat Oncol Biol Phys. 77(2):329-36, 2010
11. Watkins JM et al: Once-daily radiotherapy to > or =59.4 Gy versus twice-daily radiotherapy to > or =45.0 Gy with concurrent chemotherapy for limited-stage small-cell lung cancer: a comparative analysis of toxicities and outcomes. Jpn J Radiol. 28(5):340-8, 2010
12. Detterbeck FC et al: The new lung cancer staging system. Chest. 136(1):260-71, 2009
13. Le Péchoux C et al: Standard-dose versus higher-dose prophylactic cranial irradiation (PCI) in patients with limited-stage small-cell lung cancer in complete remission after chemotherapy and thoracic radiotherapy (PCI 99-01, EORTC 22003-08004, RTOG 0212, and IFCT 99-01): a randomised clinical trial. Lancet Oncol. 10(5):467-74, 2009
14. Vallières E et al: The IASLC Lung Cancer Staging Project: proposals regarding the relevance of TNM in the pathologic staging of small cell lung cancer in the forthcoming (seventh) edition of the TNM classification for lung cancer. J Thorac Oncol. 4(9):1049-59, 2009
15. Videtic GM et al: Report from the International Atomic Energy Agency (IAEA) consultants' meeting on elective nodal irradiation in lung cancer: small-cell lung cancer (SCLC). Int J Radiat Oncol Biol Phys. 72(2):327-34, 2008
16. Shepherd FA et al: The International Association for the Study of Lung Cancer lung cancer staging project: proposals regarding the clinical staging of small cell lung cancer in the forthcoming (seventh) edition of the tumor, node, metastasis classification for lung cancer. J Thorac Oncol. 2(12):1067-77, 2007
17. Simon GR et al: Management of small cell lung cancer: ACCP evidence-based clinical practice guidelines (2nd edition). Chest. 132(3 Suppl):324S-339S, 2007
18. De Ruysscher D et al: Systematic review and meta-analysis of randomised, controlled trials of the timing of chest radiotherapy in patients with limited-stage, small-cell lung cancer. Ann Oncol. 17(4):543-52, 2006
19. De Ruysscher D et al: Time between the first day of chemotherapy and the last day of chest radiation is the most important predictor of survival in limited-disease small-cell lung cancer. J Clin Oncol. 24(7):1057-63, 2006
20. Govindan R et al: Changing epidemiology of small-cell lung cancer in the United States over the last 30 years: analysis of the surveillance, epidemiologic, and end results database. J Clin Oncol. 24(28):4539-44, 2006
21. Beasley MB et al: The 2004 World Health Organization classification of lung tumors. Semin Roentgenol. 40(2):90-7, 2005
22. Chapet O et al: CT-based definition of thoracic lymph node stations: an atlas from the University of Michigan. Int J Radiat Oncol Biol Phys. 63(1):170-8, 2005
23. Fried DB et al: Systematic review evaluating the timing of thoracic radiation therapy in combined modality therapy for limited-stage small-cell lung cancer. J Clin Oncol. 2004 Dec 1;22(23):4837-45. Review. Erratum in: J Clin Oncol. 23(1):248, 2005
24. Jackman DM et al: Small-cell lung cancer. Lancet. 366(9494):1385-96, 2005
25. Bogart JA et al: 70 Gy thoracic radiotherapy is feasible concurrent with chemotherapy for limited-stage small-cell lung cancer: analysis of Cancer and Leukemia Group B study 39808. Int J Radiat Oncol Biol Phys. 59(2):460-8, 2004
26. Videtic GM et al: Continued cigarette smoking by patients receiving concurrent chemoradiotherapy for limited-stage small-cell lung cancer is associated with decreased survival. J Clin Oncol. 21(8):1544-9, 2003
27. Arriagada R et al: Patterns of failure after prophylactic cranial irradiation in small-cell lung cancer: analysis of 505 randomized patients. Ann Oncol. 13(5):748-54, 2002
28. Sundstrøm S et al: Cisplatin and etoposide regimen is superior to cyclophosphamide, epirubicin, and vincristine regimen in small-cell lung cancer: results from a randomized phase III trial with 5 years' follow-up. J Clin Oncol. 20(24):4665-72, 2002
29. Takada M et al: Phase III study of concurrent versus sequential thoracic radiotherapy in combination with cisplatin and etoposide for limited-stage small-cell lung cancer: results of the Japan Clinical Oncology Group Study 9104. J Clin Oncol. 20(14):3054-60, 2002
30. Argiris A et al: Staging and clinical prognostic factors for small-cell lung cancer. Cancer J. 7(5):437-47, 2001
31. Thomas CR Jr et al: Ten-year follow-up of Southwest Oncology Group 8269: a phase II trial of concomitant cisplatin-etoposide and daily thoracic radiotherapy in limited small-cell lung cancer. Lung Cancer. 33(2-3):213-9, 2001

(Left) *Axial CT shows mediastinal LN stations: Low cervical (1R/L), upper paratracheal (2R/L), preaortic (3A), retrotracheal (3P), lower paratracheal (4R/L), AP window (5), paraaortic LNs (6). Ascending aorta (Asc A), ascending azygos vein (AAV), carina (C), descending aorta (DA), superior vena cava (SVC).* **(Right)** *Same shows: Subcarinal (7), paraesophageal (8), pulmonary ligament LNs (9). Left pulmonary artery (LPA), pulmonary trunk (PT), right pulmonary artery (RPA).*

Mediastinal Anatomy

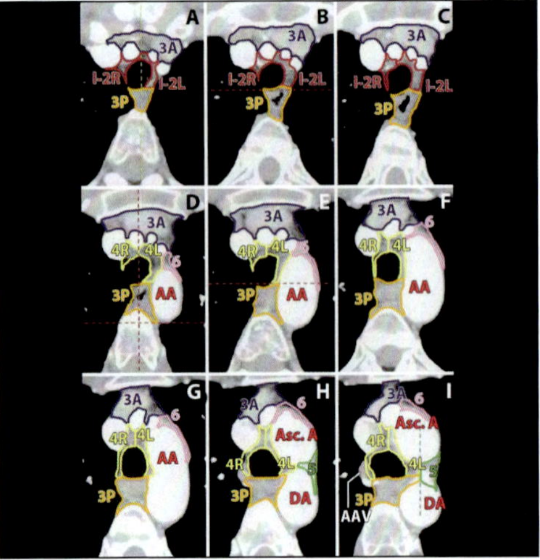

Mediastinal Anatomy

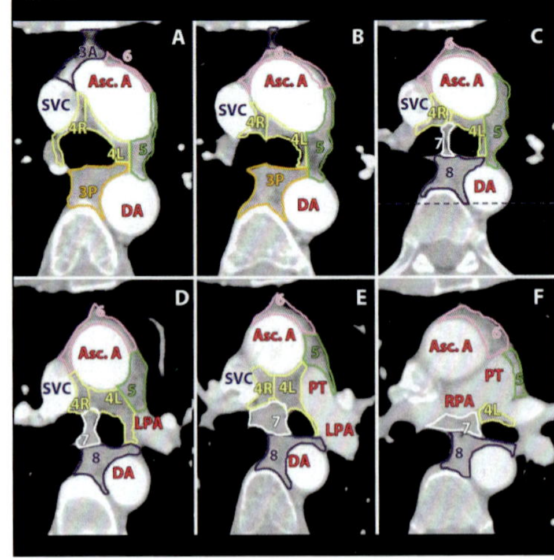

(Left) *Hilar lymph node stations are defined on axial CT in lung (A1, B1, B2) and mediastinal (A2, C, D) windows. Hilar lymph node region is outlined.* **(Right)** *Axial CECT of the same patient shows bulky confluent mediastinal and hilar lymphadenopathy with near-complete obstruction of the SVC. SVC syndrome occurs commonly in patients with SCLC. (Courtesy T. Ternes, MD.)*

Mediastinal Anatomy

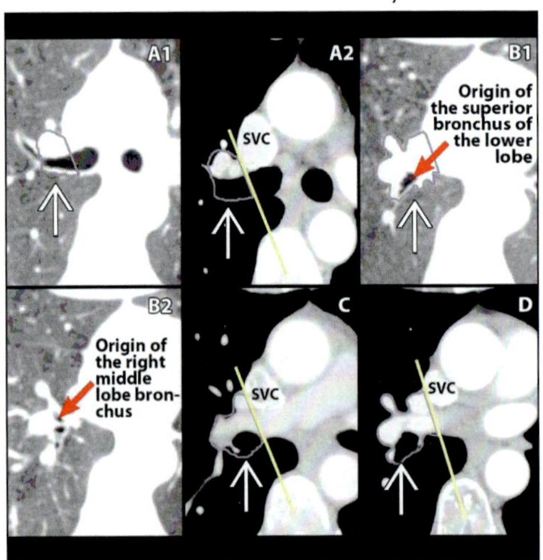

Impending SVC Syndrome

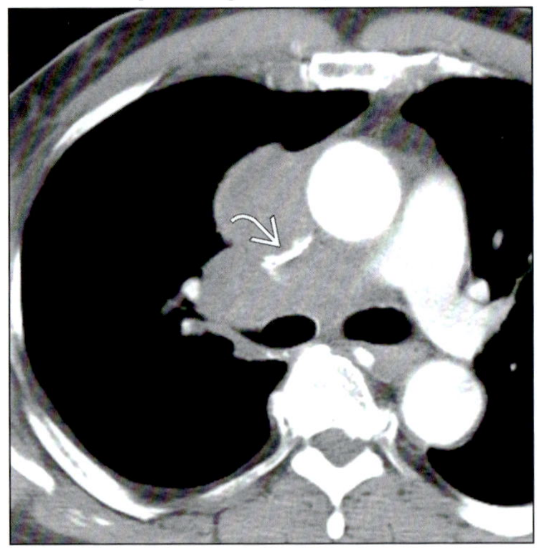

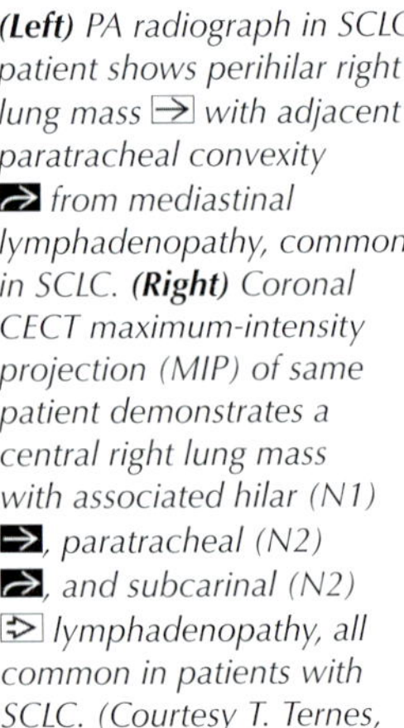

(Left) *PA radiograph in SCLC patient shows perihilar right lung mass with adjacent paratracheal convexity from mediastinal lymphadenopathy, common in SCLC.* **(Right)** *Coronal CECT maximum-intensity projection (MIP) of same patient demonstrates a central right lung mass with associated hilar (N1), paratracheal (N2), and subcarinal (N2) lymphadenopathy, all common in patients with SCLC. (Courtesy T. Ternes, MD.)*

Mediastinal Adenopathy

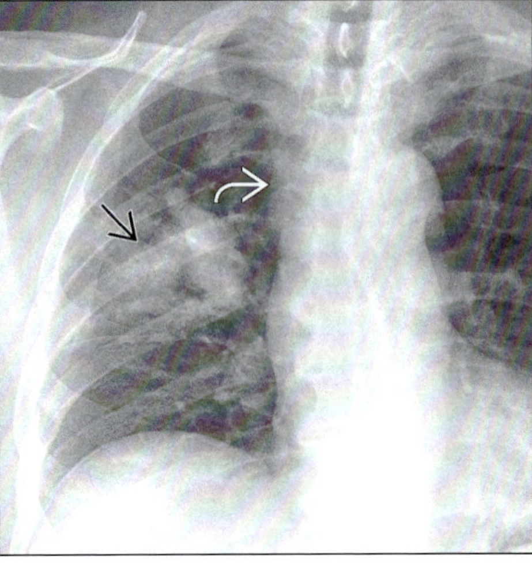

Mediastinal Adenopathy

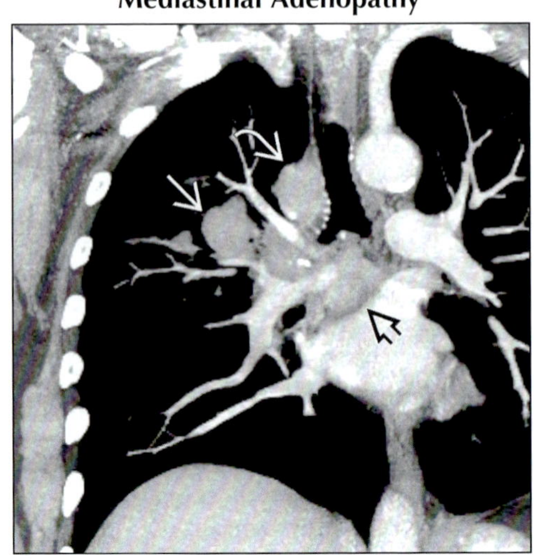

Airway Obstruction

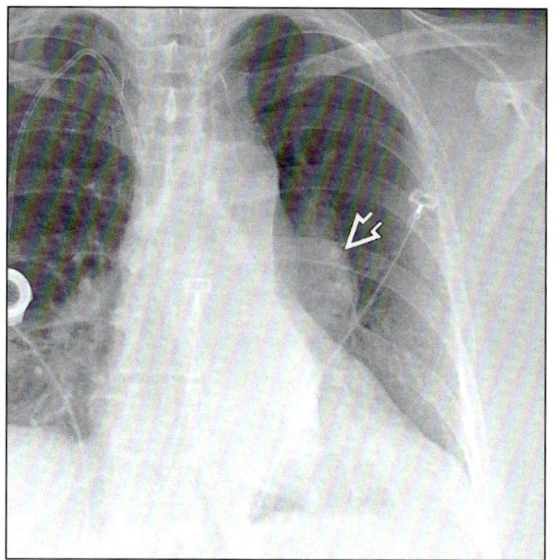

Airway Obstruction

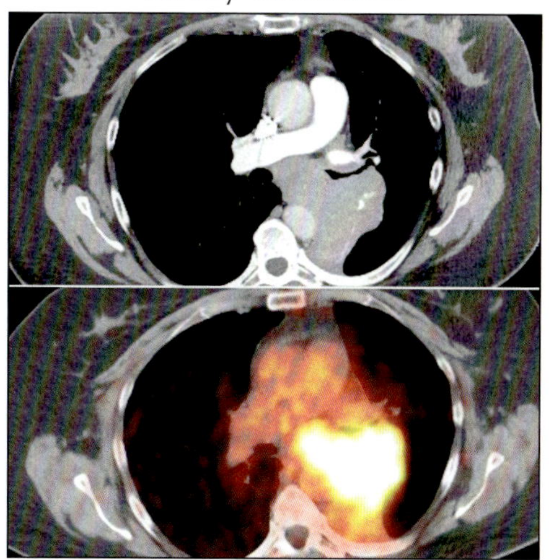

(Left) *PA chest radiograph of a patient with SCLC demonstrates a left hilar mass ➡ with left lower lobe bronchus cut-off and associated lobar atelectasis.* ***(Right)*** *Axial CECT (top) and fused PET/CT (bottom) of the same patient show a left central posterior mass with intense FDG activity encasing and obstructing the left lower lobe bronchus with associated lobar atelectasis. Central airway compression occurs often in SCLC. (Courtesy T. Ternes, MD.)*

Airway Obstruction

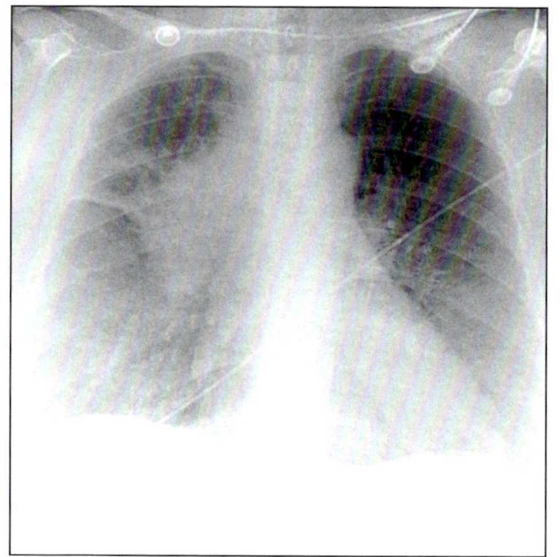

Airway Obstruction

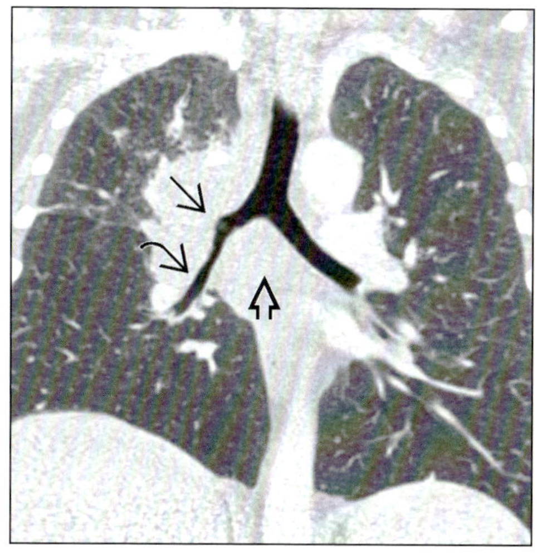

(Left) *PA chest radiograph demonstrates a large right hilar/perihilar mass in a patient presenting with dyspnea. Biopsy revealed SCLC.* ***(Right)*** *Coronal CECT of the same patient demonstrates a right hilar mass completely obliterating the right upper lobe bronchus ➡ and slightly compressing the right lower lobe bronchus ➡, with associated bulky subcarinal lymphadenopathy ➡. Central airway compression occurs commonly in SCLC patients. (Courtesy T. Ternes, MD.)*

Stage IIIA (T2a N2 M0), Limited Stage

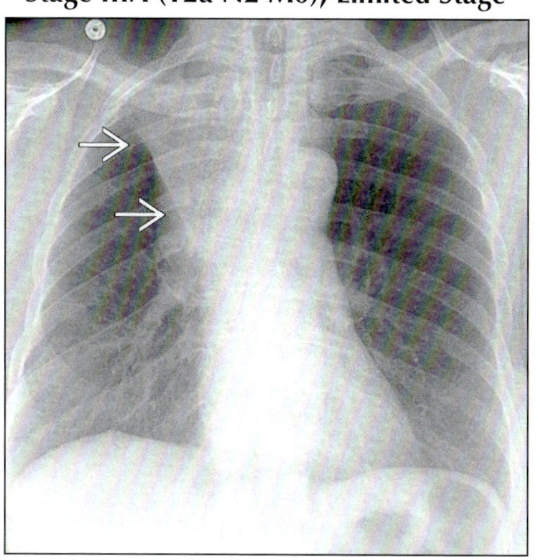

Stage IIIA (T2a N2 M0), Limited Stage

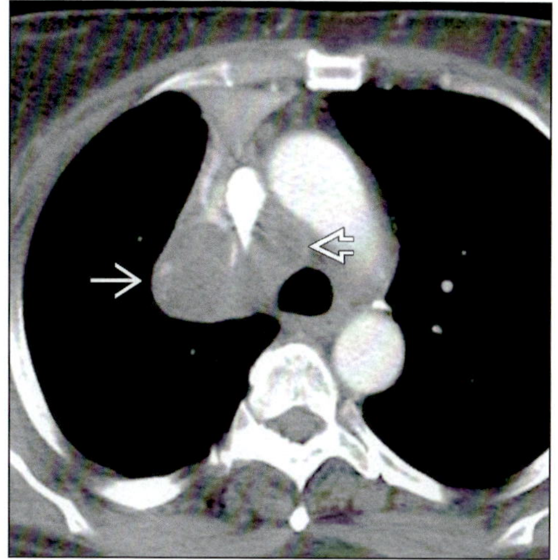

(Left) *Frontal chest x-ray shows right upper lobe collapse ➡. Any lobar collapse/atelectasis in an adult patient should raise suspicion for an endobronchial or perihilar mass.* ***(Right)*** *Axial CECT in the same patient shows a large, necrotic, right suprahilar mass ➡ as well as adjacent necrotic right paratracheal adenopathy ➡. Small cell carcinoma was diagnosed via endobronchial biopsy.*

SMALL CELL LUNG CANCER

(Left) Axial CECT demonstrated a lobulated left upper lobe mass ➡ without hilar, mediastinal, or supraclavicular lymphadenopathy. Biopsy was positive for SCLC. SCLC presents as an isolated peripheral nodule in < 5% of patients, who may be appropriate candidates for surgical resection. **(Right)** Sagittal CECT view reveals multiple sclerotic vertebral body metastases ➡, upstaging this patient to stage IV (extensive stage). (Courtesy T. Ternes, MD.)

Stage IV, Extensive Stage

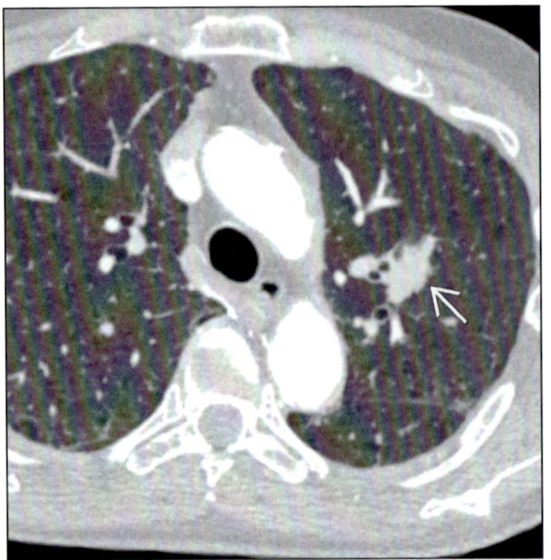

Stage IV, Extensive Stage

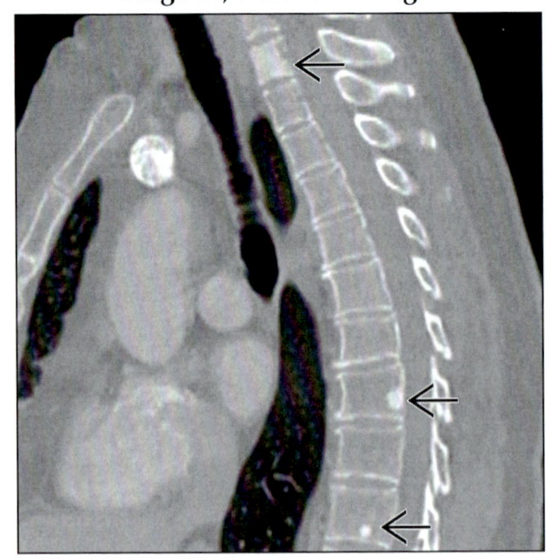

(Left) MIP PET shows advanced stage IV (extensive stage) small cell lung carcinoma, consisting of cerebellar ➡, subcutaneous ➡, right hilar, mediastinal ➡, hepatic ➡, and adrenal ➡ metastases. Brain, liver, adrenal, and bone metastases are all common in SCLC. **(Right)** Axial T1WI C+ FLAIR MR in the same patient shows multiple enhancing brain lesions ➡. Brain metastasis indicates M1b (extensive) stage.

Stage IV, Extensive Stage

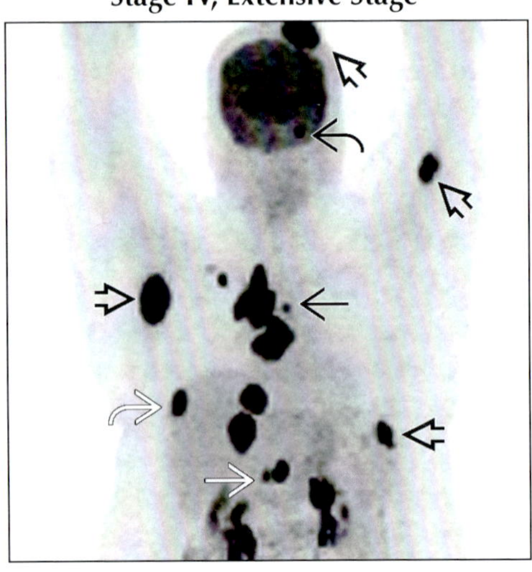

Stage IV, Extensive Stage

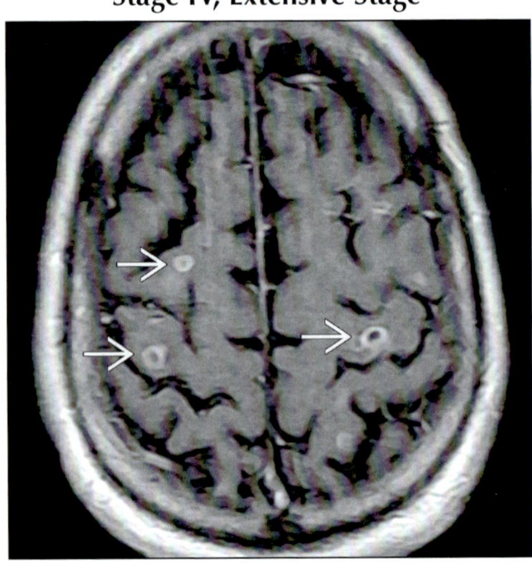

(Left) Sagittal fused PET/CT shows multiple areas of radiopharmaceutical activity, indicating thoracic vertebral metastases ➡. Distant disease to bone, liver, adrenals, and brain is common with SCLC. **(Right)** 3D reconstruction of a 3-field thoracic RT plan is shown. Great care must be taken in contouring the multiple organs at risk, including the lungs ➡, spinal cord ➡, esophagus ➡, and heart ➡.

Extensive Stage

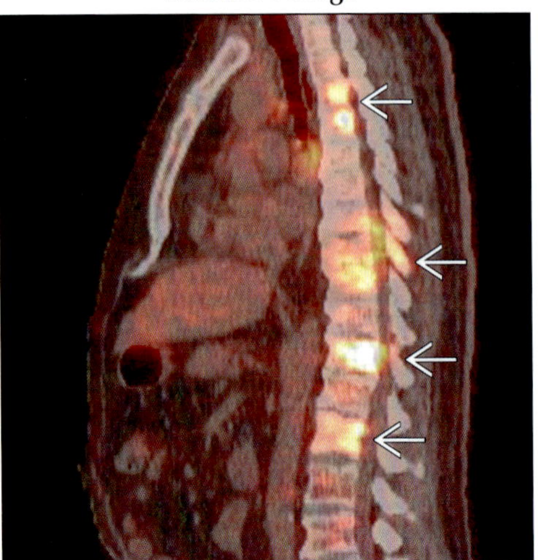

3D Planning

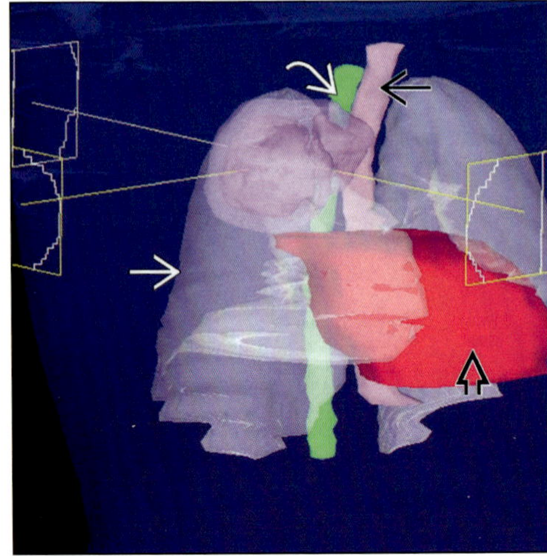

Limited Stage

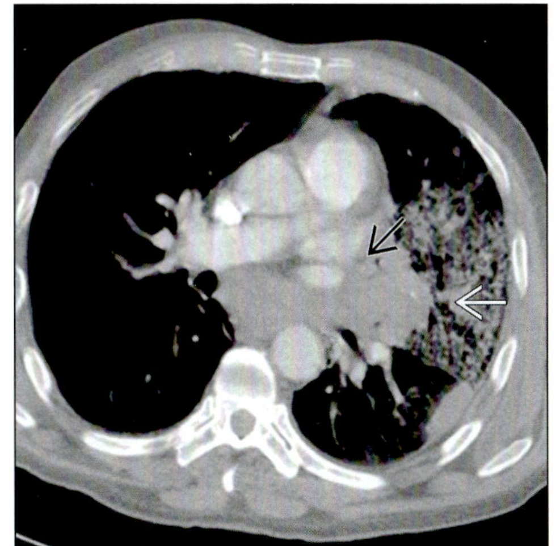

Limited Stage

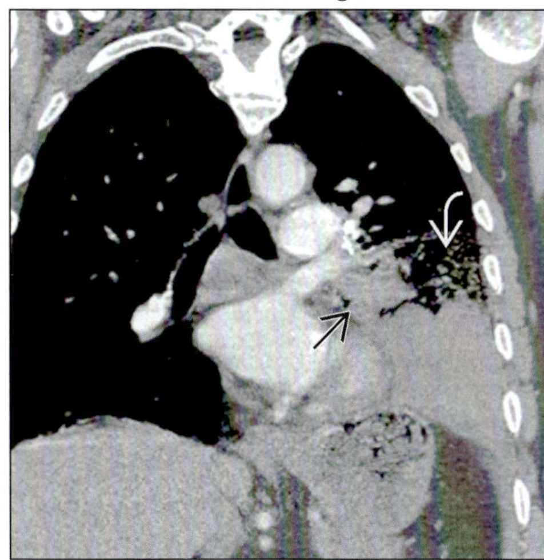

(Left) *Axial CECT shows left hilar mass → invading the mediastinum & compressing the lingular segmental bronchi causing postobstructive pneumonia ⇒, with left hilar, AP window, subcarinal, & left paraesophageal lymphadenopathy. EBUS-FNA was positive for SCLC. PET/CT was negative for distant metastases & brain MR was negative. He was staged T4 N2 M0 (IIIB, limited stage).* ***(Right)*** *Coronal CT in same patient shows adenopathy → & atelectasis ⇒.*

Limited Stage

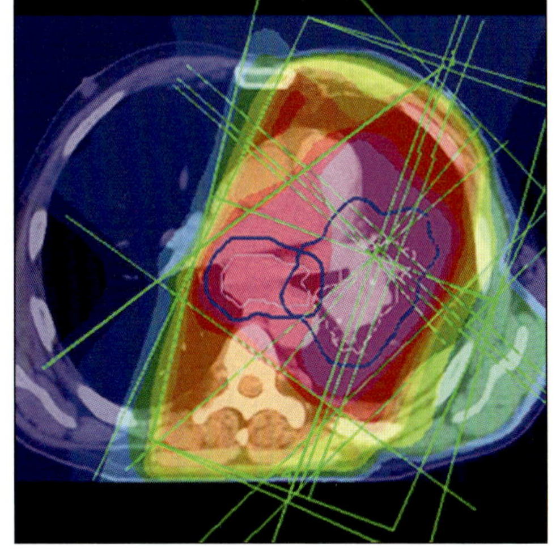

Limited Stage

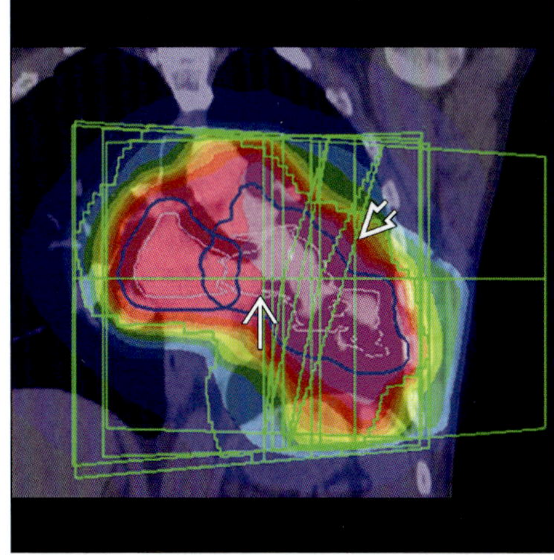

(Left) *The same patient underwent definitive CRT, receiving 45 Gy in 30 fractions of 1.5 Gy 2x daily with concurrent cisplatin and etoposide (PE). An axial slice of the RT plan shows contoured GTVs (violet) and PTVs (blue) (isodose map in % prescription dose). No elective nodal irradiation (ENI) was performed.* ***(Right)*** *Representative coronal slice of the RT plan in the same patient shows extensive subcarinal → and hilar ⇒ involvement.*

Limited Stage

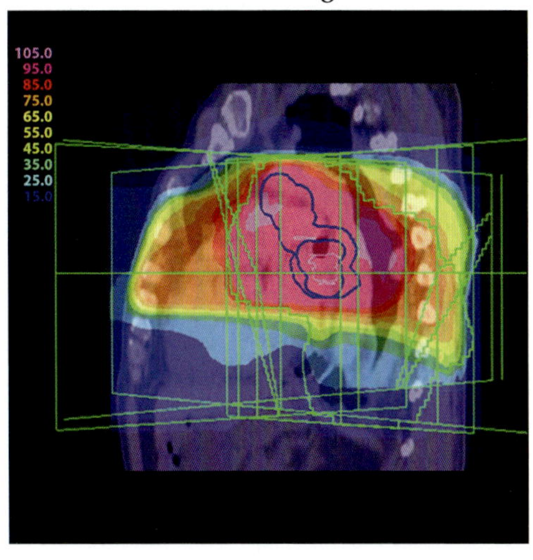

Limited Stage

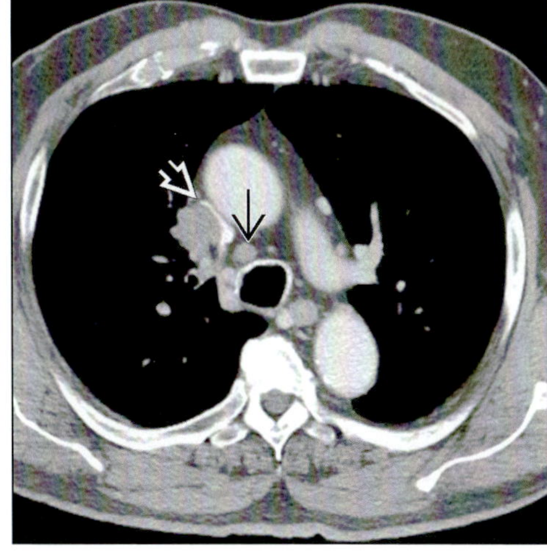

(Left) *Sagittal RT plan in same patient is shown. He completed 4 cycles of chemo with PR with no evidence of extrathoracic progression and then received PCI with 25 Gy in 10 fx.* ***(Right)*** *CT in 72-year-old man shows RUL mass with right hilar and suprahilar adenopathy compressing SVC ⇒, as well as paratracheal → and subcarinal adenopathy. PET confirmed no distant mets and brain CT was negative. EBUS-FNA returned SCLC, stage T1a N2 M0 (IIIA, limited stage).*

SMALL CELL LUNG CANCER

Limited Stage

Limited Stage

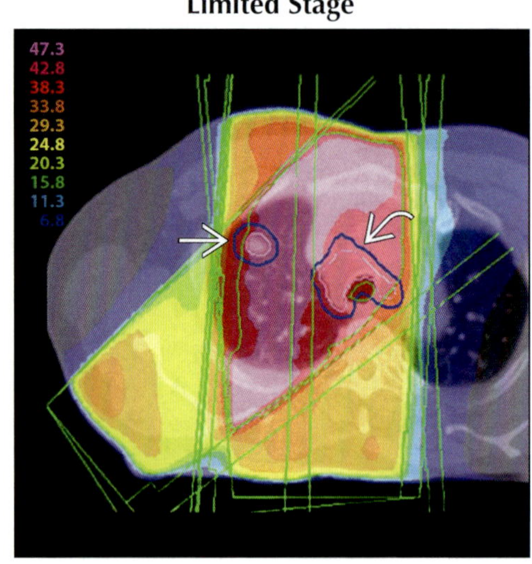

(Left) *Axial CT in the same patient shows prominent subcarinal ➔ and right hilar ➔ nodes that were FDG avid on PET.* ***(Right)*** *The same patient underwent definitive CRT, receiving 45 Gy in 30 2x-daily fractions of 1.5 Gy each with concurrent cisplatin and etoposide. RUL nodule ➔ and paratracheal ➔ GTV (violet) and PTV (blue) contours are displayed (isodose map in gray). A 4D CT simulation to account for breathing motion and permit tight margins was used to limit lung dose.*

Limited Stage

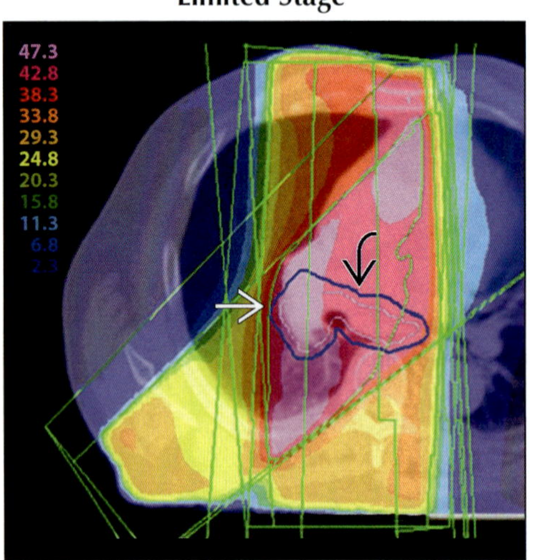

Limited Stage

ITV
ITV NODE
PTV
PTV NODE
LUNG - ITV
HEART
ESOPHAGUS
CORD

Volume [%]

Dose [Gy]

(Left) *In the same patient, GTV and PTV including the subcarinal ➔ and right hilar ➔ LNs are shown. No ENI was performed.* ***(Right)*** *In the same patient, DVH for targets and OARs is shown. Mean lung dose = 15.2 Gy, lung V20 = 32.3%, mean heart dose = 17.6 Gy, spinal cord max dose = 34.5 Gy; esophagus mean dose = 18 Gy, and esophagus max dose = 45 Gy. ITV = primary tumor internal target volume ➔; ITV NODE = nodal internal target volume ➔.*

Limited Stage

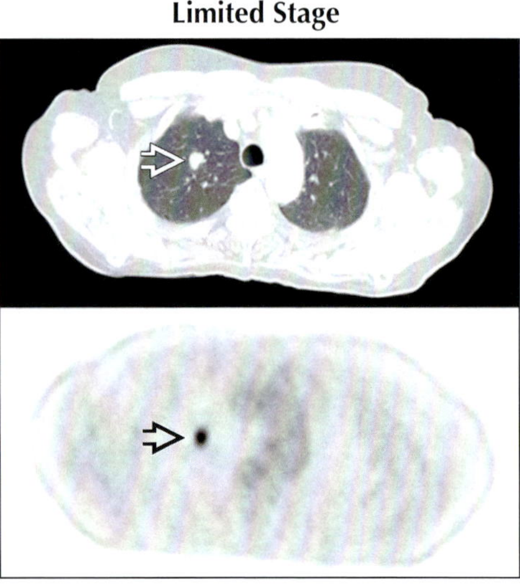

Limited Stage

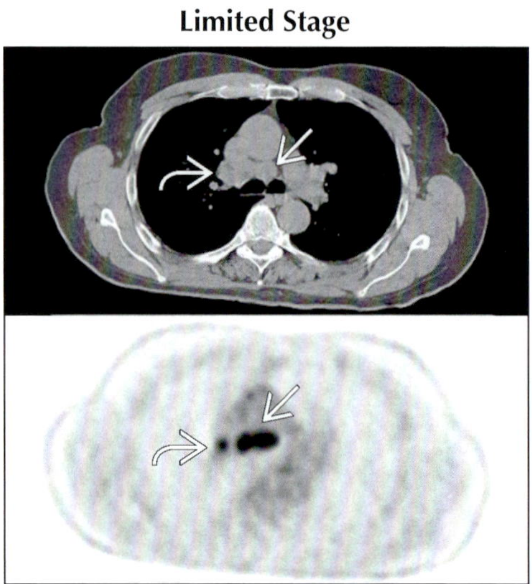

(Left) *This 67-year-old man was found to have an incidental RUL nodule on chest CT ➔ that grew on follow-up imaging. PET/ CT demonstrated intense FDG avidity in the RUL nodule ➔ and the right hilar and precarinal mediastinal lymph nodes. Brain MR was negative. A transbronchial FNA biopsy was positive for SCLC, stage T1a N2 M0 (IIIA, limited stage).* ***(Right)*** *FDG-avid precarinal ➔ and right hilar ➔ lymph nodes are shown on CT and PET scan in the same patient.*

Limited Stage

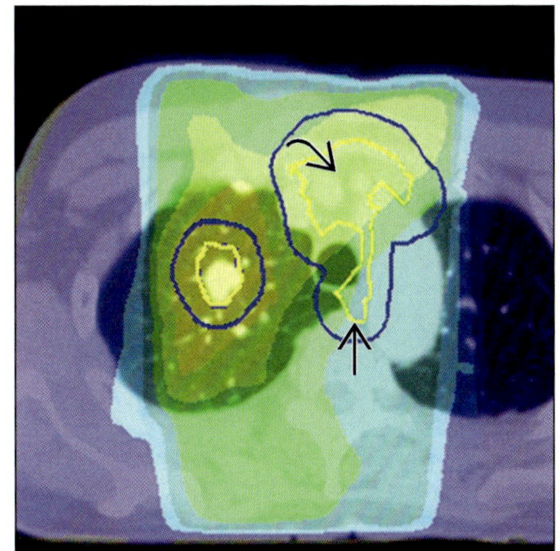

Limited Stage

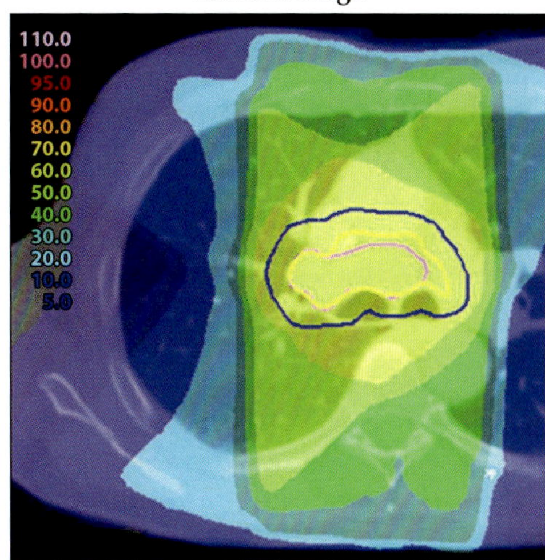

*(**Left**) The same patient received CRT on the delayed accelerated hyperfractionation arm of the CALGB 30610/RTOG 538 randomized trial. He received 61 Gy in 34 fractions over 5 weeks with concurrent PE. GTVs (violet), CTVs (yellow), and PTVs (blue) are displayed. The prevascular → and retrotracheal → nodal stations are treated with ENI. (**Right**) In the same patient, isodoses are displayed in Gy for the subcarinal GTV (pink), elective nodal CTV (yellow), and PTV (blue).*

Limited Stage

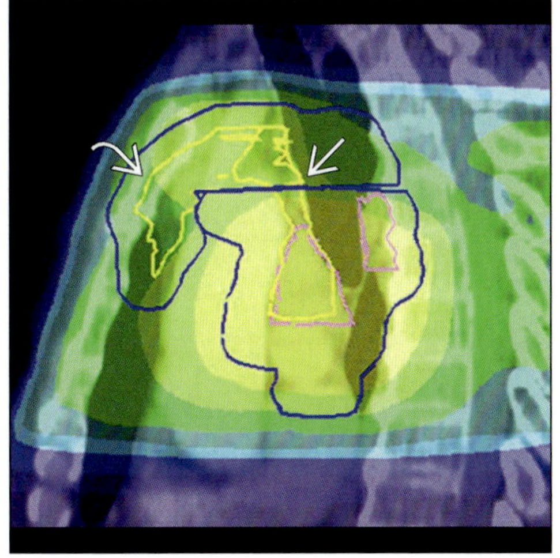

Limited Stage

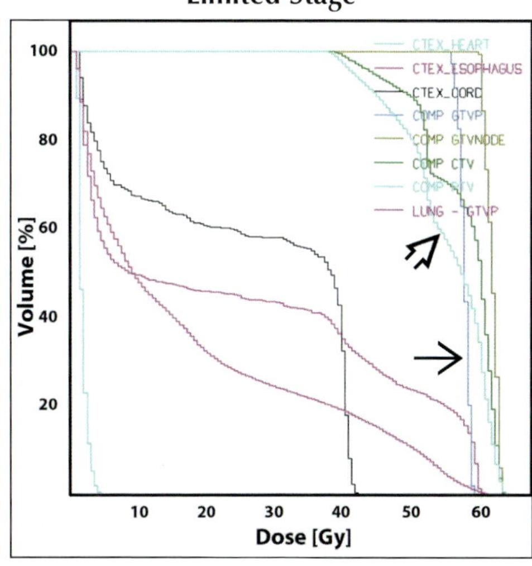

*(**Left**) Representative sagittal slice of the same plan highlights the elective nodal CTVs (yellow) coverage. The prevascular → and retrotracheal → nodal stations received ENI. (**Right**) DVH in the same patient shows coverage of targets and OARs. Mean lung dose = 18.3 Gy, lung V20 = 33.9%, mean heart dose = 1.4 Gy, and max spinal cord dose = 26.0 Gy. Note primary tumor GTV → and composite PTV →.*

Limited Stage

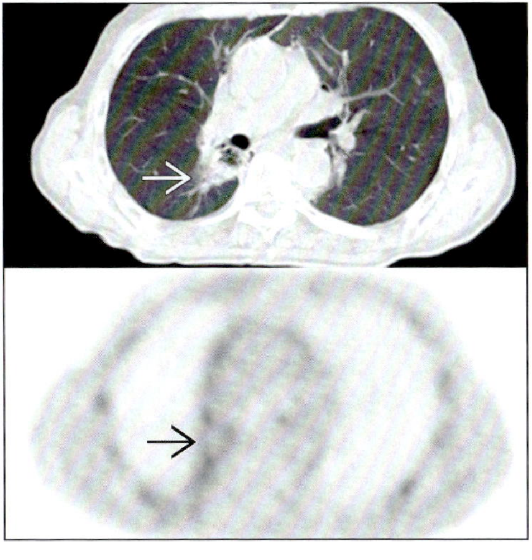

Limited Stage

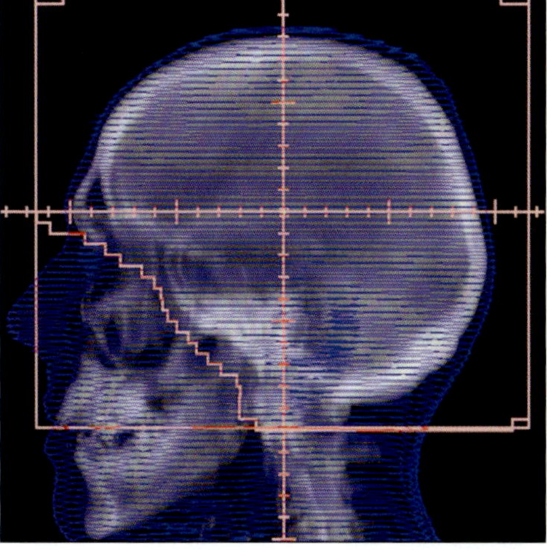

*(**Left**) Six months after CRT in the same patient, follow-up PET/CT showed complete metabolic response. Volume loss and linear and ground-glass opacities → with mild FDG uptake → along the edge of the RT portal in the medial right upper and lower lobes are seen, consistent with evolving post-RT changes. (**Right**) The same patient went on to receive prophylactic cranial irradiation with 25 Gy in 10 daily fractions. Lateral radiotherapy portal is shown.*

(Left) PET/CT demonstrates intense FDG avidity in the RLL nodule and a right hilar LN with no abnormal mediastinal or extrathoracic activity. Stage T1a N1 M0 (IIA, limited stage). Small peripheral primaries are infrequently seen in SCLC. **(Right)** The same patient underwent CRT, receiving 45 Gy b.i.d. Primary tumor and right hilar GTV (violet) and PTV (blue) contours are displayed. Isodose map is shown in gray.

Limited Stage

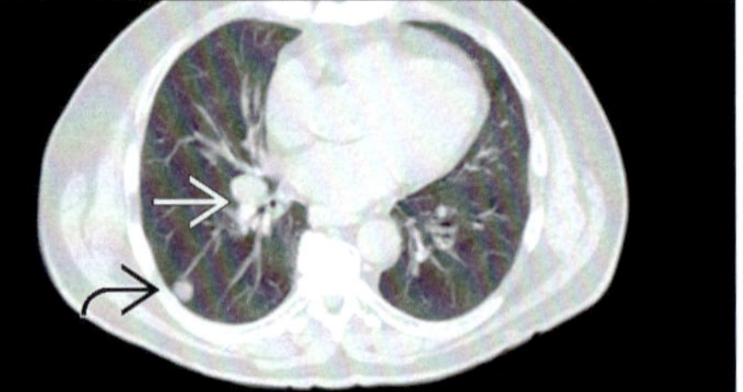

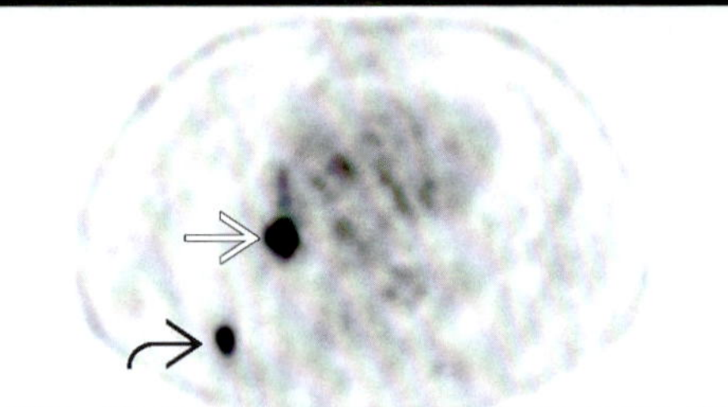

Limited Stage

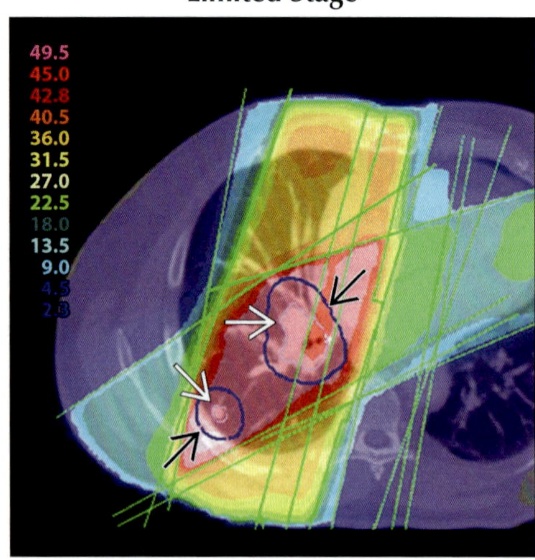

(Left) In the same patient, ENI was performed for the lower paratracheal and subcarinal mediastinal lymph node stations , designated as a CTV (yellow). **(Right)** Coronal representation of the RT plan in the same patient shows the hilar and mediastinal CTVs (yellow) and PTVs (blue). Note the relative sparing of the left ventricle of the heart and left lung .

Limited Stage

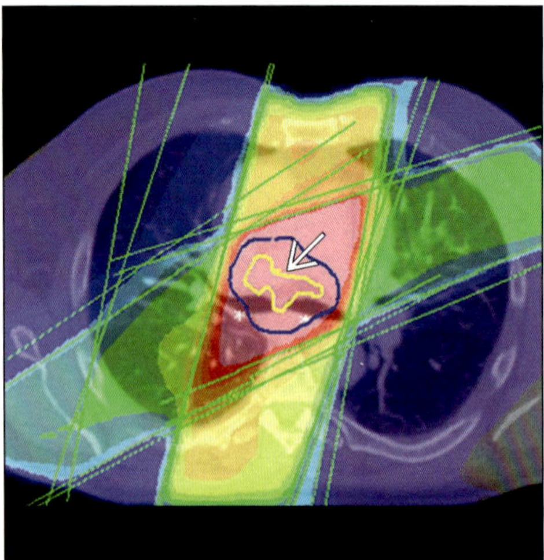

Limited Stage

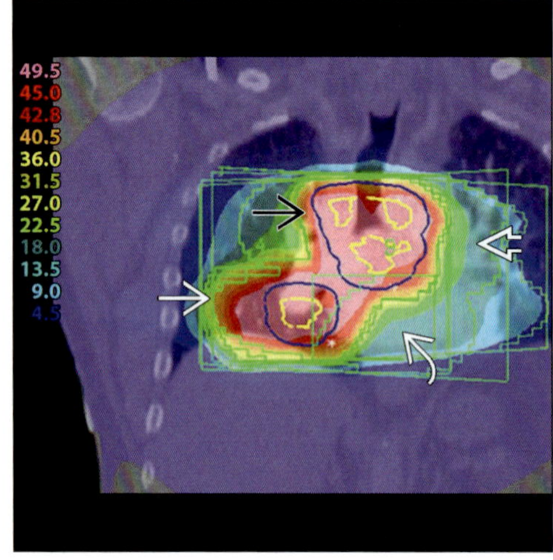

(Left) DVH in the same patient is shown for targets and OARs. Mean lung dose = 15.1 Gy, lung V20 = 30.7%, heart mean dose = 26.1 Gy, esophagus mean dose = 21 Gy, and esophagus max = 47 Gy. **(Right)** Following completion of CRT, the same patient had a CR. He remains without evidence of disease at 24 months, as shown on lung-window CT, which demonstrates stable parahilar right lower lobe lung fibrosis and scarring , consistent with postradiotherapy changes.

Limited Stage

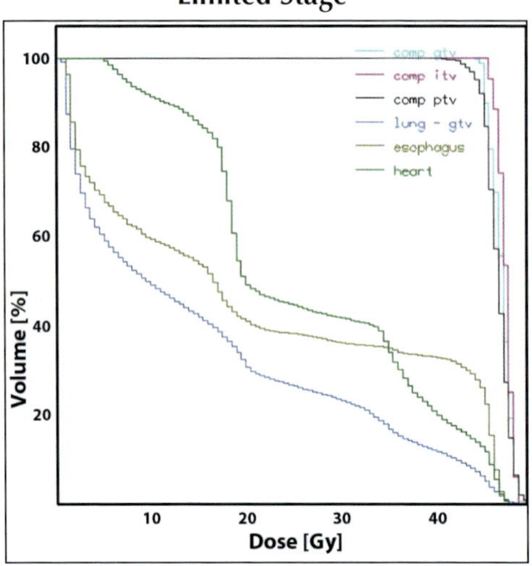

Limited Stage

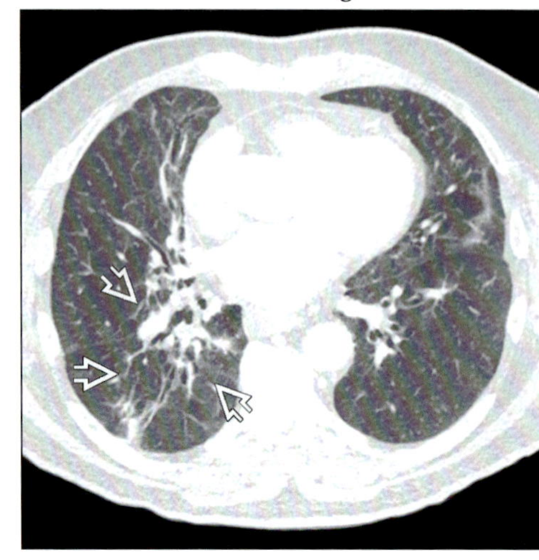

Limited Stage

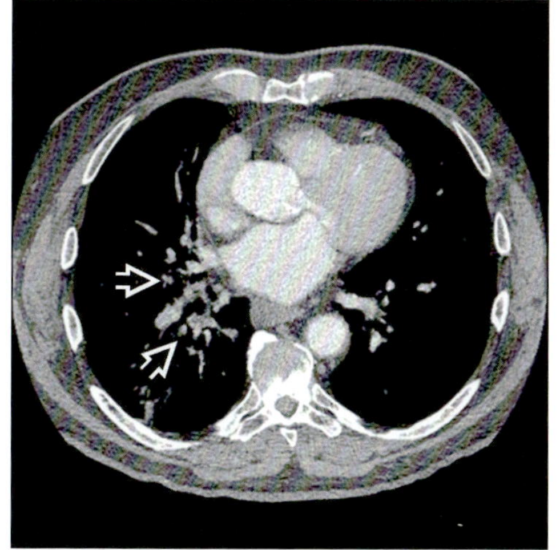

Extensive Stage

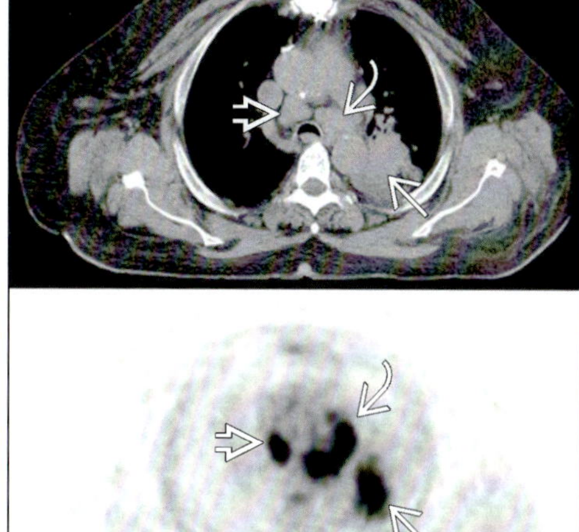

*(**Left**) Post-radiotherapy lung fibrosis is seen on CT (mediastinal window) ➡ in the same patient. (**Right**) A 58-year-old man presented with 1 year of progressive dyspnea. Chest CT shows a LUL mass ➡ with left hilar and mediastinal adenopathy in levels 2L, 3A, 4L ↷, 4R ➡, 5, 6, and 7, all with abnormal FDG avidity on PET. Thoracentesis of a left-sided pleural effusion was positive for malignant cells, upstaging him to T2 N2 M1a (stage IV, extensive stage).*

Extensive Stage

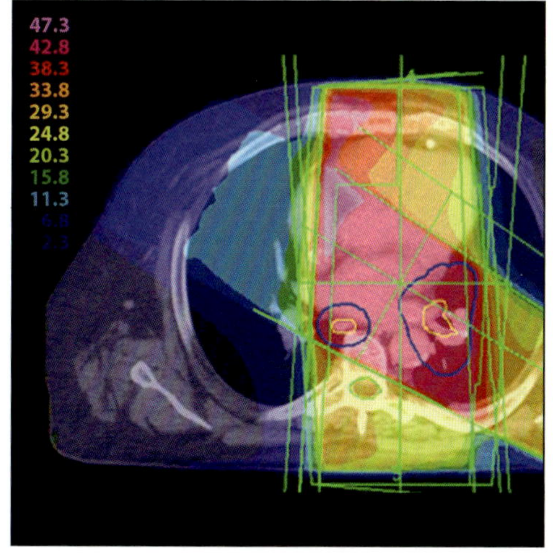

Extensive Stage

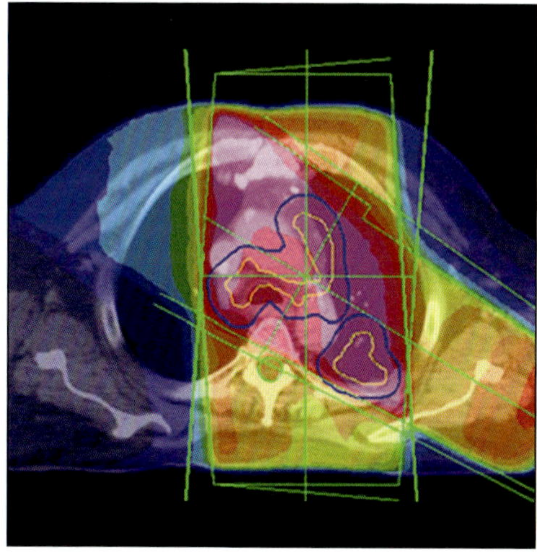

*(**Left**) After 6 cycles of carboplatin & etoposide in same patient, PET/CT showed a near CR, with mild residual FDG avidity in only the LUL lesion. He was treated with consolidative RT with 45 Gy in 15 daily 3 Gy fx. Original sites of nodal involvement were delineated as CTVs (yellow) with corresponding PTVs (blue) (isodose map in gray). No ENI was performed. PCI with 25 Gy in 10 fx was performed after completion. (**Right**) In same patient, isodose coverage is shown just above the carina.*

Extensive Stage

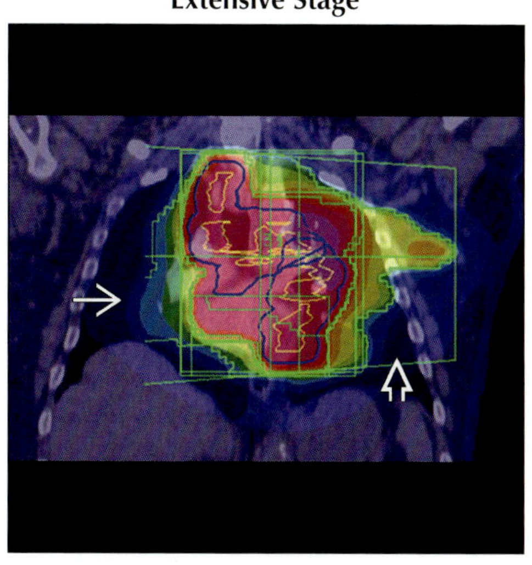

Extensive Stage

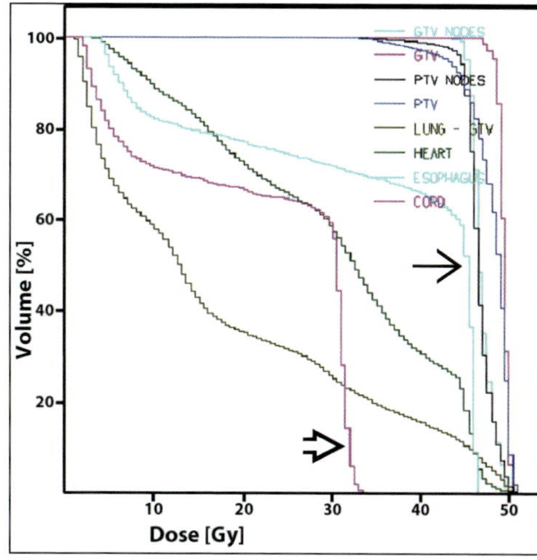

*(**Left**) Coronal representation of the consolidative RT plan in the same patient shows sparing of the right lung ➡ and lower left lung ➡ from the higher dose regions. (**Right**) DVH shows targets and OARs. Mean lung dose = 17.6 Gy, lung V20 = 35.1%, spinal cord ⇨ max = 34 Gy, esophagus → mean dose = 29.8 Gy, and esophagus max = 51 Gy. GTV = primary tumor GTV; PTV = primary tumor PTV.*

THYMUS

Masaoka Staging System

Stage	*Description*
I	Macroscopically and microscopically completely encapsulated
IIA	Microscopic transcapsular invasion
IIB	Macroscopic invasion into surrounding fatty tissue or grossly adherent to but not through mediastinal pleura or pericardium
IIIA	Macroscopic invasion into pericardium or lung without great vessel invasion
IIIB	Macroscopic invasion into pericardium or lung with great vessel invasion
IVA	Pleural or pericardial dissemination
IVB	Lymphogenous or hematogenous metastases

The Masaoka staging system is widely used to stage both thymomas and thymic carcinomas.

Spindle Cell Thymoma (WHO Type A)

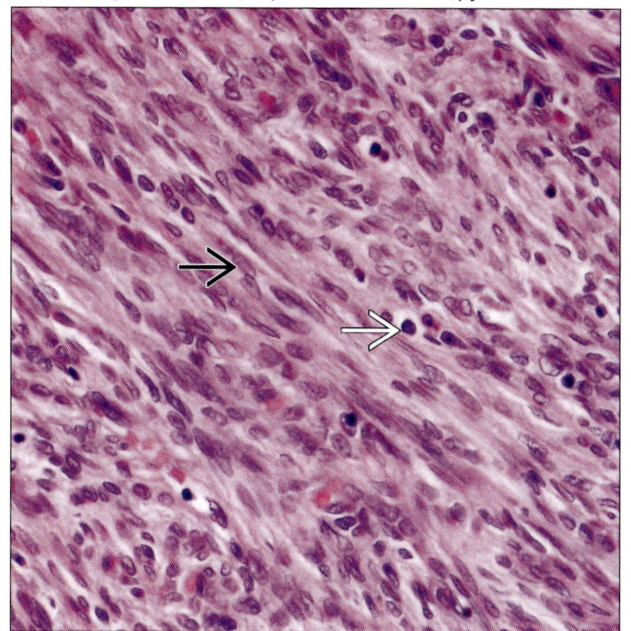

Spindle cell thymoma (WHO type A) shows fascicles of bland-appearing spindle cells ➔ admixed with a few scattered small lymphocytes ➔. (Courtesy S. Suster, MD.)

Lymphocyte-Rich Spindle Cell Thymoma (WHO Type AB)

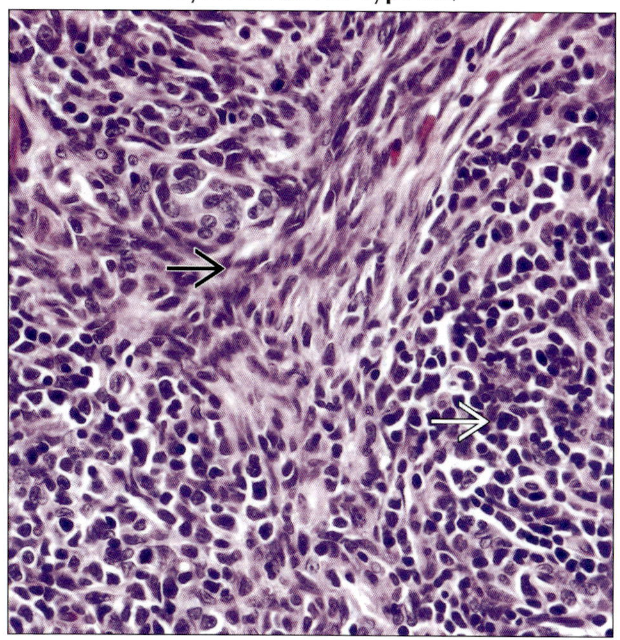

Lymphocyte-rich spindle cell thymoma (WHO type AB) shows storiform fascicle of spindle cells ➔ with few lymphocytes surrounded by areas containing scattered spindle cells admixed with numerous lymphocytes ➔. (Courtesy S. Suster, MD.)

Lymphocyte-Rich Thymoma (WHO Type B1)

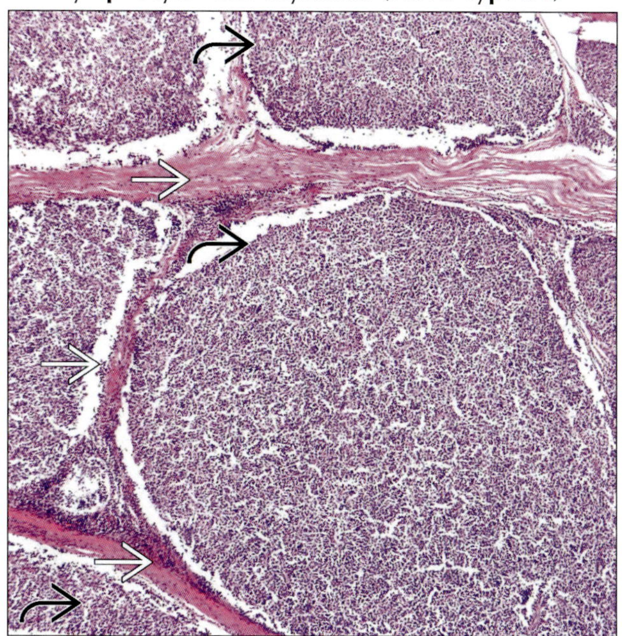

Lymphocyte-rich thymoma (WHO type B1) shows round lobules ➔ of tumor tissue containing abundant lymphocytes. The lobules are circumscribed by broad bands of fibroconnective tissue ➔. (Courtesy S. Suster, MD.)

Thymoma (WHO Type B2)

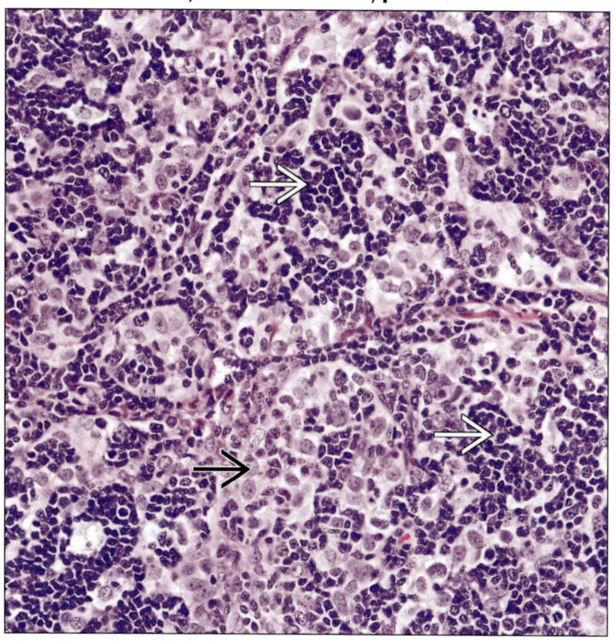

Mixed lymphoepithelial (WHO type B2) thymoma shows approximately equal admixture of lymphocytes ➔ with neoplastic epithelial cells ➔. (Courtesy S. Suster, MD.)

THYMUS

Thymoma (WHO Type B2)

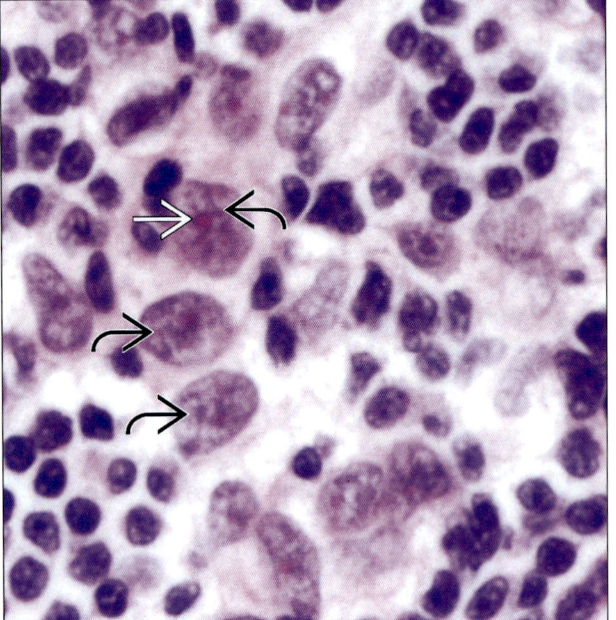

Higher magnification of mixed lymphoepithelial thymoma (WHO type B2) shows abundant large, round to oval epithelial cells ➡ displaying vesicular nuclei with prominent eosinophilic nucleoli ⇨ and indistinct rim of amphophilic cytoplasm. Note the variation in size and shape of the epithelial cells. (Courtesy S. Suster, MD.)

Thymoma (WHO Types B2 and B3)

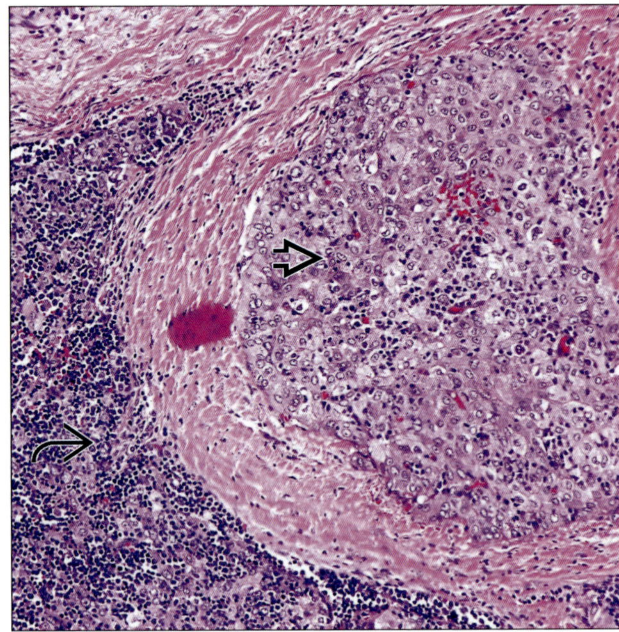

Combination of thymoma WHO types B2 (lymphoepithelial areas ⇨) and B3 (more atypical focus ⇨) is seen in approximately 30% of thymoma cases. (Courtesy S. Suster, MD.)

Microscopic Features

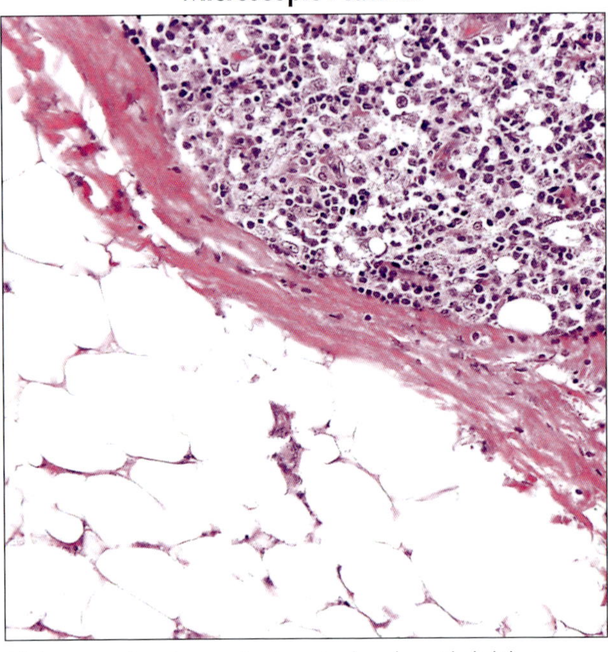

High-power view shows microinvasive lymphoepithelial thymoma infiltrating perithymic fat. (Courtesy S. Suster, MD.)

Squamous Cell Carcinoma of Thymus

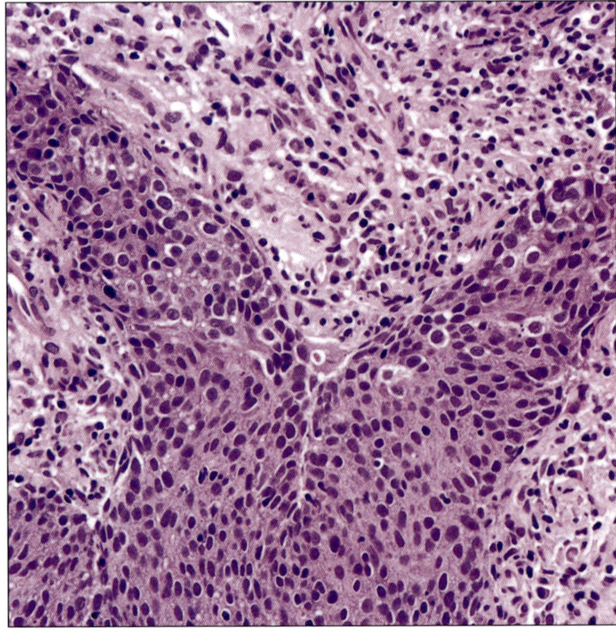

High magnification of primary squamous cell carcinoma of the thymus shows islands of large tumor cells with hyperchromatic nuclei and abundant cytoplasm and containing scattered mitotic figures. (Courtesy S. Suster, MD.)

Thymoma, Likely Stage I

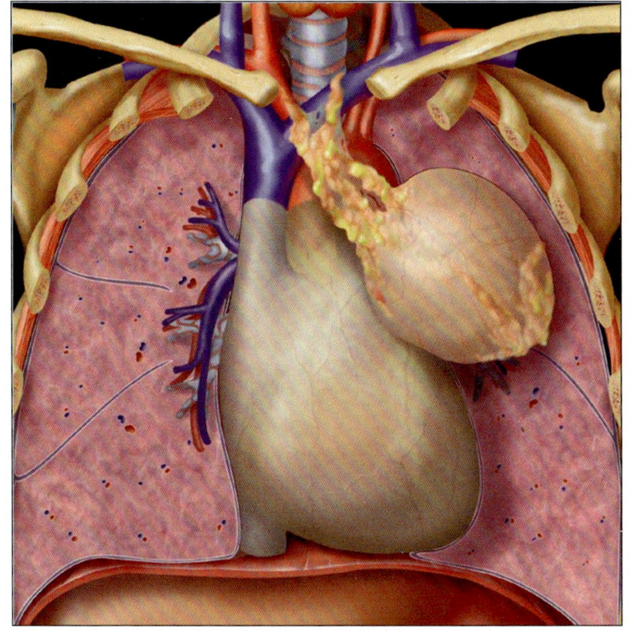

Schematic representation of the chest cavity shows a round to ovoid, well-circumscribed thymoma in the anterior mediastinal compartment on top of the pericardium and protruding onto the left hemithorax. This may be stage I, if completely encapsulated and not invasive, or stage II. Due to the smooth appearance, it is unlikely to be stage III.

Encapsulated Thymoma, Stage I or II

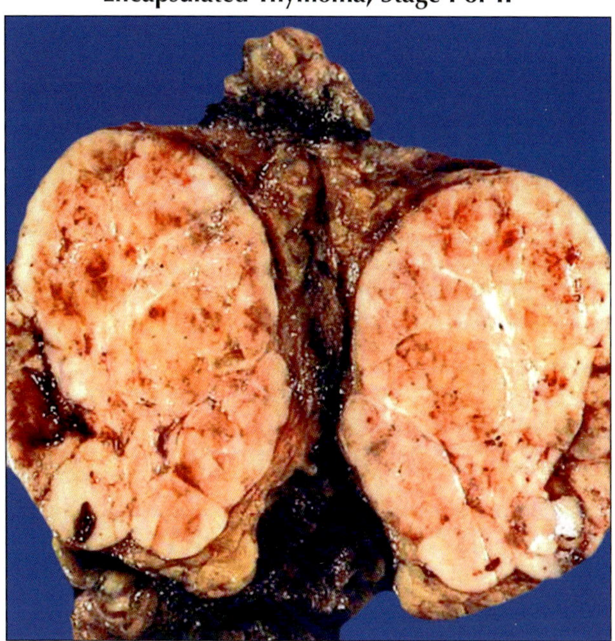

Gross appearance of bisected thymoma shows a well-circumscribed, fleshy, lobulated mass composed of tan-white, homogeneous rubbery tissue with focal areas of congestion and hemorrhage. (Courtesy S. Suster, MD.)

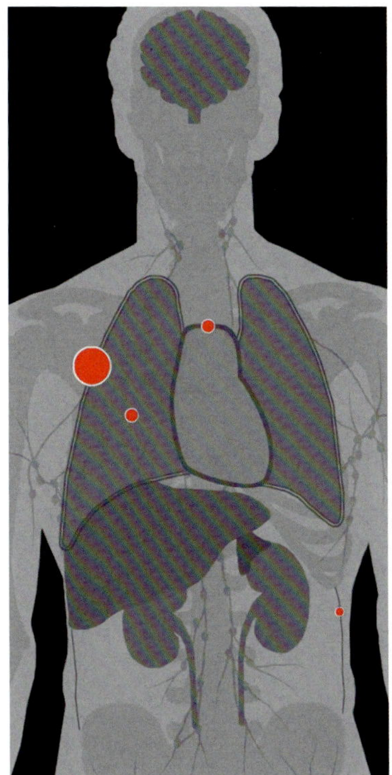

INITIAL SITE OF RECURRENCE

Pleural	90%
Mediastinum	5% (higher in some series)
Lung	5%
Extrathoracic	2%
Pericardial Metastases	Can be seen as well

Based on a Japanese series of 126 completely resected thymomas of various stages and treatments, 24 of which relapsed (22 with pleural disease, 6 with local/mediastinal recurrence, 4 with lung metastases, and 1 with bone metastases). Haniuda M et al: Recurrence of thymoma: clinicopathological features, re-operation, and outcome. J Surg Oncol. 78(3):183-8, 2001.

THYMUS

OVERVIEW

General Comments

- Epithelial neoplasm composed of thymic epithelial cells admixed in varying proportions with immature T lymphocytes
  - Thymomas generally look benign histologically and clinically but have potential for local recurrence and intrathoracic dissemination
    - Most malignant thymomas have relatively good prognosis and relatively indolent behavior
      - In contrast, thymic carcinomas have malignant clinical appearance (lymph node involvement, metastases), malignant histological appearance, and worse prognosis

Classification

- Masaoka staging system used to stage extent of disease for thymomas and thymic tumors
- No official TNM staging system

NATURAL HISTORY

General Features

- Comments
  - Invasive tumors are associated with more aggressive behavior
  - Incompletely excised tumors have tendency to recur locally and spread along chest cavity
  - Recurrences can take place many years after initial resection (i.e., > 10-15 years)
  - Most common sites for metastases are lung and pleura
  - Extrathoracic metastases are extremely rare (< 2% of cases)
- Location
  - Any part of anterior mediastinum
  - 20% of all mediastinal masses are thymomas
  - 45% of anterior mediastinal tumors are thymomas

Epidemiology & Cancer Incidence

- Number of cases in USA per year
  - 0.15 cases per 100,000 person-years
- Sex predilection
  - Slightly higher incidence in men (0.16 per 100,000) than in women (0.13 per 100,000)
- Age of onset
  - Mean age of presentation: 56 years

Genetics

- Common translocations
  - Loss of heterozygosity, typically of chromosome 6, is commonly seen

Associated Diseases, Abnormalities

- Close association with myasthenia gravis (MG) and other paraneoplastic syndromes
  - Almost 1/2 of patients with thymoma have symptoms of MG
  - MG is associated with all histological subtypes of thymoma, but not with thymic carcinoma
  - MG symptoms typically lead to diagnosis of thymoma at earlier stage as compared to patients without MG
  - MG symptoms may improve after thymectomy, although they may not resolve fully
  - Other, rarer paraneoplastic syndromes include pure red cell aplasia, hypogammaglobulinemia, or others

Gross Pathology & Surgical Features

- Early stage thymomas are encapsulated and smooth and not adherent to surrounding structures
- Thymomas should be removed en bloc to minimize risk of relapse
- Presence of adhesions is important as it may indicate thymoma beyond the capsule and at higher risk of local relapse
- Surgically, there may be concerns about invasion into lung and pericardium
  - Should be excised en bloc and carefully labeled so that pathologist can comment whether there is invasion pathologically or only adherence
- Proximity of tumor to phrenic nerve may lead to challenges in obtaining negative margins without sacrificing phrenic nerve, which should especially be avoided in patients with respiratory compromise (e.g., due to myasthenia gravis)
- Clips placed in areas of concern about close margin are very useful for radiation planning
- In more advanced cases, pleural deposits may be seen, and a few pleural deposits can be resectable; care should be taken not to contaminate pleura
- Preoperative diagnosis (e.g., fine-needle aspirate) may be hard to interpret and may potentially lead to breach of capsule and increase risk of spread
- Core biopsy may be easier to interpret but has same risk noted above
- In some centers, mediastinal masses resembling thymomas are not biopsied but are taken for surgery, especially in patients with appropriate clinical context, such as myasthenia gravis

Routes of Spread

- Local spread
  - Malignant thymomas are characterized by transcoelomic spread (along cavities), leading to tendency for recurrence within mediastinal space and risk of droplet metastases in pleura, especially when primary tumor has breached pleural surface (e.g., through invasion into lung)
  - Transcoelomic spread also leads to risk of pericardial metastases once pericardium is breached by tumor
- Lymphatic extension
  - Extremely rare to have lymph node involvement or extrathoracic metastases by malignant thymoma (much more common with thymic carcinomas)
- Metastatic sites
  - Thymomas: Pleura, pericardium, and lung
  - Thymic carcinoma: Any site, including those listed above, as well as bone, liver, and brain

IMAGING

Detection

- Common radiologic presentations
  - Anterior mediastinal mass, as seen on CXR or CT scan

Staging

- T staging
  - Masaoka staging used to stage primary tumor
- N staging
  - Rare to have nodal involvement except in thymic carcinomas
  - No formal N staging exists, although thoracic N staging used for lung cancer could be utilized if needed
- M staging
  - Pleural, pericardial, or lung metastases are considered stage IV
  - Extrathoracic metastases are very rare and would also be considered stage IV
- Nuances of staging
  - Masaoka staging is surgical staging system; impossible to accurately stage thymic tumors on basis of imaging
  - Pleural involvement may be limited to 1 or several pleural deposits or may be more widespread
  - Pericardial involvement from direct extension of tumor is stage III
  - Diffuse pericardial involvement or malignant pericardial effusion constitutes stage IV

Restaging

- Given importance of surgical resection, patients with initially unresectable thymomas should be restaged after nonsurgical treatment and considered for surgical reassessment
- Patients whose paraneoplastic syndrome (e.g., MG) improves with initial management but then relapses are usually restaged with thorax CT to rule out recurrence of thymoma, although MG can often relapse without relapse of thymoma

CLINICAL PRESENTATION & WORK-UP

Presentation

- Paraneoplastic syndromes (myasthenia gravis, hypogammaglobulinemia, pure red cell aplasia, etc.) necessitate thorax CT to rule out thymoma
- Asymptomatic in ≤ 30% of cases
- Incidental finding on routine CXR or during coronary artery bypass surgery in asymptomatic patients
- Symptoms (chest pain, shortness of breath, superior vena cava syndrome) usually indicate very bulky &/or invasive thymoma
- Patients with thymic carcinomas are more likely to exhibit chest symptoms and less likely to be asymptomatic or have paraneoplastic syndrome
- Pathology
  - Currently most widely used pathological classification is World Health Organization (WHO) classification
  - Previous pathological classifications (Bernatz, Levine and Rosai, and Muller-Hermelink) were based on appearance (spindle cell, epithelial, etc.) or area of origin (cortical, medullary)
  - WHO classification divides thymomas into
    - Type A: Previously known as medullary or spindle cell
    - Type AB
    - Type B1: Previously predominantly cortical or lymphocyte rich
    - Type B2: Cortical
    - Type B3: Previously well-differentiated thymic carcinoma or atypical thymoma
    - Type C: Thymic carcinoma
  - WHO classification has been correlated with prognosis, with types A and AB associated with excellent prognosis and considered "benign"
  - Most of A and AB thymomas are associated with Masaoka stage I or II disease
  - Type B1 is prognostically favorable, but it may be associated with stage III disease
  - Types B2 and B3 are more malignant in behavior and prognosis and more frequently associated with stage III or IV disease
  - Type C, or thymic carcinoma, has a variety of cell types, most of which are high-grade malignancies with aggressive behavior and poor prognosis

Prognosis

- Most important prognostic factor is clinical staging (Koga modification of Masaoka scheme) in association with histological subtype and completeness of resection
- Stage I is regarded as "noninvasive" or "benign"
  - Has excellent prognosis, virtually 100% cause-specific survival
- Stage II thymoma, if completely resected, usually has excellent prognosis
  - Large tumors and tumors with more malignant histological subtypes do carry risk of local relapse
- Stage III thymoma may or may not be resectable and usually requires multimodality treatment
  - Even if thymoma is completely eradicated, stage III patients are at risk of intrathoracic relapse (mediastinal, pleural, pericardial, or lung) and may live many years
  - Whether or not aggressive treatment of metastases leads to cure remains unknown
- Stage IV thymoma may be treated aggressively but usually develops further recurrences
  - Depending on histological subtype, patients may exhibit prolonged survival

Work-Up

- Clinical
  - Given paucity of extrathoracic involvement, thorax CT is only necessary imaging in cases of thymoma
  - Differential diagnosis of anterior mediastinal tumors includes lymphomas, germ cell tumors, and thyroid tumors; clinical assessment should exclude these tumors by examining neck, nodal areas, abdomen, and serum tumor markers
  - If patient presents with MG, anterior mediastinal mass is almost definitely thymoma, and may not need to be biopsied

TREATMENT

Major Treatment Alternatives

- Complete surgical excision considered mainstay of treatment for all thymomas
- Radiation therapy (RT) used postoperatively for positive margins or invasive tumors considered at high risk of mediastinal relapse
- Neoadjuvant chemo (combined with neoadjuvant radiotherapy in some centers/situations) is used for tumors that are initially considered unresectable
- Treatment of stage IV thymomas is controversial and may include surgical resection of pleural metastases, usually in combination with preoperative chemotherapy &/or radiation
- Repeat surgical excision + postop RT used for recurrent tumors in mediastinum
- Combination chemo used for tumors not considered for potential radical local management

Major Treatment Roadblocks/ Contraindications

- As thymomas are rare, and surgery plays important role, locally advanced thymoma deemed unresectable may benefit from assessment by experienced thoracic surgeon with special interest in thymoma management
- No randomized trials to guide practice
- Practice guidelines for management of thymoma do exist, although they are based on consensus (Cancer Care Ontario guidelines) or literature (NCCN guidelines)

Treatment Options by Stage

- Stage I: Complete surgical resection
  - In patients not fit for surgery, radical radiation
- Stage II: Complete surgical resection; most patients do not require any other therapy
- Stage III: If resectable, surgical resection with aim of complete resection (i.e., R0) and consideration of postop RT, either for all cases of stage III or for patients with positive margin or more aggressive histology (B2, B3, C)
  - If initially not likely resectable with R0, neoadjuvant treatment with either chemotherapy or chemoradiation, followed by reassessment for surgery
  - If surgery is not planned, radical concurrent chemoradiation
- Stage IV: With 1 or several pleural deposits, surgical resection of primary tumor and pleural deposits is a consideration
  - With multiple pleural metastases, chemotherapy is main treatment; aggressive local treatment (surgery or radiation) is less likely to be of benefit
- Recurrent local (mediastinal) disease: Surgery if possible, followed by radiation, or consideration of neoadjuvant treatment followed by surgical reassessment
- Recurrent pleural disease: Surgery if a few lesions, especially if long disease-free period and patient physically fit, or consideration of chemo, or continued observation, especially if lesions small and disease indolent

Dose Response

- Thymoma considered moderately radiosensitive

Standard Doses

- 50 Gy/25 fx postoperative radiation therapy if margins negative or close
- 60 Gy/30 fx to gross residual disease
- 45 Gy/25 fx used as preoperative dose

Organs at Risk Parameters

- Standard dose constraints from lung RT are used

Common Techniques

- Conformal RT is current standard; IMRT may be used

RECOMMENDED FOLLOW-UP

Clinical

- Due to very long natural history, with recurrences possible many years later, prolonged follow-up beyond 10 years is recommended for more advanced stages &/ or more aggressive histologies

Radiographic

- Yearly thorax CT commonly recommended in patients at risk of recurrences

SELECTED REFERENCES

1. National Comprehensive Cancer Network Guidelines. Available from www.nccn.org/professionals/physician_gls/ f_guidelines.asp. Accessed on April 17, 2012
2. Weksler B et al: The role of adjuvant radiation therapy for resected stage III thymoma: a population-based study. Ann Thorac Surg. 93(6):1822-8; discussion 1828-9, 2012
3. Detterbeck FC et al: The Masaoka-Koga stage classification for thymic malignancies: clarification and definition of terms. J Thorac Oncol. 6(7 Suppl 3):S1710-6, 2011
4. Gomez D et al: Radiation therapy definitions and reporting guidelines for thymic malignancies. J Thorac Oncol. 6(7 Suppl 3):S1743-8, 2011
5. Falkson CB et al: The management of thymoma: a systematic review and practice guideline. J Thorac Oncol. 4(7):911-9, 2009
6. Detterbeck FC: Clinical value of the WHO classification system of thymoma. Ann Thorac Surg. 81(6):2328-34, 2006
7. Masaoka A et al: Follow-up study of thymomas with special reference to their clinical stages. Cancer. 48(11):2485-92, 1981

Likely Stage I

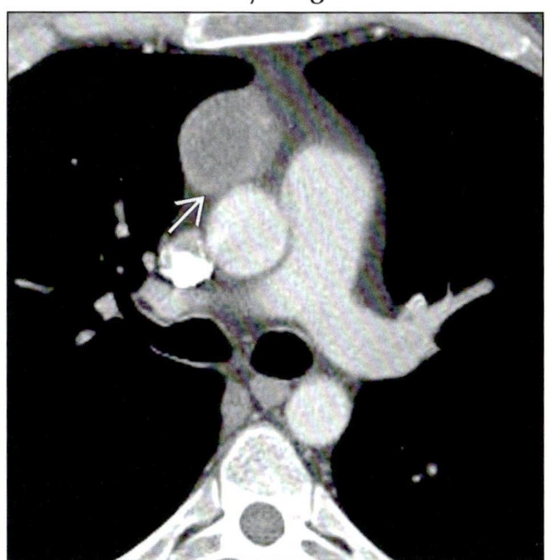

Most Likely Stage I

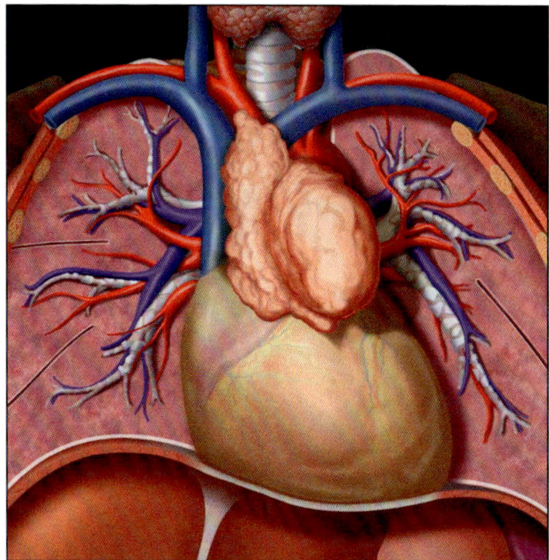

(Left) *CECT in patient with encapsulated thymoma shows rounded right anterior mediastinal mass with central low attenuation. Tissue plane ➔ with adjacent aorta is intact. (Courtesy M. Rosado-de-Christenson, MD.)* ***(Right)*** *Graphic shows the morphologic features and typical (but not sole) location of thymoma.*

Stage I, II, or III

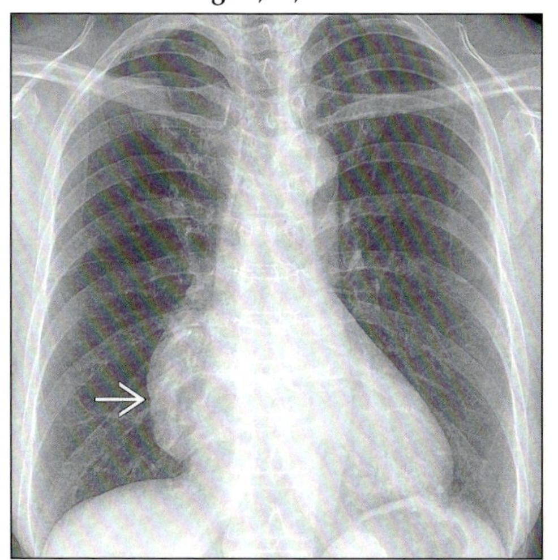

Stage I, II, or III

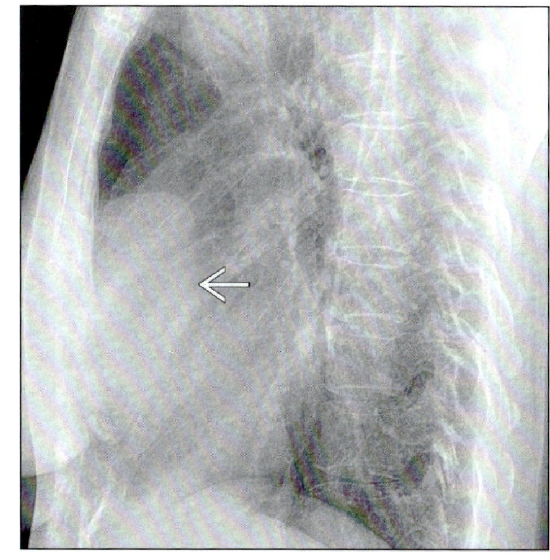

(Left) *PA chest radiograph shows a right mediastinal mass ➔ with well-defined lobular borders, typical of a thymoma. Note that thymomas can be quite inferior in the thorax. (Courtesy M. Rosado-de-Christenson, MD.)* ***(Right)*** *Lateral chest radiograph of the same patient shows the anterior mediastinal location of the mass ➔. The lateral view identifies this as an anterior mediastinal mass. (Courtesy M. Rosado-de-Christenson, MD.)*

Stage II or III

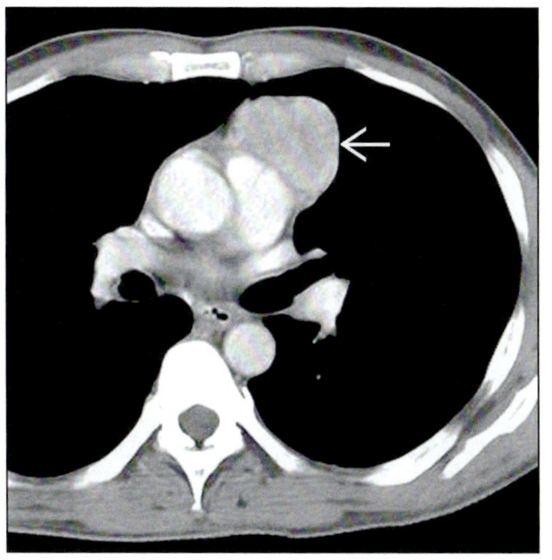

Likely Stage III

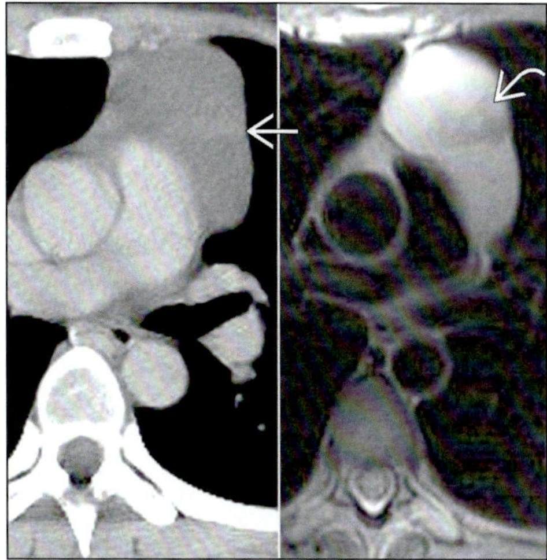

(Left) *CECT shows an anterior mediastinal mass ➔ with heterogeneous contrast enhancement. Mass abuts the adjacent pulmonary trunk without obvious vascular invasion. (Courtesy M. Rosado-de-Christenson, MD.)* ***(Right)*** *Axial T2WI (L) and axial T2WI (R) composite MR image shows left anterior mediastinal cystic mass with nodular soft tissue septum ➔, more conspicuous on right ➔. Mural nodules suggest cyst is thymoma, not benign. (Courtesy M. Rosado-de-Christenson, MD.)*

*(**Left**) CECT shows anterior mediastinal mass with irregular borders infiltrating adjacent mediastinal fat ➔. Stage IIA thymoma confirmed at surgery. (Courtesy M. Rosado-de-Christenson, MD.) (**Right**) Large, multilobular mass encases mediastinal vessels and invades SVC ➔. As this is unresectable thymoma, neoadjuvant treatment (chemo ± radiation) should be considered, followed by surgical reassessment. (Courtesy M. Rosado-de-Christenson, MD.)*

Stage II

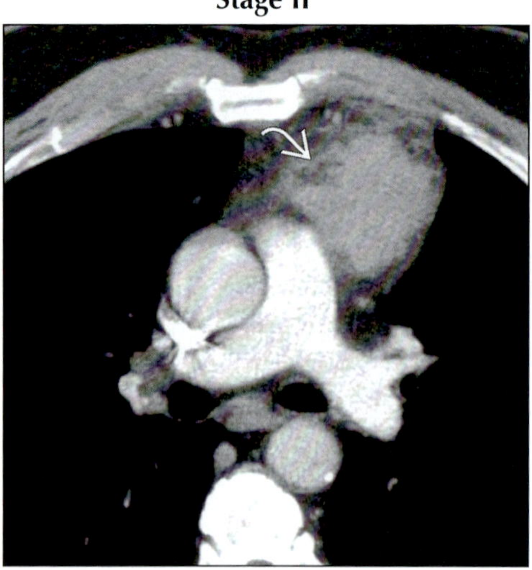

Stage III

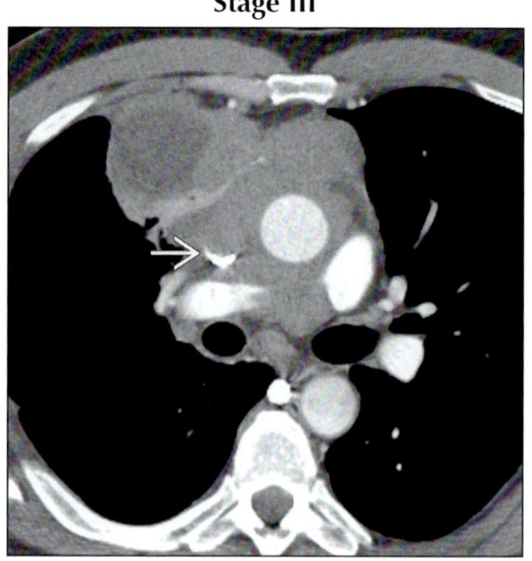

*(**Left**) Stage IVA thymoma demonstrates a large right multilobular anterior mediastinal mass with coarse calcifications ➔ (L) and multifocal ipsilateral diaphragmatic ➔ and medial pleural metastases ➔ (R). (Courtesy M. Rosado-de-Christenson, MD.) (**Right**) PET/CT of the same patient shows FDG avidity ➔ in the lesion (SUV of 4.5). The role of PET/CT in the evaluation of thymoma is not yet well defined. (Courtesy M. Rosado-de-Christenson, MD.)*

Stage IVA

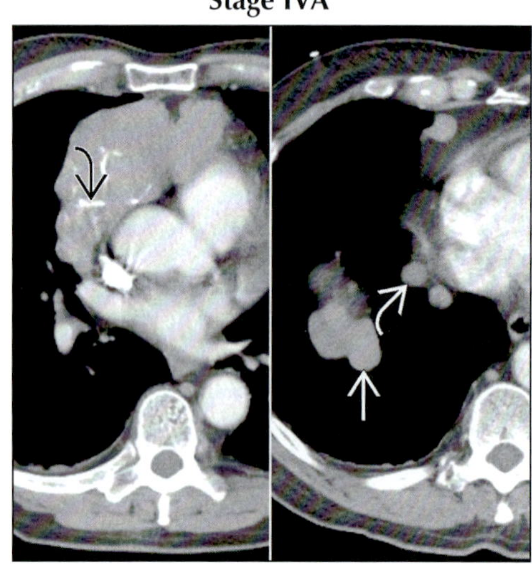

Stage IVA

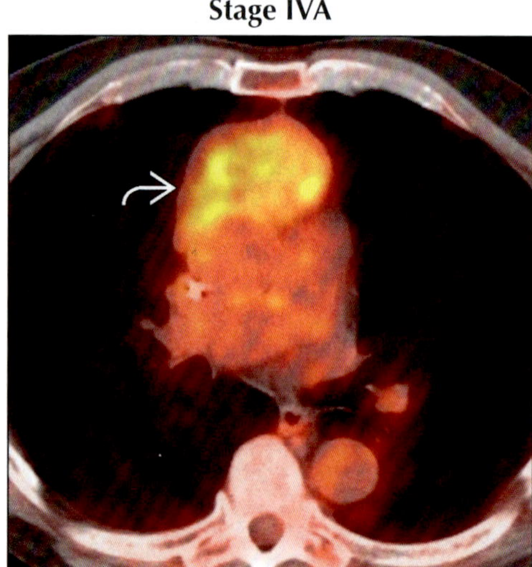

*(**Left**) Image shows heterogeneously enhancing anterior mediastinal mass ➔ with adjacent mediastinal lymph nodes ➔. Lymphadenopathy suggested thymic carcinoma, not thymoma. (Courtesy J. P. Lichtenberger III, MD.) (**Right**) CECT of a patient with thymic carcinoma shows large, heterogeneously enhancing anterior mediastinal mass invading left chest wall ➔ & compressing left pulmonary vein ➔. (Courtesy J. P. Lichtenberger III, MD.)*

Stage IV Thymic Carcinoma

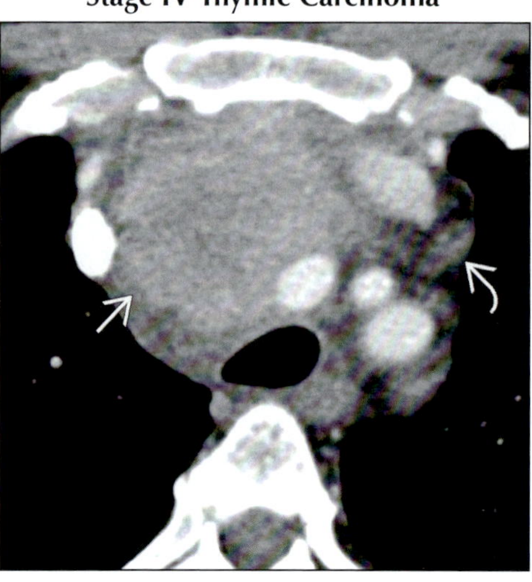

Stage III Thymic Carcinoma

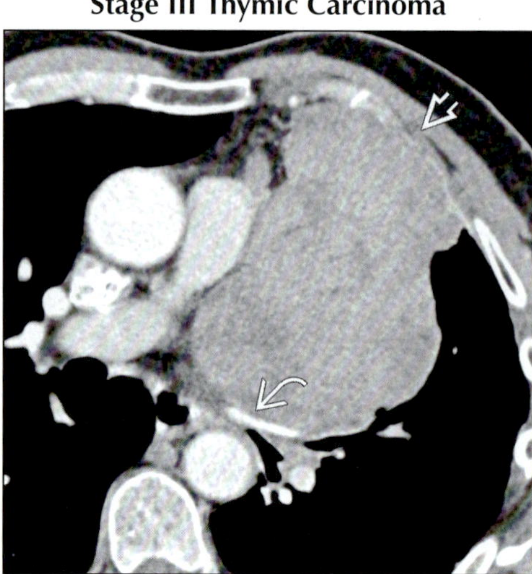

Stage III Thymoma

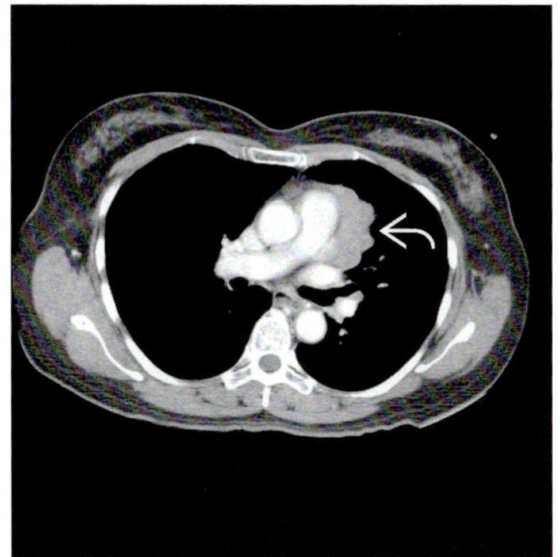

Stage III Thymoma (Resected)

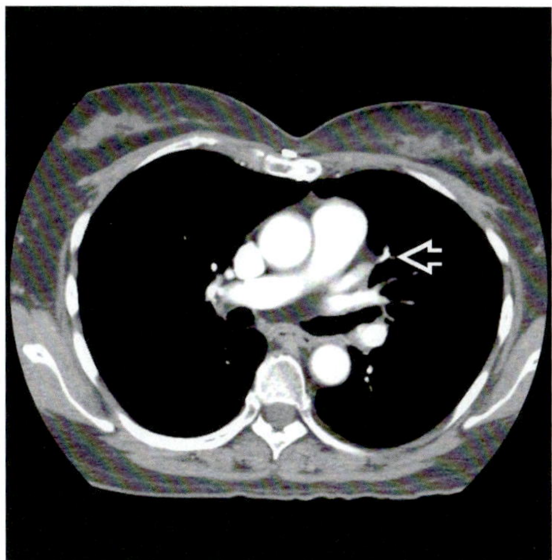

(Left) *Axial CECT of a patient with stage III thymoma shows scalloped borders, typical of high-grade thymoma (WHO type B3). The patient underwent resection with microscopic positive pericardial margin (R1).* ***(Right)*** *Restaging CECT 6 weeks post resection in the same patient shows surgical clip was used by the surgeon to denote areas of potential residual disease and thus guide planning and delivery of radiotherapy.*

Stage III Thymoma (Resected)

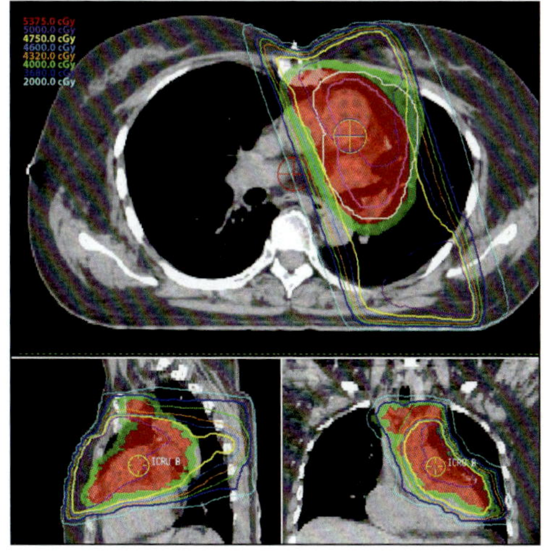

Stage III Thymoma (Resected)

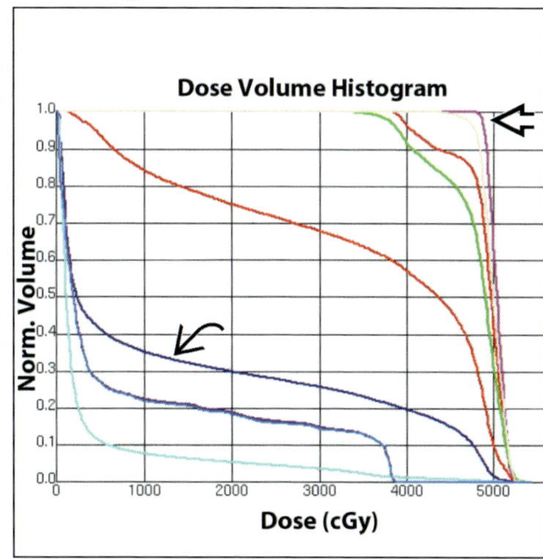

(Left) *Composite radiation plan in the same patient shows that adjuvant postoperative radiotherapy was delivered with an initial phase (40 Gy/20 fx) to cover the surgical bed, followed by a 2nd boost phase (10 Gy/5 fx) to the involved margin.* ***(Right)*** *Dose volume histogram in the same patient depicts RT doses to critical normal tissues (e.g., lung in dark blue) and the target volumes (e.g., gross target volume [GTV] in fuchsia).*

Stage III Thymoma (Resected)

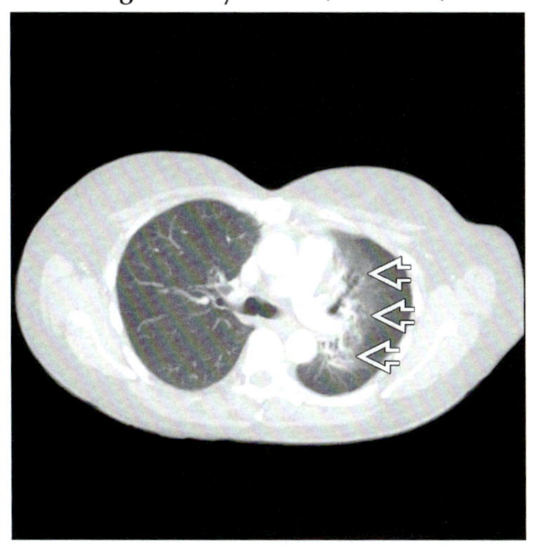

Stage III Thymoma (Resected)

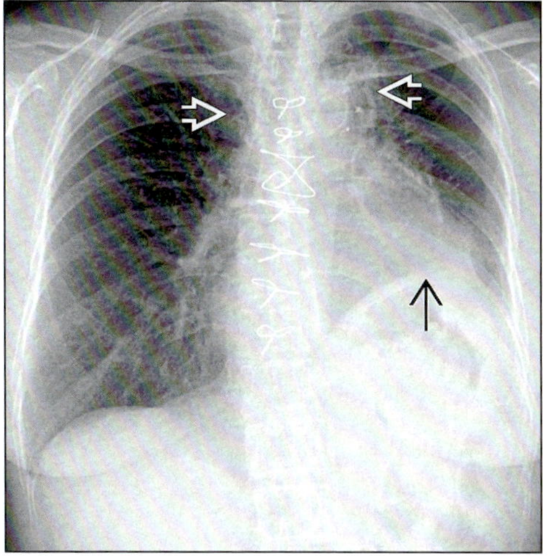

(Left) *CECT performed 5 years post surgery and RT in the same patient depicts no evidence of local recurrence but typical postradiation pulmonary fibrosis in the high-dose region.* ***(Right)*** *Chest x-ray performed 5 years post resection in the same patient depicts typical paramediastinal, postradiation fibrosis. Note the elevation of the left hemidiaphragm.*

THYMUS

(**Left**) *Baseline chest x-ray shows a bulky, locally advanced thymoma. An experienced surgeon felt that the patient required neoadjuvant therapy in order to improve likelihood of resectability.* (**Right**) *Baseline CT in the same patient demonstrates compression and intimate association of tumor with pulmonary outflow tract.*

Stage III Thymoma, Neoadjuvant

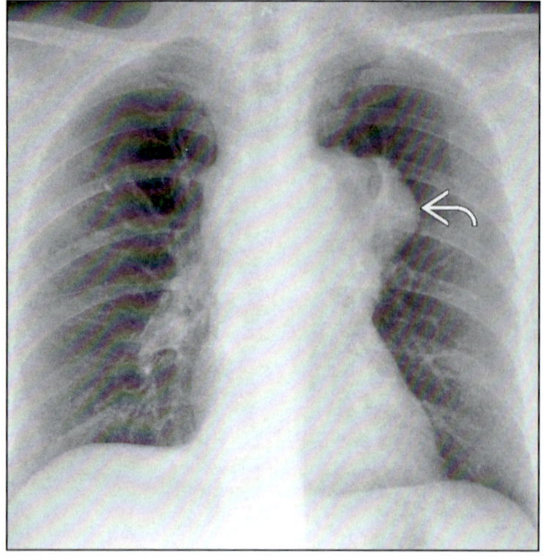

Stage III Thymoma, Neoadjuvant

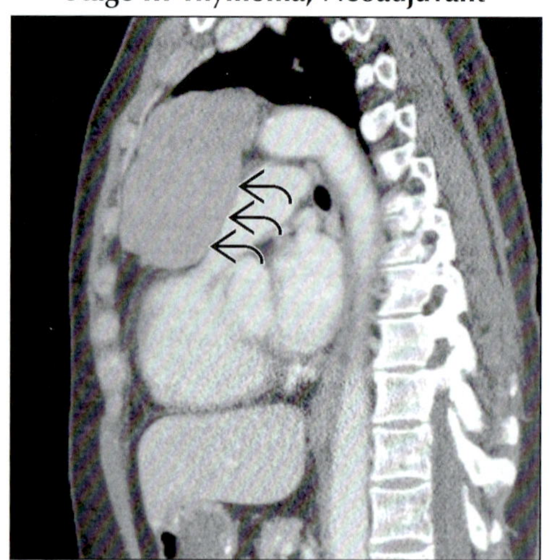

(**Left**) *CXR 3 weeks post completion of concurrent RT and chemotherapy in the same patient shows marked reduction in tumour volume compared to baseline. The patient proceeded to surgery.* (**Right**) *Same projection 3 weeks after completion of concurrent RT and chemotherapy shows marked reduction in tumor volume and complete relief of vascular compression compared to baseline CT. The patient proceeded to surgery.*

Stage III Thymoma, Neoadjuvant

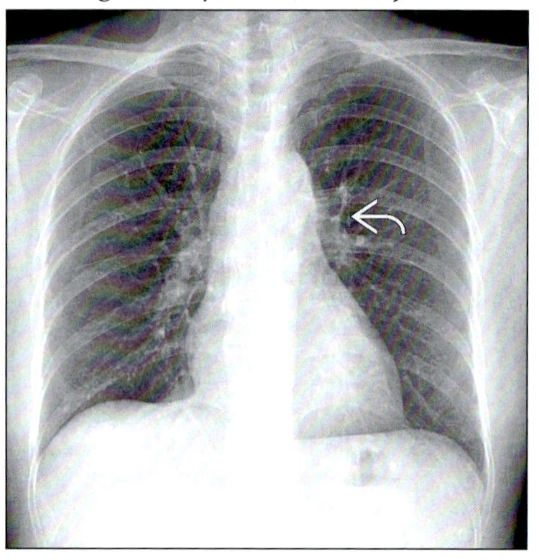

Stage III Thymoma, Neoadjuvant

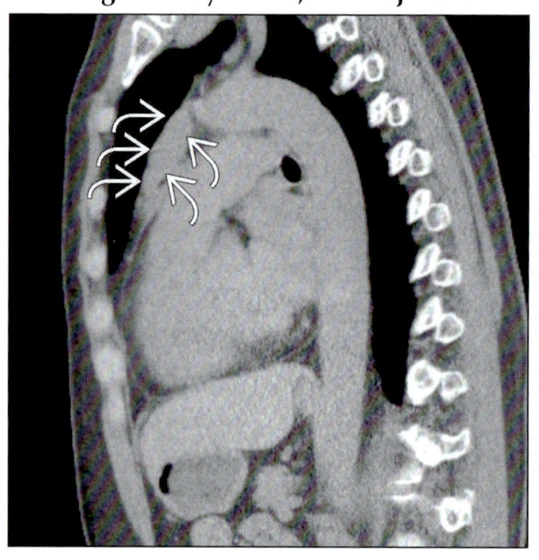

(**Left**) *Preoperative RT plan in the same patient: 45 Gy in 25 fx was prescribed, with the 95% isodose line (green) encompassing the planning target volume (yellow colorwash).* (**Right**) *Revised radiotherapy plan in the same patient: Due to rapid and significant shrinkage of tumor noted on daily cone beam imaging, the treatment was replanned after 11 fractions, administering the remaining 25.2 Gy/14 fractions to greatly reduced volumes and reduced radiation toxicity.*

Stage III Thymoma, Neoadjuvant

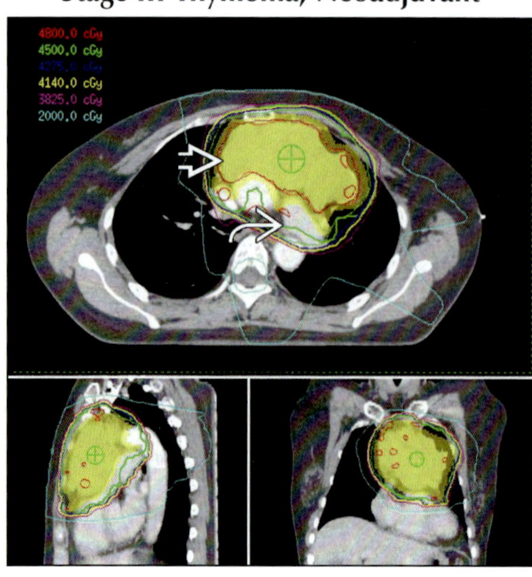

Stage III Thymoma, Neoadjuvant

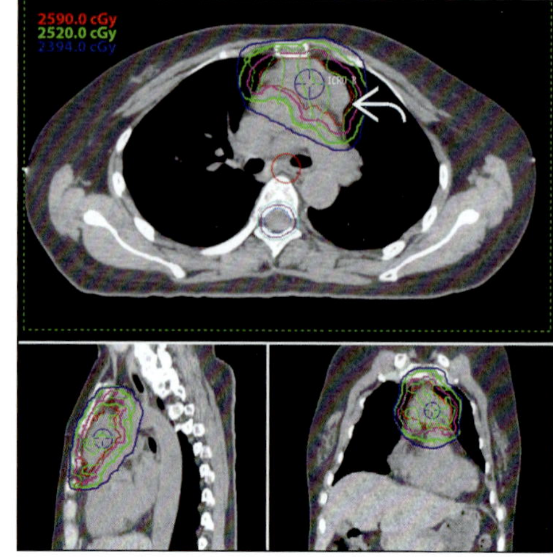

Unresectable Stage III Thymoma

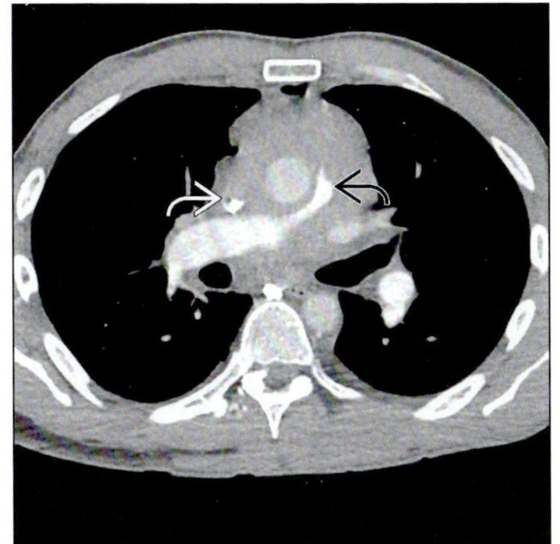

Unresectable Stage III Thymoma

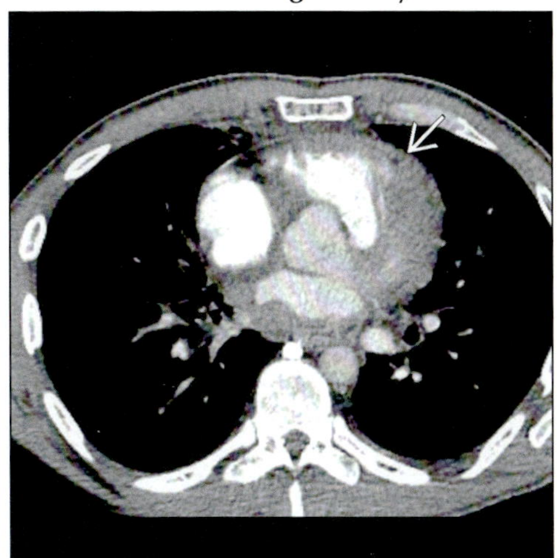

(Left) *Axial CECT in a patient with unresectable thymoma shows compression of the pulmonary trunk and superior vena cava by tumor.* ***(Right)*** *Axial CECT in the same patient (more inferior slice of the same baseline CT) demonstrates likely pericardial involvement.*

Unresectable Stage III Thymoma

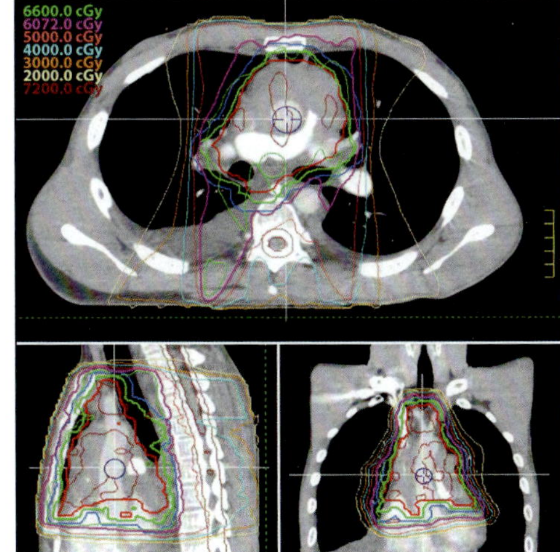

Unresectable Stage III Thymoma

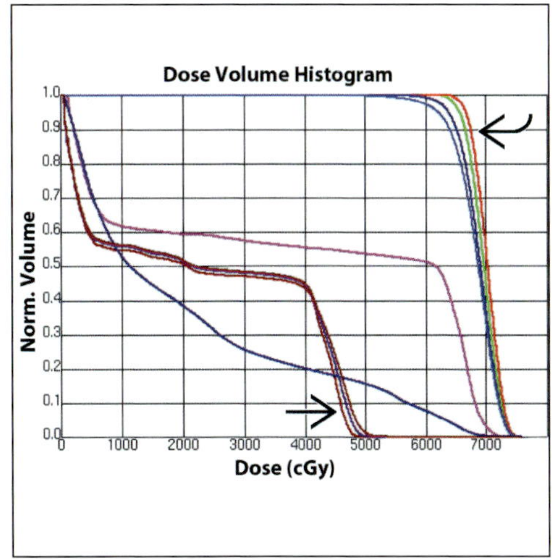

(Left) *Multifield RT plan in the same patient shows good conformality in 3 views.* ***(Right)*** *DVH of the same plan demonstrates RT dose to key normal tissues and targets, including lung (gross target volume [GTV] subtracted from total lung volume) (dark blue), esophagus (fuchsia), and spinal canal (+ 3 mm and 5 mm PRV); GTV, clinical target volume, PTV 3 mm, and PTV 5 mm.*

Unresectable Stage III Thymoma

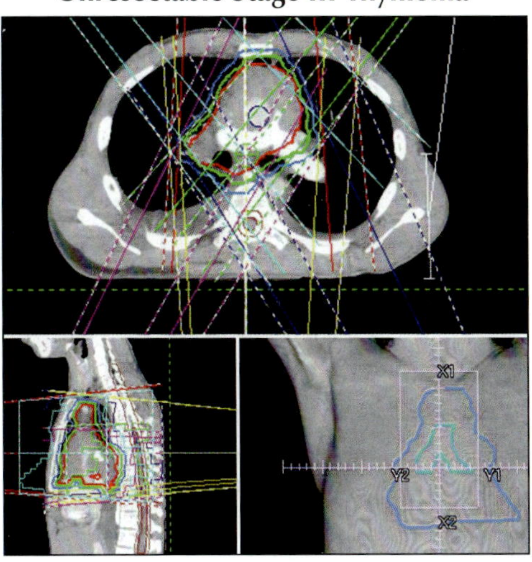

Stage III Thymic Carcinoma

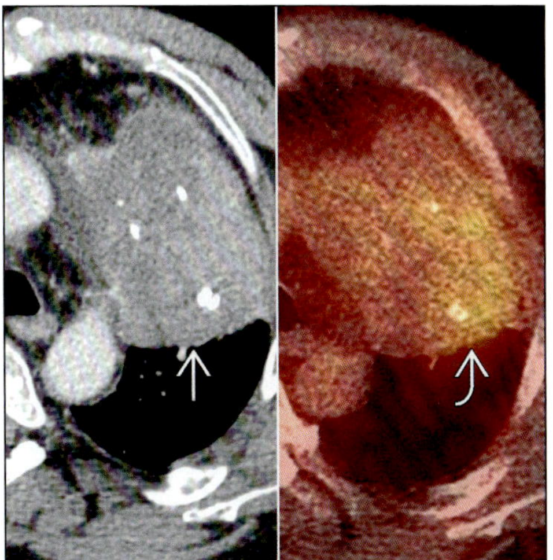

(Left) *CT in the same patient shows the 6-beam plan. The PTV 5 mm (blue), CTV (green), and GTV (red) contours are shown. The bottom right panel depicts an AP reconstruction with the skin opacified, the PTV in blue, and the reference positioning (nontreatment) field superimposed.* ***(Right)*** *Axial CECT (L) and PET/CT (R) show anterior mediastinal mass with calcification, hyperenhancement, and FDG avidity. (Courtesy J. P. Lichtenberger III, MD.)*

*(**Left**) Axial CECT of a patient with stage II, WHO type B3 thymoma shows that the mass was adherent to the phrenic nerve, which was transected at surgery and removed en bloc with the tumor. (**Right**) In the same patient, simulation fields were generated on a 2D kV simulator to deliver 40 Gy/20 fractions (10.5 x 10.5 cm fields, AP/PA, with corner shielding as marked ➩) to cover the surgical bed (guided by surgical clips ➔). Note the elevated left hemidiaphragm ➩.*

Stage II Thymoma

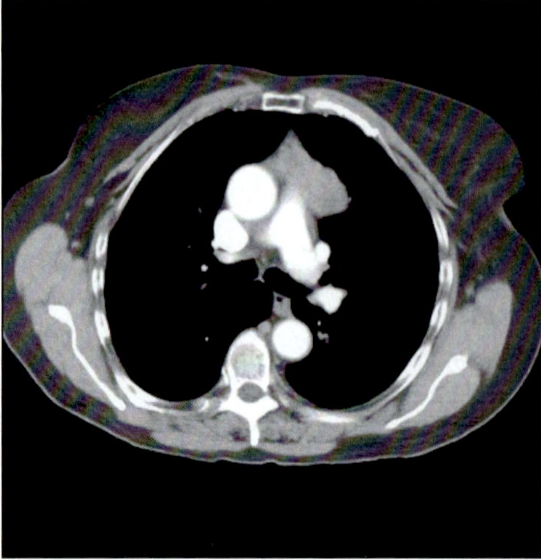

Stage II Thymoma

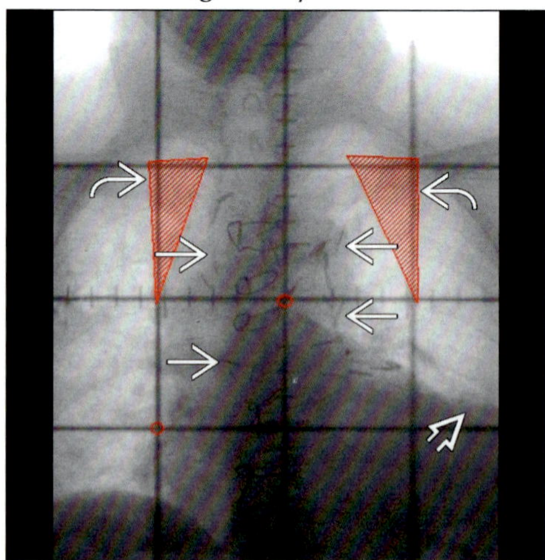

*(**Left**) In the same patient 3 years post RT, routine CT demonstrates a left upper posterior abdominal soft tissue mass ➩. Biopsy showed metastatic thymoma. The patient underwent resection of this isolated metastasis (including partial T12 vertebrectomy due to neural foramen involvement). An R0 resection was achieved, and no adjuvant treatment was given. (**Right**) Coronal slice from the same CT study shows the metastasis ➩.*

Stage IVA Recurrent Thymoma

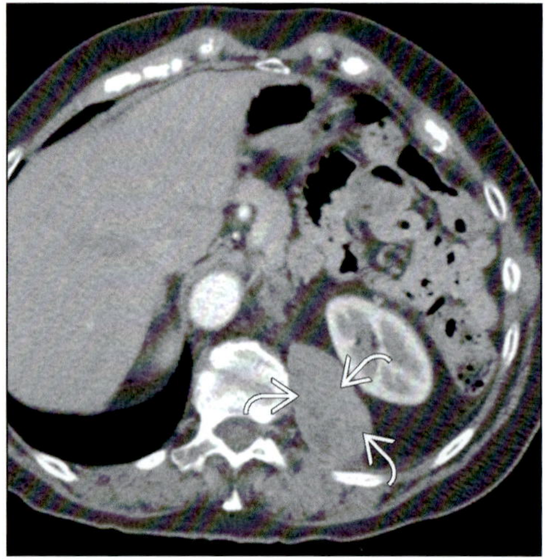

Stage IVA Recurrent Thymoma

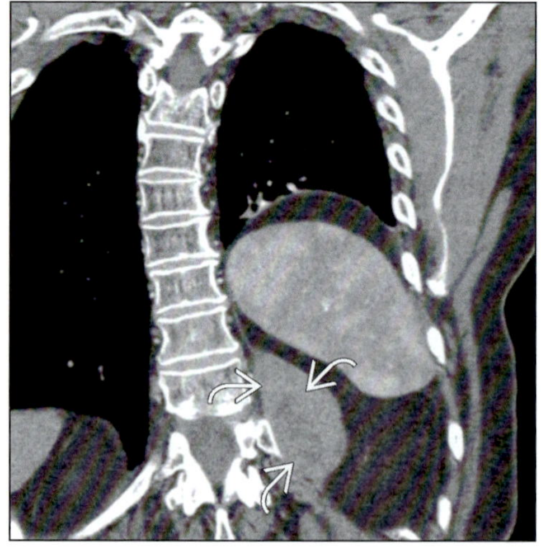

*(**Left**) Seven years post RT, the same patient developed an isolated left intrathoracic pleural mass ➩ not seen previously on CECT 1 year prior. Due to the age, frailty, and comorbidities of the patient, no chemotherapy or local treatment was recommended. The patient is lying on her side due to extreme kyphosis. (**Right**) Lung windows of CECT are depicted in left panel. Note the fibrotic changes in the lung due to previous RT ➩, anterior to the pleural mass ➩.*

Stage IVA Recurrent Thymoma

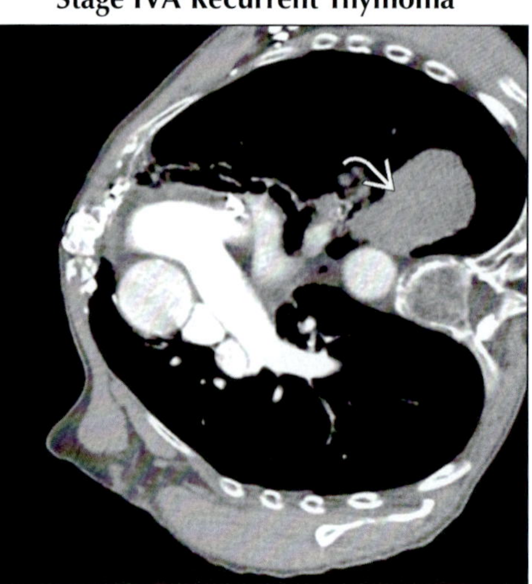

Stage IVA Recurrent Thymoma

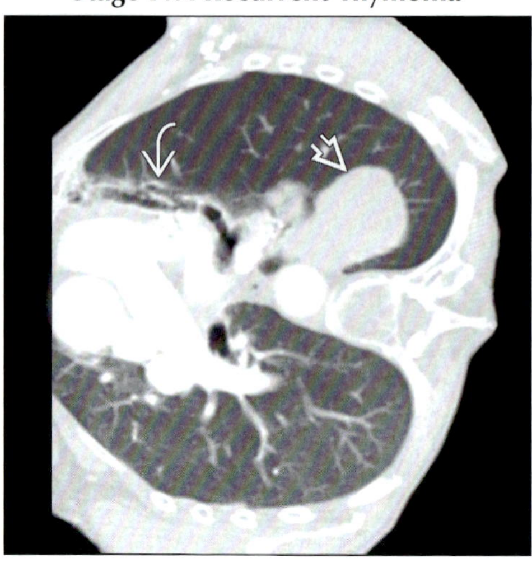

Stage III Thymoma

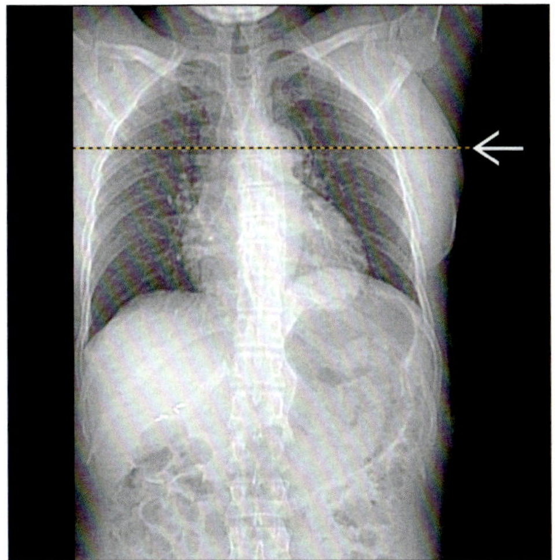

Stage III Thymoma

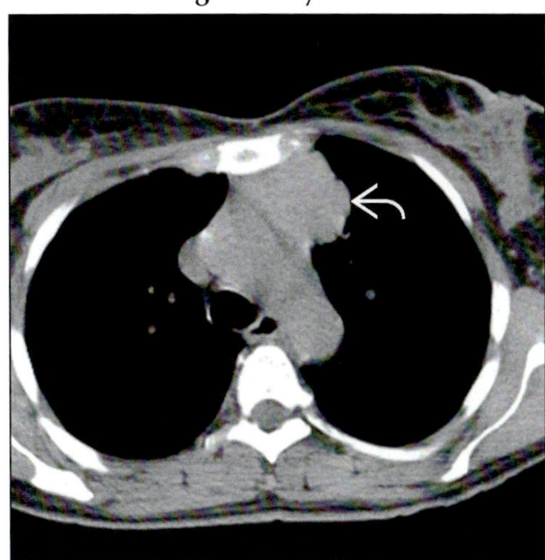

(Left) *Digitally reconstructed scout film depicts a mediastinal mass in a 43-year-old woman recently diagnosed with myasthenia gravis. Note the localizing line corresponding to an axial CT slice ➔.* ***(Right)*** *Axial CT in the same patient shows a 4 cm invasive thymoma ➔ invading the pericardium (stage III), WHO type B2. Left phrenic nerve involvement was noted at the time of surgery, necessitating resection.*

Stage III Thymoma

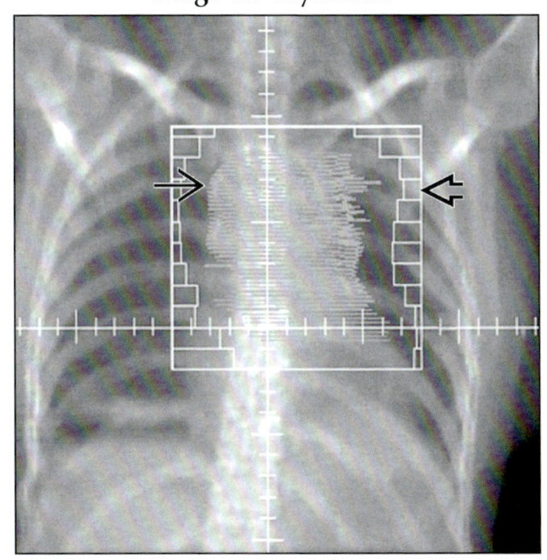

Stage III Thymoma

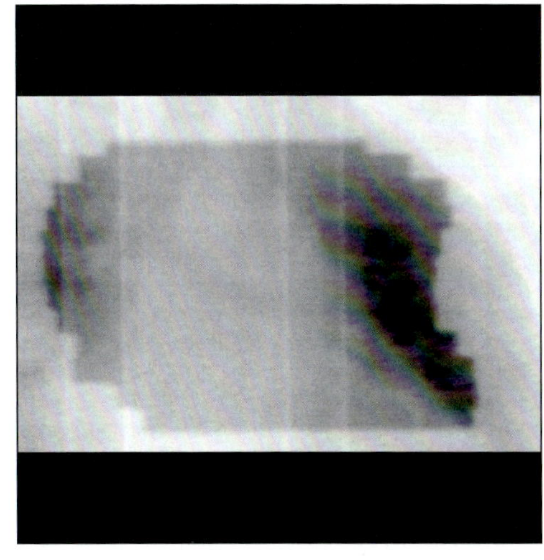

(Left) *Digitally reconstructed radiograph of a CT-planned AP field in the same patient is depicted, delivering postoperative RT (50 Gy/25 fractions). The field (for phase I, 40 Gy/20 fractions) is shaped around the clinical target volume ➔ using multileaf collimation ➲. Off-cord boost (10 Gy) is not shown.* ***(Right)*** *Megavoltage portal image of the AP field taken on the treating linear accelerator (same patient) is shown. Note the amount of lung and pericardium in the field.*

Stage III Thymoma

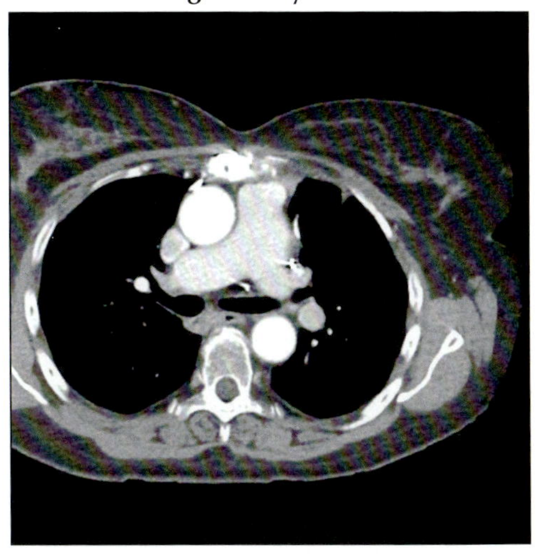

Stage III Thymoma

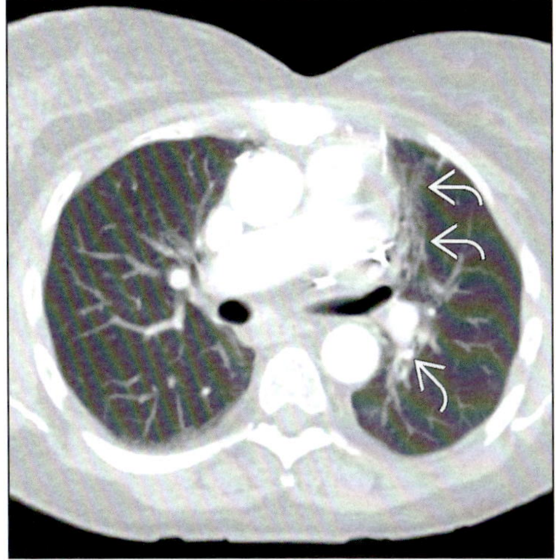

(Left) *Eight years post RT, follow-up CECT in the same patient shows no evidence of recurrence.* ***(Right)*** *Mild asymptomatic lung RT fibrosis ➔ is depicted on CT in the same patient 8 years after treatment. The patient continues to require medical management of myasthenia gravis, is diabetic, and has suffered a mild myocardial infarct.*

PLEURA

(T) Primary Tumor

Adapted from 7th edition AJCC Staging Forms.

TNM	*Definitions*
TX	Primary tumor cannot be assessed
T0	No evidence of primary tumor
T1	Tumor limited to the ipsilateral parietal pleura ± mediastinal pleura ± diaphragmatic pleural involvement
T1a	No involvement of the visceral pleura
T1b	Tumor also involving the visceral pleura
T2	Tumor involving each of the ipsilateral pleural surfaces (parietal, mediastinal, diaphragmatic, and visceral pleura) with ≥ 1 of the following: Involvement of diaphragmatic muscle, extension of tumor from visceral pleura into the underlying pulmonary parenchyma
T3	Locally advanced but potentially resectable tumor
	Tumor involving all of the ipsilateral pleural surfaces (parietal, mediastinal, diaphragmatic, and visceral pleura) with ≥ 1 of the following: Involvement of the endothoracic fascia; extension into the mediastinal fat; solitary, completely resectable focus of tumor extending into the soft tissues of the chest wall; nontransmural involvement of the pericardium
T4	Locally advanced technically unresectable tumor
	Tumor involving all of the ipsilateral pleural surfaces (parietal, mediastinal, diaphragmatic, and visceral pleura) with ≥ 1 of the following: Diffuse extension or multifocal masses of tumor in the chest wall ± associated rib destruction; direct transdiaphragmatic extension of tumor to the peritoneum; direct extension of tumor to the contralateral pleura; direct extension of tumor to mediastinal organs; direct extension of tumor into the spine; tumor extending through to the internal surface of the pericardium ± a pericardial effusion or tumor involving the myocardium

(N) Regional Lymph Nodes

NX	Regional nodes cannot be assessed
N0	No regional lymph node metastasis
N1	Metastases in the ipsilateral bronchopulmonary or hilar lymph nodes
N2	Metastases in the subcarinal or the ipsilateral mediastinal lymph nodes, including the ipsilateral internal mammary and peridiaphragmatic nodes
N3	Metastases in the contralateral mediastinal, contralateral internal mammary, ipsilateral or contralateral supraclavicular lymph nodes

(M) Distant Metastasis

M0	No distant metastasis
M1	Distant metastasis present

(G) Histologic Grade

GX	Grade cannot be assessed
G1	Well differentiated
G2	Moderately differentiated
G3	Poorly differentiated
G4	Undifferentiated

AJCC Stages/Prognostic Groups

Adapted from 7th edition AJCC Staging Forms.

Stage	*T*	*N*	*M*
I	T1	N0	M0
IA	T1a	N0	M0
IB	T1b	N0	M0
II	T2	N0	M0
III	T1, T2	N1	M0
	T1, T2	N2	M0
	T3	N0, N1, N2	M0
IV	T4	Any N	M0
	Any T	N3	M0
	Any T	Any N	M1

Desmoplastic Mesothelioma

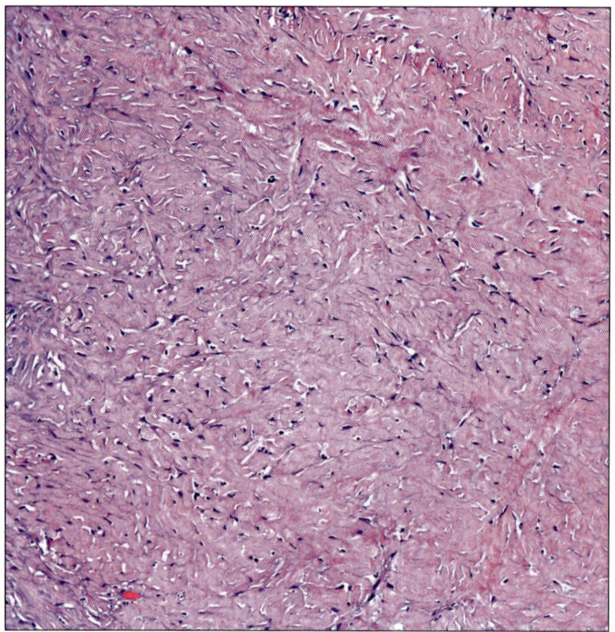

Desmoplastic mesothelioma shows prominent hyalinized stroma. (Courtesy C. Moran, MD.)

Desmoplastic Mesothelioma

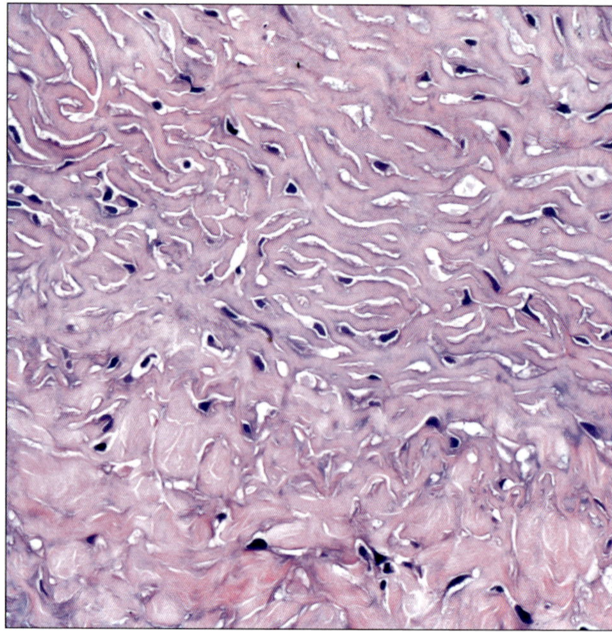

Magnified view of a desmoplastic mesothelioma shows abundant collagen deposition. (Courtesy C. Moran, MD.)

Sarcomatoid Mesothelioma

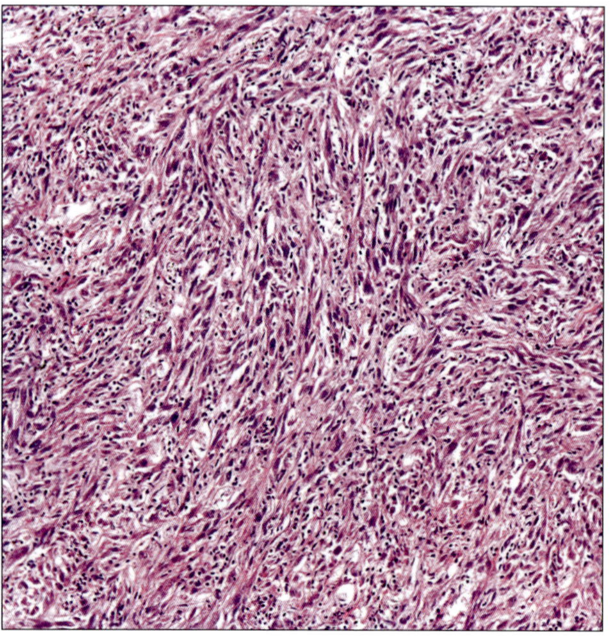

Sarcomatoid mesothelioma shows proliferation of spindle cells. (Courtesy C. Moran, MD.)

Sarcomatoid Mesothelioma

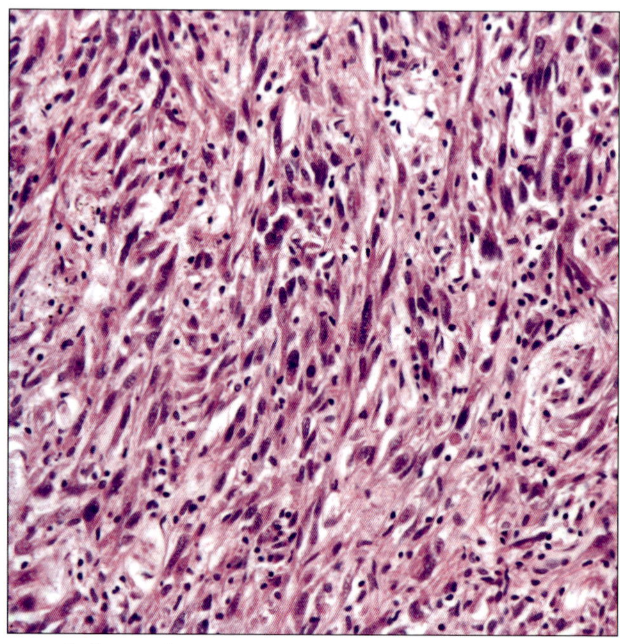

Magnified view of a sarcomatoid mesothelioma shows spindle cells with marked atypia. (Courtesy C. Moran, MD.)

Epithelioid Mesothelioma

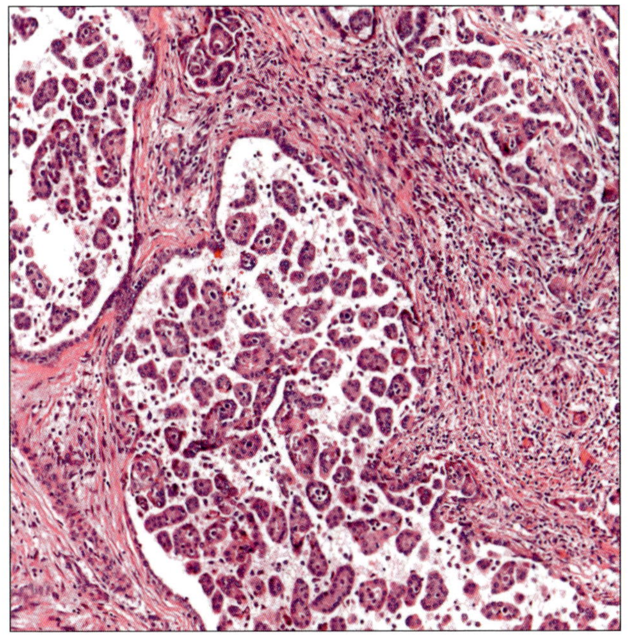

Epithelioid mesothelioma shows a papillary tumor dissecting areas of fibroconnective tissue. (Courtesy C. Moran, MD.)

Epithelioid Mesothelioma

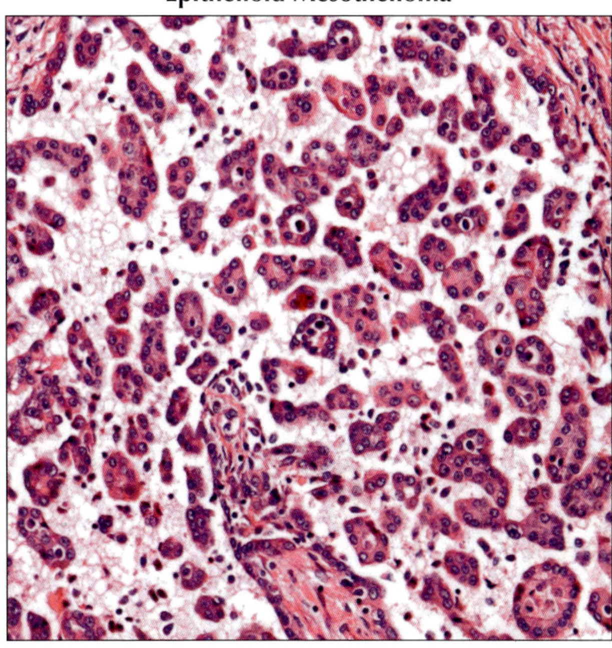

Magnified view of an epithelioid mesothelioma shows tumor cells arranged in small papillary projections. (Courtesy C. Moran, MD.)

Biphasic Mesothelioma

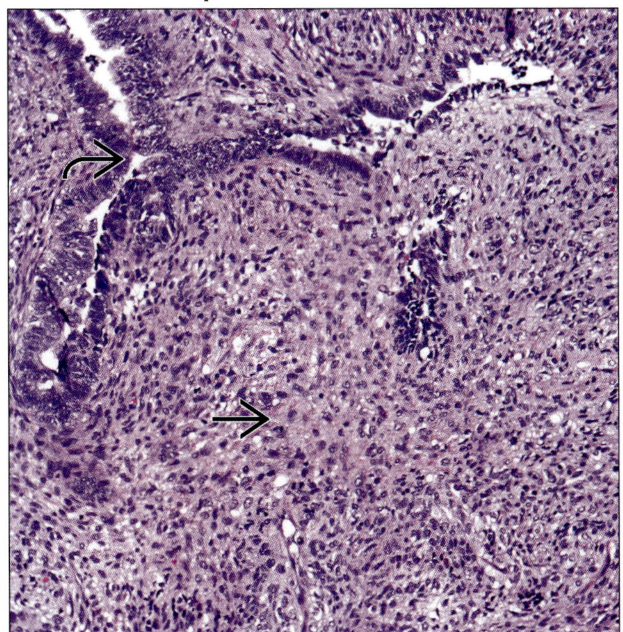

Biphasic malignant mesothelioma shows 2 distinct components: Epithelioid ⮫ and sarcomatoid →. (Courtesy C. Moran, MD.)

Biphasic Mesothelioma

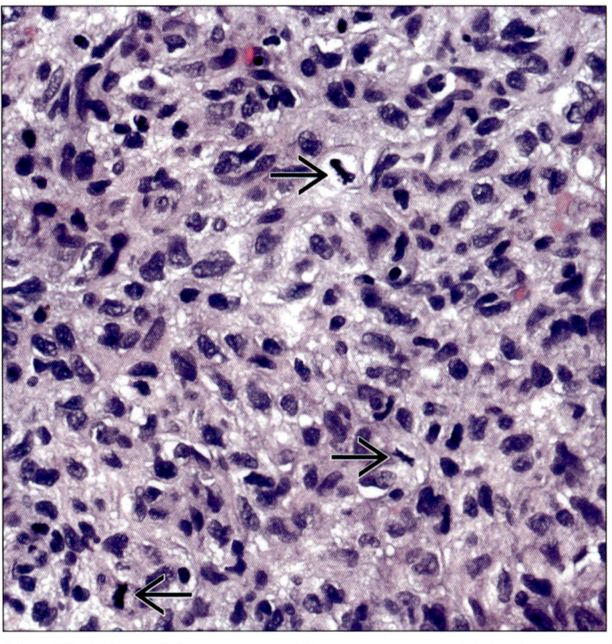

Magnified view of the sarcomatoid component in a biphasic mesothelioma shows several mitotic figures →. (Courtesy C. Moran, MD.)

PLEURA

T1

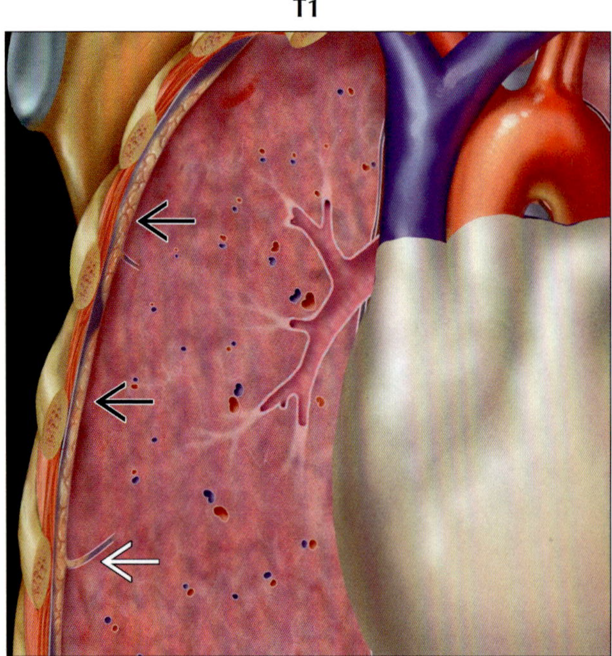

Graphic depicts tumor limited to the ipsilateral pleura ➙. Note that visceral pleural involvement ➙ is designated T1b. Without such involvement, this would be a T1a tumor.

T2

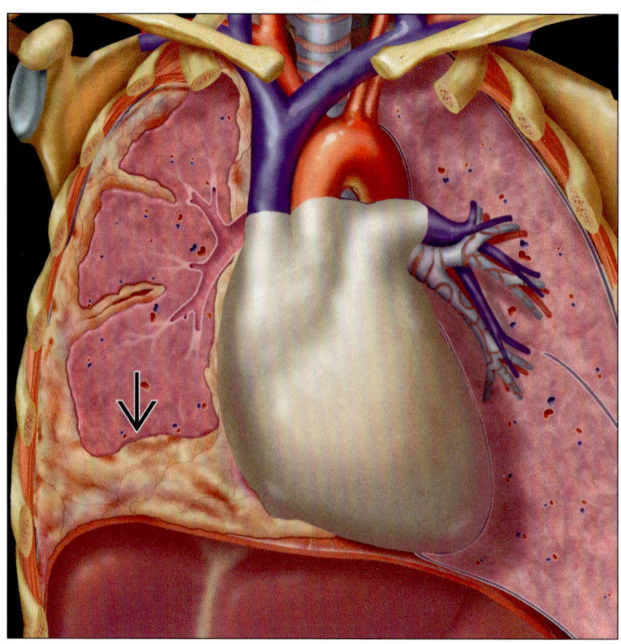

Graphic depicts tumor involving ipsilateral pleural surfaces with extension into the underlying pulmonary parenchyma ➙, making this T2 disease.

T3

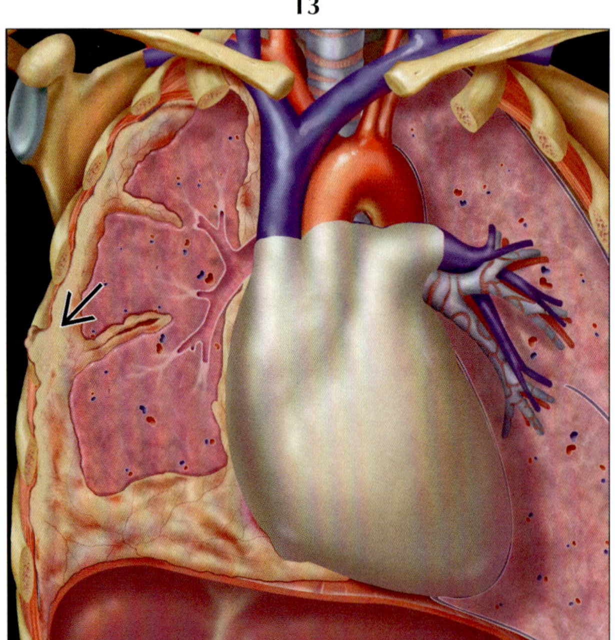

Graphic depicts invasion into the soft tissues of the chest wall ➙, making this T3 disease.

T4

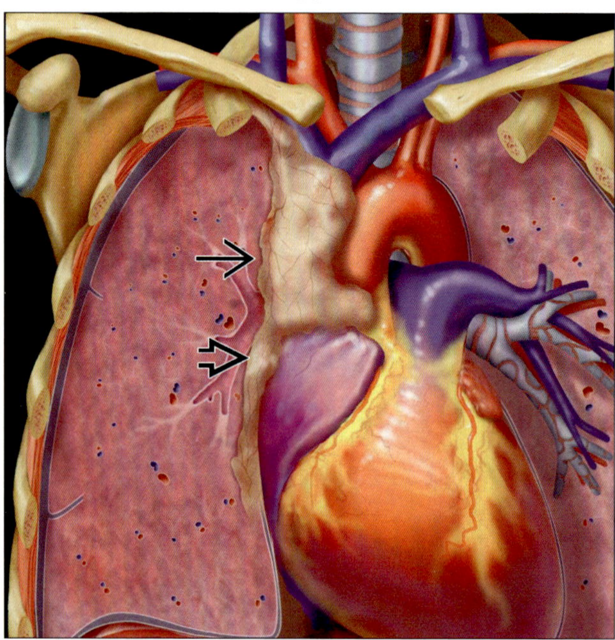

Graphic depicts tumor extending into the mediastinum to involve the great vessels ➙ and myocardium ➙, making this T4 disease.

International Association for the Study of Lung Cancer (IASLC) Lymph Node Map

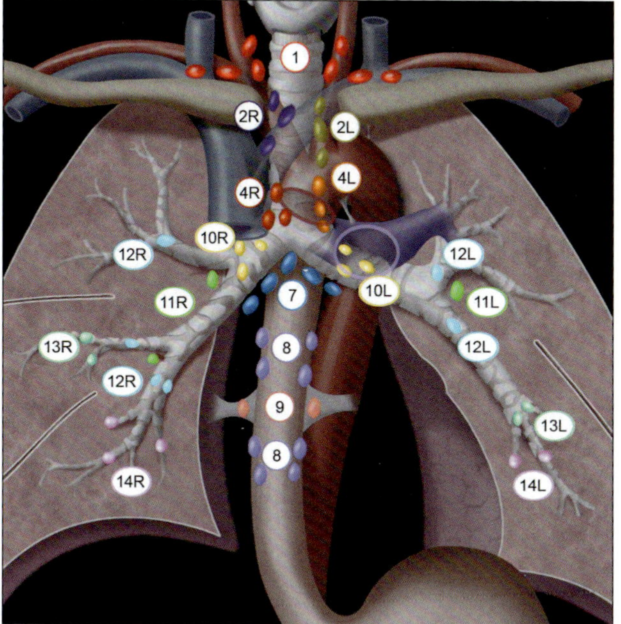

1) Supraclavicular. ***Upper zone****: 2R) Upper paratracheal (PT), right, 2L) upper PT, left, 4R) lower PT, right, 4L) lower PT, left.* ***AP zone****: 7) Subcarinal.* ***Lower zone****: 8) Paraesophageal, 9) pulmonary ligament.* ***Hilar/interlobar zone****: 10) Hilar, 11) interlobar.* ***Peripheral zone****: 12) Lobar, 13) segmental, 14) subsegmental.*

International Association for the Study of Lung Cancer (IASLC) Lymph Node Map

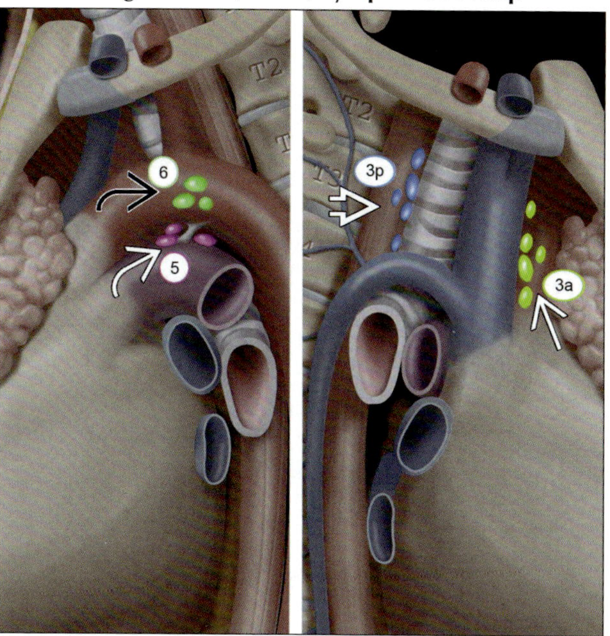

Graphic depicts 3a) prevascular ➔, 3p) retrotracheal ➔, 5) subaortic ➔, and 6) paraaortic (ascending aorta or phrenic) ➔ lymph nodes.

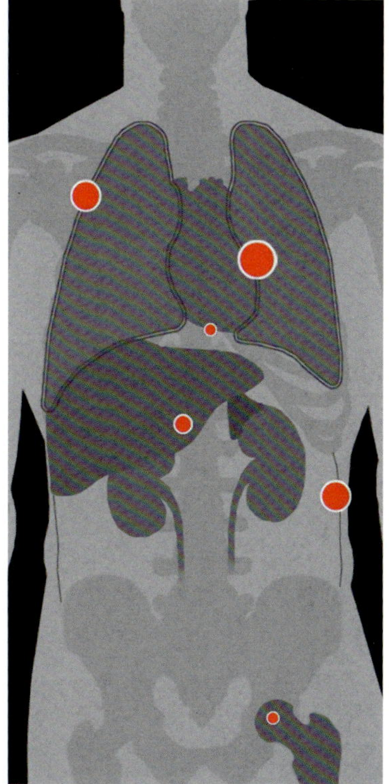

INITIAL SITE OF RECURRENCE

Site	%
Ipsilateral Chest	31%
Peritoneum	26%
Contralateral Lung/ Pleura	22%
Peritoneum and Chest	8%
Abdominal Viscera	5%
Bone	3%
Pericardium	2%
Others (Brain, Skin)	Rare

Data represent 219 patients that underwent extrapleural pneumonectomy at MSK. Distribution: Early stages I-II (25%), epithelioid histology (69%), and multimodality therapy (69%). Flores et al: J Thorac Cardiovasc Surg. 135(3):620-6, 2008.

OVERVIEW

General Comments

- Most common neoplasm arising from mesothelium
  - Mesothelioma may also arise from other serosal mesothelium
    - Peritoneum
    - Pericardium
    - Tunica vaginalis
- Uncommon neoplasm associated with asbestos exposure

Classification

- 4 subtypes
  - Epithelioid (55-65%)
    - Best prognosis
  - Sarcomatoid (10-15%)
  - Biphasic (20-35%)
  - Desmoplastic (10%)

NATURAL HISTORY

Etiology

- Inhalation of fibrous silicate materials
  - Mesothelioma: Occupational disease most commonly
  - Asbestos
    - Mineral that forms thin, fibrous crystals
    - Resistant to heat, chemical, electrical damage
    - High tensile strength, sound-absorbing properties
    - Commercial use banned in USA
  - Latency period between asbestos exposure and malignant pleural mesothelioma (MPM) is ≥ 20 years
- Agents other than asbestos are considered potential risk factors or cofactors for MPM
  - Exposure to other natural (erionite and fluoro-edenite) or man-made (refractory ceramic) fibers
    - Erionite: Mineral that forms wooly, fibrous crystals; present in sedimentary rocks; type of zeolite
  - Prior radiation therapy
    - For breast cancer or lymphoma
  - Viruses
    - SV40 virus
  - Intrapleural thorium dioxide (Thorotrast)

Epidemiology & Cancer Incidence

- Number of cases in USA per year
  - 2,200 cases per year in USA
- 15 cases per 1,000,000 in USA per year
- Rates expected to increase in developed countries until 2015, then decrease due to improved asbestos exposure regulations
- Rate increase in developing countries due to ongoing lack of asbestos exposure regulations

Associated Diseases, Abnormalities

- Asbestosis/pneumoconiosis
  - Caused by occupational exposure to asbestos (amphibole/straight more toxic than chrysotile/serpentine)
  - Slowly progressive, diffuse pulmonary fibrosis
  - Direct toxic effect on pulmonary parenchyma
  - Contribution of inflammatory mediators
  - Clinical: Dyspnea, bibasilar crackles, clubbing, cor pulmonale
  - Imaging findings: Basilar interstitial fibrosis, pleural plaques
- Other lung cancers

Gross Pathology & Surgical Features

- Firm gray plaques and nodules on visceral/parietal pleural surface
- Tumor tends to grow around lung, causing
  - Concentric thickening and contraction of pleura
  - Extension to interlobar fissures
  - Infiltration of mediastinum, chest wall, and diaphragm

Microscopic Pathology

- H&E
  - 4 subtypes
    - Epithelioid: Tubulopapillary, glandular, and epithelioid cells
    - Sarcomatoid: Spindle cells
    - Biphasic: ≥ 10% epithelial and sarcomatoid components
    - Desmoplastic: Collagenous, often paucicellular
- Special stains
  - Immunohistochemistry (IHC) markers seen in pleural mesothelioma
    - CK5/6, calretinin, mesothelin, Wilms tumor (WT1) antigen, thrombomodulin, D2-40, podoplanin
- Pleural fluid cytology
  - Not recommended to make diagnosis of mesothelioma based on cytology alone
    - High risk of diagnostic error
  - Positive in only 30-50% of patients with MPM
- Percutaneous pleural biopsy
  - Not primarily recommended for diagnosis of mesothelioma
    - Low sensitivity (30%)
- Thoracoscopy
  - Preferred method for diagnosis
    - Diagnostic in > 90%

Routes of Spread

- Local spread
  - MPM usually grows diffusely around and within pleural cavity
    - Localized MPM is rare
  - Local invasion of adjacent structures common
    - Chest wall
    - Diaphragm
    - Interlobar fissure
    - Pericardium
    - Abdominal organs
  - Seeding across tracts resulting from pleural interventions is common
- Lymphatic extension
  - Poor prognostic sign
  - Regional lymph nodes include
    - Intrathoracic
    - Scalene
    - Internal mammary
    - Peridiaphragmatic
- Metastatic sites
  - Rare hematogenous spread
  - Common sites include

- Contralateral lung
- Contralateral pleura
- Peritoneum
- Liver
- Bone
- Adrenal gland

IMAGING

Detection

- Radiography
  - Pleural effusion (95%)
  - Pleural-based mass
  - Pleural plaques ± calcification in contralateral lung
  - Small hemithorax
- CT
  - Primary imaging modality for evaluation of MPM
  - CT findings suggestive of MPM include
    - Unilateral pleural effusion
    - Rind-like tumoral encasement of lung &/or nodular pleural thickening
      - Pleural nodules may be difficult to distinguish from pleural effusions on NECT
      - Using narrow window setting and contrast improves visualization of soft tissue pleural nodules
    - Interlobar fissure thickening
    - Calcified pleural plaques are found on CT in approximately 20% of patients
      - Calcifications may become engulfed by tumor, causing tumor to mimic calcified MPM
      - Calcifications may also be seen in contralateral side
    - Volume loss affected hemithorax with
      - Ipsilateral mediastinal shift, narrowed intercostal spaces, elevation of ipsilateral hemidiaphragm
    - Nonexpansion of lung after thoracentesis for pleural fluid
  - Findings helpful in differentiating MPM from benign pleural disease
    - Rind-like pleural thickening
      - Sensitivity (54%); specificity (95%)
    - Nodular pleural thickening
      - Sensitivity (38%); specificity (96%)
    - Pleural thickness > 1 cm
      - Sensitivity (47%); specificity (64%)
    - Mediastinal pleural involvement
      - Sensitivity (70%); specificity (83%)
- MR
  - Signal characteristics
    - Iso- or slightly hyperintense on T1WI
    - Moderately hyperintense on T2WI
    - Enhances after administration of gadolinium
  - Appearance similar to CT
- PET/CT
  - MPM shows ↑ metabolic activity on FDG PET
    - Significantly higher SUV than in benign pleural diseases
      - SUV values of 7.8 ± 3.3 for malignant lesions
      - SUV values of 0.4 ± 0.8 for benign lesions
      - Suggested cut-off value of SUV 3.0 in one study yielded sensitivity and specificity of 100% for differentiation between benign and malignant pleural disease
    - Performance of PET/CT in differentiating benign from malignant pleural lesions
      - Sensitivity (94.4-96.8%); specificity (91.7%)
      - Accuracy (92.3%)
  - Help identify focal areas of ↑ metabolic activity in patients with diffuse pleural thickening to guide biopsy
- Imaging-guided biopsy
  - Imaging may be used to guide selection of sites for tissue diagnosis
    - Because blind biopsy may be diagnostic in < 50% of patients
    - Avoid use of more invasive techniques, such as thoracoscopy, video-assisted thoracoscopic surgery, or open thoracotomy
  - Techniques
    - Ultrasound-guided pleural biopsy
      - Sensitivity (77%); specificity (88%)
    - CT-guided biopsy
      - Sensitivity (83-86%)

Staging

- Imaging modalities
  - CT most commonly used modality for staging
  - MR can help assess local disease in borderline resectable tumors
    - Excellent contrast resolution of MR improves evaluation of tumor extension
      - Slightly higher sensitivity vs. CT for detecting invasion of diaphragm, fascia, chest wall
      - More accurate than CT for endothoracic fascia/ single focus of chest wall invasion (69% vs. 46%)
      - More accurate than CT for diaphragm invasion (82% vs. 55%)
  - PET/CT
    - Increased accuracy in detection of mediastinal nodal metastases
    - Identification of occult extrathoracic metastases
    - May help predict prognosis
      - Higher FDG uptake associated with significantly shorter survival time
    - Local disease
      - Limited in determining local invasion, resectability
    - PET/CT compared to CT
      - Adds value over CT for detection of regional lymph node and distant metastasis
    - PET/CT useful for directing biopsy
      - Focal pleural plaques with SUV > 2 more likely to yield diagnostic biopsy
    - Sensitivity/specificity
      - Stages II-IV > 95%
- Local spread
  - Presence of simultaneous pleural effusion, atelectasis, and chest wall invasion creates difficulties in distinguishing tumor from uninvolved adjacent tissue
  - Chest wall involvement may manifest as
    - Obliteration of extrapleural fat planes

- Irregularity of interface between tumor and chest wall is not reliable predictor of chest wall invasion
  - Invasion of intercostal muscles
  - Displacement of ribs
  - Bone destruction
- Iatrogenic chest wall extension
  - Tumor can extend into chest wall along needle biopsy tracts, surgical scars, and chest tube tracts
- Direct tumor extension into vascular structures and mediastinal organs, including heart, esophagus, and trachea
  - Usually obliteration of surrounding fat planes
  - Presence of soft tissue mass that surrounds > 50% of circumference of vascular structure is strong evidence of invasion
- Pericardial involvement
  - Nodular pericardial thickening
  - Pericardial effusion
- Transdiaphragmatic extension
  - Soft tissue mass on both sides of hemidiaphragm
- Nodal metastases
  - Staging
    - N1: Metastases to ipsilateral bronchopulmonary or hilar nodes
    - N2: Metastases in subcarinal or ipsilateral mediastinal lymph nodes, including ipsilateral internal mammary and peridiaphragmatic nodes
    - N3: Metastases in contralateral mediastinal, contralateral internal mammary, ipsilateral or contralateral supraclavicular lymph nodes
  - Imaging has poor accuracy because enlarged nodes alone do not prove nodal involvement
  - Mediastinoscopy has poor negative predictive value (50%) due to inability to sample all relevant nodes
- Pulmonary metastases
  - Nodules and masses
  - Rarely, diffuse miliary nodules
- Extrathoracic spread
  - Direct hepatic invasion
  - Retroperitoneal extension

Restaging

- CT modality of choice for evaluation of tumor response
  - Currently proposed to use modified RECIST to assess objective response in MPM
    - Measure of short diameter perpendicular to chest wall at 3 reference levels summed together
- PET/CT
  - Performance of PET/CT in differentiating benign from malignant pleural lesions
    - Sensitivity (94%)
    - Specificity (100%)
    - Positive predictive value (100%)
    - Negative predictive value (88%)
  - SUV max of recurrent MPM is 8.9 ± 4.0

CLINICAL PRESENTATION & WORK-UP

Presentation

- Dyspnea most often due to pleural effusion
- Chest pain due to local invasion
- History of occupational asbestos exposure (80%)
- Age: 50-70 years
- M:F = 4:1

Prognosis

- Untreated
  - Median survival: 4-13 months
- Treated
  - Median survival: 6-18 months
- Local extension and respiratory failure → death
- Best prognosis
  - Epithelial histology
  - Limited primary
  - No lymph node metastasis
- Worst prognosis
  - Sarcomatoid histology
  - Distant metastasis

TREATMENT

Major Treatment Alternatives

- Radical surgery
  - Extrapleural pneumonectomy (EPP) with en bloc resection of pleura, lung, pericardium, and diaphragm and systematic nodal dissection
  - Role and benefit of EPP controversial
  - Following criteria are considered for possible EPP
    - Biopsy-proven MPM of nonsarcomatoid cell type
    - Clinical &/or pathological stage T1-3 N0-1 M0
    - Patient fit for pneumonectomy by virtue of sufficient respiratory reserve and lacking other comorbidities (e.g., cardiovascular)
    - Patient fit to receive neoadjuvant/adjuvant chemotherapy
    - Patient fit to receive adjuvant radical hemithorax irradiation
  - 74% 2-year survival
  - 60% complication rate
  - Best in early stage disease in otherwise healthy patients
- Pleurectomy/decortication (P/D)
  - Not curative, but can be considered in patients to obtain symptom control
    - Symptomatic patients with entrapped lung syndrome who cannot benefit from chemical pleurodesis
  - Video-assisted thoroscopic surgery (VATS) approach is preferred
- Chemotherapy
  - First-line: Anti-folate agent (pemetrexed, raltitrexed) and cisplatin doublet
  - Second-line: Doxorubicin, cyclophosphamide
- Palliation of pleural effusion
  - Pleurodesis
    - Sterile talc is preferred to other agents
  - Pleurectomy: Not shown to increase survival
- Radiotherapy (RT)
  - Radical radiotherapy
    - Cannot give to entire pleura of intact lung due to excessive (fatal) pulmonary toxicity
  - Adjuvant radiotherapy
    - Hemithoracic RT after EPP significantly reduces risk of local relapse (< 10%)

- Adjuvant RT after P/D challenging due to risk of serious pulmonary toxicity to underlying intact lung
  - Prophylactic RT
    - Role in reducing incidence of tumor seeding at pleural intervention site debatable

Major Treatment Roadblocks/ Contraindications

- Most patients present with unresectable disease due to advanced disease, unfavorable histology, age, comorbidities

Treatment Options by Stage

- No consensus on best therapy for MPM
  - Paucity of high-quality randomized studies to guide treatment
    - Challenging pathological diagnosis
    - Difficulty assessing clinical response
      - Applying modified RECIST challenging
    - Rare tumor
      - Small sample size, slow accrual, retrospective series
    - Difficult randomization
- Stage I to resectable stage III
  - Trimodality therapy
    - Surgery alone for MPM is not curative since no oncological resection margins can be obtained
    - Includes EPP, chemotherapy, and postoperative radiation therapy
    - Neoadjuvant chemotherapy may downstage tumor and aid resectability
    - Only 1/2 of patients starting trimodality therapy finish due to attrition and disease progression
- Unresectable stage III-stage IV
  - Palliative chemotherapy
  - Palliative radiotherapy
  - Palliation of pleural effusion

Dose Response

- Thought to be radioresistant in the past since arising from mesenchymal tissue
  - Irradiated cell line studies show mesothelial radiosensitivities between non-small cell lung cancer (NSCLC) and small cell lung cancer (SCLC)
- Some studies suggest larger dose per fraction more efficacious

Standard Doses

- 45-50 Gy in adjuvant setting plus 10 Gy boost to areas of high risk (i.e., difficult dissection, positive margins)
- 20-30 Gy in palliative settings
- 7 Gy x 3 for port site prophylaxis

Organs at Risk Parameters

- Adjuvant doses to entire hemithorax with intact lung will result in fatal radiation pneumonitis
  - Can only be safely given if lung removed (i.e., EPP)
  - Conventional (bilateral) lung dose constraints dangerously high in post-pneumonectomy situation
- Keep contralateral mean lung dose < 9.5 Gy after pneumonectomy

Common Techniques

- 3D chemoradiation therapy (CRT) or intensity-modulated radiation therapy (IMRT)

Landmark Trials

- Vogelzang: Improved overall survival (OS), time to progression, response rates with cisplatin plus pemetrexed vs. cisplatin alone
- Rusch: Local recurrence dramatically reduced with adjuvant high dose hemithoracic RT following EPP
- Treasure (MARS): No difference in median OS with EPP (14.4 months) vs. no EPP (19.5 months); study criticized for excessive deaths seen in EPP arm

RECOMMENDED FOLLOW-UP

Clinical

- Follow-up exam every 3 months for 2 years, then every 6 months for 1 year, and annually thereafter per clinical discretion

Radiographic

- Chest x-ray every visit; CT of chest and abdomen every 3-6 months for 2 years then annually thereafter per clinical discretion

Laboratory

- Mesothelin, osteopontin, and CA125 not routine per clinical discretion

SELECTED REFERENCES

1. Treasure T et al: Extra-pleural pneumonectomy versus no extra-pleural pneumonectomy for patients with malignant pleural mesothelioma: clinical outcomes of the Mesothelioma and Radical Surgery (MARS) randomised feasibility study. Lancet Oncol. 12(8):763-72, 2011
2. de Perrot M et al: Trimodality therapy with induction chemotherapy followed by extrapleural pneumonectomy and adjuvant high-dose hemithoracic radiation for malignant pleural mesothelioma. J Clin Oncol. 27(9):1413-8, 2009
3. Flores RM et al: Extrapleural pneumonectomy versus pleurectomy/decortication in the surgical management of malignant pleural mesothelioma: results in 663 patients. J Thorac Cardiovasc Surg. 135(3):620-6, 626, 2008
4. Allen AM et al: Fatal pneumonitis associated with intensity-modulated radiation therapy for mesothelioma. Int J Radiat Oncol Biol Phys. 65(3):640-5, 2006
5. van Meerbeeck JP et al: Randomized phase III study of cisplatin with or without raltitrexed in patients with malignant pleural mesothelioma: an intergroup study of the European Organisation for Research and Treatment of Cancer Lung Cancer Group and the National Cancer Institute of Canada. J Clin Oncol. 23(28):6881-9, 2005
6. Vogelzang NJ et al: Phase III study of pemetrexed in combination with cisplatin versus cisplatin alone in patients with malignant pleural mesothelioma. J Clin Oncol. 21(14):2636-44, 2003
7. Rusch VW et al: A phase II trial of surgical resection and adjuvant high-dose hemithoracic radiation for malignant pleural mesothelioma. J Thorac Cardiovasc Surg. 122(4):788-95, 2001
8. Sugarbaker DJ et al: Resection margins, extrapleural nodal status, and cell type determine postoperative long-term survival in trimodality therapy of malignant pleural mesothelioma: results in 183 patients. J Thorac Cardiovasc Surg. 117(1):54-63; discussion 63-5, 1999

Stage IB (T1b N0 M0)

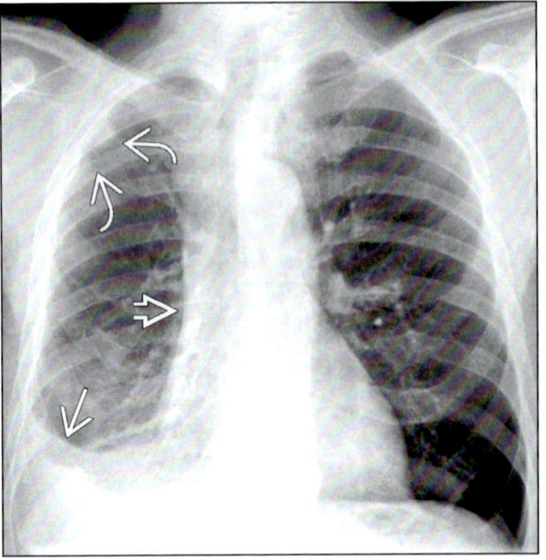

Stage IB (T1b N0 M0)

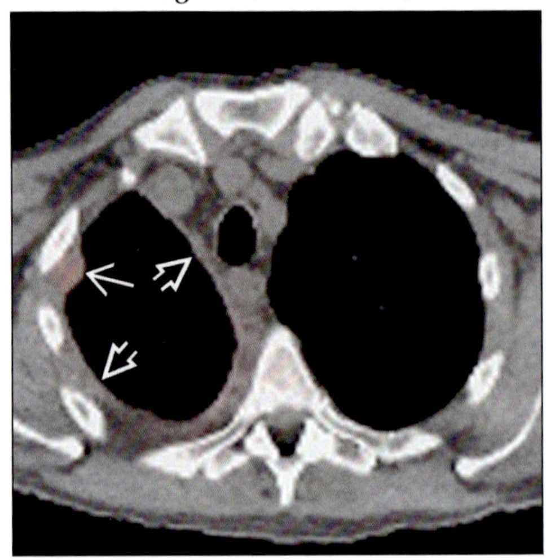

(Left) *Frontal chest x-ray in a 65-year-old man with a history of asbestos exposure shows right pleural effusion/ thickening →, mediastinal pleural thickening →, and subtle upper thoracic pleural-based nodules →. Also note the relatively low volume of the right hemithorax.* ***(Right)*** *Axial PET/CT in the same patient shows increased metabolic activity of the polypoid pleural nodule → without increased metabolic activity of the circumferential pleural thickening →.*

Stage IB (T1b N0 M0)

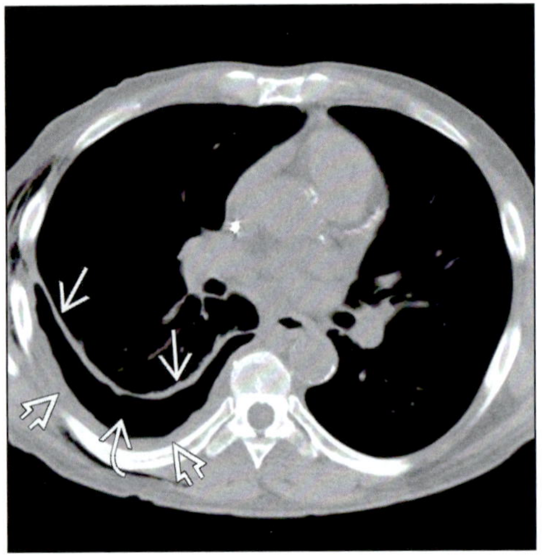

Stage IB (T1b N0 M0)

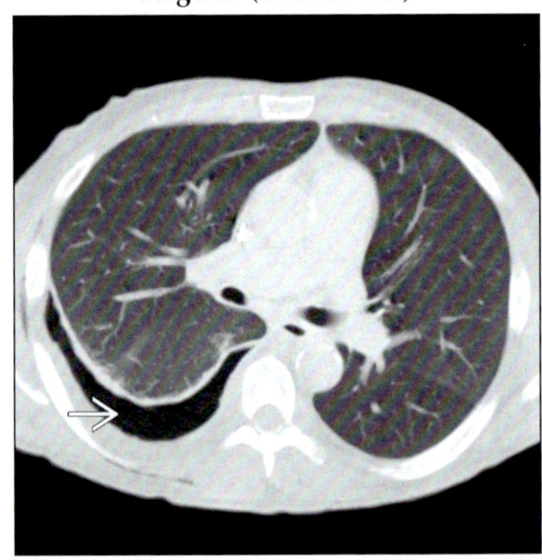

(Left) *Axial NECT following placement of a chest tube in a 45-year-old man who presented with pleural effusion shows thickening of both the visceral → and parietal → pleura. The tumor forms a rind around the lung, preventing its expansion and leading to the formation of pneumothorax →.* ***(Right)*** *Axial NECT in the same patient shows the intractable pneumothorax →. Biopsy revealed mesothelioma, and surgery confirmed T1b disease.*

Stage II (T2 N0 M0)

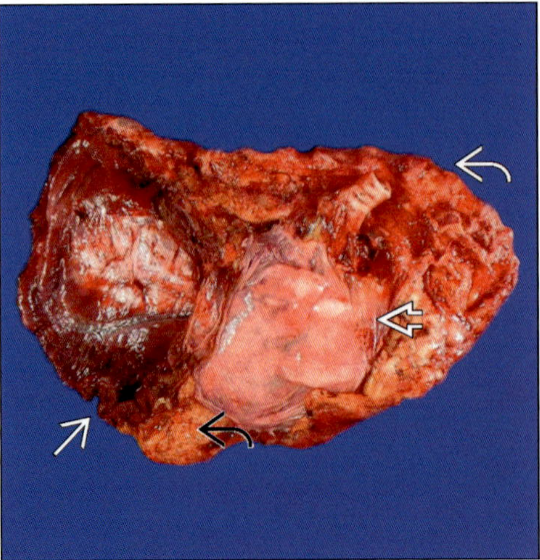

Stage II (T2 N0 M0)

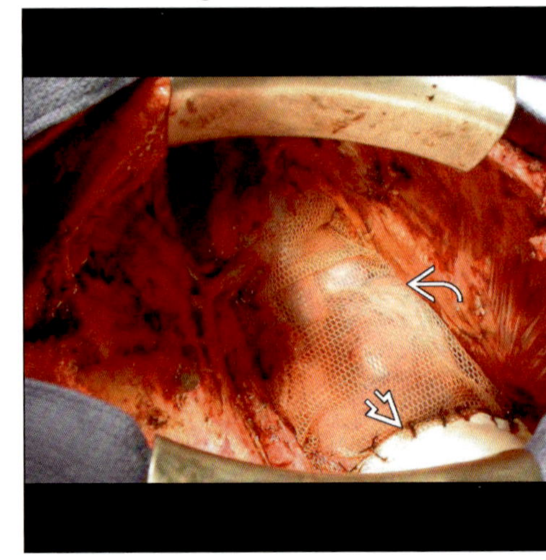

(Left) *Gross pathology specimen following right extrapleural pneumonectomy shows the en-bloc resection of pleura →, pericardium →, diaphragm →, and pleural masses →. (Courtesy M. de Perrot, MD.)* ***(Right)*** *Surgical photograph of right thoracic cavity post-extrapleural pneumonectomy shows the pericardial → and diaphragmatic → meshes in place. (Courtesy M. de Perrot, MD.)*

Stage III (T3 N0 M0)

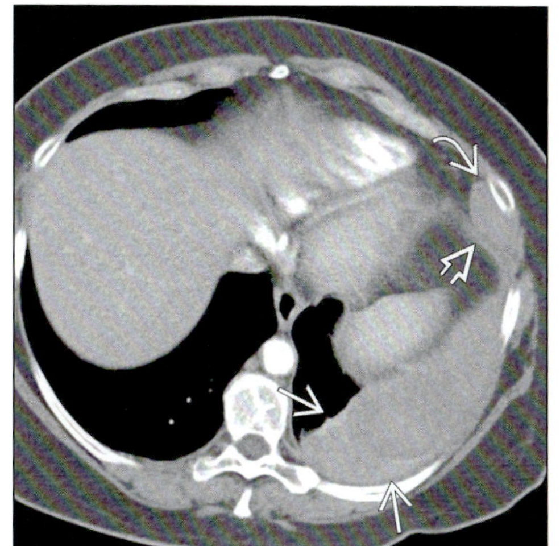

Stage III (T3 N0 M0)

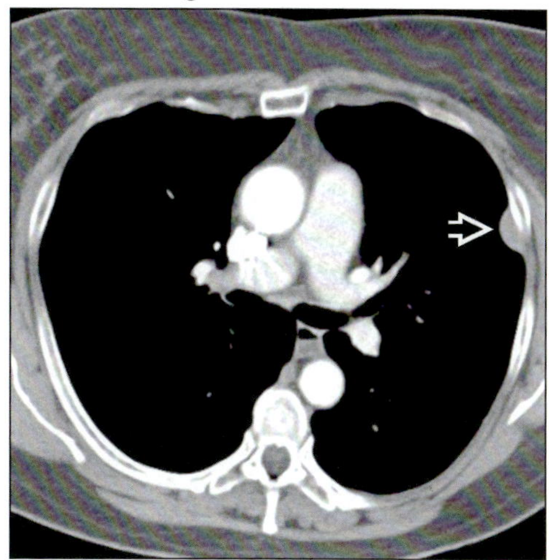

(Left) Axial CECT in a 57-year-old woman with history of asbestos exposure shows a large soft tissue mass ➡ filling the costophrenic recess. An anterior extension of the mass ↪ clearly displaces the diaphragm ⇨. *(Right)* Axial CECT in the same patient shows a separate polypoid pleural-based mass ⇨.

Stage III (T3 N0 M0)

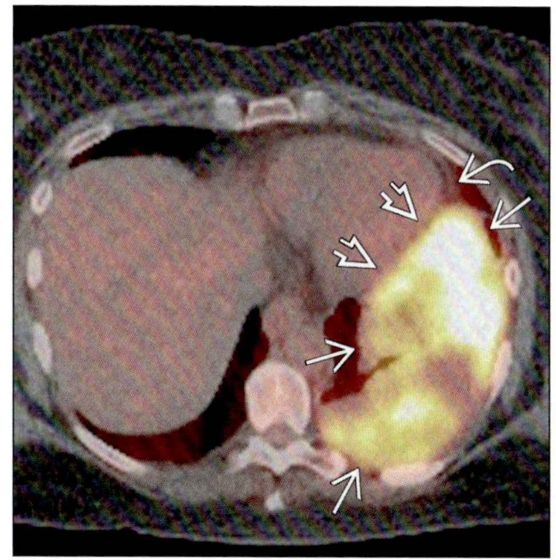

Stage III (T3 N0 M0)

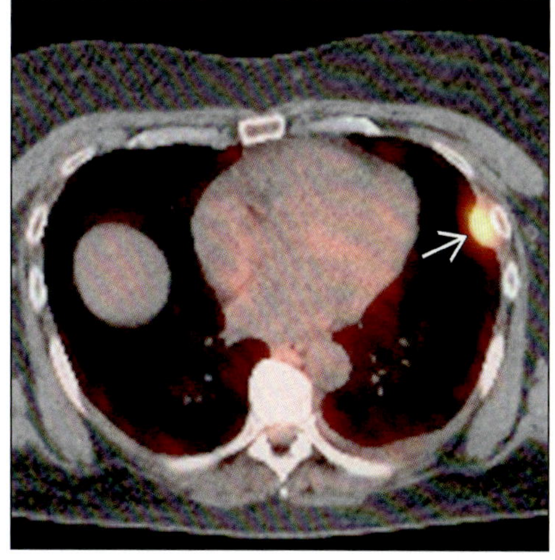

(Left) Axial PET/CT in the same patient shows high metabolic uptake in the pleural mass ➡. The tumor has significantly high SUV (range: 15-20), which helps distinguish malignant from benign pleural conditions. The tumor also has a broad interface with the heart ⇨, extending beyond the pericardium ↪. *(Right)* Axial PET/CT in the same patient shows significant increase in metabolic activity of the separate costal pleural polypoid lesion ➡.

Stage III (T3 N0 M0)

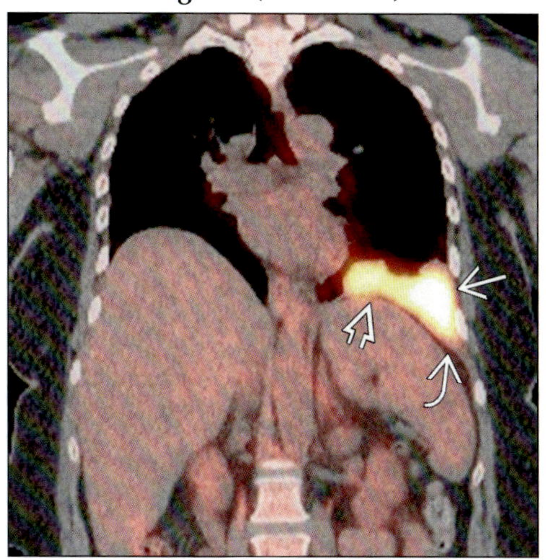

Stage III (T3 N0 M0)

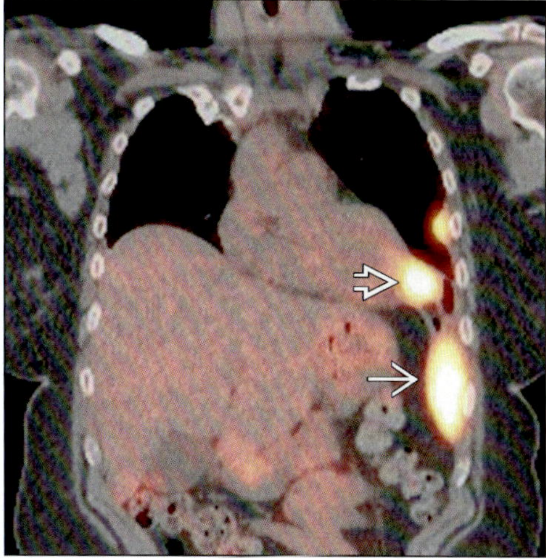

(Left) Coronal PET/CT in the same patient shows the extent of the pleural tumor involving the costal ➡ and diaphragmatic ⇨ pleura, with visible involvement of the diaphragm ↪. *(Right)* Coronal PET/CT in the same patient shows tumor extending into the deep lateral costophrenic recess ➡ and along the cardiac border ⇨. Diaphragmatic involvement constitutes T2 disease, while nontransmural pericardial involvement constitutes T3 disease.

Stage III (T3 N0 M0)

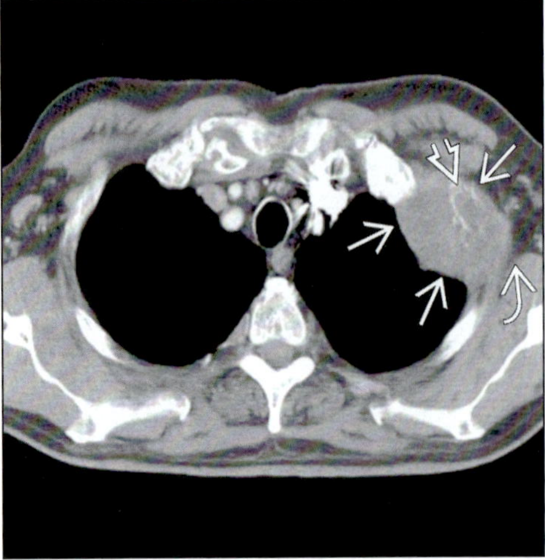

Stage III (T3 N0 M0)

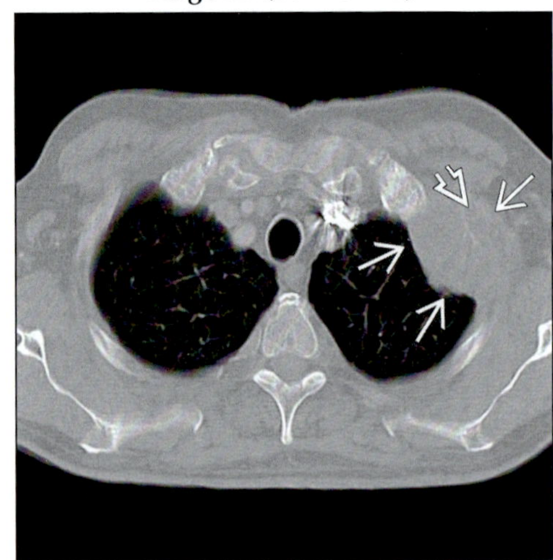

(Left) *Axial CECT in a 68-year-old man shows a left anterior chest wall mass ➔ involving the left 2nd rib ⇨ and extending beyond the chest wall to involve the fat of the left axilla ↪.* *(Right)* *Axial CECT in bone windows in the same patient shows expansion and destruction of the left 2nd rib ⇨ surrounded by the chest wall mass ➔.*

Stage III (T3 N0 M0)

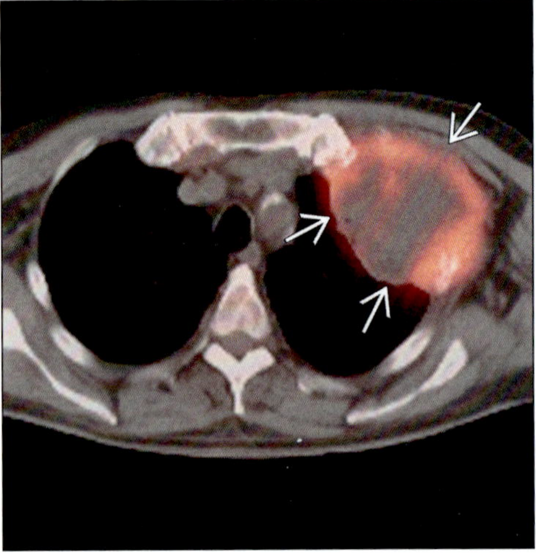

Stage III (T3 N0 M0)

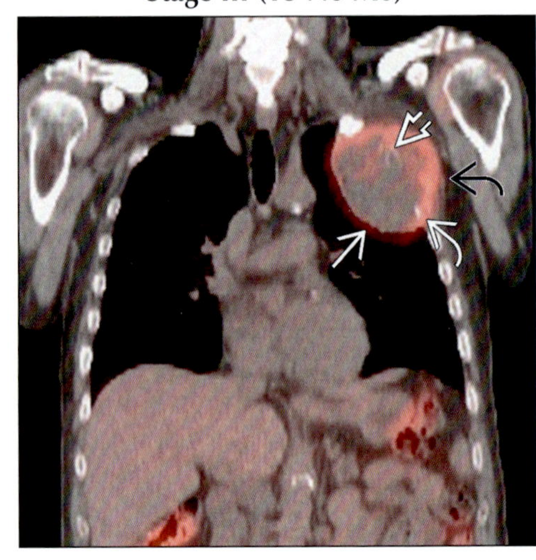

(Left) *Axial PET/CT in the same patient shows the left chest wall mass ➔ with increased metabolic activity at its periphery.* *(Right)* *Coronal PET/CT in the same patient shows the left chest wall mass ➔ involving both the 2nd ⇨ and 3rd ↪ ribs and extending into the subcutaneous fat ↪. A solitary completely resectable tumor extending into soft tissue of chest wall is classified as T3 tumor.*

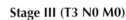

Stage III (T3 N0 M0)

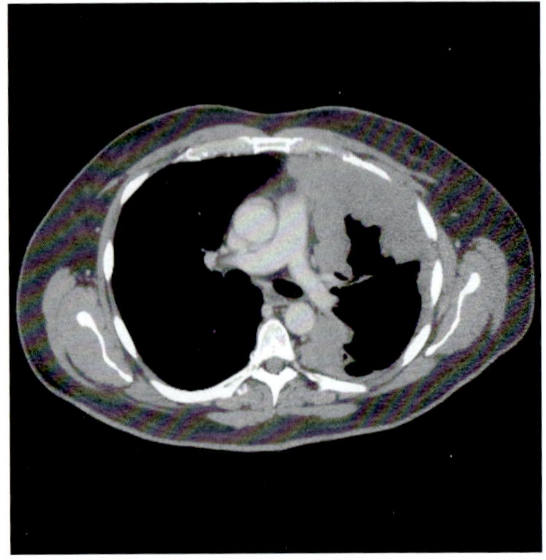

Stage III (T3 N0 M0)

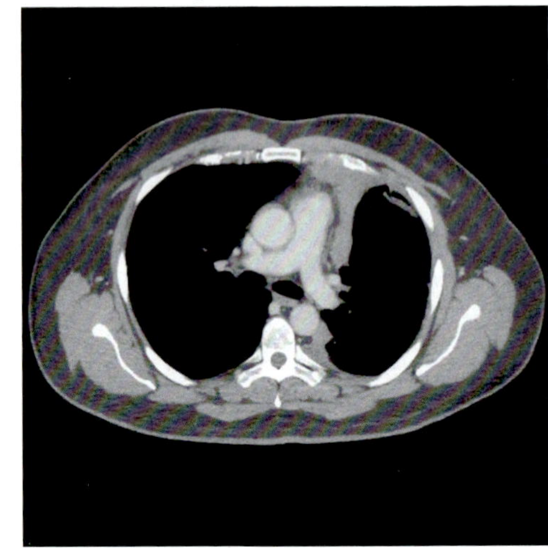

(Left) *Axial CECT of a bulky left epithelioid mesothelioma patient prior to neoadjuvant chemotherapy (cisplatin plus raltitrexed) is shown.* *(Right)* *Axial CECT of the same patient after 3 cycles of neoadjuvant chemotherapy shows significant partial response.*

Stage III (pT3 N0 M0)

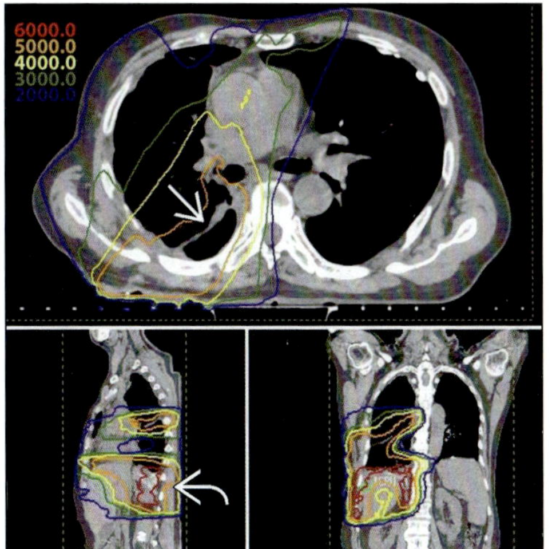

Stage III (pT3 N0 M0)

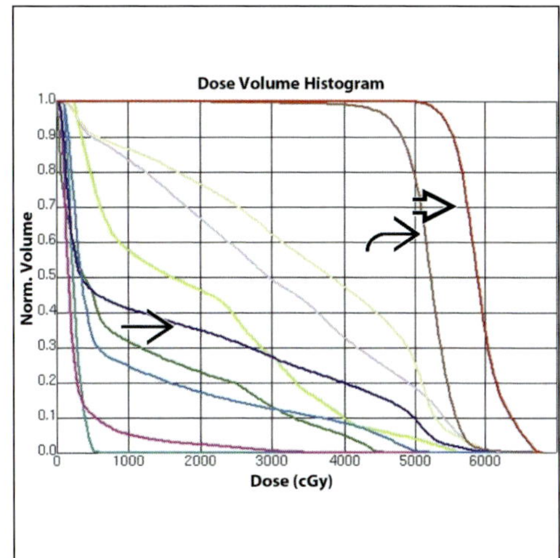

(Left) *Orthogonal CT views of adjuvant IMRT plan for right biphasic mesothelioma after pleurectomy/decortication shows coverage of lower hemithorax, including oblique fissure, with boost to diaphragmatic crus. The red, orange, yellow, green, and blue represent the 120%, 100%, 80%, 60%, and 20% isodoses.* ***(Right)*** *DVH of the same patient shows coverage of hemithorax, boost, and bilateral nontarget lung volumes.*

Stage III (pT3 N0 M0)

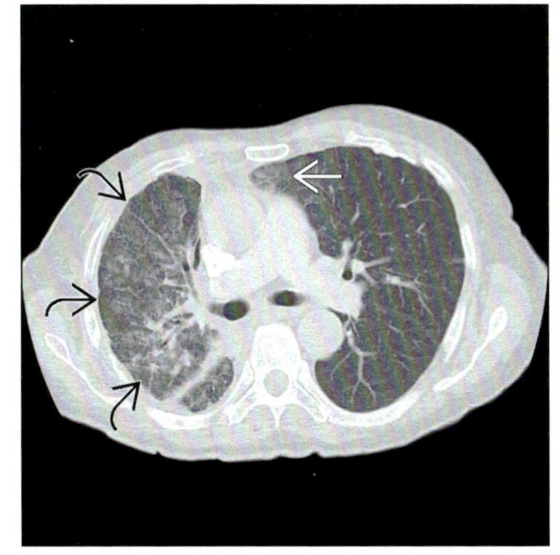

Stage III (pT3 N0 M0) Recurrent Tumor

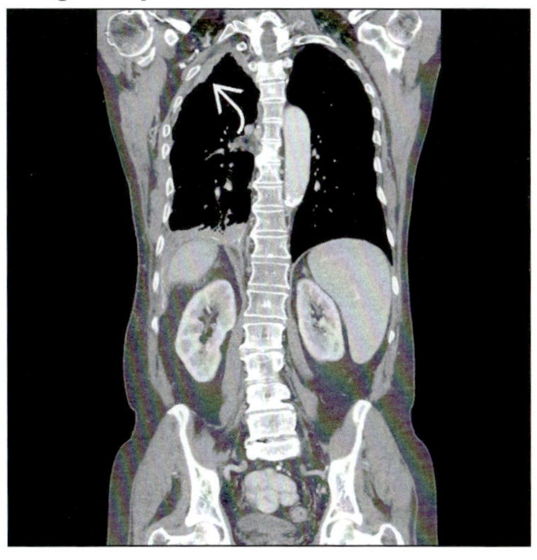

(Left) *Axial CECT of the same patient approximately 5 weeks after starting adjuvant partial hemithoracic radiotherapy shows radiation pneumonitis, including irradiated area of contralateral lung. Patient presented with cough, fever, and dyspnea and required admission and steroids.* ***(Right)*** *Coronal CECT of same patient shows out-of-field recurrence and control of disease within irradiated volume.*

Stage IV (pT4 pN2 M0)

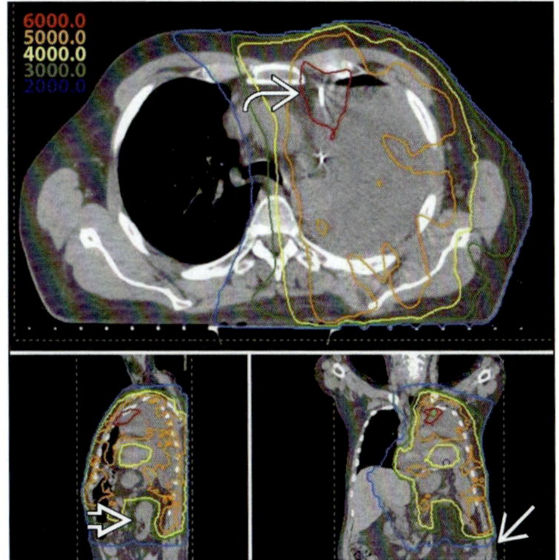

Stage IV (pT4 pN2 M0)

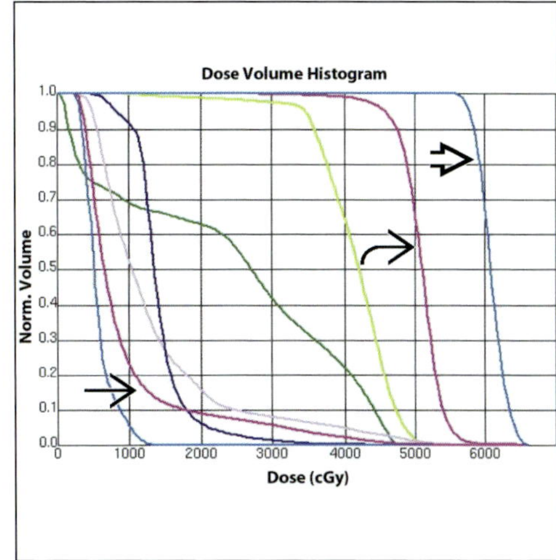

(Left) *Orthogonal CT views of IMRT plan for left epithelioid mesothelioma shows coverage of entire hemithorax with parasternal boost to a localized area of chest wall invasion. Note the sparing of left kidney and coverage to lower ribs to insertion of diaphragm. The red, orange, yellow, green, and blue represent the 120%, 100%, 80%, 60%, and 20% isodoses.* ***(Right)*** *DVH of same patient shows coverage of hemithorax, boost, and right lung volumes.*

PLEURA

(Left) Axial CECT in a 62-year-old man shows concentric thickening of the right pleura ➔, involving mainly the costal pleura at this level, and measuring > 2 cm. Pleural thickening > 1 cm helps differentiate malignant from benign disease. (Right) Axial CECT in the same patient shows pleural thickening ➔ with extension into the azygoesophageal recess ➔. An ipsilateral hilar node ➔ is present.

Stage IV (T4 N2 M0)

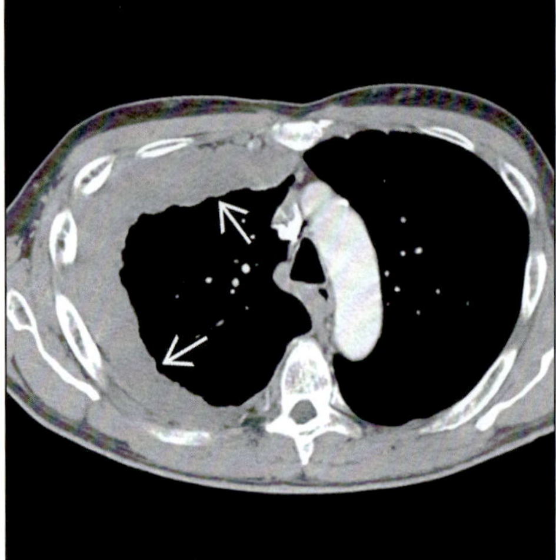

Stage IV (T4 N2 M0)

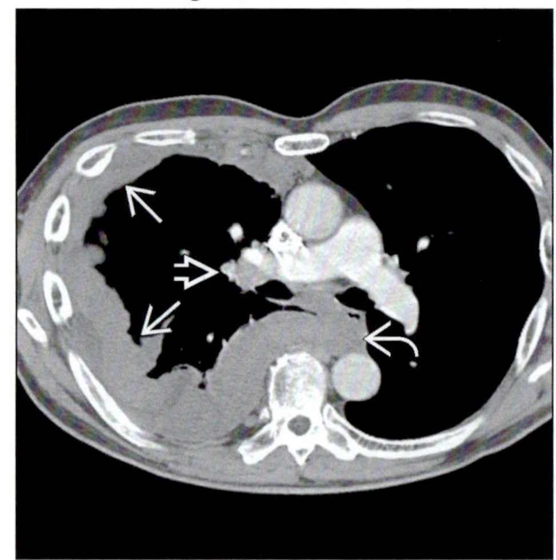

(Left) Axial CECT in the same patient shows bulky disease involving the contralateral pleura ➔ with tumor extension into the minor interlobar fissure ➔ and into the anterior mediastinal fat ➔. Contralateral pleural involvement is T4. (Right) Coronal CECT in the same patient shows pleural tumor invading the diaphragm ➔. Thickening of the diaphragmatic crus ➔ due to tumor invasion is also seen.

Stage IV (T4 N2 M0)

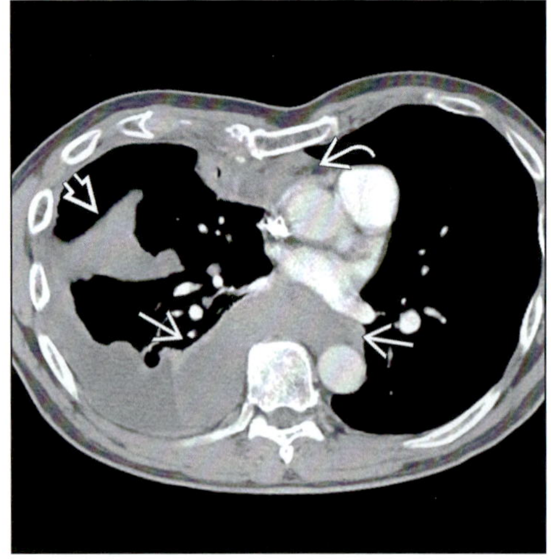

Stage IV (T4 N2 M0)

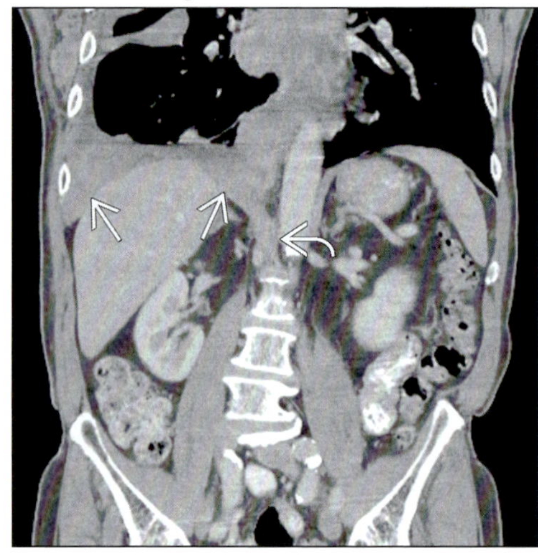

(Left) Axial CECT shows a massive right biphasic mesothelioma ➔ invading through chest wall. (Right) Coronal CECT of same patient shows invasion ➔ through chest wall.

Stage IV (T4 N2 M0)

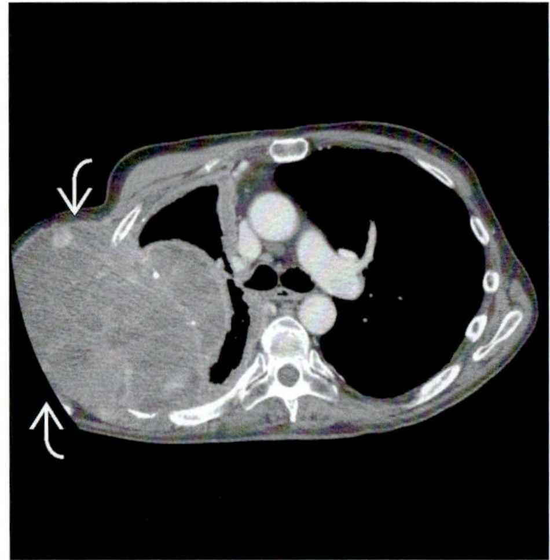

Stage IV (T4 N2 M0)

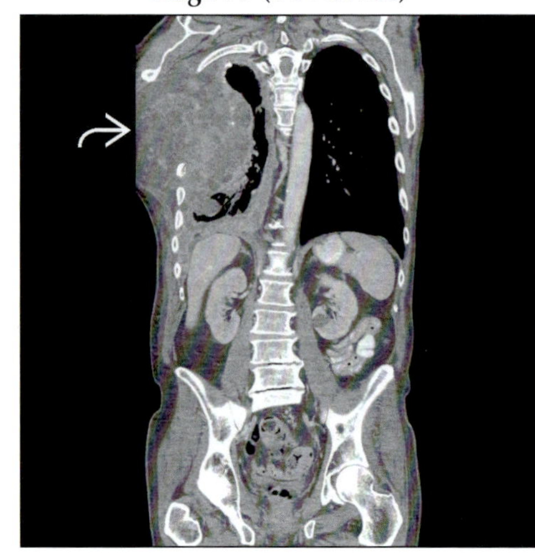

Stage IV (T4 N3 M1)

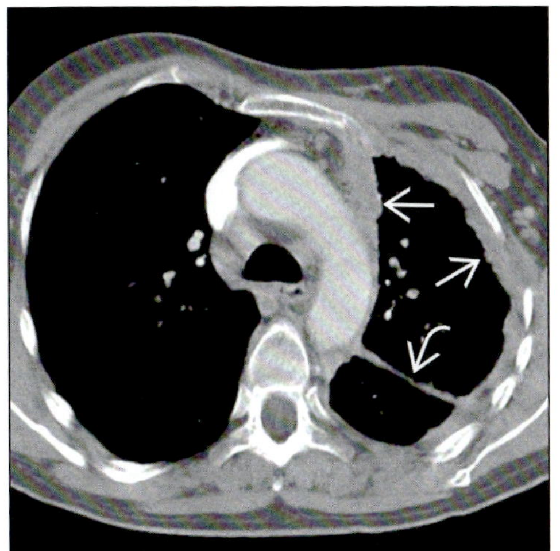

Stage IV (T4 N3 M1)

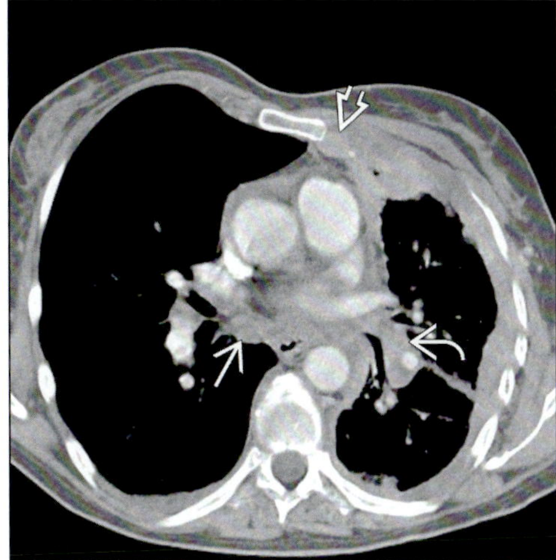

(Left) *Axial CECT in a 52-year-old woman with mesothelioma shows concentric pleural thickening ➔ and involvement of interlobar fissure ➔. This indicates involvement of the visceral pleura, since the parietal pleura is not a component of the pleura lining the interlobar fissures.* ***(Right)*** *Axial CECT in same patient shows, in addition to pleural thickening, enlarged subcarinal ➔, ipsilateral internal mammary ➔, and ipsilateral hilar ➔ nodes.*

Stage IV (T4 N3 M1)

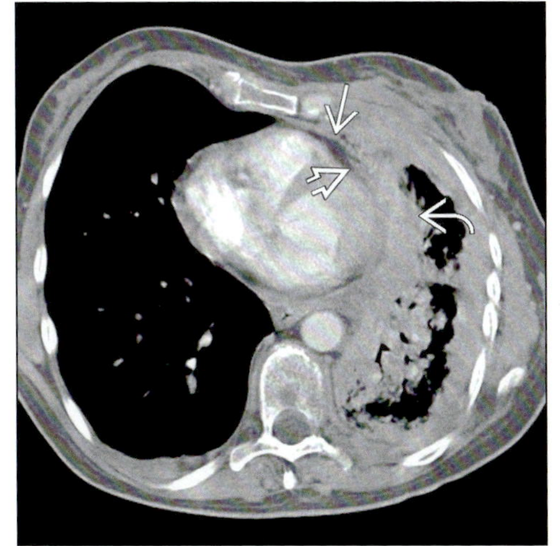

Stage IV (T4 N3 M1)

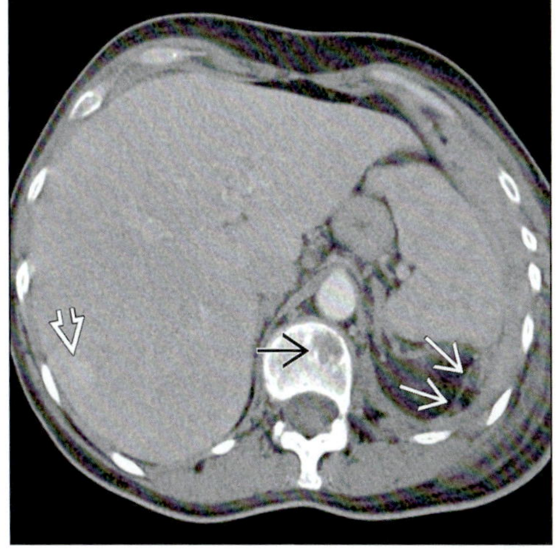

(Left) *Axial CECT in the same patient shows tumor ➔ infiltrating through the pericardium ➔ into the epicardial fat ➔.* ***(Right)*** *Axial CECT in the same patient shows distant metastases to the vertebral body ➔ and liver ➔. There is also transdiaphragmatic extension to the peritoneum ➔. Transdiaphragmatic extension to the peritoneum constitutes T4 disease.*

Stage IV (T3 N2 M1)

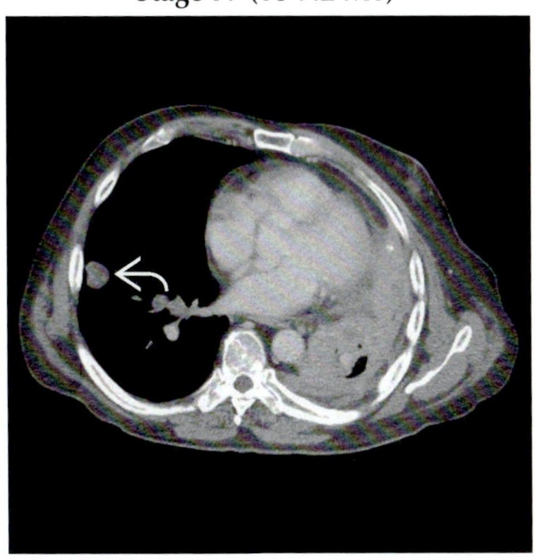

Stage IV (T3 N2 M1)

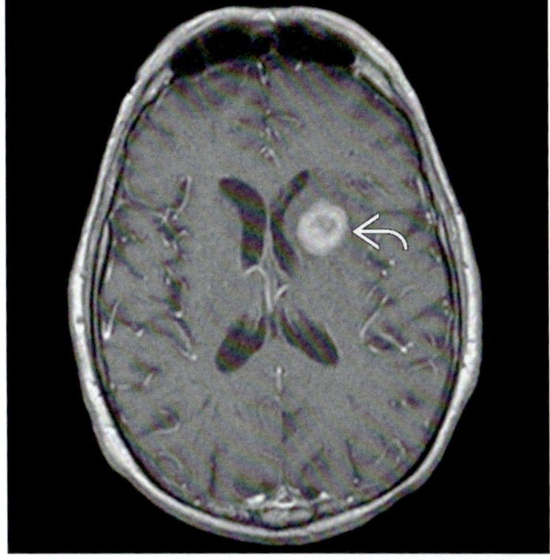

(Left) *Axial CECT of left epithelioid mesothelioma shows a right pulmonary metastasis ➔ (M1) and progressive restriction of left chest wall.* ***(Right)*** *Axial T1WI C+ MR of the same patient shows a brain metastasis ➔, which is an uncommon late presentation for mesothelioma.*

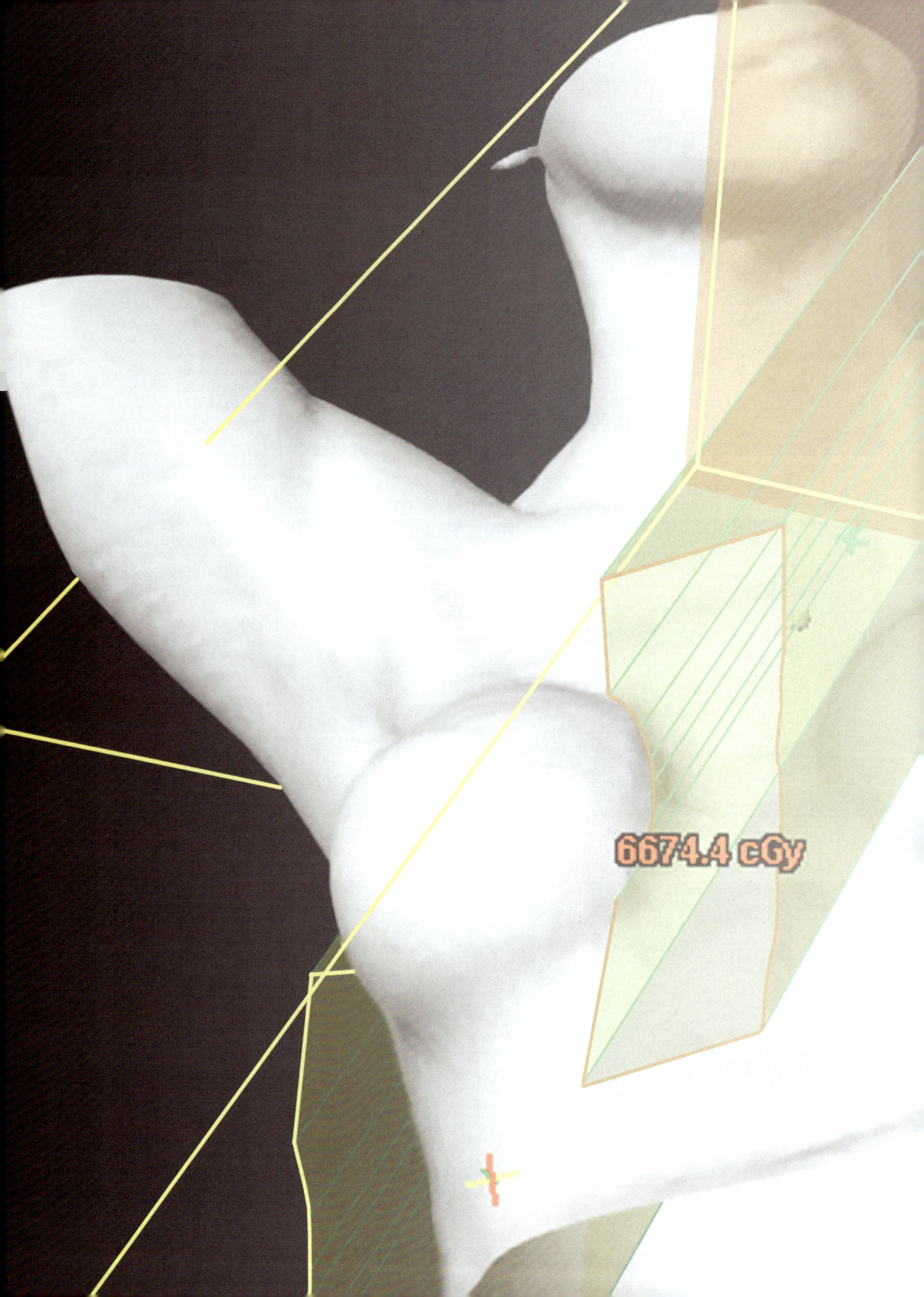
6674.4 cGy

SECTION 4
Breast

BREAST

(T) Primary Tumor

Adapted from 7th edition AJCC Staging Forms.

TNM	*Definitions*
TX	Primary tumor cannot be assessed
T0	No evidence of primary tumor
Tis	Carcinoma in situ
Tis (DCIS)	Ductal carcinoma in situ
Tis (LCIS)	Lobular carcinoma in situ
Tis (Paget)	Paget disease of the nipple **not** associated with invasive carcinoma &/or carcinoma in situ (DCIS &/or LCIS) in the underlying breast parenchyma; carcinomas in the breast parenchyma associated with Paget disease are categorized based on the size and characteristics of the parenchymal disease, although the presence of Paget disease should still be noted
T1	Tumor ≤ 20 mm in greatest dimension
T1mi	Tumor ≤ 1 mm in greatest dimension
T1a	Tumor > 1 mm but ≤ 5 mm in greatest dimension
T1b	Tumor > 5 mm but ≤ 10 mm in greatest dimension
T1c	Tumor > 10 mm but ≤ 20 mm in greatest dimension
T2	Tumor > 20 mm but ≤ 50 mm in greatest dimension
T3	Tumor > 50 mm in greatest dimension
T4	Tumor of any size with direct extension to the chest wall &/or to the skin (ulceration or skin nodules); invasion of the dermis alone does not qualify as T4
T4a	Extension to the chest wall, not including only pectoralis muscle adherence/invasion
T4b	Ulceration &/or ipsilateral satellite nodules &/or edema (including peau d'orange) of the skin, which do not meet the criteria for inflammatory carcinoma
T4c	Both T4a and T4b
T4d	Inflammatory carcinoma

The T classification of the primary tumor is the same regardless of whether it is based on clinical or pathologic criteria, or both. Size should be measured to the nearest millimeter. If the tumor size is slightly less than or greater than a cutoff for a given T classification, it is recommended that the size be rounded to the millimeter reading that is closest to the cutoff. For example, a reported size of 1.1 mm is reported as 1 mm or a size of 2.01 cm is reported as 2.0 cm. Designation should be made with the subscript "c" or "p" modifier to indicate whether the T classification was determined by clinical (physical examination or radiologic) or pathologic measurements, respectively. In general, pathologic determination should take precedence over clinical determination of T size.

(N) Regional Lymph Nodes, Clinical Classification

Adapted from 7th edition AJCC Staging Forms.

TNM	*Definitions*
NX	Regional lymph nodes cannot be assessed (e.g., previously removed)
N0	No regional lymph node metastases
N1	Metastases to movable ipsilateral level I, II axillary lymph node(s)
N2	Metastases in ipsilateral level I, II axillary lymph nodes that are clinically fixed or matted; or in clinically detected* ipsilateral internal mammary nodes in the **absence** of clinically evident axillary lymph node metastases
N2a	Metastases in ipsilateral level I, II axillary lymph nodes fixed to one another (matted) or to other structures
N2b	Metastases only in clinically detected* ipsilateral internal mammary nodes and in the **absence** of clinically evident level I, II axillary lymph node metastases
N3	Metastases in ipsilateral infraclavicular (level III axillary) lymph node(s) with or without level I, II axillary lymph node involvement; or in clinically detected[1] ipsilateral internal mammary lymph node(s) with clinically evident level I, II axillary lymph node metastases; or metastases in ipsilateral supraclavicular lymph node(s) with or without axillary or internal mammary lymph node involvement
N3a	Metastases in ipsilateral infraclavicular lymph node(s)
N3b	Metastases in ipsilateral internal mammary lymph node(s) and axillary lymph node(s)
N3c	Metastases in ipsilateral supraclavicular lymph node(s)

**"Clinically detected" is defined as detected by imaging studies (excluding lymphoscintigraphy) or by clinical examination and having characteristics highly suspicious for malignancy or a presumed pathologic macrometastasis based on fine needle aspiration biopsy with cytologic examination. Confirmation of clinically detected metastatic disease by fine need aspiration without excision biopsy is designated with an (f) suffix, for example, cN3a(f). Excisional biopsy of a lymph node or biopsy of a sentinel node, in the absence of assignment of a pT, is classified as a clinical N, for example, cN1. Information regarding the confirmation of the nodal status will be designated in site-specific factors as clinical, fine needle aspiration, core biopsy, or sentinel lymph node biopsy. Pathologic classification (pN) is used for excision or sentinel lymph node biopsy only in conjunction with a pathologic T assignment.*

BREAST

(pN) Pathologic Lymph Node Classification[1]

Adapted from 7th edition AJCC Staging Forms.

TNM	*Definitions*
pNX	Regional lymph nodes cannot be assessed (e.g., previously removed, or not removed for pathologic study)
pN0	No regional lymph node metastasis identified histologically
pN0(i-)	No regional lymph node metastases histologically, negative IHC[2]
pN0(i+)	Malignant cells in regional lymph node(s) ≤ 0.2 mm (detected by H&E or IHC including ITC[3])
pN0(mol-)	No regional lymph node metastases histologically, negative molecular findings (RT-PCR)[4]
pN0(mol+)	Positive molecular findings (RT-PCR),[4] but no regional lymph node metastases detected by histology or IHC
pN1	Micrometastases; or metastases in 1-3 axillary lymph nodes; &/or in internal mammary nodes with metastases detected by sentinel lymph node biopsy but not clinically detected[5]
pN1mi	Micrometastases (> 0.2 mm &/or > 200 cells, but none > 2.0 mm)
pN1a	Metastases in 1-3 axillary lymph nodes, ≥ 1 metastasis > 2.0 mm
pN1b	Metastases in internal mammary nodes with micrometastases or macrometastases detected by sentinel lymph node biopsy but not clinically detected[5]
pN1c	Metastases in 1-3 axillary lymph nodes and in internal mammary lymph nodes with micrometastases or macrometastases detected by sentinel lymph node biopsy but not clinically detected[5]
pN2	Metastases in 4-9 axillary lymph nodes; or in clinically detected[6] internal mammary lymph nodes in the **absence** of axillary lymph node metastases
pN2a	Metastases in 4-9 axillary lymph nodes (≥ 1 tumor deposit > 2.0 mm)
pN2b	Metastases in clinically detected[6] internal mammary lymph nodes in the **absence** of axillary lymph node metastases
pN3	Metastases in ≥ 10 axillary lymph nodes; or in infraclavicular (level III axillary) lymph nodes; or in clinically detected[6] ipsilateral internal mammary lymph nodes in the **presence** of ≥ 1 positive level I, II axillary lymph nodes; or in > 3 axillary lymph nodes and in internal mammary lymph nodes with micrometastases or macrometastases detected by sentinel lymph node biopsy but not clinically detected[5]; or in ipsilateral supraclavicular lymph nodes
pN3a	Metastases in ≥ 10 axillary lymph nodes (≥ 1 tumor deposit > 2.0 mm); or metastases to infraclavicular (level III axillary lymph) nodes
pN3b	Metastases in clinically detected[6] ipsilateral internal mammary lymph nodes in the **presence** of ≥ 1 positive axillary lymph nodes; or in > 3 axillary lymph nodes and internal mammary lymph nodes with micrometastases or macrometastases detected by sentinel lymph node biopsy but not clinically detected[5]
pN3c	Metastases in ipsilateral supraclavicular lymph nodes

[1]*Classification is based on axillary lymph node dissection with or without sentinel lymph node biopsy. Classification based solely on sentinel lymph node biopsy without subsequent axillary lymph node dissection is designated (sn) for "sentinel node."*

[2]*IHC: Immunohistochemistry.*

[3]*Isolated tumor cell clusters (ITC) are defined as small clusters of cells not greater than 0.2 mm, or single tumor cells, or a cluster of fewer than 200 cells in a single histologic cross section. ITCs may be detected by routine histology or by immunohistochemical methods. Nodes containing only ITCs are excluded from the total positive node count for purposes of N classification but should be included in the total number of nodes evaluated.*

[4]*RT-PCR: Reverse transcriptase/polymerase chain reaction.*

[5]*"Not clinically detected" is defined as not detected by imaging studies (excluding lymphoscintigraphy) or by clinical examination.*

[6]*"Clinically detected" is defined as detected by imaging studies (excluding lymphoscintigraphy) or by clinical examination and having characteristics highly suspicious for malignancy or a presumed pathologic macrometastasis based on fine needle aspiration biopsy with cytologic examination.*

(M) Distant Metastases

Adapted from 7th edition AJCC Staging Forms.

TNM	*Definitions*
M0	No clinical or radiographic evidence of distant metastases
cM0(i+)	No clinical or radiographic evidence of distant metastases, but deposits of molecularly or microscopically detected tumor cells in circulating blood, bone marrow, or other nonregional nodal tissue that are ≤ 0.2 mm in a patient without symptoms or signs of metastases
M1	Distant detectable metastases as determined by classic clinical and radiographic means &/ or histologically proven > 0.2 mm

AJCC Stages/Prognostic Groups

Adapted from 7th edition AJCC Staging Forms.

Stage	*T*	*N*	*M*
0	Tis	N0	M0
IA	T1[1]	N0	M0
IB	T0	N1mi	M0
	T1[1]	N1mi	M0
IIA	T0	N1[2]	M0
	T1[1]	N1[2]	M0
	T2	N0	M0
IIB	T2	N1	M0
	T3	N0	M0
IIIA	T0	N2	M0
	T1[1]	N2	M0
	T2	N2	M0
	T3	N1	M0
	T3	N2	M0
IIIB	T4	N0	M0
	T4	N1	M0
	T4	N2	M0
IIIC	Any T	N3	M0
IV	Any T	Any N	M1

Notes: M0 includes M0(i+). The designation pM0 is not valid; any M0 should be clinical. If a patient presents with M1 prior to neoadjuvant systemic therapy, the stage is considered IV and remains stage IV regardless of response to neoadjuvant therapy. Stage designation may be changed if postsurgical imaging studies reveal the presence of distant metastases, provided that the studies are carried out within 4 months of diagnosis in the absence of disease progression and provided that the patient has not received neoadjuvant therapy. Post-neoadjuvant therapy is designated with a "yc" or "yp" prefix. Of note, no stage group is assigned if there is a complete pathologic response (CR) to neoadjuvant therapy, for example, ypT0ypN0cM0.

[1]*T1 includes T1mi.*

[2]*T0 and T1 tumors with nodal micrometastases only are excluded from stage IIA and are classified stage IB.*

Invasive Adenocarcinoma

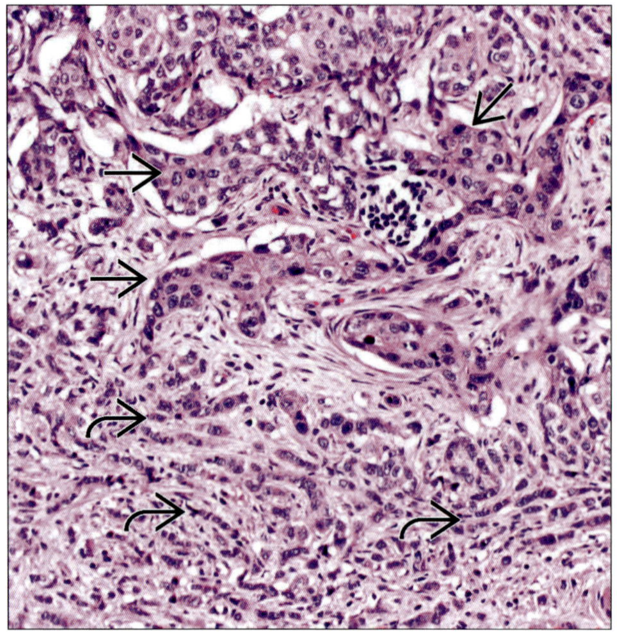

This graphic has examples of both invasive ductal carcinoma ➔ and lobular carcinoma ➔. The grading system for ductal carcinoma evaluates nuclear pleomorphism, tubule formation, and mitotic activity, with each feature getting a score of 1-3. (Courtesy D. Hicks, MD.)

Invasive Lobular Carcinoma

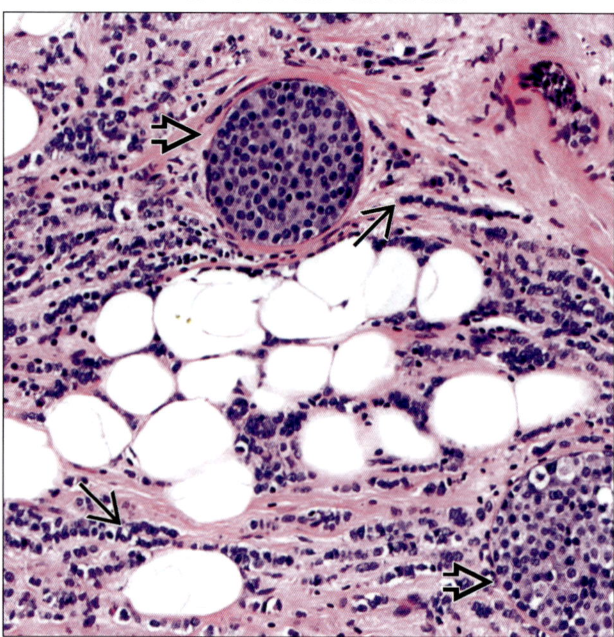

Invasive lobular carcinoma is characterized by dyscohesive cells ➔ with little stromal reaction, often in a single file. LCIS ➔ is often present. (Courtesy D. Hicks, MD.)

Tis (Paget)

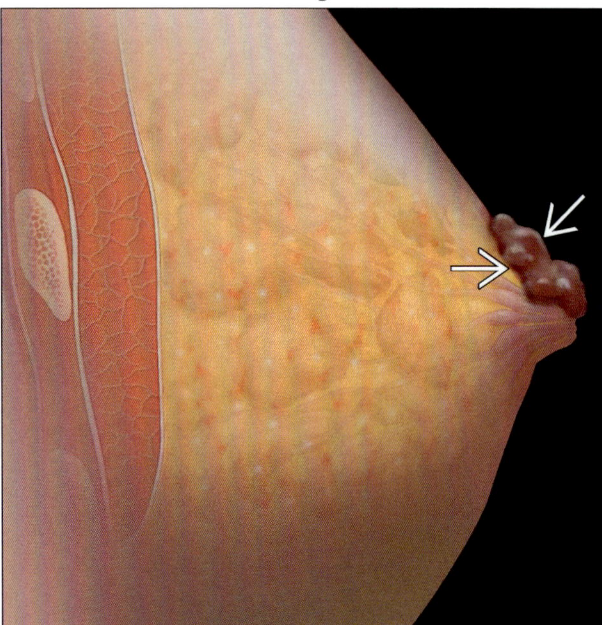

Tis (Paget) is defined as skin changes ➔ of the nipple without an underlying mass. The skin findings associated with Paget disease are caused by an infiltration of noninvasive breast cancer epithelial cells.

T1mi

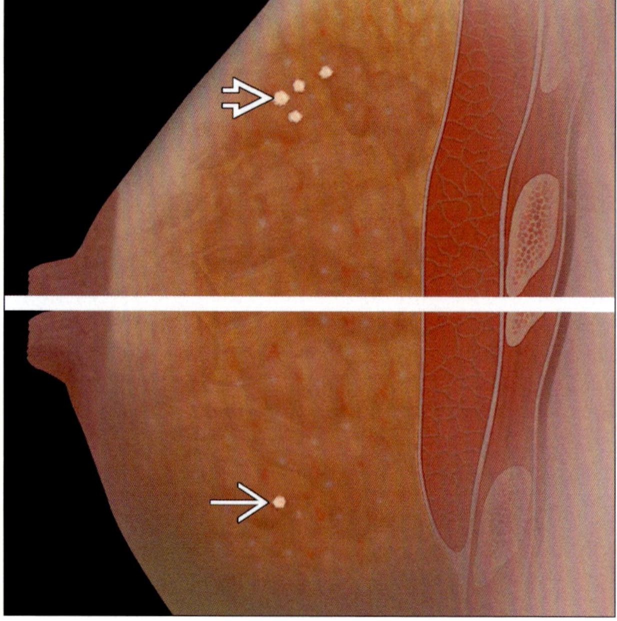

Graphic shows T1mi, defined as a microinvasion ➔ ≤ 0.1 cm in greatest dimension. The presence of multiple tumor foci of microinvasion ➔ should be noted.

T1a-T1c

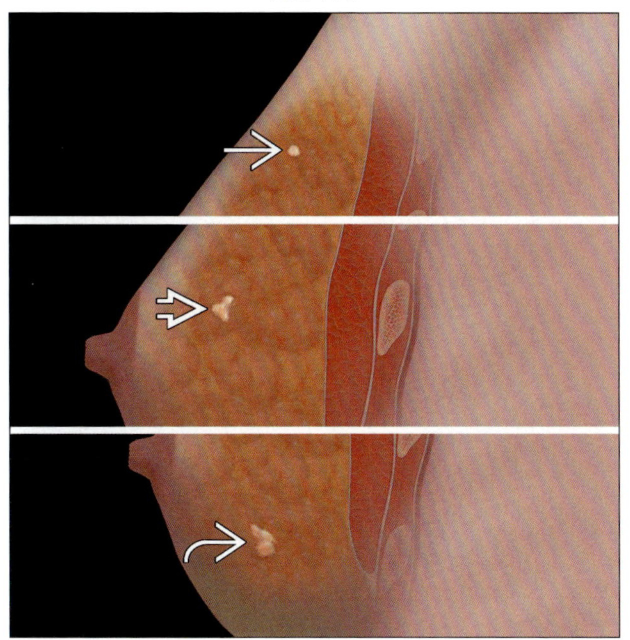

Graphic shows examples of T1 lesions, defined as a tumor ≤ 2 cm in greatest dimension. T1a is defined as a tumor ➡ > 0.1 cm but not > 0.5 cm. T1b is defined as a tumor ➡ > 0.5 cm but not > 1 cm. T1c is defined as a tumor ➡ > 1 cm but not > 2 cm.

T2 and T3

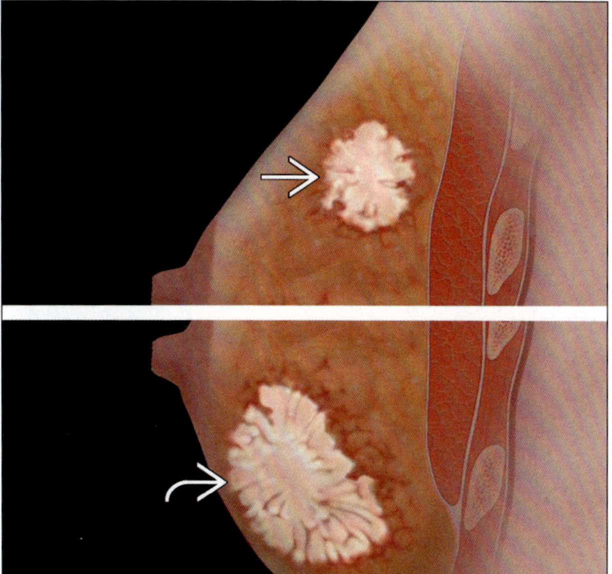

Graphic shows examples of T2 and T3 lesions. T2 is defined as a tumor ➡ > 2 cm but not > 5 cm in greatest dimension. T3 is defined as a tumor ➡ > 5 cm in greatest dimension.

T4b

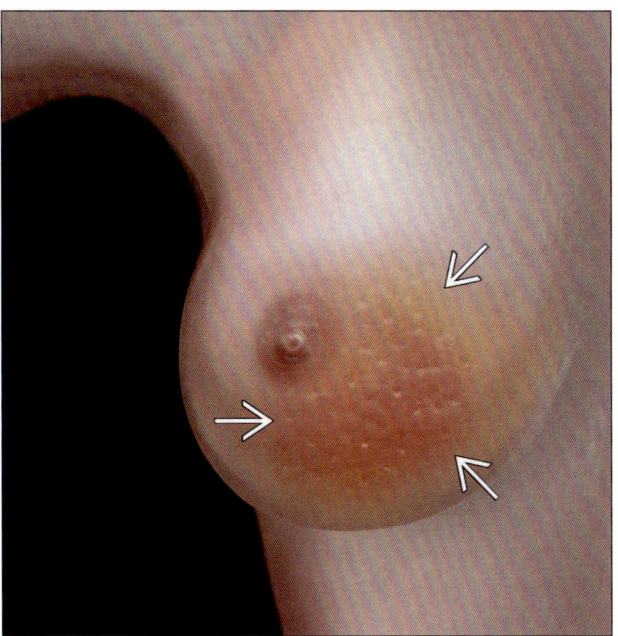

Graphic shows a T4b lesion ➡, illustrated here as skin edema, redness, and thickening or peau d'orange. Inflammatory breast cancer (T4d) is primarily a clinical diagnosis characterized by rapid growth and involvement of ≥ 1/3 of the skin of the breast. The pathologic correlate is tumor emboli in dermal lymphatics. Imaging often reveals skin thickening.

T4c

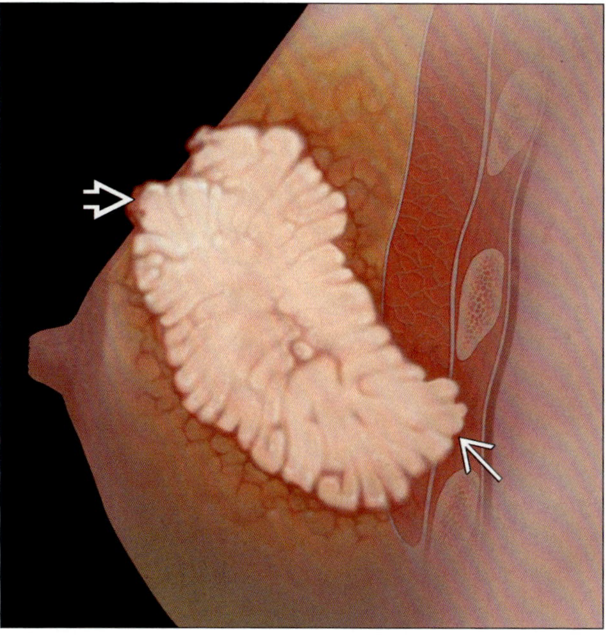

Graphic shows a T4c lesion, which by definition meets the requirements for both T4a ➡ (invasion of the chest wall not including the pectoralis muscle) and T4b (invasion of the skin) ➡. T4b lesions may have edema (including peau d'orange) or ulceration of the skin of the breast or satellite skin nodules, confined to the same breast.

Clinical N1

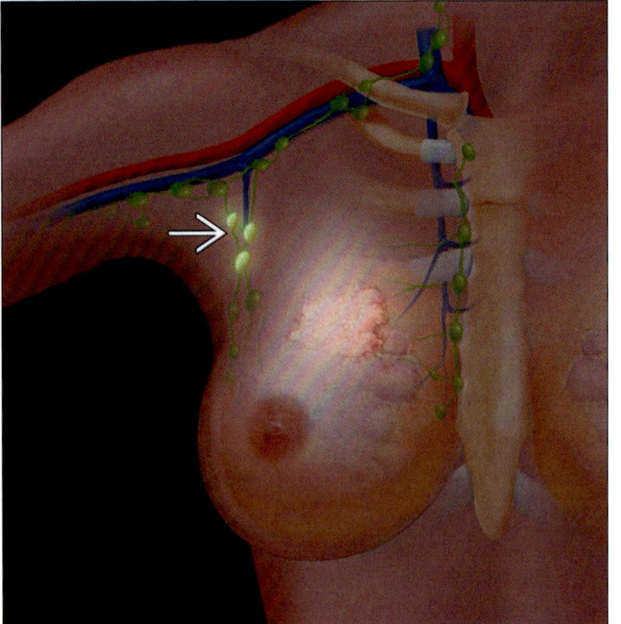

Graphic shows N1, defined as metastasis in movable ipsilateral axillary lymph node(s) ➡.

Clinical N2a

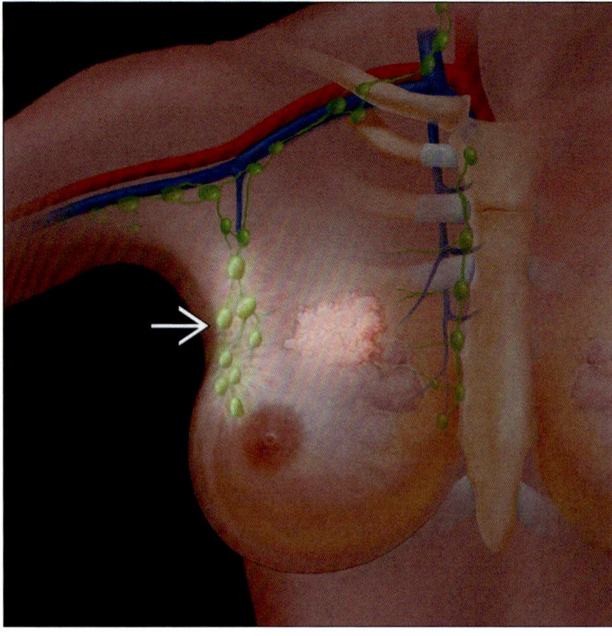

Graphic shows N2a, defined as metastasis in ipsilateral axillary lymph nodes ➡ fixed to each other (matted) or to other structures.

Clinical N3a

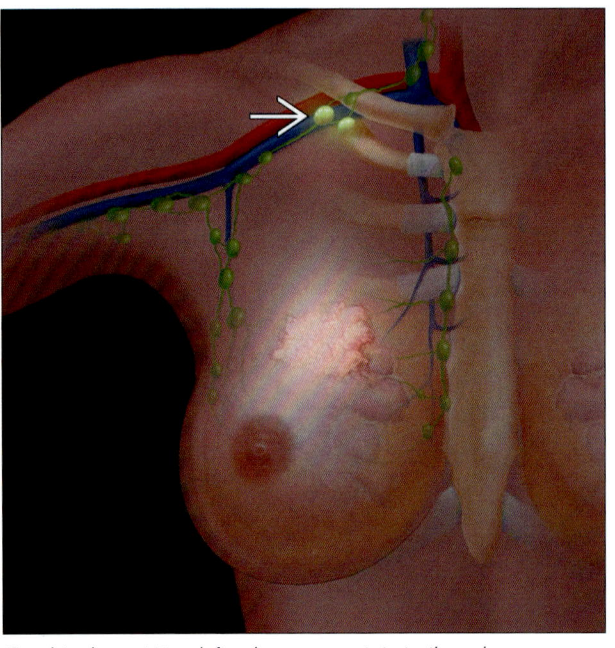

Graphic shows N3a, defined as metastasis in ipsilateral infraclavicular lymph node(s) ➡ without axillary or internal mammary lymph node involvement.

Clinical N3c

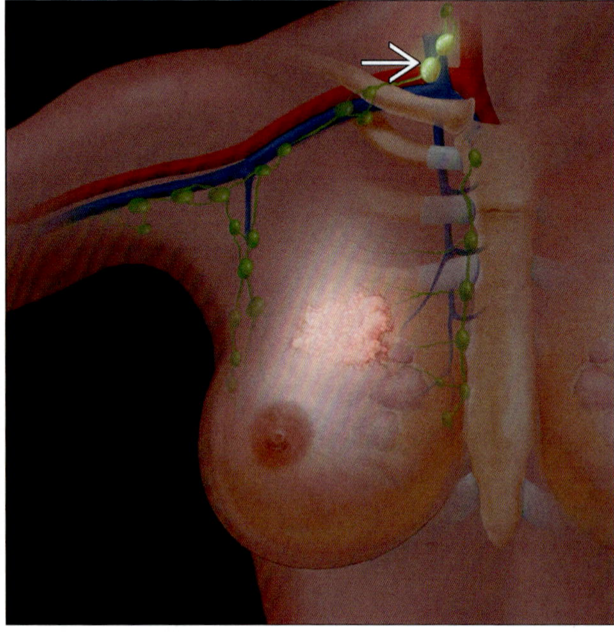

Graphic shows N3c, defined as metastasis in ipsilateral supraclavicular lymph node(s) ➡.

pN0(i+)

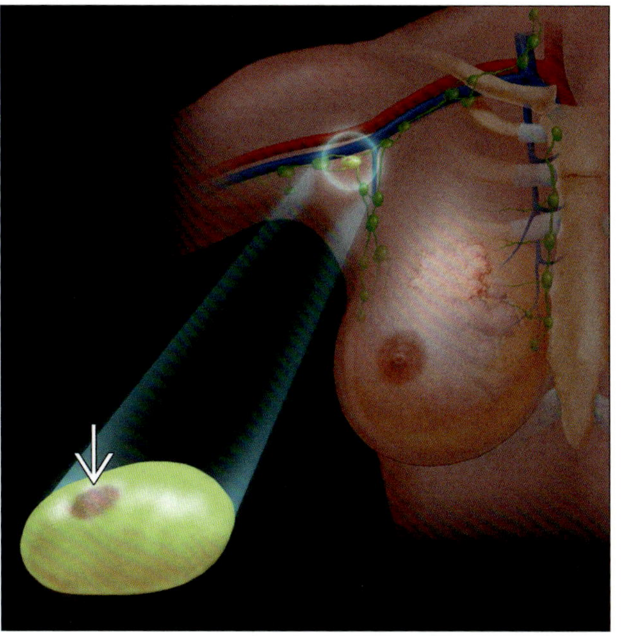

Graphic shows pN0(i+), defined as malignant cells in regional node(s) detected by H&E stains or immunohistochemistry (IHC). No isolated tumor cell cluster (ITC) is larger than 0.2 mm →.

pN1mi

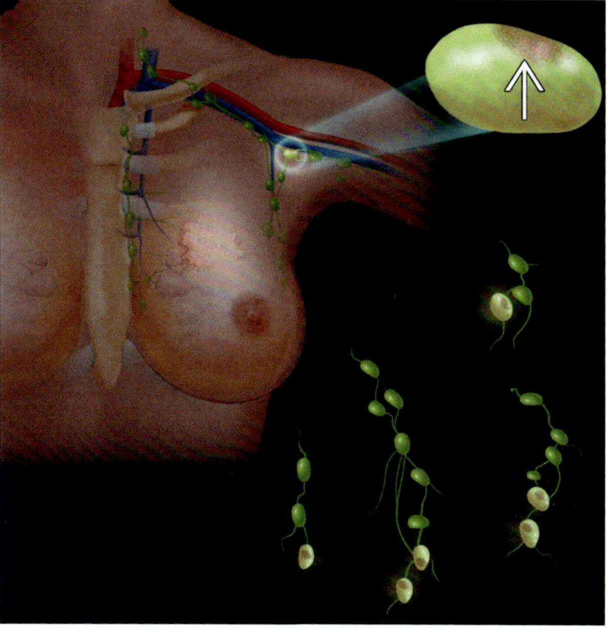

Graphic illustrates the pN1mi, defined as micrometastasis → > 0.2 mm &/or > 200 cells, but with none > 2.0 mm.

INITIAL SITE OF RECURRENCE

Site	%
Bone	71%
Lung	69%
Liver	65%
Pleura	51%
Adrenals	49%
Skin	30%
Thyroid	24%
Brain	22%
Ovaries	20%
Pericardium	19%
Intestine	18%
Kidneys, Spleen, Pancreas	17%
Uterus, Heart, Diaphragm	≤15%

Most common metastatic sites of breast cancer at autopsy in 100 cases. Haagensen C: Disease of the Breast, ed 3. Philadelphia: WB Saunders. 686, 1986

BREAST

OVERVIEW

General Comments

- Cancer of mammary ducts and glands (ductal carcinoma) or of lobules and terminal ducts (lobular carcinoma)
- **Ductal carcinoma in situ (DCIS)**
  - Entirely confined to duct system of breast
  - Both smaller ductolobular units and larger extralobular ducts
  - Noninvasive
  - Considered direct precursor of invasive ductal carcinoma, with magnitude of risk being variable and dependent on
    - Histological grade
    - Lesion size
    - Age
  - DCIS increases chance of developing invasive cancer in ipsilateral or contralateral breast
- **Invasive ductal carcinoma**
  - Most rapidly growing subgroup of breast cancer
  - ~ 80% of all invasive breast cancers
- **Lobular carcinoma in situ (LCIS)**
  - Noninvasive lesion that arises from lobules and terminal ducts of breast
  - Almost always represents incidental finding
  - Not usually identified clinically, mammographically, or by gross pathologic examination
  - Not direct precursor lesion for invasive breast cancer, although new studies are challenging this belief
  - Associated with increased risk of developing invasive ductal or lobular carcinoma in either breast
- **Infiltrating lobular carcinoma**
  - 2nd most common type of invasive breast cancer
  - Accounts for about 5-10% of invasive lesions
  - Incidence rates of lobular cancer are rising faster than rates of ductal carcinoma in United States

Classification

- Ductal carcinoma traditionally classified according to architectural pattern
  - Comedo
  - Cribriform
  - Micropapillary
  - Papillary
  - Solid
- **Grade classification**
  - Scarff-Bloom-Richardson scoring system
    - 1-3 points are given for nuclear pleomorphism, mitotic rate, and tubule formation
      - Low grade: 3-5
      - Intermediate grade: 6-7
      - High grade: 8-9
  - Reflects potential of lesion to recur within breast or to progress to invasive breast cancer
  - Architectural and cytologic features
    - **Well differentiated (grade 1)**
      - Infiltration of stroma as solid nests of glands
      - Nuclei are relatively uniform with little or no evidence of mitotic activity
    - **Moderately differentiated (grade 2)**
      - Infiltration as solid nests with some glandular differentiation
      - Nuclear pleomorphism and moderate mitotic rate
    - **Poorly differentiated (grade 3)**
      - Composed of solid nests of neoplastic cells without evidence of gland formation
      - Marked nuclear atypia and considerable mitotic activity

NATURAL HISTORY

General Features

- Comments
  - DCIS represents heterogeneous group of proliferative lesions with diverse malignant potential
    - Proliferation of presumably malignant epithelial cells within mammary ductal system
    - No evidence of invasion into surrounding stroma on routine light microscopic examination

Etiology

- Risk factors
  - Gender
    - Females have 100x higher risk than males
  - Age
    - Incidence rates rise sharply with age until about 45-50 years
  - Benign breast conditions
    - Multiple nonproliferative lesions with cytologic atypia
  - Personal history
    - Invasive or in situ breast cancer
  - Family history
  - Dietary factors
    - Alcohol
      - Moderate alcohol intake is associated with increased risk of hormone receptor-positive breast cancer
    - Fat, red meat intake
  - Smoking
  - Exposure to endogenous estrogens for prolonged period
  - Younger age at menarche
    - For every 2-year delay in onset of menarche, approximately 10% reduction in cancer risk
  - Later age of menopause
    - Relative risk increases by 1% for each year older at menopause
  - Nulliparity
  - Older age at 1st full-term pregnancy
    - Women with 1st full-term pregnancy at age 35 have 1.6x higher risk than women who bear 1st child at age 26-27
  - Long-term use of postmenopausal hormone replacement therapy (HRT)
  - Ionizing radiation of chest at young age

Epidemiology & Cancer Incidence

- Number of cases in USA per year
  - > 229,000 cases expected in USA in 2012
    - > 39,000 deaths
- Widespread adoption of mammographic screening dramatically altered number of cases of DCIS
  - Increased detection led to increased number of cases

- DCIS now accounts for approximately 21% of all new breast cancers diagnosed in USA
  - Over 90% of new cancers are detected only on imaging studies

Genetics

- Inherited breast-ovarian cancer syndrome defined by mutations in *BRCA* genes
  - Mutations in *BRCA1* and *BRCA2* genes
  - 5-10% of women with family history of breast cancer have germline mutations of *BRCA* genes
    - Lifetime risk of developing breast cancer is 40-85%
  - Common in Jewish ancestry
  - DCIS occurs at younger age
- Other genes related to breast cancer include mutations of
  - *p53*
  - *ATM*
  - *PTEN*

Associated Diseases, Abnormalities

- ***BRCA* mutation**
  - Carriers have higher risk of breast and ovarian cancers
  - *BRCA1* carriers have 2-3x increased risk of additional malignancies
    - Melanoma
    - Pancreatic
    - Prostate
    - Colon
  - *BRCA2* mutation carriers also have increased risk of additional malignancies
    - Pancreatic
    - Gastric
    - Male breast cancer
    - Melanoma
  - Lifetime risk of developing breast cancer is 40-85%
- **Li-Fraumeni syndrome**
  - Autosomal dominant
  - Multiple tumors associated with syndrome
    - Soft tissue sarcomas
    - Osteosarcomas
    - Leukemias
    - Brain tumors
    - Early onset breast cancer
  - 50% of carriers develop some form of cancer by age 30; 90% do so by age 70
- ***CHEK2* mutations**
  - 2-3x increased risk of breast cancer
- **Ataxia-telangiectasia**
  - Autosomal recessive
  - 2x increased risk of breast cancer was identified in many epidemiologic studies of ataxia-telangiectasia families
- **Cowden syndrome**
  - Rare autosomal dominant
  - Germline mutations in *PTEN*
  - Multiple hamartomas and increased risk of early onset breast and thyroid cancer
  - Breast cancer develops in 25-50% of female carriers
- **Peutz-Jeghers syndrome**
  - Autosomal dominant
  - Relative risk for breast &/or gynecologic cancer in affected women is 20
- **Hereditary diffuse gastric cancer syndrome**
  - Autosomal dominant
  - Mutations in E-cadherin gene
  - Cumulative risk of lobular breast cancer ranges from 20-54%
  - 50% of patients with sporadic lobular breast cancers have E-cadherin mutations

Gross Pathology & Surgical Features

- Invasive ductal carcinoma on gross pathologic evaluation
  - Typically hard, gray-white, gritty masses
  - Tumor invades surrounding tissue in haphazard fashion to create characteristic irregular, stellate shape
- Malignant cells induce fibrous response as they infiltrate breast parenchyma, resulting in
  - Clinically and grossly palpable mass
  - Radiologic density
  - Solid sonographic characteristics
- Lobular carcinoma
  - Firm, irregularly marginated tumors
  - Often infiltrate to point where tumor margin cannot be identified

Microscopic Pathology

- H&E
  - **Comedo**
    - Prominent necrosis in center with calcification
    - Cells are large and show nuclear pleomorphism
    - Mitotic activity may be prominent
  - **Cribriform**
    - Formation of back-to-back glands without intervening stroma
    - Small to medium-sized cells with relatively uniform hyperchromatic nuclei
    - Mitoses are infrequent, and necrosis is limited to single cells or small cell clusters
  - **Micropapillary**
    - Small tufts of cells oriented perpendicular to basement membrane of involved spaces and projecting into lumina
    - Club-shaped cells
    - Micropapillae lack fibrovascular cores
    - Nuclei show diffuse hyperchromasia
    - Mitoses are infrequent
  - **Papillary**
    - Intraluminal projections of tumor cells demonstrate fibrovascular cores and thereby constitute true papillations
    - Intracystic papillary carcinoma, a variant of papillary DCIS, is characterized by cells in a single cystically dilated space
  - **Solid**
    - Not as well defined as other subtypes
    - Tumor cells fill and distend involved spaces and lack significant necrosis, fenestrations, or papillations
  - **Ductal carcinoma**
    - Small epithelial cells in single file growing around ducts and lobules; clusters and sheets also possible
    - Signet ring cells are frequently seen
    - Often concentric rings of tumor cells surround normal ducts
    - Cytology: Small cells containing oval or round nuclei with nonadherent, small nucleoli

  - Cells of atypical lobular hyperplasia, LCIS, and invasive lobular carcinoma are identical

Routes of Spread

- Primary route of dissemination of breast cancer is via axillary lymphatics
  - Reported incidence of axillary lymph node involvement in patients with DCIS with microinvasion averages ≤ 5%
  - Lymph node involvement strongly correlated with tumor size in invasive lesions
- Other routes of spread
  - Supraclavicular node or internal mammary nodes
  - Direct tumor extension through chest wall
- Common sites of metastasis include
  - Bone
  - Lung
  - Liver
- Lobular carcinoma
  - More likely than ductal carcinoma to spread to abdomen
    - Peritoneum
    - Retroperitoneum
    - Gastrointestinal tract
    - Ovaries
    - Uterus
  - Less likely to metastasize to pleura and lungs

IMAGING

Detection

- Common radiologic presentations
  - May present with palpable thickening/lump or abnormality seen on mammogram
  - Classic findings are dense mass with spiculated margins with possible associated calcifications
  - Mammography and ultrasound establish diagnosis
  - T1-weighted, post-contrast fat-saturated MR is ideal for mapping extent of disease after diagnosis
- **Ultrasound**
  - Preferred modality for determining cystic vs. solid nature of mass found on mammography
  - DCIS
    - Sensitivity is 50%
    - Findings include
      - Dilated ducts
      - Indistinct walls
      - Echogenic calcification
    - On power Doppler, increased vascularity is common
  - Infiltrating ductal carcinoma
    - Irregular hypoechoic shadowing mass
    - Taller-than-wide or perpendicular to skin
    - Architectural distortion, may have echogenic halo
- **Mammography**
  - Screening mammography ± clinical breast examination is recommended annually for women age 40 and older
  - Mass densities and calcification are most sensitive findings
  - Sensitivity increases during follicular phase of menstrual cycle
  - Majority of ductal breast carcinoma cases are detected on mammography screening
  - Microcalcifications have sensitivity of 70-80% for DCIS
  - Breast imaging-reporting and data system (BI-RADS): Quality assurance reporting system
    - 0: Incomplete
    - 1: Negative
    - 2: Benign finding(s)
    - 3: Probably benign
    - 4: Suspicious abnormality
    - 5: Highly suggestive of malignancy
    - 6: Known biopsy proven malignancy

Staging

- **Mammography**
  - DCIS: Calcifications are more common finding
  - Fine, linear, or branching calcifications are highly suggestive of DCIS
  - Most cases of breast cancer detected on screening are stage I
    - Dense mass with spiculated margins
    - Focal asymmetric density ± distortion
    - Associated with calcifications
- **CT**
  - More useful for assessment of spread than for imaging of primary lesions
  - **CECT**
    - Useful for mediastinal and organ metastases, especially for liver metastases
    - Malignancy typically measures above water attenuation
      - When large, appears as discrete mass and may be spiculated
    - Tumors appear as dense lesions and show early contrast enhancement
  - **NECT**
    - Useful for lung and pleural metastases, detecting lymphatic spread
- **MR**
  - DCIS: Sensitivity is 88-95%
    - T1WI C+ FS: Linear or segmental clumped enhancement
  - Infiltrating ductal carcinoma
    - T2WI FS: Usually hypointense focal mass
    - T1WI C+ FS: 90% enhance rapidly and intensely, may have rim enhancement, internal enhancing septations
  - Useful for evaluation of brain and hepatic metastases
  - Used in some high-risk patients to look for bilateral breast involvement
- **PET/CT**
  - Can be used to assess distant metastases, local recurrence, and treatment response
  - Sensitivity is 80-90% for evaluation of primary tumors
  - Positive axillary lymph nodes on PET/CT has high positive predictive value for malignancy despite relative insensitivity (80%)
  - Patients with suspected advanced disease or deemed "high risk" should be considered for PET/CT for overall staging evaluation
  - Not usually recommended for initial diagnosis but may help in patients with implants or dense breast tissue
  - 80-95% sensitivity for detecting distant metastases at time of initial diagnosis

- Helpful for detecting hepatic and osseous metastases
- N staging
  - **Ultrasound**
    - Useful for lesion characterization and to guide biopsy
    - Can identify and biopsy axillary or supraclavicular nodes which, if positive, may obviate sentinel lymph node (SLN) procedure
      - Globular shape and increased cortical thickness are among suspicious features
      - Often can be done at time of breast biopsy
  - **CT**
    - Staging CT can show enlarged or abnormal lymph nodes in axilla or mediastinum
    - Involved nodes may show abnormal enhancement; necrotic lymph nodes will be hypodense
  - **MR**
    - MR also may show enlarged axillary nodes
    - < 1% present as occult cancers (adenocarcinoma in axillary lymph nodes without identified primary source)
    - Useful in occult breast cancers to evaluate for a primary; in one study, MR found primary in 21 of 35 cases
  - **PET/CT**
    - If lymph nodes are (+) on PET/CT, high probability of being malignant
    - Has advantage of screening mediastinum
    - Superior to MR or CT in detecting internal mammary or mediastinal lymph nodes
    - PET/CT has sensitivity of 60-80% for axillary lymph nodes
    - Limited in detecting lesions < 8 mm
  - **Nuclear medicine**
    - Sentinel lymph node mapping intraoperatively using vital blue dye and filtered technetium-labeled sulfur colloid
      - Reflects histologic characteristics of remainder of axillary lymph nodes
- M staging
  - **General**
    - Most common route of local spread is through axillary lymph node
    - Common sites of organ metastases
      - Bone
      - Lung
      - Liver
  - **CT**
    - Useful for mediastinal and organ metastases, especially for liver metastases
    - Hepatic metastases will be low density on CT
    - Will visualize lung, pleural, and lymphatic spread (axillary, supraclavicular)
  - **MR**
    - Superior at screening high-risk patients
    - Best for evaluating extent of disease in ipsilateral breast
    - Can also be used to monitor treatment response
    - MR has also been shown to detect synchronous malignancy in contralateral breast in approximately 3-4% of patients
    - CT or PET/CT are generally preferred in evaluation of distant metastases
  - **PET/CT**
    - Overall, limit of detection is ~ 8 mm
    - 80-95% sensitivity for detecting distant metastases at time of initial diagnosis
    - Negative predictive value of PET/CT is 70-90%
    - Concurrent infection/inflammation may give false positives
    - Either bone scan or PET/CT should be considered to evaluate skeleton in high-risk patients
    - Lytic and trabecular metastases are detected with > 90% sensitivity on PET
    - PET/CT has been shown to change management in a high fraction of cases
  - **Nuclear medicine**
    - Useful for osseous metastases
    - Bone scan is preferred to PET for detecting cortical blastic metastases
    - Poor sensitivity for lytic metastases

Restaging

- **General**
  - Risk of recurrence is highest during 1st 5 years after treatment
  - History and physical
    - Every 3-6 months for the 1st 3 years, every 6-12 months for years 4-5, then annually
  - Patient education regarding symptoms of recurrence
    - New lumps
    - Bone pain
    - Chest pain
    - Abdominal pain
    - Dyspnea
    - Persistent headaches
    - Other neurologic symptoms
- **Mammography**
  - 1st post-treatment mammogram 1 year after initial mammogram that leads to diagnosis
  - No earlier than 6 months after definitive radiation therapy
  - Best diagnostic clue: New suspicious calcifications &/ or increased density/mass in treated breast
  - In patients getting regular mammograms, recurrent tumors are usually detected between 5 and 20 mm
- **CT**
  - Used to follow patient to assess treatment response and for recurrent disease
  - Intravenous contrast increases sensitivity for metastatic lesions
- **MR**
  - Screening MR for women with personal history of breast cancer still controversial
  - Linear enhancement is suspicious for DCIS on T1WI post-contrast MR
  - Enhancing irregular mass suspicious for invasive carcinoma
  - Decreased parenchymal enhancement is commonly seen after radiation
  - Fat necrosis can enhance for years
  - Seromas will show thin rim enhancement
- **PET/CT**
  - Overall, FDG PET has equal or better accuracy for restaging compared to conventional imaging
  - Combined PET/CT offers higher sensitivity and specificity than PET alone
  - Surgical site may remain avid for 3-12 months

- Also may see inflammation around clips or sutures
- In patients with rising tumor markers or asymptomatic breast cancer, FDG PET is superior to conventional imaging for diagnosis of metastatic disease
- SUV is accurate indicator of treatment response; ideally 50-60% reduction in SUV following 2 cycles of chemotherapy
- Detection of poor response may be useful as a guide to change therapies

- **Nuclear medicine**
  - Bone scan useful for skeletal metastases, particularly blastic metastases

CLINICAL PRESENTATION & WORK-UP

Presentation

- Widespread adoption of mammographic screening dramatically altered clinical presentation of DCIS
  - 90% present with microcalcifications on mammogram during screening
  - 10% present with palpable mass
- **Mastodynia or mastalgia**
  - Most common symptom but nonspecific
  - 10% of painful masses are malignant
- **Palpable mass**
  - 2nd most common symptom
  - Likelihood of malignancy of palpable mass increases with age
  - Average size of invasive carcinomas that present with palpable mass is 2.4 cm
- **Nipple discharge**
  - More specific as indicator of malignancy with increasing patient age
  - Galactorrhea is associated with hormonal changes, both pathologic and physiologic
  - Bloody discharge can be induced by pregnancy-related changes
  - Solitary large duct papilloma, cyst, and carcinoma are most common causes of solitary discharge
- **Paget disease**
  - Skin changes involving nipple or areola

Prognosis

- **Prognostic factors**
  - Age and menopausal status of patient
  - Stage of disease
  - Histologic and nuclear grade of primary tumor
  - ER and PR status of tumor
  - Measures of proliferative capacity of tumor
  - *HER-2/neu* gene amplification
- **5-year survival rates**
  - Stage I: 88%
  - Stage IIA: 81%
  - Stage IIB: 74%
  - Stage IIIA: 67%
  - Stage IIIB: 41%
  - Stage IIIC: 49%
  - Stage IV: 15%

Work-Up

- Clinical
  - H&P with attention to family history
  - Genetic counseling if high risk
- Radiographic
  - Diagnostic bilateral mammogram, cone down views as needed
  - US may be useful for primary and nodal staging
  - Breast MR optional for invasive disease
    - Contralateral breast cancers are diagnosed in 3% of patients with MR
  - For laboratory abnormalities or symptoms, consider CECT of chest/abdomen/pelvis
  - For stage III and higher, stage with BS, CECT, or PET/CT
- Laboratory
  - CBC, alkaline phosphatase, LFTs, ER for DCIS, ER/PR/HER2neu for invasive disease

TREATMENT

Major Treatment Alternatives

- **Surgical removal**
  - **Breast conserving therapy (BCT)**
    - Surgical removal of tumor without removing excessive amounts of normal breast tissue
    - Followed by radiation therapy; either whole breast or partial breast irradiation
  - **Modified radical mastectomy**
    - Removal of entire breast with level I-II axillary dissection
- **Radiation therapy (RT)**
  - Standard component of BCT and may also be indicated after mastectomy
  - Intent of RT delivery is to eradicate subclinical residual disease and minimize local recurrence rates
  - Whole breast RT
    - Standard fractionation: ~ 50 Gy in 5 weeks
    - Hypofractionation: Multiple trials have shown equivalence for ipsilateral control compared with standard fractionation
    - Accelerated partial breast irradiation (APBI)
      - External beam: 3D or IMRT, 38.5 Gy commonly delivered bid in 5 treatment days
      - Balloon or interstitial brachytherapy: 34 Gy commonly delivered bid in 5 treatment days
    - Regional nodal RT
      - Treat axilla, paraclavicular, and IMN if 4 or more
      - Consider paraclavicular and IMN nodal RT in patients with 1-3 + axillary lymph nodes
      - Supraclavicular fields in absence of gross disease should cover corresponding vessels as surrogates for the nodes; depth depends on patient size
      - IMN: If positive, treat; IM artery and vein should be used as surrogates for the nodes
      - Post axillary boost should be individualized to cover deep regions, may result in more complications
    - Intraoperative RT
      - Different techniques used; 20 Gy given to lumpectomy surface is one protocol
    - Boost
      - Improved local control, no OS difference

- EORTC trial showed fibrosis rates of 1.6%, 3.3%, 4.4%, and 14.4% for 0, 10, 16, and 26 Gy boosts, respectively
  - Post-mastectomy RT
    - Trials showed survival benefit for lymph node (LN) positive patients
    - 1-3 LNs controversial; clear consensus for 4 or more
    - Controversial for T3 N0
    - T1-2 N0 with positive margins often treated, especially if LVSI &/or if margin involvement is more than focal
- **Management of regional lymph nodes**
  - Status of axillary nodes is single most important prognostic factor in women with early stage disease
  - Axillary metastases are important indicator of need for adjuvant systemic therapy and post-mastectomy RT
  - Lymph nodes can be assessed through sentinel node biopsy (preferred) or dissection
    - US may be helpful in staging axilla or guiding FNA, particularly for neoadjuvant cases
- **Adjuvant systemic therapy**
  - Administration of hormone therapy or chemotherapy after definitive local therapy for breast cancer
  - Chemotherapy precedes RT except in cases of APBI
  - Patients with node-positive breast cancer and those with tumor size ≥ 1 cm should receive adjuvant systemic therapy
  - Obtain 21 gene assay for ≥ 5 mm ER/PR(+) and Her2(-), node-negative lesions
- **Hormone therapy**
  - Often used as component of adjuvant therapy
  - Only effective toward cancer cells that produce estrogen or progesterone receptors
  - Examples include tamoxifen, anastrozole, and goserelin
- **Neoadjuvant therapy**
  - NSABP B-18: No difference in OS; statistically significant 8% ↑ in breast conservation in neoadjuvant arm
- **Trastuzumab**
  - Humanized anti-HER2 monoclonal antibody
  - Effective in treatment of HER2-overexpressing metastatic breast cancer, both as monotherapy and in combination regimens

Major Treatment Roadblocks/ Contraindications

- **Contraindications to BCT**
  - Persistently positive resection margins after reasonable reexcision attempts
  - Multicentric disease in which there are ≥ 2 primary tumors in separate breast quadrants
  - History of prior RT to breast or chest wall
  - Pregnancy: Defer breast RT until after delivery

Treatment Options by Stage

- **DCIS**
  - BCT (unless contraindicated) and RT
  - Axillary node dissection is not necessary at this stage
- **LCIS**
  - Observation: No evidence to support reexcision to document clear margins
  - Tamoxifen has been shown to reduce chance of subsequent invasive carcinoma by 56%
  - Bilateral prophylactic mastectomy without axillary lymph node dissection
- **Early stage invasive breast cancer (stages I and II)**
  - BCT (unless contraindicated) and RT
  - Radiation therapy
    - Consider nodal RT to IMN and paraclavicular regions
  - Axillary lymph node dissection or sentinel node biopsy
  - Adjuvant therapy with hormone therapy or chemotherapy
  - Modified radical mastectomy ± breast reconstruction
- **Locally advanced and inflammatory breast cancer (stage III)**
  - Multimodality treatment: Induction (neoadjuvant) chemotherapy followed by locoregional therapy: Surgery, then radiation
- **Metastatic breast cancer (stage IV)**
  - Patients with metastatic breast cancer are unlikely to be cured of their disease by any means
  - Complete remission from chemotherapy, which is prerequisite for cure, is uncommon
  - Weigh likelihood of achieving palliation with available therapies and establish treatment priorities
  - Therapy choices include local vs. systemic treatments, hormone therapy, chemotherapy, radiation therapy

Dose Response

- 50 Gy in 5 weeks was established by Fletcher as dose needed to control microscopic disease
- Boost vs. no boost trials showed increasing local control with increasing dose

Standard Doses

- ~ 50 Gy in 5 weeks to whole breast or chest wall and regional nodes
  - Boost to lumpectomy site: 10-16 Gy
- 42.6 Gy in 16 fractions for whole breast
- APBI
  - External beam: 3D or IMRT, 38.5 Gy commonly delivered bid in 5 treatment days
  - Balloon or interstitial brachytherapy: 34 Gy commonly delivered bid in 5 treatment days

Organs at Risk Parameters

- Great care should be taken in simulation and treatment planning to limit dose to heart, lung, thyroid, and contralateral breast

Common Techniques

- Tangents
- Modified wide tangents (blocking used to shield heart/ lung)
- Comprehensive breast RT
  - Monoisocentric: Limits field length to 1/2 field or 20 cm
  - Couch kick technique
  - Supplemental posterior axillary boost (PAB)
    - Use for gross disease or highly contaminated axilla
- Post-mastectomy RT
  - Tangents or modified wide tangents

- Tangents with separate electron/photon IMN field (5° steeper than tangents)
- Danish technique
  - Electrons to chest wall matched to anterior photons to paraclavicular ± axillary LNs and lateral chest wall
- Electrons (multiple stationary or arc)

Landmark Trials

- DCIS: Surgery ± RT
  - 4 trials all showed significant local control advantage of RT with HR ranging 0.40-0.57
- Early breast cancer and DCIS: Surgery and RT ± tamoxifen
  - B24 and UK trial: Tam ↓ DCIS in both trials, but no ↓ in invasive lesions in UK trial
- Extent of surgery
  - B-04: Modified radical mast vs. simple mast + RT vs. simple mast
    - No difference in OS, DFS, or distant mets; no advantage to removal or RT of occult axillary LNs
- Breast conserving surgery ± RT
  - 15 trials showed ↓ ipsilateral recurrences and no difference in survival
  - In B-06, local recurrence was 39.2% vs. 14.3% at 20 years for no RT vs. RT, respectively
- Hypofractionation vs. standard fractionation
  - 6 trials show no difference in local control
  - START A trial showed that breast cancer and normal breast tissue responded similarly to different fractionation
- RT boost vs. no boost
  - Improved local control with boost; no difference in OS
- Preop vs. postop chemo
  - NSABP B-18: No difference in OS; statistically significant 8% ↑ in breast conservation in neoadjuvant arm

RECOMMENDED FOLLOW-UP

Clinical

- H&P every 4-6 months, then annually after 5 years
- Annual gyn exam for women on tamoxifen
- Monitor bone health for women with ovarian failure or on aromatase inhibitors
- Encourage active lifestyle and maintain ideal body weight (BMI 20-25)

Radiographic

- Annual diagnostic mammogram

Laboratory

- As needed to work-up symptoms

SELECTED REFERENCES

1. Siegel R et al: Cancer statistics, 2012. CA Cancer J Clin. 62(1):10-29, 2012
2. American Joint Committee on Cancer: AJCC Cancer Staging Manual. 7th ed. New York: Springer. 347-76, 2010
3. Vieira CC et al: Microinvasive ductal carcinoma in situ: clinical presentation, imaging features, pathologic findings, and outcome. Eur J Radiol. 73(1):102-7, 2010
4. Whelan TJ et al: Long-term results of hypofractionated radiation therapy for breast cancer. N Engl J Med. 362(6):513-20, 2010
5. Basu S et al: Comparison of triple-negative and estrogen receptor-positive/progesterone receptor-positive/HER2-negative breast carcinoma using quantitative fluorine-18 fluorodeoxyglucose/positron emission tomography imaging parameters: a potentially useful method for disease characterization. Cancer. 112(5):995-1000, 2008
6. DeMartini W et al: Breast MRI for cancer detection and characterization: a review of evidence-based clinical applications. Acad Radiol. 15(4):408-16, 2008
7. Poortmans PM et al: The addition of a boost dose on the primary tumour bed after lumpectomy in breast conserving treatment for breast cancer. A summary of the results of EORTC 22881-10882 "boost versus no boost" trial. Cancer Radiother. 12(6-7):565-70, 2008
8. Rastogi P et al: Preoperative chemotherapy: updates of National Surgical Adjuvant Breast and Bowel Project Protocols B-18 and B-27. J Clin Oncol. 2008 Feb 10;26(5):778-85. Erratum in: J Clin Oncol. 26(16):2793, 2008
9. START Trialists' Group et al: The UK Standardisation of Breast Radiotherapy (START) Trial A of radiotherapy hypofractionation for treatment of early breast cancer: a randomised trial. Lancet Oncol. 9(4):331-41, 2008
10. Weaver DL et al: Pathologic findings from the Breast Cancer Surveillance Consortium: population-based outcomes in women undergoing biopsy after screening mammography. Cancer. 106(4):732-42, 2006
11. Byrne AM et al: Positron emission tomography in the staging and management of breast cancer. Br J Surg. 91(11):1398-409, 2004
12. Kumar R et al: Fluorodeoxyglucose-PET in the management of breast cancer. Radiol Clin North Am. 42(6):1113-22, ix, 2004
13. Luciani A et al: Simultaneous bilateral breast and high-resolution axillary MRI of patients with breast cancer: preliminary results. AJR Am J Roentgenol. 182(4):1059-67, 2004
14. Houghton J et al: Radiotherapy and tamoxifen in women with completely excised ductal carcinoma in situ of the breast in the UK, Australia, and New Zealand: randomised controlled trial. Lancet. 362(9378):95-102, 2003
15. Michaelson JS et al: Gauging the impact of breast carcinoma screening in terms of tumor size and death rate. Cancer. 98(10):2114-24, 2003
16. Peterson JJ et al: Diagnosis of occult bone metastases: positron emission tomography. Clin Orthop Relat Res. (415 Suppl):S120-8, 2003
17. Fisher B et al: Twenty-five-year follow-up of a randomized trial comparing radical mastectomy, total mastectomy, and total mastectomy followed by irradiation. N Engl J Med. 347(8):567-75, 2002
18. Fisher B et al: Twenty-year follow-up of a randomized trial comparing total mastectomy, lumpectomy, and lumpectomy plus irradiation for the treatment of invasive breast cancer. N Engl J Med. 347(16):1233-41, 2002
19. Ichizawa N et al: Long-term results of T1a, T1b and T1c invasive breast carcinomas in Japanese women: validation of the UICC T1 subgroup classification. Jpn J Clin Oncol. 32(3):108-9, 2002
20. Fisher B et al: Prevention of invasive breast cancer in women with ductal carcinoma in situ: an update of the National Surgical Adjuvant Breast and Bowel Project experience. Semin Oncol. 28(4):400-18, 2001
21. Overgaard M et al: Postoperative radiotherapy in high-risk premenopausal women with breast cancer who receive adjuvant chemotherapy. Danish Breast Cancer Cooperative Group 82b Trial. N Engl J Med. 337(14):949-55, 1997

Stage IA (T1a N0 M0)

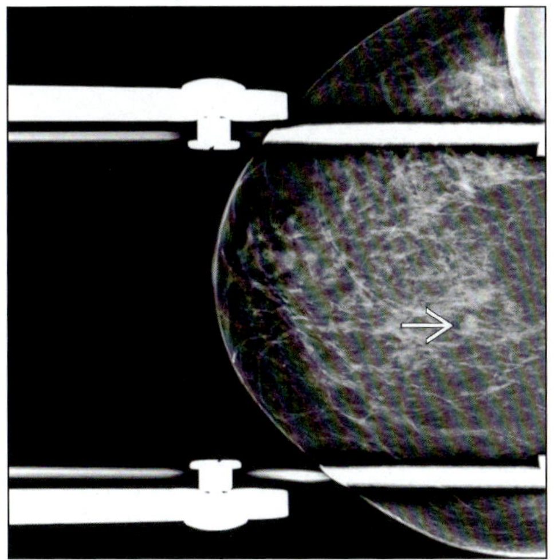

Stage IA (T1a N0 M0)

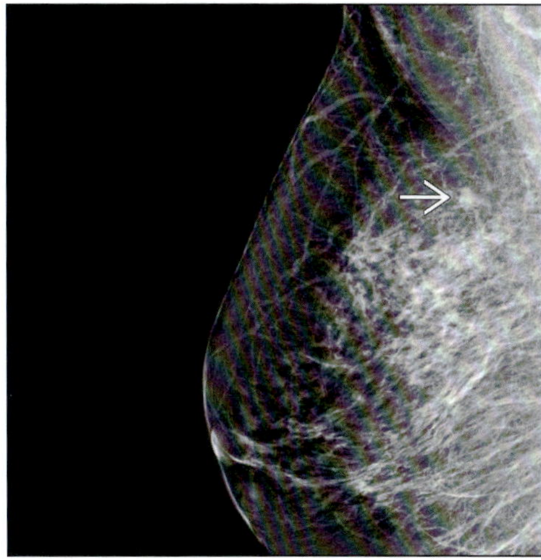

(Left) *Right CC mammogram shows a small density* ➡ *in the right breast that measures 4 mm, compatible with a T1a lesion, which is defined as a lesion > 1 mm but ≤ to 5 mm in greatest dimension.* ***(Right)*** *Right ML mammogram in the same patient shows the 4 mm mass* ➡*, compatible with a T1a lesion, to be superior to the nipple line.*

Stage IA (T1a N0 M0)

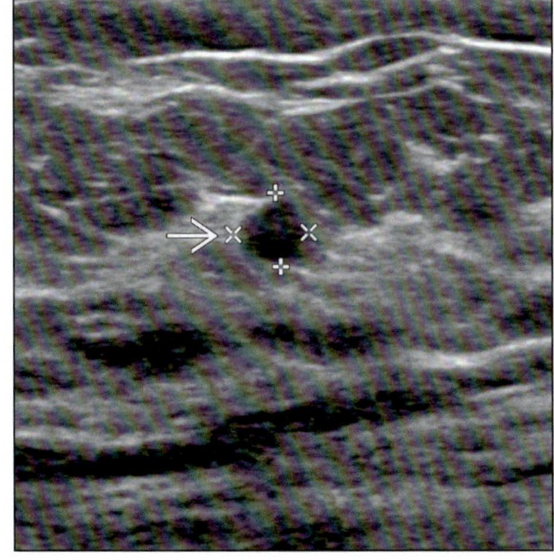

Stage IA (T1a N0 M0)

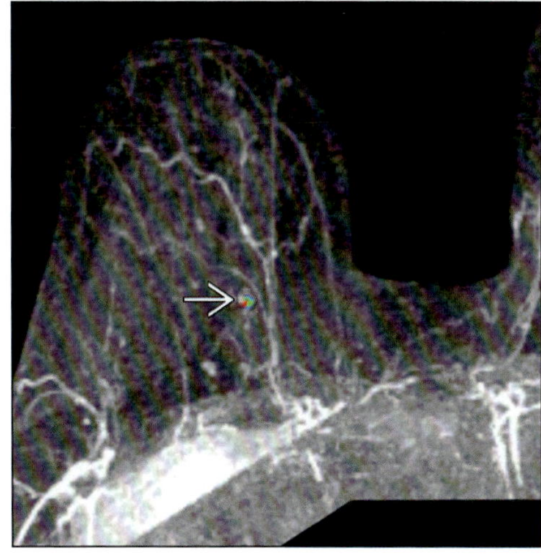

(Left) *Grayscale ultrasound in the same patient shows a hypoechoic lesion* ➡ *that corresponds to the abnormal mammographic finding.* ***(Right)*** *Breast MR in the same patient shows that the lesion* ➡ *in the right breast demonstrates increased enhancement, shown with abnormal color.*

Stage IA (T1a N0 M0)

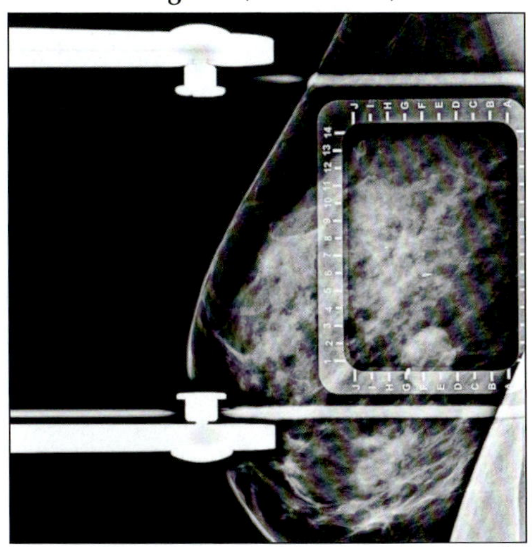

Stage IA (T1a N0 M0)

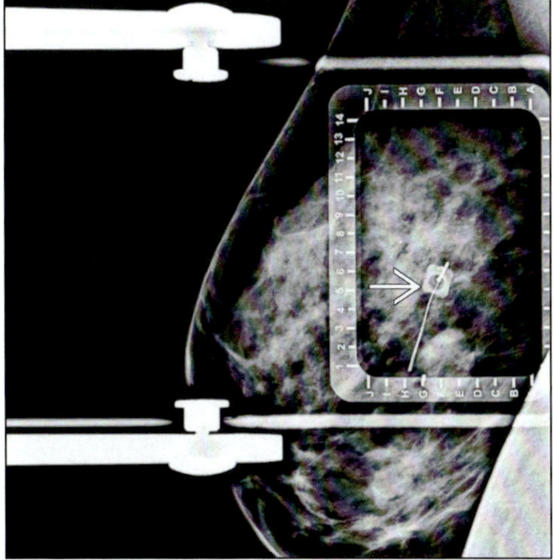

(Left) *Right CC mammogram shows no mammographic abnormalities in a patient with a palpable breast lesion that showed enhancement on MR and was subsequently biopsied under MR.* ***(Right)*** *Right ML mammogram in the same patient shows a localization needle* ➡ *placed at the point of prior clip following an MR-guided biopsy. Subsequent resection showed a 5 mm (T1a) ductal carcinoma.*

BREAST

(Left) *Image from a left MCC mammogram shows a questionable rounded density ➡ within an area of glandular tissue in this patient with a palpable breast mass.* **(Right)** *Left MLO mammogram in the same patient shows the rounded mass ➡ to be slightly more conspicuous on this view.*

Stage IA (T1b N0 M0)

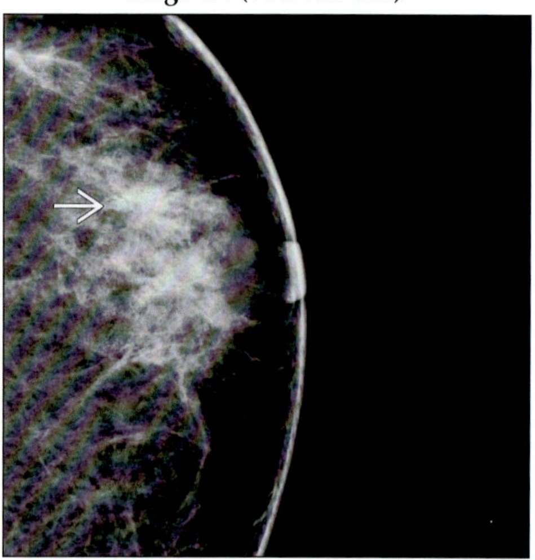

Stage IA (T1b N0 M0)

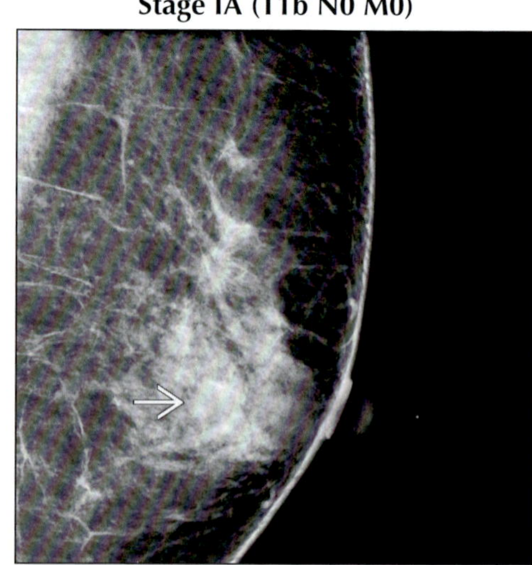

(Left) *Grayscale ultrasound shows a hypoechoic lesion ➡ that was subsequently biopsied and shown to be ductal carcinoma.* **(Right)** *Breast MR in the same patient shows an 8 mm enhancing lesion ➡. Lesions > 5 mm but ≤ to 10 mm are classified as T1b lesions.*

Stage IA (T1b N0 M0)

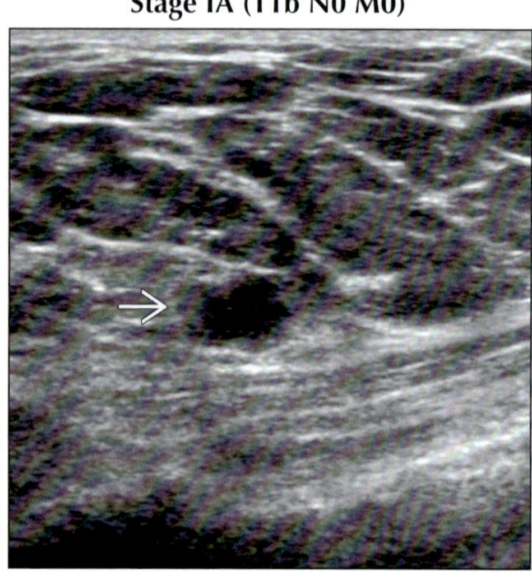

Stage IA (T1b N0 M0)

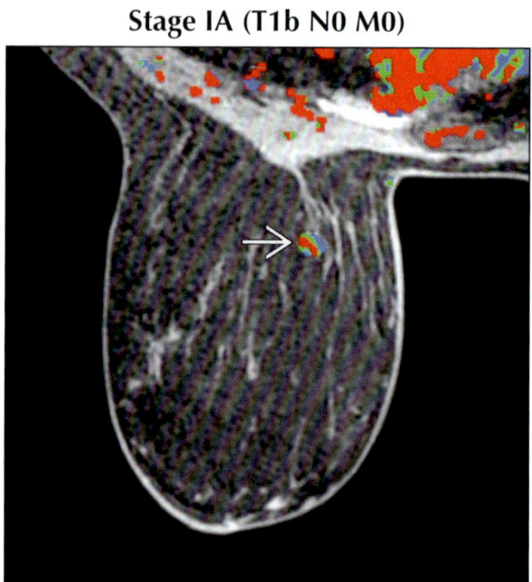

(Left) *Axial CECT shows an incidental enhancing nodule ➡ in the left breast of this patient with a history of non-Hodgkin lymphoma.* **(Right)** *Axial fused PET/CT in the same patient shows focal intense FDG activity ➡ within the left breast nodule. Patient was referred for mammography, ultrasound, and biopsy. Following a positive biopsy, the patient was taken to surgery and a 10 mm or T1b ductal carcinoma was resected.*

Stage IA (T1b N0 M0)

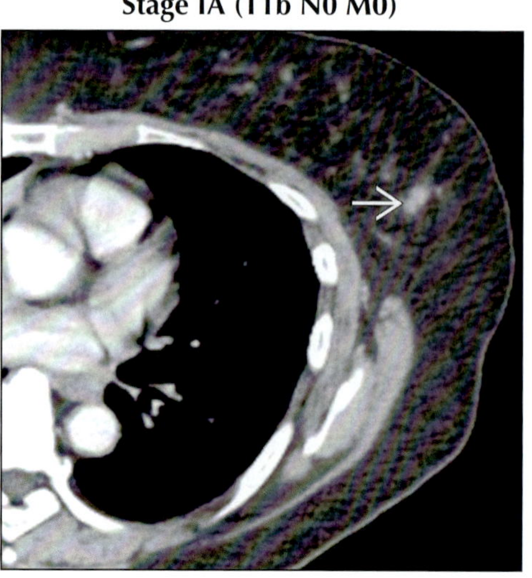

Stage IA (T1b N0 M0)

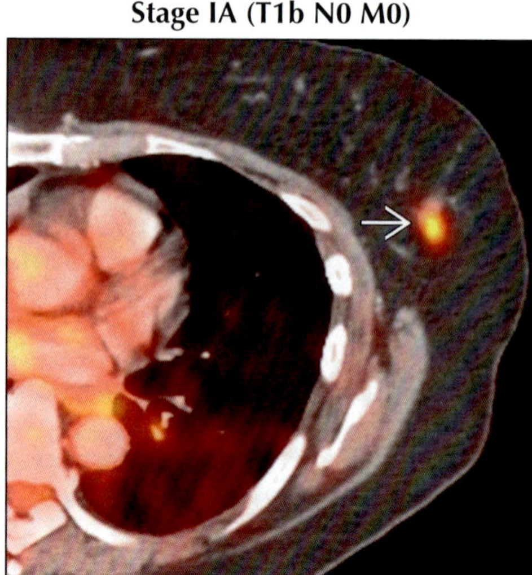

Partial Breast Irradiation

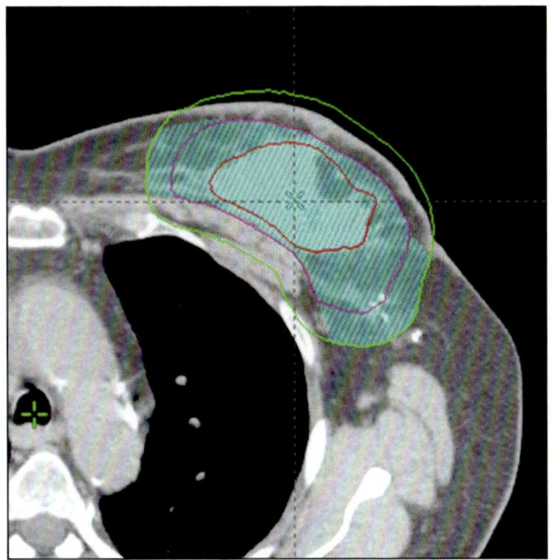

Partial Breast Irradiation

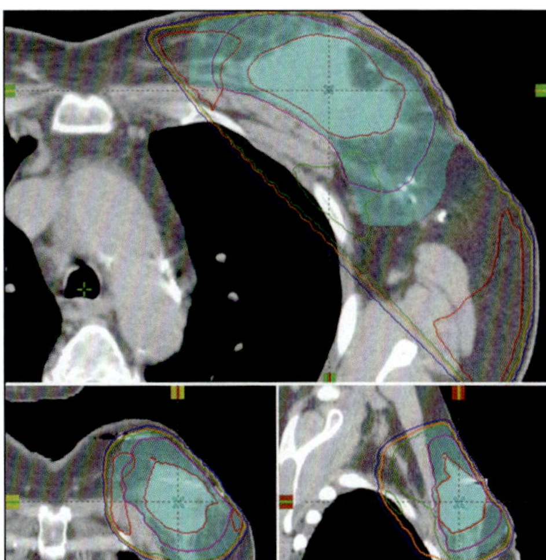

(Left) *Axial CT demonstrates lumpectomy cavity contoured in red. The CTV is the purple line. 1 cm is added to CTV to yield PTV (green line), and the PTV evaluation is shown in the blue stippled volume.* ***(Right)*** *3D conformal external beam radiotherapy (EBRT) is shown in 3 cardinal planes in the same patient. Beams are non-coplanar and the red, green, orange, and blue lines represent the 105%, 98%, 95%, and 85% isodose lines, respectively.*

Partial Breast Irradiation

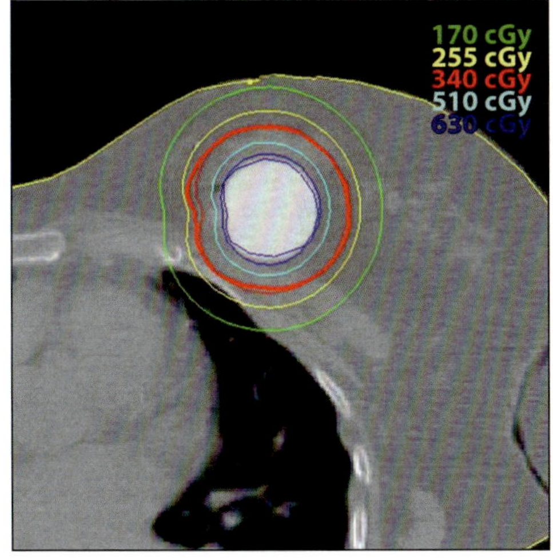

Partial Breast Irradiation

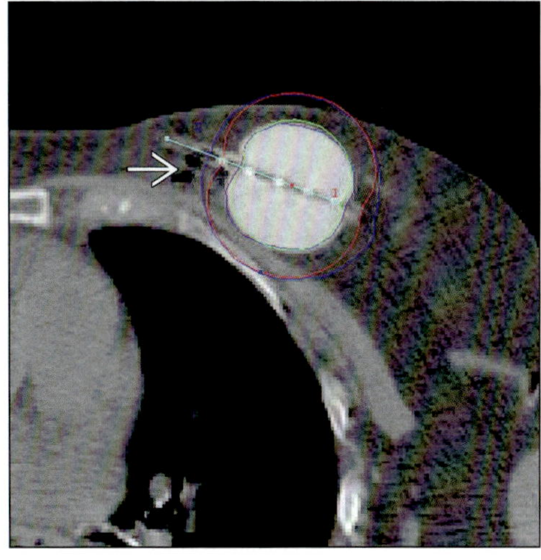

(Left) *Axial CT shows spherical balloon brachytherapy in an ideal case: A deep lesion in a large breast. The light blue, red, yellow, and green lines represent the 150%, 100%, 75%, and 50% isodose lines, respectively.* ***(Right)*** *An unacceptable implant demonstrates a skin dose > 100% (100% isodose line shown in red), balloon skin distance < 5 mm, trapped air ➔, and a nonspherical balloon. This patient was not treated with balloon brachytherapy.*

Partial Breast Irradiation

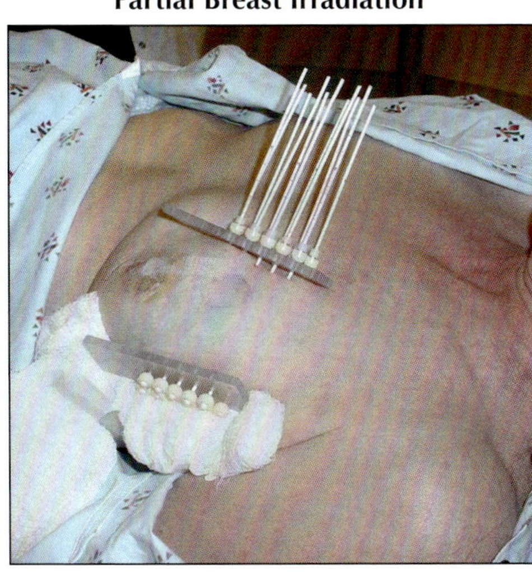

Partial Breast Irradiation

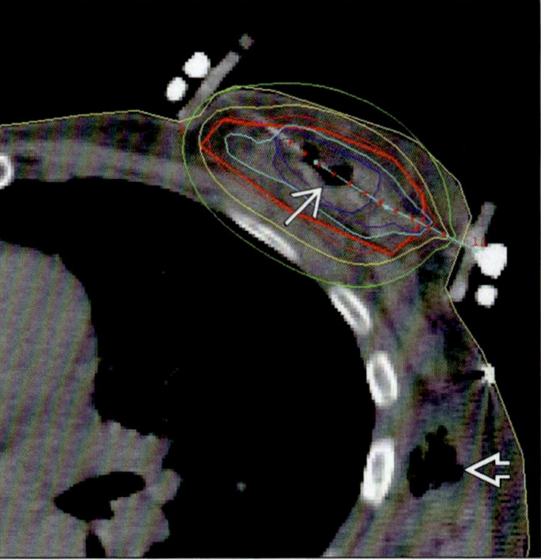

(Left) *HDR interstitial breast brachytherapy shows 12 catheters secured via templates. Multiple dwell positions permit excellent conformality.* ***(Right)*** *Dual plane implant shows good conformality of the 100% isodose line in red to the PTV shown in the bold red line. The green line shows the 50% isodose surface. Note the trapped air ➔ and air in the axillary dissection cavity ⇨.*

(Left) Axial CT shows the Savi® applicator. Nonspherical dose distributions are possible due to the multiple dwell positions. The PTV (here and on the right) is shown in red, and the orange, yellow, and blue lines represent the 150%, 100%, and 50% isodose lines, respectively. *(Right)* Axial CT shows the Contura® applicator. Multichannel applicators aid in reducing dose to skin, chest wall, and lung. (Courtesy C. Yashar, MD.)

Partial Breast Irradiation

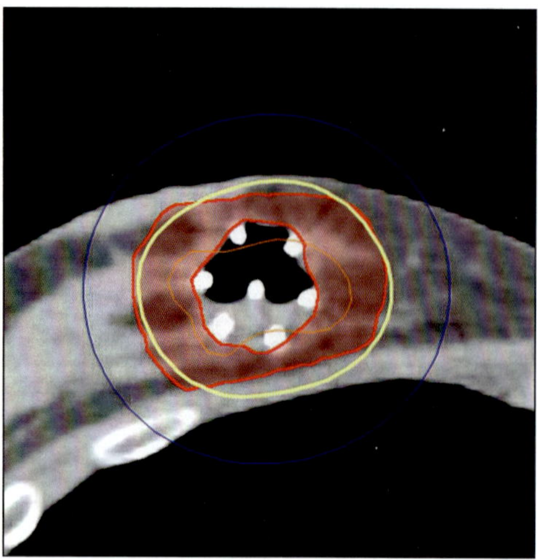

Partial Breast Irradiation

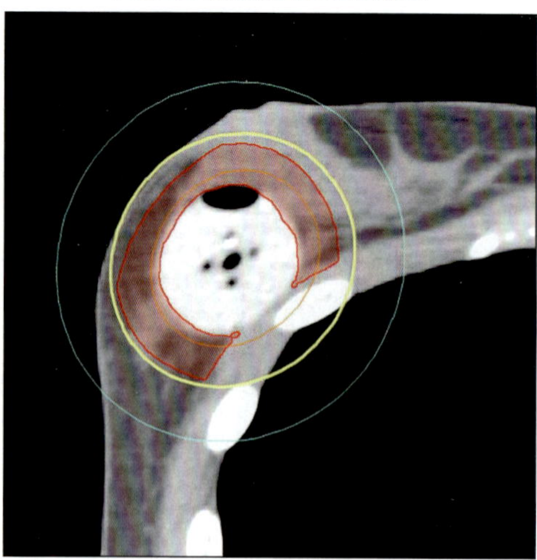

(Left) Grayscale ultrasound shows a hypoechoic lesion ➔ with a linear hyperechoic structure representing the needle traversing the lesion. Pathology revealed invasive ductal carcinoma. *(Right)* Breast MR in the same patient shows a hyperenhancing lesion ➔ in the left breast, correlating with the mammographic abnormality. Resection of the lesion showed an 18 mm or T1c invasive ductal carcinoma.

Stage IA (T1c N0 M0)

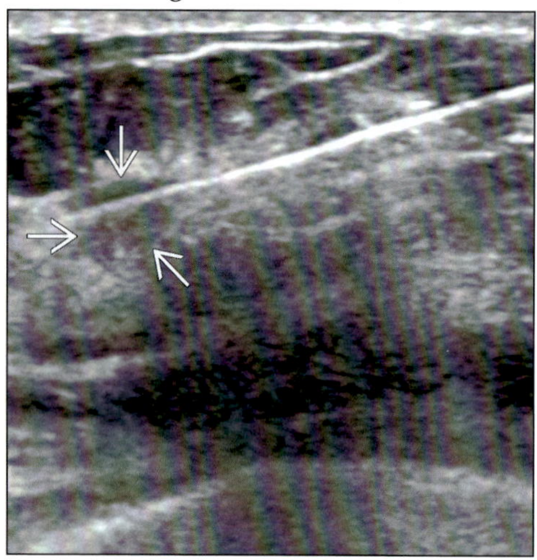

Stage IA (T1c N0 M0)

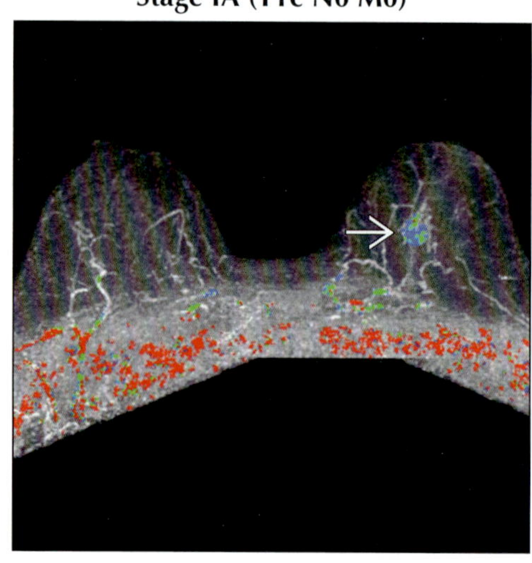

(Left) Grayscale ultrasound in the same patient shows a poorly defined hypoechoic lesion ➔, a typical appearance for an invasive ductal carcinoma. *(Right)* Coronal PET in the same patient shows focal, mild, moderately increased FDG activity ➔ in the area of the left breast. This degree of FDG activity would be typical for a breast cancer of this size. Also note multiple foci of brown fat ➔.

Stage IA (T1c N0 M0)

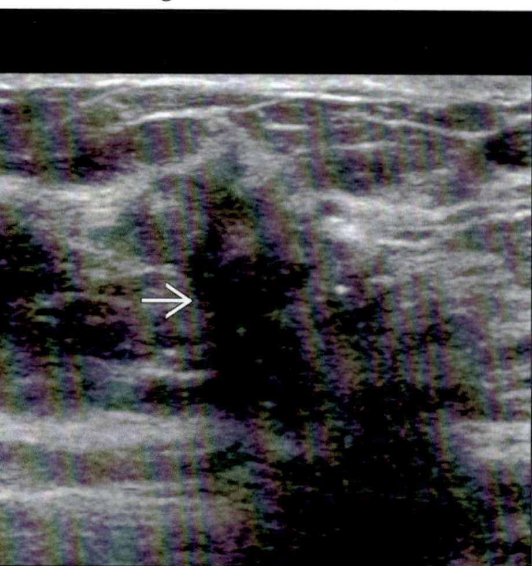

Stage IA (T1c N0 M0)

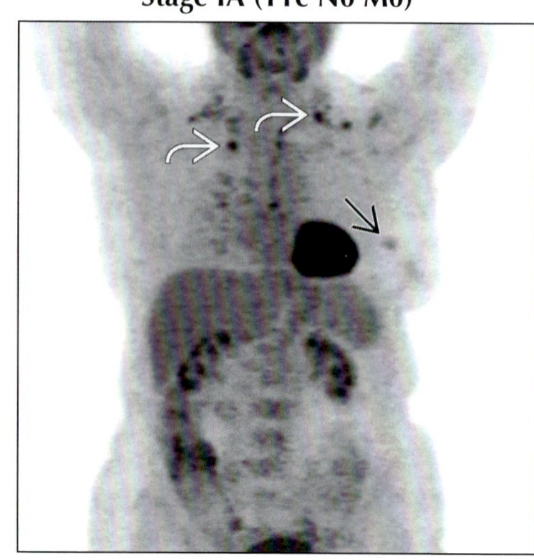

Stage IA (T1c N0 M0)

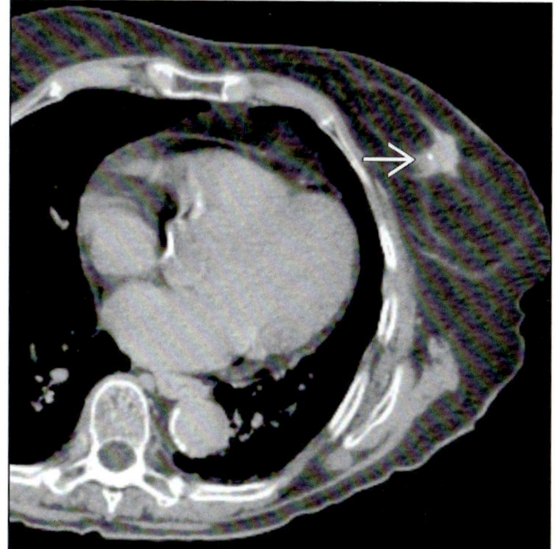

Stage IA (T1c N0 M0)

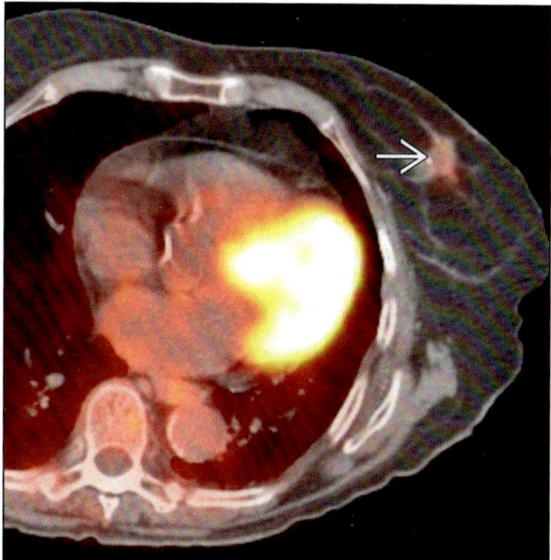

(Left) *Axial CECT in the same patient shows a nonspecific, slightly hyperenhancing mass ➔ in the left breast with a focus of high attenuation, which represents the clip from a recent biopsy.* ***(Right)*** *Axial fused PET/CT in the same patient shows mildly increased FDG activity ➔ correlating with the left breast mass. Approximately 20-40% of primary breast masses up to 2 cm are only mildly if not at all FDG avid.*

Stage IA (T1c N0 M0)

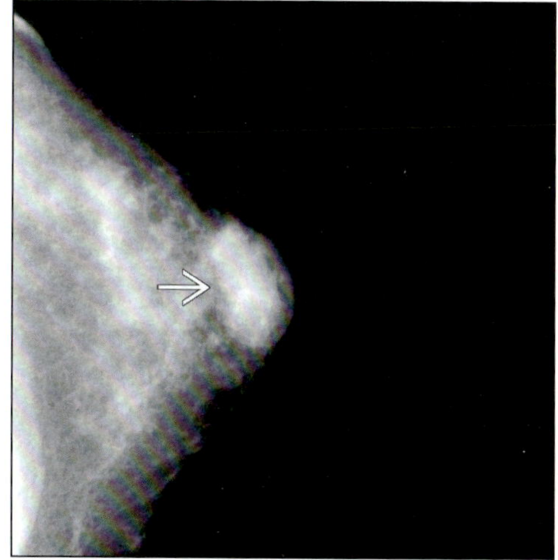

Stage IA (T1c N0 M0)

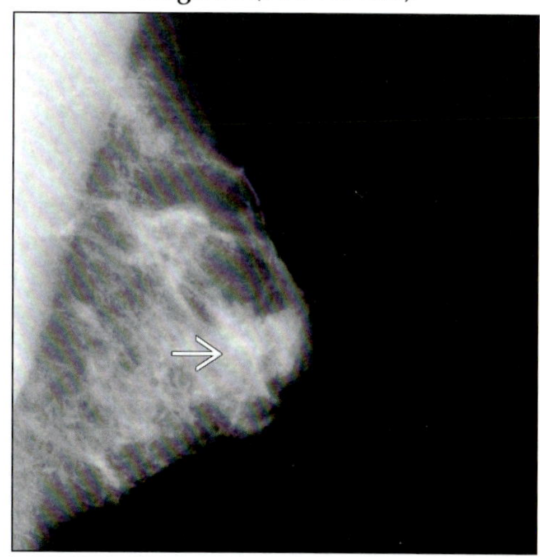

(Left) *Left CC mammogram shows a retroareolar abnormal density ➔, which was new from the patient's previous mammogram (not shown).* ***(Right)*** *Left MLO mammogram in the same patient shows the mass ➔ slightly inferior in the retroareolar region.*

Stage IA (T1c N0 M0)

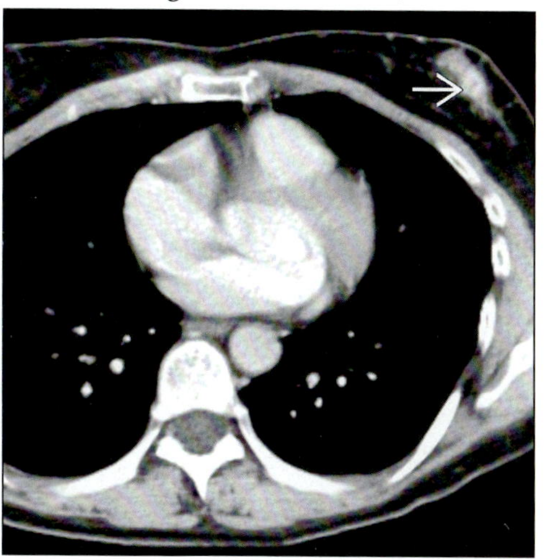

Stage IA (T1c N0 M0)

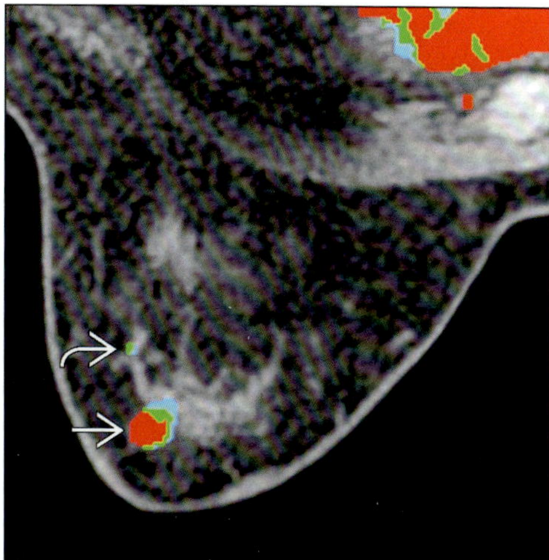

(Left) *Axial CECT in the same patient shows a relatively nonspecific, enhancing, nodular lesion ➔ in the left breast, subsequently shown to be a 17 mm carcinoma.* ***(Right)*** *Breast MR from the same patient shows that the mass ➔ correlating to the mammographic study demonstrates marked abnormal enhancement and identifies a 2nd focus ➔ of abnormal enhancement more posteriorly, representing an additional focus of carcinoma.*

BREAST

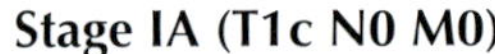

Stage IA (T1c N0 M0)

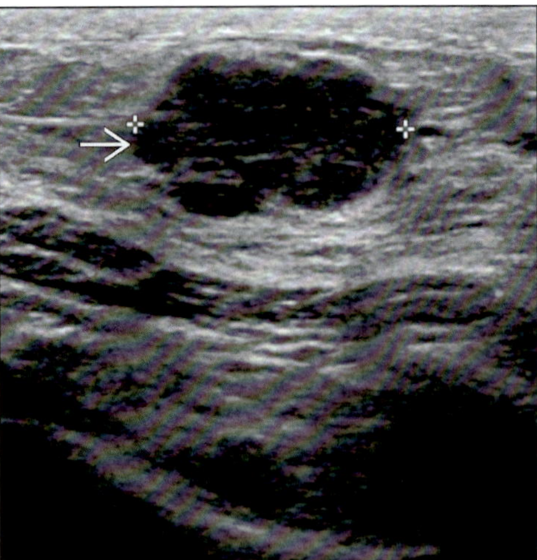

Stage IA (T1c N0 M0)

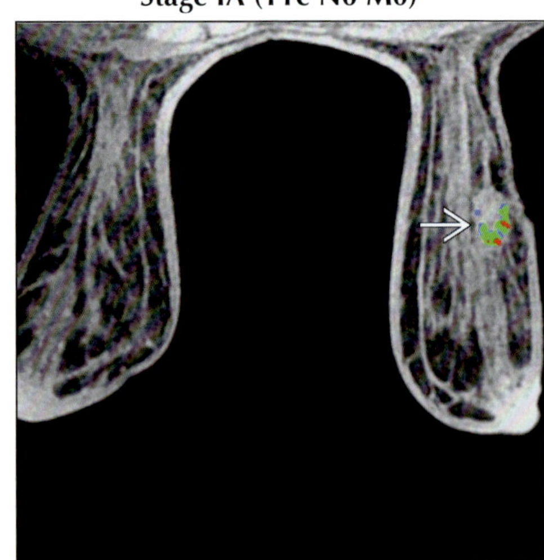

(Left) *Grayscale ultrasound in the same patient shows a fairly well-circumscribed hypoechoic lesion ➔ that was subsequently biopsied and shown to be invasive ductal carcinoma.* ***(Right)*** *Breast MR in the same patient shows the lesion ➔ to measure approximately 1.4 cm and demonstrate heterogeneous areas of increased enhancement. This lesion would be classified as a T1c lesion.*

Tangential EBRT

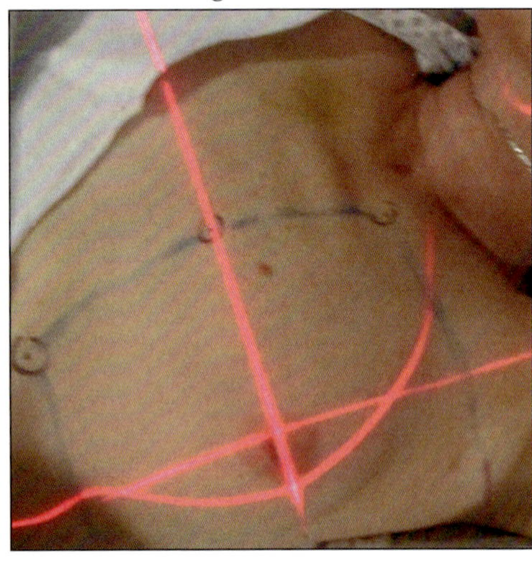

Tangential EBRT

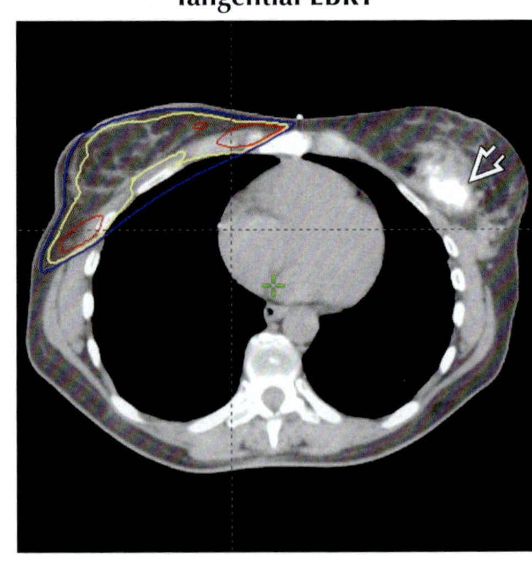

(Left) *Lasers are indispensable for proper positioning and reproducible breast setups.* ***(Right)*** *Optimal dosimetry is influenced by many factors, including the patient's separation and breast size. The red, yellow, and blue lines represent the 105%, 100%, and 90% isodose lines, respectively. In the contralateral breast, the edge of a calcified implant ⇨ is seen.*

Tangential EBRT, 6 MV

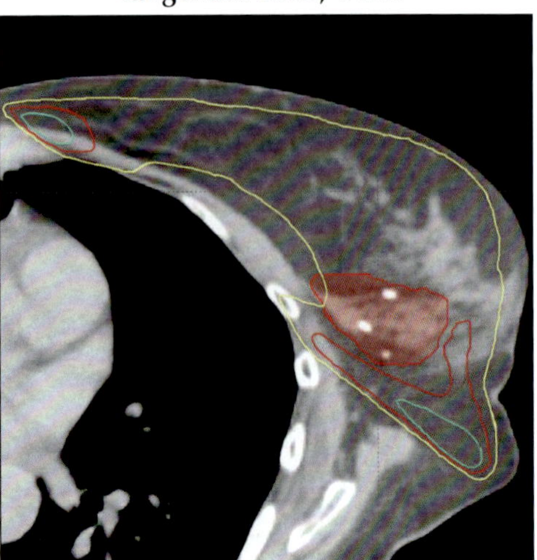

Tangential EBRT, 10 MV

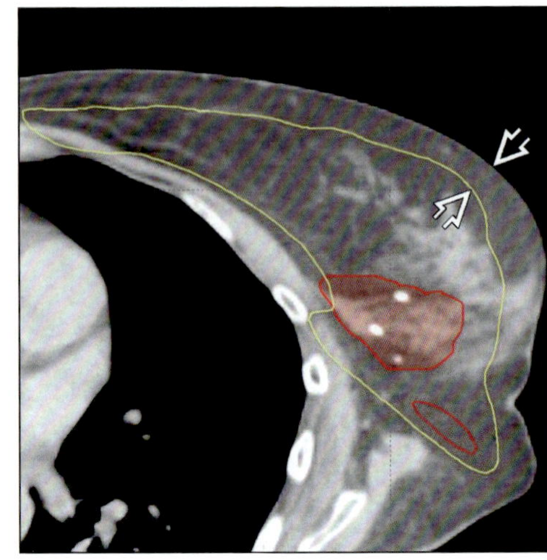

(Left) *Standard tangents with a 6 MV beam show the lumpectomy cavity in red. The yellow, red, and blue lines represent the 100%, 105%, and 108% isodose lines, respectively. The near-complete coverage with the 100% isodose line and the symmetric hot spots are desirable.* ***(Right)*** *A 10 MV beam in the same patient demonstrates greater skin sparing ⇨ with reduced hot spots. Yellow and red represent the 100% and 105% isodose lines, respectively.*

Tangential EBRT

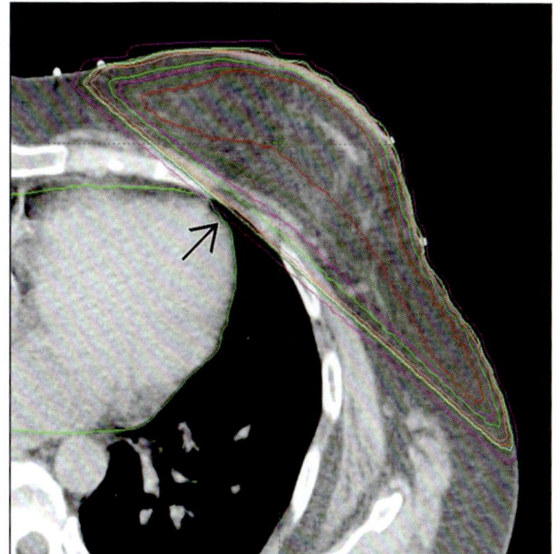

Tangential EBRT

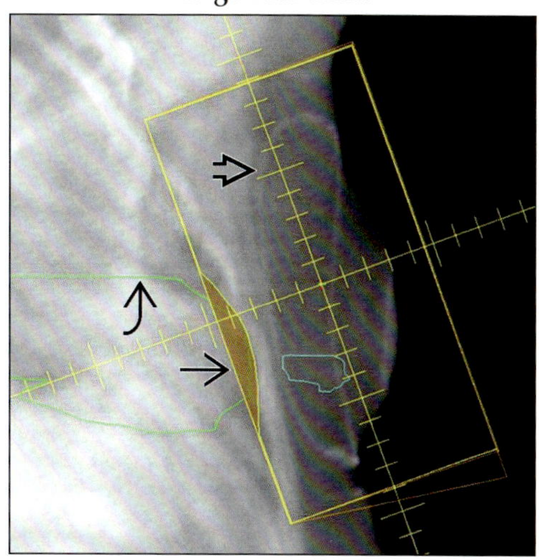

*(**Left**) Simulation CT shows standard open left-sided tangents. Note the anterior aspect of the heart ⇒ in this case. With careful placement of gantry and collimator angles, the heart can be excluded from the beam in most cases. (**Right**) DRR shows left-sided tangents with a heart block ⇒. The lumpectomy cavity is shown in blue, and the breast ⇒ was wired at simulation to ensure complete clinical coverage. The heart ⇒ is contoured in green.*

Tangential EBRT

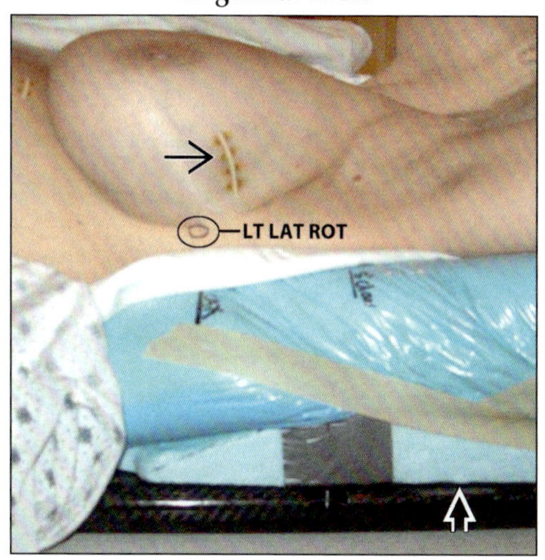

Breast Boost

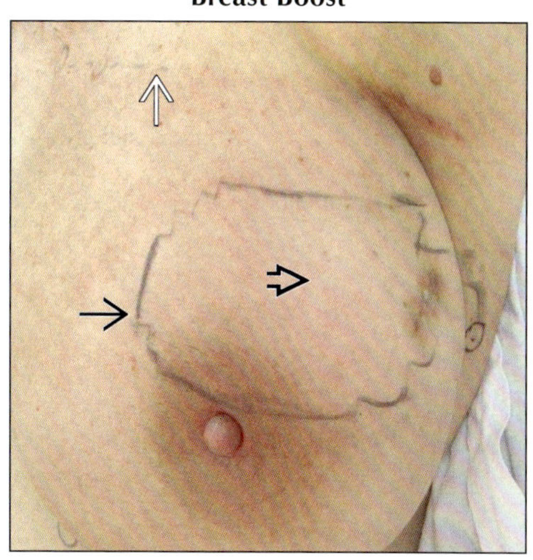

*(**Left**) In large or pendulous breasts, a wedge or breast board ⇒ can be used to elevate the shoulders to allow the breast to lay flat, reducing axillary skin folds. Wire ⇒ is placed on the scar. (**Right**) Verification simulation after 50 Gy shows 1 of 2 photon breast boost fields ⇒. There is minimal erythema ⇒ of the tangent ports and slight cutaneous edema ⇒.*

Breast Boost

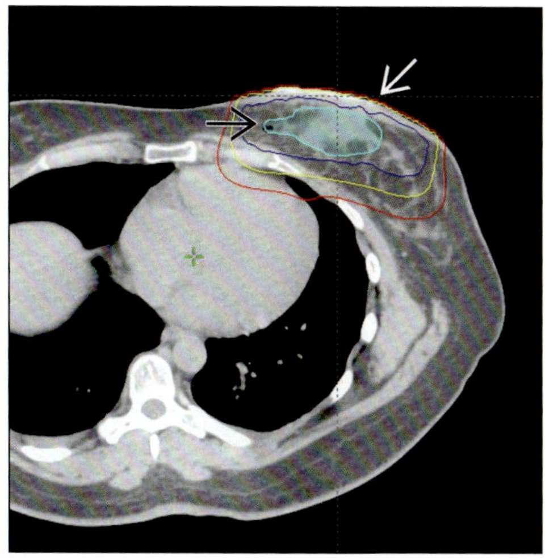

Breast Boost

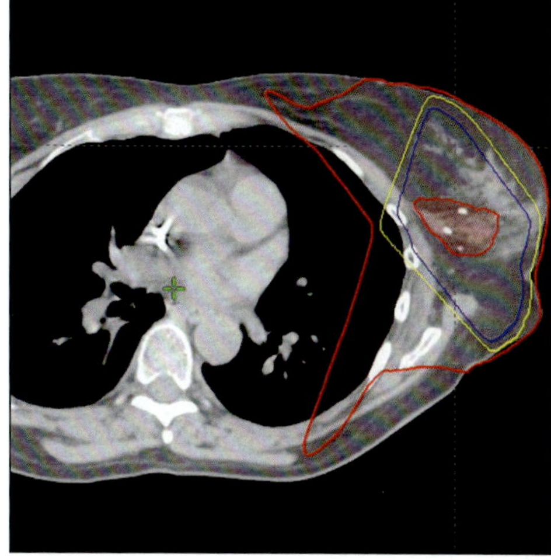

*(**Left**) En face 12 MEV electron plan shows good coverage of the lumpectomy cavity. The blue, yellow, and red lines represent the 95%, 70%, and 30% isodose lines, respectively. Air ⇒ is present in the lumpectomy cavity, and skin thickening ⇒ is secondary to postsurgical induration. (**Right**) In this case, the lumpectomy cavity is too deep for electrons and hence a wedge pair photon plan is used. The blue, yellow, and red lines represent the 95%, 70%, and 30% isodose lines, respectively.*

BREAST

(**Left**) *Spot mammographic image in a patient with heavily dense breasts shows an area of architectural distortion ➔ posteriorly with suspicious calcifications.* (**Right**) *Grayscale ultrasound in the same patient shows an irregular hypoechoic lesion ➔ with posterior acoustic shadowing. The lesion was subsequently biopsied, and pathology showed invasive lobular carcinoma.*

Stage IIA (T2 N0 M0)

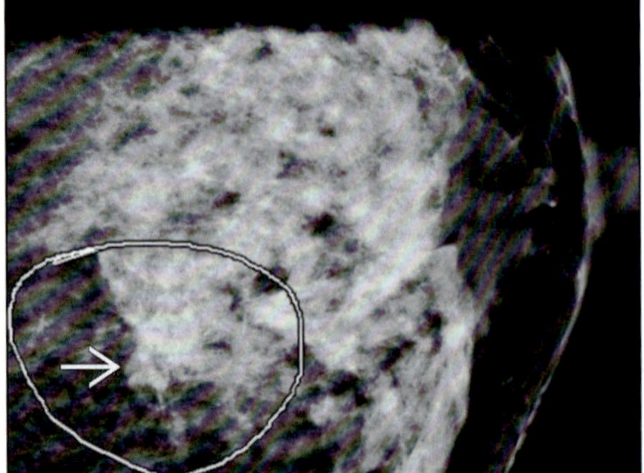

Stage IIA (T2 N0 M0)

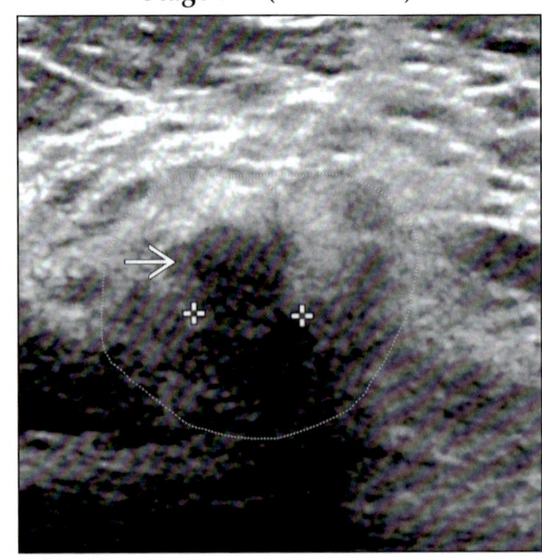

(**Left**) *Breast MR in the same patient shows a lesion with marked enhancement ➔, compatible with the patient's known invasive lobular carcinoma. Surgical resection showed the lesion to measure 21 mm, compatible with a T2 lesion, which is defined as > 20 mm but ≤ to 50 mm in greatest dimension.* (**Right**) *Left CC mammogram image in a different patient shows a large, well-circumscribed, posterior left breast mass ➔, very worrisome for malignancy.*

Stage IIA (T2 N0 M0)

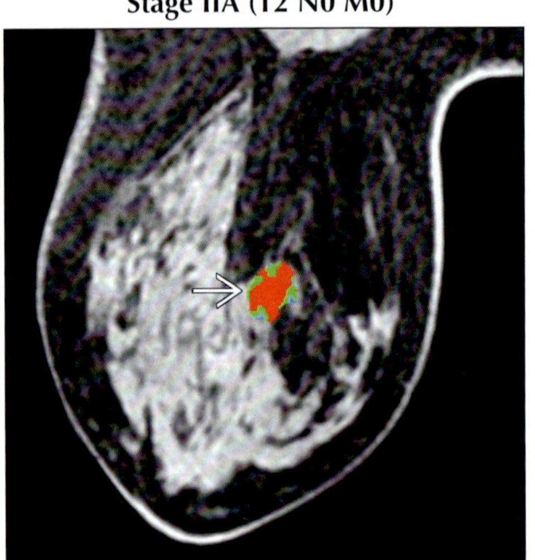

Stage IIA (T2 N0 M0)

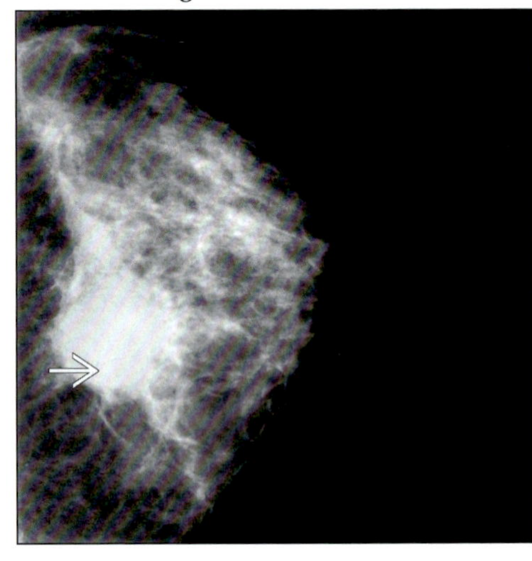

(**Left**) *Breast MR shows a 3.8 cm or T2 mass ➔ with marked abnormal enhancement in the medial aspect of the left breast, compatible with the patient's known invasive lobular carcinoma.* (**Right**) *Axial PET/CT in the same patient shows only minimally increased FDG activity ➔ in the area of pathologically proven invasive lobular carcinoma. Approximately 65% of lobular carcinomas may be relatively non-FDG avid.*

Stage IIA (T2 N0 M0)

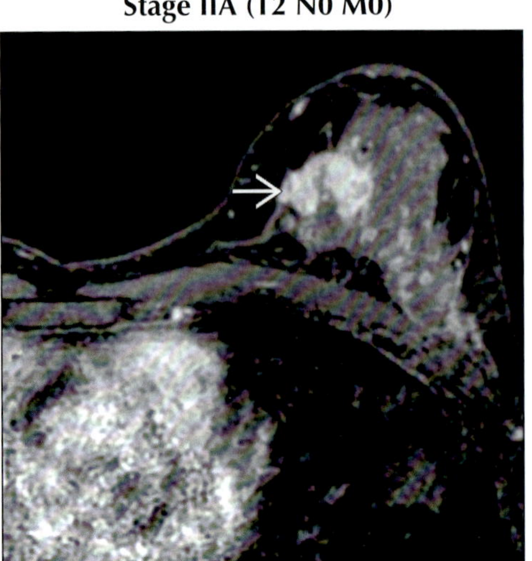

Stage IIA (T2 N0 M0)

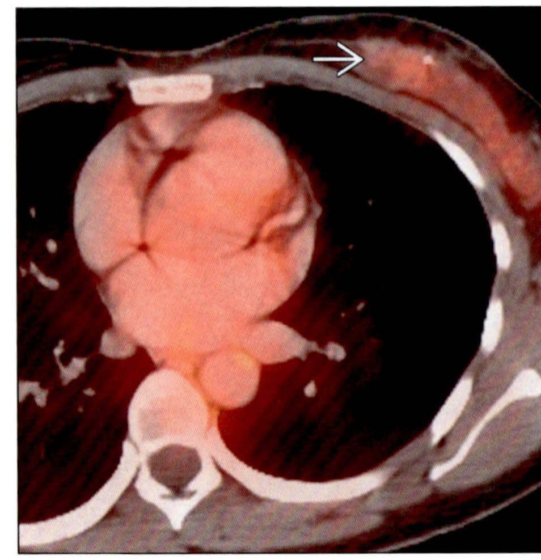

Prone vs. Supine

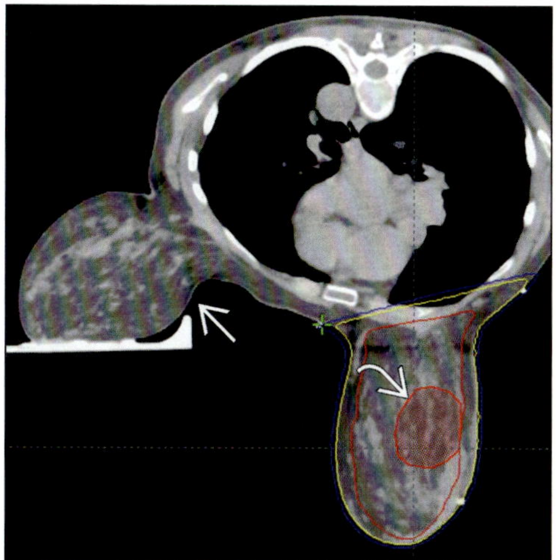

Prone vs. Supine

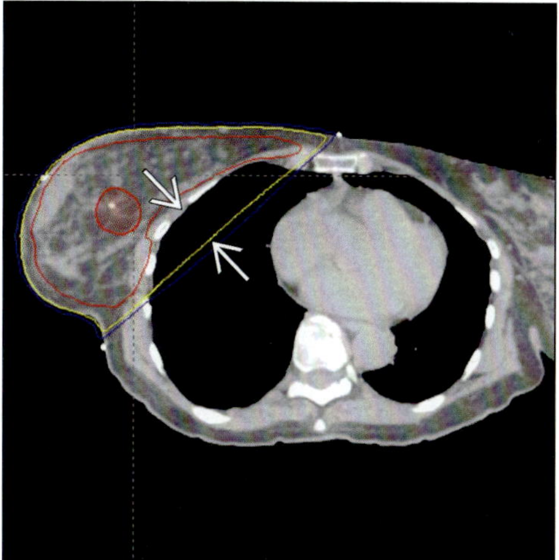

(Left) *Axial CT shows prone tangential breast plan with the lumpectomy cavity shown. The red, yellow, and blue lines indicate the 100%, 70%, and 30% isodose lines, respectively. The contralateral breast is carefully positioned away from the tangential beam.* ***(Right)*** *Supine setup in the same patient reveals a significant central lung distance. Due to the large size of the breast, a significant portion of liver was in field.*

Prone vs. Supine

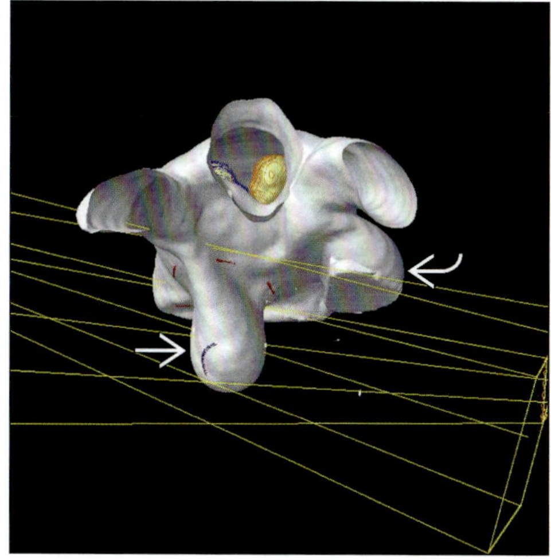

Prone vs. Supine

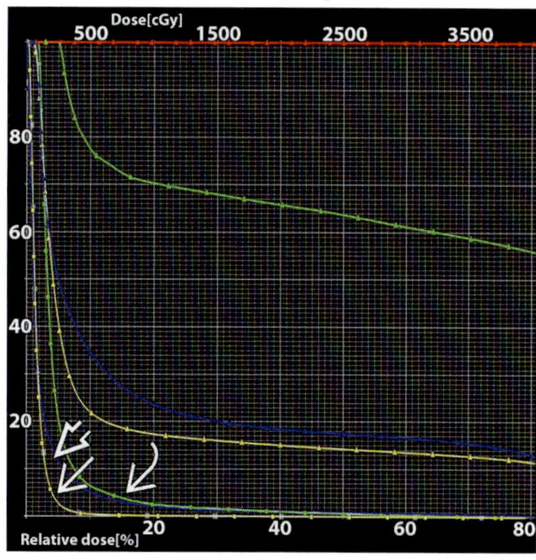

(Left) *DRR shows the pendulous right breast and the laterally displaced left breast. In many cases, patient postioning is less reproducible, but a reduction in dose to OAR is achieved.* ***(Right)*** *DVH shows a marked reduction in dose to level 1 lymph nodes (green), right lung (blue), and liver (yellow) in the prone position compared to supine (matched colors). Target coverage for the lumpectomy cavity is identical (red).*

Stage IIA (T2 N0 M0)

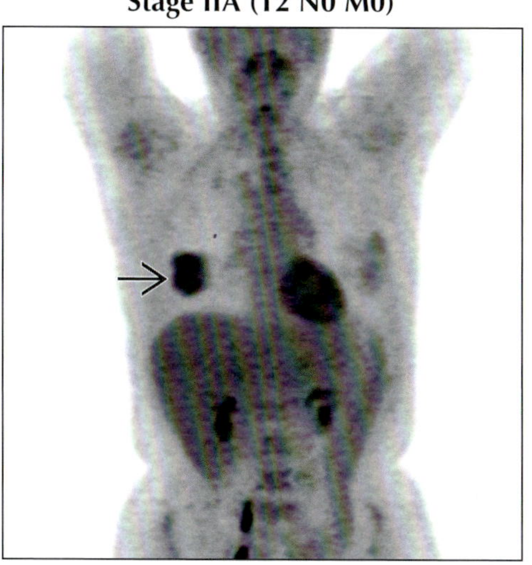

Stage IIA (T2 N0 M0)

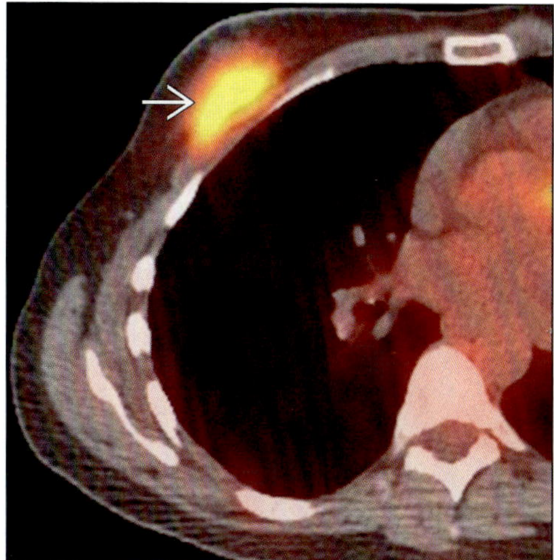

(Left) *Coronal PET image shows asymmetric moderate to intense FDG activity corresponding to a 3.3 cm or T2 right breast invasive carcinoma.* ***(Right)*** *Axial PET/CT in the same patient shows intense FDG activity corresponding to the right breast carcinoma. In general, invasive ductal carcinoma tends to be more FDG avid than lobular carcinomas.*

Stage IIA (T2 N0 M0)

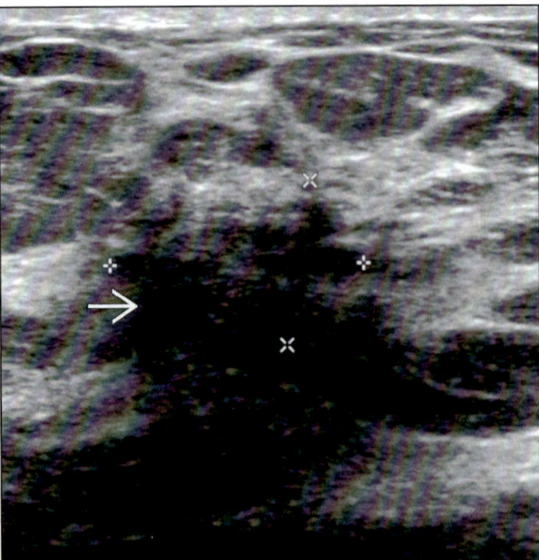

Stage IIA (T2 N0 M0)

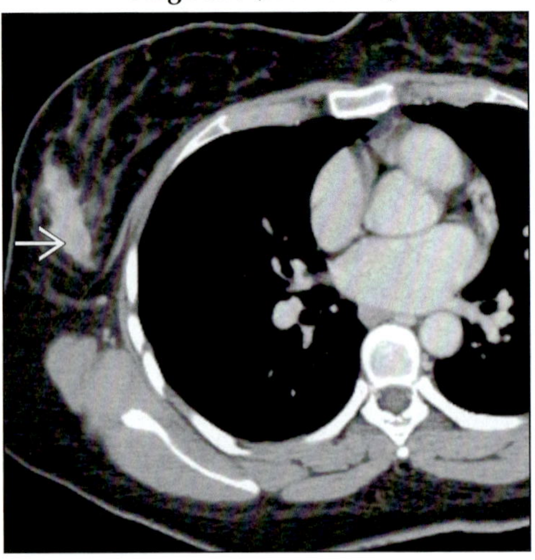

(Left) Grayscale ultrasound of a patient with a newly diagnosed 3.6 cm or T2 invasive ductal carcinoma shows an invasive breast carcinoma with an atypical appearance, manifesting here as a hypoechoic lesion ➔ with ill-defined margins. (Right) Axial CECT in the same patient shows an abnormally enhancing right breast mass ➔ in the lateral aspect of the breast.

Stage IIA (T2 N0 M0)

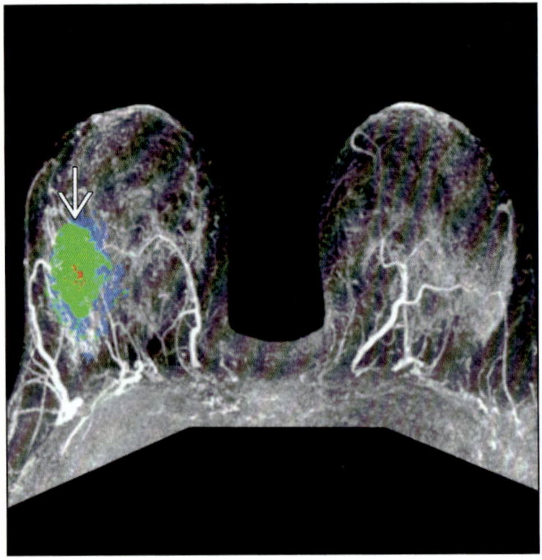

Stage IIA (T2 N0 M0)

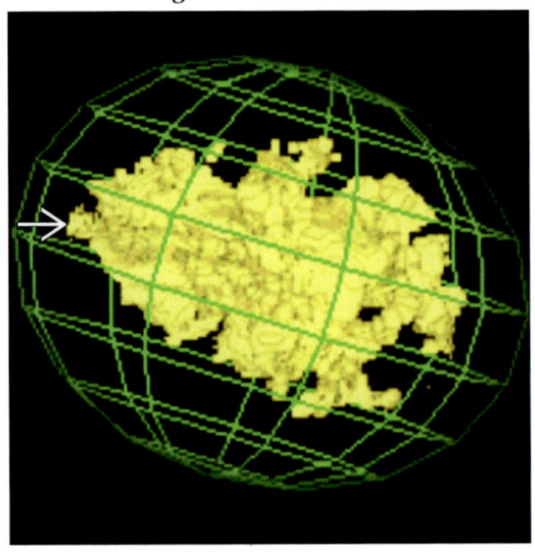

(Left) Breast MR from the same patient shows the oval-shaped carcinoma ➔ in the lateral aspect of the right breast with abnormal enhancement. (Right) Reconstructed view from a breast MR shows the tumor volume ➔. The lack of axillary nodal involvement is compatible with an overall stage of IIA.

Internal Mammary Nodal (IMN) Treatment

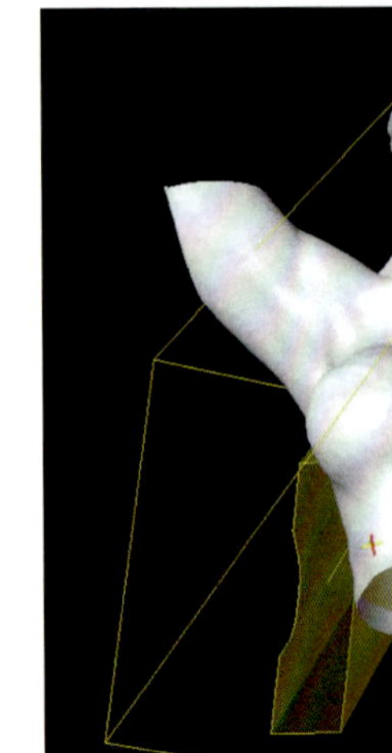

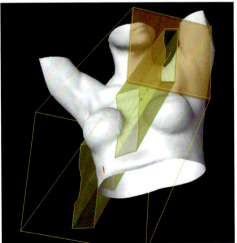

IMN Treatment

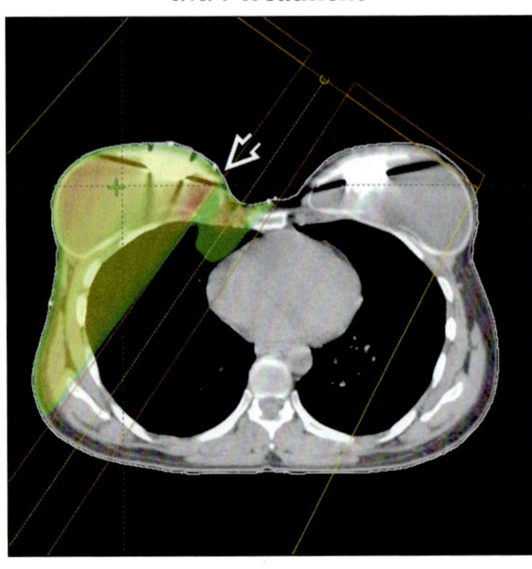

(Left) In bilateral breast reconstruction, standard gantry angles can be precluded by the contralateral breast. A separate IMN electron field can be used to reduce dose to the lung. (Right) The IMN gantry angle is 5° less than the breast tangents. Green is 30 Gy and yellow is 50 Gy in the colorwash. Hot spots need to be checked carefully at the match ➔, particularly since electron beams display greater side scatter.

IMN Treatment

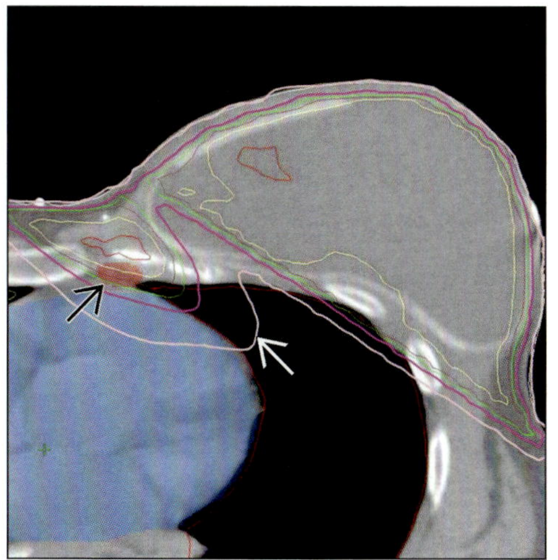

IMN Treatment

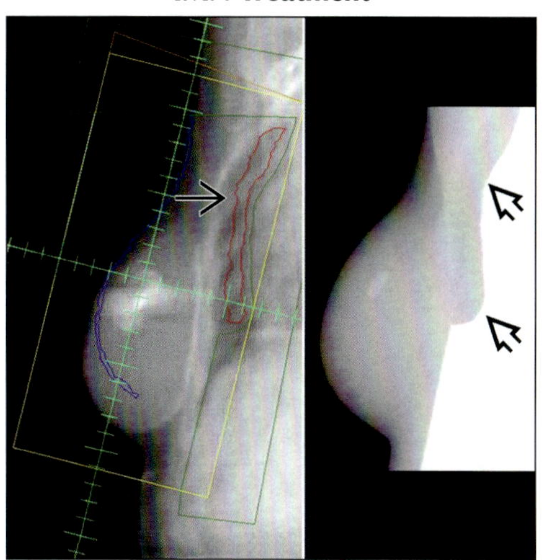

(Left) *A separate IMN electron field can be utilized to reduce dose to heart and lung. The IMN region is shown in red ⇨ and the heart in blue. The yellow, green, and light pink ➡ lines represent the 50, 45, and 25 Gy isodose lines, respectively.* ***(Right)*** *DRR on the left and port film on the right indicate that shaping ⇨ can be easily used to encompass IMNs ⇨ (shown in red) and limit extraneous dose to the lung.*

Stage IIA (T2 N0 M0)

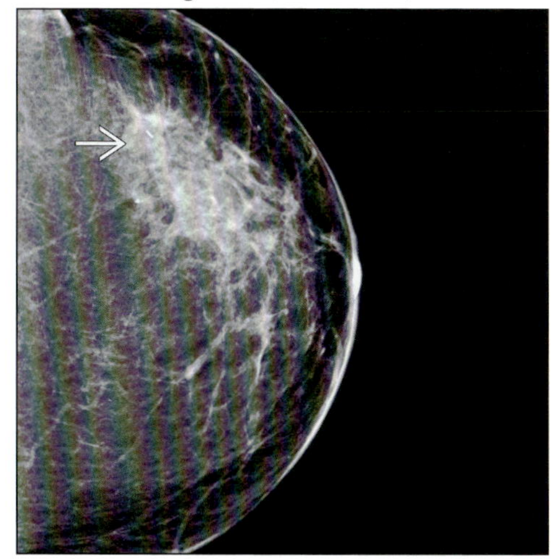

Stage IIA (T2 N0 M0)

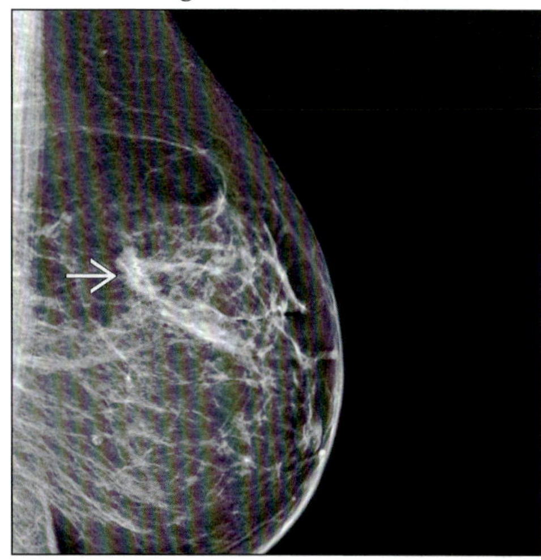

(Left) *Left CC mammogram shows an ill-defined mass ➡ or area of architectural distortion.* ***(Right)*** *Left ML mammogram shows the same area of architectural distortion ➡. Primary breast lesions > 2 cm but ≤ 5 cm are classified as T2 lesions. This lesion was subsequently biopsied and shown to be a 4.2 cm invasive ductal carcinoma.*

Stage IIA (T2 N0 M0)

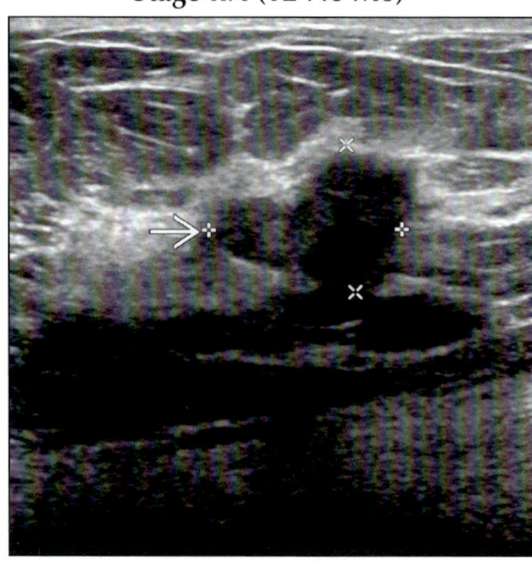

Stage IIA (T2 N0 M0)

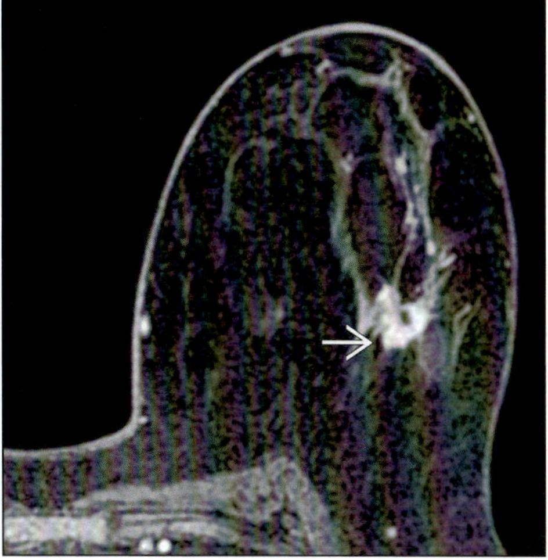

(Left) *Grayscale ultrasound in the same patient shows a T2 breast carcinoma as a hypoechoic lesion ➡ with fairly well-circumscribed margins. The lack of spread to regional lymph nodes or distant metastatic lesions makes this stage IIA.* ***(Right)*** *Subsequent breast MR in the same patient shows the lesion ➡ to have abnormal enhancement, a finding characteristic of breast carcinoma.*

BREAST

(**Left**) *Survival is improved with RT after mastectomy in node-positive patients, and multiple techniques can be used. Anatomic considerations may determine the optimal technique. Electrons can be well suited to treat the chest wall. Shown is an electron arc RT with blue, red, orange, and pink lines representing the 100%, 90%, 60%, and 30% isodose lines, respectively.* (**Right**) *After 50 Gy, this patient has brisk erythema. The scar is wired and the electron boost field is drawn.*

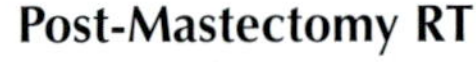

Post-Mastectomy RT

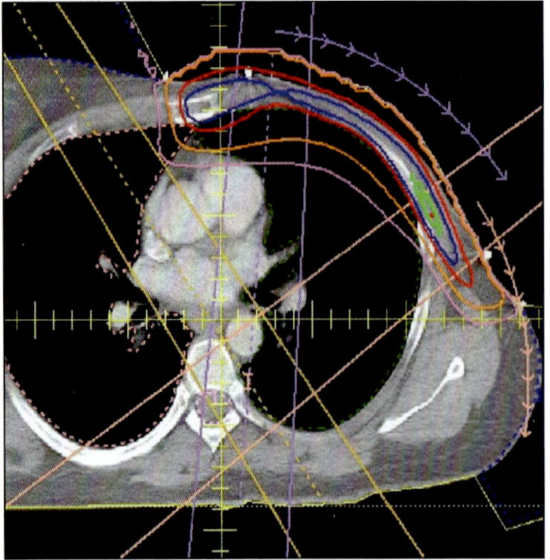

Post-Mastectomy Boost

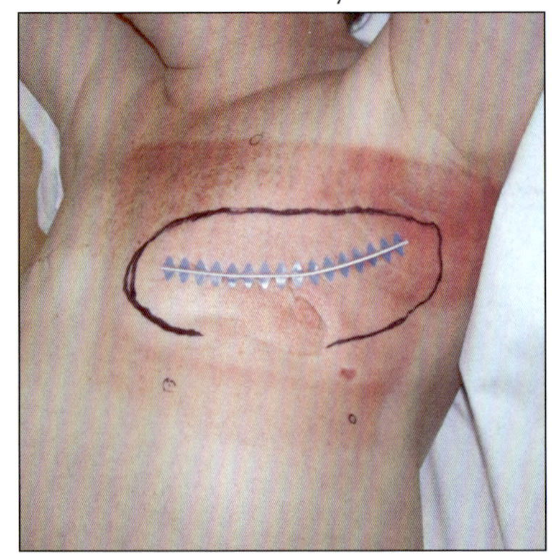

(**Left**) *Breast MR in the same patient shows a large mass ➔ in the medial left breast along with abnormal enhancement. The lesion was subsequently shown to be a large invasive ductal carcinoma. Note an enlarged axillary node ➔.* (**Right**) *3D reconstructed fused PET/CT shows intense FDG activity ➔ corresponding to the the patient's primary breast carcinoma. A T2 primary lesion and a single lymph node seen in the left axilla (not shown) makes this stage IIB.*

Stage IIB (T2 N1 M0)

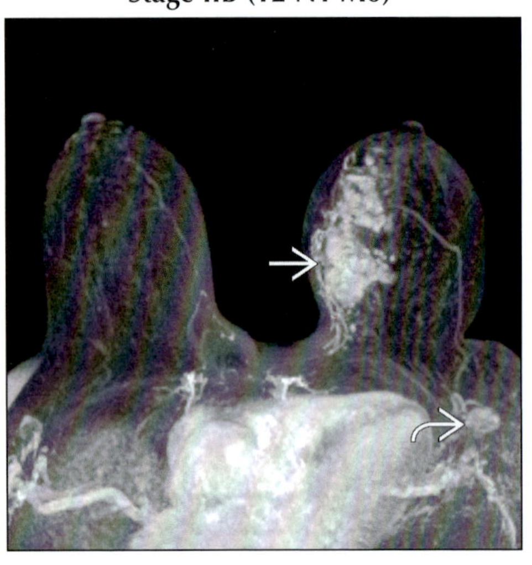

Stage IIB (T2 N1 M0)

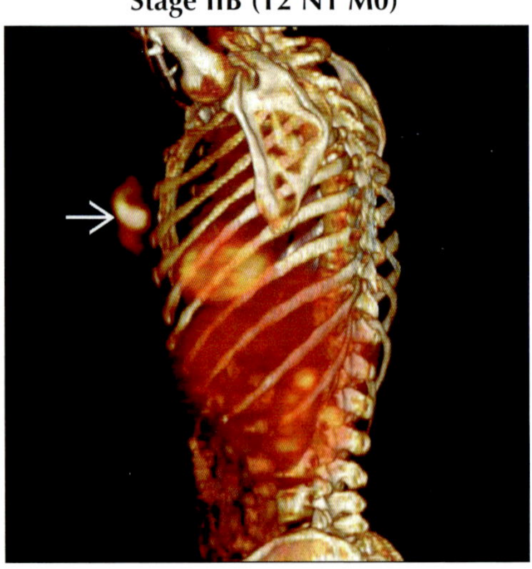

(**Left**) *Axial CECT MIP in same patient shows large area of abnormally enhancing tissue ➔ in the left breast, compatible with breast carcinoma.* (**Right**) *Axial PET/CT MIP in same patient shows intense FDG activity ➔ in left breast mass, compatible with carcinoma. Enhancing tissue more centrally ➔ demonstrates only mild FDG activity, although it is still carcinoma. Small lymph node ➔ in left axilla with mildly increased FDG activity proved to be a metastatic node.*

Stage IIB (T2 N1 M0)

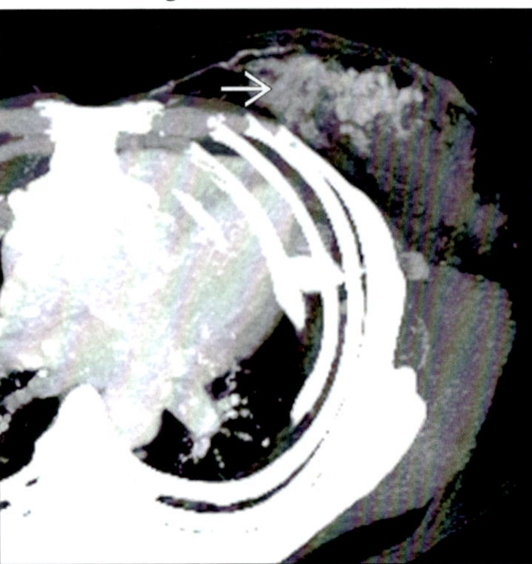

Stage IIB (T2 N1 M0)

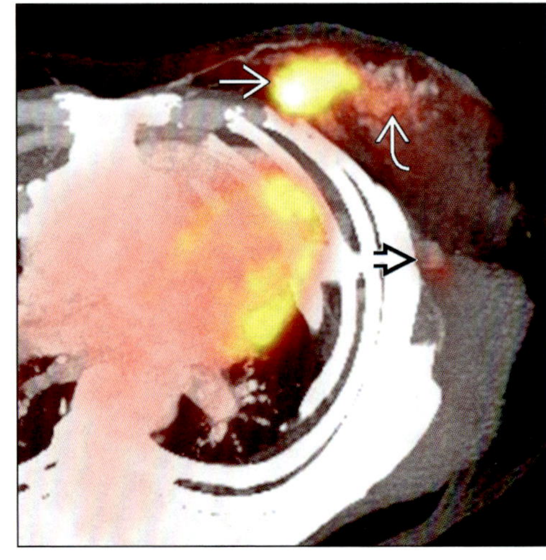

Comprehensive Nodal Radiation

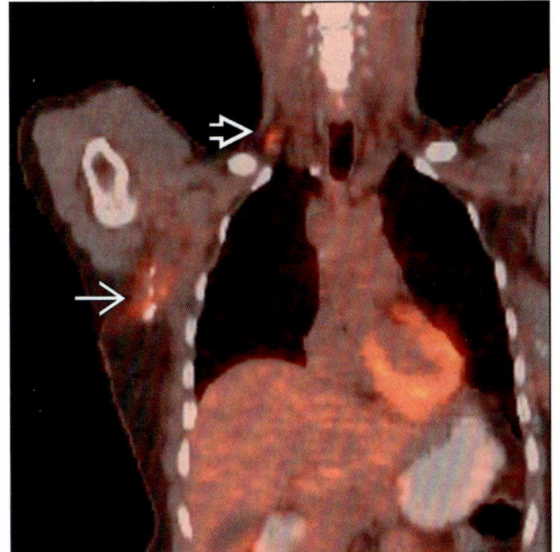

Comprehensive Nodal Radiation

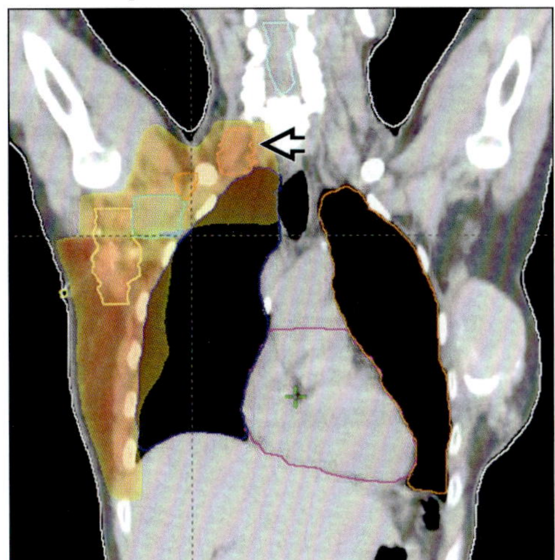

*(**Left**) PET/CT shows the level I/II axillary dissection site ➔ and an avid supraclavicular node (N3) ➔. Ten of 10 axillary lymph nodes contained metastases. (**Right**) Coronal CT in the same patient has levels I, II, III, and supraclavicular nodes ➔ contoured. Contouring regional nodes is essential to determine adequate coverage. The anterior supraclavicular field is matched to the tangent fields intersecting levels I and II. The colorwash indicates the 50 Gy surface.*

Comprehensive Nodal Radiation

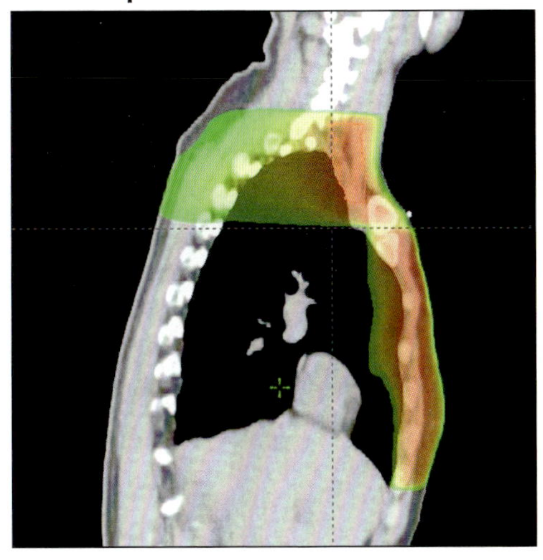

Comprehensive Nodal Radiation

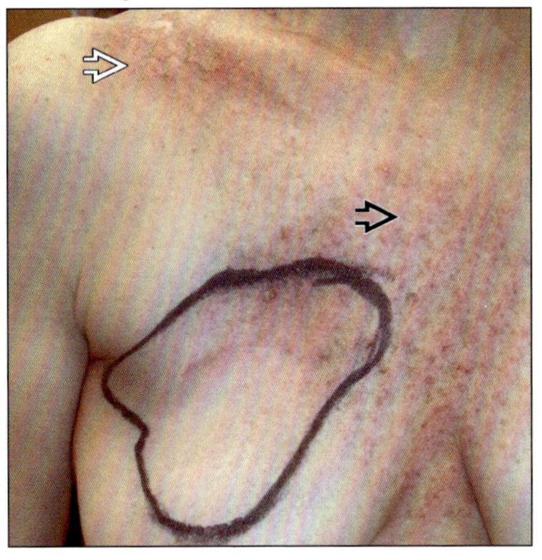

*(**Left**) Sagittal CT in the same patient shows the match plane at the base of the clavicular head. The colorwash indicates the 50 Gy surface and shows fall off from the anterior supraclavicular field. (**Right**) Skin reaction in the same patient after 50 Gy shows a typical follicular erythematous rash in the upper medial quadrant ➔ and the supraclavicular fossa ➔.*

Comprehensive Nodal Radiation

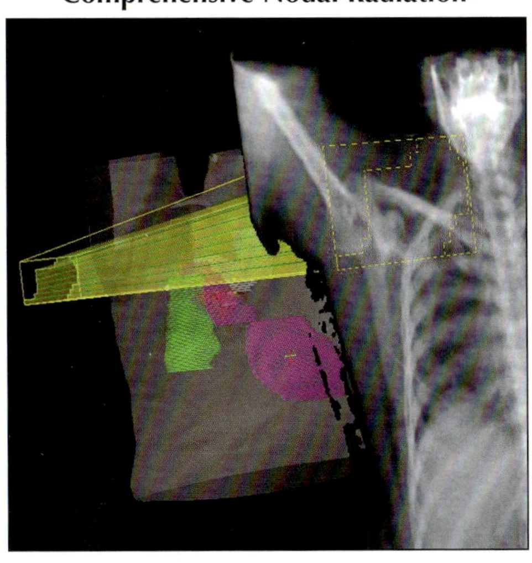

Comprehensive Nodal Radiation

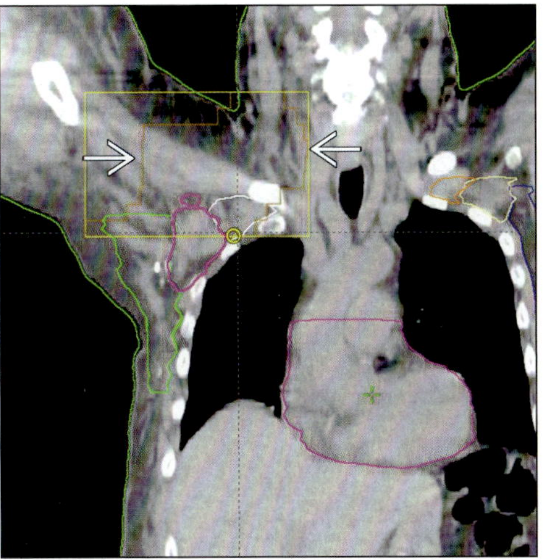

*(**Left**) DRR shows a posterior axillary boost (PAB), which is used to supplement dose to the midplane or deep aspects of the axilla. A PAB may increase morbidity, and it should be used in high-risk cases where dose from an anterior beam is not sufficient. (**Right**) PAB ➔ in the same patient is unusually large due to the patient's large size and gross disease in the low neck (not shown). Axillary levels I, II, and III on the right are contoured in green, pink, and white, respectively.*

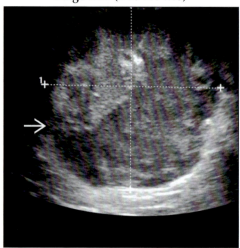

*(**Left**) Axial post-contrast MR of the breast shows a large mass ➡ with markedly abnormal enhancement and central necrosis. Also note skin thickening laterally. Involvement of the skin ➡ makes this a T4b lesion. (**Right**) Grayscale ultrasound in the same patient shows a heterogeneous hypoechoic lesion ➡ that was subsequently biopsied and shown to be invasive ductal carcinoma.*

Stage IIIB (T4b N1 M0)

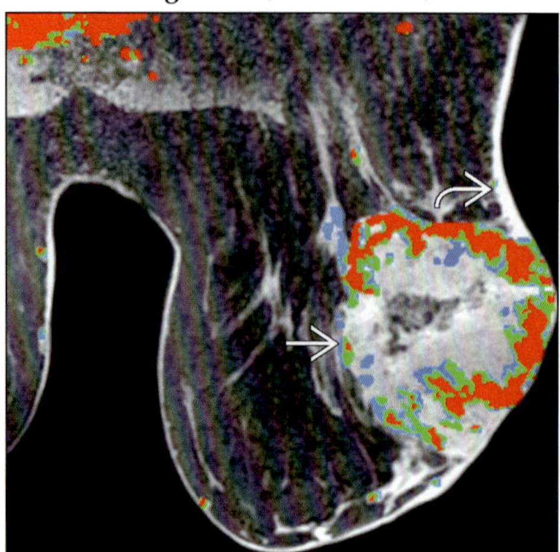

Stage IIIB (T4b N1 M0)

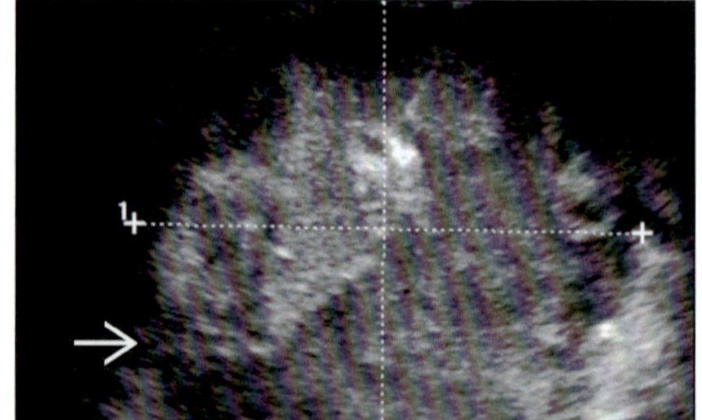

*(**Left**) Axial CECT in the same patient shows a borderline-enlarged right axillary lymph node ➡, but with a partial fatty hilum. (**Right**) Axial fused PET/CT in the same patient shows intense FDG activity ➡ within the slightly enlarged right axillary lymph node, compatible with metastatic disease. Due to the single involved lymph node, the overall stage would be IIIB (T4b N1 M0).*

Stage IIIB (T4b N1 M0)

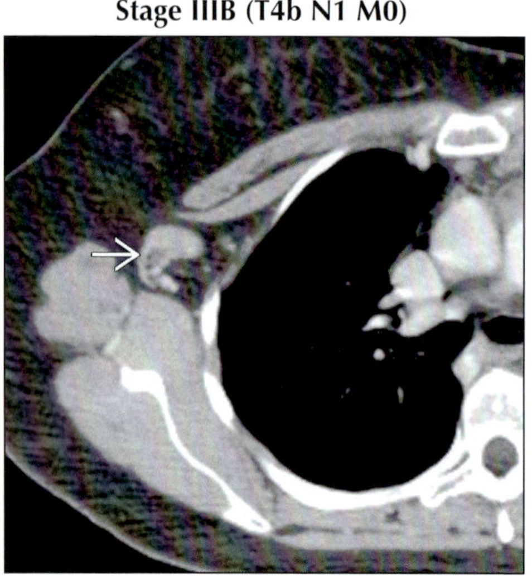

Stage IIIB (T4b N1 M0)

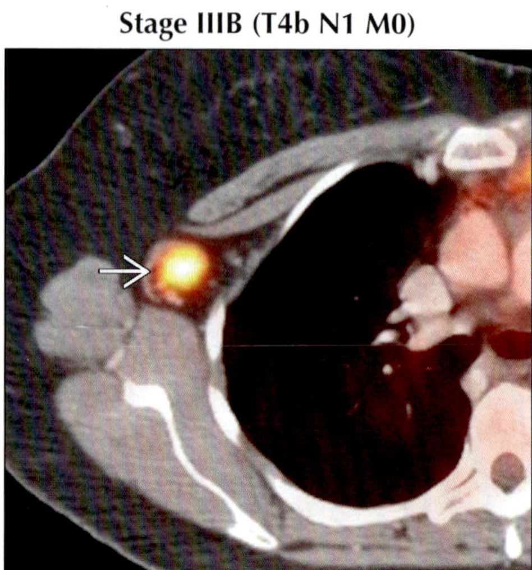

*(**Left**) Left CC mammogram shows a large lobulated mass ➡ measuring 5.4 cm in this patient with recently diagnosed breast carcinoma. By size, this would be T3. However, there was also skin dimpling and nodularity, making this a T4b mass. (**Right**) Grayscale ultrasound in the same patient shows a heterogeneously echogenic mass ➡ that subsequently biopsied positive for invasive ductal breast carcinoma.*

Stage IIIB (T4b N1 M0)

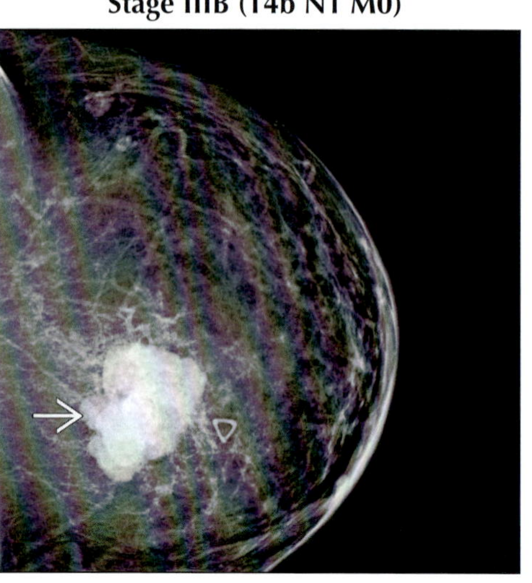

Stage IIIB (T4b N1 M0)

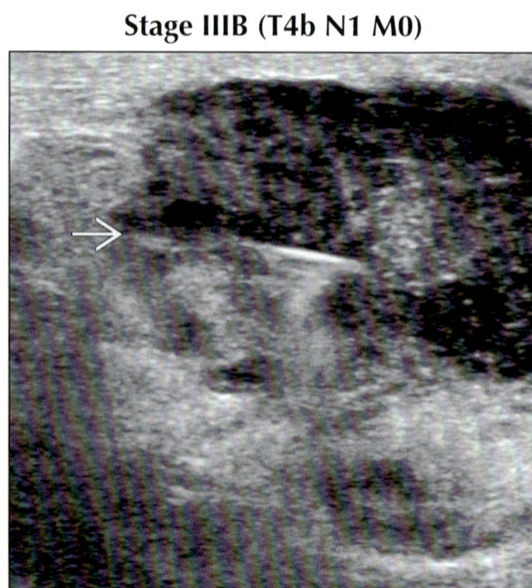

Stage IIIB (T4b N1 M0)

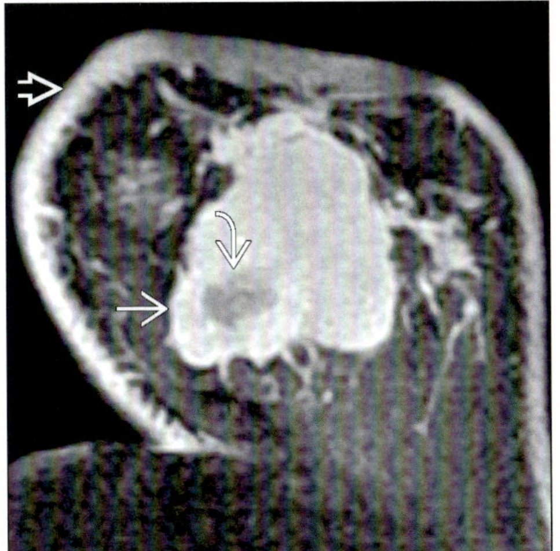

Inflammatory Breast Cancer

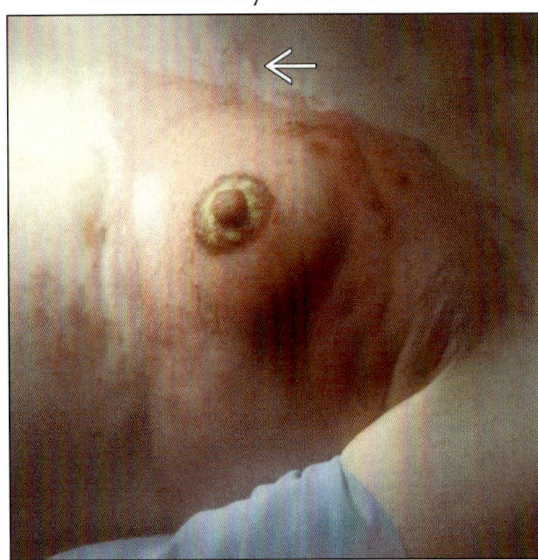

*(**Left**) Contrast-enhanced breast MR in the same patient shows a large mass ➡ with central necrosis ➡ and overlying skin thickening ➡. (**Right**) Inflammatory breast cancer (T4d) is characterized by rapid growth, erythema, warmth, peau d'orange skin, and an erysipeloid edge. The pathologic hallmark is tumor emboli in dermal lymphatics. The standard paradigm is chemo, mastectomy, and RT. Satellite lesions ➡ are evident near the contralateral breast. (Courtesy D. Hicks, MD.)*

Recurrent Breast Cancer

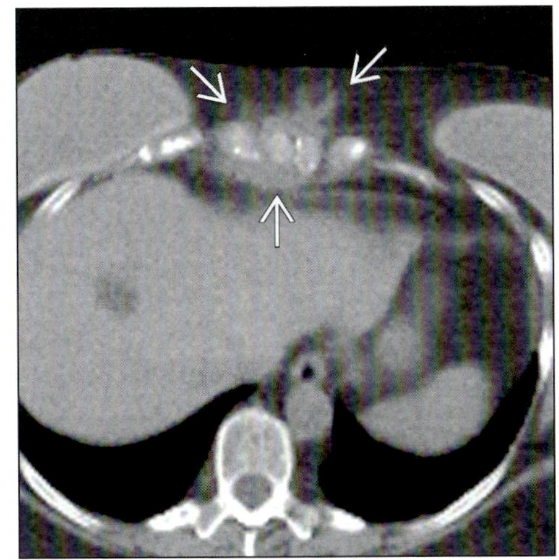

Recurrent Breast Cancer

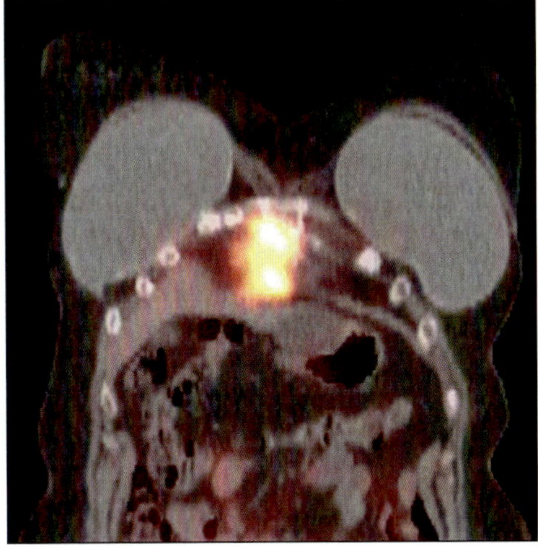

*(**Left**) Axial CT in a patient who underwent mastectomy and reconstruction 15 years earlier showed xiphoid recurrence ➡. (**Right**) Coronal fused PET/CT in the same patient shows avid sternal and xiphoid mass.*

Recurrent Breast Cancer

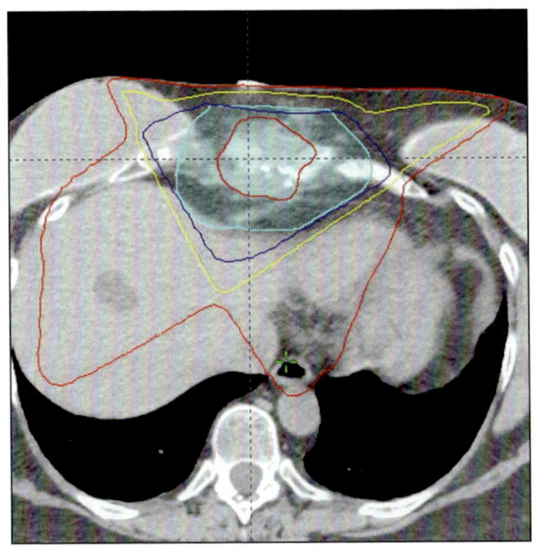

Recurrent Breast Cancer

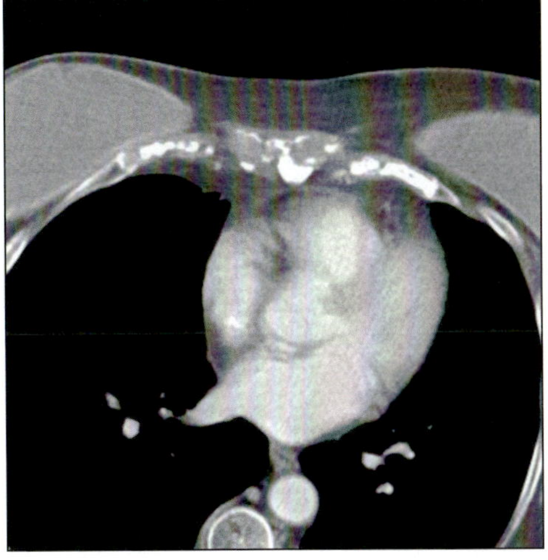

*(**Left**) Planning CT in the same patient shows PTV outlined in blue and GTV in red. A wedge pair technique was used to 50 Gy, and the blue, yellow, and red lines indicate the 95%, 70%, and 30% isodose lines, respectively. Following this, a mixed electron/photon anterior beam was used to a reduced PTV to a total of 64 Gy. (**Right**) The same patient demonstrates continued freedom from recurrence 6 years later.*

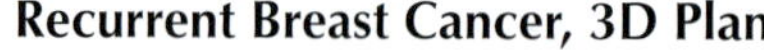

(**Left**) *Axial CECT shows aortopulmonary ➔ and anterior tracheal adenopathy ➔ from metastatic breast cancer in a patient that previously had comprehensive left radiotherapy. Patient also recurred simultaneously in the right supraclavicular fossa.* (**Right**) *The same patient was treated with an oblique 4-field plan to the mediastinum. Colorwash represents 50 Gy. The red volume is the CTV and the blue line indicates the PTV.*

Recurrent Breast Cancer, 3D Plan

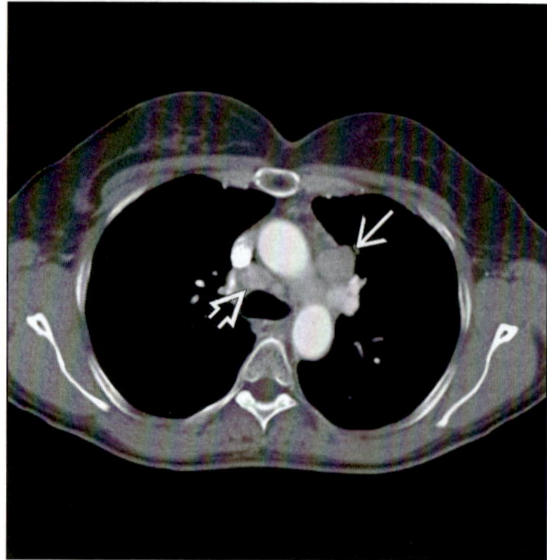

Recurrent Breast Cancer, 3D Plan

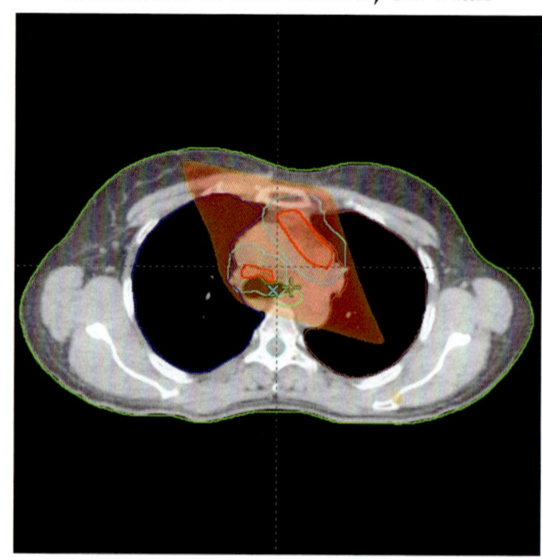

(**Left**) *Coronal CT in the same patient shows a beam split plan was used: 4 field to the mediastinum and an oblique anterior beam to the right supraclavicular region. Blue, yellow, and red represent 15, 50, and 55 Gy, respectively.* (**Right**) *Sagittal CT in the same patient shows good coverage of both anterior ➔ and posterior mediastinal adenopathy ➔. Follow-up imaging in ensuing months demonstrates local control.*

Recurrent Breast Cancer, 3D Plan

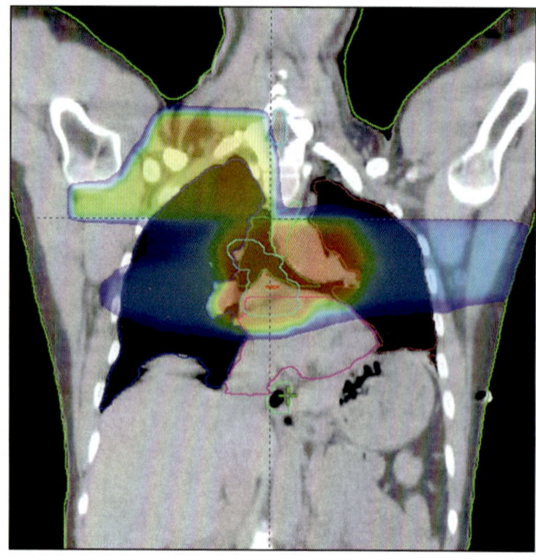

Recurrent Breast Cancer, 3D Plan

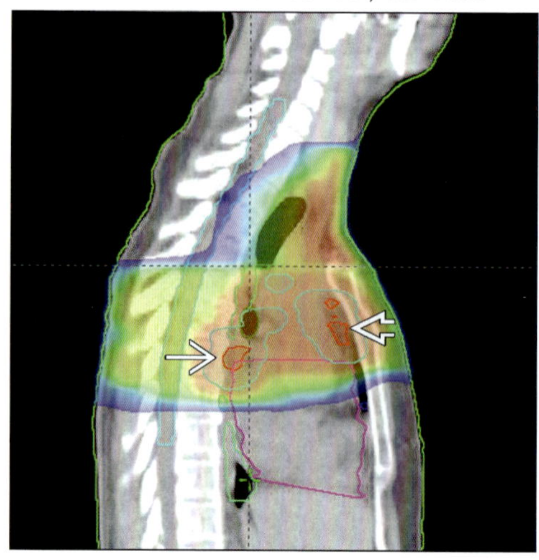

(**Left**) *This NECT shows a patient with a massive recurrence ➔ in the chest wall, thorax, and abdomen 18 years after lumpectomy and RT. The tumor extensively involves the pericardium ➔.* (**Right**) *PET/CT in the same patient (lower plane, in abdomen) shows extensive disease involving a broad portion of the chest wall ➔. The patient was initially treated with chemotherapy with a limited response.*

Recurrent Breast Cancer, IMRT Plan

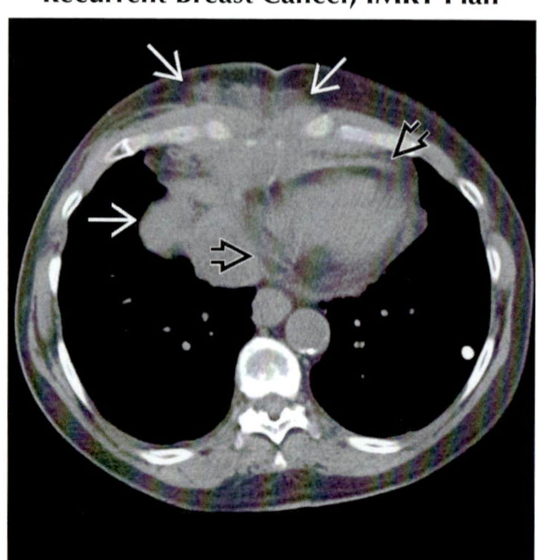

Recurrent Breast Cancer, IMRT Plan

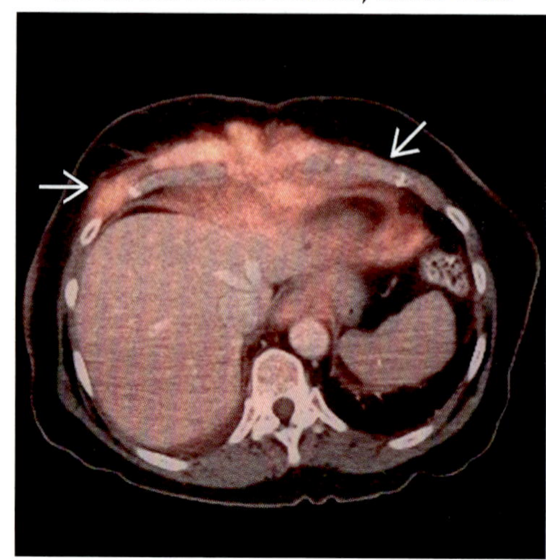

Recurrent Breast Cancer, IMRT Plan

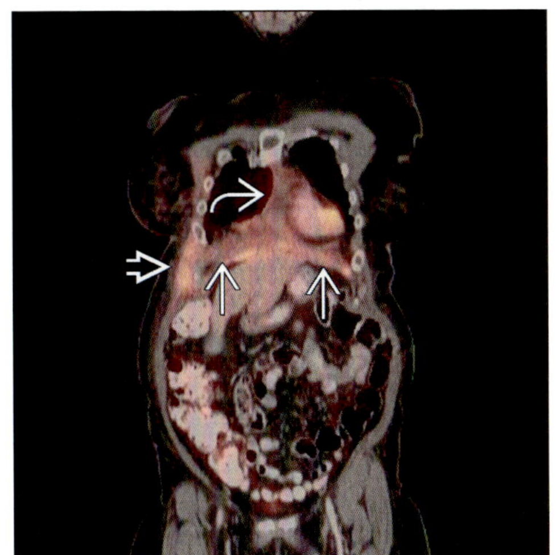

Recurrent Breast Cancer, IMRT Plan

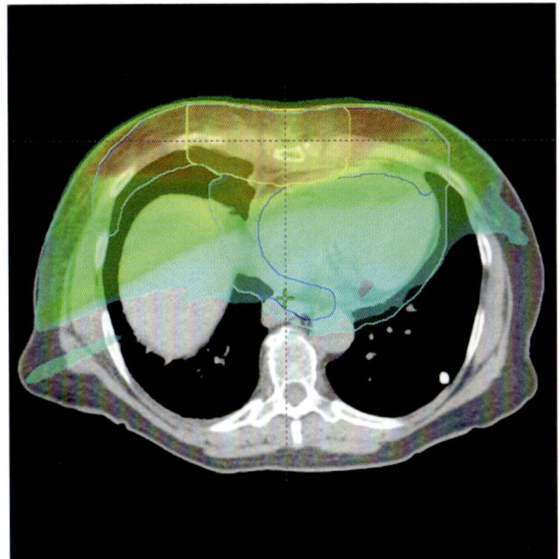

(Left) Coronal PET/CT in the same patient shows increased avidity along the diaphragm ➡, chest wall ➡, and anterior mediastinum ➡. *(Right)* Axial CT in the same patient shows PTV1, PTV2, and PTV3 displayed by the light blue, dark blue, and yellow lines, respectively. An IMRT plan was generated to treat these volumes to 25 Gy, 45 Gy, and 64.8 Gy, respectively. The colorwash shows the 25 Gy, 45 Gy, and 64 Gy surface in light blue, green, and orange, respectively.

Recurrent Breast Cancer, IMRT Plan

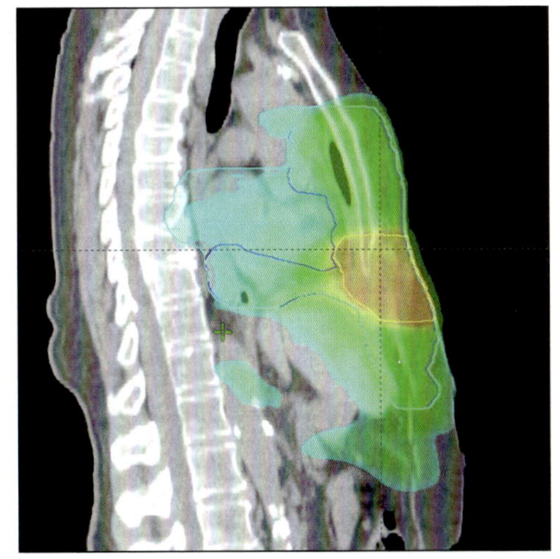

Recurrent Breast Cancer, IMRT Plan

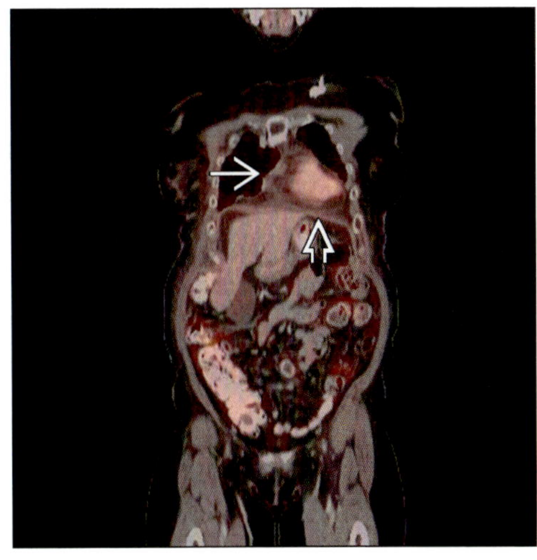

(Left) Sagittal view in the same patient shows sparing of posterior structures by the IMRT plan. *(Right)* 6 months after RT, the same patient shows a complete metabolic response. Note lack of avidity in mediastinum ➡ and diaphragm ➡.

Contralateral Breast Cancer Recurrence

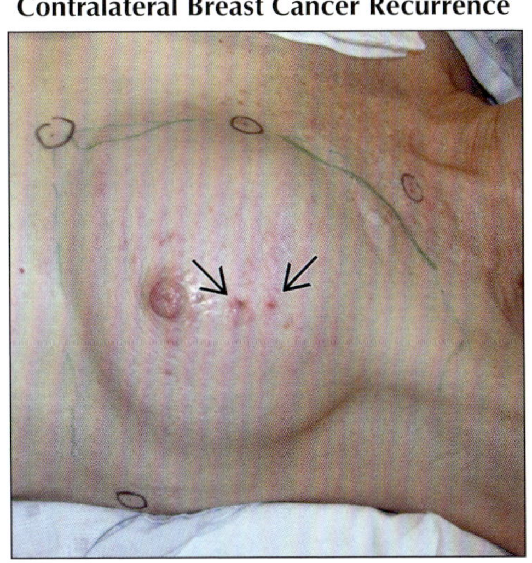

Contralateral Breast Cancer Recurrence

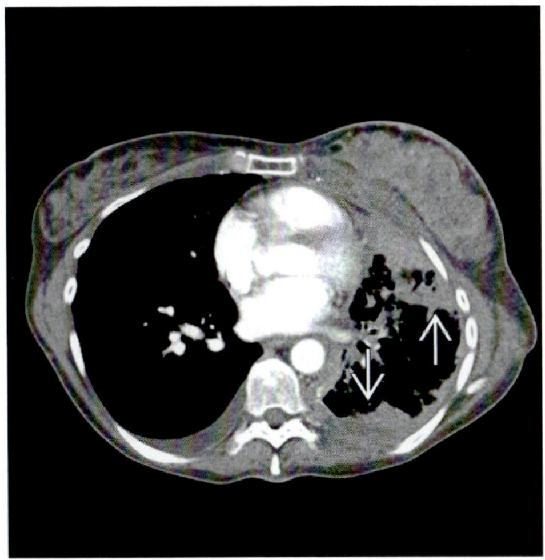

(Left) This patient with a 9-year history of breast cancer developed skin involvement ➡ and pain in the left breast after multiple different treatments with chemotherapy. RT was used for palliation. *(Right)* Axial CECT shows enlargement of the left breast and extensive pleural disease ➡.

BREAST

(Left) In the same patient, customized bolus is used to prevent air gaps. Note use of tape to keep bolus in contact with skin. *(Right)* In the same patient, chain mail bolus can be used to increase skin dose. Chain mail is more deformable than standard tissue equivalent bolus.

Contralateral Breast Cancer Recurrence

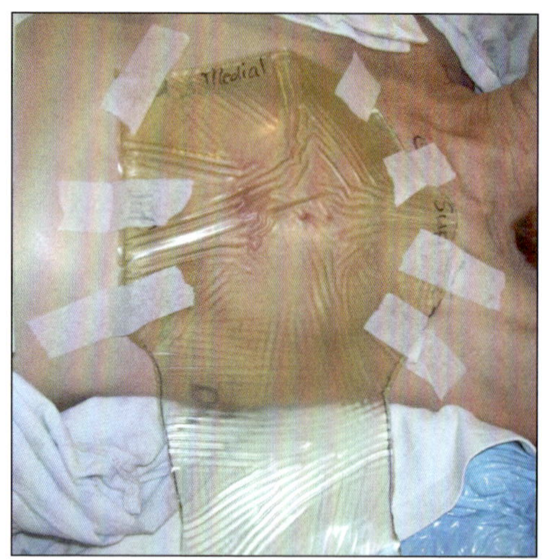

Contralateral Breast Cancer Recurrence

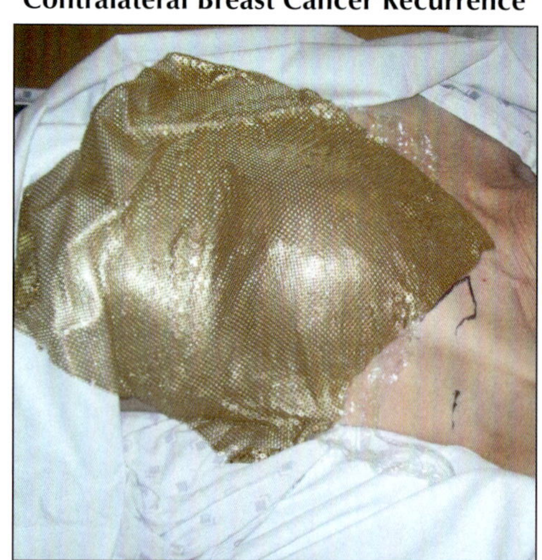

(Left) Neglected breast cancer demonstrates severe contraction (automastectomy) and skin ulceration. Patient was treated with electrons to central chest and anterior photons to lateral chest wall and supraclavicular region. *(Right)* Same patient shows contraction of breast ➔ and disease extending to pleural surface ⮚. Bolus is used as a range modifier to reduce dose to heart. Yellow, cyan, green, and red lines represent 100%, 90%, 80%, and 60% isodose lines, respectively.

Neglected Breast Cancer

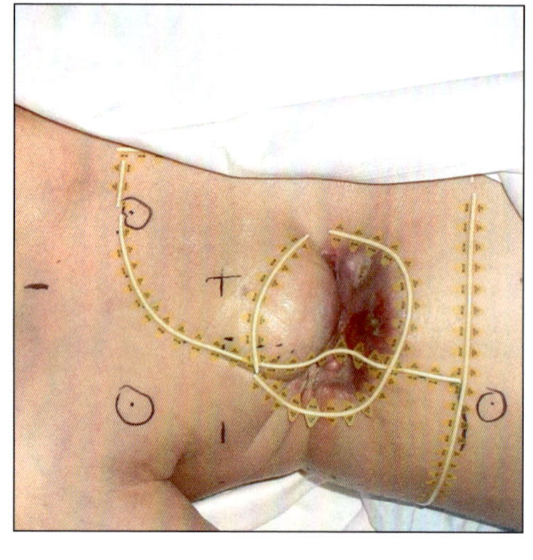

Neglected Breast Cancer

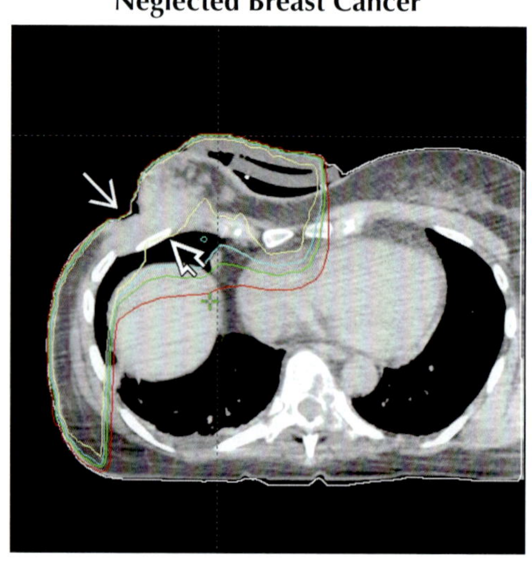

(Left) The same patient in the sagittal plane shows approximately the 90% isodose line ➔ conforming to the pleural surface. *(Right)* This image shows extensive cutaneous chest wall and arm disease being treated for palliation. The margins are very narrow since the patient had previously received RT. Clear delineation of previous tattoos is essential for accurate daily treatments.

Neglected Breast Cancer

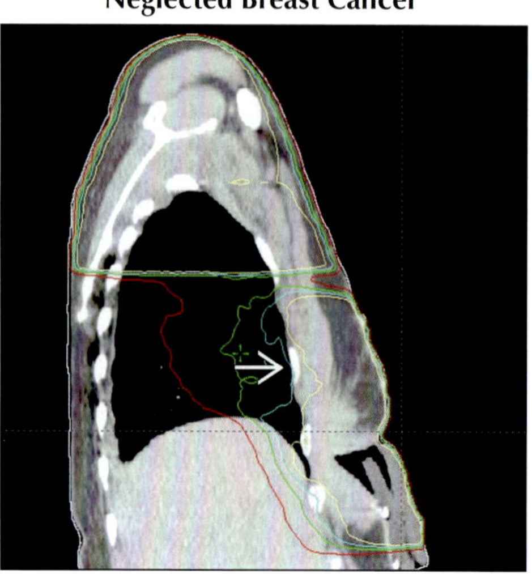

Recurrent Breast Cancer

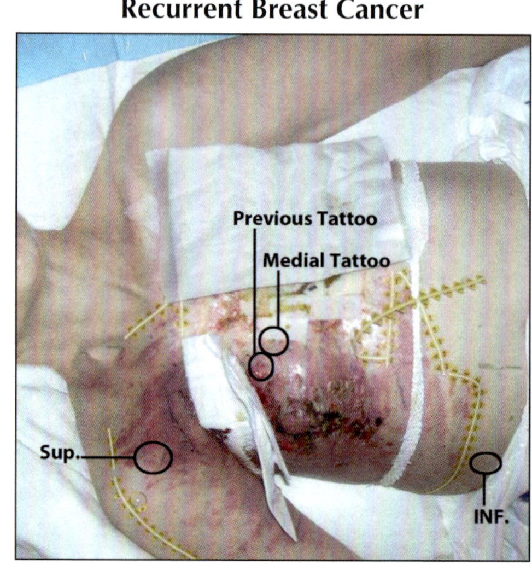

Neglected Breast Cancer, T4c N3 M0

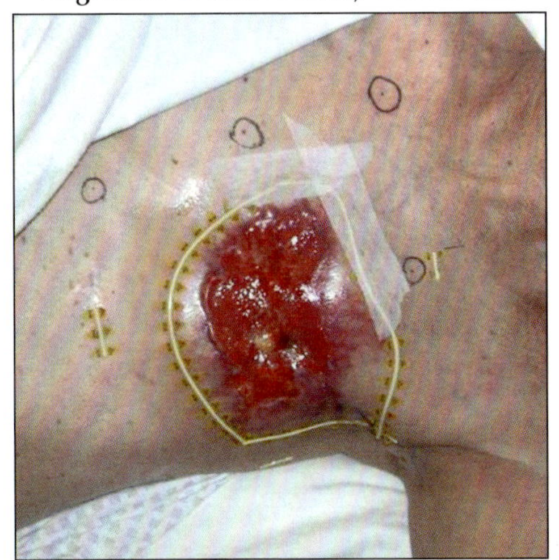

Neglected Breast Cancer, T4c N3 M0

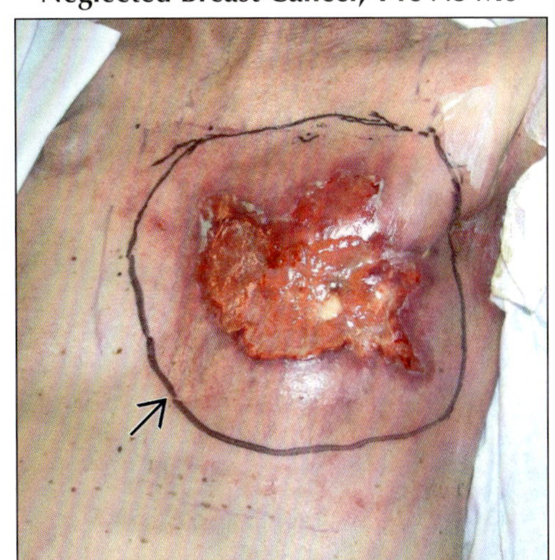

(Left) *This patient presented with a left breast mass that had been present for years. Severe contraction causing auto-mastectomy was evident. The patient underwent neoadjuvant chemotherapy and continued to have a large area of ulceration.* ***(Right)*** *The same patient was treated with comprehensive chest wall and nodal RT. Clinical photo was obtained at 50 Gy. Areas of healing of the epithelium have already begun. The patient then underwent an 18 Gy electron boost ➙.*

Neglected Breast Cancer, T4c N3 M0

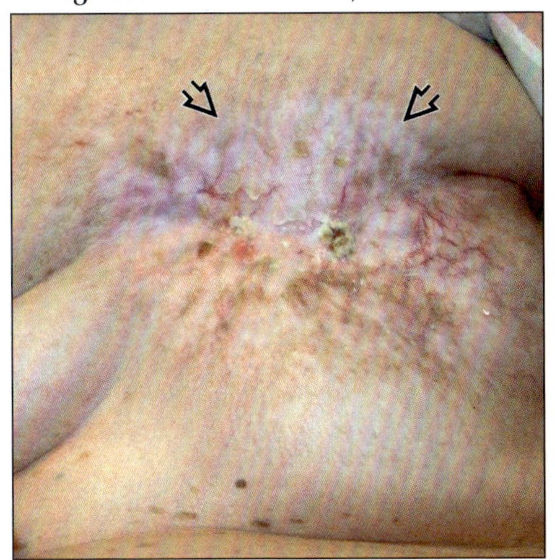

Stage IV (T3 N2 M1)

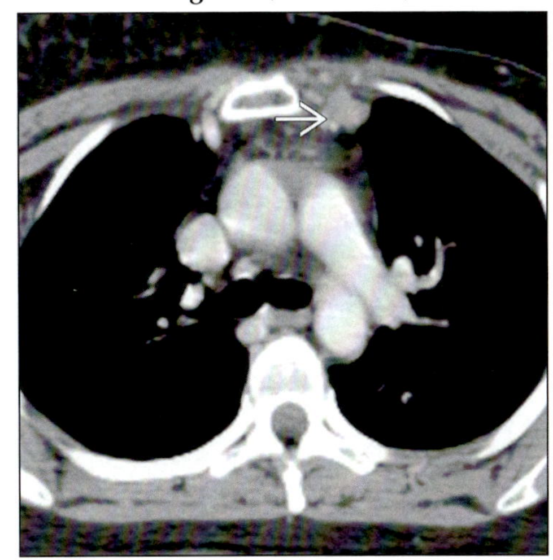

(Left) *The same patient 1 year later exhibits dense scarring ➪ but complete healing of the open ulcer.* ***(Right)*** *Axial CECT shows an enlarged left internal mammary lymph node ➡, worrisome for additional metastatic disease. This was markedly avid on PET.*

Stage IV (T3 N2 M1)

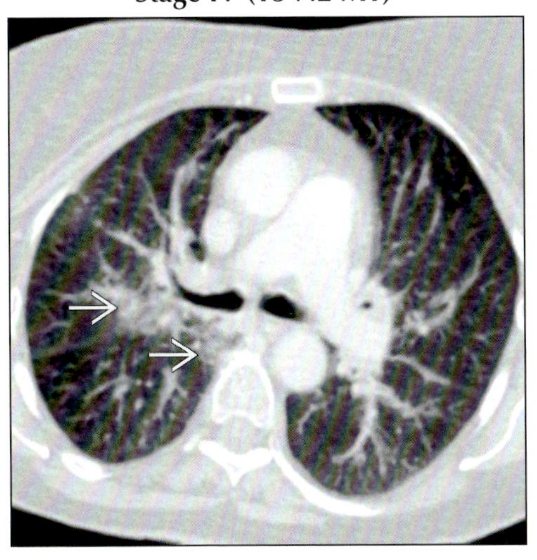

Stage IV (T3 N2 M1)

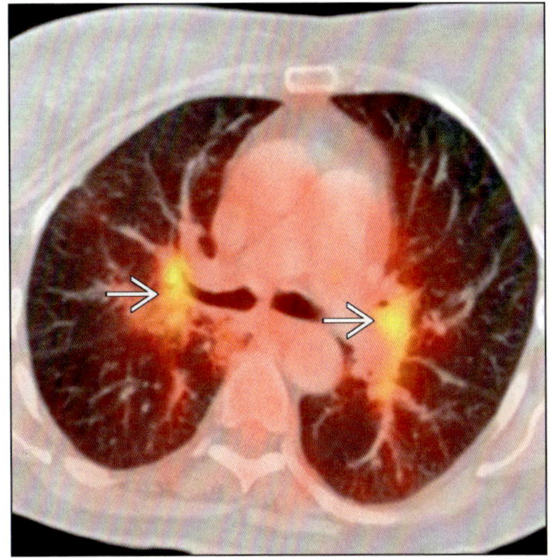

(Left) *Axial CECT in the same patient shows central nodularity ➡ along the interlobular pulmonary septum, worrisome for lymphangitic spread of tumor.* ***(Right)*** *Axial fused PET/CT shows abnormally increased FDG activity ➡ along the inferior perihilar areas, corresponding to the nodularity along the septa, compatible with lymphangitic spread of tumor. The overall stage of this patient would be IV (T3 N2 M1).*

*(**Left**) Coronal bone scan in a patient with a history of breast cancer shows a focal area of increased tracer activity ➔ in the skull, compatible with recurrent metastatic disease. (**Right**) Coronal bone scan in a patient with a history of breast cancer shows widespread recurrent metastatic disease ➔ involving the majority of the vertebral bodies, ribs, and bones of the pelvis.*

Recurrent Breast Cancer

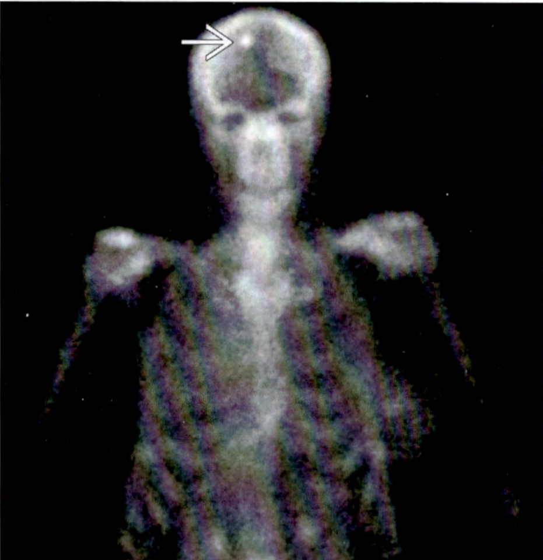

Recurrent Breast Cancer

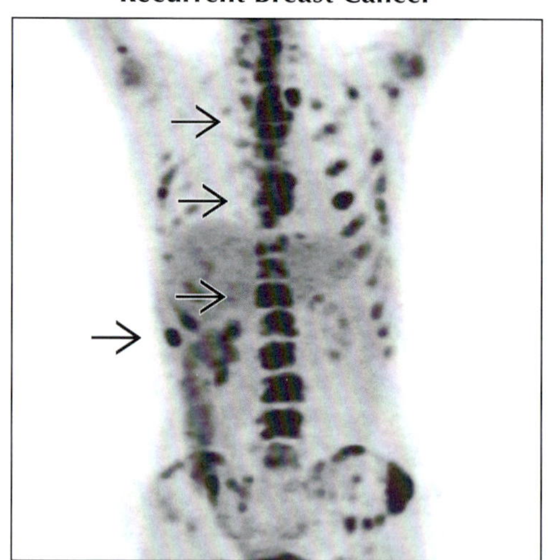

*(**Left**) Axial CECT in a patient with a history of breast cancer status post left mastectomy shows superficial and subcutaneous nodularity ➔, worrisome for local regional recurrence of breast cancer. (**Right**) Axial fused PET/CT in the same patient shows intense FDG activity ➔ corresponding to the superficial and subcutaneous nodular lesions, confirming local recurrence.*

Recurrent Breast Cancer

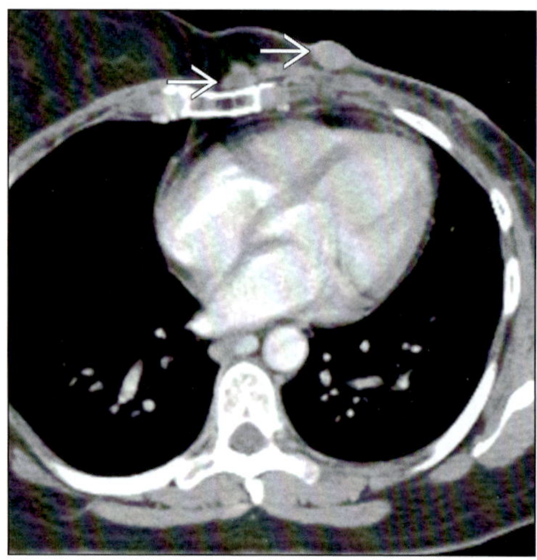

Recurrent Breast Cancer

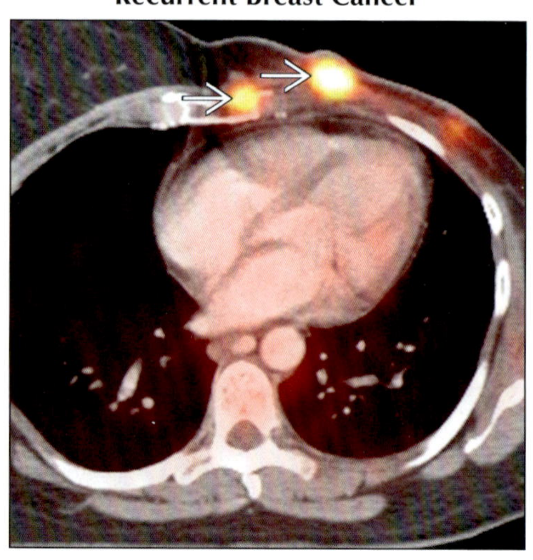

*(**Left**) The most common retinal tumor ➔ is metastatic carcinoma. This patient had vision loss and MR with contrast showed small brain parenchymal lesions (not shown). She was treated to 37.5 Gy in 15 fractions and vision returned. (**Right**) Follow-up axial MR with gadolinium shows a CR after RT. Brain parenchymal lesions regrew after 17 months, and the patient underwent stereotactic radiosurgery.*

Metastatic Disease

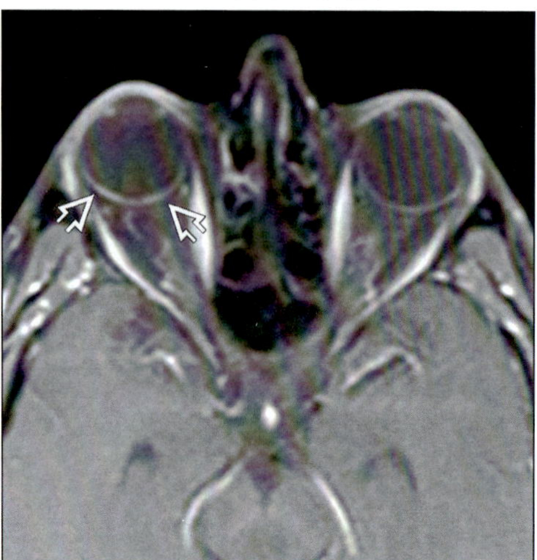

Metastatic Disease

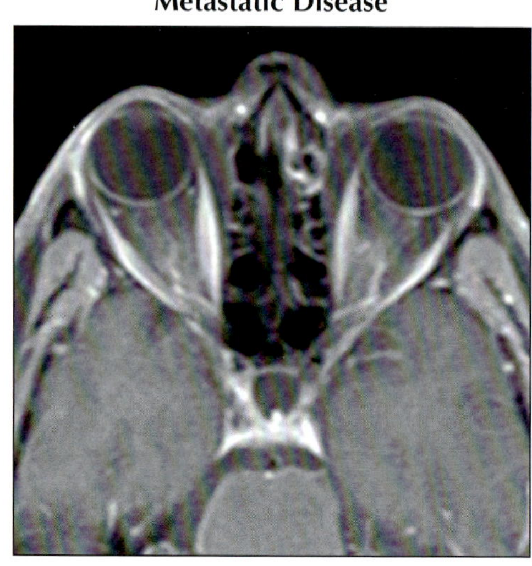

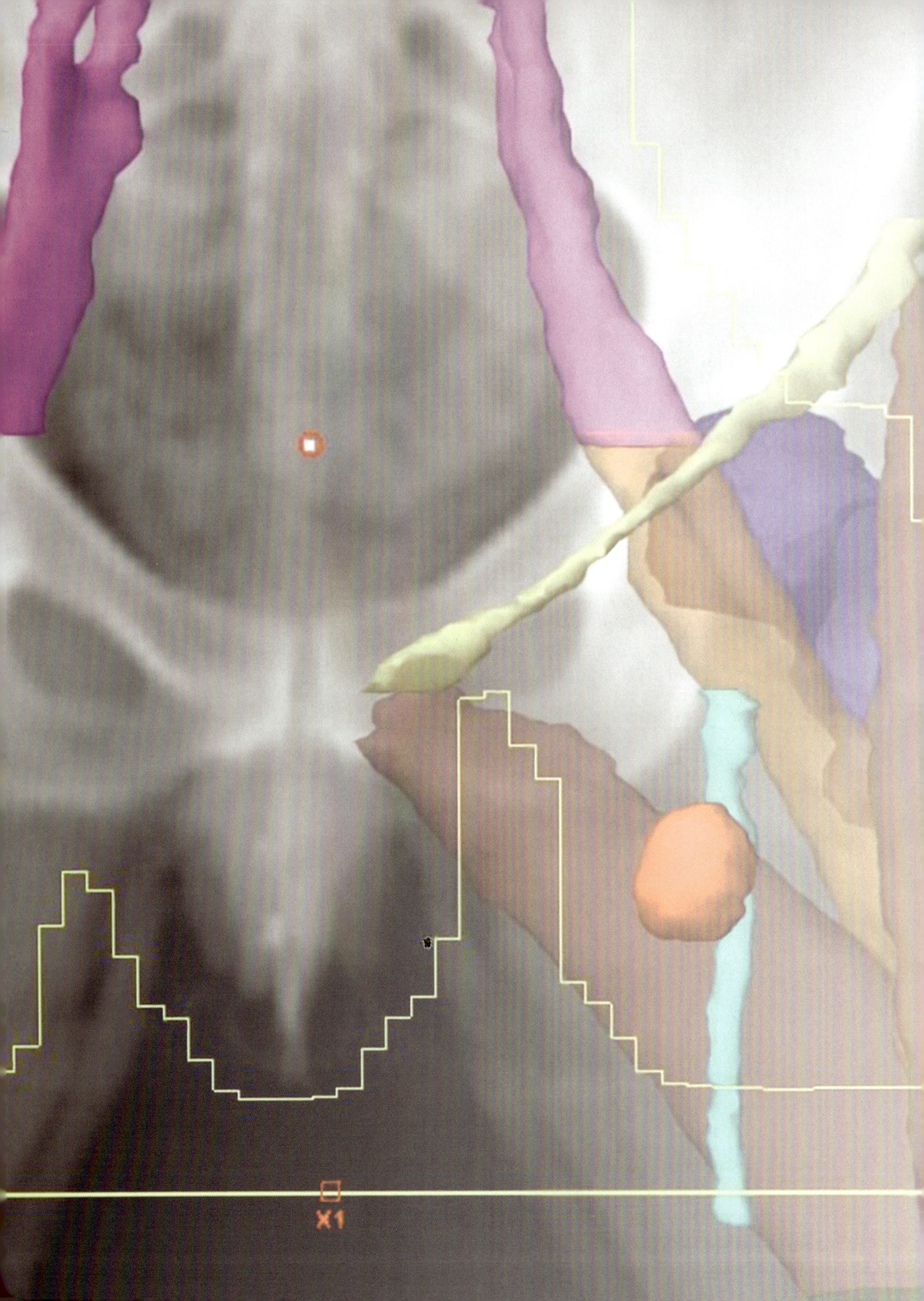
X1

SECTION 5
Gastrointestinal System

ESOPHAGUS

(T) Primary Tumor

Adapted from 7th edition AJCC Staging Forms.

TNM	*Definitions*
TX	Primary tumor cannot be assessed
T0	No evidence of primary tumor
Tis	High-grade dysplasia*
T1	Tumor invades lamina propria, muscularis mucosae, or submucosa
T1a	Tumor invades lamina propria or muscularis mucosae
T1b	Tumor invades submucosa
T2	Tumor invades muscularis propria
T3	Tumor invades adventitia
T4	Tumor invades adjacent structures
T4a	Resectable tumor invading pleura, pericardium, or diaphragm
T4b	Unresectable tumor invading other adjacent structures, such as aorta, vertebral body, trachea, etc.

(N) Regional Lymph Nodes

NX	Regional lymph nodes cannot be assessed
N0	No regional lymph node metastasis
N1	Metastasis in 1-2 regional lymph nodes
N2	Metastasis in 3-6 regional lymph nodes
N3	Metastasis in ≥ 7 regional lymph nodes

(M) Distant Metastasis

M0	No distant metastasis
M1	Distant metastasis

(G) Histologic Grade

GX	Grade cannot be assessed; stage grouping as G1
G1	Well differentiated
G2	Moderately differentiated
G3	Poorly differentiated
G4	Undifferentiated; stage grouping as G3 squamous

At least maximal dimension of the tumor must be recorded; multiple tumors require the T(m) suffix. Number must be recorded for total number of regional nodes sampled and total number of reported nodes with metastasis.

**High-grade dysplasia includes all noninvasive neoplastic epithelia that were formerly called carcinoma in situ, a diagnosis that is no longer used for columnar mucosae anywhere in the gastrointestinal tract.*

ESOPHAGUS

AJCC Stages/Prognostic Groups for Adenocarcinoma

Adapted from 7th edition AJCC Staging Forms.

Stage	*T*	*N*	*M*	*G*
0	Tis	N0	M0	G1, GX
IA	T1	N0	M0	G1-2, GX
IB	T1	N0	M0	G3
	T2	N0	M0	G1-2, GX
IIA	T2	N0	M0	G3
IIB	T3	N0	M0	Any G
	T1-2	N1	M0	Any G
IIIA	T1-2	N2	M0	Any G
	T3	N1	M0	Any G
	T4a	N0	M0	Any G
IIIB	T3	N2	M0	Any G
IIIC	T4a	N1-2	M0	Any G
	T4b	Any N	M0	Any G
	Any T	N3	M0	Any G
IV	Any T	Any N	M1	Any G

AJCC Stages/Prognostic Groups for Squamous Cell Carcinoma[1]

Adapted from 7th edition AJCC Staging Forms.

Stage	*T*	*N*	*M*	*G*	*Location*[2]
0	Tis	N0	M0	G1, GX	Any location
IA	T1	N0	M0	G1, GX	Any location
IB	T1	N0	M0	G2-3	Any location
	T2-3	N0	M0	G1, GX	Lower, X
IIA	T2-3	N0	M0	G1, GX	Upper, middle
	T2-3	N0	M0	G2-3	Lower, X
IIB	T2-3	N0	M0	G2-3	Upper, middle
	T1-2	N1	M0	Any G	Any location
IIIA	T1-2	N2	M0	Any G	Any location
	T3	N1	M0	Any G	Any location
	T4a	N0	M0	Any G	Any location
IIIB	T3	N2	M0	Any G	Any location
IIIC	T4a	N1-2	M0	Any G	Any location
	T4b	Any N	M0	Any G	Any location
	Any T	N3	M0	Any G	Any location
IV	Any T	Any N	M1	Any G	Any location

[1]*Or mixed histology including a squamous component or NOS.*

[2]*Location of the primary cancer site is defined by the position of the upper (proximal) edge of the tumor in the esophagus.*

T1a

High magnification shows malignant cells ➔ with gland formation invading into bundles of muscularis mucosae ➔.

T2

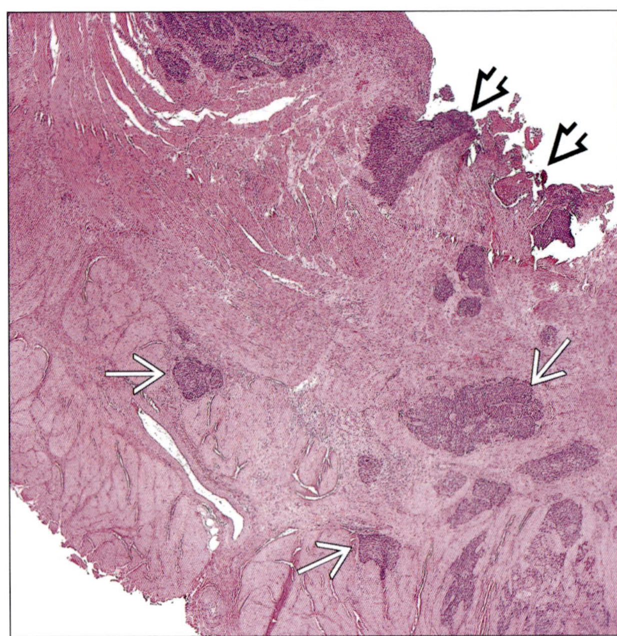

H&E stained section of an esophageal resection specimen shows denuded esophageal mucosa at the luminal aspect ➔. The invasive esophageal carcinoma cells ➔ invade through, but not beyond, the muscularis propria.

T3

H&E stained section shows esophageal carcinoma → extending beyond the muscularis propria ➔ into the fibrofatty tissue ↗ of the adventitia. The inset shows a higher magnification of the invasive neoplastic cells arranged in gland formation.

T4b

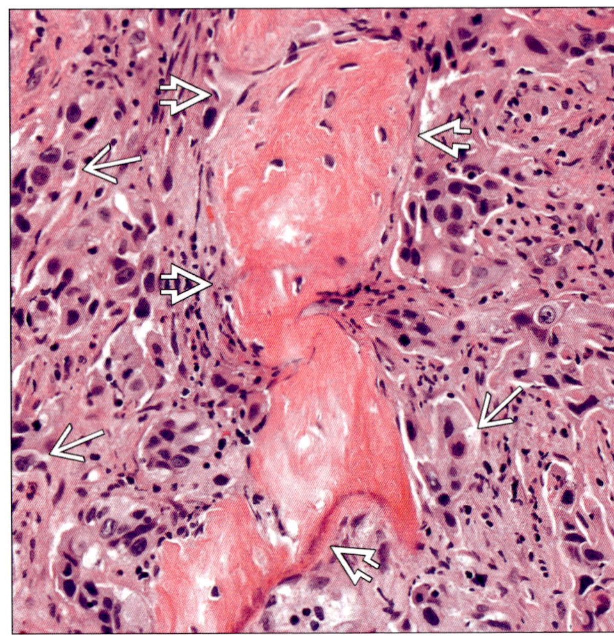

Photomicrograph shows esophageal carcinoma ➔ extending to invade a vertebral body. Bony trabecula ➔ is seen surrounded by tumor. Unresectable tumor invading other adjacent structures is classified as T4b.

T1a

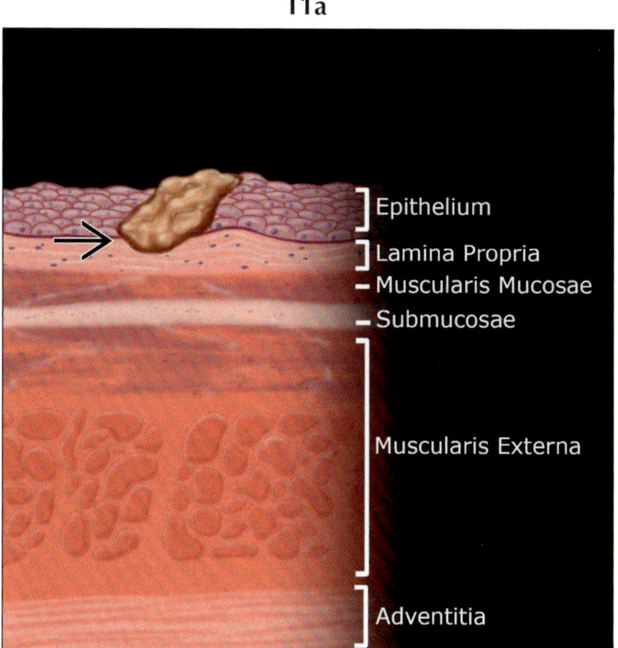

Graphic shows tumor invading lamina propria ➙.

T1b

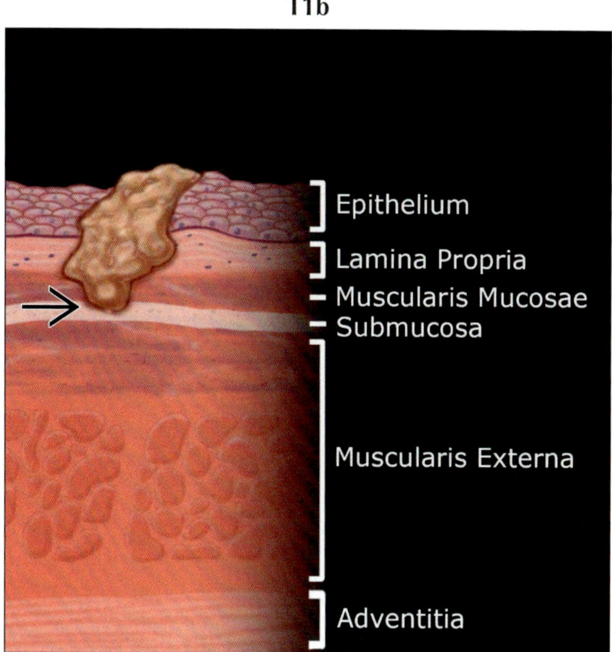

Graphic shows tumor extending into submucosa ➙.

T2

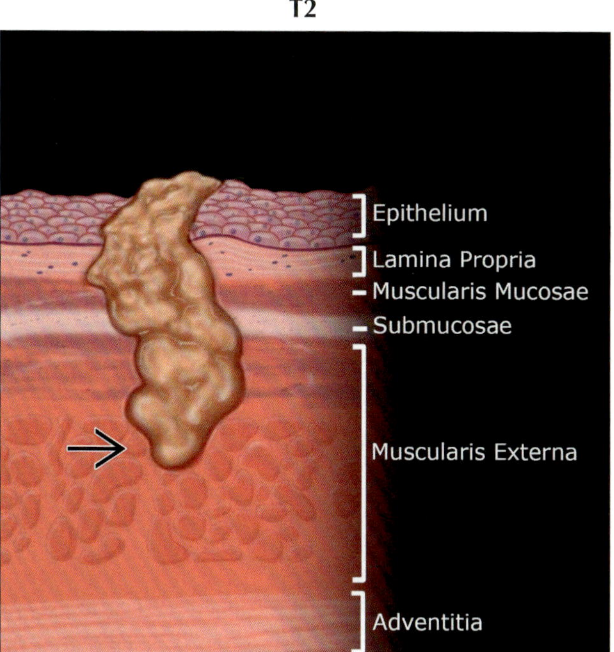

Graphic shows tumor invading muscularis propria ➙.

T3

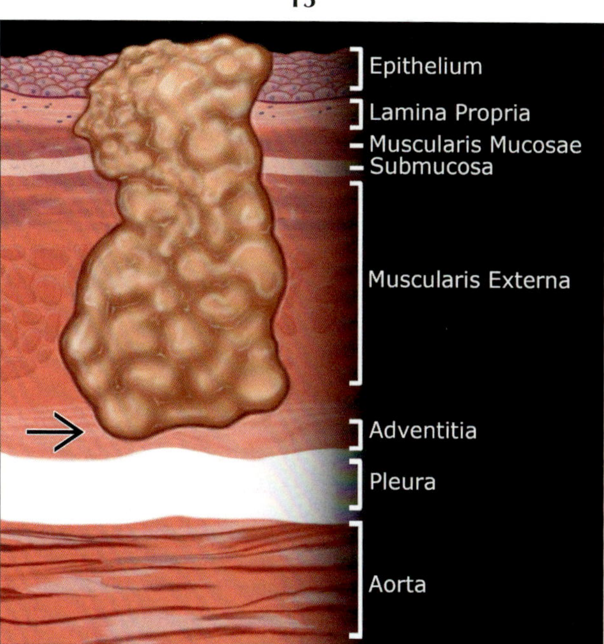

Graphic shows tumor extending to adventitia ➙.

T3

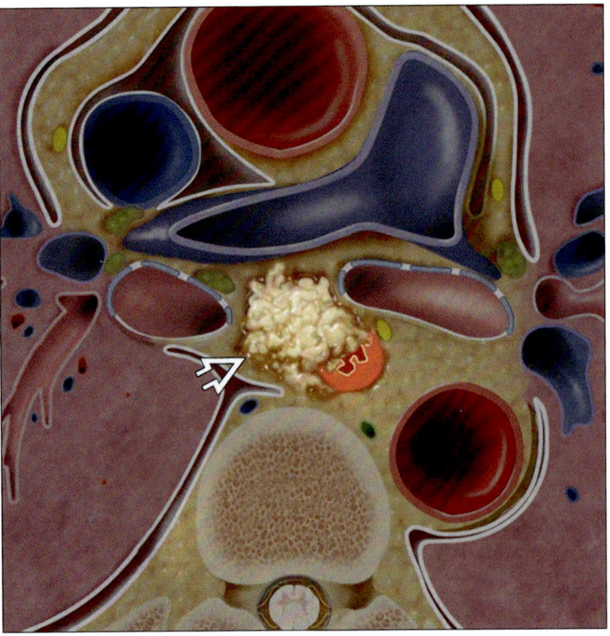

Graphic illustrates T3 tumor ➔ invading through the adventitia and into the mediastinal fat, without invading the surrounding mediastinal structures.

T4a

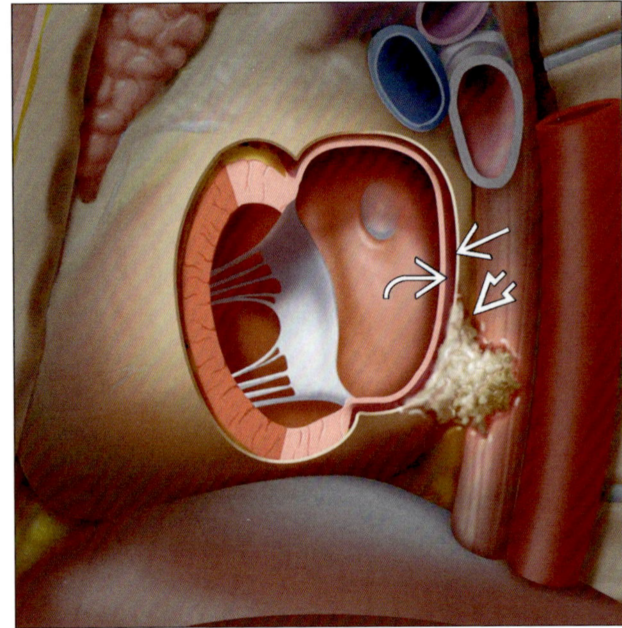

Graphic illustrates T4a tumor ➔ invading the pericardium →, separated from the heart by a thin epicardial fat layer ↪. T4a tumors are potentially resectable.

T4b

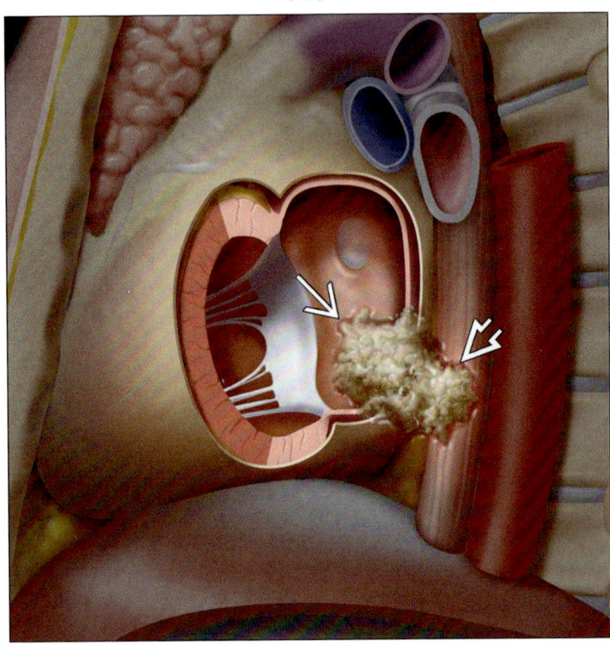

Graphic illustrates T4b tumor ➔ invading the heart →. Tumors that invade aorta, carotid vessels, azygos vein, trachea, left main bronchus, and vertebral body are also T4b. T4b tumors are unresectable.

Regional Drainage of Esophageal Carcinoma

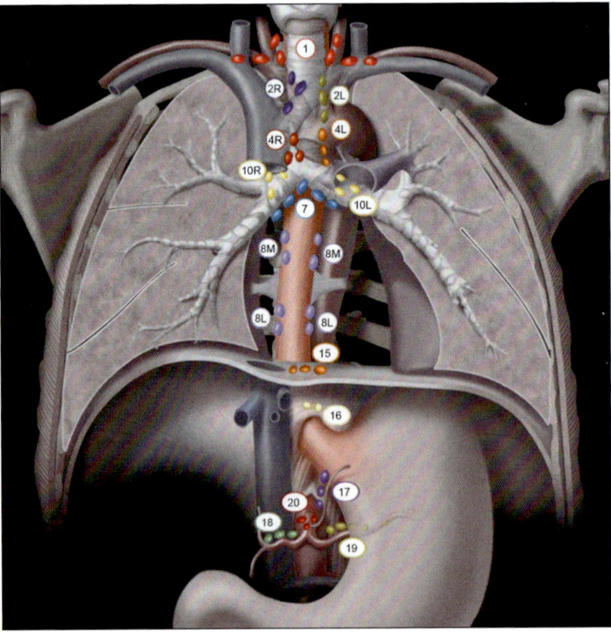

1: Supraclavicular; 2R: Right upper paratracheal; 2L: Left upper paratracheal; 4R: Right lower paratracheal; 4L: Left lower paratracheal; 7: Subcarinal; 8: Paraesophageal; 9: Pulmonary ligament; 10R: Right tracheobronchial; 10L: Left tracheobronchial; 15: Diaphragmatic; 16: Paracardial; 17: Left gastric; 18: Common hepatic; 19: Splenic; 20: Celiac.

Regional Nodal Drainage of Esophageal Carcinoma (Right Side)

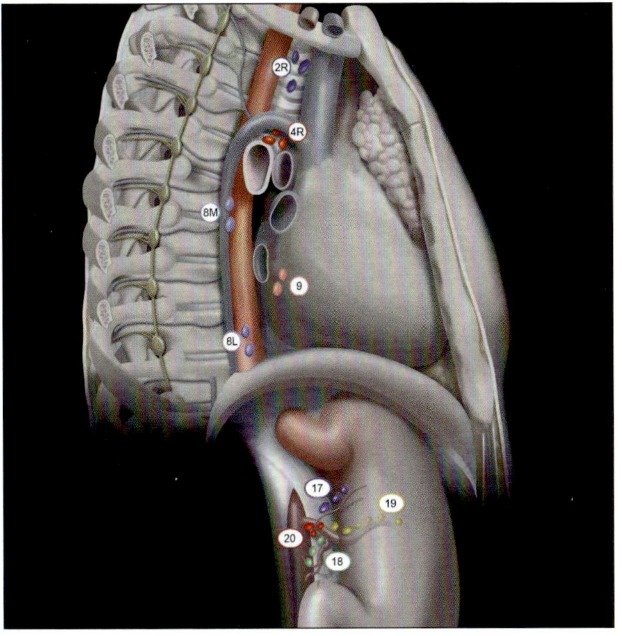

2R: Right upper paratracheal; 4R: Right lower paratracheal; 8M: Middle paraesophageal; 8L: Right lower paraesophageal; 9: Pulmonary ligament; 17: Left gastric; 18: Common hepatic; 19: Splenic; 20: Celiac nodes.

Regional Nodal Drainage of Esophageal Carcinoma (Left Side)

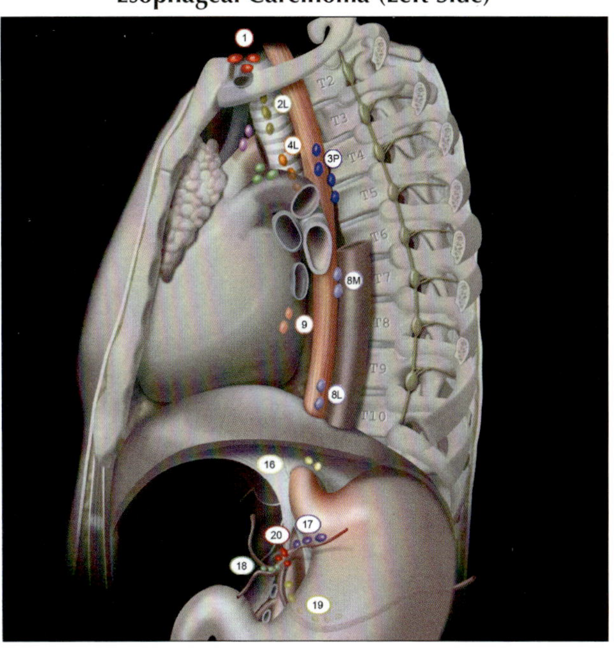

1: Supraclavicular; 2L: Left upper paratracheal (PT); 3P: Posterior mediastinal; 4L: Left lower PT; 8M: Middle paraesophageal (PE); 8L: Left lower PE; 9: Pulmonary ligament; 16: Paracardial; 17: Left gastric; 18: Common hepatic; 19: Splenic; 20: Celiac nodes.

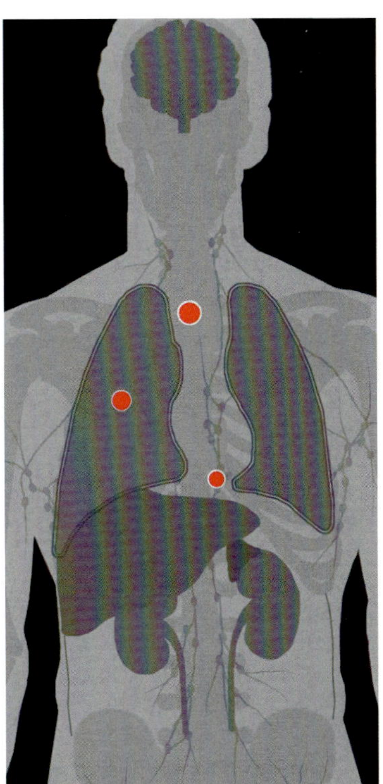

INITIAL SITE OF RECURRENCE

Persistent Disease	26%
Local Regional Failure	17%
Distant Failure	12%
Local Regional and Distant Failure	9%

Data represent 130 patients from the randomized and nonrandomized definitive CRT arms of RTOG 8501 (Herskovic). The most common sites for distant disease in decreasing order include liver, lung, bone, adrenals, peritoneum, and brain.

ESOPHAGUS

OVERVIEW

Classification

- Adenocarcinoma (AC) 60-80% of esophageal cancers in United States; rapid ↑ in past 2 decades
- Squamous cell carcinoma (SCC) ~ 20-40%
  - SCC variants
    - Basaloid carcinoma
    - Spindle cell carcinoma
    - Verrucous carcinoma
    - Lymphoepithelioma-like carcinoma
- Other esophageal cancers
  - Melanoma
  - Malignant stromal tumors
  - Carcinoid
  - Lymphoma
  - Other rare carcinomas

NATURAL HISTORY

General Features

- Comments
  - Determination of tumor location is important
    - Surgical planning is affected
    - Site of primary tumor can affect tumor stage in case of SCC
      - T2-3 N0 M0 tumor in lower esophagus is stage IB whereas similar tumor in upper or middle esophagus is stage IIA
  - Tumor location is best expressed as distance from incisors as measured endoscopically
  - Esophageal anatomical divisions
    - Cervical esophagus
      - Bordered superiorly by hypopharynx and inferiorly by thoracic outlet (at level of sternal notch)
      - Typically 15-20 cm from incisors
      - Thickening of esophageal wall begins above sternal notch
      - Related to trachea, carotid sheath, and vertebrae
    - Upper thoracic esophagus
      - Bordered superiorly by thoracic outlet (at level of sternal notch) and inferiorly by lower border of azygos vein
      - Typically 20-25 cm from incisors
      - Thickening of esophageal wall begins between sternal notch and azygos vein
      - Related to trachea, arch vessels, great veins, and vertebrae
    - Middle thoracic esophagus
      - Bordered superiorly by lower border of azygos vein and inferiorly by inferior pulmonary vein
      - Typically 25-30 cm from incisors
      - Thickening of esophageal wall begins between azygos vein and inferior pulmonary vein
      - Related to pulmonary hilum, descending thoracic aorta, pleura, and vertebrae
    - Lower thoracic esophagus
      - Bordered superiorly by inferior pulmonary vein and inferiorly by stomach, including gastroesophageal junction (GEJ)
      - Typically 30-40 cm from incisors
      - Thickening of esophageal wall begins below inferior pulmonary vein
      - Related to pericardium, descending thoracic aorta, and vertebrae
    - Abdominal esophagus
      - Tumors of GEJ or those with epicenter in proximal stomach (5 cm of gastric cardia) with extension to GEJ are grouped with esophageal carcinoma

Etiology

- AC
  - Associated with gastroesophageal reflux
    - Obesity may contribute by increasing intraabdominal pressure
    - Weekly symptoms = 8x increased risk of AC
  - Barrett esophagus
    - Associated with development of > 95% of ACs
    - Normally mucosa changes from squamous to columnar at GEJ
    - Progressive columnar metaplasia of distal esophagus
    - Overall prevalence of AC in patients with Barrett esophagus is 5-28%
  - Associated with prior radiation therapy (RT) (breast, mediastinal cancer)
- SCC
  - Esophagus normally lined with stratified squamous epithelium
    - Carcinoma develops from progression of premalignant or dysplastic precursor lesions
    - Carcinomas associated with dysplasia more likely to be multifocal
  - Tobacco use
    - Tobacco carcinogens in saliva contact esophageal mucosa
    - Higher quantity and duration of smoking → higher risk
  - Alcohol abuse
    - Chronic irritation of esophageal mucosa
  - Synergetic effect of alcohol and tobacco use
  - Associated with low socioeconomic status, chronic irritation (tobacco, alcohol, chemicals, bacteria), caustic injury, prior radiation (breast, mediastinum)
  - Increased incidence in patients with esophageal achalasia

Epidemiology & Cancer Incidence

- Number of cases in USA per year
  - Increasing incidence and mortality since 1975, with dramatic increase in AC
  - Estimated 17,460 new cases of esophageal AC and SCC diagnosed in USA in 2012
  - 6th leading cause of cancer death worldwide
    - Estimated 15,070 deaths in USA in 2012
  - Esophageal AC more common than SCC in USA
    - Incidence of AC is rapidly increasing since 1970s
    - Incidence of SCC is stable to declining
- Esophageal SCC more common worldwide than AC
  - Responsible for as much as 90% of cases
- Large geographic variation in incidence: High incidence in northern China
- Sex predilection
  - Lifetime risk: 0.8% for men; 0.3% for women
    - AC: M:F = 7:1

- SCC: M:F = 3:1
- Highest incidence in USA among African-American men
  - 13 per 100,000
- Age of onset
  - Mean age at diagnosis is 67 years old

Genetics

- AC
  - Probable with Barrett esophagus
    - Frequent chromosome loss/gain/amplification
- SCC
  - High predisposition in patients with nonepidermolytic palmoplantar keratoderma (tylosis)
    - Rare
    - 95% risk of esophageal SCC by 70 years of age
    - Autosomal dominant
    - Abnormal 17q25 chromosome

Associated Diseases, Abnormalities

- Predisposing conditions
  - Chronic stasis
  - Lye strictures
  - Head and neck tumors
  - Celiac disease
- Complications
  - Tracheoesophageal fistula
  - Bleeding from erosions

Gross Pathology & Surgical Features

- AC
  - Masses or nodules in esophageal mucosa, usually in distal 1/3 of esophagus
  - Patterns
    - Polypoid (5-10%)
    - Infiltrating (40-50%)
    - Fungating (20-25%)
    - Flat (10-15%)
- SCC
  - Superficial lesions
    - White/gray plaques on mucosal surface
  - 3 patterns found in deeper lesions
    - Polypoid (60%)
      - Protrudes into esophageal lumen
    - Ulcerative (25%)
      - May erode into aorta, trachea, pericardium
    - Infiltrative (15%)
      - Causes luminal narrowing of esophagus, may ulcerate
  - Location
    - Proximal 1/3 (10-20%)
    - Middle 1/3 (50-60%)
    - Distal 1/3 (30%)

Microscopic Pathology

- H&E
  - AC
    - Well differentiated
      - Cells cuboidal to columnar in shape, irregular nucleoli, and variable amount of eosinophilic or clear cytoplasm
    - Moderately differentiated
      - Cells arranged in solid nests or clusters; may display cribriform pattern and show stratification
    - Poorly differentiated
      - Often diffusely infiltrates esophageal wall in sheets of cells with poorly formed glands
  - SCC
    - Well differentiated
      - Intracellular bridges and abundant keratinization
    - Moderately differentiated
      - ↑ in primitive basaloid cells, only focal keratinization
    - Poorly differentiated
      - No keratinization, contains large pleomorphic cells
    - May see various degrees of differentiation within single tumor
- Special stains
  - Lugol iodine may identify areas of dysplasia

Routes of Spread

- Local spread
  - No anatomic barrier to prevent local extension of tumor into mediastinum
    - Esophageal wall lacks serosa, attached to neighboring structures by only loose connective adventitia
  - Esophageal cancer can invade adjacent structures in neck or thorax, including
    - Upper esophagus: Trachea, thyroid gland, larynx
    - Middle esophagus: Trachea, bronchi, aorta, lung, pericardium
    - Lower esophagus: Aorta, lung, pericardium, diaphragm
- Lymphatic extension
  - Rich lymphatic plexus → early lymph node involvement
  - Flow of lymph in upper 2/3 of esophagus tends to be upward; in distal 1/3 tends to be downward
    - Tumors in upper esophagus more likely to spread to cervical or mediastinal nodes
    - Tumors in distal esophagus more likely to spread to abdominal lymph nodes
  - All lymphatic channels intercommunicate
    - Lymphatic fluid from any portion of esophagus allows spread to any draining regional nodes
  - Nodal stations as described by AJCC
    - 1: Supraclavicular nodes (paraesophageal)
      - Above suprasternal notch and clavicles
    - 2R: Right upper paratracheal nodes
      - Between intersection of caudal margin of innominate artery with trachea and lung apex
    - 2L: Left upper paratracheal nodes
      - Between top of aortic arch and lung apex
    - 3P: Posterior mediastinal nodes
      - Upper paraesophageal nodes, above tracheal bifurcation
    - 4R: Right lower paratracheal nodes
      - Between intersection of caudal margin of innominate artery with trachea and cephalic border of azygous vein
    - 4L: Left lower paratracheal nodes
      - Between top of aortic arch and carina
    - 7: Subcarinal nodes
      - Caudal to tracheal carina
    - 8M: Middle paraesophageal nodes

- From tracheal bifurcation to caudal margin of inferior pulmonary vein
- 8L: Lower paraesophageal nodes
  - From caudal margin of inferior pulmonary vein to esophagogastric junction
- 9: Pulmonary ligament nodes
  - Within inferior pulmonary ligament
- 10R: Right tracheobronchial nodes
  - From cephalic border of azygous vein to origin of right upper lung bronchus
- 10L: Left tracheobronchial nodes
  - Between carina and left upper lung bronchus
- 15: Diaphragmatic nodes
  - Lying on dome of diaphragm and adjacent to or behind its crura
- 16: Paracardial nodes
  - Immediately adjacent to GEJ
- 17: Left gastric nodes
  - Along course of left gastric artery
- 18: Common hepatic nodes
  - Along course of common hepatic artery
- 19: Splenic nodes
  - Along course of splenic artery
- 20: Celiac nodes
  - At base of celiac artery

- Hematogenous spread
  - Most common sites, in descending order
    - Liver
    - Lungs
    - Bones
    - Adrenal glands
    - Peritoneum
    - Brain
- Pleural or peritoneal seeding
  - Pleural seeding follows tumor extension to parietal pleura
  - Peritoneal seeding is usually secondary to abdominal or retroperitoneal lymph node metastases

IMAGING

Detection

- Endoscopy
  - Gold standard for diagnosis
  - Endoscopic biopsy establishes histologic diagnosis
- Esophagogram (barium swallow)
  - Imaging appearances
    - Annular constriction
      - Irregular stricture
    - Polypoid
      - Intraluminal filling defect
    - Infiltrative
      - May cause luminal narrowing
    - Ulcerated mass
      - Central collection of barium
- CECT
  - Irregular, thick, enhancing esophageal wall
    - Normal distended esophageal wall is usually < 3 mm thick
    - Any wall thickness > 5 mm is considered abnormal
    - Wall thickening is usually asymmetric
  - Luminal narrowing, usually eccentric
  - Proximal esophageal dilatation
- PET/CT
  - Higher sensitivity than CT
    - Helpful in patients with metastases of unknown origin

Staging

- T staging
  - **Endoscopic ultrasound (EUS)**
    - Most accurate modality for T staging
      - Accurately predicts depth of invasion in 80-90% of patients
      - Can differentiate between T1, T2, and T3 disease
    - 7.5 and 12 MHz
      - Esophageal wall seen as 5 alternating layers of differing echogenicity
      - 1st hyperechoic layer: Interface between balloon and superficial mucosa
      - 2nd hypoechoic layer: Lamina propria and muscularis mucosae
      - 3rd hyperechoic layer: Submucosa
      - 4th hypoechoic layer: Muscularis propria
      - 5th hyperechoic layer: Interface between serosa and surrounding tissues
    - 20 MHz
      - 9 layers can be distinguished
    - Improved accuracy with higher T stage
      - T1: 75-82%
      - T2: 64-82%
      - T3: 89-94%
      - T4: 88-100%
    - Limitations
      - Operator dependent
      - Stenotic tumors may prevent passage of endoscope
      - Risk of perforation with malignant stricture
      - Insensitive for deep lymph nodes
  - CECT
    - Limited in determining depth of esophageal wall infiltration
    - Unable to adequately differentiate between T1, T2, and T3 disease
    - Accuracy of CT for T stage less than EUS
      - Accuracy of 49-59% for CECT vs. 76-89% for EUS
    - Exclusion or confirmation of T4 disease is most important role of CT in evaluating local disease
    - CT criteria for local invasion include
      - Loss of fat planes with adjacent mediastinal structures
      - Displacement or indentation of other mediastinal structures
    - Aortic invasion is suggested by
      - ≥ 90° of aorta in contact with tumor
      - Obliteration of triangular fat space between esophagus, aorta, and spine next to primary
    - Tracheobronchial invasion is suggested by
      - Displacement of trachea or bronchus
      - Indentation of tracheal or bronchial posterior wall
      - Tracheobronchial fistula or tumor extension into airway lumen
    - Pericardial invasion is suspected if there is
      - Pericardial thickening
      - Pericardial effusion
      - Heart indentation with loss of pericardial fat plane

- Performance of CECT for detection of mediastinal invasion
  - Sensitivity (88-100%)
  - Specificity (85-100%)
- PET/CT
  - Limited value in assessing T stage
    - Depth of tumor invasion cannot be resolved
- N staging
  - Nodal staging depends on number of involved nodes
    - In 6th edition of AJCC cancer staging manual, locoregional lymph nodes were defined on basis of location of primary esophageal tumor
      - Nodes away from primary tumor were metastatic disease
      - Supraclavicular nodes: M1a if primary tumor in cervical esophagus
      - Celiac nodes: M1a disease if primary tumor in lower thoracic esophagus or GEJ
    - In 7th edition of AJCC cancer staging manual
      - Regional nodes are redefined as extending from periesophageal supraclavicular nodes to celiac nodes
      - N stage is subclassified according to number of involved regional nodes
  - **EUS**
    - Criteria for involved nodes on EUS
      - Short axis > 10 mm
      - Round
      - Homogeneous, hypoechoic, central echo
      - Clear border
    - Superior to CT in detecting lymph node metastases
      - Accuracy ranges from 72-80%
      - Sensitivity (79%) & specificity (74%)
    - Improved accuracy with EUS-guided biopsy
  - **CECT**
    - Less accurate than EUS and biopsy
    - Determining involvement of nodes depends on nodal size
      - Intrathoracic and abdominal lymph nodes > 1 cm in diameter
      - Supraclavicular lymph nodes with short axis > 5 mm
    - Limitations
      - Micrometastasis may be found in normal-sized nodes
      - Some enlarged nodes may be reactive
    - Performance of CECT for detection of regional adenopathy
      - Sensitivity (30-60%)
      - Specificity (60-80%)
      - Accuracy (46-58%)
    - Performance of CECT for detection of abdominal nodes
      - Sensitivity (42%)
      - Specificity (93%)
  - **PET/CT**
    - Performance depends on location of lymph nodes in relation to primary tumor
      - Intense uptake of FDG by primary tumor may obscure uptake in adjacent regional lymph nodes
    - Better performance for nodes away from primary tumor
      - Accuracy (86%)
      - Sensitivity of up to 90%
    - PET may confirm that enlarged node is likely metastatic
    - Sensitivity and specificity: 30-57% and 85-90%
      - FDG PET is more sensitive than CT for depicting nodal metastases in patients with esophageal SCC
      - FDG PET is slightly less specific than CT for depicting metastases
      - Low specificity of FDG PET for depiction of nodal metastasis compared with that of CT is caused mainly by high rate of false-positive hilar node interpretations
- M staging
  - **EUS**
    - No role in evaluation of distant metastases
  - **CECT**
    - Liver metastases
      - Ill-defined hypoattenuating lesions
    - Lung metastases
      - Single or multiple nodules
      - Presence of primary lung carcinoma needs to be ruled out in patients with a solitary pulmonary metastasis
  - **PET/CT**
    - Added value for staging over CECT alone
      - In patients with no metastases suspected, PET/CT detects metastases in up to 15%
    - Hypermetabolic activity in liver, lung, bone, peritoneum, nonregional lymph nodes, brain
- **Pleural or peritoneal seeding**
  - Pleural seeding is usually unilateral, may also be bilateral
  - CT demonstrates pleura-based nodules, pleural effusion, and irregular pleural thickening
  - Peritoneal seeding is usually secondary to abdominal or retroperitoneal lymph node metastases
    - Should be suspected when ascites or nodular peritoneal lesions develop

Restaging

- Imaging recommendations
  - PET/CT
    - Added value in differentiating tumor recurrence from post-treatment changes
      - Post-treatment changes may include fibrosis and inflammation, making CT appearance nonspecific
    - Most sensitive method of differentiating chemotherapy responders from nonresponders
    - Perform no sooner than 5 weeks after completion of chemoradiation
- Restaging important after neoadjuvant chemotherapy to determine if patient is surgical candidate
- Esophagectomy not recommended if metastases found on PET/CT restaging

CLINICAL PRESENTATION & WORK-UP

Presentation

- Most common: Dysphagia for solids
- Later: Dysphagia for liquids, odynophagia, weight loss

- If local invasion: Aspiration (tracheoesophageal fistula), bleeding (aortoesophageal fistula)
- If metastases: Lymphadenopathy (Virchow node, left supraclavicular fossa), hepatomegaly, pleural effusion

Prognosis

- More than 1/2 of patients present with unresectable disease/metastases
- Survival rates at 5 years
  - Overall: 14%
  - Stage 0: > 95%
  - Stage I: 50-80%
  - Stage IIA: 30-40%
  - Stage IIB: 10-30%
  - Stage III: 10-15%
  - Stage IV: Median survival < 1 year
- Predictors of poor prognosis
  - Higher stage
  - Older age
  - Weight loss > 10% body mass
  - Dysphagia
  - Large tumors
  - Lymphatic micrometastases
  - Esophageal AC has better long-term prognosis after resection than does SCC
    - Overall 5-year survival rate is 47% for AC vs. 37% for SCC group

TREATMENT

Major Treatment Alternatives

- Endoscopic mucosal resection (EMR) for superficial cancer controversial
  - Mostly used with < 2 cm, flat mucosal lesions arising in Barrett esophagus
  - Requires close follow-up with endoscopy
  - Long-term outcomes unknown
- Photodynamic therapy (PDT)
  - Photosensitizing drug injected into tumor or IV
  - Tumor exposed to specific wavelength of light through endoscope
  - Nonthermal phototoxic reaction → cell death
- RT
  - Used for palliation
- Perioperative chemotherapy
  - Probable small survival benefit vs. surgery alone
- Concurrent chemoradiation (CRT)
  - Chemotherapy helps sensitize cancer to RT and treats micrometastases
  - Doublets include cisplatin & 5-fluorouracil or carboplatin & taxol
  - Higher toxicity than RT alone
  - Increases survival over RT alone
  - 5-year survival ~ 26%
  - Consider as definitive nonoperative treatment (data better for SCC vs. AC)
- Neoadjuvant CRT + esophagectomy
  - Standard of care in USA for AC
  - Increased disease-free survival over CRT alone for SCC
- Esophagectomy
  - Resectable: Invasion of pericardium, pleura, or diaphragm
  - Unresectable: Invasion of heart, great vessels, trachea, liver, lung, pancreas, and spleen
- Transthoracic esophagectomy (Ivor-Lewis)
  - Laparotomy plus right thoracotomy to create anastomosis in upper chest or neck
  - Lymphadenectomy under direct visualization
  - Complications: Anastomosis leak, cardiopulmonary complications
- Transhiatal esophagectomy
  - Anastomosis created in neck, avoids thoracotomy
  - Fewer complications vs. transthoracic esophagectomy

Major Treatment Roadblocks/ Contraindications

- Patient may not be a candidate for esophagectomy
  - Operative mortality (8-20%)
    - Lower end of mortality rate in centers that perform > 19 per year; 2% in high-volume centers

Treatment Options by Stage

- Tis N0
  - EMR or ablation
- T1a N0
  - EMR and ablation
  - Esophagectomy
- T1b, any N
  - Esophagectomy (for noncervical lesions)
  - Chemoradiation (for cervical lesions)
- T2 or higher, any N
  - Preoperative chemoradiation
  - Definitive chemoradiation
  - Esophagectomy
    - If Tis-T2 & N0 may observe
    - If node positive
      - Proximal or mid esophagus: Observe or chemoradiation
      - Distal esophagus or GEJ: Chemoradiation
- M1
  - Palliative treatment, may include RT &/or chemotherapy
  - Palliative interventional techniques include stents, balloon dilatation, and brachytherapy
    - Improvement in tumor-related dysphagia is faster with stents, but more durable with brachytherapy

Dose Response

- Beyond 50.4 Gy with chemo, no benefit to higher doses of external beam RT (EBRT) or brachytherapy boost
- Doses ≥ 60 Gy with chemo may be appropriate to improve control in unresectable SCC of the cervical esophagus

Standard Doses

- Definitive/preop: 45-50.4 Gy in 25-28 fractions
- Palliative brachytherapy: 12 Gy x 1 or 7 Gy x 3 over 2-3 weeks

Organs at Risk Parameters

- Lungs: V5 < 60%, V10 < 40%, V20 < 25% (up to 30%), V30 < 20%; mean < 20 Gy
- Heart: D100 < 30 Gy, D50 < 40 Gy
- Kidney: 70% combined kidney volume ≤ 20 Gy
- Liver: V60 < 30 Gy; mean < 25 Gy

Common Techniques

- 3D CRT is standard for all stages
- 4D assessment of tumor movement is recommended
  - Distal tumors have significantly greater motion than proximal or mid-esophageal tumors
- IMRT may be appropriate to ↓ dose to the heart and lungs, but area receiving lower doses may ↑
  - Long-term outcome studies needed for IMRT
- Volume definition
  - GTV is delineated using information from endoscopy and PET/CT
  - CTV primary is defined as the primary tumor plus 3-4 cm expansion superiorly and inferiorly along the length of esophagus and cardia and a 1 cm radial expansion
    - For SCC, pathologic data shows 3 cm margin from GTV would cover proximal and distal microscopic disease in 94% of patients
    - For AC of GEJ, pathologic data shows a 3 cm margin would cover microscopic disease in 100% of patients when extended proximally
      - If extended distally, 3 cm margin would only cover microscopic disease in 84% of patients
      - Distal margin of 5 cm would cover microscopic disease in 94% of patients, but the added toxicity from such a large expansion may be prohibitive
  - CTV nodal should be defined by 0.5-1.5 cm expansion from nodal GTV
  - PTV expansion should be 0.5-1 cm and may be non-uniform

Landmark Trials

- RTOG 8501: ↑ local control (LC), distant metastasis free survival, and overall survival (OS) with chemo added to RT
- RTOG 9207: Compared to historic controls, no ↑ LC or survival and ↑ toxicity with 15-20 Gy brachytherapy boost after 50 Gy EBRT
- RTOG 9405/INT 0123: No ↑ in LC or OS with EBRT dose ↑ from 50.4 Gy to 64.8 Gy
- Stahl: In SCC, improved LC but ↑ treatment-related mortality and equivalent survival if esophagectomy follows CRT vs. definitive CRT
- CROSS trial: Adding neoadjuvant CRT (involving carboplatin & paclitaxel concurrent with 41.4 Gy) to resection improved survival from 24.0 to 49.4 months

RECOMMENDED FOLLOW-UP

Clinical

- H&P every 3-6 months for 1-2 years, every 6-12 months for 3-5 years, and then annually
- Upper GI endoscopy with biopsy as clinically indicated
- Nutritional counseling

Radiographic

- Imaging as clinically indicated

Laboratory

- CBC and chemistry profile as clinically indicated

SELECTED REFERENCES

1. van Hagen P et al: Preoperative chemoradiotherapy for esophageal or junctional cancer. N Engl J Med. 366(22):2074-84, 2012
2. Ajani JA et al: Esophageal and esophagogastric junction cancers. J Natl Compr Canc Netw. 9(8):830-87, 2011
3. Wang D et al: 3D-conformal RT, fixed-field IMRT and RapidArc, which one is better for esophageal carcinoma treated with elective nodal irradiation. Technol Cancer Res Treat. 10(5):487-94, 2011
4. American Joint Committee on Cancer: AJCC Cancer Staging Manual. 7th ed. New York: Springer. 103-15, 2010
5. Rice TW et al: 7th edition of the AJCC Cancer Staging Manual: esophagus and esophagogastric junction. Ann Surg Oncol. 17(7):1721-4, 2010
6. Kim TJ et al: Multimodality assessment of esophageal cancer: preoperative staging and monitoring of response to therapy. Radiographics. 29(2):403-21, 2009
7. Patel AA et al: Implications of respiratory motion as measured by four-dimensional computed tomography for radiation treatment planning of esophageal cancer. Int J Radiat Oncol Biol Phys. 74(1):290-6, 2009
8. Stahl M et al: Phase III comparison of preoperative chemotherapy compared with chemoradiotherapy in patients with locally advanced adenocarcinoma of the esophagogastric junction. J Clin Oncol. 27(6):851-6, 2009
9. van Vliet EP et al: Staging investigations for oesophageal cancer: a meta-analysis. Br J Cancer. 98(3):547-57, 2008
10. Gao XS et al: Pathological analysis of clinical target volume margin for radiotherapy in patients with esophageal and gastroesophageal junction carcinoma. Int J Radiat Oncol Biol Phys. 67(2):389-96, 2007
11. Bergquist H et al: Stent insertion or endoluminal brachytherapy as palliation of patients with advanced cancer of the esophagus and gastroesophageal junction. Results of a randomized, controlled clinical trial. Dis Esophagus. 18(3):131-9, 2005
12. Downey RJ et al: Whole body 18FDG-PET and the response of esophageal cancer to induction therapy: results of a prospective trial. J Clin Oncol. 21(3):428-32, 2003
13. Gaspar LE et al: A phase I/II study of external beam radiation, brachytherapy, and concurrent chemotherapy for patients with localized carcinoma of the esophagus (Radiation Therapy Oncology Group Study 9207): final report. Cancer. 88(5):988-95, 2000
14. Cooper JS et al: Chemoradiotherapy of locally advanced esophageal cancer: long-term follow-up of a prospective randomized trial (RTOG 85-01). Radiation Therapy Oncology Group. JAMA. 281(17):1623-7, 1999
15. Herskovic A et al: Combined chemotherapy and radiotherapy compared with radiotherapy alone in patients with cancer of the esophagus. N Engl J Med. 326(24):1593-8, 1992

ESOPHAGUS

Adenocarcinoma, Stage IA (T1 N0 M0 G2)

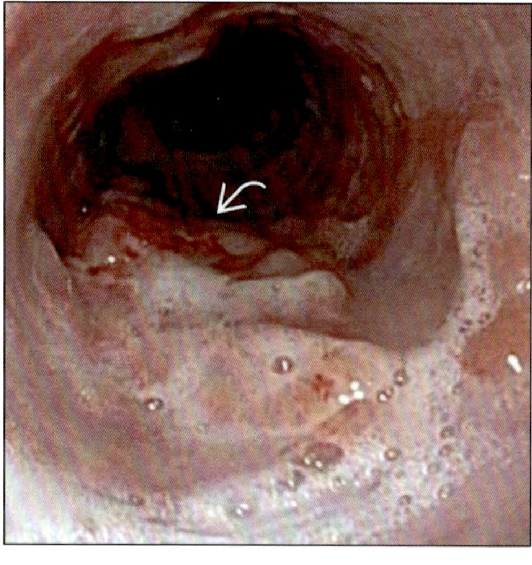

Adenocarcinoma, Stage IA (T1 N0 M0 G2)

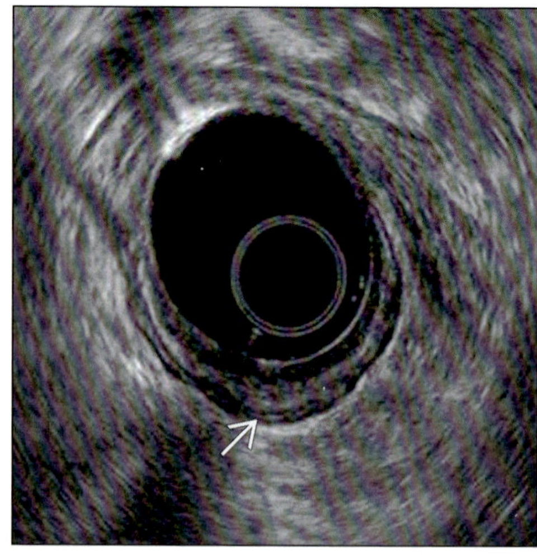

(Left) *Endoscopic photograph shows fungating, nonobstructive, 1 cm wide mass* ➔ *extending 35-40 cm from the incisors.* ***(Right)*** *Radial EUS in the same patient performed at 10 MHz shows a heterogeneous lesion extending to but not involving the muscularis propria (MP). Hyperechoic line separates the inner circular and outer longitudinal layers of the MP* ➔*. Mini-probes are often required to distinguish T1a from T1b. (Courtesy D. G. Adler, MD.)*

Adenocarcinoma, Stage IB (T2 N0 M0 G2)

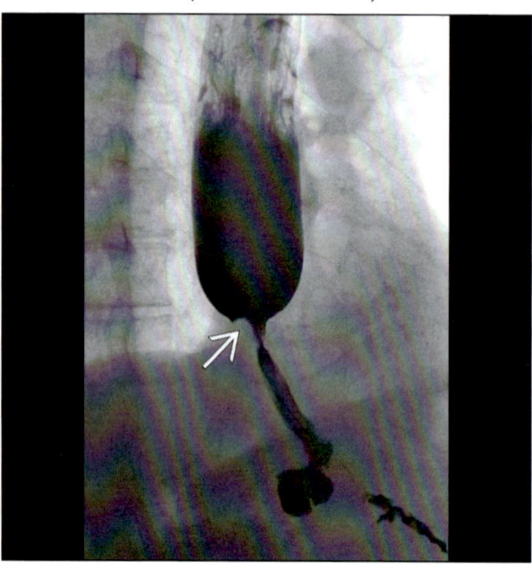

Adenocarcinoma, Stage IB (T2 N0 M0 G2)

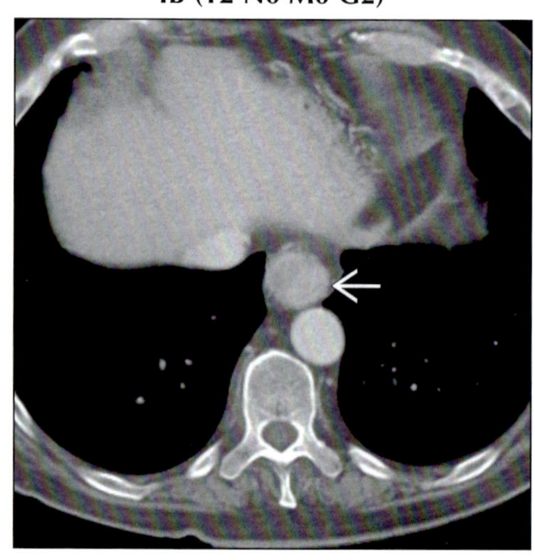

(Left) *Esophagram in a 57-year-old man shows abrupt narrowing* ➔ *in distal thoracic esophagus. EUS with biopsy revealed G2 adenocarcinoma 32-36 cm from the incisors. If this tumor were G3, the stage would be IIA.* ***(Right)*** *In the same patient, axial CECT following administration of PO barium shows obliteration of the esophageal lumen* ➔ *of the diffusely thickened lower thoracic esophagus.*

Adenocarcinoma, Stage IIB (T3 N0 M0)

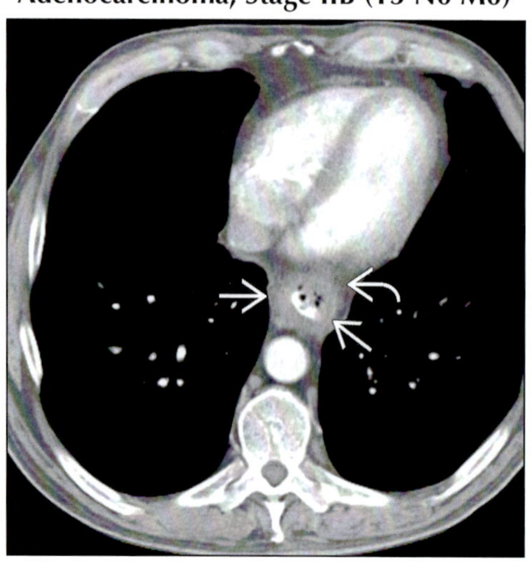

Adenocarcinoma, Stage IIB (T3 N0 M0)

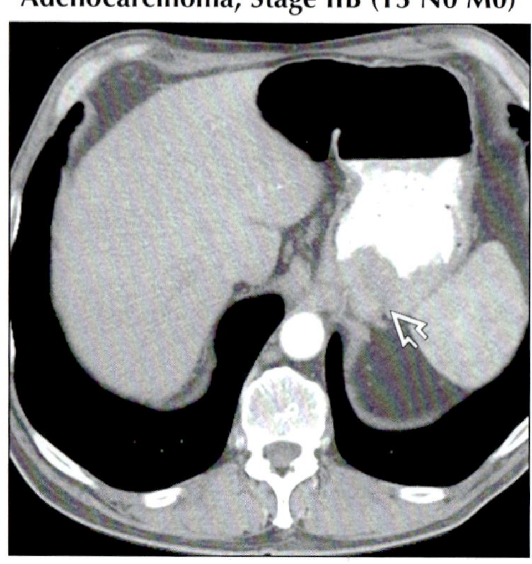

(Left) *Axial CECT in a 55-year-old man with history of reflux shows distal thoracic esophageal circumferential wall thickening* ➔*. Hazy interface with the periesophageal fat* ➔ *suggests adventitial invasion.* ***(Right)*** *Axial CECT in the same patient shows tumor invading the gastric cardia* ➔*. A T3 N0 M0 lower esophageal adenocarcinoma is stage IIB, regardless of histological grade, whereas T3 N0 M0 squamous cell carcinoma is stage IB if G1 and stage IIA if G2-3.*

Adenocarcinoma, Stage IIA (T2 N0 M0 G3)

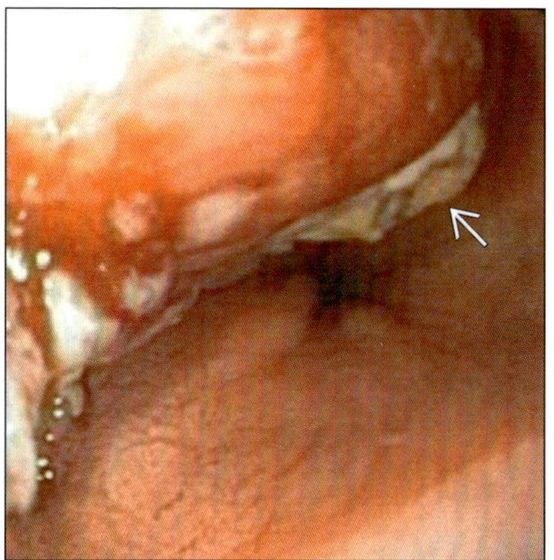

Adenocarcinoma, Stage IIA (T2 N0 M0 G3)

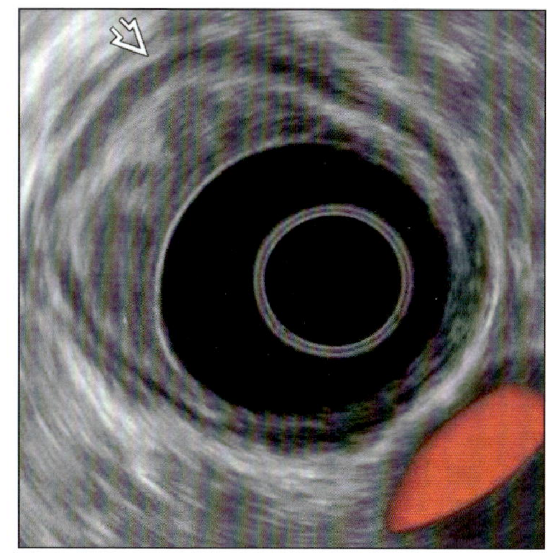

(Left) *Endoscopic photograph in a 72-year-old man shows a fungating mass ➔ involving 1/3 of the esophageal lumen, which extends 35-39 cm from the incisors.* ***(Right)*** *Radial EUS in the same patient performed at 10 MHz with Doppler reveals hypoechoic/heterogeneous polypoid mass invading the hypoechoic MP, consistent with T2 disease and manifested by thickening and wavy appearance of the MP ➲. (Courtesy D. G. Adler, MD.)*

Adenocarcinoma, Stage IIA (T2 N0 M0 G3)

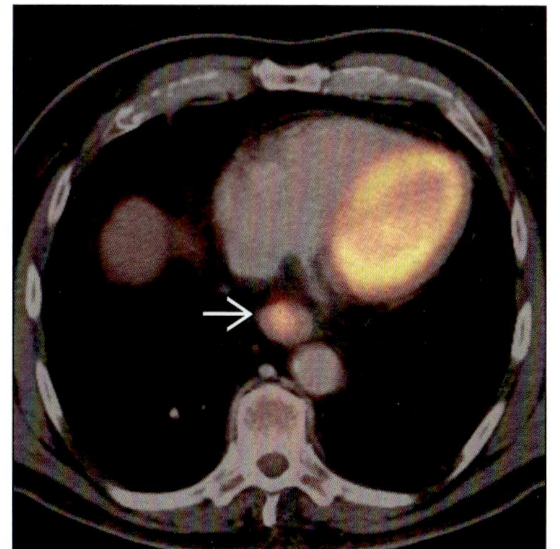

Adenocarcinoma, Stage IIA (T2 N0 M0 G3)

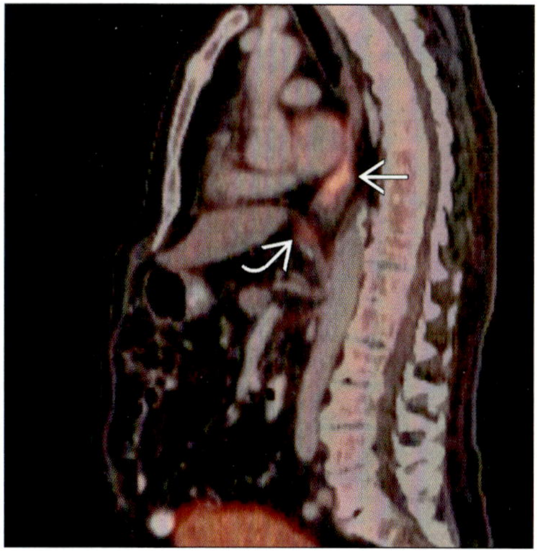

(Left) *In the same patient, axial PET/CT shows hypermetabolic activity ➔ predominantly on thickened right side of the lower thoracic esophagus.* ***(Right)*** *Sagittal PET/CT in the same patient shows increased metabolic activity of the primary tumor spanning 5 cm of the distal thoracic esophagus ➔ as well as in region of prior esophageal hiatal surgery ➚.*

Adenocarcinoma, Stage IA (T1 N0 M0 G2)

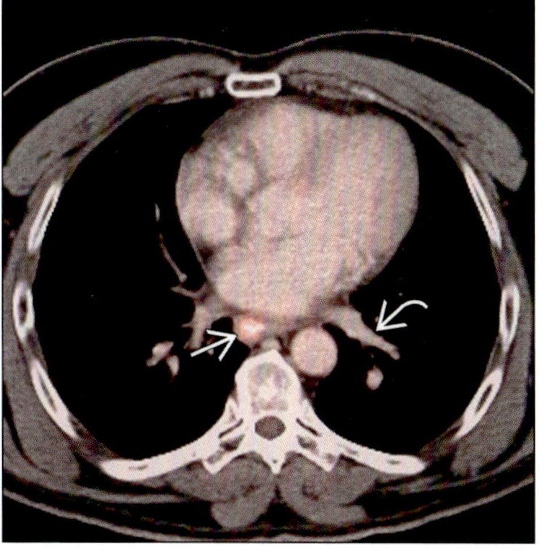

Adenocarcinoma, Stage IIIA (T3 N1 M0)

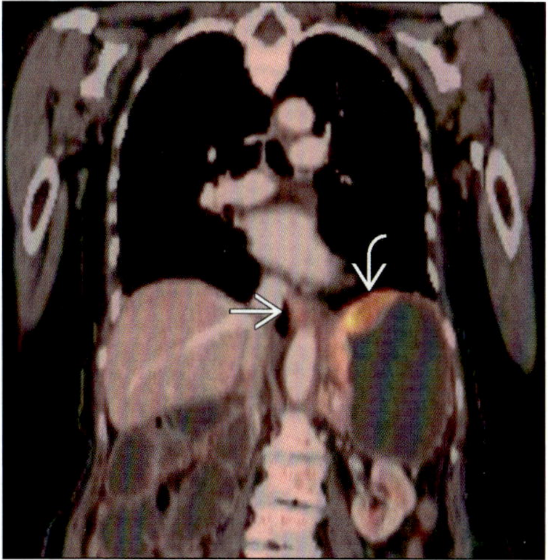

(Left) *Axial PET/CT shows an eccentric area of increased metabolic activity ➔. The upper end of the lesion is above the level of the lower border of the inferior pulmonary vein ➚, making this a middle thoracic lesion.* ***(Right)*** *Coronal PET/CT in an 80-year-old woman shows tumor extending from GE junction ➔ to the gastric cardia ➚. Epicenter is within proximal 5 cm of gastric cardia and is therefore defined as an abdominal esophageal adenocarcinoma.*

Adenocarcinoma, Stage IIIA (T3 N1 M0)

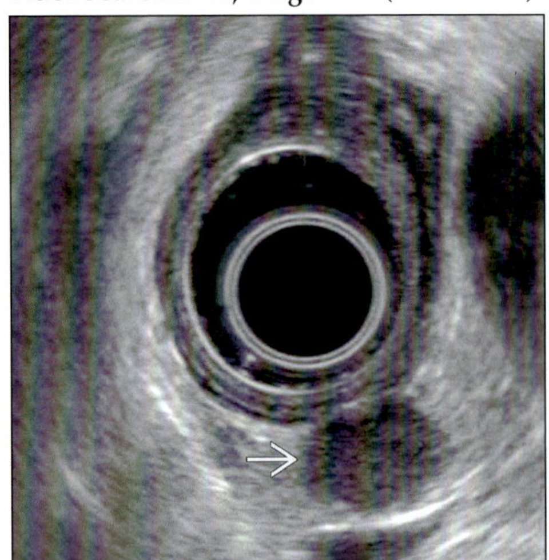

Adenocarcinoma, Stage IIIA (T3 N1 M0)

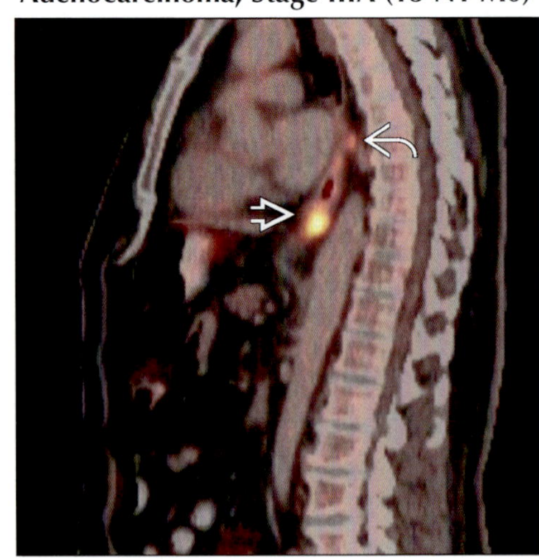

(Left) *Ultrasound shows a hypoechoic, round, 9 x 10 mm lymph node with well-defined borders. Biopsy was consistent with adenocarcinoma.* ***(Right)*** *Sagittal PET/CT in the same patient shows distance of 3 cm from primary tumor to biopsy-proven involved node.*

Adenocarcinoma, Stage IIIA (T3 N1 M0)

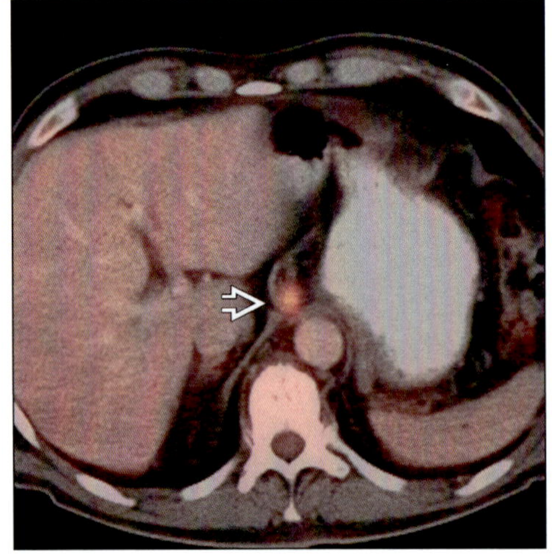

Adenocarcinoma, Stage IIIA (T3 N1 M0)

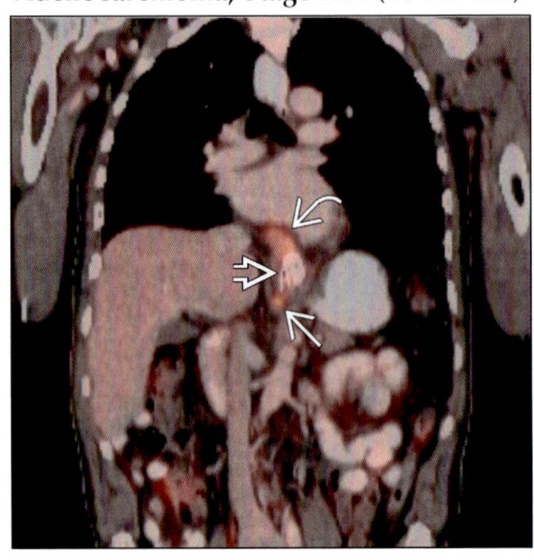

(Left) *Axial PET/CT shows a hypermetabolic 1.6 x 1.6 cm gastrohepatic ligament lymph node (SUV 9.2) in a patient with a GE junction adenocarcinoma.* ***(Right)*** *Coronal PET/CT in the same patient shows location of the gastrohepatic node (SUV 9.2) relative to distal thoracic/ GE junction primary, located 33-41 cm from the incisors. Stent was placed to relieve dysphagia.*

Adenocarcinoma, Stage IIIB (T3 N2 M0)

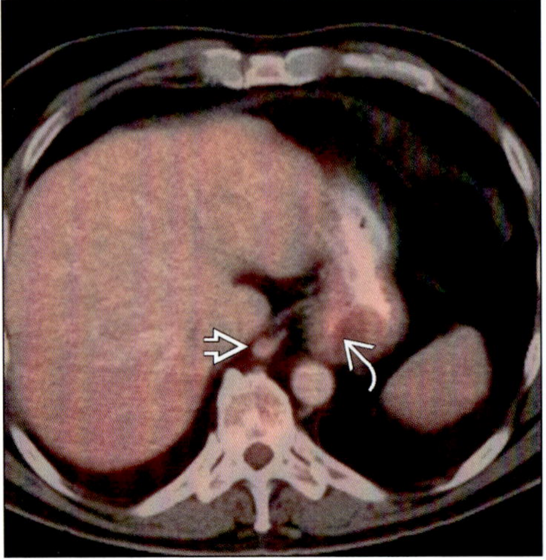

Adenocarcinoma, Stage IIIB (T3 N2 M0)

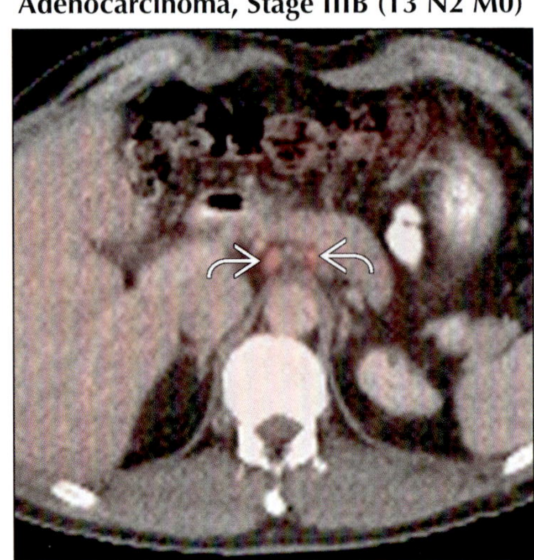

(Left) *Axial PET/CT in a 63-year-old man shows hypermetabolic retrocrural node measuring 10 x 22 mm (SUV 3.1). SUV of the primary tumor is 17.5, and mild hypermetabolic activity (SUV 5.8) is concerning for gastric extension.* ***(Right)*** *Axial PET/CT shows increased metabolic activity within 2 small celiac nodes. Celiac nodes are considered regional lymph nodes in the 7th edition AJCC staging system (2010).*

Adenocarcinoma, Stage IIIB (T3 N2 M0)

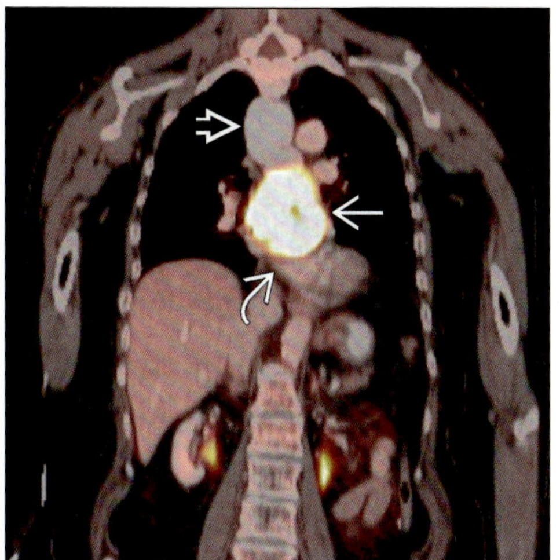

Adenocarcinoma, Stage IIIB (T3 N2 M0)

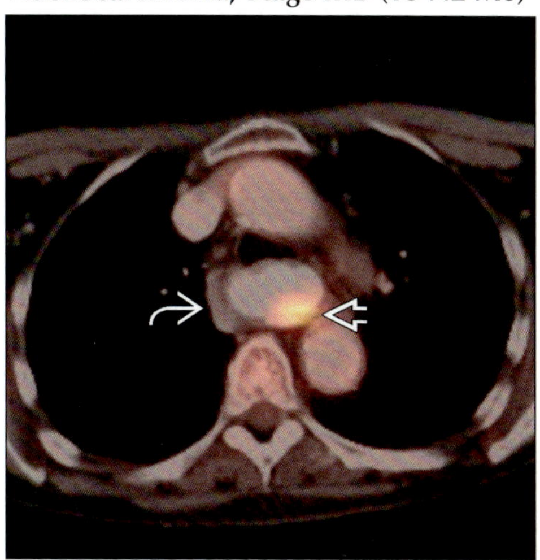

(Left) *Coronal PET/CT in a 78-year-old woman shows an upper thoracic mass ➡ (SUV 8.4) causing proximal dilatation ➡ and left atrium compression ➡. Endoscopy revealed extension of disease 25-29 cm from the incisors.* **(Right)** *Axial PET/CT in the same patient shows extension of the primary ➡ above the inferior portion of the azygous vein ➡, making this an upper thoracic lesion. Bronchoscopy showed tracheal luminal narrowing without invasion.*

Adenocarcinoma, Stage IIIB (T3 N2 M0)

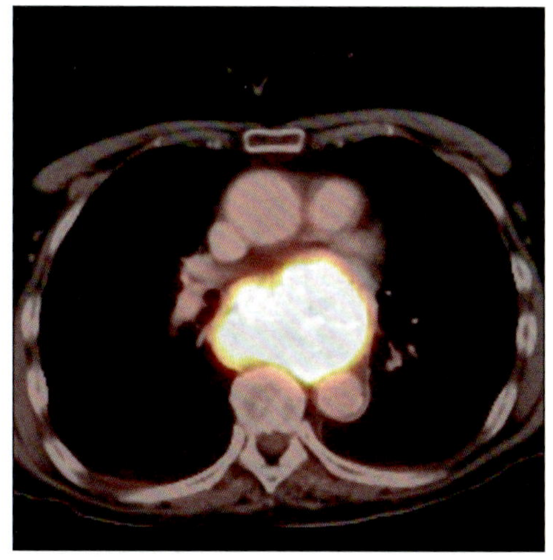

Adenocarcinoma, Stage IIIB (T3 N2 M0)

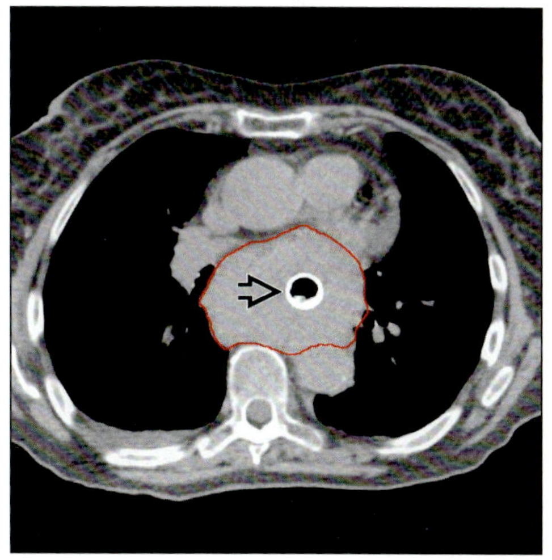

(Left) *Axial PET/CT in the same patient shows a massive 7 cm esophageal adenocarcinoma displacing mediastinal structures.* **(Right)** *Axial NECT in the same patient shows stent placement ➡ before radiation therapy due to dysphagia to liquids (red = GTV).*

Adenocarcinoma, Stage IIIC (T1b N3 M0)

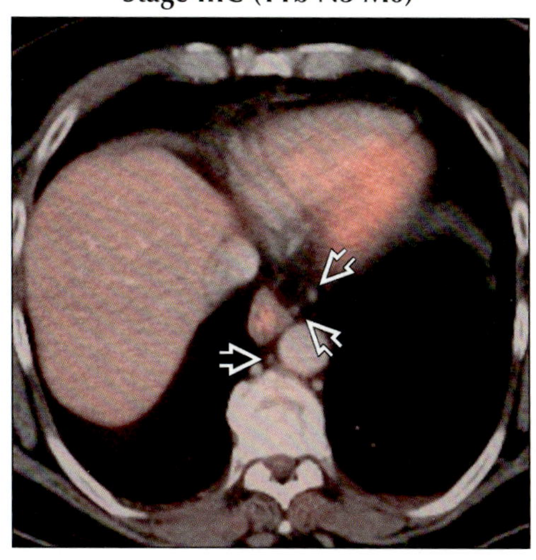

Adenocarcinoma, Stage IIIC (T3 N3 M0)

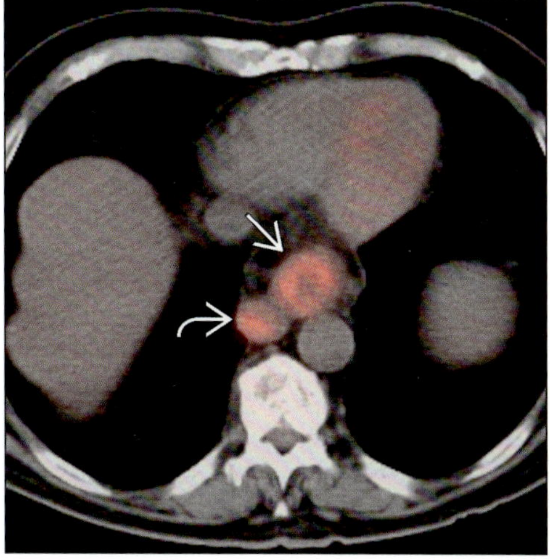

(Left) *Axial PET/CT shows 3 subcentimeter nonmetabolically active nodes ➡ surrounding the esophageal tumor (SUV 5.1). EUS showed hypoechoic, well-demarcated round nodes concerning for malignancy.* **(Right)** *Axial PET/CT shows hypermetabolic, diffuse thickening (up to 1.4 cm) of the distal esophageal wall ➡ (SUV 17.6). A large hypermetabolic lymph node at the gastroesophageal junction ➡ measures 2.6 x 1.9 cm (SUV 14.7).*

Adenocarcinoma, Stage IIIC (T4b N0 M0)

Adenocarcinoma, Stage IIIC (T4b N0 M0)

(Left) Axial CECT shows circumferential esophageal wall thickening ➡ and abnormal paraesophageal soft tissue ➡ with > 90° contact with the descending thoracic aorta ➡ suggesting aortic involvement. This was confirmed at surgery. (Right) Radial EUS performed at 10 MHz reveals loss of muscularis propria between esophageal tumor and aorta ➡. (Courtesy D. G. Adler, MD.)

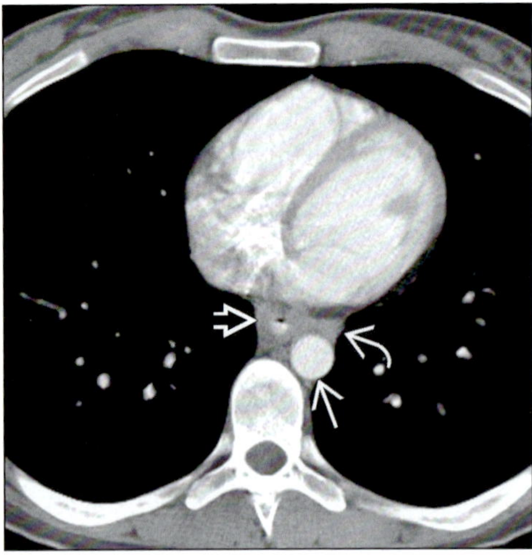

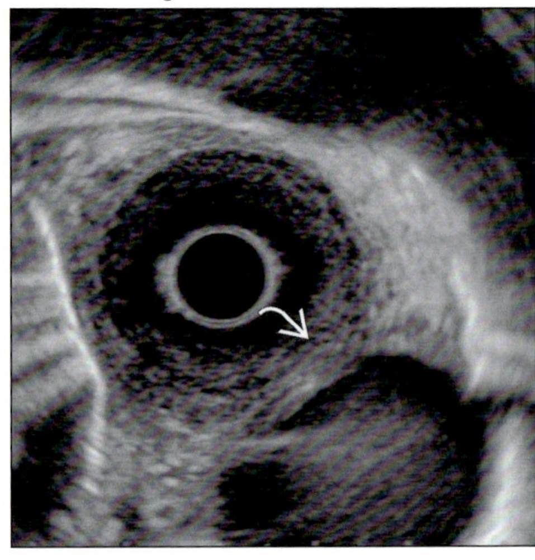

Adenocarcinoma, Stage IIIC (T4b N1 M0)

Adenocarcinoma, Stage IIIC (T4b N1 M0)

(Left) Coronal CECT in a 41-year-old woman shows invasion of the diaphragm surrounding the hiatus ➡ and the liver ➡, confirmed at the time of surgery. The tumor was also noted to invade the posterior pericardium and aorta posteriorly. (Right) Axial CECT in the same patient shows fat plane loss between the esophageal mass and the liver ➡.

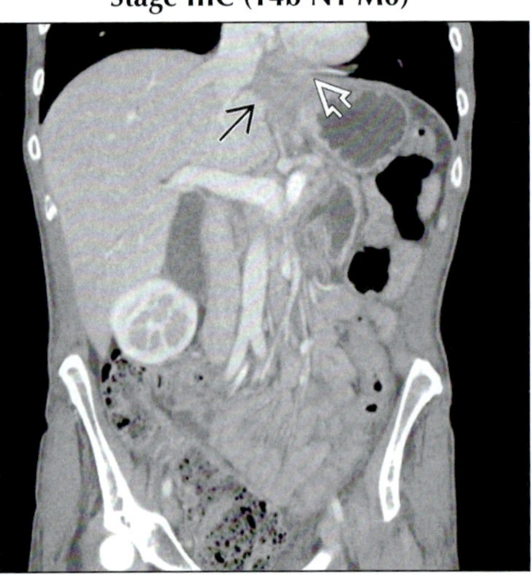

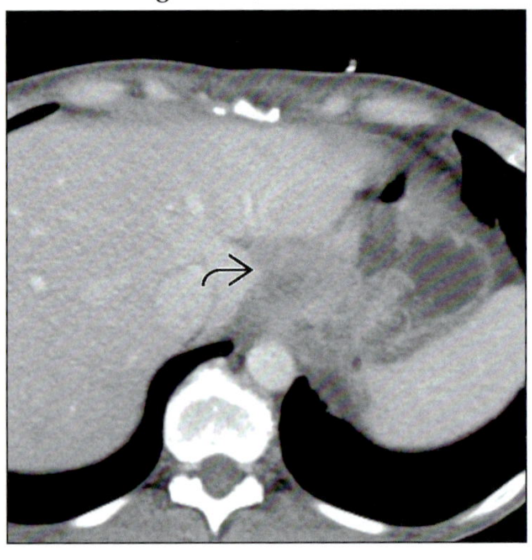

Squamous Cell Carcinoma, Stage IIIC (T4b N3 M1)

Squamous Cell Carcinoma, Stage IIIC (T4b N3 M1)

(Left) Axial PET/CT in a 63-year-old man with a history of 50 pack-years and significant alcohol consumption, presenting with increasing shortness of breath and dysphagia, shows invasion of the posterior trachea ➡ by the hypermetabolic mass (SUV 21). (Right) Axial PET/CT in the same patient shows involvement of prevascular nodes ➡ (level 3A). These nonparaesophageal mediastinal nodes are considered M1 disease.

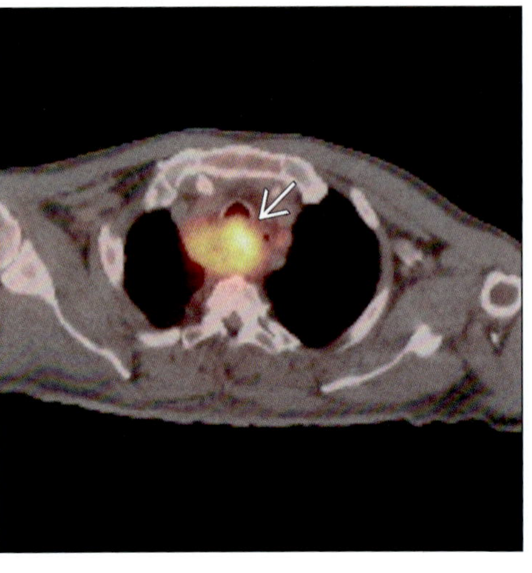

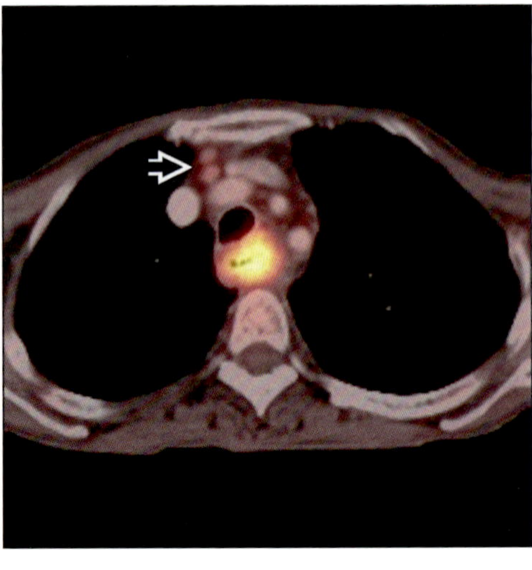

Squamous Cell Carcinoma, Stage IIIC (T4b N3 M1)

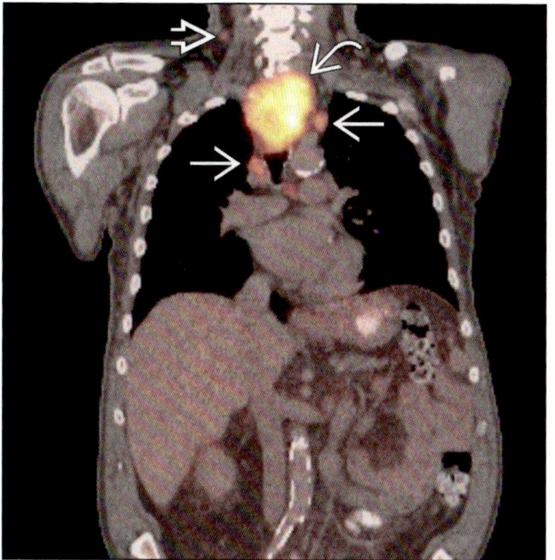

Squamous Cell Carcinoma, Stage IIIC (T4b N3 M1)

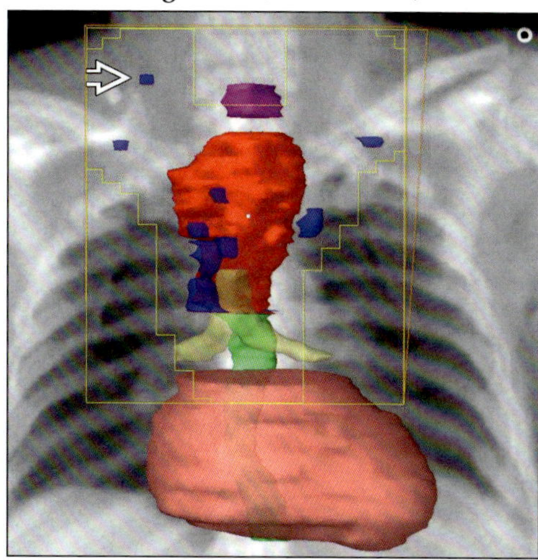

(Left) *Coronal PET/CT in the same patient shows the primary ➔ and mediastinal nodes ➔. The nonparaesophageal supraclavicular node (SUV 5) ➔ is considered M1 disease.* **(Right)** *AP DRR in the same patient shows radiation field including the supraclavicular node ➔. GTV = red, involved nodes = blue, esophagus = green, larynx = magenta, carina = yellow, and heart = pink.*

Adenocarcinoma, Stage IIIC (T3 N3 M0)

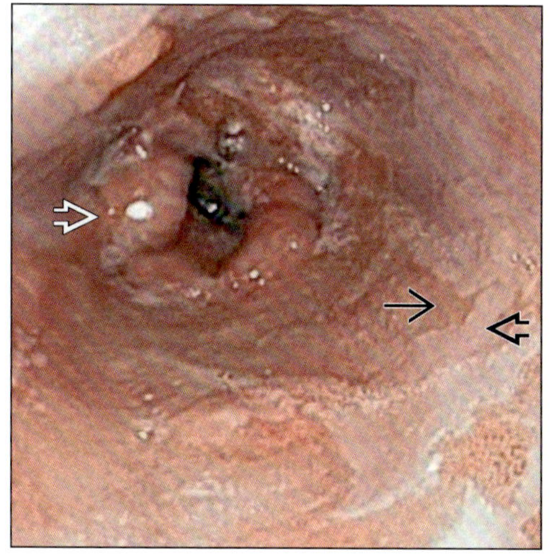

Adenocarcinoma, Stage IIIC (T3 N3 M0)

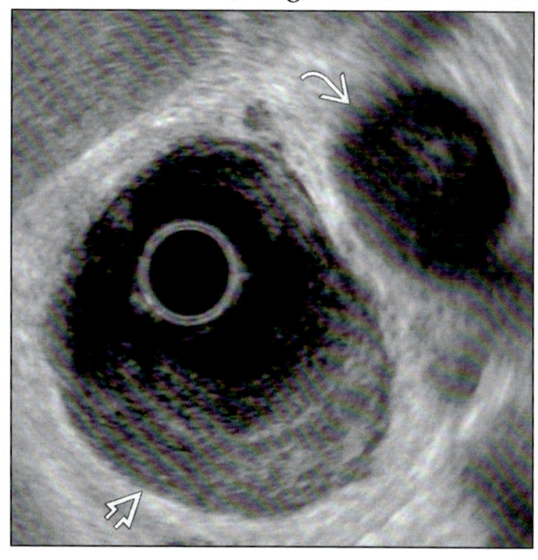

(Left) *Endoscopic photograph shows a circumferential, partially obstructing mass ➔, which extends 32-40 cm from the incisors. It is arising from a field of circumferential Barrett esophagus (salmon-colored tongues → extending into normal, lighter colored mucosa ➔). (Courtesy D. G. Adler, MD.)* **(Right)** *Radial EUS performed in the same patient at 10 MHz reveals circumferential mass invading through the MP ➔. Note aorta ➔. (Courtesy D. G. Adler, MD.)*

4D CT Simulation

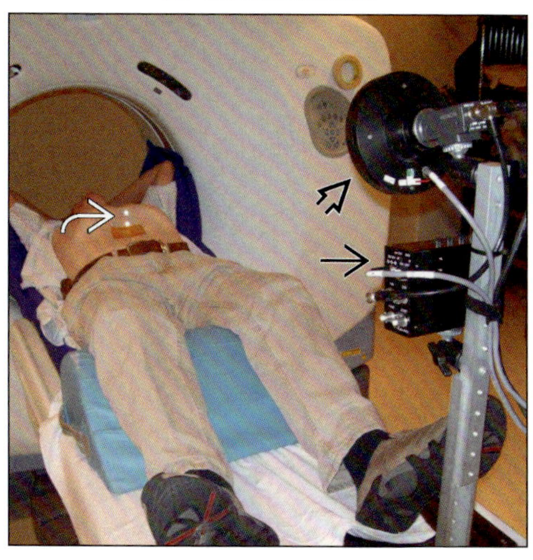

4D Software

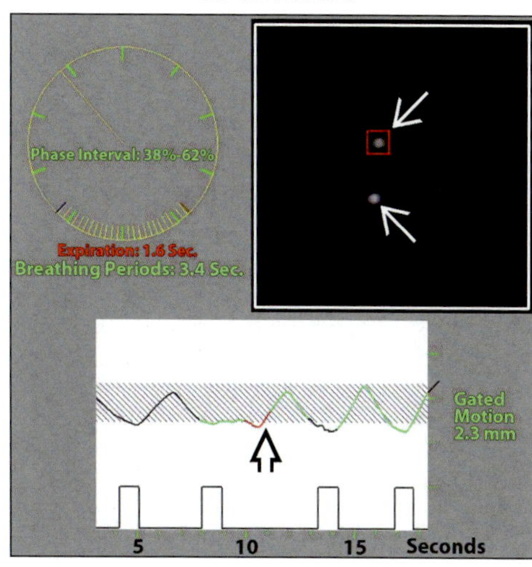

(Left) *This is a 4D CT simulation during which the apparatus ➔ emits and then receives infrared light reflected off markers ➔. Display screen → shows marker motion. 4D cine data are acquired at multiple couch positions.* **(Right)** *Real-time position management (RPM) system software shows respiratory trace curve ➔. GE advantage 4D program processes raw cine data into 10 respiratory phase scans via this curve. Respiratory marker ➔ is seen.*

T1b N2 M0 4D EBRT Planning

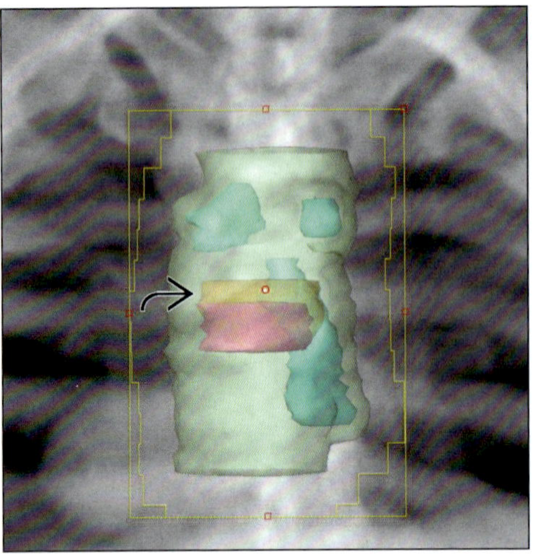

T1b N2 M0 4D EBRT Planning

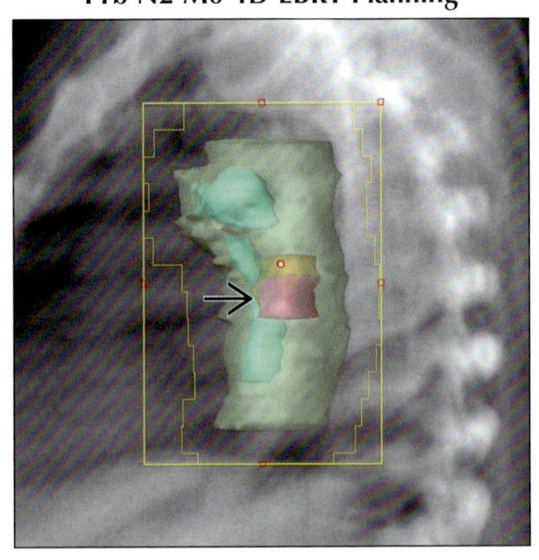

(Left) *AP DRR shows GTV (magenta), ITV (orange), involved nodes (cyan), and CTV (light green) for a mid-thoracic lesion. Note that almost all GTV movement for this particular patient is in the superior direction ↪, indicating a non-uniform expansion may more accurately delineate target volumes.* ***(Right)*** *Lateral DRR in the same patient shows minimal AP movement → of the GTV. Note that treatment of the SCV or celiac regions is unnecessary for this tumor location.*

T2 N0 M0 4D EBRT Planning

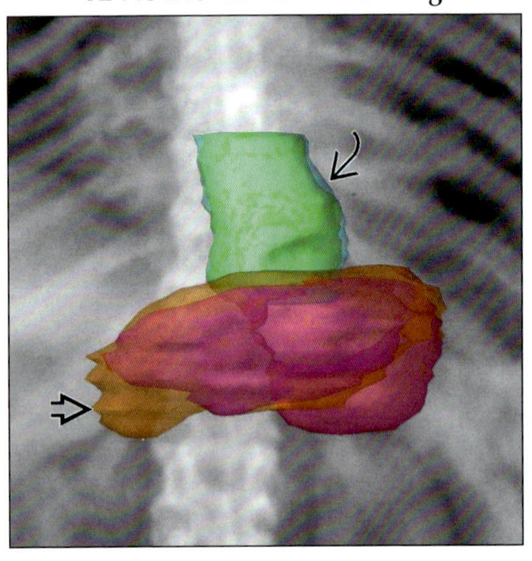

T2 N0 M0 4D EBRT Planning

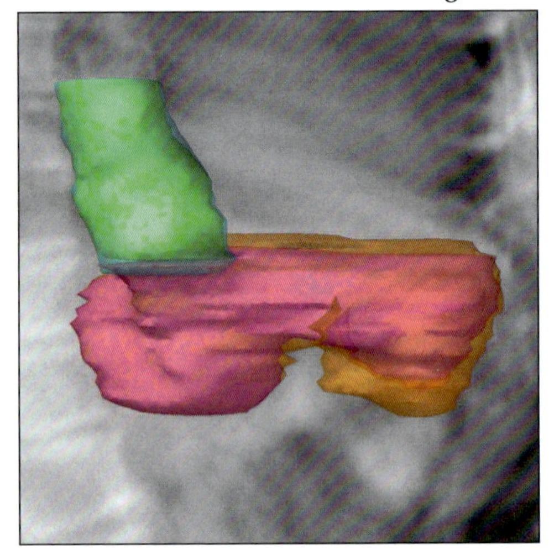

(Left) *AP DRR shows GTV (green), ITV (cyan) ↪, stomach (magenta), and ITV stomach (orange) ⇨ for a GE junction lesion. Note almost all GTV movement is directed inferiorly and to the left. Stomach motion may be significant in areas, indicating creation of an ITV stomach when delineating CTV expansions into this organ may decrease the chance of marginal misses.* ***(Right)*** *Lateral DRR in the same patient delineates GTV and stomach motion with respiration.*

Effect of Magin Expansion

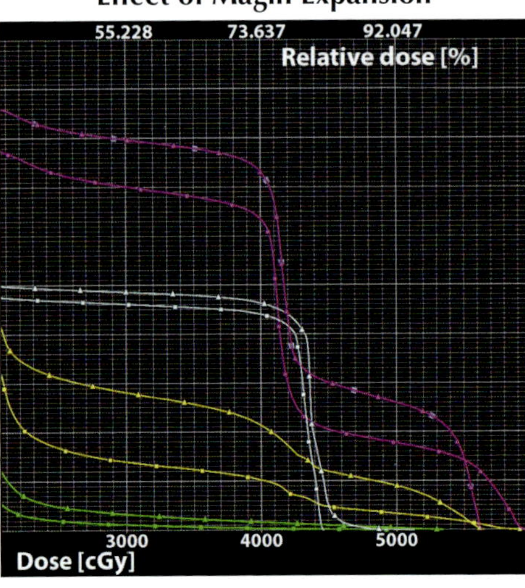

T3 N0 M0 Cone Down Boost

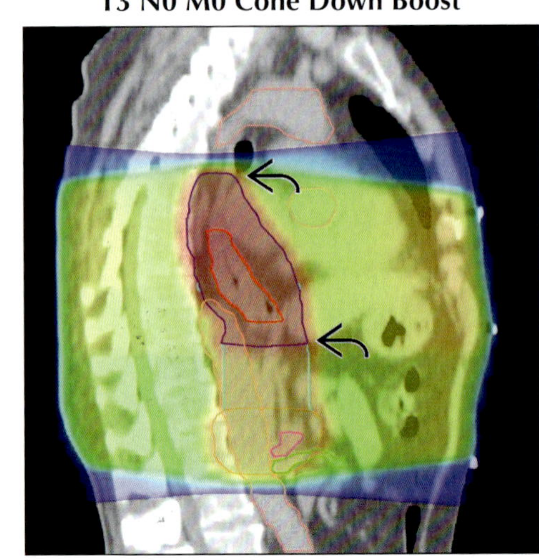

(Left) *DVH shows reduction in dose to heart (magenta), lungs (yellow), kidneys (green), and spinal cord (cyan) when the PTV margin is decreased from 1-0.5 cm. Therefore, consider methods to decrease PTV margin such as by a 4D simulation.* ***(Right)*** *NECT shows method to decrease dose to OARs. Initial field was treated to 45 Gy, with final 5.4 Gy ↪ excluding the elective celiac nodal region. CTV = cyan, CTV boost = blue, aorta = pink, celiac art = magenta, and SMA = green.*

EBRT Planning Distal Lesion

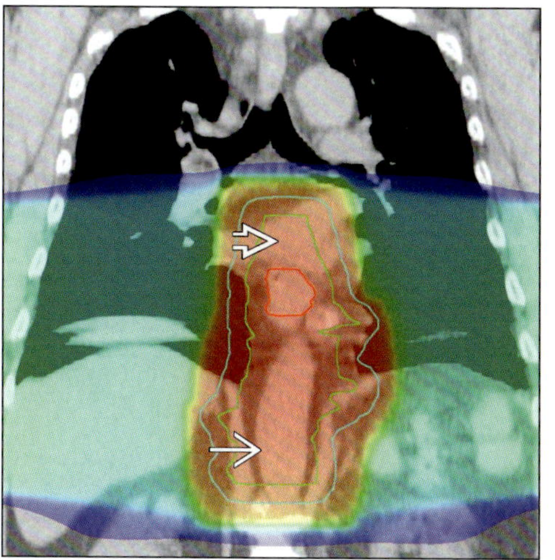

EBRT Planning Distal Lesion

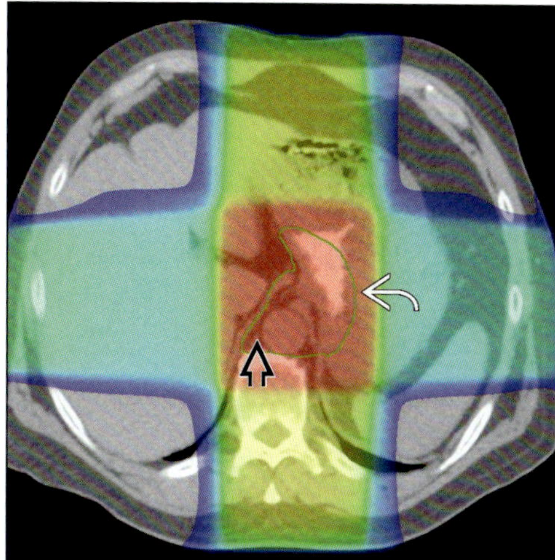

(Left) *Coronal NECT dose colorwash indicates coverage of GTV (red), CTV (green), and PTV (blue). Volumes seen are typical of most distal esophageal cancers. The lowest dose shown is 10% of the prescription of 50.4 Gy (dark blue). Note 4 cm proximal expansion of CTV from GTV and elective coverage of the celiac region.* ***(Right)*** *Axial NECT in the same patient shows CTV expansion into the stomach as well as elective coverage of the retrocrural area.*

EBRT Planning Distal Lesion

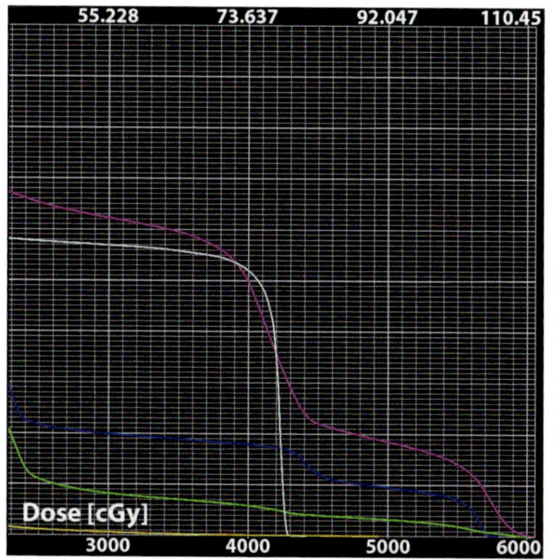

EBRT Planning Distal Lesion, Follow-Up

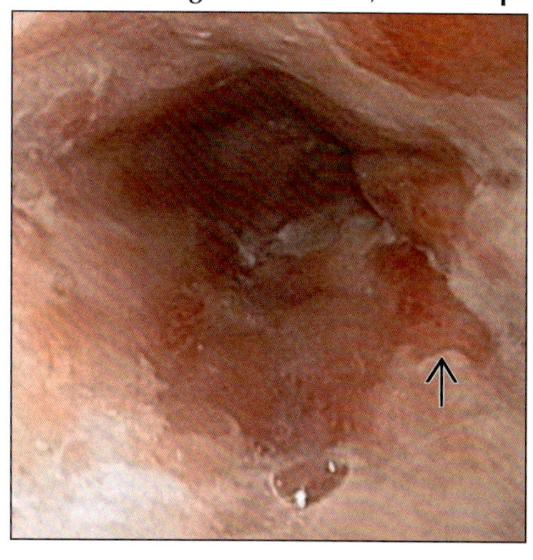

(Left) *DVH in the same patient shows heart (magenta), spinal cord (cyan), liver (blue), total lung (green), and bilateral kidneys (orange), all within acceptable dose limits.* ***(Right)*** *Endoscopic photograph taken 6 weeks after chemoradiation shows mucosal erosions, consistent with radiation esophagitis.*

T3 N1 M0 Cervical Lesion

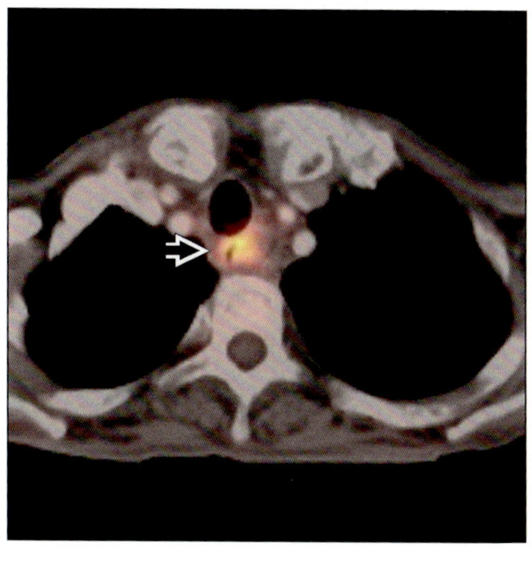

T3 N1 M0 Cervical Lesion

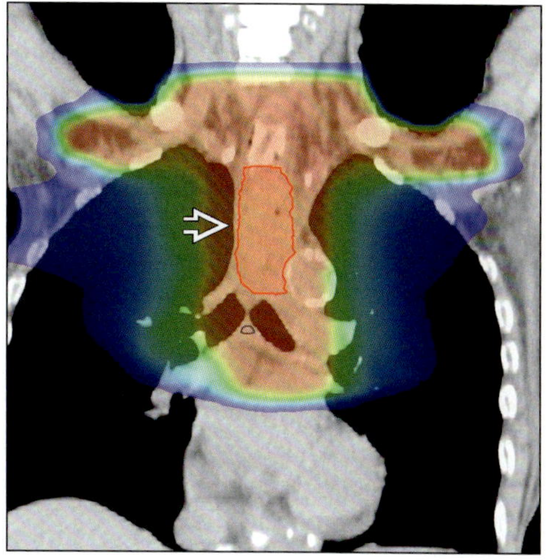

(Left) *Axial PET/CT shows superior extent of hypermetabolic adenocarcinoma (SUV 24) above the sternal notch, consistent with a cervical location. Endoscopy revealed a tumor 19-24 cm from the incisors.* ***(Right)*** *Coronal NECT in the same patient shows the dose colorwash covering the supraclavicular nodal basin, which is recommended for cervical and upper thoracic lesions. Note GTV in red.*

T3 N2 M0, Lung Injury

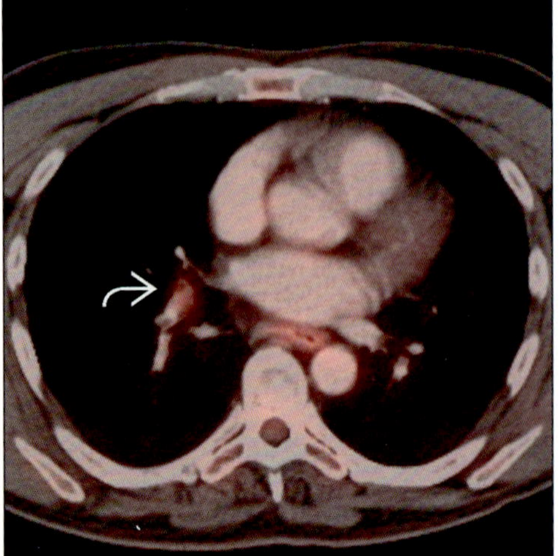

T3 N2 M0, Lung Injury

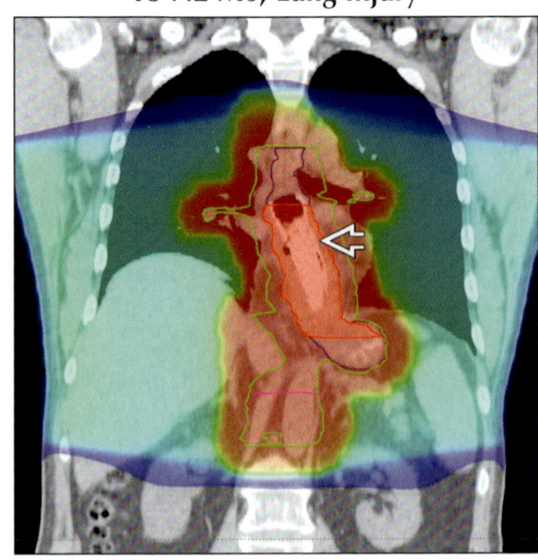

(Left) *Axial PET/CT in a distal thoracic adenocarcinoma (SUV 18) shows mildly increased activity in the bilateral hila (SUV 3.1) ➢, concerning for disease.* ***(Right)*** *Coronal NECT in the same patient shows dose colorwash. A large amount of lung receives a high dose when treating the bilateral hilum. GTV is in red, CTV is in blue, and PTV is in green. Note stent ⇨. Consider not treating hilum if low level of suspicion since the false-positive rate in PET/CT is high.*

T3 N2 M0, Lung Injury

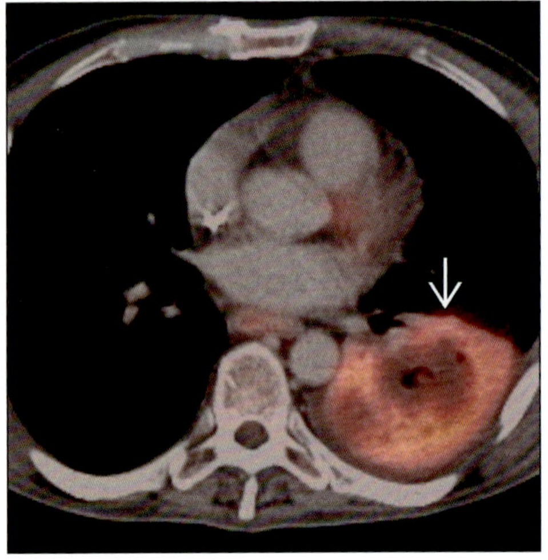

Radiation Pneumonitis

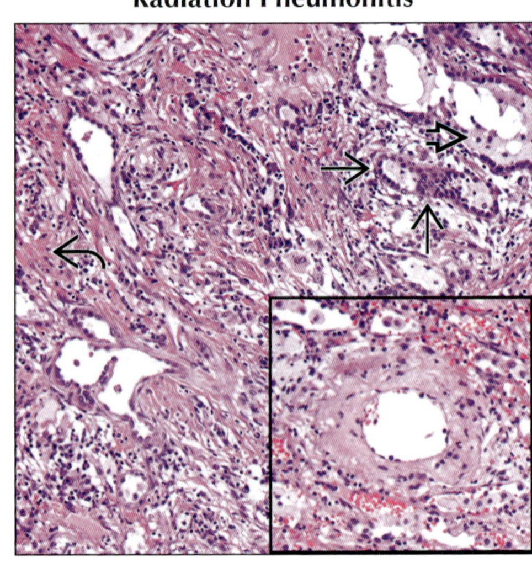

(Left) *Axial PET/CT in the same patient 1 year since finishing CRT shows development of necrotizing pneumonia refractory to antibiotics ➡.* ***(Right)*** *H&E from lobectomy revealed an abscess cavity arising in a background of inflammation. Features consistent with radiation pneumonitis include interstitial fibrosis ➢, atypical hyperplasia of type II pneumocytes ➡, intraalveolar macrophages ⇨, & arteriole sclerosis (inset). (Courtesy C. A. Garcia, MD.)*

T3 N0 M0 Postop EBRT

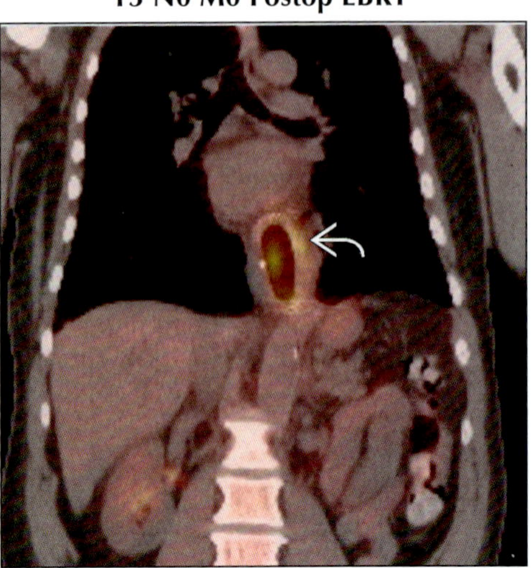

T3 N0 M0 Postop EBRT

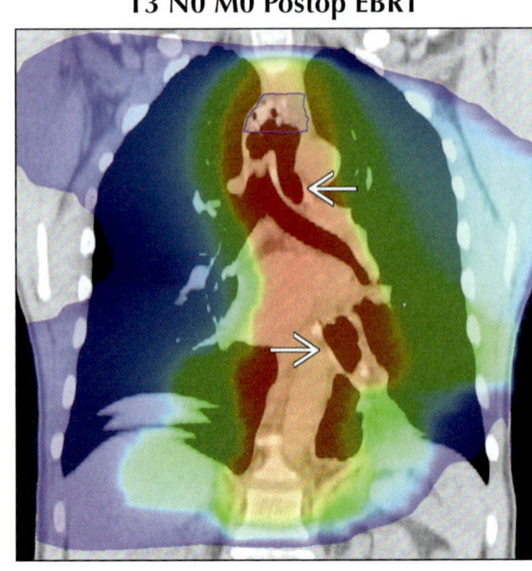

(Left) *Coronal PET/CT in a 63-year-old patient shows hypermetabolic region in distal esophagus ➢. Endoscopic biopsies were nondiagnostic.* ***(Right)*** *Coronal NECT with dose colorwash in the same patient shows anastomosis (blue) and gastric conduit ➡ status post transhiatal esophagectomy. Pathology showed T3 N0 disease and CRT was recommended. Note very large field size due to need to treat anastomosis, gastric conduit, operative bed, and nodal regions.*

T3 N1 M0 Distal Lesion

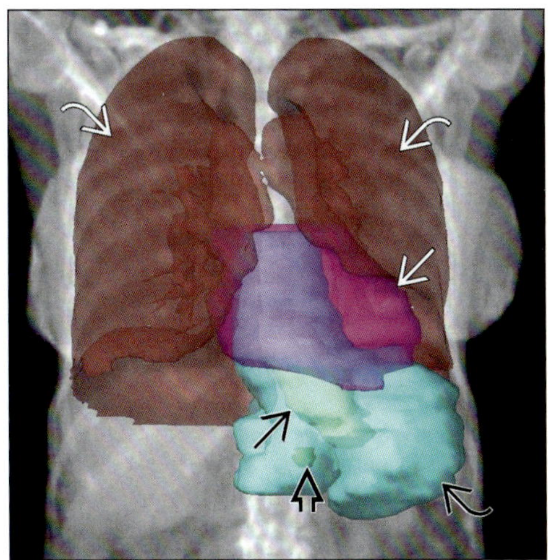

T3 N1 M0 Distal Lesion

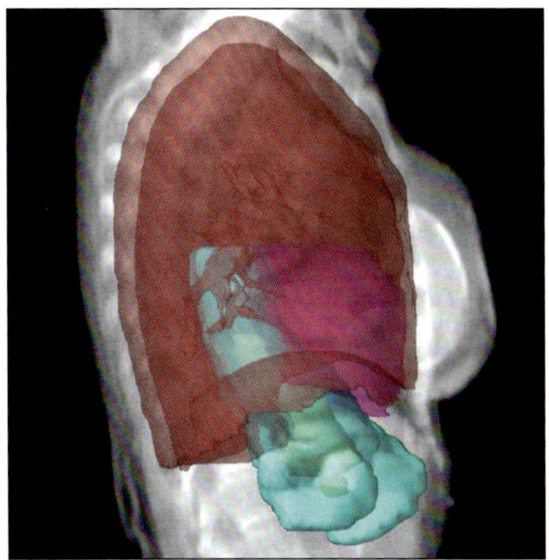

(Left) *AP DRR shows treatment volumes and OARs for distal esophageal cancer extending into gastric cardia. GTV = yellow, PTV = cyan, celiac artery = green, heart = magenta, and lungs = brown.* ***(Right)*** *AP DRR shows treatment volumes and OARs.*

T3 N1 M0 Distal Lesion, 4 Field

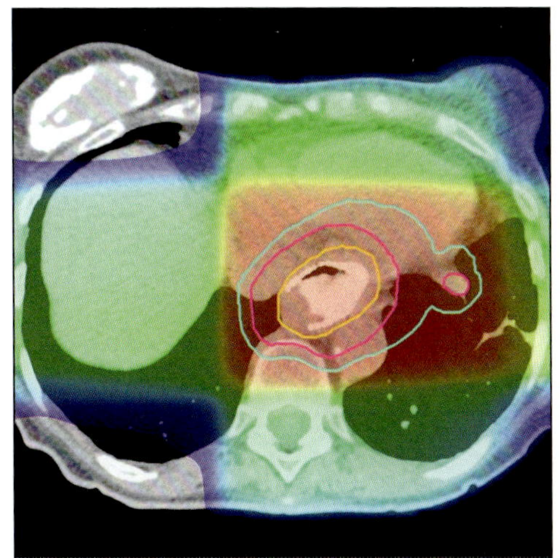

T3 N1 M0 Distal Lesion, 6 Field

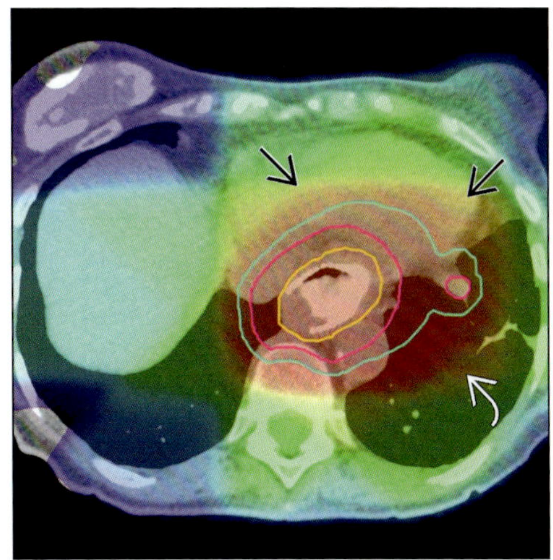

(Left) *Axial NECT shows colorwash dose distribution for a 4-field plan.* ***(Right)*** *Axial NECT shows dose distribution for a 6-field plan. Note reduction in heart and lung high-dose regions.*

T3 N1 M0 Distal Lesion, IMRT

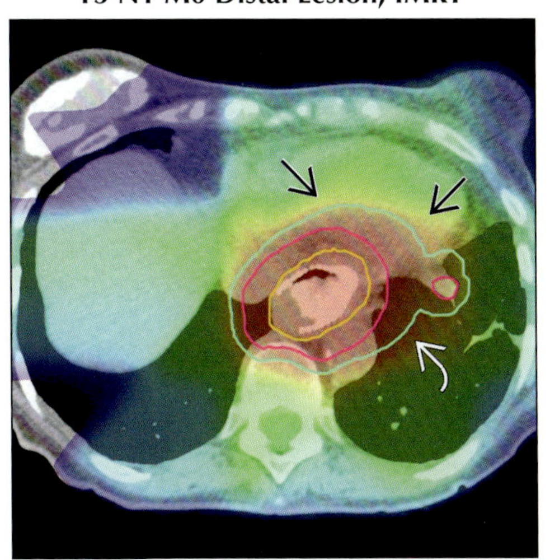

T3 N1 M0 Distal Lesion, DVH

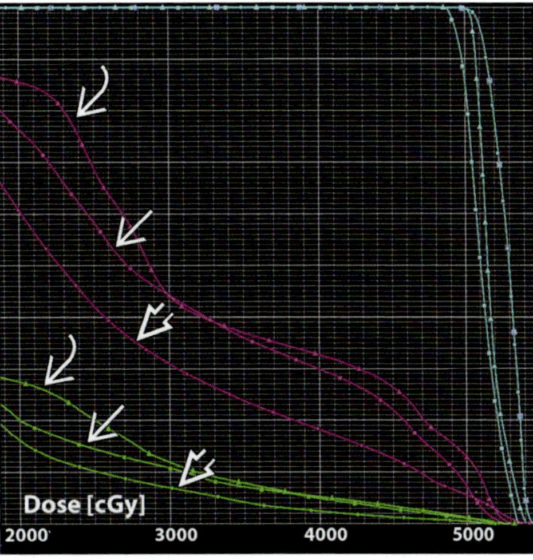

(Left) *Axial NECT shows dose distribution for an IMRT plan. Note further reduction in heart and lung high-dose regions.* ***(Right)*** *Comparison of DVHs for the 3 plans (green = total lung, magenta = heart, and cyan = PTV) shows a reduction in dose to OARs with IMRT and 6 fields compared to 4 fields.*

(Left) *AP DRR shows noncontiguous fields used to decrease treatment volumes due to large distance between primary and concerning proximal nodes. Lower field includes primary (GTV = red; SUV 18 on PET) and regional nodes (paraesophageal = blue; SUV 15) and celiac region (yellow = celiac artery). Upper field includes rounded, suspicious paraesophageal nodes (magenta, SUV 3).* ***(Right)*** *Sagittal DRR in the same patient shows noncontiguous fields.*

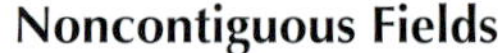

Noncontiguous Fields

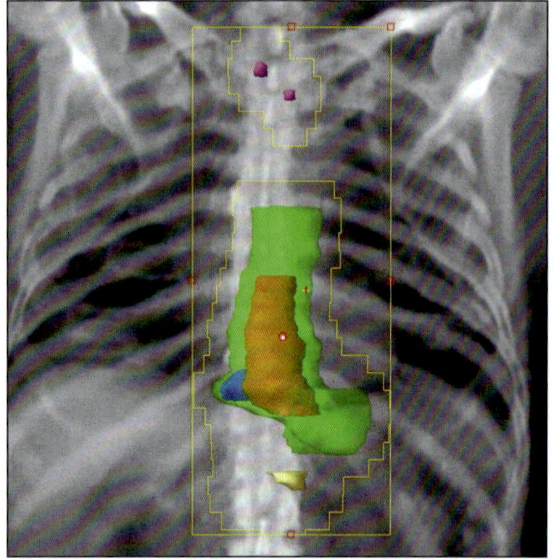

Noncontiguous Fields

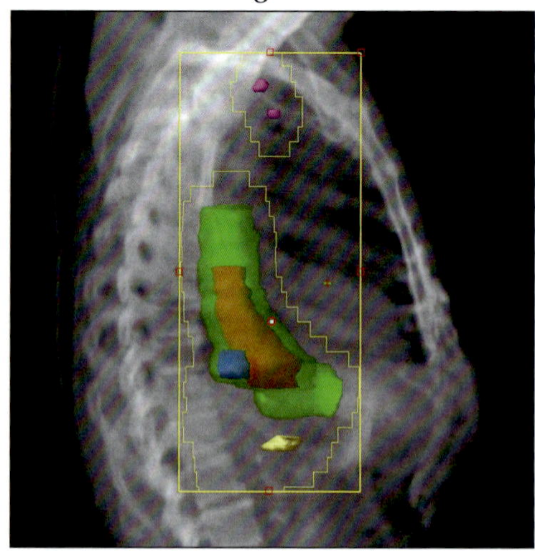

(Left) *Axial NECT in the same patient shows 3D conformal plan. 6 fields were used to decrease heart and lung doses compared to 4. Note large paraesophageal node (blue), GTV (red), and CTV (green).* ***(Right)*** *Axial PET/CT in the same patient 6 weeks after CRT shows large paraesophageal node dramatically reduced in size (to 9 mm) → and hypermetabolic activity resolved (SUV 2.2). Elevated SUV of the primary resolved at the subsequent scan done 5 months post CRT.*

Noncontiguous Fields

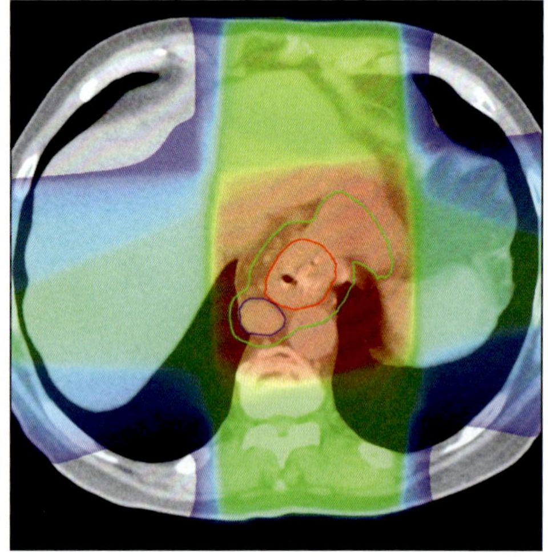

Noncontiguous Fields, Follow-Up

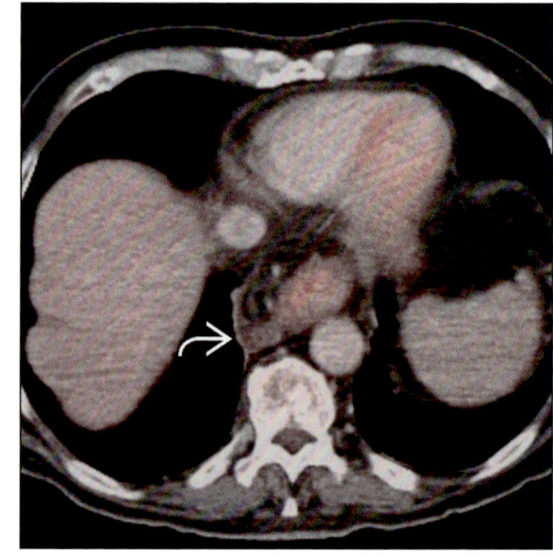

(Left) *Coronal PET/CT in an 80-year-old man shows distal esophageal mass with elevated SUV of 26 →. Due to his age and cardiac comorbidities, he was not an operative candidate.* ***(Right)*** *Coronal PET/CT in the same patient 6 weeks following definitive chemoradiation shows complete PET response →. The tumor recurred locally 1 year post treatment and the patient died from brain metastases 7 months afterward.*

T3 N1 M0 CRT

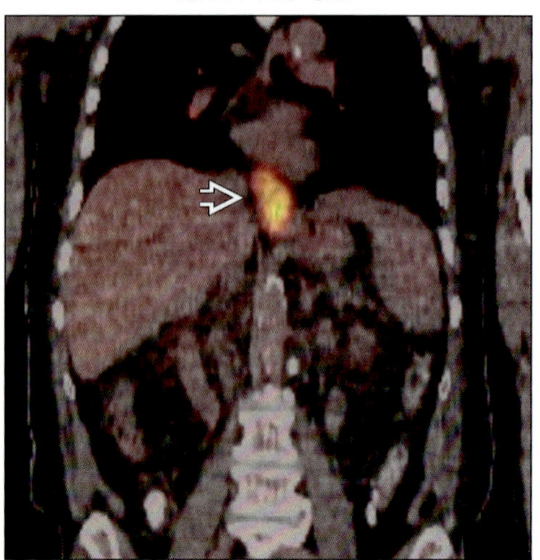

T3 N1 M0 CRT

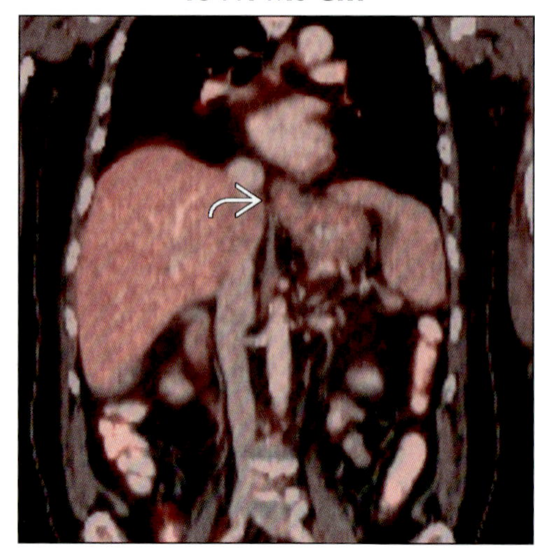

Anastamotic Recurrence

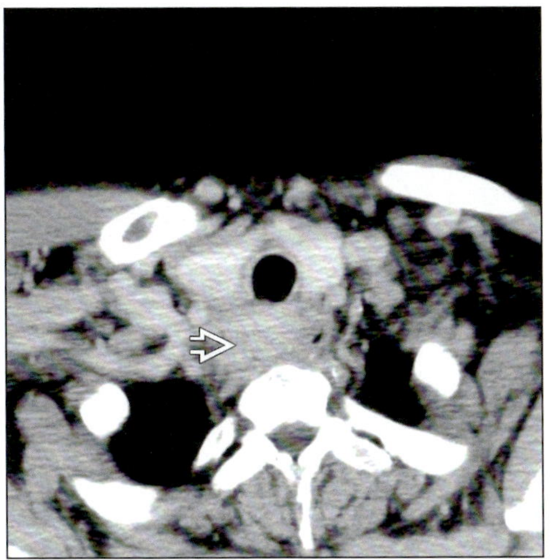

Anastamotic Recurrence

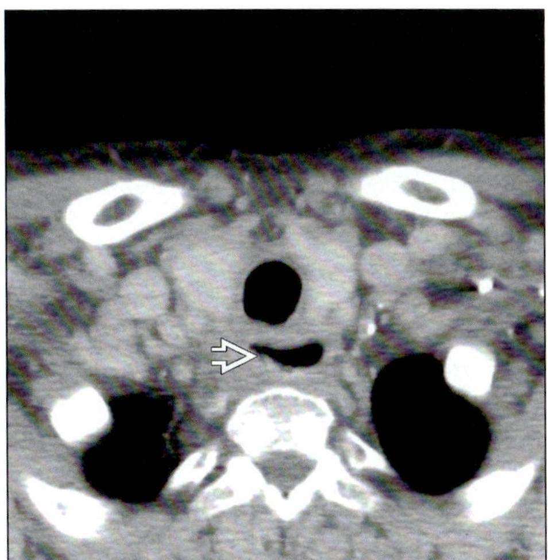

*(**Left**) Four years following neoadjuvant CRT and transhiatal esophagectomy for a stage IIIA (T3 N1 M0) AC, axial CECT in this 48-year-old man shows an enhancing, obstructive mass at the anastomosis ➡. (**Right**) Axial CECT in the same patient was done 2 months after 49.2 Gy in 41 fractions of 1.2 Gy given b.i.d., concurrent with cisplatin and 5-FU. Note the excellent response with opening of the esophageal lumen ➡, allowing for resolution of his dysphagia.*

Anastamotic Recurrence With Stenosis

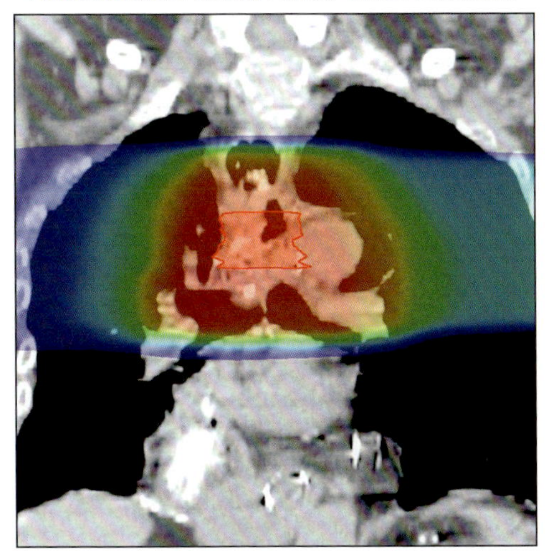

Anastamotic Recurrence With Stenosis

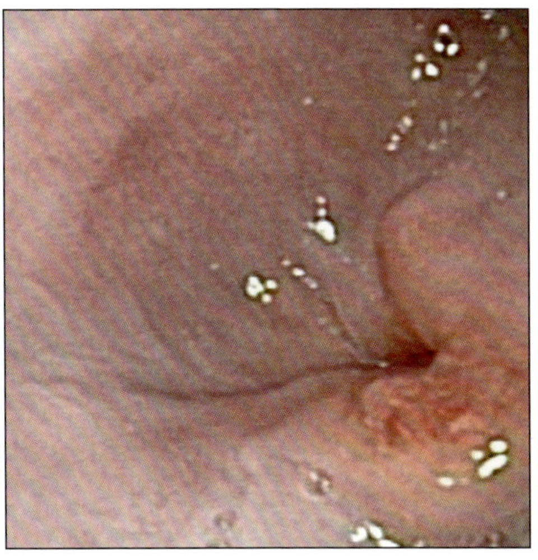

*(**Left**) Coronal NECT shows anastomotic recurrence in a 75-year-old man with a history of stage IIIA disease. 4.5 years prior he received 50.4 Gy with chemotherapy followed by esophagectomy. For his repeat course of concurrent chemoradiation, he received 32 Gy in 28 fractions. (**Right**) Endoscopic photograph in the same patient 1 year later shows a stricture 22 cm from the incisors at the esophagogastric anastomosis.*

Anastamotic Recurrence With Stenosis

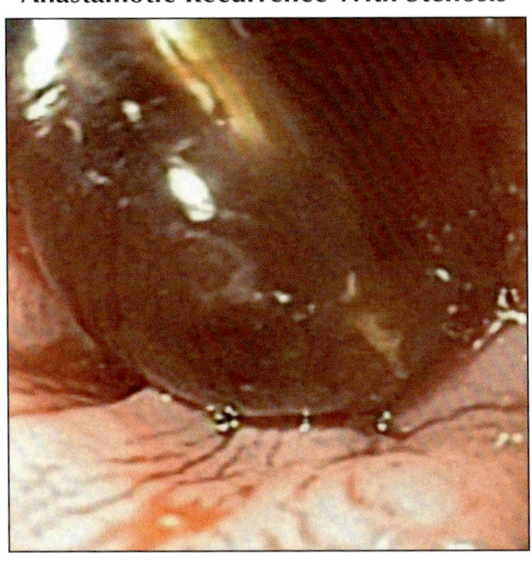

Anastamotic Recurrence With Stenosis

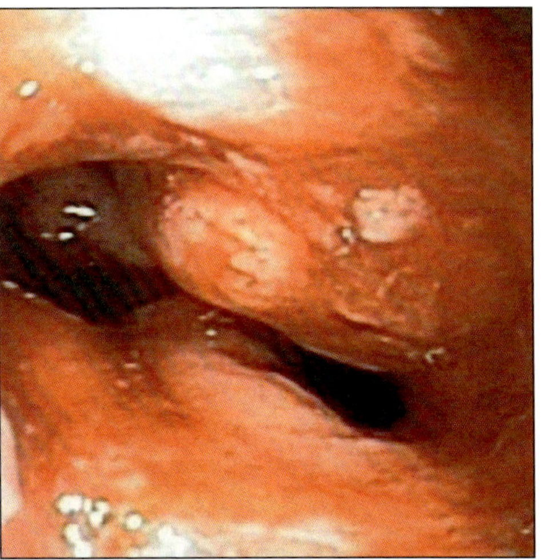

*(**Left**) Endoscopic photograph in the same patient shows esophageal balloon dilating esophagus to 16.5 mm, following placement of a 0.035" guidewire. (**Right**) Endoscopic photograph in the same patient shows successful dilation and luminal opening. Biopsies were positive for disease.*

Anastamotic Recurrence With Stenosis

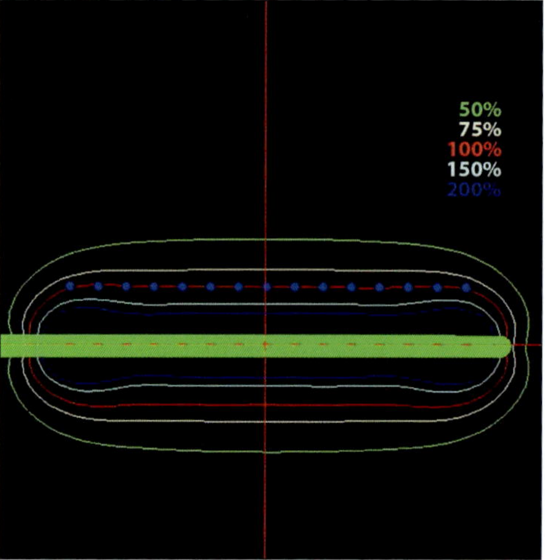

Anastamotic Recurrence With Stenosis

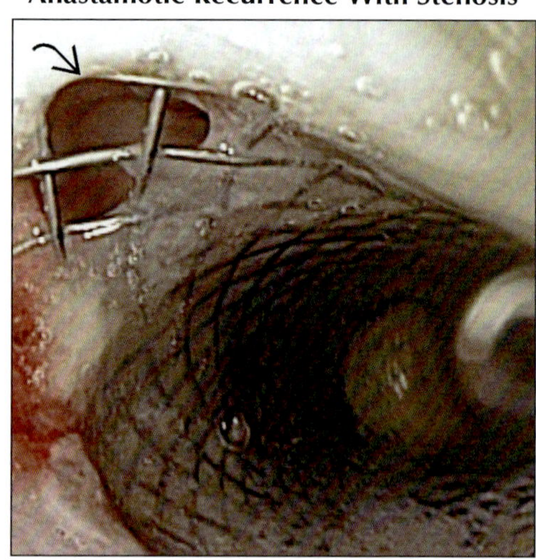

(Left) *For this 2nd recurrence at the anastomosis, the same patient received brachytherapy to 8 Gy in a single fraction, prescribed at 1 cm from the source. This brachytherapy dose was lower than usual because of the prior EBRT.* ***(Right)*** *Endoscopic photograph 5 months later shows tracheoesophageal fistula that formed in the multiply radiated area. It can be seen behind the proximal uncovered portion of an Ultraflex 1.8 x 10 cm covered esophageal stent ➘.*

Anastamotic Recurrence With Stenosis

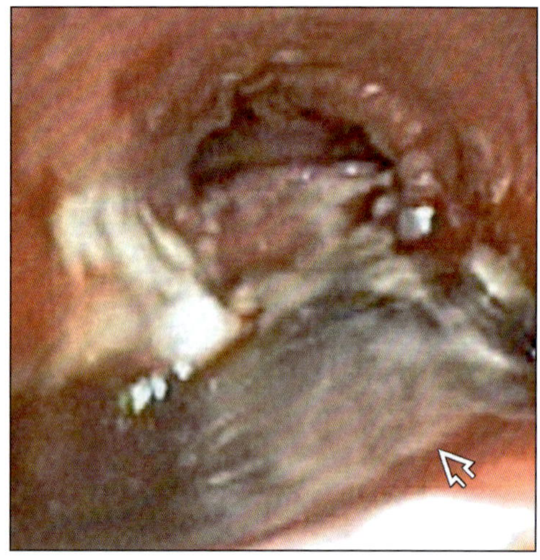

Anastamotic Recurrence With Stenosis

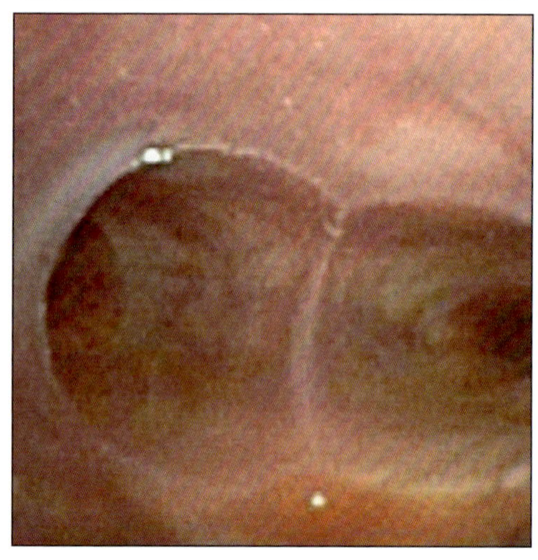

(Left) *Bronchoscopy in the same patient reveals the esophageal stent ➡ behind a 4 cm defect along the membranous trachea, starting 1 cm proximal to the carina.* ***(Right)*** *In the same patient, a silicone Y stent was placed to cover the tracheal side of the fistula.*

Anastamotic & Nodal Recurrence

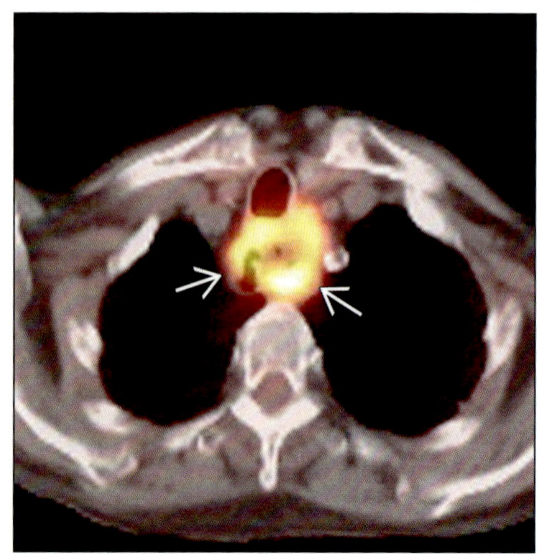

Anastamotic & Nodal Recurrence

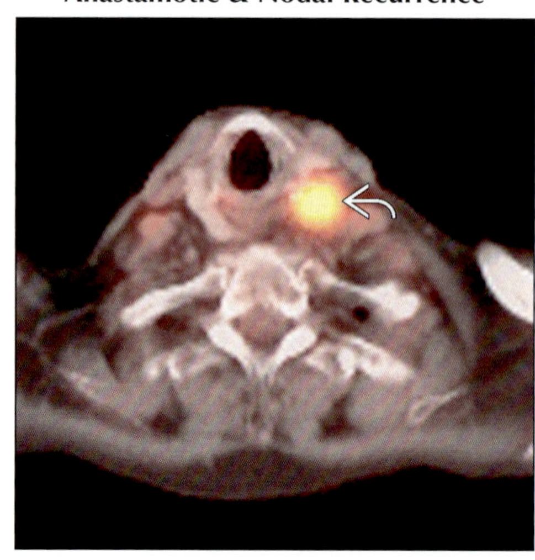

(Left) *Axial PET/CT in the same patient shows a hypermetabolic mass ➡ arising at the site of esophagogastric anastomosis.* ***(Right)*** *Axial PET/CT in the same patient at the level of the lower neck shows a metastatic, hypermetabolic, left-side neck lymph node ➡.*

T3 N2 M0 CRT

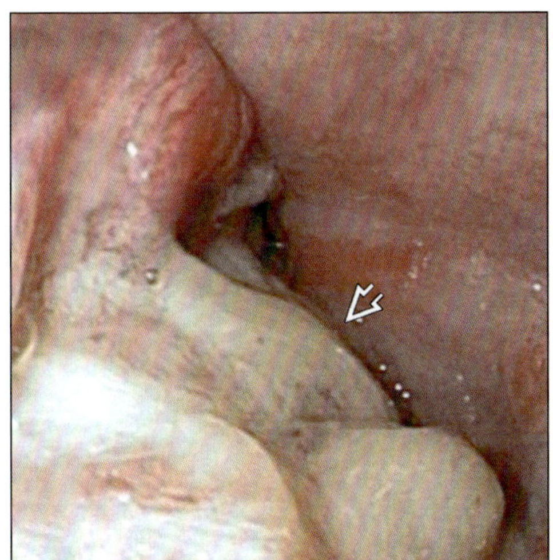

T3 N2 M0 CRT

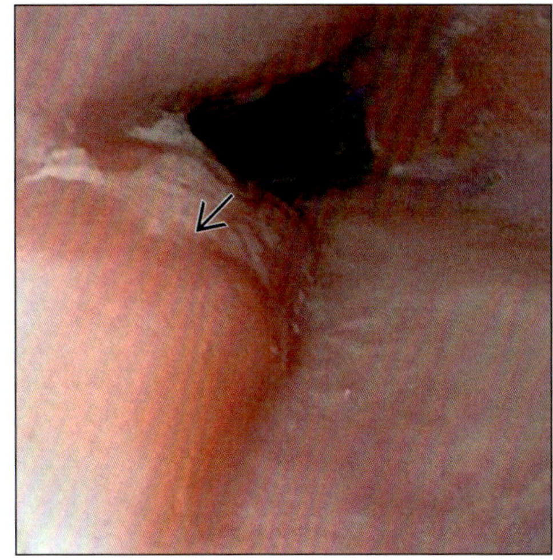

(Left) *Endoscopic photograph in a 61-year-old-man shows a large, fungating mass ➡ 31-37 cm from the incisors involving 2/3 of the lumen circumference.* ***(Right)*** *Endoscopic photograph in the same patient shows marked shrinkage of the fungating tumor ➡ 6 weeks post chemoradiation. Corresponding PET/CT showed decrease in SUV from 57.4 to 4.7. Biopsy was negative for disease.*

T3 N2 M0 CRT

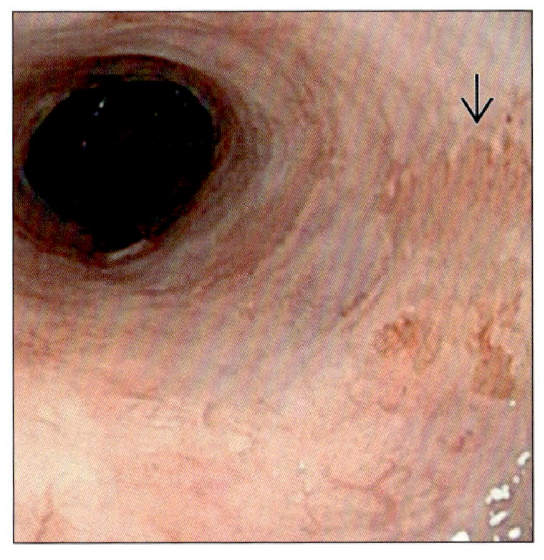

T3 N2 M0 CRT, Pericardial Effusion

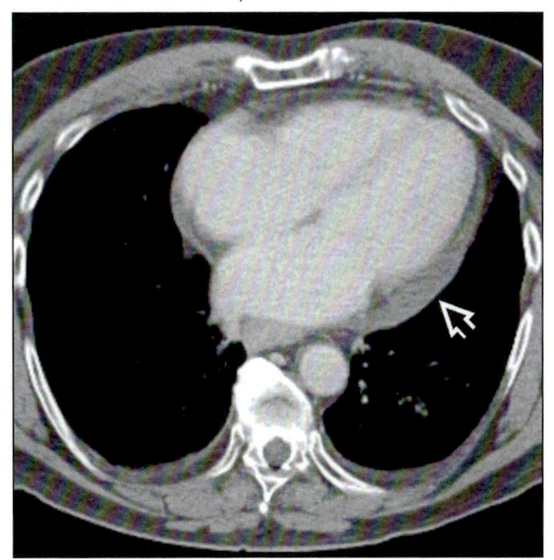

(Left) *Endoscopic photograph in the same patient 10 months post treatment shows mucosal abnormality ➡ characterized by atrophy, texture change, and decreased vascular pattern. Although biopsy was consistent with adenocarcinoma, the esophagectomy specimen did not show any residual disease.* ***(Right)*** *Axial CECT in the same patient shows mild, asymptomatic pericardial effusion ➡ 10 months out from chemoradiation.*

Recurrent Disease Following Esophagectomy

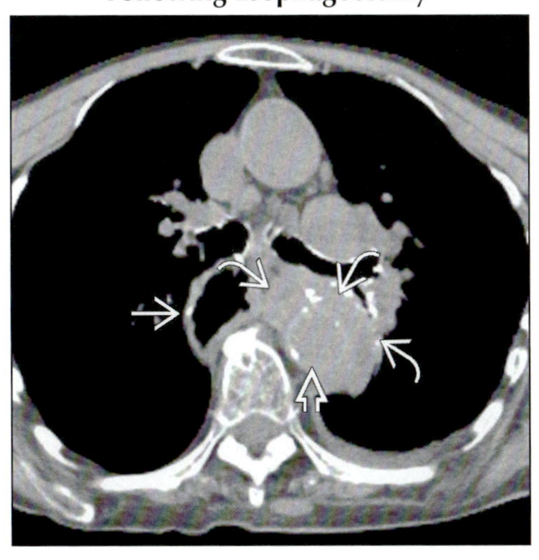

Recurrent Disease Following Esophagectomy

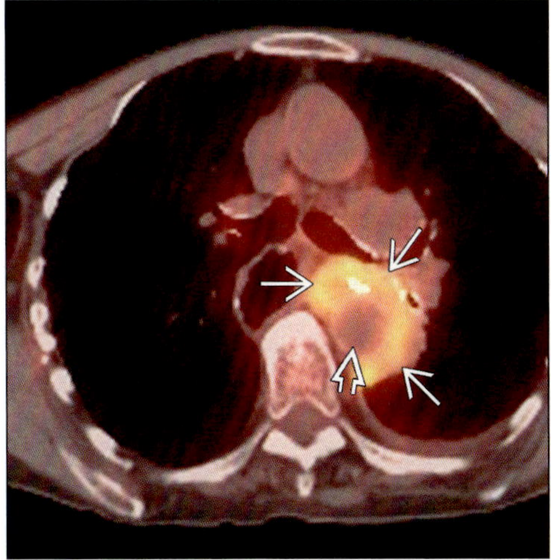

(Left) *Axial NECT in a 77-year-old woman, 12 months after esophagectomy for stage IIB esophageal adenocarcinoma (T3 N0 M0), shows gastric pull-up ➡ and abnormal soft tissue ➡ encasing the thoracic aorta ➡.* ***(Right)*** *Axial PET/CT in the same patient shows increased metabolic activity of the abnormal soft tissue ➡ encasing the descending thoracic aorta ➡.*

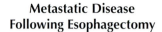

ESOPHAGUS

(**Left**) *Axial CECT in the same patient 6 months after esophagectomy shows a metastatic low-attenuation lesion within the left pectoralis muscle ➡ and destructive lesion of the left scapula ➡.* (**Right**) *Axial CECT in the same patient shows widespread low-attenuation, ill-defined metastatic lesions within the liver ➡, a large metastatic lesion of the right adrenal gland ➡, and a hypoattenuating lesion within the spleen ➡.*

Metastatic Disease Following Esophagectomy

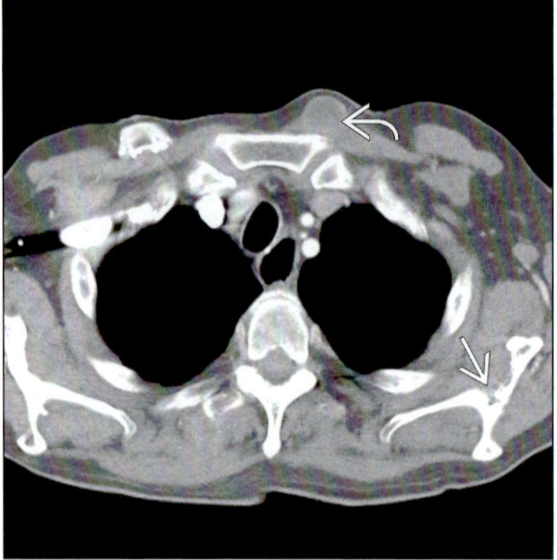

Metastatic Disease Following Esophagectomy

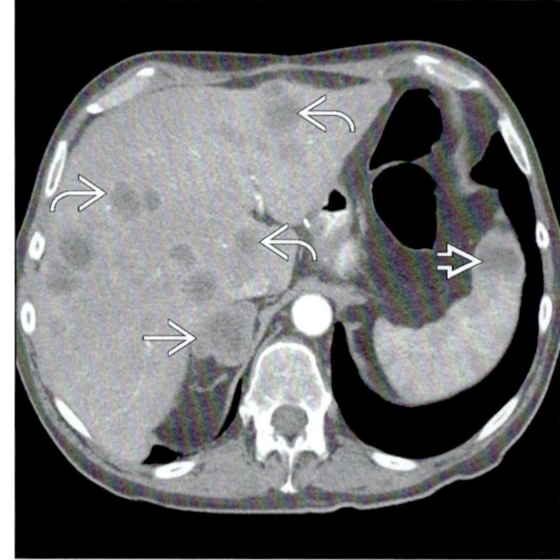

(**Left**) *Axial PET/CT in a 67-year-old woman with GE junction tumor shows extension to gastric cardia (SUV 31) ➡, gastrohepatic lymph nodes (SUV 17) ➡, and a retrocrural node (SUV 26) ➡.* (**Right**) *Axial PET/CT shows mildly suspicious 6 mm node ➡ with minimal PET avidity (SUV 1.6) adjacent to the left renal artery.*

Distant Nodal Recurrence

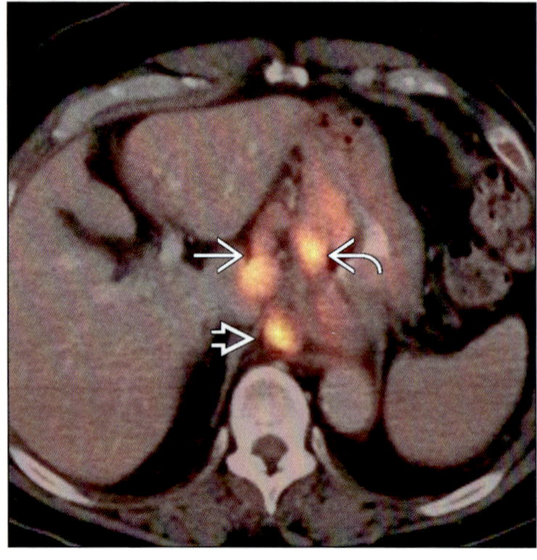

Distant Nodal Recurrence

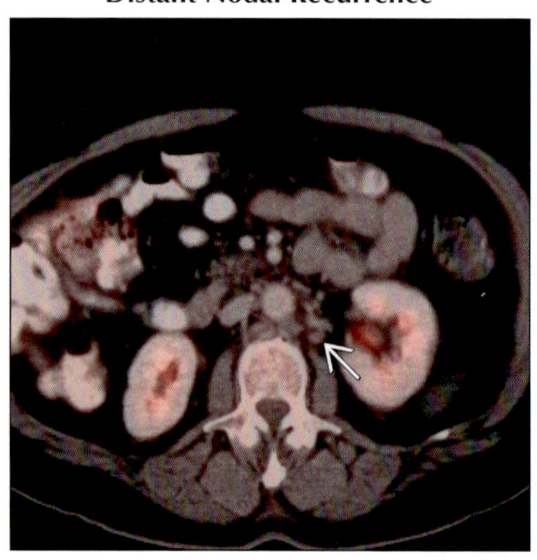

(**Left**) *Axial PET/CT 5 months after CRT shows massive retroperitoneal nodal progression ➡ in area of prior suspicious node. Biopsy confirmed recurrent AC.* (**Right**) *Coronal PET/CT shows extensive lymphadenopathy involving the SCV, mediastinal, retrocrural, retroperitoneal ➡, gastrohepatic, and common iliac regions ➡. SUV of the primary ➡ has increased, there is a new lung met, and the pleural effusion ➡ was confirmed as malignant on cytology.*

Distant Nodal Recurrence

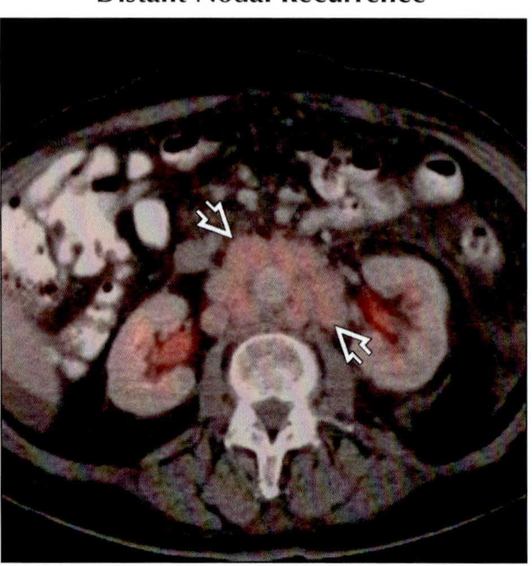

Distant Nodal Recurrence

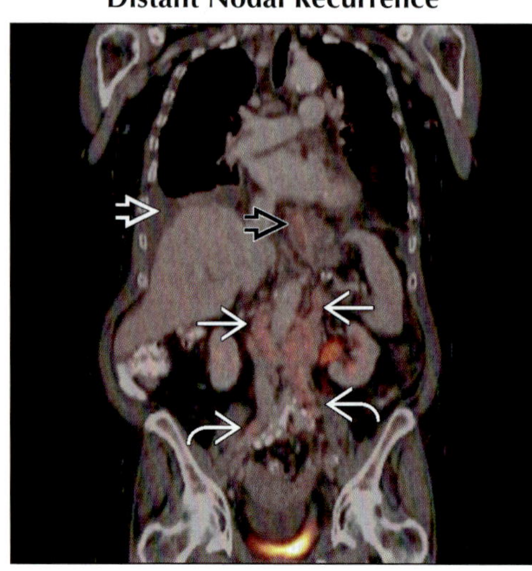

Carcinomatosis

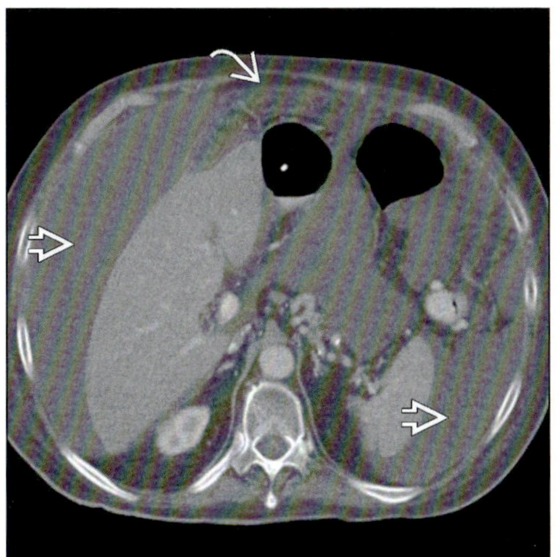

Distant Recurrence

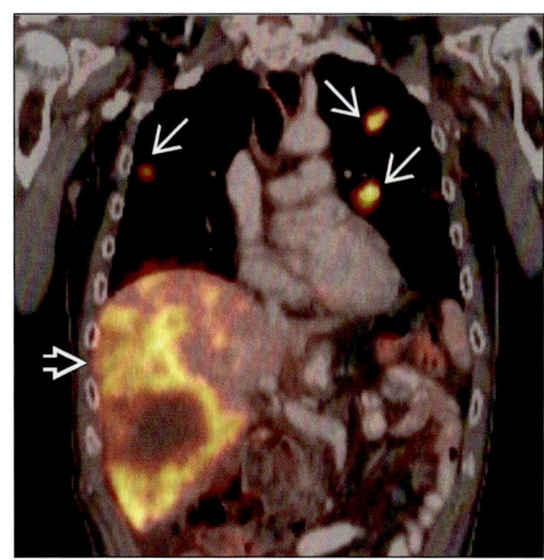

(Left) *Axial CECT in a 65-year-old patient 4 months after definitive chemoradiation shows abnormal induration and nodularity of the omentum, suggestive of peritoneal carcinomatosis ⮫. Note extensive ascites in abdominal cavity ➲.* ***(Right)*** *Coronal PET/CT was performed on a 64-year-old-man for fatigue 16 months following neoadjuvant chemoradiation and esophagectomy. Recurrence is noted in the liver ➲ and lungs bilaterally ➔.*

Transient Hepatitis

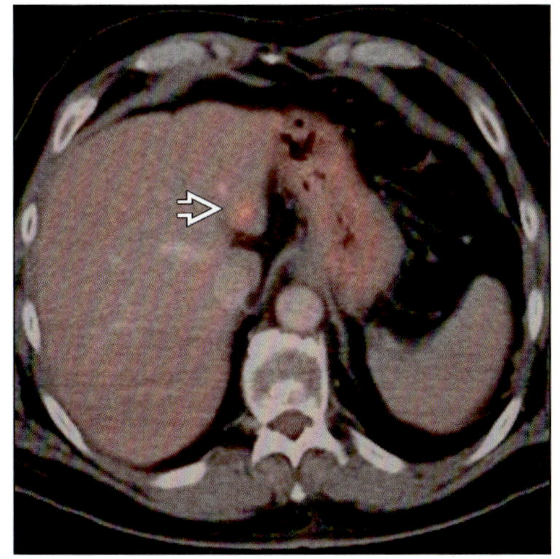

Transient Hepatitis

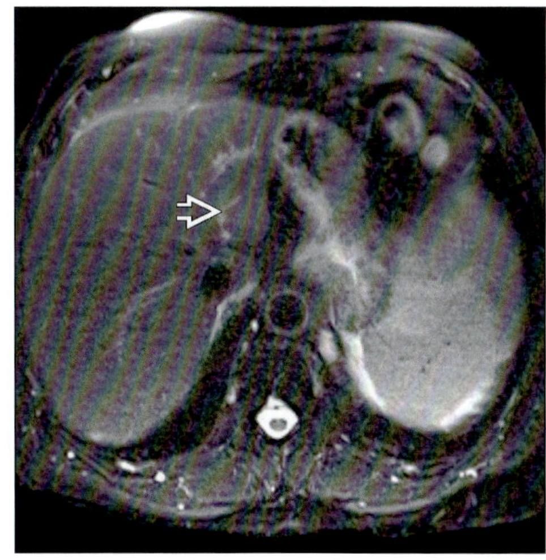

(Left) *Axial PET/CT in a 59-year-old man 6 weeks after definitive chemoradiation shows hypermetabolic activity (SUV 5.6) within a hypoattenuating lesion in segment 2 of the liver ➲, concerning for metastasis.* ***(Right)*** *Axial T2WI FSE MR in the same patient shows the mass with slightly increased T2 signal intensity ➲ compared to the remainder of the liver. It had decreased T1 intensity and enhanced heterogeneously, concerning for metastasis.*

Transient Hepatitis

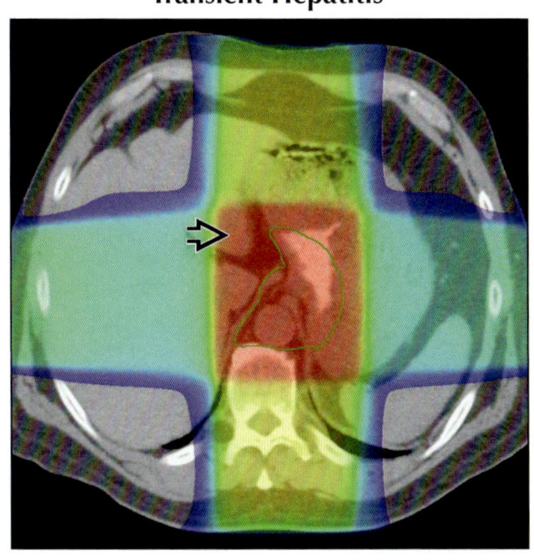

Transient Hepatitis

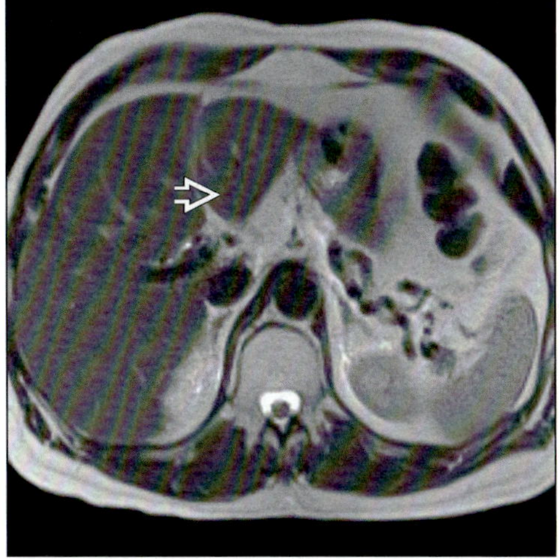

(Left) *Axial NECT in the same patient shows area of liver abnormality ➲ was previously included in the high-dose region of 50.4 Gy.* ***(Right)*** *Axial T2WI MR in the same patient 2 months after initial MR shows resolution of the segment 2 abnormality ➲, indicating that radiation hepatitis was the likely cause.*

STOMACH

(T) Primary Tumor

Adapted from 7th edition AJCC Staging Forms.

TNM	*Definitions*
TX	Primary tumor cannot be assessed
T0	No evidence of primary tumor
Tis	Carcinoma in situ: Intraepithelial tumor without invasion of the lamina propria
T1	Tumor invades lamina propria, muscularis mucosae, or submucosa
T1a	Tumor invades lamina propria or muscularis mucosae
T1b	Tumor invades submucosa
T2	Tumor invades muscularis propria[1]
T3	Tumor penetrates subserosal connective tissue without invasion of visceral peritoneum or adjacent structures[2]
T4	Tumor invades serosa (visceral peritoneum) or adjacent structures[2]
T4a	Tumor invades serosa (visceral peritoneum)
T4b	Tumor invades adjacent structures

(N) Regional Lymph Nodes

NX	Regional lymph node(s) cannot be assessed
N0	No regional lymph node metastasis[3]
N1	Metastasis in 1-2 regional lymph nodes
N2	Metastasis in 3-6 regional lymph nodes
N3	Metastasis in ≥ 7 regional lymph nodes
N3a	Metastasis in 7-15 regional lymph nodes
N3b	Metastasis in ≥ 16 regional lymph nodes

(M) Distant Metastasis

M0	No distant metastasis
M1	Distant metastasis

[1]*A tumor may penetrate the muscularis propria with extension into the gastrocolic or gastrohepatic ligaments, or into the greater or lesser omentum, without perforation of the visceral peritoneum covering these structures. In this case, the tumor is classified T3. If there is perforation of the visceral peritoneum covering the gastric ligaments or the omentum, the tumor should be classified T4.*

[2]*The adjacent structures of the stomach include the spleen, transverse colon, liver, diaphragm, pancreas, abdominal wall, adrenal gland, kidney, small intestine, and retroperitoneum. Intramural extension to the duodenum or esophagus is classified by the depth of the greatest invasion in any of these sites, including the stomach.*

[3]*A designation of pN0 should be used if all examined lymph nodes are negative, regardless of the total number removed and examined.*

STOMACH

AJCC Stages/Prognostic Groups

Adapted from 7th edition AJCC Staging Forms.

Stage	*T*	*N*	*M*
0	Tis	N0	M0
IA	T1	N0	M0
IB	T2	N0	M0
	T1	N1	M0
IIA	T3	N0	M0
	T2	N1	M0
	T1	N2	M0
IIB	T4a	N0	M0
	T3	N1	M0
	T2	N2	M0
	T1	N3	M0
IIIA	T4a	N1	M0
	T3	N2	M0
	T2	N3	M0
IIIB	T4b	N0	M0
	T4b	N1	M0
	T4a	N2	M0
	T3	N3	M0
IIIC	T4b	N2	M0
	T4b	N3	M0
	T4a	N3	M0
IV	Any T	Any N	M1

T1

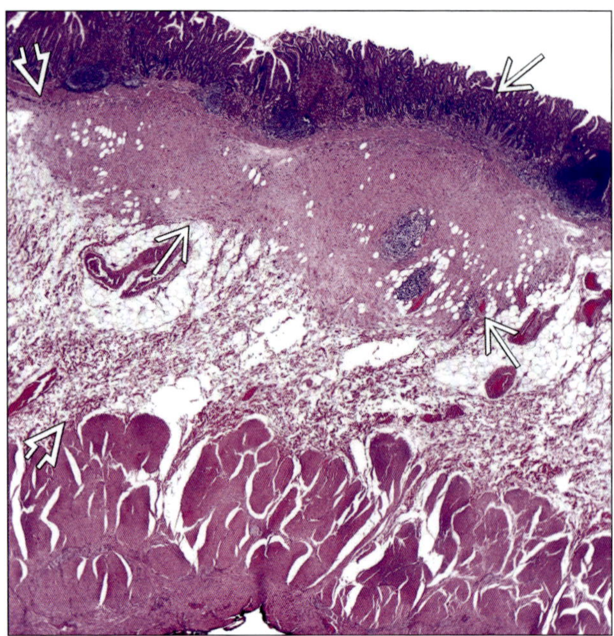

H&E stained section shows invasive gastric carcinoma ➡ that involves lamina propria and extends to invade the upper portion of the submucosa ➡.

T1

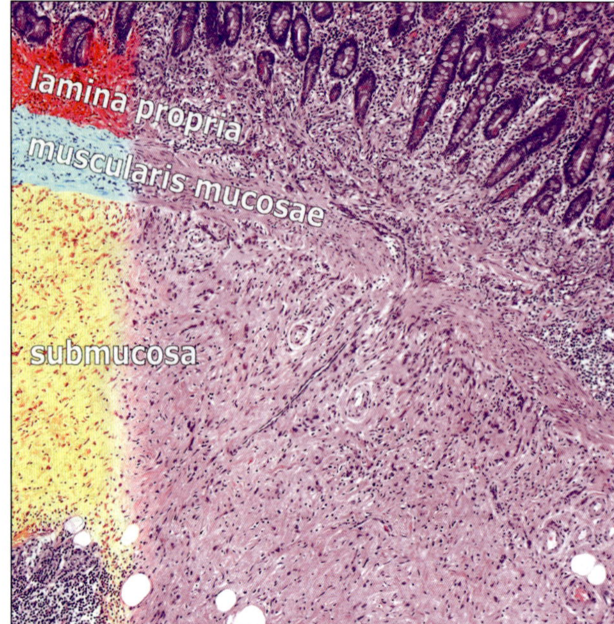

Higher magnification of H&E stained section of invasive gastric adenocarcinoma shows the neoplastic cells in the lamina propria extending through the muscularis mucosae and into the submucosa.

T2

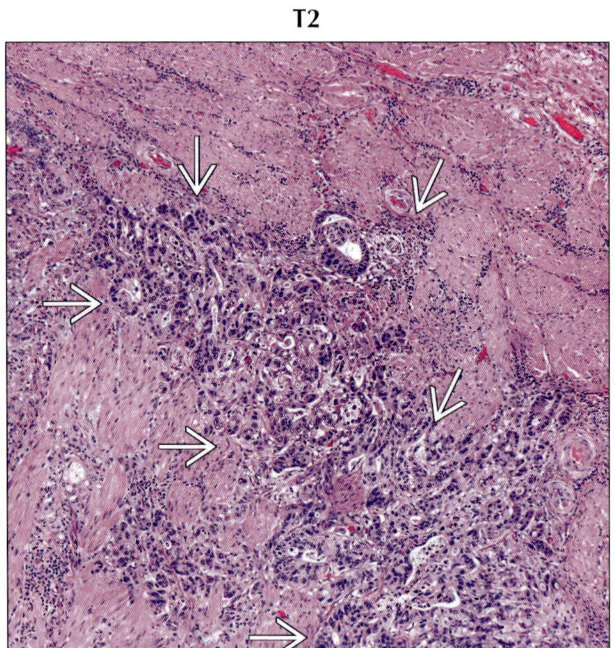

H&E stained section shows invasive gastric adenocarcinoma ➡ extending into the muscle bundles of the muscularis propria.

T4

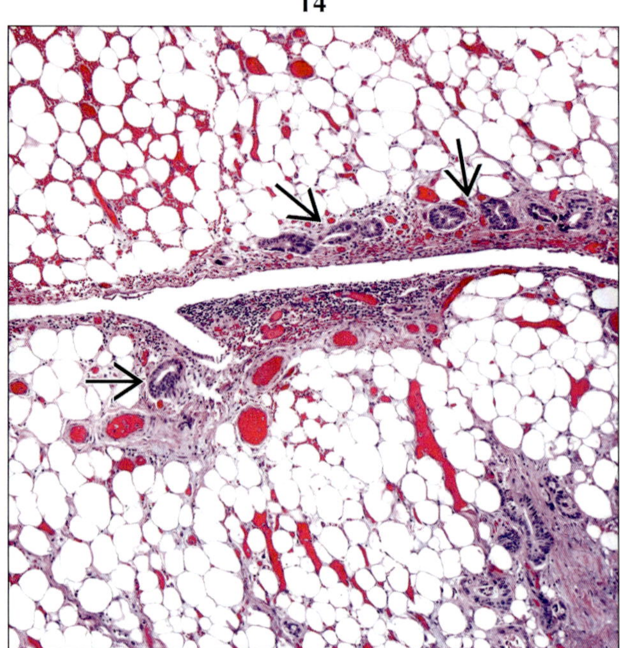

H&E stained section from invasive gastric adenocarcinoma shows the neoplastic glands ➡ invading serosa and extending to involve the fibrofatty connective tissue of the omentum. The fat cells are the round (clear/white) spaces.

T1a

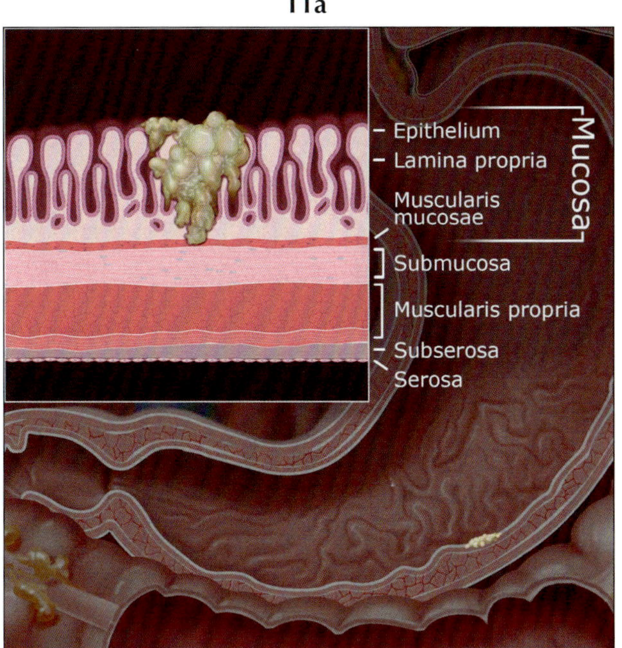

Graphic illustrates T1a tumor, which invades lamina propria or muscularis mucosae.

T1b

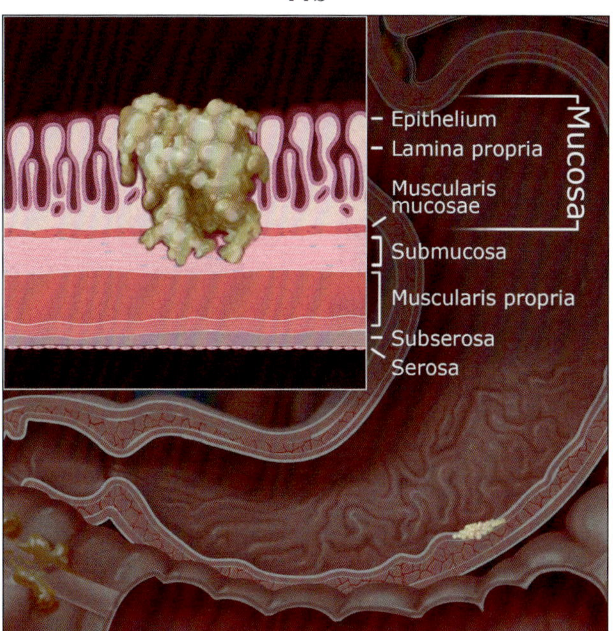

Graphic illustrates T1b tumor, which invades the submucosal layer.

T2

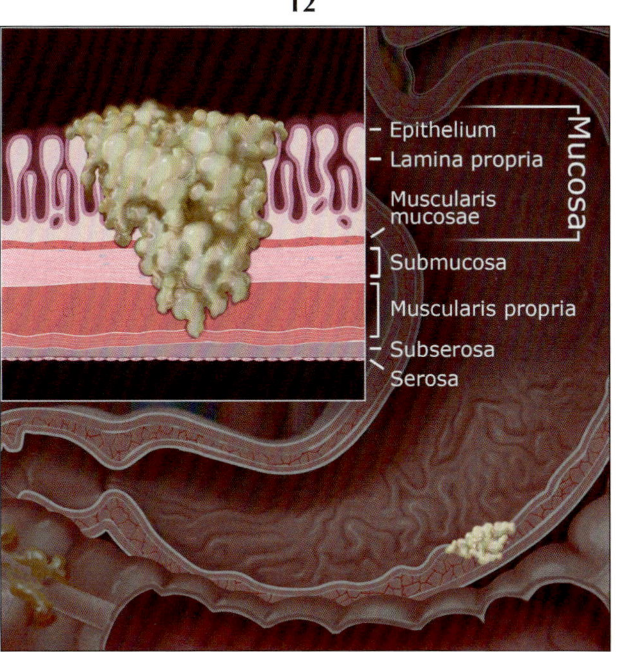

Graphic illustrates T2 tumor, which invades muscularis propria.

T3

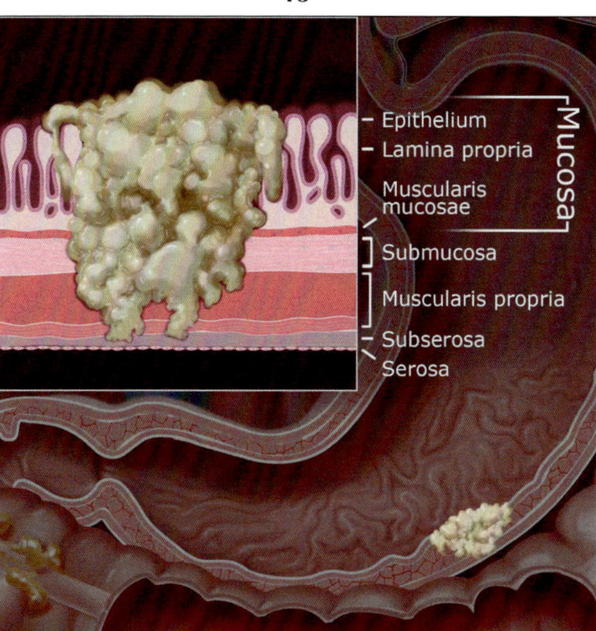

Graphic illustrates T3 tumor, which invades subserosal connective tissue without invasion of visceral peritoneum or adjacent structures.

T4a

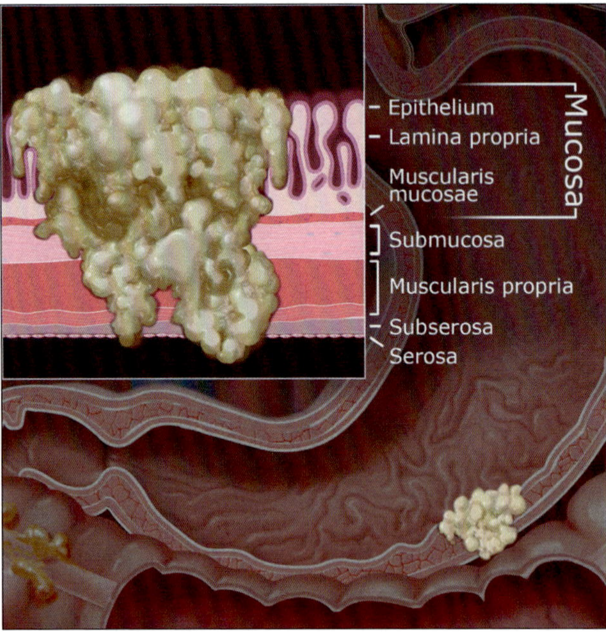

Graphic illustrates tumor that invades serosa (visceral peritoneum) without extension to adjacent structures, consistent with T4a disease.

T4b

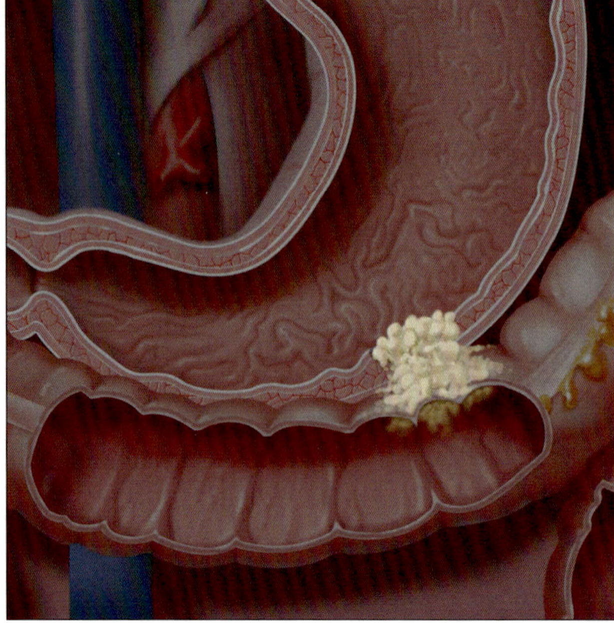

Graphic illustrates tumor invading the transverse colon. Invasion of adjacent structures, which also include the spleen, liver, diaphragm, pancreas, abdominal wall, adrenal gland, kidney, small intestine, and retroperitoneum, constitutes T4b disease.

N1

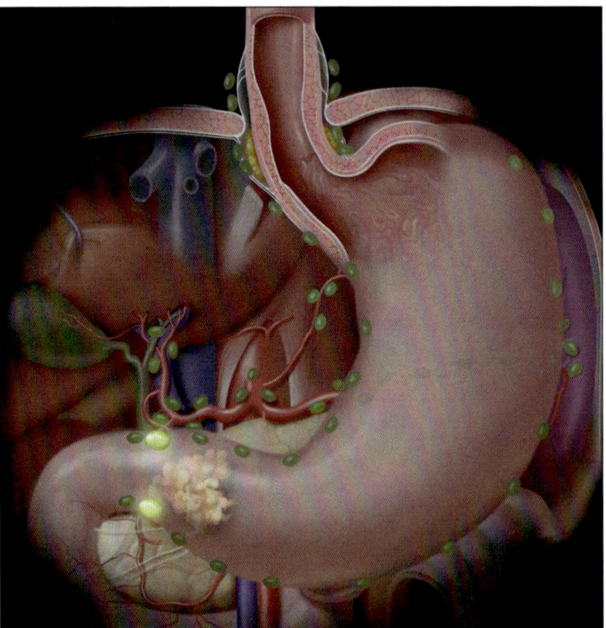

Graphic illustrates N1 disease, defined as metastases in 1-2 regional nodes.

N2

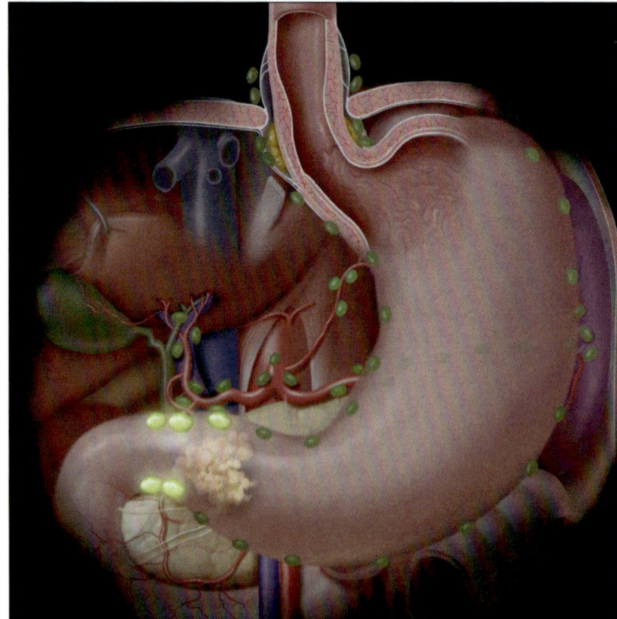

Graphic illustrates N2 disease, defined as metastases in 3-6 regional nodes.

N3

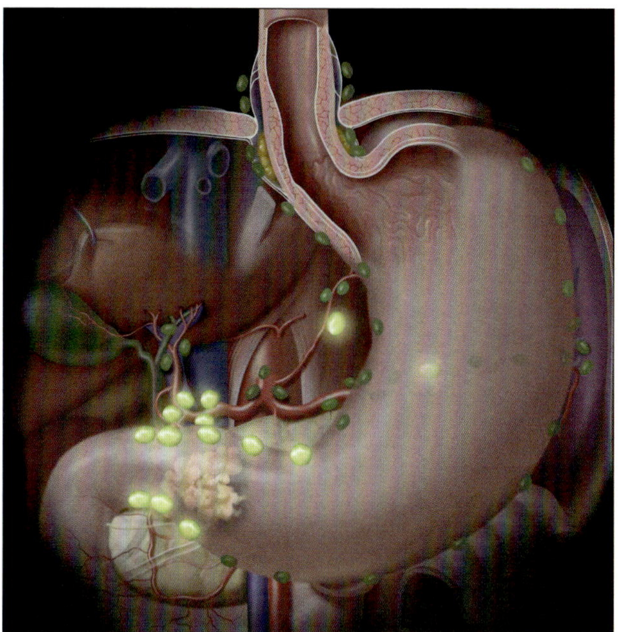

Graphic illustrates N3 disease, defined as metastases in at least 7 regional nodes.

Nodal Stations of the Stomach

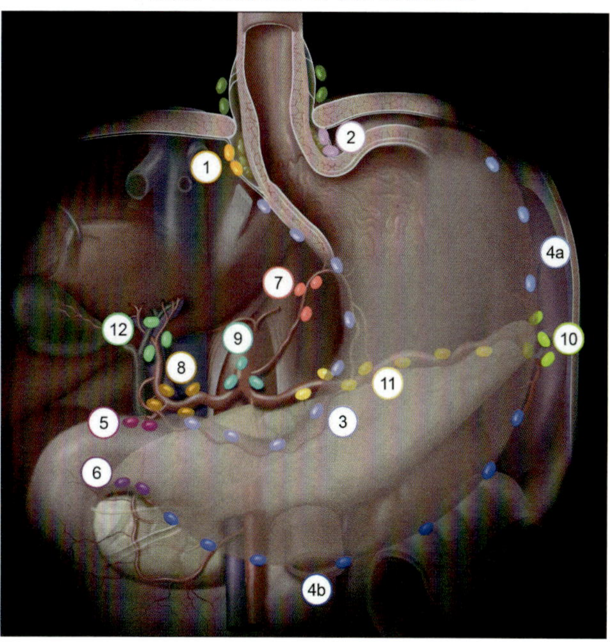

Graphic shows nodal stations of stomach: Perigastric nodes of lesser curvature (1, 3, and 5); perigastric nodes of greater curvature (2, 4, and 6); left gastric nodes (7); nodes along common hepatic artery (8); nodes along celiac artery (9); nodes along splenic artery (10-11); and hepatoduodenal nodes (12).

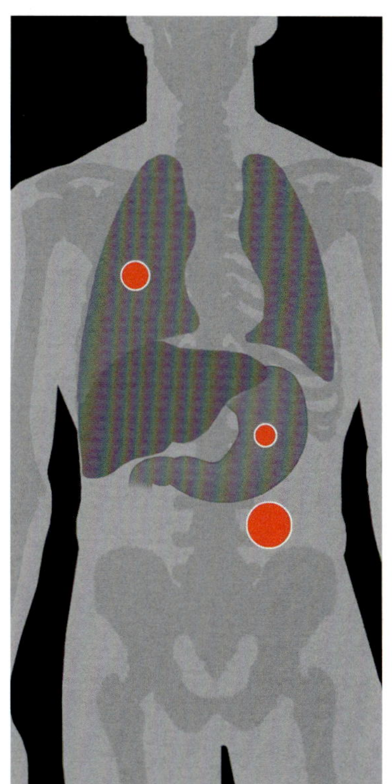

INITIAL SITE OF RECURRENCE

Regional (Including Carcinomatosis)	65%
Distant	33%
Local	19%

Data represent 120 patients treated with surgery and postoperative chemoradiation in the randomized Intergroup trial. Macdonald JS et al: Chemoradiotherapy after surgery compared with surgery alone for adenocarcinoma of the stomach or gastroesophageal junction. N Engl J Med. 345:725-730, 2001.

STOMACH

OVERVIEW

General Comments

- Tumors arising at gastroesophageal junction (GEJ) or arising in stomach ≤ 5 cm from and crossing GEJ are staged with esophageal carcinoma

Classification

- Histological classification
  - Adenocarcinoma
    - Intestinal type
    - Diffuse type
  - Papillary adenocarcinoma
  - Tubular adenocarcinoma
  - Mucinous adenocarcinoma
    - Substantial amount of extracellular mucin (> 50% of tumor) is retained within tumor
  - Signet ring cell carcinoma (> 50% signet ring cells)
  - Adenosquamous carcinoma
  - Squamous cell carcinoma
  - Small cell carcinoma
  - Undifferentiated carcinoma
  - Other

NATURAL HISTORY

General Features

- Comments
  - Incidence of gastric cancer ↓ markedly over the last 80 years in the United States; however, incidence of GEJ adenocarcinoma ↑ in the last few decades, especially for white males

Etiology

- Risk factors
  - *Helicobacter pylori* gastric infection
    - 6x increase in risk
  - Advanced age
  - Male gender
  - Diet low in fruits and vegetables
  - Diet high in salted, smoked, or preserved foods
  - Chronic atrophic gastritis
  - Intestinal metaplasia
  - Pernicious anemia
  - Gastric adenomatous polyps
  - Family history of gastric cancer
  - Cigarette smoking
  - Ménétrier disease (giant hypertrophic gastritis)
  - Familial adenomatous polyposis
    - 0.5% risk of developing gastric carcinoma
  - Previous gastric surgery
    - Rationale is that previous gastric surgery alters normal pH of stomach

Epidemiology & Cancer Incidence

- Median age at diagnosis is 71 years
- Age-adjusted incidence rate is 7.9 per 100,000 per year
  - 11.0 per 100,000 men
  - 5.5 per 100,000 women
- 4th most common cancer worldwide
  - Estimated 21,320 cases of gastric carcinoma diagnosed in USA in 2012
    - 13,020 men and 8,300 women
- 2nd leading cause of cancer death worldwide
  - Estimated 10,540 patient deaths from gastric carcinoma in USA in 2012
- Highest rates of gastric carcinoma in Asia and Eastern Europe

Associated Diseases, Abnormalities

- Chronic atrophic gastritis
- Pernicious anemia
- Gastric adenomatous polyps
- Ménétrier disease (giant hypertrophic gastritis)

Gross Pathology & Surgical Features

- Borrmannthis morphological classification
  - Type I (polypoid): Well-circumscribed polypoid tumors
  - Type II (fungating): Polypoid tumors with marked central infiltration
  - Type III (ulcerated): Ulcerated tumors with infiltrative margins
  - Type IV (infiltrating): Linitis plastica

Microscopic Pathology

- Gastric adenocarcinoma
  - Intestinal type
    - Characterized by cohesive neoplastic cells forming gland-like tubular structures
  - Diffuse type
    - Cell cohesion is absent so that individual cells infiltrate and thicken stomach wall without forming discrete mass
- Papillary adenocarcinoma
  - Exophytic lesions with elongated slender or plump, finger-like processes in which fibrovascular cores and connective tissue support cells
- Tubular carcinoma
  - Well-defined glandular lumina
- Mucinous carcinoma
  - Sometimes also referred to as colloid carcinoma
  - Contain abundant mucin secreted by tumor cells, creating mucous lakes
- Signet ring cell carcinoma
  - Composed of cells containing unsecreted mucus in cytoplasm to compress nucleus to edge of cell
  - Often demonstrate infiltrative gross appearance
  - Some signet ring tumors appear to form a linitis plastica-type tumor by spreading intramurally, usually not involving mucosa

Routes of Spread

- Submucosal spread
  - Main mechanism of transpyloric spread of tumor into duodenum
    - Brunner glands believed to prevent direct cancer invasion from gastric mucosa to duodenal mucosa
- Subperitoneal spread
  - Tumor may penetrate muscularis propria with extension within subperitoneal space without perforation of visceral peritoneum
    - Such tumor is classified T3
  - Tumor may spread to adjacent organs between peritoneal layers forming ligaments around stomach
    - Spread to left lobe of liver via gastrohepatic ligament (GHL)
      - GHL stretches from cardia and lesser curvature to insert into fissure of ligamentum venosum

- GHL identified by presence of left and right gastric vessels
    - Spread to liver via hepatoduodenal ligament (HDL)
        - HDL is free edge of gastrohepatic ligament; extends from upper aspect of proximal duodenum to liver hilum
        - HDL contains hepatic artery, bile duct, and portal vein
    - Spread to spleen via gastrosplenic ligament (GSL)
        - GSL attaches posterolateral wall of fundus and greater curvature to splenic hilum
        - GSL carries short gastric and leftmost parts of left gastroepiploic vessels
    - Spread to transverse colon via gastrocolic ligament (GCL)
        - GCL extends from greater curvature to transverse colon and extends anteriorly to form greater omentum, which covers colon and small intestine
        - GCL contains right and most of left gastroepiploic vessels
    - Spread to pancreas via lesser sac
- Peritoneal spread
    - Tumor invading serosa can seed into peritoneal cavity
    - Krukenberg tumors
        - Metastatic tumor to ovaries through peritoneal seeding
        - Usually bilateral
- Nodal spread
    - Perigastric lymph nodes are involved early and later drain into central nodes around celiac axis and superior mesenteric artery
        - Tumors along lesser curvature of body and GEJ (area supplied by left gastric artery) → GHL nodes → left gastric nodes → suprapancreatic nodes → celiac nodes
        - Tumors along lesser curvature of antrum and pylorus (area supplied by right gastric artery) → hepatoduodenal ligament nodes → nodes along hepatic artery → celiac nodes
        - Tumors along greater curvature (area supplied by right gastroepiploic artery) → nodes accompanying right gastroepiploic vessels → nodes at gastrocolic trunk or gastroduodenal nodes → superior mesenteric or celiac nodes
        - Tumors along greater curvature of body (area supplied by left gastroepiploic artery) → nodes along left gastroepiploic vessels → splenic hilum nodes → celiac nodes
    - Risk factors for lymph node metastasis include
        - Lymphovascular invasion
        - Depth of invasion (submucosa)
        - Tumor diameter > 20 mm
        - Ulcer or ulcer scar
        - Mucinous adenocarcinoma histological type
- Hematogenous spread
    - Usually involves liver, lungs, and bones

IMAGING

Detection

- Endoscopy
    - Most sensitive and specific diagnostic method in patients suspected of having gastric cancer
    - Allows direct visualization of tumor location, extent of mucosal involvement, and biopsy (or cytologic brushings) for tissue diagnosis
- Double-contrast upper gastrointestinal series
    - 3 major radiographic patterns
        - Malignant ulcer: Radiographic findings include
            - Irregular ulcer crater
            - Distortion or obliteration of surrounding normal areae gastricae
            - Presence of nodular, irregular, radiating folds, which may stop well short of ulcer crater
            - Fused, clubbed, or amputated tips of folds
            - Does not project beyond expected gastric contour when viewed in profile
            - Presence of tumor mass forming an acute angle with gastric wall
        - Polypoid or nodular thickening of gastric wall
        - Diffuse infiltrative pattern (linitis plastica)
            - Diffuse, decreased distensibility of stomach
            - Diffuse fold thickening
- CT
    - MDCT has improved detection of gastric carcinoma compared to single-slice CT
        - Improved detection rate on thin-sliced MPR images compared to 5 mm slice axial images
        - MDCT allows 3D volume rendering and virtual endoscopic imaging
            - Detection rate of early gastric cancer increases up to 96% when using 3D MDCT
    - Water-filling method with gastric CT allows clear depiction of gastric wall and gastric tumor without overshooting artifacts by air in lumen
    - Appearance on CT parallels gross pathological types
        - Well-circumscribed polypoid tumors
        - Ulcerated tumors with infiltrative margins
        - Linitis plastica
        - Patients with nonvisualized primary lesions on MDCT with optimized imaging protocol have early gastric cancers
            - 98% have stage pT1 confined to mucosa or involving submucosal layer
- FDG PET
    - Water intake just before PET imaging is effective method for suppressing physiological FDG uptake in stomach
    - Variable levels of FDG uptake have been found
    - Mucinous adenocarcinoma, signet ring cell carcinoma, and poorly differentiated adenocarcinomas tend to show significantly lower FDG uptake than do other histologic types

Staging

- T staging
    - Endoscopic ultrasound (EUS), MDCT, and MR have comparable diagnostic accuracy in T staging and in assessing serosal involvement
    - EUS
        - Regarded as imaging modality of choice in assessing local invasion of gastric cancer
        - Invasive technique
            - Requires sedation
            - Has recognized procedure- and sedation-related complications, morbidity, and mortality

- Has limited depth of penetration
  - Well suited for evaluation of local invasion
- Diagnostic accuracy of EUS for overall T staging varies (65-92.1%)
- Sensitivity and specificity for assessing serosal involvement varies (77.8-100% and 67.9-100%, respectively)

- CT
  - MDCT has better diagnostic performance than single-row CT scanner
    - Faster scanning overcomes breathing artifacts
    - Thinner slices avoid partial volume effect and allow multiplanar reformats
    - Reported accuracy in tumor staging ranges from 43-86% for single-detector-row CT scanners and from 77-89% for MDCT
  - Advantages of MDCT over EUS
    - Ability to demonstrate regional perigastric disease beyond reach of EUS
    - Ability to demonstrate distant regions like paraaortic lymph nodes and abdominal organs, such as liver
  - Diagnostic accuracy of MDCT for overall T staging varies (73.8-88.9%)
  - Diagnostic accuracy is higher with advanced T disease
    - T1: 45.93%
    - T2: 53.03%
    - T3: 86.49%
    - T4: 85.79%
  - Sensitivity and specificity for assessing serosal involvement varies (82.8-100% and 80-96.8%, respectively)
- MR
  - Diagnostic accuracy of MR for overall T staging varies (71.4-82.6%)
  - Sensitivity and specificity for assessing serosal involvement varies (89.5-93.1% and 94.1-100%, respectively)
- PET/CT
  - Not helpful for local staging

- Imaging criteria for T staging
  - T1
    - Tumor invades lamina propria, muscularis mucosae, or submucosa
    - Tumor shows focal thickening of inner gastric wall
    - Visible low-attenuation stripe along outer layer of gastric wall
  - T2 and T3
    - Different articles in literature describe imaging findings differentiating T2 and T3
      - Articles are based on 6th edition of AJCC staging system
      - Difficult to radiologically distinguish between T2 and T3 in 7th edition
    - T2
      - Tumor invades muscularis propria
      - Thickened gastric wall with loss or disruption of low-attenuation stripe
      - Smooth outer border and clear fat plane around tumor
    - T3
      - Tumor penetrates subserosal connective tissue without invasion of visceral peritoneum or adjacent structures
      - Tumor shows focal or diffuse transmural thickening of gastric wall
      - Tumor penetrating muscularis propria with extension into gastric ligaments without perforation of visceral peritoneum covering these structures would be classified as T3
  - T4a
    - Tumor invades visceral peritoneum
    - Irregular or nodular outer border &/or infiltration of epigastric fat
      - Tumor perforating visceral peritoneum covering gastric ligaments or omenta is classified as T4a
  - T4b
    - Tumor invades adjacent structures
      - Loss of intervening fat plane between tumor and adjacent structures does not necessarily imply invasion
      - Structures adjacent to stomach are spleen, transverse colon, liver, diaphragm, pancreas, abdominal wall, adrenal gland, kidney, small intestine, and retroperitoneum
- **Local disease**
- N staging
  - Regional lymph nodes are
    - Perigastric nodes, found along lesser and greater curvatures
    - Nodes located along left gastric, common hepatic, splenic, and celiac arteries
  - Involvement of other intraabdominal lymph nodes, such as hepatoduodenal, retropancreatic, mesenteric, and paraaortic is classified as distant metastasis
  - Regional nodes are considered involved when
    - Short axis diameter is > 6 mm for perigastric nodes
    - Short axis diameter is > 8 mm for extraperigastric nodes
    - Nearly round shape
    - Fatty hilum is absent or eccentric
    - Marked or heterogeneous enhancement
  - Overall accuracy of MDCT in preoperative N staging is 75.22%
  - Regional lymphadenectomy specimen will ordinarily contain at least 16 lymph nodes
- M staging
  - Common sites are liver, lungs, and bones

Restaging

- CT is modality of choice for restaging and follow-up after curative surgery
  - Allows detection of local recurrence, peritoneal implants, and metastatic disease
    - Sensitivity is 89%
    - Specificity is 64%
  - Recurrence at gastric stump or anastomosis appears as nonspecific localized bowel wall thickening
- EUS can be used for local and nodal restaging following neoadjuvant therapy
- PET/CT
  - Sensitivity is 68-75%
  - Specificity is 71-77%
  - Accuracy is 75-83%
  - Negative predictive value is 55-78%
  - Positive predictive value is 86-89%

- Limitations of PET/CT include
  - Low FDG uptake in signet ring cell carcinoma and mucinous carcinoma
  - Poor spatial resolution for detection of small peritoneal nodules
  - Variability among patients in terms of physiologic peritoneal uptake

CLINICAL PRESENTATION & WORK-UP

Presentation

- Early gastric carcinoma often produces no specific symptoms when it is superficial and potentially surgically curable
  - Up to 50% of patients may have nonspecific gastrointestinal complaints, such as dyspepsia
    - However, gastric cancer is found in only 1-2% of patients with dyspepsia
- Patients may present with
  - Anorexia and weight loss (95%)
  - Vague and insidious abdominal pain
  - Nausea, vomiting, and early satiety
    - May occur with
      - Tumors obstructing gastrointestinal lumen (gastric outlet obstruction)
      - Infiltrative tumors impairing gastric distension
  - Ulcerated tumors may cause bleeding
    - Hematemesis
    - Melena
    - Massive upper gastrointestinal hemorrhage
  - Patients with advanced disease
    - Palpable abdominal mass
    - Cachexia
    - Bowel obstruction
    - Ascites
    - Hepatomegaly
    - Lower extremity edema
- Carcinoembryonic antigen (CEA) and CA-19.9 serum levels may be elevated in patients with advanced gastric cancers
  - Only approximately 1/3 of all patients with stomach carcinoma have abnormal CEA &/or CA-19.9 levels

Prognosis

- Stage of gastric carcinoma at diagnosis
  - Stage I: 20%
  - Stage II: 19%
  - Stage III: 34%
  - Stage IV: 27%
- Survival depends on tumor stage
  - Overall survival rate for gastric carcinoma is approximately 15-20%
  - 5-year survival for gastric carcinoma
    - Stage IA: 70.8%
    - Stage IB: 57.4%
    - Stage IIA: 45.5%
    - Stage IIB: 32.8%
    - Stage IIIA: 19.8%
    - Stage IIIB: 14.0%
    - Stage IIIC: 9.2%
    - Stage IV: 4.0%

Work-Up

- Clinical
  - History and physical examination
  - Endoscopy with biopsies
  - Laparoscopic staging should be considered for patients undergoing preoperative chemoradiation or chemotherapy
- Radiographic
  - Chest and abdominal CT
  - PET or PET/CT
    - Some gastric cancers may show low FDG uptake
  - Endoscopic ultrasound
- Laboratory
  - CBC and chemistry
  - HER-2 neu in patients with metastatic disease
  - Testing for *H. pylori*

TREATMENT

Major Treatment Alternatives

- Surgery is the primary treatment for nonmetastatic gastric cancer
  - Patients with proximal gastric cancer should undergo total gastrectomy, while those with distal gastric cancer may undergo total or subtotal gastrectomy
  - Appropriate extent of lymph node dissection is controversial
    - D2 lymphadenectomy (perigastric, celiac, left gastric, hepatic, splenic) is regarded as a standard in many institutions and countries
    - Randomized trials have not shown a benefit for D2 over D1 (perigastric) lymphadenectomy
    - Current AJCC staging system recommends evaluation of at least 16 lymph nodes
- Postoperative chemoradiation improves survival compared to surgery alone
- Perioperative chemotherapy improves survival compared to surgery alone
- Postoperative chemotherapy: Recent trials indicate that postoperative chemotherapy improves survival and disease-free survival compared to surgery alone
- Preoperative chemoradiation has been evaluated in phase II trials

Major Treatment Roadblocks/ Contraindications

- Patients with poor performance status or comorbidities may not be candidates for surgical resection
- Patients with poor performance status or nutritional status may not be candidates for adjuvant therapy

Treatment Options by Stage

- T1a N0: Endoscopic mucosal resection (EMR) in selected cases or surgery
- T1b N0: Surgery
- T2 N0: Surgery or surgery with postoperative chemoradiation (CRT) or surgery with perioperative chemotherapy
- T2-4 &/or N+: Surgery with postoperative chemoradiation or surgery with perioperative chemotherapy
- M1: Chemotherapy, with radiotherapy for palliation

Standard Doses

- 45-50.4 Gy

Organs at Risk Parameters

- Spinal cord: Dmax < 45 Gy
- Kidneys: V20 < 33% for at least 1 kidney
- Liver: V30 < 33%

Common Techniques

- 3D treatment planning and CT-based simulation should be used
  - Intensity-modulated radiation therapy (IMRT) may be used in selected cases
    - For IMRT, careful attention must be given to accurate contouring of target volume and uncertainties, such as organ motion arising from respiration and gastric filling
- For postoperative chemoradiation, tumor bed, anastomosis, and gastric remnant should be included in the field
- Nodal regions should be included based on location of gastric tumor
  - Proximal 1/3 of stomach: Perigastric, celiac, splenic hilum, ± porta hepatis
    - Include distal periesophageal region for tumors involving GE junction
  - Mid 1/3 of stomach: Perigastric, celiac, splenic hilum, porta hepatis, pancreaticoduodenal
  - Distal 1/3 of stomach: Perigastric, celiac, splenic hilum, porta hepatis, pancreaticoduodenal

Landmark Trials

- Intergroup trial
  - 556 patients with stages IB-IV, randomized to
    - Surgery alone
    - Surgery and postop CRT (45 Gy radiation, fluorouracil, and leucovorin: 1 cycle before, 2 cycles during, and 2 cycles after radiation)
  - ↑ overall survival for CRT (3-year survival 50% vs. 41%)
- MAGIC trial
  - 503 patients with ≥ stage II, randomized to
    - Surgery alone
    - Surgery with perioperative chemotherapy (ECF, epirubicin, cisplatin, and fluorouracil: 3 cycles before and 3 cycles after surgery)
  - Perioperative chemo had significantly ↑ overall survival (5-year survival 36% vs. 23%)

RECOMMENDED FOLLOW-UP

Clinical

- History and physical examination q. 3-6 months for 1-2 years, then q. 6-12 months for years 3-5, then annually
- Endoscopy may be useful in selected patients

Radiographic

- Chest and abdominal CT as indicated

Laboratory

- CBC and chemistry
  - B12 and iron levels to evaluate for deficiencies after surgery

SELECTED REFERENCES

1. Bang YJ et al: Adjuvant capecitabine and oxaliplatin for gastric cancer after D2 gastrectomy (CLASSIC): a phase 3 open-label, randomised controlled trial. Lancet. 379(9813):315-21, 2012
2. Siegel R et al: Cancer statistics, 2012. CA Cancer J Clin. 62(1):10-29, 2012
3. American Joint Committee on Cancer: AJCC Cancer Staging Manual. 7th ed. New York: Springer. 117-26, 2010
4. Catalano V et al: Gastric cancer. Crit Rev Oncol Hematol. 71(2):127-64, 2009
5. Kim YH et al: Staging of T3 and T4 gastric carcinoma with multidetector CT: added value of multiplanar reformations for prediction of adjacent organ invasion. Radiology. 250(3):767-75, 2009
6. Kunisaki C et al: Risk factors for lymph node metastasis in histologically poorly differentiated type early gastric cancer. Endoscopy. 41(6):498-503, 2009
7. Namikawa T et al: Clinicopathological features of early gastric cancer with duodenal invasion. World J Gastroenterol. 15(19):2309-13, 2009
8. Sim SH et al: The role of PET/CT in detection of gastric cancer recurrence. BMC Cancer. 9:73, 2009
9. Yan C et al: Value of multidetector-row computed tomography in the preoperative T and N staging of gastric carcinoma: a large-scale Chinese study. J Surg Oncol. 100(3):205-14, 2009
10. Sakuramoto S et al: Adjuvant chemotherapy for gastric cancer with S-1, an oral fluoropyrimidine. N Engl J Med. 2007 Nov 1;357(18):1810-20. Erratum in: N Engl J Med. 358(18):1977, 2008
11. Sun L et al: Clinical role of 18F-fluorodeoxyglucose positron emission tomography/computed tomography in post-operative follow up of gastric cancer: initial results. World J Gastroenterol. 14(29):4627-32, 2008
12. Chen CY et al: Gastric cancer: preoperative local staging with 3D multi-detector row CT--correlation with surgical and histopathologic results. Radiology. 242(2):472-82, 2007
13. Kwee RM et al: Imaging in local staging of gastric cancer: a systematic review. J Clin Oncol. 25(15):2107-16, 2007
14. Cunningham D et al: Perioperative chemotherapy versus surgery alone for resectable gastroesophageal cancer. N Engl J Med. 355(1):11-20, 2006
15. D'Angelica M et al: Patterns of initial recurrence in completely resected gastric adenocarcinoma. Ann Surg. 240(5):808-16, 2004
16. Smalley SR et al: Gastric surgical adjuvant radiotherapy consensus report: rationale and treatment implementation. Int J Radiat Oncol Biol Phys. 52(2):283-93, 2002
17. Fuchs CS et al: Gastric carcinoma. N Engl J Med. 333(1):32-41, 1995

Stage IA (T1a N0 M0)

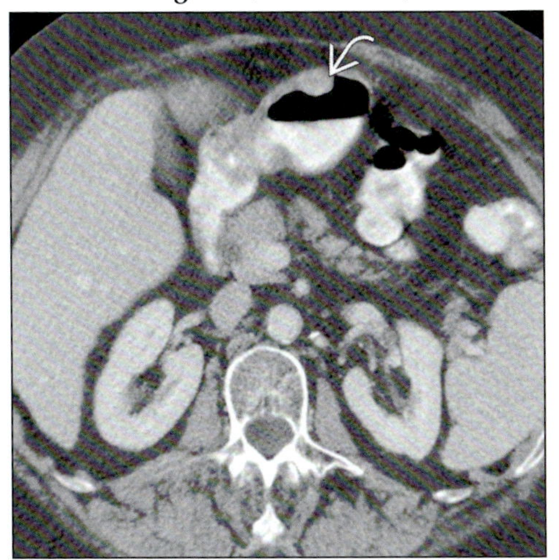

Stage IA (T1a N0 M0)

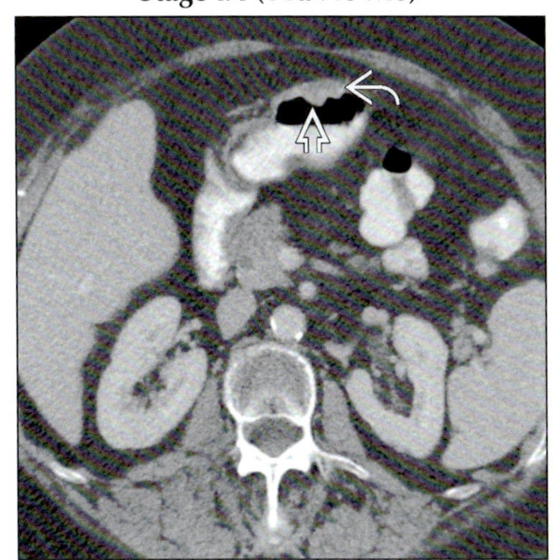

(Left) *Axial CECT in a 35-year-old asymptomatic woman who requested to have a CT of the abdomen because of a strong family history of gastric carcinoma shows a focal mass along the anterior wall of the stomach.* ***(Right)*** *Axial CECT in the same patient shows focal thickening of the anterior wall of the stomach with a hypoattenuating stripe at the base of the mass. A T1a lesion invading the submucosa was found on histologic examination.*

Stage IB (T1b N1 M0)

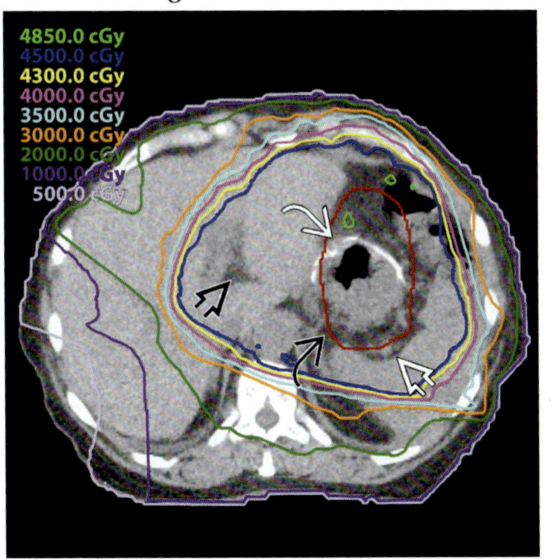

Stage IB (T1b N1 M0)

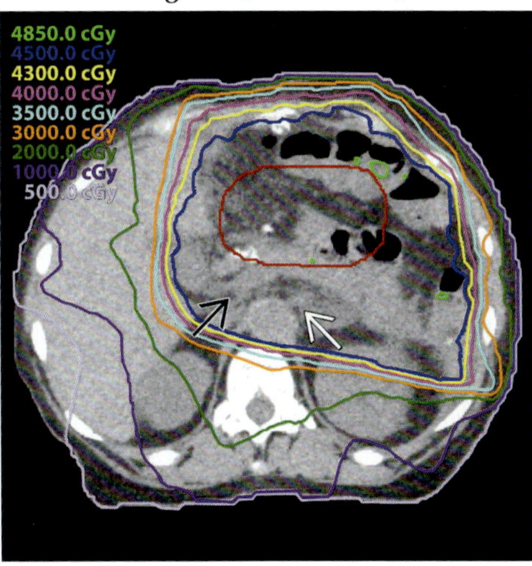

(Left) *This 56-year-old woman underwent a subtotal gastrectomy for a T1b N1 adenocarcinoma of the gastric body. She was treated with postop chemoradiation, a dose of 45 Gy, using IMRT. The 45 Gy isodose line (blue) covers the tumor bed (red), gastric remnant, anastomosis, porta hepatis, and splenic hilum.* ***(Right)*** *In the same patient, the 45 Gy isodose (blue) covers the tumor bed (red), celiac axis, and pancreaticoduodenal region.*

Stage IB (T1b N1 M0)

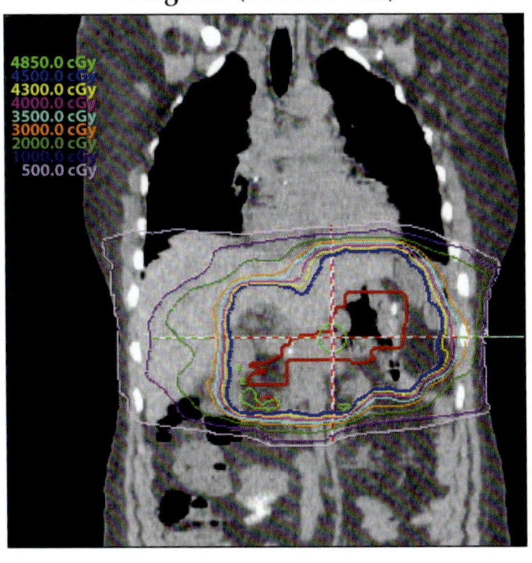

Stage IB (T1b N1 M0)

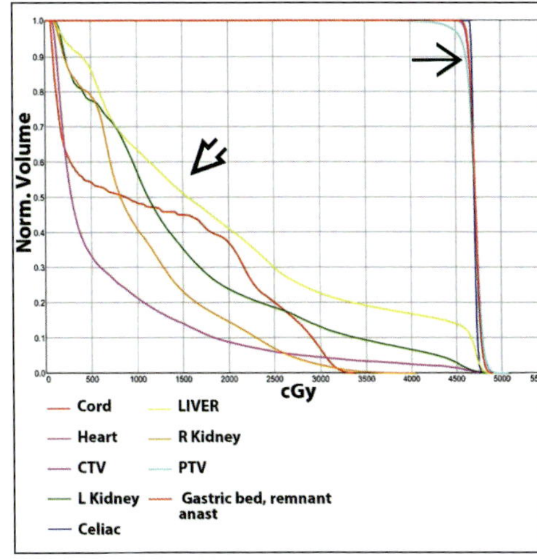

(Left) *This is a coronal view of the 45 Gy (blue) and other isodose lines in the same patient.* ***(Right)*** *Dose volume histogram (DVH) in the same patient demonstrates sparing of OARs with an IMRT technique while achieving good target coverage.*

Stage IIA (T3 N0 M0)

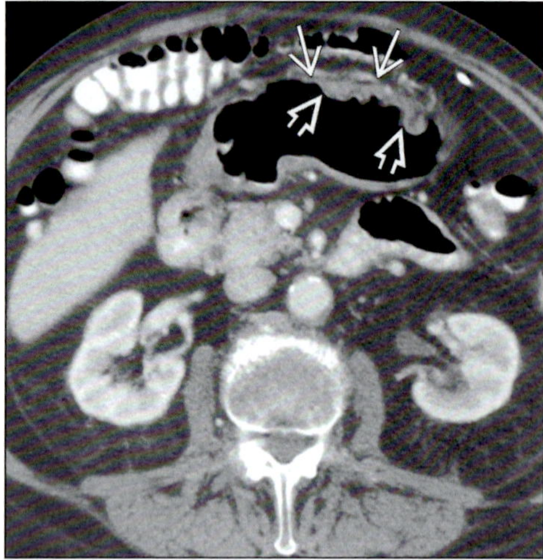

Stage IIA (T3 N0 M0)

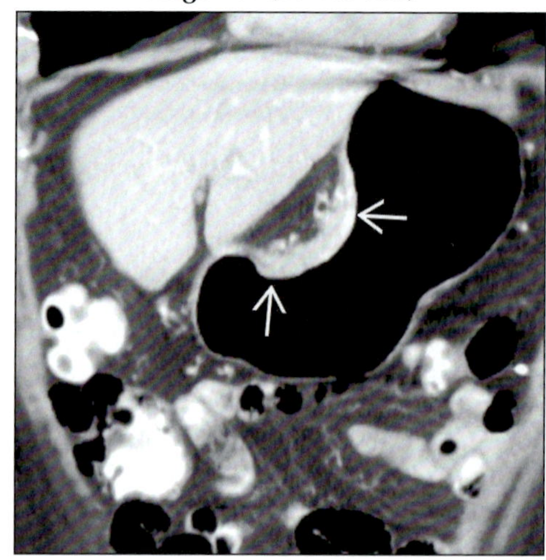

***(Left)** Axial CECT in an 82-year-old man who had an abnormal EGD shows an infiltrating polypoid gastric mass ➡ along the anterior wall of the stomach with transmural enhancement. Note the sharp gastric contour at the base of the mass ➡. **(Right)** Coronal CECT in the same patient shows extension of the tumor ➡ along the lesser curvature of the stomach without evidence of invasion beyond the gastric wall.*

Stage IIA (T2 N1 M0)

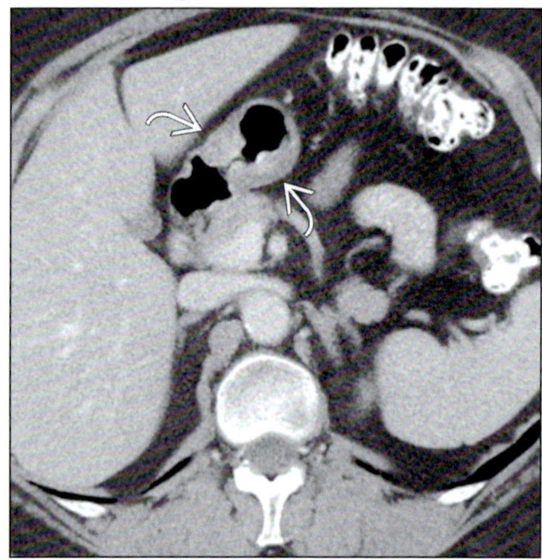

Stage IIA (T2 N1 M0)

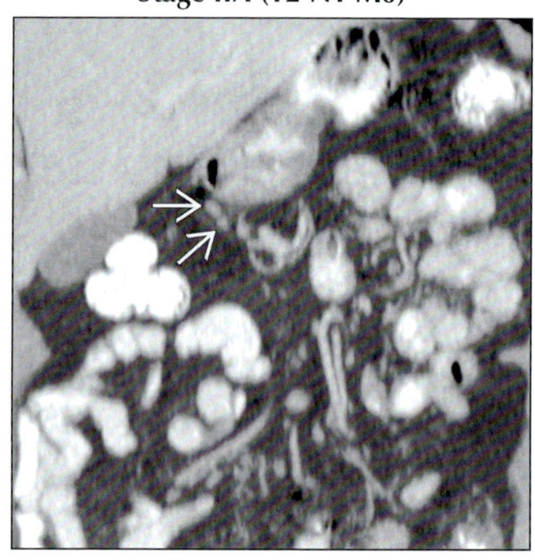

***(Left)** Axial CECT in a patient who presented with epigastric pain demonstrates circumferential thickening of the antrum ➡. The outer contour of the stomach appears smooth. **(Right)** Coronal CECT in the same patient shows 2 pathologic perigastric lymph nodes ➡. Pathological examination confirmed muscularis propria invasion without involvement of the subserosal connective tissue or T2 category.*

Stage IIA (T3 N0 M0)

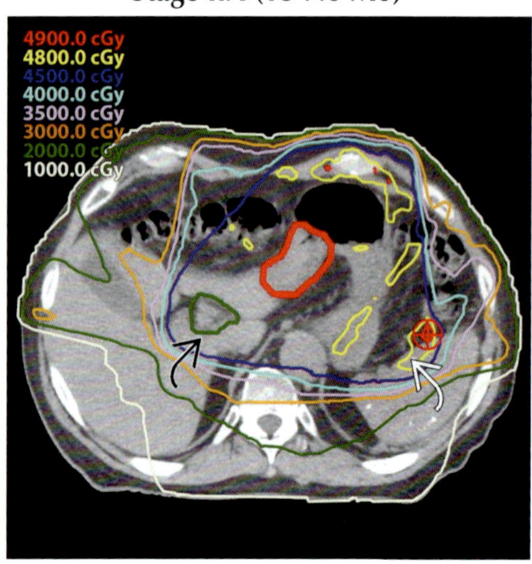

Stage IIA (T3 N0 M0)

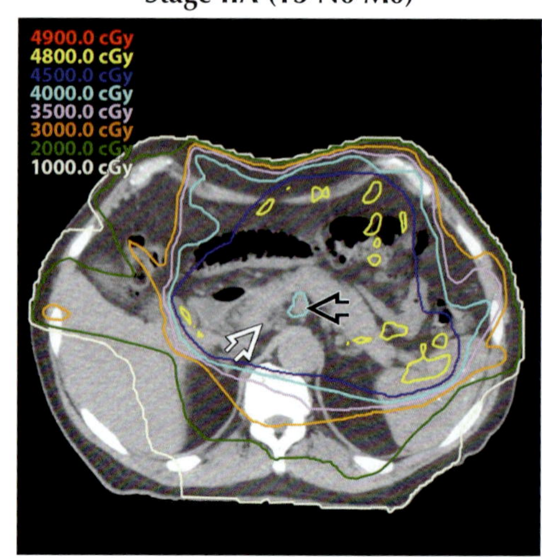

***(Left)** This 74-year-old man with T3 N0 adenocarcinoma of the gastric antrum was treated with preoperative chemoradiation, with a radiation dose of 45 Gy, using IMRT. The 45 Gy isodose line (blue) covers the tumor (red), the porta hepatis ➡, and the splenic hilum ➡. **(Right)** In the same patient, the 45 Gy isodose line (blue) covers the celiac axis ➡ and the pancreaticoduodenal ➡ region.*

Stage IIIA (T4a N1 M0)

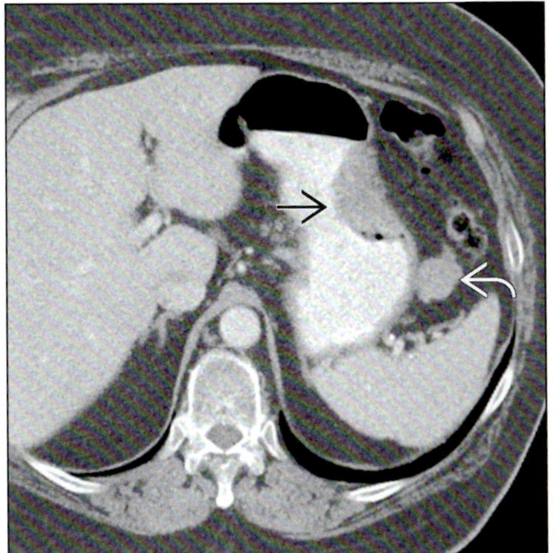

Stage IIIA (T4a N1 M0)

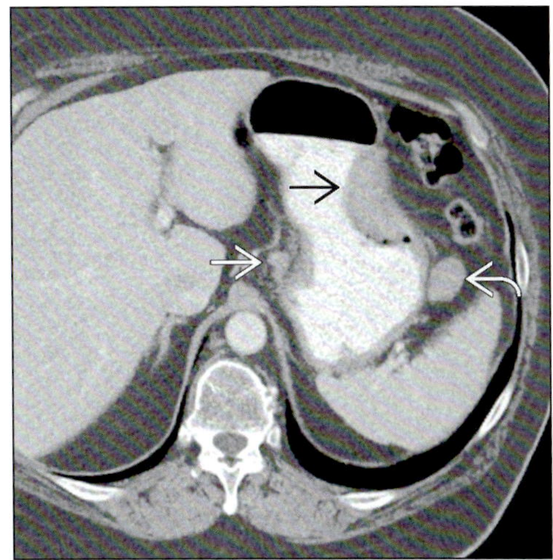

(Left) *A 69-year-old man presented with dysphagia and was found to have a gastric mass on EGD. Axial CECT in this patient shows a mass → along the greater curvature with an enlarged greater curvature lymph node ↷.* ***(Right)*** *Axial CECT in the same patient reveals a gastrohepatic ⇨ lymph node as well as the mass → along the greater curvature and the enlarged greater curvature lymph node ↷.*

Stage IIIA (T4a N1 M0)

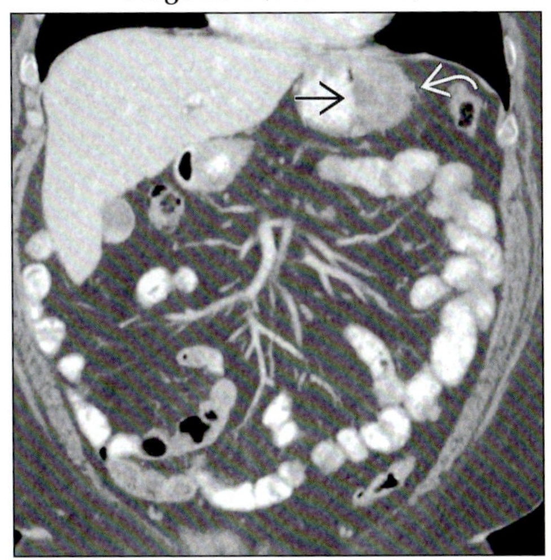

Stage IIIA (T4a N1 M0)

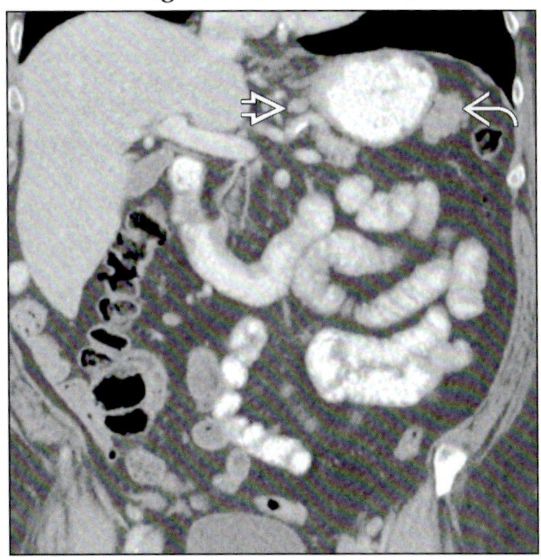

(Left) *Coronal CECT in the same patient shows a mass → along the greater curvature with irregular gastric outer contour ↷, indicating serosal invasion.* ***(Right)*** *Coronal CECT in the same patient shows the greater curvature lymph node ↷ as well as the enlarged lymph node ⇨ within the gastrohepatic ligament.*

Stage IIIC (T4b N2 M0)

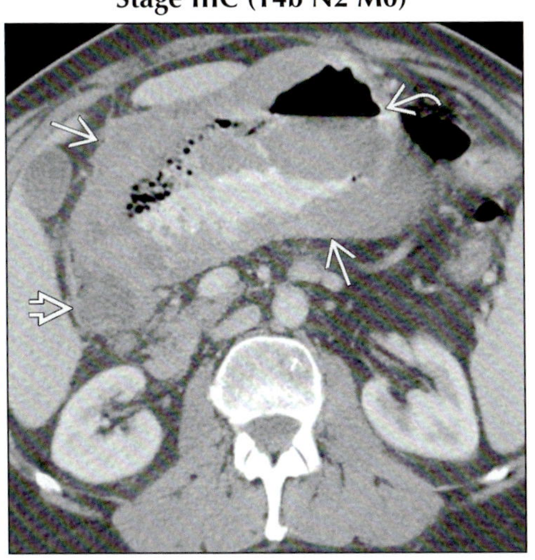

Stage IIIC (T4b N2 M0)

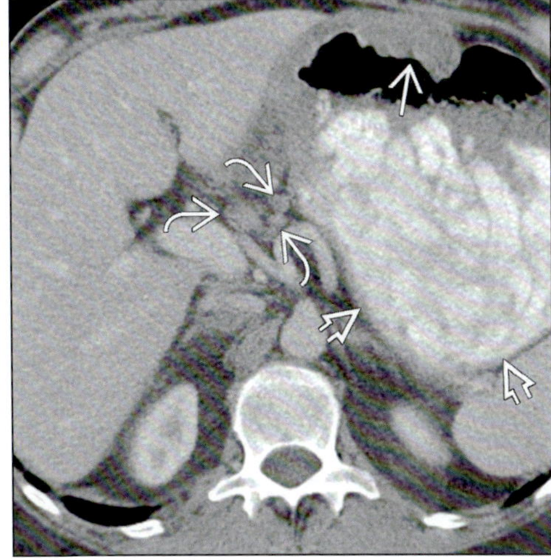

(Left) *Axial CECT in a 56-year-old man who presented with symptoms of gastric outlet obstruction shows a distended stomach ↷ with diffuse gastric wall thickening → involving the gastric body and antrum. The tumor also involves the proximal duodenum ⇨.* ***(Right)*** *Axial CECT in the same patient shows gastric wall thickening → and distension ⇨. Three enlarged gastrohepatic lymph nodes ↷ are present on this image.*

(Left) *This 64-year-old woman underwent a subtotal gastrectomy for a T3 N2 carcinoma of the gastric body. She was treated with postop chemoradiation, with a dose of 45 Gy, using IMRT. The 45 Gy isodose line (blue) covers the gastric remnant (red), splenic hilum, and porta hepatis.* ***(Right)*** *In the same patient, the 45 Gy isodose line (blue) covers the tumor bed (red), celiac axis, and pancreaticoduodenal region.*

Stage IIIA (T3 N2 M0)

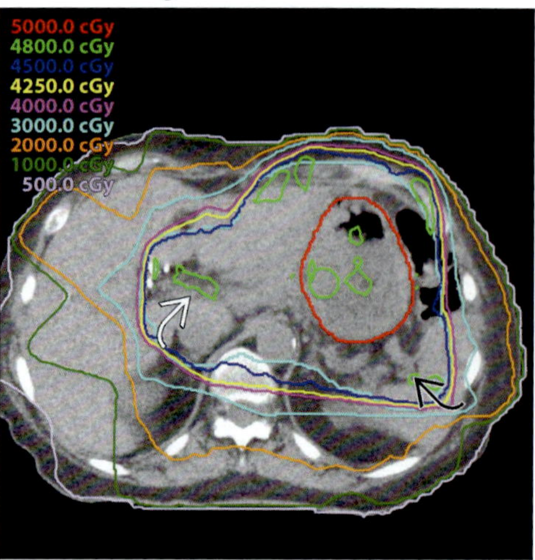

Stage IIIA (T3 N2 M0)

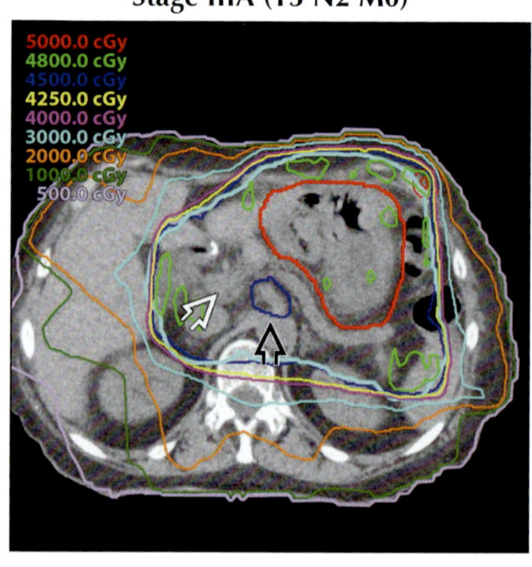

(Left) *This is a coronal view of the 45 Gy (blue) and other isodose lines in the same patient.* ***(Right)*** *This 67-year-old man underwent a total gastrectomy for a T3 N3 carcinoma of the gastric body and antrum. He was treated with postop chemoradiation with a dose of 45 Gy, using a 3-field (AP, RAO, LPO) 3D conformal technique. The 45 Gy isodose line (blue) covers the tumor bed (red), anastomosis (green), porta hepatis, and splenic hilum.*

Stage IIIA (T3 N2 M0)

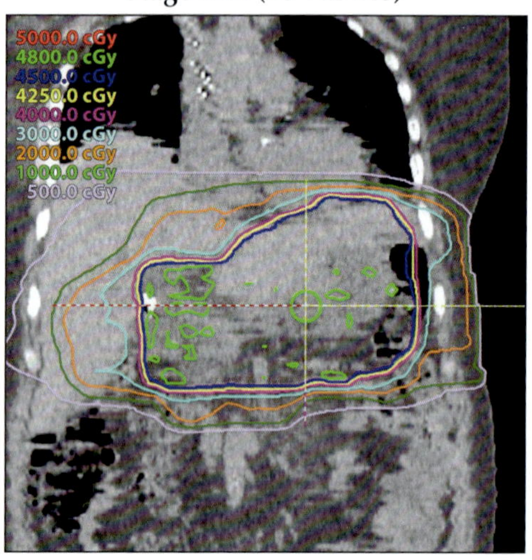

Stage IIIB (T3 N3 M0)

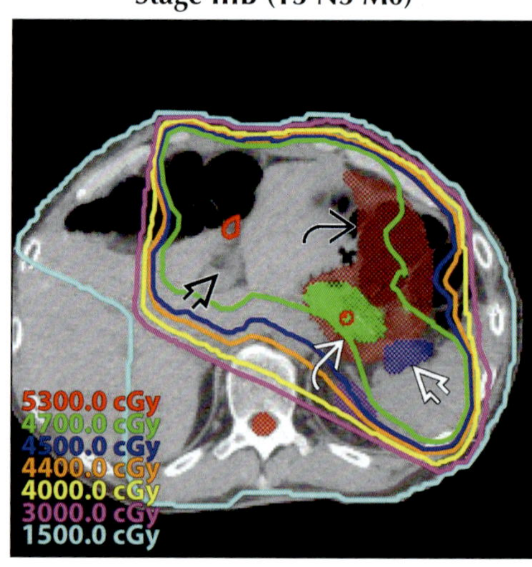

(Left) *In the same patient, the 45 Gy isodose line (blue) covers the tumor bed (red), porta hepatis, and retropancreatic regions.* ***(Right)*** *In the same patient, the 45 Gy isodose line (blue) covers the celiac axis.*

Stage IIIB (T3 N3 M0)

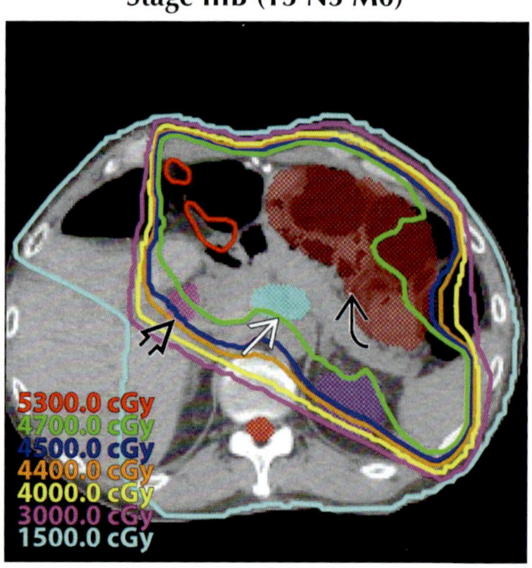

Stage IIIB (T3 N3 M0)

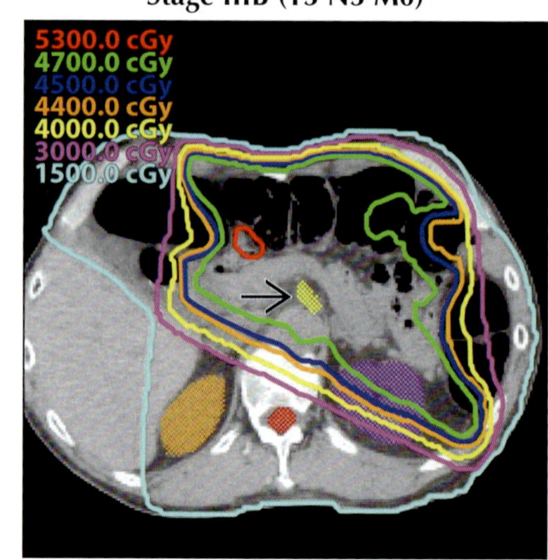

Stage IIB (T2 N2 M0)

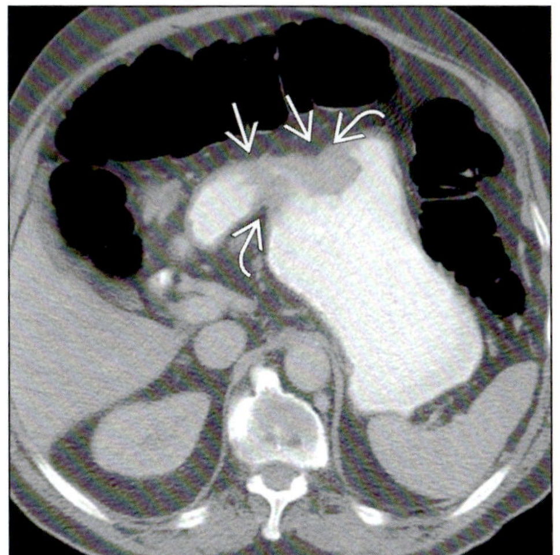

Stage IIB (T2 N2 M0)

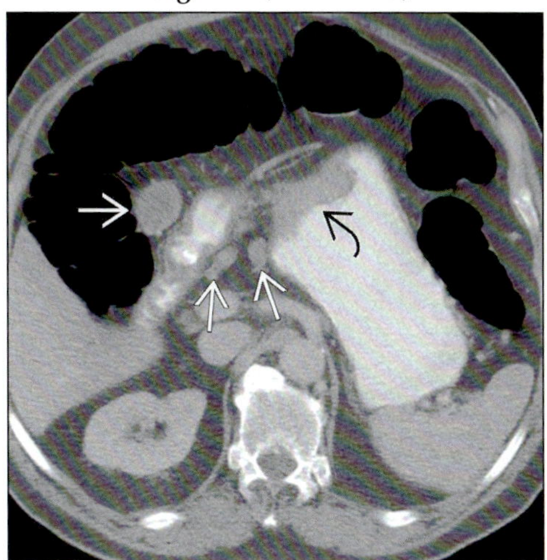

(Left) *Axial CECT in a patient who presented with melena shows a circumferential antral mass causing narrowing of the gastric antrum. The mass exhibits marked scirrhous reaction with flattening and decreased distensibility of the anterior gastric wall.* ***(Right)*** *Axial CECT in the same patient shows the antral mass. Multiple pathologic perigastric nodes are seen. A total of 5 pathologic nodes were found during surgery, making this N2 disease.*

Stage IIB (T4a N0 M0)

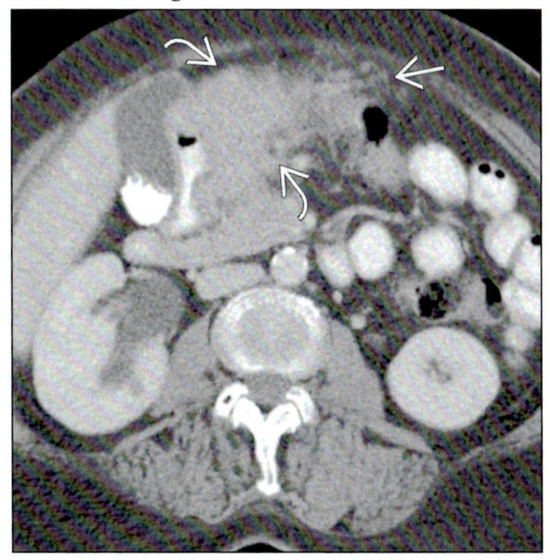

Stage IIB (T4a N0 M0)

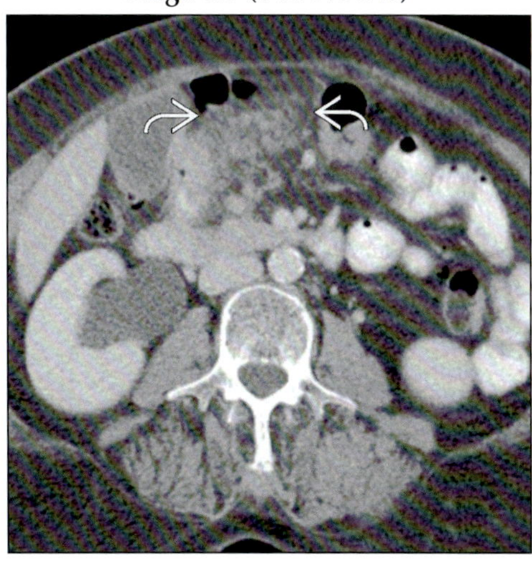

(Left) *Axial CECT shows a fungating circumferential mass involving the gastric antrum and pylorus. The mass significantly narrows the stomach at the antrum. Haziness and nodularities are seen involving the gastrocolic ligament adjacent to the mass. The ligament stretches from the greater curvature of stomach to the transverse colon.* ***(Right)*** *Axial CECT in the same patient shows the gastrocolic ligament studded with multiple small nodules.*

Stage IIB (T4a N0 M0)

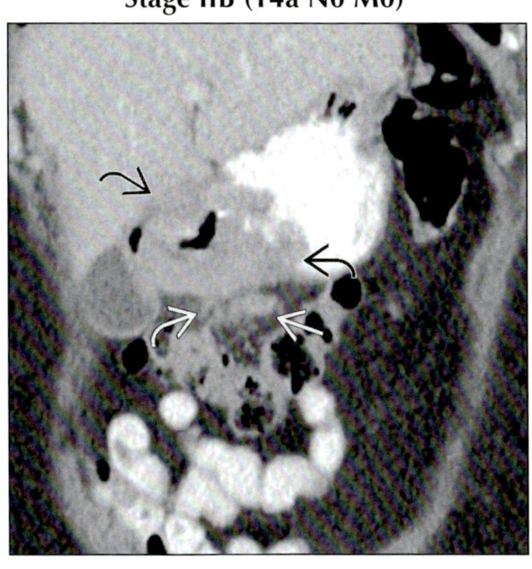

Stage IIB (T4a N0 M0)

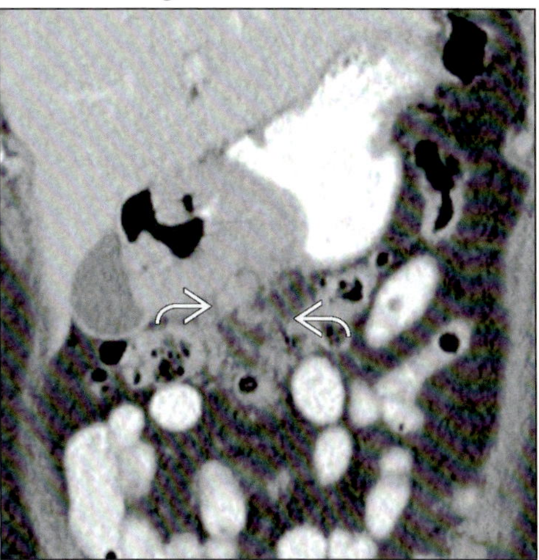

(Left) *Coronal CECT in the same patient shows diffuse circumferential thickening of the gastric antrum. Irregularity of the gastric contour suggests serosal invasion. Haziness and nodularity of the gastrocolic ligament is again seen.* ***(Right)*** *Coronal CECT in the same patient shows nodularity of the gastrocolic ligament. Tumor extending to the gastrocolic ligament without invading the transverse colon is categorized as T4a.*

(Left) Axial CECT in the same patient shows tumor invading the gastrocolic ligament. The landmarks of the ligament are the gastroepiploic vessels. (Right) Coronal CECT in the same patient shows tumor along the greater curvature with invasion through the gastrocolic ligament into the transverse colon.

Stage IIIC (T4b N2 M0)

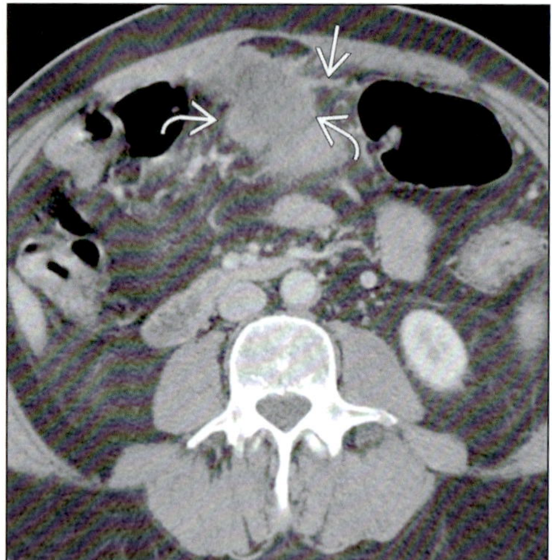

Stage IIIC (T4b N2 M0)

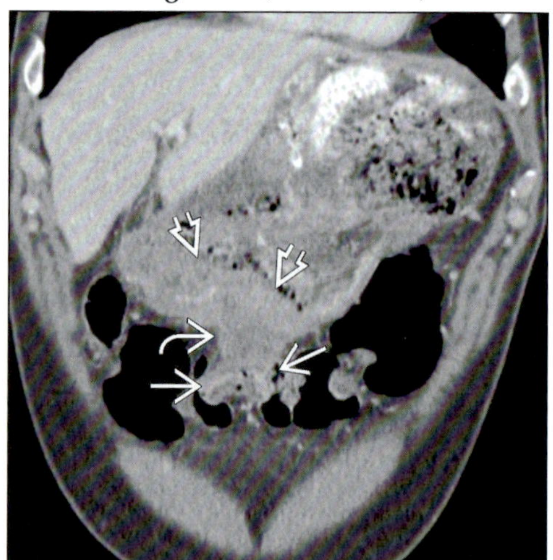

(Left) Axial T1WI C+ FS MR in the same patient shows gastrohepatic lymph nodes and enhancing tumor along the anterior wall. The interface between the tumor and the left lobe of the liver is sharp, indicating absence of hepatic invasion. (Right) Axial T1WI C+ FS MR in the same patient shows the extensive thickening of the gastric wall (linitis plastica) and invasion of the duodenum.

Stage IIIC (T4b N2 M0)

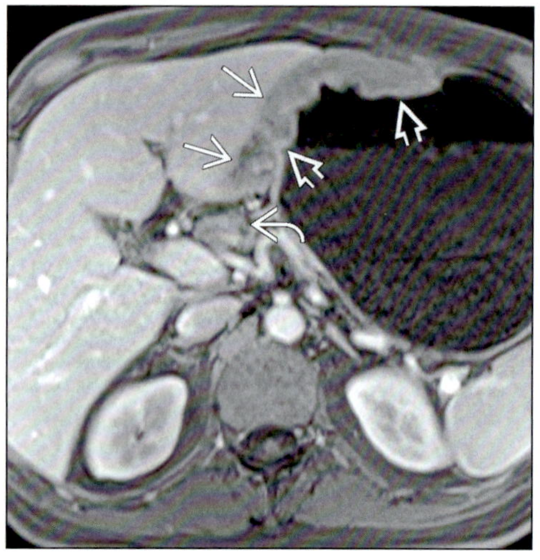

Stage IIIC (T4b N2 M0)

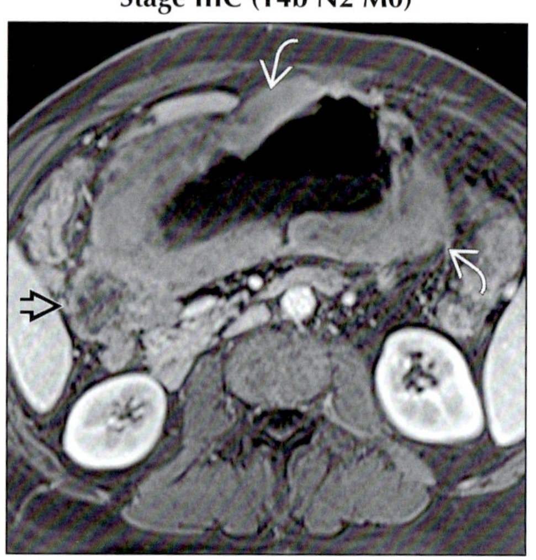

(Left) Axial T1WI C+ FS MR in the same patient shows gastric wall thickening and invasion of the gastrocolic ligament marked by the gastroepiploic vessels. (Right) Axial T1WI C+ FS MR in the same patient shows tumor extending inferiorly through the gastrocolic ligament and reaching to the transverse colon.

Stage IIIC (T4b N2 M0)

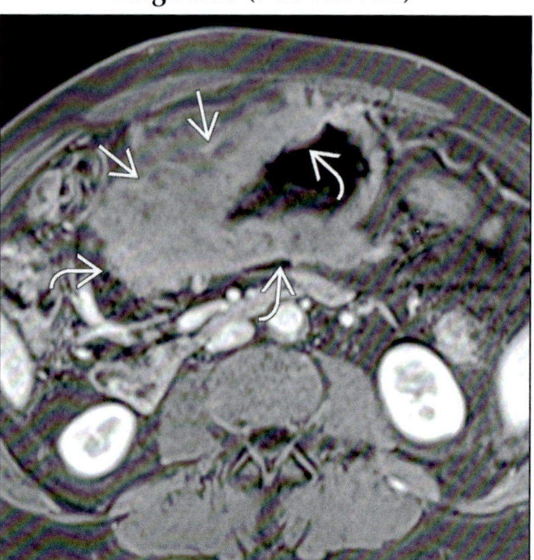

Stage IIIC (T4b N2 M0)

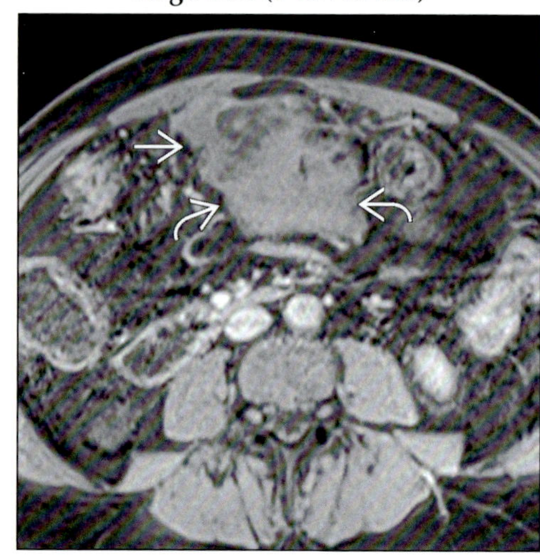

Stage IV (T3 N0 M1)

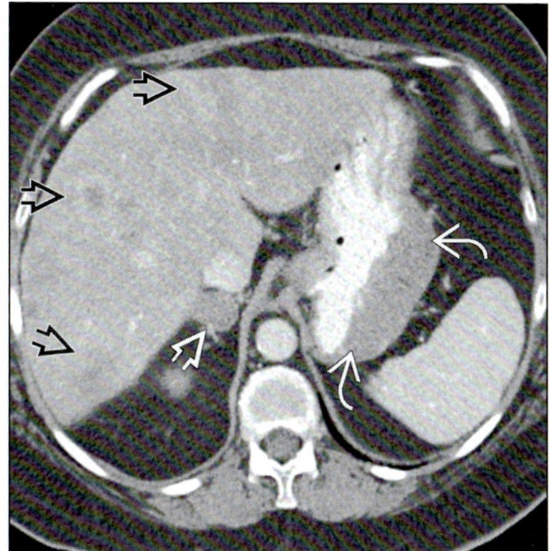

Stage IV (T3 N0 M1)

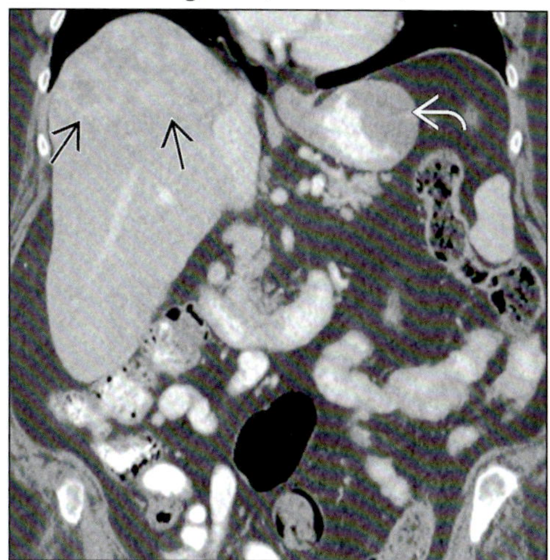

(Left) *Axial CECT in a 72-year-old man who presented with right upper quadrant pain shows a mass along the greater curvature of the stomach, multiple hepatic metastatic lesions, and right adrenal mass.* ***(Right)*** *Coronal CECT in the same patient shows the greater curvature gastric mass and the enhancing hepatic metastatic lesions.*

Stage IV (T3 N2 M1)

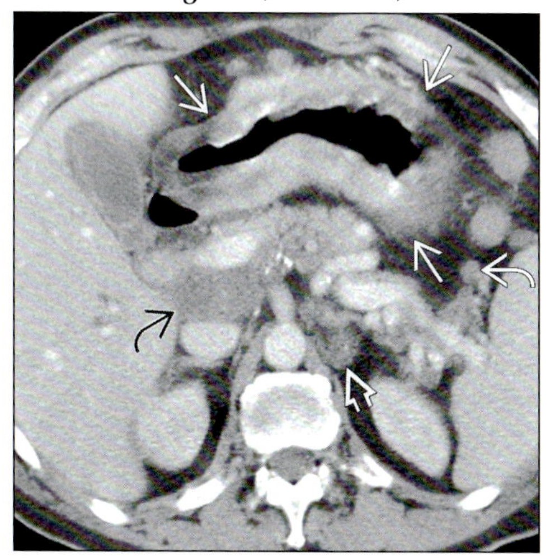

Stage IV (T3 N2 M1)

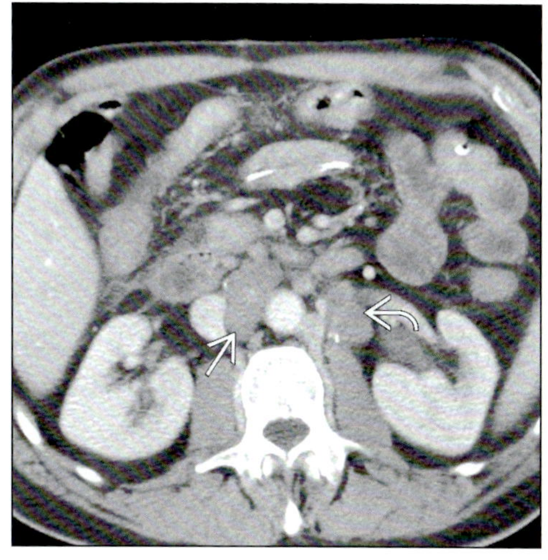

(Left) *Axial CECT in a patient with mucinous adenocarcinoma shows diffuse thickening of stomach wall. Multiple calcified enlarged nodes are seen, including portocaval, paraaortic, and splenic nodes.* ***(Right)*** *Axial CECT in same patient shows enlarged aortocaval and paraaortic lymph nodes. Involvement of intraabdominal lymph nodes, such as hepatoduodenal, mesenteric, and paraaortic, is classified as distant metastasis (M1).*

Stage IV (T4a N1 M1)

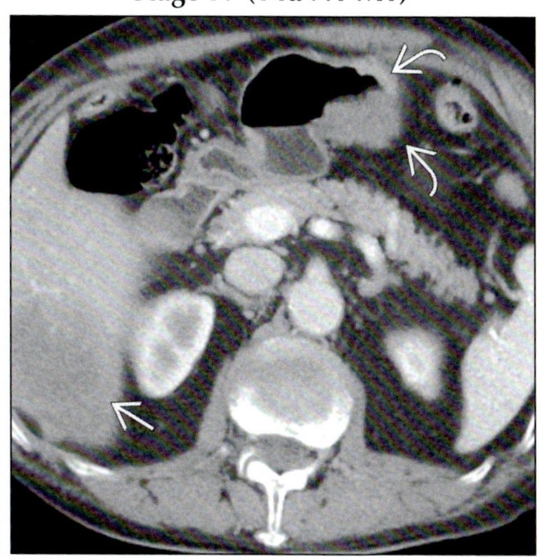

Stage IV (T4a N1 M1)

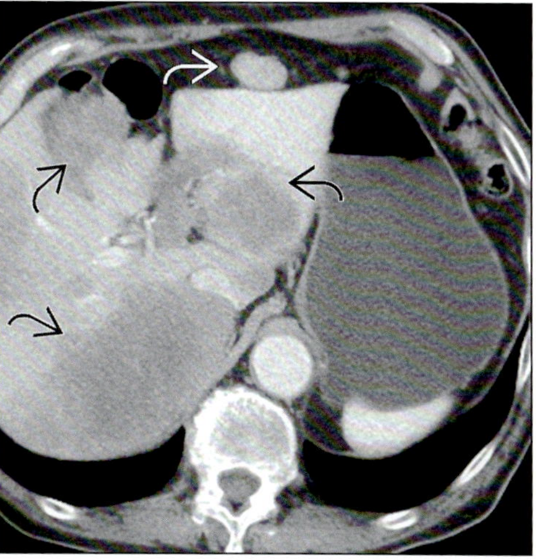

(Left) *Axial CECT in a 44-year-old man who presented with hematemesis shows a fungating mass along the greater curvature. There is no evidence of perigastric involvement on this image. A large metastatic lesion occupies most of segment 6 of the right lobe of the liver.* ***(Right)*** *Axial CECT in the same patient shows an enhancing peritoneal mass anterior to the left lobe of the liver. Large hepatic metastatic lesions involve both right and left lobes.*

COLON AND RECTUM

Adapted from 7th edition AJCC Staging Forms.

(T) Primary Tumor

TNM	*Definitions*
TX	Primary tumor cannot be assessed
T0	No evidence of primary tumor
Tis	Carcinoma in situ: Intraepithelial or invasion of lamina propria[1]
T1	Tumor invades submucosa
T2	Tumor invades muscularis propria
T3	Tumor invades through muscularis propria into pericolorectal tissue
T4a	Tumor penetrates to surface of visceral peritoneum[2]
T4b	Tumor directly invades or is adherent to other organs or structures[2-3]

(N) Regional Lymph Nodes

NX	Regional lymph nodes cannot be assessed
N0	No regional lymph node metastasis
N1	Metastasis in 1-3 regional lymph nodes
N1a	Metastasis in 1 regional lymph node
N1b	Metastasis in 2-3 regional lymph nodes
N1c	Tumor deposit(s) in subserosa, mesentery, or nonperitonealized pericolic or perirectal tissues without regional nodal metastasis
N2	Metastasis in ≥ 4 regional lymph nodes
N2a	Metastasis in 4-6 regional lymph nodes
N2b	Metastasis in ≥ 7 lymph nodes

(M) Distant Metastasis

M0	No distant metastasis
M1	Distant metastasis
M1a	Metastasis confined to 1 organ or site (e.g., liver, lung, ovary, nonregional node)
M1b	Metastases in > 1 organ/site or the peritoneum

[1]*Tis includes cancer cells confined within the glandular basement membrane (intraepithelial) or mucosal lamina propria (intramucosal) with no extension through the muscularis mucosae into the submucosa.*

[2]*Direct invasion in T4 includes invasion of other organs or other segments of the colorectum as a result of direct extension through the serosa, as confirmed on microscopic examination (for example, invasion of the sigmoid colon by a carcinoma of the cecum) or, for cancers in a retroperitoneal or subperitoneal location, direct invasion of other organs or structures by virtue of extension beyond the muscularis propria (i.e., respectively, a tumor on the posterior wall of the descending colon invading the left kidney or lateral abdominal wall; or a mid or distal rectal cancer with invasion of prostate, seminal vesicles, cervix, or vagina).*

[3]*Tumor that is adherent to other organs or structures, grossly, is classified cT4b. However, if no tumor is present in the adhesion, microscopically, the classification should be pT1-4a depending on the anatomical depth of wall invasion. The V and L classifications should be used to identify the presence or absence of vascular or lymphatic invasion whereas the PN site-specific factor should be used for perineural invasion.*

(G) Histologic Grade*

Adapted from 7th edition AJCC Staging Forms.

TNM	*Definitions*
GX	Grade cannot be assessed
G1	Well differentiated
G2	Moderately differentiated
G3	Poorly differentiated
G4	Undifferentiated

**The terms "low-grade" (G1-G2) and "high-grade" (G3-G4) should be applied as they may be associated with outcome independently of TNM staging.*

AJCC, Dukes, and MAC Stages/ Prognostic Groups

Adapted from 7th edition AJCC Staging Forms.

AJCC	*T*	*N*	*M*	*Dukes*[1]	*MAC*[2]
0	Tis	N0	M0	-	-
I	T1	N0	M0	A	A
	T2	N0	M0	A	B1
IIA	T3	N0	M0	B	B2
IIB	T4a	N0	M0	B	B2
IIC	T4b	N0	M0	B	B3
IIIA	T1-T2	N1/N1c	M0	C	C1
	T1	N2a	M0	C	C1
IIIB	T3-T4a	N1/N1c	M0	C	C2
	T2-T3	N2a	M0	C	C1/C2
	T1-T2	N2b	M0	C	C1
IIIC	T4a	N2a	M0	C	C2
	T3-T4a	N2b	M0	C	C2
	T4b	N1-N2	M0	C	C3
IVA	Any T	Any N	M1a	D	D
IVB	Any T	Any N	M1b	D	D

[1]*Dukes B is a composite of better (T3 N0 M0) and worse (T4 N0 M0) prognostic groups, as is Dukes C (any T N1 M0 and any T N2 M0).*

[2]*MAC is the modified Astler-Coller classification. Description of MAC: B1 is defined as invasion into the muscularis propria without nodal disease; B2 is invasion into the perirectal or pericolic fat without nodal disease; B3 represents involvement of adjacent structures; C1 is B1 with nodal disease; C2 is B2 with nodal disease; and C3 is B3 with nodal metastasis.*

COLON AND RECTUM

T1

H&E stained section of an adenomatous polyp shows an invasive adenocarcinoma → involving the lamina propria and the submucosa.

T2

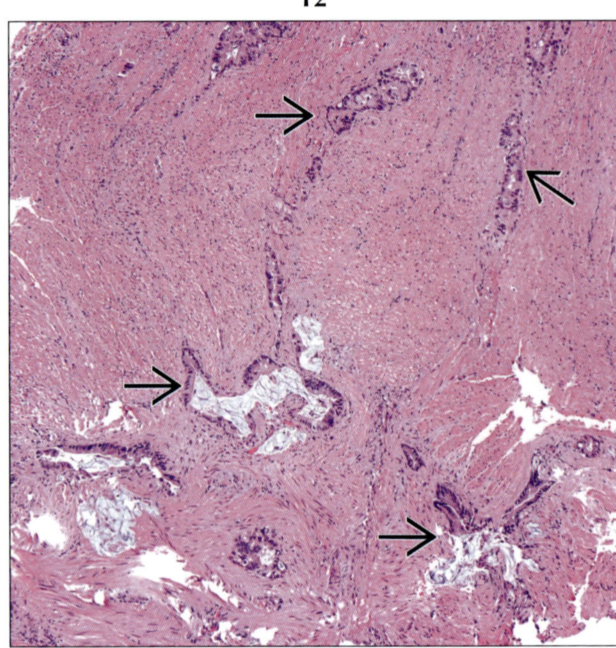

H&E stained section shows invasive adenocarcinoma that involves muscularis propria. The neoplastic cells are arranged in irregular well-formed glands → that dissect through the muscle bundles of the muscularis mucosa.

T3

H&E stained section shows adenocarcinoma that invades through the pink muscularis propria → and extends to involve the pericolorectal tissue ⇨. The tumor is surrounded by extensive desmoplastic reaction ➡.

T4a

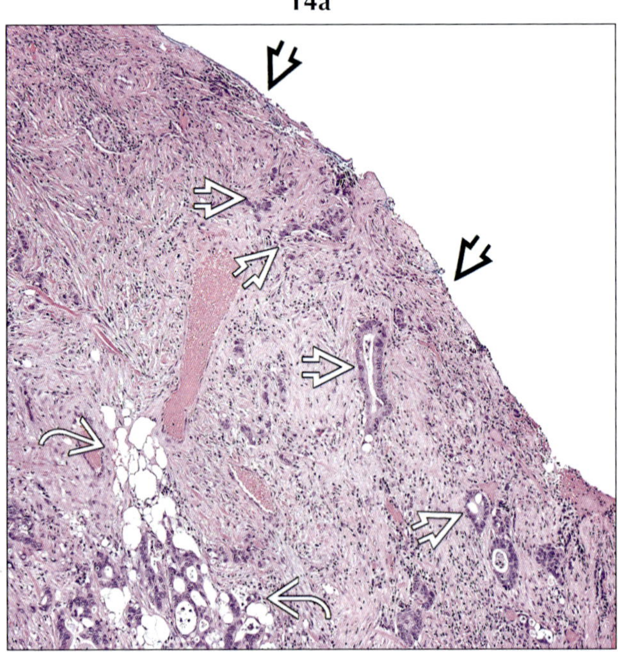

H&E stained section shows invasive colonic adenocarcinoma that extends to the serosal surface ⇨. The neoplastic glands ➡ invade the pericolonic fat ➡ and extend to involve the serosal surface without extension to adjacent organs.

T1

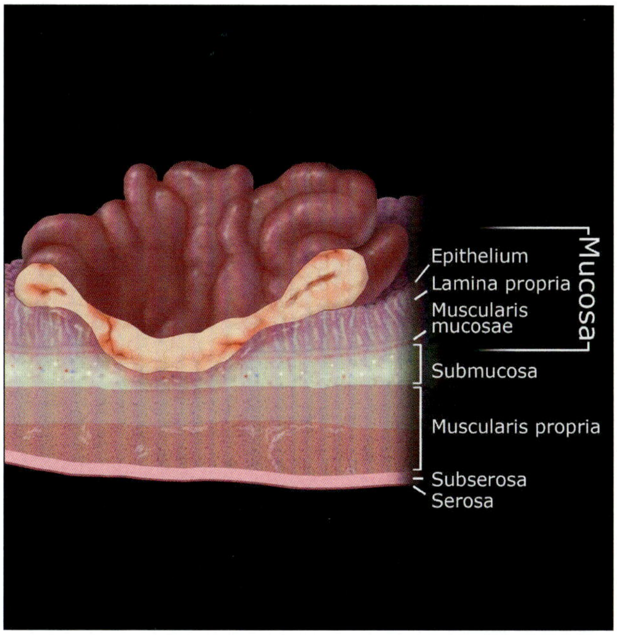

Graphic shows an ulcerating mass invading into the submucosa, classified as T1 disease.

T2

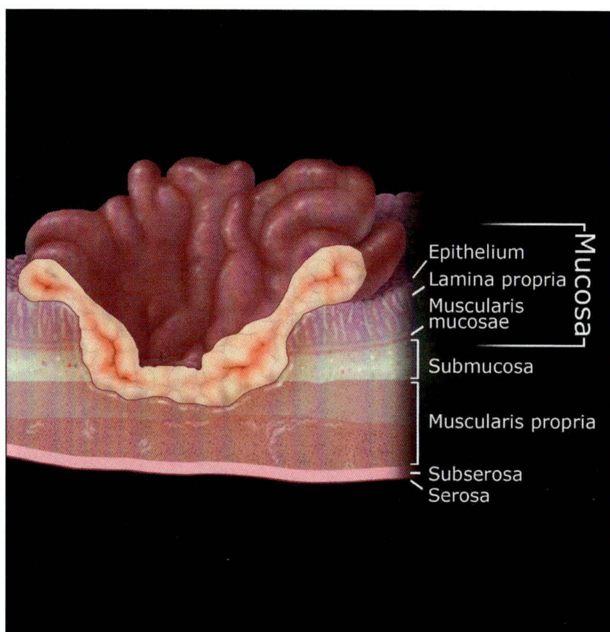

Graphic demonstrates an ulcerating mass invading into the muscularis propria, consistent with T2 disease.

T3

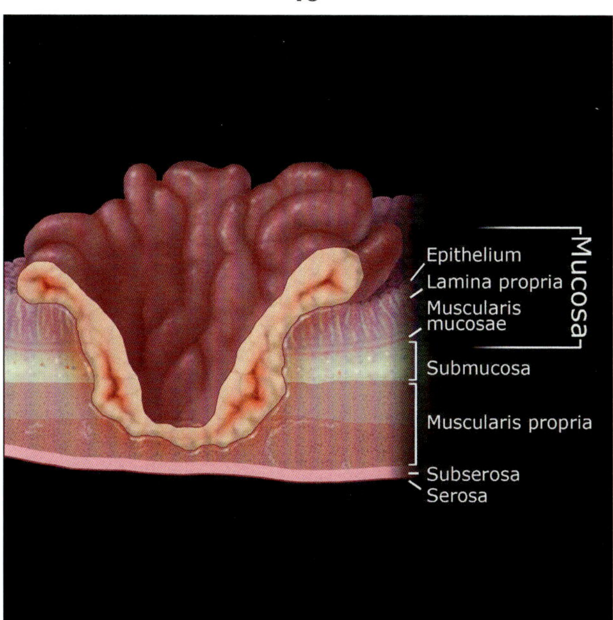

Graphic shows an ulcerating mass invading through the muscularis propria into the subserosa or the nonperitonealized pericolorectal tissue.

T4a

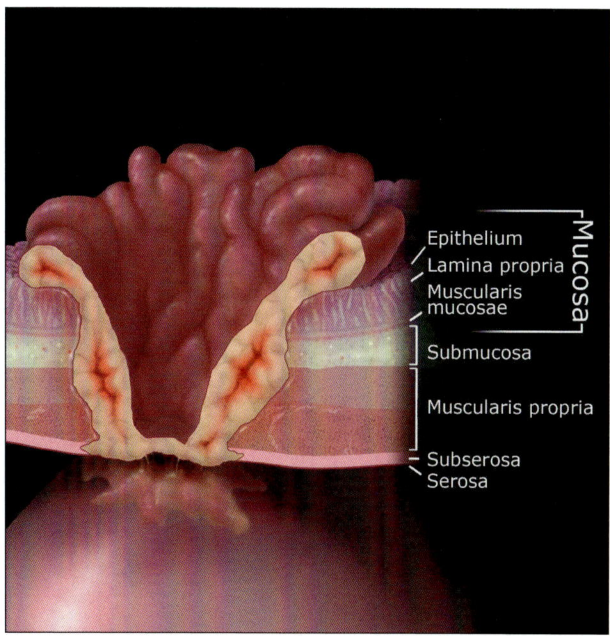

Graphic reveals an ulcerating mass penetrating to the surface of the serosa (visceral peritoneum), indicative of T4a disease. Direct invasion through the serosa is confirmed on microscopic examination.

T4b

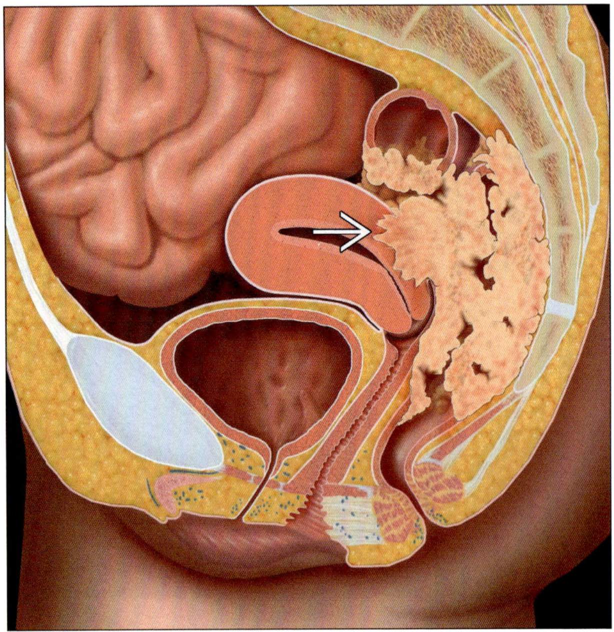

Graphic demonstrates appearance of T4b tumor ➔ that invades or is adherent to adjacent structures. For tumors in a retroperitoneal or subperitoneal location such as the mid or distal rectum, this includes direct invasion of the sacrum, prostate, seminal vesicles, cervix, or vagina.

Nodal Drainage of Cecum, Ascending and Transverse Colon

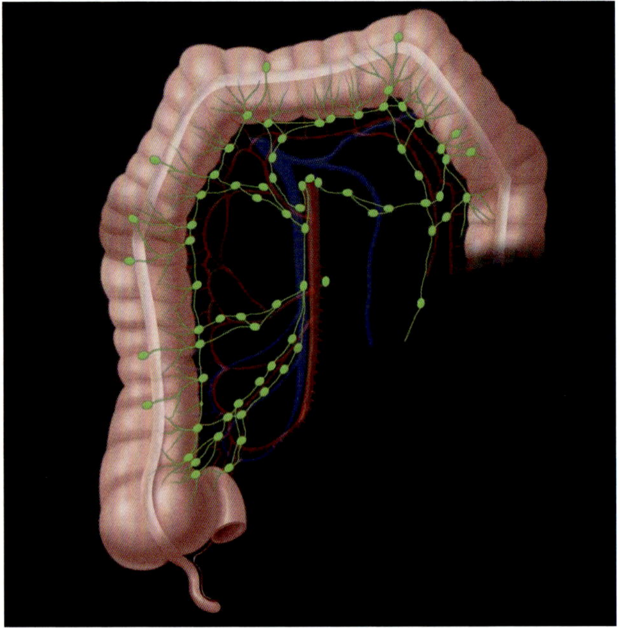

Regional nodes include pericolic nodes (located along the mesocolic border of the colon), nodes along the vascular arcades of the marginal arteries, and nodes along the ileocolic and right colic vessels for the ascending colon and along the middle colic vessels for the transverse colon.

Nodal Drainage of Desending and Rectosigmoid Colon

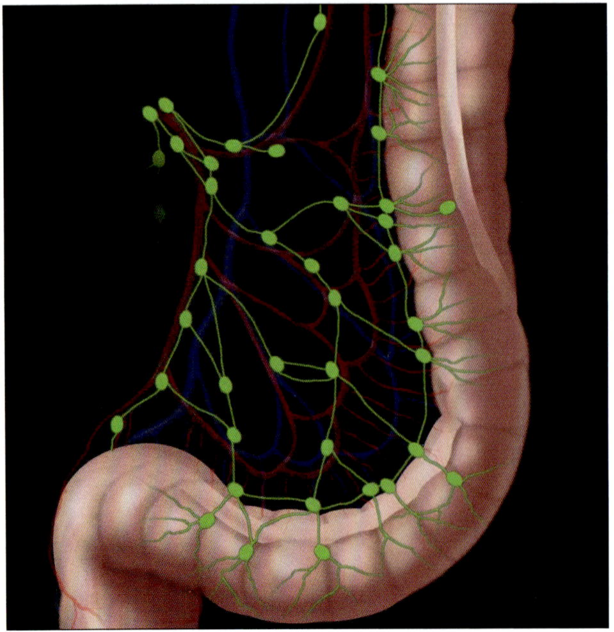

Regional nodes include pericolic nodes (located along the mesocolic border of the colon), nodes along vascular arcades of the marginal arteries, and nodes along the left colic and inferior mesenteric arteries.

Nodal Drainage of Rectum

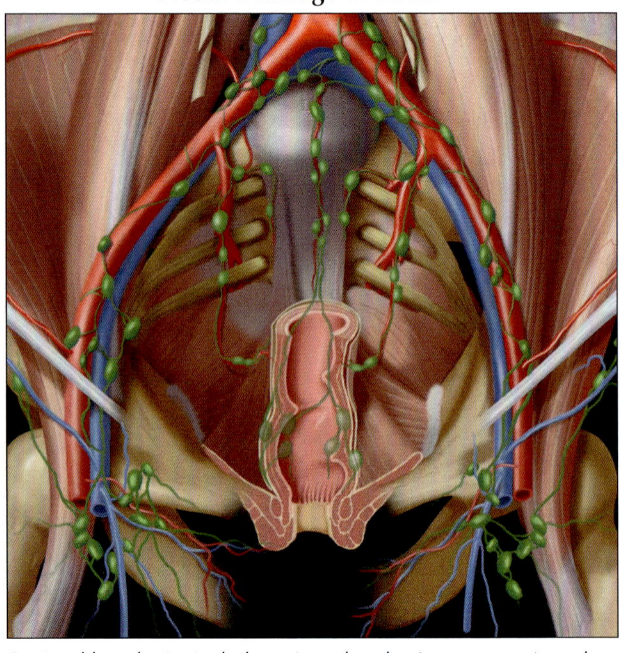

Regional lymphatics include perirectal nodes (mesorectum), nodes along the sigmoid mesenteric and inferior mesenteric arteries, nodes around the sacrum (such as the lateral sacral & sacral promontory regions), nodes along the internal iliac arteries, and nodes along the superior, middle, and inferior rectal arteries.

N1

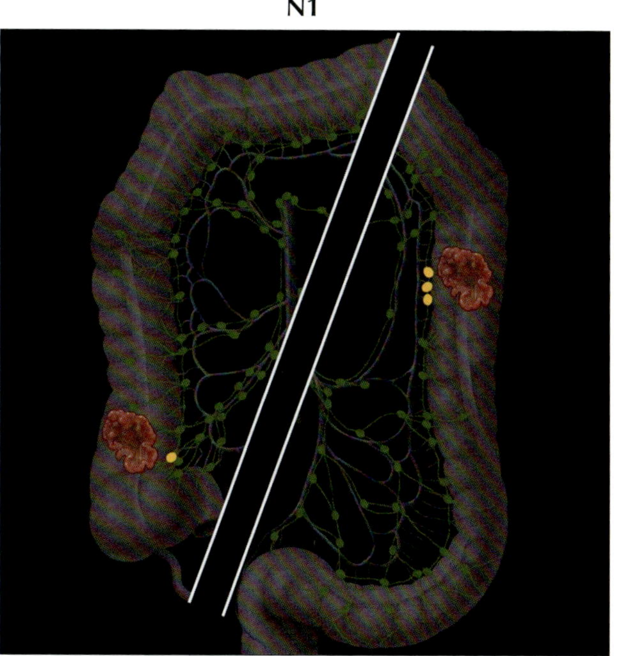

N1 disease involves metastases in 1-3 regional lymph nodes: N1a describes metastasis in a single node (left); N1b describes metastases in 2-3 regional lymph nodes (right); N1c (not shown) describes tumor deposit(s) in the subserosa, mesentery, or nonperitonealized pericolic or perirectal tissues without regional nodal metastasis.

N2

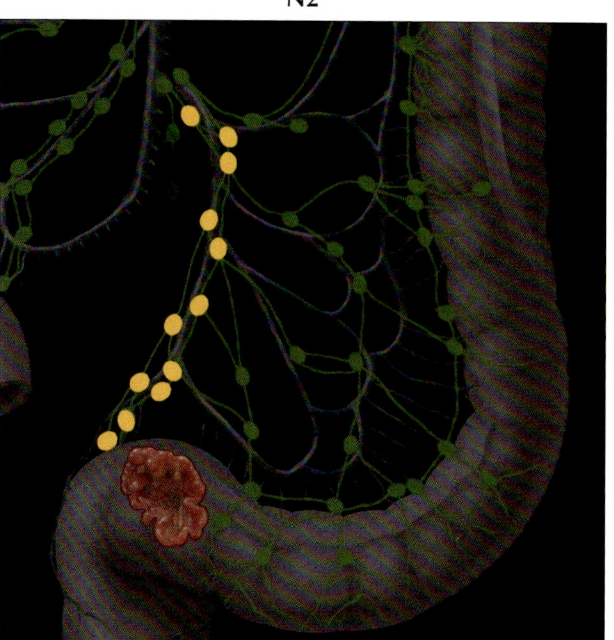

N2 disease denotes metastasis in ≥ 4 regional lymph nodes: N2a involves metastases in 4-6 regional lymph nodes; N2b involves metastases in ≥ 7 regional lymph nodes.

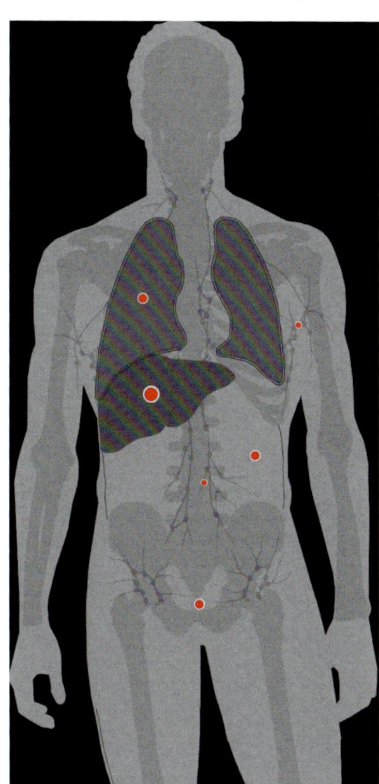

INITIAL SITE OF RECURRENCE

Site	%
Liver	14%
Lung	9%
Local Regional	9%
Intraabdominal	8%
Retroperitoneal	4%
Peripheral Lymph Node	2%

Data represent 818 patients with Duke B2-C colorectal cancer who had surgery alone. The overall recurrence rate was 43%. Galandiuk S. et al. Surg Gynecol Obstet. 174(1):27-32, 1992.

COLON AND RECTUM

OVERVIEW

General Comments

- Rectal and colon cancers constitute the 3rd most common new cancer diagnosis and cause of cancer-related deaths in USA
- Accurate staging and tumor localization are critical in guiding primary and adjuvant treatments
- Rectal and colon cancers are treated differently based on different patterns of failure after surgery
  - Tumor at or below the posterior peritoneal reflection is considered rectal cancer
    - Clinically defined as lesion located within 12-16 cm of the anal verge by rigid proctoscopy
    - Rectum is approximately 12 cm in length, from fusion of the taenia to the puborectalis ring
  - Tumor above the posterior peritoneal reflection is considered colon cancer
    - Transition from sigmoid colon to rectum is approximately at level of sacral promontory

Classification

- Histology
  - Adenocarcinoma in situ (pTis)
    - Synonymous with "high-grade dysplasia" or "severe dysplasia"
  - Adenocarcinoma (90-95%)
  - Medullary carcinoma
  - Signet ring cell carcinoma
    - > 50% signet ring cells
  - Mucinous (colloid type)
  - Others (5-10%)
    - Squamous cell (epidermoid)
    - Adenosquamous
    - Small cell (oat cell) carcinoma
    - Undifferentiated
    - Carcinoma, NOS
- Staging system applies to cancers of the rectum and colon
  - Separate staging system for appendiceal, anal, and carcinoid carcinomas

NATURAL HISTORY

General Features

- Conventional adenoma-carcinoma sequence
  - Multistep progression → in situ dysplasia → adenomatous polyps → invasive carcinoma
  - Adenomatous polyps
    - Estimated 5% risk of finding invasive carcinoma in polyps
    - ↑ risk of cancer in
      - Polyps > 1 cm
      - Polyps with high-grade dysplasia
      - Polyps with > 25% villous histology
    - Histologic classification
      - Tubular (80%)
      - Villous (5-15%)
      - Tubulovillous (5-15%)
    - Morphology
      - Sessile
      - Pedunculated
      - Depressed
    - Size and risk of dysplasia/cancer
      - < 1 cm (1-10%)
      - 1-2 cm (10%)
      - > 2 cm (30-50%)
- Sessile serrated adenomas (SSA)
  - Premalignant flat or sessile lesions
  - Predominantly found in cecum and ascending colon
  - Histologic classification
    - SSA with cytological dysplasia
    - SSA without cytological dysplasia
  - ↑ risk of cancer
    - Multiple SSAs confer higher risk
    - SSAs with high-grade dysplasia

Etiology

- Risk factors
  - Greatest risk factor is advanced age
  - Genetic syndromes
  - Family history
  - Modifiable risk factors
    - Alcohol consumption
    - Obesity
    - Diet low in fiber or calcium, high in fat or phosphate
    - Diabetes mellitus and insulin resistance
  - Inflammatory bowel disease
    - With Crohn disease, 2% developed colorectal cancer at 10 years, 8% at 20 years
    - With ulcerative colitis, 20% developed colorectal cancer at 10 years
      - After 8-10 years, chronic pancolitis increases risk by 5-15% above general population
- Protective factors
  - NSAIDs, calcium, vitamin D may decrease risk

Epidemiology & Cancer Incidence

- Number of cases in USA per year
  - In 2012, estimated 40,290 new cases of rectal cancer
  - In 2012, estimated 103,170 new colon cancer cases
- Sex predilection
  - Estimated 23,500 new cases of rectal cancer in men and 16,790 new cases in women
  - Estimated 49,920 new cases of colon cancer in men and 53,250 new cases in women
  - Lifetime probability of colorectal cancer diagnosis is higher for men (5.27%) than for women (4.91%)
- Age of onset
  - Median age at diagnosis is 7th decade
  - At age 70 or older, men have 1 in 23 (women have 1 in 25) chance of developing colorectal cancer
- Estimated death rate in USA per year
  - ~ 51,690 deaths, or 9% of all cancer-related deaths, in 2012
    - 3rd most common cause of death, after prostate and lung in men and breast and lung in women
  - 50% of patients with colorectal cancer die within 5 years of diagnosis and curative surgical resection
- Trends
  - Incidence per 100,000 has decreased from 60.5 in 1976 to 46.4 in 2008
    - Decline in incidence rates largely attributed to screening for precancerous polyps
  - Mortality ↓ by almost 35% from 1990 to 2007
    - Decline in death rates largely reflects improvements in early detection &/or treatment

Genetics

- Majority of colorectal cancers are sporadic
- 10% of patients have inherited predisposition, 25% have familial predisposition without clear heritable pattern
  - Family history in 2 or more first-degree relatives increases risk 2-3x that of general population
- Genetic syndromes
  - Familial adenomatous polyposis (FAP)
    - 1% of colorectal cancers
    - Syndromes include Gardner, Turcot, and attenuated adenomatous polyposis coli
    - Multiple (100-1,000) adenomas appear in childhood, often symptomatic by teens to 20s
    - 90% of untreated patients will progress to colorectal cancer by 45 years of age
    - Germline mutation in *APC* gene
  - Hereditary nonpolyposis colorectal cancer (Lynch syndrome)
    - Autosomal dominant syndrome
    - 1-5% of colorectal cancers; more common than FAP
    - Germline mutations in mismatch repair genes such as *hMLH1*, *hMSH2*, *hMSH6*, or *PMS2*
    - Synchronous tumors in 10% of patients, with increased risk for endometrial cancer and other malignancies
  - Juvenile polyposis
  - Peutz-Jeghers syndrome
- Multiple overlapping pathways to carcinogenesis
  - Conventional adenoma-carcinoma sequence (~ 60%)
    - Initiating *APC* gene mutation leads to formation of conventional adenomas
      - Mutations in Wnt/APC/β-catenin signaling pathway can be germline or acquired
    - Additional mutations (*TP53*, *PTEN*, *KRAS*, *DCC*, etc.) lead to microsatellite stable (MSS) carcinomas
      - Multistep progression to MSS carcinoma takes ~ 10 years
  - Alternate serrated pathway (~ 40%)
    - Activating mutation in *BRAF* gene leads to sessile serrated adenomas
    - Additional mutations and epigenetic changes lead to microsatellite unstable (MSI-H) carcinomas
      - Methylation of *hMLH1* and errors in DNA mismatch repair lead to microsatellite instability
      - MSI-H carcinomas have better prognosis than MSS carcinomas (stage for stage)
- Molecular genetic prognostic markers
  - Microsatellite instability and 18qLOH are predictive markers in patients with high-risk stage II colon cancer
  - Epidermal growth factor receptor (EGFR) overexpression occurs in colorectal cancers
    - Anti-EGFR antibodies (cetuximab or panitumumab) inhibit EGFR signaling and are effective in some patients
    - *KRAS* mutations (codons 12 and 13 of exon 2) predict lack of response to EGFR antibody therapy
  - *BRAF* V600E mutation confers a poorer prognosis than wild type *BRAF*

Gross Pathology & Surgical Features

- Fungating or exophytic
- Stenosing
- Constricting (annular, circumferential)
- Ulcerating
  - Ulcerating tumors may have worse prognosis than exophytic tumors

Microscopic Pathology

- Surgical pathologic evaluation
  - Histologic grade
    - High-grade tumors have < 50% gland formation, poorly differentiated with loss of nuclear polarity
    - Intermediate-grade tumors are moderately differentiated with irregular tubules
    - Low-grade tumors have well-differentiated glands and uniform nuclei that maintain polarity
    - Histologic grade has not proven to be an independent factor in overall prognosis
  - Depth of penetration and extension to adjacent structures (T stage)
    - In cases of neoadjuvant therapy, T stage is based on viable, residual tumor
  - Number of regional lymph nodes evaluated
    - NCCN recommends minimum of 12 nodes; AJCC recommends 10-14 nodes
  - Number of positive regional lymph nodes (N stage)
  - Number of extranodal tumor deposits in perirectal fat
    - Tumor deposits outside the leading edge of tumor, with no residual lymphatic tissue but within primary lymphatic drainage
    - Associated with worse disease-free and overall survival
    - Staged as pN1c, if no positive nodes
  - Distant metastases to nonregional lymph nodes or other organs (M stage)
  - Status of resection margins
    - Proximal
    - Distal
    - Circumferential (radial)
      - Closest margin between deepest penetration of tumor and edge of resected perirectal soft tissue or edge of a lymph node
      - Positive margin = tumor ≤ 1 mm from the transected margin
      - Strong predictor of local recurrence and overall survival, especially with neoadjuvant therapy
      - Important in recommending postoperative treatments
  - Treatment effects of neoadjuvant therapy
    - Prefix "yp" denotes pathologic staging after neoadjuvant therapy
  - Lymphovascular space invasion (LVI)
  - Perineural invasion (PNI)
    - Associated with worse disease-free and overall survival

Routes of Spread

- Local spread
  - Penetration of bowel wall and invasion of adjacent organs
    - Rectal
      - Sacrum; genitourinary structures (e.g., prostate, seminal vesicles, uterus, cervix, vagina, bladder)
    - Colon

- Abdominal wall; adjacent organs (e.g., bowel, stomach, kidney, spleen, liver, pancreas)
- Perineural invasion
  - Local spread may be as far as 10 cm from primary tumor
- Retroperitoneal invasion
  - Most of rectum is extraperitoneal
    - Upper 1/3 of rectum is covered by peritoneum anteriorly and laterally
    - Middle 1/3 of rectum is covered by peritoneum anteriorly
    - Lower 1/3 and posterolateral middle 1/3 of rectum are not covered by peritoneum
  - Posterior walls of ascending and descending colon are retroperitoneal
- Peritoneal spread
  - Ascending and descending colon are covered by peritoneum anteriorly
  - Transverse colon is suspended by transverse mesocolon
  - Sigmoid and cecum are covered by peritoneum
  - Peritoneal spread to ovaries (Krukenberg tumor)
- Lymphatic extension
  - Regional lymph node involvement in 20-40% of patients at presentation
  - Different regional nodes by tumor location
    - Rectum
      - Initial tumor spread to perirectal nodes in mesorectum
      - Upper 1/3 → superior rectal nodes → sigmoid mesenteric nodes → inferior mesenteric nodes
      - Middle and lower 1/3 → middle and inferior rectal nodes → internal iliac nodes
      - Other nodes include obturator, lateral sacral, presacral, sacral promontory nodes
      - Common iliac, external iliac, paraaortic and inguinal nodes are nonregional and are considered metastatic disease
    - Rectosigmoid
      - Pericolic, perirectal, left colic, sigmoid mesenteric, sigmoidal inferior mesenteric, superior rectal, middle rectal nodes
    - Sigmoid colon
      - Pericolic, superior rectal, sigmoidal, sigmoid mesenteric, inferior mesenteric nodes
    - Descending colon
      - Pericolic, left colic, inferior mesenteric, sigmoid nodes
    - Splenic flexure
      - Pericolic, middle colic, left colic, inferior mesenteric nodes
    - Transverse colon
      - Pericolic and middle colic nodes
    - Hepatic flexure
      - Pericolic, middle colic, right colic
    - Ascending colon
      - Pericolic, ileocolic, right colic, middle colic
    - Cecum
      - Pericolic, anterior cecal, posterior cecal, ileocolic, right colic
- Metastatic sites
  - Liver and lungs are main sites of hematogenous metastases
    - Liver-only metastases are seen in 40% of autopsies
  - Seeding of other segments of colon, small intestine, or peritoneum can occur

IMAGING

Detection

- Colonoscopy
  - High sensitivity for detecting mucosal lesions
  - Allows biopsy and polypectomy during visualization
    - Complications include perforation and bleeding from polypectomy
  - Detects synchronous lesions and other pathologic conditions of rectum and colon
    - Synchronous tumors have same prognosis as solitary tumors according to standard staging
    - Up to 15% of patients present with obstructing proximal lesion that impedes complete colonoscopy
    - Metachronous tumors develop in 1-3% of patients within 5 years of initial diagnosis
      - Location: Cecum (10%), ascending colon (15%), transverse colon (15%), descending colon (5%), sigmoid colon (25%), rectosigmoid (10%), rectum (20%)
- Flexible sigmoidoscopy
  - Evaluation up to splenic flexure only
  - Up to 66% of tumors can be missed due to incomplete bowel evaluation
- Capsule endoscopy
  - Ingested capsule provides photographic evaluation of colon and rectum
  - Sensitivity 64% & specificity 84% for polyps ≥ 6 mm
- Double contrast barium enema (DCBE)
  - Useful in patients with incomplete colonoscopy
  - Requires additional procedure for intervention or biopsy
  - Detects only 20% of polyps found on colonoscopy
    - Rate of detection is related to size
      - ≤ 0.5 cm (21% rate of detection)
      - 0.6-1.0 cm (42% rate of detection)
      - > 1.0 cm (46% rate of detection)
- Contrast-enhanced CT (CECT)
  - Not useful for early tumor detection
  - CT imaging findings
    - Intraluminal polypoid mass
    - Asymmetric mural thickening ± luminal narrowing
      - Wall thickness: 3-6 mm = indeterminate
      - Wall thickness: > 6 mm = abnormal
  - CT colonography (CTC)
    - Noninvasive technique to evaluate obstructive lesions and cases of incomplete colonoscopy
    - Can simultaneously evaluate disease spread outside rectum and colon
    - Reported rates of detection are comparable to conventional colonoscopy
    - Reported sensitivity up to 90% in patients with lesions ≥ 10 mm in diameter
    - Radiation exposure
      - Radiation dose of CTC is about 1/2 that used for standard body CT examination
      - Minimum average dose of ~ 5 mSv
      - Less radiation exposure than barium enema

COLON AND RECTUM

Staging

- Standard evaluation of rectal cancer includes endorectal ultrasound, chest/abdominal/pelvic CT, or pelvic MR
- PET/CT is not routinely indicated but can be considered in potentially surgically curable M1 disease
- **Tumor staging of rectal cancer**
  - Endorectal ultrasound (EUS)
    - High specificity in evaluating depth of invasion into muscularis propria
    - Allows tumor and nodal biopsy at time of evaluation
    - High degree of operator dependence
  - Pelvic MR with endorectal coil
    - Improved field of view and visualization of mesorectal fascia compared to EUS
    - Less operator dependence than EUS
    - Best imaging modality to predict circumferential resection margins prior to surgery
    - Assess feasibility of sphincter-sparing surgery
  - CECT
    - Unable to detect T1 or T2 tumors reliably
    - Not optimal for evaluating invasion depth or differentiating stages of tumor confined to bowel wall
    - Reported sensitivity and specificity for size of primary lesion are highly variable
  - Comparisons
    - Endorectal US: 80-95% sensitivity; 86% specificity
    - CECT: 65-75% sensitivity; 50% specificity
    - MR: 75-85% sensitivity; 69% specificity
    - Digital rectal exam: 62% sensitivity; 80-90% specificity
  - Radiographic features
    - Tis-T2
      - Sessile or pedunculated lesions
      - Well-defined peripheral wall with clear adjacent fat
      - Luminal narrowing without extension through serosa
    - T3
      - Invasion into subserosa of peritonealized organs
      - Poorly defined peripheral wall with nodular margin and pericolonic fat infiltration
      - Extension to nonperitonealized surfaces
      - Retroperitoneal extension from posterior walls of ascending colon and descending colon, as well as rectum distal to peritoneal reflections
    - T4
      - Loss of fat planes between colon and adjacent structures
      - Pericolonic mass
      - Stranding of pericolic fat indicates extension through serosal or peritoneal surfaces
- **Nodal staging of rectal cancer**
  - Accuracy is a challenge in preop staging of rectal cancer
    - Endorectal US: 67% sensitivity; 78% specificity; cannot evaluate iliac, mesenteric, or retroperitoneal nodes
    - CECT: 55% sensitivity; 74% specificity
    - MR: 66% sensitivity; 76% specificity
    - None of the 3 standard imaging modalities is significantly superior
  - Radiographic features
    - Nodes ≥ 10 mm in short axis
    - Involved nodes may have hazy outer margins, round to oval appearance, with loss of fatty hilum
    - Found along bowel surface and associated vascular pedicle
- **Metastasis staging**
  - Chest/abdominal/pelvic CT is the standard evaluation
    - Sensitivity for detecting distant metastases (75-87%)
    - Highly variable sensitivity for detecting peritoneal implants
    - Higher accuracy for detecting liver metastases than nodal metastases
  - PET/CT has high sensitivity (76-95%) in detecting metastatic lesions
    - Changes clinical stage in ~ 31% and changes management in ~ 14% of rectal cancer patients
  - Liver metastases
    - Intrabiliary growth with intrahepatic bile duct dilatation (more than noncolorectal metastases or hepatocellular carcinoma)
    - CT appearance
      - Calcifications may be seen initially or following chemo
      - Portal venous phase is most reliable
      - Hypoattenuating with occasional faint ring of enhancement
    - MR appearance of liver metastases
      - T1WI: Usually slightly hypointense relative to normal liver
      - T2WI: Slightly hyperintense relative to normal liver
      - Gadolinium-enhanced T1WI
      - Metastases are best seen on portal venous phase
      - Thin peripheral ring of strong enhancement that persists through all phases of enhancement
      - Metastases > 3 cm in size show cauliflower-like appearance
    - Ultrasound appearance of liver metastases
      - Usually hypoechoic relative to liver parenchyma
      - May be hyperechoic if calcified or hemorrhagic
  - Lung metastases
    - 2nd most common site of metastatic disease
    - Evaluate with CT of chest
  - Bone metastases
    - Lytic or blastic osseous lesion depending on histologic subtype
    - Evaluate with x-ray plain films, CT, or PET/CT
  - Brain metastases
    - Multiple or solitary; not frequently evaluated preoperatively
    - MR is preferred method of diagnosis and evaluation

CLINICAL PRESENTATION & WORK-UP

Presentation

- Common symptoms
  - Abdominal pain (44%)
  - Change in bowel habits (43%)

- GI bleeding (40%)
- Isolated anemia (11%)
- Weight loss (6%)
- Rectal cancer
  - Palpable mass
  - Painless bleeding
  - Changes in stool caliber or constipation
  - Locally advanced: Tenesmus, urgency, urinary symptoms, sciatic pain, perineal pain
- Right-sided colon cancer
  - Bleeding and anemia
- Left-sided colon cancer
  - Constipation, diarrhea, bowel obstruction

Prognosis

- 5-year survival rates by stage
  - Rectum
    - Stage I: 74.1%
    - Stage IIA: 64.5%
    - Stage IIB: 51.6%
    - Stage IIC: 32.3%
    - Stage IIIA: 74.0%
    - Stage IIIB: 45.0%
    - Stage IIIC: 33.4%
    - Stage IV: 6%
  - Colon
    - Stage I: 74.0%
    - Stage IIA: 66.5%
    - Stage IIB: 58.6%
    - Stage IIC: 37.3%
    - Stage IIIA: 73.1%
    - Stage IIIB: 46.3%
    - Stage IIIC: 28.0%
    - Stage IV: 5.7%
- Prognostic factors
  - Lymphatic and venous invasion are independent adverse factors regardless of T stage
  - Patients with tumors arising around peritoneal reflections, either rectosigmoid or rectal, have worse 5-year survival rate regardless of stage
  - Presenting with obstruction or perforation increases mortality risk
    - 5-year survival rate for patients with symptomatic disease 49% vs. 71% for asymptomatic patients
  - Serum CEA levels
    - ≥ 5.0 ng/mL has adverse impact on survival independent of stage
    - Elevated levels serve as marker for recurrent disease after resection
  - Tumor deposits
    - Number of satellite tumor deposits discontinuous from leading edge of primary carcinoma
  - Tumor regression grade
    - Pathologic features that allow response to adjuvant therapies to be assessed
    - Complete pathologic response predicts improved overall survival (OS)
  - Circumferential resection margin
  - *KRAS* mutation status
  - Microsatellite instability
  - Perineural invasion

Work-Up

- Clinical
  - Colonoscopy, rigid proctoscopy, biopsy
- Radiographic
  - Chest/abdominal/pelvic CT, endorectal ultrasound &/or pelvic MR
- Laboratory
  - CEA, LFTs, CBC

TREATMENT

Major Treatment Alternatives

- Surgical resection of rectal cancer
  - Abdominal perineal resection (APR)
    - For distal (low) tumors involving anal sphincter or levator muscles, or when resection would compromise sphincter function
    - Total mesorectal excision (TME) is standard treatment for draining lymphatics
    - Abdominal and perineal incisions; en block resection of rectosigmoid, rectum, anus, mesorectum, perianal tissues
    - Complete proctectomy and creation of permanent colostomy
  - Low anterior resection (LAR)
    - Used for invasive tumors of proximal (mid to upper) rectum
      - Generally sphincter sparing depending on distal margins (need ≥ 2 cm below tumor)
    - Dissection and anastomosis below peritoneal reflection, with ligation of superior and middle hemorrhoidal arteries
    - Additional dissection along prostate gland or plane of anterior rectal wall
    - TME is standard
    - Coloanal anastomosis
      - Allows sphincter preservation for distal cancers
      - J-pouch is created by folding distal bowel back on itself, creating neorectum
      - Requires temporary diverting ostomy
  - Local procedures (i.e., polypectomy, transanal endoscopic microsurgery, or transanal excision)
    - T1, N0, grades 1-2, < 3 cm, < 8 cm from anal verge, < 30% circumference, clear margins (> 3 mm), no LVI/PNI, mobile, normal CEA
- Neoadjuvant/adjuvant chemoradiation therapy (CRT) in rectal cancer
  - Concurrent 5-FU-based chemotherapy with RT
  - RT field to include tumor or tumor bed with 2 cm margin, mesorectum, presacral nodes, internal iliac nodes
    - Include external iliac nodes for T4b tumors involving anterior structures
  - Preoperative CRT
    - Stage II (T3-4 N0) or stage III (N+ disease)
    - High risk of locoregional recurrence
    - Outcomes associated with improved local control, less treatment-related toxicity, higher rates of sphincter preservation compared to postop
  - Postoperative CRT
    - Clinical stage I that has been upstaged to stages II or III after surgery
    - 5-FU-based chemo before and after CRT
    - After APR, field should include the perineal scar
- Adjuvant chemotherapy
  - Stages II or III rectal cancer

  - Total of ~ 6 months of perioperative chemotherapy
  - 5-FU/LV, FOLFOX, capecitabine ± oxaliplatin
- Resection of liver metastases
  - Criteria for resectability
    - Limited number of lesions
    - Lack of major vascular involvement
    - Absent or limited extrahepatic disease
    - Ability to achieve R0 resection
      - > 1 cm surgical margin and absence of portal lymph node involvement
    - Sufficient functional liver reserve (remnant volume)
      - Involvement of > 70% of liver precludes resection
  - Outcomes
    - 5-year relapse-free survival rates of 24-38% for patients with < 4 liver lesions treated with surgical resection
    - 5-year survival of patients with resected liver metastases averages 40%; 10-year survival 25%

Major Treatment Roadblocks/ Contraindications

- Widespread metastatic disease
- Primary tumors invading adjacent organs
- Perforation and obstruction upon presentation
- Lack of adequate resection margins
  - Higher rate of rectal cancer recurrence due to confined anatomy within bony pelvis, adjacent organs, inadequate nodal sampling

Treatment Options by Stage

- **Rectal cancer**
  - Stage I (cT1 N0 M0) if fits criteria for local procedure
    - Transanal excision
    - Transanal endoscopic microsurgery increasingly utilized in T1 tumors
  - Stage I (cT1-T2 N0 M0)
    - TME with APR for low lesions or LAR for mid-upper lesions
      - If pT3 N0 or pT1-3 N1-2, then postop CRT followed by adjuvant chemotherapy
      - If pT1-2 N0, then observation
  - Stage II-III (cT3 N0 M0, cN1-2)
    - Preop 5-FU-based CRT
    - TME with APR for low lesions or LAR for mid-upper lesions (e.g., ≥ 5 cm from anal verge)
      - En bloc resection of tumor, vascular pedicle, and lymphatic drainage
      - ≥ 2 cm surgical margins desired
    - Adjuvant chemotherapy
  - T4b or locally unresectable tumors
    - CRT then assess for resection
      - Consider IORT at time of surgery
    - Definitive CRT
    - Adjuvant chemotherapy
  - Stage IVA
    - Combination chemotherapy
    - Consider resection of rectal primary following neoadjuvant CRT with liver or lung metastasectomy
    - Tumor palliation
      - EBRT for symptomatic primary lesions
      - For unresectable liver metastases, consider radiofrequency ablation, chemoembolization, yttrium-90, SBRT, or 3D CRT
- Colon cancer
  - Stage I
    - Colectomy with en block resection of regional lymph nodes
  - Stage II
    - Colectomy with en block resection of regional lymph nodes
    - Consider adjuvant chemotherapy
  - Stage III
    - Colectomy with en block resection of regional lymph nodes
    - Adjuvant chemotherapy
  - T4b, tumor penetrating or adherent to a fixed structure
    - Colectomy with en block resection of regional lymph nodes
    - Consider adjuvant CRT to tumor bed
  - Stage IVA
    - Combination chemotherapy FOLFOX or FOLFIRI ± bevacizumab
    - Consider colectomy with liver or lung metastasectomy
    - For unresectable liver metastases, consider radiofrequency ablation, chemoembolization, yttrium-90, SBRT, or 3D CRT

Standard Doses

- Rectal: 45 Gy in 25 fractions to pelvis
  - Rectal/mesorectum boost of 5.4 Gy in 3 fractions in preoperative CRT
    - Consider 9 Gy boost for T4b tumors
  - Tumor bed boost of 5.4-9.0 Gy in 3-5 fractions in postoperative CRT
- Colon: 45 Gy in 25 fractions to operative bed
  - Consider boost of 5.4 Gy in 3 fractions if minimal small bowel in RT field

Organs at Risk Parameters

- Minimize volume of small bowel in RT field, especially bowel receiving > 45 Gy

Common Techniques

- Standard is 3D conformal, 3 or 4 field
- Ability of IMRT to decrease toxicity under investigation
  - Potential benefit for T4b tumors if external iliac regions require treatment
    - May decrease dose to small bowel located between external iliac regions

Landmark Trials

- Benefit of postop RT/CRT in rectal cancer
  - GITSG 7175: Surgery vs. postop chemo vs. postop RT vs. postop CRT
    - Postop CRT improved 5-year LC, DFS, and OS compared to surgery alone
  - NSABP R-01 and R-02 showed that postop RT improved LC whereas postop chemo improved DFS and OS compared to surgery alone
  - NCCTG 79-47-51 showed that postop CRT improved LC, DM, & OS compared to postop RT
- Benefit of preop RT/CRT in rectal cancer
  - Swedish trial: Non-TME surgery vs. preop RT 25 Gy in 5 fx + non-TME surgery

- Preop RT reduced LR and improved OS compared to surgery alone
- Dutch trial: TME surgery alone vs. preop RT 25 Gy in 5 fx + TME surgery
  - Preop RT improved LC but not OS; RT increased perineal complications if APR done & bleeding during operation
- Preop CRT vs. postop CRT
  - German trial: Preop CRT improved LR, decreased acute and late toxicity, increased sphincter preservation
- Reirradiation for recurrent tumors
  - Multi-institution phase II: Hyperfractionated RT (1.2 Gy b.i.d. to 40.8 Gy) with 5-FU
    - Outcomes: Palliation of pain (83%) and bleeding (100%) with acceptable rates of acute and late toxicity
  - If b.i.d. treatment not feasible, consider daily treatment to ≥ 36 Gy/20 fractions

RECOMMENDED FOLLOW-UP

Clinical

- Goals are detection of early recurrence and new metachronous lesions
  - Local recurrences in rectal cancer continue to occur after 5 years
  - Long-term survival possible (5-year survival rate of 15.6%) in patients treated for local recurrence of rectal cancer
  - 80% of recurrences were in 1st 3 years after surgical resection of primary tumor
- H&P every 3-6 months for 1st 2 years, every 6 months for 5 years, then annually
- Surveillance colonoscopy
  - Initial colonoscopy at ~ 1 year following resection; 3-6 months post resection if incomplete colonoscopy initially
  - Repeat colonoscopy at 3 years, then every 5 years thereafter
    - Repeat colonoscopy in 1 year if advanced adenoma (villous, > 1 cm, or high-grade dysplasia)
- Proctoscopy
  - Every 6 months for 5 years
  - Evaluate local recurrence at rectal anastomosis after LAR

Radiographic

- CT of chest/abdomen/pelvis
  - Used to monitor response to therapy and detect recurrent disease
  - Annually for 1st 3-5 years in stages II and III patients
- PET/CT
  - Not routinely recommended in absence of other evidence of recurrent or metastatic disease
  - Useful in asymptomatic patients with rising CEA levels to exclude recurrent disease
  - More sensitive than conventional CT in post-treatment surveillance
  - Overall specificity and sensitivity for detection of recurrent cancer is 97% and 76%, respectively

Laboratory

- Post-treatment CEA at baseline, every 3-6 months for 2 years, then every 6 months for 5 years

SELECTED REFERENCES

1. Sauer R et al: Preoperative Versus Postoperative Chemoradiotherapy for Locally Advanced Rectal Cancer: Results of the German CAO/ARO/AIO-94 Randomized Phase III Trial After a Median Follow-Up of 11 Years. J Clin Oncol. 30(16):1926-33, 2012
2. American Joint Committee on Cancer: AJCC Cancer Staging Manual. 7th ed. New York: Springer. 143-64, 2010
3. Das P et al: Hyperfractionated accelerated radiotherapy for rectal cancer in patients with prior pelvic irradiation. Int J Radiat Oncol Biol Phys. 77(1):60-5, 2010
4. Engstrom PF et al: NCCN Clinical Practice Guidelines in Oncology: colon cancer. J Natl Compr Canc Netw. 7(8):778-831, 2009
5. Engstrom PF et al: NCCN Clinical Practice Guidelines in Oncology: rectal cancer. J Natl Compr Canc Netw. 7(8):838-81, 2009
6. Myerson RJ et al: Elective clinical target volumes for conformal therapy in anorectal cancer: a radiation therapy oncology group consensus panel contouring atlas. Int J Radiat Oncol Biol Phys. 74(3):824-30, 2009
7. Greenberg JA et al: Local excision of distal rectal cancer: an update of cancer and leukemia group B 8984. Dis Colon Rectum. 51(8):1185-91; discussion 1191-4, 2008
8. Valentini V et al: Preoperative hyperfractionated chemoradiation for locally recurrent rectal cancer in patients previously irradiated to the pelvis: A multicentric phase II study. Int J Radiat Oncol Biol Phys. 64(4):1129-39, 2006
9. Taylor A et al: Mapping pelvic lymph nodes: guidelines for delineation in intensity-modulated radiotherapy. Int J Radiat Oncol Biol Phys. 63(5):1604-12, 2005
10. Gunderson LL et al: Impact of T and N stage and treatment on survival and relapse in adjuvant rectal cancer: a pooled analysis. J Clin Oncol. 22(10):1785-96, 2004
11. Myerson R et al: Technical aspects of image-based treatment planning of rectal carcinoma. Semin Radiat Oncol. 13(4):433-40, 2003
12. Mohiuddin M et al: Long-term results of reirradiation for patients with recurrent rectal carcinoma. Cancer. 95(5):1144-50, 2002
13. Taylor N et al: Elective groin irradiation is not indicated for patients with adenocarcinoma of the rectum extending to the anal canal. Int J Radiat Oncol Biol Phys. 51(3):741-7, 2001
14. Willett CG et al: Postoperative radiation therapy for high-risk colon carcinoma. J Clin Oncol. 11(6):1112-7, 1993
15. Gunderson LL et al: Areas of failure found at reoperation (second or symptomatic look) following "curative surgery" for adenocarcinoma of the rectum. Clinicopathologic correlation and implications for adjuvant therapy. Cancer. 34(4):1278-92, 1974

Stage IIA (T3 N0 M0)

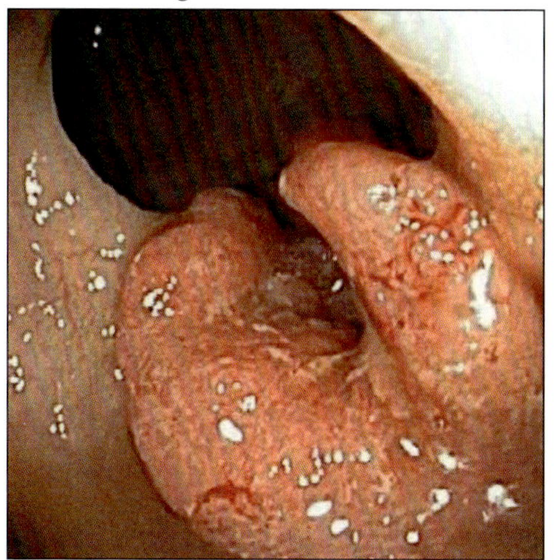

Stage IIA (T3 N0 M0)

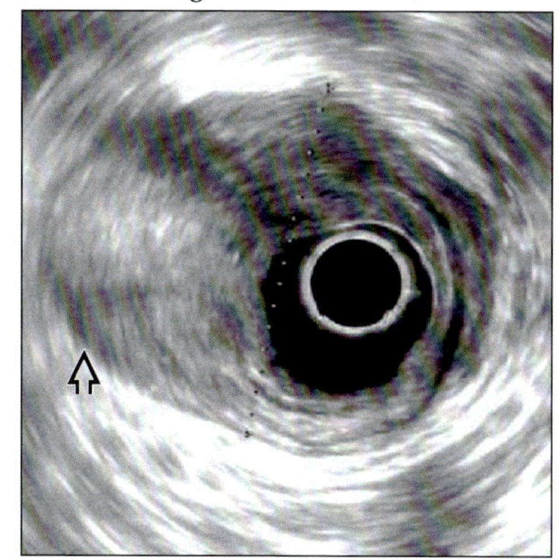

(Left) *Colonoscopy shows a nonobstructing polypoid mass in the distal, anterior rectum in a 36-year-old woman who presented with hematochezia. On rigid proctoscopy, it is 6.5 cm from the anal verge. Biopsy revealed a moderately differentiated adenocarcinoma.* ***(Right)*** *Endorectal ultrasound (7.5 and 10 Mhz) shows a 4 cm lesion extending through the rectal wall into adventitia ➩ (T3). No peritumoral adenopathy was identified.*

Stage IIA (T3 N0 M0)

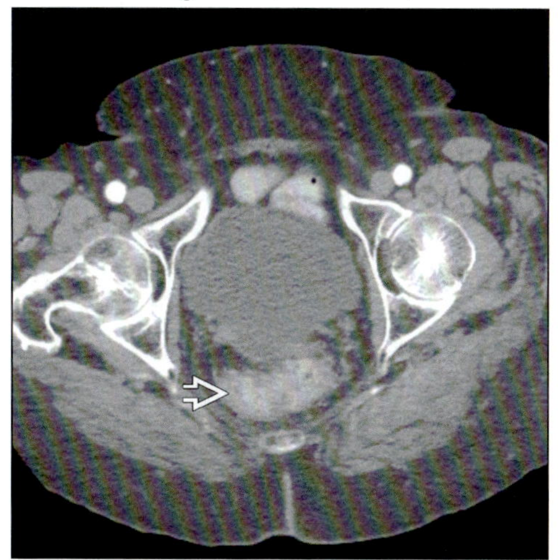

Stage IIA (T3 N0 M0)

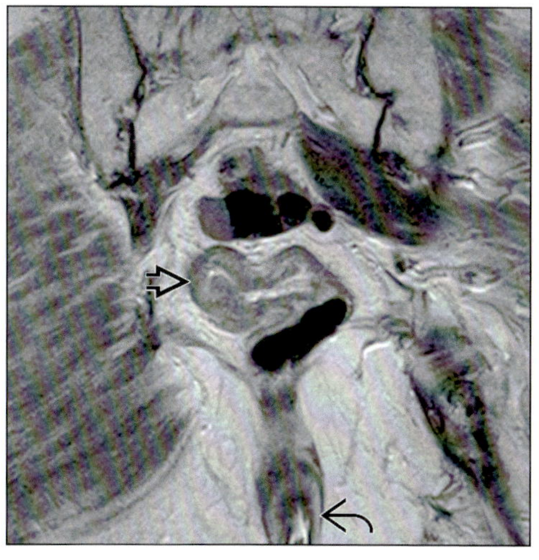

(Left) *Axial CECT shows concentric wall thickening with tumor ➡ extending into perirectal tissues in a patient with tumor located 8 cm from the anal verge based on rigid proctoscopy.* ***(Right)*** *Coronal T2WI FS MR shows a partially obstructing tumor ➩ starting approximately 8 cm from the anal verge ↷ and extending over approximately 5.1 cm of rectum. The tumor is hyperintense on diffusion-weighted imaging.*

Stage IIA (T3 N0 M0)

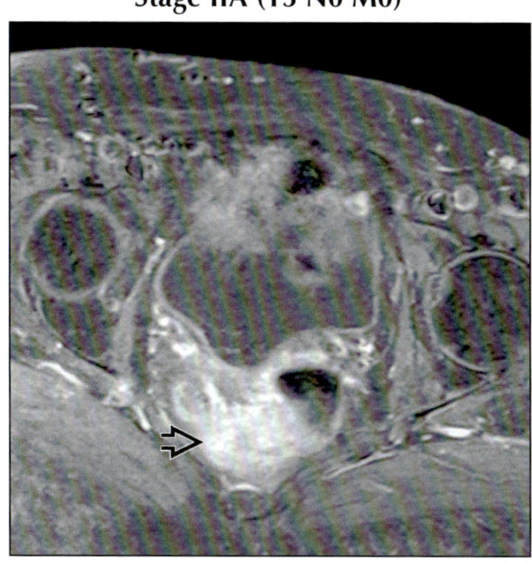

Stage IIA (T3 N0 M0)

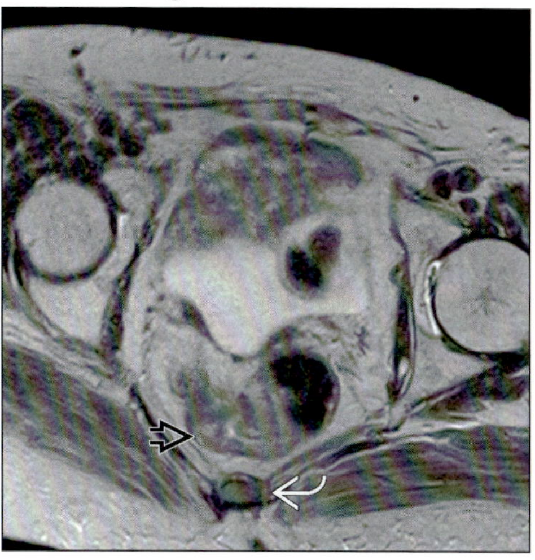

(Left) *Axial T1WI C+ MR shows an enhancing rectal tumor ➩ predominantly in the posterior wall but circumferential in areas causing luminal narrowing.* ***(Right)*** *Axial T2WI FSE MR in the same patient shows a T3 N0 rectal tumor extending into perirectal fat, which directly abuts the mesorectal fascia on the right ➩. There is no evidence of invasion of the coccyx ➡.*

COLON AND RECTUM

(Left) Axial CECT shows concentric rectal wall thickening ➡ with tumor extending into perirectal tissues ➡ below the peritoneal reflection. (Right) Axial CECT in the same patient shows large infiltrative lymph node ➡ along superior rectal vessels. Two adjacent nodes ➡ are also present, and all 3 were found to contain metastatic deposits on pathological examination following chemoradiation.

Stage IIIB (T3 N1b M0)

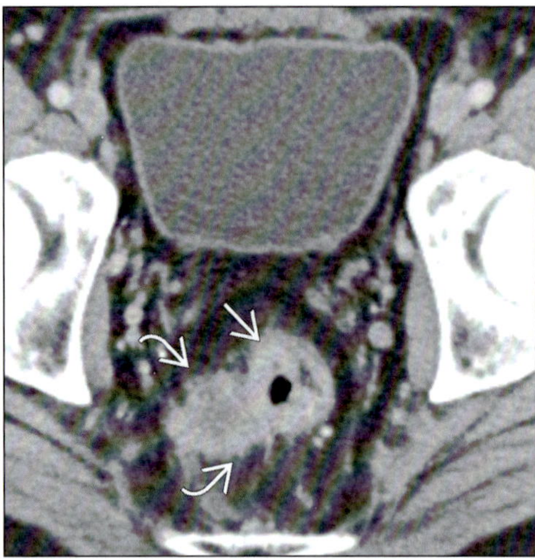

Stage IIIB (T3 N1b M0)

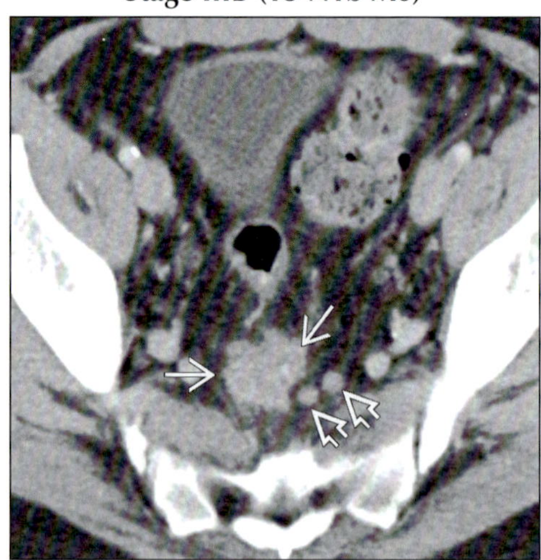

(Left) During simulation, patient lies prone with arms up, on a belly board ➡ with downsloped back edge, pubic symphysis ➡ at edge of board aperture, and alpha cradle indexed to bottom of board. (Right) Sagittal CT shows the same patient, with full (350 mL) bladder (yellow), anal marker (green) at the verge, and rectal contrast in place. Small bowel ➡ (pink) is displaced superiorly and anteriorly by bladder distension and the belly board.

EBRT Simulation

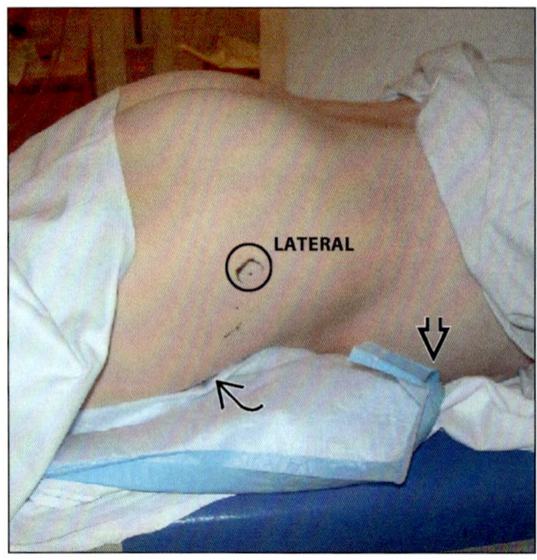

EBRT Simulation

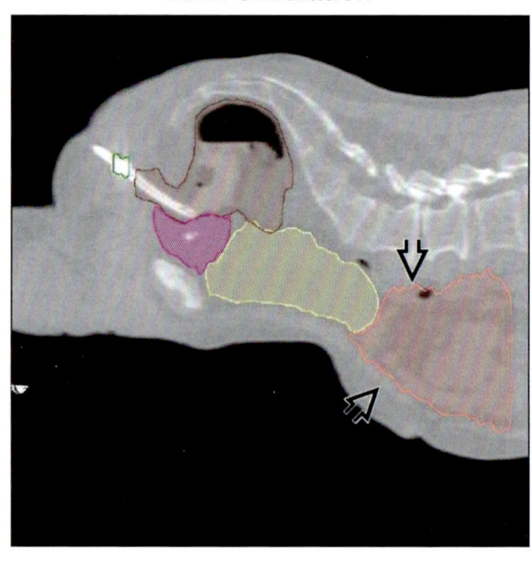

(Left) PA DRR shows preop pelvic field with CTVs for presacral LN (orange), internal iliac LN (green), mesorectum (red), and pelvic floor (cyan). Classic field borders are sup.: L5-S1 junction, inf.: 3 cm below GTV (or below obturator foramina, whichever is most inf.), laterally: 1.5 cm from pelvic inlet. (Right) Lateral DRR in same patient shows CTVs. Classic borders are ant.: base of pubis for T3 (1 cm ant. to pubis for T4b) & post.: 1 cm behind ant. sacrum.

Pelvic EBRT

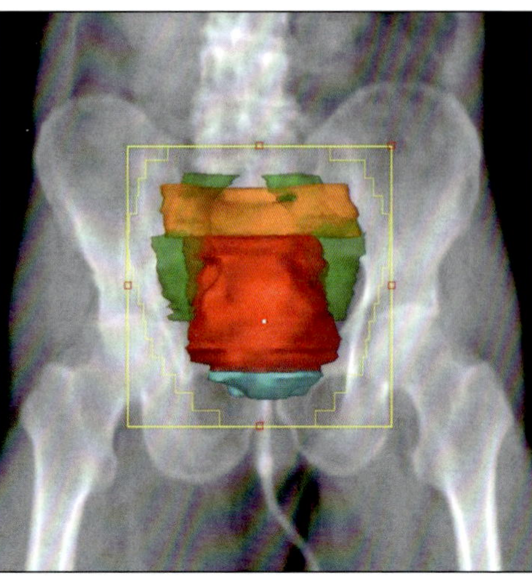

Pelvic EBRT

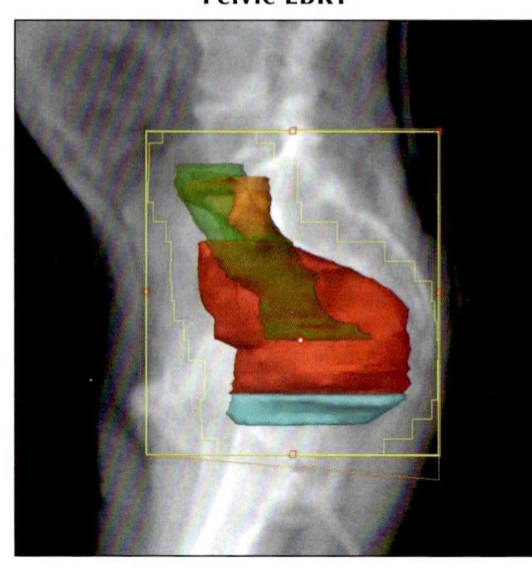

T3 N0 Proximal Rectal Tumor

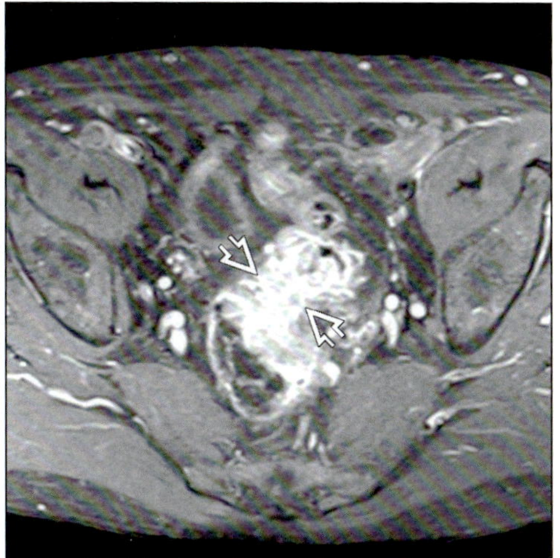

T3 N0 Proximal Rectal Tumor

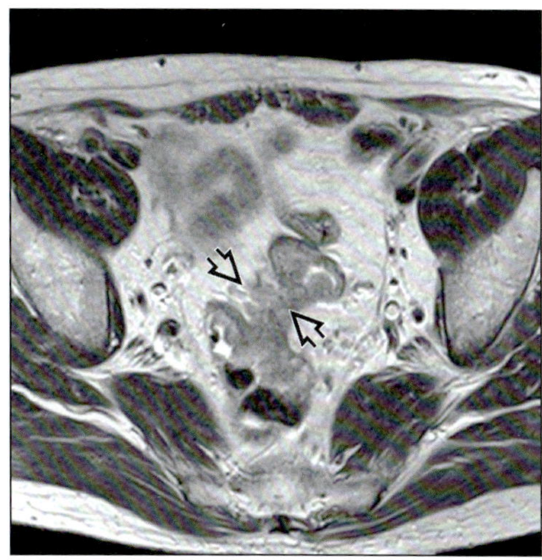

*(**Left**) Axial T1WI C+ FS MR shows an enhancing proximal rectal mass ➡ in a 61-year-old man who presented with hematochezia and diarrhea. (**Right**) Axial T2WI MR in the same patient shows circumferential mass with low T2 signal ➡ extending into the mesorectal fat, extending minimally beyond the expected margin of the muscularis layer. This is consistent with endorectal ultrasound (EUS) findings of penetration through all layers of the rectal wall (uT3 N0).*

T3 N0 Proximal Rectal Tumor

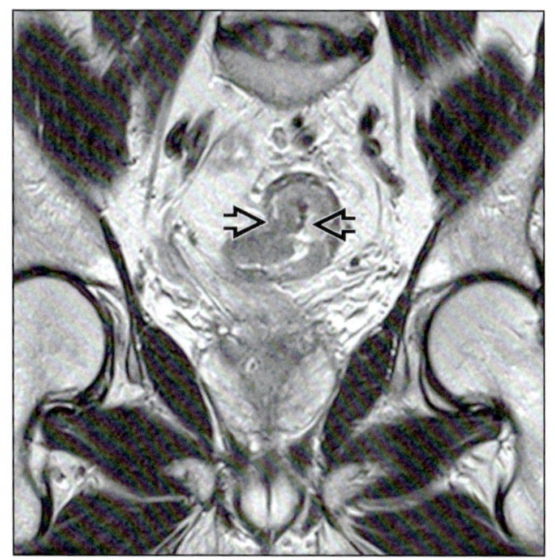

T3 N0 Proximal Rectal Tumor

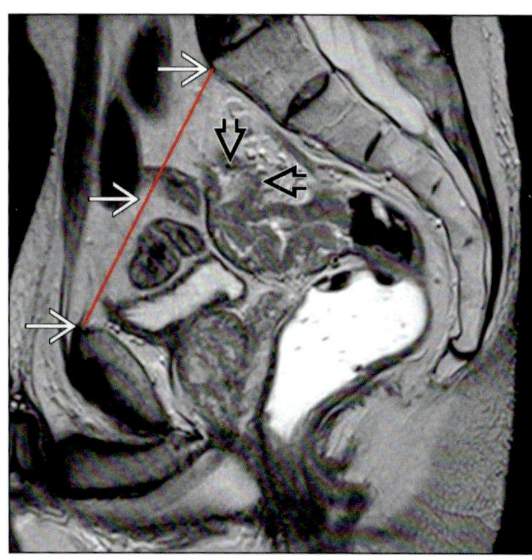

*(**Left**) Coronal T2WI MR in the same patient shows a T2 hypointense tumor ➡ near the rectosigmoid junction. Colonoscopy locates the tumor at 12 cm from the anal verge. Rigid proctoscopy notes mass extends from 9 to 14 cm above dentate line. (**Right**) Sagittal T2WI FS MR shows location of the same mass ➡. The rectosigmoid junction should be below the pelvic inlet ➡, approximated by a line drawn from the sacral promontory to the superior pubic symphysis.*

T3 N0 Proximal Rectal Tumor

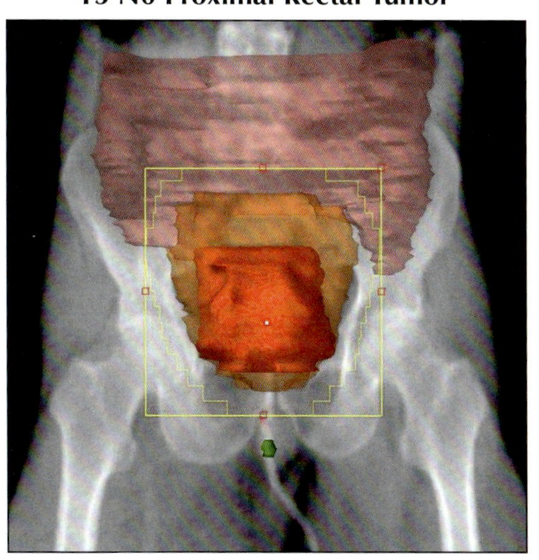

T3 N0 Proximal Rectal Tumor

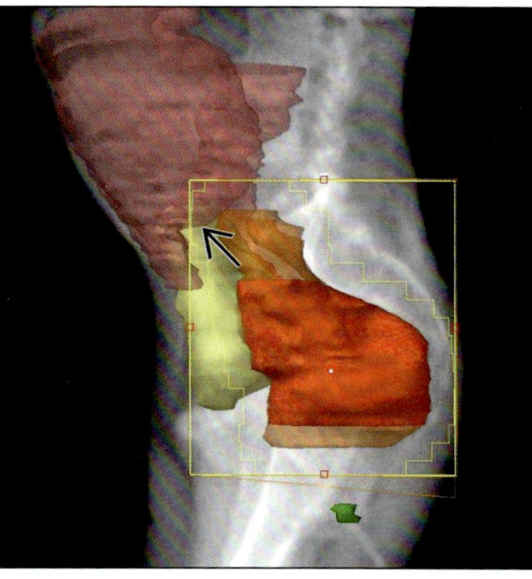

*(**Left**) PA DRR shows pelvic preop RT field in the same patient. The initial CTV (orange) was treated with 4 fields to 45 Gy. Boost CTV (red) covers the GTV plus 2 cm including the mesorectum, prescribed to an additional 5.4 Gy. Distally, the anal verge (marker in green) and perineum are outside the field. (**Right**) Lateral DRR shows same initial and boost CTVs. Small bowel ➡ (pink) is excluded from field due to effective setup. Patient subsequently underwent LAR.*

T3 N0 Distal Rectal Tumor

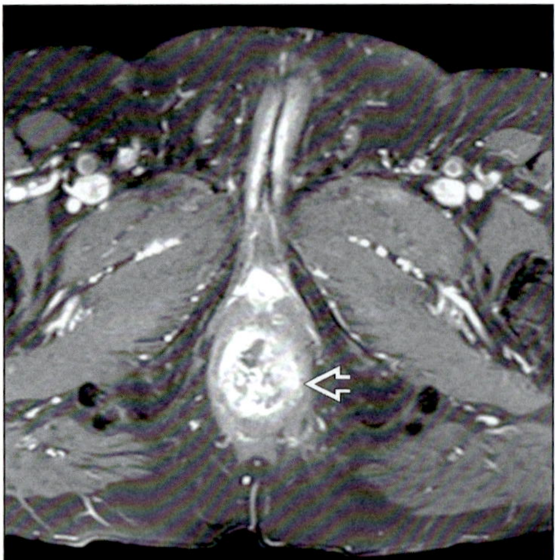

T3 N0 Distal Rectal Tumor

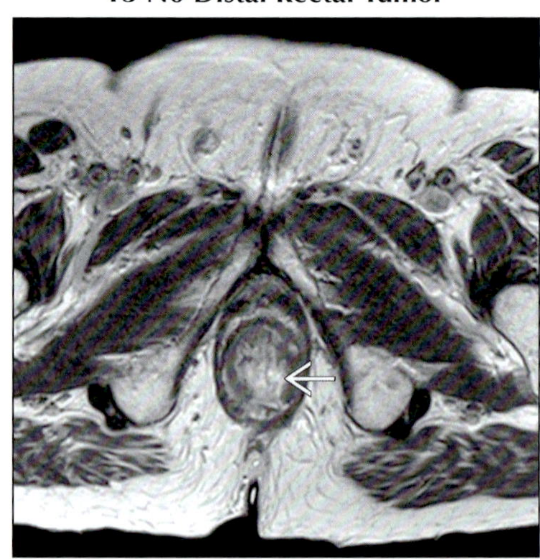

(Left) *Axial T1WI C+ FS MR shows an enhancing tumor ➔ in the distal rectum approaching the anal canal in a 70-year-old man with rectal pain. DRE reveals a 2 cm fixed mass at the left posterolateral sphincter. Biopsy shows mucinous adenocarcinoma.* ***(Right)*** *Axial T2WI MR in the same patient shows focal T2 hyperintensity ➔ in the left posterolateral distal rectum, with extension into perirectal tissue, with no enlarged perirectal, inguinal, or iliac nodes.*

T3 N0 Distal Rectal Tumor

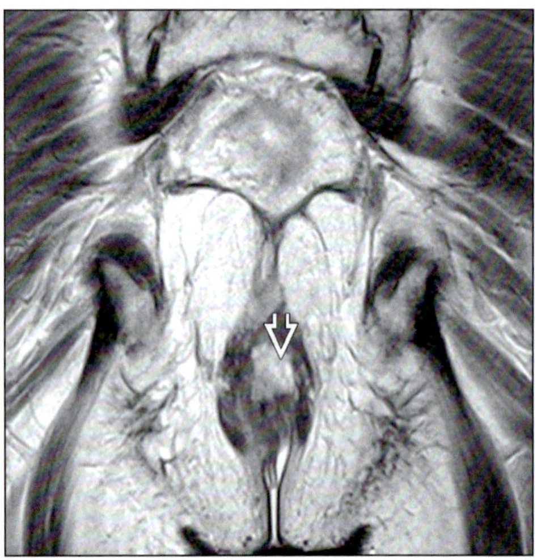

T3 N0 Distal Rectal Tumor

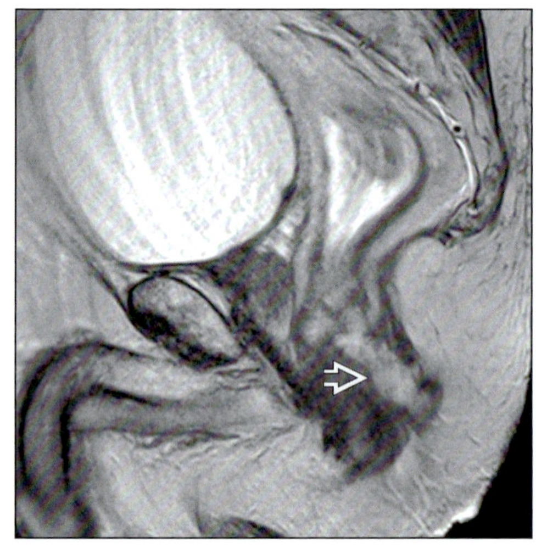

(Left) *Coronal T2WI MR of the same patient shows a T2 hyperintense tumor ➔ located in the posterior and midline distal rectum. The tumor measures 2.0 x 0.8 x 2.5 cm.* ***(Right)*** *Sagittal T2WI FSE MR shows same rectal mass ➔ that appears to involve the anal canal. The puborectalis sling appears intact. There is no invasion outside the mesorectal fat or into the prostate or seminal vesicles. This is consistent with exam and EUS findings.*

T3 N0 Distal Rectal Tumor

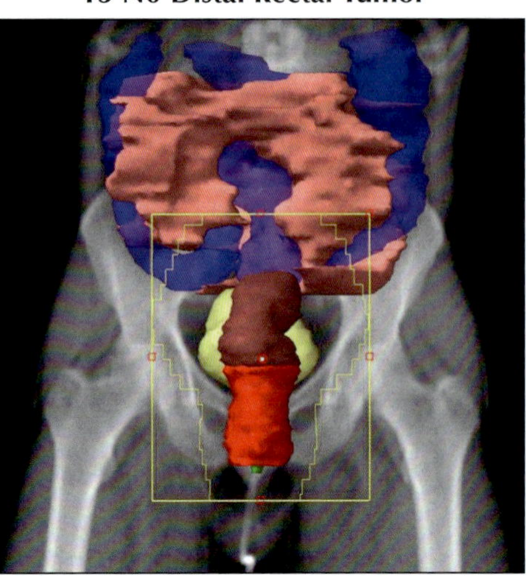

T3 N0 Distal Rectal Tumor

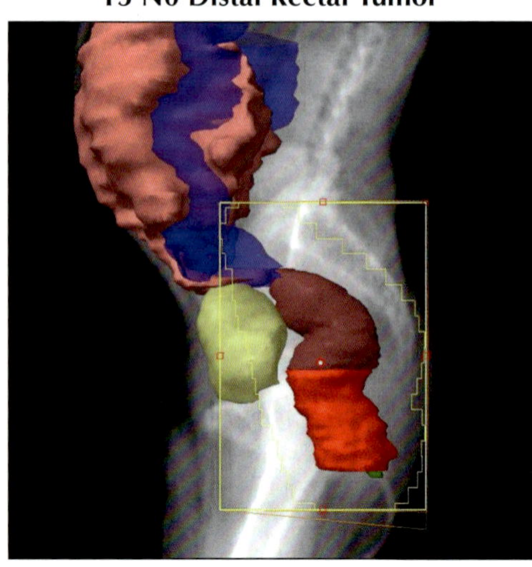

(Left) *PA DRR shows pelvic field for the same patient. CTV is expanded 2 cm beyond GTV (red) to include the anal verge (green). Elective groin RT is not indicated since inguinal failure rates are low (< 5%) and treating this region would cause significant morbidity.* ***(Right)*** *Lateral DRR shows distal extent of CTV coverage. The uninvolved colon (blue), small bowel (pink), and anterior bladder are blocked. This patient then underwent an APR.*

Pelvic EBRT, 4 Field

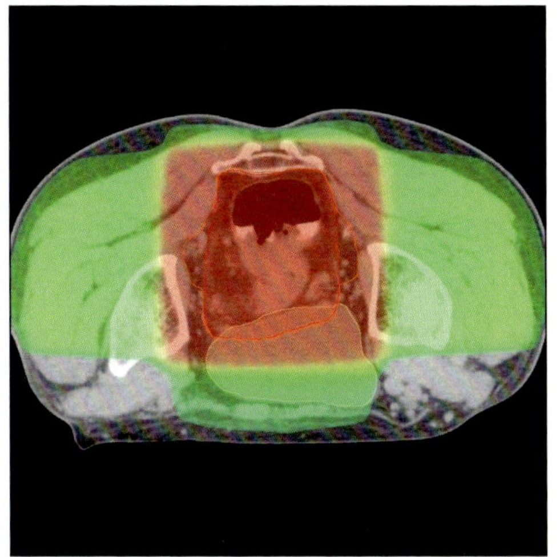

Pelvic EBRT, 3 Field

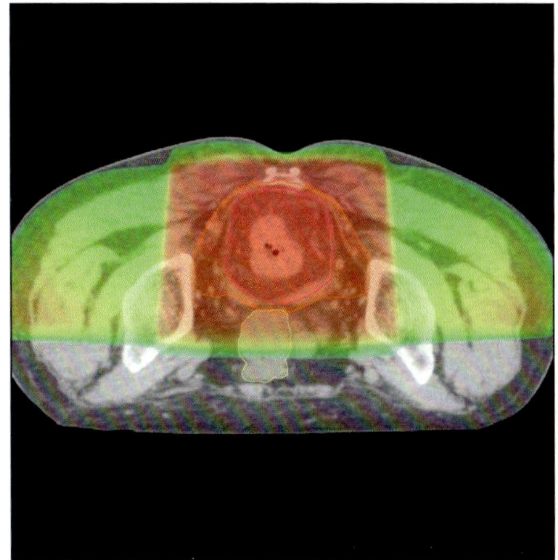

*(**Left**) Axial CT shows 3D treatment planning for preop RT using 4-field technique. Dose colorwash shows the 45 Gy volume as a square area covering initial (orange) and boost (red) CTVs. Anterior field improves anterior CTV coverage in this patient. (**Right**) Axial CT shows treatment plan in a thinner patient using a 3-field technique. The 45 Gy red colorwash encompasses initial and boost CTVs. Anterior structures are spared from low dose exposure in this case.*

Mesorectum

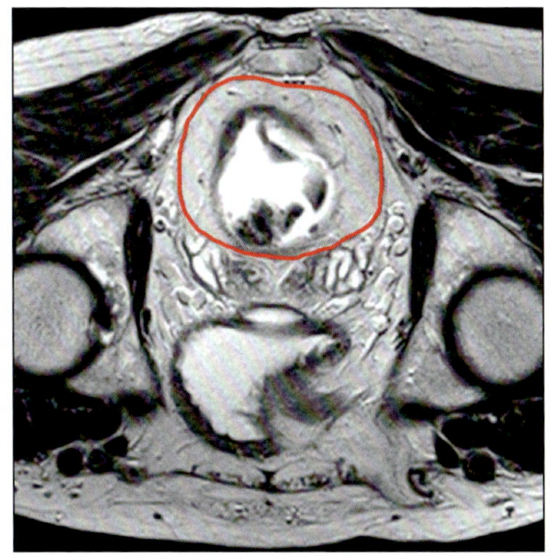

Mesorectum

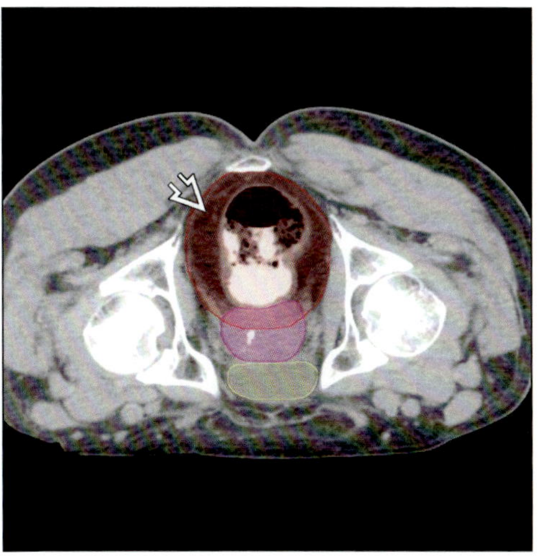

*(**Left**) Axial T2WI MR shows a well-defined mesorectum in red. Distal tumors likely have both upward and lateral mesorectal drainage. Proximal tumors likely only have upward drainage. (**Right**) Axial simulation CT shows CTV (orange) coverage of a well-defined mesorectum ⇨. This includes a 1 cm expansion into the immediately anterior GU structure (e.g., prostate = magenta) to account for variations in bladder and rectal filling, which could affect mesorectum shape.*

Pelvic EBRT

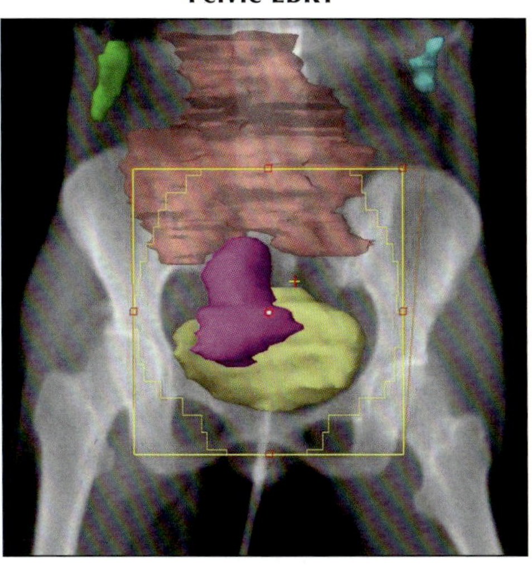

Pelvic EBRT

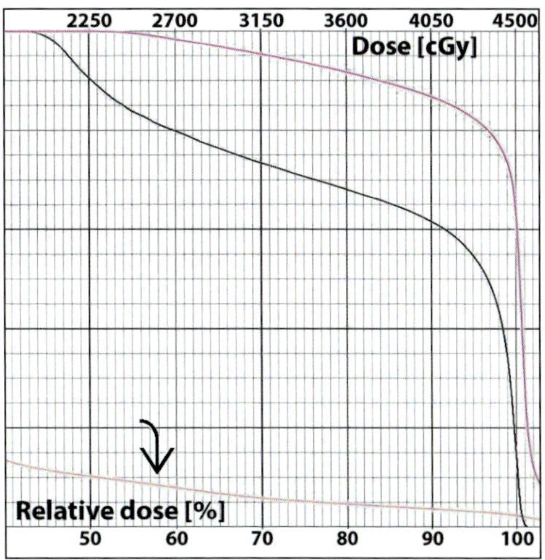

*(**Left**) PA DRR shows RT field and location of ovaries (green and cyan), bladder (yellow), small bowel (pink), and uterus (purple). This 36-year-old woman's ovaries were surgically repositioned in an attempt to preserve ovarian function and fertility. (**Right**) DVH shows small bowel ⤳, uterus (purple), and bladder (black). Transposed ovaries receive < 2 Gy each (not shown). The uterus receives near full dose and thus may not be able to carry a pregnancy to term.*

(Left) Surgical pathology photograph shows a resected rectal adenocarcinoma with an ulcerated center ➔ and residual adenoma ➔ present at the raised border. *(Right)* H&E stained section shows a pathologic complete response (ypCR) after preop CRT. There is a thickened fibrous wall, inflammation with giant cell reaction ➔, crypt distortion ➔, and no viable cancer cells. ypCR occurs in 8-20% of cases after CRT. (Courtesy K. E. Affolter, MD.)

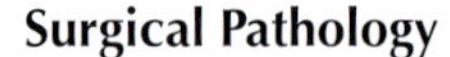

Surgical Pathology

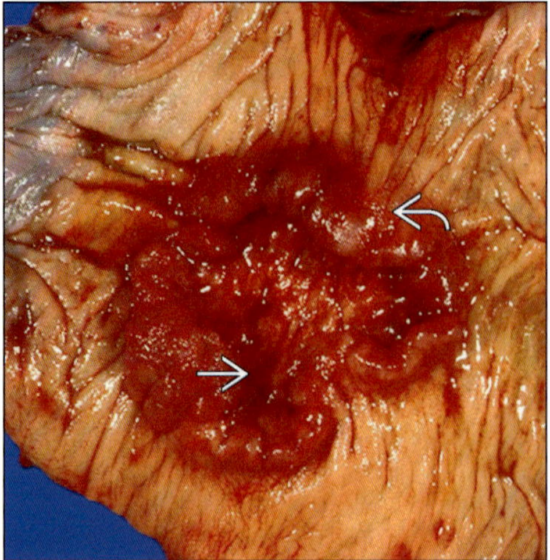

Surgical Pathology

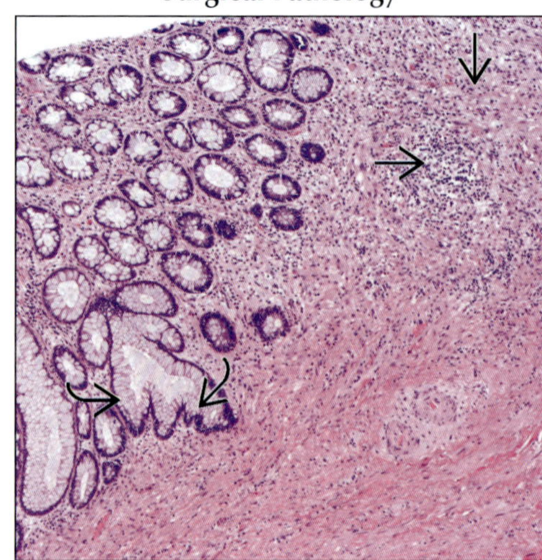

(Left) Screening colonoscopy shows a 3 cm mass at the mid rectum extending to the rectosigmoid junction in a 67-year-old woman. Biopsy reveals adenocarcinoma. *(Right)* Sagittal CECT in the same patient shows a 3 cm apple core lesion ➔ in the mid rectum about 10 cm from the anal verge. Low anterior resection (LAR) removed a 2.5 x 3.0 x 1.0 cm adenocarcinoma with invasion through the muscularis propria. Two out of 14 lymph nodes contained carcinoma.

Stage IIIB (pT3 N1b M0)

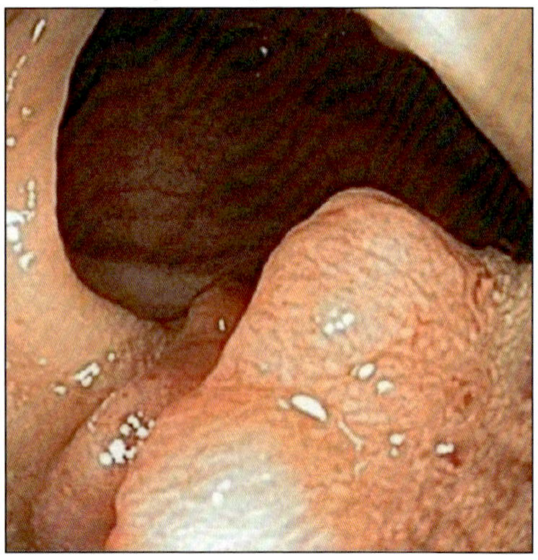

Stage IIIB (pT3 N1b M0)

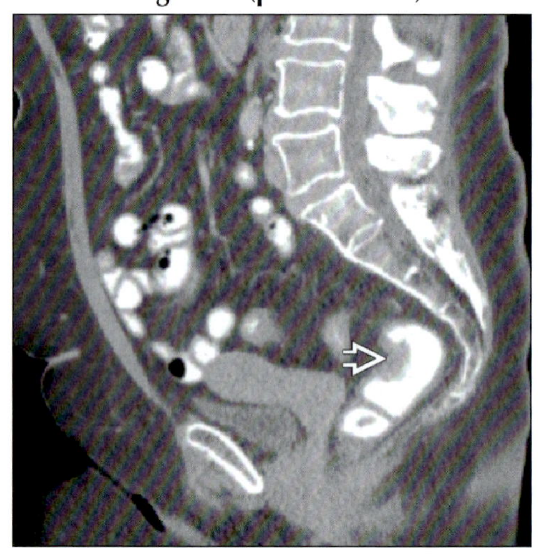

(Left) PA DRR shows postop RT field in this woman who underwent LAR. Initial CTV (orange) received 45 Gy. Boost CTV (red) received additional 5.4 Gy to cover 2 cm margins above and below the anastomosis. Distal rectum and perineum are blocked. *(Right)* Sagittal NECT shows 50.4 Gy dose colorwash covering boost CTV (red) that was expanded from the GTV anastomosis (black), which is the entire rectal circumference at the site delineated by surgical staples ➔.

Post-LAR EBRT

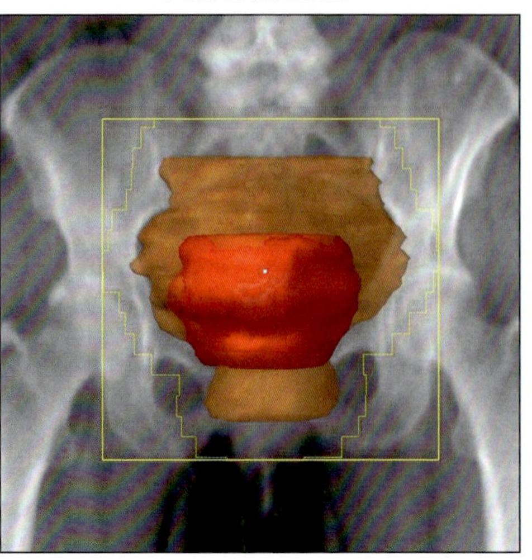

Post-LAR EBRT

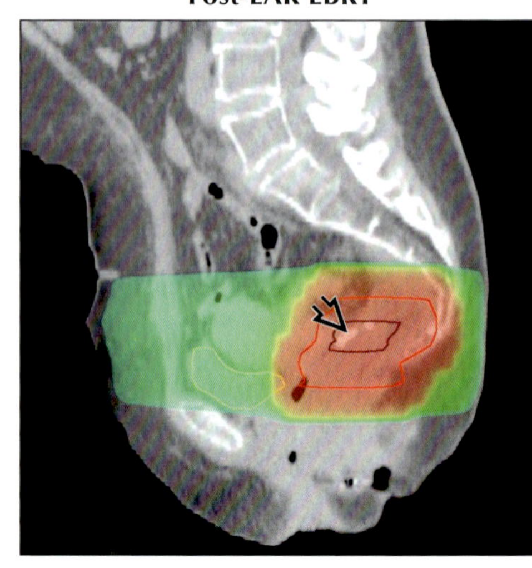

Stage I (uT1 N0 M0)

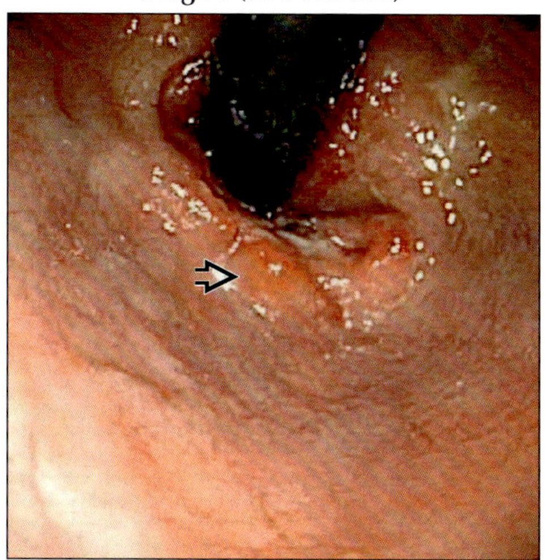

Stage IIIC (pT3 N2b M0)

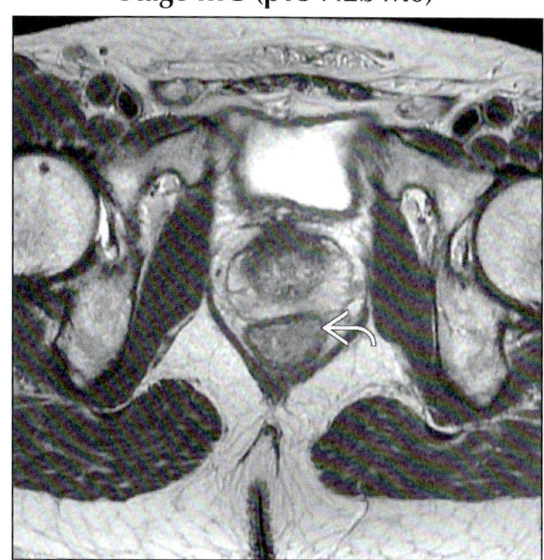

(Left) *Colonoscopy shows a 2.5 cm tumor ⇨. Biopsy confirmed adenocarcinoma. Rigid proctoscope noted mass extending 2-4 cm from the anal verge. EUS shows no invasion of muscularis propria (uT1).* ***(Right)*** *Axial T2WI FSE MR in same patient shows mass ➡ along anorectal junction, with intact muscularis propria agreeing with EUS staging. He underwent an APR, which upstaged him from stage I to IIIC, with tumor extension into perirectal fat and 10/13 positive LNs.*

Post-APR EBRT

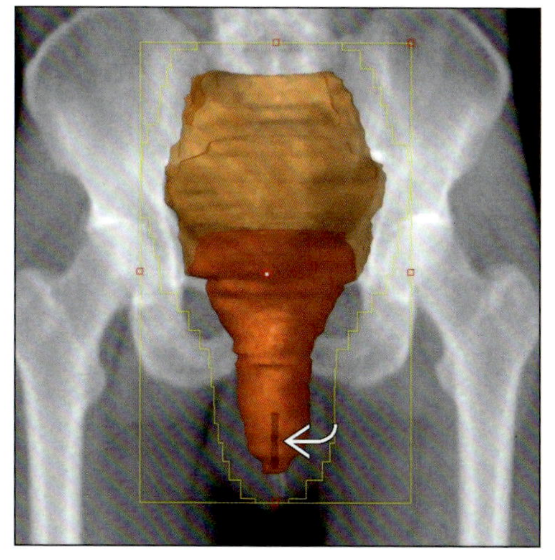

Post-APR EBRT

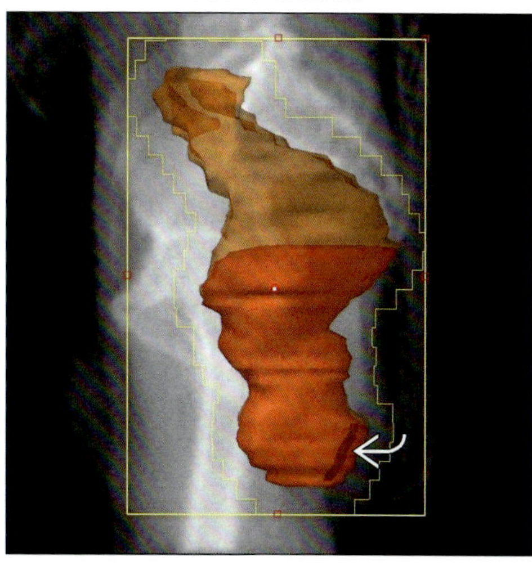

(Left) *PA DRR shows postop RT field in the same patient with tumor located 2 cm from anal verge. This patient was placed supine due to the ostomy. Initial CTV (orange) includes presacral LN, internal iliac LN, and boost CTV (red), which includes the preop GTV and APR scar (delineated by wire ➡).* ***(Right)*** *Lateral DRR shows sagittal projection of initial and boost CTVs. Inferior border is below the APR scar ➡. Perineal scar was bolused every other day.*

Pretreatment

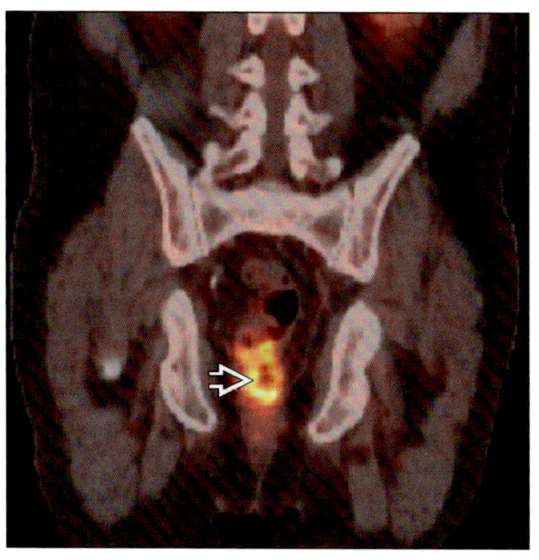

Post Treatment

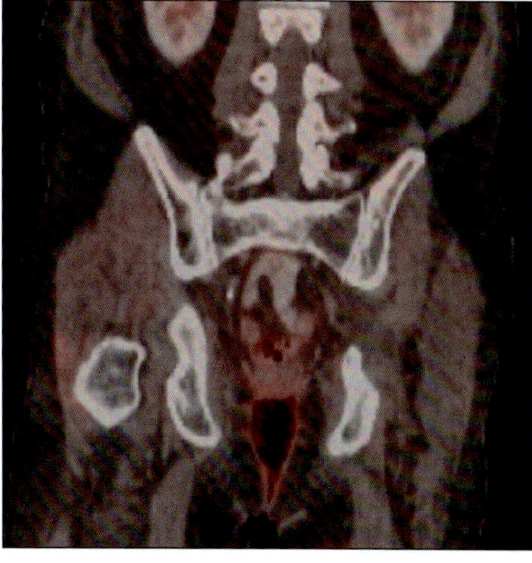

(Left) *Coronal fused PET/CT shows a hypermetabolic mass ➡ located in the lower rectum in a 56-year-old man who presented with rectal pain and hematochezia. EUS reveals a uT3 N1 tumor at the dentate line. This patient received preop CRT to 50.4 Gy followed by an APR.* ***(Right)*** *Follow-up PET/CT shows no evidence of recurrent disease in the pelvis.*

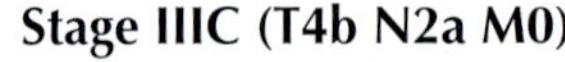

Stage IIIC (T4b N2a M0)

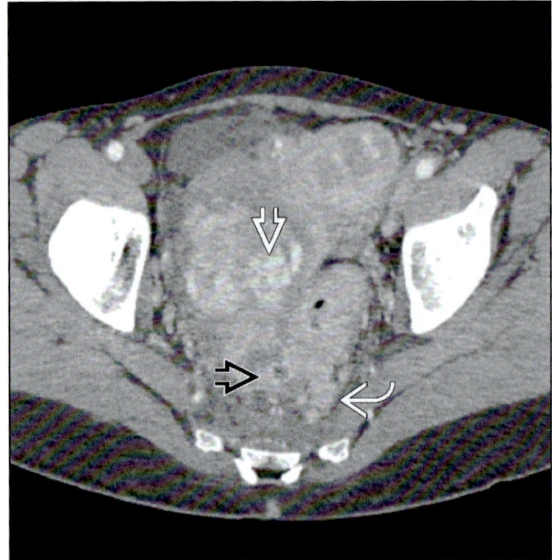

Stage IIIC (T4b N2a M0)

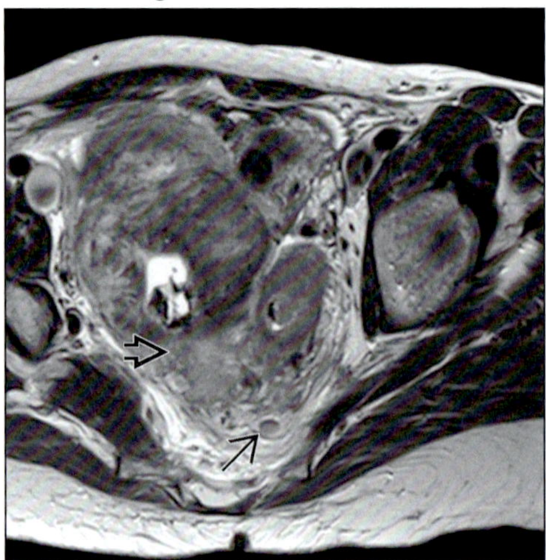

(Left) *Axial CECT shows rectal wall thickening with perirectal fat stranding, presacral thickening, and multiple enlarged nodes in a 58-year-old woman who presented with hematochezia. Leiomyoma is seen anteriorly.* ***(Right)*** *Axial T2WI MR in the same patient shows bulky, polypoid mass extending beyond mesorectal fascia, into the posterior uterine serosa. On exam, the mass is fixed anteriorly. Concerning LNs are noted in mesorectal fat.*

Stage IIIC (T4b N2a M0)

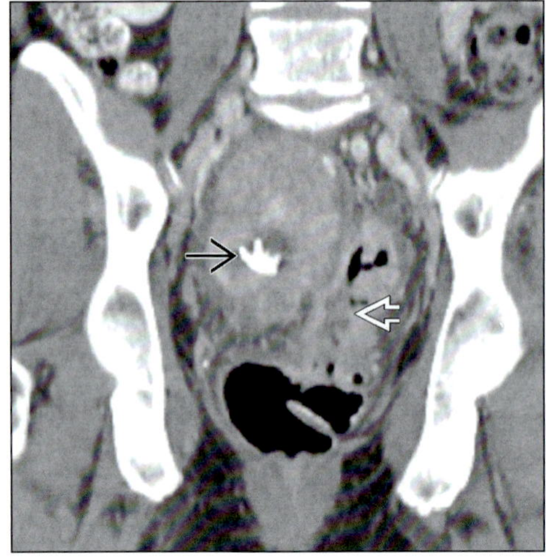

Stage IIIC (T4b N2a M0)

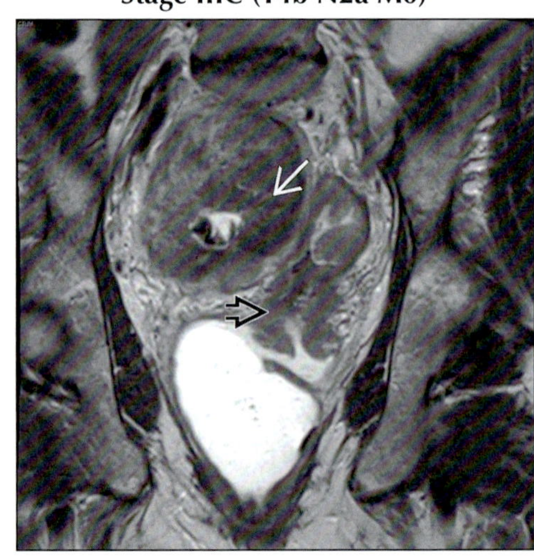

(Left) *Coronal CECT in the same patient shows a long segment of circumferential wall thickening involving the rectum and distal sigmoid colon. On rigid proctoscopy, the mass was 8 cm from the anal verge. The dominant uterine fibroid has central coarse calcifications .* ***(Right)*** *Coronal T2WI MR in the same patient shows a 10 cm long segment of an irregular, nodular mass involving the proximal rectum, next to a large uterine fibroid .*

Stage IIIC (T4b N1b M0)

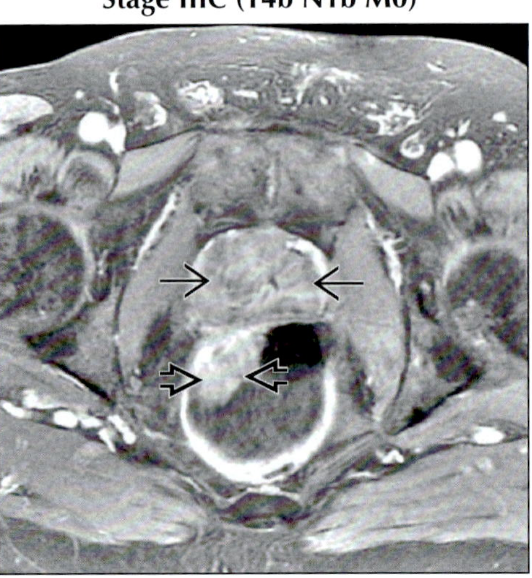

Stage IIIC (T4b N1b M0)

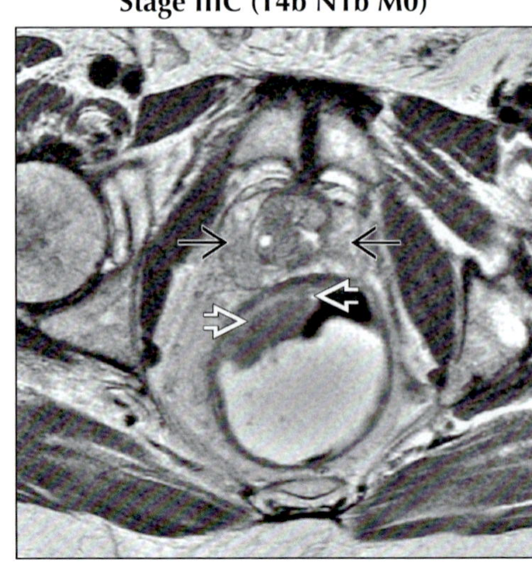

(Left) *Axial T1WI C+ FS MR shows a circular, lobulated, partially obstructing, enhancing tumor at lower rectal wall, abutting the prostate . On endorectal ultrasound, there was loss of the fat plane between rectum and prostate.* ***(Right)*** *Axial T2WI FSE MR in the same patient shows a T2 hypointense rectal mass with obliteration of fat plane between rectum and posterior prostate , suggesting adherence to, but not definite invasion of, the prostate.*

Stage IIIC (T4b N1b M0)

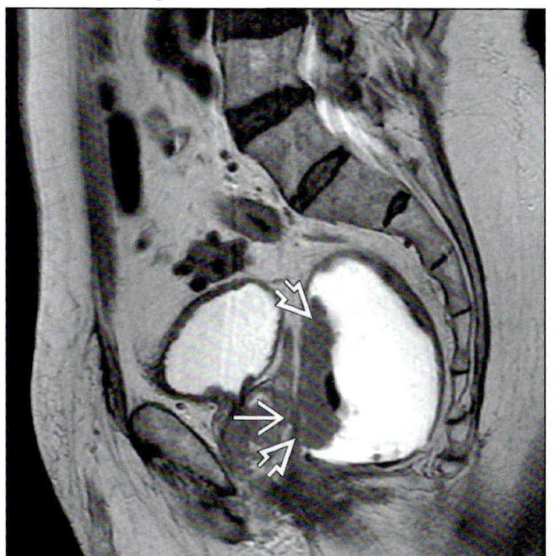

EBRT Planning

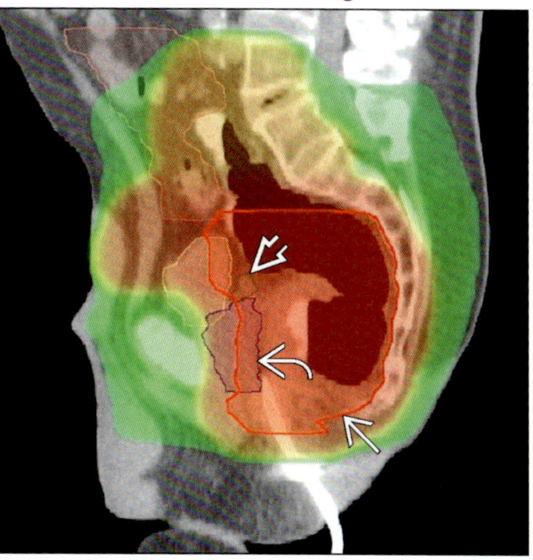

*(**Left**) Sagittal T2WI FSE MR in the same patient shows a 6 cm T2 hypointense mass ➡. There is loss of fat plane between rectum and prostate but no direct invasion ➡. (**Right**) Sagittal NECT shows 50 Gy colorwash (red) covering boost CTV ➡ including posterior prostate ➡ and seminal vesicles ➡. Small bowel and bladder are shown. 45 Gy (orange) coverage includes external iliac LNs. Following preop CRT, the patient underwent APR and prostatectomy.*

Stage IIIC (T4b N2a M0)

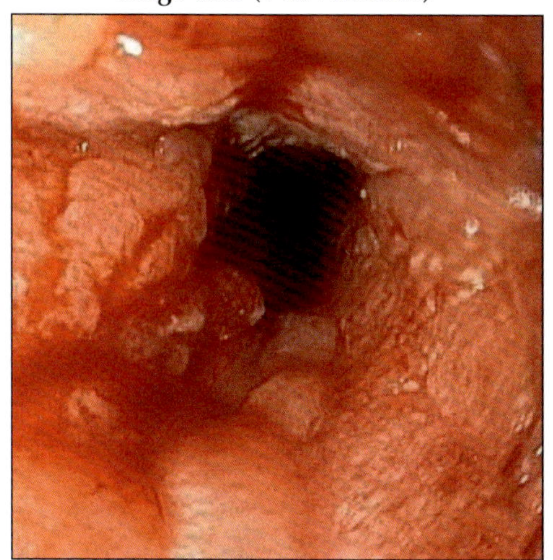

Stage IIIC (T4b N2a M0)

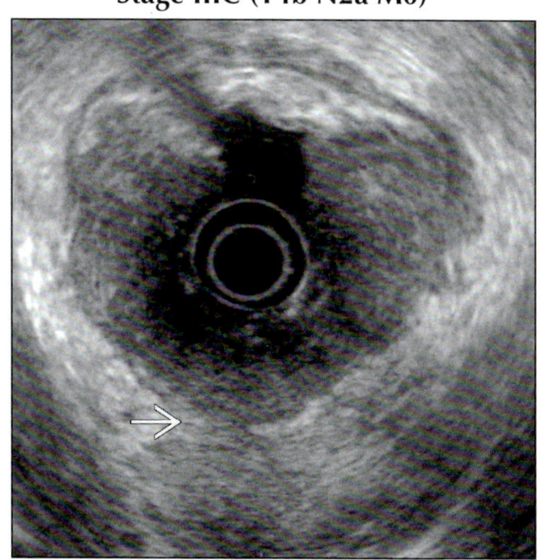

*(**Left**) Flexible sigmoidoscopy in a 26-year-old man who presents with rectal pain and bleeding shows friable, infiltrated mucosa in the rectum, extending proximally from the anorectal junction. Biopsy confirmed adenocarcinoma. (**Right**) Endorectal ultrasound (7.5 and 10 MHz) shows a large rectal mass invading into the prostate, evidenced by the loss of the fat plane between the structures ➡.*

Stage IIIC (T4b N2a M0)

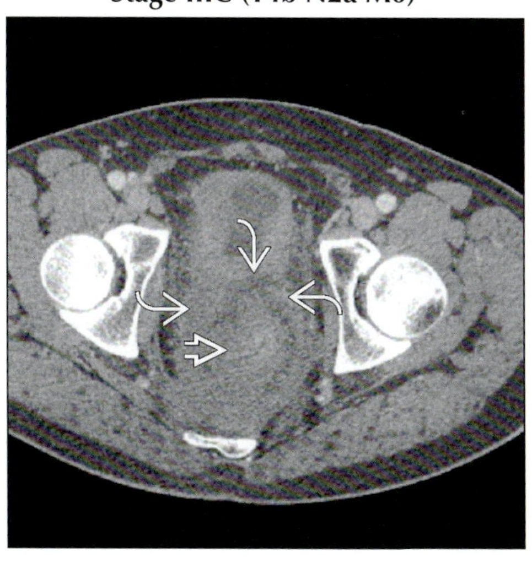

Stage IIIC (T4b N2a M0)

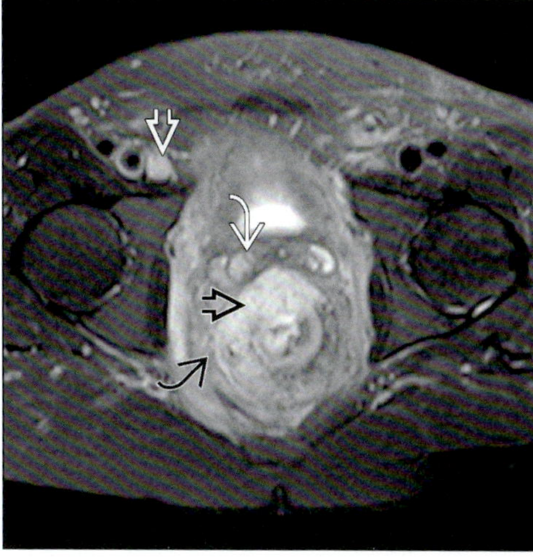

*(**Left**) Axial CECT in same patient shows circumferential thickening of distal rectum ➡ and anal canal. Note the perirectal stranding ➡ with fat plane loss between posterior bladder, prostate, and right seminal vesicle with the mass. (**Right**) Axial T2WI FSE MR in same patient shows T2 hyperintense tumor ➡ at the right anterolateral anorectum with invasion of perirectal musculature ➡ and seminal vesicles ➡. There is an enlarged node of Cloquet ➡.*

*(**Left**) Axial CT in the prone position shows 54 Gy boost dose colorwash (red) covering boost CTV (orange), which includes primary tumor (red) and the large 5 cm right pelvic lymph node (magenta). The tumor was deemed unresectable. A 4-field technique was used. (**Right**) Axial CT in the same patient shows 54 Gy colorwash covering the CTV (green) expanded from primary rectal GTV (red) and the enlarged right node of Cloquet ➪ that measured > 1 cm in short axis.*

Stage IIIC (T4b N2a M0)

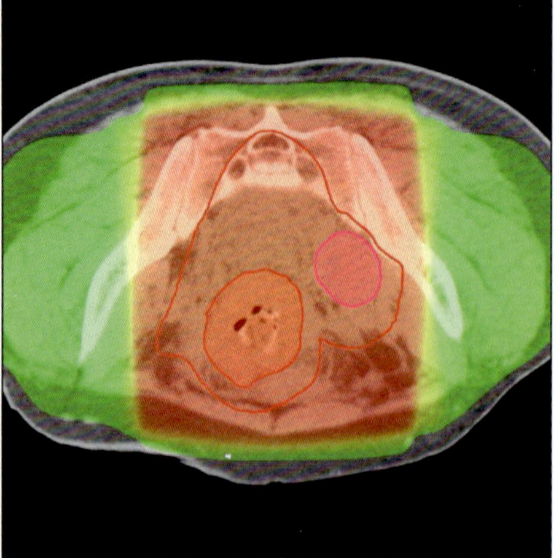

Stage IIIC (T4b N2a M0)

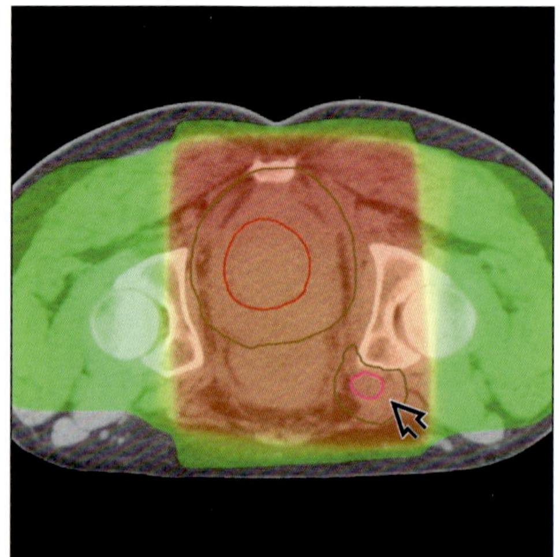

*(**Left**) Sagittal T2WI FS MR in the same patient shows T2 hyperintense tumor ➪ invading into the prostate ➡ and seminal vesicles ➡ anteriorly and the sacrum posteriorly ↗. Circumferential wall thickening from the tumor extended approximately 13 cm. (**Right**) Sagittal CT shows 95% dose colorwash (red) covering the CTV (orange) including the sacrum, prostate (magenta), posterior 1 cm of bladder (yellow), presacral, internal, and external iliac LNs.*

Stage IIIC (T4b N2a M0)

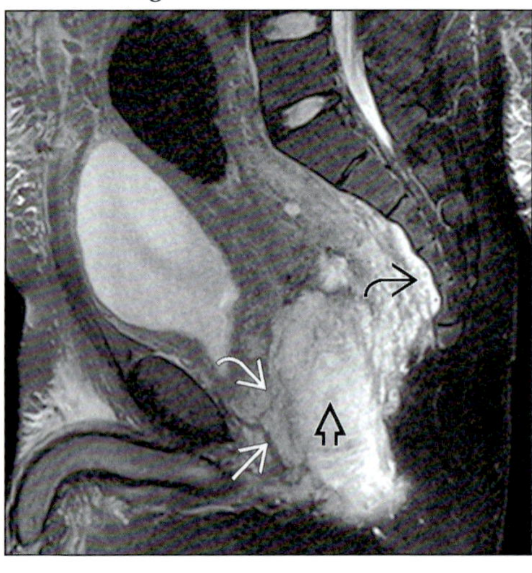

Stage IIIC (T4b N2a M0)

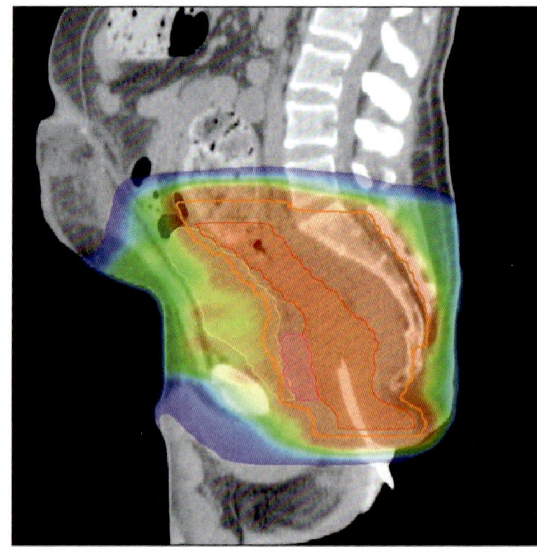

*(**Left**) Axial PET/CT 6 weeks after CRT shows residual hypermetabolic activity (SUV 8.7) associated with rectal thickening ➡. The right node of Cloquet ➡ has minimal activity and decreased size. (**Right**) Sagittal PET/CT shows residual hypermetabolic activity in rectal mass ➡ at the level of quadrilateral plates, inferior to the ischial tuberosities. Small, left-sided external iliac chain lymph nodes are mildly hypermetabolic.*

Stage IIIC (T4b N2a M0)

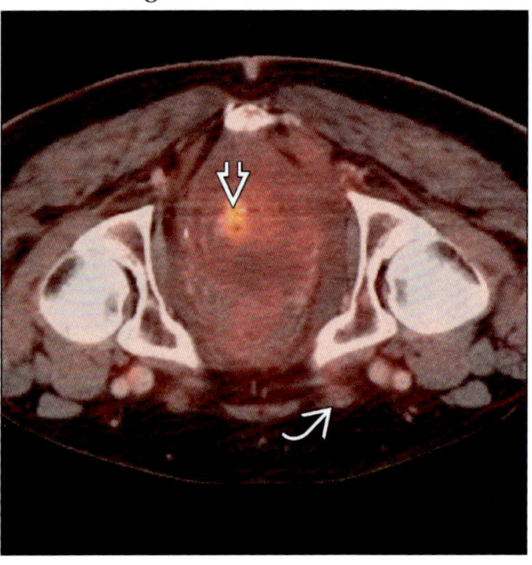

Stage IIIC (T4b N2a M0)

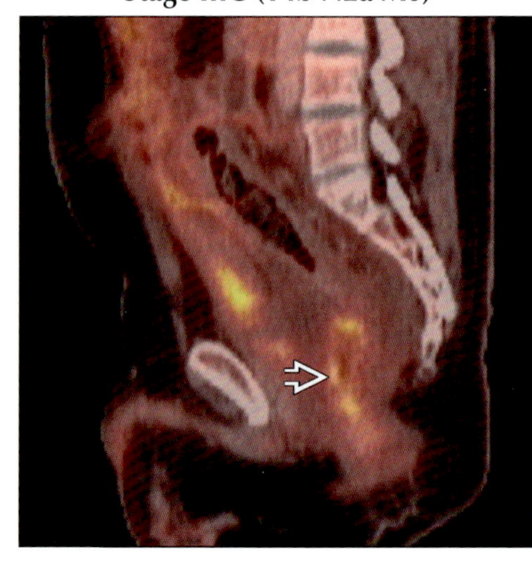

Iliac Nodes: T3 Rectum

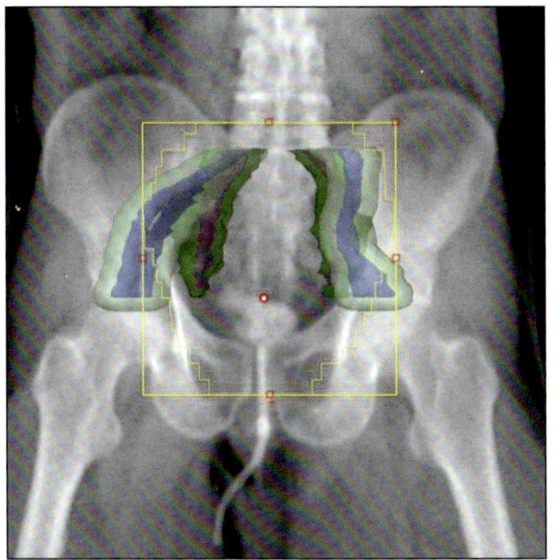

Iliac Nodes: T3 Rectum

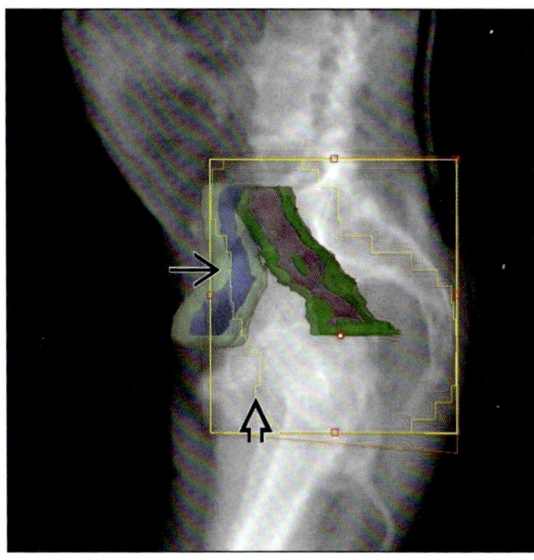

(Left) *PA DRR showing the pelvic field for treatment of T3 rectal cancer includes coverage of internal iliac vessels (magenta) within the expanded CTV (dark green) and not the external iliac CTV (light green).* **(Right)** *Lateral DRR shows T3 rectal pelvic field indicating coverage of internal iliac vessels (magenta) with CTV margin without intentional coverage of the external iliac CTV ➔ (light green). Classically, the anterior border is the base of pubis ⇨.*

Iliac Nodes: T4b Rectum

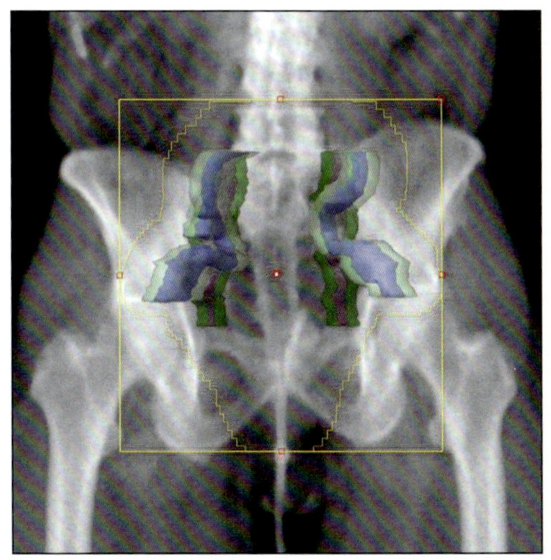

Iliac Nodes: T4b Rectum

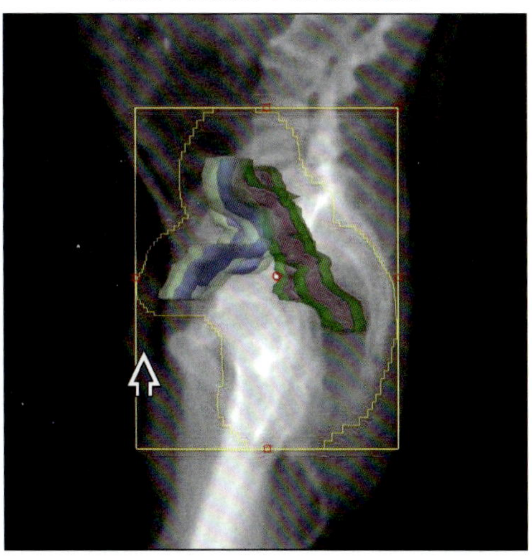

(Left) *PA DRR showing the pelvic field for a T4b rectal cancer involving an anterior structure shows coverage of both the external (light green) and internal (dark green) iliac LN CTVs.* **(Right)** *Lateral DRR showing the pelvic field for a T4b rectal cancer shows CTV coverage of both the external iliac LNs (light green) and internal iliac LNs (dark green). Classically, the anterior border is 1 cm anterior to the pubis ⇨.*

T4b Rectum: 3D CRT

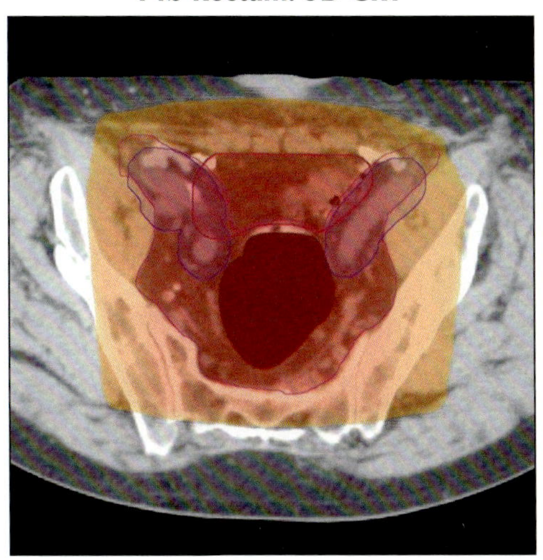

T4b Rectum: IMRT

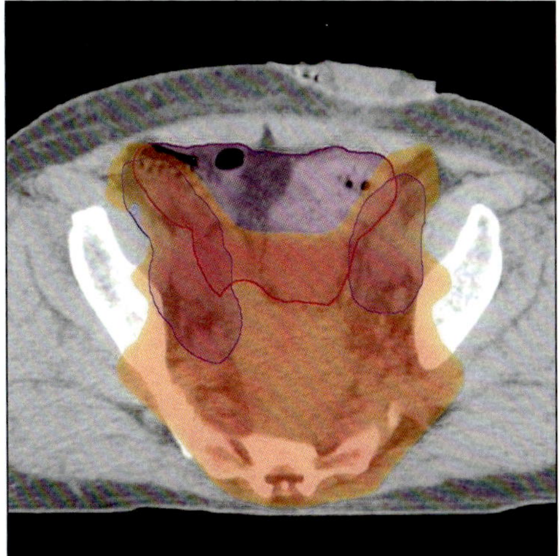

(Left) *Axial NECT shows 3D CRT plan with 95% dose colorwash (red) square box coverage of external iliac node CTV (blue) and inclusion of bowel (magenta) in a patient with rectal cancer invading the prostate. Patient is prone.* **(Right)** *Axial NECT in a different patient with T4b rectal cancer shows IMRT plan with 95% dose wash (red) covering external iliac node CTV (blue) with sparing of the small bowel (magenta) from the high-dose region. Patient is supine.*

Stage IIIC (T4b N2a M0) Colon

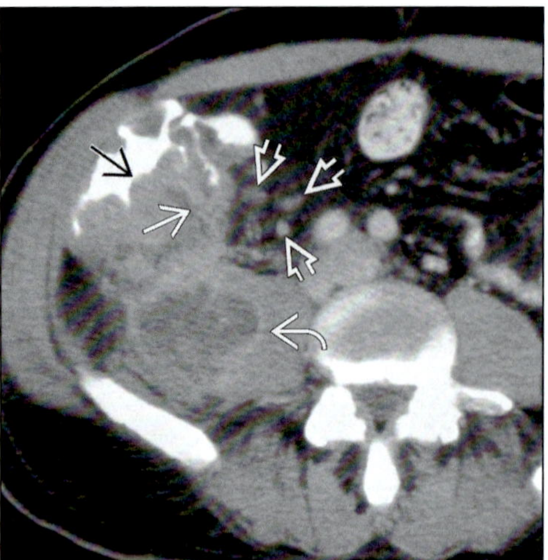

Stage IIIC (T4b N2a M0) Colon

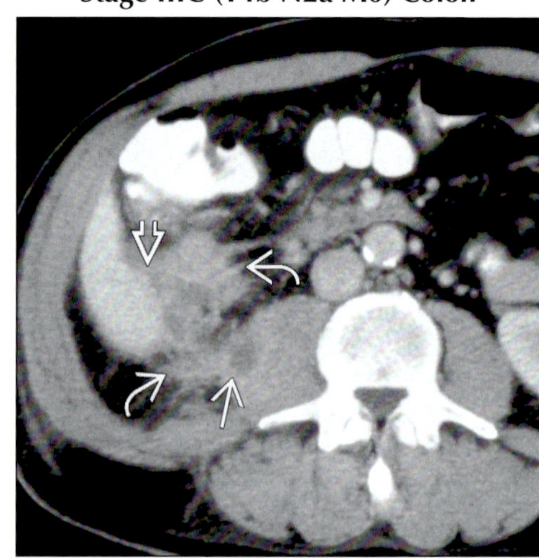

(Left) *Axial CECT shows polypoid thickening of cecum wall ⇨ with tumor invading through the retroperitoneum into the psoas muscle ➨. Tumor also invades the terminal ileum ➨. Note multiple concerning lymph nodes ➨.* ***(Right)*** *Axial CECT in the same patient shows tumor extending superiorly to invade through the retroperitoneum ➨ into the psoas muscle ➨. The tumor also invades the lowermost aspect of the right lobe of the liver ➨.*

Stage IIIC (T4b N1b M0) Colon

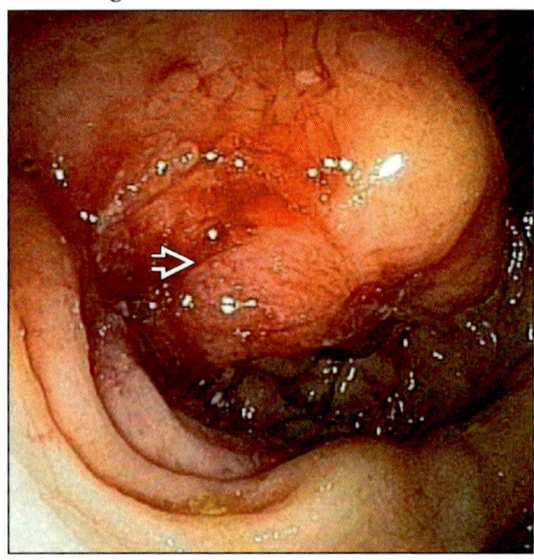

Stage IIIC (T4b N1b M0) Colon

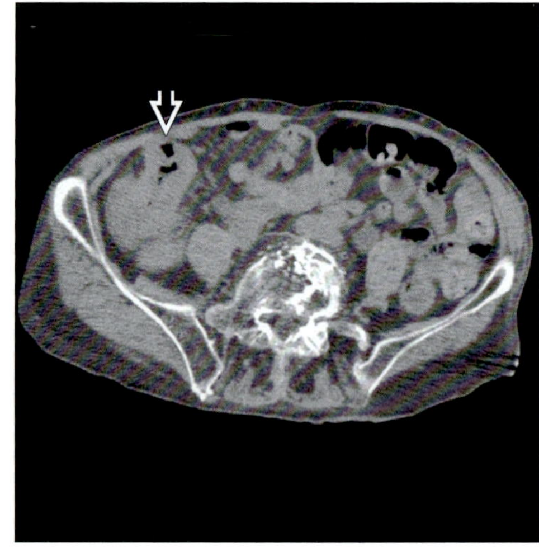

(Left) *Colonoscopy shows an ulcerated, friable, partially obstructing mass ➨ in the cecum of an 87-year-old man who presented with iron-deficiency anemia. Biopsy confirmed adenocarcinoma.* ***(Right)*** *Axial NECT in the same patient shows a large cecal mass ➨ with dense adherence to the right abdominal wall. Right colectomy removed a 6 cm adenocarcinoma invading the abdominal wall musculature and retroperitoneum, with positive radial margins.*

Stage IIIC (T4b N1b M0) Colon

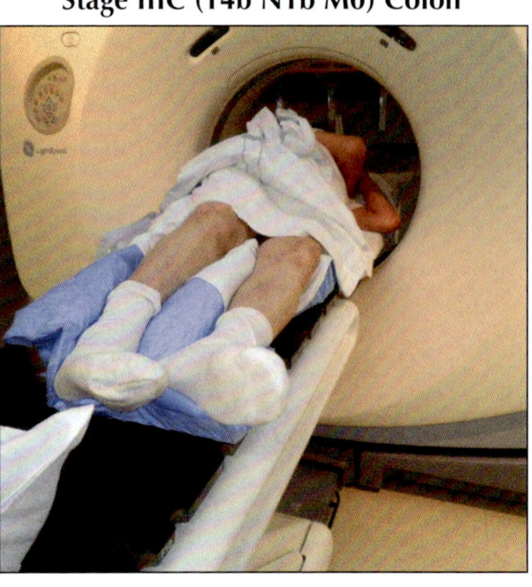

Stage IIIC (T4b N1b M0) Colon

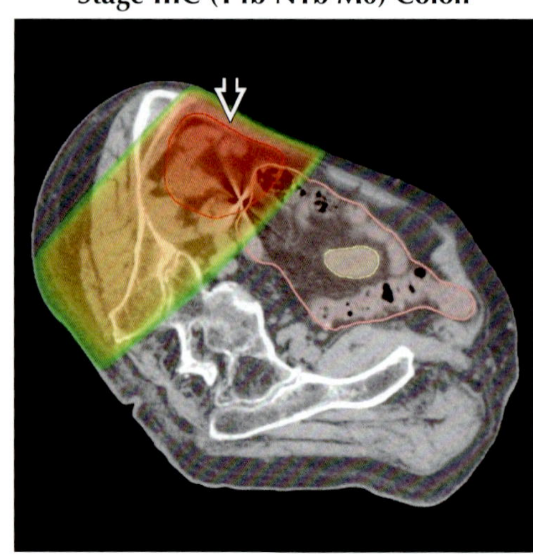

(Left) *Simulation photograph shows the same patient lying in left lateral decubitus position, with his pelvis and abdomen set in an alpha cradle.* ***(Right)*** *Axial CT shows treatment plan in the same patient in a partial left lateral decubitus position, effectively displacing bowel (pink) and bladder (yellow) away from the CTV (red) covering the operative bed and right abdominal wall ➨. Postop RT 45 Gy was delivered with unequally weighted parallel opposed fields.*

Stage IIC (T4b N0 M0) Colon

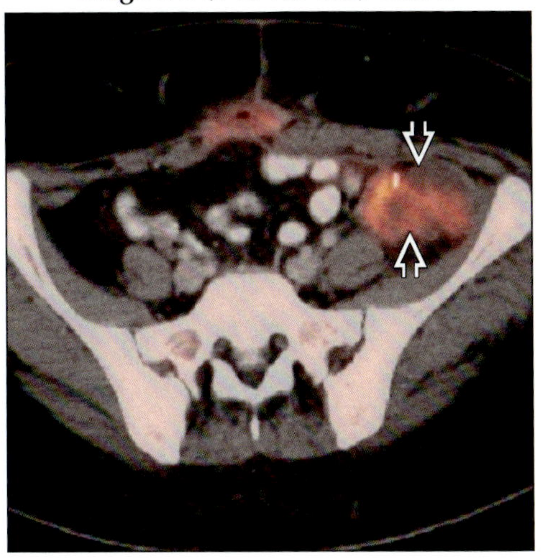

Stage IIC (T4b N0 M0) Colon

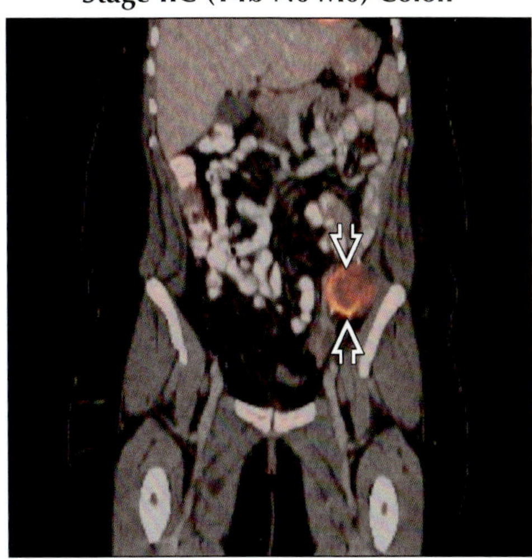

*(**Left**) Axial PET/CT shows hypermetabolic (SUV 20) gross residual disease ➡ in left lower quadrant, adherent to abdominal musculature in a 34-year-old woman with stage IIC descending colon cancer S/P left colectomy and colostomy. Intraoperatively, there was bowel perforation. (**Right**) Coronal PET/CT shows the hypermetabolic residual mass ➡ that perforated the bowel wall and adhered to the anterior abdominal wall. None of 20 resected LNs contained disease.*

EBRT Planning

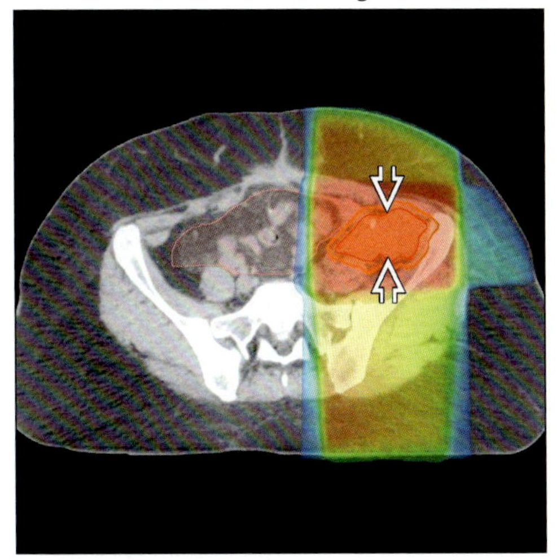

EBRT Planning

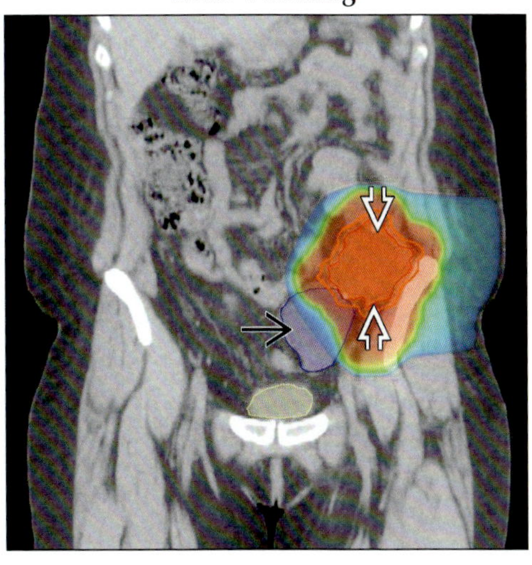

*(**Left**) The residual mass ➡ was initially deemed unresectable due to abdominal wall invasion. The patient received FOLFOX x 6 followed by CRT to 50.4 Gy with 5-FU. Axial NECT shows 50 Gy dose colorwash (red) covering GTV (red) and CTV (orange). A 3-field technique was used. (**Right**) Coronal NECT shows 50 Gy dose (red) covering gross tumor ➡ and CTV (orange) with relative sparing of the bowel, even from low dose. A cystic hydrosalpinx ➔ was noted.*

Post Treatment

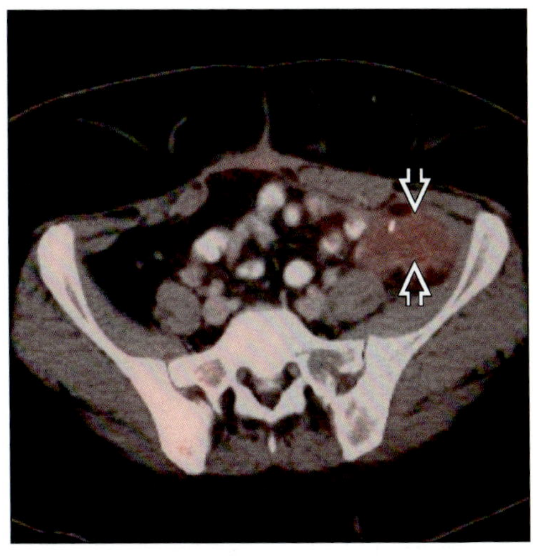

Post Treatment

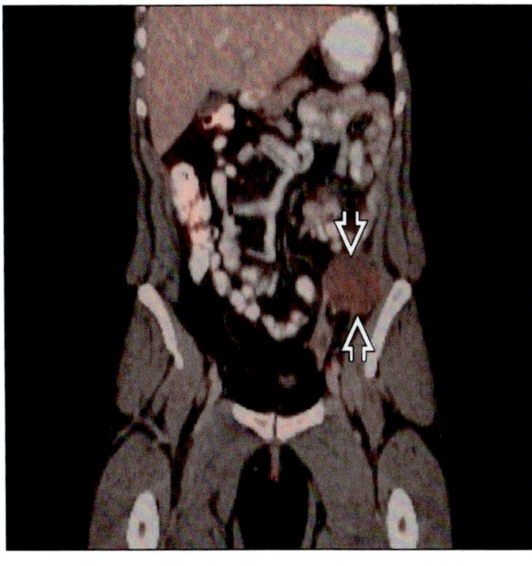

*(**Left**) Axial PET/CT 1 month after CRT shows persistent residual mass ➡ invading left pelvic side wall with markedly decreased metabolic activity (SUV 4.2). There was no evidence of distant metastases. (**Right**) Coronal PET/CT shows residual mass ➡. The patient underwent radical en bloc resection, partial colectomy, TAH-BSO, resection of left superior iliac crest and psoas, and sacrifice of left femoral nerve. Follow-up scan at 6 months shows she is NED.*

*(**Left**) Flexible sigmoidoscopy shows an ulcerated, fixed mass ➡ at site of previous colorectal anastomosis ➡ in a patient who underwent preop CRT followed by LAR for a mid-rectal cancer 4 years ago. Biopsies confirmed recurrent adenocarcinoma. (**Right**) Axial CECT in the same patient shows an enhancing 2.8 cm ill-defined tumor ➡ at the left posterior rectum at the anastomotic site, with invasion of the left seminal vesicle and ischiorectal ligament.*

Recurrent Rectal Adenocarcinoma

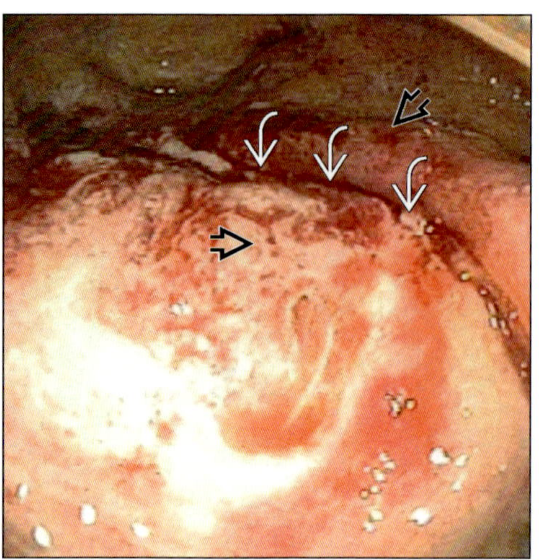

Recurrent Rectal Adenocarcinoma

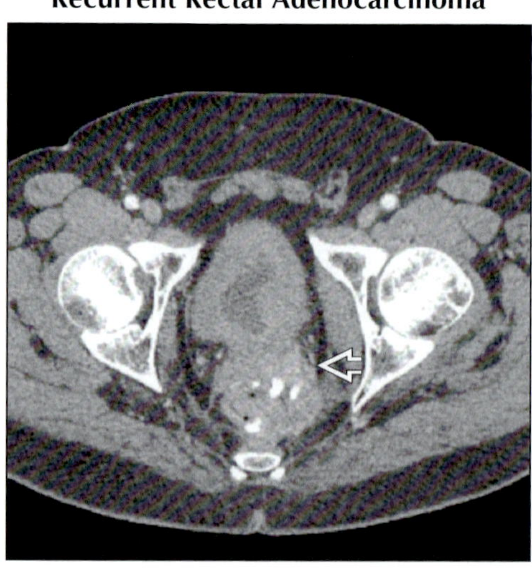

*(**Left**) Coronal T1WI C+ FS MR in the same patient shows enhancement of recurrent tumor ➡ extending into ➡ perirectal fat. (**Right**) Because the recurrent mass was fixed and invaded seminal vesicles, it was deemed unresectable. The patient underwent salvage CRT using 3-field technique. Axial NECT shows GTV (red) at level of anastomosis. CTV (orange) is 2 cm margin on GTV plus prostate and seminal vesicles (magenta). 95% (red) and 50% (green) dose wash are shown.*

Recurrent Rectal Adenocarcinoma

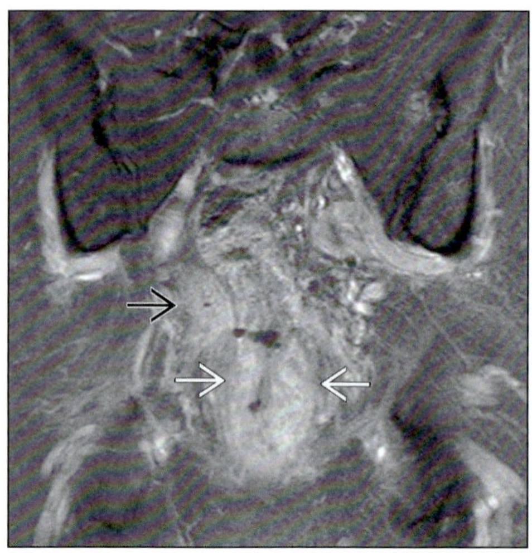

Recurrent Rectal Adenocarcinoma

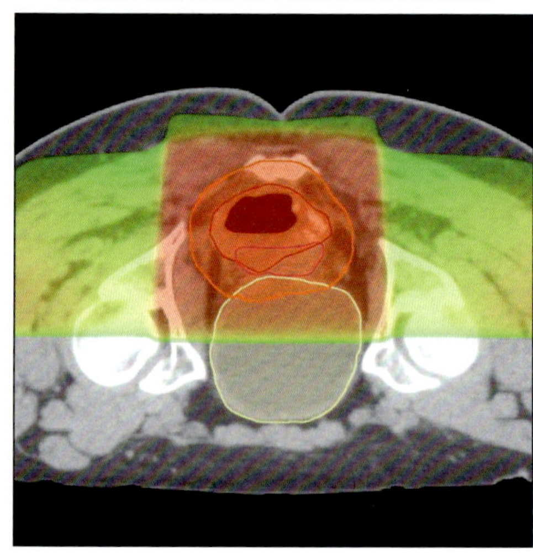

*(**Left**) Sagittal NECT shows 95% (red) and 50% (green) dose cloud covering GTV (red) and CTV (orange) with inclusion of prostate/seminal vesicles. The recurrent tumor was treated to 40.8 Gy at 1.2 Gy b.i.d. with chemo. (**Right**) Axial CECT shows treatment effect with significant reduction in size of mass ➡ 3 months after reirradiation. There is residual thickening of rectal wall and presacral soft tissue. Clinically, the patient had palliation of pain and bleeding.*

Recurrent Rectal Adenocarcinoma

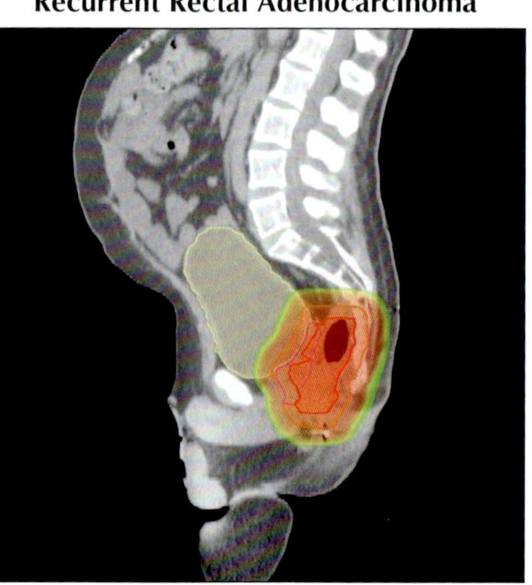

Recurrent Rectal Adenocarcinoma

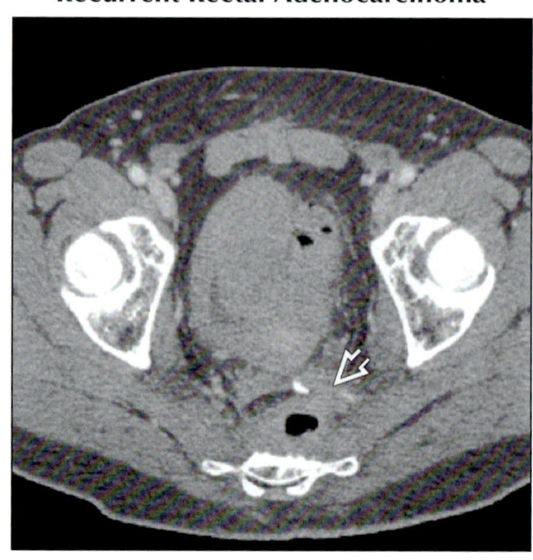

Stage IIA Rectal Cancer in Crohn

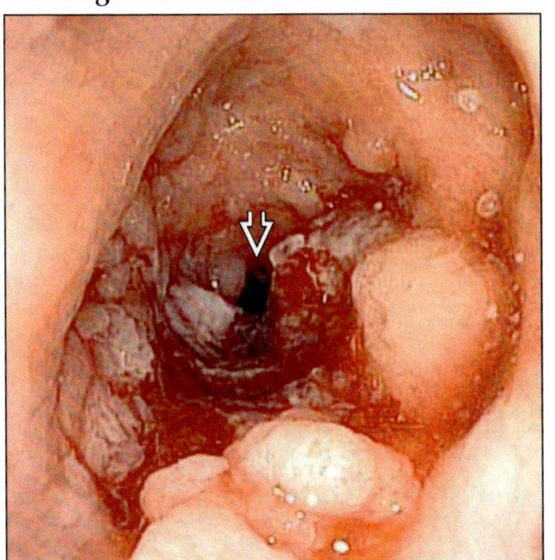

Stage IIA Rectal Cancer in Crohn

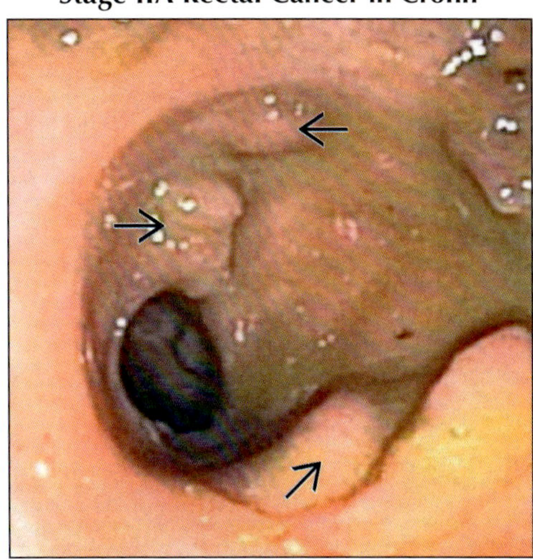

(Left) *Colonoscopy in a 55-year-old man with history of Crohn disease shows a polypoid, ulcerated adenocarcinoma in the rectum 5 cm from the anal verge. The colon lumen* ⇨ *is partially obstructed by the tumor, allowing passage of only a pediatric colonoscope.* ***(Right)*** *Colonoscopy in the same patient shows inflammation, congestion, and erythema throughout entire colon with multiple pedunculated inflammatory polyps* → *. Random biopsies of colon were normal.*

Stage IIA Rectal Cancer in Crohn

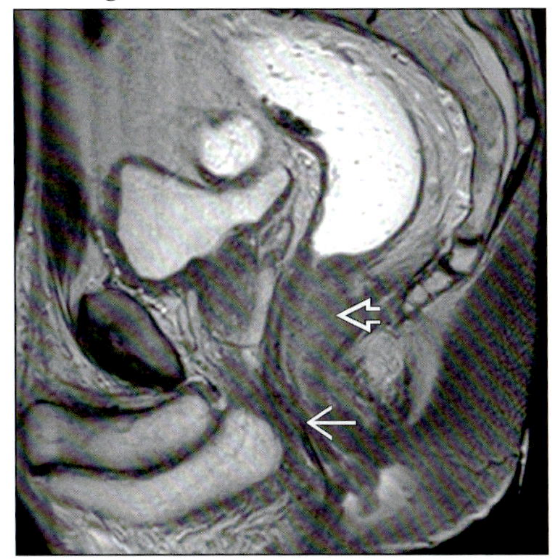

Stage IIA Rectal Cancer in Crohn

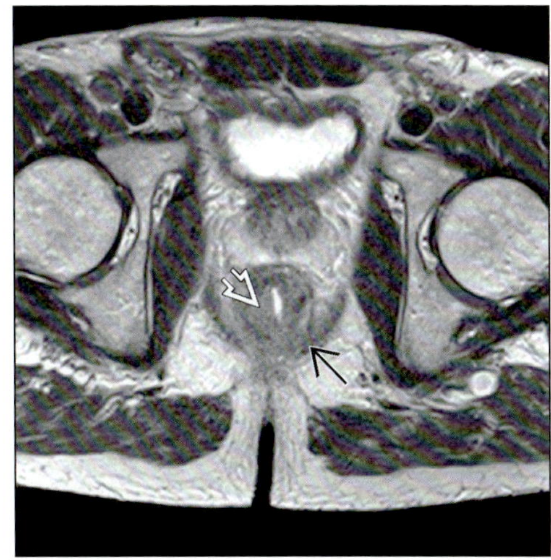

(Left) *Sagittal T2WI MR in the same patient shows T2 hypointense mass* ⇨ *involving a segment of distal rectum and proximal anal canal 5.8 cm in length, with thickening posteriorly. The mass is causing stenosis of the anorectum* → *. No pelvic adenopathy is seen.* ***(Right)*** *Axial T2WI MR shows a 5.8 cm distal circumferential T2 hypointense rectal mass* ⇨ *with extension into perirectal fat abutting the levator ani muscles* → *. He is stage IIA (cT3 N0 M0).*

Stage IIA Rectal Cancer in Crohn

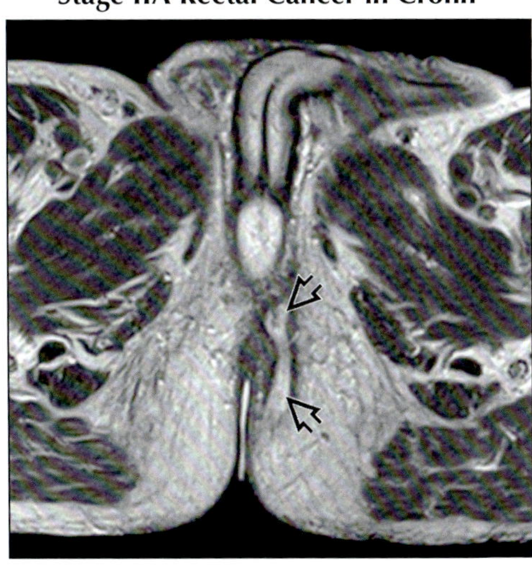

Stage IIA Rectal Cancer in Crohn

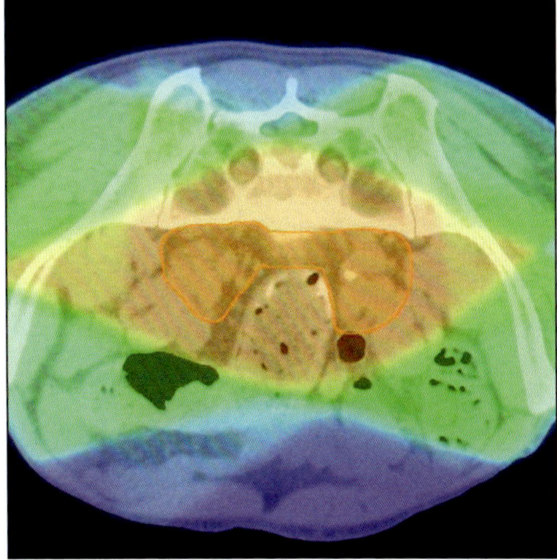

(Left) *Axial T2WI MR shows a T2 hyperintense fistula tract* ⇨ *that extends superiorly from the cutaneous surface of the left buttock to connect with the anal canal. It measures approximately 7.6 cm in length.* ***(Right)*** *Axial NECT shows CTV (orange) at the level of presacral and internal iliac nodes. 45 Gy dose colorwash (orange) covers the pelvic CTV. A 5-field arrangement was used to spare bowel and genitalia from high-dose regions.*

(**Left**) *Axial NECT in the same patient shows 50 Gy dose colorwash (red) after additional 5.4 Gy boost to the primary tumor ➡ and fistula tract (red). The 5-field arrangement also spared genitalia ⇨ from high-dose RT regions.* (**Right**) *Restaging PET/CT was performed to rule out distant metastases before surgery. Axial view at the level of perineum shows fistula tract ➡ as a linear focus of increased metabolic activity tracking from the rectum to the skin.*

Crohn EBRT Planning

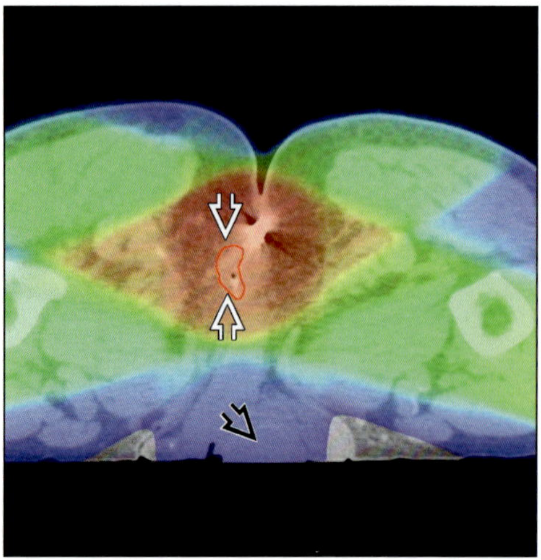

Crohn Post Treatment

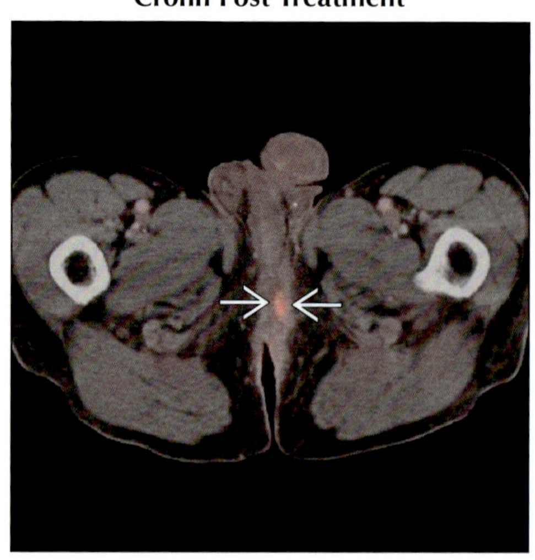

(**Left**) *Sagittal view of restaging PET/CT shows that the wall of distal sigmoid colon ➡ and rectum ➦ are mildly thickened and hypermetabolic. The patient then underwent a total proctocolectomy, permanent end ileostomy, resection of fistulas, and perineal reconstruction.* (**Right**) *H&E section shows a pathologic CR with ulcerated rectum containing chronic inflammation, denuded epithelium, and no residual carcinoma. (Courtesy K. E. Affolter, MD.)*

Crohn Post Treatment

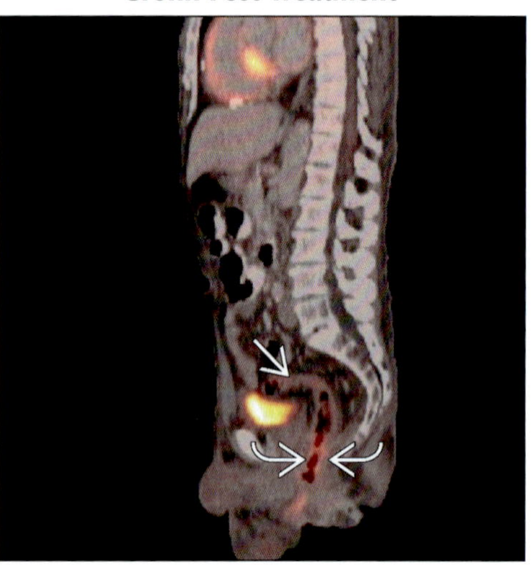

Crohn Treatment Effect

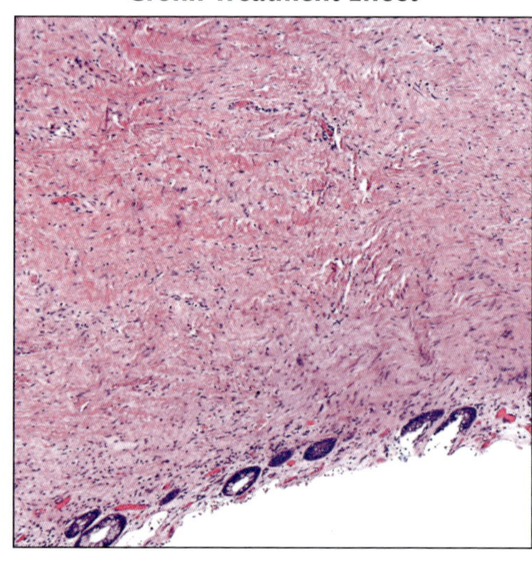

(**Left**) *Axial CECT shows thickening of the wall of the rectum ➡ with tumor infiltrating into the perirectal fat ➦ and reaching posteriorly almost to the sacrum ➡. An enlarged perirectal node ⇨ is also present.* (**Right**) *Axial CECT in the same patient shows loss of the fat plane between the rectal mass ➡ and the lower uterus ➦ due to local tumor invasion.*

Stage IVB (T4b N2b M1b)

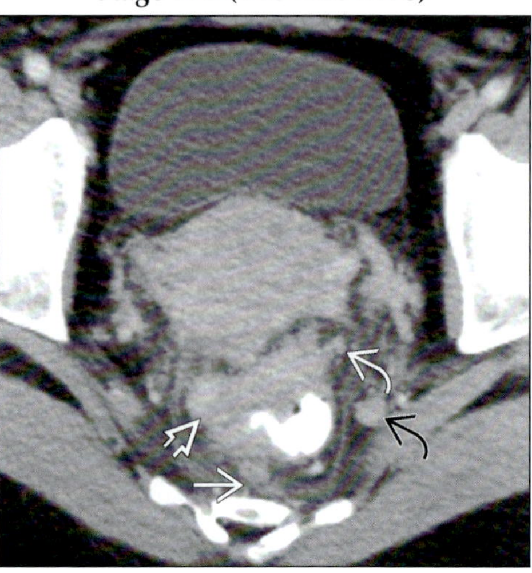

Stage IVB (T4b N2b M1b)

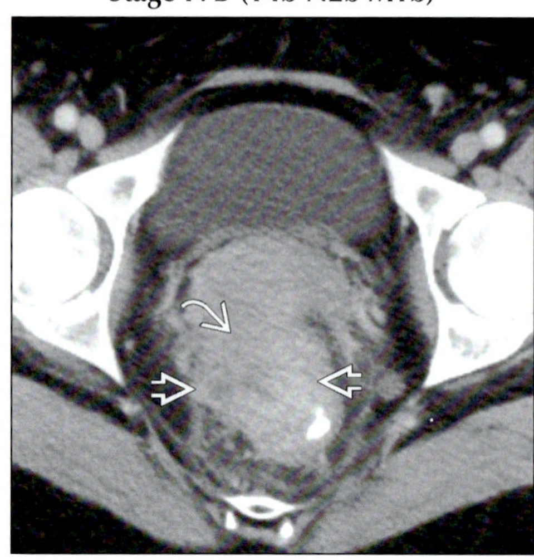

Stage IVB (T4b N2b M1b)

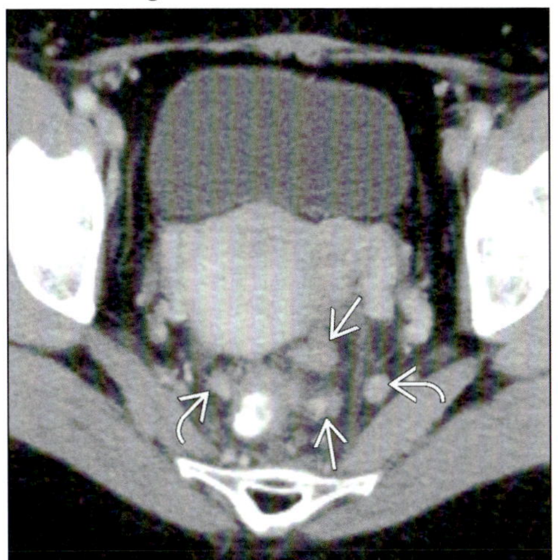

Stage IVB (T4b N2b M1b)

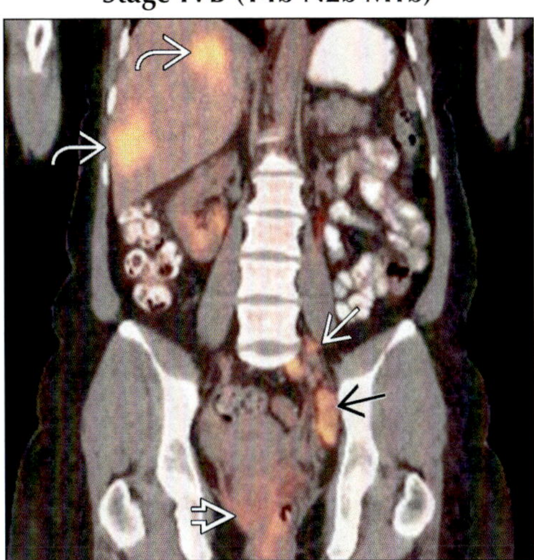

(Left) Axial CECT in the same patient shows multiple enlarged perirectal lymph nodes ➢ in addition to tumor deposits in the perirectal fat ➡. *(Right)* Coronal PET/CT in the same patient shows increased metabolic activity in the rectum ➨, metastatic internal ➞ and common ➡ iliac lymph nodes, and multiple liver metastases ➢.

Stage IVA (T3 N1a M1a)

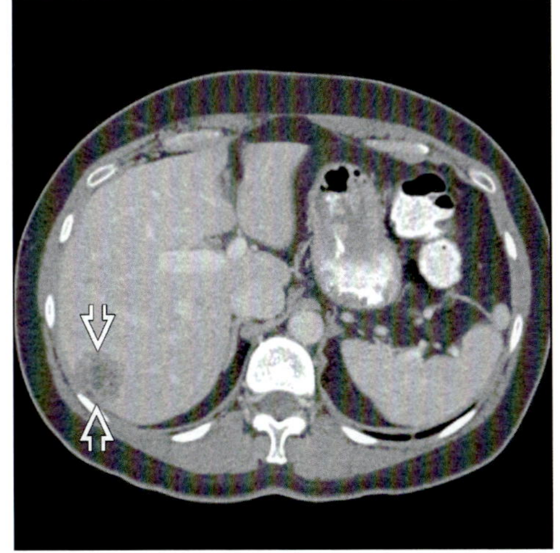

Stage IVA (T3 N1a M1a)

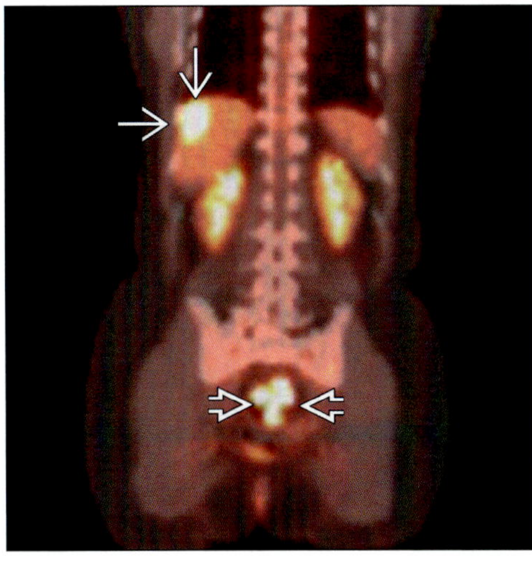

(Left) Axial CECT shows a 3.2 cm hypodense liver lesion ➨ in the right posterolateral lobe (segment 7) in a patient with rectal adenocarcinoma 11 cm from the anal verge on rigid proctoscopy. EUS shows a uT3 N1 primary. Pretreatment CEA is 7.4. *(Right)* Coronal PET/CT shows a hypermetabolic tumor ➨ in the proximal rectum with thickened bowel wall. In addition, there is a hypermetabolic lesion ➡ in segment 7 of the liver, consistent with a single metastasis.

Stage IVA (T3 N1a M1a)

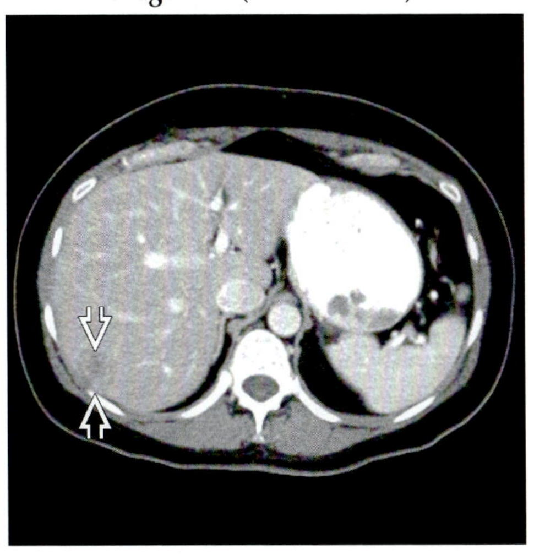

Stage IVA (T3 N1a M1a)

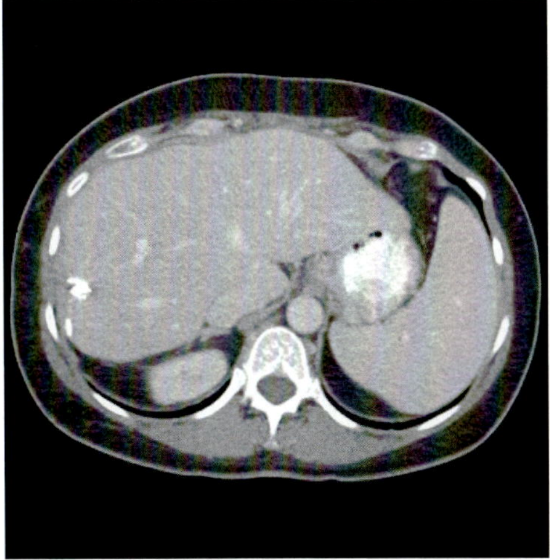

(Left) The same patient was treated with preop pelvic CRT to 50.4 Gy, followed by 2 cycles of FOLFOX. Axial CECT shows a stable 3.0 cm hypodense lesion ➨ in segment 7 of the liver. *(Right)* The same patient underwent LAR, diverting loop ileostomy, and partial hepatectomy with resection of segment 7. Pathology shows a ypT2 N0 primary and a 3.2 cm liver metastasis with clear margins. Axial CECT at 9 months postop shows the patient to be NED & CEA < 1.

ANUS

(T) Primary Tumor

Adapted from 7th edition AJCC Staging Forms.

TNM	*Definitions*
TX	Primary tumor cannot be assessed
T0	No evidence of primary tumor
Tis	Carcinoma in situ (Bowen disease, high-grade squamous intraepithelial lesion [HSIL], anal intraepithelial neoplasia II-III [AIN II-III])
T1	Tumor ≤ 2 cm in greatest dimension
T2	Tumor > 2 cm but ≤ 5 cm in greatest dimension
T3	Tumor > 5 cm in greatest dimension
T4	Tumor of any size invading adjacent organ(s), e.g., vagina, urethra, bladder*

(N) Regional Lymph Nodes

NX	Regional lymph nodes cannot be assessed
N0	No regional lymph node metastasis
N1	Metastasis in perirectal lymph node(s)
N2	Metastasis in unilateral internal iliac &/or inguinal lymph node(s)
N3	Metastasis in perirectal and inguinal lymph nodes &/or bilateral internal iliac &/or inguinal lymph nodes

(M) Distant Metastasis

M0	No distant metastasis
M1	Distant metastasis

**Direct invasion of the rectal wall, perirectal skin, subcutaneous tissue, or the sphincter muscle(s) is not classified as T4.*

AJCC Stages/Prognostic Groups

Adapted from 7th edition AJCC Staging Forms.

Stage	*T*	*N*	*M*
0	Tis	N0	M0
I	T1	N0	M0
II	T2	N0	M0
	T3	N0	M0
IIIA	T1	N1	M0
	T2	N1	M0
	T3	N1	M0
	T4	N0	M0
IIIB	T4	N1	M0
	Any T	N2	M0
	Any T	N3	M0
IV	Any T	Any N	M1

Tis (AIN)

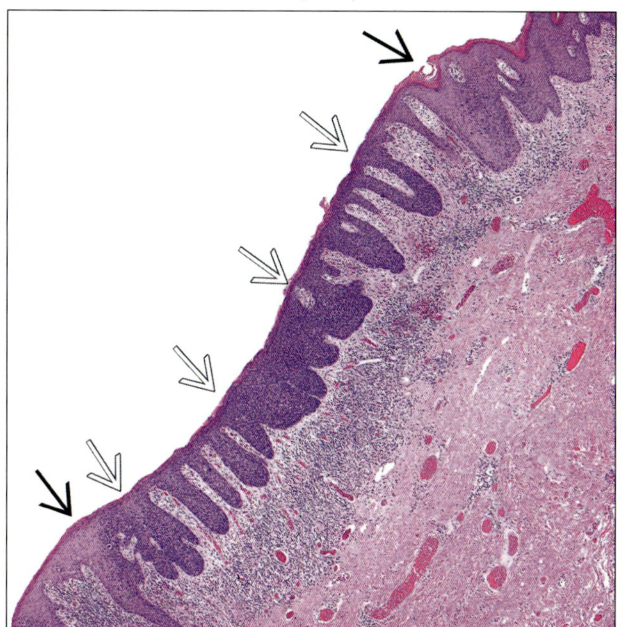

Low-power H&E section of hemorrhoidectomy specimen shows incidental anal intraepithelial neoplasia (AIN). AIN ➡ involves most of the thickness of the squamous epithelium and has a darker color with abrupt demarcation from the normal squamous epithelium ⇨.

Tis (AIN)

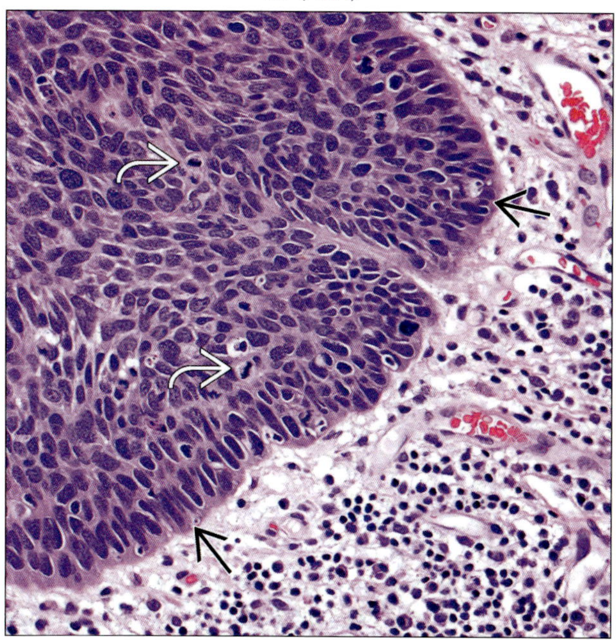

Higher magnification of AIN depicted in the previous image shows crowded neoplastic cells (upper left corner) with increased nuclear:cytoplasmic ratio and numerous mitotic figures ↪. The cells respect the basement membrane ⇨ with no evidence of invasion.

T1

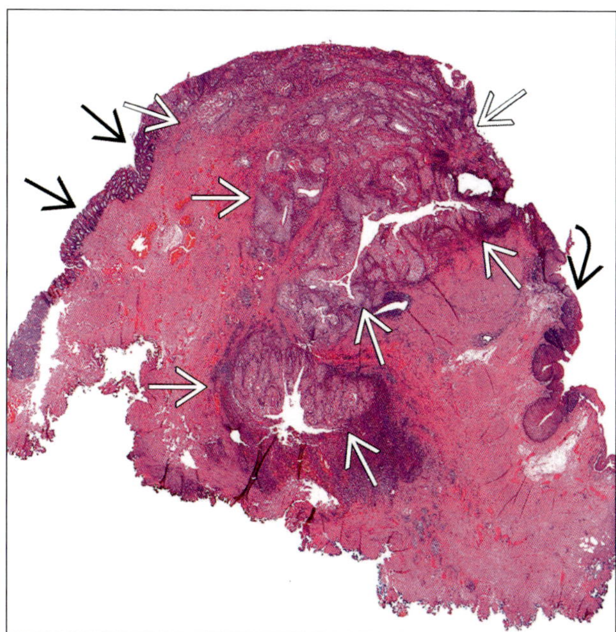

Scanned whole mount of H&E section shows invasive squamous cell carcinoma ➡ of the anus arising from the squamous epithelium and invading into the submucosa. The tumor measures 12 mm. Compare with normal glandular mucosa on the left side ⇨ and the uninvolved squamous epithelium on the right ↪.

T1

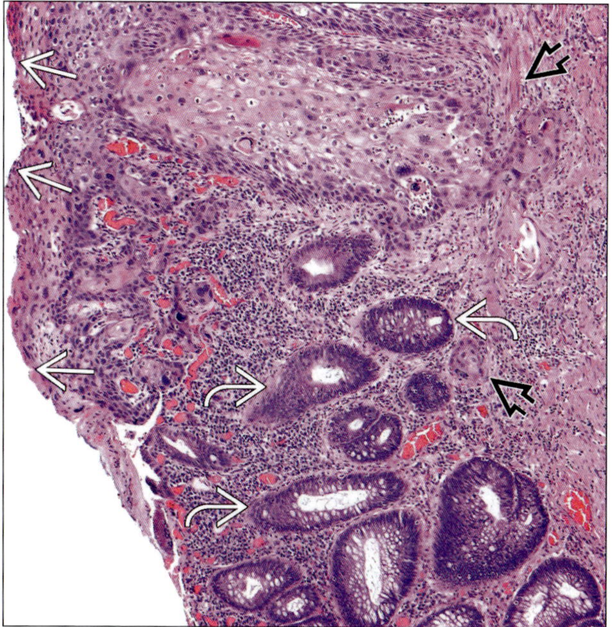

Higher magnification of the right upper part of the prior image shows the invasive squamous cell carcinoma extending from the surface ➡ and invading into the submucosa ⊳. Note the adjacent uninvolved glands of the colorectal mucosa ↪.

T1

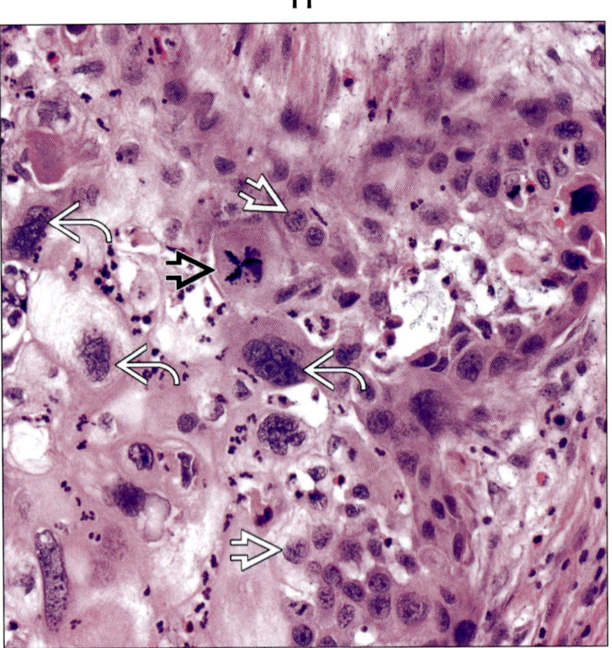

Higher magnification of the previous image shows the pleomorphic atypical cells with numerous large cells ➦, intermediate to small neoplastic cells ➡, and a tripolar mitotic figure ⇨.

T2

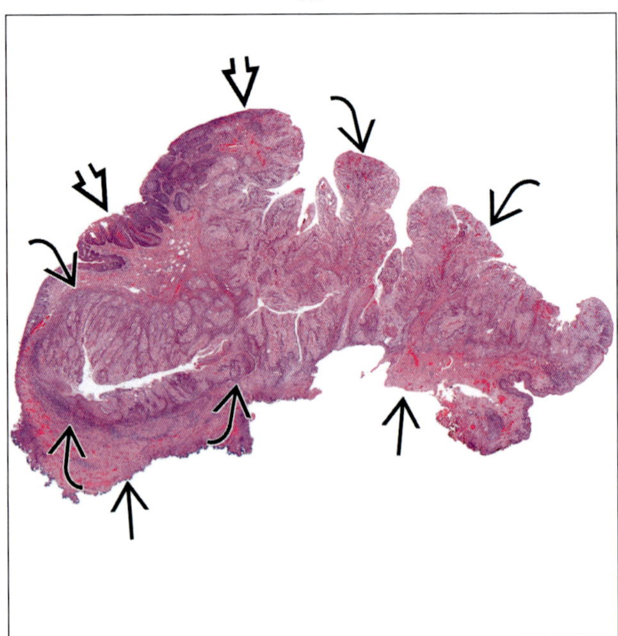

Scanned whole mount of H&E section of invasive squamous cell carcinoma of the anus shows a 2.9 cm tumor ➦. Note the resection margin → and the surface mucosa ⇨.

T2

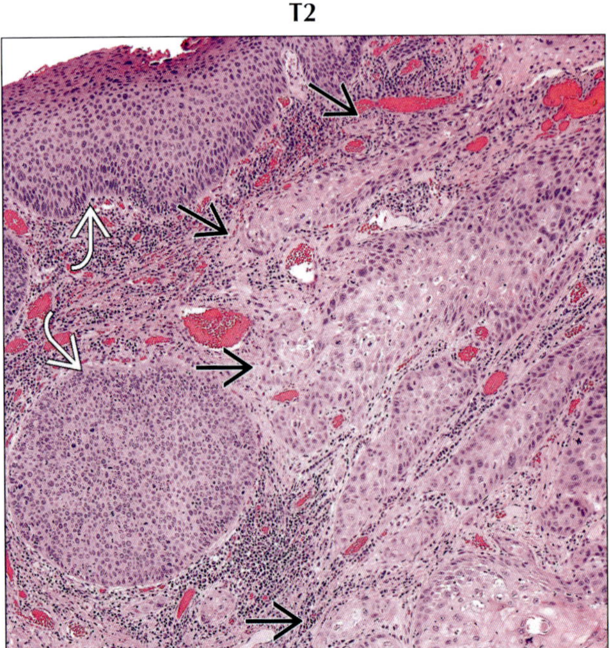

Higher magnification of the previous image shows the invasive squamous carcinoma → in close proximity to intraepithelial carcinoma ➦.

T2

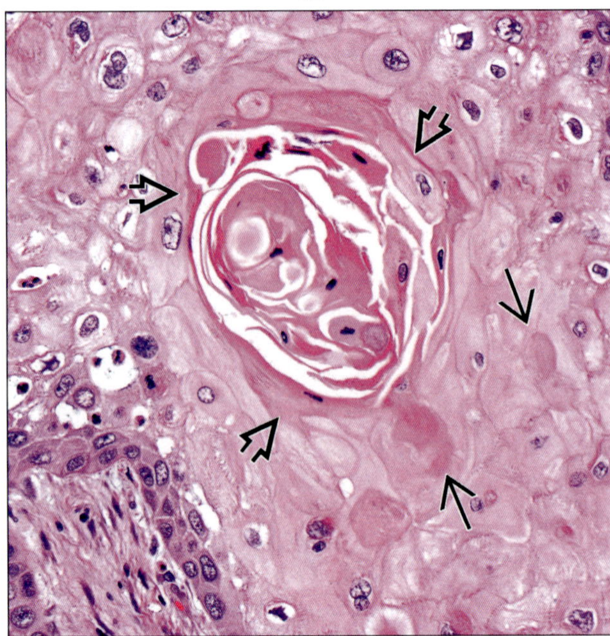

Higher magnification of the invasive squamous cell carcinoma cells shows cytoplasmic eosinophilic pink materials (keratin) → as well as keratin pearl formation ⇨, indicating a well-differentiated squamous cell carcinoma.

T1

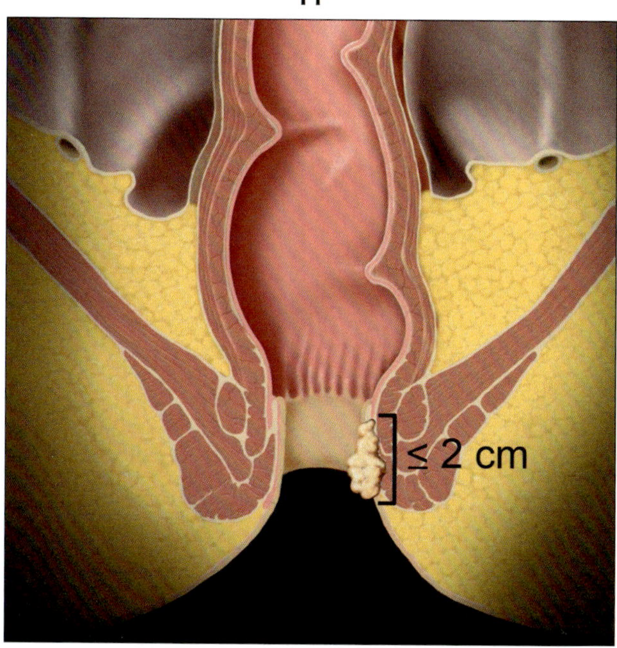

Graphic illustrates an anal canal tumor 2 cm or less in greatest dimension, consistent with T1 disease.

T2

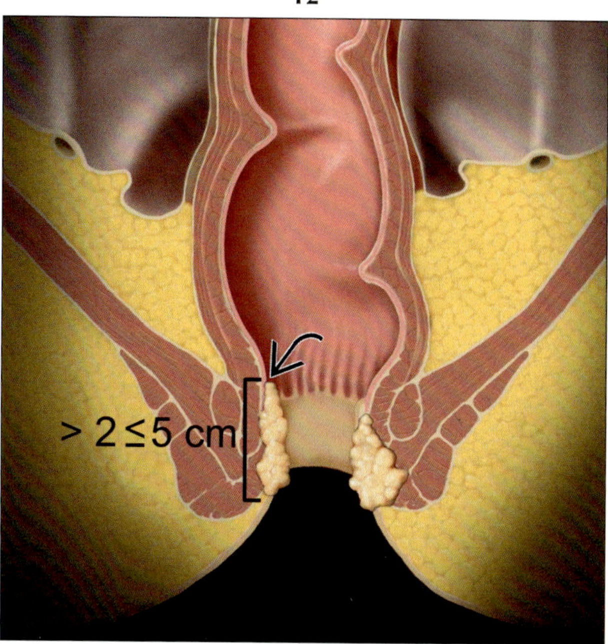

Graphic illustrates an anal canal tumor > 2 cm but not > 5 cm in greatest dimension. On the left side of the graphic, tumor extends above the dentate line ➙.

T3

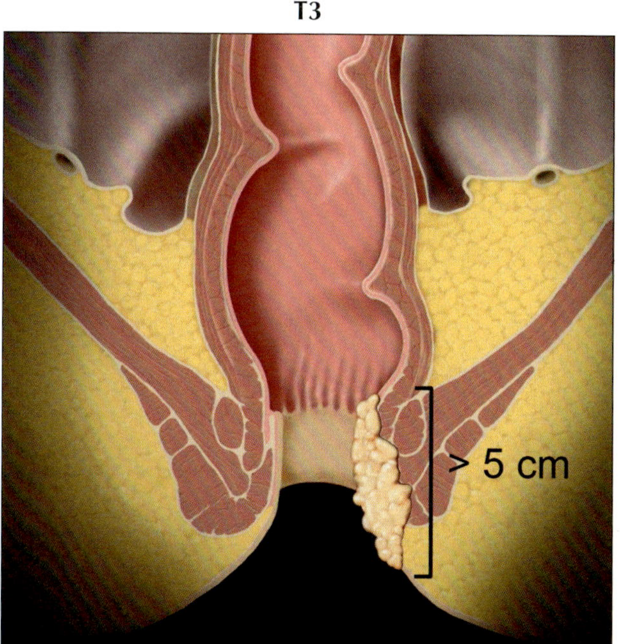

Graphic illustrates an anal canal tumor > 5 cm in greatest dimension, which is classified as T3 disease.

T4

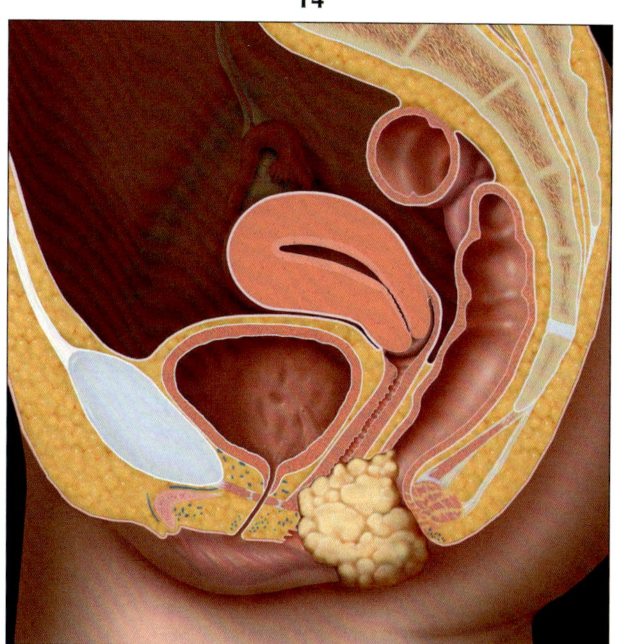

Graphic illustrates an anal canal tumor invading the vagina. T4 tumor is defined as tumor of any size invading adjacent organs or structures, such as vagina, urethra, or urinary bladder.

N1

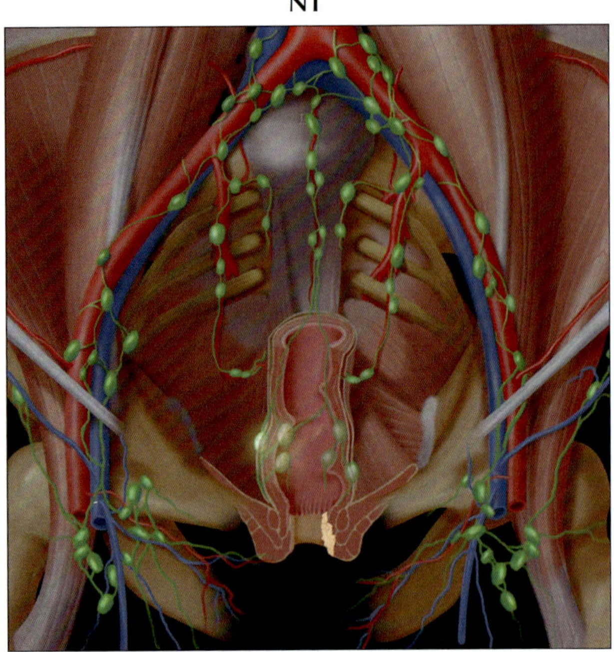

Graphic shows metastasis in a perirectal lymph node, consistent with N1 disease. Even if multiple perirectal lymph nodes were affected, the N classification would still be N1.

N2

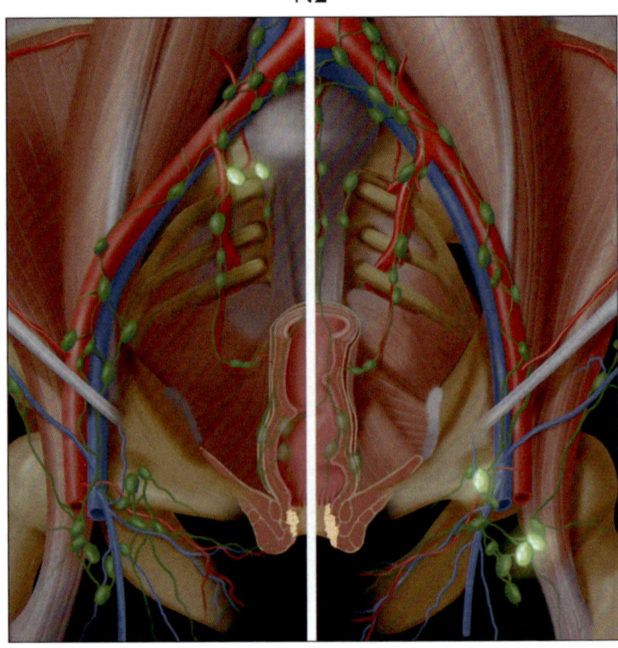

Graphics show metastases to a single group of nodes, internal iliac (left) or inguinal (right). N2 is defined as metastases in unilateral internal iliac &/or inguinal lymph nodes.

N2

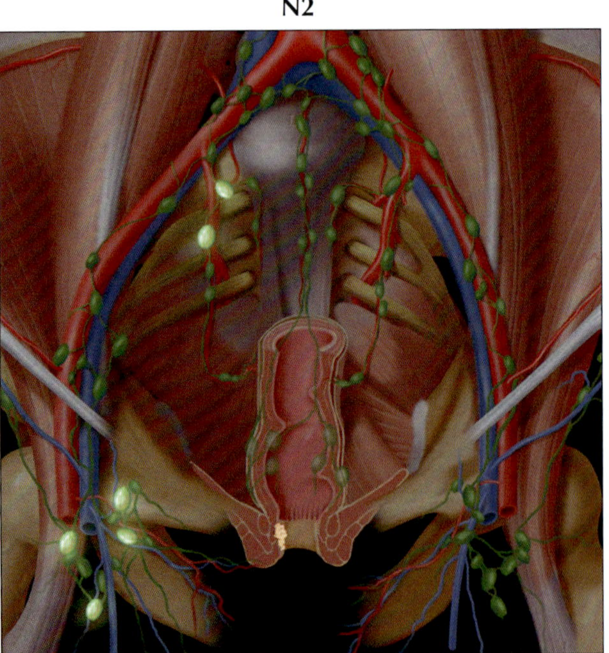

Graphic shows unilateral metastases to both internal iliac and inguinal lymph nodes, another scenario that is considered N2.

N3

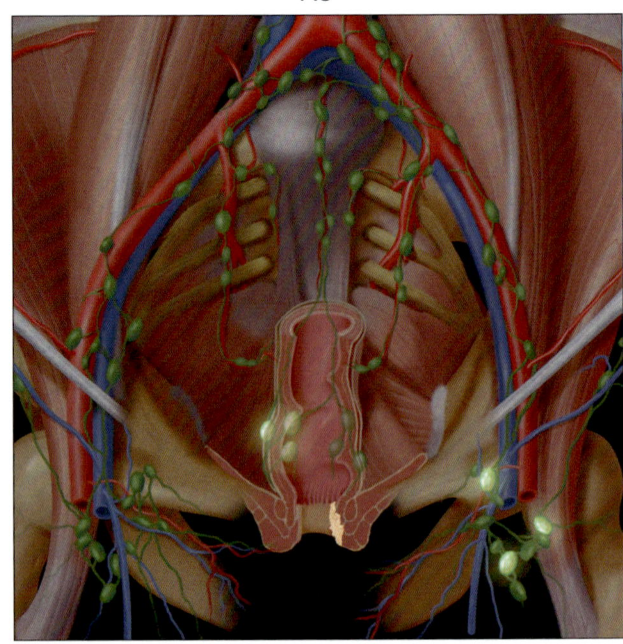

Graphic illustrates metastases to perirectal and inguinal lymph nodes. N3 is defined as metastases in perirectal and inguinal lymph nodes &/or bilateral internal iliac &/or inguinal lymph nodes.

N3

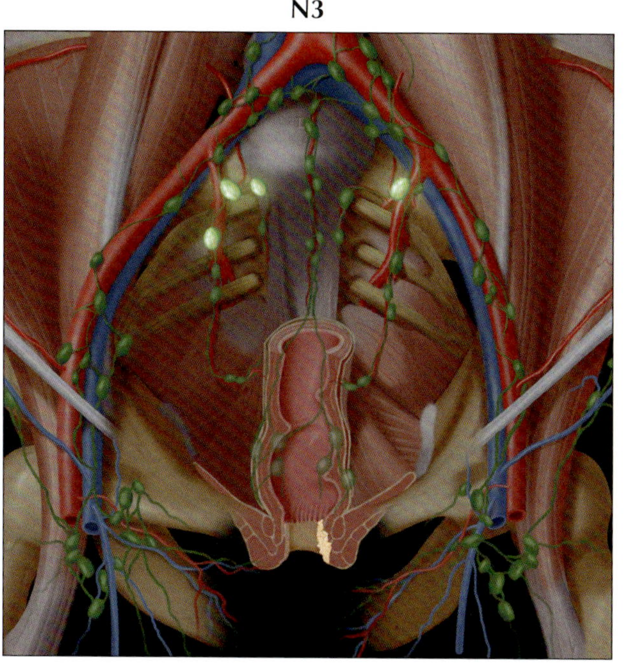

Graphic illustrates metastases to bilateral internal iliac lymph nodes, consistent with N3 disease.

N3

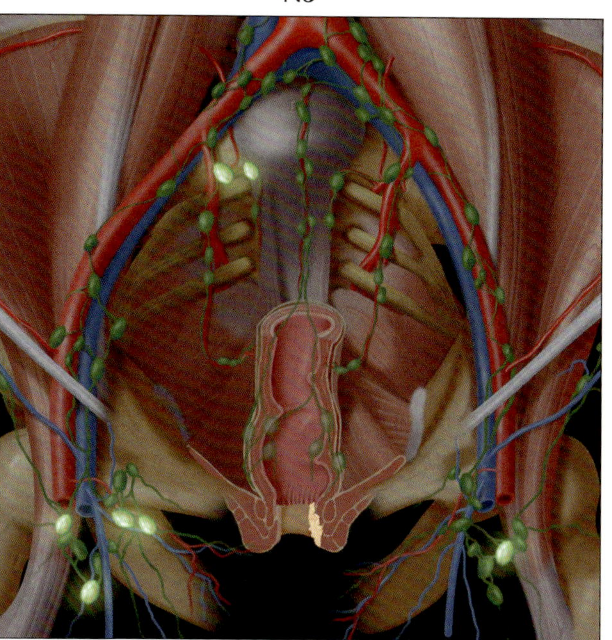

Graphic illustrates metastases to bilateral inguinal and unilateral internal iliac lymph nodes, which is also N3 disease.

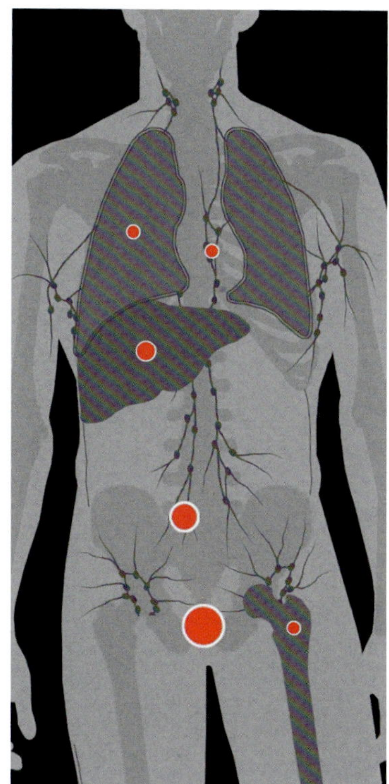

INITIAL SITE OF RECURRENCE

Primary Site	50%
Inguinal Nodes	22%
Pelvic Nodes	17%
Multiple Distant Sites	15%
Liver	9%
Distant Nodes	4%
Lungs	2%
Bone	2%

Tomaszewski JM et al: Twenty-five-year experience with radical chemoradiation for anal cancer. Int J Radiat Oncol Biol Phys. 83(2):552-8, 2012.

ANUS

OVERVIEW

General Comments

- Tumors that develop from anal mucosa are termed anal canal carcinomas
  - True anal mucosa is glandular, transitional, or squamous epithelium (from proximal to distal)
  - Superior border is anorectal ring
    - Palpable upper border of anal sphincter complex and puborectalis muscles
    - Dentate line is visible zone of transitional mucosa from anal to rectal epithelium
      - Superior border of anal canal is ~ 1-2 cm proximal to dentate line
    - Tumors with epicenter > 2 cm proximal to dentate line or anorectal ring are rectal cancers
    - Tumors with epicenter ≤ 2 cm from dentate line are classified as anal canal cancers
  - Inferior border is where modified squamous epithelium transitions to epidermis (anal verge)
    - Roughly coincides with palpable intersphincteric groove
  - Typically staged clinically according to size and extent of untreated primary tumor
    - Pathologic staging is not done in most cases due to nonoperative treatments
- Tumors that develop from perianal skin ≤ 5-6 cm from anal verge are anal margin carcinomas
  - Not included in this staging scheme
    - Staged with skin cancers
  - Anal verge to perianal skin at or distal to squamous mucocutaneous junction
    - Covered by epidermis, not mucosa
- Tumors can involve both anal canal and anal margin

Classification

- WHO classification of anal canal carcinoma
  - Squamous cell carcinomas (SCCs): 80% of cases
    - Cloacogenic (basaloid) and transitional cell are considered variants of SCC
      - Exhibit similar natural history & response to treatment, but higher distant metastasis rates
      - All are associated with human papilloma virus (HPV) infection
      - Subtypes: Large cell keratinizing, large cell nonkeratinizing, and less differentiated
  - Adenocarcinomas (10%)
    - Rectal type
    - Adenocarcinomas of anal glands
    - Adenocarcinomas within anorectal fistula
  - Mucinous adenocarcinoma
  - Small cell carcinoma
  - Undifferentiated carcinoma
- Perianal or anal margin carcinoma
  - SCC
  - Verrucous carcinoma (giant condyloma)
  - Basal cell carcinoma
  - Bowen disease
  - Paget disease
- Melanomas, carcinoid tumors, and sarcomas are excluded from anus staging system

NATURAL HISTORY

Etiology

- Risk factors
  - History of persistent high-risk HPV infection
    - High-risk genotype are HPV-16 and HPV-18
    - Infection with multiple HPV genotypes
    - HPV may be an etiologic agent in anal carcinoma
  - History of cervical dysplasia or cancer
  - History of vulvar or vaginal cancer
  - Anoreceptive intercourse
  - High lifetime number of sexual partners
  - Anogenital warts
    - Present in approximately 50% of homosexual men with anal cancer
    - Present in only 20% of women and heterosexual men with anal cancer
  - History of sexually transmitted disease
  - Immunosuppression after solid organ transplant
  - HIV seropositivity
    - Low CD4 count
    - Highly active antiretroviral therapy (HAART) lacks impact on progression of anal precursors
  - Cigarette smoking
  - Long-term use of corticosteroids
  - Crohn disease
- Protective factors
  - Prevention or treatment of high-grade anal intraepithelial neoplasia
    - Quadrivalent HPV vaccine

Epidemiology & Cancer Incidence

- Uncommon malignancy
  - 1.5% of gastrointestinal malignancies in USA
  - 4-5% of anorectal malignancies
- Number of cases in USA per year
  - An estimated 6,230 new cases of anal cancer in 2012
  - Incidence rate increased 1.9x for men and 1.5x for women from 1973 to 2000
- Sex predilection
  - 2,250 new cases in men and 3,980 in women in 2012
  - Marked female predominance
- Age of onset
  - Wide age range
  - Median age of onset ~ 62 years
- Mortality
  - Estimated 780 deaths in USA in 2012

Gross Pathology & Surgical Features

- Anal carcinomas are usually nodular and often ulcerated

Microscopic Pathology

- High-grade anal intraepithelial neoplasia (AIN)
  - Precursor to anal cancer
- Majority of anal canal carcinomas are SCC
  - Variants include
    - Large cell keratinizing
    - Large cell nonkeratinizing
    - Basaloid
- Other less common types include adenocarcinoma, melanoma, and small cell carcinoma

Routes of Spread

- Local spread

- Local spread can occur to adjacent structures, including vagina, urethra, and urinary bladder
- Lymphatic extension
  - Regional nodes
    - Superficial inguinal
    - Anorectal, perirectal, and lateral sacral
    - Internal iliac (hypogastric)
  - Distant nodes
    - External iliac (still included in standard RT field)
    - Common iliac
  - Lymphatic drainage depends on location of tumor in relation to dentate line
    - Tumors below dentate line → superficial inguinal and deep femoral nodes
    - Tumors above dentate line → anorectal, perirectal, paravertebral, and internal iliac nodes
      - Similar to rectal cancers
    - Lymphatics are not isolated; therefore, inguinal node mets can occur in proximal anal cancer
  - Incidence of nodal metastasis ~ 10% at diagnosis
    - May be as high as 60% for T4 lesions
- Hematogenous spread
  - Occurs in ~ 10% of anal carcinoma cases
- Metastatic sites
  - Mainly to liver, distant nodes, and lungs

IMAGING

Detection

- Because of their location, anal canal cancers are easy to evaluate clinically
  - Digital rectal exam (DRE) can gauge primary tumor size and degree of fixation
  - All lesions are within easy reach of biopsy
- CT
  - Difficult to detect anal carcinoma due to poor tissue contrast
  - Only large lesions causing significant contour deformity can be seen
- MR
  - Majority of tumors are heterogeneously hyperintense on T2 and STIR images
  - Sensitivity 89% in primary tumor detection
- PET/CT
  - Sensitivity 91-100% for nonexcised primary tumors

Staging

- T staging
  - Clinical exam
    - DRE: Emphasis on assessing size of primary
    - Anoscopy: Allows direct visual assessment of tumor extent within anal canal
  - Endorectal ultrasound
    - Not used or recommended in staging
  - MR
    - Good agreement in T staging of tumor by MR imaging and clinical assessment
    - Clinical examination may actually underestimate degree of local invasion in T4 tumors
    - Good correlation between tumor size as determined by MR imaging and clinical assessment
  - CT
    - Not useful for local staging due to poor tissue contrast
  - PET/CT
    - Can be used to show extent of primary tumor and tissue involvement
    - Sensitivity 93%, specificity 81%
- N staging
  - CT
    - Can detect enlarged perirectal and inguinal lymph nodes
    - Sensitivity 62%, specificity 60%
  - PET/CT
    - Detection of nodes: Sensitivity 100%, specificity 83%, positive predictive value 43%
    - Upstages or changes management in 15-20% cases
- M staging
  - CT is useful for detection of metastatic disease to liver and lungs
  - PET/CT
    - Appears more useful than CT in detection of nodes & metastases
      - Sites of metastases not observed on CT scan were identified in 24% of patients

Restaging

- CT
  - Can be used for detection of liver and lung metastases
  - Not useful for detection of local recurrence
- MR
  - Useful in follow-up after chemoradiation
    - MR criteria for tumor response
      - Reduction in tumor size
      - Decreased tumor signal intensity on T2WI
- PET/CT
  - Post-treatment PET scans appear to be of little value in predicting durability of local response
    - Minimal residual PET activity at primary site on 1-month follow-up PET can be seen in patients without recurrence
    - Recurrences possible in patients who had negative post-treatment PET studies

CLINICAL PRESENTATION & WORK-UP

Presentation

- Most initially thought to have benign anorectal conditions
- Rectal bleeding (45%)
  - Diagnosis can be delayed because bleeding is often ascribed to hemorrhoids
- Rectal pain or mass sensation (30%)
- Palpable inguinal mass (20%)
  - Usually unilateral
  - Up to 50% of enlarged nodes are reactive
  - Additional 10-25% have subclinical positive inguinal nodes
- No symptoms or nonspecific symptoms (20%)
- Incontinence (< 5%)
- Pruritus ani
- Anal discharge

Prognosis

- Stage at diagnosis
  - Stage I: 25.3%

- Stage II: 51.8%
- Stage III: 17.1%
- Stage IV: 5.7%
- 5-year observed survival by stage
  - Stage I: 69.5%
  - Stage II: 61.8%
  - Stage IIIA: 45.6%
  - Stage IIIB: 39.6%
  - Stage IV: 15.3%
- Tumor size is most important prognostic factor
- Histologic type
  - Improved survival seen in patients with SCC vs. nonsquamous tumors, stage-for-stage

Work-Up

- Clinical
  - H&P
    - Focus on sexual history & HPV/HIV risk
    - Digital rectal exam, gynecologic exam, screen for cervix cancer, inguinal node evaluation
  - Anoscopy
  - Biopsy of primary tumor
    - Consider biopsy of suspicious nodes
- Radiographic
  - CT or MR of abdomen/pelvis
  - CXR or chest CT
  - Consider PET/CT
- Laboratory
  - CBC, LFTs, renal function, consider HIV

TREATMENT

Major Treatment Alternatives

- Abdominoperineal resection (APR) was standard treatment until late 1970s
  - APR now reserved for salvage treatment
- Chemoradiation therapy (CRT) (sphincter preservation)
  - Replaced APR as treatment of choice
  - CRT with 5-fluorouracil (5-FU) + mitomycin C (MMC) more effective than RT alone
    - Improved complete response (CR) rates, local control (LC), colostomy-free survival (CFS), progression-free survival (PFS), but not overall survival (OS)
  - Survival and recurrence rates equivalent to those achieved with APR
  - Preserves sphincter function
- Local excision of anal margin carcinomas
  - Consider for T1 N0 well-differentiated tumors

Major Treatment Roadblocks/ Contraindications

- HIV(+) status is not a contraindication to standard chemoradiation
- Consider lowering dose or withholding mitomycin-C if active HIV/AIDS-related complications

Treatment Options by Stage

- Stage 0
  - Surgical resection for perianal lesions not involving anal sphincter
  - Consider radiotherapy for lesions not amenable to local excision
- Stages I, II, & III
  - Chemoradiation (5-FU/MMC or 5-FU/CDDP)
    - Target volumes
      - Perianal region
      - Anal canal
      - Distal rectum
      - Perirectal, inguinal, presacral, internal iliac, and external iliac lymph nodes
      - Consider omitting inguinal radiation for T1 N0 patients (< 2% risk of failure)
- Stage IV
  - Palliative surgery
  - Palliative radiation therapy
  - Palliative chemotherapy + radiation therapy
- Recurrent disease
  - Salvage APR for residual or recurrent disease after nonoperative therapy
    - Salvage rates: 5-year disease-free survival (DFS) 37%, OS 47%
    - High risk of perineal breakdown
    - Consider unilateral or bilateral superficial and deep inguinal node dissection
  - Consider additional chemoradiation
  - Salvage chemotherapy with 5-FU/CDDP + RT boost
    - May avoid permanent colostomy in selected patients with small residual tumor after initial nonoperative therapy

Dose Response

- All regimens with concurrent chemotherapy
- 30 Gy: Nigro protocol; 5/6 patients had pCR at APR; 26/28 had clinical CR
- 45-50 Gy: 70-80% LC
- > 54 Gy: Retrospective studies suggest ↑ OS, response rates, and LC
  - Prospective studies show no clinical difference between 54 Gy and 59.4 Gy
- 59.4 Gy: Split course, no clinical benefit

Standard Doses

- 3D CRT
  - 30.6 Gy to entire pelvis
  - 36 Gy to node-negative inguinal nodes
  - 45 Gy to pelvis below inferior SI joints
  - 54-59 Gy for T3/T4, node-positive disease, or T2 residual disease after 45 Gy
- IMRT
  - If T1/T2 & N0, 50.4 Gy to primary anorectum and 42 Gy to elective nodes in 28 fractions
  - If T3/T4 & N0, 54 Gy to primary anorectum and 45 Gy to elective nodes in 30 fractions
  - Node-positive disease
    - 50.4 Gy to nodes ≤ 3 cm
    - 54 Gy to nodes > 3 cm

Organs at Risk Parameters

- Following guidelines from RTOG 0529, evaluate IMRT in anal cancer
  - Small bowel
    - ≤ 200 mL > 30 Gy; ≤ 150 mL > 35 Gy; ≤ 20 mL > 45 Gy; none > 50 Gy
  - Femoral heads
    - ≤ 50% > 30 Gy; ≤ 35% > 40 Gy; ≤ 5% > 44 Gy
  - Iliac crests
    - ≤ 50% > 30 Gy; ≤ 35% > 40 Gy; ≤ 5% > 50 Gy

- External genitalia
  - ≤ 50% > 20 Gy; ≤ 35% > 30 Gy; ≤ 5% > 40 Gy
- Bladder
  - ≤ 50% > 35 Gy; ≤ 35% > 40 Gy; ≤ 5% > 50 Gy
- Large bowel
  - ≤ 200 mL > 30 Gy; ≤ 150 mL > 35 Gy; ≤ 20 mL > 45 Gy

Common Techniques

- IMRT or 3D CRT

Landmark Trials

- Nigro protocol: 30 Gy with 5-FU/MMC; 26/28 had clinical CR
- UK CCCR ACT I: RT vs. CRT (5-FU/MMC), 45 Gy + 15 Gy EBRT or 25 Gy brachy boost
  - CRT ↑ 3-year LC, cause-specific survival, but ↑ acute morbidity; no difference in OS
- EORTC: RT vs. CRT (5-FU/MMC), 45 Gy + 15-20 Gy boost
  - CRT ↑ 3-year LC, CFS, PFS, and CR rates; no difference in OS
- RTOG 87-04: CRT (5-FU) vs. CRT (5-FU/MMC), 45 Gy + 5.4 Gy boost + 9 Gy salvage RT to biopsy-positive residual
  - CRT (5-FU+MMC) ↑ 4-year CFS, LC, and DFS, but ↑ grade 4-5 toxicity; no difference in OS
- RTOG 98-11: CRT (5-FU/MMC) vs. induction 5-FU/cisplatin + CRT (5-FU/cisplatin)
  - CRT (5-FU/MMC) ↑ 5-year CFS; trend improvement in DFS and OS
- RTOG 0529: IMRT for anal cancer vs. RTOG 98-11 standard arm
  - IMRT ↓ grade 3 acute GI/GU/skin toxicity and duration of treatment breaks
- UK CCCR ACT II: CRT (5-FU/MMC) vs. (5-FU/CDDP) ± maintenance 5-FU/CDDP, 50.4 Gy
  - No difference in colostomy rate, CR rate, relapse-free survival, or OS between all 4 arms; more acute hematologic toxicities with MMC

RECOMMENDED FOLLOW-UP

Clinical

- Mean time to tumor regression is 3 months although CR may take up to 1 year
- Reevaluate with exam & DRE in 8-12 weeks S/P CRT
- Classify as complete remission, persistent disease, or progressive disease
  - If complete remission, then anoscopy, DRE, inguinal node palpation q. 3-6 months x 5 years; annual CT chest/abdomen/pelvic x 3 years
  - If persistent disease without progression, then reevaluate in 4 weeks and serial exams to monitor regression
    - If no regression on multiple serial exams, then biopsy + restaging scans; if positive biopsy, then APR if no metastasis
  - If progressive disease, then biopsy + restaging scans; if positive biopsy, then APR if no metastasis

SELECTED REFERENCES

1. Mistrangelo M et al: Role of positron emission tomography-computed tomography in the management of anal cancer. Int J Radiat Oncol Biol Phys. 84(1):66-72, 2012
2. Tomaszewski JM et al: Twenty-five-year experience with radical chemoradiation for anal cancer. Int J Radiat Oncol Biol Phys. 83(2):552-8, 2012
3. Engledow AH et al: The role of ^{18}fluoro-deoxy glucose combined position emission and computed tomography in the clinical management of anal squamous cell carcinoma. Colorectal Dis. 13(5):532-7, 2011
4. American Joint Committee on Cancer: AJCC Cancer Staging Manual. 7th ed. New York: Springer. 165-73, 2010
5. Northover J et al: Chemoradiation for the treatment of epidermoid anal cancer: 13-year follow-up of the first randomised UKCCCR Anal Cancer Trial (ACT I). Br J Cancer. 102(7):1123-8, 2010
6. Bilimoria KY et al: Outcomes and prognostic factors for squamous-cell carcinoma of the anal canal: analysis of patients from the National Cancer Data Base. Dis Colon Rectum. 52(4):624-31, 2009
7. Myerson RJ et al: Elective clinical target volumes for conformal therapy in anorectal cancer: a radiation therapy oncology group consensus panel contouring atlas. Int J Radiat Oncol Biol Phys. 74(3):824-30, 2009
8. Ajani JA et al: Fluorouracil, mitomycin, and radiotherapy vs fluorouracil, cisplatin, and radiotherapy for carcinoma of the anal canal: a randomized controlled trial. JAMA. 299(16):1914-21, 2008
9. Cotter SE et al: FDG-PET/CT in the evaluation of anal carcinoma. Int J Radiat Oncol Biol Phys. 65(3):720-5, 2006
10. Ortholan C et al: Anal canal carcinoma: early-stage tumors < or =10 mm (T1 or Tis): therapeutic options and original pattern of local failure after radiotherapy. Int J Radiat Oncol Biol Phys. 62(2):479-85, 2005
11. Taylor A et al: Mapping pelvic lymph nodes: guidelines for delineation in intensity-modulated radiotherapy. Int J Radiat Oncol Biol Phys. 63(5):1604-12, 2005
12. Papagikos M et al: Chemoradiation for adenocarcinoma of the anus. Int J Radiat Oncol Biol Phys. 55(3):669-78, 2003
13. Bartelink H et al: Concomitant radiotherapy and chemotherapy is superior to radiotherapy alone in the treatment of locally advanced anal cancer: results of a phase III randomized trial of the European Organization for Research and Treatment of Cancer Radiotherapy and Gastrointestinal Cooperative Groups. J Clin Oncol. 15(5):2040-9, 1997
14. Epidermoid anal cancer: results from the UKCCCR randomised trial of radiotherapy alone versus radiotherapy et al: UKCCCR Anal Cancer Trial Working Party. UK Co-ordinating Committee on Cancer Research. Lancet. 348(9034):1049-54, 1996
15. Flam M et al: Role of mitomycin in combination with fluorouracil and radiotherapy, and of salvage chemoradiation in the definitive nonsurgical treatment of epidermoid carcinoma of the anal canal: results of a phase III randomized intergroup study. J Clin Oncol. 14(9):2527-39, 1996

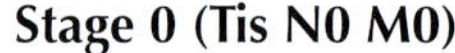

(**Left**) *Pretreatment photo shows bilateral perianal ulcerations with heaped-up edge at the anus in an HIV(+) man. Repeat biopsies showed carcinoma in situ with no evidence of invasion.* (**Right**) *Axial T1WI C+ FS MR to evaluate for osteomyelitis shows ulceration in the perianal soft tissue and a small, enhancing rectocutaneous fistula tract passing through the right gluteal fold. There is no abscess or involvement of bone or muscle.*

Stage 0 (Tis N0 M0)

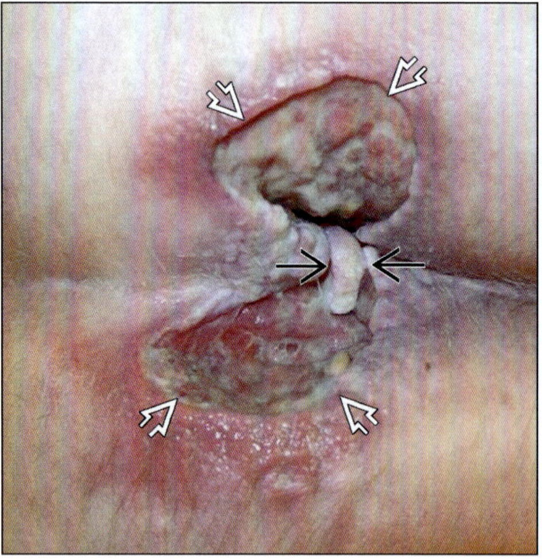

Stage 0 (Tis N0 M0)

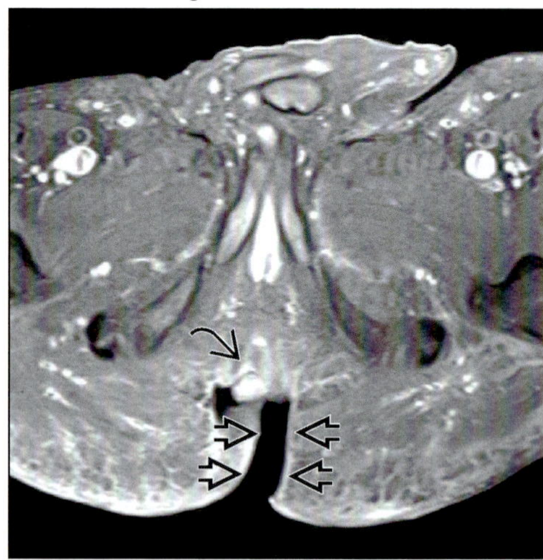

(**Left**) *The same patient was not a candidate for local excision or acetic acid due to CD4 count of 8. RT was prescribed to 59.4 Gy. He was simulated in prone position with 1 cm bolus.* (**Right**) *Skin rendering shows relation of GTV (red) to bladder (yellow), prostate (green), and small bowel (pink). CTV includes anorectum, mesorectum, and perianal tissue. Wire was placed around bilateral skin involvement and covered with bolus (blue) to increase skin dose.*

Simulation

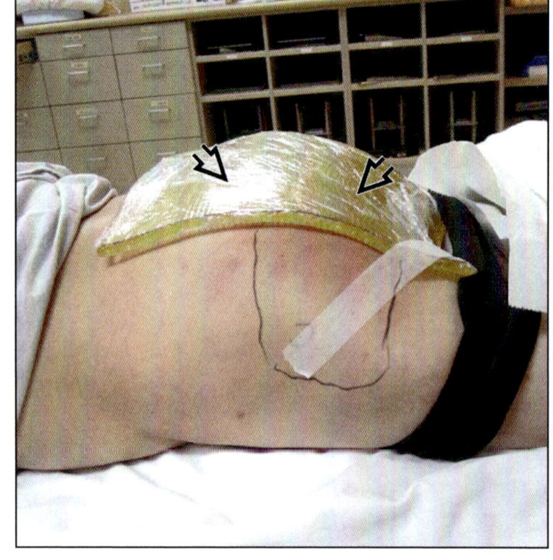

EBRT Planning

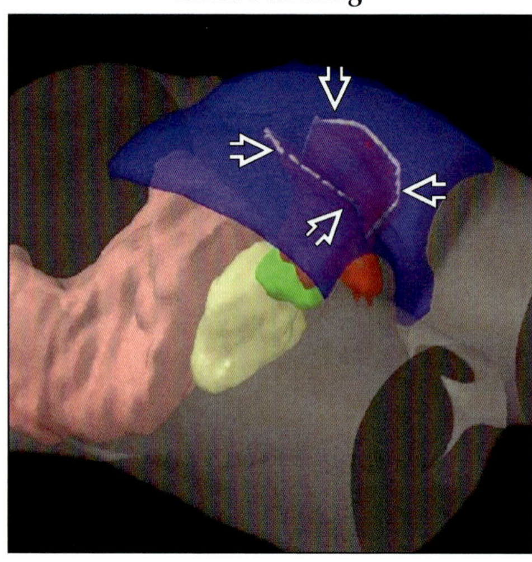

(**Left**) *Sagittal NECT with dose colorwash (50% in green) shows coverage of the initial CTV (orange), which includes the anal canal, distal rectum, and perirectal tissue. A 3-field technique spares the bladder (yellow) and small bowel (pink). Lincolnshire bolus was used to fill in crevices, and 1 cm bolus was placed over entire target area.* (**Right**) *Axial NECT shows dose covering CTV, which was expanded beyond the skin involvement marked by wire.*

EBRT Planning

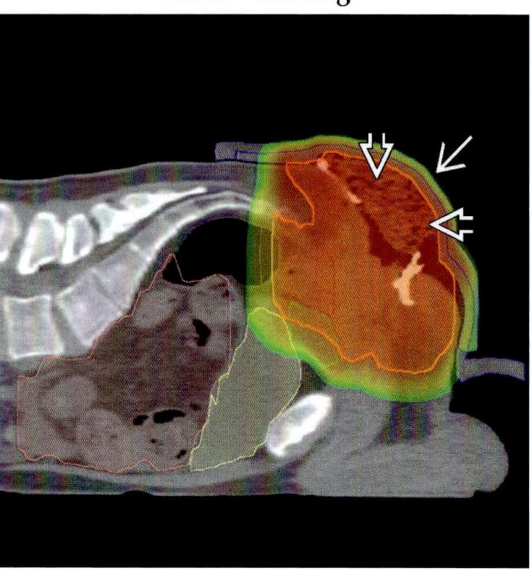

EBRT Planning

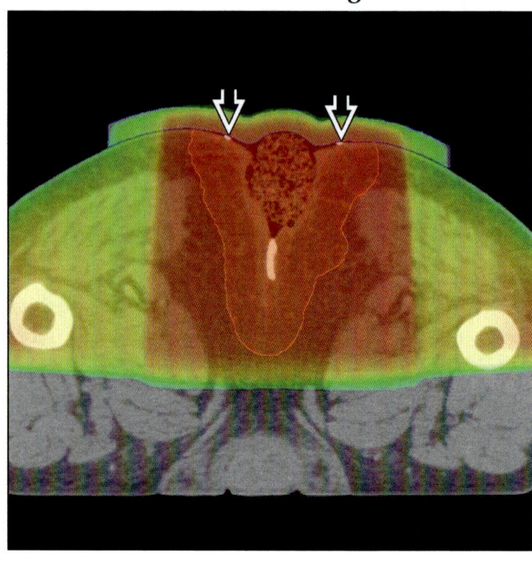

Stage 0 (Tis N0 M0)

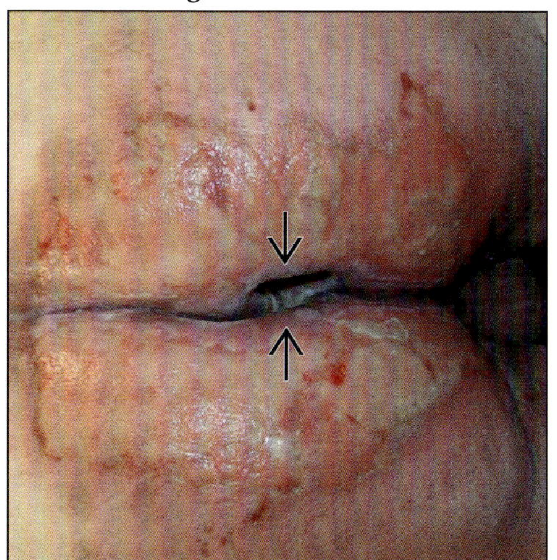

Stage 0 (Tis N0 M0)

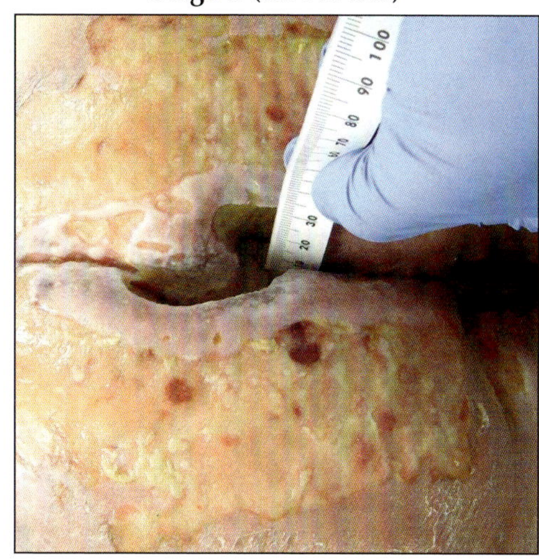

(Left) *Photo of same patient's perianal skin during treatment (at 43.2 Gy/24 fractions) shows decrease in size of bilateral ulcerations ⇨ but grade 3 dermatitis with moist desquamation. Patient required a 6-day treatment break. The final 9 Gy boost after 50.4 Gy was delivered to the focal area plus a 2 cm margin.* ***(Right)*** *Photo taken at 1 month post treatment shows healing skin and surrounding epithelium formation and granulation.*

Stage I (T1 N0 M0)

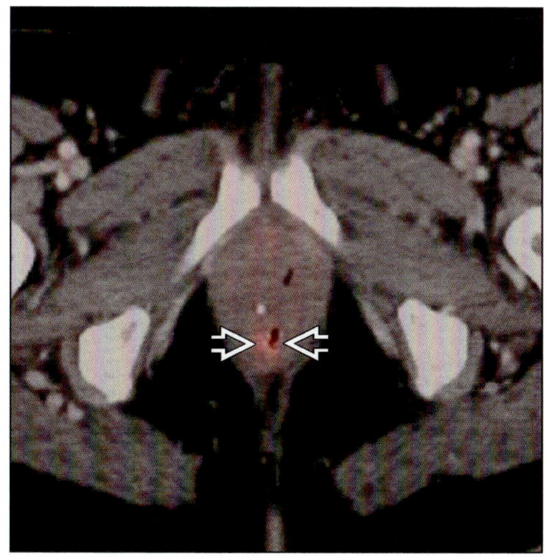

Stage I (T1 N0 M0)

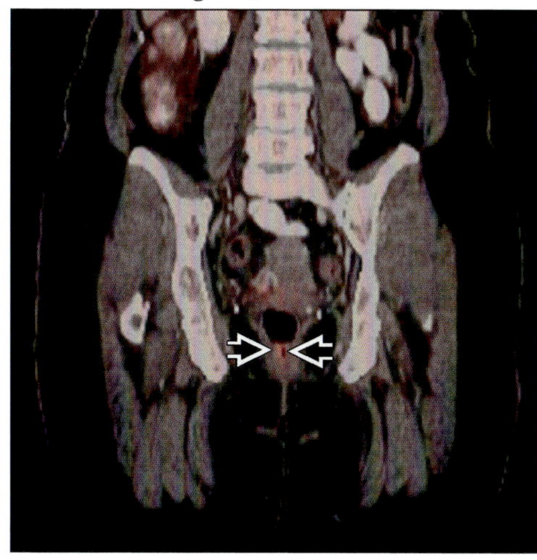

(Left) *Axial PET/CT shows increased metabolic activity (SUV 6.6) in the anus ⇨ of a 59-year-old asymptomatic woman with irregular anorectal mucosa on colonoscopy. Biopsy showed . DRE revealed firmness at the right anal verge. Anoscopy showed a 6 mm mass in anal canal, consistent with T1 disease.* ***(Right)*** *Coronal PET/CT shows same lesion ⇨ in the posterior anal canal to the right of midline, with no evidence of nodal or distant metastases.*

CT Simulation

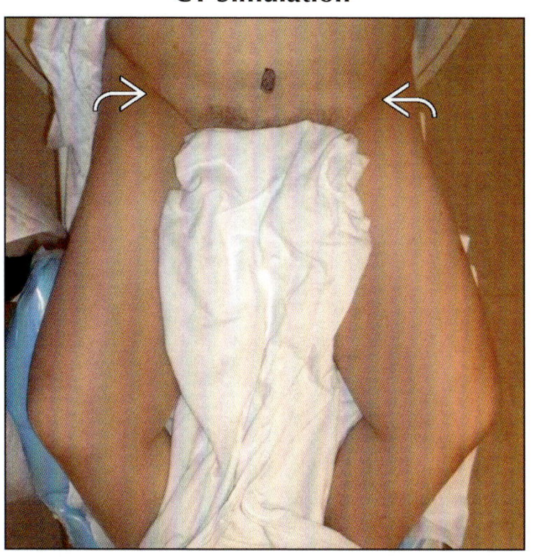

CT Simulation

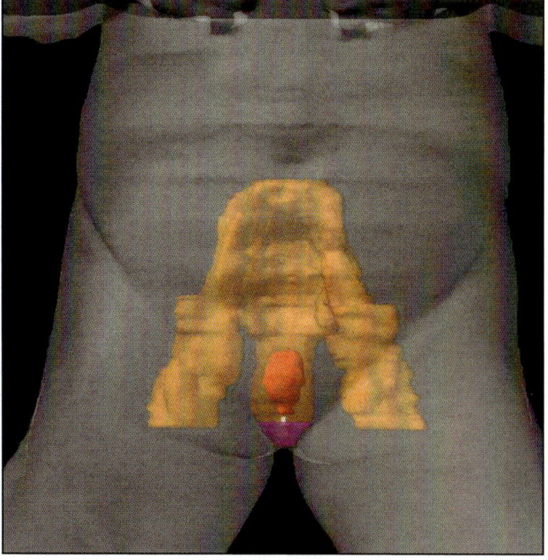

(Left) *Photo shows same patient simulated in supine, frog-leg position to decrease inguinal skin folds ⇨, in alpha cradle, with non-empty bladder and marker at the anal verge.* ***(Right)*** *AP skin rendering shows elective nodal CTV (orange) covering mesorectum, presacral space, internal & external iliac, obturator, and inguinal nodes. The GTV is in red, with an anal verge marker (white) below. External genitalia (magenta) is anterior to the inferiormost part of the CTV.*

(Left) Axial NECT of the same patient shows 50.4 Gy dose colorwash (red), coverage of primary CTV (orange), and 42 Gy (yellow) coverage of the elective nodal CTV (blue) using a dose-painting, simultaneous-integrated boost IMRT technique. *(Right)* Coronal NECT in the same patient shows cranial-caudal extent of 42 Gy dose coverage from the bifurcation of the common iliac vessels at L5/S1 ➔ to below the pelvic diaphragm ➔.

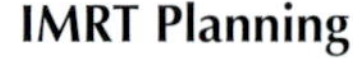

IMRT Planning

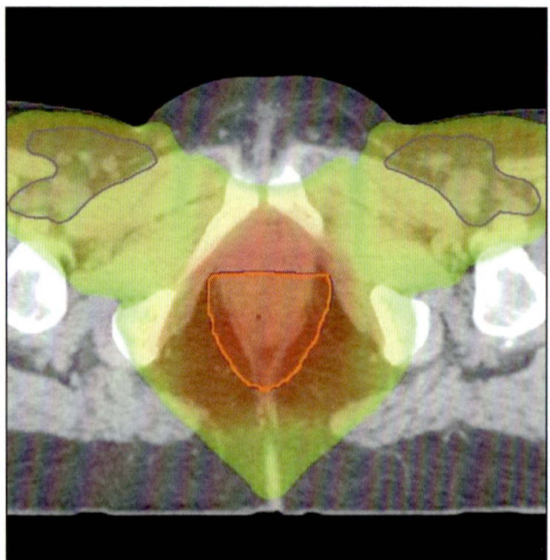

IMRT Planning

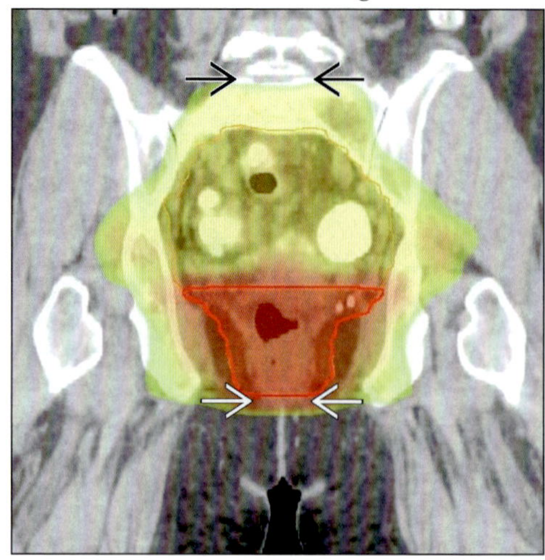

(Left) Axial NECT shows the elective CTV (orange), which should extend beyond the mesorectal fascia to the pelvic sidewalls ➔ laterally and ~ 1 cm into anterior structures ➔. The mesorectum should extend to the presacral space posteriorly, to the rectosigmoid junction cranially, and to the levators caudally. *(Right)* Below the pelvic diaphragm, the CTV (green) should extend only 3-5 mm into fat surrounding the levator ani muscles ➔, unless the tumor extends into the ischiorectal fossa.

Elective CTV

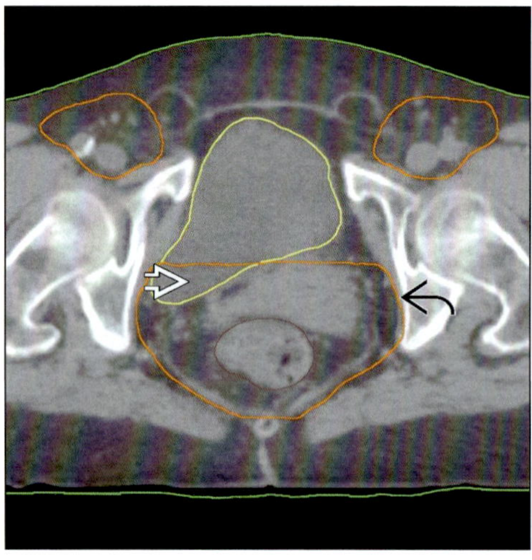

Pelvic Diaphragm

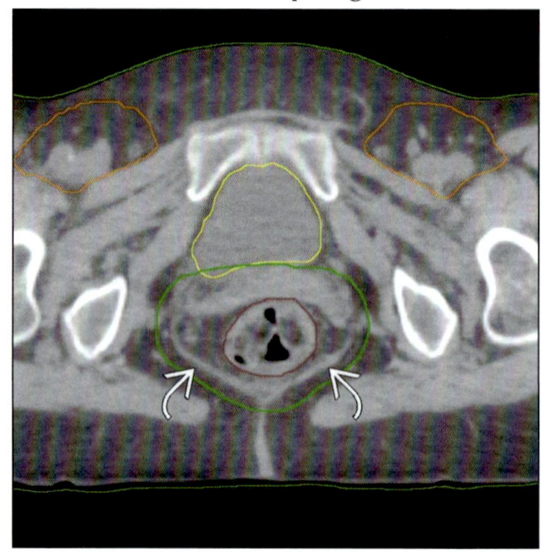

(Left) Axial NECT shows primary GTV (red) contained within the puborectalis muscles ➔. The primary CTV (green) extends 3 mm beyond the muscles. *(Right)* Coronal NECT shows the contour of CTV from the entire mesorectum to the pelvic floor ➔. Note 2 cm expansion cranially & caudally from the GTV to make the primary CTV, which also extends laterally to include the rectum and mesorectum within the expansion.

Pelvic Diaphragm

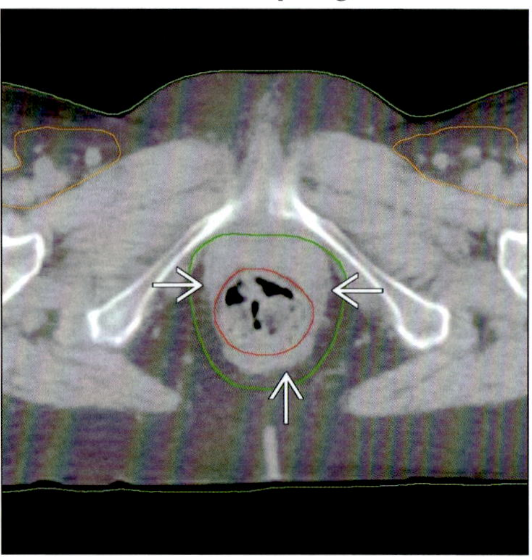

IMRT Planning

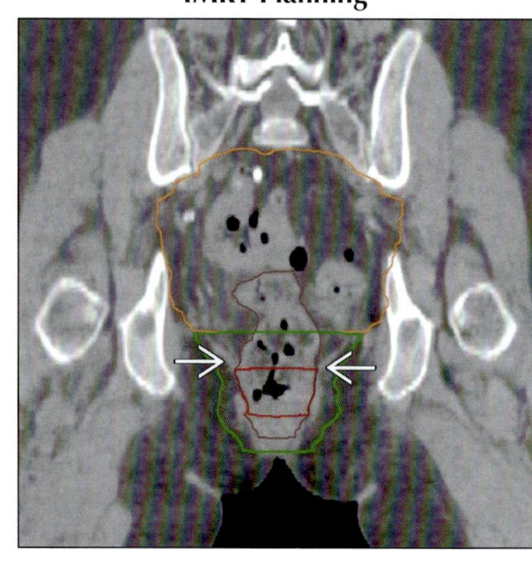

External Iliac Nodes

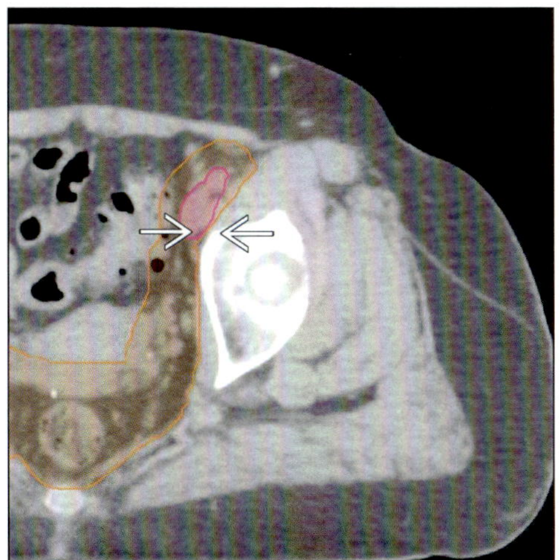

Inguinal Nodes

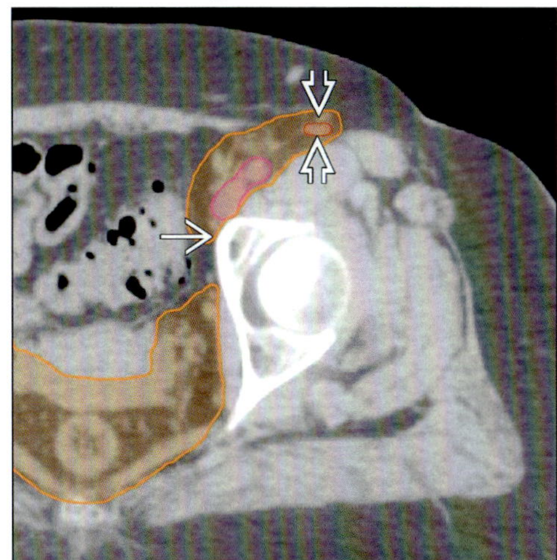

(Left) *Axial NECT shows inferiormost external iliac region (magenta) extent, almost having exited the bony pelvis ➡. CTV (orange) extends 7 mm from vessels, except 1 cm anterolaterally.* ***(Right)*** *When vessels exit the bony pelvis ➡, they become femoral vessels (magenta), approximately at the top of the femoral heads or the superior aspect of the pubic rami. The inguinal CTV should be contoured as a region including femoral vessels and any identified nodes ➡.*

Superficial Inguinal Nodes

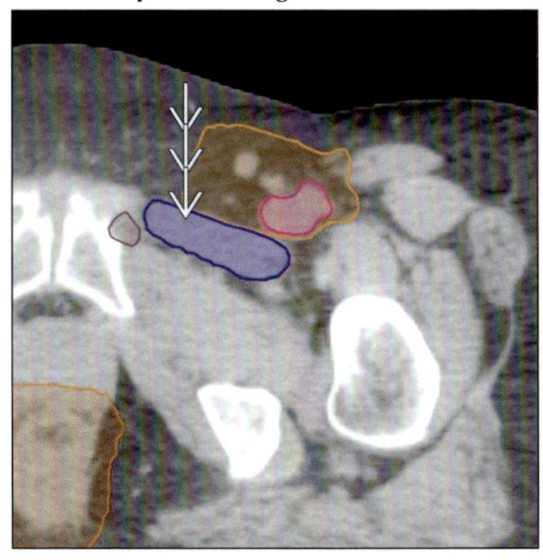

Inguinal Nodes

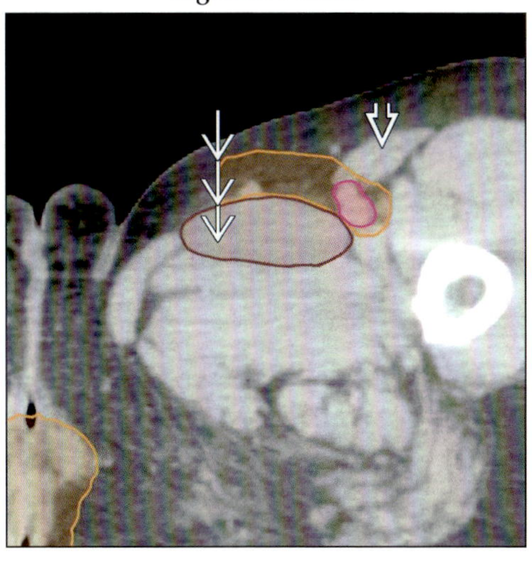

(Left) *Axial NECT shows the inguinal nodal CTV (orange) with a ≥ 1 cm margin around the femoral vessels (magenta), with the medial border at vertical line ➡ transecting the medial 1/2 to 1/3 of pectineus muscle (blue).* ***(Right)*** *A more caudal slice of the axial CT shows the medial border of inguinal nodal CTV (orange) at vertical line ➡ transecting the medial 1/3 of the adductor longus (brown). The lateral border extends to below the sartorius muscle ➡.*

Inguinal Nodes

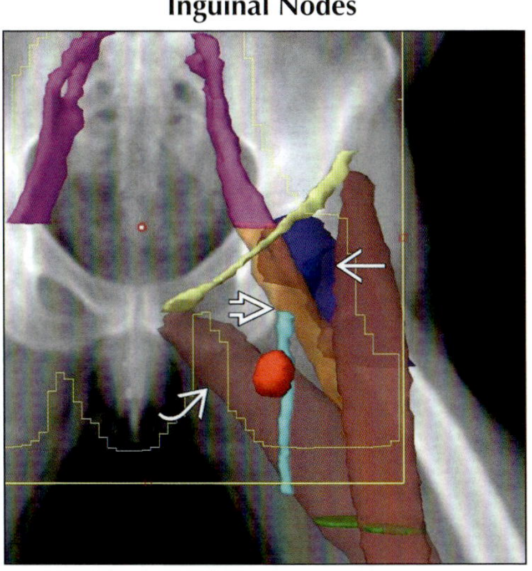

Regional Nodes

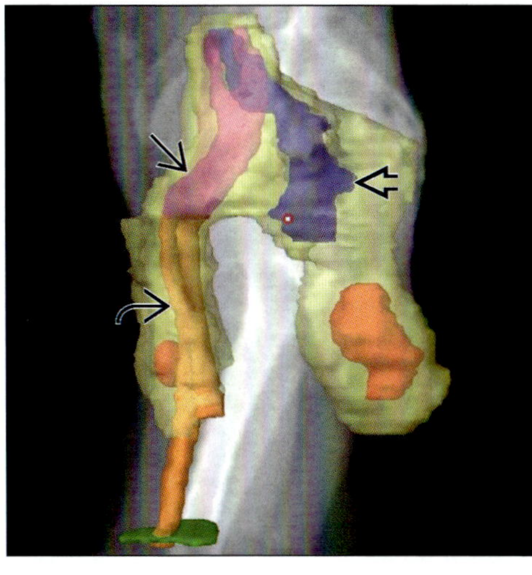

(Left) *AP DRR shows femoral triangle bordered by inguinal ligament (yellow) and medial edges of sartorius ➡ and adductor longus ➡. Caudal inguinal border recommendations include 2 cm below the saphenous (cyan)/femoral (orange) vessel junction ➡. Here, a 2 cm involved node (red) extends 6 cm below this junction.* ***(Right)*** *Sagittal DRR shows entire CTV (yellow) including external iliac ➡, femoral ➡, and internal iliac/ presacral regions ➡ at risk.*

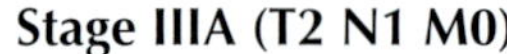

Stage IIIA (T2 N1 M0)

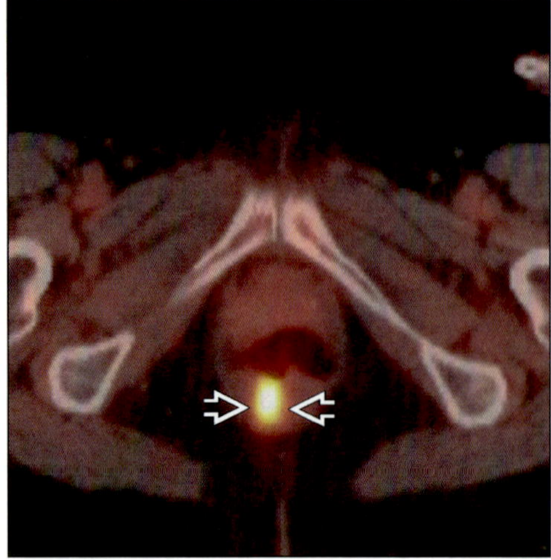

Stage IIIA (T2 N1 M0)

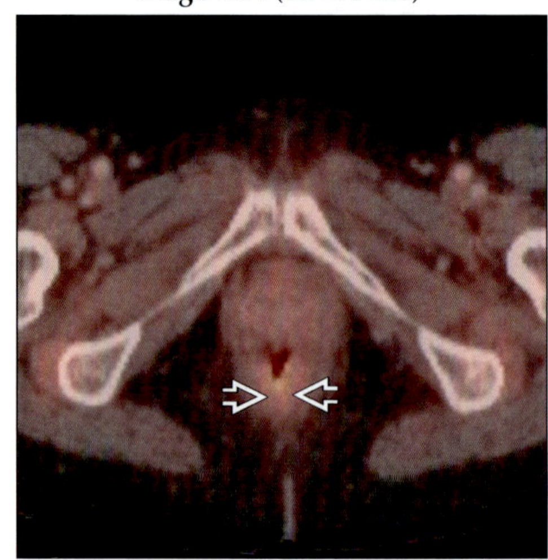

(Left) *Axial PET/CT shows a 4.5 x 2.7 cm hypermetabolic (SUV 13.6) lesion ➡ in right posterior wall of distal rectum and anal canal in a 68-year-old woman presenting with rectal bleeding. Biopsy showed keratinizing SCC. Suspicious subcentimeter, mildly active perirectal nodes make this N1 disease.* ***(Right)*** *Axial PET/CT 9 months after CRT shows resolution of hypermetabolic activity and residual nodularity ➡ in posterior distal rectum and anus.*

3D CRT Planning

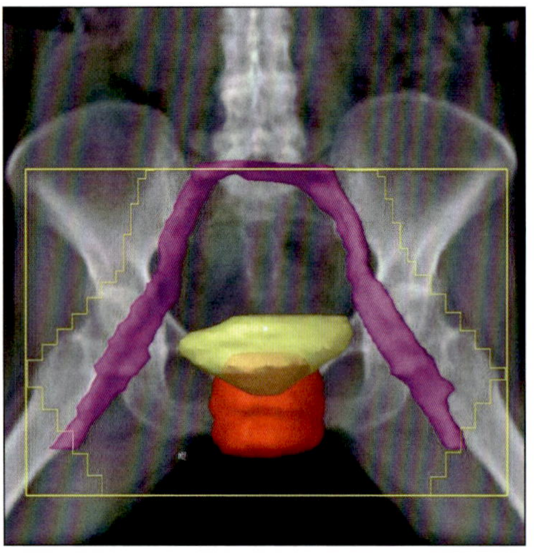

3D CRT Planning

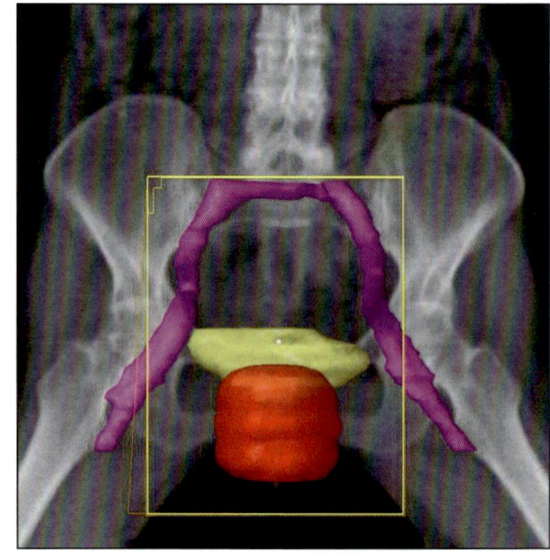

(Left) *DRR shows wide AP field to include bilateral inguinals, internal and external iliacs, and primary GTV (red). The iliofemoral vessels (magenta) guide inguinal fields. Consider adding electrons or photons to cover inguinals, depending on target depth. For AP/PA treatments, match anterior electrons or photons to the PA beam's divergence to bring the inguinal dose to ≥ 36 Gy.* ***(Right)*** *DRR shows narrow PA field. Borders are lateral to the greater sciatic notch.*

3D CRT Planning

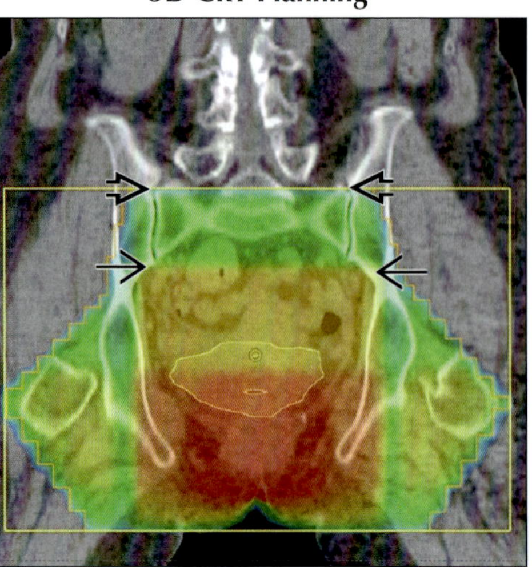

3D CRT Planning

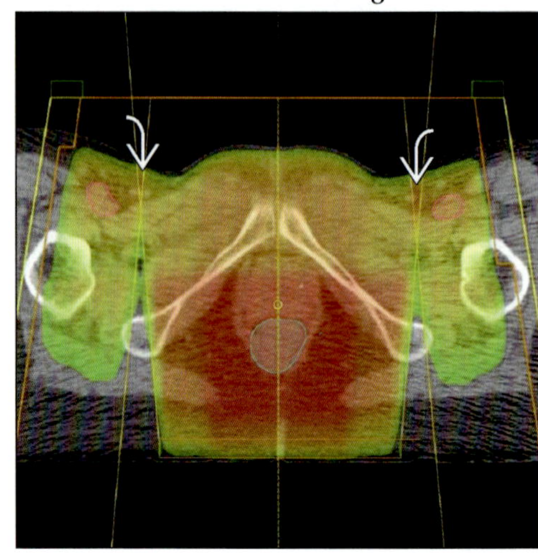

(Left) *Coronal NECT shows dose wash based on the prescriptions: 30.6 Gy to initial field with cranial border at L5/S1 ➡; superior border dropped to inferior SI joints for next 14.4 Gy →. Inguinal and pelvic regions received 45 Gy due to suspicious nodes. DRE showed 75% size reduction but 2.5 cm residual anal mass at 45 Gy, so gross tumor received 9 Gy boost.* ***(Right)*** *Axial NECT shows divergence of PA field into inguinal regions, which can create hotspots ➡.*

Stage IIIB (T3 N2 M0)

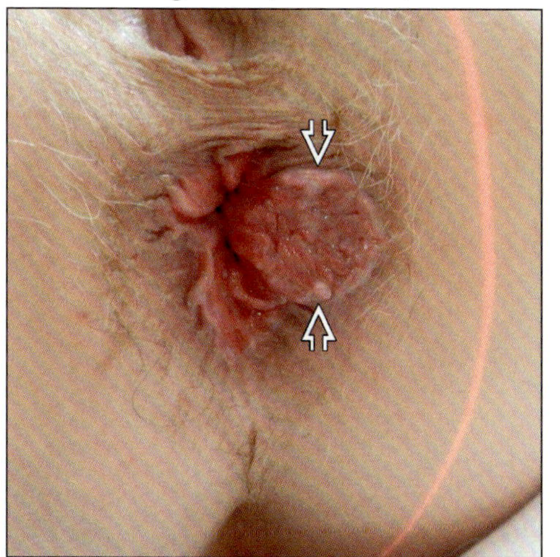

Stage IIIB (T3 N2 M0)

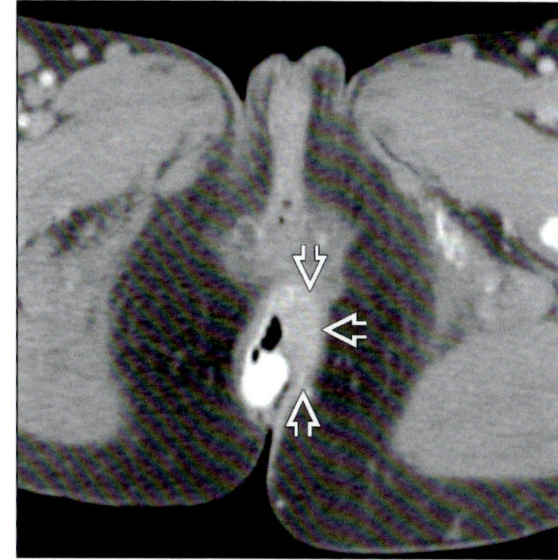

*(**Left**) Photo of a 54-year-old woman shows an exophytic 3 x 2 cm anal margin mass ➡, which extended 3 cm into the anal canal. The total size of the primary tumor is > 5 cm and is therefore a T3 lesion. Biopsy showed SCC. (**Right**) Axial CECT of the same patient shows thickening and increased soft tissue density ➡ in the left anal canal, measuring 2.9 x 1.5 cm. This lesion extends inferiorly to the left levator ani, with involvement of the anal sphincter.*

Stage IIIB (T3 N2 M0)

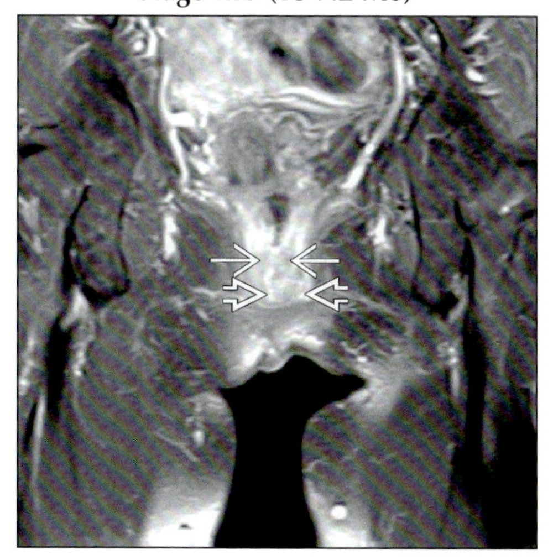

Stage IIIB (T3 N2 M0)

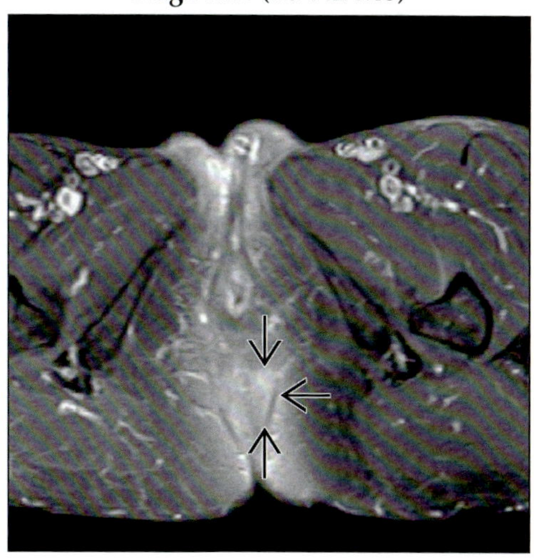

*(**Left**) Coronal T1WI C+ FS MR in the same patient shows an enhancing lesion ➡ located mostly superficially to the anal sphincter ➡ and inferiorly to the levators, but extending into the anal canal. (**Right**) Axial T1WI C + FS MR in the same patient confirms enhancement ➡ in the left anal verge next to the sphincter. There is no involvement of vulva or distal vagina. A concerning 14 mm enhancing left lateral inguinal node (not shown) makes the nodal stage N2.*

Tumor Regression

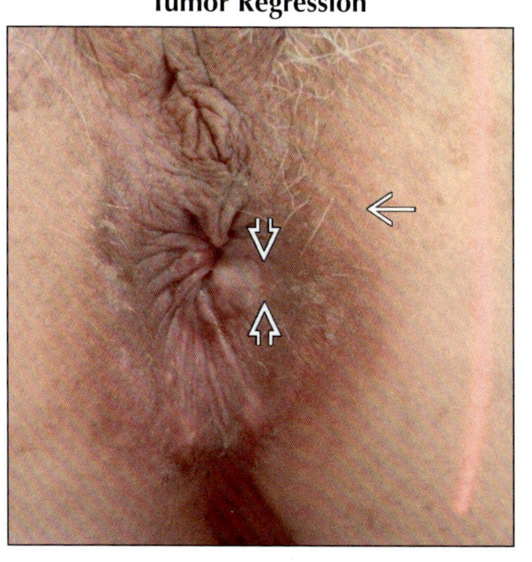

Tumor Regression

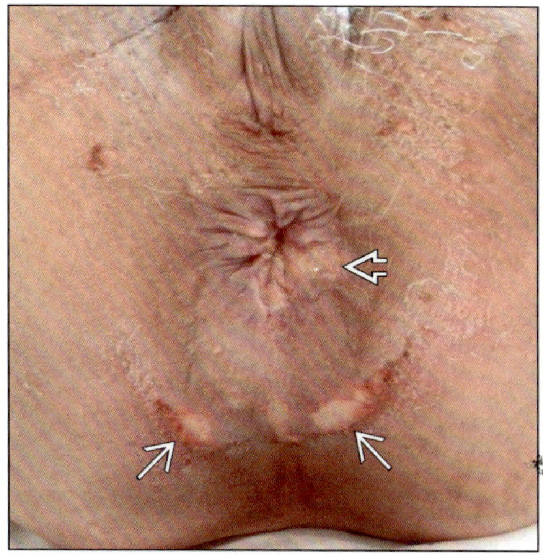

*(**Left**) Same patient was treated with definitive CRT. Photo shows significant regression of anal mass with small residual ulceration ➡ after receiving 34.2 Gy of the 54 Gy prescription dose to primary tumor. Only trace skin erythema is noted ➡. (**Right**) Photo of the same patient at the end of treatment shows grade 2 dermatitis (moist desquamation in areas of skin folds ➡). There is only an ulcer ➡ present where the tumor used to be.*

*(**Left**) 3D CRT plan was generated for the same patient using AP/PA technique. Axial NECT in the plane inferior to the SI joints shows 45 Gy dose colorwash (yellow) encompassing at-risk nodal areas as well as small bowel. (**Right**) The same patient was treated with IMRT using the following prescriptions: 54 Gy to the primary PTV, 50.4 Gy to the suspicious inguinal node, and 45 Gy to elective nodes, all in 30 fractions. Axial NECT shows small bowel sparing →.*

3D CRT Planning

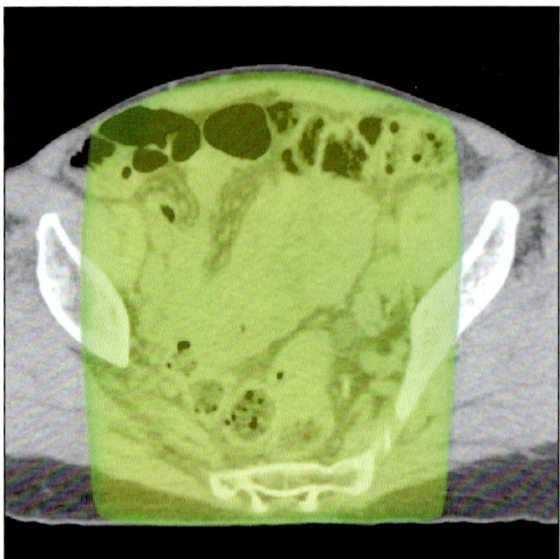

IMRT Planning

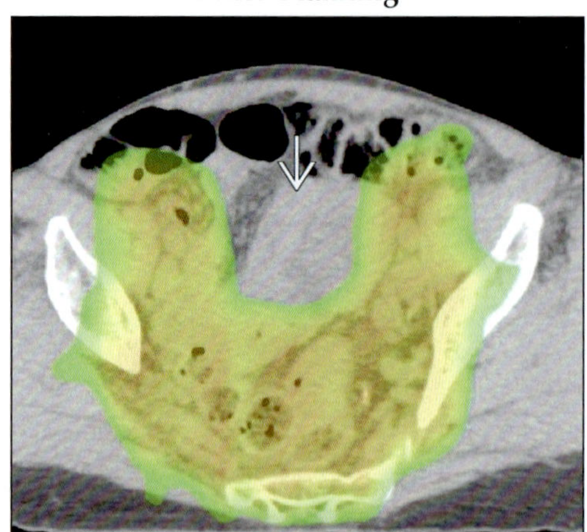

*(**Left**) Coronal NECT of the 3D CRT plan in same patient shows 30.6 Gy (green) → covering the pelvis above the inf. SI joints, 45 Gy (yellow) → covering the pelvis below SI joints and the inguinal regions, and 54 Gy (red) covering the primary tumor. External genitalia → receives full prescription dose. (**Right**) Coronal NECT in the same patient shows the IMRT dose-painting technique providing relative sparing of external genitalia → and small bowel →.*

3D CRT Planning

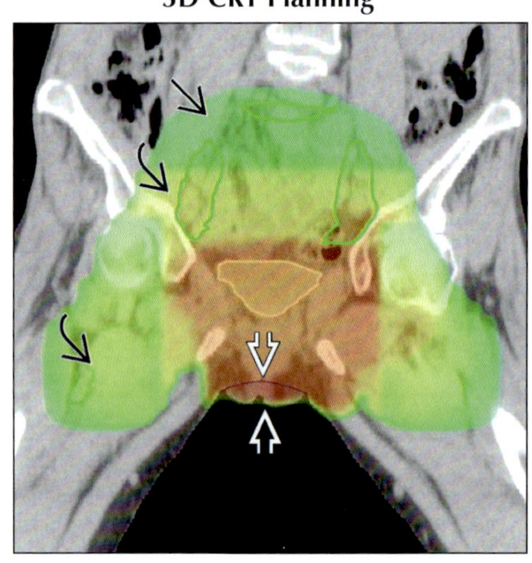

IMRT Planning

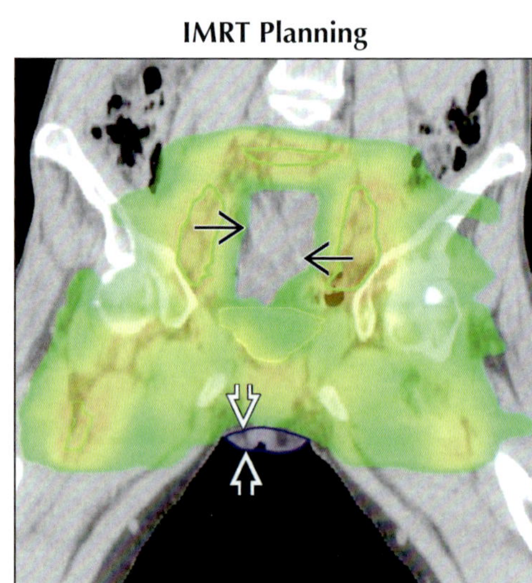

*(**Left**) Sagittal NECT in the same patient shows different field reductions with area above inferior SI joint receiving 30.6 Gy, low sacrum receiving 45 Gy, and pelvic floor structures receiving 54 Gy. (**Right**) Sagittal view in the same patient shows relative sparing of small bowel →, bladder (yellow), and external genitalia (blue) →. IMRT reduces dose to anterior structures and is associated with lower acute grade 3 GI/GU & skin toxicity compared to 3D CRT.*

3D CRT Planning

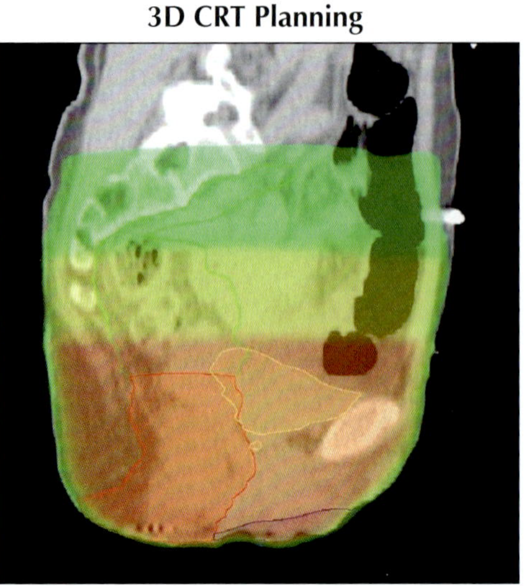

IMRT Planning

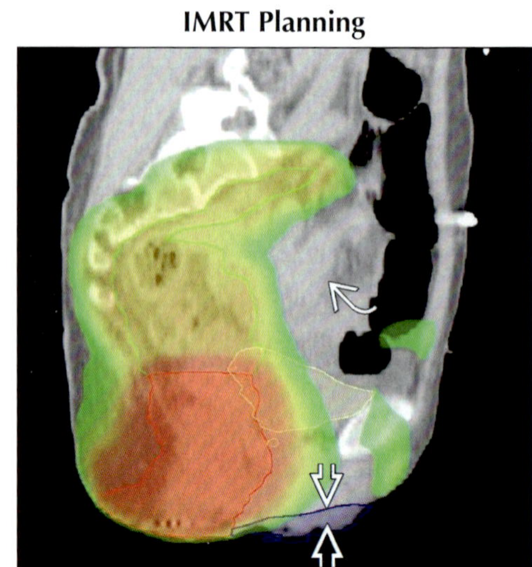

Stage IIIB (T2 N3 M0)

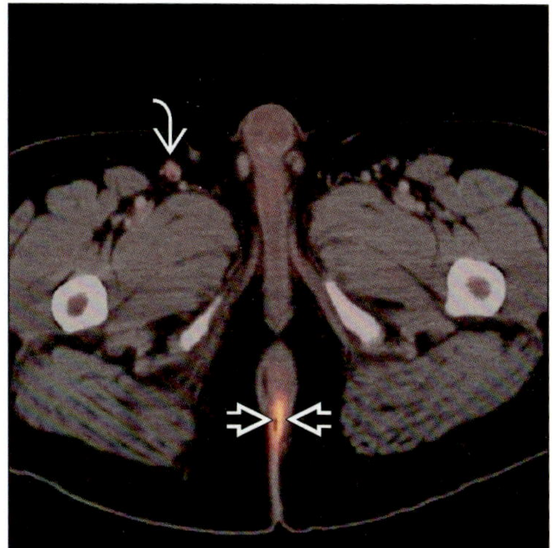

IMRT Planning

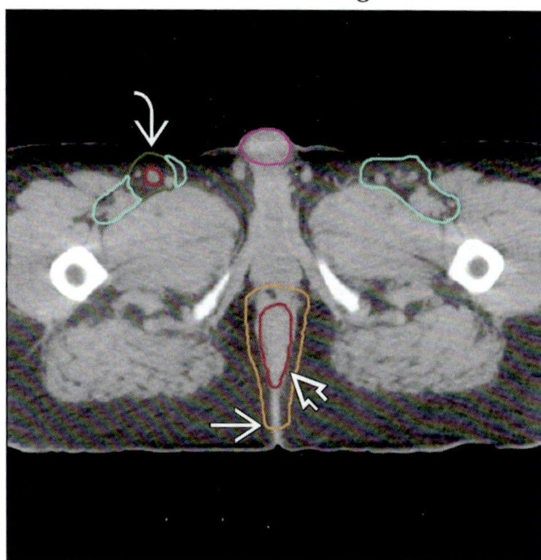

*(**Left**) Axial PET/CT in a male patient shows a 2.8 x 1.0 cm hypermetabolic nodule (SUV 16.7) ➡ along the left anus and a 1.2 cm right inguinal node ➡ (SUV 3.3). Bilateral inguinal nodes make this N3 disease. (**Right**) Same patient was treated with IMRT. Primary CTV (orange) receives 54 Gy and extends 5 mm into the ischiorectal fat ➡ and 2 cm along the perianal skin from the GTV (red) ➡. Elective CTV (cyan) receives 45 Gy. 1 cm around nodes ≤ 3 cm ➡ receives 50.4 Gy (green).*

Post Treatment

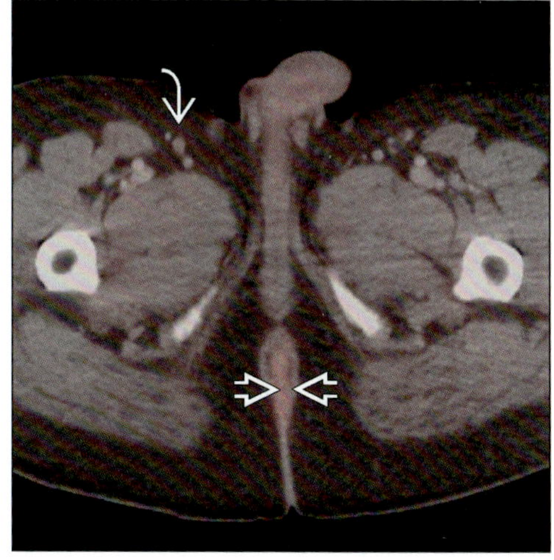

Post Biopsy

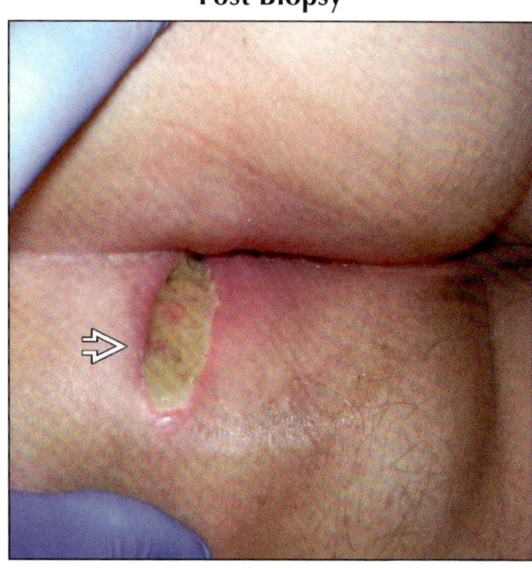

*(**Left**) Axial PET/CT in the same patient 3 months after CRT shows a marked decrease in FDG activity of the anal lesion (SUV 4.7) ➡ and the right inguinal node ➡. (**Right**) After CRT, a 1 cm ulcer at the left anal margin persisted in the same patient. Serial exams showed no regression. Therefore, at 5 months, the anal ulcer was excised, with pathology showing no residual carcinoma. Photo shows biopsy site ➡ 2 weeks postop. The ulcer took 6 months to completely heal.*

Stage IIIC (T3 N3 M0)

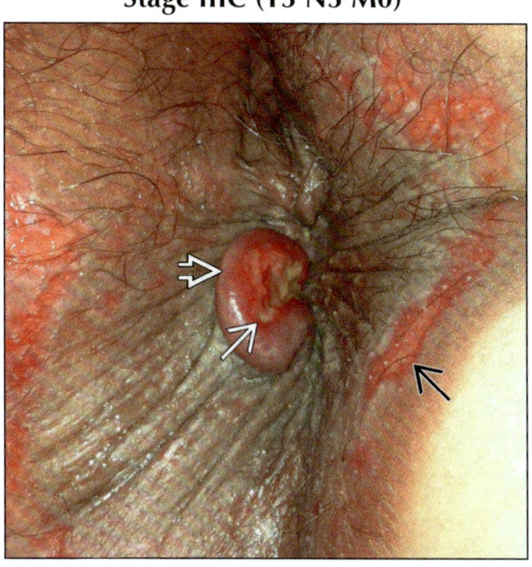

Stage IIIC (T3 N3 M0)

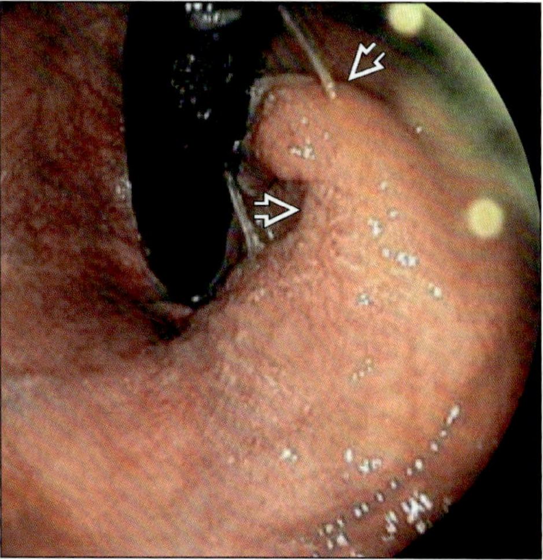

*(**Left**) Photo of a 55-year-old woman shows 2.5 cm external skin tag ➡ at right posterolateral position. Underlying the skin tag is a visible ulceration ➡, with a contiguous palpable mass extending 4 cm into the anal canal. Biopsy shows SCC. After discontinuation of a topical cream, allergic contact dermatitis ➡ resolved. (**Right**) Retroflexed view from colonoscopy in the same patient shows an area of heaped-up ulceration ➡ in the distal rectum near the anus.*

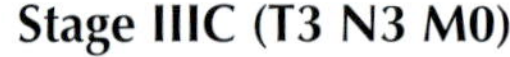

Stage IIIC (T3 N3 M0)

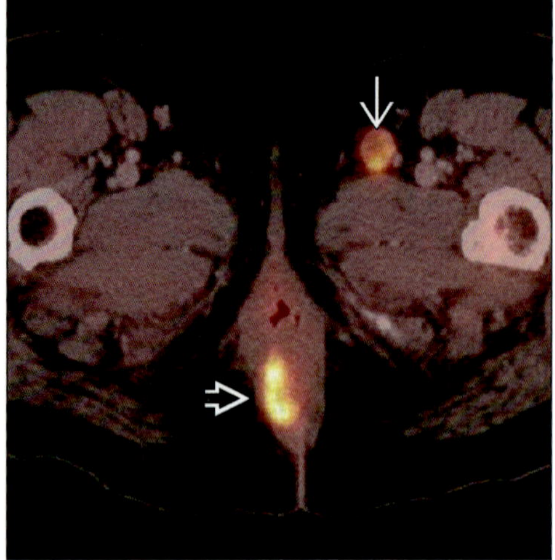

Stage IIIC (T3 N3 M0)

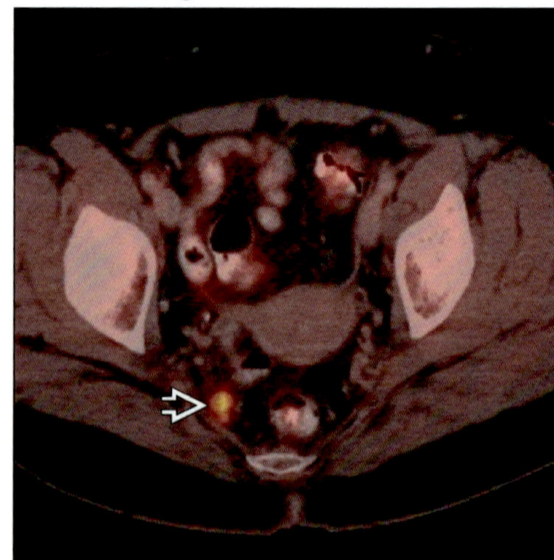

(Left) *Axial PET/CT in the same patient shows the right-sided lesion at the anal verge with increased FDG activity (SUV 16.2) extending into the anal canal ⇨. There is a 2.3 cm, necrotic left inguinal node → with peripheral enhancement and central hypoattenuation (SUV 8.2).* ***(Right)*** *Additionally, there is a 1.3 x 1.1 cm, hypermetabolic (SUV 9.8) right perirectal node ⇨. Simultaneous metastases in perirectal and inguinal nodes are N3 disease.*

Stage IIIA (T4 N0 M0)

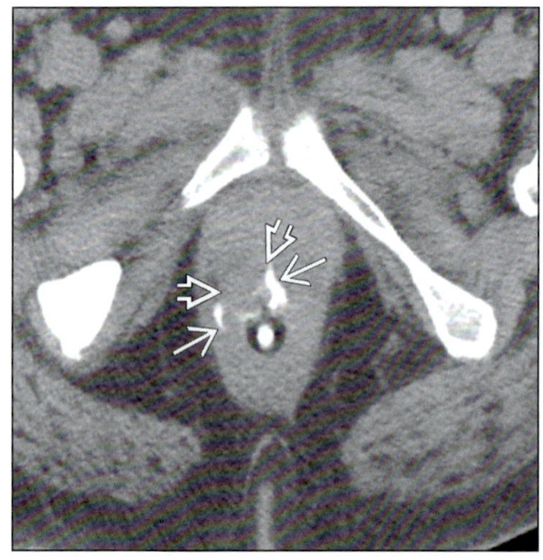

Stage IIIA (T4 N0 M0)

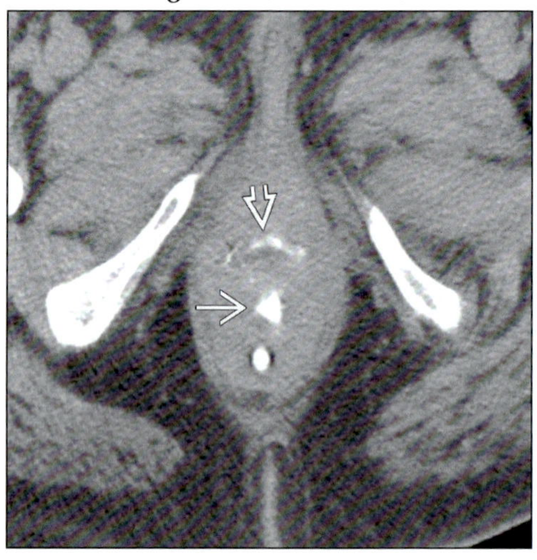

(Left) *Axial NECT after administration of rectal contrast in a 54-year-old woman, who presented due to passage of stool through the vagina, shows the contrast within the anal canal → and a filling defect ⇨ representing an anal carcinoma.* ***(Right)*** *Axial NECT in the same patient shows contrast both within the anal canal → and vagina ⇨ due to anovaginal fistula resulting from the anal carcinoma. Invasion of vagina makes this T4 disease.*

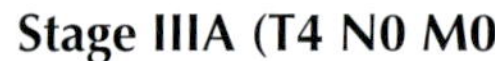

Stage IIIA (T4 N0 M0)

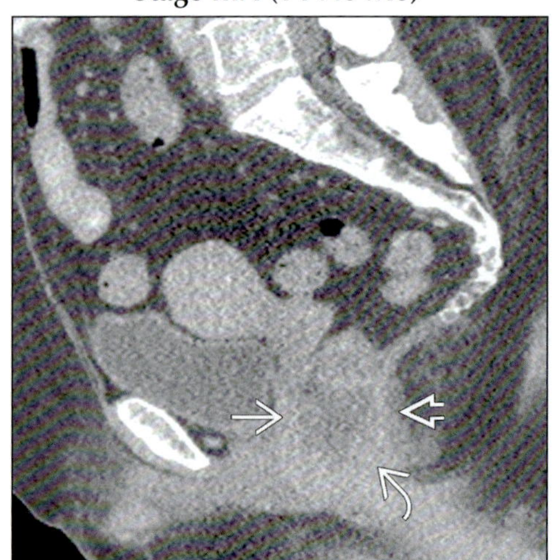

Stage IIIA (T4 N0 M0)

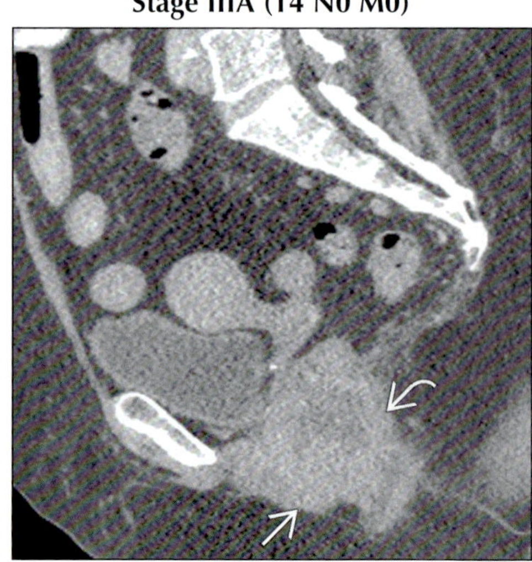

(Left) *Sagittal CECT in the same patient shows the anal mass ↗ invading the distal vagina → and the levator ani muscle ⇨.* ***(Right)*** *Sagittal CECT in the same patient shows the anal mass ↗ invading the skin of the perineum →.*

Stage IV (T4 N3 M1)

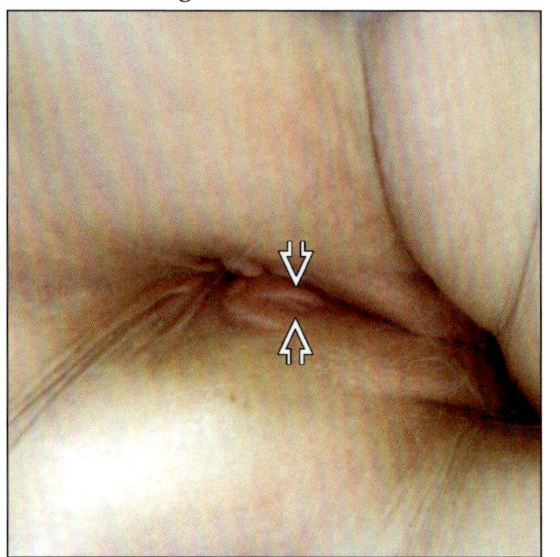

Stage IV (T4 N3 M1)

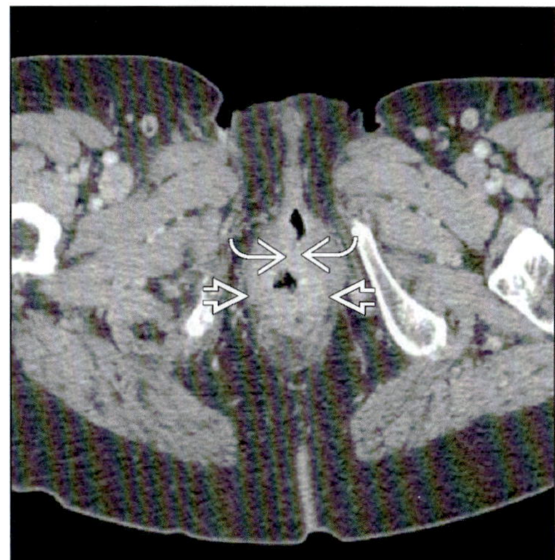

(Left) *Photo shows a polypoid lesion ➡ extending into the left anterior anal canal in a 68-year-old woman presenting with vaginal spotting and vaginal fecal discharge. EUA shows a 4 cm anal mass invading the posterior vagina, forming an anovaginal fistula. Biopsy of anal mass and vaginal wall show basaloid SCC.* ***(Right)*** *Axial CECT in the same patient shows the mass in the distal rectum and anus ➡, with an irregular lumen extending anteriorly to form an anovaginal fistula ➡.*

Stage IV (T4 N3 M1)

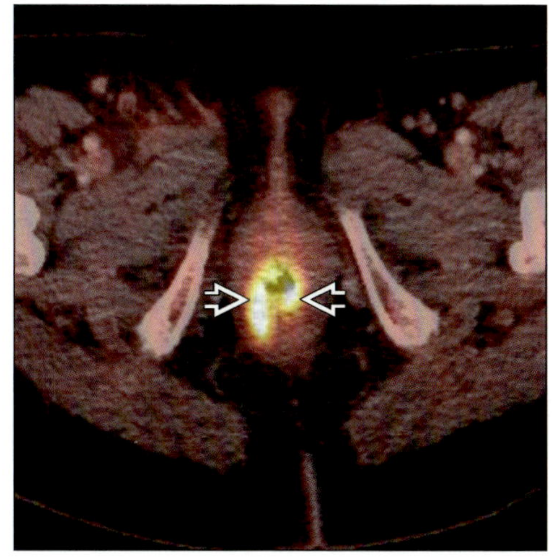

Stage IV (T4 N3 M1)

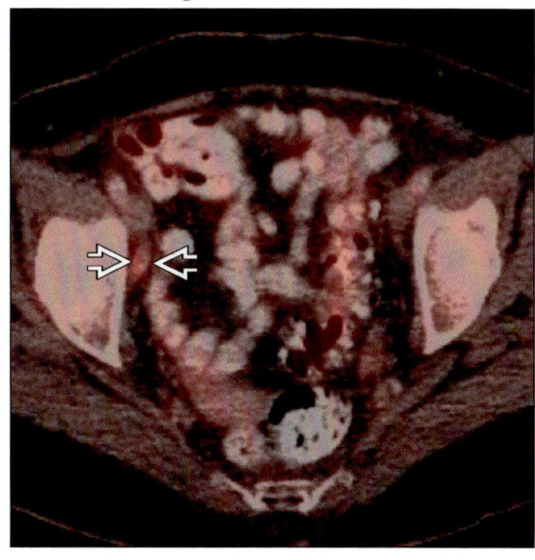

(Left) *Axial PET/CT in the same patient shows that the lobulated mass ➡ is hypermetabolic (SUV 22.5) with activity extending from the anal verge to the distal rectum, with anterior extension to the vagina.* ***(Right)*** *Axial PET/CT in the same patient shows a mildly hypermetabolic (SUV 3.5), 1.9 x 2.8 cm, right external iliac node ➡. This is considered a nonregional node in anal cancer and is therefore M1 disease.*

Stage IV (T4 N3 M1)

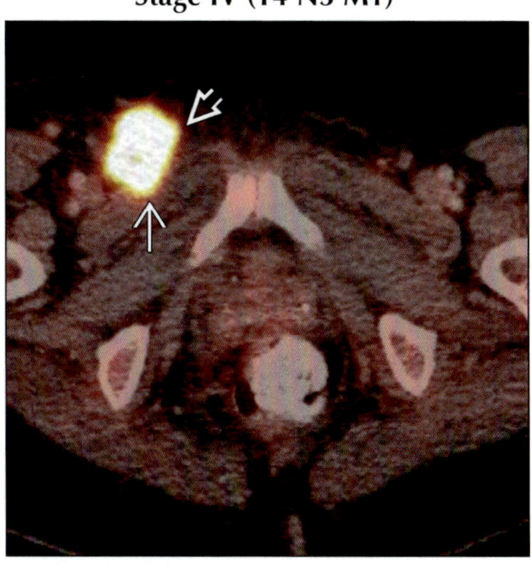

Stage IV (T4 N3 M1)

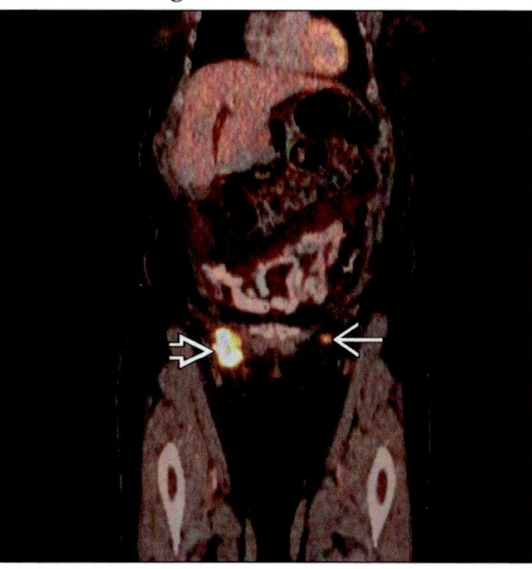

(Left) *Pretreatment axial PET/CT in the same patient shows a 4.2 x 3.6 cm, necrotic, hypermetabolic right inguinal node (SUV 25.6) ➡ with surrounding stranding, invasion of pectineus muscle ➡, and thickening of dermis.* ***(Right)*** *Coronal PET/CT in the same patient shows hypermetabolic right inguinal node ➡ and a small (13 mm), metabolically active (SUV 5.8) left inguinal node ➡. Bilateral inguinal adenopathy represents N3 disease.*

(Left) Axial NECT in the same patient with dose colorwash shows coverage of the primary CTV (orange) to 54 Gy. Extended margins beyond the levator muscles ➡ & into the vagina ➡ were used due to her T4 status. Note sparing of high-dose region to genitalia (blue) & femora. *(Right)* Axial PET/CT in the same patient 6 months after CRT shows marked decrease in FDG uptake of primary tumor ➡ (SUV 3.7) & vagina ➡. A vaginal dilator was recommended post RT to prevent stenosis.

IMRT Planning

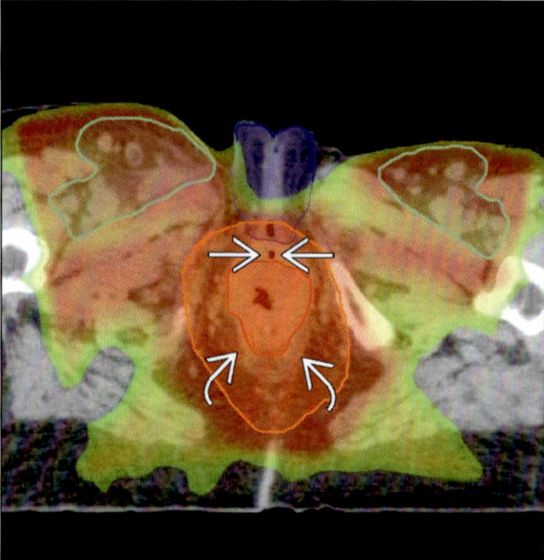

Tumor Regression

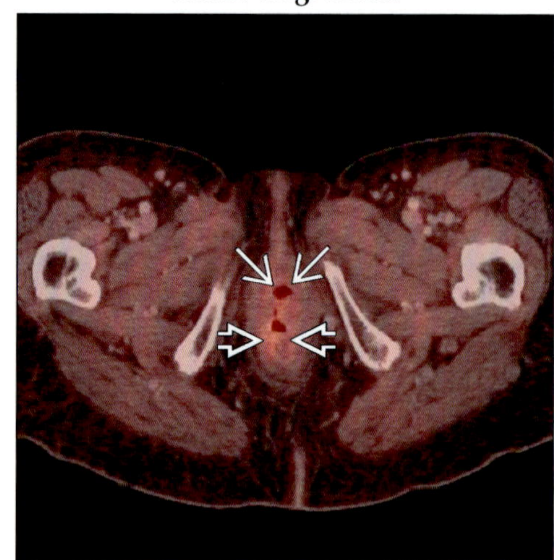

(Left) Axial CT in same patient shows node > 3 cm (red) ➡ receiving 54 Gy. Nodes ≤ 3 cm (green) ➡ should receive 50.4 Gy. Elective nodes should receive 45 Gy, with doses delivered in 30 fractions via IMRT dose-painting technique. *(Right)* Coronal NECT in same patient shows high-dose coverage of bilateral inguinal nodal regions and a boost to the large right node ➡. IMRT allows sparing of the small bowel and genitalia ➡ from the high-dose regions.

IMRT Planning

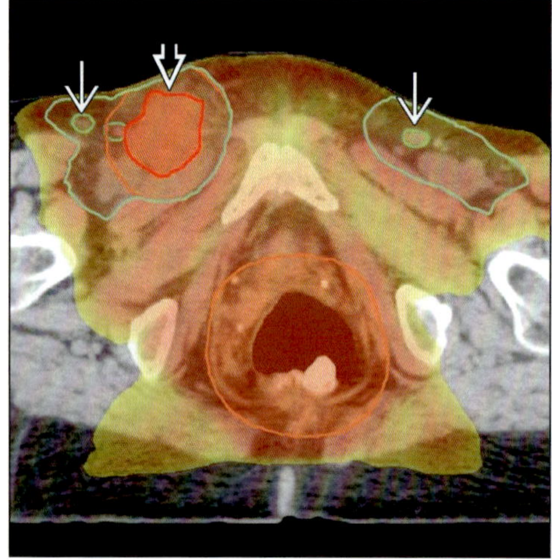

IMRT Planning

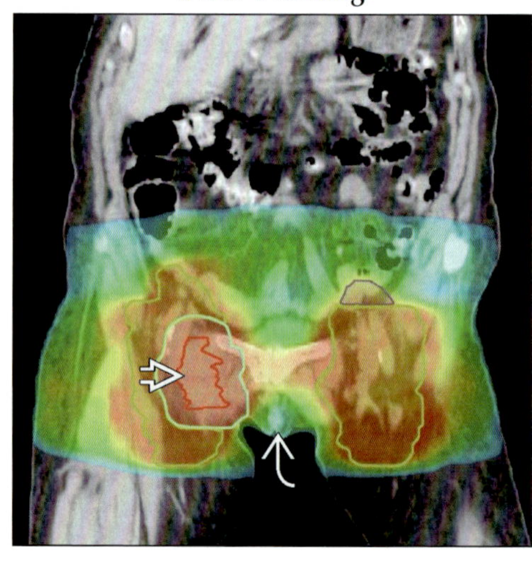

(Left) Axial PET/CT in the same patient 6 months after CRT shows that the large, metabolically active lymph node in the right inguinal region ➡ has resolved. *(Right)* In addition to resolution of the right inguinal node ➡ in the same patient, the previously demonstrated left hypermetabolic inguinal lymph node has significantly decreased in size to 8 mm ➡ and is no longer metabolically active after CRT.

Tumor Regression

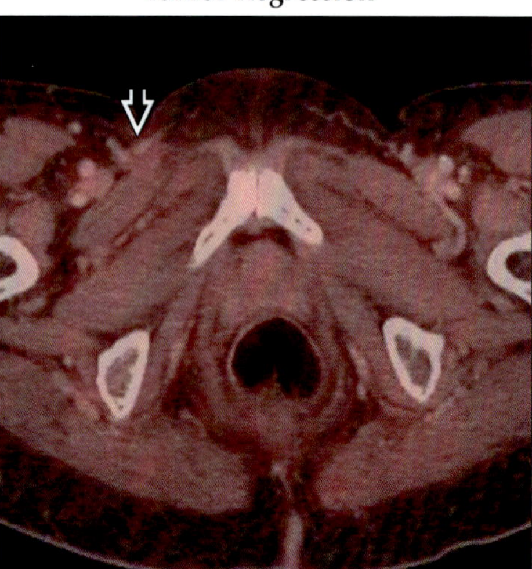

Tumor Regression

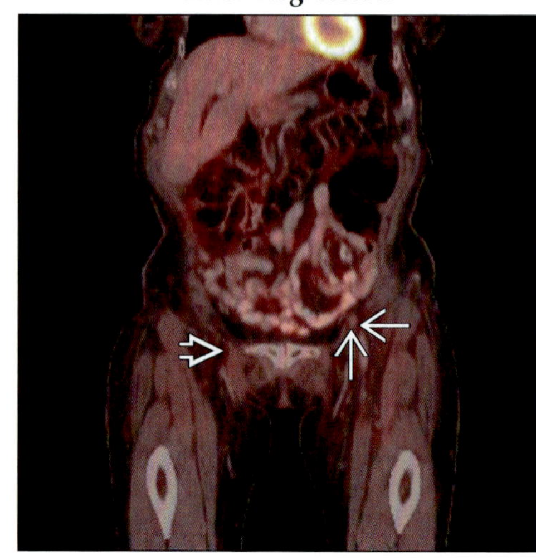

Stage IV (T3 N3 M1)

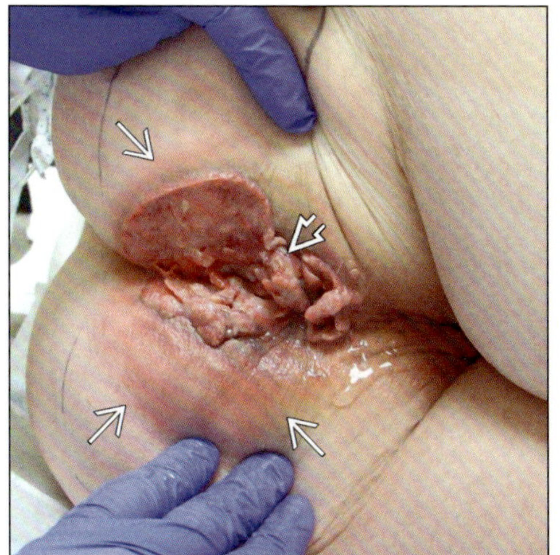

Stage IV (T3 N3 M1)

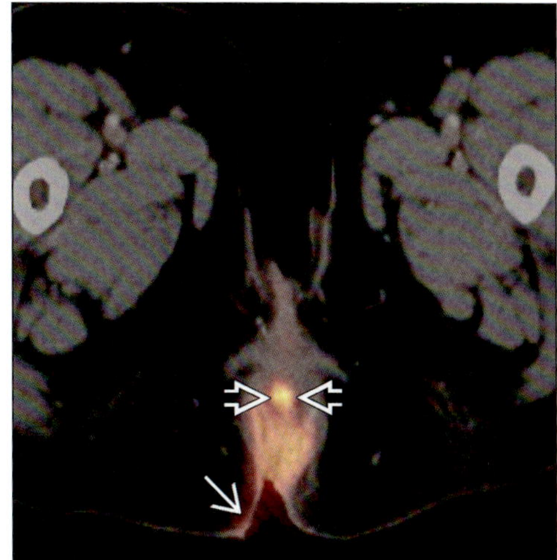

(Left) Photo shows a 6 cm ulcerating and fungating lesion ➔ involving the bilateral perianal skin, which also extends to the left perianal region and anal canal. There is extensive area of skin erythema ➔ surrounding the lesion. Biopsy confirms SCC. **(Right)** Axial fused PET/CT in the same patient shows an ill-defined (SUV 21.5) lesion in the anal canal ➔. Diffuse metabolic activity extensively involving the anal margin skin ➔ likely represents tumor.

Stage IV (T3 N3 M1)

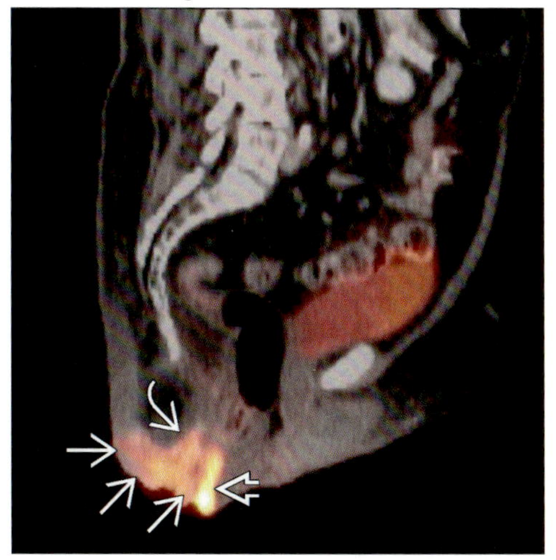

Stage IV (T3 N3 M1)

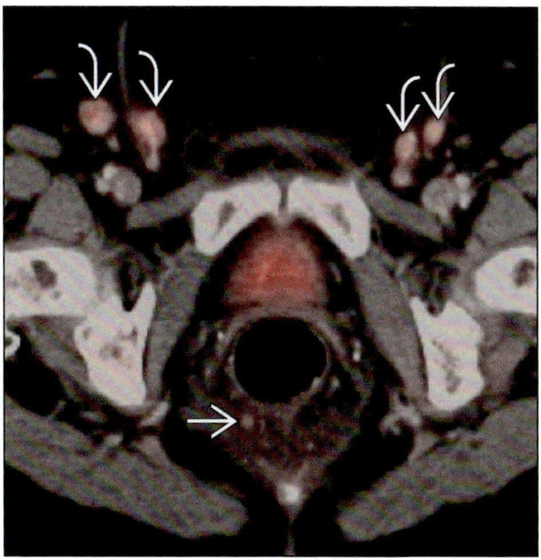

(Left) Sagittal PET/CT in the same patient shows the ~ 2.3 x 3 cm anal canal lesion ➔. Increased FDG uptake of perianal skin ➔ corresponds to the area of erythema. In addition, there is hazy opacity and metabolic activity in the perirectal fat ➔. **(Right)** Axial PET/CT (same patient) shows bilateral enlarged, hypermetabolic inguinal lymph nodes ➔, the largest at 1.5 cm (SUV 8.7). Also note many small hypermetabolic perirectal ➔, internal, & external iliac nodes.

IMRT Planning

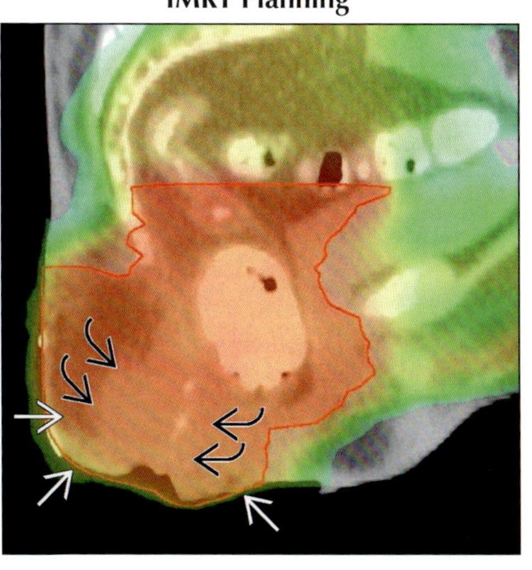

IMRT Planning

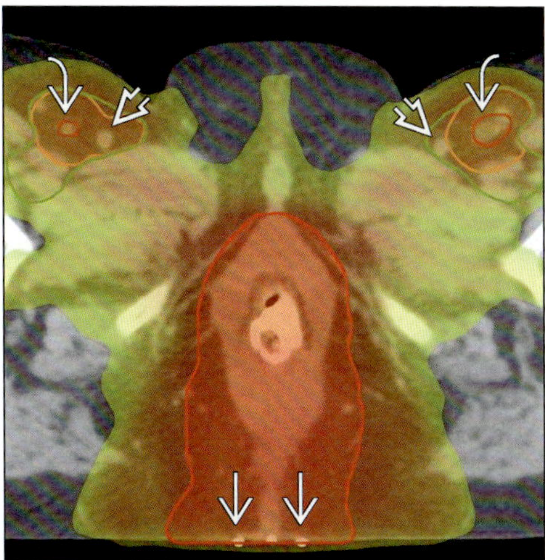

(Left) The same patient was treated with IMRT. Sagittal NECT shows the 54 Gy red dose colorwash covering the primary CTV (red), which includes perianal skin ➔, anorectum, and perirectal thickening ➔. **(Right)** Axial NECT in the same patient shows the primary CTV (red) extending 2 cm beyond areas of skin erythema as marked by wire ➔. Involved nodes ➔ receive 50.4 Gy, and elective nodes receive 45 Gy (green). Note the saphenous vein medially ➔.

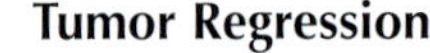

Tumor Regression

(Left) Photo of the same patient taken on last day of treatment shows significant tumor regression and grade 2 dermatitis. Patchy moist desquamation ➡ was confined to skin folds. White plaques in perianal area were treated with nystatin cream. *(Right)* Photo of the same patient at the 3-week follow-up shows further significant tumor regression and significant healing of the radiation dermatitis. There is a residual 3.5 cm ulcer ➡.

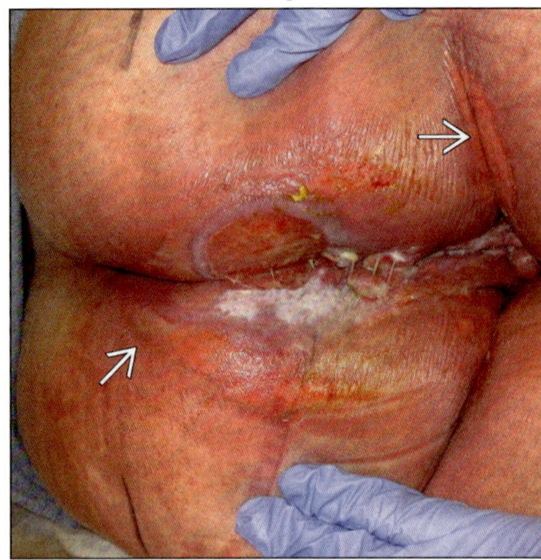

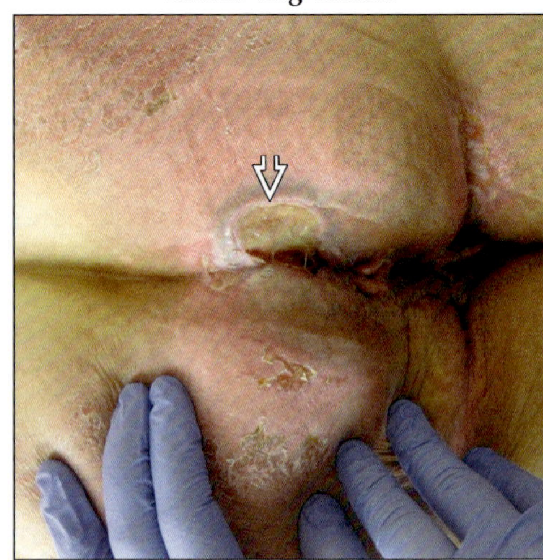

Local Recurrence

(Left) This 56-year-old woman had transanal excision of a T2 N0 proximal anal canal SCC 3 years ago. Surveillance anoscopy showed a polypoid lesion at the left posterolateral anal canal. Excisional biopsy showed recurrent SCC. Axial PET/CT shows focal asymmetric thickening of the posterior anus (SUV 6.6) ➡. *(Right)* Sagittal PET/CT in the same patient shows craniocaudal extent of the focal lesion in the posterior anal canal ➡, with no involved lymph nodes.

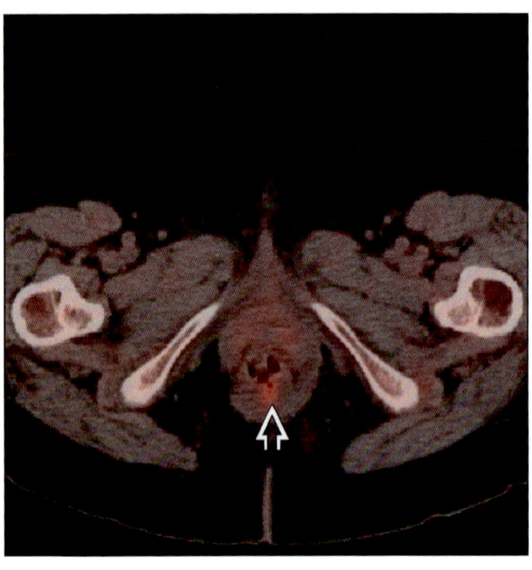

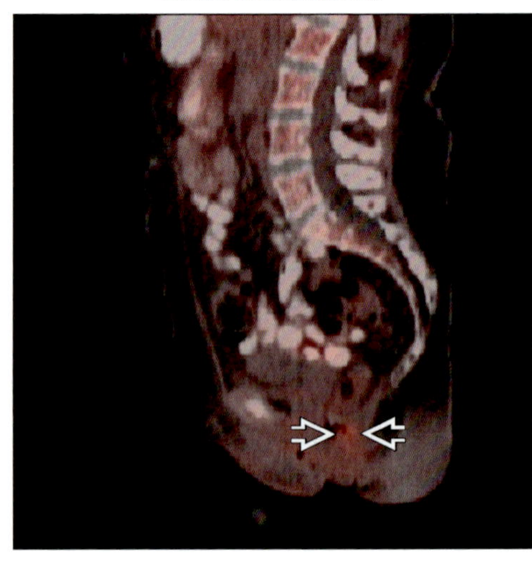

Polycystic Kidney Disease

(Left) Axial PET/CT in same patient shows enlarged liver parenchyma with multiple cysts ➡ without focal hypermetabolic activity. The native kidneys are nearly completely replaced with cysts ➡ and calcifications. *(Right)* Sagittal PET/CT in the same patient shows multiple liver cysts predominantly in the left lobe. Although lymph nodes and liver are common sites of spread in anal cancer, there is no evidence of nodal or distant metastases in this patient.

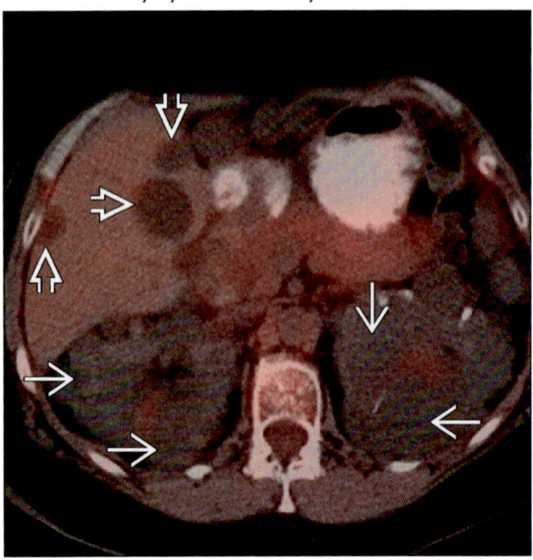

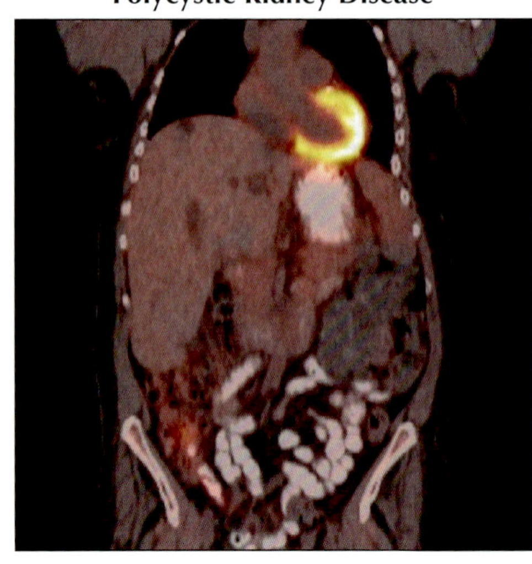

IMRT Planning

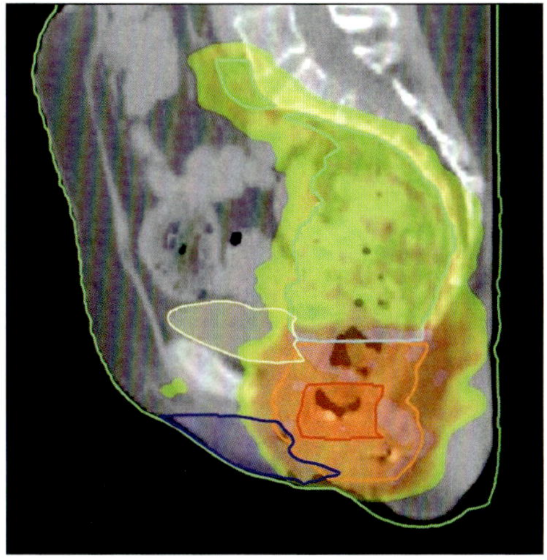

IMRT Planning

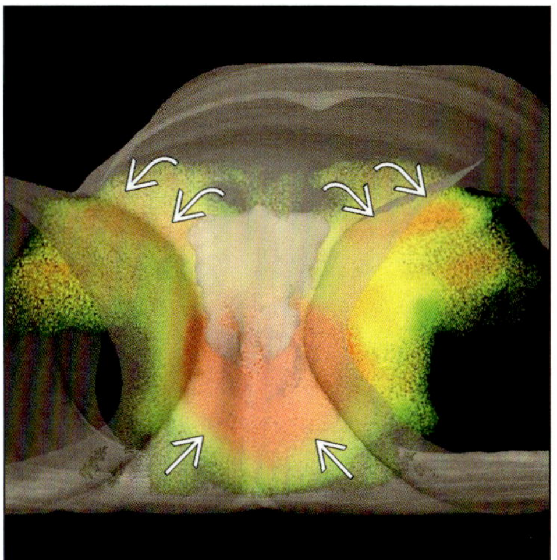

*(**Left**) The same patient underwent definitive CRT for locally recurrent anal cancer. Sagittal NECT with colorwash shows coverage of primary CTV (orange) with 50.4 Gy (red) and elective nodal CTV (cyan) with 42 Gy (yellow). Primary GTV (red) includes entire anorectum at level of recurrent tumor. (**Right**) Skin rendering in same patient shows high-dose colorwash (red) covering perianal skin ➔ and inguinal skin folds ➔ but sparing external genitalia (white).*

Grade 3 Dermatitis

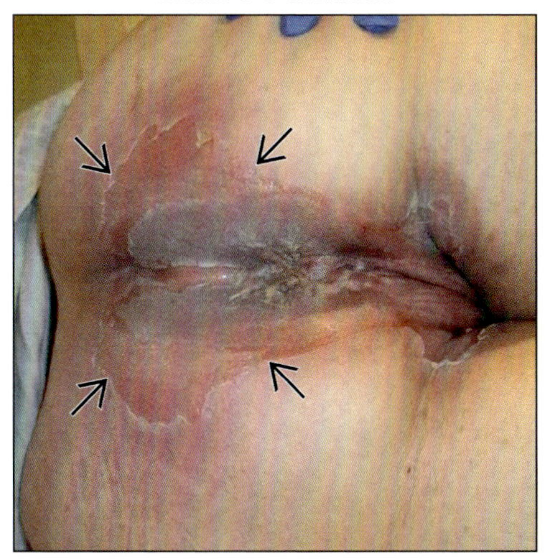

Grade 3 Dermatitis

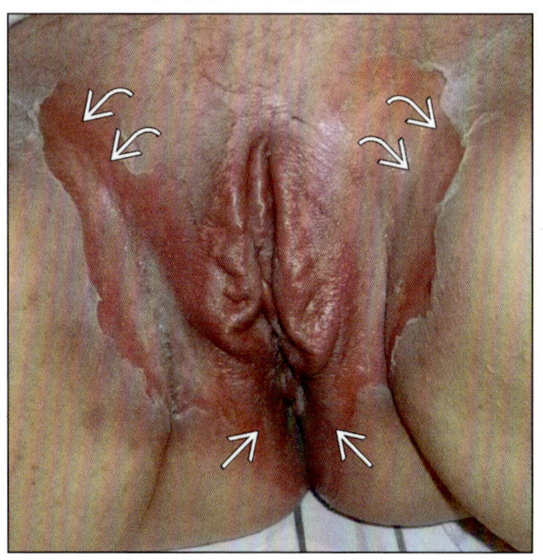

*(**Left**) Photo of same patient taken at 46.8 of 50.4 Gy shows grade 3 dermatitis on perianal skin, defined as moist desquamation ➔ in areas other than skin folds and creases. (**Right**) Photo of the perineum (same patient at same time) shows moist desquamation of inguinal skin creases ➔ and perianal skin ➔.*

Follow-Up

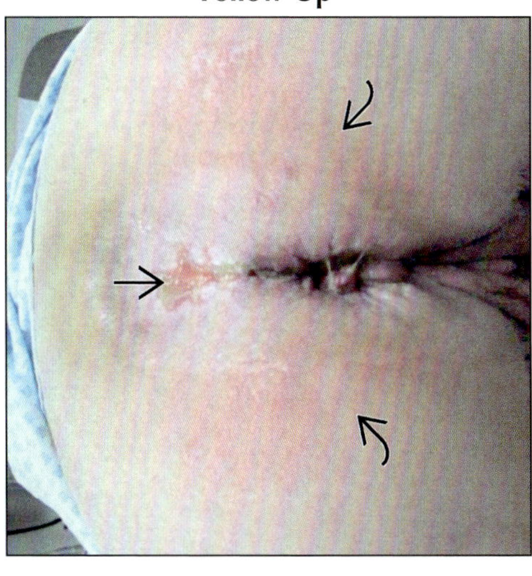

Follow-Up

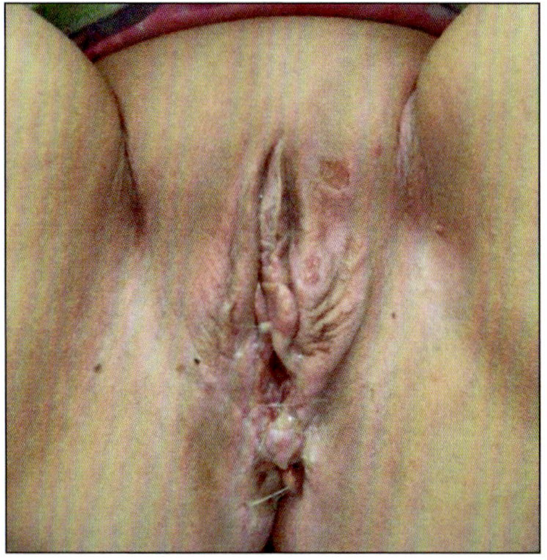

*(**Left**) Photo of the same patient 1 month after completion of CRT shows improvement to predominately grade 1 dermatitis (mild erythema ➔) in the perianal skin. Grade 2 dermatitis (moist desquamation ➔) in the gluteal crease is resolving. (**Right**) Photo of the perineum in the same patient shows reepithelialization and predominant healing of skin at 1-month follow-up.*

Stage II (T2 N0 M0) Adenocarcinoma

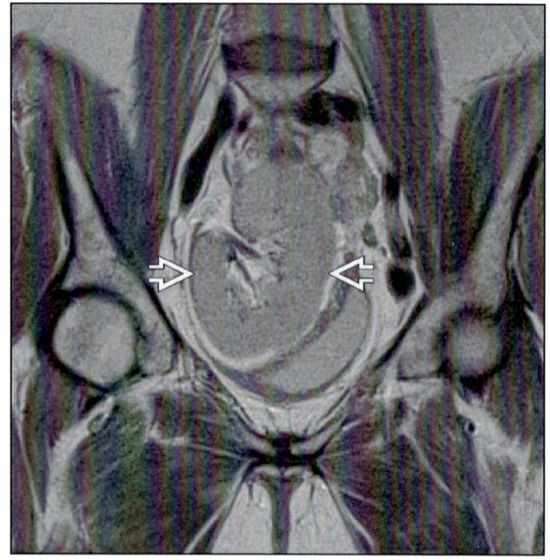

IMRT Planning

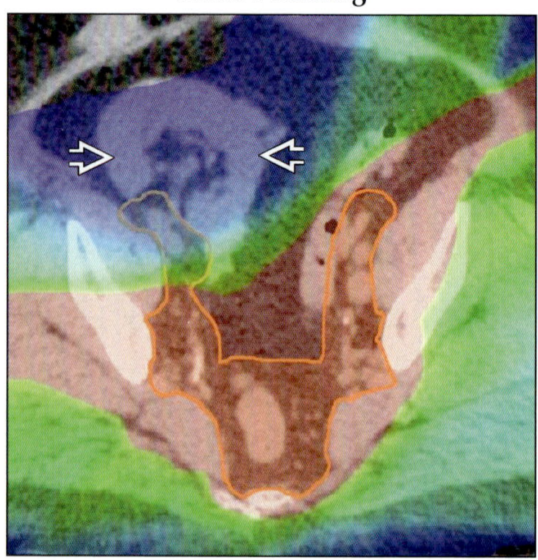

(Left) *Coronal T2WI MR shows right pelvic renal allograft* ➡ *in a woman with Lynch syndrome presenting with rectal bleeding. DRE revealed a 3 cm anal margin mass extending into anal canal. Biopsy confirmed adenocarcinoma.* ***(Right)*** *The same patient was treated with neoadjuvant CRT using IMRT, 50.4 Gy to primary CTV, and 45 Gy to nodal CTV (orange). Axial NECT with colorwash shows sparing of the kidney* ➡ *with < 5% receiving > 18 Gy and mean dose of 9.3 Gy.*

Follow-Up

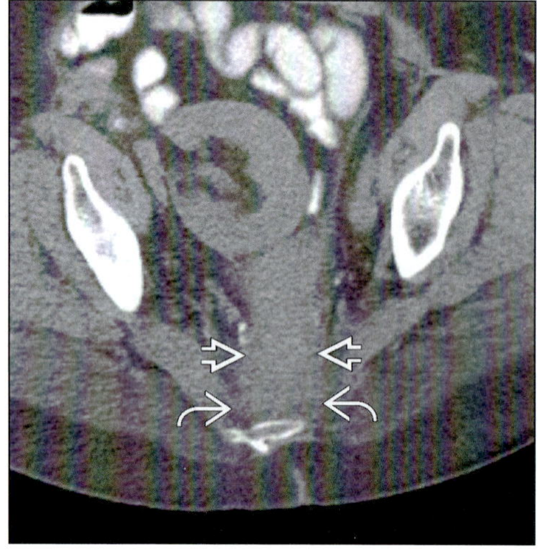

Follow-Up

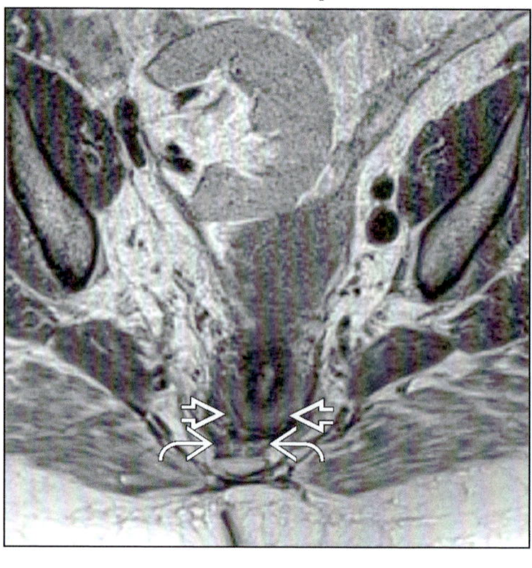

(Left) *APR in the same patient 3 months after CRT revealed 1.2 cm of residual adenocarcinoma and 0/11 involved nodes. Axial NECT 1 year later shows rectal thickening* ➡ *with obliteration of sacral fat planes* ➡*.* ***(Right)*** *Axial T2WI MR in the same patient shows soft tissue stranding of perirectal fat* ➡ *with no invasion of the presacral space* ➡*. This is a common benign finding after surgery and radiation therapy.*

Recurrent Anal Carcinoma

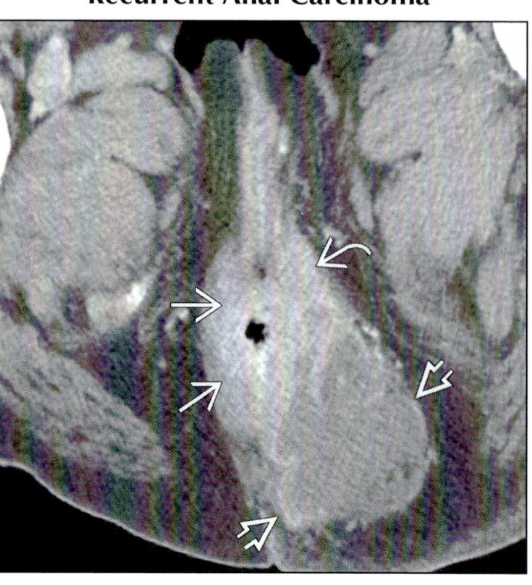

Recurrent Anal Carcinoma

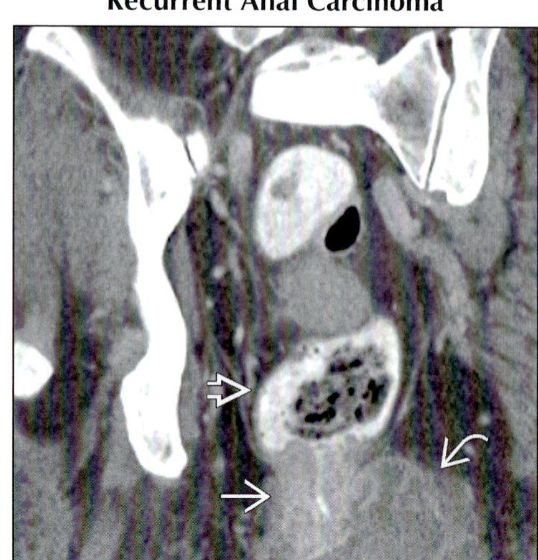

(Left) *Axial CECT in a 61-year-old woman presenting with fever and septic shock, who has a history of anal carcinoma 2 years earlier treated with CRT, shows circumferential thickening of anal canal* ➡ *with perianal tumor extension* ➡ *and a large fluid density perianal abscess* ➡*.* ***(Right)*** *Coronal CECT in the same patient shows circumferential thickening of anal canal* ➡ *with mild dilatation of the proximal rectum* ➡ *and perianal abscess* ➡*.*

Stage II (T2 N0 M0)

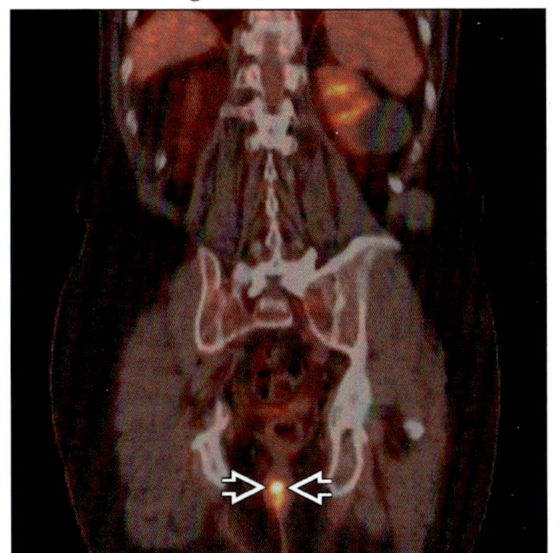

IMRT Planning

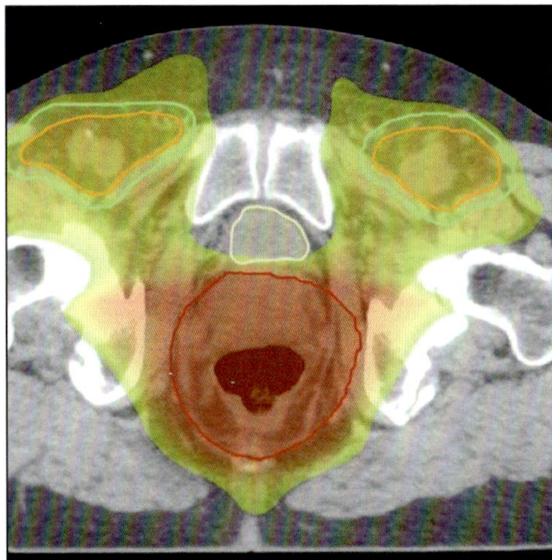

(Left) *Coronal PET/CT shows a hypermetabolic anal lesion ➡ (SUV 10.9) with no evidence of nodal metastases in a 77-year-old man. The 2 cm anal canal lesion is contiguous with a 2 cm anal margin lesion.* ***(Right)*** *Same patient was treated with IMRT plus concurrent 5-FU/MMC. Axial NECT shows dose colorwash with coverage of the primary PTV (red) to 50.4 Gy. Elective nodal CTV (orange) and PTV (cyan) were covered with 42 Gy.*

Post Treatment

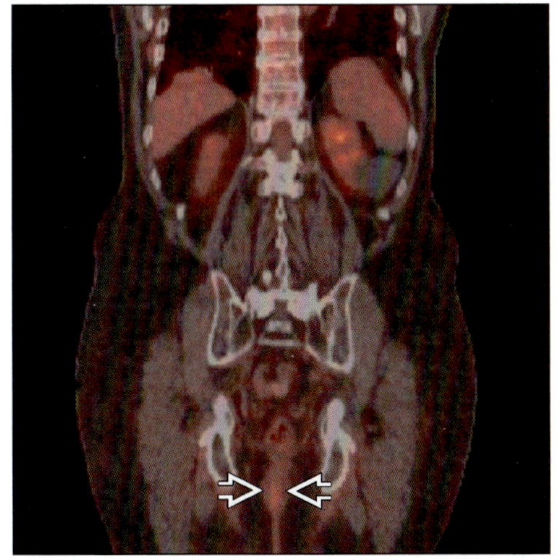

Nodal Recurrence

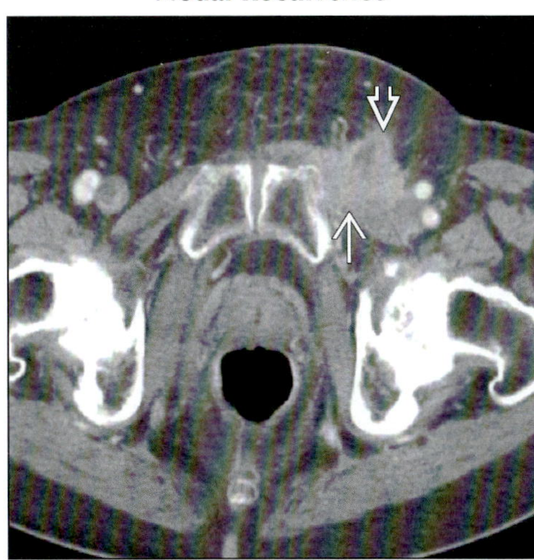

(Left) *Coronal view of post-treatment PET/CT in the same patient shows decrease in FDG activity of the anal lesion ➡ (SUV 2.8). Repeat exam revealed no visible or palpable lesion.* ***(Right)*** *Six months after CRT, the same patient developed a painful, palpable groin mass. Axial CECT shows exophytic nodal conglomerate ➡ in the previously irradiated region lateral to the pubic symphysis with invasion of pectineus ➡. Biopsy confirmed metastatic SCC.*

Nodal Recurrence

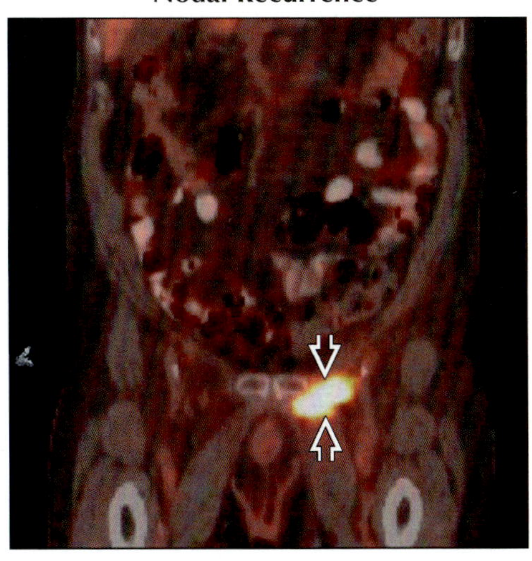

Distant Metastases

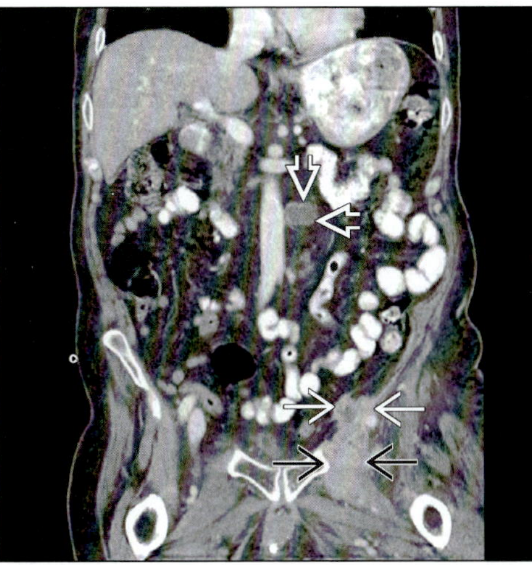

(Left) *Coronal PET/CT in same patient shows FDG uptake (SUV 17.1) in left inguinal mass ➡ with no other areas of concern. After chemo and repeat PET showing no progression, he underwent left groin radical lymph node dissection, revealing SCC in 11/13 nodes with ECE and multiple positive margins.* ***(Right)*** *Coronal CECT at 1 month post surgery shows paraaortic ➡, left external iliac ➡, & left inguinal → lymphadenopathy, plus lung nodules (not shown).*

LIVER

(T) Primary Tumor

Adapted from 7th edition AJCC Staging Forms.

TNM	*Definitions*
TX	Primary tumor cannot be assessed
T0	No evidence of primary tumor
T1	Solitary tumor without vascular invasion
T2	Solitary tumor with vascular invasion or multiple tumors, none > 5 cm
T3a	Multiple tumors > 5 cm
T3b	Single tumor or multiple tumors of any size involving a major branch of the portal vein or hepatic vein
T4	Tumor(s) with direct invasion of adjacent organs other than the gallbladder or with perforation of visceral peritoneum

(N) Regional Lymph Nodes

NX	Regional lymph nodes cannot be assessed
N0	No regional lymph node metastasis
N1	Regional lymph node metastasis

(M) Distant Metastasis

M0	No distant metastasis
M1	Distant metastasis

(G) Histologic Grade

G1	Well differentiated
G2	Moderately differentiated
G3	Poorly differentiated
G4	Undifferentiated

AJCC Stages/Prognostic Groups

Adapted from 7th edition AJCC Staging Forms.

Stage	*T*	*N*	*M*
I	T1	N0	M0
II	T2	N0	M0
IIIA	T3a	N0	M0
IIIB	T3b	N0	M0
IIIC	T4	N0	M0
IVA	Any T	N1	M0
IVB	Any T	Any N	M1

T1 N0 M0

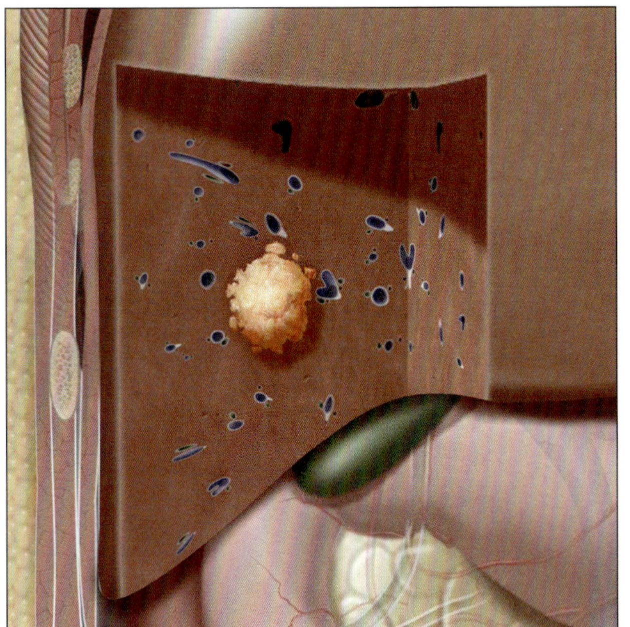

Graphic shows a solitary tumor without vascular invasion, consistent with T1 disease.

T2 N0 M0

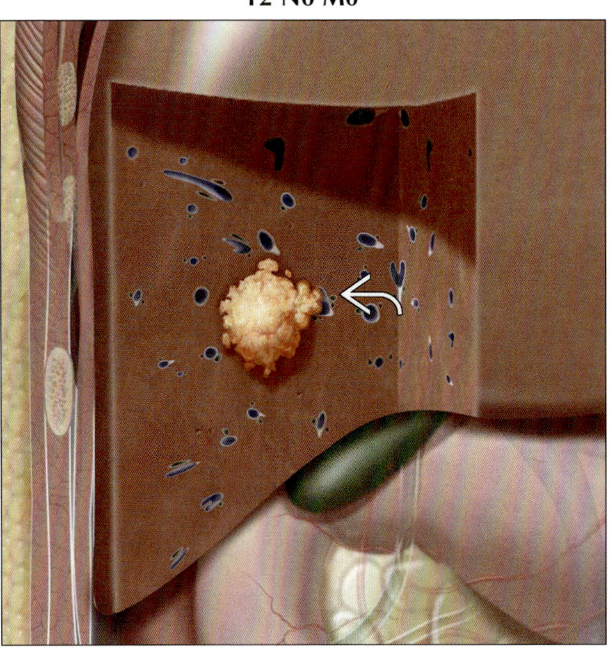

Graphic shows a solitary tumor with small vessel invasion ⮫, consistent with T2 disease.

T2 N0 M0

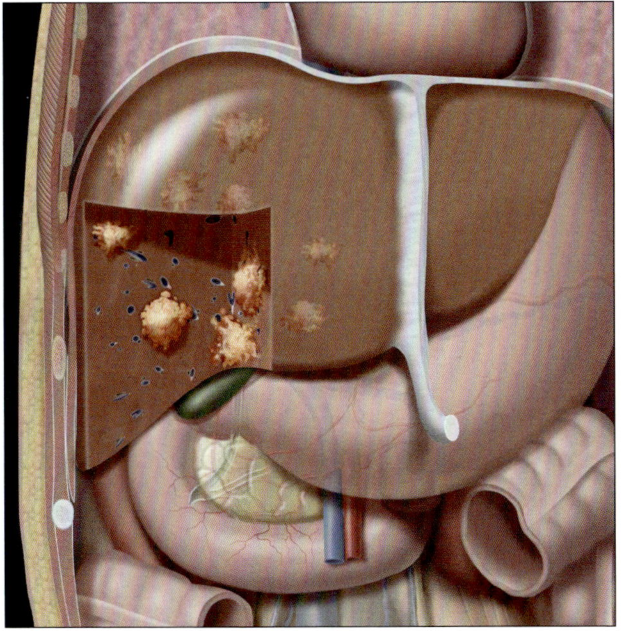

Graphic shows multiple tumors throughout the liver, all of which are smaller than 5 cm. No vascular invasion is seen, consistent with T2 disease.

T3a N0 M0

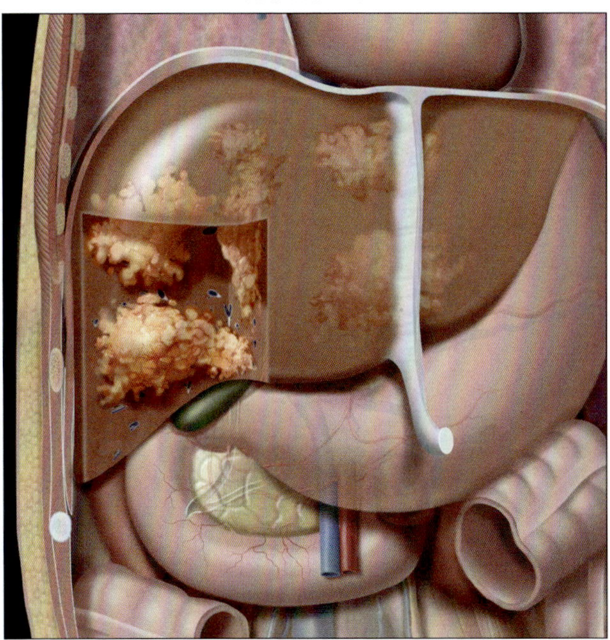

Graphic shows multiple tumors throughout the liver measuring more than 5 cm, consistent with T3a disease.

LIVER

T3b N0 M0

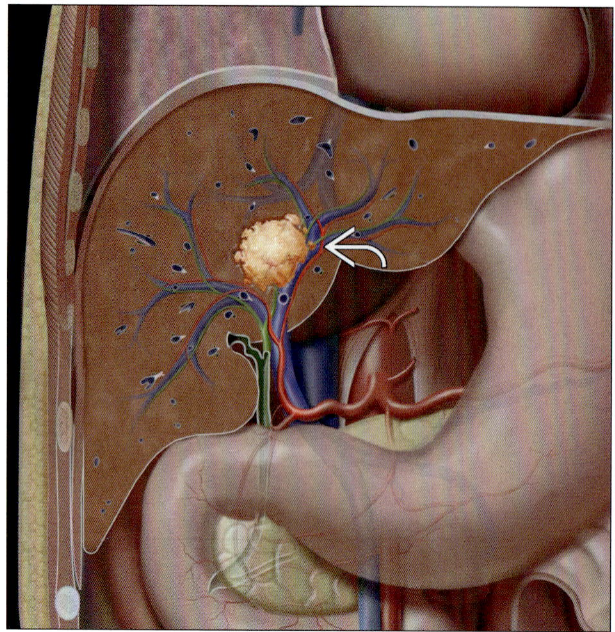

Graphic shows a solitary tumor with adjacent invasion of the portal vein ➲, consistent with T3b disease.

T3b N0 M0

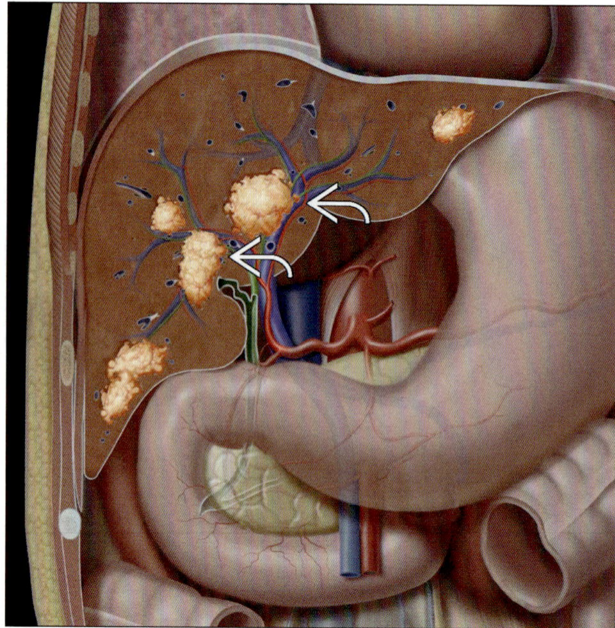

Graphic shows multiple tumors throughout the liver with portal venous invasion ➲. The presence of major vascular invasion, whether associated with a single tumor or multiple tumors, is considered T3b disease.

T4 N0 M0

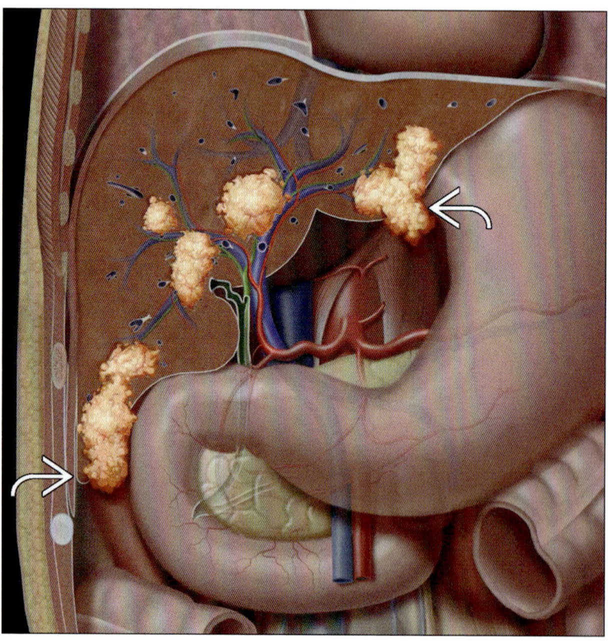

Graphic shows multiple tumors throughout the liver, some of which demonstrate extracapsular extension ➲. Extracapsular tumoral extension with perforation of the visceral peritoneum is consistent with T4 disease.

Liver Segments

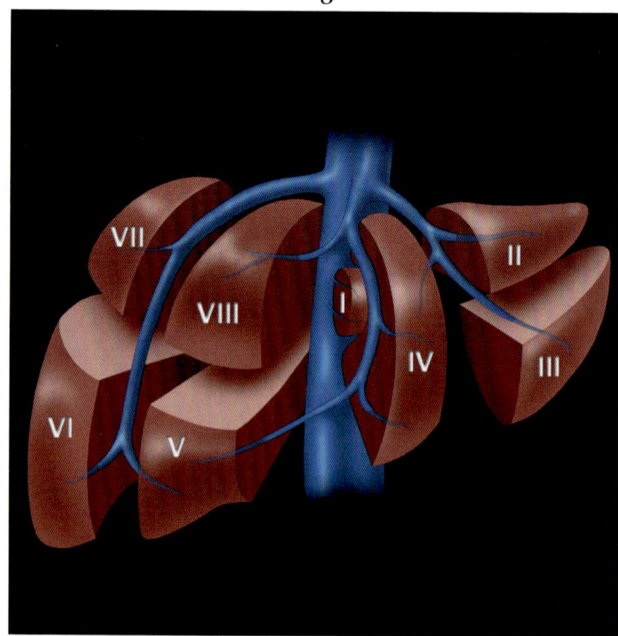

Graphic demonstrates the various liver segments.

Regional Lymphadenopathy

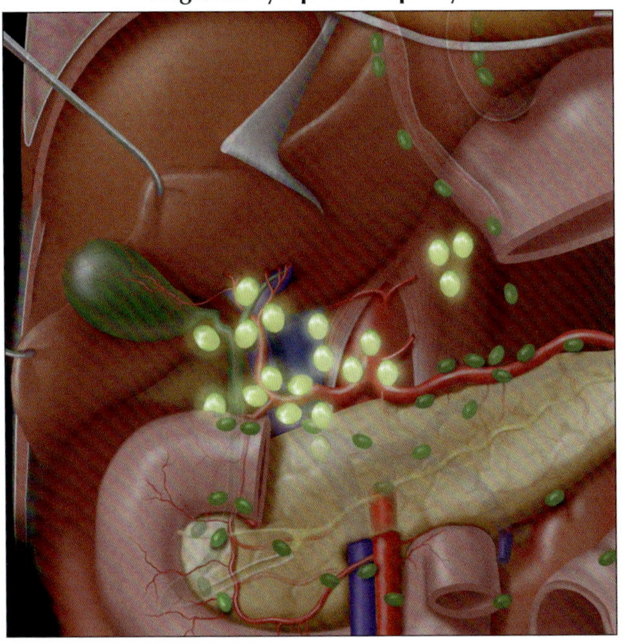

Graphic shows regional lymphadenopathy for metastatic hepatocellular carcinoma. These include paraceliac, hilar (common bile duct, hepatic artery, portal vein, and cystic duct), paraaortic, and portocaval lymph nodes.

Thoracic Lymphadenopathy

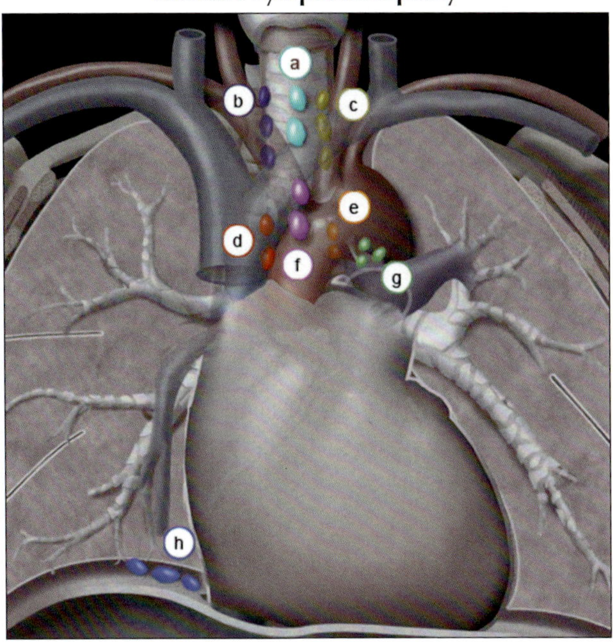

Graphic shows thoracic lymph nodes in metastatic hepatocellular carcinoma. These include a) pretracheal, b) right paratracheal, c) left paratracheal, d) right hilar, e) aortopulmonary, f) anterior mediastinal, g) left hilar, and h) cardiophrenic lymph nodes.

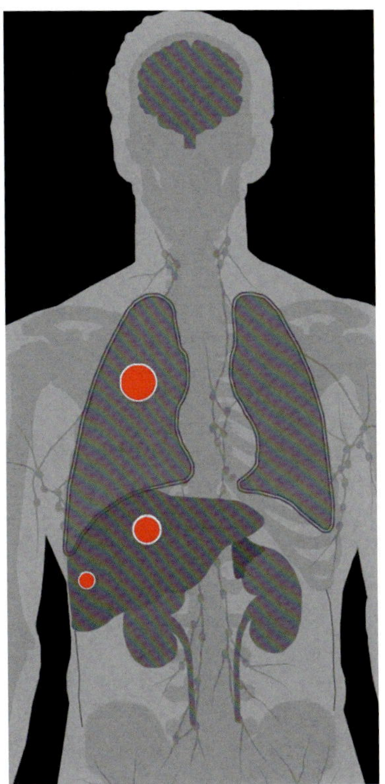

INITIAL SITE OF RECURRENCE

Extrahepatic	51%
Isolated Hepatic	33%
Intratumoral Hepatic	12%

Data obtained from an SBRT study of liver metastases in 67 assessable patients. Local control at 1 year was 71%. There were no isolated local failures, and 71% of extrahepatic failures previously had systemic metastases. Lee MT et al: Phase I study of individualized stereotactic body radiotherapy of liver metastases. J Clin Oncol. 27(10):1585-91, 2009.

OVERVIEW

General Comments

- Most common primary hepatic malignant tumor
- Synonymous with hepatoma

Classification

- Hepatocellular carcinoma (HCC)
  - Usually occurs in setting of cirrhosis
  - Poor prognosis
- Fibrolamellar carcinoma
  - Relatively rare variant of HCC
  - Does not occur in setting of cirrhosis
  - Better prognosis than conventional HCC

NATURAL HISTORY

General Features

- Comments
  - Carcinogenesis of HCC in cirrhosis
    - Commonly described as multistep evolution of cirrhotic nodules
  - International Working Party describes 2 types of cirrhotic nodules
    - Regenerative nodules
      - Localized proliferation of hepatocytes and supporting stroma
      - Response to local hepatocellular damage
      - Hyperplasia secondary to deficient portal venous perfusion → early arterial neovascularity
    - Dysplastic nodules
      - Hepatocytes that undergo abnormal growth due to genetic alteration
      - Histologic precursor to HCC
      - Small HCCs (< 2 cm) are often histologically indistinguishable from dysplastic nodules
      - ↑ arterial neovascularity compared to regenerative nodules

Etiology

- Risk factors
  - HCC usually occurs in setting of cirrhosis (90%)
  - Common causes of cirrhosis include
    - Viral hepatitis (individuals with chronic hepatitis are at 20x greater risk of developing HCC)
      - Hepatitis C virus (accounts for 55% of cirrhosis)
      - Hepatitis B virus (accounts for 16% of cirrhosis)
    - Alcoholism
    - Carcinogens
      - Aflatoxins: Particular populations found in sub-Saharan Africa and China have a mutated hepatic enzyme that fails to deactivate aflatoxin
      - Activated aflatoxin interacts with specific sites within *p53* gene contributing to high incidence of HCC
      - Thorotrast (particularly in development of cholangiocarcinoma)
      - Androgens
      - Hemosiderosis (from repeated blood transfusions)
    - Metabolic disorders
      - α-1-antitrypsin deficiency
      - Hemochromatosis
      - Wilson disease
      - Tyrosinosis
- Protective factors
  - Universal vaccination of children against HBV in endemic areas (began in Taiwan in 1984 and has markedly decreased HBV infection rate)

Epidemiology & Cancer Incidence

- Number of cases in USA per year
  - 35,557 (2011)
- Sex predilection
  - M:F = 8:1 (in countries with high incidence); 2-3:1 (in countries with low incidence)
- Age of onset
  - Median age of diagnosis is 63 years
- 3rd leading cause of death from cancer worldwide
- Accounts for 250,000 deaths worldwide each year
- Incidence of HCC in developing nations is more than double that of developed countries
  - Incidence of HCC is highest in Asia and Africa due to high prevalence of hepatitis B and C
- Frequency in United States
  - Incidence in USA has more than doubled in last 20 years from 2.6 to 7.5 per 100,000 population
  - There is an increased incidence in USA amongst Asian/Pacific Islander men (22:100,000)
  - 75% of cases occur in men compared to women (11.6 vs. 3.9 per 100,000)
  - Racial distribution
    - Caucasian (48%)
    - Hispanic (15%)
    - African American (14%)
    - Other, predominantly Asian (24%)

Genetics

- Common translocations
  - Aflatoxin acts on guanosine base in codon 249 of *p53* tumor suppressor gene leading to a G to T transversion
    - This is often identified in HCC found in regions of sub-Saharan Africa and China, contributing to high incidence in these regions
- HBV
  - Viral DNA integrates into host's genomic DNA in tumor cells
  - HBV X protein acts as a transactivator of cellular and viral promoters
    - Disrupts normal cell growth
    - Also binds to *p53* tumor suppressor gene
- Cirrhosis
  - Repeated cycles of cell death and regeneration lead to accumulation of mutations
  - Important component of the pathogenesis of HCV- and HBV-associated liver cancer

Associated Diseases, Abnormalities

- Fibrolamellar carcinoma
  - Variant of hepatocellular carcinoma
  - Relatively rare neoplasm with better prognosis than conventional HCC
  - Occurs most commonly in absence of cirrhosis
  - Affects younger age group with peak incidence at 24.8 ± 8 years
  - Higher incidence among Caucasians
  - No gender predilection

- Cholangiocarcinoma
  - 15-20% of primary liver tumors
  - 2nd most common primary liver tumor (80% extrahepatic subtype)
  - 30-50% have nodal spread at presentation
  - 10-20% have distant metastasis at presentation
  - Similar risk factors as hepatocellular, but also
    - Primary sclerosing cholangitis, tobacco smoke, chronic ulcerative colitis in Western countries, and endobiliary infections in Asia (liver flukes)
  - Incidence ↑ in USA (0.7 per 100,000)
  - Average age of diagnosis is 73 years
- Metastatic disease
  - Secondary liver cancer is ~ 20x more common than primary
  - Most commonly secondary to colorectal cancer
  - 5-year survival < 5% with hepatic failure most common cause of death
  - Surgical resection may achieve 5-year survival of 37-58% but only 20-25% are eligible
  - Most metastatic cancers are adenocarcinomas that quickly outgrow blood supply and thus have a central necrotic region on imaging

Gross Pathology & Surgical Features

- Classic macroscopic classification proposed by Eggle in 1901 is still used today
  - Nodular
    - Smaller and more distinct than massive lesions
    - Sharper margins
  - Massive: 2 dominant forms
    - Composed of confluent small tumors
    - 1 large lesion occupying almost entire liver
  - Diffuse
    - Multiple infiltrating lesions occupying large part of liver

Microscopic Pathology

- H&E
  - Edmondson grading system widely used to grade histology of HCC
    - Grade I
      - Tumor cells similar in size to normal hepatocytes
      - Arranged in relatively thin trabeculae
      - Acini containing bile are rare
    - Grade II
      - Cells larger than normal hepatocytes
      - Hyperchromatic nuclei occupy greater proportion of cells
      - Thicker trabeculae
      - Acini containing bile are common
    - Grade III
      - Hepatocytes with large nuclei that occupy > 50% of cytoplasm
      - Trabeculae still dominant although isolated cells may be present
      - Giant and bizarre cells common
      - Bile is rarely present
    - Grade IV
      - Cells contain nuclei that occupy most of cytoplasm
      - Predominantly solid areas with little or no bile
      - Intravascular and intrasinusoidal growth common
- Special stains
  - Reticulin stain commonly used to visualize reticular fibers
  - Hep-Par 1
    - Commonly used immunostain for suspected HCC
    - Highly sensitive and specific for hepatocytic differentiation

Routes of Spread

- Local spread
  - 3 distinct intrahepatic forms have been commonly described
    - Solitary massive tumor
    - Multiple nodules scattered throughout liver
    - Diffuse infiltration of liver
  - Vascular invasion commonly seen
    - Hepatic vein invasion may lead to Budd-Chiari syndrome
    - Portal venous invasion
- Lymphatic extension
  - Regional lymphadenopathy implies N1 disease by TNM criteria
  - Regional nodal involvement (in order of prevalence)
    - Periceliac
    - Portohepatic
    - Paraaortic
    - Portocaval
    - Peripancreatic
    - Aortocaval
    - Retrocaval
  - Distant lymphadenopathy (in order of prevalence)
    - Mediastinal
    - Cardiophrenic
    - Mesenteric
    - Internal mammary
    - Perirectal
    - Retrocrural
    - Iliac
    - Paraspinal
- Hematogenous spread
  - Hematogenous spread is relatively uncommon despite obvious vascular invasion
- Metastatic sites
  - Distant metastases (in order of prevalence)
    - Lungs
    - Musculoskeletal sites
    - Adrenal gland
    - Peritoneum &/or omentum

IMAGING

Detection

- Cirrhosis alters normal liver morphology with variable degree of
  - Fibrosis
  - Scarring
  - Nodular regeneration
  - Altered hepatic perfusion
    - Portal hypertension
    - Portal venous occlusion ± reversal of flow
- **Regenerative nodules**
  - Ultrasound
    - Plays little role in detection of discrete liver nodules

- Liver margins may demonstrate nodular contour in setting of macronodular cirrhosis
  - CT
    - Nodules poorly visualized on NECT
    - Enhancement similar to background parenchyma on CECT
    - Siderotic nodules may be occasionally seen as hyperdense on NECT
  - MR
    - T1WI
      - Nonsiderotic nodules can occasionally be detected as slightly hyperintense
      - Siderotic nodules well visualized on gradient-echo images, but rarely seen on spin-echo images
    - T2WI
      - Nonsiderotic nodules rarely seen
      - Siderotic nodules well visualized as discrete hypointense foci
    - T1 C+
      - Nonsiderotic nodules poorly visualized (may very rarely demonstrate arterial phase enhancement)
      - Siderotic nodules commonly seen as hypointense foci
- **Dysplastic nodules**
  - Ultrasound
    - Plays little role in detection of liver nodules
  - CT
    - Nodules may occasionally be seen as hyperdense on NECT
    - Generally isodense to liver on CECT
  - MR
    - T1WI
      - Large nodules may be homogeneously hyperintense
    - T2WI
      - Large nodules may be homogeneously hypointense
    - T1 C+
      - Enhancement rare
      - Mimics HCC when seen
- **Hepatocellular carcinoma**
  - Ultrasound
    - Usual modality of choice for screening of HCC in cirrhotic patient
      - Most affordable imaging modality
      - No ionizing radiation
    - Echogenicity of HCC highly variable
    - Small lesions (< 5 cm) are usually hypoechoic
      - Thin hypoechoic halo corresponding to fibrous capsule commonly seen
    - Larger lesions (> 5 cm) are generally mixed echogenicity
      - Hyperechoic areas can be seen in setting of intratumoral fat
      - Hypoechoic regions commonly seen in setting of necrosis
    - Color Doppler
      - Neovascularity and arteriovenous shunting may be seen
      - High-velocity waveforms characteristic, albeit nonspecific
      - Power Doppler signal variable; cannot be used to reliably distinguish HCC from metastatic disease
- CT
  - NECT
    - Visualization generally limited without IV contrast
    - Lesions are usually hypodense if detected
      - Patchy fat attenuation may be seen in lesions with intratumoral fat
      - Fluid attenuation may be seen with tumoral necrosis
  - CECT
    - Arterial phase
      - Avid homogeneous enhancement in small lesions
      - Heterogeneous enhancement in larger lesions
      - Transient hepatic attenuation difference may be seen as wedge-shaped region of ↑ perfusion from local portal vein occlusion
      - Some advocate both early and late arterial phases to overcome differences in blood flow kinetics and tumor characteristics
    - Portal venous phase
      - Small lesions usually not detectable due to washout
      - Larger lesions may retain variable degree of enhancement
    - Delayed phase
      - Both small and large lesions generally not well visualized
    - Hepatic artery catheter CT ("coned-beam CT")
- MR
  - Most sensitive and specific imaging modality for detection of HCC
  - Considered gold standard for characterization of liver nodules in setting of cirrhosis
  - T1WI
    - Variable signal, depending on degree of fatty metaplasia, fibrosis, and necrosis
    - Generally iso- to hypointense
    - Rarely hyperintense in presence of fat, copper, or glycoproteins
  - T2WI
    - Variable signal although generally hyperintense
    - "Nodule within nodule" occasionally seen (small T2 hyperintense focus within uniformly T2 hypointense dysplastic nodule)
  - T1 C+
    - Small lesions (< 2 cm) generally show rapid arterial enhancement with rapid washout in portal venous and delayed phases
    - Large lesions (> 2 cm) demonstrate heterogeneous nodular enhancement during both arterial and later phases
  - Diffusion-weighted imaging (DWI)
    - Evolving technology used in conjunction with other imaging sequences
    - Useful tool for lesion detection
    - DWI presently limited for lesion characterization; good for follow-up post TACE and radioembolization
- Arteriography
  - Enlarged arterial feeders
  - Coarse neovascularity
  - Arterioportal shunts
  - "Threads and streaks"

    - Linear parallel vascular channels coursing along portal venous radicles
    - Seen in setting of portal venous involvement
  - 3D C-arm cone-beam CT
    - Hepatic arteriography with concomitant 3D cross-sectional imaging
    - May decrease overall radiation dose during angiographic procedures by providing real-time 3D information for therapeutic planning
    - More sensitive than conventional CT for lesion identification
- Nuclear medicine
  - Technetium sulfur colloid
    - Focal defect in cirrhotics
    - Heterogeneous uptake in non-cirrhotics
  - Hepatobiliary scan
    - Variable uptake (roughly 50% of lesions)
  - Gallium scan
    - Avid uptake in 90% of cases

Staging

- Nuances of staging
  - T staging system based on factors affecting prognosis after resection
- Multiple staging systems for HCC are currently employed
- Surgical staging
  - American Joint Committee on Cancer/Union Internationale Contre le Cancer (AJCC/UICC) system (7th edition)
    - Most widely used surgical system
    - Incorporates anatomic and histologic findings at tumor resection
    - Based on standard system of tumor, node, and metastasis classification
    - System can be applied after liver resection or transplantation
- Medical and clinical staging
  - Okuda system
    - Earliest medical classification system
    - 1st system to incorporate both tumor size and liver function parameters
    - Has been largely replaced with newer Cancer of the Liver Italian Program (CLIP) and Barcelona Clinic Liver Cancer (BCLC) systems
    - System parameters include
      - Tumor size
      - Ascites
      - Jaundice
      - Serum albumin
    - Individuals are assigned to stages 1-3 based on above parameters
      - 1 implies best prognosis
      - 3 implies worst prognosis
    - Limitations of Okuda system
      - Does not categorize tumor as unifocal, multifocal, or diffuse
      - Does not specify presence or absence of vascular invasion
  - CLIP system
    - Scoring system designed to classify
      - Extent and severity of HCC
      - Clinical parameters of underlying liver disease
    - Generally regarded as easier to implement and more accurate than Okuda classification
    - Parameters of CLIP system include
      - Child-Pugh score
      - Tumor morphology
      - α-fetoprotein (AFP)
      - Portal vein patency
    - Individuals are assigned score from 0-6 according to CLIP system
      - 0 implies best prognosis
      - 6 implies worst prognosis
  - BCLC staging
    - Regarded as highly reliable staging system that includes the following parameters
      - Tumor stage
      - Underlying liver function
      - Physical status
- Assessment of underlying liver disease
  - Child-Turcotte-Pugh score
    - Not a scoring system for HCC
      - Used to assess severity of cirrhosis
    - Originally used to predict mortality during surgery
    - Often employed in patients with HCC for establishing prognosis, treatment options, including the utility of transplantation
    - Scoring is based on 5 clinical measures
      - Total bilirubin
      - Serum albumin
      - INR
      - Ascites
      - Hepatic encephalopathy
    - Liver disease is stratified into Child-Pugh classes A-C based on Child-Turcotte-Pugh scoring system
      - Class A associated with 100% 1-year survival and 85% 2-year survival
      - Class B associated with 81% 1-year survival and 57% 2-year survival
      - Class C associated with 45% 1-year survival and 35% 2-year survival
  - Model of end-stage liver disease (MELD) score
    - Additional scoring system for assessing severity of chronic liver disease
    - Used to predict mortality for patients with chronic end-stage disease
    - United Network for Organ Sharing (UNOS) and Eurotransplant use for allocating liver transplants
    - Scoring is based on 3 clinical parameters
      - Serum bilirubin
      - INR
      - Serum creatinine
  - Fibrosis score
    - Often employed as additional prognostic indicator in setting of HCC
    - Scoring system uses 0-6 scale
    - F0: 0-4 (none to moderate fibrosis)
    - F1: 5-6 (severe fibrosis or cirrhosis)
- Imaging techniques for local staging
  - Ultrasound
    - Useful tool for HCC screening
      - Wide availability
      - Low cost
      - Lack of ionizing radiation
    - Plays little role in staging of HCC
  - CT
    - Preferred imaging modality for staging of widespread metastatic disease

- Useful tool for local staging if MR not feasible
  - Implanted medical devices that are MR incompatible
  - Lack of MR availability
  - Patient claustrophobia
- Multiplanar capability significantly improved with ongoing evolution of robust post-processing software

- MR
  - Imaging modality of choice for local staging of HCC
  - Continual evolution of faster pulse sequences provides high-quality imaging
  - Excellent intrinsic soft tissue contrast
  - Superb multiplanar capability
  - Multiple available contrast agents allow for greater flexibility of liver imaging
    - Extracellular fluid agents (conventional gadolinium)
    - Hepatobiliary-specific agents
    - Reticuloendothelial agents
    - Blood pool agents
  - Permits serial evaluation of liver lesions following IV contrast administration

Restaging

- Whole-body 18F FDG PET/CT may be useful for metabolic restaging of HCC
- In advanced HCC, CT perfusion
  - Sensitive biomarker for monitoring early effects of antiangiogenic and liver-directed therapies
  - Sensitive biomarker for predicting progression free survival (PFS) compared with RECIST

CLINICAL PRESENTATION & WORK-UP

Presentation

- Clinical signs and symptoms vary depending on degree of underlying cirrhosis
  - Right upper quadrant fullness
  - Abdominal pain
  - Weight loss
  - Jaundice
  - Ascites
  - Tumoral rupture with hemoperitoneum
    - More common in Africa and Southeast Asia
- Systemic metabolic complications can include
  - Hypoglycemia
  - Erythrocytosis
  - Hypercalcemia
  - Hyperlipidemia
- Abnormal lab values
  - Elevated AFP
    - Signifies dedifferentiation of hepatocytes
    - Elevated AFP levels (> 400 μg/mL) seen in 40-65% of patients with HCC
    - RTOG-8301 found serum AFP levels to be prognostic
      - Negative serum AFP levels indicate longer survival
  - Abnormal liver function tests (LFTs)

Prognosis

- 5-year survival < 5% without treatment

Work-Up

- Clinical
  - Multidisciplinary approach to care is essential
  - Evaluate age, performance status (ECOG), labs, Child-Pugh class, comorbidities, staging
- Radiographic
  - Contrast-enhanced CT or MR
- Laboratory
  - LFTs, CBC, coagulation profile, tumor markers (AFP)

TREATMENT

Major Treatment Alternatives

- Transplantation
- Surgical resection
- Ablation
  - RFA
  - Microwave
  - Chemical
- Chemoembolization
- Radioembolization
- SBRT
- Sorafenib (oral multikinase inhibitor)

Treatment Options by Stage

- Transplantation
  - Preferred treatment for cirrhotic patients with low volume disease
  - BCLC stage 0-A
  - 75% 4-year survival if within Milan
    - Milan criteria
      - 1 HCC up to 5 cm
      - 2 or 3 HCC, each up to 3 cm
      - No vascular invasion
      - No extrahepatic disease
  - Few patients are eligible for transplant at time of diagnosis
  - Waiting period for transplantation varies depending on region (2-14 months)
- Surgical resection
  - (Selected T1 and T2; N0, M0), BCLC stage 0-A
  - Treatment of choice in non-cirrhotic patients and select Child-Pugh class A cirrhotics
    - Normal bilirubin and no portal hypertension
  - 5-year survival up to 70% in early solitary HCC
  - Must have a liver remnant at least 40% of total liver volume in cirrhotic patients and at least 20% in non-cirrhotic patients
  - Few patients are eligible for surgery at time of diagnosis (10-15%)
- Ablation (radiofrequency and microwave)
  - BCLC stage 0-B
  - Potentially curative modality with excellent tumor control in small tumors
  - Treatment of choice in nonoperative candidates with early HCC tumors up to 5 cm, no vascular invasion, no extrahepatic spread, and Child-Pugh class A or B
  - May be limited by intrahepatic disease location and proximity to major vessels

- Chemical (dehydrated alcohol, acetic acid) ablation performed infrequently after advent of thermal ablative technologies
- Chemoembolization
  - BCLC stage 0-C
  - First-line noncurative therapy for nonsurgical patients with large or multifocal HCC
  - Reduces mortality in HCC compared to symptomatic therapy
  - 3-year survival approximately 25-30%
  - May treat high-performing BCLC stages B and C patients (portal vein invasion, Child-Pugh class B) with selective drug-eluting bead chemoembolization
  - May be used to "downstage" patients for surgery
  - Limited in patients with poor performance status and advanced liver disease
- Yttrium-90 radioembolization
  - BCLC stage 0-C
  - Response rate and survival appear similar to transarterial chemoembolization (TACE) in cohort studies; no randomized controlled trials to date
  - Low embolic effect and mild side effects make yttrium-90 a good option for elderly patients, those with decreased performance status, and in patients with portal venous invasion
  - May be used to "downstage" patients for surgery
  - Limited use in patients with advanced liver disease
- Stereotactic body radiation
  - Limited data to recommend as part of the standard HCC treatment paradigm
  - Noninvasive and has demonstrated effectiveness against small and medium-sized HCC
  - 73% partial response rate
  - 60% 2-year survival
  - Promising treatment option for small HCC in patients ineligible for locoregional treatment
  - Narrow therapeutic window of liver (< 15 Gy) limits external beam RT
- Sorafenib
  - Oral multikinase inhibitor
  - ↑ survival from 7.9-10.7 months in advanced HCC
  - Diarrhea, weight loss, hand-foot syndrome are common side effects
  - Expensive (approximately $4,000/month)

Dose Response

- SBRT: Local control ↑ with > 42 Gy total dose or > 75 Gy biologically equivalent dose (BED)

Standard Doses

- SBRT: 30-60 Gy in 3-6 fractions
- 3D/IMRT: 30-60 Gy in conventional fractions depending on volume of untreated liver and intent

Organs at Risk Parameters

- For 3-fraction SBRT
  - Liver: > 700 mL, < 15 Gy
  - Bowel: 100%, < 30 Gy
  - Cord: Maximum dose, < 18 Gy
  - Kidney (bilateral): < 33%, < 15 Gy
  - Chest wall: < 5 mL, < 40 Gy

Common Techniques

- SBRT most effective for smaller lesions
- IMRT/3D mostly palliative

Landmark Trials

- SHARP (sorafenib HCC assessment randomized protocol)
  - Phase 3, randomized, placebo-controlled trial
  - Advanced HCC, Child-Pugh A, ECOG 0-1
  - OS of 10.7 months (sorafenib) vs. 7.9 months (placebo)
- Liver transplantation for small HCC (N Engl J Med, 1996)
  - Curative in patients with no vessel invasion, ≤ 3 nodules, no lymph node involvement
- Arterial embolization or chemoembolization vs. symptomatic treatment in patients with unresectable HCC
  - Established chemoembolization as the treatment of choice for nonsurgical patients

RECOMMENDED FOLLOW-UP

Clinical

- Depending on treatment modality (RFA, TACE, SBRT)
  - Clinical follow-up at 1 month, 3 months, and 6 months post treatment, then yearly thereafter

Radiographic

- Depending on treatment modality (RFA, TACE, SBRT)
  - MR, CT

Laboratory

- Depending on treatment modality (RFA, TACE, SBRT)
  - CBC, CMP, PT/INR, AFP, CA19-9

SELECTED REFERENCES

1. Salem R et al: Radioembolization for hepatocellular carcinoma using Yttrium-90 microspheres: a comprehensive report of long-term outcomes. Gastroenterology. 138(1):52-64, 2010
2. Seale MK et al: Hepatobiliary-specific MR contrast agents: role in imaging the liver and biliary tree. Radiographics. 29(6):1725-48, 2009
3. Lencioni R et al: Guidelines for imaging focal lesions in liver cirrhosis. Expert Rev Gastroenterol Hepatol. 2(5):697-703, 2008
4. Llovet JM et al: Sorafenib in advanced hepatocellular carcinoma. N Engl J Med. 359(4):378-90, 2008
5. Willatt JM et al: MR imaging of hepatocellular carcinoma in the cirrhotic liver: challenges and controversies. Radiology. 247(2):311-30, 2008
6. Clark HP et al: Staging and current treatment of hepatocellular carcinoma. Radiographics. 25 Suppl 1:S3-23, 2005
7. Llovet JM et al: Arterial embolisation or chemoembolisation versus symptomatic treatment in patients with unresectable hepatocellular carcinoma: a randomised controlled trial. Lancet. 359(9319):1734-9, 2002
8. Katyal S et al: Extrahepatic metastases of hepatocellular carcinoma. Radiology. 216(3):698-703, 2000

(**Left**) *Hepatocellular carcinoma is typically composed of neoplastic cells resembling hepatocytes with a high nuclear to cytoplasmic ratio, which are organized into thick, disordered trabeculae. (Courtesy J. Misdraji, MD.)* (**Right**) *In this pseudoglandular pattern of hepatocellular carcinoma, dilated spaces in the centers of trabeculae ⇨ mimic glands. (Courtesy J. Misdraji, MD.)*

Hepatocellular Carcinoma

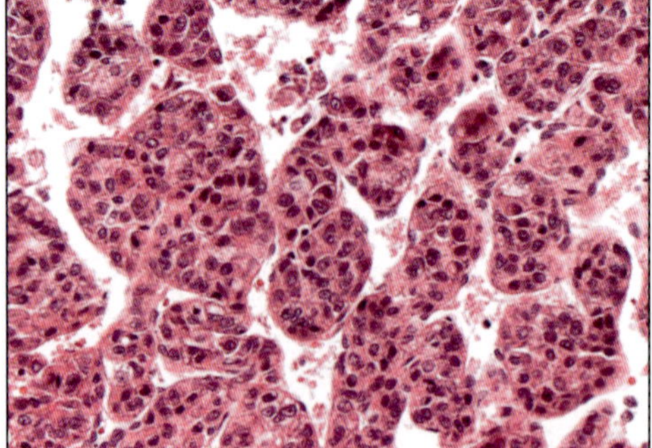

Hepatocellular Carcinoma

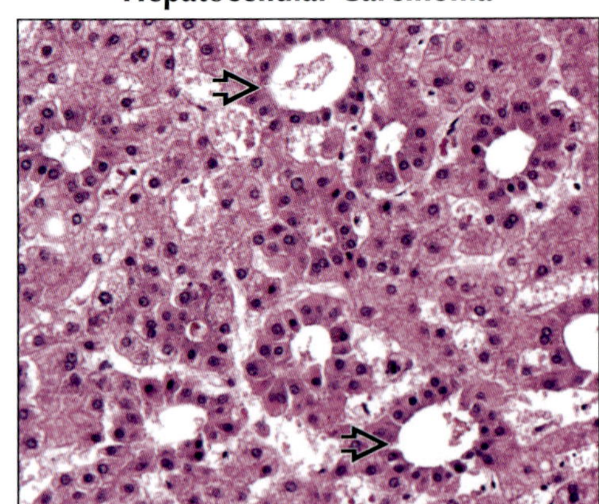

(**Left**) *Fine needle aspiration shows smooth contours → of this group of HCC cells created by endothelial wrapping. Note increased nuclear density. (Courtesy J. Misdraji, MD.)* (**Right**) *Fibrolamellar HCC shows fibrous septae of parallel collagen fibers ↷ separating tumor cells. (Courtesy J. Misdraji, MD.)*

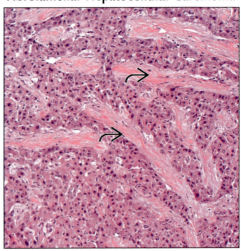

Hepatocellular Carcinoma

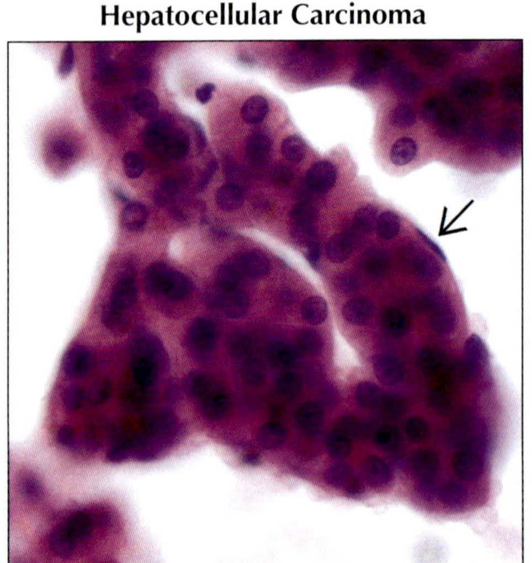

Fibrolamellar Hepatocellular Carcinoma

(**Left**) *Well-differentiated intrahepatic bile duct carcinoma demonstrates well-formed glands ⇨ infiltrating into fibrotic stroma. (Courtesy M. Rezvani, MD.)* (**Right**) *Immunohistochemical stain with antibody against cytokeratin (CK7) demonstrates positive brown staining → supporting a diagnosis of cholangiocarcinoma. Various stains can differentiate primary from metastatic tumors. (Courtesy M. Rezvani, MD.)*

Intrahepatic Bile Duct Carcinoma

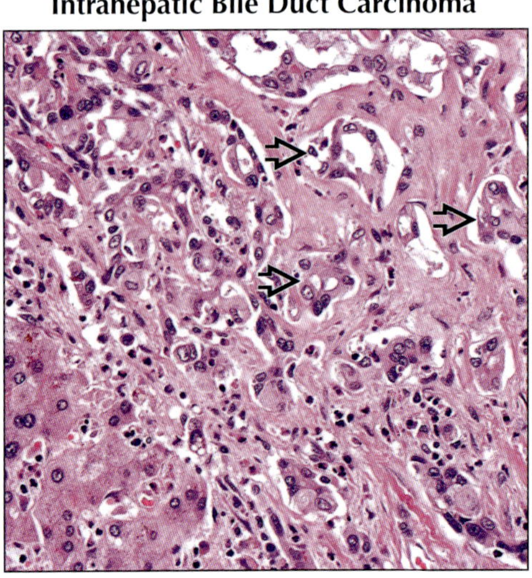

Cholangiocarcinoma

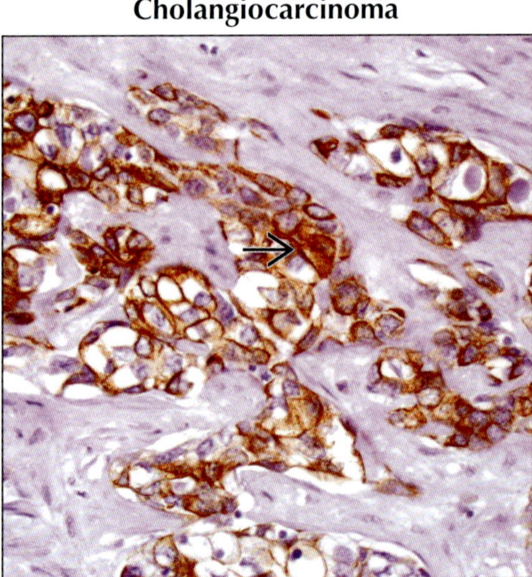

T1

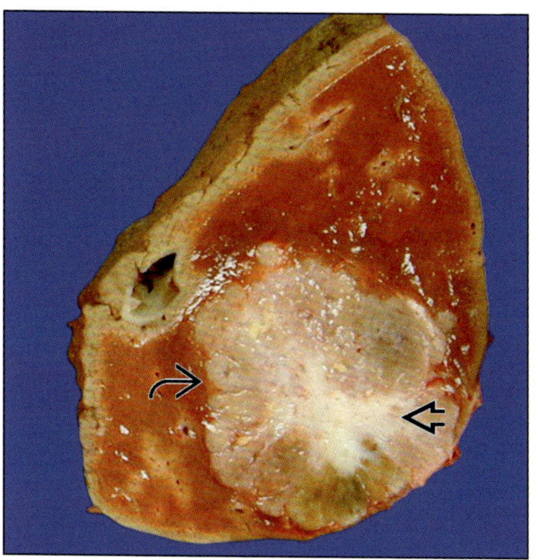

Stage I (T1 N0 M0)

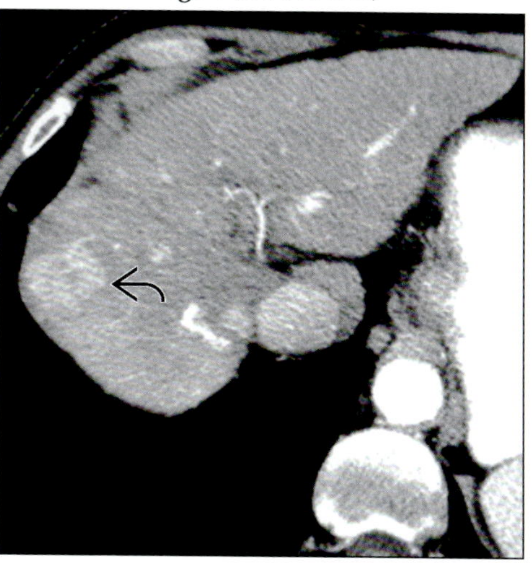

(Left) Gross specimen shows a solitary fibrolamellar hepatocellular carcinoma without vascular invasion. Note the well-circumscribed tumor ➡ with radiating fibrous septa that merge to form a central scar ➡. *(Right)* Axial CECT in the late arterial phase in a cirrhotic patient shows an enhancing mass ➡ within the anterior segment of the right hepatic lobe, which is consistent with HCC.

Stage I (T1 N0 M0)

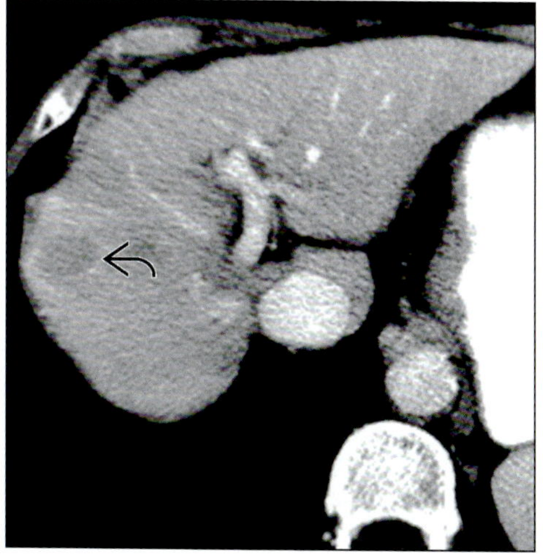

Stage I (T1 N0 M0)

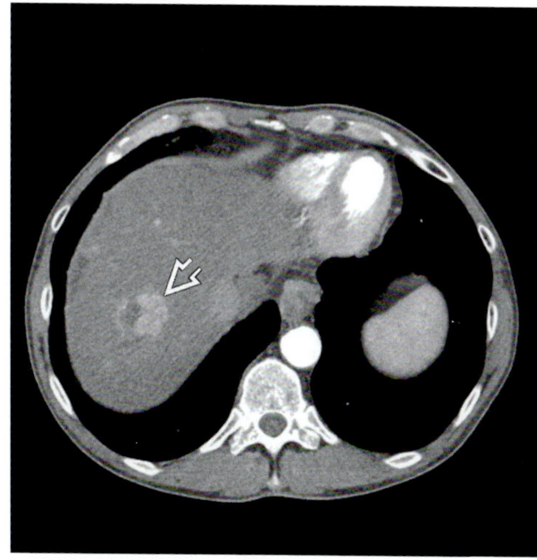

(Left) Axial CECT in the portal venous phase in the same patient shows washout of contrast from the mass ➡ within the anterior segment of the right lobe. *(Right)* Axial CECT of a 60-year-old man with hepatitis C cirrhosis demonstrates a heterogeneously enhancing HCC ➡ in segment 8. The patient was not a surgical candidate based on his multiple medical comorbidities.

Stage I (T1 N0 M0)

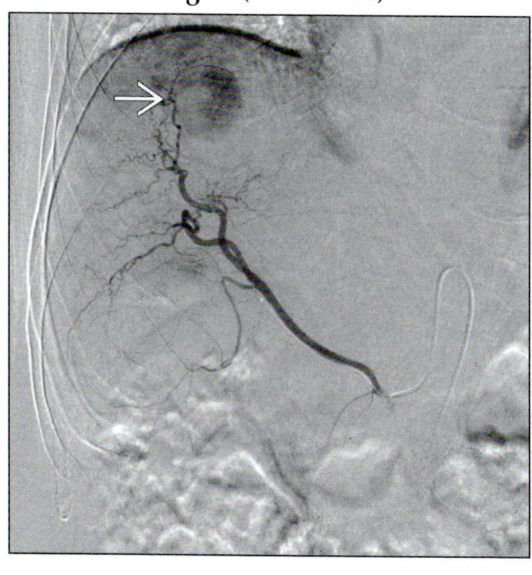

Stage I (T1 N0 M0)

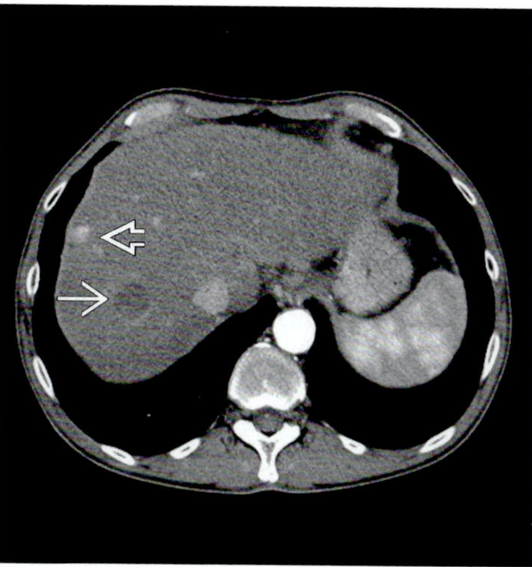

(Left) Hepatic arteriogram in the same patient via a replaced right hepatic artery demonstrates tumor blush ➡ in segment 8. Chemoembolization was performed, delivering 50 mg of doxorubicin loaded on 100-300 μm drug-eluting beads. *(Right)* Axial CECT in the same patient performed 1 month later demonstrates complete necrosis of the segment 8 lesion ➡. An arterial portal shunt is noted peripherally ➡.

(**Left**) *Gross specimen shows multiple small tumor nodules ➔, none measuring > 5 cm.* (**Right**) *Axial CECT in the arterial phase shows multiple enhancing masses throughout the liver; all of the masses measure < 5 cm. These findings are consistent with stage II multifocal HCC.*

Stage II (T2 N0 M0)

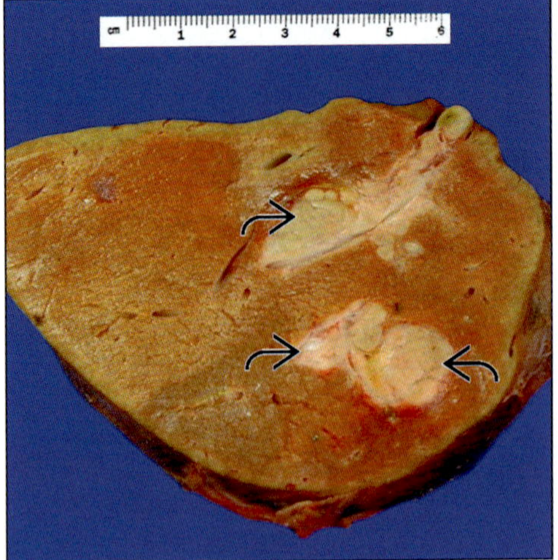

Stage II (T2 N0 M0)

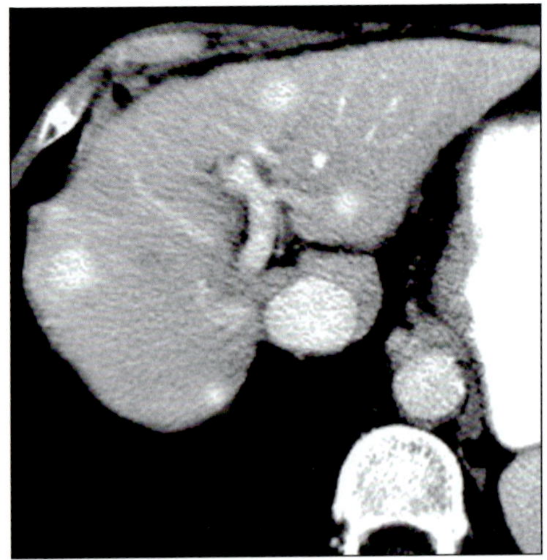

(**Left**) *Coronal CECT in a 55-year-old man with hepatitis C cirrhosis demonstrates an enhancing 3.0 cm lesion in segment 6 ➔. Two other lesions in segment 8 are not shown.* (**Right**) *Coronal CBCT in the same patient performed during chemoembolization demonstrates 2 hypervascular lesions in segment 8 ➔.*

Stage II (T2 N0 M0)

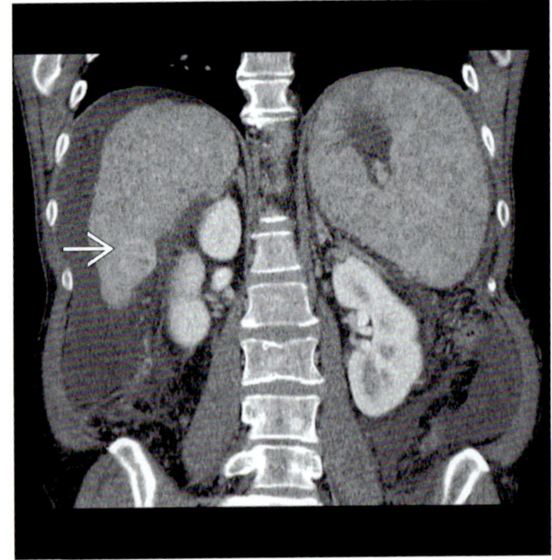

Stage II (T2 N0 M0)

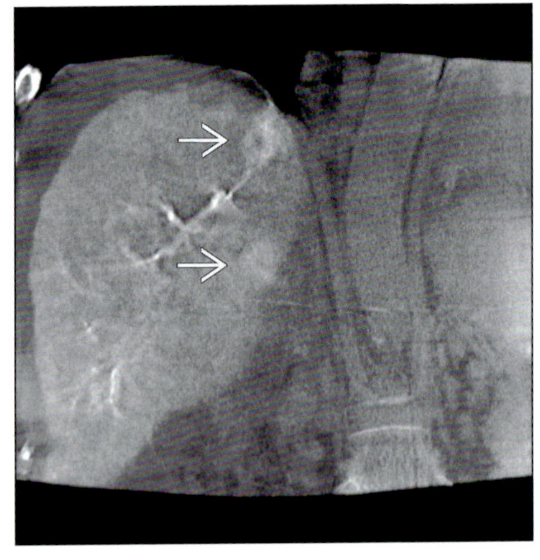

(**Left**) *Coronal angiography in the same patient demonstrates hypervascular lesions in segments 6 ➔ and 8 ➔.* (**Right**) *Axial T1WI C+ MR shows evidence of prior right hepatectomy for a solitary HCC within the right lobe ➔. Heterogeneously enhancing masses are noted at the resection margin ➔, consistent with disease recurrence.*

Stage II (T2 N0 M0)

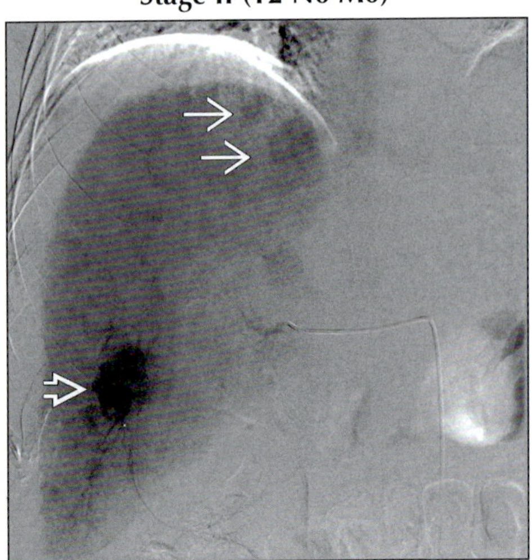

Stage II (T2 N0 M0)

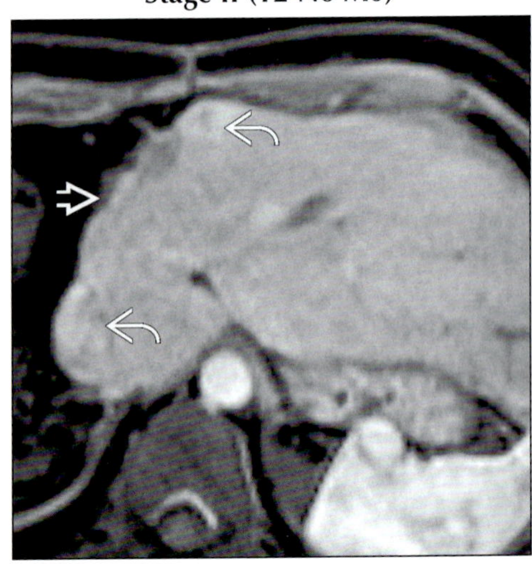

Fibrolamellar HCC, Stage IIIA (T3a N0 M0)

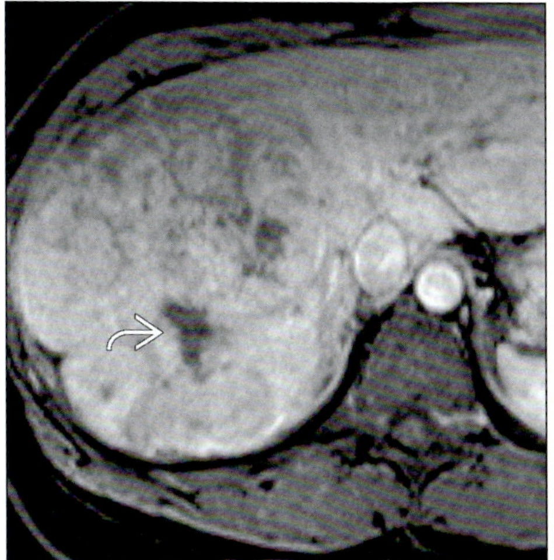

Stage IIIA (T3a N0 M0)

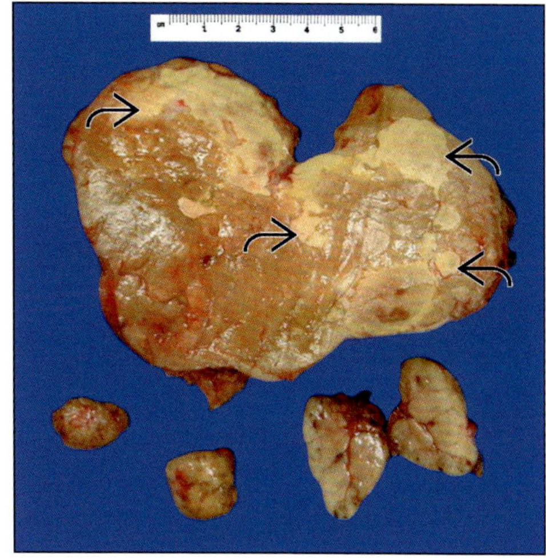

(Left) *Axial T1WI C+ MR in the arterial phase shows avid heterogeneous enhancement of the mass, consistent with fibrolamellar HCC. There is no enhancement of the central scar* ➔. ***(Right)*** *Gross specimen in the same patient shows multiple discrete tumor nodules* ➔*, some of which measure > 5 cm.*

Stage IIIA (T3a N0 M0)

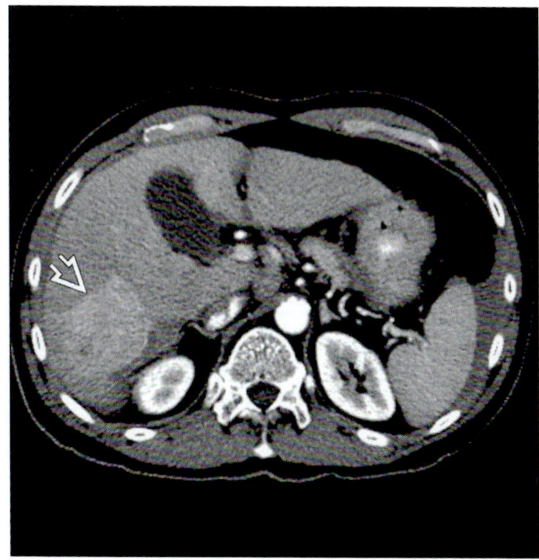

Stage IIIA (T3a N0 M0)

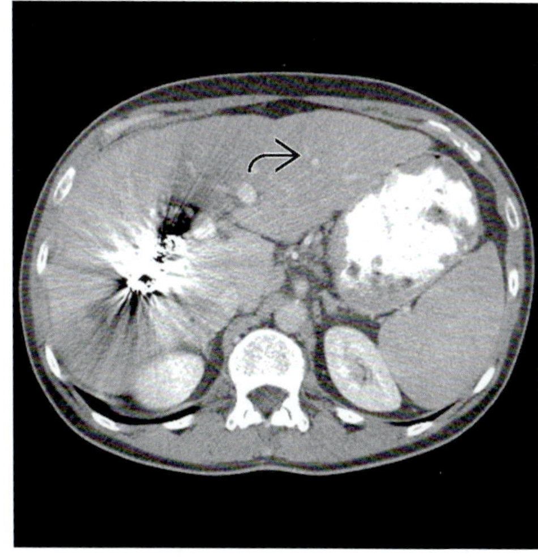

(Left) *Axial CECT in a 60-year-old man with alcoholic cirrhosis shows a 6.7 cm hypervascular lesion in segment 8* ➔. ***(Right)*** *Axial CECT in the same patient 6 weeks post portal vein embolization of segments 5-8. The patient had a 46% increase in the size of segments 2-4* ➔ *and subsequently underwent successful right hepatectomy.*

Stage IIIB (T3b N0 M0)

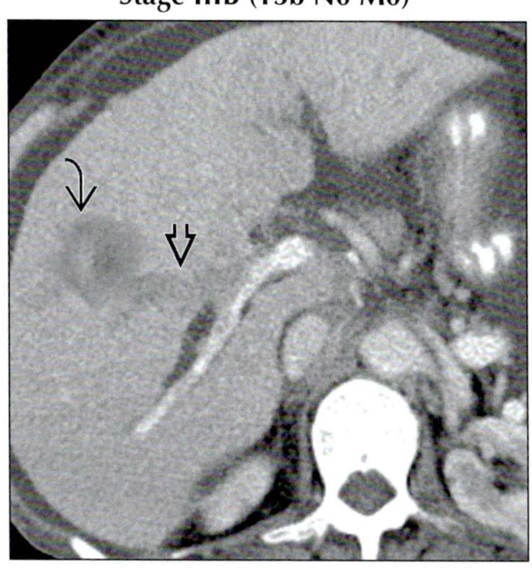

Stage IIIB (T3b N0 M0)

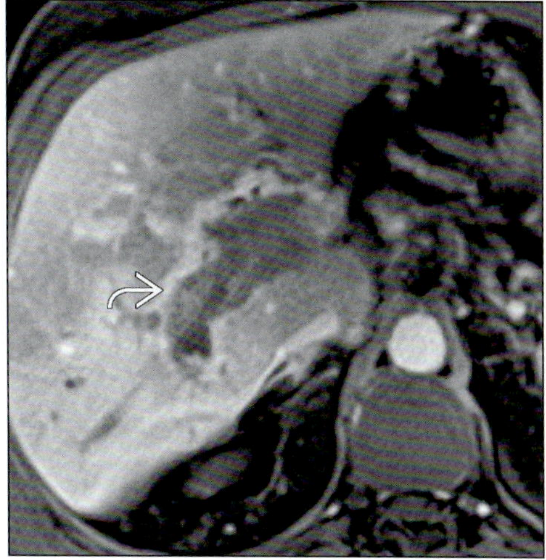

(Left) *Axial CECT in the portal venous phase shows an ill-defined mass within the anterior segment of the right hepatic lobe* ➔. *There is direct tumoral extension into the anterior division of the right portal vein* ➔. ***(Right)*** *Axial T1WI C+ MR in the portal venous phase shows extensive tumoral thrombus expanding the right portal vein* ➔ *and main portal vein.*

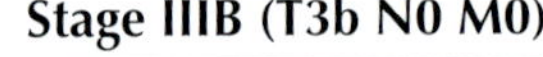

Stage IIIB (T3b N0 M0)

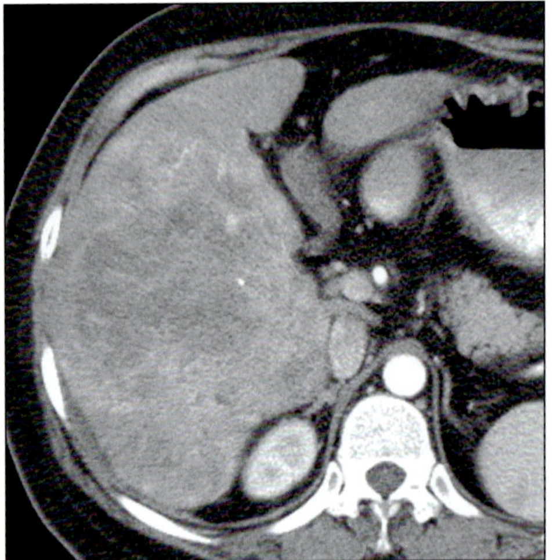

Stage IIIB (T3b N0 M0)

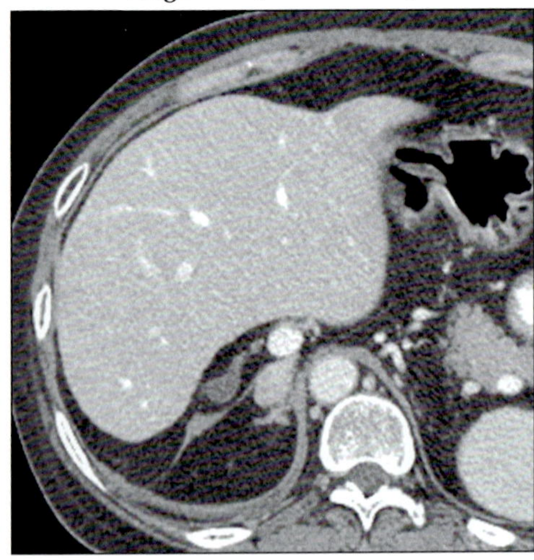

(Left) *Axial CECT reveals a large hepatoma encompassing most of the liver in a 34 year old. Presenting symptoms were pain and nausea, and AFP was > 1,000,000. The patient was treated palliatively using cisplatin and 40 Gy with shaped fields AP/PA. Due to a prompt response, a 10 Gy boost was delivered.* ***(Right)*** *Axial CECT in the same patient performed 10 years later shows a complete response. AFP had normalized.*

Stage IIIC (T4 N0 M0)

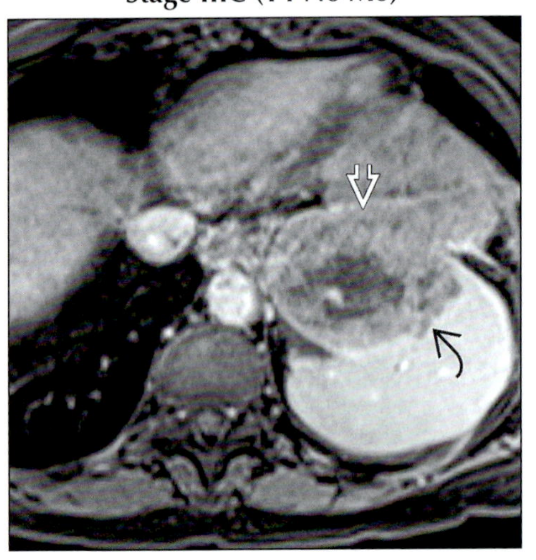

Stage IIIC (T4 N0 M0)

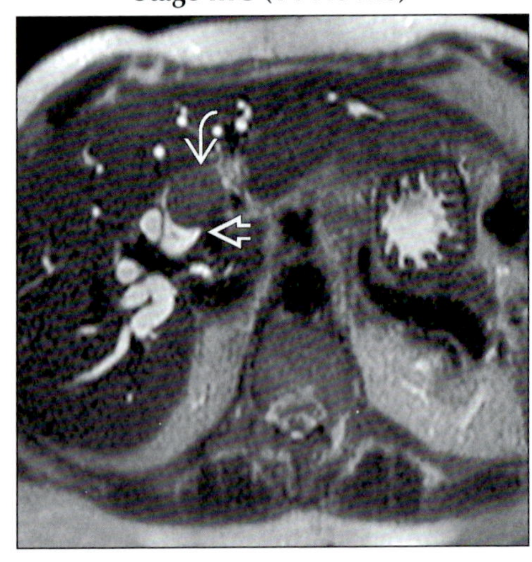

(Left) *Axial T1WI C+ MR shows a large exophytic HCC arising from the lateral segment of the left lobe and invading the splenic hilum.* ***(Right)*** *Axial T2WI FS MR shows a mass arising from the posterior aspect of segment 2 and extending beyond the visceral peritoneum. There is direct tumoral extension into the left main bile duct.*

Stage IVB (T2 N1 M1)

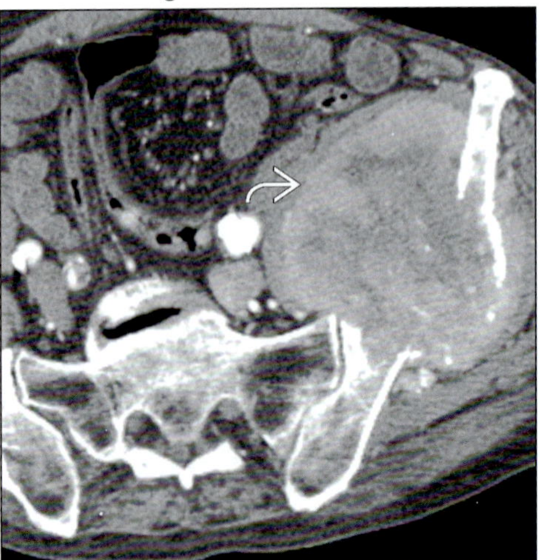

Stage IVB (T2 N1 M1)

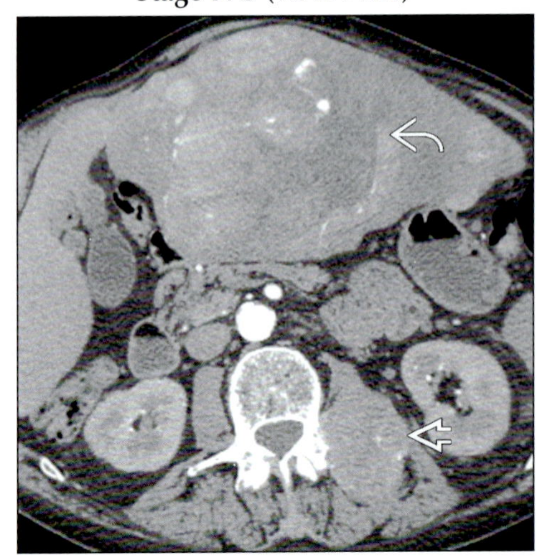

(Left) *Axial CECT shows a very large, lytic soft tissue mass arising from the left iliac bone. Biopsy of the lesion was positive for HCC.* ***(Right)*** *Axial CECT shows a heterogeneously enhancing mass expanding the left lobe of the liver, consistent with HCC. Note the left paraspinal mass with associated destructive changes of the L2 transverse process. Percutaneous CT-guided biopsy of the paraspinal mass confirmed osseous metastatic HCC.*

Stage IVA (T3 N1 M0) Cholangiocarcinoma

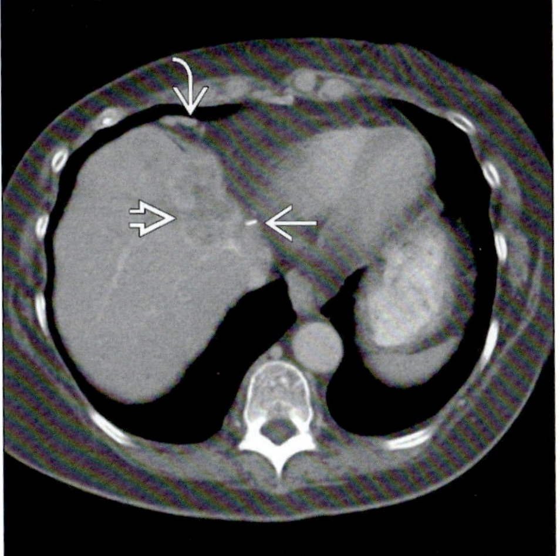

Stage IVA (T3 N1 M0) Cholangiocarcinoma

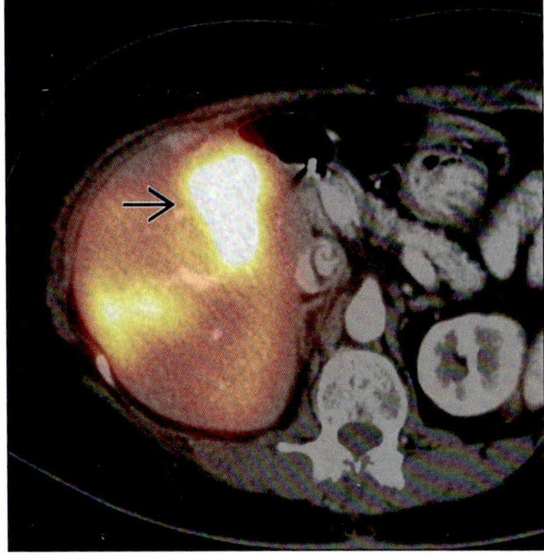

(Left) Axial oblique CECT in a 69-year-old woman with cholangiocarcinoma demonstrates a 5.4 cm enhancing lesion in segment 8 ➡. A 2 cm lymph node is seen anteriorly ➡. Note the surgical clip post left hepatic lobectomy ➡. (Right) Axial SPECT in the same patient post right hepatic arterial injection of 4 mCi Tc-99m MAA for radioembolization planning demonstrates activity in the segment 8 lesion ➡.

Stage IVA (T3 N1 M0) Cholangiocarcinoma

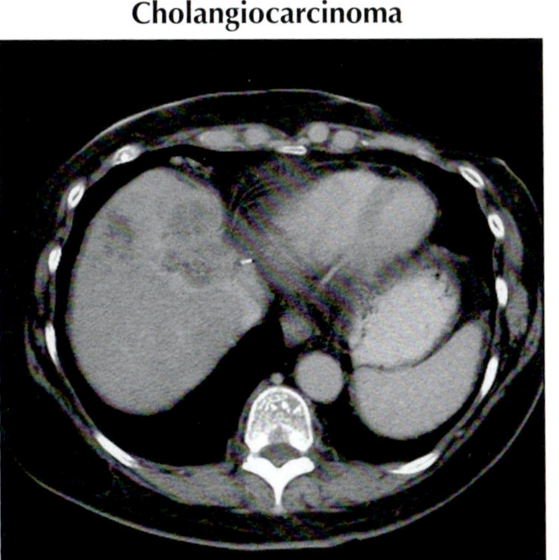

Stage IVA (T3 N1 M0) Cholangiocarcinoma

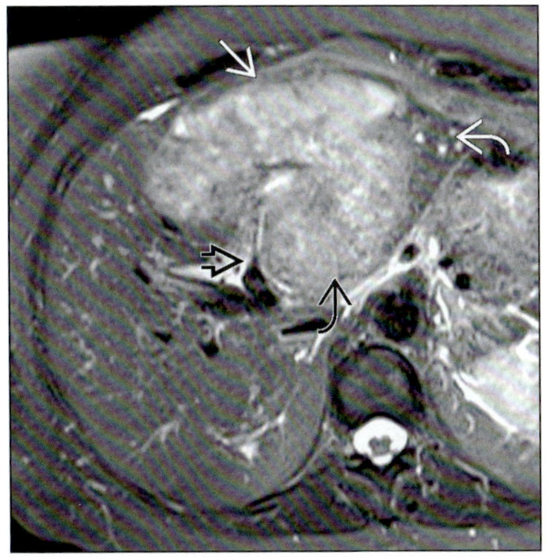

(Left) Axial CECT in the same patient 1 month post right hepatic arterial delivery of 1.42 GBq (38.25 mCi) yttrium-90 demonstrates no enhancing residual disease. (Right) Axial T2WI FS MR shows recurrence several months later. Hyperintense areas ➡ correspond to necrosis. Intermediate signal areas ➡ represent viable tumor. Note left portal vein occlusion ➡. Biliary dilatation ➡ is more common with CCA than metastasis. (Courtesy M. Rezvani, MD.)

Stage IVA (T3 N1 M0) Cholangiocarcinoma

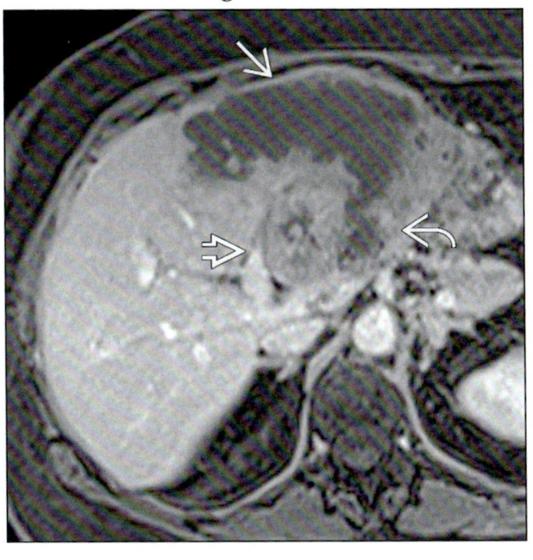

Stage IVB (T3a N1 M1)

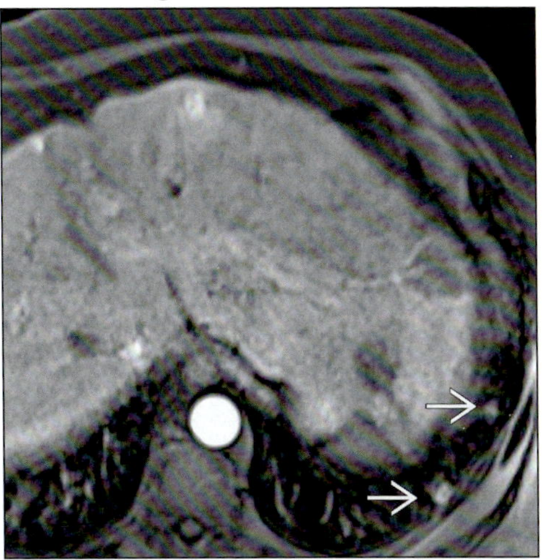

(Left) Axial T2WI C+ FS MR in the same patient shows lack of enhancement in areas of necrosis ➡, enhancing viable tumor ➡, and left portal vein obstruction ➡. (Courtesy M. Rezvani, MD.) (Right) Axial T1WI C+ MR shows multiple masses throughout the liver that demonstrate variable enhancement, consistent with multifocal HCC. Two lung nodules are noted within the left lower lobe ➡, consistent with metastatic disease.

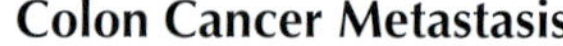

Colon Cancer Metastasis

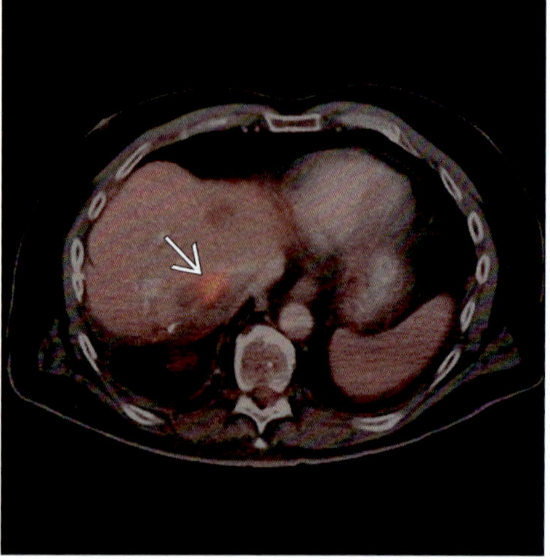

Colon Cancer Metastasis

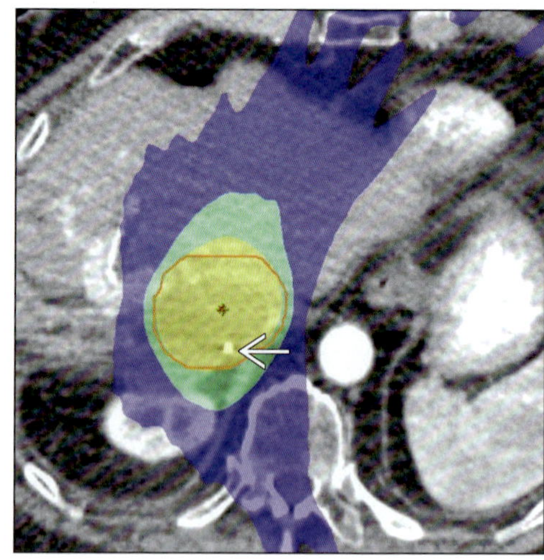

*(**Left**) Axial FDG PET/CT in a 72-year-old man demonstrates a hypermetabolic lesion in the caudate lobe ➔, consistent with metastatic colon cancer. (**Right**) Axial CT in the same patient shows the PTV outlined in red. Note the fiducial marker ➔. Yellow, green, and blue represent the 100%, 70%, and 40% isodose lines, respectively. 4D planning scans permit complete inclusion of the tumor regardless of the respiratory phase.*

Colon Cancer Metastasis

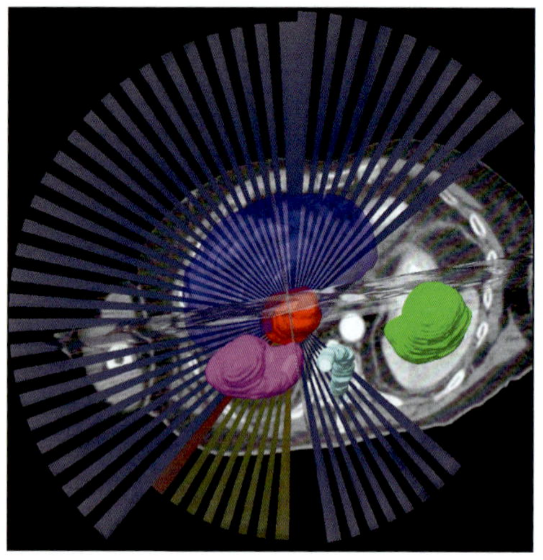

Colon Cancer Metastasis

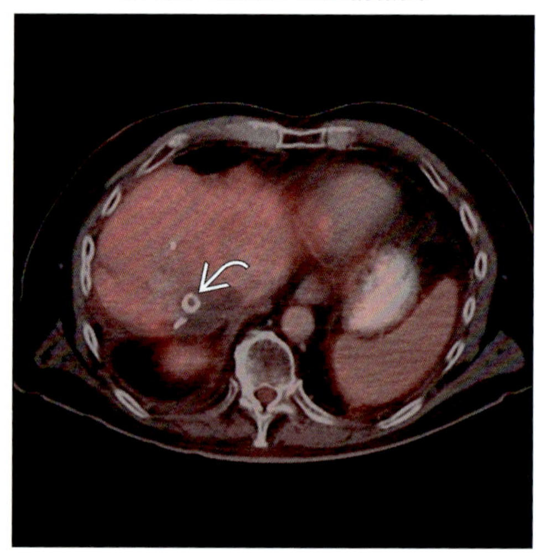

*(**Left**) Axial CT in the same patient shows the dynamic arcs were separated into 4 segments. The patient was treated to 55 Gy in 5 fractions prescribed to the 95% line. (**Right**) FDG PET/CT in the same patient 4 months post therapy demonstrates no residual disease. The patient had biliary stenosis requiring stenting ➔ but otherwise continues to do well 1 year later. SBRT should be used with caution in central/hilar lesions.*

Colon Cancer Metastasis

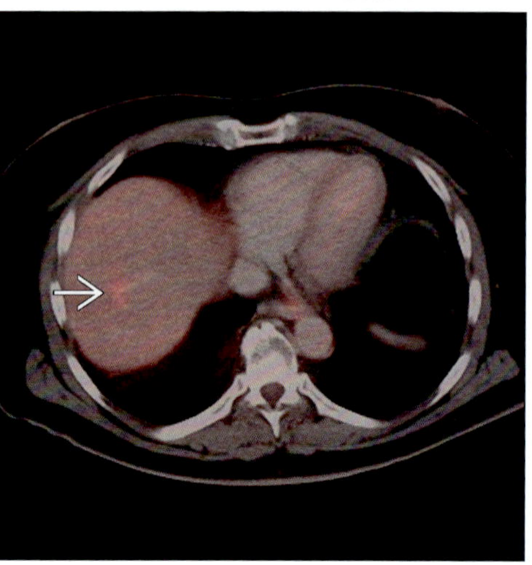

Colon Cancer Metastasis

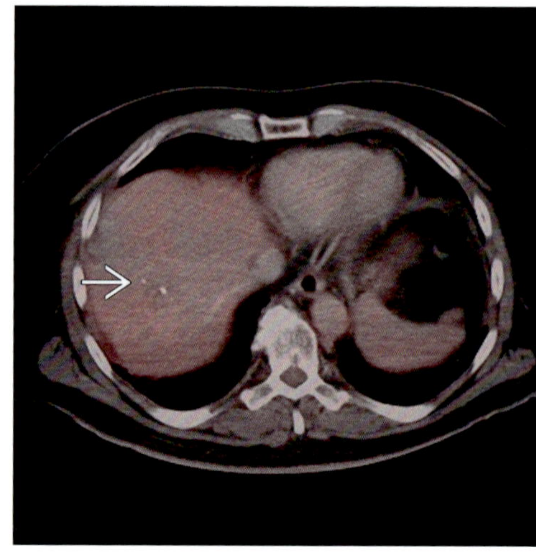

*(**Left**) FDG PET/CT in a 60-year-old man with metastatic colorectal cancer status post multiple cycles of systemic chemotherapy. A hypermetabolic focus with an SUV of 5.43 is seen in segment 8 ➔. (**Right**) FDG PET/CT in the same patient 7 months after SBRT demonstrates no evidence of residual disease. Note the fiduciary markers in the tumor bed ➔. Unfortunately, the tumor recurred 12 months later.*

Metastatic Ocular Melanoma

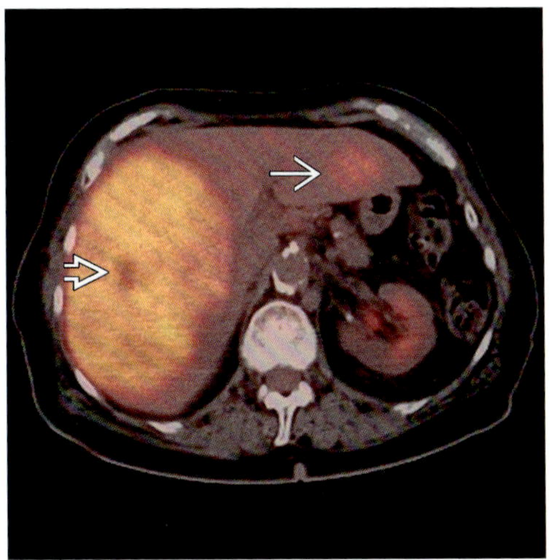

Metastatic Ocular Melanoma

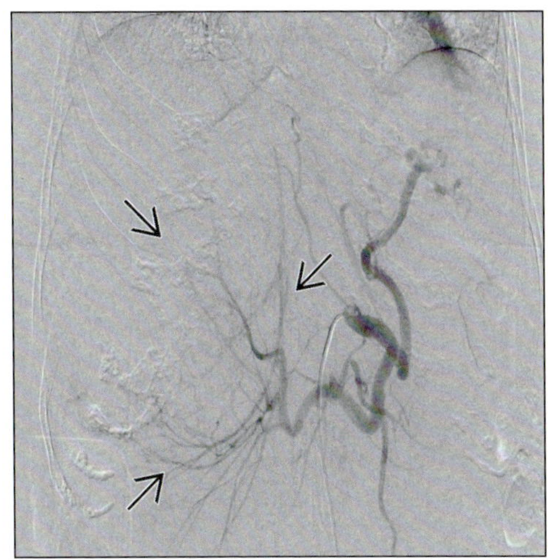

*(**Left**) Axial FDG PET/CT in a 64-year-old woman with metastatic ocular melanoma shows a large hypermetabolic mass in the right hepatic lobe ➡ and segment 3 of the left hepatic lobe ➡. (**Right**) Angiography in the same patient demonstrates displacement of the hepatic vasculature in the right hepatic lobe secondary to the mass ➡. Chemoembolization was performed delivering 200 mg of 1,3-bis(2-chloroethyl)-1-nitrosourea (BCNU) dissolved in Ethiodol.*

Metastatic Ocular Melanoma

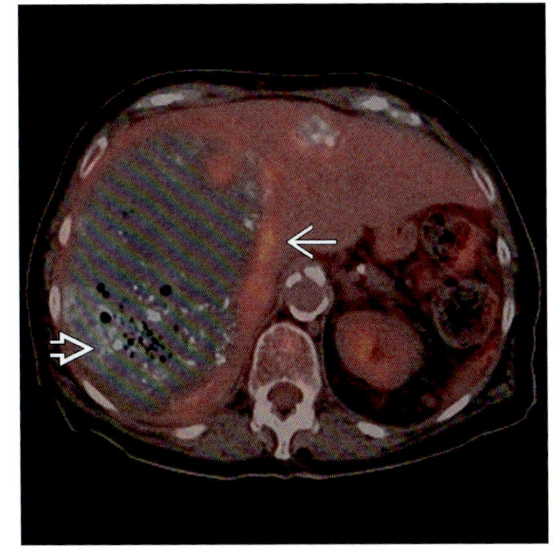

Metastatic Pancreatic Cancer

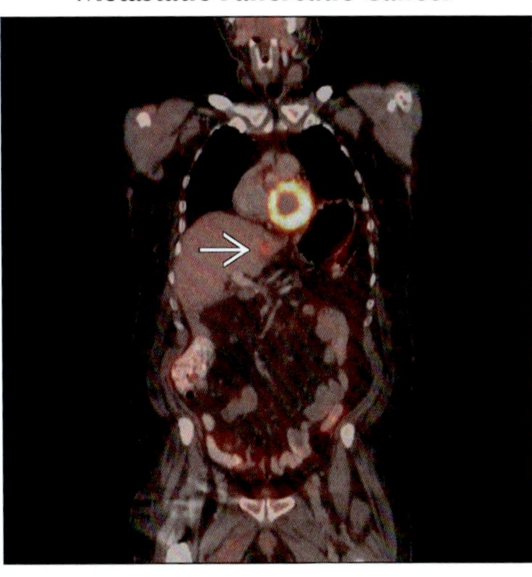

*(**Left**) Axial FDG PET/CT in the same patient 1 month later demonstrates almost complete necrosis of the right hepatic lobe tumor. Note nodular peripheral areas of hypermetabolism ➡. Areas of hyperdensity ➡ represent areas of residual Ethiodol. The patient continues to do well at 6 months. (**Right**) Coronal FDG PET/CT shows a 72-year-old man with metastatic pancreatic cancer and a solitary lesion in segment 2 ➡. He has completed multiple cycles of chemotherapy.*

Metastatic Pancreatic Cancer

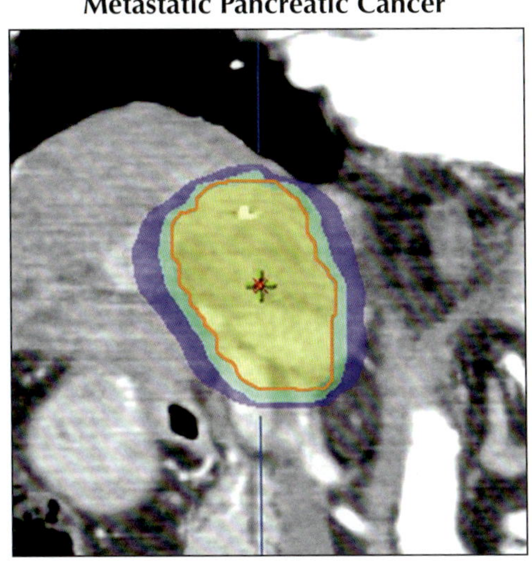

Metastatic Pancreatic Cancer

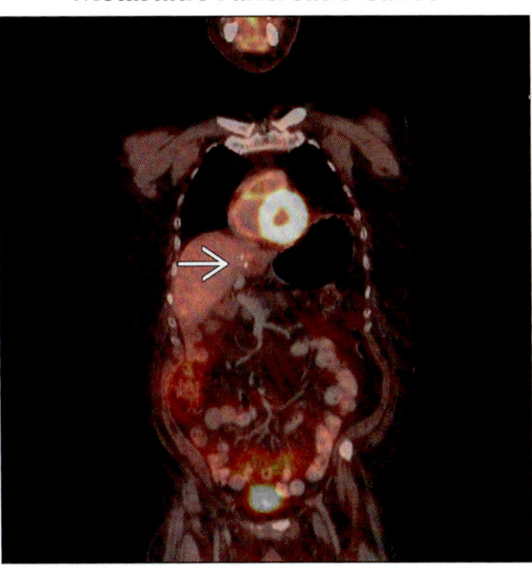

*(**Left**) Coronal CT in the same patient demonstrates conformality to the PTV. He received a total of 25 Gy in 5 fractions. (**Right**) PET/CT in the same patient 15 months later shows no evidence of residual disease ➡.*

PANCREAS

(T) Primary Tumor

Adapted from 7th edition AJCC Staging Forms.

TNM	*Definitions*
TX	Primary tumor cannot be assessed
T0	No evidence of primary tumor
Tis	Carcinoma in situ*
T1	Tumor limited to pancreas, ≤ 2 cm in greatest dimension
T2	Tumor limited to pancreas, > 2 cm in greatest dimension
T3	Tumor extends beyond pancreas but without involvement of celiac axis or superior mesenteric artery
T4	Tumor involves celiac axis or superior mesenteric artery (unresectable primary tumor)

(N) Regional Lymph Nodes

NX	Regional lymph nodes cannot be assessed
N0	No regional lymph node metastasis
N1	Regional lymph node metastasis

(M) Distant Metastasis

M0	No distant metastasis
M1	Distant metastasis

**This also includes the "PanIN-3" classification.*

AJCC Stages/Prognostic Groups

Adapted from 7th edition AJCC Staging Forms.

Stage	*T*	*N*	*M*
0	Tis	N0	M0
IA	T1	N0	M0
IB	T2	N0	M0
IIA	T3	N0	M0
IIB	T1	N1	M0
	T2	N1	M0
	T3	N1	M0
III	T4	Any N	M0
IV	Any T	Any N	M1

Tis

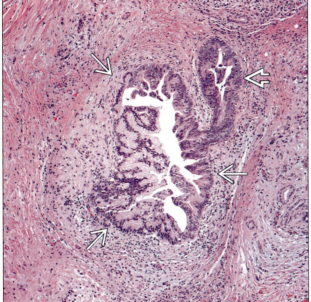

H&E stained section shows carcinoma in situ (Tis) involving an interlobular duct with surrounding fibrosis. The portion of the duct in the upper right portion of the image demonstrates high-grade dysplasia without invasion of the basement membrane.

Tis

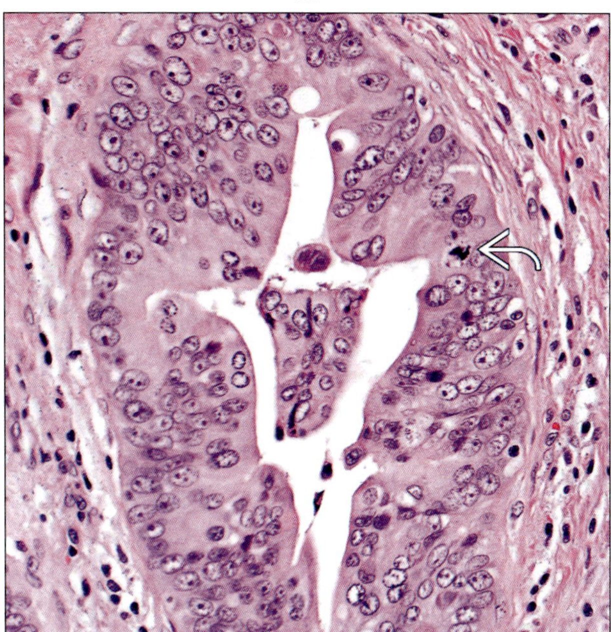

High-power view of the right upper portion of the previous image shows neoplastic epithelial cells, which are characterized by increased nuclear to cytoplasmic ratio and haphazard arrangement of atypical nuclei. Additionally, the atypical nuclei are conspicuous, vesicular, and chromatic. Mitotic figures are easily found.

T1

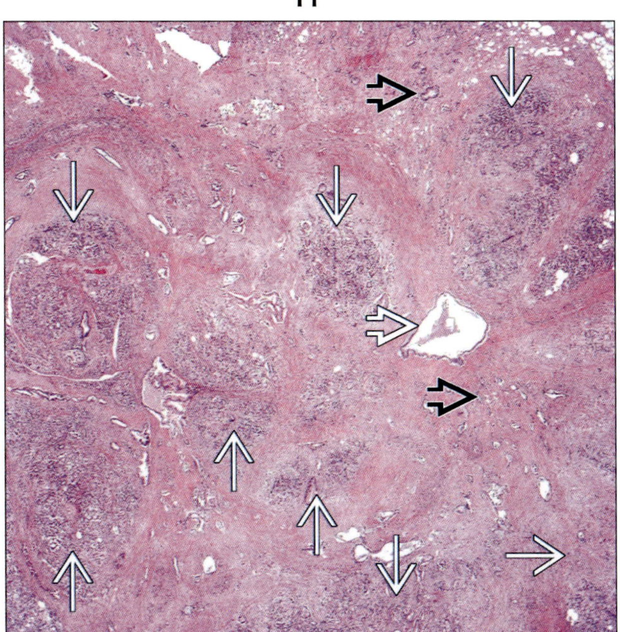

H&E stained section shows chronic pancreatitis with considerable loss of unevenly distributed acinar tissue with intervening fibrosis and a few dilated ducts with inspissated secretions. Scattered foci of well-differentiated ductal adenocarcinoma are present.

T1

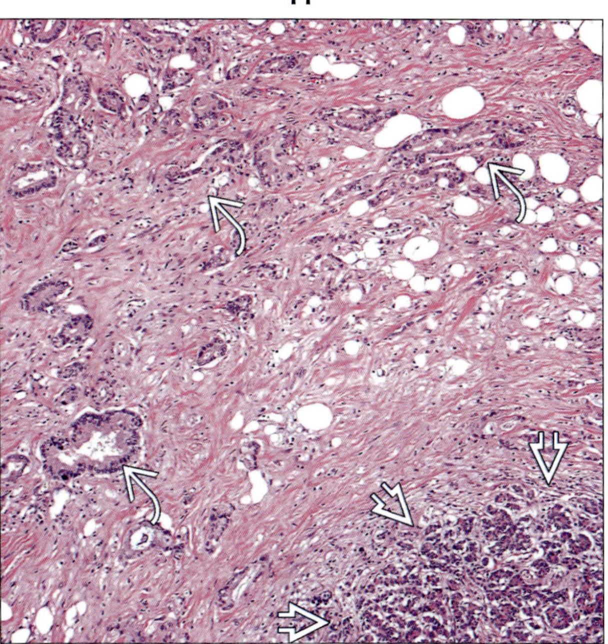

Higher magnification shows the right upper portion of the previous image. The left upper portion of this image demonstrates invasive well-differentiated ductal adenocarcinoma. Pancreatic islet cells are seen in the lower right portion of this image.

PANCREAS

T1

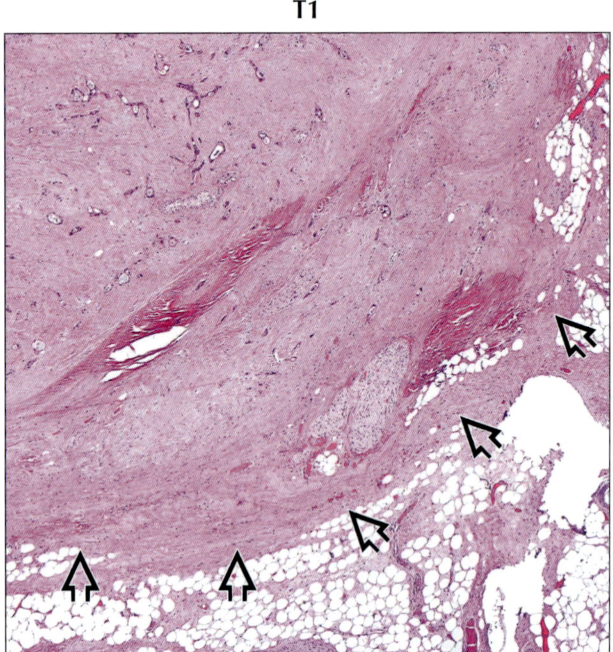

H&E stained section shows a ≤ 2 cm pancreatic adenocarcinoma in the left upper portion of the image that is confined to the pancreas, consistent with T1 disease. Note the interface between the pancreas and the peripancreatic fat ⇨.

T1

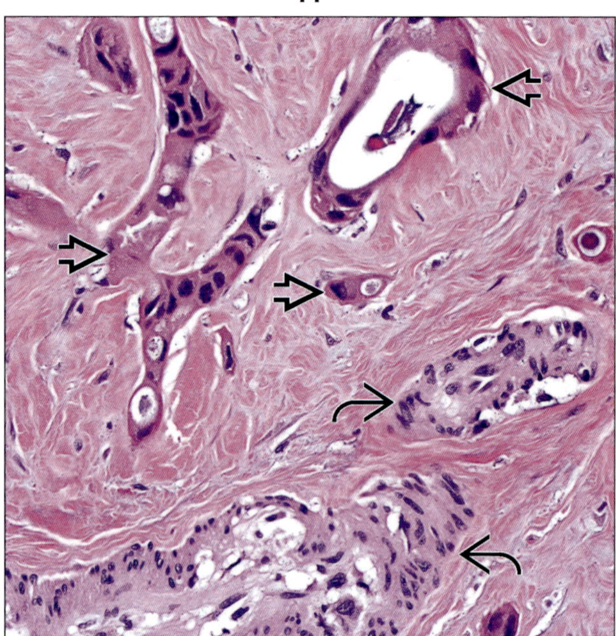

Higher power view of the previous image shows neoplastic cells arranged in irregular glands ⇨ invading into a densely fibrotic stroma (wavy pink areas). Several nerves are seen in the lower portion of the image ↗.

T3

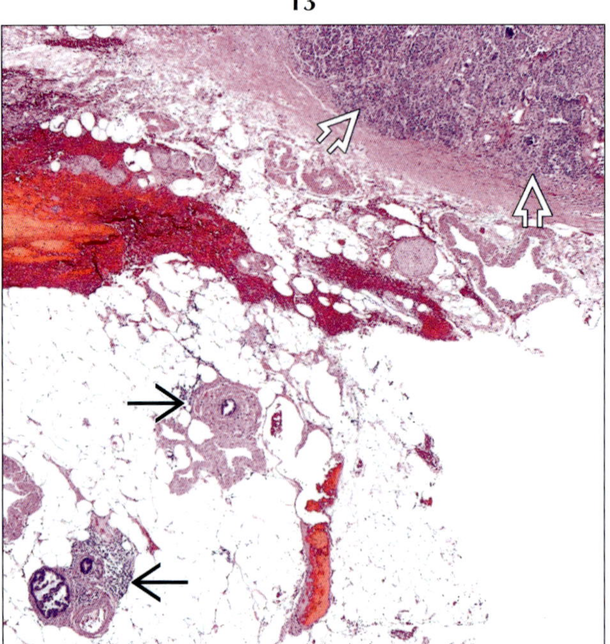

Low-power H&E stained section shows pancreatic tissue ➡ in the right upper portion of the image. Two small foci of pancreatic adenocarcinoma → are present in the peripancreatic fat.

TX

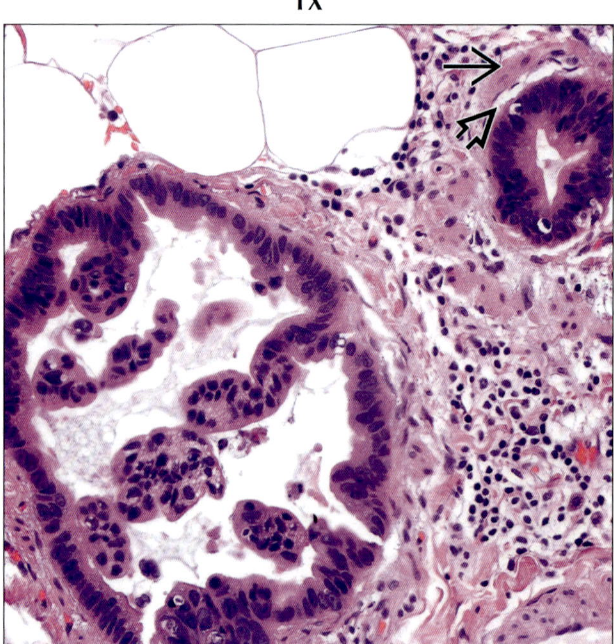

High-power view of pancreatic adenocarcinoma shows neoplastic glands expanding the lumina of 2 vessels. A slit-like space ⇨ represents a portion of the lumen lined by endothelial cells →. Lymphatic and venous invasion have been combined into lymphovascular invasion for collection by cancer registrars.

T1

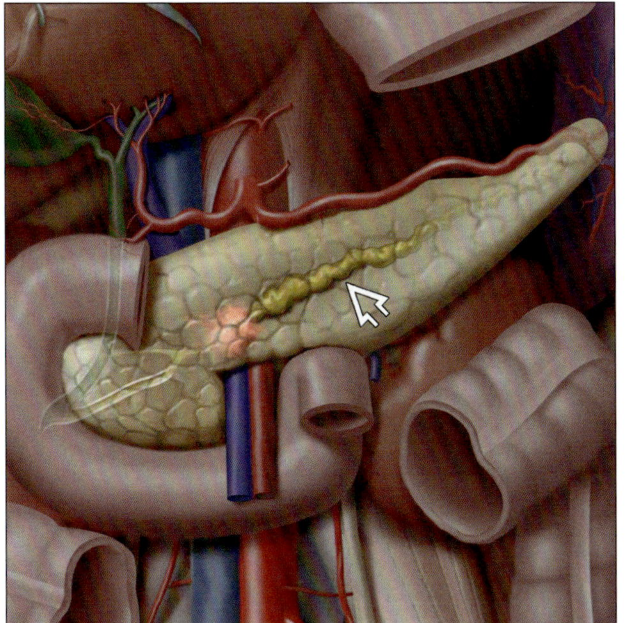

Graphic depicts a tumor ≤ 2 cm without extension beyond the pancreas, consistent with T1 disease. In this case, there is upstream pancreatic dilation ⇨. This is a resectable tumor.

T2

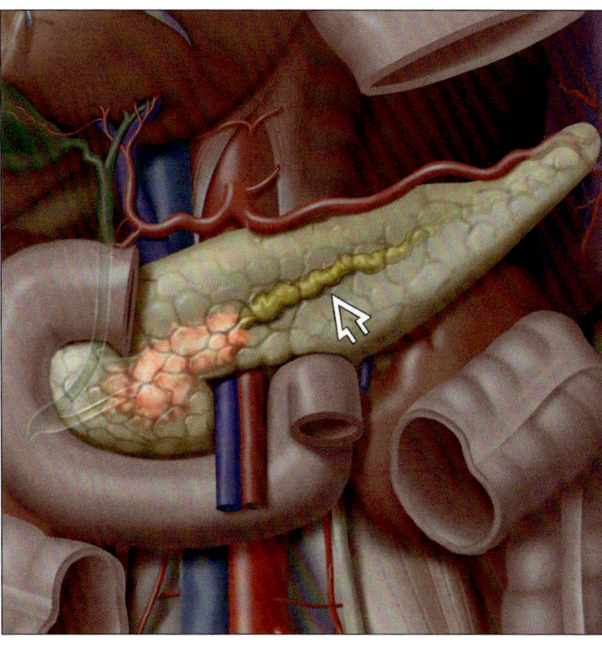

Graphic depicts a tumor measuring > 2 cm confined to the pancreas, consistent with T2 disease. Note upstream pancreatic ductal dilation ⇨. This is a resectable tumor.

T3

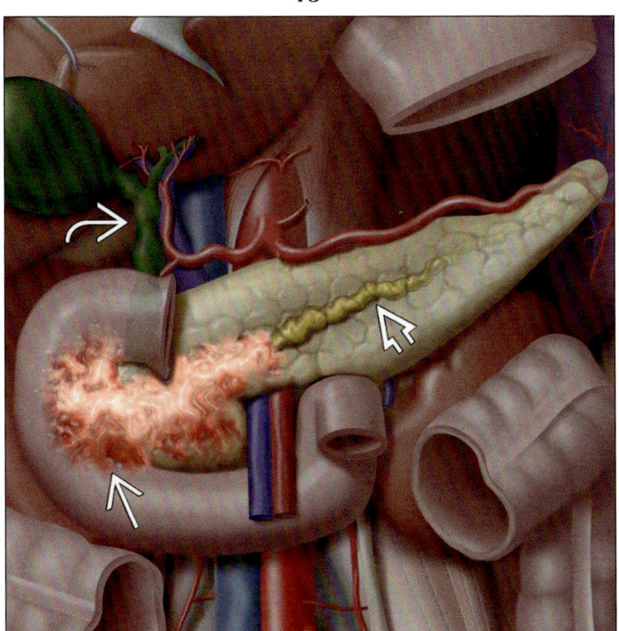

Graphic depicts a resectable tumor that invades into the duodenum → and produces a "double duct" sign by obstructing and distending the pancreatic ⇨ and common bile ducts ↷. Tumors that extend beyond the pancreas but do not involve the superior mesenteric or celiac arteries are designated T3.

T3

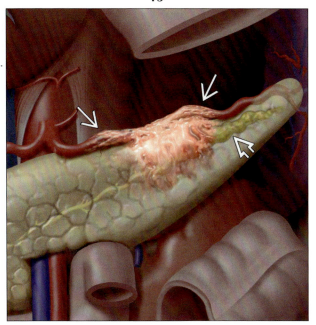

This pancreatic tail tumor extends beyond the pancreas and invades the splenic artery. The tumor tracks along the perivascular, perineural, &/or perilymphatic tissues toward the splenic hilum and celiac axis →. There is upstream pancreatic ductal dilation ⇨. This is a borderline resectable tumor.

T3

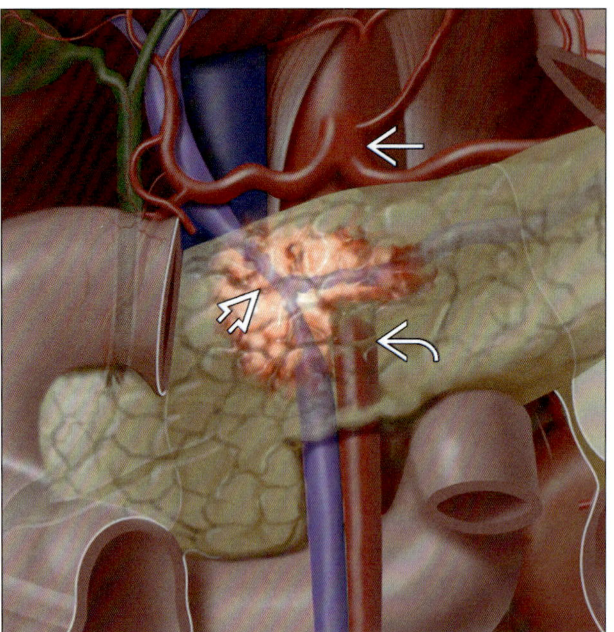

Graphic depicts tumor that extends beyond the pancreas posteriorly and invades the confluence of the superior mesenteric, splenic, and main portal veins ➡. Tumors that extend beyond pancreas but do not involve the superior mesenteric ➡ or celiac ➡ arteries, such as this borderline resectable tumor, are designated T3.

T3

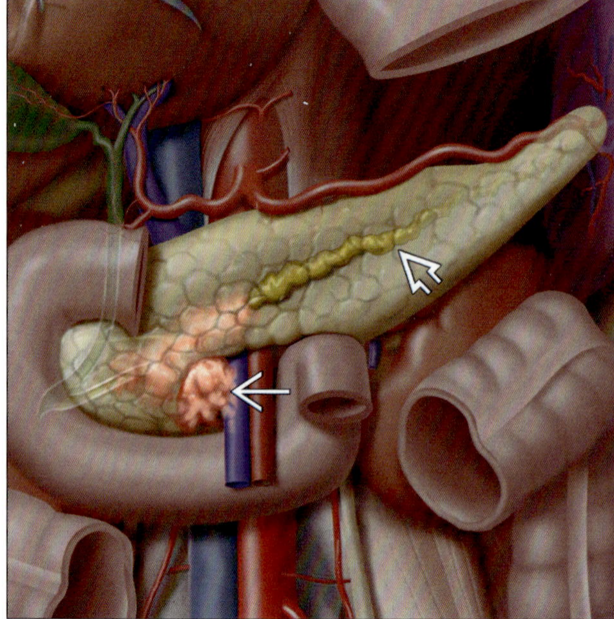

This pancreatic head tumor extends beyond the pancreas and invades the upper superior mesenteric vein ➡. However, because the superior mesenteric and celiac arteries are spared, this borderline resectable tumor is classified as T3. Upstream pancreatic ductal dilation is present ➡.

T4

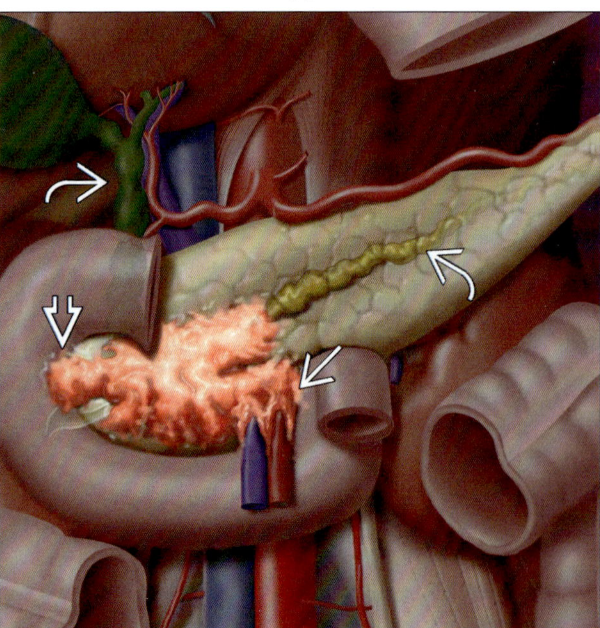

Graphic depicts a tumor invading the superior mesenteric artery and vein ➡. Additionally, there is invasion of the duodenum ➡ and a "double duct" sign ➡. This unresectable tumor is classified as T4, as any tumor that invades the superior mesenteric or celiac arteries is designated as T4.

T4

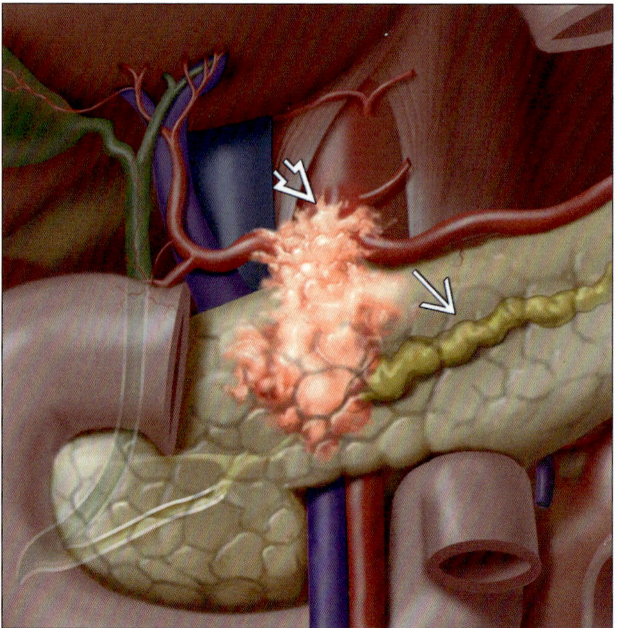

Graphic depicts a tumor that extends beyond the pancreas and invades the celiac axis ➡, as well as the proximal common hepatic and splenic arteries. Upstream pancreatic ductal dilation is present ➡. Involvement of the celiac axis results in a T4 classification. This is an unresectable tumor.

Peripancreatic Lymph Node Groups

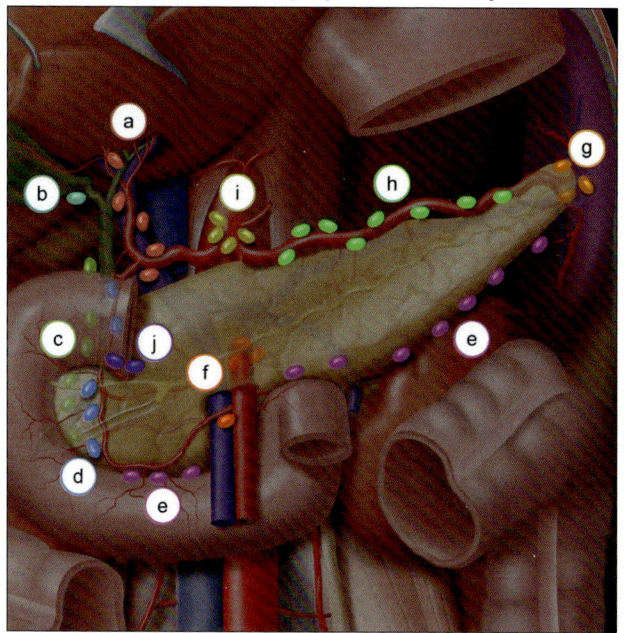

Graphic depicts peripancreatic lymph node groups: a) Hepatic, b) cystic duct, c) posterior pancreaticoduodenal, d) anterior pancreaticoduodenal, e) inferior pancreaticoduodenal, f) superior mesenteric, g) splenic hilar, h) superior, i) celiac, and j) pyloric.

Whipple Anatomy

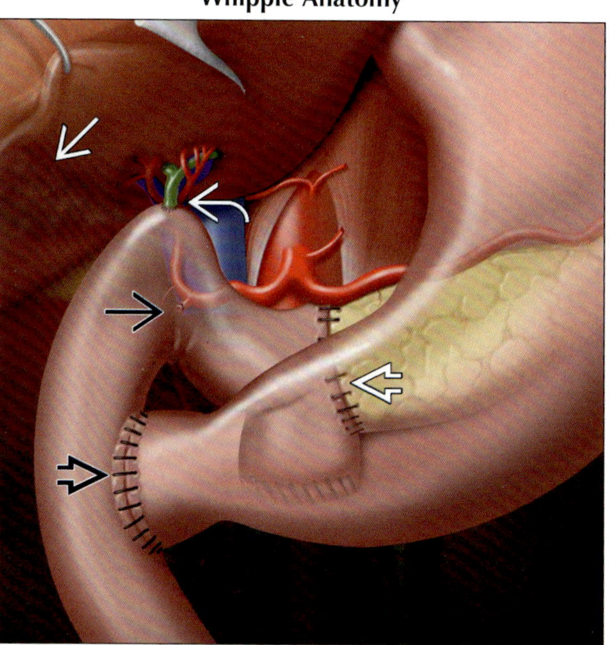

Graphic depicts Whipple anatomy: Pancreaticojejunostomy ⇨, choledochojejunostomy ⇨, gastrojejunostomy or duodenojejunostomy ⇨, and cholecystectomy ⇨. The pylorus may be removed or preserved, depending on extent of disease and surgeon preference. Note the ligated gastroduodenal artery →.

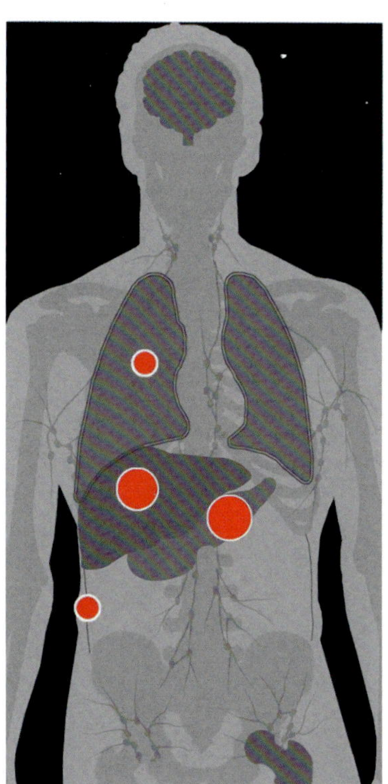

INITIAL SITE OF RECURRENCE

Local	70-80%
Liver	50-60%
Peritoneum	10-40%
Other (Lung, Pleura, Bone, Adrenal, Brain, etc.)	25-50%

These percentages represent data from patients that underwent curative resection. Hishinuma et al: J Gastrointest Surg 10(4):511-8, 2006; Sperti et al: World J Surg 21(2):195-200, 1997; Griffin et al: Cancer 66(1):56-61, 1990.

PANCREAS

OVERVIEW

General Comments

- > 95% of pancreas malignancies are classified as exocrine tumors
  - Histopathologically a heterogeneous group of carcinomas
  - Lowest median survival rate of all cancers
    - Often diagnosed at advanced stage
- Endocrine pancreatic tumors originate from islet cells of Langerhans that make up endocrine pancreas
  - Pancreatic neuroendocrine tumors (PNETs) are also called islet cell tumors
    - < 5% of total pancreatic mass consists of endocrine cells
  - High rate of malignancy (60-92%)
    - Malignant potential of insulinoma is low
    - Other syndromic tumors are more frequently malignant

Classification

- Exocrine tumors
  - Ductal origin (> 95%)
    - Ductal adenocarcinoma (> 85%)
    - Cystic mucinous carcinoma
    - Noncystic mucinous carcinoma (colloid carcinoma)
      - Associated with more protracted course
    - Undifferentiated carcinoma
      - Sarcomatoid (spindle cell)
      - Anaplastic giant cell
      - Carcinosarcoma
      - Undifferentiated carcinoma with osteoclast-like giant cells
    - Adenosquamous carcinoma
    - Intraductal papillary mucinous carcinoma
    - Signet ring cell carcinoma
    - Serous cystadenocarcinoma (very rare)
    - Medullary carcinoma (very rare)
  - Acinar origin (1-2%)
    - Acinar cell carcinoma
  - Mixed origin
    - Mixed ductal-endocrine carcinoma (rare)
      - Behaves similar to ductal carcinoma
    - Mixed ductal-acinar carcinoma (rare)
      - Behaves similar to ductal carcinoma
    - Mixed acinar-endocrine carcinoma
      - Behaves similar to acinar carcinoma
    - Pancreatoblastoma
      - Typically includes all 3 cell types (endocrine, ductal, acinar) but composed of cells of acinar origin
      - Typically in children (peak age: 4 years) with small 2nd peak in 4th decade of life
  - Supportive element origin
    - Squamous cell carcinoma (very rare)
  - Unknown origin
    - Solid pseudopapillary carcinoma
  - Borderline, indolent, or premalignant neoplasms
    - Up to 2% of exocrine pancreatic cancers arise from these
      - Intraductal papillary mucinous neoplasm (IPMN)
      - Pancreatic intraepithelial neoplasia III (PanInIII)
      - Mucinous cystadenoma
      - Intraductal oncocytic papillary neoplasm (very rare)
      - Solid pseudopapillary tumor
- Endocrine tumors
  - Typically divided depending on clinical and biochemical manifestations
  - Syndromic (hyperfunctioning, 65-70%)
    - Insulinoma
      - Arises from islet β cells
      - Most common functioning PNET
      - Usually solitary
      - 6-10% are malignant
      - 10% of patients with clinical syndrome will have "islet cell hyperplasia" rather than discrete insulinoma
    - Gastrinoma
      - 2nd most common syndromic PNET
      - Many patients will have Zollinger-Ellison syndrome (excess production of gastrin)
      - 60-90% are malignant
    - Glucagonoma
      - Uncommon PNET
      - 60% are malignant
    - VIPoma
      - 80% are malignant
      - Secretes variety of hormones, including vasoactive intestinal peptide (VIP)
    - Somatostatinoma
      - Arises from delta cells
      - Majority are malignant
    - Others
  - Nonsyndromic (nonhyperfunctioning, 30-35%)
  - Carcinoid tumors
    - Carcinoid tumor
    - Atypical carcinoid
    - Composite carcinoid (combined with adenocarcinoma)
    - Adenocarcinoid
- According to 2010 AJCC staging guidelines, pancreatic exocrine and endocrine tumors now utilize same staging system

NATURAL HISTORY

General Features

- Comments
  - Majority of pancreatic tumors arise from ductal structures
    - Ductal tissue represents 15% of volume of pancreas
      - Remaining 85% is acinar tissue
    - Ductal tissue is only pancreatic tissue exposed to external carcinogens
- Location
  - Exocrine tumors
    - Head (60%)
    - Body (20%)
    - Tail (5%)
    - Diffuse (15%)
  - Endocrine tumors
    - Insulinoma
      - Equal distribution in head, body, and tail
    - Gastrinoma

- Located in gastrinoma triangle
- Formed by cystic duct confluence, junction of pancreatic neck and body, and junction of 2nd and 3rd parts of duodenum
- VIPoma
  - Located in tail of pancreas in 75% of cases
  - Can be extrapancreatic in 20% of cases
- Somatostatinoma
  - Duodenal in 50% cases

Etiology

- Risk factors
  - Exocrine tumors
    - Tobacco
      - 2-3x increased risk
      - Smoking responsible for 20-35%
    - Increased BMI
    - Diets high in animal fat
    - Occupational exposure
      - β-naphthylamine, benzidine (used in dye production)
      - Metal-refining chemicals
      - Gasoline
    - Heavy alcohol consumption
    - Chronic pancreatitis
    - New-onset diabetes mellitus (type 2)
    - Family history of pancreatitis or pancreatic cancer
  - Endocrine tumors
    - Usually arise sporadically
    - Family history of multiple endocrine neoplasia type 1 (MEN1)

Epidemiology & Cancer Incidence

- Exocrine tumors
  - Number of cases in USA per year
    - Estimated 43,920 new cases and 37,390 deaths in 2012
    - 10th most common malignancy in USA
      - 4th leading cause of cancer death in USA (after lung, breast/prostate, and colorectal cancer)
  - Median age at diagnosis: 72 years
  - M = F
  - Racial incidence
    - African-American: 14.9/100,000
    - Caucasian-American: 11.2/100,000
    - Native-American: 10.8/100,000
    - Hispanic-American: 10.3/100,000
    - Asian-American: 9.0/100,000
- Endocrine tumors
  - Rare tumors
    - Up to 5% of all primary pancreatic malignancies
    - Crude annual incidence of 0.22 per 100,000 in USA
    - PNETs can be found in 0.8-10% of autopsies
      - Discrepancy between incidence in population and incidence at autopsy suggests that people frequently harbor asymptomatic PNETs
    - Slightly higher incidence among males
    - Incidence increases with age and peaks in 6th and 7th decade
      - Earlier age of onset in patients with genetic syndromes

Genetics

- Exocrine tumors
  - Hereditary syndromes
    - *BRCA2*
    - Peutz-Jeghers (*STK1* gene)
    - Atypical multiple mole-melanoma syndrome (*p16* gene)
    - Hereditary nonpolyposis colorectal cancer (*MLH1* and *MSH2* genes)
    - Familial pancreatic cancer (*PALLD* gene)
    - Familial chronic pancreatitis (40-75% lifetime risk)
    - Beckwith-Wiedemann or familial polyposis coli syndromes (pancreatoblastoma)
  - Other genes related to pancreatic cancer include mutations of
    - *K-ras* (70-100%)
    - *p53* (50%)
- Endocrine tumors
  - Hereditary syndromes
    - MEN1
      - Inherited condition characterized by synchronous or metachronous tumors of parathyroid glands, anterior pituitary, pancreas, and gastrointestinal tract
      - 75% gastrinomas, 25% insulinomas
      - 40-70% of MEN1 patients develop PNET
      - Germline mutation in 1 copy of gene located on centromeric portion of long arm of chromosome 11 (11q13)
    - von Hippel-Lindau (VHL) disease
      - PNETs develop in 10-17% of patients with VHL
      - Almost invariably nonsyndromic PNETs
    - Neurofibromatosis type 1
    - Tuberous sclerosis

Gross Pathology & Surgical Features

- Exocrine tumors
  - Scirrhous mass with ill-defined borders
  - Difficult to differentiate macroscopically from benign scar tissue within pancreas (i.e., chronic pancreatitis)
- Endocrine tumors
  - Tumor size is variable
    - 90% of insulinomas are smaller than 2 cm in diameter
      - Most patients with insulinoma present early with relatively small tumors
    - Glucagonomas are usually large
      - Mean diameter is 6.5 cm
  - Small tumors
    - Homogeneous
    - Unencapsulated
  - Larger tumors
    - Cystic
    - Necrotic
    - Hemorrhagic
    - Contain fibrous pseudocapsule
      - Pseudocapsule is often incomplete and should not be mistaken for invasive behavior
  - Well demarcated
  - Soft to firm or rubbery in consistency, depending on relative content of fibrous stroma
  - Calcifications may be found in larger tumors

Microscopic Pathology

- H&E
  - Ductal adenocarcinoma

PANCREAS

- Often well differentiated with recognizable ductal structures that are occasionally difficult to distinguish from benign ductal epithelium
  - May be poorly differentiated with no recognizable ductal structures
- Ductal adenocarcinoma cells are usually cuboidal with nuclear atypia and form duct-like structures
- Highly infiltrative
  - Desmoplastic stroma with abundant fibrosis and inflammation is characteristic
  - Tumors often have more stromal than ductal tissue
- Up to 80% have microscopic perineural invasion
- Vascular invasion is common
  - May manifest as well-formed ductal elements within vascular spaces, which is rare with other tumors
- Squamous differentiation may rarely occur in ductal adenocarcinoma
  - Pure squamous cell carcinoma without ductal elements is very rare
- Undifferentiated carcinomas may be composed of epithelioid &/or spindle cells
  - May rarely include bone or cartilage components
  - May include nonneoplastic osteoclast-like giant cells

- Acinar cell carcinoma
  - Monotonous and highly cellular tumor arranged in solid sheets and nests with foci of acinar or glandular cells
  - Lacks desmoplastic stroma seen in ductal adenocarcinoma
  - Cells classically demonstrate apical eosinophilic granularity secondary to zymogen granules (trypsin, lipase, and chymotrypsin)
- Polyphenotypic carcinoma
  - Rare tumors include
    - Mixed acinar-endocrine
    - Mixed ductal-acinar
    - Mixed ductal-endocrine
    - Pancreatoblastoma
  - Pancreatoblastoma is predominantly composed of cells of acinar lineage
    - "Squamoid nest" is a characteristic finding
- Both benign and malignant PNETs have similar appearance
  - Determination of benign vs. malignant is primarily by finding additional metastatic sites in liver and lymph nodes
  - Majority show histologic patterns that reflect relatively high level of cellular differentiation
    - Trabecular ± gyriform arrangement
    - Acinar or glandular pattern, often surrounding lumen
    - Medullary or solid pattern
  - Nuclei are relatively uniform in size and shape with dispersed chromatin and inconspicuous nucleoli
    - Mitoses are unusual, even in tumors that behave aggressively
  - Rare type of PNET appears as poorly differentiated neoplasms that are virtually identical to small cell carcinoma of the lung
    - More likely to exhibit infiltrative growth pattern similar to pancreatic adenocarcinoma

- Special stains
  - Exocrine pancreas
    - Immunohistochemical stains are useful for diagnosing acinar cell carcinoma
      - Trypsin
      - Lipase
      - Chymotrypsin
  - Endocrine pancreas
    - Chromogranin appears to be the most consistent general marker for pancreatic neuroendocrine tumors
    - Other commonly used immunohistochemical markers include
      - Synaptophysin
      - Vasoactive monoamine transporter 2
      - Serotonin
      - Substance P

Routes of Spread

- **Lymphatic spread**
  - Pancreatic head and uncinate tumors
    - Anterior and superior pancreatic head
      - Drain along anterior superior pancreaticoduodenal vessels to pyloric and celiac axis nodes
    - Posterior and superior pancreatic head
      - Drain along posterior superior pancreaticoduodenal vessels to pyloric and celiac axis nodes or along common bile duct to portal vein and to hepatic hilar nodes
    - Inferior pancreatic head and uncinate
      - Drain along inferior pancreaticoduodenal vessels to superior mesenteric and paraaortic nodes
  - Pancreatic body and tail tumors
    - Drain either along splenic artery to celiac axis nodes or splenic hilar nodes
- **Perineural/perivascular spread**
  - Pathways similar to lymphatic spread of tumor
  - 80% of pancreatic carcinomas demonstrate perineural invasion on pathology
- **Hematogenous spread**
  - Common for patients to have hematogenous metastases at time of presentation
  - Hepatic metastases are common
    - Pancreas drained by portal venous structures
    - Hepatic sinusoids lack basement membrane and are relatively porous, which is thought to allow metastases to permeate into space of Disse
  - Distant hematogenous metastases are less common
    - Generally only seen in advanced disease
      - Lung
      - Pleura
      - Adrenal glands
      - Brain
      - Bone
      - Other
- **Peritoneal spread**
  - Common location of metastatic disease

IMAGING

Detection

- **Abdominal ultrasound**
  - Primary tumor

- Exocrine tumors
  - Generally ill defined and hypoechoic but can be heterogeneous or echogenic
  - May have increased color Doppler signal
  - May efface or obliterate normal planes between pancreas and vessels in setting of vascular invasion
  - Enlarged lymph nodes may be present
  - May present as pancreatic &/or biliary ductal dilation without mass
- Endocrine tumors
  - Small lesions are usually homogeneous and hypoechoic
  - Larger lesions are more heterogeneous, reflecting presence of hemorrhage, necrosis, and calcifications

- **NECT**
  - Exocrine tumors
    - Generally isodense to normal pancreatic parenchyma unless extensive necrosis or cystic changes are present
    - Cystic changes are uncommon
      - Occasionally pseudocysts may be present
    - Calcifications are rare
  - Endocrine tumors
    - Can be homogeneous, heterogeneous, or cystic in appearance
    - Cystic degeneration, calcification, and necrosis are more common in larger syndromic PNETs
- **Pancreatic protocol CECT**
  - Primary tumor: Exocrine tumors
    - Typically ill-defined margins and delayed enhancement
      - Isoenhancing or avid early arterial enhancing lesions are less common
    - Detection rate for tumors ≤ 2 cm (71%), > 2 cm (89%)
    - Invasion of extrapancreatic structures
    - "Double duct" sign
      - Simultaneous dilatation of the common bile and pancreatic ducts, generally secondary to contiguous obstruction or encasement of both ducts
      - Nonspecific for pancreatic mass
      - Suggestive of pancreatic head or ampullary mass
      - Pancreatic ductal dilation may be absent in setting of pancreas divisum
    - Distended pancreatic duct distal to tumor
      - Tumor itself may be difficult to appreciate if isoattenuating &/or small
      - Often seen in conjunction with pancreatic atrophy distal to tumor
    - Courvoisier sign suggests malignancy
      - Enlarged nontender gallbladder
      - Mild jaundice
    - Disruption of normal pancreatic architecture or contour abnormalities
      - Abnormal focal increased tissue density in patients with fatty atrophy of pancreas
    - Diffuse pancreatic carcinoma can mimic acute pancreatitis
    - Acinar cell carcinoma imaging characteristics
      - Well marginated (90%)
      - Partially or completely exophytic (80%)
      - Typically homogeneously hypoenhancing to pancreas on venous phase imaging; reports of early arterial enhancement
      - Oval or round
      - Solid when small, can have large areas of cystic necrosis if tumor is large
      - May have calcifications
      - Often larger than ductal adenocarcinoma at time of diagnosis
  - Primary tumor: Endocrine tumors
    - Most tumors show increased enhancement in at least 1 phase of enhancement
    - Syndromic PNETs
      - Tumor detection is difficult because of their small size
      - Typically intense and prolonged enhancement
      - Some are hypoattenuating relative to enhancing pancreas, best seen during portal venous or pancreatic phase
      - Cystic degeneration, calcification, and necrosis are more common in larger syndromic PNETs
    - Nonsyndromic PNETs
      - Tend to be large at initial presentation (average tumor size is 5.2 cm)
      - May show calcifications, cysts, and necrosis
      - Hypervascular, enhancing during both arterial and venous phases
    - Cystic neuroendocrine tumors
      - Uncommon appearance of PNET
      - May be syndromic or nonsyndromic
      - Typically solid and well vascularized with central cystic component
      - Cystic components found in 17% of PNETs
      - More likely to occur in patients with MEN1
      - Predominantly well circumscribed
  - Vascular involvement
    - Distended mesenteric venous collaterals in setting of superior mesenteric, portal, or splenic venous obstruction or occlusion
    - Perivascular soft tissue cuffs indicating perineural, perivascular, or lymphatic disease
    - Irregular narrowing of normal contours of arteries or veins
      - SMA
      - Celiac
      - Portal vein
      - SMV (teardrop morphology of SMV implies venous involvement)
      - Gastroduodenal artery (GDA)
      - Hepatic arteries
  - Local nodal involvement
    - Should be identified, but CT is poor at prognosticating presence of metastatic disease
    - Hepatic artery lymph node (at origin of gastroduodenal artery) is important to identify if present, regardless of size
      - If involved, survival rate is similar to patients with liver or peritoneal metastases
  - Metastatic disease
    - Regional lymphadenopathy
      - Lymphadenopathy beyond surgical bed is considered metastatic disease
    - Hepatic metastases
    - Peritoneal metastases

- Other distant metastases are uncommon
  - Lung
  - Brain
  - Pleura
  - Adrenal gland
  - Bone
- **MR**
  - Exocrine tumors
    - T1WI: Hypointense relative to bright pancreas
    - T2WI: Variable signal relative to pancreas but often hypointense and difficult to visualize unless there is substantial necrosis
    - "Duct penetrating" sign to distinguish inflammatory mass from pancreatic cancer
      - Seen more often in pancreatitis (85%) than pancreatic cancer (4%)
      - Defined as either normal or stenotic main pancreatic duct without ductal wall irregularity penetrating pancreatic mass
      - Pancreatic cancer tends to obstruct duct or demonstrate ductal irregularity of intratumoral main pancreatic duct
    - Post-contrast images: Similar enhancement characteristics to CT
      - Tumor margins are generally ill defined and infiltrative
      - Typically tumors demonstrate delayed enhancement compared to pancreatic parenchyma secondary to extensive desmoplastic reaction
  - Endocrine tumors
    - T1WI
      - Low signal intensity compared to bright pancreas
      - May be best sequence to detect subtle tumors
    - T2WI
      - Usually bright
      - Lesions with intermediate or low T2W signal intensity may be seen
    - Gadolinium-enhanced T1WI
      - Typical hyperenhancing during arterial phase
      - Degree, uniformity, and timing of enhancement can be highly variable
      - Larger, more malignant lesions usually show more heterogeneous enhancement
    - Diffusion-weighted imaging (DWI)
      - Can be added to MR imaging protocol to detect lesions in patients with clinical suspicion for PNET with negative or suspicious imaging findings
      - Restricted water diffusion leads to ↓ signal on ADC maps and ↑ signal intensity on DWI
- **Endoscopic ultrasound (EUS)**
  - Useful in cases where pancreatic or biliary ductal dilation is present but no mass is identified on CT or MR
  - More sensitive than CT for small masses
    - EUS reported to have nearly 100% detection of tumors < 1.6 cm whereas CT may miss up to 33%
- **PET/CT**
  - Exocrine tumors
    - Generally demonstrates increased FDG uptake, although highly mucinous tumors may have areas without significant uptake
    - False-negatives with lesions < 8 mm
    - Blood glucose > 150 mg/dL may result in false-negatives
  - Endocrine tumors
    - Standard PET scans using fluorodeoxyglucose (FDG) are not useful in diagnosis of pancreatic neuroendocrine tumors
    - Gallium-68 receptor PET/CT is much more sensitive than OctreoScan™
    - C-5-hydroxyl-L-tryptophan PET has very high sensitivity
- **ERCP**
  - Exocrine tumors
    - Irregular, nodular, rat-tailed eccentric obstruction
    - "Double duct" sign
    - Generally used for stenting and biliary decompression
    - Intraductal brushings can provide tissue diagnosis, but yield is significantly lower than EUS
  - Endocrine tumors
    - Useful for differentiating between benign and malignant pancreatic neuroendocrine tumors
- **Octreotide scintigraphy** (endocrine tumors)
  - Somatostatin receptor scintigraphy is useful for localization of PNET
  - Not all neuroendocrine tumors express enough somatostatin receptors to be detected
    - Negative scan cannot exclude gastrinoma or insulinoma
  - Diagnostic sensitivity of In-111 DTPA-octreotide scans is 80-90% and varies among different types of PNETs
    - Glucagonomas (100%)
    - VIPomas (88%)
    - Carcinoids (87%)
    - Gastrinomas (73%)
    - Insulinomas (< 25%)
  - Single photon emission tomography (SPECT imaging) is essential to achieve high sensitivity
    - To isolate possible lesions from renal background
  - Octreotide scan has been used for prediction of octreotide therapeutic response
- **Percutaneous transhepatic portal venous sampling (PTPVS)** (endocrine tumors)
  - Performed by transhepatic catheterization of portal vein
  - Invasive procedure with significant complication rate
  - Samples for hormonal analysis are obtained from
    - Splenic vein
    - Superior and inferior mesenteric veins
    - Portal and pancreatic veins
  - Exact location of tumor cannot be pinpointed in same way as in imaging study
- **Arterial stimulation with venous sampling (ASVS)** (endocrine tumors)
  - Invasive technique for detection of insulinomas and gastrinomas
  - Should only be used if noninvasive techniques fail to reveal tumor
  - Catheter placed selectively in splenic, superior mesenteric, and gastroduodenal arteries with infusion of calcium gluconate followed by venous sampling from hepatic vein

- Localized discrete insulin-secreting PNETs to regions of pancreas
- ≥ 2x step-up in right hepatic vein insulin concentration from baseline at 20, 40, &/or 60 seconds after arterial calcium injection constitutes positive response
- Sensitivity > 90% for detection and localization of insulinoma

Staging

- General principles
  - Based on
    - Size of primary tumor
    - Extrapancreatic invasion
    - Local nodal involvement
    - Vascular invasion
    - Distant metastatic disease
  - Designated by modality (CT, EUS, MR, surgical) to convey inherent advantages and limitations of each method
  - Biopsy proof is not necessary prior to surgical resection if there is high index of suspicion and should not delay definitive therapy
  - Biopsy of metastatic lesion is preferred over sampling of primary tumor, if possible
  - Endoscopic ultrasound-guided FNA tissue sampling is preferred to percutaneous biopsy to decrease risk of peritoneal seeding
- **Pancreatic protocol CT**
  - Primary method of staging due to wide availability and ability to assess local tumor invasion, presence of lymph nodes, vascular involvement, and distal metastases
  - Excellent at determining unresectability of tumors (89-100%), but less accurate for predicting tumor resectability (45-79%)
  - Good for identifying regional lymph nodes
    - Poor at prognosticating whether they are malignant
  - Allows for concurrent evaluation of metastatic disease
    - However, CT is unable to resolve low-volume peritoneal or hepatic metastatic disease
      - Found intraoperatively in up to 20% of cases deemed resectable by CT
    - If distant metastases are present, there is no need for diagnostic EUS
  - CT angiography can by used for presurgical planning and to identify variant vascular anatomy
  - Pancreatic protocol CECT for staging should ideally be performed prior to biliary decompression
    - Eliminate confounding post-procedure inflammatory findings that can mimic local invasion or lymphatic/perineural spread of tumor
- **EUS**
  - Complementary with CT or MR for diagnosis and staging
  - Allows for fine needle aspiration to establish tissue diagnosis
  - Limited availability and operator dependent
  - Good for evaluation of venous involvement
    - 80% sensitive and 85% specific for involvement of portal and superior mesenteric veins
  - Limited evaluation of superior mesenteric artery and uncinate process of pancreas in some patients
  - Good for discriminating between benign and malignant strictures or stenosis
  - Good for characterizing cystic pancreatic lesions
  - Better at prognosticating malignancy in regional lymph nodes than CT
    - Size (> 1 cm)
    - Distinct margins
    - Hypoechogenicity
    - Round shape
    - If all 4 findings are present in same lymph node, there is 80% likelihood of malignant involvement
  - Therapeutic interventions, such as celiac plexus neurolysis and removal of ascites, can be performed
- **Pancreatic protocol MR**
  - Used for staging if MRCP desired
  - Used as problem-solving tool
    - Improved tissue contrast may identify primary tumor in cases where it is isoattenuating to pancreas on CT
    - MR is slightly more accurate (94%) than CT (87%) in identifying hepatic metastases
  - Poor at evaluating peritoneal metastases
- **PET/CT**
  - Rarely used as primary staging tool but may be used for evaluating for recurrence
  - Increased sensitivity for detection of metastatic disease when performed after pancreatic protocol CT
  - Generally used as problem-solving tool
  - Good for evaluating regional lymphadenopathy and findings suspicious for distant metastasis
- **Staging laparoscopy ± ultrasound**
  - Occasionally performed to rule out subradiologic metastatic disease in patients at high risk of disseminated disease, as indicated by
    - Borderline resectable disease
    - Markedly elevated CA19-9 (> 150)
    - Body or tail tumors
    - Large primary tumor
  - Can be used to further evaluate questionable hepatic or peritoneal lesions on cross-sectional imaging or in setting of low-volume ascites
  - Malignant cytology from peritoneal washings is considered M1 disease
  - Detects occult metastases not seen on staging CT in 24-31%
    - 7% had positive cytology from intraoperative peritoneal washings as only evidence of occult metastatic disease
- **Exploratory laparotomy**
  - Performed if tumor deemed resectable or following neoadjuvant therapy for borderline resectable tumors
  - Allows for palliative procedures in tumors deemed unresectable at time of laparotomy

Restaging

- Exocrine tumors
  - Following resection and adjuvant therapy, surveillance recommended every 3-6 months for 2 years and yearly thereafter
    - Surveillance includes
      - CECT (controversial)
      - CA19.9 levels (controversial)
      - History and physical exam
      - PET/CT or MR may be used for problem solving in certain cases

- Findings of recurrence
  - Local tumor recurrence in surgical bed
  - Metastatic disease (regional lymphadenopathy, liver, and peritoneum are most common)
  - Increasing periarterial soft tissue
    - Must distinguish from post-treatment scarring
    - May represent recurrent local tumor or perineural/lymphatic disease progression
- Endocrine tumors
  - CT or MR can be used for follow-up of patients following tumor resections
    - Detection of local recurrence
    - Detection of hepatic metastases
    - Detection of new tumors in patients with MEN1
  - Variable enhancement pattern of liver metastases can make it difficult to assess treatment response
    - Unenhanced images on CT and MR can be useful for measuring lesions

Criteria for Resectability

- **Resectable**
  - Clean fat planes surrounding superior mesenteric artery, hepatic artery, and celiac axis
  - Patency of superior mesenteric and portal veins
  - No distant metastatic disease
- **Borderline resectable**
  - If high likelihood of tumor resection resulting in R1 (microscopic disease at surgical margins) or R2 (gross disease at margins), neoadjuvant chemoradiation is recommended prior to attempted resection
  - Head or body tumors
    - Tumor abuts (< 180°) SMA
      - More likely to be resectable if this abutment manifests as soft tissue stranding or has convex margin with SMA
    - GDA encased up to origin from common hepatic artery with either short segment encasement or direct abutment of the hepatic artery, without extension to the celiac axis
    - Short segment occlusion of SMV, portal vein (PV), or SMV-PV confluence if involvement is amenable to vascular reconstruction
      - Criterion is used at some high-volume centers
      - Venous structures proximal and distal to occlusion must be patent and amenable to reconstruction
      - If primary anastomosis cannot be performed, interposition graft (internal jugular vein) may be placed
    - Colon or mesocolon invasion
  - Tail tumors
    - Adrenal, colon, mesocolon, or renal invasion
- **Unresectable**
  - Pancreatic head tumors
    - Distant metastases
    - Tumor encases SMA (> 180°) or abuts celiac axis
    - SMV &/or PV occlusion that is unreconstructable
    - Aortic invasion or encasement
  - Pancreatic body tumors
    - Distant metastases
    - Tumor encases SMA or celiac axis (> 180°)
    - SMV &/or PV occlusion that is unreconstructable
    - Aortic invasion
  - Pancreatic tail tumors
    - Distant metastases
    - Tumor encases SMA or celiac axis (> 180°)
  - Nodal status
    - Metastatic disease to lymph nodes beyond field of resection

CLINICAL PRESENTATION & WORK-UP

Presentation

- Exocrine tumors
  - Jaundice
    - Courvoisier sign: Jaundice and nontender palpable gallbladder
    - Common with pancreatic head lesions
  - Sharp midepigastric abdominal pain radiating to the back
    - Due to direct tumor extension posteriorly to 1st and 2nd celiac ganglia
    - Common with unresectable pancreatic body or tail lesions
  - Weight loss
    - Due to anorexia and malabsorption from exocrine insufficiency
  - Dark urine
  - Light or floating stools
  - Nausea
  - Venous thromboembolic disease
  - Lipase hypersecretion syndrome
    - May be seen in acinar cell carcinoma secondary to lipase secretion
    - Subcutaneous fat necrosis, polyarthralgia, and eosinophilia
  - Glucose intolerance
  - Trousseau sign: Migratory thrombophlebitis
  - Depression
- Endocrine tumors
  - Insulinoma
    - Classic clinical triad (Whipple triad) includes
      - Fasting serum glucose levels < 50 mg/dL
      - Symptoms of hypoglycemia
      - Relief of symptoms after glucose administration
    - Symptoms related to catecholamine release
      - Palpitations, sweating, and headache
  - Gastrinoma
    - Most patients present with epigastric pain
      - Due to recurrent or intractable peptic ulcer disease
      - Ulcers in unusual locations (e.g., postbulbar)
    - Patients may also have diarrhea due to excessive delivery of acid to small bowel
      - ↑ serum gastrin levels
  - Glucagonoma
    - Characteristic migratory rash called necrolytic migratory erythema
      - Usually affects genitals
    - Stomatitis, diarrhea, anemia, weight loss, depression, and deep vein thrombosis
      - 4D syndrome: **D**ermatitis, **d**iarrhea, **d**epression, and **d**eep vein thrombosis
    - ↑ glucagon level
    - Levels of associated hormones may also be elevated, such as
      - Insulin

- Serotonin
- Gastrin
- VIPoma
  - WDHA syndrome
    - **W**atery **d**iarrhea
    - **H**ypokalemia
    - **A**chlorhydria

Prognosis

- Exocrine tumors
  - Pancreatic adenocarcinoma
    - Overall median survival is 3-6 months with 5-year survival rate of 3-6%
    - Resected patients: Median survival is 15-19 months with 5-year survival rate of 10-25%
    - Only 10-15% of patients have resectable tumors
    - Only 15-30% of patients with resectable tumors have surgical margins free of disease
      - In general, median survival for patients with positive surgical margins are similar to those for patients treated with chemoradiation alone (9-11 months)
      - Exception is in patients with R1 resection after neoadjuvant chemoradiation who have median survival similar to patients with R0 resection (20 months)
    - Unresected patients: Median survival is 11-17 months with 3-year survival rate of 7% and 5-year survival rate of 3-4%
  - Acinar cell carcinoma
    - More indolent course than ductal carcinomas
    - Tend to present at younger age (56 vs. 70 years)
    - Overall 5-year survival rate: 43%
    - Resected 5-year survival rate: 72%
    - Unresectable disease 5-year survival rate: 22%
  - Prognostic factors
    - Pathologic variables
      - Tumor size (< 2 cm)
      - Presence or absence of perineural invasion
      - Lymph node status
    - Treatment-related variables
      - Complete surgical resection of primary tumor
      - R1 and R2 resections are not curative
      - Use of adjuvant CRT
- Endocrine tumors
  - Better survival compared to pancreatic adenocarcinoma
    - Overall 5-year survival rate is 29% for all patients
      - 55% for patients with resected tumors
      - 16% for patients with unresected tumors

Work-Up

- Clinical
  - History and physical
- Radiographic
  - Pancreatic protocol CECT &/or MR
    - Multiphase imaging technique is optimal
      - Noncontrast phase plus arterial, pancreatic parenchymal, and portal venous phases of contrast enhancement
    - Thin cuts (3 mm or less) through abdomen
  - EUS
  - Chest CT
- Laboratory
  - Exocrine tumors
    - CA19-9
      - 70% sensitivity and 87% specificity when using cutoff of 70 U/mL
      - Preoperative measurement should be performed after biliary decompression and normalization of bilirubin
      - Post-resection CA19-9 levels are prognostic in patients receiving adjuvant therapy
    - Liver function tests
  - Endocrine tumors
    - Laboratory evaluation should include biochemical assessment for a functional endocrine syndrome, if suspected
    - Markers of neuroendocrine tumors, such as chromogranin A, may also be helpful as baseline

TREATMENT

Major Treatment Alternatives

- Exocrine tumors
  - Surgical resection
    - Resection is primary potentially curative treatment
  - Chemoradiation
    - Cytologic confirmation of malignancy should be obtained prior to RT
  - Systemic chemotherapy
- Endocrine tumors
  - Surgical resection
    - Patients with localized, regional, and metastatic PNETs who are reasonable operative candidates should be considered for resection of their primary tumors
      - Survival benefit has been demonstrated even for patients with metastatic disease
    - Choice of procedure depends on tumor location, number of tumors, and risk of malignancy based on parameters such as type, size, and tumor features
      - Enucleation
      - Distal pancreatectomy
      - Pancreaticoduodenectomy
      - Resection of hepatic metastases whenever possible
      - Debulking in locally advanced tumors
  - Interventional procedures
    - Mainly directed at treatment of hepatic or extrahepatic metastases
    - Possible interventions include
      - Transcatheter arterial embolization (TAE)
      - Transcatheter arterial chemoembolization (TACE)
      - Radiofrequency ablation (RFA)
  - Stereotactic radiosurgery is being explored as an ablative technique for hepatic or extrahepatic metastases
  - Medical treatment
    - Gastrinoma
      - Symptoms of acid hypersecretion can be controlled by proton pump inhibitors in virtually all patients with Zollinger-Ellison syndrome
      - Histamine H2 receptor antagonists or somatostatin analogues are also effective

- Insulinoma
  - Prior to surgery and for rare patients with malignant disease
  - Treatment for hypoglycemia
  - Frequent small feedings
  - Diazoxide, a benzothiadiazide, directly inhibits insulin release through α-adrenergic stimulation and promotes glycogenolysis in liver
- Glucagonoma
  - Combination chemotherapy for unresectable tumor
  - Somatostatin analogue therapy
  - Necrotizing erythema of glucagonoma: Somatostatin analogue, with nearly complete disappearance within 1 week

- Because endocrine tumors are less common and the role of radiotherapy has yet to be determined, radiotherapeutic management of these tumors is not discussed further here

Major Treatment Roadblocks/ Contraindications

- Unresectable at diagnosis (80-95% of cases)
- Medical comorbidities
- Advanced age

Treatment Options by Stage

- Stage I or II: Resectable or borderline resectable
  - Treatment is guided by resectability
  - Resectable: Surgical resection followed by adjuvant therapy **or** neoadjuvant therapy on a clinical trial
    - Surgical resection
      - Whipple (pancreaticoduodenectomy) for pancreatic head and uncinate tumors
      - Distal pancreatectomy ± splenectomy for pancreatic body and tail tumors
      - Total pancreatectomy is rarely necessary to achieve negative margins
    - Adjuvant therapy following resection
      - Clinical trial **or** chemotherapy ± chemoradiation
      - Ideally should be initiated within 4-8 weeks postop
    - Neoadjuvant therapy
      - Clinical trial **or** chemoradiation **or** chemotherapy followed by chemoradiation
      - Approximately 25% of patients who are restaged after neoadjuvant therapy are found to have progression of disease
      - Ideally, surgical resection should be attempted 6-8 weeks following chemoradiation
  - Borderline resectable: Neoadjuvant therapy prior to laparotomy with intent to resect
    - Induction chemotherapy followed by chemoradiation **or** neoadjuvant chemoradiation
      - Generally achieves disease downstaging in 8-19% cases
- Stage III: Locally unresectable disease
  - Clinical trial **or** chemoradiation (5-FU or capecitabine or gemcitabine-based) **or** induction chemotherapy followed by chemoradiation (5-FU or gemcitabine-based) **or** chemotherapy alone (gemcitabine or combination)
  - Maintenance chemotherapy should be considered
  - Endoscopic biliary stenting, surgical bypass, &/or celiac neurolysis as needed
- Stage IV: Metastatic disease
  - Clinical trial **or** chemotherapy (gemcitabine or combination)
  - Endoscopic biliary stenting, surgical bypass, celiac neurolysis, &/or RT as needed
- Recurrent disease
  - Treatment is guided by tumor resectability status
    - Resectable
    - Borderline
    - Unresectable
  - Therapy choices include local vs. systemic treatments: Chemotherapy, RT surgery

Dose Response

- Optimal dose and scheduling of RT has not been determined
- Radiation dose-response relationship seems to exist for local tumor control, possibly leading to modest improvements in median survival times
- Multiple dose-escalation studies with hyperfractionation, brachytherapy, IORT, radiosurgery, hypofractionation, and other methods are under investigation
  - RT that is gated to the respiratory cycle is necessary for dose-escalation studies > 60 Gy

Standard Doses

- Neoadjuvant
  - 45-54 Gy in 1.8-2.5 Gy fractions
  - **Or** 36 Gy in 2.4 Gy fractions
- Definitive: 45-54 Gy in 1.8 Gy fractions **or** 36 Gy in 2.4 Gy fractions to gross tumor and clinically enlarged lymph nodes
  - Consider dose escalation with boost to gross tumor volume
  - No standard dose-fractionation has been established for SBRT
- Postoperative
  - 45 Gy in 1.8 Gy fractions to the tumor bed, surgical anastomoses, and adjacent lymph node regions, followed by
    - 5.4 Gy in 1.8 Gy fractions boost to
      - Tumor bed
      - Superior mesenteric vessels
      - Celiac axis
      - Anastomoses
      - Consider boost to areas of gross residual disease
- Palliative: 30-36 Gy in 2.4-3 Gy fractions to primary tumor plus a margin for local palliation for obstruction or pain

Organs at Risk Parameters

- Liver: Mean ≤ 25 Gy
- Bilateral kidneys: D50% < 18 Gy
- Stomach and small intestine: Max dose ≤ 54 Gy; D15% < 45 Gy
- Spinal cord: Max dose < 45 Gy

Common Techniques

- General
  - CT simulation and 3D treatment planning with IV and oral contrast

    - When IV contrast cannot be used, fusion of the planning CT with diagnostic CT should be used
  - In postoperative cases, treatment volumes should be based on preoperative CT and surgical clips
  - RT that is gated to the respiratory cycle is necessary for dose-escalation studies > 60 Gy
- 3D conformal radiotherapy
  - 4- or 5-beam arrangement
- Intensity-modulated radiotherapy (IMRT)
  - May allow for dose escalation to gross tumor/tumor bed while minimizing toxicity to surrounding tissue
- Stereotactic body radiotherapy (SBRT)
  - May allow for dose escalation to gross tumor/tumor bed while minimizing toxicity to surrounding tissue
  - May be used alone as definitive therapy or as a boost after EBRT
  - Should be done on clinical trial
- Intraoperative radiation therapy (IORT)
  - May allow for dose escalation to gross tumor/tumor bed while minimizing toxicity to surrounding tissue
  - Used when resection may result in close or involved margins
  - Techniques include electron beam radiation therapy (EBRT) or HDR brachytherapy
- Brachytherapy
  - May allow for dose escalation to gross tumor/tumor bed while minimizing toxicity to surrounding tissue
  - Iodine-125 implant is most commonly used isotope
- Proton beam therapy
  - May allow for dose escalation to gross tumor/tumor bed while minimizing toxicity to surrounding tissue
  - Consider clinical trial

Landmark Trials

- Resectable disease
  - Postoperative chemoradiation
    - GITSG 9173
      - Suboptimal chemo (in dose and schedule) and inadequate RT dose and schedule
      - Median survival 20 months with postop CRT (5-FU) vs. 11 months with no adjuvant treatment (NAT)
      - 2-year survival 43% with CRT vs. 18% with NAT
      - 5-year survival 19% with postop CRT vs. 0% with NAT
    - EORTC 40891
      - Median survival 17 months with adjuvant CRT (5-FU) vs. 13 months with NAT
      - 2-year survival 34% with adjuvant CRT vs. 26% with NAT
      - 5-year survival 20% with adjuvant CRT vs. 10% with NAT
    - ESPAC-1
      - No survival benefit with adjuvant CRT vs. NAT
      - Lack of attention to quality control for RT
    - RTOG 97-04
      - Concurrent chemo was 5-FU in both arms; gemcitabine vs. 5-FU given before and after chemoradiation
      - Median survival 21 months with gemcitabine vs. 17 months with 5-FU
      - 3-year survival 31% with gemcitabine vs. 22% with 5-FU
  - Postoperative chemotherapy
    - ESPAC-1
      - Median survival 22 months with adjuvant 5-FU vs. 17 months with NAT
    - CONKO-001
      - Median DFS 13.4 months with adjuvant gemcitabine vs. 11.5 months with NAT
      - No difference in OS
      - No central surgical or pathologic quality control; unrecognized incomplete surgical resections may have confounded results
  - Neoadjuvant chemoradiation (no completed phase III studies)
    - MDACC (Evans, prospective trial)
      - 85% of patients → surgery after CRT
      - Median survival 34 months with CRT followed by surgery vs. 7 months with CRT alone
    - FCCC (Pingpank, retrospective trial)
      - Negative margins in 51% with neoadjuvant CRT vs. 26% without neoadjuvant CRT
      - OS ↑ in negative margin vs. positive margin
    - Northwestern (Talamonti, prospective trial): All patients went on to surgery after CRT
      - 85% underwent resections
      - 94% had negative margins
      - 65% had negative lymph nodes
- Borderline resectable disease
  - Neoadjuvant chemoradiation (no completed phase III studies)
    - Harvard (Jessup, prospective)
      - 13% of patients went on to surgical resection after chemoradiation
      - Mean survival 8 months with neoadjuvant CRT → surgery
    - Germany (Wilkowski, prospective)
      - 19% of patients → surgery after neoadjuvant therapy
      - Type and schedule of chemo did not change survival
    - Brown (Safran, prospective)
      - 10% of patients → surgery after neoadjuvant therapy
      - Median survival 8 months with concurrent paclitaxel and RT
- Unresectable disease
  - Concurrent CRT vs. RT alone
    - Mayo clinic (Moertel)
      - Median survival 10.4 months with CRT vs. 6.3 months with RT alone
      - 1-year overall survival (OS) 22% with CRT vs. 6% with RT alone
    - GITSG 9273
      - Median survival 9.7 months with CRT (40 Gy) vs. 9.3 months with CRT (60 Gy) vs. 5.3 months with RT alone (60 Gy)
      - 1-year OS 46% with concurrent CRT (40 Gy) vs. 35% with concurrent CRT (60 Gy) vs. 10% with RT alone
  - Concurrent chemoradiation vs. chemotherapy alone
    - GITSG 9283
      - Median survival 9.7 months with CRT vs. 7.4 months with chemo alone
    - ECOG (Klaassen)
      - No difference in median survival, 8.3 months with CRT vs. 8.2 months with chemo alone

- Lower RT dose; included patients with recurrence or residual disease after resection
    - ECOG E4201
        - Median survival 11.1 months with EBRT + concurrent/adjuvant gemcitabine vs. 9.2 months with gemcitabine
        - Grade 4 or 5 toxicity 41% with EBRT + gemcitabine vs. 9% with gemcitabine
    - FFCD-SFRO
        - Median survival 8.6 months with CRT (5-FU and cisplatin) vs. 13 months with gemcitabine alone
        - Grades 3-4 toxicity 36% with CRT vs. 22% with gemcitabine
        - Toxicity may be due to dose intensity of radiation (60 Gy), regional lymph node irradiation, and use of concurrent cisplatin
  - Induction chemotherapy followed by chemoradiation (no completed phase III studies)
    - MDACC (Krishnan, retrospective)
        - Median survival 9 months with CRT vs. 12 months with chemo followed by CRT
        - Survival improvement may be achieved by eliminating patients who have micrometastases that progress during induction phase
- Prophylactic hepatic irradiation
  - Johns Hopkins (Abrams, phase I/II)
    - Site of 1st failure was liver in 43% of patients treated
    - Postop doses 50.4-57.6 Gy of EBRT to operative bed and regional lymphatics, and 23.4-27 Gy to liver with concurrent 5-FU plus leucovorin
  - RTOG 88-01
    - Local progression in 73%, and abdominal spread in 27%
    - Prophylactic hepatic irradiation may reduce frequency of hepatic metastasis
        - However, survival remains poor because of local failure and intraabdominal spread

RECOMMENDED FOLLOW-UP

Clinical

- History and physical for symptom assessment every 3-6 months for 2 years
  - Then every 6 months or annually

Radiographic

- Consider CT scan every 3-6 months for 2 years
  - Then every 6 months or annually

Laboratory

- Consider CA19-9 level every 3-6 months for 2 years
  - Then every 6 months or annually

SELECTED REFERENCES

1. Goodman KA et al: Radiation Therapy Oncology Group consensus panel guidelines for the delineation of the clinical target volume in the postoperative treatment of pancreatic head cancer. Int J Radiat Oncol Biol Phys. 83(3):901-8, 2012
2. Loehrer PJ Sr et al: Gemcitabine alone versus gemcitabine plus radiotherapy in patients with locally advanced pancreatic cancer: an Eastern Cooperative Oncology Group trial. J Clin Oncol. 29(31):4105-12, 2011
3. Small W Jr et al: Phase II trial of full-dose gemcitabine and bevacizumab in combination with attenuated three-dimensional conformal radiotherapy in patients with localized pancreatic cancer. Int J Radiat Oncol Biol Phys. 80(2):476-82, 2011
4. American Joint Committee on Cancer: AJCC Cancer Staging Manual. 7th ed. New York: Springer. 241-9, 2010
5. Khrizman P et al: The use of stereotactic body radiation therapy in gastrointestinal malignancies in locally advanced and metastatic settings. Clin Colorectal Cancer. 9(3):136-43, 2010
6. Anaye A et al: Successful preoperative localization of a small pancreatic insulinoma by diffusion-weighted MRI. JOP. 10(5):528-31, 2009
7. Hill JS et al: Pancreatic neuroendocrine tumors: the impact of surgical resection on survival. Cancer. 115(4):741-51, 2009
8. Wilkowski R et al: Chemoradiotherapy with concurrent gemcitabine and cisplatin with or without sequential chemotherapy with gemcitabine/cisplatin vs chemoradiotherapy with concurrent 5-fluorouracil in patients with locally advanced pancreatic cancer--a multi-centre randomised phase II study. Br J Cancer. 101(11):1853-9, 2009
9. Chauffert B et al: Phase III trial comparing intensive induction chemoradiotherapy (60 Gy, infusional 5-FU and intermittent cisplatin) followed by maintenance gemcitabine with gemcitabine alone for locally advanced unresectable pancreatic cancer. Definitive results of the 2000-01 FFCD/SFRO study. Ann Oncol. 19(9):1592-9, 2008
10. Evans DB et al: Preoperative gemcitabine-based chemoradiation for patients with resectable adenocarcinoma of the pancreatic head. J Clin Oncol. 26(21):3496-502, 2008
11. Halfdanarson TR et al: Pancreatic neuroendocrine tumors (PNETs): incidence, prognosis and recent trend toward improved survival. Ann Oncol. 19(10):1727-33, 2008
12. Metz DC et al: Gastrointestinal neuroendocrine tumors: pancreatic endocrine tumors. Gastroenterology. 135(5):1469-92, 2008
13. Regine WF et al: Fluorouracil vs gemcitabine chemotherapy before and after fluorouracil-based chemoradiation following resection of pancreatic adenocarcinoma: a randomized controlled trial. JAMA. 2008 Mar 5;299(9):1019-26. Erratum in: JAMA. 299(16):1902, 2008
14. Small W Jr et al: Full-dose gemcitabine with concurrent radiation therapy in patients with nonmetastatic pancreatic cancer: a multicenter phase II trial. J Clin Oncol. 26(6):942-7, 2008
15. Cordera F et al: Significance of common hepatic artery lymph node metastases during pancreaticoduodenectomy for pancreatic head adenocarcinoma. Ann Surg Oncol. 14(8):2330-6, 2007
16. Krishnan S et al: Induction chemotherapy selects patients with locally advanced, unresectable pancreatic cancer for optimal benefit from consolidative chemoradiation therapy. Cancer. 110(1):47-55, 2007
17. Oettle H et al: Adjuvant chemotherapy with gemcitabine vs observation in patients undergoing curative-intent resection of pancreatic cancer: a randomized controlled trial. JAMA. 297(3):267-77, 2007
18. Tamm EP et al: Imaging of neuroendocrine tumors. Hematol Oncol Clin North Am. 21(3):409-32; vii, 2007
19. Falconi M et al: Surgical strategy in the treatment of pancreatic neuroendocrine tumors. JOP. 7(1):150-6, 2006
20. Talamonti MS et al: A multi-institutional phase II trial of preoperative full-dose gemcitabine and concurrent radiation for patients with potentially resectable pancreatic carcinoma. Ann Surg Oncol. 13(2):150-8, 2006

21. Neoptolemos JP et al: A randomized trial of chemoradiotherapy and chemotherapy after resection of pancreatic cancer. N Engl J Med. 2004 Mar 18;350(12):1200-10. Erratum in: N Engl J Med. 351(7):726, 2004
22. Debray MP et al: Imaging appearances of metastases from neuroendocrine tumours of the pancreas. Br J Radiol. 74(887):1065-70, 2001
23. Pingpank JF et al: Effect of preoperative chemoradiotherapy on surgical margin status of resected adenocarcinoma of the head of the pancreas. J Gastrointest Surg. 5(2):121-30, 2001
24. Wick MR et al: Pancreatic neuroendocrine neoplasms: a current summary of diagnostic, prognostic, and differential diagnostic information. Am J Clin Pathol. 115 Suppl:S28-45, 2001
25. Treatment of locally unresectable carcinoma of the pancreas: comparison of combined-modality therapy (chemotherapy plus radiotherapy) to chemotherapy alone: Gastrointestinal Tumor Study Group. J Natl Cancer Inst. 80(10):751-5, 1988
26. Klaassen DJ et al: Treatment of locally unresectable cancer of the stomach and pancreas: a randomized comparison of 5-fluorouracil alone with radiation plus concurrent and maintenance 5-fluorouracil--an Eastern Cooperative Oncology Group study. J Clin Oncol. 3(3):373-8, 1985
27. National Comprehensive Cancer Network. NCCN Clinical Practice Guidelines in Oncology. Pancreatic Adenocarcinoma. Version 2.2012. Accessed June 6, 2012. http://www.nccn.org/professionals/physician_gls/pdf/pancreatic.pdf

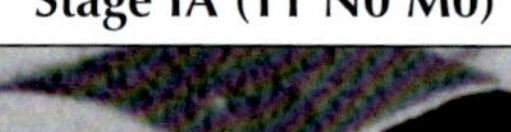

Stage IA (T1 N0 M0)

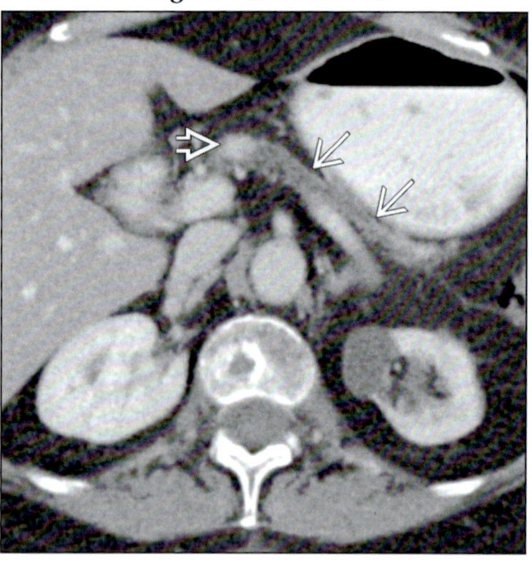

Stage IA (T1 N0 M0)

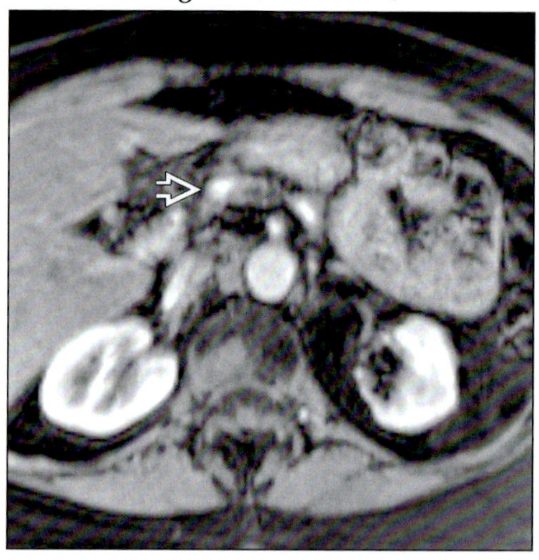

(Left) *Axial CECT demonstrates a ≤ 2 cm early arterial enhancing mass and distal pancreatic atrophy. There is no extrapancreatic extension, local lymph nodes, metastatic disease, or vascular involvement.* ***(Right)*** *Axial T1WI C+ FS MR in the same patient and plane shows similar findings. Distinct margins and early arterial enhancement are atypical for ductal adenocarcinoma. Surgical pathology was acinar cell carcinoma.*

Stage IB (T2 N0 M0)

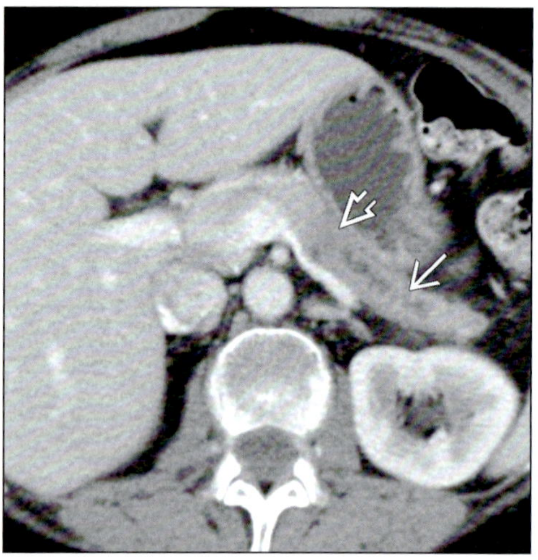

Stage IB (T2 N0 M0)

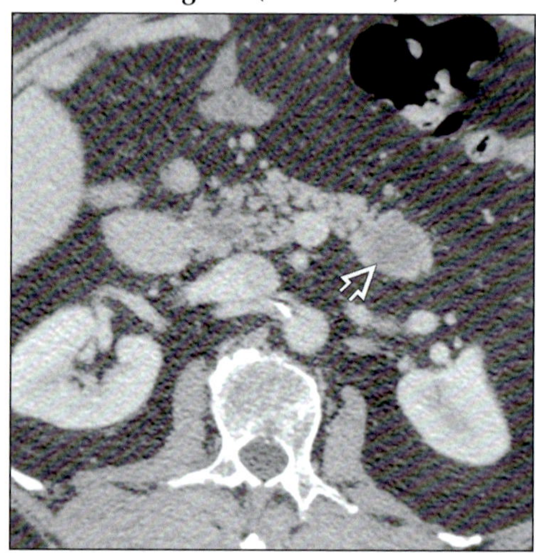

(Left) *Axial CECT shows a > 2 cm, poorly marginated, mildly hypoenhancing pancreatic body mass with distal ductal dilation. Abrupt distal pancreatic ductal dilation, even in the absence of a definite lesion, is highly suspicious for a pancreatic mass. Pathology was ductal adenocarcinoma.* ***(Right)*** *Axial CECT shows a well-marginated, hypoenhancing acinar cell carcinoma in the pancreatic tail. These are characteristic features for this pathology.*

Stage IB (T2 N0 M0)

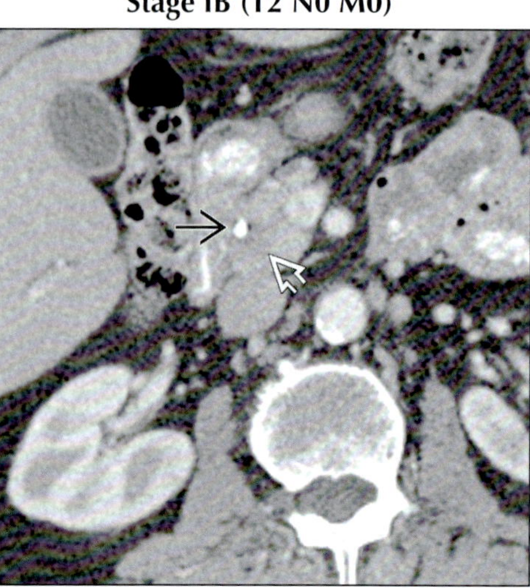

Stage IB (T2 N0 M0)

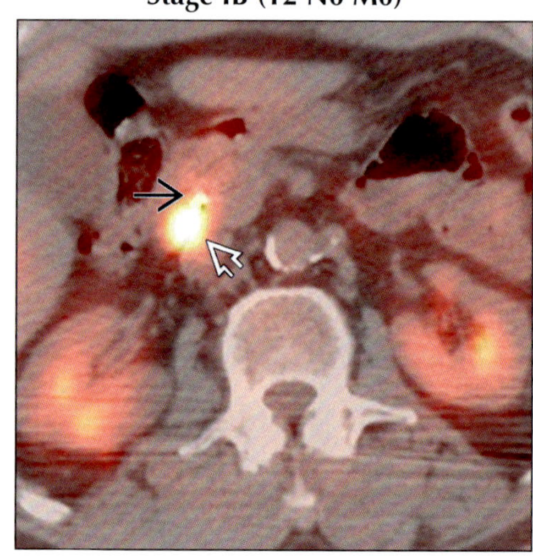

(Left) *Axial CECT shows a subtle, nearly isoenhancing > 2 cm ductal adenocarcinoma in the pancreatic head. Note the temporary biliary stent within the common bile duct.* ***(Right)*** *Axial PET/CT at the same level shows prominent FDG uptake in the pancreatic head. PET can be used to identify subtle tumors, metabolic nodes, or metastatic lesions. Biliary stents produce local inflammatory changes and confound interpretation of PET and CT findings.*

Neoadjuvant CRT

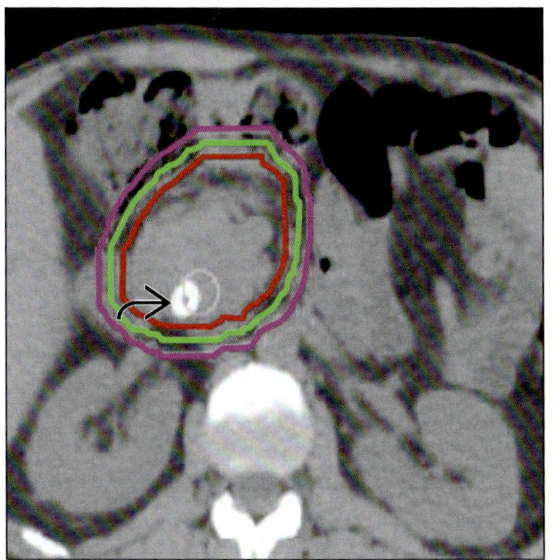

Neoadjuvant CRT

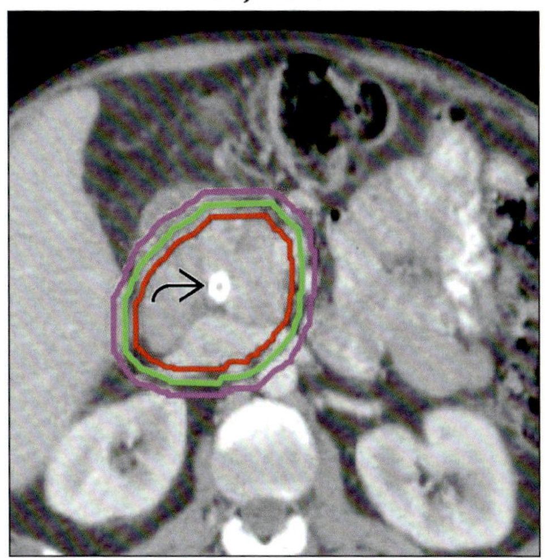

(Left) *Planning CT (pre-contrast) in a patient receiving neoadjuvant chemoradiotherapy for a pancreatic head tumor shows the GTV, CTV, and PTV. Note the biliary stent within the common bile duct.* ***(Right)*** *Planning CT (post contrast) in the same patient shows the GTV, CTV, and PTV. Note the biliary stent within the common bile duct and the respiratory motion between the pre-contrast and post-contrast scans.*

Neoadjuvant CRT

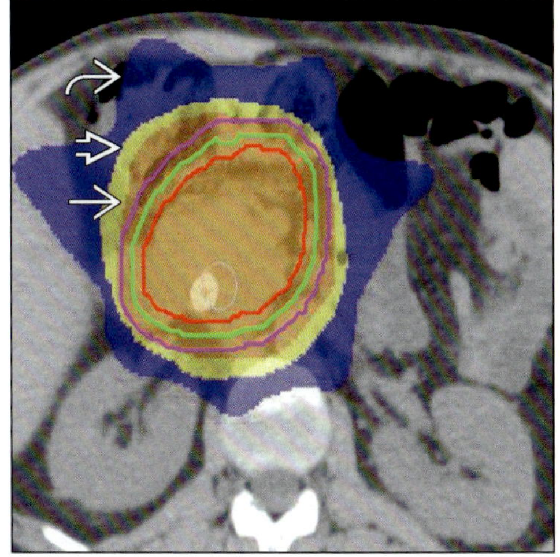

Neoadjuvant CRT

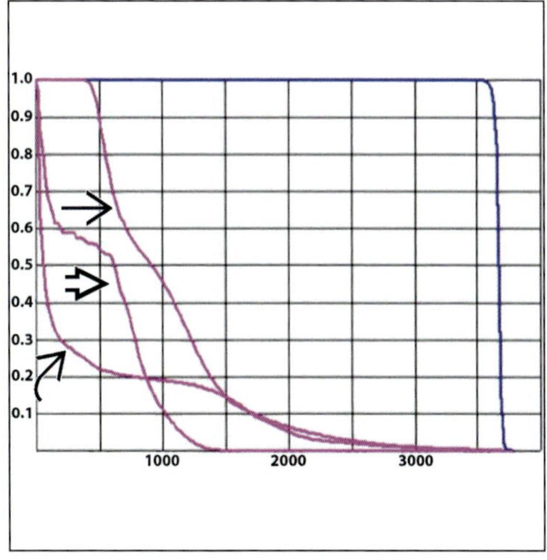

(Left) *5-field IMRT was used to deliver 36 Gy in 15 fractions in the same patient. The dose colorwash is shown. 20 Gy isodose line is shown in blue; 30 Gy isodose line in yellow; and 36 Gy isodose line in orange. Note the dose wrapping around to avoid the right kidney and spinal cord.* ***(Right)*** *DVH shows target coverage in the same patient. Liver was limited to mean < 30 Gy; spinal cord to < 15 Gy, and right kidney to D50% < 20 Gy.*

Stage IIA (T3 N0 M0)

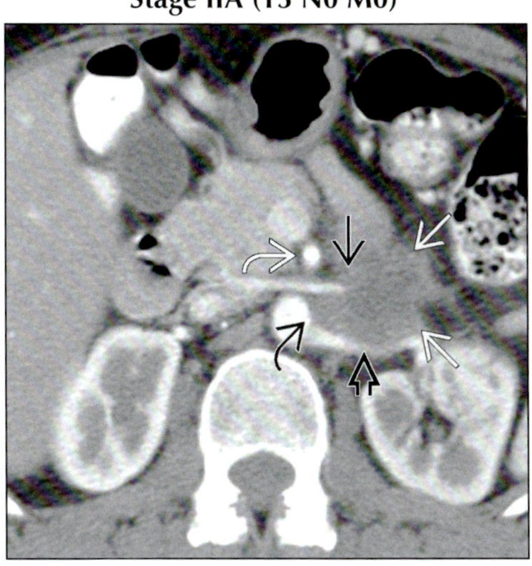

Stage IIA (T3 N0 M0)

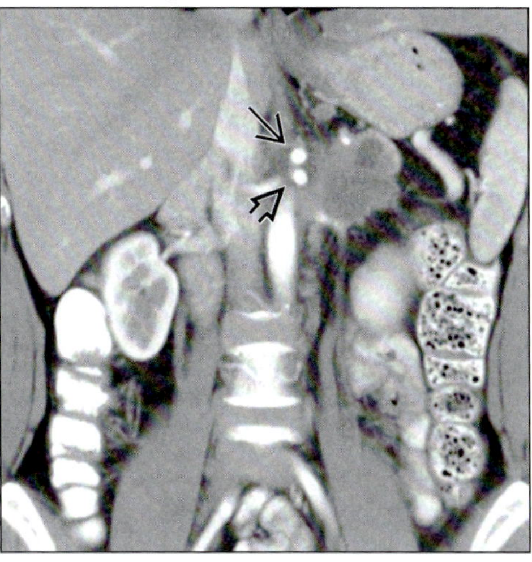

(Left) *Axial CECT shows an infiltrative ductal adenocarcinoma in the pancreatic tail invading the left renal vein, aorta, and left renal artery. The superior mesenteric artery (SMA) and celiac axis were not involved. Presence of aortic involvement makes this locally unresectable.* ***(Right)*** *Coronal CECT in the same patient shows the SMA and celiac axis with some surrounding fat stranding but no clear encasement or abutment.*

*(**Left**) Axial CECT shows a > 2 cm ductal adenocarcinoma abutting (< 180°) the SMV. The SMA is not involved, evidenced by presence of a circumferentially intact fat plane. This is a borderline resectable lesion. (**Right**) Coronal CECT from the same study shows the tumor abutting the SMV with short segment narrowing. Patency of the SMV proximal and distal to the abutment is important in resections requiring venous reconstruction.*

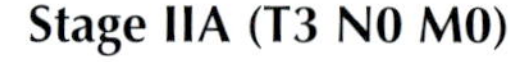

Stage IIA (T3 N0 M0)

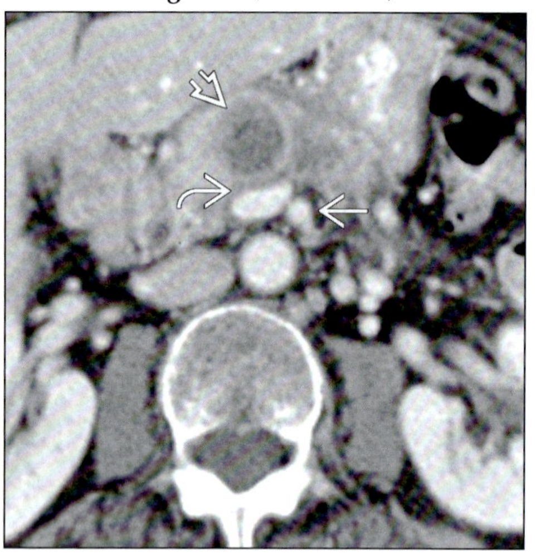

Stage IIA (T3 N0 M0)

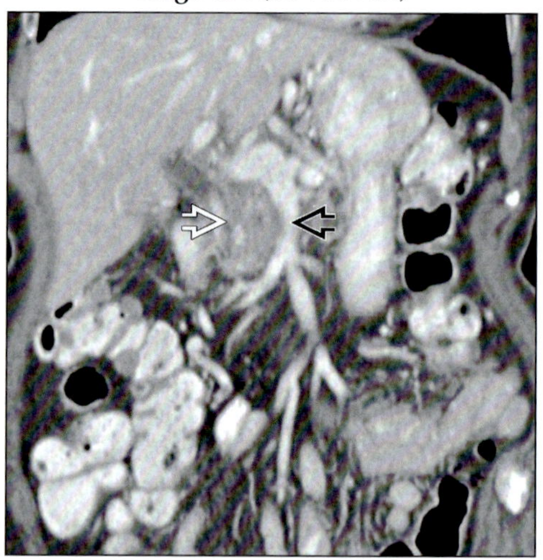

*(**Left**) Planning CT in a patient with resected pancreatic adenocarcinoma shows the preoperative tumor volume, CTV and PTV. The PTV is a 5 mm expansion from the CTV. Note the postoperative clips included in the CTV. (**Right**) Planning CT with 3D conformal 4-field beam arrangement is displayed in the same patient.*

Postop 4 Field

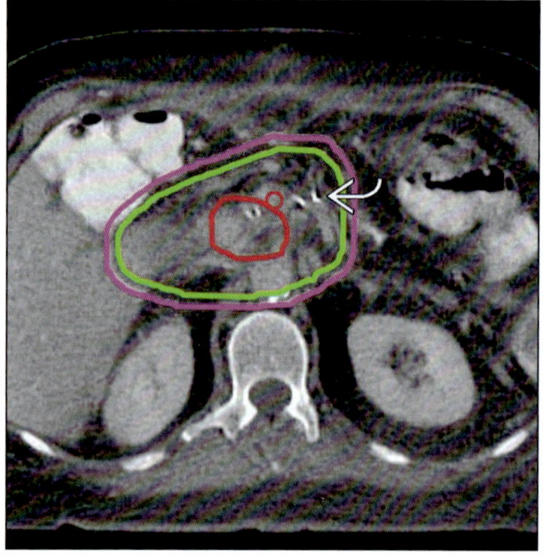

Postop 4 Field

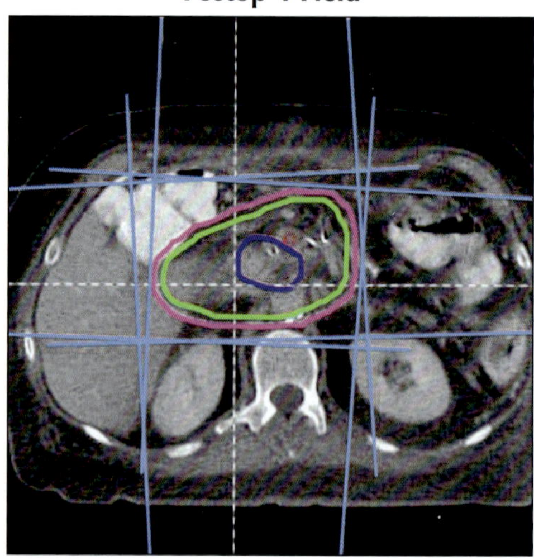

*(**Left**) Sequential 3D conformal 4-field plans were used to deliver a total of 59.4 Gy in 33 fractions. The composite dose colorwash is shown. 30 Gy isodose line is in blue; 45 Gy in yellow; 50.4 Gy in orange; and 59.4 Gy in green. (**Right**) DVH shows target coverage in the same patient. Liver was limited to mean < 30 Gy; spinal cord to < 45 Gy, and right kidney to D50% < 20 Gy.*

Postop 4 Field

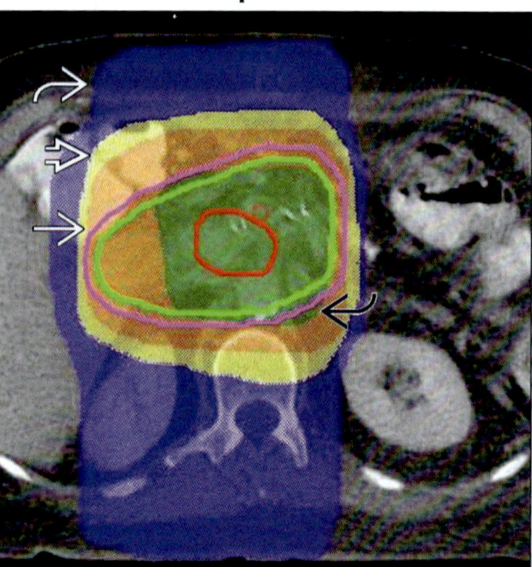

Postop 4 Field

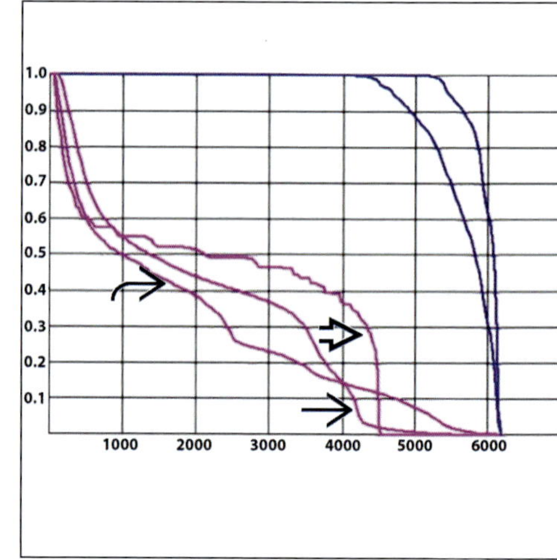

Postop IMRT

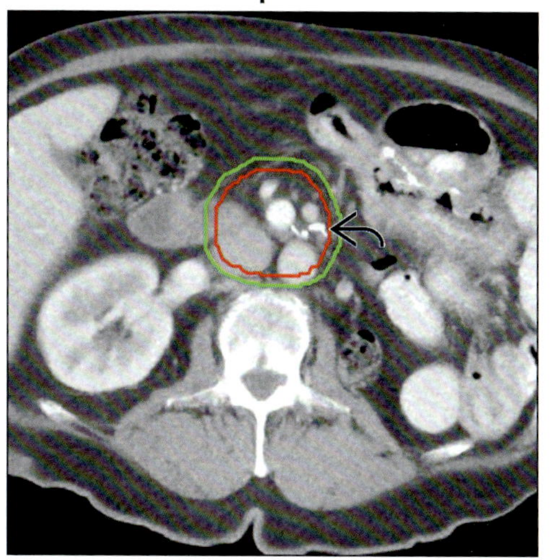

Postop IMRT

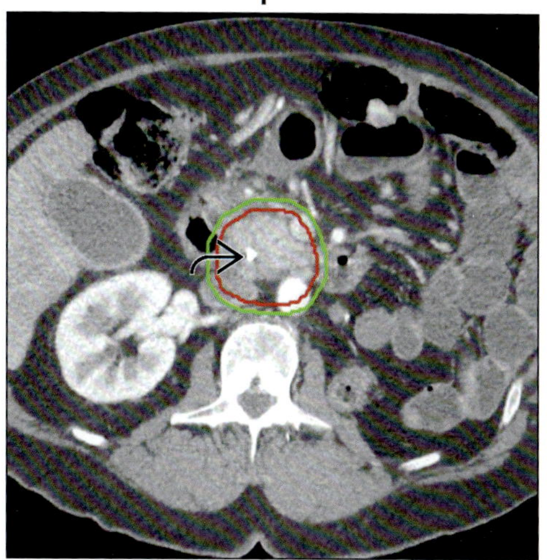

(Left) *Planning CT in a patient with resected pancreatic adenocarcinoma shows the CTV and PTV. The PTV is a 5 mm expansion from the CTV. Note the postoperative clips included in the CTV. Also note the left kidney is surgically absent.* ***(Right)*** *Preoperative CT was fused to planning CT in the same patient. The CTV encompasses preoperative gross tumor. The PTV is a 5 mm expansion from the CTV. Note the plastic biliary stent within the common bile duct.*

Postop IMRT

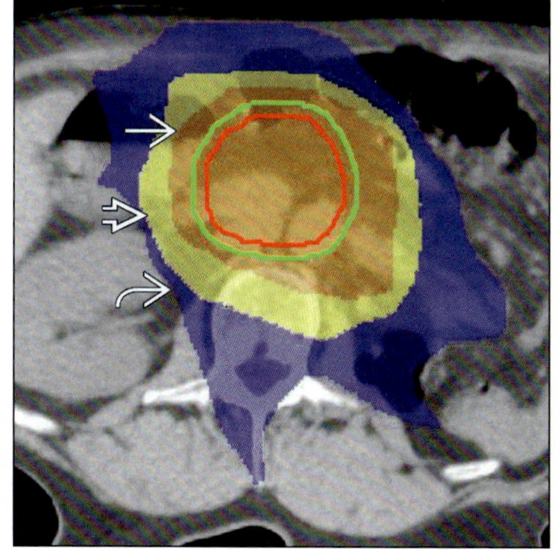

Postop IMRT

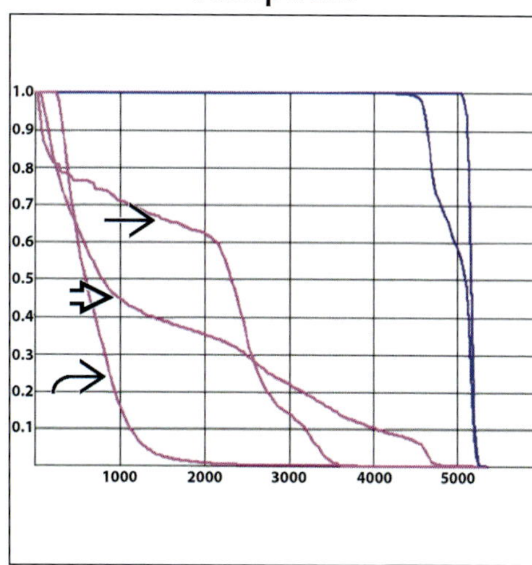

(Left) *7-field IMRT was used to deliver 45 Gy in 25 fractions in the same patient. This was followed by a 5.4 Gy boost. The composite dose colorwash is shown. 30 Gy isodose line is in blue; 45 Gy in yellow; and 50.4 Gy in orange. Note the dose wrapping around to avoid the kidney.* ***(Right)*** *DVH shows target coverage in the same patient. The kidney was limited to < 30 Gy and D15% < 20 Gy, liver mean < 30 Gy, and spinal cord < 50 Gy.*

Stage IIB (T3 N1 M0)

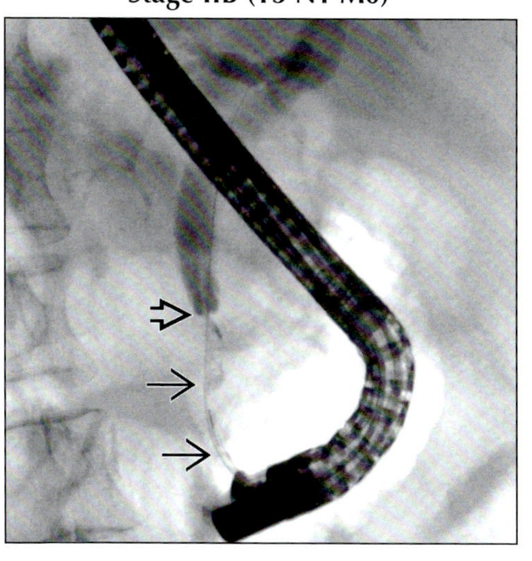

Stage IIB (T3 N1 M0)

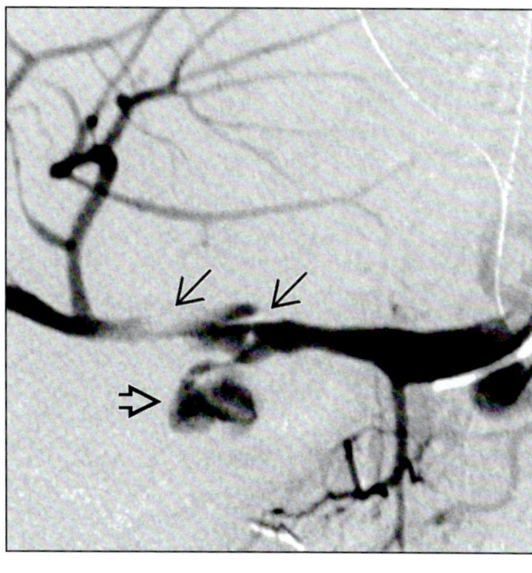

(Left) *ERCP shows irregularity of the distal common bile duct with associated shouldering. This is concerning for malignancy. ERCP is generally performed for biliary decompression, but brushings can provide a diagnosis.* ***(Right)*** *Coronal digital subtraction angiography (DSA) after Whipple shows extravasation from the gastroduodenal artery stump. Dissection of the hepatic artery is noted. The stump was coiled and the artery stented.*

PANCREAS

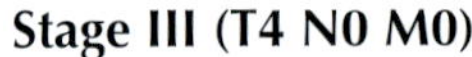

Stage III (T4 N0 M0)

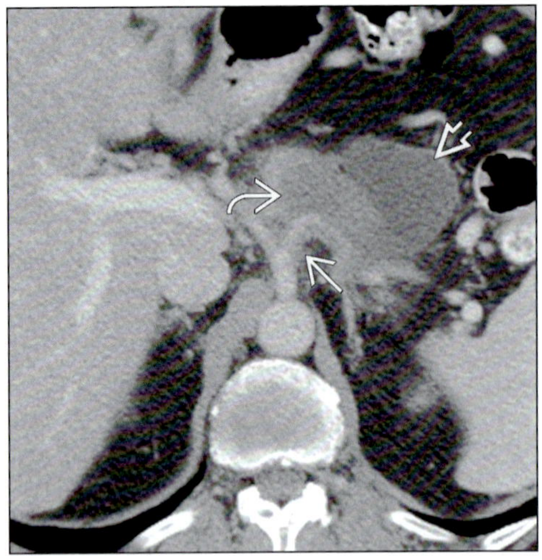

Stage III (T4 N0 M0)

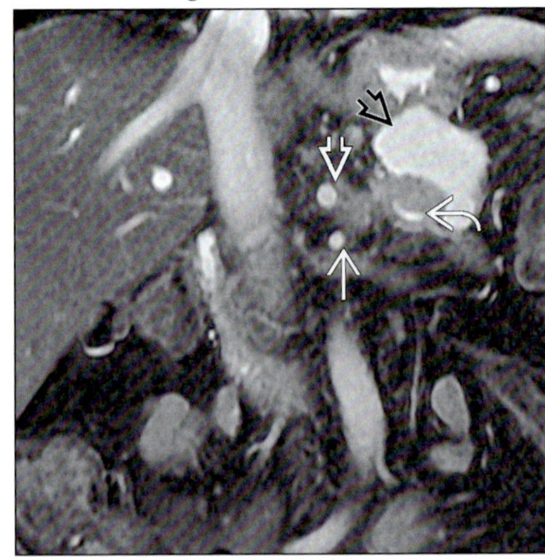

(Left) *Axial CECT shows a hypoenhancing ductal adenocarcinoma invading the splenic, hepatic, and celiac arteries. A large cystic component is seen anterior to the body. Cystic tumor components can be present in pancreatic cancer.* ***(Right)*** *Coronal T2WI MR in the same patient shows tumor abutting (< 180°) the celiac axis and SMA and encasing the splenic artery. The cystic component seen on the previous image is T2 bright.*

Stage IV (T4 N1 M1)

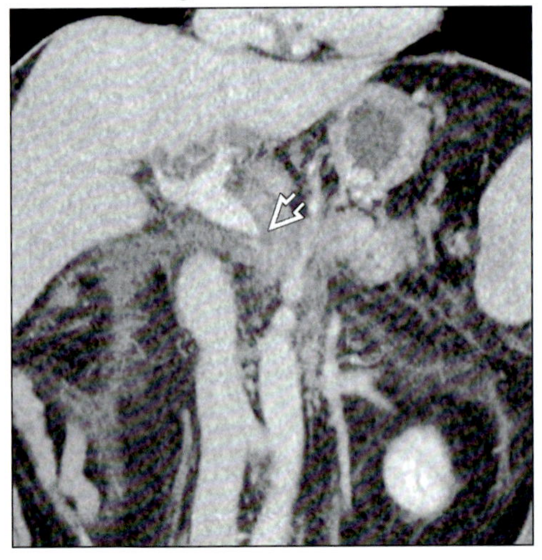

Stage IV (T4 N1 M1)

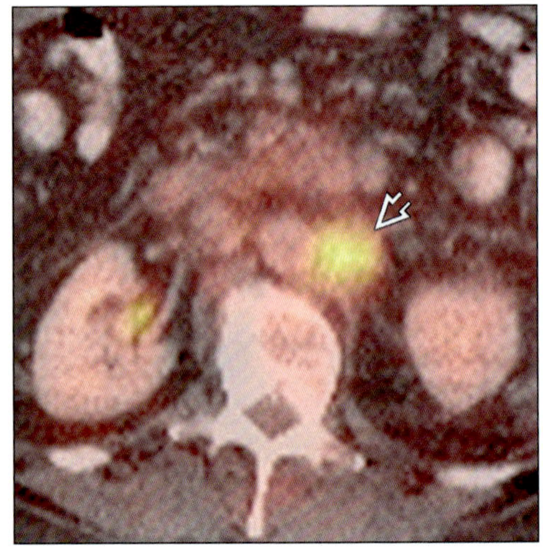

(Left) *Coronal CECT shows encasement of the portal vein. The confluence of superior mesenteric vein and portal vein is nearly occluded by tumor invasion.* ***(Right)*** *Axial PET/CT in the same patient shows an FDG-avid paraaortic lymph node. Biopsy showed adenocarcinoma. Diseased lymph nodes beyond the surgical field are considered metastatic (M1). Biopsy of a metastatic lesion is preferred to biopsy of the primary tumor.*

Stage IV (T4 N1 M1)

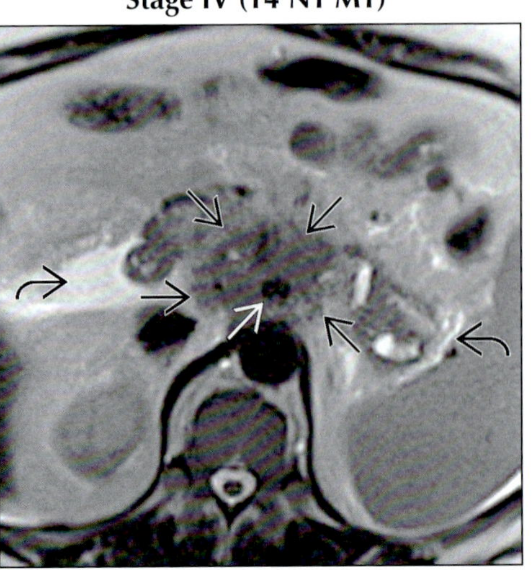

Stage IV (T4 N1 M1)

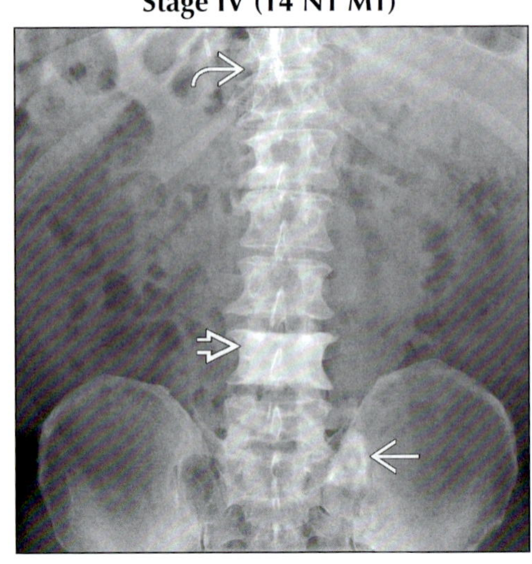

(Left) *Axial T2WI MR shows a diffusely infiltrative T2 hypointense mass encasing (> 180°) the celiac axis. Areas of peripancreatic inflammation and edema are present.* ***(Right)*** *Coronal radiograph shows blastic metastases including an ivory L4 vertebrae and a left sacral lesion. Distant hematogenous metastases usually occur after hepatic or peritoneal metastases, late in the disease process. A permanent common bile duct stent is also seen.*

Stage IV (T4 NX M1)

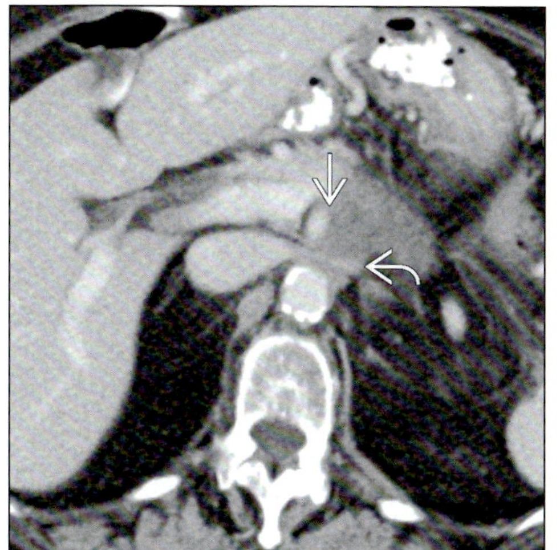

Stage IV (T4 NX M1)

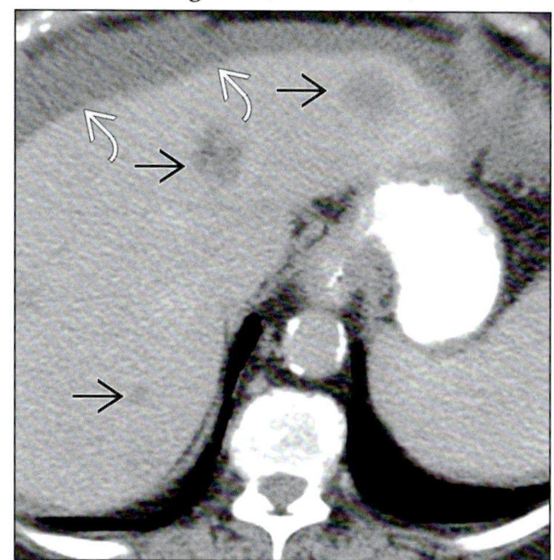

(Left) *Axial CECT shows an infiltrative mucinous cystadenocarcinoma encasing the SMA* ➡ *and left renal vein* ➡*.* ***(Right)*** *Axial CECT shows multiple hypoattenuating, ill-defined hepatic metastatic lesions* ➡*. Liver and peritoneum are the most common sites of metastatic pancreatic cancer. Note the presence of perihepatic ascites* ➡*, which is suspicious for subradiological peritoneal metastases.*

Stage IV (T4 NX M1)

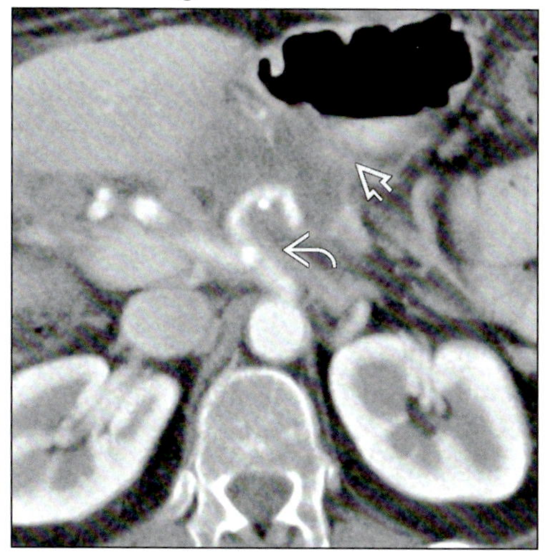

Stage IV (T4 NX M1)

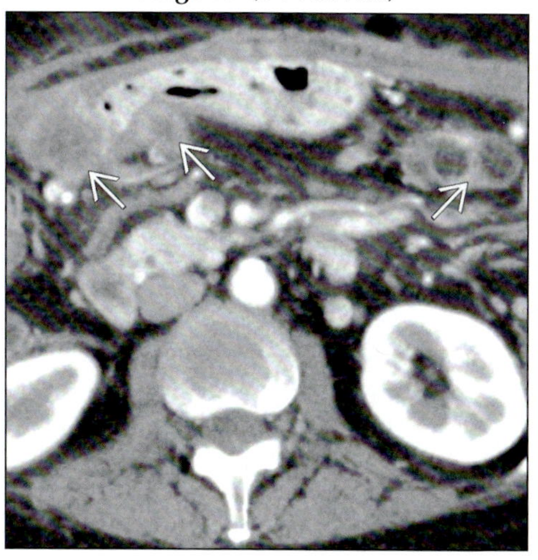

(Left) *Axial CECT shows an infiltrative ductal adenocarcinoma encasing (> 180°) the splenic, common hepatic, and celiac arteries* ➡*. Additionally, there is invasion of the posterior wall of the gastric body* ➡*. This is an unresectable primary tumor.* ***(Right)*** *Axial CECT in the same patient shows multiple peripherally enhancing peritoneal metastases* ➡*. Along with the liver, the peritoneum is the most common site of metastatic disease in pancreatic cancer.*

Stage IV (T3 N1 M1)

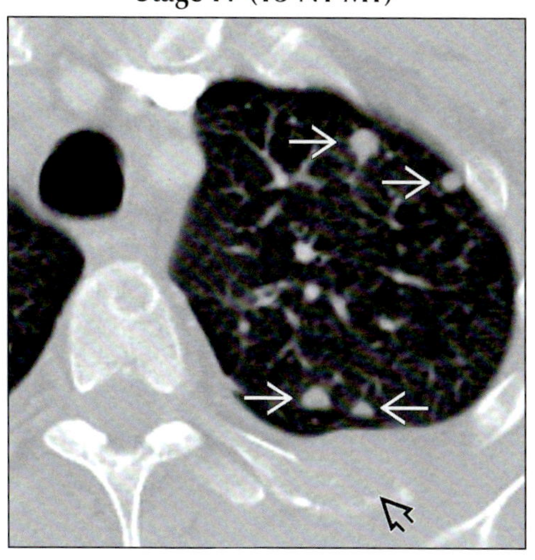

Stage IV (T3 N1 M1)

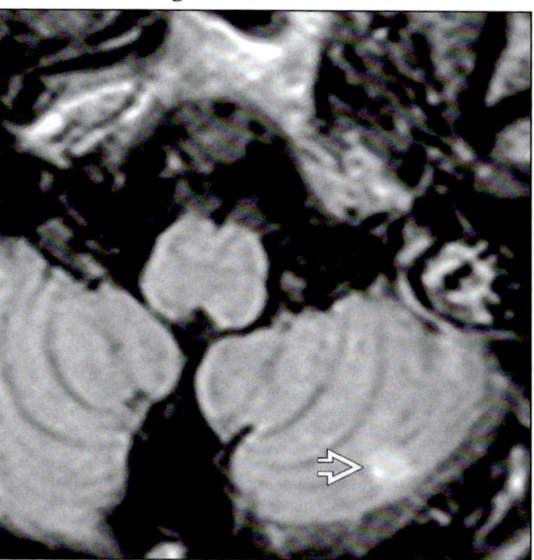

(Left) *Axial NECT shows multiple pulmonary metastases* ➡ *and a large destructive osseous lesion in a posterior left-sided rib* ➡*. Distant hematogenous metastases are rarely seen in the absence of either hepatic or peritoneal metastases and occur late in the disease process.* ***(Right)*** *Axial T1WI C+ MR in the same patient shows an enhancing metastasis to the left cerebellum* ➡*. Brain metastases are rare.*

(Left) *Axial CECT shows a hypoattenuating lesion in the pancreatic head and associated ductal dilation, consistent with a mixed type intraductal papillary mucinous neoplasm (IPMN). Note the unremarkable appearance of the pancreatic body at this time.* **(Right)** *Axial CECT in the same patient 12 months after the initial CT shows an infiltrative hypoenhancing mass in the pancreatic body, consistent with ductal adenocarcinoma. The IPMN is again seen.*

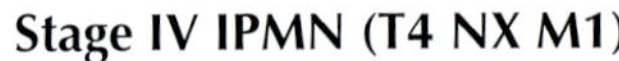

Stage IV IPMN (T4 NX M1)

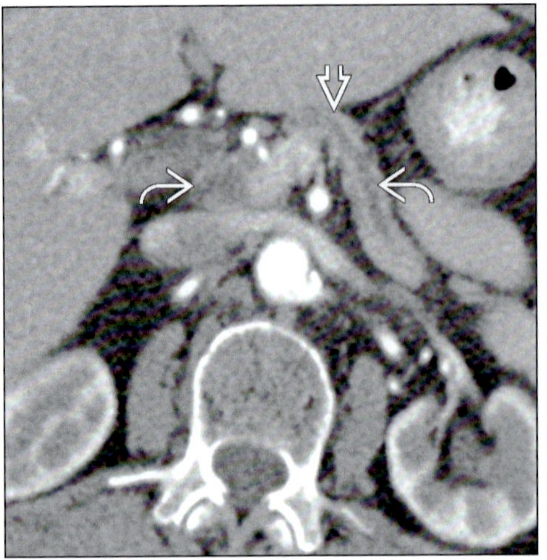

Stage IV IPMN (T4 NX M1)

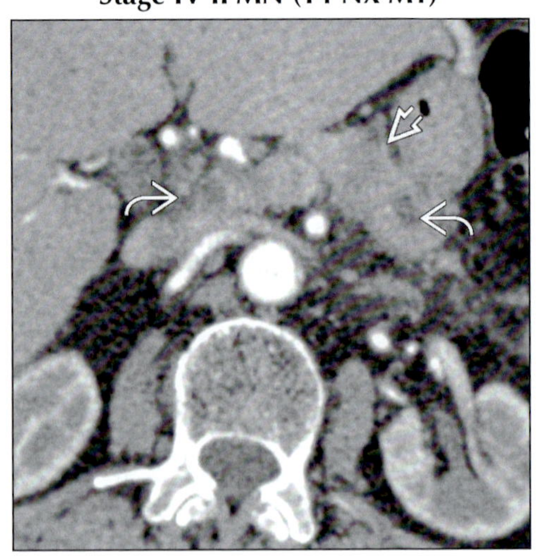

(Left) *Axial CECT in the same patient shows encasement of the celiac axis and proximal splenic and common hepatic arteries, consistent with T4 disease. This is unresectable.* **(Right)** *Axial CECT from the same study shows the invasive ductal adenocarcinoma invading the portal vein and abutting the SMA. Small, ill-defined, hypoattenuating metastatic lesions are seen in the periphery of the liver.*

Stage IV IPMN (T4 NX M1)

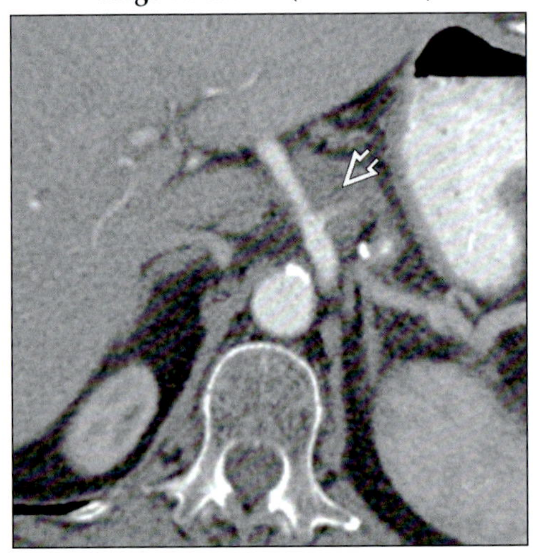

Stage IV IPMN (T4 NX M1)

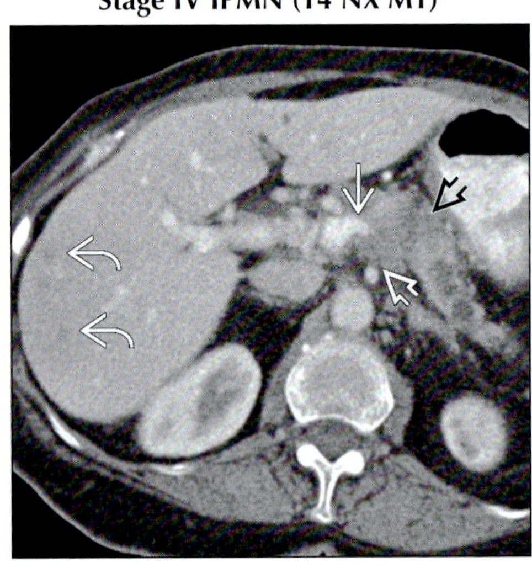

(Left) *Axial CECT shows a "double duct" sign with distention of the common bile duct and pancreatic duct due to a tumor located in the uncinate process. The presence of a subcentimeter celiac lymph node is important to note.* **(Right)** *Chest x-ray from the same patient shows a cavitary mass in the left lung, and a 2nd solid mass is seen on the right. Biopsy revealed lung metastases. Cavitary lung masses from pancreatic cancer are rare.*

Stage IV (T3 NX M1)

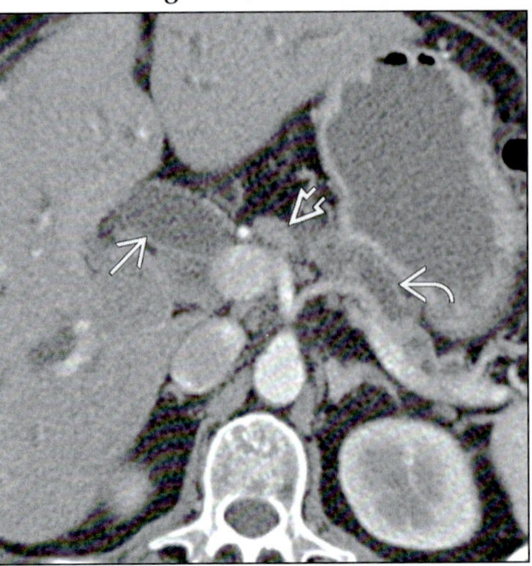

Stage IV (T3 NX M1)

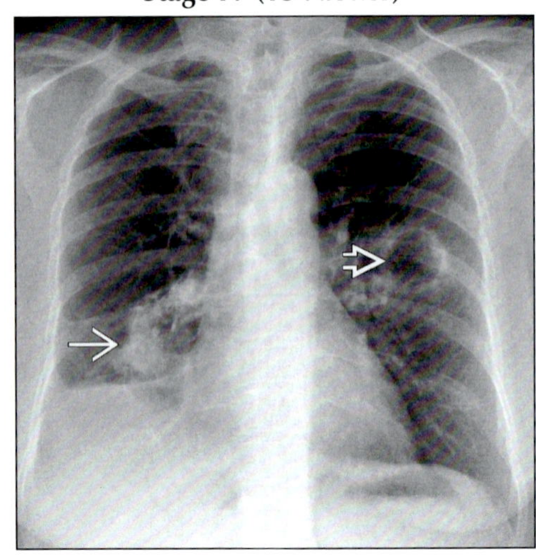

Stage IV (T3 N0 M1)

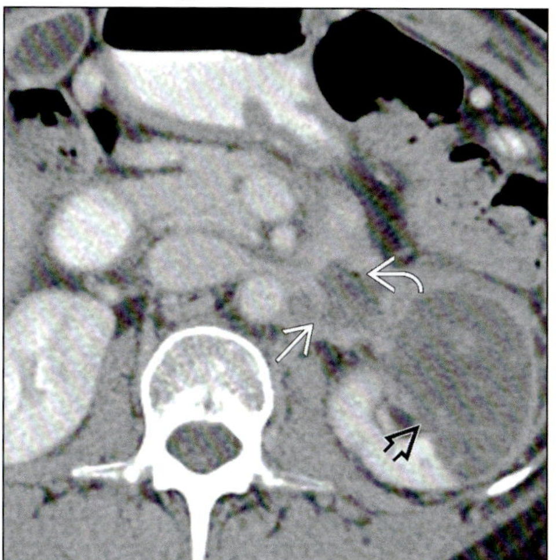

Stage IV (T3 N0 M1)

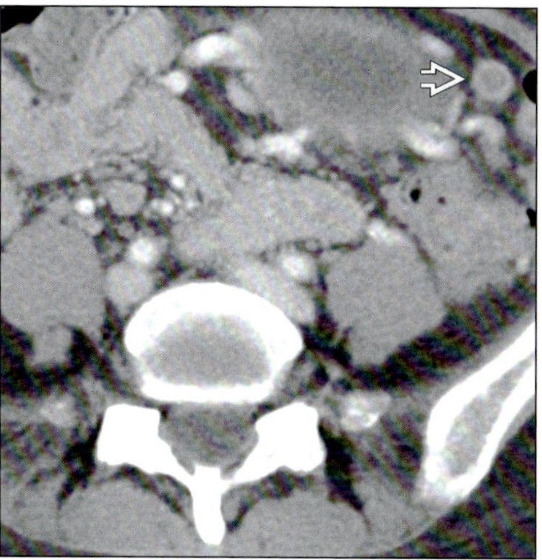

*(**Left**) Axial CECT following neoadjuvant chemotherapy for a T3 cancer shows progression of disease. At the time of diagnosis, the mass encased the left renal artery and abutted the aorta. Now the mass has invaded the left renal artery, resulting in infarction of the left kidney. A small focus of gas within the mass was secondary to fistulization with the duodenum. (**Right**) Axial CECT shows a peritoneal metastasis in the same patient.*

Stage IV Postop

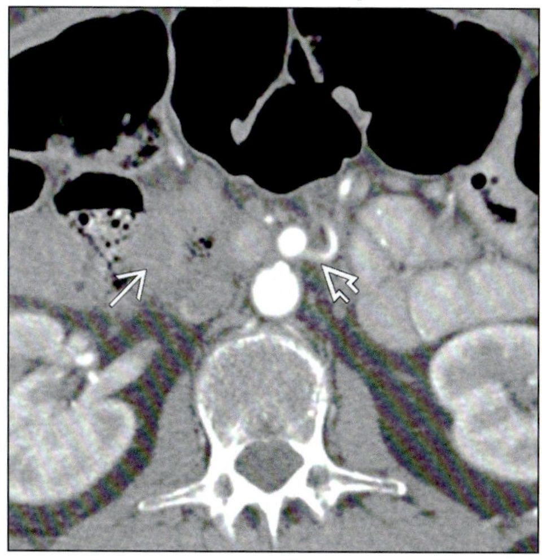

Stage IV Recurrence

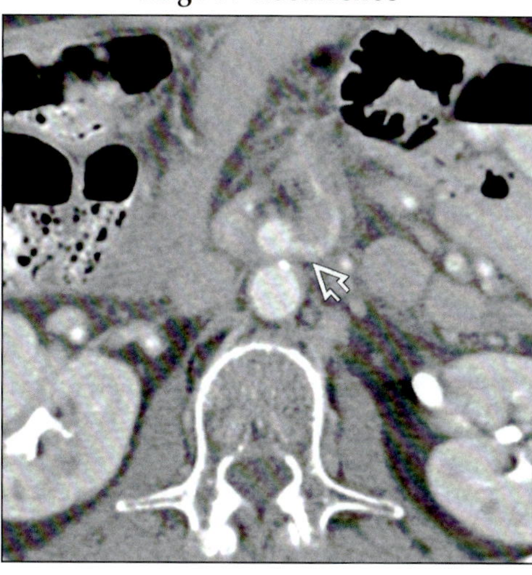

*(**Left**) Axial CECT in a different patient shows a study performed soon after surgical resection (Whipple). Note the postoperative changes and clean fat planes around the SMA and proximal jejunal branch. (**Right**) Axial CECT in the same patient at follow-up shows development of encasement of the proximal jejunal branch to the level of the SMA. This is consistent with local perineural, perivascular, or lymphatic disease recurrence.*

Stage IV Recurrence

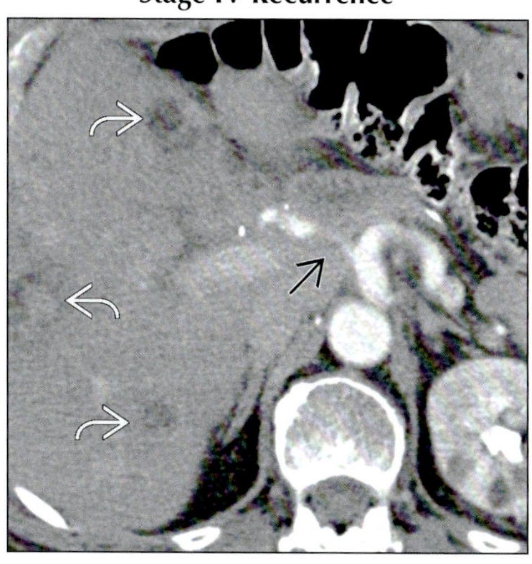

Stage IV Recurrence

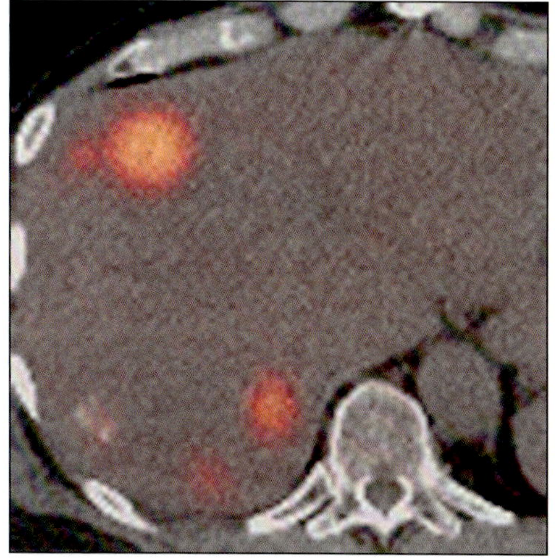

*(**Left**) Axial CECT in the same patient demonstrates development of multiple hypoattenuating liver metastases and encasement and narrowing of the proximal common hepatic artery following Whipple resection of the primary tumor. (**Right**) Axial PET/CT in the same patient shows multiple FDG-avid liver metastases. The most common patterns of failure in pancreatic cancer are local recurrence or development of peritoneal or hepatic metastatic disease.*

INTRA- AND EXTRAHEPATIC BILIARY

(T) Primary Tumor

Adapted from 7th edition AJCC Staging Forms.

TNM	*Definitions*
Intrahepatic bile ducts	
TX	Primary tumor cannot be assessed
T0	No evidence of primary tumor
Tis	Carcinoma in situ (intraductal tumor)
T1	Solitary tumor without vascular invasion
T2a	Solitary tumor with vascular invasion
T2b	Multiple tumors ± vascular invasion
T3	Tumor perforating the visceral peritoneum or involving the local extrahepatic structures by direct invasion
T4	Tumor with periductal invasion
Extrahepatic bile ducts (perihilar)	
TX	Primary tumor cannot be assessed
T0	No evidence of primary tumor
Tis	Carcinoma in situ
T1	Tumor confined to the bile duct, with extension up to the muscle layer or fibrous tissue
T2a	Tumor invades beyond the wall of the bile duct to surrounding adipose tissue
T2b	Tumor invades adjacent hepatic parenchyma
T3	Tumor invades unilateral branches of the portal vein or hepatic artery
T4	Tumor involves main portal vein or its branches bilaterally; or the common hepatic artery; or the second-order biliary radicals bilaterally; or unilateral second-order biliary radicals with contralateral portal vein or hepatic artery involvement

(N) Regional Lymph Nodes

NX	Regional lymph nodes cannot be assessed
N0	No regional lymph node metastasis
N1	Regional lymph node metastasis (including nodes along cystic duct, common bile duct, hepatic artery, and portal vein)
N2	Metastasis to periaortic, pericaval, superior mesenteric artery, &/or celiac artery lymph nodes (for extrahepatic tumors only)

(M) Distant Metastasis

M0	No distant metastasis
M1	Distant metastasis

AJCC Stages/Prognostic Groups

Adapted from 7th edition AJCC Staging Forms.

Stage	*T*	*N*	*M*
0	Tis	N0	M0
I	T1	N0	M0
II	T2a, T2b	N0	M0
IIIA	T3	N0	M0
IIIB	T1, T2, T3	N1	M0
IVA	T4	N0, N1	M0
IVB	Any T	N2	M0
	Any T	Any N	M1

T1

Most cholangiocarcinomas are extrahepatic (EHCC), and the majority of EHCCs (80%) are perihilar. Graphic shows hepatic hilum with infiltrative tumor confined to wall of bile duct (stage T1) at confluence of right and left hepatic ducts. Inset shows tumor invasion up to muscle layer or fibrous tissue of bile duct wall.

T1

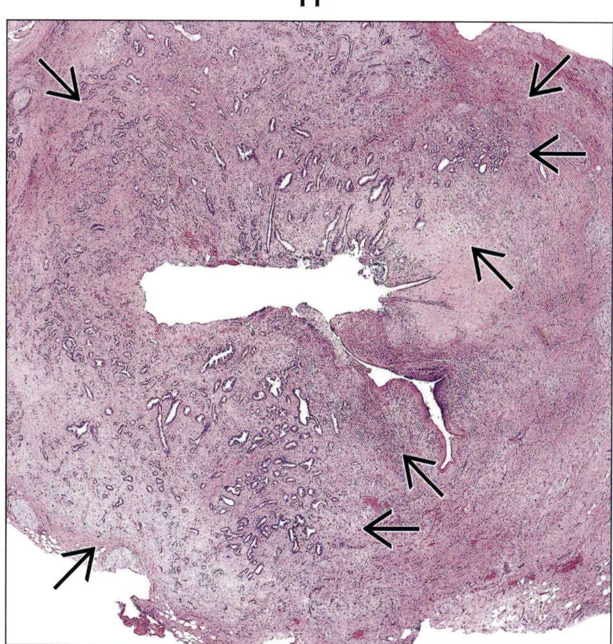

H&E stained section of a perihilar bile duct shows invasive carcinoma involving the duct wall. There is a patent central lumen with carcinoma → confined to the muscle and fibrous layer of the bile duct.

T2

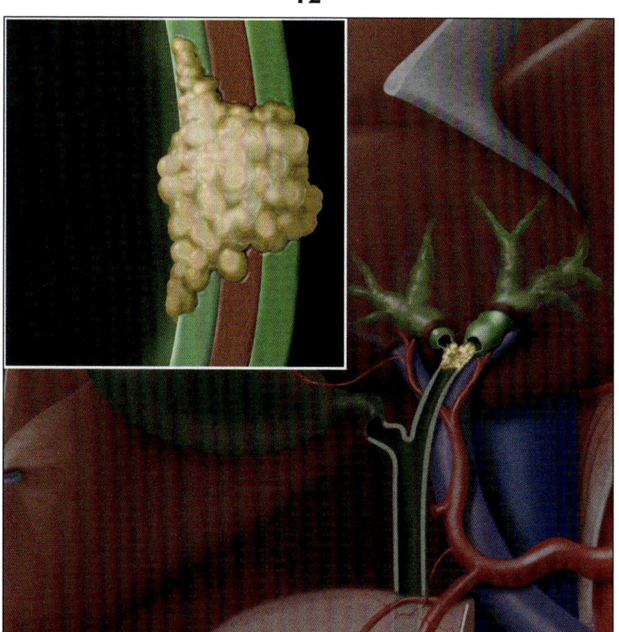

EHCCs extending beyond the wall of the bile duct are T2. Inset shows tumor invasion beyond the bile duct wall into surrounding adipose tissue.

T2

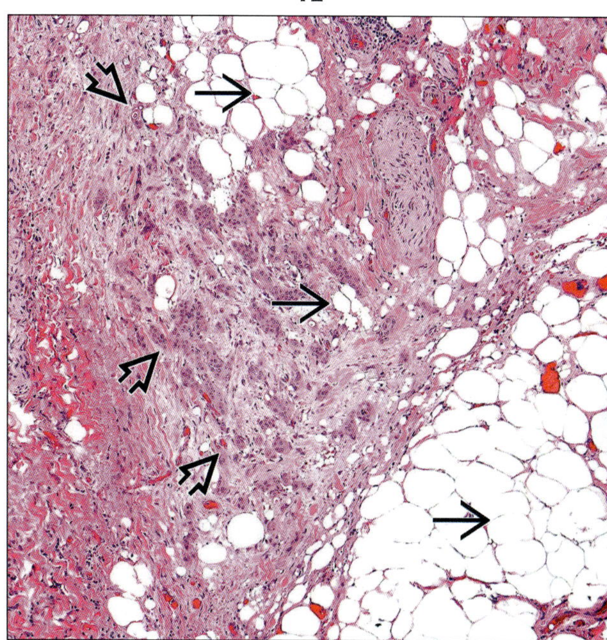

H&E stained section shows invasive carcinoma of the perihilar bile duct. The neoplastic cells are arranged in nests ⇨, are surrounded with fibrotic stroma, and infiltrate the surrounding adipose tissue →.

T3

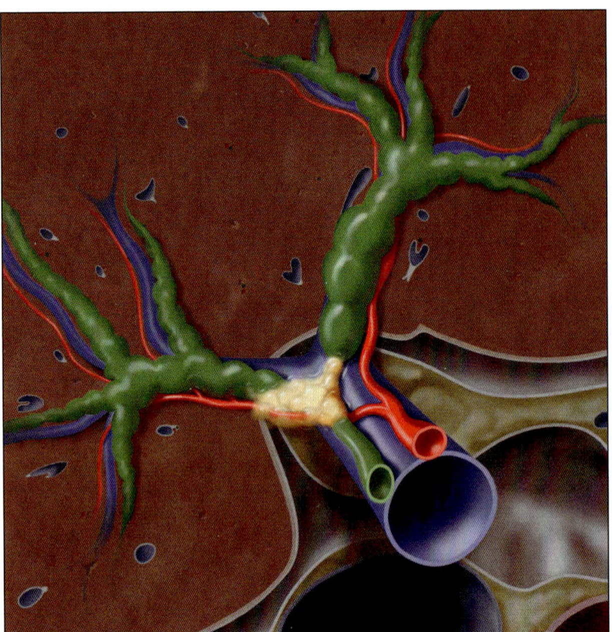

Axial graphic depicts the hepatic hilum with perihilar tumor encasing the right hepatic artery. Unilateral invasion of the portal vein or hepatic artery is classified as a T3 primary tumor.

T3

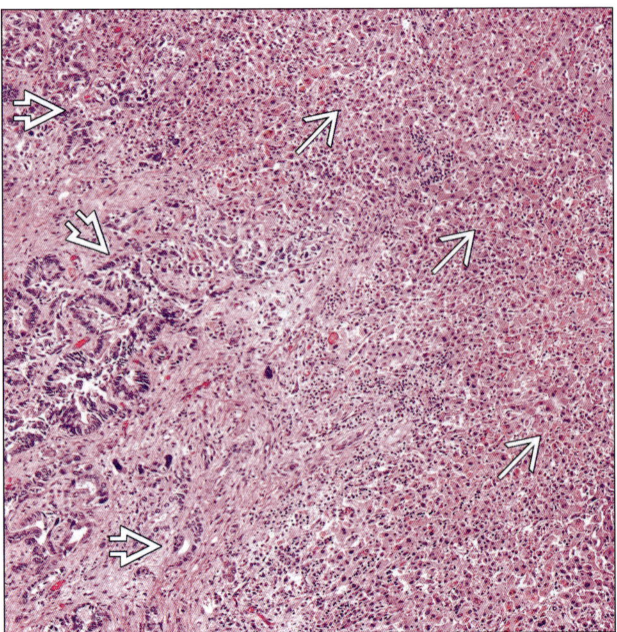

H&E stained section shows invasive carcinoma ➡ of the perihilar bile duct that extends beyond the wall of the bile duct to involve the hepatic parenchyma ➡. The right portal vein was also found to be involved.

T4

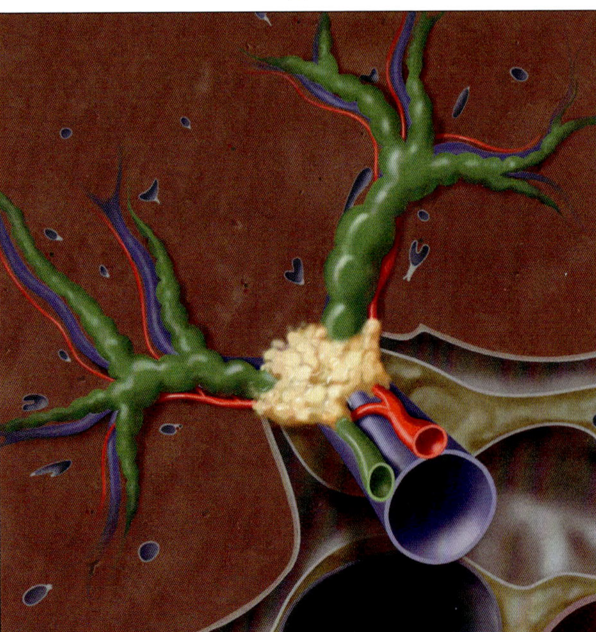

Axial graphic depicts the hepatic hilum with perihilar tumor encasing the right and left hepatic arteries.

T4

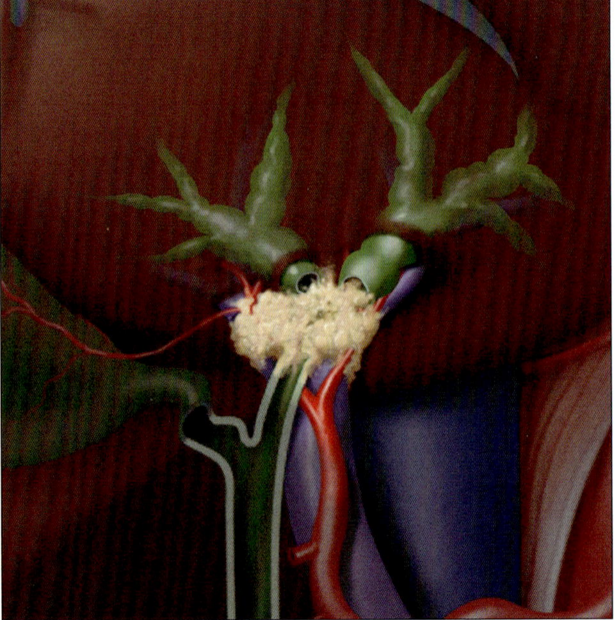

Graphic depicts the hepatic hilum with infiltrative tumor at the confluence of the right and left hepatic ducts with an exophytic mass-forming component invading bilateral portal veins and hepatic arteries. Invasion of the common hepatic artery, main portal vein, or bilateral branches constitutes stage T4 tumor.

N1

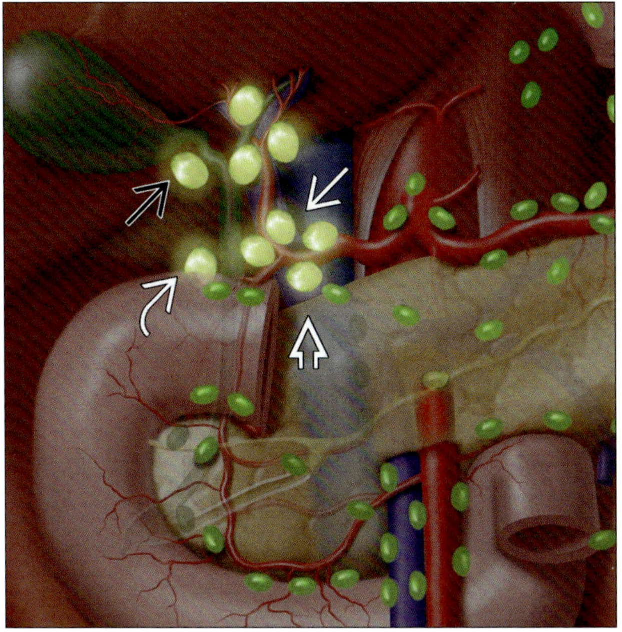

N1 nodes include cystic ➔, common bile ➔, hepatic artery ➔, and portal vein ➔ nodes.

N2

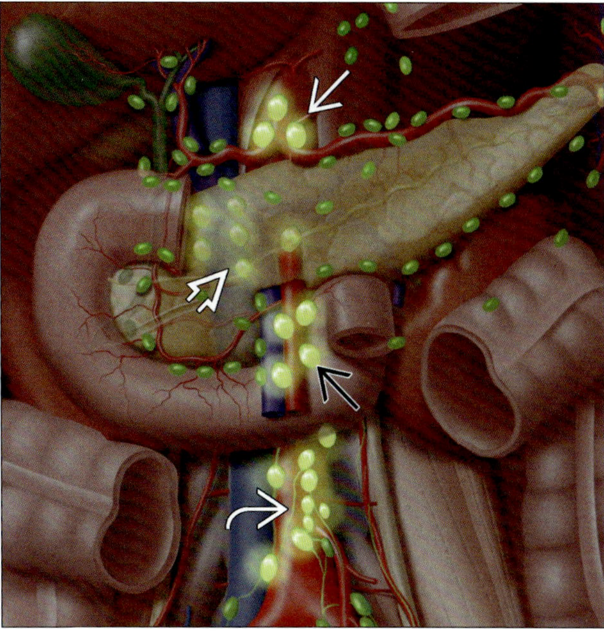

Graphic highlights N2 regional lymph nodes. These include periaortic ➔, pericaval ➔, superior mesenteric artery ➔, and celiac artery ➔ lymph nodes.

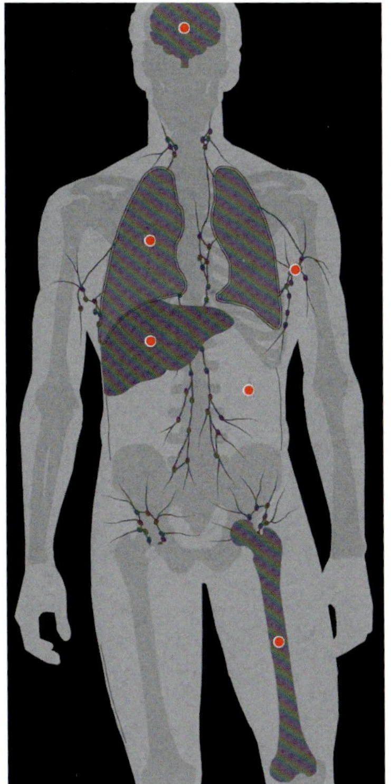

INITIAL SITE OF RECURRENCE

Local	41%
Distant	36%
Regional	24%

Data was obtained from 80 patients with hilar cholangiocarcinoma. Most common distant sites for metastases were lung, liver, and peritoneum. Jarnagin WR et al: Patterns of initial disease recurrence after resection for gall bladder carcinoma and hilar cholangiocarcinoma. Cancer 98(8):1689-1700, 2003.

INTRA- AND EXTRAHEPATIC BILIARY

OVERVIEW

General Comments

- Tumor arising in extrahepatic bile duct upstream to cystic duct origin
  - Klatskin tumor: Tumor at biliary confluence of right and left hepatic ducts
- ~ 70% of cholangiocarcinomas (CCAs) are perihilar

Classification

- Histologic types
  - Adenocarcinoma
    - Adenocarcinoma, intestinal type
    - Clear cell adenocarcinoma
  - Mucinous carcinoma
  - Signet ring cell carcinoma
  - Squamous cell carcinoma
  - Adenosquamous carcinoma
  - Small cell (oat cell) carcinoma
  - Undifferentiated carcinoma
  - Papillomatosis
  - Papillary carcinoma, noninvasive
  - Papillary carcinoma, invasive
  - Carcinoma, not otherwise specified (NOS)

NATURAL HISTORY

General Features

- Comments
  - 80% of cholangiocarcinomas are extrahepatic
    - 70-80% are perihilar
    - 20-30% are distal bile duct

Etiology

- Risk factors
  - Age
  - Primary sclerosing cholangitis (PSC)
  - Chronic ulcerative colitis
  - Hepatolithiasis
  - Caroli disease
  - Choledochal cysts
  - Tobacco abuse (in association with PSC)
  - Bile duct adenoma & biliary papillomatosis
  - Hepatobiliary flukes
  - Chronic typhoid carriers
  - Exposure to thorotrast
  - Familial polyposis
- Additional risk factors in USA and Europe
  - Cirrhosis
  - Chronic hepatitis C infection
  - Alcohol abuse

Epidemiology & Cancer Incidence

- Incidence is 1-2 per 100,000 in USA
- Increasing incidence worldwide

Genetics

- Gene mutations suggest possible genetic link
  - Inactivation of tumor suppressor genes
  - Mutations in oncogenes
  - Chromosomal aneuploidy
- No established clinical role for molecular profiling at this time

Associated Diseases, Abnormalities

- Primary sclerosing cholangitis
  - Common risk factor in Western countries
  - Prevalence of cholangiocarcinoma in this setting is 5-15%
  - Risk not associated with duration or severity of PSC or inflammatory bowel disease
- Hepatobiliary flukes
  - *Opisthorchis viverrini* and *Clonorchis sinensis*
  - Endemic in east Asia
  - Ingested in undercooked fish
  - Infest biliary tree ± gallbladder
- Choledochal cysts
  - 10-15% lifetime risk of developing CCA
  - Malignant degeneration uncommon if cyst excised early in life
  - 15-20% ↑ incidence if not treated until > 20 years of age
- Hepatolithiasis
  - Risk factor in parts of Asia
  - ≤ 10% complicated by cholangiocarcinoma
  - In endemic areas, 70% of tumors manifest with hepatolithiasis

Gross Pathology & Surgical Features

- Patterns of tumor growth
  - Mass-forming (exophytic)
    - Most common at intrahepatic location
    - Radial growth pattern invading liver
  - Periductal (infiltrating)
    - Most common in perihilar tumors
    - Tendency to extend submucosally
    - Sclerotic lesion with abundant fibrous tissue
  - Mixed (mass-forming and periductal)
  - Intraductal (polypoid)
    - Usually papillary adenocarcinoma
    - Intraluminal polypoid mass
    - Uncommon except tumors arising in choledochal cysts
- Macroscopic subtypes
  - Sclerosing
    - Majority of tumors
    - Perihilar > distal bile duct
    - Firm tumor → annular thickening of bile duct
    - Often diffuse infiltration & fibrosis of periductal tissues
  - Nodular
    - Firm, irregular nodule projecting into duct lumen
  - Papillary
    - 10% of cholangiocarcinomas
    - Distal bile duct > perihilar
    - Soft, friable tumor
    - May have little transmural invasion
    - Tends to be polypoid mass expanding duct
    - Can be quite large and arising from well-defined stalk with majority of tumor mobile within duct

Microscopic Pathology

- H&E
  - 90% are adenocarcinomas
  - Usually well to moderately differentiated
  - Exhibit glandular or acinar structures
  - Cuboidal or low columnar cells resembling biliary epithelium

- Intracytoplasmic mucin is common
- Mitotic figures are rare
- Dense, sparsely cellular fibrous stroma
- Tendency to invade lymphatics, blood vessels, perineural & periductal spaces, and portal tracts

Routes of Spread

- **Contiguous spread**
  - Predilection for longitudinal submucosal spread in duct wall
    - May have substantial extension of tumor beneath intact epithelial lining
      - Up to 2 cm proximally and 1 cm distally
    - Perihilar tumor tends to infiltrate intrahepatic ducts
  - Spread along periductal tissues
    - Neural and perineural involvement
  - Direct invasion of adjacent structures
    - Invasion of hepatic parenchyma in 85%
    - Invasion of vasculature
      - Portal vein is common
      - Hepatic artery
    - Invasion of adjacent organs
      - Pancreas
      - Stomach, duodenum, or colon
      - Omentum and abdominal wall
- **Lymphatic spread**
  - Prevalence of 30-53%
  - ↑ prevalence of lymph node metastases with ↑ in primary tumor stage
  - Most commonly involves hepatoduodenal nodes
    - Hilar nodes
    - Pericholedochal nodes
  - N1 regional nodes
    - Cystic duct
    - Common bile duct
    - Hepatic artery
    - Portal vein
  - N2 regional nodes
    - Periaortic
    - Pericaval
    - Superior mesenteric artery
    - Celiac artery
  - Incidence of N2 nodal metastases is 14-50% in patients with lymphatic spread
- **Hematogenous spread**
  - 10-20% have distant metastases at presentation
  - 50% have metastatic disease at autopsy
  - Liver is common site of metastases
  - Spread to other organs, especially extraabdominal, is uncommon
- **Peritoneal spread**
  - 10-20% have peritoneal involvement

IMAGING

Detection

- **Ultrasound**
  - Excellent for identifying biliary obstruction
  - Poor sensitivity & specificity for identifying mass
    - Difficult to see intraductal or infiltrating lesions
    - Mass-forming tumors have variable echogenicity
    - Advanced stage when seen on US
  - Findings
    - Segmental dilation with abrupt cut-off of right and left hepatic ducts at porta hepatis
    - Lobar atrophy results in crowding of dilated ducts
    - Hypovascular mass → poor color Doppler signal
    - May detect portal vein occlusion or infiltration
- **CT**
  - Findings
    - NECT
      - Hypodense bile duct wall thickening
      - Mass at confluence of right & left hepatic ducts
    - CECT
      - Thickened bile duct wall continues to enhance on delayed images
      - Mass showing progressive and persistent enhancement on delayed images
  - Atrophy-hypertrophy complex
    - Bile duct dilation in an atrophic hepatic lobe with compensatory hypertrophy of contralateral lobe
  - Mass may not be visible; however, biliary dilation abruptly terminates at biliary confluence
  - No extrahepatic biliary dilation
  - Diffuse intrahepatic biliary ductal dilation
- **PET/CT**
  - FDG accumulates in tumor cells but limited if large fibrotic component
  - Mucinous carcinoma → no FDG uptake
  - Higher rate of tumor detection for mass-forming growth pattern than for infiltrative
  - Some report better detection of intrahepatic tumor than perihilar or distal bile duct tumor
  - Efficacy of PET in setting of PSC is controversial
  - Focal FDG uptake with ↑ CA19-9 is more sensitive & specific
- **MR/MRCP**
  - Findings
    - T1WI
      - Hypointense to isointense mass
    - T2WI
      - Bile duct wall thickening and obliteration of lumen at biliary confluence
      - Hyperintense to isointense mass
      - Signal intensity depends on fibrotic, mucinous, and necrotic components of tumor
      - Fat saturation improves conspicuity of hyperintense masses
    - Dynamic post-contrast images
      - Progressive and persistent enhancement on delayed images
    - DWI
      - Malignant lesions tend to have lower absolute diffusion coefficients
      - Lesion conspicuity is enhanced due to suppression of vascular high signal
    - MRCP
      - Abrupt occlusion of bile ducts at level of biliary confluence
      - Intrahepatic biliary dilation
      - No extrahepatic biliary dilation
      - Delineates level of obstruction, longitudinal extent, or multifocality of tumor
  - Atrophy-hypertrophy complex
    - Atrophy of 1 hepatic lobe with crowding of dilated bile ducts
    - Compensatory hypertrophy of contralateral lobe

- Often indicates concomitant portal vein occlusion of atrophic lobe
- Tissue-specific contrast agents
  - Iron oxide particles may improve tumor detection
  - Increase lesion-liver contrast & lesion conspicuity
- Primary sclerosing cholangitis
  - Findings of superimposed CCA
    - Progressive stricture formation (most common)
    - Upstream bile duct dilation
    - Polypoid intraductal mass

Staging

- Primary tumor may be staged by multiple modalities
- **Ultrasound**
  - Limited in detection of mass and vascular invasion
  - No role in staging
- **CT**
  - Multidetector CT allows rapid acquisition in multiple phases of contrast enhancement
    - Arterial & portal venous phase
      - Arterial & venous anatomy, invasion, encasement
    - Delayed phase (10-15 minutes)
      - Characterization of tumors with dominant fibrous component
  - Isotropic data allows multiplanar reformation
    - Minimum intensity projection
      - Visualization of biliary anatomy
      - Determination of level of obstruction
      - Morphology of stricture
      - Presence of intraductal mass
    - Reconstruction of arterial & portal venous phases
      - Visualization of vascular anatomy, tumor encasement, occlusion, or invasion
  - Criteria for vascular involvement
    - Vessel occlusion or stenosis
    - Vessel contour deformity associated with tumor contact
    - > 50% perimeter contact with tumor
  - Limited in defining longitudinal tumor extent
- **PET/CT**
  - Not superior to CT or MR/MRCP for detection of primary lesion
  - Limitations for primary tumor
    - Assessment of longitudinal tumor extent
    - Evaluation of vascular invasion
    - Detection of hepatic invasion
- **MR/MRCP**
  - Optimal initial examination for suspected CCA
    - Liver and biliary anatomy
    - Tumor extent along bile ducts
    - Liver metastasis
    - Vascular invasion or encasement
  - Superior to CT for detection of intraductal lesions
  - Comparable to conventional angiography for evaluation of vascular invasion
  - MR
    - Helpful for visualization of
      - Exophytic component
      - Invasion of adjacent organs & vasculature
      - Satellite nodules
    - In conjunction with MRCP, allows better estimation of longitudinal extent of tumor
    - Dynamic 3D IV contrast-enhanced images
      - Multiphasic acquisition and improved spatial resolution
      - Vascular invasion
      - Direct invasion of adjacent structures
  - MRCP
    - Ideally, performed prior to biliary drainage
    - Localizes level of obstruction
    - Defines morphology & longitudinal extent of strictures
    - Can evaluate biliary tree upstream to obstruction
    - Navigator triggered isotropic 3D FSE
      - ↑ signal to noise ratio and spatial resolution
      - Allows reformation and isolation of biliary tree
    - Limitations
      - Not able to perform cytologic evaluation and bile duct sampling
      - Not able to relieve obstruction
      - Evaluation of intraductal lesions limited post stent placement
      - Limited in periampullary region
  - 3 tesla
    - Higher spatial resolution
    - Improved signal to noise ratio
- **Direct cholangiography** (ERCP or percutaneous transhepatic cholangiography)
  - Invasive
  - Useful for defining extent of infiltrating lesions
  - Allows bile duct sampling
    - Brush cytology has low reported accuracy (9-24%)
    - In patients with PSC, sensitivity is 60-73%
    - Negative result does not exclude malignancy
  - Allows stent placement to relieve obstruction
  - May not be able to evaluate bile ducts past obstruction
  - Altered anatomy due to prior surgery may preclude ERCP
  - Percutaneous transhepatic cholangiography is performed if
    - Lumen obliterated by tissue
    - Proximal lesion
    - Biliary tree not well visualized with ERCP
- **Endoscopic ultrasound**
  - Invasive
  - Can visualize distal extrahepatic bile duct, gallbladder, regional lymph nodes, and vasculature
  - Assesses depth of intraductal lesions
  - Localizes stricture for accurate FNA
    - FNA of perihilar mass is not recommended due to risk of peritoneal seeding
- **Bismuth-Corlette**
  - Cholangiographic classification to delineate longitudinal extent of perihilar tumor
  - MRCP may be used in place of conventional cholangiography except in setting of PSC
  - Classification
    - Type I: Involvement of common hepatic duct distal to confluence
    - Type II: Involvement of biliary confluence
    - Type IIIa: Involvement of biliary confluence and right hepatic duct
    - Type IIIb: Involvement of biliary confluence and left hepatic duct
    - Type IV: Involvement of right and left hepatic ducts or multifocal tumor

- **Regional lymph nodes**
  - Anatomic imaging (CT & MR)
    - Low sensitivity for lymph node metastasis
    - Findings
      - Size: ≥ 10 mm short axis
      - Central necrosis
  - Metabolic imaging (PET/CT)
    - Can be complementary to CT for nodal metastasis
    - Sensitivity: 32%; specificity: 88%
    - Higher specificity and accuracy than CT alone
    - Findings
      - Relative increase in FDG uptake compared to normal nodes
  - Limitations of anatomic & metabolic imaging
    - Differentiation of reactive from malignant adenopathy
    - Micrometastasis
  - Fine-needle aspiration biopsy may be performed with endoscopic ultrasound
    - 5-15% of those with negative CT have involved nodes with FNA at endoscopic ultrasound
  - Enlarged periportal lymph nodes are common in PSC, not necessarily indicative of metastasis
- **Metastatic disease**
  - Common in liver
    - Intrahepatic ductal extension
    - Perineural
    - Periductal lymphatics
  - Extraabdominal sites are uncommon
    - Peritoneal cavity, lung, brain, bone
  - Metabolic imaging may be valuable in detection of unsuspected distant metastasis
    - Sensitivity of PET: 65%; sensitivity of PET/CT: 56%; specificity: 88-92%
    - May also be helpful for indeterminate lesions seen on conventional imaging

CLINICAL PRESENTATION & WORK-UP

Presentation

- Age usually > 65 years (peak in 8th decade)
- Early symptoms are nonspecific (present in 30%)
  - Abdominal pain, anorexia, weight loss
- Later symptoms of biliary obstruction
  - Jaundice, pale stool, dark urine, pruritus
- Prolonged obstruction
  - Decrease in fat-soluble vitamins
  - Increase in prothrombin time
- Cholangitis is rare without biliary intervention
  - Right upper quadrant pain, fever, chills
- Liver function tests → obstructive pattern
  - ↑ alkaline phosphatase & bilirubin
  - Aminotransferases are often normal, unless acute obstruction or cholangitis
- Serum tumor markers
  - No specific tumor marker for cholangiocarcinoma
  - Used in conjunction with other diagnostic tests
  - CA19-9
    - ↑ in ≤ 85% of patients
    - ↑ in absolute level (> 100 U/mL) or change over time
    - Obstructive jaundice without malignancy can cause ↑ but should not persist after decompression
    - Nonspecific, can also be elevated in
      - Pancreatic malignancy
      - Gastric malignancy
      - Severe hepatic injury
    - Lewis phenotype must be positive (10% of population is Lewis negative)
  - CEA
    - ↑ in 30% of patients
    - Nonspecific, can be elevated in
      - Inflammatory bowel disease
      - Biliary obstruction
      - Severe hepatic injury
      - Other malignancies
  - CA125
    - ↑ in 40-50% of patients
    - May signify peritoneal involvement
    - Nonspecific, can be elevated in other GI and gynecologic malignancies

Prognosis

- Most important stage-independent prognostic factor: Extent of resection & microscopic margin evaluation
- Factors negatively impacting survival
  - High tumor grade
  - Perineural invasion
  - Vascular invasion
  - Lobar atrophy
  - Lymph node metastasis
- Hepatic parenchymal invasion has better prognosis than vascular invasion
- Papillary tumor has better prognosis

Work-Up

- Clinical
  - Pertinent history (jaundice, pruritus, fat malabsorption, weight loss) and physical examination
- Radiographic
  - Abdomen CT, abdomen MR, ERCP with needle biopsy, metastatic work-up with chest CT or PET/CT
- Laboratory
  - CBC, liver panel, tumor markers (CA19-9, CEA)

TREATMENT

Major Treatment Alternatives

- Resection is only curative treatment option
  - 20% resectable at diagnosis
  - High operative mortality (5-10%)
  - 5-year survival rate: 9-18%
- High local recurrence rates even with curative resection
- Goals of surgery
  - Complete tumor excision
  - Negative histologic margins
  - Relief of biliary obstruction
  - Reestablishment of biliary-enteric communication
- Localized resectable tumor
  - Eligibility for resection depends on
    - Biliary and vascular anatomy
    - Location and extent of tumor
    - Hepatic parenchymal invasion
    - Relationship to vessels

- Extended hepatectomy improves negative margin rate and overall survival
    - Higher morbidity and mortality
- Resection strategy depends on Bismuth-Corlette (BC) classification of longitudinal tumor extent
    - BC types I, II, IIIa → extended right hepatectomy with resection of segment 4
    - BC type IIIb → left hepatectomy including segment 4
- Removal of caudate lobe is controversial
    - High % of resected specimens contain tumor
    - Most common site of hepatic recurrence
- Portal vein resection & reconstruction if gross invasion
- Must assess lymph node metastases at surgery
    - Important predictor of survival postop
- External beam radiation therapy (EBRT) has been used in conjunction with surgery
- Radiation therapy may improve local control

- Unresectable tumor (e.g., BC type IV)
    - Involves majority of patients with bile duct cancer
    - Management directed at palliation
    - Relief of biliary obstruction
        - Surgical biliary-enteric anastomosis
        - Endoscopic stent
        - Percutaneous stent
    - Options under investigation
        - Chemotherapy: Gemcitabine/cisplatin, other gemcitabine-based regimen, or fluoropyrimidine
        - Chemoradiation with fluoropyrimidine
        - Transarterial chemo or radioembolization
        - Radiofrequency ablation (mass-forming lesion)
        - Photodynamic therapy
- Liver transplantation
    - Considered for select cases following regimen of
        - High-dose external beam radiation
        - Chemotherapy
        - Brachytherapy
    - Must exclude stage III or greater disease and regional adenopathy

Major Treatment Roadblocks/ Contraindications

- Findings precluding surgical resection
    - Longitudinal and radial tumor extent
        - Tumor invasion of right and left hepatic ducts to level of secondary biliary radicles
        - Multifocal tumor
        - Lobar atrophy with involvement of contralateral secondary biliary radicles
        - Invasion of secondary biliary radicles with contralateral vascular invasion
    - Vascular invasion
        - Lobar atrophy + contralateral vascular invasion
        - Main portal vein involvement
        - Common or proper hepatic artery encasement
        - Bilateral hepatic artery involvement
    - Remnant liver volume
        - Remaining liver following resection needs to be sufficient to sustain hepatic function
        - Small remnant liver volume is associated with high morbidity due to liver failure
        - Minimum recommended volume of remnant liver is 25% of total preop volume for healthy liver, 40% of total preop volume in chronic disease
    - Lymph node metastasis
    - Distant metastasis
    - Comorbidities
        - Significant liver disease, cirrhosis, cardiovascular, or other systemic disease

Treatment Options by Stage

- Localized extrahepatic cholangiocarcinoma, resected; negative margin and negative nodes
    - Observation or adjuvant chemotherapy (gemcitabine-based regimen or fluoropyrimidine) ± chemoradiation with fluoropyrimidine
- Localized extrahepatic cholangiocarcinoma, resected; positive margin with infiltrative disease (R1) or (R2) or carcinoma in situ at margin or positive nodes
    - Adjuvant chemotherapy gemcitabine-based regimen & chemoradiation with fluoropyrimidine ± high dose rate intracavitary brachytherapy (HDRIB), or chemotherapy alone
- Localized extrahepatic cholangiocarcinoma, unresectable
    - Stenting or surgical procedure to decompress bile duct followed by chemotherapy gemcitabine-based regimen ± chemoradiation with fluoropyrimidine ± HDRIB
- Localized intrahepatic cholangiocarcinoma, resected; negative margin and negative nodes
    - Observe or adjuvant chemotherapy (gemcitabine-based regimen or fluoropyrimidine) ± chemoradiation with fluoropyrimidine
- Localized intrahepatic cholangiocarcinoma, resected; positive margin with infiltrative disease (R1) or (R2) or carcinoma in situ at margin or positive nodes
    - Adjuvant chemotherapy gemcitabine-based regimen & chemoradiation with fluoropyrimidine, or chemotherapy alone
- Localized intrahepatic cholangiocarcinoma, unresectable
    - Chemotherapy gemcitabine-based regimen ± chemoradiation with fluoropyrimidine
- M1 disease (intra- or extrahepatic cholangiocarcinoma)
    - Palliative chemotherapy gemcitabine-based regimen ± radiation therapy to control local symptoms
        - Retrospective data indicates that radiation, either external beam or endocavitary brachytherapy, might prolong stent patency
- Experience from Mayo clinic showed promising results using neoadjuvant chemoradiation therapy and high dose rate (HDR) followed by liver transplantation for selected population of patients with hilar cholangiocarcinoma

Dose Response

- Data are from single institution retrospective studies, but all seem to support dose > 54 Gy using either external beam alone or combination of external beam and HDR intracavitary brachytherapy (IB)
- Unresectable extrahepatic cholangiocarcinoma: Trend toward improved median time to local progression with external beam radiation doses > 54 Gy in 30 fractions

- Unresectable extrahepatic cholangiocarcinoma: Trend toward improved median survival when dose of combined external beam radiation (45 Gy in 25 fx) and HDRIB was 66 Gy vs. 52-59 Gy
  - Trend toward improved median survival when dose of combined external beam radiation (45 Gy in 25 fx) and HDRIB was 66 Gy vs. 52-59 Gy
  - Median survival of 4.5, 9, 18, and 25 months for patients who received < 45, 45-55, 55-65, and 66-70 Gy, respectively, using combination of external beam and endoluminal brachytherapy

Standard Doses

- Adjuvant setting: External beam radiation 45-50.4 Gy in 25-28 fx ± concomitant chemotherapy
  - If residual disease in bile duct, add HDRIB 7 Gy (prescribed to 1 cm) 1-2 weekly fraction
- Inoperable tumors
  - External beam radiation 45 Gy in 25 fractions with HDRIB 7 Gy (prescribed to 1 cm) weekly fraction x 3
  - Or external beam radiation ≤ 57.6 Gy in 32 fx

Organs at Risk Parameters

- Liver mean dose: < 30 Gy
- Kidney mean dose: < 18 Gy
- Bowel maximum dose: < 54 Gy, 45 Gy to < 200 mL
- Stomach and duodenum maximum dose: < 54 Gy, D15 < 45 Gy
- Cord maximum dose: < 45 Gy

Common Techniques

- 3D EBRT, IMRT, and HDRIB

RECOMMENDED FOLLOW-UP

Clinical

- Physical examination every 3 months for 1 year, then every 6 months

Radiographic

- Radiological control with abdominal CT to be done every 6 months post treatment

Laboratory

- Liver panel, tumor markers CA19-9, CEA

SELECTED REFERENCES

1. Moon CM et al: The role of (18)F-fluorodeoxyglucose positron emission tomography in the diagnosis, staging, and follow-up of cholangiocarcinoma. Surg Oncol. 20(1):e10-7, 2011
2. American Joint Committee on Cancer: AJCC Cancer Staging Manual. 7th ed. New York: Springer. 219-25, 2010
3. Momm F et al: Stereotactic fractionated radiotherapy for Klatskin tumours. Radiother Oncol. 95(1):99-102, 2010
4. Anderson C et al: Adjuvant therapy for resected extrahepatic cholangiocarcinoma: a review of the literature and future directions. Cancer Treat Rev. 35(4):322-7, 2009
5. Blechacz BR et al: Cholangiocarcinoma. Clin Liver Dis. 12(1):131-50, ix, 2008
6. Kim JY et al: Clinical role of 18F-FDG PET-CT in suspected and potentially operable cholangiocarcinoma: a prospective study compared with conventional imaging. Am J Gastroenterol. 103(5):1145-51, 2008
7. Li J et al: Preoperative assessment of hilar cholangiocarcinoma by dual-modality PET/CT. J Surg Oncol. 98(6):438-43, 2008
8. Park HS et al: Preoperative evaluation of bile duct cancer: MRI combined with MR cholangiopancreatography versus MDCT with direct cholangiography. AJR Am J Roentgenol. 190(2):396-405, 2008
9. Sainani NI et al: Cholangiocarcinoma: current and novel imaging techniques. Radiographics. 28(5):1263-87, 2008
10. Walker SL et al: Diagnosing cholangiocarcinoma in primary sclerosing cholangitis: an "evidence based radiology" review. Abdom Imaging. 33(1):14-7, 2008
11. Lee HY et al: Preoperative assessment of resectability of hepatic hilar cholangiocarcinoma: combined CT and cholangiography with revised criteria. Radiology. 239(1):113-21, 2006
12. Lim JH et al: Early bile duct carcinoma: comparison of imaging features with pathologic findings. Radiology. 238(2):542-8, 2006
13. Parikh AA et al: Operative considerations in resection of hilar cholangiocarcinoma. HPB (Oxford). 7(4):254-8, 2005
14. Rea DJ et al: Liver transplantation with neoadjuvant chemoradiation is more effective than resection for hilar cholangiocarcinoma. Ann Surg. 242(3):451-8; discussion 458-61, 2005
15. Gores GJ: Cholangiocarcinoma: current concepts and insights. Hepatology. 37(5):961-9, 2003
16. Crane CH et al: Limitations of conventional doses of chemoradiation for unresectable biliary cancer. Int J Radiat Oncol Biol Phys. 53(4):969-74, 2002
17. Han JK et al: Cholangiocarcinoma: pictorial essay of CT and cholangiographic findings. Radiographics. 22(1):173-87, 2002
18. Khan SA et al: Guidelines for the diagnosis and treatment of cholangiocarcinoma: consensus document. Gut. 51 Suppl 6:VI1-9, 2002
19. Lu JJ et al: High-dose-rate remote afterloading intracavitary brachytherapy for the treatment of extrahepatic biliary duct carcinoma. Cancer J. 8(1):74-8, 2002
20. Gores GJ: Early detection and treatment of cholangiocarcinoma. Liver Transpl. 6(6 Suppl 2):S30-4, 2000
21. Jarnagin WR: Cholangiocarcinoma of the extrahepatic bile ducts. Semin Surg Oncol. 19(2):156-76, 2000
22. Eschelman DJ et al: Malignant biliary duct obstruction: long-term experience with Gianturco stents and combined-modality radiation therapy. Radiology. 200(3):717-24, 1996
23. Alden ME et al: The impact of radiation dose in combined external beam and intraluminal Ir-192 brachytherapy for bile duct cancer. Int J Radiat Oncol Biol Phys. 28(4):945-51, 1994

T2a N1 M0

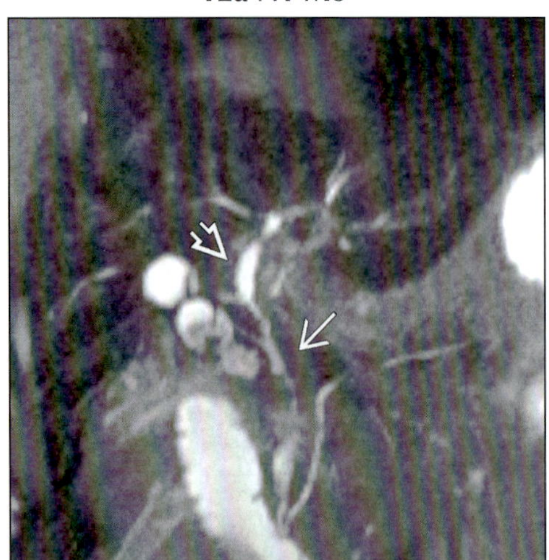

T2a N1 M0

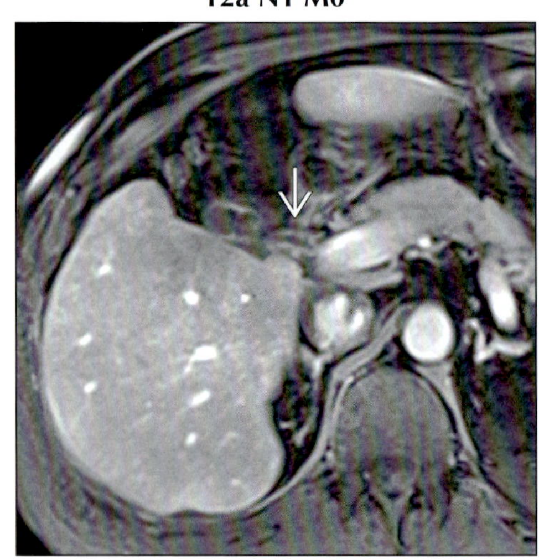

(Left) *A 67-year-old woman presented with history of jaundice and right upper quadrant pain. Coronal MRCP shows irregularity of the common hepatic and common bile duct ➔ with long segment narrowing. Note the mild upstream biliary ductal dilation ➲.* ***(Right)*** *Axial T1WI C+ FS MR in the same patient shows common hepatic duct ➔ wall thickening with mild enhancement in the arterial phase.*

T2a N1 M0

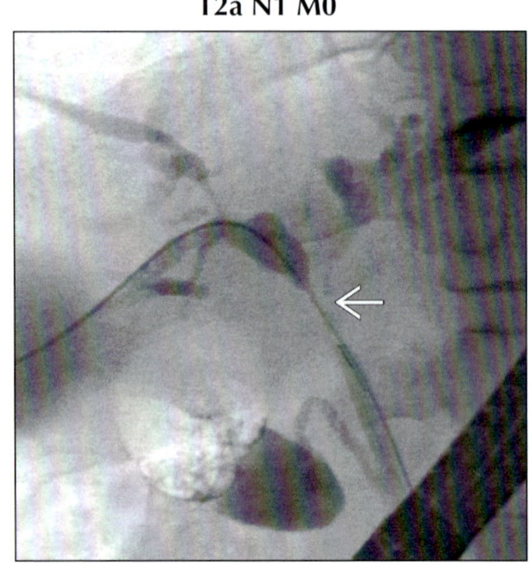

T2a N1 M0

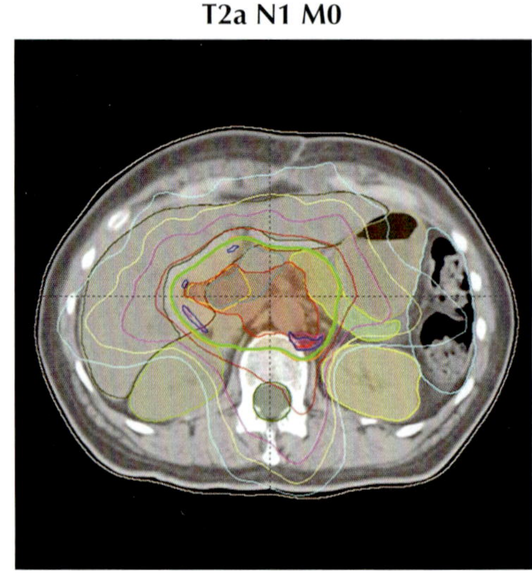

(Left) *ERCP in the same patient shows obstruction at the confluence ➔ of the hepatic ducts with upstream biliary duct dilation.* ***(Right)*** *Patient underwent surgery and was found to have pT2 N1 (2/12) M0 adenocarcinoma. Regional lymph nodes (periductal) were found to be involved. PTV for adjuvant external beam radiation includes initial tumor bed, the anastomosis, and the positive nodal area with a margin for organ motion (assessed by 4D CT) and setup uncertainty.*

T2a N1 M0

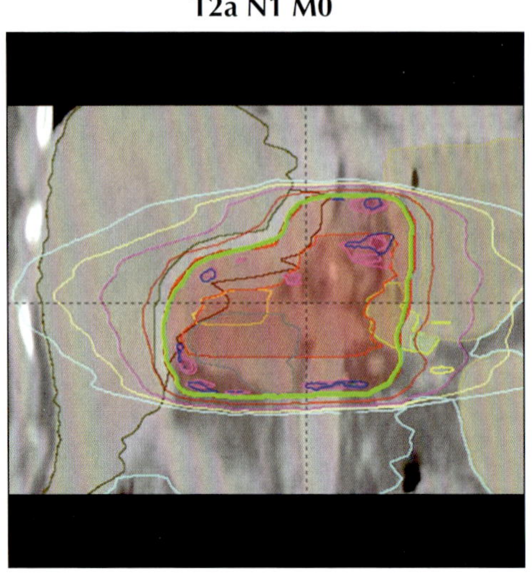

T2a N1 M0

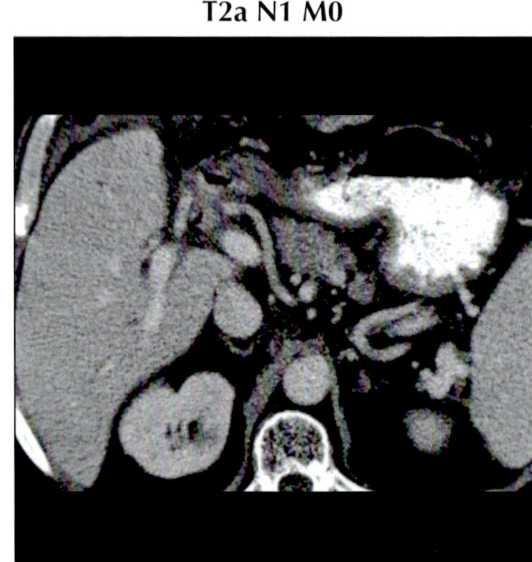

(Left) *IMRT plan of adjuvant external beam radiation of an extrahepatic cholangiocarcinoma delivers a dose of 50.4 Gy in 28 fractions to the PTV with concomitant 5-FU. IMRT permits very conformal plans.* ***(Right)*** *Follow-up axial CECT scan 12 months post treatment shows absence of local recurrence of metastatic disease.*

pT3 N1 M0

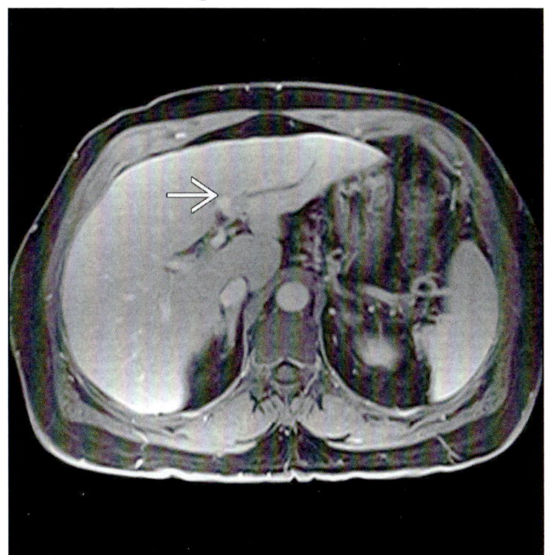

pT3 N1 M0

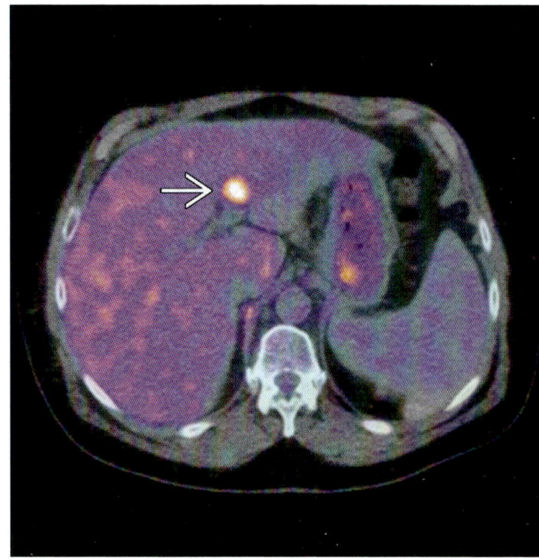

(Left) *Incidentally, biliary duct dilatation in a 65-year-old man was found. A small mass adjacent to the medial aspect of the left portal vein ➔ was seen. Greater contrast retention of segment 3 is due to associated transient high intensity difference caused by compression of the left portal vein.* **(Right)** *On PET/CT, there was abnormal FDG accumulation in the left lobe of the liver ➔, segment 3 with an SUV value of 6.23, corresponding to the small mass seen on MR.*

pT3 N1 M0

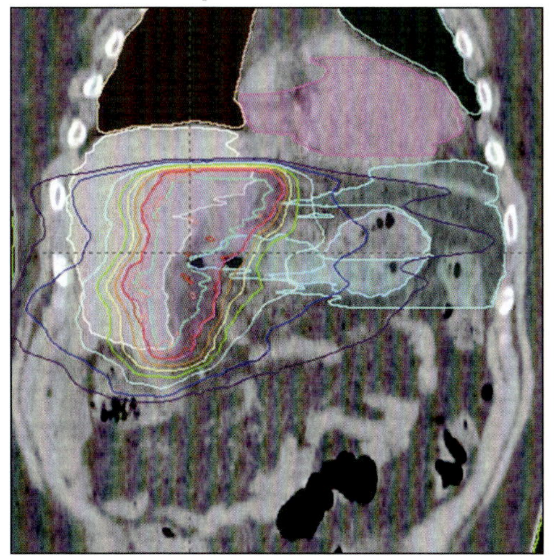

pT3 N1 M0

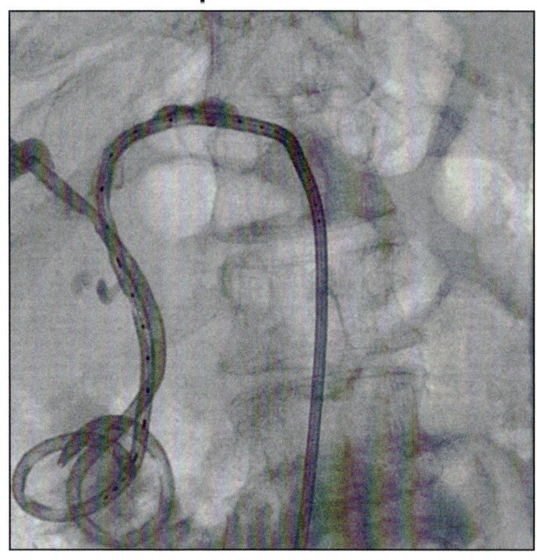

(Left) *Patient underwent surgery, and pathology showed a pT3 N1 M0, R1 (positive bile duct margin) adenocarcinoma. Adjuvant chemoradiation was delivered. External beam was delivered using IMRT to a dose of 45 Gy in 25 fractions. Planning was done with a 4D planning CT to assess tumor motion.* **(Right)** *High dose rate brachytherapy (HDRBT) was used to deliver a boost to the positive ductal margin. A dose of 21 Gy in 3 fractions was delivered to 1 cm from center.*

pT3 N1 M0

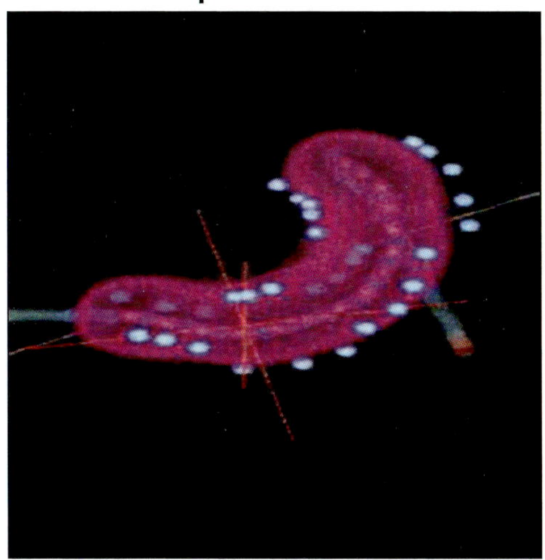

pT3 N1 M0

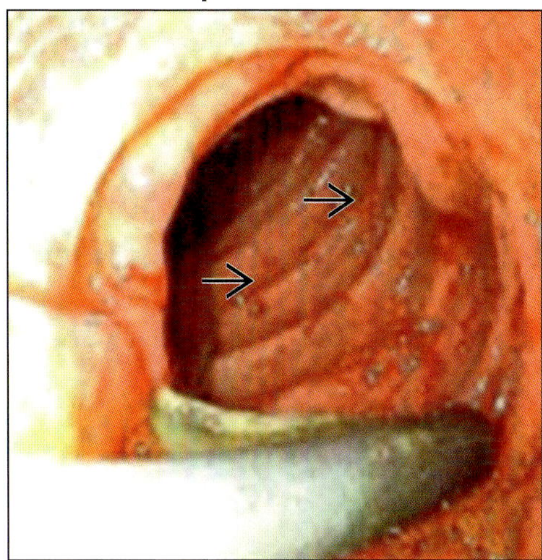

(Left) *Diagram shows the dose distribution from HDRIB treatment for a patient with cholangiocarcinoma receiving adjuvant treatment for a pT3 N1 M0, R1 cancer. Most series show an increase in local control with a higher dose of RT.* **(Right)** *One of the long-term treatment side effects is duodenitis →, seen here, which can be associated with gastrointestinal bleeding.*

T4 N2 M0

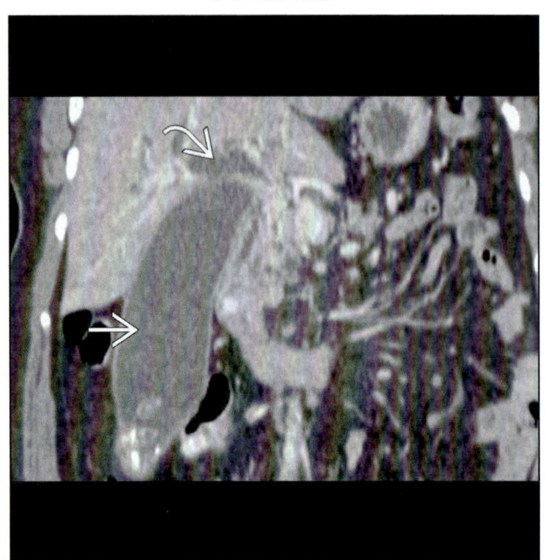

T4 N2 M0

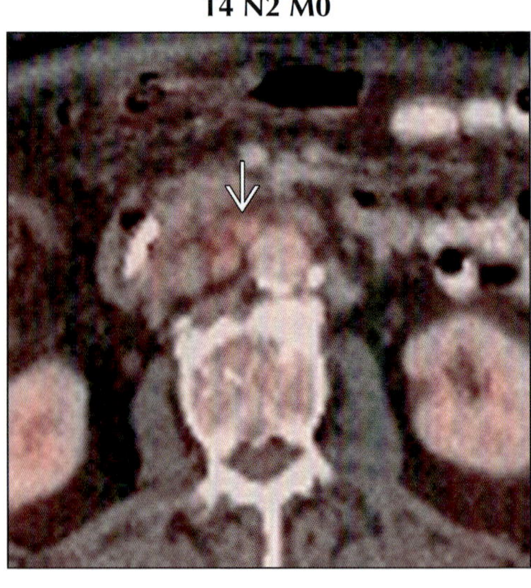

(Left) *A 64-year-old woman presented with a history of weight loss, pruritus, jaundice, and right upper quadrant pain. A CT of the abdomen showed a dilated gall bladder ➔ and intrahepatic bile duct ➔.* ***(Right)*** *Axial fused PET/CT in the same patient shows hypermetabolic interaortocaval adenopathy ➔. Although small in size, these lymph nodes demonstrate increased FDG accumulation, consistent with N2 lymph node metastases.*

T4 N2 M0

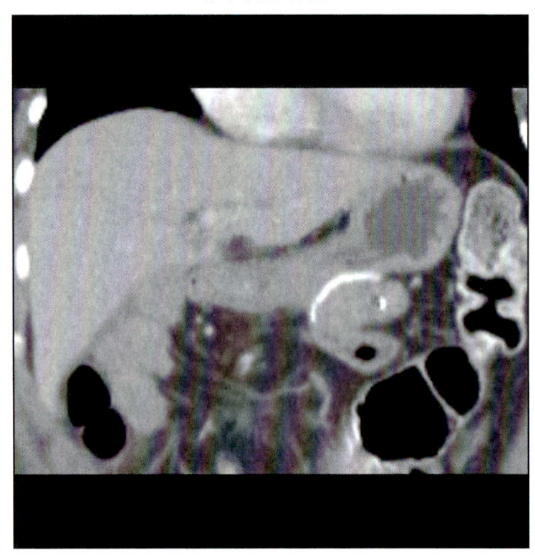

T4 N2 M0, Unresectable

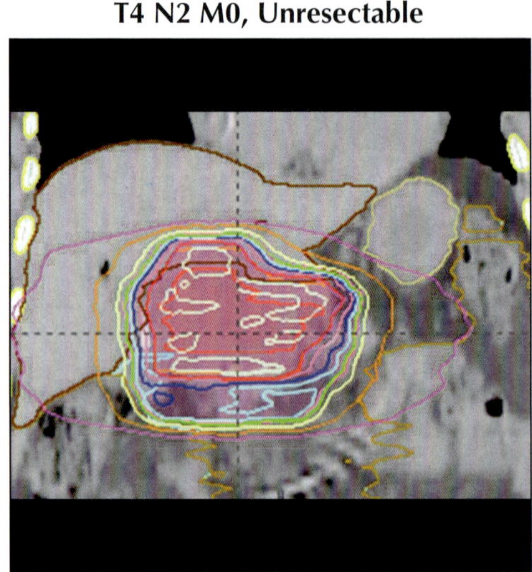

(Left) *The tumor was deemed unresectable. Same patient underwent a cholecystectomy and a gastrojejunal diversion. Her case was reviewed at the multidisciplinary tumor board, and she was offered a course of chemotherapy followed by combined chemoradiation therapy.* ***(Right)*** *IMRT treatment for an unresectable extrahepatic cholangiocarcinoma is shown. In this setting, when possible, the dose to the PTV primary should be higher than 55 Gy.*

T4 N2 M0, Unresectable

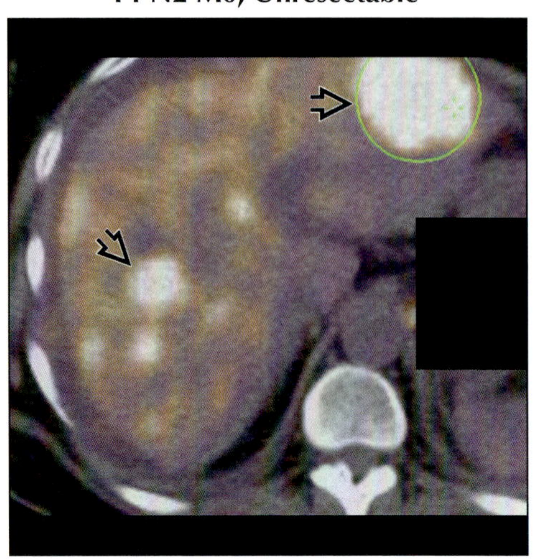

T4 N2 M0, Unresectable

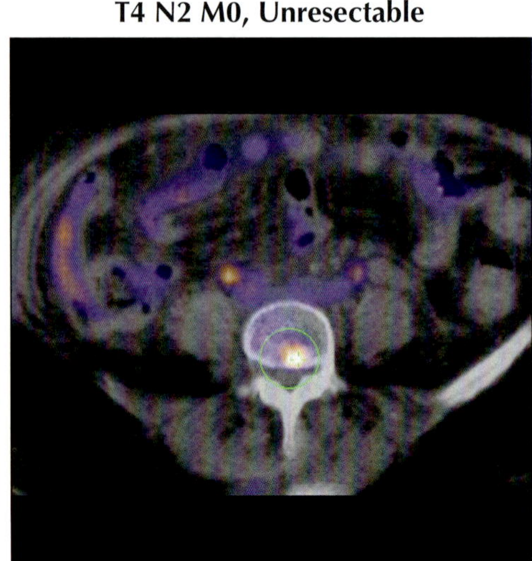

(Left) *On follow-up PET/CT imaging, 8 months after diagnosis, patient was found to have multiple liver metastases ➲.* ***(Right)*** *On further follow-up, 12 months after diagnosis, patient was found on PET/CT to have a bone metastasis at L4. She received a short course of palliative radiation with good pain control.*

Bismuth-Corlette Type I

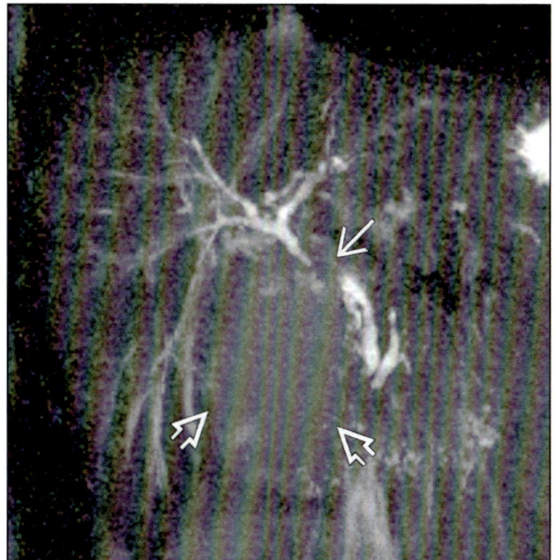

Bismuth-Corlette Type II

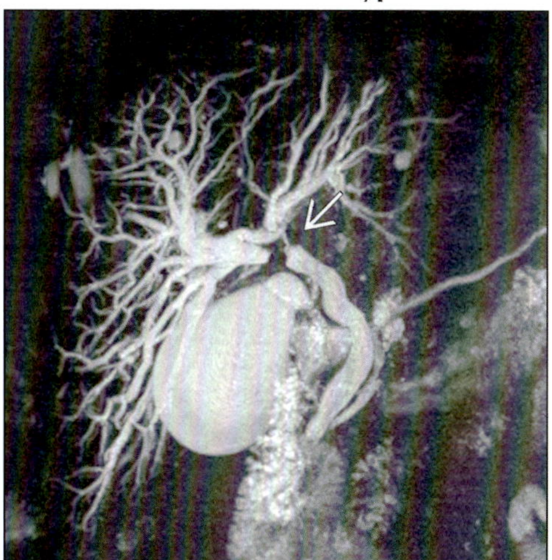

(Left) *Coronal MRCP shows occlusion of the common hepatic duct ➔ due to infiltrative tumor with upstream biliary dilation. The gallbladder ➔ is distended due to occlusion of the cystic duct.* ***(Right)*** *Coronal MRCP shows complete occlusion at the confluence ➔ of the right and left hepatic ducts with resulting intrahepatic biliary ductal dilation.*

Bismuth-Corlette Type IIIa

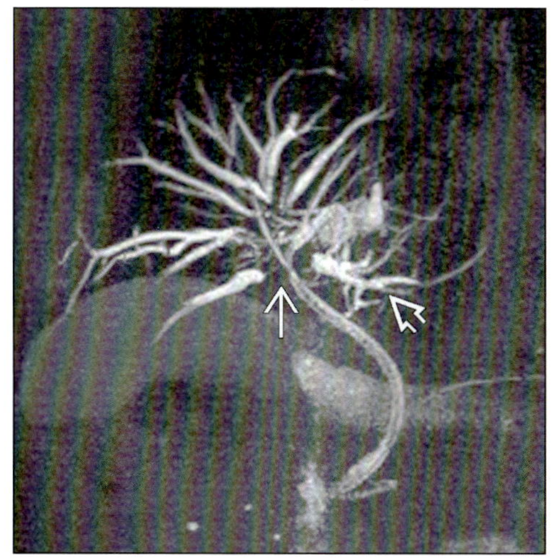

Bismuth-Corlette Type IV

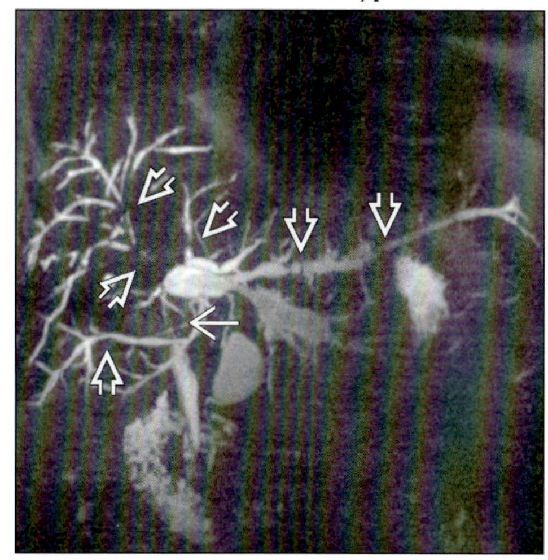

(Left) *Coronal MRCP shows tumor at the confluence ➔ of the right and left ➔ hepatic ducts, resulting in diffuse biliary dilation despite bilateral biliary stents. The branches of the right hepatic duct abruptly terminate upstream to the confluence, indicating intrahepatic extension of tumor on the right.* ***(Right)*** *Coronal MRCP shows multifocal strictures ➔ and occlusion involving the right and left intrahepatic bile ducts as well as the common hepatic duct ➔.*

Recurrence

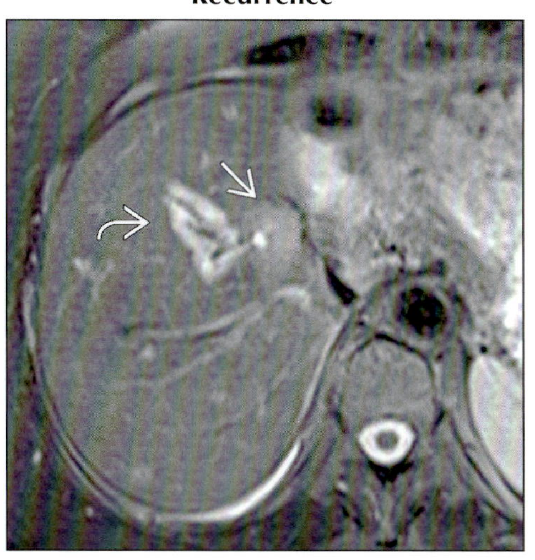

Stage IVB (T4 N0 M1)

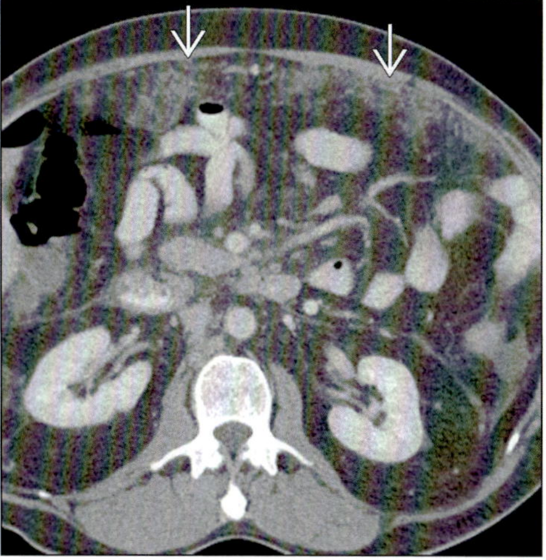

(Left) *Axial T2WI FS MR obtained at the level of biliary obstruction shows a hyperintense perihilar mass ➔ and intrahepatic biliary ductal dilation ➔, consistent with recurrence.* ***(Right)*** *Axial CECT shows soft tissue infiltration ➔ of the greater omentum, consistent with peritoneal metastatic disease.*

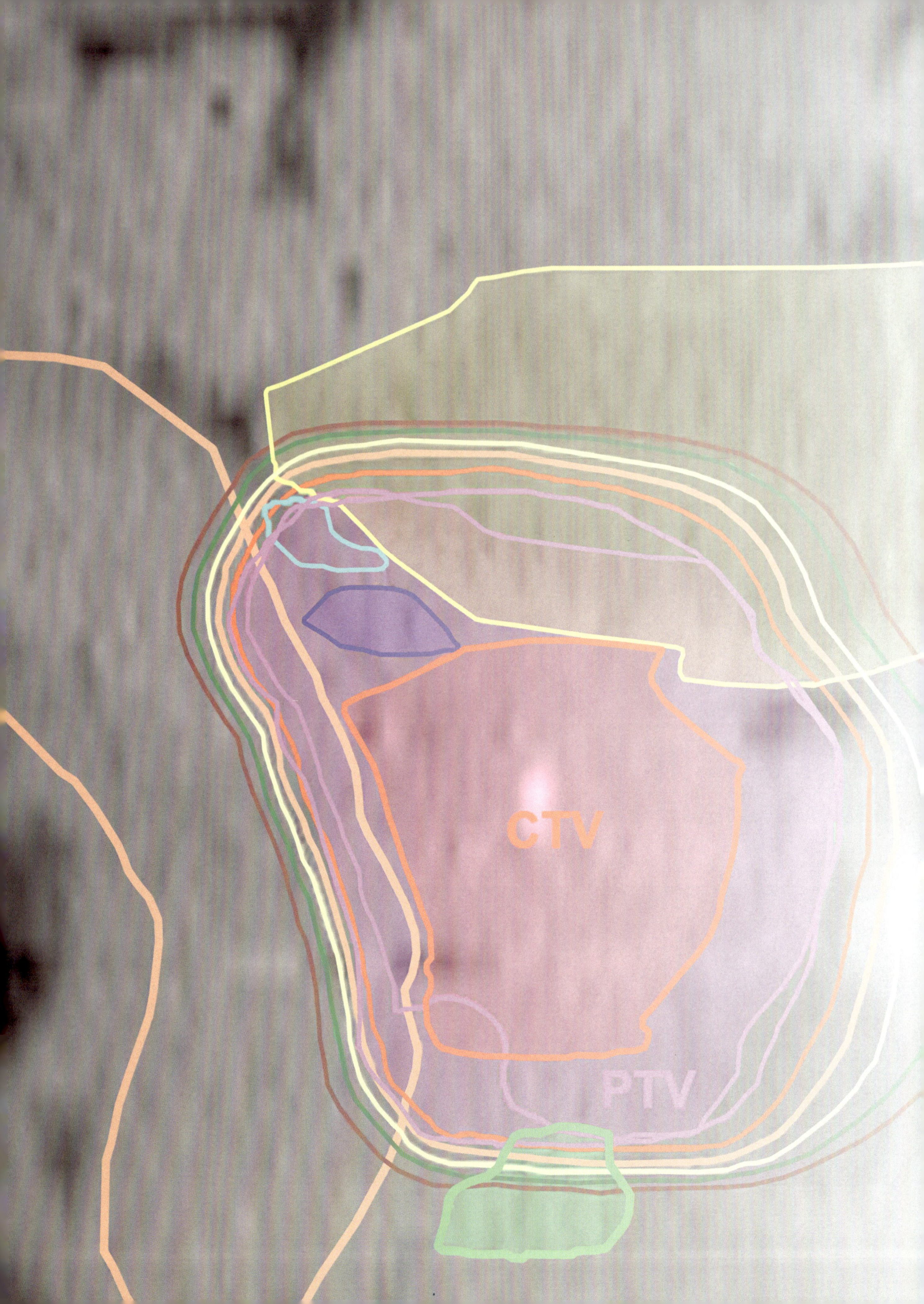
CTV
PTV

SECTION 6
Genitourinary System

KIDNEY

(T) Primary Tumor

Adapted from 7th edition AJCC Staging Forms.

TNM	*Definitions*
TX	Primary tumor cannot be assessed
T0	No evidence of primary tumor
T1	Tumor ≤ 7 cm in greatest dimension, limited to the kidney
T1a	Tumor ≤ 4 cm in greatest dimension, limited to the kidney
T1b	Tumor > 4 cm but ≤ 7 cm in greatest dimension, limited to the kidney
T2	Tumor > 7 cm in greatest dimension, limited to the kidney
T2a	Tumor > 7 cm but ≤ 10 cm in greatest dimension, limited to the kidney
T2b	Tumor > 10 cm, limited to the kidney
T3	Tumor extends into major veins or perinephric tissues but not into the ipsilateral adrenal gland and not beyond Gerota fascia
T3a	Tumor grossly extends into the renal vein or its segmental (muscle containing) branches, or tumor invades perirenal &/or renal sinus fat but not beyond Gerota fascia
T3b	Tumor grossly extends into the vena cava below the diaphragm
T3c	Tumor grossly extends into the vena cava above the diaphragm or invades the wall of the vena cava
T4	Tumor invades beyond Gerota fascia (including contiguous extension into the ipsilateral adrenal gland)

(N) Regional Lymph Nodes

NX	Regional lymph nodes cannot be assessed
N0	No regional lymph node metastasis
N1	Metastasis in regional lymph node(s)

(M) Distant Metastasis

M0	No distant metastasis
M1	Distant metastasis

AJCC Stages/Prognostic Groups

Adapted from 7th edition AJCC Staging Forms.

Stage	*T*	*N*	*M*
I	T1	N0	M0
II	T2	N0	M0
III	T1 or T2	N1	M0
	T3	N0 or N1	M0
IV	T4	Any N	M0
	Any T	Any N	M1

Wilms Tumor Staging

Stage	*Definitions*
I	Tumor limited to kidney, completely resected; no rupture or prior biopsy; vessel of sinus uninvolved and margin negative
II	Tumor extends beyond kidney, but completely excised; negative margins
III	Node positive, peritoneal implants, unresectable, biopsy, rupture or removed > 1 piece
IV	Hematogenous metastases (nonadrenal), lymph node (+) outside abdomen or pelvis
V	Bilateral Wilms at diagnosis; each kidney staged separately for treatment decision

Normal Kidney Medulla

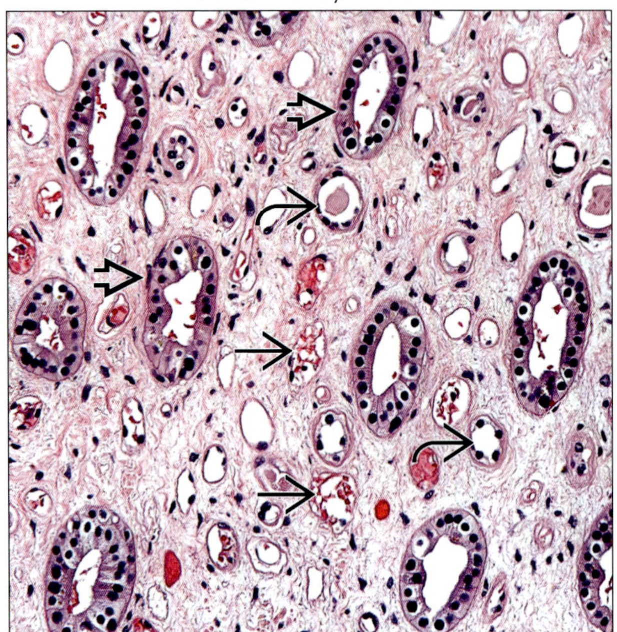

H&E stain demonstrating a cross section of the inner medulla shows prominent collecting ducts ➭ and thin loops of Henle ➦ embedded in abundant interstitial stroma. The peritubular capillaries → in the medulla form a network of vasa recta. (Courtesy N. Kambham, MD.)

Clear Cell Renal Carcinoma

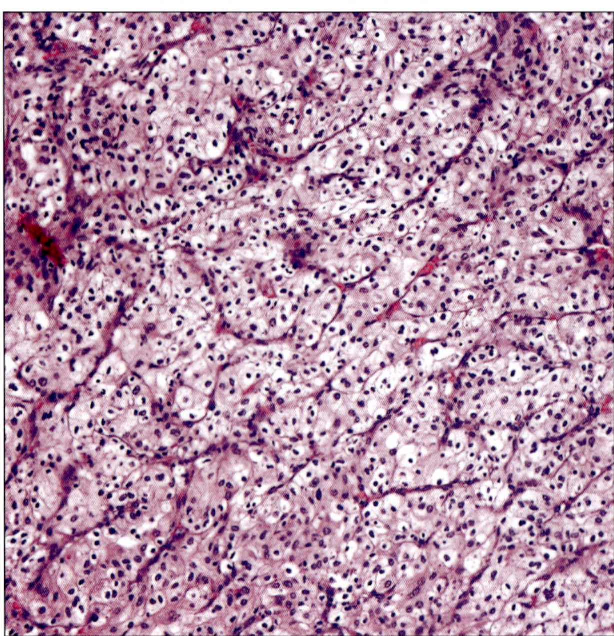

H&E stain of a nephrectomy specimen demonstrates clear cell renal carcinoma. (Courtesy A. Matynia, MD.)

Normal Kidney and Wilms Tumor

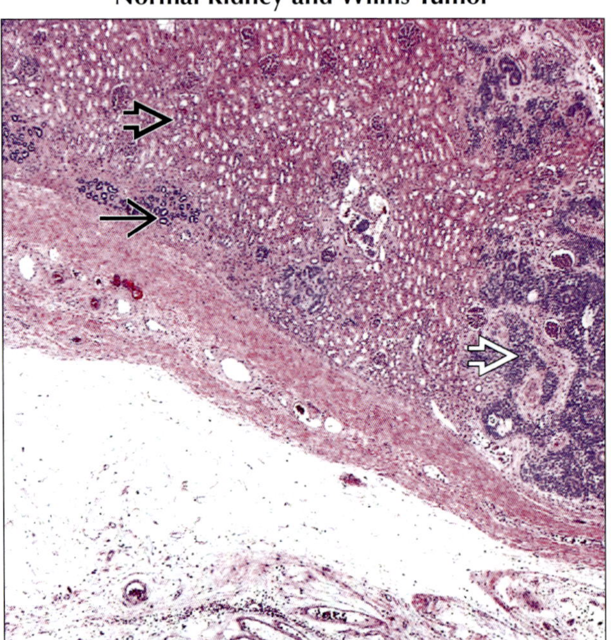

H&E stain demonstrates the contrast of normal kidney ➭, nephrogenic rests →, and Wilms tumor ➡. (Courtesy A. Putnam, MD.)

Favorable Histology Wilms Tumor

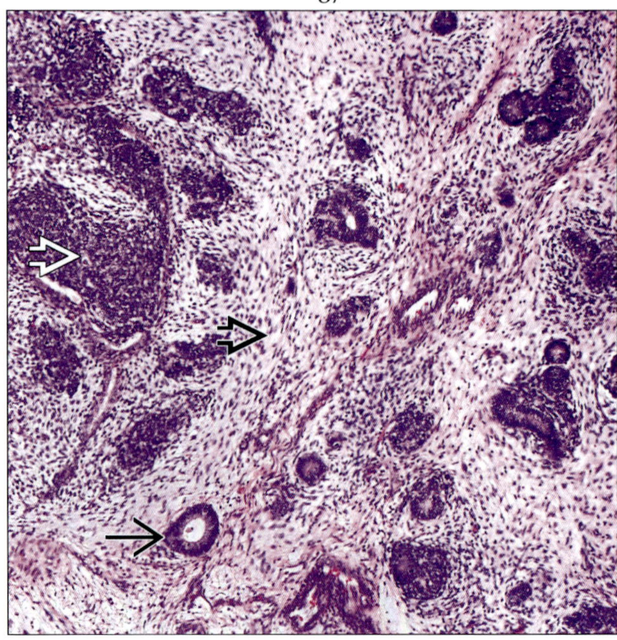

H&E stain demonstrates the classic triphasic nephroblastoma of Wilms tumor with blastemal ➭, stromal ➡, and epithelial components →. (Courtesy A. Putnam, MD.)

T1a

Coronal graphic shows a typical T1a lesion ➔, defined as ≤ 4 cm and confined to the kidney.

T1b

Coronal graphic shows a typical T1b lesion ➔, defined as > 4 cm but ≤ 7 cm and confined to the kidney.

T2a

Coronal graphic shows a T2a renal cell carcinoma ➔, defined as > 7 cm but ≤ 10 cm and confined to the kidney. These lesions may also be described as exophytic but do not invade outside of the kidney.

T2b

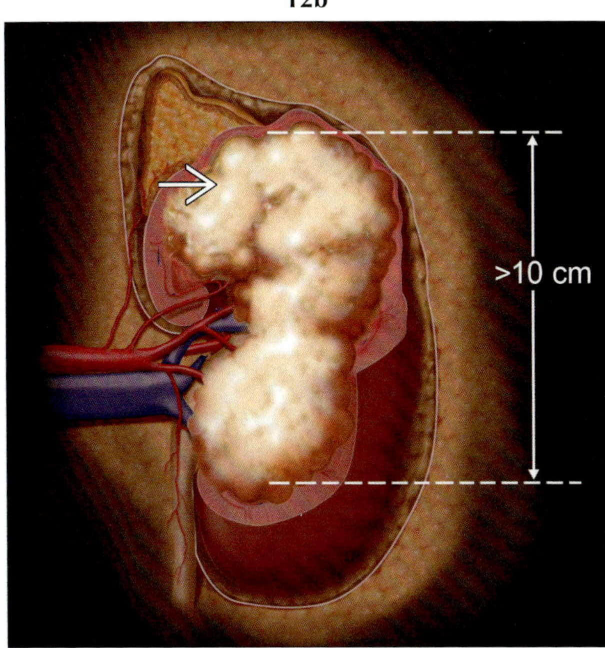

Coronal graphic shows a typical T2b renal cell carcinoma ➔, defined as > 10 cm but confined to the kidney.

T3a

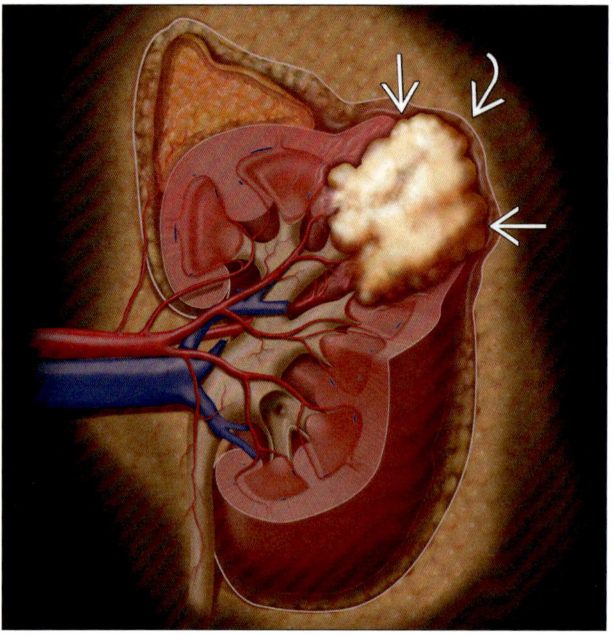

Coronal graphic shows a T3a renal cell carcinoma with tumor extension ➡ into the perirenal fat but not beyond the confines of Gerota fascia ↪.

T3a

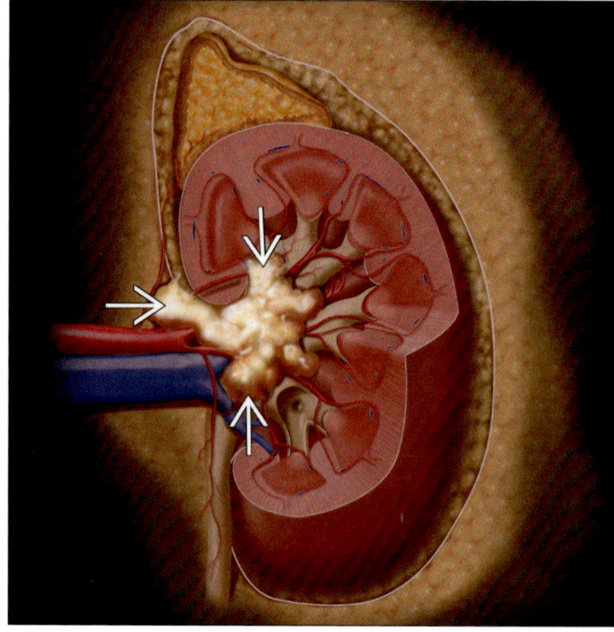

Coronal graphic shows another example of a T3a lesion with extension into the perirenal or renal sinus fat ➡. Again, the tumor is limited by the confines of Gerota fascia.

T3b

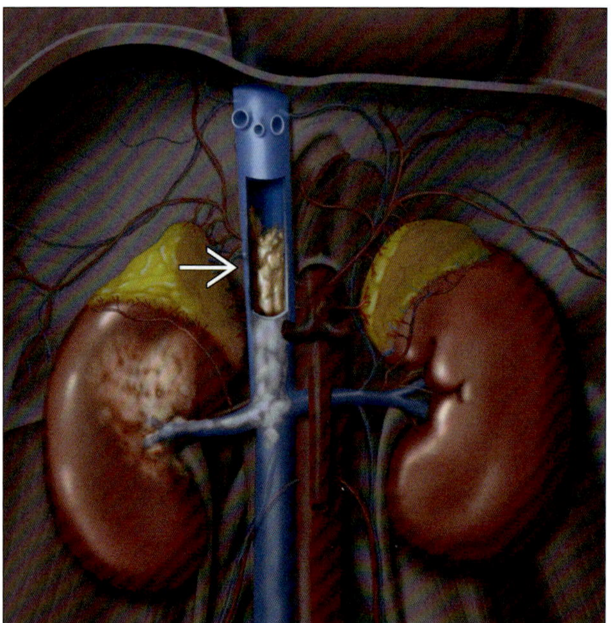

Coronal graphic shows a T3b renal cell carcinoma with extension of tumor not only into the renal vein but also into the inferior vena cava ➡. T3b lesions do not extend above the diaphragm.

T3c

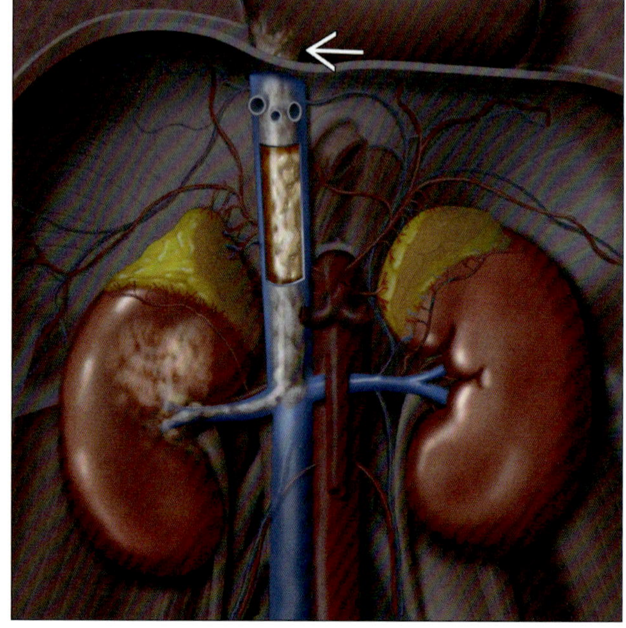

Coronal graphic shows a T3c renal cell carcinoma with involvement of tumor in the renal vein and inferior vena cava, as well as extension of tumor within the inferior vena cava above the diaphragm ➡.

T4

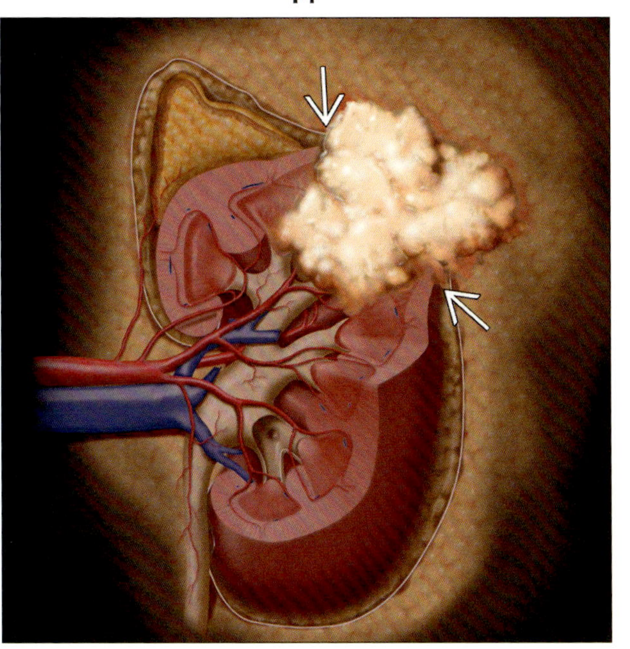

Coronal graphic shows another example of a T4 lesion with invasion into not only the perirenal fat but also with extension beyond the Gerota fascia ➔.

N1 Disease (Stage III or IV)

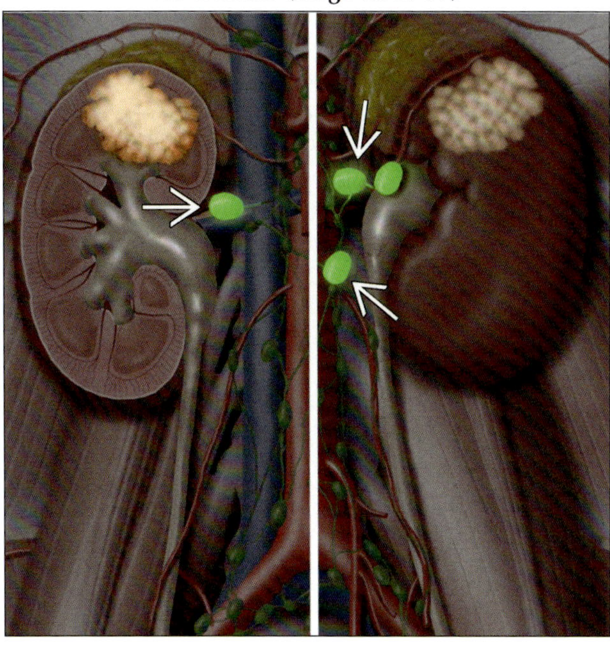

Coronal graphic shows retroperitoneal adenopathy on both sides of midline ➔. N0 disease is classified as no regional lymph node metastasis whereas N1 disease is classified as metastatic disease in regional lymph nodes.

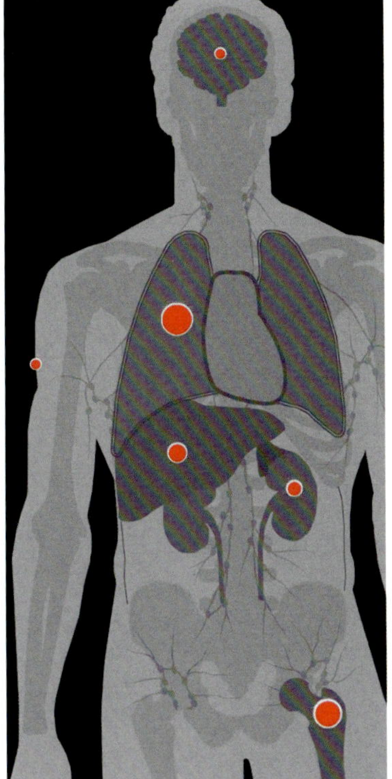

INITIAL SITE OF RECURRENCE

Site	%
Lung	38%
Bone	25%
Liver	11%
Others	9%
Local	7%
Brain	4%
Skin	3%

25-40% of patients present with metastatic disease. After initial nephrectomy from 187 patients reviewed prospectively from 1982-1997, 56 patients developed recurrence in 98 sites. Risk of recurrence increased with initial stage. Median time to recurrence is 14.5 months with 80% occurring within 3 years. Ljungberg B et al: Follow-up guidelines for nonmetastatic renal cell carcinoma based on the occurrence of metastases after radical nephrectomy. BJU Int. 84(4):405-11, 1999.

OVERVIEW

General Comments

- Represents 2-3% of all adult cancers
- Only 2-4% occur in inherited syndromes
- Bilateral involvement
  - 2% synchronous and 6-8% asynchronous
- 85% renal cell carcinoma (RCC)
  - Others: Transitional cell carcinoma (TCC) and Wilms tumor

Classification

- **4 major histopathologic subtypes of renal cell carcinoma**
  - Clear cell carcinoma
  - Papillary carcinoma
  - Collecting duct carcinoma
  - Chromophobe renal carcinoma

NATURAL HISTORY

General Features

- Comments
  - Renal cell carcinoma arises from renal tubular epithelium
- Location
  - At time of diagnosis, 45% localized, 25% regional, and 30% metastatic (50% eventually metastatic)

Etiology

- Genetic and environmental causes
  - Genetic
    - Tuberous sclerosis
    - von Hippel-Lindau
    - Birt-Hogg-Dubé syndrome
    - Hereditary papillary RCC
  - Environmental
    - Cigarette smoking: Dose dependent
    - Obesity
    - Hypertension
    - Acquired cystic disease from chronic dialysis
    - Environmental exposure
      - Phenacetin
      - Benzene
      - Cadmium
      - Asbestos
      - Thorium dioxide
      - Petroleum products
    - Occupational
      - Leather tanners
      - Shoe workers
      - Asbestos workers

Epidemiology & Cancer Incidence

- Number of cases in USA per year
  - 64,700 cases with 13,570 deaths (per NCI)
  - Wilms tumor: 450-540 new cases
    - 90% unifocal, 12% multifocal, 7% bilateral
- Sex predilection
  - M:F = 3:2
  - Wilms tumor: F > M
- Age of onset
  - Highest incidence in 6th-8th decade
  - Average age at diagnosis is 55-60 years
  - Wilms tumor: Majority present < age 5
- Black > white

Genetics

- **Hereditary papillary RCC**
  - Multiple
  - Bilateral
  - Papillary renal tumors
  - Autosomal dominant
  - *C-met* oncogene on chromosome 7
- **Hereditary leiomyoma and renal cell cancer syndrome**
  - Cutaneous leiomyomas
  - Uterine fibroids
  - Renal cell cancer
  - Suspected mutation of fumarate hydratase gene
- **von Hippel-Lindau**
  - Retinal angioma
  - Hemangioblastomas
  - Pheochromocytomas and others
  - Mutation of *VHL* gene on chromosome 3p25
  - Clear cell renal cancer develops in approximately 40% of patients with von Hippel-Lindau
  - Major cause of mortality
- **Birt-Hogg-Dubé syndrome**
  - Fibrofolliculomas on head and neck
  - Chromophobic RCC or oncocytoma
  - Mutation of *BDH* gene on chromosome 17p
- **Wilms tumor**
  - 10% congenital anomalies
    - WAGR
      - Wilms, aniridia, GU malformations, retardation
      - Deletion of 11p13 and *WT1* gene
    - Beckwith-Wiedemann
      - Hemihypertrophy, GU abnormalities, macroglossia, gigantism
      - *WT2* 11p15 abnormality
    - Denys-Drash
      - Renal mesangial sclerosis, renal failure, pseudohermaphroditism
      - *WT1* gene mutation
    - LOH 1p &/or 16q have worse outcomes per NWTS-5

Associated Diseases, Abnormalities

- Multiple paraneoplastic disorders associated with RCC usually caused by tumor release of various cytokines
  - Hypercalcemia
  - Erythrocytosis
  - Polyneuropathy
  - Amyloidosis
  - Hypertension
  - Dermatomyositis
- Syndromes may resolve after successful treatment of tumor

Gross Pathology & Surgical Features

- Varies from solid to cystic mass
- Yellow areas are due to lipid-rich tumor cells
- May have gray or black areas of necrosis or hemorrhage

Microscopic Pathology

- H&E
  - **Clear cell carcinoma**
    - Have clear or granular cytoplasm in round cells

- Tumors may have solid, trabecular, or tubular pattern
  - **Papillary carcinoma**
    - Tumor cells are cuboidal or low columnar
    - Tumor pattern is papillary
  - **Chromophobe RCC**
    - Tumor cell morphology varies, but cells are lightly eosinophilic stained
    - Tumor pattern is solid sheets
- Wilms tumor histology
  - Small round blue cell tumor
    - 90% favorable
      - No anaplasia or sarcoma components
    - 10% unfavorable
      - Anaplastic (focal or diffuse), rhabdoid, or clear cell

Routes of Spread

- Hematogenous, lymphatic, &/or direct invasion
- 25% may be multifocal in the same kidney
- Found incidentally at autopsy, in some series in up to 25% of cases
- 25-40% RCC present with metastatic disease
  - Lung (75%)
  - Soft tissue (35%)
  - Bone (20%)
  - Liver (20%)
  - Cutaneous tissues (8%)
  - CNS (8%)

IMAGING

Detection

- **General T staging imaging characteristics**
- Accuracy ~ 80% with noted difficulty in imaging some retroperitoneal and perinephric areas
  - **T1**: Tumor ≤ 7 cm in greatest dimension, limited to kidney
    - No evidence of perinephric fat or renal fascial involvement
    - Exophytic tumors may not be reliably classified into T1a, T1b, or T2
    - Solid enhancing lesion
  - **T2**: Tumor > 7 cm in greatest dimension, limited to kidney
    - Imaging may be useful for distinguishing between T2a and T2b lesions
  - **T3**: Tumor extends into major veins or perinephric tissues but not into ipsilateral adrenal gland and not beyond Gerota fascia
    - Ultrasound and MR very useful to demonstrate venous thrombus and to evaluate possible tumor thrombus
      - In general, thrombi that contain enhancing vessels are tumor
    - Can be used to identify thrombi in renal veins or inferior vena cava (IVC) with accuracy of 87%
  - **T4**: Tumor invades beyond Gerota fascia or invades IVC above diaphragm
    - Chest CT is recommended for large or aggressive primary tumors
    - Brain MR and bone scans are often performed in patients with suggestive signs or symptoms
    - PET/CT may be useful for identifying possible distant metastases in patients with large primary lesions
      - Debated whether to use for primary detection of metastases or only to verify equivocal CT findings
- **Ultrasound**
  - Primary method for differentiating a cyst from a solid lesion
  - Primary tumor may be variably echogenic relative to background renal cortex
    - Isoechoic
      - May be missed on ultrasound, as tumor may be indistinguishable from background renal parenchyma
      - Look for border contour deformity
    - Hypoechoic
      - Differentiated from a cyst by lack of through transmission
    - Hyperechoic
      - Tend to be smaller
      - May look similar to angiomyolipomas
  - Large lesions often heterogeneous in echotexture
- **CT**
  - NECT and parenchymal phase CECT are necessary for all patients unless contraindicated
  - **NECT**
    - Variable appearance
      - Small lesions may be homogeneous in attenuation
      - Larger lesions often show central necrosis
      - May have calcifications
      - Almost never contain macroscopic fat
      - May also be primarily cystic
    - Low attenuation
      - Papillary RCCs
    - Moderate attenuation
      - May be chromophobe RCC or angiomyolipoma (soft tissue component of mass, lipomatous areas will be low density)
    - High attenuation
      - Clear cell RCC lesions often have mixed pattern
      - High-attenuation regions represent soft tissue areas while low-attenuation regions are necrotic or cystic
      - Oncocytomas may have a similar appearance on CT
    - Pseudocapsule may be seen as high-density ring surrounding tumor
  - **CECT**
    - Renal mass protocol includes
      - Thin slice 1.25-2.5 mm
      - Noncontrast and contrast-enhanced acquisitions
      - Arterial phase with 20-second delay helpful for evaluating arterial vessels
      - Nephrographic phase with 60-70-second delay best for evaluating parenchyma
      - Delayed phase with 5-10-minute delay best for evaluating collecting system
      - Coronal reformatted images also helpful for better defining relationship of tumor to other structures
    - Enhancement pattern during nephrographic phase is most useful for determining type of tumor

    - Gold standard for detection and staging is CT
    - RCCs have variable enhancement patterns
      - Some will enhance briskly
      - Papillary RCCs may have very little enhancement (can be mistaken for a hyperdense cyst with pseudoenhancement)
      - Solid enhancing mass in the kidney is RCC until proven otherwise
- **MR**
  - In general, similar findings to CT
  - Variable signal characteristics and enhancement pattern
  - Typically iso- to hypointense compared to normal renal cortex on T1-weighted images
  - Typically hyperintense on T2-weighted images
  - Cystic RCCs will generally have enhancing septa or mural nodularity
- **PET/CT**
  - RCCs have variable FDG avidity
    - More helpful when intensely FDG avid
    - Solid mass without FDG activity can still be RCC
    - Not generally used to differentiate benign from malignant renal masses
- **Image-guided biopsies**
  - Not routinely done
  - Can be performed for problem solving
    - e.g., for differentiating metastasis from primary renal malignancy in a patient with a primary malignancy other than renal

Staging

- **Nodal**
  - **Ultrasound**
    - Not used for nodal or metastatic evaluation
    - Can be used for problem solving with lesions seen in other organs, e.g., liver
    - Can be used to evaluate renal vessels and IVC for patency
      - CT with contrast likely better to look for vascular invasion
  - **CT**
    - Gold standard for detection of nodes and for evaluation of vascular structures
    - Nodes may hyperenhance
    - Smaller nodes may appear normal
    - Larger nodal metastases may be heterogeneous or have central necrosis
    - Best modality for looking at invasion of perinephric fat and other local structures
  - **MR**
    - Typically reserved for patients with renal insufficiency or contraindications for CT contrast
    - Particularly useful for determining invasion and extent of involvement into IVC
  - **PET/CT**
    - For RCC metastases using FDG PET
      - Sensitivity (63%), specificity (100%), PPV (100%)
      - Higher than CT alone
    - For identification and characterization of primary RCC tumors
      - Sensitivity (47%), specificity (80%), accuracy (51%)
      - Lower than CT alone
      - False negatives are due to urinary excretion of tracer in some tumors
    - Lesions ≤ 1 cm have far lower sensitivity due to scanner limitations
  - **CTA or MRA**
    - Can be helpful in establishing tumor relation to vascular supplies
    - Also potentially useful for nephron sparing or laparoscopic procedures
- **Metastatic disease**
  - **CT**
    - Tumor extension or thrombus via renal vein (23%), inferior vena cava (7%)
    - Usually seen as hypervascular metastases
  - **MR**
    - On T1 post-contrast imaging, RCC usually enhances less than renal tissue
    - Multiplanar capacity of MR allows ideal assessment of renal vein and IVC
    - Preferred to evaluate for intracranial metastases
    - Staging with MR is equal or better to CT
  - **PET/CT**
    - FDG uptake by RCC primary or metastatic lesion is variable
    - PET and PET/CT are more clinically helpful when positive
    - Negative exam may be true negative or non-FDG-avid RCC
    - 80-100% specific for bony metastases

Restaging

- **Ultrasound**
  - Risk increases without clean surgical margins
  - Small bowel occupying nephrectomy bed can be mistaken for recurrence
  - Ultrasound is not acceptable for monitoring nephrectomy bed
- **CT**
  - Useful to follow patients after treatment
  - 20-30% of patients with apparent localized renal cell carcinoma at time of surgery relapse following radical nephrectomy
    - Majority are distant metastases
    - Usually relapse within 3 years
  - Lung metastases are most common late relapse finding
    - May appear as hemorrhagic metastases, show lymphatic invasion, or produce consolidation
  - Bone metastases are less common
  - Rarely, pancreatic lesions are identified
- **MR**
  - MR is superior to CT in assessing venous involvement
  - CT is currently preferred to MR in following patients for disease recurrence after surgery
- **PET/CT**
  - Nephrectomy bed has highest area of recurrence (20-40%)
  - Partial nephrectomy patients should have remnant carefully evaluated
    - Recurrence rates in remnant are 4-6% within 2-4 years, depending on stage
    - Some recurrence may be from incomplete margins whereas others represent multifocal disease
  - Thoracic involvement should be evaluated by CT
  - Bone scan and brain MR may be performed with appropriate clinical indications

- PET/CT has been shown useful for both local recurrence and metastases
- Metastatic frequency by tumor stage
  - T1 disease: 7.1%
  - T2 disease: 26.5%
  - T3 disease: 39.4%

CLINICAL PRESENTATION & WORK-UP

Presentation

- "Classic" triad
  - Hematuria
  - Flank pain
  - Abdominal mass
- < 15% of patients present with classic triad
- Other signs and symptoms include
  - Weight loss
  - Fever
  - Hypercalcemia
  - Night sweats
  - Malaise
  - Hypertension
- Roughly 1/2 of cases are identified as incidental finding on imaging
- Remainder are suspected based on
  - Various symptoms of paraneoplastic syndromes
  - Direct effects of tumor metastasis
  - Identification of palpable renal mass
- Wilms tumor presentation
  - Abdominal mass
  - Pain
  - Hematuria
  - Fever
  - Hypertension
  - Malaise
  - Calcifications < 10% of cases vs. neuroblastoma > 90%

Prognosis

- 5-year survival by stage
  - I: 81%
  - II: 74%
  - III: 53%
    - Invasion of perinephric fat, T3a N0 M0 (60-80%)
    - Venous involvement, T3b-T3c N0 M0 (40-65%)
  - IV: 8%
    - Adrenal involvement, T4 N0 M0 (0-30%)
    - Locally advanced, T4 N0 M0 (0-20%)
    - Lymph involvement, any T, N+ M0 (0-20%)
    - Systemic metastases, any T, any N, M1 (0-10%)
- 4-year OS Wilms tumor based on NWTS 3/4
  - Favorable histology
    - I: 96-97%
    - II: 90-95%
    - III: 85-91%
    - IV: 78-87%
    - V: 78%
  - Anaplastic
    - Stages II-III: 49%
    - Stage IV: 18%
  - Rhabdoid: 25%
  - Clear cell: 75%

Additional Predictors of Short Survival

- ≥ 3 of the following
  - LDH > 1.5x normal
  - Hb < lower limit normal
  - Corrected serum Ca > 10 mg/dL
  - < 1 year diagnosis to development of metastatic disease
  - Karnofsky performance score (KPS) ≤ 70
  - ≥ 2 sites of organ metastasis

Work-Up

- Clinical
  - History and physical
- Radiographic
  - RCC: Abdominal and pelvic CT (or MR) with contrast, chest imaging
    - Bone scan and brain MR if clinically indicated
  - Wilms: Abdominal US, CT (or MR) of the primary, CXR or chest CT
    - Clear cell: Add bone scan and MR brain
    - Rhabdoid: Add MR brain (10-15% CNS PNET)
- Laboratory
  - RCC
    - CBC, CMP, UA, and biopsy if indicated (small lesion in which therapy less than nephrectomy is being considered)
      - If urothelial carcinoma suspected, consider urine cytology and ureteroscopy
  - Wilms
    - No biopsy (unless unresectable or bilateral), CBC, UA, Bun:Cr, LFT
      - Bone marrow for clear cell histology

TREATMENT

Major Treatment Alternatives

- Radical nephrectomy is treatment of choice for RCC if resectable
- Alternative treatments of RCC
  - Partial nephrectomy
  - Radiofrequency ablation
  - Cryoablation
  - Ultrasound ablation
  - Microwave radiotherapy
- Currently no recommendation for adjuvant therapy after resection of RCC with no metastasis

Major Treatment Roadblocks/ Contraindications

- RCCs typically have high levels of MDR protein, making chemotherapy difficult

Treatment Options by Stage

- Stage I
  - Partial nephrectomy, nephrectomy, or ablative therapy
- Stages II-III
  - Radical nephrectomy
- Stage IV
  - Nephrectomy + metastasectomy (individualized)
- Unresectable or poor surgical candidate
  - Chemo at stage IV, or RT
- Relapse or stage IV

- First-line agents: Sunitinib, temsirolimus, bevacizumab + interferon-α, pazopanib, or high-dose IL-2
- RT for local control relapse or palliation of metastatic site

Dose Response

- RCC generally considered radioresistant, although large hypofractionated doses appear to overcome this "resistance"

Standard Doses

- Unresectable lesions or high-risk postoperative bed, 45-50 Gy to tumor and regional lymphatics
- Metastatic lesions: When practical, there is evidence emerging that SBRT or SRS may improve local control over conventional fractionation

Organs at Risk Parameters

- Contralateral kidney
  - Uninvolved whole kidney < 1,440 cGy, V20 < 32%
- Small bowel
  - Minimize volume > 45 Gy (ideally < 195 cc)
- Liver
  - Mean < 30-32 Gy

Common Techniques

- Multiple beam arrangements possible to minimize dose to contralateral kidney, normal bowel, and liver

Landmark Trials

- OS ↑ by nephrectomy in stage IV RCC

Wilms Tumor Treatment

- Surgery: 95% resectable at diagnosis; radical nephrectomy in 1 piece is standard practice
  - Bilateral or unresectable: Chemotherapy followed by resection
- Chemotherapy: Combination based on risk group
  - May include
    - Vincristine (V)
    - Actinomycin (A)
    - Doxorubicin (D)
    - Cyclophosphamide (C)
    - Etoposide (E)
    - Carboplatin (P)
    - Irinotecan (I)
  - Actinomycin not given during RT
- Radiation
  - Start day 9 postop
    - Based on
      - Stage
      - Histology
      - Operative findings
      - Presence of metastasis
  - No RT: Stages I-II favorable histology
  - Flank RT: Stage III 10.8-19.8 Gy per histology
  - Whole abdominal RT: Tumor spillage, peritoneal seeding; 10.5 Gy with boost to residual
  - Lung mets: Whole lung RT to 9-12 Gy (based on age)
  - Other mets: As appropriate with dosage per COG guidelines
- Possible treatment complications
  - Scoliosis
  - Kyphosis
  - Renal failure
  - Pneumonitis
  - Congestive heart failure
  - Secondary malignancy

RECOMMENDED FOLLOW-UP

Clinical

- Physical exam every 4-6 months for 2 years
  - Then annually for 5 years

Radiographic

- PT1-2: Annual CXR for 5 years
- PT3: q. 6-month CXR with abdominal CT @ 6, 12, 24, and 36 months, then every 2 years

Laboratory

- CMP (including LDH) every 6 months for 2 years
  - Then annually for 5 years

SELECTED REFERENCES

1. Jhaveri PM et al: A dose-response relationship for time to bone pain resolution after stereotactic body radiotherapy (SBRT) for renal cell carcinoma (RCC) bony metastases. Acta Oncol. 51(5):584-8, 2012
2. Zelefsky MJ et al: Tumor control outcomes after hypofractionated and single-dose stereotactic image-guided intensity-modulated radiotherapy for extracranial metastases from renal cell carcinoma. Int J Radiat Oncol Biol Phys. 82(5):1744-8, 2012
3. American Joint Committee on Cancer: AJCC Cancer Staging Manual. 7th ed. New York: Springer. 479-89, 2010
4. Dawson LA et al: Radiation-associated kidney injury. Int J Radiat Oncol Biol Phys. 76(3 Suppl):S108-15, 2010
5. Kavanagh BD et al: Radiation dose-volume effects in the stomach and small bowel. Int J Radiat Oncol Biol Phys. 76(3 Suppl):S101-7, 2010
6. Zhang J et al: Imaging of kidney cancer. Radiol Clin North Am. 45(1):119-47, 2007
7. Reznek RH: CT/MRI in staging renal cell carcinoma. Cancer Imaging. 4 Spec No A:S25-32, 2004
8. Stephenson AJ et al: Guidelines for the surveillance of localized renal cell carcinoma based on the patterns of relapse after nephrectomy. J Urol. 172(1):58-62, 2004
9. Israel GM et al: Renal imaging for diagnosis and staging of renal cell carcinoma. Urol Clin North Am. 30(3):499-514, 2003
10. Mirels H: Metastatic disease in long bones: A proposed scoring system for diagnosing impending pathologic fractures. 1989. Clin Orthop Relat Res. (415 Suppl):S4-13, 2003
11. Flanigan RC et al: Nephrectomy followed by interferon alfa-2b compared with interferon alfa-2b alone for metastatic renal-cell cancer. N Engl J Med. 345(23):1655-9, 2001
12. Mickisch GH et al: Radical nephrectomy plus interferon-alfa-based immunotherapy compared with interferon alfa alone in metastatic renal-cell carcinoma: a randomised trial. Lancet. 358(9286):966-70, 2001
13. Vasselli JR et al: Lack of retroperitoneal lymphadenopathy predicts survival of patients with metastatic renal cell carcinoma. J Urol. 166(1):68-72, 2001
14. Coll DM et al: 3-dimensional volume rendered computerized tomography for preoperative evaluation and intraoperative treatment of patients undergoing nephron sparing surgery. J Urol. 161(4):1097-102, 1999
15. Bechtold RE et al: Imaging approach to staging of renal cell carcinoma. Urol Clin North Am. 24(3):507-22, 1997

16. Jamis-Dow CA et al: Small (< or = 3-cm) renal masses: detection with CT versus US and pathologic correlation. Radiology. 198(3):785-8, 1996
17. Curry NS: Small renal masses (lesions smaller than 3 cm): imaging evaluation and management. AJR Am J Roentgenol. 164(2):355-62, 1995
18. Newhouse JH: The radiologic evaluation of the patient with renal cancer. Urol Clin North Am. 20(2):231-46, 1993
19. Yamashita Y et al: Small renal cell carcinoma: pathologic and radiologic correlation. Radiology. 184(2):493-8, 1992
20. McClennan BL: Oncologic imaging. Staging and follow-up of renal and adrenal carcinoma. Cancer. 67(4 Suppl):1199-208, 1991
21. Fein AB et al: Diagnosis and staging of renal cell carcinoma: a comparison of MR imaging and CT. AJR Am J Roentgenol. 148(4):749-53, 1987
22. Hricak H et al: Magnetic resonance imaging in the diagnosis and staging of renal and perirenal neoplasms. Radiology. 154(3):709-15, 1985

(Left) Axial CECT shows an exophytic, enhancing, solid mass → in the posterior aspect of the right kidney, measuring approximately 2 cm and compatible with a T1a lesion. *(Right)* Axial CECT shows a heterogeneously enhancing exophytic mass → with areas of central low attenuation or necrosis arising off the lateral aspect of the right kidney, compatible with a renal cell carcinoma.

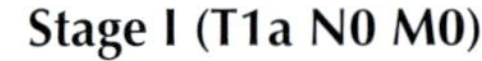

Stage I (T1a N0 M0)

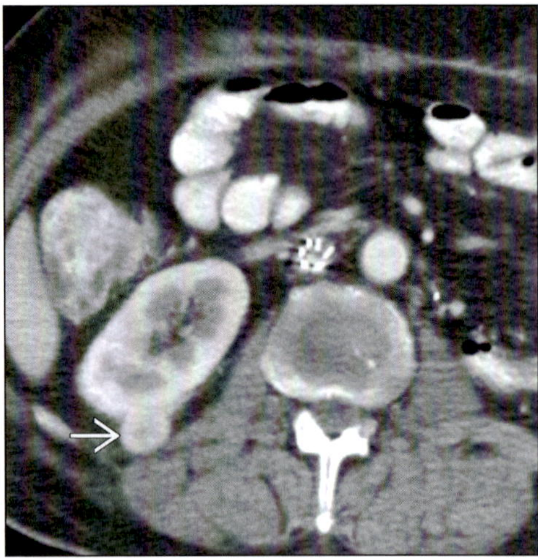

Stage I (T1a N0 M0)

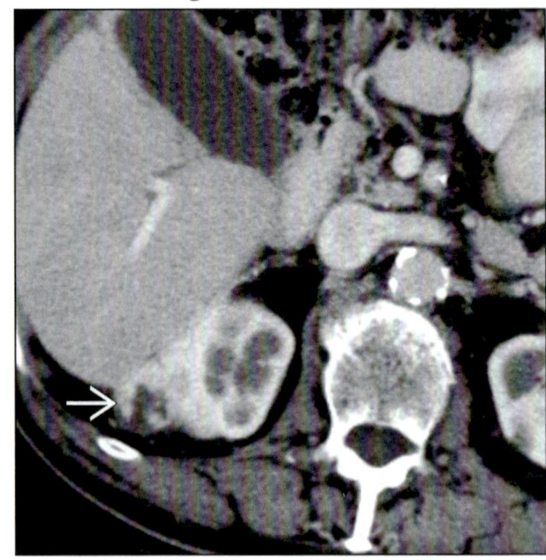

(Left) Axial PET/CT shows focal FDG within the pathologically confirmed T1a renal cell carcinoma → in the right kidney. Renal cell carcinomas have variable FDG uptake, but intensely FDG-avid lesions should be viewed as very suspicious. Note the gallstones ↪. *(Right)* Transverse transabdominal ultrasound shows a 1.7 cm T1a renal cell carcinoma (calipers) that is iso- to slightly hyperechoic compared to normal background renal cortical tissue.

Stage I (T1a N0 M0)

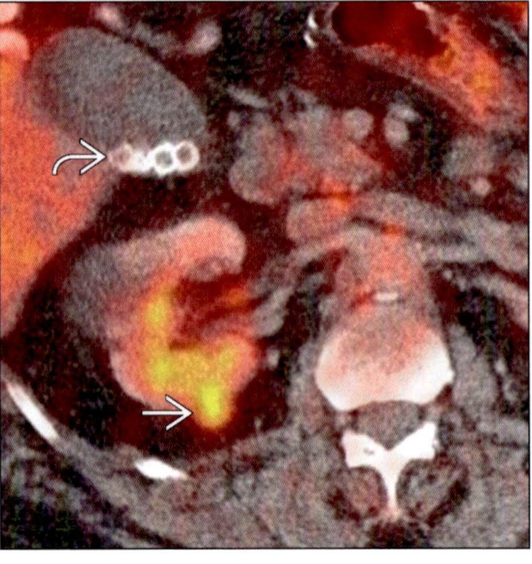

Stage I (T1a N0 M0)

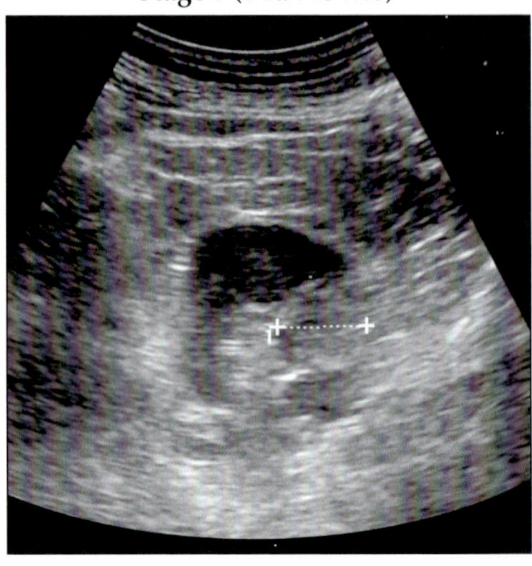

(Left) Bisected correlative pathologic specimen from the same patient shows the mass → in the inferior pole of the left kidney to be 2.8 cm, confined to the kidney, and without positive nodes, compatible with a stage I (T1a N0 M0) lesion. *(Right)* Gross pathologic specimen in the same patient shows the large resected mass →. Final pathology demonstrated a stage II (T2b N0 M0) lesion.

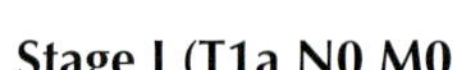

Stage I (T1a N0 M0)

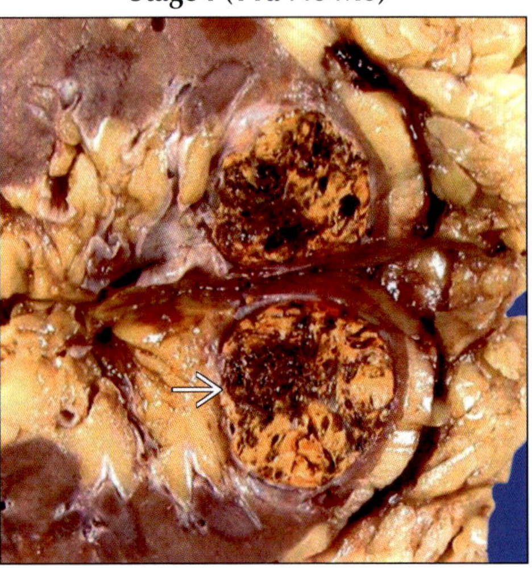

Stage II (T2b N0 M0)

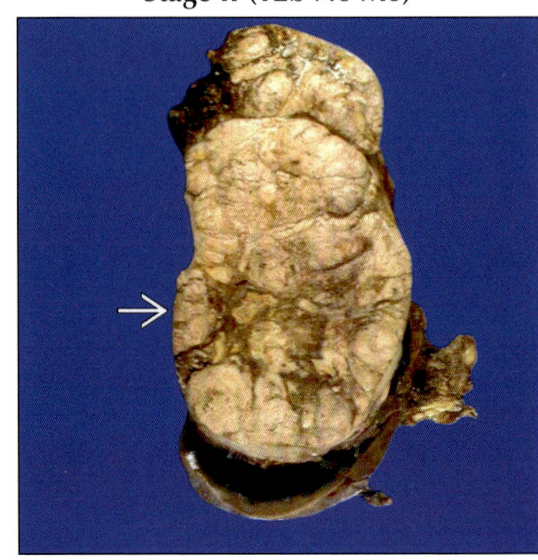

Stage I (T1b N0 M0)

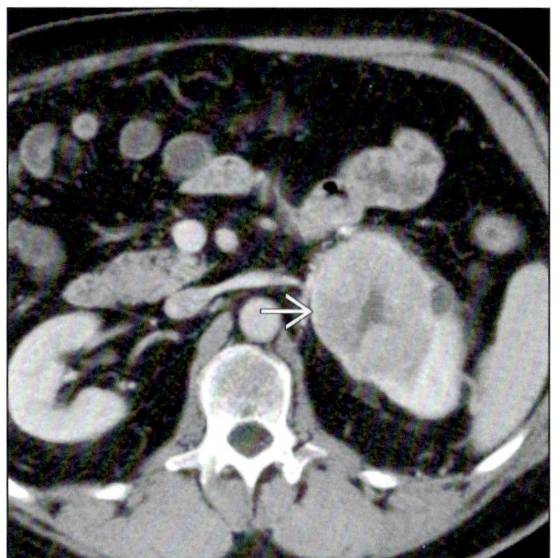

Stage I (T1b N0 M0)

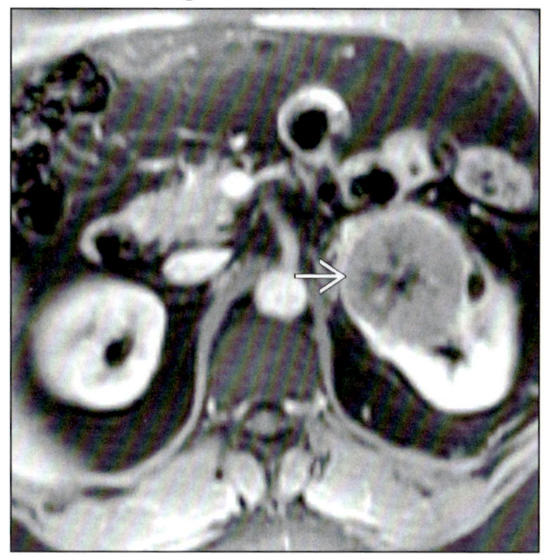

(Left) *Axial CECT shows a 5 cm mass ➔ in the left kidney with heterogeneous enhancement and central low attenuation, compatible with a renal cell carcinoma. The differential diagnosis may include an oncocytoma, which also characteristically has a central scar.* ***(Right)*** *Axial T1WI C+ FS MR in the same patient shows a correlative MR image of an enhancing solid mass ➔ in the left kidney, most compatible with a renal cell carcinoma.*

Stage I (T1b N0 M0)

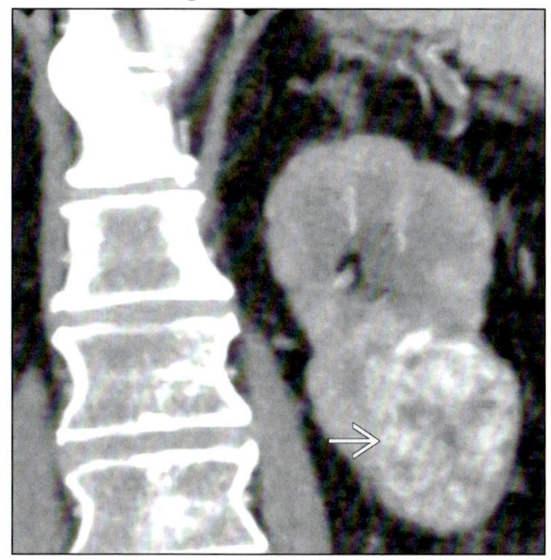

Stage I (T1b N0 M0)

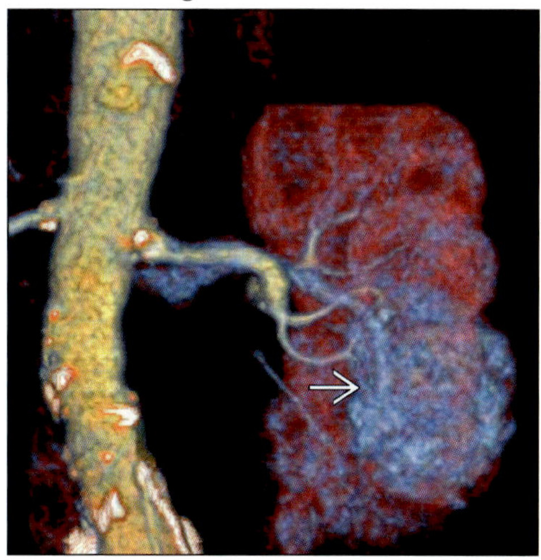

(Left) *Coronal CECT in the same patient shows the renal cell carcinoma to be relatively vascular ➔ compared to the background renal parenchyma.* ***(Right)*** *Reconstructed image from an abdominal CTA in the same patient shows the relative vascularity of the inferior pole renal cell carcinoma ➔ compared to the background renal vascularity.*

Stage I (T1b N0 M0)

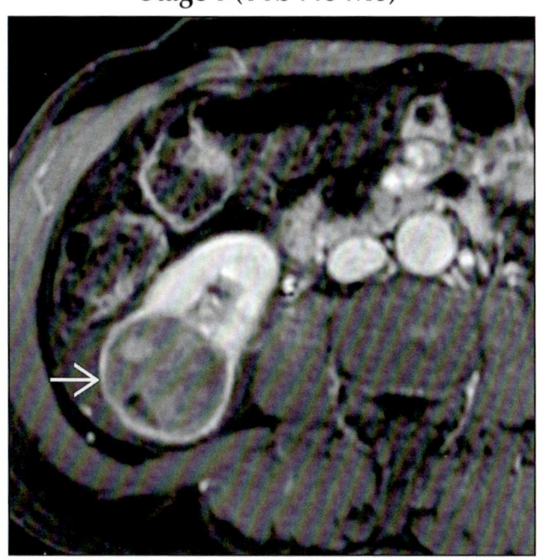

Stage I (T1b N0 M0)

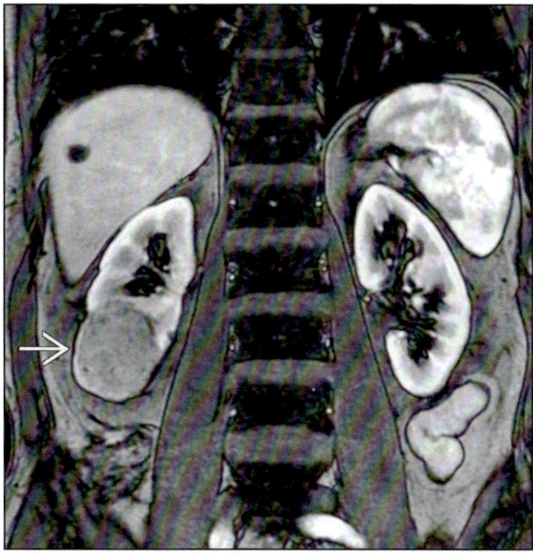

(Left) *Axial T1WI C+ FS MR shows an example of a T1b lesion ➔ in the posterior aspect of the inferior pole of the right kidney. In this case, the margins of the tumor are fairly well circumscribed, and the internal signal of the lesion is somewhat complex.* ***(Right)*** *Coronal T1WI C+ FS MR shows a 5.5 cm enhancing mass ➔ in the inferior pole of the right kidney, subsequently confirmed pathologically as a renal cell carcinoma.*

KIDNEY

(**Left**) *Axial T1WI C+ FS MR shows a 7.9 cm mass ➔ in the left kidney with complex internal signal, the overall appearance of which is very worrisome for renal cell carcinoma.* (**Right**) *Coronal T1WI C+ FS MR in the same patient shows the large exophytic mass ➔ arising from the inferior pole of the left kidney. Subsequent nephrectomy revealed a stage II (T2a N0 M0) renal cell carcinoma.*

Stage II (T2a N0 M0)

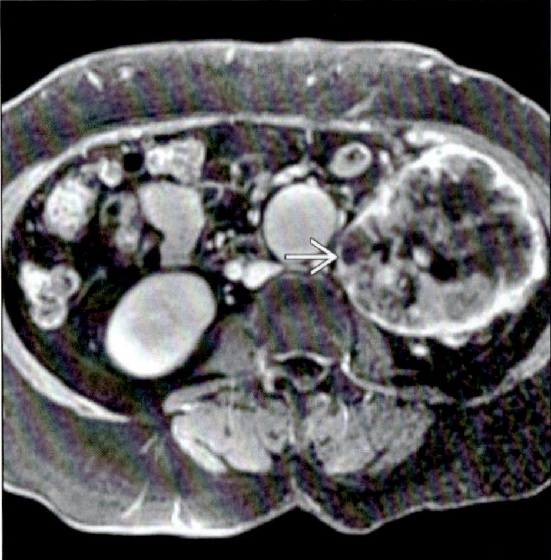

Stage II (T2a N0 M0)

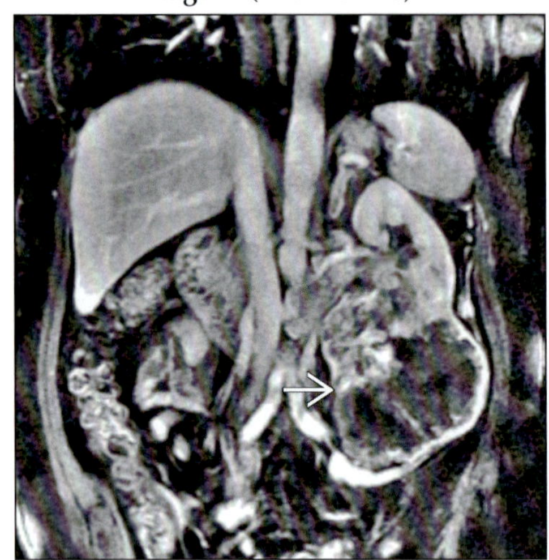

(**Left**) *Axial fused PET/CT in the same patient shows almost no increased metabolic activity within the large left renal mass ➔.* (**Right**) *This 65-year-old woman is considered a nonoperative candidate. Initial fields ➔ include the kidney and urethra but may also include the paracaval and paraaortic lymph nodes, depending on nodal risk. Field reductions reduce toxicity with CT urography to identify the renal pelvis and spare parenchyma.*

Stage II (T2a N0 M0)

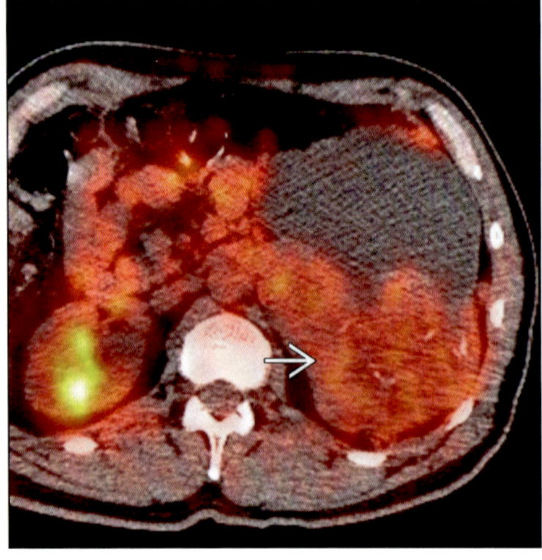

Stage II TCC Renal Pelvis and Urethra

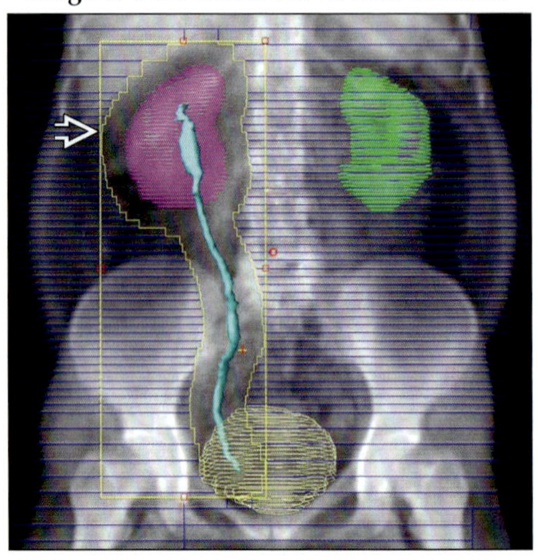

(**Left**) *CECT shows a renal cell carcinoma ➔ in the right kidney.* (**Right**) *The tumor is invading the right renal vein ➔. Tumor extending into the renal vein or its segmental branches constitutes a T3a lesion, extension of tumor in the IVC is staged as T3b, and extension above the diaphragm constitutes a T3c lesion. The low attenuation within the IVC ➔ is the result of mixing of opacified with nonopacified blood and should not be mistaken for tumor invasion.*

Stage III (T3a N0 M0)

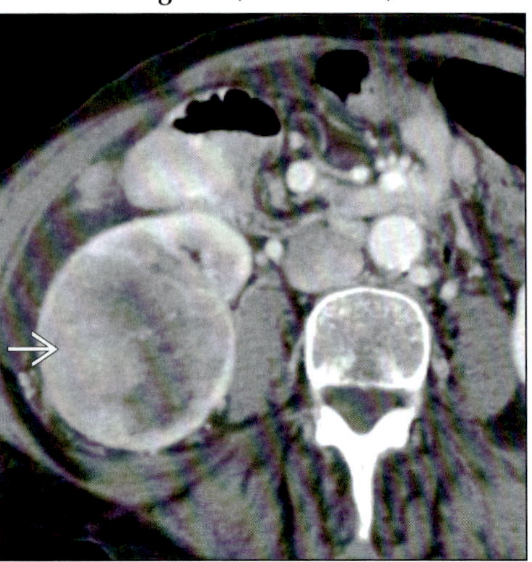

Stage III (T3a N0 M0)

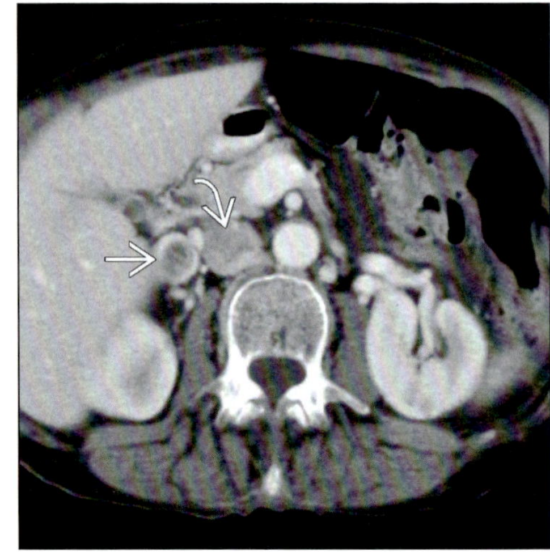

T3a N0 M0 RCC

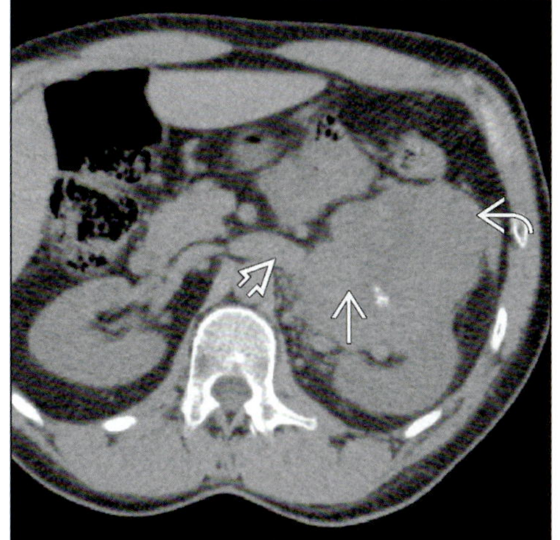

T3a N0 M0 RCC

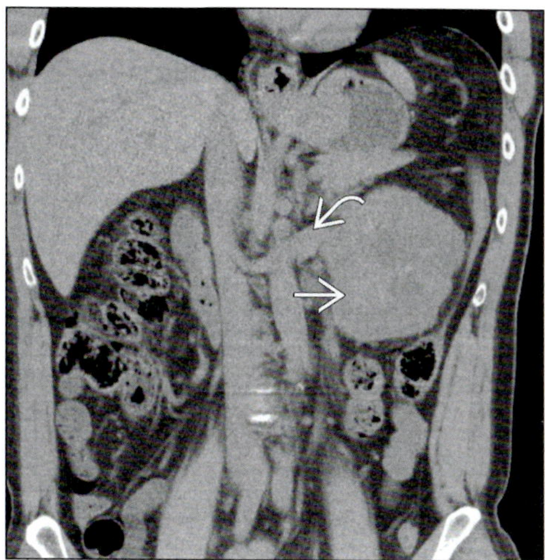

*(**Left**) Axial NECT shows a RCC of 10 cm in the left kidney ➡ with enlargement of the renal vein ➡ due to tumor infiltration. Surgery confirmed invasion into perinephric fat (T3a disease), but not through Gerota fascia ➡. (**Right**) Coronal NECT of the same patient demonstrates T3a RCC ➡ with renal vein enlargement ➡.*

T3a N0 M0 RCC Nodal Recurrence

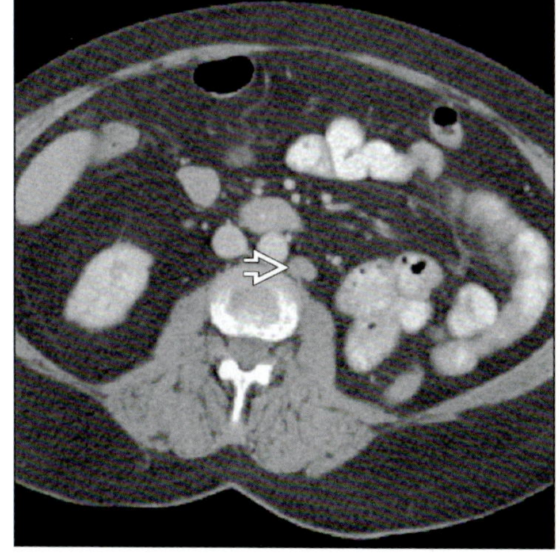

T3a N0 M0 RCC Nodal Recurrence

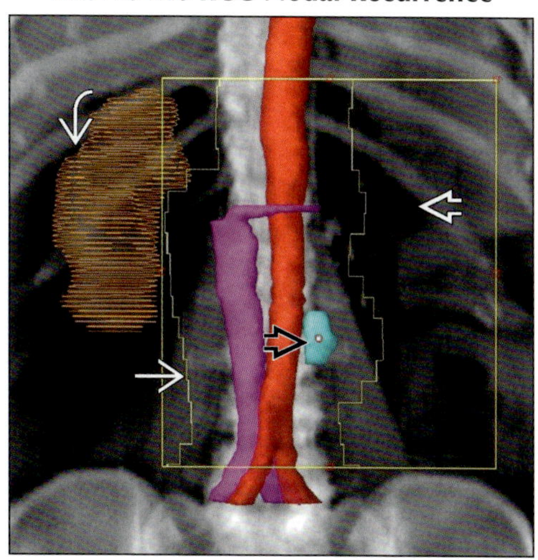

*(**Left**) Two years later, axial CT demonstrates a paraaortic nodal recurrence ➡. (**Right**) Digitally reconstructed radiograph (DRR) demonstrates nodal recurrence ➡ and absence of left kidney ➡. Paraaortic nodal field includes a 2.0 cm margin from the artery, vein, and involved lymph node, as shown by the multileaf collimator ➡ block edge. 45 Gy in 25 fractions was delivered AP:PA with maximal sparing of the remaining kidney ➡.*

Stage IV (T1a N1 M0)

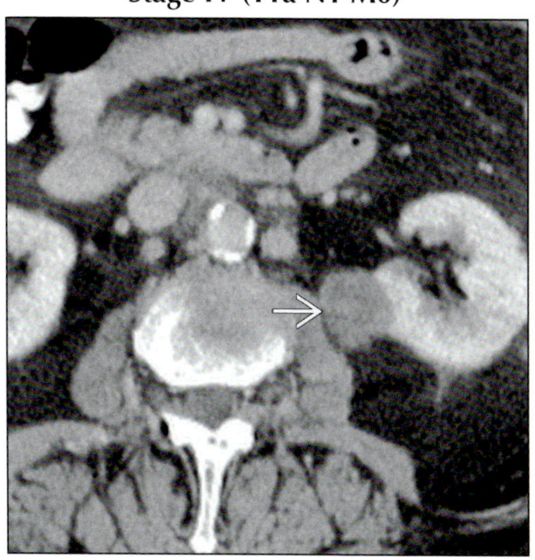

Stage IV (T1a N1 M0)

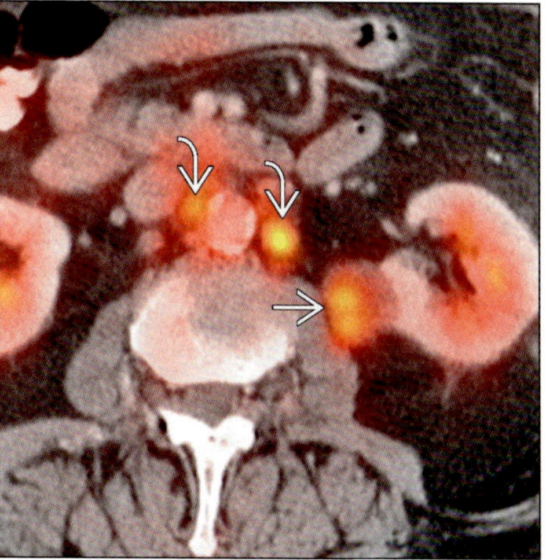

*(**Left**) Axial CECT shows a low-attenuation enhancing mass ➡ within the left kidney. (**Right**) Axial fused PET/CT in the same patient shows moderate increased FDG activity along the medial border of this renal cell carcinoma ➡. In addition, the left paraaortic and aortocaval nodes ➡ demonstrate increased metabolic activity compatible with metastatic nodes, making this N1 disease.*

Stage IV (T1b N0 M1)

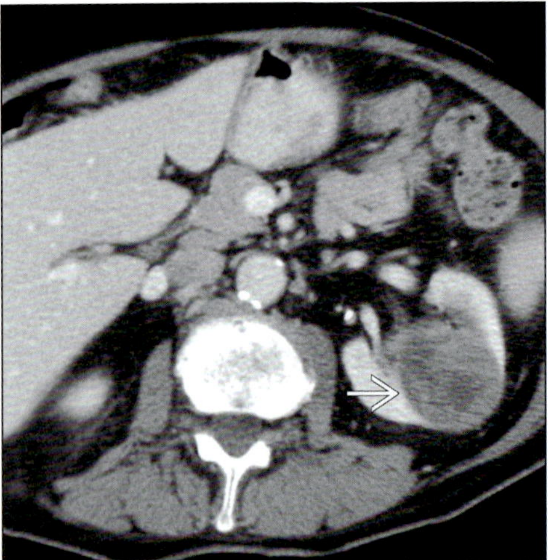

Stage IV (T1b N0 M1)

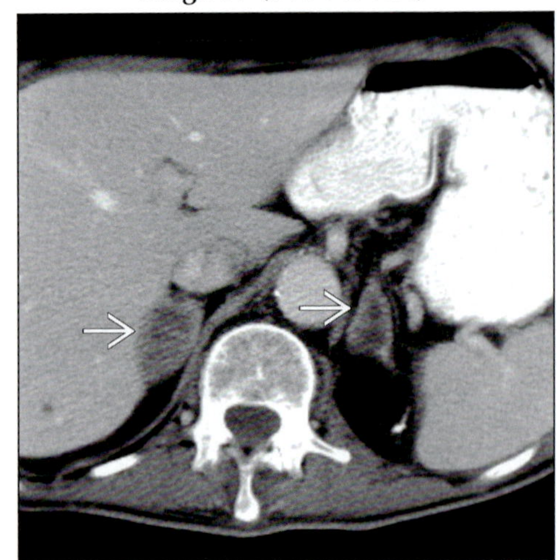

(Left) *Axial CECT shows a 4.3 cm, mixed attenuation, and heterogeneously enhancing mass ➔ in the left kidney, compatible with a T1b lesion.* ***(Right)*** *Axial CECT in the same patient shows bilateral adrenal masses ➔. These masses are indeterminate on this single contrast-enhanced CT. The patient was referred for a CT-guided biopsy of the right adrenal gland mass, which showed metastatic renal cell carcinoma.*

Stage IV Recurrent RCC

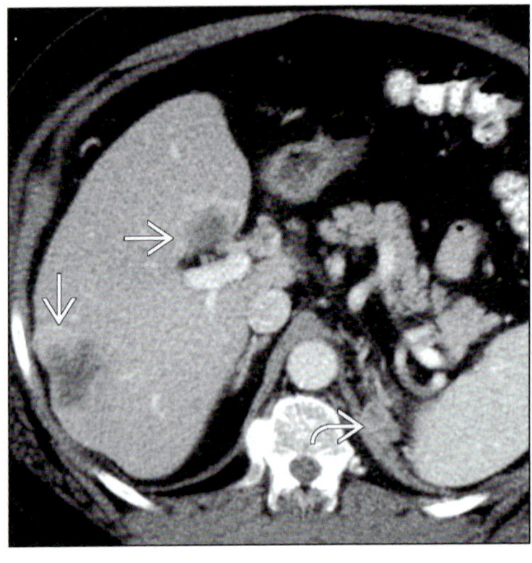

Stage IV Recurrent RCC

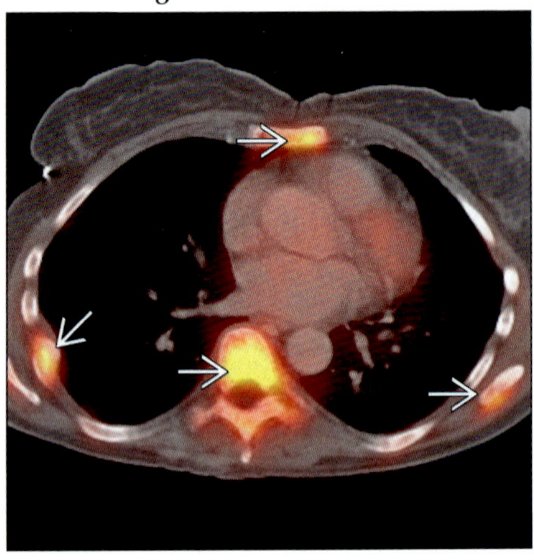

(Left) *Axial CECT shows multiple low-attenuation lesions ➔ in the liver in this patient with a history of renal cell carcinoma, compatible with recurrent stage IV disease. In addition, there is recurrent disease ↪ in the left renal fossa.* ***(Right)*** *Axial fused PET/CT in the same patient shows multiple hypermetabolic bone lesions ➔, compatible with osseous metastases from renal cell carcinoma.*

Stage IV (T1b N0 M1)

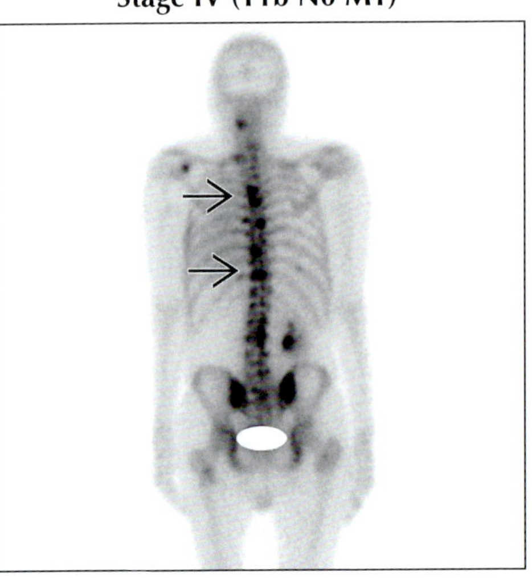

Stage IV (T3 N1 M1)

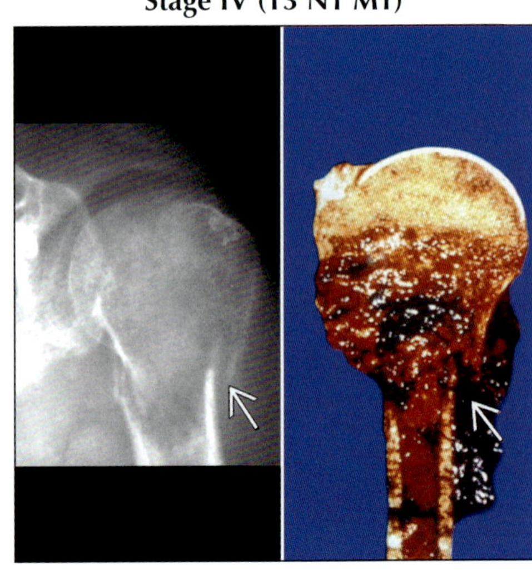

(Left) *Coronal posterior bone scan in a patient who underwent a nephrectomy for a 6 cm RCC (T1b) shows multiple abnormal foci of increased tracer activity throughout the spine ➔, compatible with metastatic disease.* ***(Right)*** *Composite image shows a pathologic fracture ➔ of the humerus with corresponding specimen (autopsy). The patient presented with acute arm pain after minor trauma. Work-up revealed T3 tumor of the kidney and metastasis elsewhere.*

Stage IV Recurrent RCC

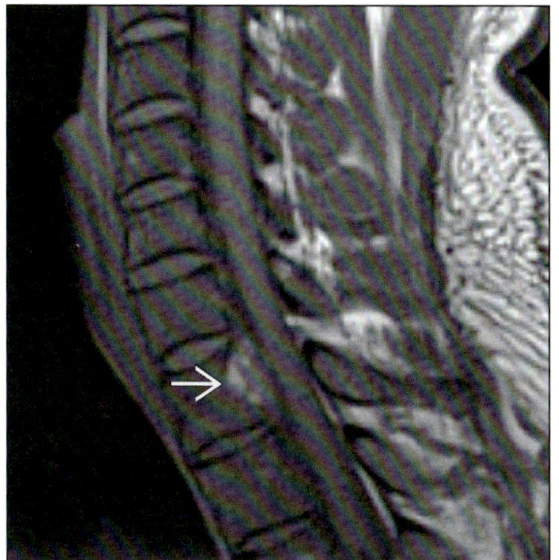

Stage IV Recurrent RCC

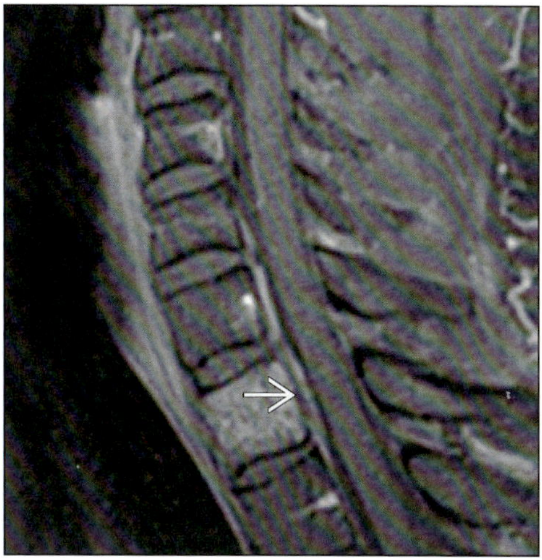

*(**Left**) Sagittal T1WI MR demonstrates T1 vertebral body metastasis ➔ without evidence of spinal cord compression in a 35-year-old patient presenting with acute neck pain (8 out of 10), 2 years after nephrectomy for a T2b N0 RCC. (**Right**) Sagittal T1WI C+ MR in the same patient demonstrates signal replacement of the T1 vertebral body ➔ with minimal retropulsion or bulging into the epidural space.*

Stage IV Recurrent RCC

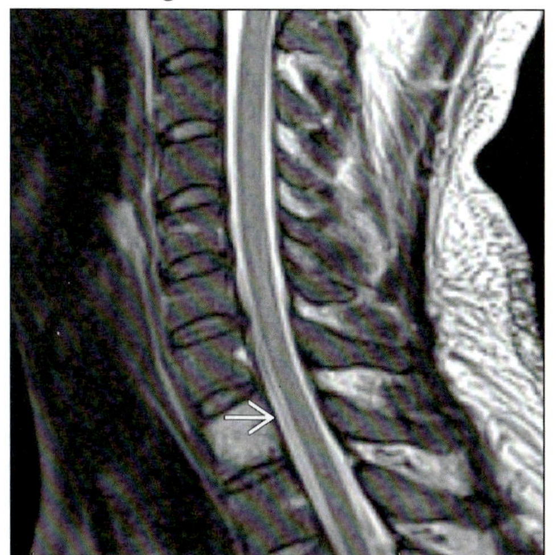

Stage IV Recurrent RCC

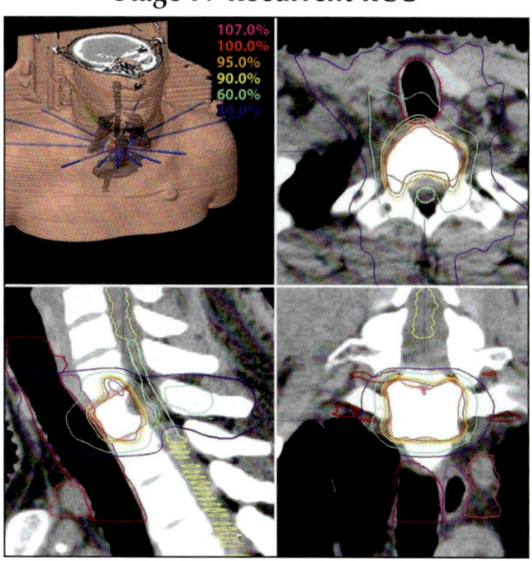

*(**Left**) Sagittal T2WI MR in the same patient demonstrates CSF ➔ anterior to the spinal cord with no evidence of cord compression. (**Right**) The same patient was treated with stereotactic body radiation therapy (SBRT) delivering 16 Gy in a single fraction. His pain score went from 8/10 to 2/10 in a few weeks. SBRT is currently being compared to fractionated radiation therapy of the spine in a randomized RTOG trial.*

Stage IV Recurrent RCC

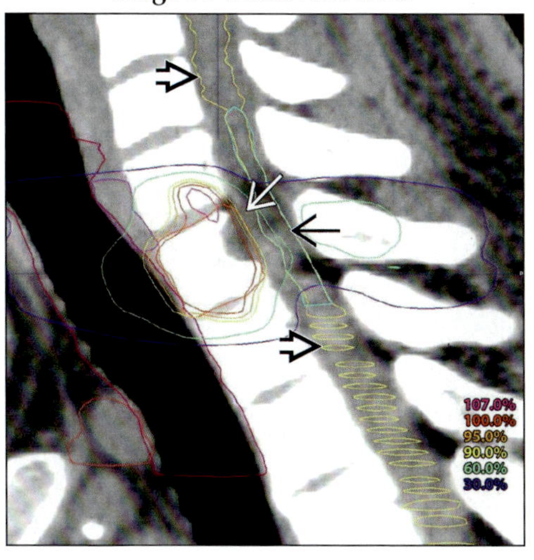

Stage IV Recurrent RCC

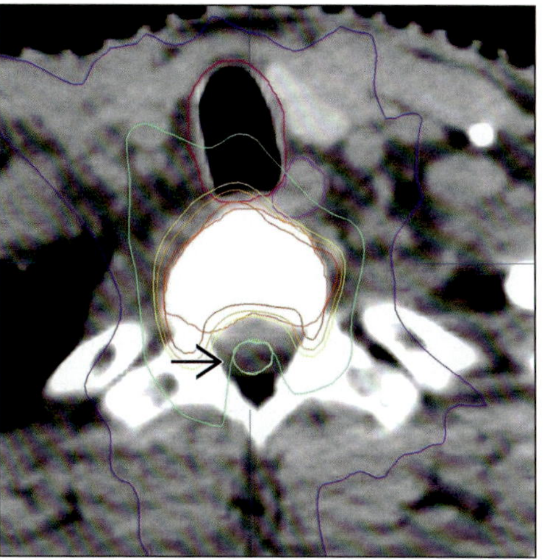

*(**Left**) IMRT creates isodose curves ➔ with a rapid dose fall-off. With SBRT, spinal cord behind involved vertebral body ⇨ is limited to < 10% receiving more than 10 Gy. Spinal cord outside this area ⇨ is limited to < 0.35 mL receiving a dose greater than 10 Gy with a maximum volume of < 0.03 mL receiving over 14 Gy. (**Right**) In the same patient, isodose curves ⇨ conform to a concave volume using IMRT, thus limiting the dose to spinal cord.*

T4 N1 M1 RCC

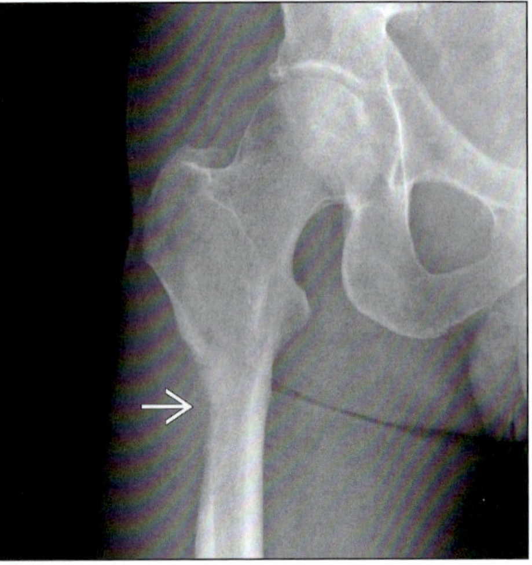

T4 N1 M1 RCC

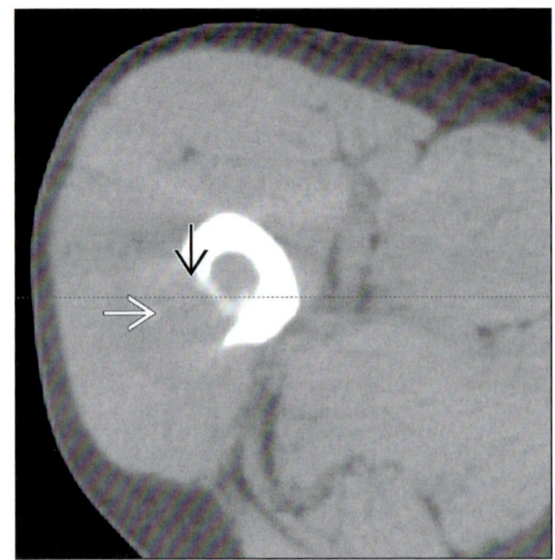

(Left) *AP radiograph of a 60-year-old male presenting with right hip pain demonstrates cortical disruption and resulting femoral instability* ➔*. Biopsy revealed RCC. Mirels criteria for prophylactic fixation include: Site, pain, type of lesion (blastic/ lytic), and % of cortex involved.* ***(Right)*** *Axial NECT demonstrates cortical disruption* → *in the same patient. The soft tissue mass* ➔ *associated with the metastasis has poorly defined borders without contrast.*

T4 N1 M1 RCC

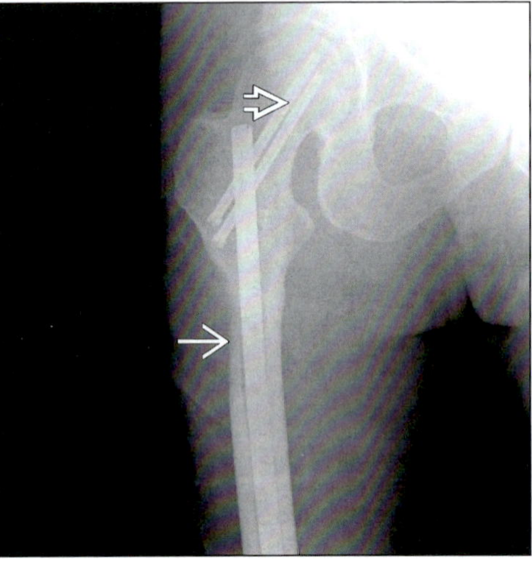

T4 N1 M1 RCC

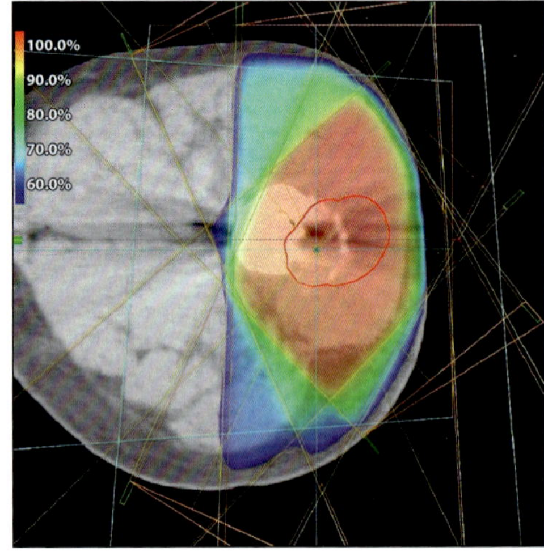

(Left) *AP radiograph shows the presence of an intramedullary rod* ➔ *and 2 reconstruction screws* ➔*, placed prophylactically to prevent a pathological fracture. Postop RT is routinely used.* ***(Right)*** *Axial NECT demonstrates a postoperative radiation plan of 24 Gy delivered in 3 fractions. 8 Gy fractions were selected to overcome the inherent radiation resistance seen with clear cell RCC. Some institutions report improved outcomes with single dose SBRT.*

Stage III Wilms Tumor

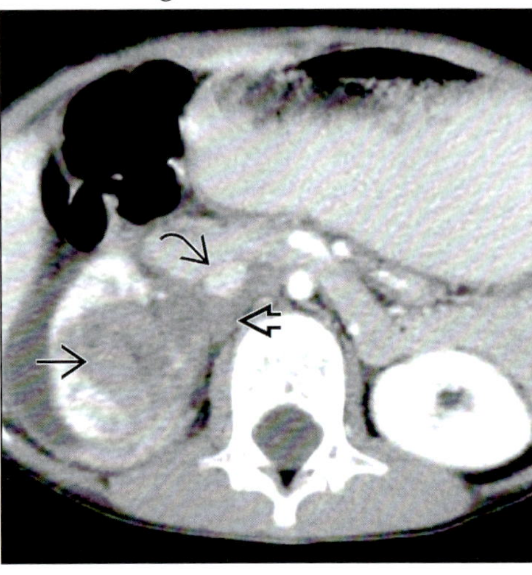

Stage III Wilms Tumor

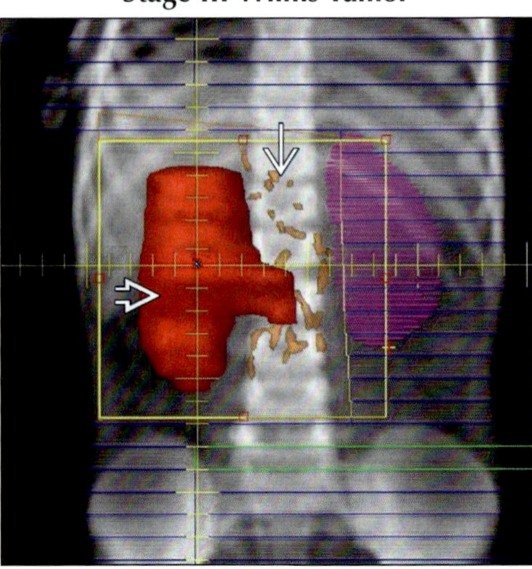

(Left) *CECT shows a right renal mass* → *with heterogeneity. Medial to the mass are enlarged lymph nodes* ⇨ *posterior to the IVC* ↗*.* ***(Right)*** *In the same patient, the tumor was dissected off of the vena cava (surgical clips* ➔*). The margins were negative and 5/18 lymph nodes were positive. Preop kidney and tumor* ➔ *are shown. The flank was given 10.8 Gy, avoiding the residual kidney, while vertebral bodies were treated with uniform dose to prevent scoliosis.*

Stage IV Wilms Tumor

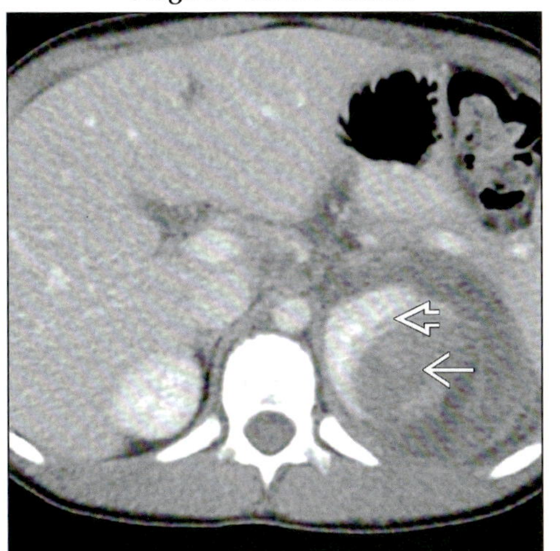

Stage IV Wilms Tumor

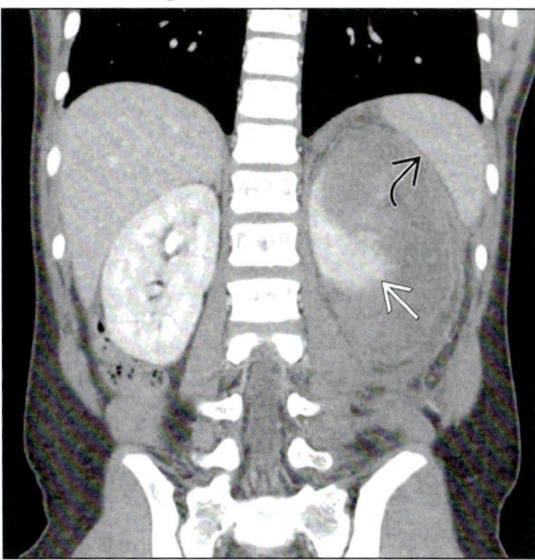

(Left) *Four-year-old patient presents with an 18 cm heterogeneous mass ➔ in the left renal fossa. This mass causes some deformity in renal contours ⇨ and extends to but does not cross the midline. The patient has stage IV disease based on lung metastasis.* ***(Right)*** *Coronal CECT in the same patient demonstrates the mass distorting the normal renal contour ➔ and compressing the spleen ↗.*

Stage IV Wilms Tumor

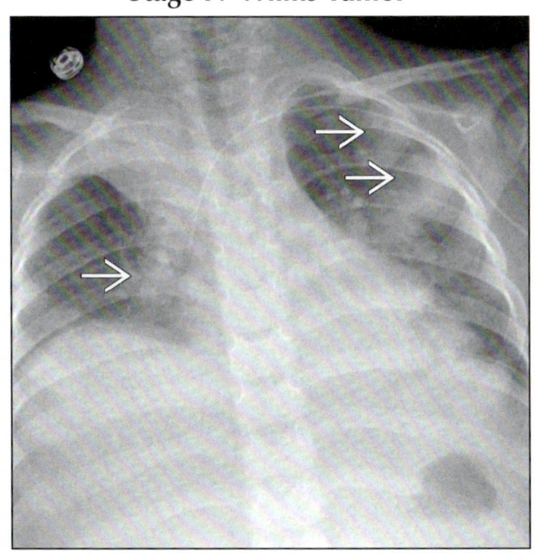

Stage IV Wilms Tumor

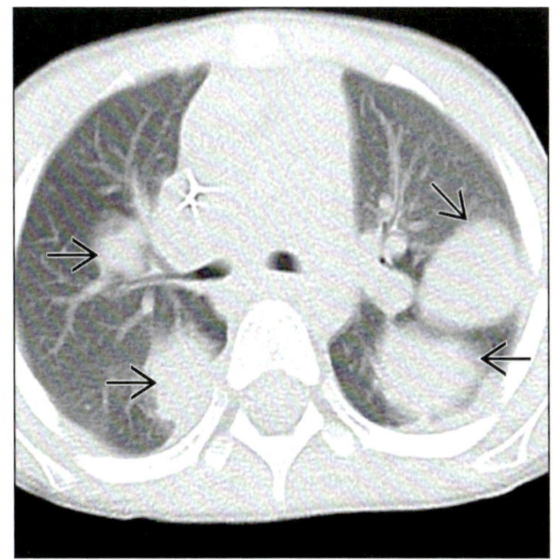

(Left) *AP chest x-ray in the same patient demonstrates multiple large bilateral lung masses ➔. Staging and treatment of lung masses seen on CT alone is currently an area of controversy.* ***(Right)*** *Chest CT in the same patient demonstrates numerous bilateral pulmonary masses ➔ of varying size, ranging from subcentimeter to > 4 cm. 4-year OS with stage IV favorable histology Wilms is > 80%, and for unfavorable histology it is < 20%.*

Stage IV Wilms Tumor

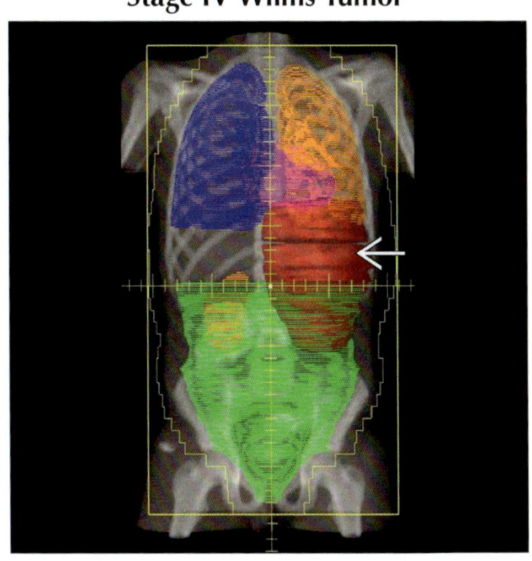

Stage IV Wilms Tumor

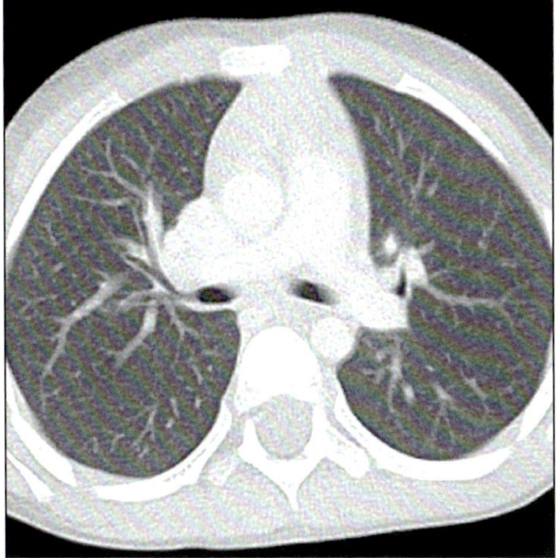

(Left) *In the same patient, renal mass ➔ ruptured into peritoneal cavity. Histology was unfavorable and whole abdominal RT (10.5 Gy) and whole lung RT (12 Gy) were given simultaneously at 1.5 Gy per day. Whole abdominal RT rather than flank RT was used due to the intraoperative rupture.* ***(Right)*** *NECT in same patient shows no masses 2 years after treatment: 30+ weeks of chemotherapy (revised UH-1), surgical resection of primary, and whole lung/ abdominal RT.*

ADRENAL GLAND

(T) Primary Tumor

Adapted from 7th edition AJCC Staging Forms.

TNM	*Definitions*
TX	Primary tumor cannot be assessed
T0	No evidence of primary tumor
T1	Tumor ≤ 5 cm in greatest dimension, no extraadrenal invasion
T2	Tumor > 5 cm, no extraadrenal invasion
T3	Tumor of any size with local invasion but not invading adjacent organs*
T4	Tumor of any size with invasion of adjacent organs*

(N) Regional Lymph Nodes

NX	Regional lymph nodes cannot be assessed
N0	No regional lymph node metastasis
N1	Metastasis in regional lymph node(s)

(M) Distant Metastasis

M0	No distant metastasis
M1	Distant metastasis

**Adjacent organs include kidney, diaphragm, great vessels, pancreas, spleen, and liver.*

AJCC Stages/Prognostic Groups

Adapted from 7th edition AJCC Staging Forms.

Stage	*T*	*N*	*M*
I	T1	N0	M0
II	T2	N0	M0
III	T1	N1	M0
	T2	N1	M0
	T3	N0	M0
IV	T3	N1	M0
	T4	N0	M0
	T4	N1	M0
	Any T	Any N	M1

T1

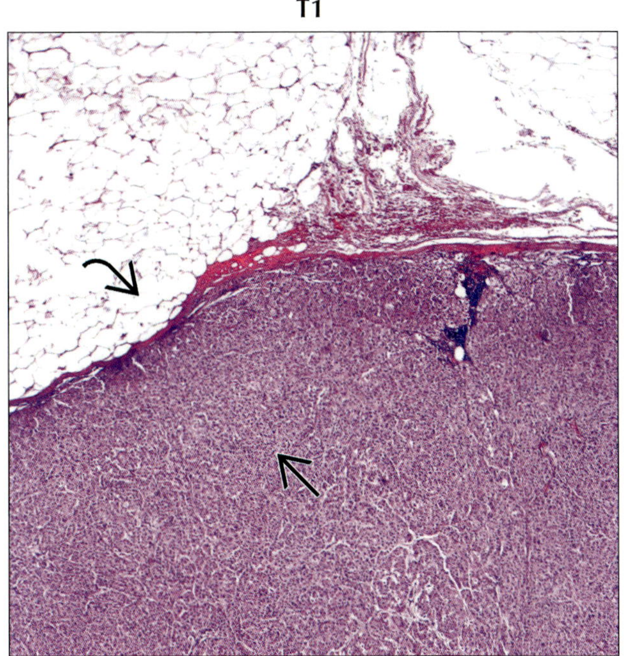

Low-power magnification of an H&E section shows sheets of adrenal cortical neoplastic cells ⇒ that are limited to the adrenal gland (T1). Adipose tissue ↗ surrounding the adrenal gland is negative for tumor.

T2

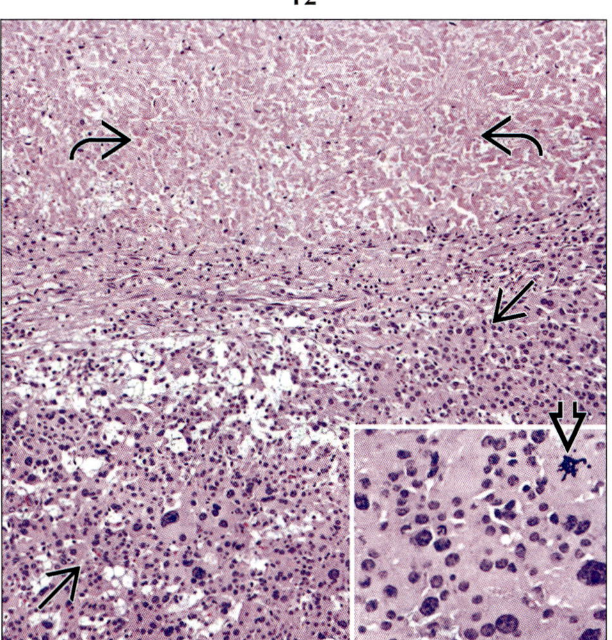

Photomicrograph shows an H&E section from adrenal cortical carcinoma ⇒ with large areas of necrosis in the upper aspect of the slide ↗. The inset shows the particularly striking nuclear pleomorphism (large vs. small nuclei) as well as a mitotic figure ⇨.

T3

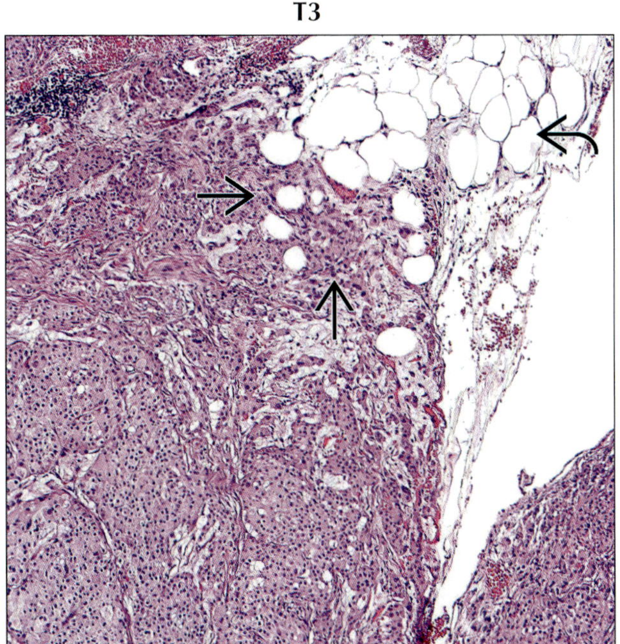

H&E stain shows tumor with local invasion but no extension into adjacent organs, consistent with T3 disease. The adrenal cortical carcinoma ⇒ invades locally into the surrounding adrenal fat ↗.

T4

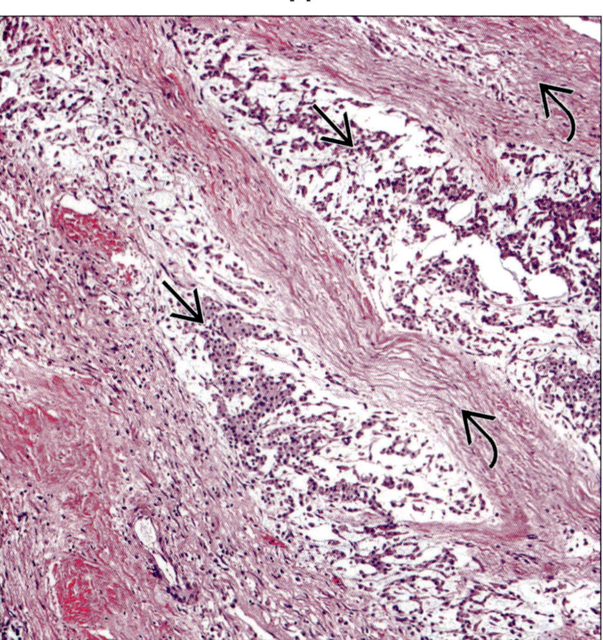

In T4 disease, tumor invades into adjacent organs. This tumor extends to involve the diaphragm. This photomicrograph shows the neoplastic tumor cells ⇒ extending into surrounding fibrotic connective tissue ↗.

ADRENAL GLAND

T1

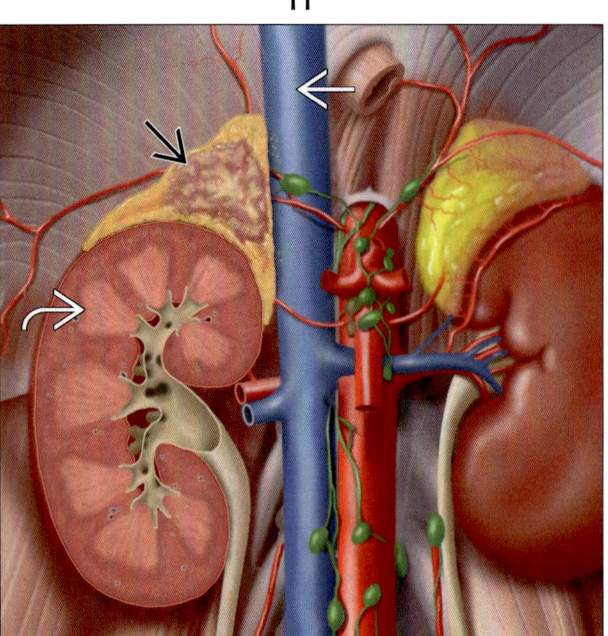

Coronal graphic demonstrates T1 disease. The primary tumor → is ≤ 5 cm in greatest dimension without invasion of adjacent organs, including kidney ➦ or inferior vena cava ➡.

T2

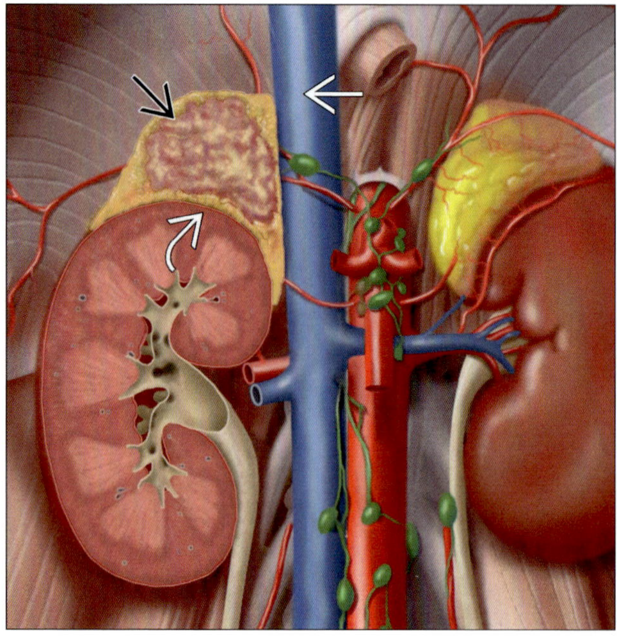

Coronal graphic demonstrates T2 disease. The primary tumor → is > 5 cm in greatest dimension without invasion of adjacent organs, including kidney ➦ or inferior vena cava ➡.

T3

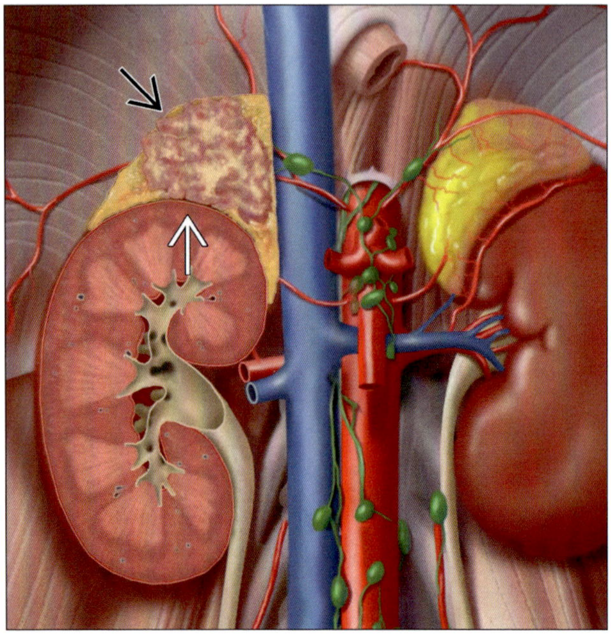

Coronal graphic demonstrates T3 disease. The primary tumor may be any size with local invasion beyond the confines of the adrenal capsule, shown in the superolateral margin →, but no involvement of adjacent organs such as the kidney ➡.

T4

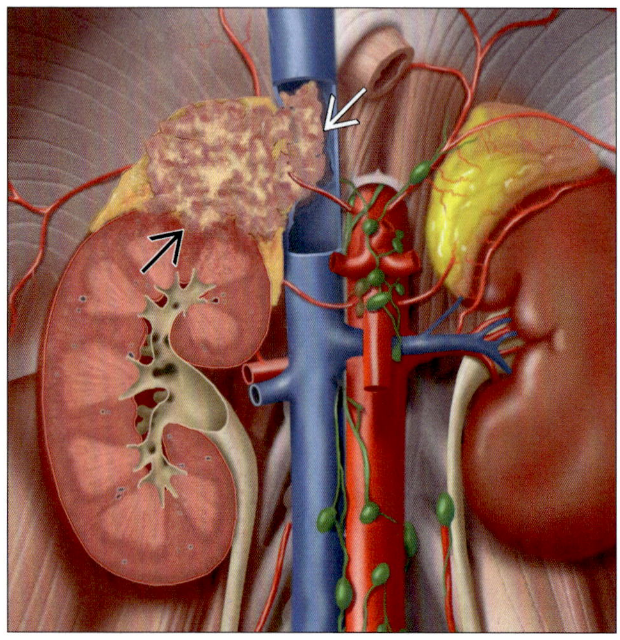

Coronal graphic demonstrates T4 disease. The primary tumor can be any size with local invasion beyond the confines of the adrenal capsule and into adjacent organs, including the kidney →. Direct extension into the inferior vena cava is illustrated ➡.

T4

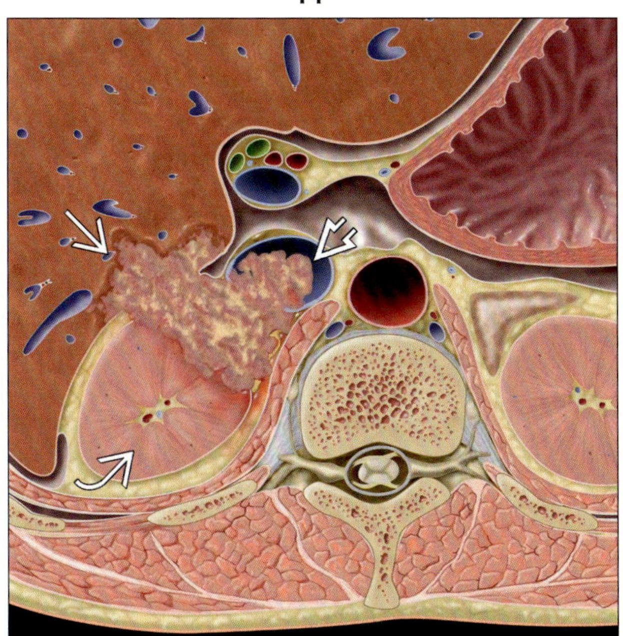

Axial graphic demonstrates right-sided adrenal cortical carcinoma invading adjacent organs including the right kidney ➔, the liver ➔, and the inferior vena cava ➔.

N1 and M1

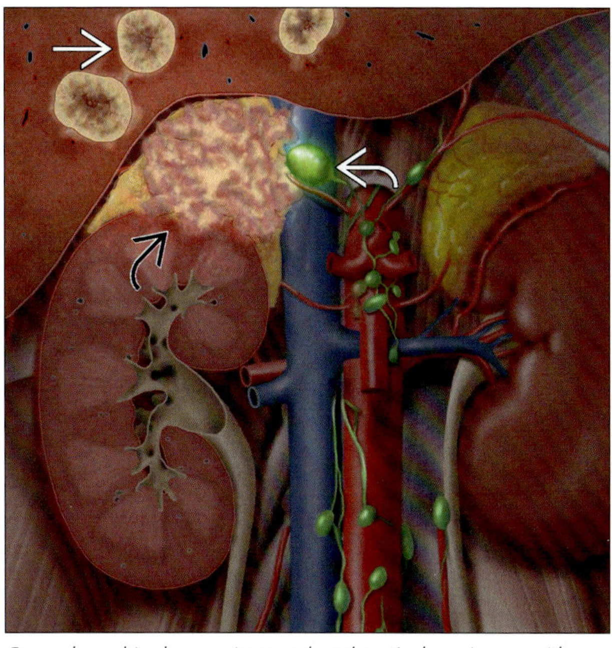

Coronal graphic shows primary adrenal cortical carcinoma with invasion into the adjacent kidney ➔. N1 and M1 disease with an enlarged paraaortic lymph node ➔ and multifocal hepatic metastases ➔ are also illustrated.

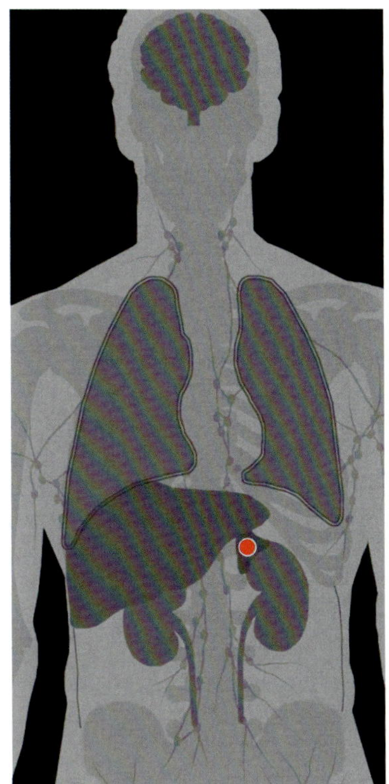

INITIAL SITE OF RECURRENCE

Local Failure (no RT)	79% (11/14)
Local Failure (RT)	14% (2/14)

Data from Fassnacht M et al: Efficacy of adjuvant radiotherapy of the tumor bed on local recurrence of adrenocortical carcinoma. J Clin Endocrinol Metab. 91(11):4501-4, 2006.

ADRENAL GLAND

OVERVIEW

General Comments

- AJCC staging system applies only to adrenal cortical carcinoma (ACC)
  - Adrenal medullary tumors such as pheochromocytoma and neuroblastoma are not included in this staging system

Classification

- Central: Catecholamine-producing medulla
- Peripheral: Steroid-secreting cortex functionally separate from medulla (different embryologic origin)
- Histological classification
  - Differentiated are usually functioning tumors
  - Anaplastic are rarely hormone producing
- Hormonal: ~ 60% hormone producing
  - Clinical syndromes with functioning tumors
    - Hypercortisolism: Cushing syndrome (30-40%, most common)
    - Adrenogenital syndrome
    - Virilization in females
    - Feminization in males
    - Precocious puberty
    - Hyperaldosteronism
    - Primary hyperaldosteronism: Conn syndrome

NATURAL HISTORY

General Features

- Comments
  - Large, solid, unilateral suprarenal mass
    - < 10% present bilaterally
      - Metastases may be bilateral in up to 50%
  - Poorly defined or invasive margins
  - Very heterogeneous lesions
    - Usually contain hemorrhagic, cystic, and calcific areas
  - Functioning tumors
    - Usually ≤ 5 cm at presentation
  - Nonfunctioning tumors
    - May be ≥ 10 cm at presentation
  - ACC
    - 95% are functioning
    - Aggressive; invades capsule and surrounding tissue
- Location
  - Adrenals are between kidney and diaphragmatic crura
  - Cortex or medulla (separate function and epidemiology)

Etiology

- Adrenal cortical
  - Unknown for sporadic adrenal carcinoma
  - Benign lesions and metastases much more common than primary adrenal cortical carcinoma
- Adrenal medullary
  - Chromaffin cells

Epidemiology & Cancer Incidence

- Rare malignant tumors, benign more common
  - Affects 1-2 persons/1,000,000 population
- Responsible for only 0.2% of annual cancer deaths in USA
- M:F approximately 1:1 (functional > women, nonfunctional > men)
- Median age
  - Bimodal occurrence
    - 1st peak < age 5
    - 2nd peak in 4th-5th decades of life
- Median age of ganglioneuroma and neuroblastoma 17 months

Genetics

- ACC
  - ↑ incidence of tumor in genetic syndromes
    - Beckwith-Wiedemann syndrome
      - Hemihypertrophy, neuroblastoma, Wilms tumor
      - ↑ secretion of insulin-like growth factor 2 (IGF-2)
    - Li-Fraumeni syndrome (breast Ca, soft tissue sarcoma (STS), brain tumors, and ACC)
      - ↑ breast Ca, STS, brain tumors, and ACC
      - Caused by mutations of tumor suppressor gene *p53*
    - Carney complex
      - Autodominant triad: Myxomas of heart and skin, hyperpigmentation, and endocrine overactivity
    - Multiple endocrine neoplasia 1 (MEN1) syndrome
      - ACC occurs in 25-40% of patients
      - Born 1 mutated *MEN1* gene, other copy becomes mutated allowing cells to form tumors
- Adrenal medullary tumors
  - Most MEN2 caused by a mutation in *RET* proto-oncogene, specific for neuronal crest cells, autosomal dominant
  - MEN2A
    - Bilateral pheochromocytoma, medullary thyroid Ca, and parathyroid hyperplasia
  - MEN2B
    - Pheochromocytoma, marfanoid, mucosal neuromas, medullary thyroid Ca
  - von Hippel-Lindau (VHL)
    - 25% have pheochromocytoma
    - Mutation in *VHL* gene results alters hypoxia inducible factor 1A

Gross Pathology & Surgical Features

- Usually large & predominantly yellow on cut surface
- Necrotic, hemorrhagic, calcific, lipoid, & cystic areas

Microscopic Pathology

- H&E
  - No absolute histologic criteria for malignancy
    - Documented distant metastases &/or local invasion required for definitive diagnosis
  - Weiss histopathologic system is most commonly used; ≥ 3 of the 9 criteria predict malignant clinical behavior
    - Nuclear grade III or IV, based on Fuhrman criteria
    - Mitotic rate > 5 per 50 high-power fields (HPF)
    - Atypical mitotic figures
    - ≥ 25% clear cells
    - > 1/3 diffuse architecture
    - Necrosis
    - Venous invasion
    - Sinusoid invasion
    - Invasion of tumor capsule
- Special stains

- MIB-1: Cell cycle-associated marker ↑ in ACC

Routes of Spread

- Local invasion
  - Only 30% confined to adrenal gland at presentation
    - Almost 20% present with IVC involvement
  - Common to spread via extracapsular infiltration locally into adjacent organs, including
    - Kidney
    - Diaphragm
    - Great vessels
      - Commonly extends into IVC
      - May occlude adjacent vessels
    - Pancreas
    - Spleen
    - Liver
    - Bone
- Lymphatic metastases
  - Regional lymph nodes
    - Paraaortic/retroperitoneal nodes
- Hematogenous metastases
  - > 30% present with metastases, commonly to
    - Liver
    - Lung

IMAGING

Detection

- **CT**
  - Study of choice to differentiate benign from malignant adrenal mass
  - Solid > 5 cm adrenal mass
    - If < 5 cm, ACC is usually functioning
    - < 3 cm lesions are probably benign, if no history of primary malignancy
  - Irregular margins
  - ± necrosis and calcification
    - Calcification seen in up to 30%
    - Variable enhancement due to necrosis & hemorrhage
  - Usually unilateral, may be bilateral
  - On NECT, mean attenuation of adrenal carcinoma tends to be > mean attenuation of adenoma
    - Some overlap in attenuation between carcinoma and adenoma on NECT and 60-sec CECT
  - 10-minute delayed CECT
    - Significantly less washout of adrenal carcinomas than that seen in adenomas
      - Typically < 40% washout in carcinomas compared to > 50% washout for adenomas
- **MR**
  - T1WI: Hypointense adrenal mass compared to liver
    - T1 (in phase and out of phase [OOP]): No significant loss of signal on OOP imaging to suggest adrenal adenoma
      - Pitfall: ACC may contain foci of intracytoplasmic lipid
      - Loss of signal may be seen in small portions of mass
    - Hemorrhagic byproducts may produce ↑ T1 signal intensity (SI)
  - T2WI: Hyperintense heterogeneous adrenal mass compared to liver
    - Necrosis may contribute to ↑ T2 SI
  - T1 C+: Heterogeneous enhancement due to variable necrosis
    - Multiplanar imaging shows vascular invasion into renal vein, IVC, and adjacent solid organs such as kidney
    - Coronal imaging very good for showing IVC invasion
- **Ultrasound**
  - Best imaging tool for initial screening
  - Grayscale ultrasound
    - Small tumors: Echo pattern similar to renal cortex
    - Large tumors: Mixed heterogeneous echo pattern with hypoechoic/anechoic areas (due to necrosis & hemorrhage)
    - "Scar" sign: Complex, predominately echogenic pattern with radiating linear echoes
      - When seen in large adrenal mass, suggestive of adrenal carcinoma
    - Enlarged regional and paraaortic lymph nodes are reliable sign of malignancy
    - Large tumor may cause compression/mass effect on upper pole and anterior surface of adjacent kidney
    - US cannot reliably differentiate between adrenal carcinoma, adrenal adenoma, & neuroblastoma
  - Color Doppler
    - Invasion or occlusion of adrenal vein, renal vein, and IVC
    - Visualization of intraluminal tumor thrombus ± vascularity
- **Nuclear medicine**
  - FDG PET
    - Increased FDG uptake in adrenal carcinoma
    - Adenoma demonstrates limited FDG uptake
    - Not useful to differentiate ACC from mets, lymphoma, or pheochromocytoma
- **Angiography**
  - Historically used to assess renal vein and IVC involvement
  - Replaced by noninvasive imaging including Doppler US, MR, and CT angiography

Staging

- CT
  - T stage
    - Cross-sectional diameter
    - Extracapsular tumor invasion
    - Patency of adjacent vessels
    - IVC extension
  - N stage
    - Assess local nodal size
  - M stage
    - Liver, bone, and lung lesions
  - Important to perform venous-phase imaging through base of heart
    - Evaluate for renal vein and IVC invasion
- MR
  - Best contrast resolution to determine local extension to adjacent organs and vascular involvement
  - Adds specificity to CT characterization

Restaging

- CT
  - Local recurrence, liver and lung metastases

- Because liver and lung are most common sites for metastases, may be able to image chest and abdomen only with CECT
- Contrast-enhanced ultrasound
  - Microbubble enhancement may add sensitivity for detection of hepatic metastases < 1 cm
    - Early enhancement compared to normal liver parenchyma
  - Hypoechoic and sharply marginated lesions
- MR
  - May have increased sensitivity for small hepatic metastases
- FDG PET/CT
  - May be very useful for detection of local recurrence and distant metastases

CLINICAL PRESENTATION & WORK-UP

Presentation

- Non-hormonally active
  - Abdominal pain, fullness, and palpable mass
  - Early satiety, pain, weakness, fever
  - Incidentally discovered mass on imaging study
  - Presence of metastases
- Hormonally active
  - ~ 60% of patients present with symptoms of excessive hormone secretion
  - Cushing syndrome due to ↑ cortisol
    - Most common presentation in symptomatic patients
      - Moon facies
      - Truncal obesity
      - Purple skin striae
      - Buffalo hump
  - Female virilization or male feminization due to ↑ androgens or estrogens
    - Most common presentation in children
    - Virilization present in 95% of functioning childhood tumors
  - Conn syndrome (primary hyperaldosteronism)
    - Hypertension & weakness
  - Other clinical syndromes
    - Hypoglycemia, polycythemia, & non-glucocorticoid-related insulin resistance
  - Pheochromocytoma
    - Labile hypertension, MI, CVA
    - Headache, diaphoresis, tachycardia
    - Pallor, palpitations, panic attacks, weakness

Prognosis

- All stages ACC 5-year overall survival (OS) 20-25%
- Radical surgical excision only method by which long-term disease-free survival achieved
  - Recurrence in 70-80% after resection
  - Overall 5-year survival for tumors resected with curative intent ~ 40%
- Stage IV survival usually < 9 months
- Poor prognostic factors
  - Age > 55 at presentation
  - Positive resection margins
  - Lymph node positive disease
  - Tumor size and stage
  - Poorly differentiated primary tumor
  - Distant metastases at presentation
  - Invasion of contiguous organ requiring resection

Work-Up

- Clinical
  - H&P look for abdominal mass and evidence hormone or catecholamine secretion
- Radiographic
  - CT or MR abdomen with thin cuts through adrenal
  - PET may help distinguish benign versus malignant
  - Chest CT
  - MIBG if suspect neuroblastoma
- Laboratory
  - CBC, CMP, UA, serum and urine cortisol and catecholamines
  - Bone marrow biopsy for neuroblastoma

TREATMENT

Major Treatment Alternatives

- Radical surgical excision for early stage disease with curative intent
- If metastatic and functioning, removal of primary tumor and metastatic disease for palliation of symptoms

Major Treatment Roadblocks/ Contraindications

- 30% metastatic at presentation

Treatment Options by Stage

- Stage I & II: Radical surgical excision
  - Adjuvant radiation or chemotherapy not demonstrated to improve survival
  - Adjuvant RT recommended for positive margins
- Stage III: Radical surgical excision ± lymph node dissection
  - Clinical trial enrollment recommended for patients with regional lymphadenopathy
  - Possible role for radiation therapy in localized but unresectable disease
  - Adjuvant RT recommended
  - Mitotane may be indicated if radiographically measurable metastases identified
- Stage IV
  - Radical surgical excision
  - Mitotane
  - Radiation therapy (local control)
  - Surgical resection of functioning localized metastases
  - Clinical trials using cisplatin and other agents
- RT adrenal CA or metastasis
  - 50-60 Gy gross disease, 45-54 Gy high-risk microscopic disease (regional nodes, positive margins), palliative 30-40 Gy 2.5-3 Gy fx, SBRT dose/ fx being studied (various schedules published)
- Neuroblastoma, based on Children's Oncology Group (COG) risk grouping
  - Low risk, 3-year OS > 90%
    - Surgery
      - GTR = observation
      - STR or recurrence = multi-agent chemo
      - Stable 4S patients = observation after biopsy
  - Intermediate risk, 3-year OS 70-90%

- Maximal safe resection with lymphadenectomy
  - Chemo
  - Partial response to chemo then 2nd-look surgery
- High risk, 3-year OS 30%
  - High-dose chemo, maximal safe resection, high-dose chemo followed by bone marrow transplant (± total body irradiation [TBI])
  - RT to postchemo presurgical tumor with 2 cm margin + metastatic sites
    - RT typically 21.6 Gy to areas at risk and metastatic sites, with 14.4 Gy boost to gross disease at primary site
  - 13-cis retinoic acid given for 6 months
  - Current COG protocol evaluating addition of anti-GD2 monoclonal antibody therapy

Dose Response

- Considered a radiation sensitive tumor

Organs at Risk Parameters

- Adults
  - Liver mean < 30-32 Gy, and < 28 Gy if Child-Pugh class A, or HCC
  - Kidney (bilateral) mean < 15-18 Gy, V20 < 32%
  - Small bowel (peritoneal cavity) V45 < 195 mL
- Peds
  - Liver 50% < 9 Gy and 75% < 18 Gy
  - Kidney ipsilateral 100% max = 14.4 Gy and 50% < 19.8 Gy; contralateral kidney 50% < 8 Gy and 80% < 12 Gy
  - Total lung max 2/3 < 15 Gy

RECOMMENDED FOLLOW-UP

Clinical

- Exam every 3 months x 1 year, then every 6 months until year 5, then annually; PFTs at year 1 (NB)

Radiographic

- Adrenal tumors
  - Consider 2 years of CT imaging after removal of adrenal nodules
    - Every 3 months for 1st year
    - Every 6 months for 2nd year
- Neuroblastoma
  - Tumor imaging (CT or MR), bone scan, and MIBG (NB); MUGA years 1 and 5 if Adriamycin used

Laboratory

- Urine/serum catecholamines, CBC every 3 months x 1 year, then every 6 months until years 3-5; TSH/T4 at year 1

SELECTED REFERENCES

1. American Joint Committee on Cancer: AJCC Cancer Staging Manual. 7th ed. New York: Springer. 515-20, 2010
2. Bauditz J et al: Improved detection of hepatic metastases of adrenocortical cancer by contrast-enhanced ultrasound. Oncol Rep. 19(5):1135-9, 2008
3. Bilimoria KY et al: Adrenocortical carcinoma in the United States: treatment utilization and prognostic factors. Cancer. 113(11):3130-6, 2008
4. Fareau GG et al: Diagnostic challenges in adrenocortical carcinoma: recommendations for surveillance after surgical resection of selected adrenal nodules. Endocr Pract. 13(6):636-41, 2007
5. Leboulleux S et al: Diagnostic and prognostic value of 18-fluorodeoxyglucose positron emission tomography in adrenocortical carcinoma: a prospective comparison with computed tomography. J Clin Endocrinol Metab. 91(3):920-5, 2006
6. Mackie GC et al: Use of [18F]fluorodeoxyglucose positron emission tomography in evaluating locally recurrent and metastatic adrenocortical carcinoma. J Clin Endocrinol Metab. 91(7):2665-71, 2006
7. Szolar DH et al: Adrenocortical carcinomas and adrenal pheochromocytomas: mass and enhancement loss evaluation at delayed contrast-enhanced CT. Radiology. 234(2):479-85, 2005
8. Elsayes KM et al: Adrenal masses: mr imaging features with pathologic correlation. Radiographics. 24 Suppl 1:S73-86, 2004
9. Marcus KJ et al: Primary tumor control in patients with stage 3/4 unfavorable neuroblastoma treated with tandem double autologous stem cell transplants. J Pediatr Hematol Oncol. 25(12):934-40, 2003
10. Aubert S et al: Weiss system revisited: a clinicopathologic and immunohistochemical study of 49 adrenocortical tumors. Am J Surg Pathol. 26(12):1612-9, 2002
11. Lockhart ME et al: Imaging of adrenal masses. Eur J Radiol. 41(2):95-112, 2002
12. Matthay KK et al: Treatment of high-risk neuroblastoma with intensive chemotherapy, radiotherapy, autologous bone marrow transplantation, and 13-cis-retinoic acid. Children's Cancer Group. N Engl J Med. 341(16):1165-73, 1999

*(**Left**) Axial T2WI MR demonstrates a well-circumscribed T2 dark adrenal nodule ➔, measuring < 3 cm. (**Right**) Coronal T1WI MR shows a T1 dark, well-circumscribed right adrenal nodule ➔. There is a clear fat plane between the nodule and the adjacent kidney ➔ and liver ➔.*

Stage I (T1 N0 M0)

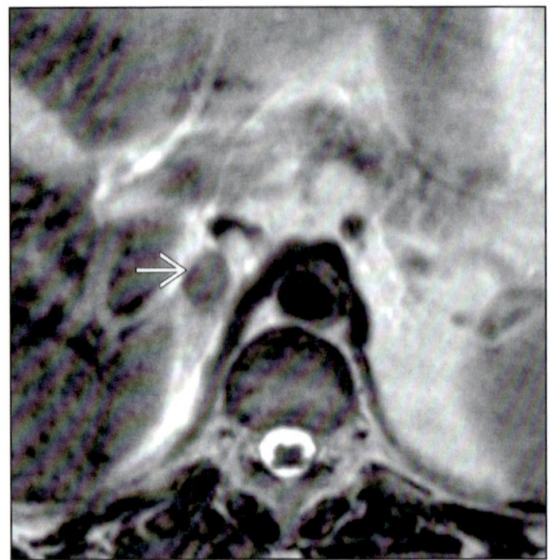

Stage I (T1 N0 M0)

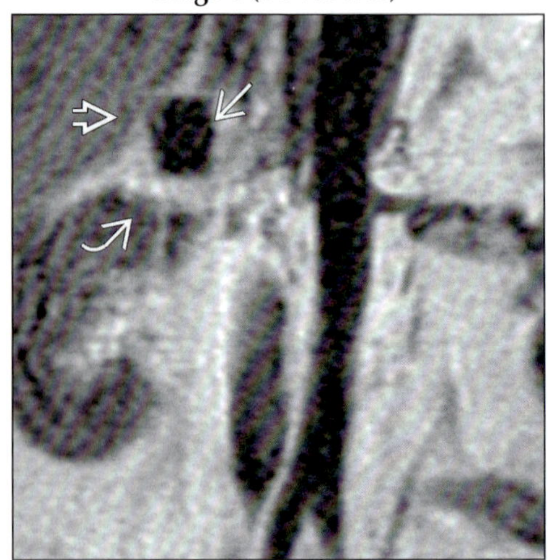

*(**Left**) Axial T1WI MR in the same patient demonstrates that the nodule gains signal intensity ➔ on the out-of-phase imaging (bottom) compared to the in-phase ➔ imaging (top). A benign adrenal nodule would lose signal on the out-of-phase imaging. (**Right**) Gross image shows the well-circumscribed rubbery adrenal mass ➔ corresponding to the lesion seen in the preceding MR images.*

Stage I (T1 N0 M0)

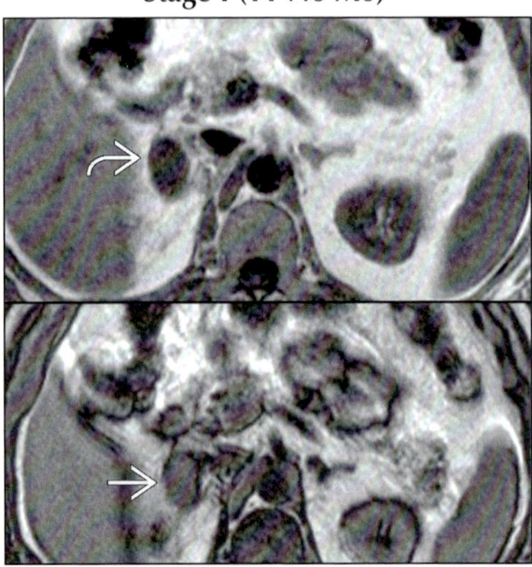

Stage I (T1 N0 M0)

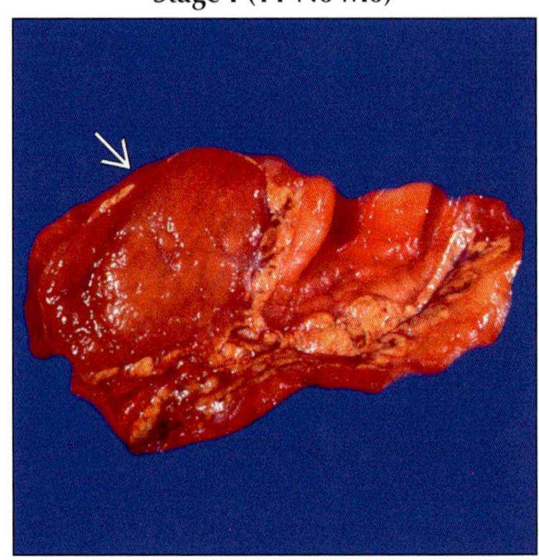

*(**Left**) Multimodality imaging can be very helpful for characterizing tumor margins for preoperative staging. This CECT demonstrates a large (> 5 cm), heterogeneous left adrenal mass ➔ that appears very well circumscribed in a 30-year-old woman presenting with Cushing syndrome. (**Right**) Coronal T1WI C+ MR in the same patient suggests that an intact plane is present between the mass and the adjacent kidney ➔. This was confirmed on resection.*

Stage II (T2 N0 M0)

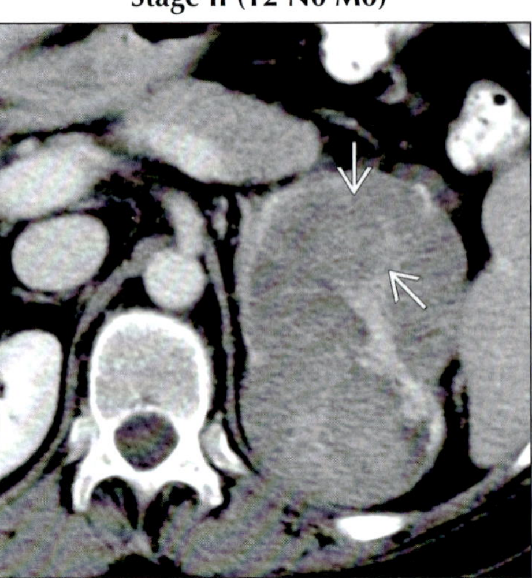

Stage II (T2 N0 M0)

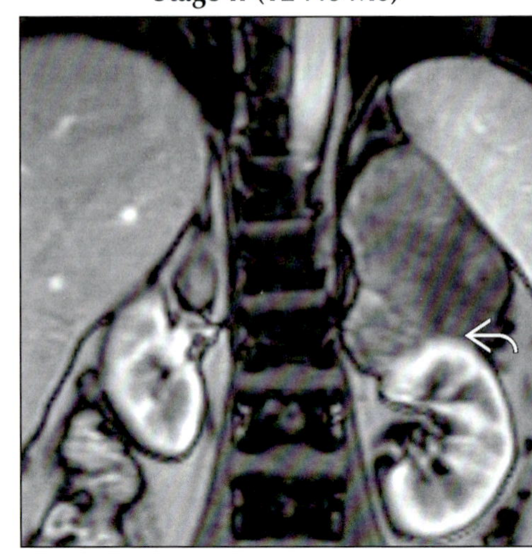

Stage III (T3 N0 M0)

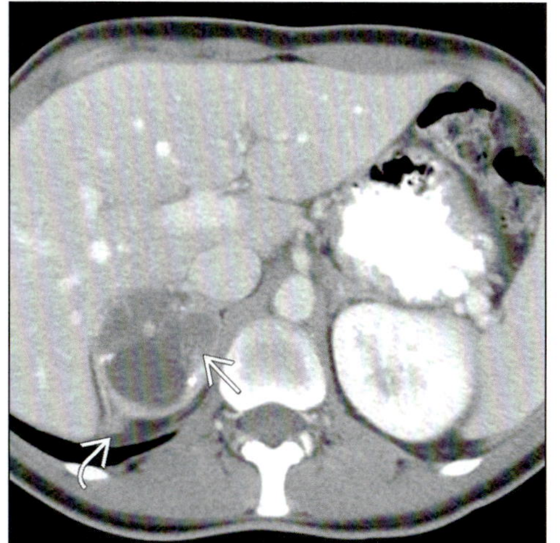

Stage III (T3 N0 M0)

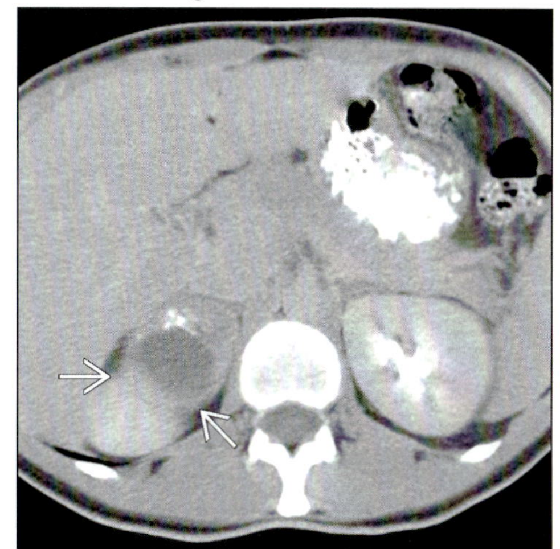

*(**Left**) Axial CECT in the same patient shows a suggestion of soft tissue nodularity and infiltration in the adjacent fat, which would indicate T3 disease. An intact plane is difficult to appreciate, but it is present between the mass ➔ and the liver ➔. (**Right**) Delayed CECT in the same patient illustrates the difficulty of documenting an intact plane between the mass and the kidney ➔, especially on delayed CECT.*

Stage III (T3 N0 M0)

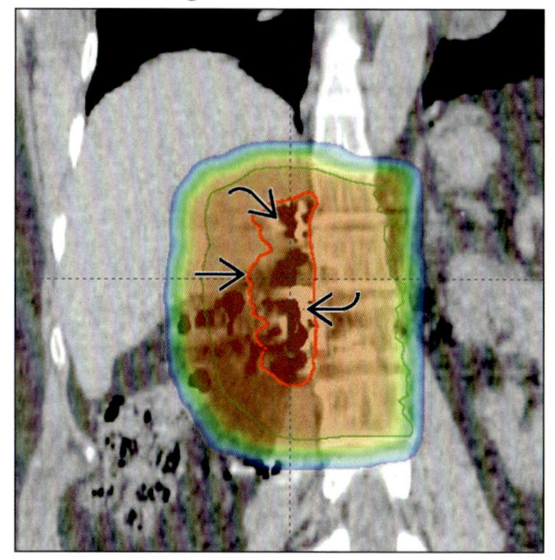

Stage III (T3 N0 M0)

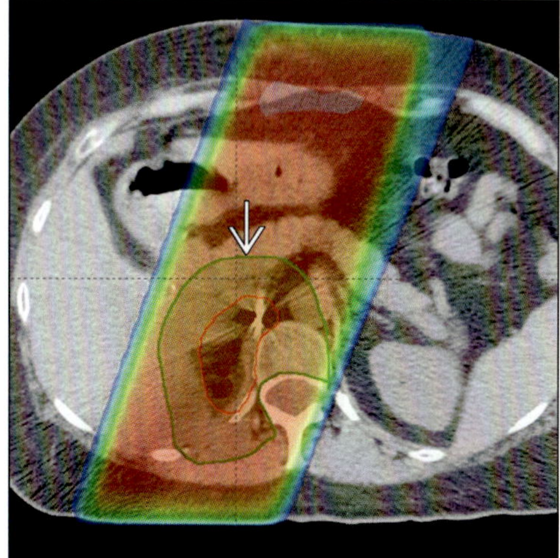

*(**Left**) Coronal CT demonstrates the CTV ➔ outlining the resection bed in a 62 year old after removal of an 8 cm adrenal cortical tumor with positive margins. Surgical clips are seen within the CTV ➔. Patient received 45 Gy in 25 fractions. (**Right**) Axial CT shows the PTV in green ➔. Oblique fields were used to reduce dose to liver. Since the spinal cord was treated to tolerance, an image-guided boost was performed with SBRT for an additional 15 Gy in 6 fractions.*

Stage III (T3 N0 M0)

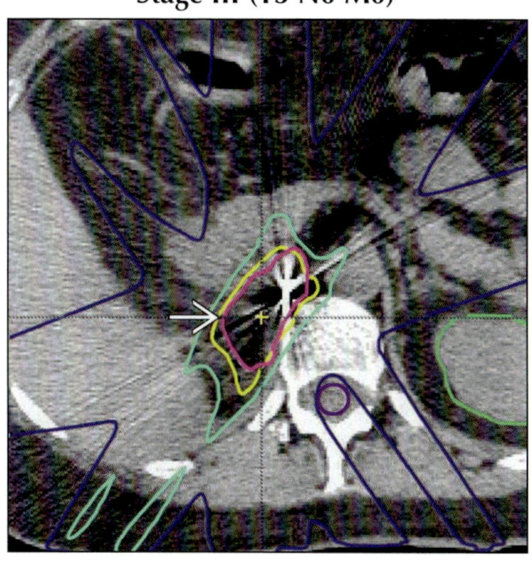

Stage IV (T4 NX M1)

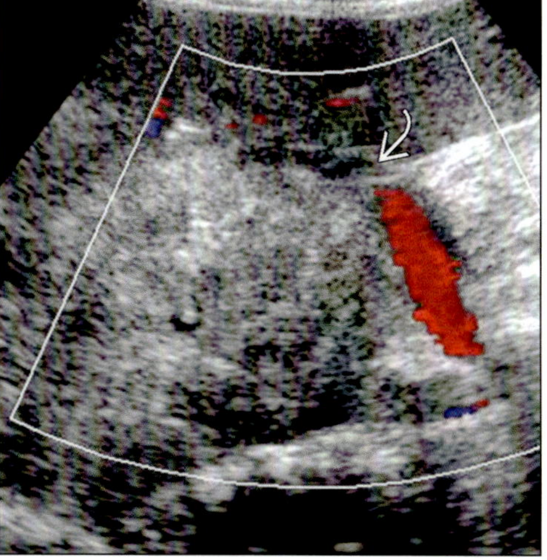

*(**Left**) Axial CT in the same patient demonstrates image-guided boost. Total dose was 60 Gy. PTV ➔ is shown along with the 95%, 70%, and 10% isodose lines. (**Right**) Longitudinal color Doppler ultrasound reveals the extrinsic compression of the inferior vena cava ➔. US can also be useful for identifying hepatic metastases.*

*(**Left**) Axial CECT shows large, partially necrotic, heterogeneous adrenal mass with infiltration beyond the adrenal capsule into perinephric space. Infiltration into the right diaphragm makes this T4 disease. No distinct plane is between the mass and adjacent liver. (**Right**) More caudal axial CECT demonstrates inferior extension of intraluminal tumor thrombus within the IVC. Small nodes do not meet CT criteria for pathologic enlargement.*

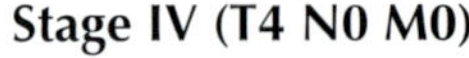

Stage IV (T4 N0 M0)

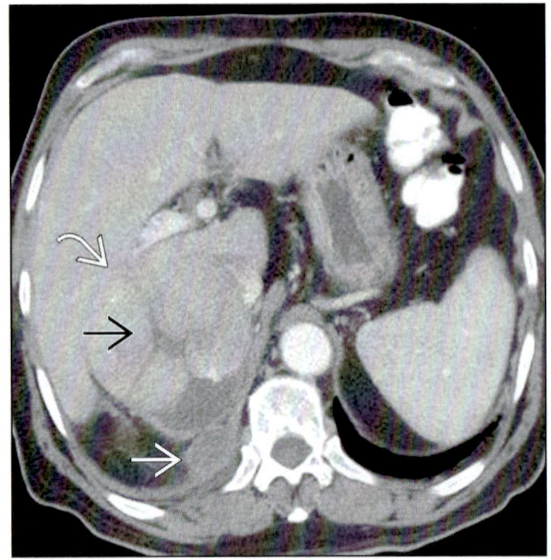

Stage IV (T4 N0 M0)

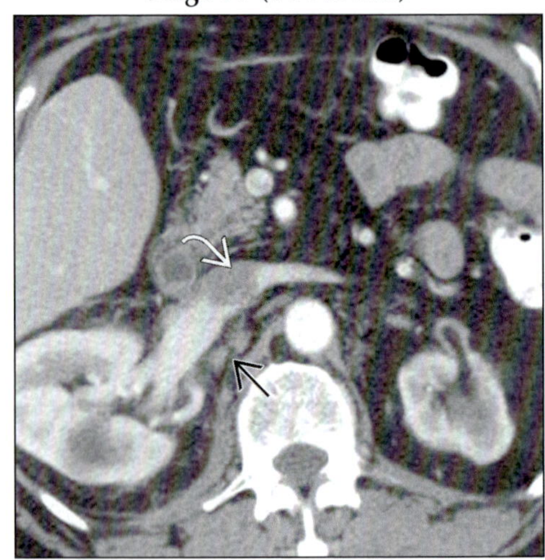

*(**Left**) Scout image from CT demonstrates calcifications in a right upper quadrant mass. Hepatic flexure is inferiorly displaced by the inferior displacement of the right kidney. (**Right**) Axial arterial phase CECT demonstrates the very large, well-circumscribed right adrenal mass with central calcifications. An enlarged paraaortic lymph node is consistent with N1 disease, upstaging this patient's disease to stage IV.*

Stage IV (T3 N1 M0)

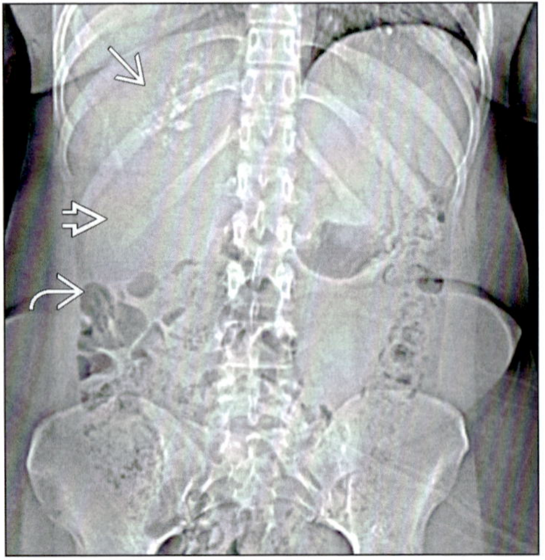

Stage IV (T3 N1 M0)

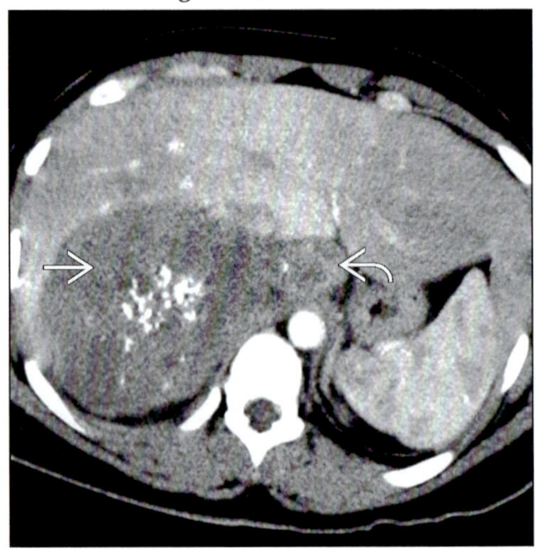

*(**Left**) Coronal MIP image in the same patient demonstrates the inferior displacement of the right kidney. Intact planes are present between the mass and adjacent organs, but large local nodal metastases are present. (**Right**) Gross image demonstrates the clean plane between the mass and adjacent kidney, as well as the metastatic lymph nodes.*

Stage IV (T3 N1 M0)

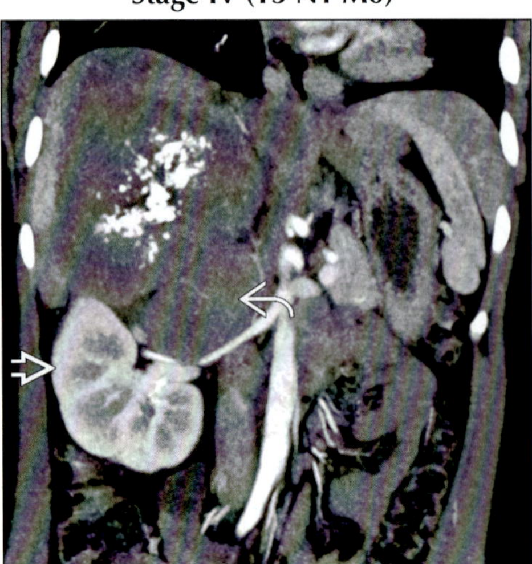

Stage IV (T3 N1 M0)

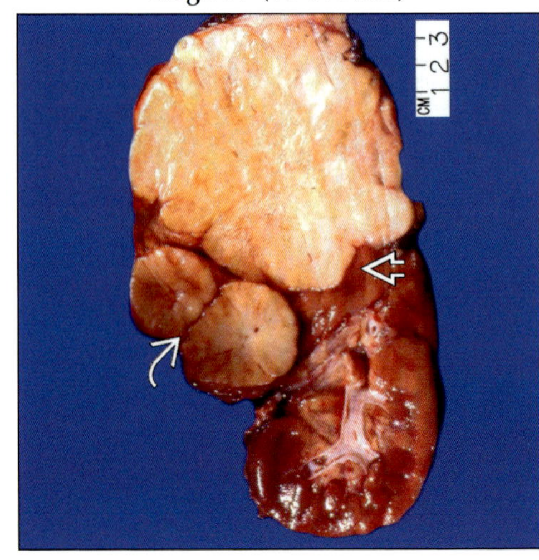

Stage IV (T4 N1 M0)

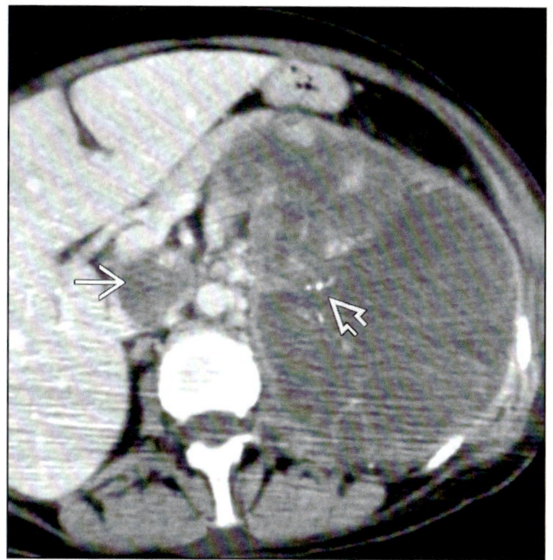

Stage IV (T4 N1 M0)

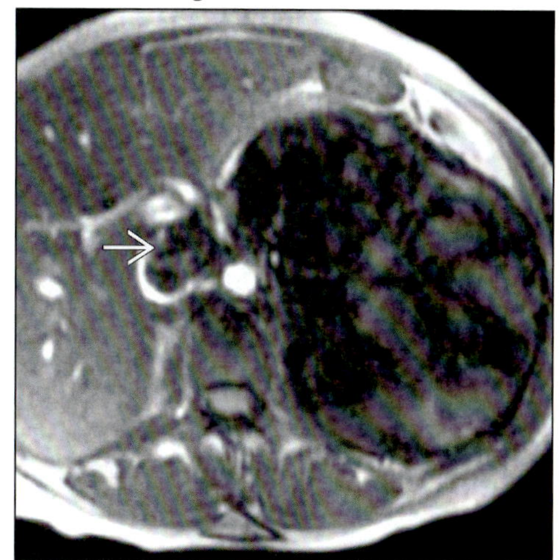

(Left) *This axial CECT demonstrates a large tumor in the left pararenal space. The center of the mass is low attenuation, with calcifications* ➨*. Tumor thrombus* ➨ *in the infrahepatic inferior vena cava makes this a T4 lesion.* ***(Right)*** *Axial T1WI C+ MR in the same patient demonstrates the large, heterogeneously low T1 signal intensity mass in the left perirenal space with IVC thrombus* ➨ *of the same low signal intensity.*

Stage IV (T4 N1 M0)

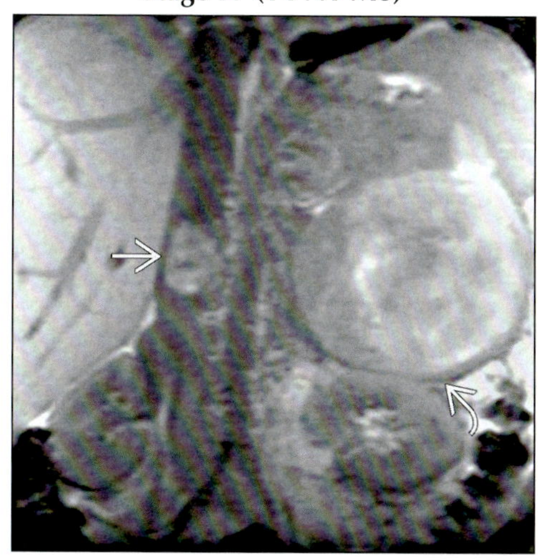

Stage IV (T4 N1 M0)

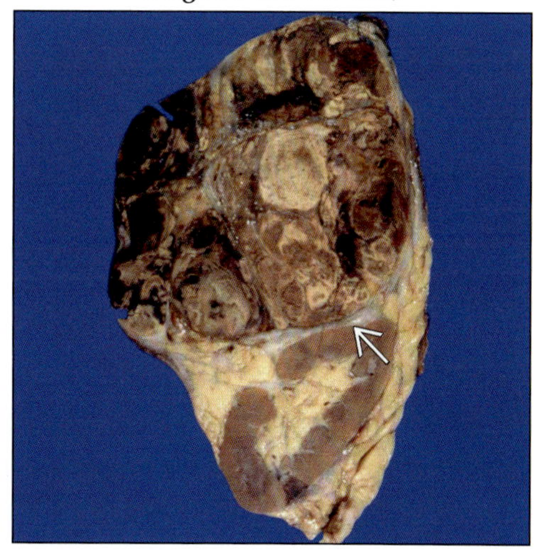

(Left) *Coronal T1WI MR in the same patient shows, more convincingly, the tumor thrombus* ➨ *in the IVC. The left kidney is displaced inferiorly; however, there appears to be an intact plane* ➨ *between the mass and the kidney.* ***(Right)*** *Gross image shows the heterogeneously solid and necrotic left adrenal carcinoma. A fibrous capsule* ➨ *separates the mass from the adjacent kidney, corresponding to the findings on MR. The IVC invasion was confirmed at resection.*

Stage IV (T4 N1 M1)

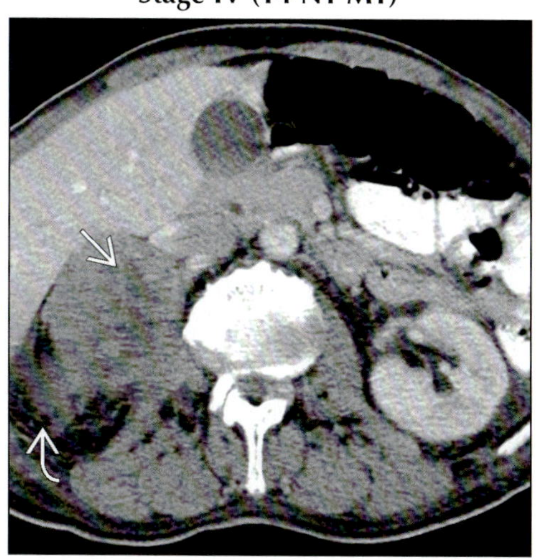

Stage IV (T4 N1 M1)

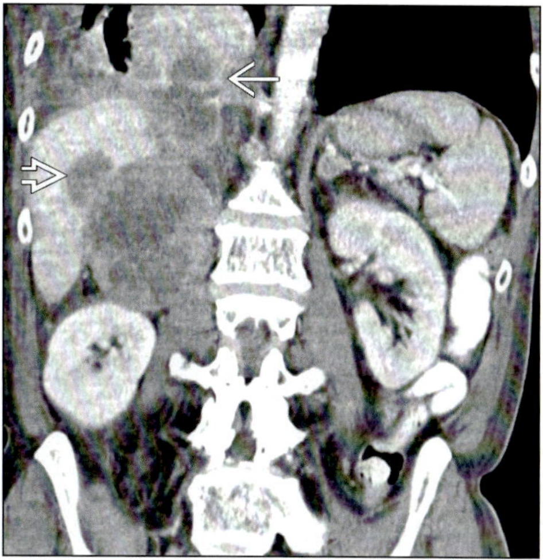

(Left) *Axial CECT reveals a large, heterogeneous right adrenal mass* ➨ *with infiltration* ➨ *of the surrounding fat, well demonstrated on the CT.* ***(Right)*** *Coronal image shows both the hepatic metastasis* ➨ *that may have arisen from direct tumor invasion and invasion of the tumor through the diaphragm to involve the right lung base* ➨*. This constitutes unresectable disease.*

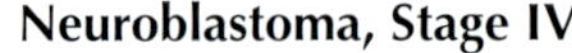

Neuroblastoma, Stage IV

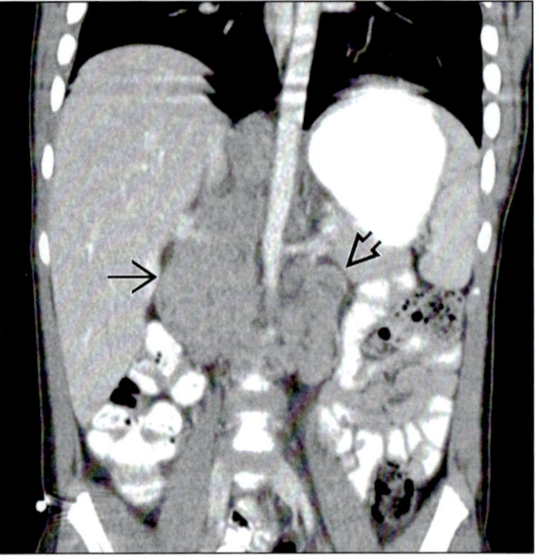

Neuroblastoma, Stage IV

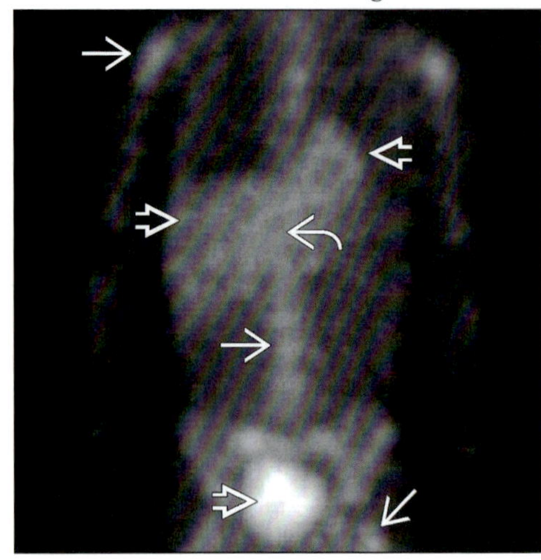

(Left) *Coronal CECT shows a large neuroblastoma arising from the right adrenal gland and spreading across midline in a 4 year old with positive bone marrow and MIBG.* ***(Right)*** *MIBG SPECT demonstrates abnormal radionuclide in proximal humeri, bony pelvis, entire spine, and proximal femurs. Physiologic uptake is seen in the myocardium, liver, spleen and urinary tract. There is abnormal uptake in the right suprarenal and mid abdominal mass.*

Neuroblastoma, Stage IV

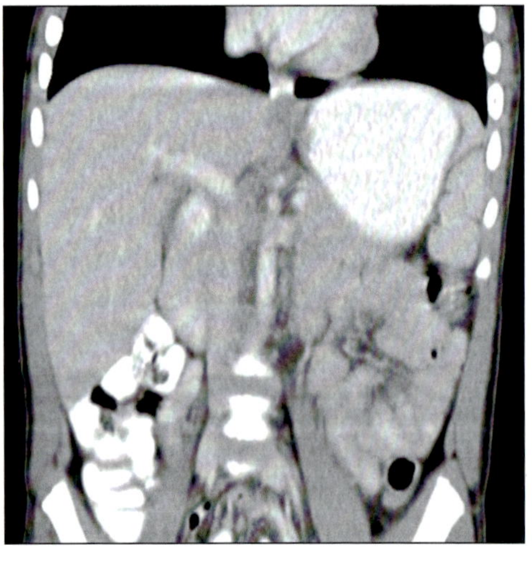

Neuroblastoma, Stage IV

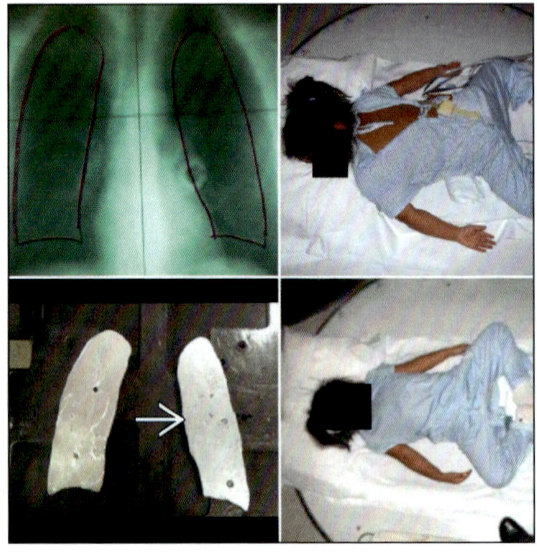

(Left) *Coronal CT 3 months after induction chemotherapy shows a good response. Patient underwent high-dose chemotherapy with stem cell transplant, 12 Gy total body irradiation in 6 fx b.i.d. followed by a "tandem" transplant, and 10.8 Gy postop radiation to the surgical bed.* ***(Right)*** *This patient is positioned for AP/PA total body irradiation at an extended distance from the head of the accelerator. Custom lung blocks are designed to partially attenuate the dose to the lungs.*

Neuroblastoma, Stage IV

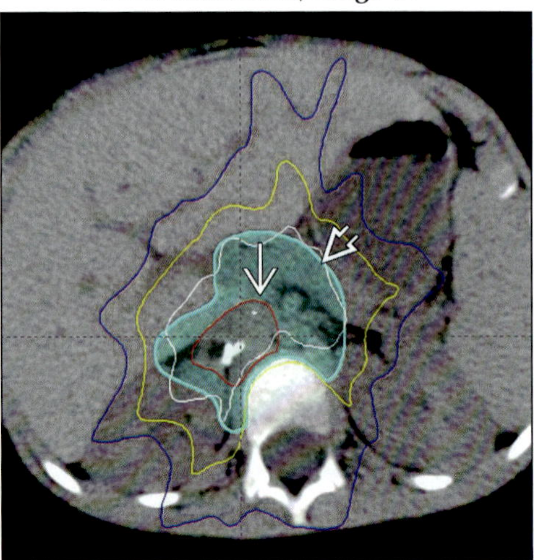

Neuroblastoma, Stage IV

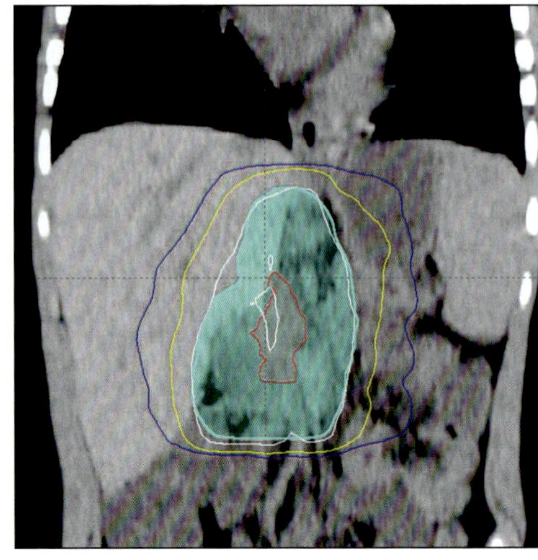

(Left) *Axial CT shows a 7-field IMRT boost plan delivering 10.8 Gy in 6 fractions. The GTV and PTV are shown, as well as the 95%, 70%, and 50% isodose lines, respectively. Note the dose uniformity delivered to the vertebral body to minimize the risk of an abnormal curvature later in life.* ***(Right)*** *Coronal CT shows good conformality of the 95% isodose line to the PTV. In children, it is particularly important to limit dose to OAR.*

SBRT: Isolated Metastasis

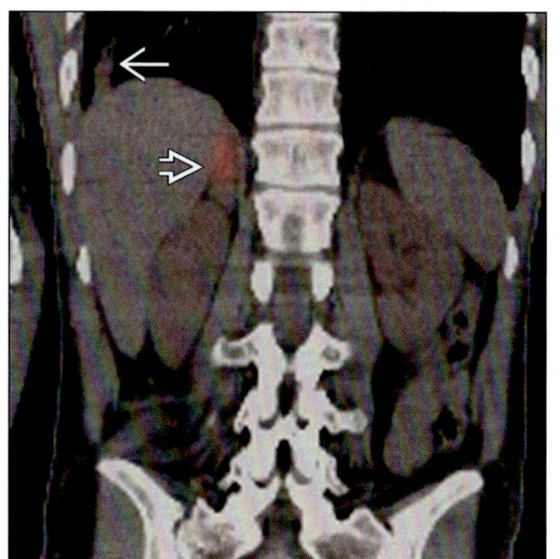

SBRT: Isolated Metastasis

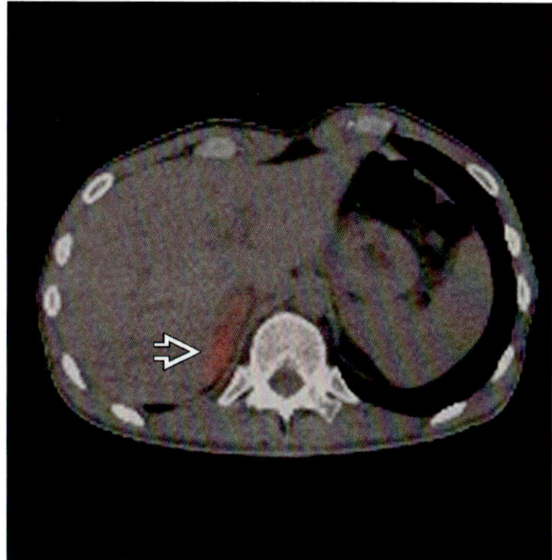

(Left) *Coronal fused PET/CT reveals a 4.7 cm adrenal metastasis ➡ from non-small cell lung cancer (NSCLC) with an SUV of 12.5. The patient had previously been treated to the left lower lung (LLL) with RT, and fibrosis ➡ is evident that is not FDG avid.* ***(Right)*** *Axial fused PET/CT shows diffuse replacement of the right adrenal gland ➡.*

SBRT: Isolated Metastasis

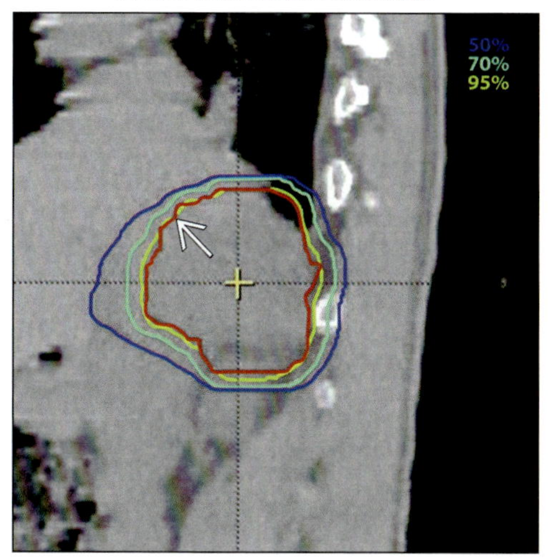

SBRT: Isolated Metastasis

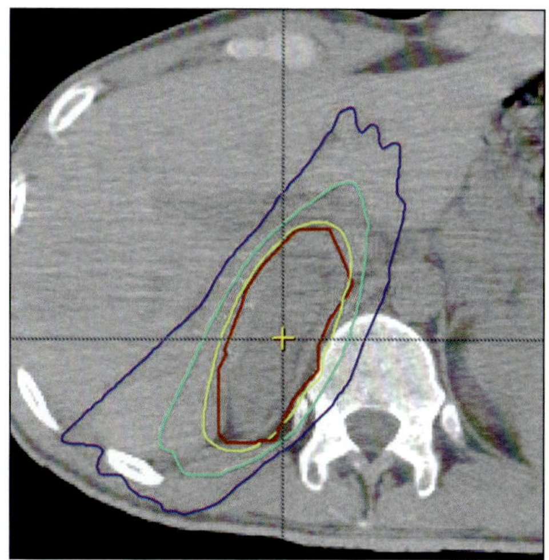

(Left) *Coronal CT shows the PTV and coverage by the 95%, 70%, and 50% isodose lines ➡. Excellent conformality was achieved in the coronal plane. Total dose was 36 Gy in 3 fractions.* ***(Right)*** *Axial CT displays the dynamic conformal co-planar arc plan. The arc was divided into 3 segments to minimize dose to the liver and kidneys.*

Isolated Metastasis from NSCLC

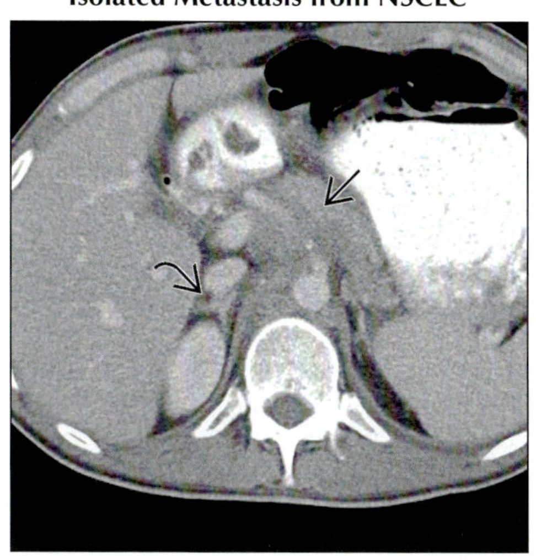

Stage IV (T4 NX M1)

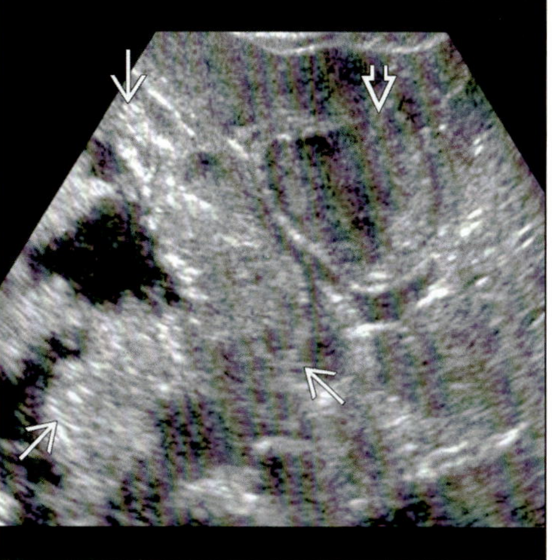

(Left) *Axial CECT 4 months later reveals a complete response to the adrenal lesion ➡; however, extensive retroperitoneal adenopathy ➡ was identified.* ***(Right)*** *Transverse transabdominal ultrasound demonstrates both the large, centrally necrotic adrenal carcinoma ➡ and a well-defined hepatic metastasis ➡ adjacent to the carcinoma.*

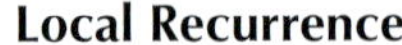

Local Recurrence

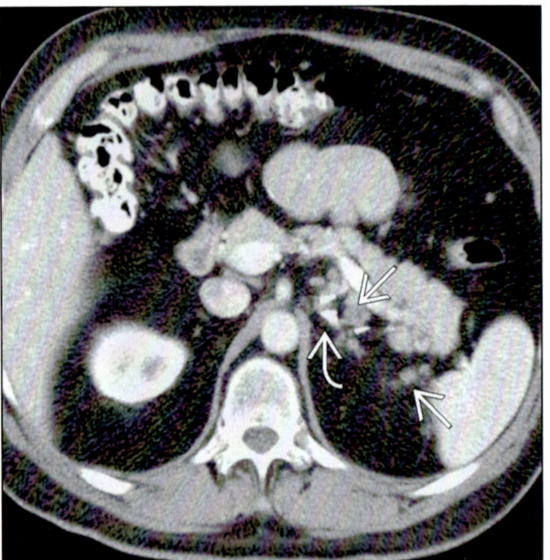

Local Recurrence

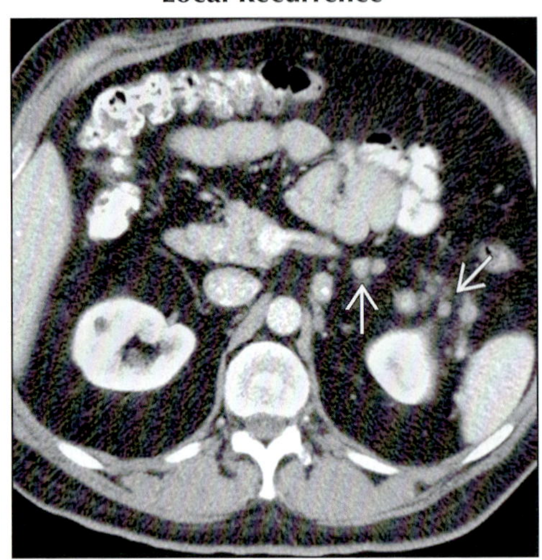

(Left) *CECT demonstrates surgical clips ➔ in the region of the left adrenal gland. Soft tissue nodules stud the surgical bed and left perinephric space ➔. This patient had undergone a left adrenalectomy 1 year prior for a 3 cm lesion.* ***(Right)*** *More inferior image demonstrates numerous soft tissue nodules ➔ studding the left perinephric space. When the patient's serum cortisol began rising, repeat imaging was obtained, demonstrating the recurrence.*

Local Recurrence

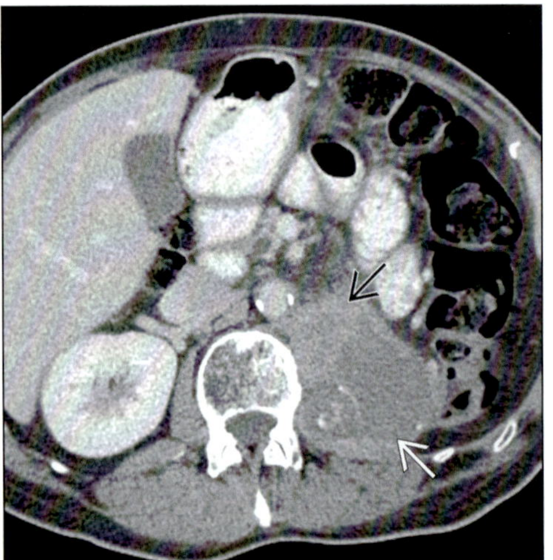

Local Recurrence

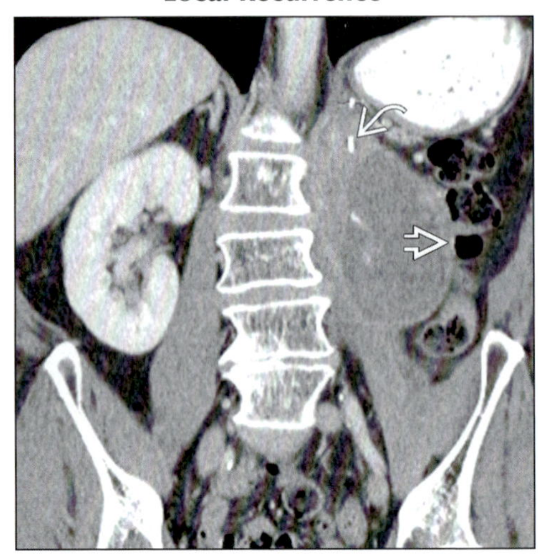

(Left) *CECT shows a cystic ➔ and solid ➔ mass in the left adrenal bed. Recurrence developed 1 year after adrenalectomy for a 5 cm lesion. After an uncomplicated postoperative course, back pain developed prompting further work-up.* ***(Right)*** *Coronal CECT in the same patient shows the extensive local recurrence. No discernible tissue plane is identified between the mass and the adjacent descending colon ➔. Surgical clips ➔ from adrenalectomy are present.*

Local Recurrence

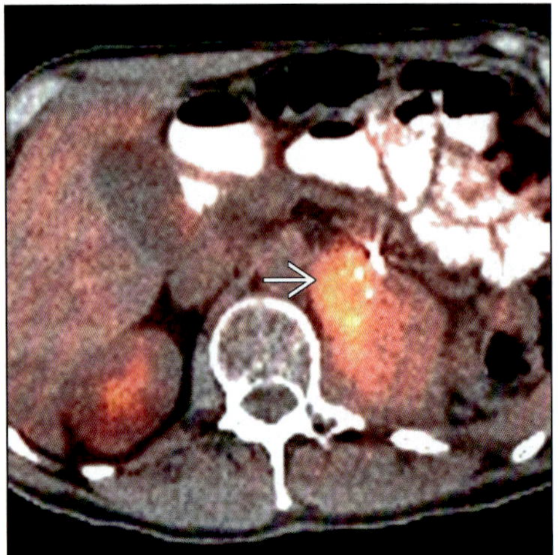

Local Recurrence

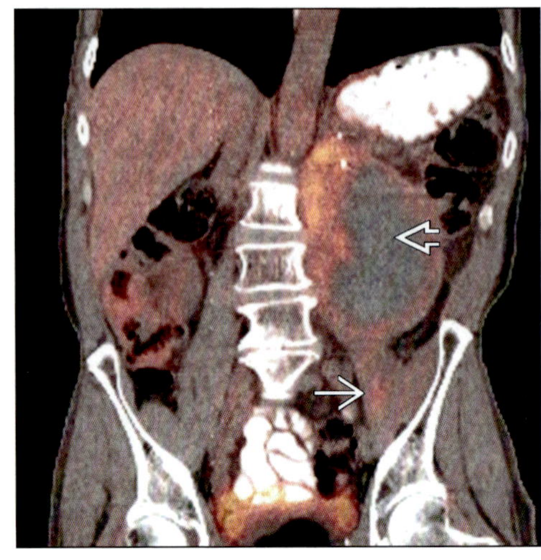

(Left) *PET/CT in the same patient demonstrates high metabolic activity in the solid components of the tumor ➔. Streak artifact is present from the adrenalectomy clips. PET/CT was obtained to evaluate for metastases distant from the surgical bed, none of which were found.* ***(Right)*** *The necrotic center ➔ of the recurrent tumor is not metabolically active. There is mild increased F18 FDG activity in the left psoas muscle ➔, raising a concern for local infiltration.*

Metastatic Disease

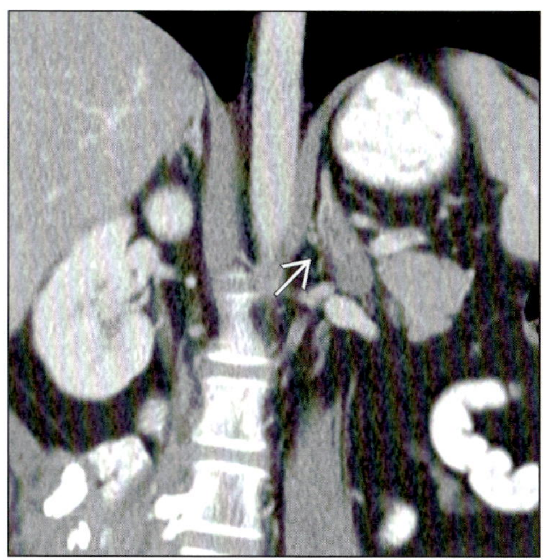

Metastatic Disease

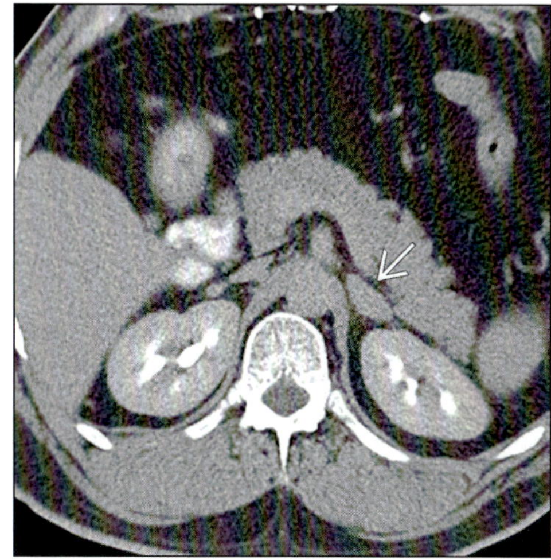

(Left) *Coronal CECT shows an enlarged left adrenal gland ➔ that was too dense on precontrast images and displayed late enhancement. Hence, metastatic disease was highly suspected. Patient had previously undergone a hip disarticulation for an epithelioid hemangioendothelioma. Biopsy confirmed recurrence.* ***(Right)*** *Axial CECT in the same patient shows enlarged adrenal gland ➔ measuring 3 cm x 4.3 cm.*

Metastatic Disease

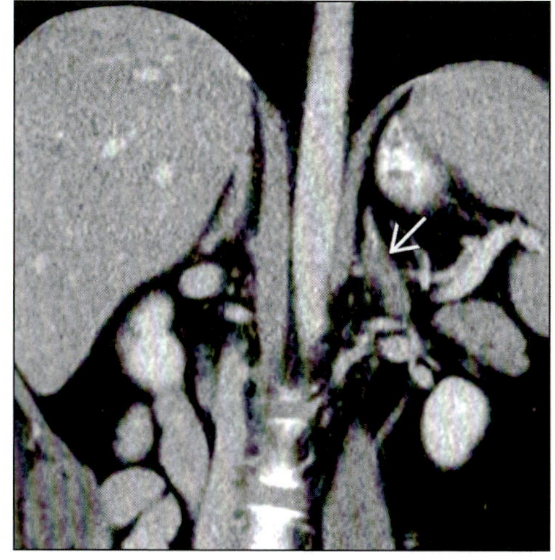

Metastatic Disease

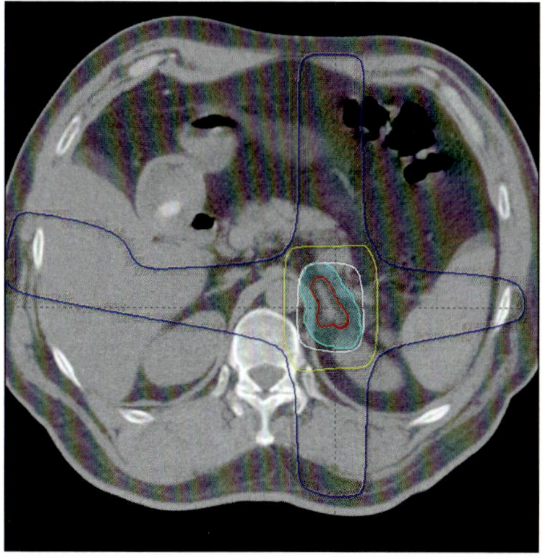

(Left) *Axial CECT in the same patient shows a good partial response of the left adrenal gland ➔ to gemcitabine chemotherapy.* ***(Right)*** *The same patient was treated with palliative intent to 37.5 Gy in 15 fractions. The CTV is shown in red and the PTV in blue. The white, yellow, and blue lines represent the 100%, 70%, and 50% isodose lines, respectively.*

Metastatic Disease

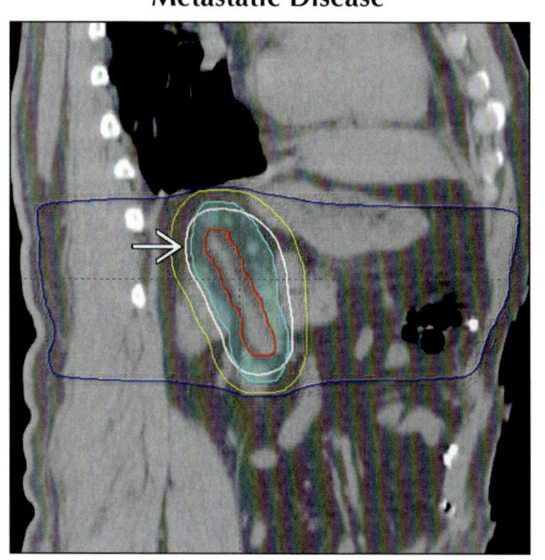

Metastatic Disease

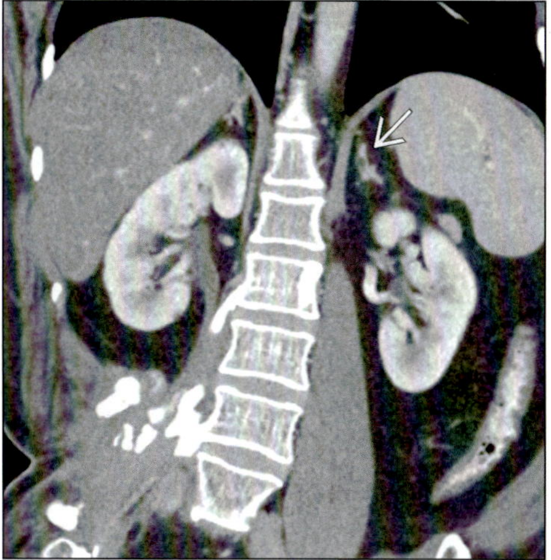

(Left) *Sagittal CT in the same patient shows good conformality of the 100% isodose line ➔ to the PTV.* ***(Right)*** *Coronal CECT in the same patient shows a complete response obtained 21 months after RT. The left adrenal is misshapen and has a small stable cyst ➔.*

BLADDER

(T) Primary Tumor

Adapted from 7th edition AJCC Staging Forms.

TNM	*Definitions*
TX	Primary tumor cannot be assessed
T0	No evidence of primary tumor
Ta	Noninvasive papillary carcinoma
Tis	Carcinoma in situ: "Flat tumor"
T1	Tumor invades subepithelial connective tissue
T2	Tumor invades muscularis propria
pT2a	Tumor invades superficial muscularis propria (inner half)
pT2b	Tumor invades deep muscularis propria (outer half)
T3	Tumor invades perivesical tissue
pT3a	Tumor invades perivesical tissue microscopically
pT3b	Tumor invades perivesical tissue macroscopically (extravesical mass)
T4	Tumor invades any of the following: Prostatic stroma, uterus, vagina, pelvic wall, abdominal wall
T4a	Tumor invades prostatic stroma, uterus, vagina
T4b	Tumor invades pelvic wall, abdominal wall

(N) Regional Lymph Nodes

NX	Regional lymph nodes cannot be assessed
N0	No regional lymph node metastasis
N1	Single regional lymph node metastasis in true pelvis (hypogastric, obturator, external iliac, or presacral lymph node)
N2	Multiple regional lymph node metastases in true pelvis (hypogastric, obturator, external iliac, or presacral lymph node)
N3	Lymph node metastasis to common iliac lymph nodes

(M) Distant Metastasis

M0	No distant metastasis
M1	Distant metastasis

Regional lymph nodes include both primary and secondary drainage regions. All other nodes above the aortic bifurcation are considered distant lymph nodes.

AJCC Stages/Prognostic Groups

Adapted from 7th edition AJCC Staging Forms.

Stage	*T*	*N*	*M*
0a	Ta	N0	M0
0is	Tis	N0	M0
I	T1	N0	M0
II	T2a	N0	M0
	T2b	N0	M0
III	T3a	N0	M0
	T3b	N0	M0
	T4a	N0	M0
IV	T4b	N0	M0
	Any T	N1-3	M0
	Any T	Any N	M1

T Staging of Urinary Bladder Carcinoma

T2a T2b T1 T3 Tis T4

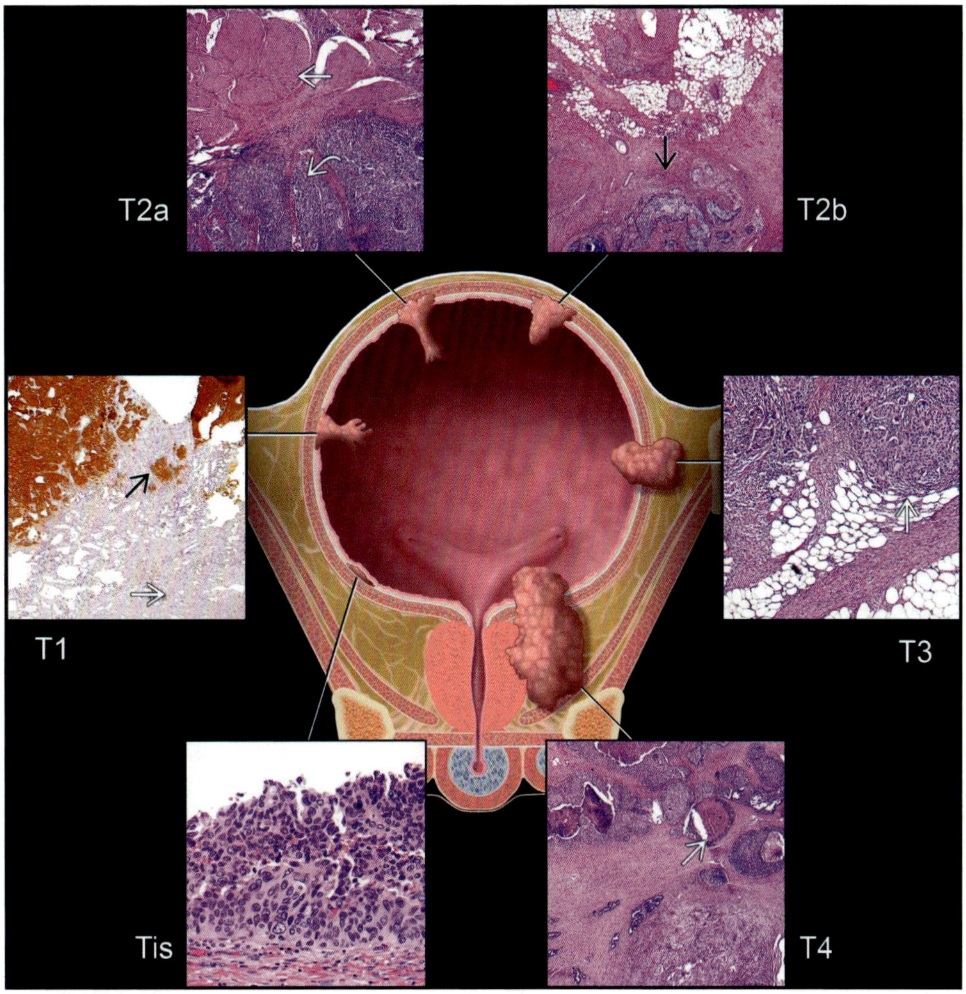

Graphics show the T stages of urinary bladder carcinoma with histologic correlation.

***Tis**, or carcinoma in situ, refers to a nonpapillary (flat) mucosa in which the normal urothelium has been replaced by cancer cells that have not invaded through the basement membrane. The carcinoma in situ is a high-grade lesion and essentially recognized because of cytologic abnormalities similar to those noted in high-grade papillary tumors. The neoplastic cells are pleomorphic, hyperchromatic, and occupy a portion of the thickness of the urothelium. They lack polarity in relation to the basement membrane.*

***T1** describes urothelial tumor invasion through the basement membrane into the subepithelial connective tissue. In this photomicrograph, cytokeratin immunohistochemical stain is used to highlight the tumor ⇨ invading into the subepithelial connective tissue but not to the muscularis propria ➡.*

***T2** designates tumor that invades the muscularis propria. **T2a**: H&E stain shows tumor cell invading superficial/inner half of the muscularis propria ➦. Note that the outer half of the muscularis propria is not involved ➡. **T2b**: H&E stain shows tumor cells ⇨ invading the outer half of the muscularis propria.*

***T3** applies to tumor invading perivesical tissue. H&E stain shows tumor cells ➡ invading perivesical fat tissue. Tumor is considered T3a if perivesical fat involvement is microscopic (not evident by imaging) and T3b if macroscopic (potentially detected by imaging).*

***T4** describes tumor invading any of the following: Prostate, uterus, vagina, pelvic wall, or abdominal wall. It is T4a when tumor invades the prostate, uterus, and vagina; the tumor is T4b when it invades the pelvic wall and abdominal wall. H&E stain demonstrates neoplastic transitional cell carcinoma cells ➡ invading the prostate.*

T4a: Male

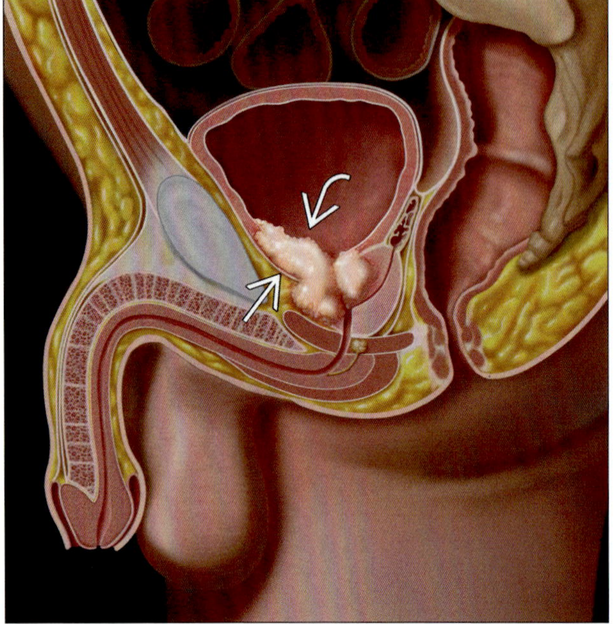

Graphic shows a bladder neck tumor ➲ in a male patient; the tumor invades the prostate ➡, constituting stage T4a. To be considered T4a disease, the tumor should have prostatic stromal invasion directly from the bladder tumor. Subepithelial invasion of prostatic urethra will not constitute T4 staging status.

T4a: Female

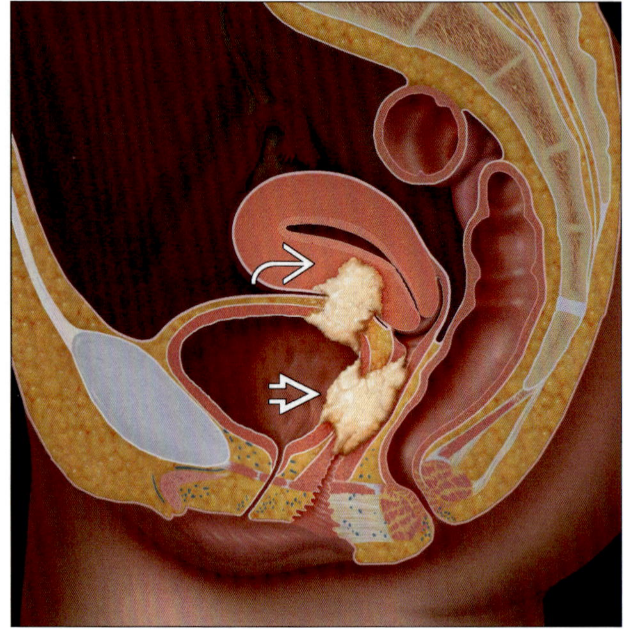

Graphic shows posterior wall bladder tumors in a female patient invading the uterus ➲ and vagina ⇨. Invasion of the uterus &/or vagina constitutes stage T4a.

T4b: Male

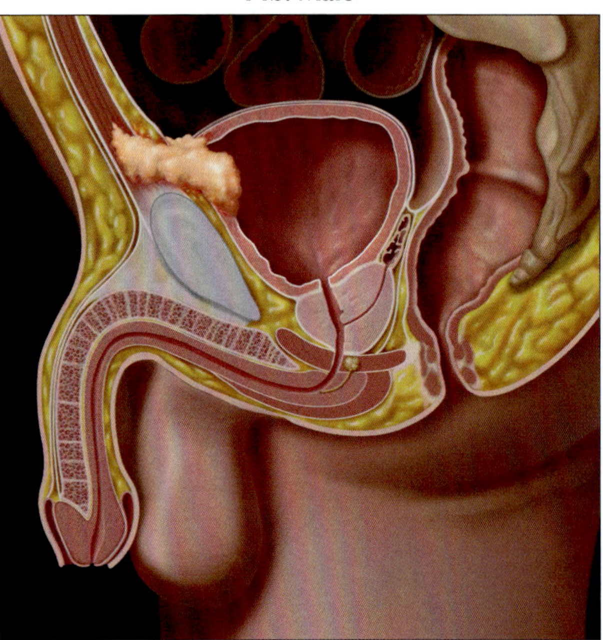

Graphic shows a tumor of the anterior wall of the urinary bladder that invades into the extraperitoneal prevesical fat (space of Retzius) and eventually the muscles of the anterior abdominal wall, constituting stage T4b.

T4b: Female

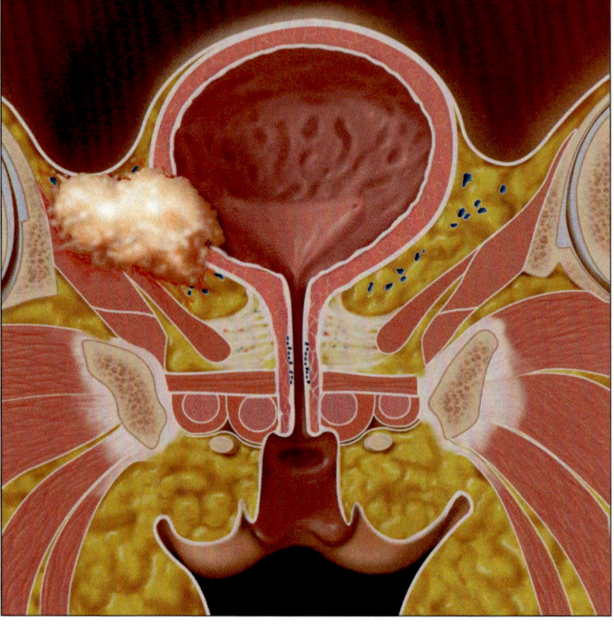

Graphic shows a lateral wall bladder tumor invading the muscles of the lateral pelvic wall, constituting stage T4b.

N1 and N2

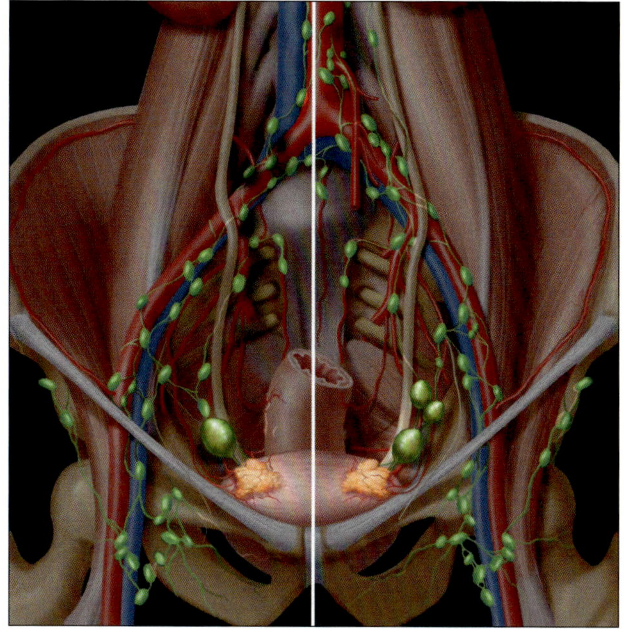

Graphics show N1 and N2 disease in urinary bladder carcinoma. Both classifications describe nodal metastases confined to the true pelvis. N1 (left) is a single metastatic pelvic lymph node, whereas N2 (right) is defined as multiple metastatic pelvic lymph nodes.

N3 and Distant Nodal Metastases

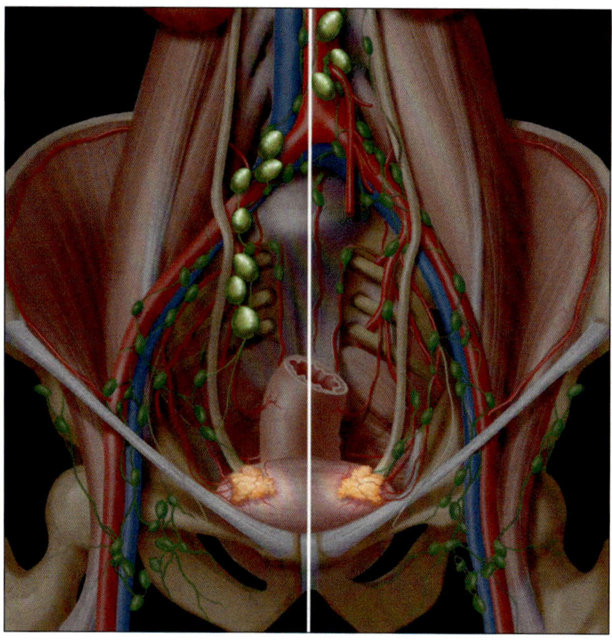

The graphic on the left shows N3 disease, which describes involvement of the common iliac lymph nodes. The graphic on the right shows involvement of paraaortic lymph nodes, which constitute distant metastases and M1 staging.

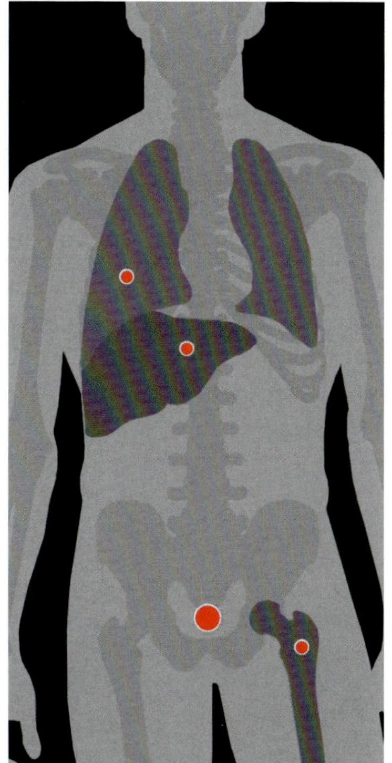

INITIAL SITE OF RECURRENCE	
Local Failure	20.3%
Bone	13.9%
Liver	10.7%
Lung	9.9%

Adapted from Volkmer BG et al: Oncological followup after radical cystectomy for bladder cancer-is there any benefit? J Urol. 181(4):1587-93, 2009.

BLADDER

OVERVIEW

Classification

- Uroepithelial (95%)
  - Transitional cell carcinoma (TCC) (90%)
  - Squamous cell carcinoma (6-8%)
  - Adenocarcinoma (2%)
    - Urachal origin
    - Nonurachal origin (usually chronic irritation)
  - Neuroendocrine (1%)
  - Mixed
- Mesenchymal (5%) includes
  - Neurofibrosarcoma
  - Pheochromocytoma
  - Lymphoma
  - Angiosarcoma
  - Leiomyosarcoma
  - Rhabdomyosarcoma
  - Liposarcoma
  - Chondrosarcoma
  - Osteosarcoma
  - Plasmacytoma

NATURAL HISTORY

Etiology

- Direct prolonged contact with excreted carcinogens
  - Smoking is most important risk factor
    - Smokers' risk is 2x that of nonsmokers
  - Industrial carcinogens (aniline, benzidine, arylamine, naphthylamines)
  - High level of arsenic in drinking water
  - Cytoxan exposure
- Recurrent urinary tract infections and stone disease
  - Squamous cell carcinoma
- *Schistosoma hematobium* infection
  - Squamous cell carcinoma
- Chronic indwelling catheter

Epidemiology & Cancer Incidence

- 4th most common cancer in men
- 10th most common cancer in women
- Median age at diagnosis is 73 years
- Incidence differs by sex and race
  - 4x more common in men than women
  - 2x more common in whites than in African-Americans
- Lifetime incidence of 1 in 42 Americans
  - Estimated 69,250 new cases in USA in 2011
- Age-adjusted death rate of 4.4/100,000 Americans per year
  - Estimated 14,990 deaths in USA in 2011

Associated Diseases, Abnormalities

- Metaplastic changes can involve extensive areas of bladder epithelium
- 30% present with multifocal urinary bladder disease
  - Often widespread bladder squamous metaplasia and carcinoma in situ
- 50% of patients presenting with upper urinary tract carcinoma will develop metachronous tumors in urinary bladder
- 5% of patients presenting with urinary bladder carcinoma will develop metachronous tumors in upper urinary tract
  - More likely in patients with multiple bladder lesions

Gross Pathology & Surgical Features

- Urothelial neoplasms of urinary bladder may be subdivided into
  - Papillary
    - Papillomas
    - Low malignant potential papillary tumors
    - Papillary carcinoma
  - Nonpapillary
    - Urothelial carcinoma in situ
    - Invasive carcinoma
      - Invasive urothelial carcinoma may present as polypoid, sessile, ulcerated, or infiltrative lesion

Microscopic Pathology

- H&E
  - Carcinoma in situ (CIS)
    - Malignant urothelial cells within nonpapillary urothelial lining
      - Characterized by extensive (often full thickness) replacement of urothelium by cells demonstrating severe cytologic atypia
  - Papillary lesions
    - Microscopic appearance
      - Contain well-defined fibrovascular cores
      - Lining urothelium may vary from indistinguishable from normal (papilloma) to markedly anaplastic (high-grade urothelial carcinoma)
    - Papillary urothelial neoplasia of low malignant potential (PUNLMP)
      - Papillary tumor characterized by cytologically bland, yet thickened, epithelium when compared to papilloma
      - Lower rate of recurrence than low-grade urothelial carcinoma
    - Papillary lesions with cytological atypia
      - Low-grade papillary urothelial carcinoma (LGPUC)
      - High-grade papillary urothelial carcinoma (HGPUC)
  - Invasive carcinoma
    - Neoplastic cells invade bladder wall as nests, cords, trabeculae, small clusters, or single cells that are usually separated by desmoplastic stroma

Routes of Spread

- Local spread
  - Extension through layers of bladder wall into perivesical fat
  - Invasion of local pelvic organs
    - Seminal vesicles
    - Prostate
    - Uterus
    - Ovaries
    - Rectum
    - Perineum
  - Later spread to pelvic side wall or anterior abdominal wall
- Lymphatic spread

- Depends on depth of invasion of bladder wall, overall 20%
  - Superficial tumors (< T2): 5% risk of nodal metastases
  - Muscle invasion (T2-T3a): 30% risk of nodal metastases
  - Perivesical extension (T3): 50-60% risk of nodal metastases
  - Organ invasion (T4): 50%
- Initially to perivesical, presacral, and sacral nodes
- Later to internal iliac, obturator, and external iliac nodes, and eventually to common iliac and paraaortic nodes
- Regional lymph node metastases are those confined to true pelvis (hypogastric, obturator, external iliac, or presacral lymph node)
  - N1: Single regional lymph node
  - N2: Multiple regional lymph nodes
- Common iliac nodes are defined as N3 disease
- All other nodes above aortic bifurcation are considered distant metastases (M1 disease)

- Hematogenous spread
  - Occurs late and with recurrent disease
  - Common sites are bones, lung, brain, and liver
    - Bone metastases occur mainly to pelvic bones and spine (perivesical venous plexus → Batson paravertebral plexus → vertebral bodies)
    - Direct extension to pelvic bones is also common

IMAGING

Detection

- **Cystoscopy** is considered gold standard for detection of bladder cancer
- **Intravenous urography (IVP)**
  - Traditionally modality of choice in evaluating hematuria
  - Largely replaced by CT IVP
  - Used primarily to access upper urinary tract + cystoscopy
  - Only 60% of bladder cancers are detected by IVP
    - Small tumors may be obscured in contrast-filled urinary bladder
  - Tumors appear as sessile or pedunculated filling defects
- **Ultrasound**
  - Bladder tumors may be found incidentally or during work-up for hematuria
  - Sonographic features include
    - Focal hypoechoic or mixed echogenicity nonmobile mass projecting into bladder lumen
    - No posterior shadowing
    - Focal bladder wall thickening
    - Color Doppler shows ↑ vascularity (differentiate bladder masses from blood clots)
  - Sonographic detection of bladder tumors depends on size and location
    - Difficult to detect tumors < 5 mm in size and tumors located in neck or dome of bladder
  - Transrectal US can be useful in differentiating bladder neck from prostatic tumor
- **NECT**
  - Modality of choice in patients presenting with painful hematuria to assess for stones
  - Polypoid bladder tumors, isodense to bladder wall, may be seen against background of fluid density urine
    - Changing window settings can make it easier to detect bladder tumors
  - Factors that can make tumor easier to detect against isodense urine
    - Presence of tumor calcifications
      - Tumoral calcifications in approximately 5% of cases of transitional cell carcinoma
      - Calcification typically encrusts tumor surface
    - Presence of high-density hemorrhage in bladder lumen
- **CT IVP**
  - Modality of choice in evaluating patients presenting with painless hematuria
  - Evaluation of upper urinary tract for synchronous tumors in patients with known or suspected carcinoma
  - Consistent performance in detection of bladder tumors
    - Sensitivity (79%)
    - Specificity (94%)
    - Accuracy (91%)
    - Positive predictive value (75%)
    - Negative predictive value (95%)
  - Imaging features
    - Tumors appear as polypoid or flat lesions of similar attenuation compared to bladder wall
    - Larger tumors tend to be more heterogeneous with areas of low density due to necrosis
    - Urachal carcinoma
      - Midline mass anterosuperior to bladder dome
      - Low-attenuation components, which represent pools of mucin at pathologic examination
      - Peripheral calcifications in masses of soft tissue attenuation occur in 50-70% of cases (pathognomonic for urachal adenocarcinoma)
- **MR**
  - Not used routinely for tumor detection
    - Tumors may be detected during pelvic imaging for other indications
  - As good as CT IVP for detection of bladder tumors
    - Sensitivity and positive predictive value > 90%
  - Imaging features
    - T1WI
      - Intermediate signal intensity, isointense to bladder wall, higher than urine and lower than perivesical fat
    - T2WI
      - Slightly hyperintense to bladder wall and hypointense to urine
    - Dynamic gadolinium-enhanced T1WI
      - Earlier and more pronounced enhancement than bladder wall
    - Diffusion-weighted imaging (DWI) under free breathing is very promising in detection of urinary bladder carcinoma
      - ADC values of urinary bladder carcinoma are lower compared to urine, normal bladder wall, prostate, and seminal vesicles

- Sensitivity (98.1%); specificity (92.3%); positive predictive value (100%); negative predictive value (92.3%); and accuracy (97.0%)
- Dynamic contrast-enhanced MR parameters: Peak time enhancement in 1st minute (E[max/1]) after contrast administration and steepest slope
  - E(max/1) and steepest slope correlate with histologic grade

Staging

- Determined by depth of invasion of bladder wall during cystoscopic examination, which includes
  - Deep biopsy, encompassing all layers of bladder wall
  - Examination under anesthesia to assess
    - Size and mobility of palpable masses
    - Degree of induration of bladder wall
    - Presence of extravesical extension or invasion of adjacent organs
- Unfortunately, clinical staging is not perfect
  - Errors reported in 25-50% of cases
- Patients shown to have muscle-invasive disease following cystoscopy are referred for imaging, usually CT or MR, for complete staging
- **Imaging techniques for local staging**
  - **MR** is imaging modality of choice in local staging of urinary bladder carcinoma
    - Sensitivity and positive predictive value > 90% and overall diagnostic accuracy of 62-75%
    - Inherent high soft tissue contrast
    - Multiplanar capabilities
    - Nonnephrotoxic contrast
    - Superior to CT in assessing depth of muscular invasion
    - Diffusion-weighted MR improves specificity for detection of invasive urinary bladder tumors
  - **CT** is useful to distinguish tumors confined to bladder wall from those spreading into perivesical fat
    - Cannot determine depth of wall invasion to differentiate T2a from T2b disease
  - **Transabdominal US** is not useful for staging
  - **Transurethral US** can be used for staging
    - Can distinguish between T2 and T3 disease
    - Invasive
    - Does not provide more staging information than CT or MR
  - **FDG PET** has limited role in local staging
    - Increased tumor uptake may be obscured by radioisotope excretion into bladder
    - Early results suggest promising role of tracer 11C-choline in evaluation of bladder cancer because of its minimal urinary excretion
- **Local staging**
  - Urinary bladder carcinoma stages
    - Not possible to differentiate Ta from T1 by imaging
    - **T1**: Intraluminal filling defect with normal underlying wall
    - **T2**: Localized wall thickening and retraction indicate muscle involvement
    - **T3a**: Microscopic perivesical invasion cannot be resolved with CT or MR
    - **T3b**: Loss of clear interface between bladder wall and perivesical fat → perivesical fat stranding and nodularity
    - **T4**: Tumor invading adjacent organs, abdominal or pelvic wall, and perineum → distortion and irregularity between tumor and adjacent organs
      - T4 disease includes prostatic stromal invasion; subepithelial invasion of prostatic urethra does not constitute T4 disease
  - Presence of ureteral obstruction strongly suggests muscle invasion
  - MR imaging tends to overestimate local extent of tumor
    - Improved detection of perivesical fat stranding, which may be reactive or inflammatory rather than metastatic
  - MR is particularly helpful to differentiate muscle-invasive from noninvasive disease
    - T2WI
      - Interrupted low signal intensity muscle layer → muscle invasion (T2 disease)
    - Dynamic gadolinium-enhanced T1WI
      - Can differentiate T2a from T2b by showing depth of muscle invasion
    - Improved accuracy of T stage diagnosis from 67% for T2WI alone to 88% for T2W + DW images
  - Staging CT or MR should be delayed > 7 days after transurethral resection (TUR) because focal wall thickening and perivesical fat stranding can be seen following TUR → overstaging
  - Tumors arising in bladder diverticula are challenging from staging point of view
    - Tend to invade perivesical fat early due to absence of muscle layer in diverticular wall
    - Thinner wall makes accurate staging difficult
    - Omission of T2 has been suggested
      - Tumor either confined to diverticulum (T1) or extradiverticular tumor (T3)
- **Nodal metastases**
  - Nodal size and morphology criteria
    - Nodal metastases in oval nodes > 10 mm and round nodes > 8 mm
  - CT and routine MR have similar accuracy for detection of nodal disease
    - Reported accuracy (73-92%)
    - Sensitivity (83%) and specificity (98%)
  - Improved detection of nodal metastases using ultrasmall superparamagnetic iron oxide (ferumoxtran-10) particles
    - Can detect metastases in normal-sized nodes and exclude metastases in enlarged reactive nodes
    - Normal nodal tissue shows contrast material uptake → ↓ signal intensity on T2- or T2*-weighted images
    - Nodal metastases lack ferumoxtran-10 uptake and retain high signal intensity on ferumoxtran-10-enhanced images
  - PET can be used for detection of nodal metastases
- **Distant metastases**
  - Lung metastases are common and can present as
    - Solitary nodule
    - Multiple nodules
    - Cavitary nodules
    - Diffuse multinodular opacities
  - Bony metastases are usually lytic, although sclerotic and mixed lesions are also common

- Bone scan may be used if there is suspicion of bone metastases
- T1WI MR is useful to assess pelvic bone marrow involvement

- Brain metastases
  - Rare manifestation of metastatic bladder carcinoma
  - Usually occurs with advanced metastatic disease
  - May present as single or multiple enhancing parenchymal masses
  - Can rarely present as leptomeningeal carcinomatosis
- PET can be used for detection of distant metastases

Restaging

- Routine imaging follow-up is **not** indicated for patients with superficial TCC and no additional risk factors
  - Cystoscopy every 3 months for 2 years, then every 6 months for 2 years, and then yearly thereafter
- Patients with invasive TCC, especially those with risk factors, should have CT IVP every 1-2 years
- Patients requiring cystectomy for invasive bladder cancer should have
  - Abdominal and pelvic CT (or MR) at 6, 12, and 24 months
    - Local recurrence can present as
      - Pelvic lymphadenopathy
      - Well-defined or poorly defined pelvic soft tissue masses
      - Tumor invading adjacent structures, such as vagina, urethra, pelvic sidewall, anterior abdominal wall, seminal vesicle, and spermatic cord
  - Chest x-ray at 6, 12, 18, 24, 36, 48, and 60 months postoperatively

CLINICAL PRESENTATION & WORK-UP

Presentation

- Macroscopic painless hematuria
  - 80% of cases of bladder carcinoma present with painless hematuria
  - Bladder carcinoma is detected in up to 13-28% of patients presenting with macroscopic hematuria
- Urinary frequency, urgency, and dysuria
- Urinary tract infections
- Urinary obstruction
- Urinary bladder rupture is rare; can result
  - Spontaneously
  - Following biopsy
  - From endovesical chemotherapy with mitomycin C
  - As long-term complication of radiotherapy

Prognosis

- Approximately 70% of newly diagnosed cases of bladder cancer represent superficial disease
  - High risk of local recurrence
  - Rarely progress to invasive or metastatic disease
- Risk of disease relapse following radical cystectomy may be as high as 70%
- As many as 50% of patients who have muscle-invasive tumors will have occult metastases that will present within 5 years of diagnosis
- 78% of patients who developed metastases did so within 1 year of cystectomy
  - Suggests that metastases must be present at time of cystectomy
- Presence of ≥ 1 of the following risk factors ↑ likelihood of recurrent or metastatic disease in TCC
  - Extent of bladder wall invasion
  - Tumor size
    - Tumors > 3 cm have up to 35% chance of progression
  - Pathological tumor grade (i.e., degree of differentiation)
    - 5-year survival of patients with grade I tumors is 94% and only 40% for patients with grade III tumors
    - < 10% of grade I tumors, 50% of grade II tumors, and > 80% of grade III tumors are invasive at time of initial diagnosis
  - Adjacent or remote bladder mucosal changes
    - CIS in patients with low-grade, low-stage lesions may be associated with progression to muscle invasion (> 80% within 4 years of diagnosis)
  - Multiplicity of foci
    - Recurrence rate is almost 1/3 higher in patients with multiple lesions than in patients with single lesions
  - Upper tract obstruction
    - 5-year survival for patients with bilateral hydronephrosis: 31%
    - 5-year survival for patients with unilateral hydronephrosis: 45%
    - 5-year survival for patients with no hydronephrosis: 63%
  - Lymphatic invasion in lamina propria
    - Very poor prognostic sign
    - Most patients die within 6 years
  - Involvement of prostate
    - Increased risk of urethral recurrence
- 70-80% present with superficial bladder tumors (i.e., stage Ta, Tis, or T1)
  - Complete cure is expected
- 5-year survival rate for bladder cancer by stage
  - Stage 0: 95%
  - Stage I: 85%
  - Stage II: 55%
  - Stage III: 38%
  - Stage IV: 16%

Work-Up

- Clinical
  - H&P, cystoscopy with bladder mapping and EUA
- Radiographic
  - CT chest, abdomen, and pelvis considered standard
    - MR may be optimal at delineating primary tumor
    - Consider PET/CT
- Laboratory
  - CBC, BUN, Cr, alkaline phosphatase, UA, urine cytology, bladder biopsy

TREATMENT

Major Treatment Alternatives

- Ta, Tis, and T1 lesions are treated with TURBT with consideration of adjuvant intravesicular therapy
- High-grade T1 lesions can be considered for definitive chemoradiation (controversial)
- Muscle invasive (T2-T4) options include radical cystectomy, definitive chemoradiation, partial cystectomy, radical radiation
- Role of neoadjuvant and adjuvant chemo is unclear and evolving

Major Treatment Roadblocks/ Contraindications

- Limitations to bladder preservation success
  - Hydronephrosis
  - T4 lesions
  - Invasive tumors not associated with in situ component
  - Inability to tolerate chemotherapy
  - Lesion > 5 cm
  - Poor bladder function at baseline

Treatment Options by Stage

- **Stage 0 and I**
  - TUR and fulguration
  - TUR with fulguration followed by intravesical bacille Calmette-Guérin (BCG)
  - TUR with fulguration followed by intravesical chemotherapy
  - Segmental cystectomy (rarely indicated)
  - Radical cystectomy in selected patients with extensive or refractory superficial tumor
  - External beam radiotherapy ± chemotherapy
- **Stage II and III**
  - Radical cystectomy ± pelvic lymph node dissection
  - Urinary diversion becomes necessary and can be accomplished through
    - Cutaneous ureterostomy
    - Ileal conduit with ureteroileocutaneostomy
    - Ureterosigmoidostomy
    - Orthotopic neobladder reconstruction with ileal or ileocecal segments
  - Neoadjuvant platinum-based combination chemotherapy followed by radical cystectomy
  - Maximal TURBT if possible and EBRT ± concurrent chemotherapy
    - Cisplatin-containing regimen is standard
    - 5-FU and mitomycin C acceptable, nonnephrotoxic alternative
    - Gemcitabine emerging as a high-response modality
  - Interstitial implantation of radioisotopes uncommonly used
  - TUR with fulguration (in selected patients)
  - Segmental cystectomy (in selected patients)
- Locally advanced stage IV
  - Radical cystectomy + pelvic lymph node dissection
  - Maximal TURBT if possible followed by EBRT ± chemotherapy
  - Urinary diversion or cystectomy for palliation
  - Chemotherapy as an adjunct to local treatment
- Stage IV with distant metastases
  - Chemotherapy ± adjunct to local treatment
  - EBRT ± chemotherapy for palliation
  - Urinary diversion or cystectomy for palliation

Standard Doses

- Pure small cell carcinoma of bladder: 45-50 Gy to pelvis and whole bladder with chemo
- Transitional cell carcinomas, squamous cell and adenocarcinomas
  - Node negative: 45-50 Gy to pelvic lymph nodes, boost primary or whole bladder to 60-66 Gy
  - Node positive: 50 Gy to uninvolved pelvic nodes and bladder, 56-60 Gy to positive nodes, boost primary or whole bladder to 60-66 Gy

Organs at Risk Parameters

- Rectum: V50 < 50%, V60 < 35%, V65 < 25%, V70 < 20%, and V75 < 15%
- Small bowel: V45 < 195 mL
- Femoral head: Maximum dose < 50 Gy

Common Techniques

- Cystectomy candidates, definitive bladder preservation, node negative
  - 40-45 Gy to pelvic nodes and bladder with concurrent chemo
    - If complete response at 2nd look cystectomy, boost whole bladder or primary to 60-66 Gy
      - Otherwise, perform radical cystectomy
- Noncystectomy candidates, definitive
  - Pelvic nodal basins and bladder to 50 Gy with concurrent chemo
  - Boost whole bladder 60-66 Gy
- Noncystectomy candidates, palliative
  - Consider 39 Gy in 13 fractions or 45 Gy in 18 fractions to bladder alone
  - Definitive chemoradiotherapy also acceptable to achieve greatest chance of local control
- Node positive, definitive
  - 50 Gy to pelvis and bladder with chemo
  - Boost positive nodes 54-60 Gy
  - Boost whole bladder or primary 60-66 Gy
- Preoperative radiotherapy
  - Doses of 40-50 Gy conventionally or hyperfractionated without chemo have been tried in older series
    - Meta-analysis reveals no benefit to preoperative radiotherapy
    - Single institutional reports claim disease-free survival advantage for T3-T4 tumors
    - Some experts argue that with newer image-guided techniques, and concurrent chemo, benefits could outweigh potential toxicity
- Postoperative radiotherapy
  - Doses of 40-50 Gy conventionally fractionated or hyperfractionated without chemo have been tried in older series
  - DFS advantage seen for radiation over cystectomy in randomized trials
    - High intestinal morbidity reports have limited the adoption of routine postoperative radiation therapy (PORT)
- Simulation and special considerations

  - Intravesicle contrast 30-70 mL introduced via catheter, ± additional air (15-30 mL), has historically been used to delineate lesion
  - Most common practice for 3D conformal radiotherapy is to add 2.5 cm for CTV to the bladder GTV
  - IMRT useful when pelvic lymph nodes will be irradiated
  - Daily cone-beam CT demonstrates that margins of 1.5-2 cm are inadequate to account for target coverage in 65% of patients
  - Intrafractional bladder wall volume demonstrated to range from 19-108% over 28-minute period
  - Several strategies have been tried to accommodate organ motion/deformation
    - CBCT daily with choice of 1 of 3 different PTV margin plans daily to account for variability
    - Simulation with bladder full and treatment with empty bladder
    - Simulation with bladder full and then empty fused to create ITV to attempt to decrease PTV
    - Adaptive radiotherapy planning
    - Gating of treatment beam with fiducials
    - Composite volume reconstruction after 1st 5 fractions to determine maximum excursions
      - CTV to PTV margin shown to be reducible by 40%

Landmark Trials

- No randomized trials comparing cystectomy to definitive chemoradiation have been performed
- RTOG 8512, 8802, 8903, 9506, 9706, and 9906
  - Phases II and III bladder preservation protocols
  - Differing combinations of neoadjuvant or concurrent chemotherapy with various radiation fractionation regimens
  - Cystectomy reserved to salvage patients without CR at "2nd look" cystoscopy
  - ChemoRT bladder preservation protocols have same control rates as radical cystectomy with good bladder function in most patients
- NCIC trial
  - ± concurrent cisplatin to preoperative or definitive RT in locally advanced bladder cancer
  - Cisplatin may improve pelvic control
  - No improvement in OS or distant metastasis free survival

RECOMMENDED FOLLOW-UP

Clinical

- Cystoscopy every 3-4 months with urine cytology required

Radiographic

- CT scan of chest, abdomen, and pelvis considered every 6 months for 1st 2 years for muscle-invasive cancers

SELECTED REFERENCES

1. American Joint Committee on Cancer: AJCC Cancer Staging Manual. 7th ed. New York: Springer. 497-505, 2010
2. Zaghloul MS: Adjuvant and neoadjuvant radiotherapy for bladder cancer: revisited. Future Oncol. 6(7):1177-91, 2010
3. Takeuchi M et al: Urinary bladder cancer: diffusion-weighted MR imaging--accuracy for diagnosing T stage and estimating histologic grade. Radiology. 251(1):112-21, 2009
4. Volkmer BG et al: Oncological followup after radical cystectomy for bladder cancer-is there any benefit? J Urol. 181(4):1587-93; discussion 1593, 2009
5. Canter D et al: Hydronephrosis is an independent predictor of poor clinical outcome in patients treated for muscle-invasive transitional cell carcinoma with radical cystectomy. Urology. 72(2):379-83, 2008
6. Zhang J et al: Imaging of bladder cancer. Radiol Clin North Am. 45(1):183-205, 2007
7. Wong-You-Cheong JJ et al: From the Archives of the AFIP: neoplasms of the urinary bladder: radiologic-pathologic correlation. Radiographics. 26(2):553-80, 2006
8. Wallmeroth A et al: Patterns of metastasis in muscle-invasive bladder cancer (pT2-4): An autopsy study on 367 patients. Urol Int. 62(2):69-75, 1999
9. Coppin CM et al: Improved local control of invasive bladder cancer by concurrent cisplatin and preoperative or definitive radiation. The National Cancer Institute of Canada Clinical Trials Group. J Clin Oncol. 14(11):2901-7, 1996

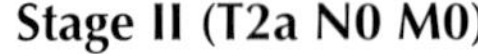

Stage II (T2a N0 M0)

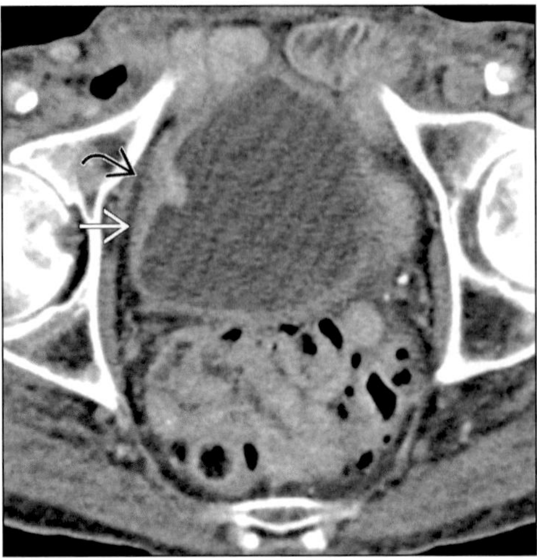

Stage II (T2a N0 M0)

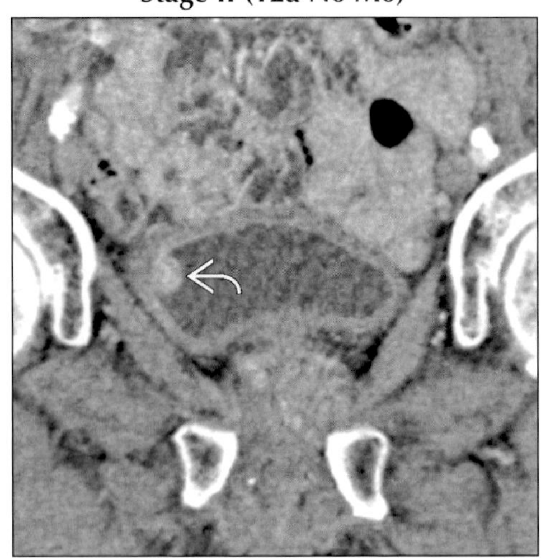

(Left) *Axial CECT shows an enhancing polypoid mass arising from the right lateral wall of the urinary bladder. There is associated thickening of the adjacent bladder wall.* ***(Right)*** *Coronal CECT in the same patient shows the enhancing urinary bladder mass. Enhancement is limited to the mass without involvement of the underlying wall, suggesting the absence of muscle invasion, although CT is not adequate to definitely make this distinction. This was found to be a T2a tumor.*

Stage II (T2b N0 M0)

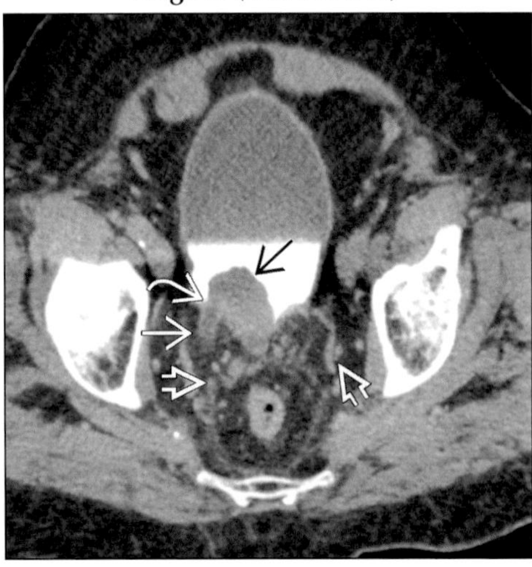

Stage III (T3b N0 M0)

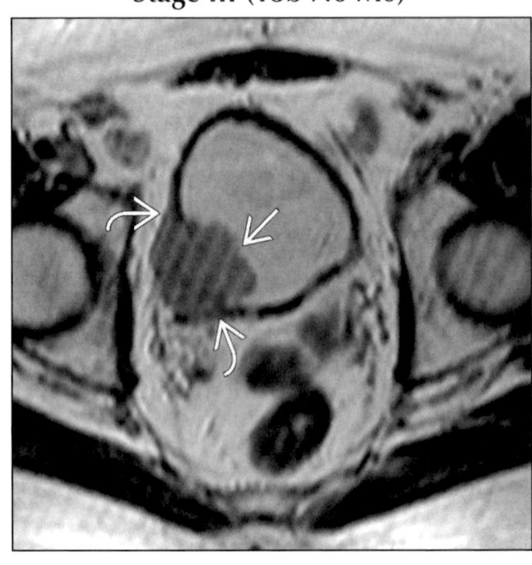

(Left) *Axial CECT in a patient with hematuria shows a posterior wall bladder mass that involves the ureteric orifice. The ureter is slightly dilated. Small nodular densities in the perivesical fat represent dilated veins.* ***(Right)*** *Axial T2WI MR shows a bladder mass that is hyperintense relative to the dark bladder wall and hypointense relative to urine and perivesical fat. Note the interruption of the dark bladder wall signal where the mass extends into the perivesical fat.*

Stage III (T3b N0 M0)

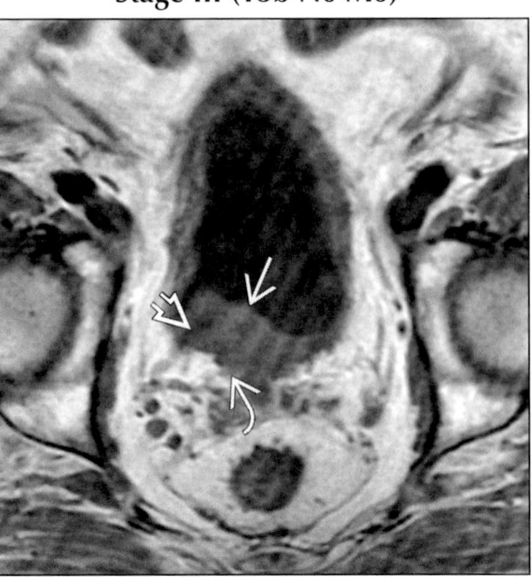

Stage III (T3b N0 M0)

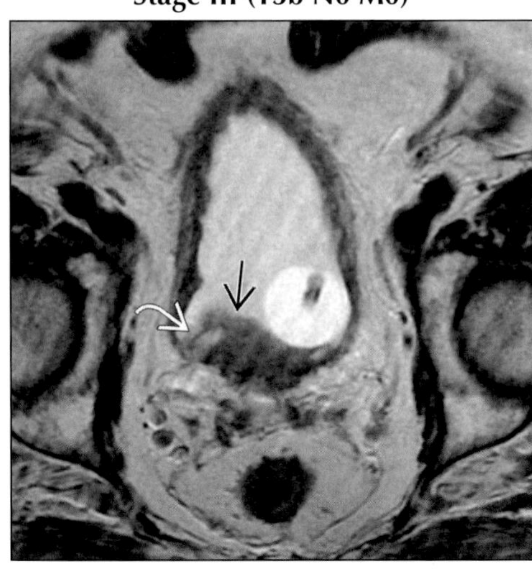

(Left) *Axial T1WI MR shows an intermediate signal intensity posterior wall bladder mass that is hyperintense to urine, hypointense to fat, and isointense to muscle. Tumor nodules extend into high signal perivesical fat. The ureteric orifice is embedded in the mass.* ***(Right)*** *Axial T2WI MR in the same patient shows an intermediate signal bladder mass that is hypointense to the urine and perivesical fat. Note also involvement of the ureteric orifice.*

Small Cell (T2a N0 M0)

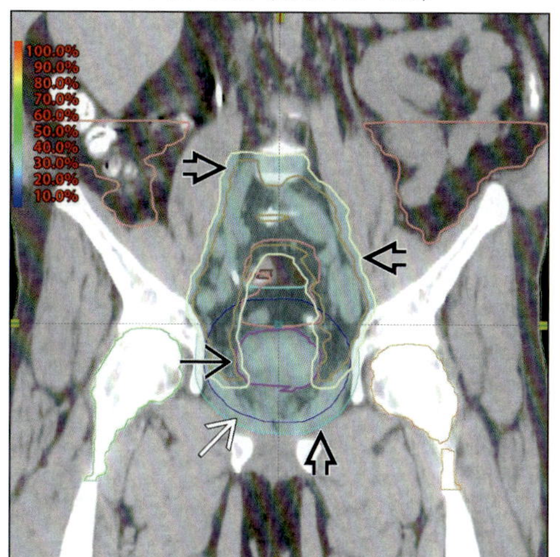

Small Cell (T2a N0 M0)

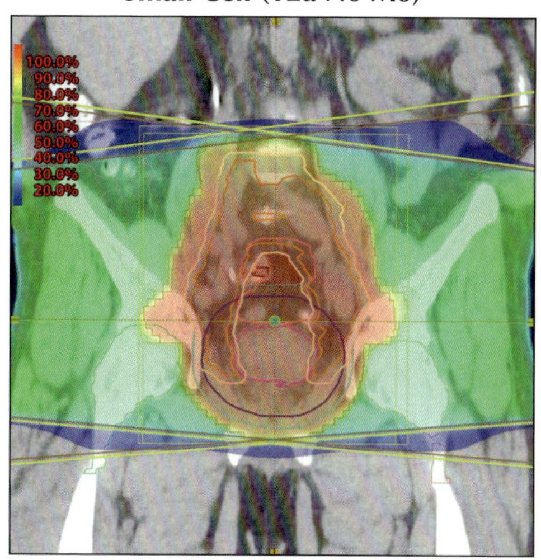

(Left) Coronal CT scan shows pelvic volumes for a T2a N0 M0 small cell bladder cancer in a 63-year-old man who was not a surgical candidate. The empty bladder ➔ and the 2.5 cm CTV bladder margin ➔ are shown. The cyan wash is the nodal and bladder PTV volume ➔. *(Right)* Dose colorwash is shown in the same patient on a coronal CT. A conventional 4-field technique was used to 45 Gy.

Small Cell (T2a N0 M0)

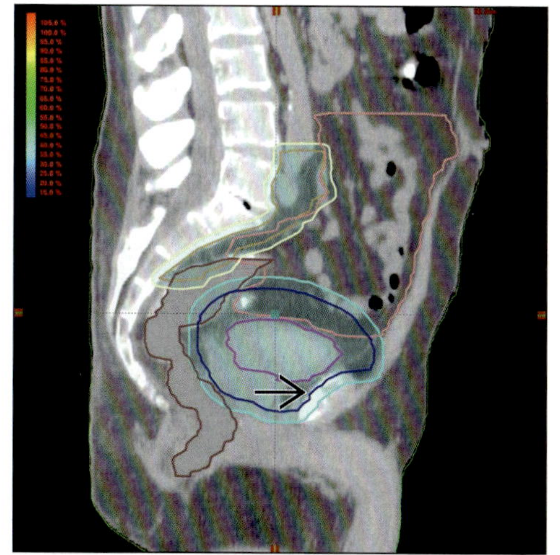

Small Cell (T2a N0 M0)

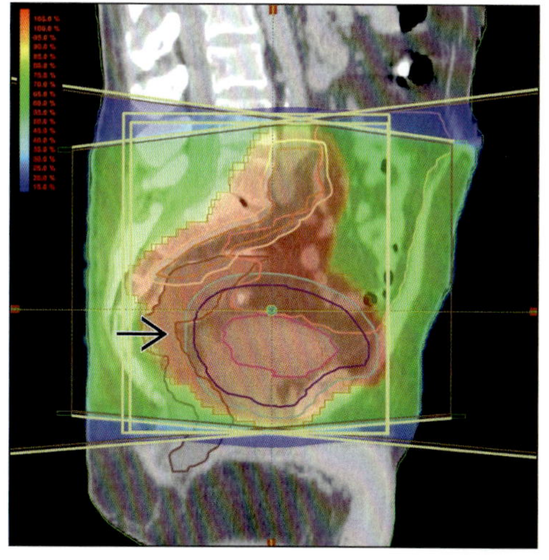

(Left) Sagittal CT view in the same patient shows the field design. Note that the CTV ➔ need not extend into the pubic symphysis anteriorly. *(Right)* Sagittal CT shows the dose distribution in the same patient. Note the full dose to the rectum ➔ in this non-IMRT treatment plan. With a 4-field conventional design, it is challenging to spare the rectum in order to ensure good dosimetric coverage to the internal iliac vessels.

Small Cell (T2a N0 M0)

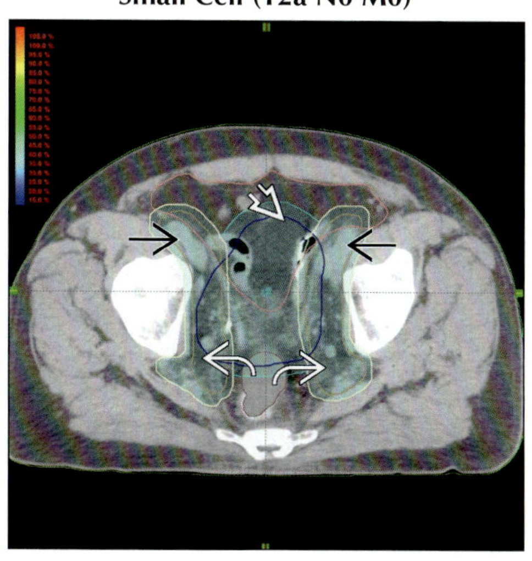

Small Cell (T2a N0 M0)

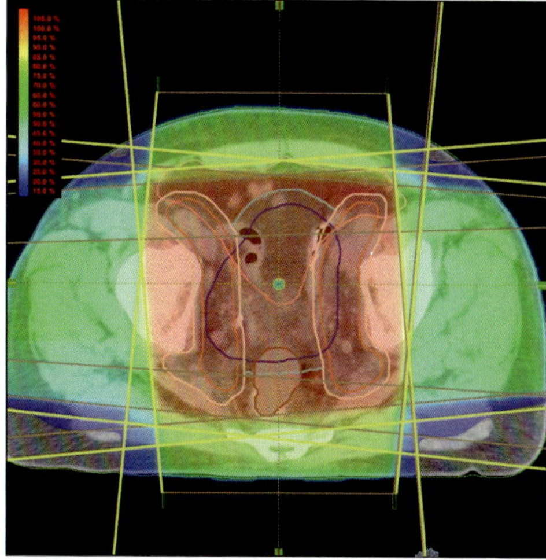

(Left) Axial CT in the same patient shows the field design of the internal ➔ and external ➔ iliac lymph node chains. The cyan color represents the 45 Gy PTV ➔ designed to encompass the nodal basins and bladder. *(Right)* Axial CT in the same patient shows the dose colorwash with a 4-field conventional technique. Because patient was only being prescribed 45 Gy total, a 4-field technique was deemed acceptable, and IMRT was not employed.

(Left) *Axial CT shows bladder TCC in a 57-year-old man. Planning CT shows a tumor along the right lateral bladder wall. The patient was simulated with full bladder (green contour) and then asked to empty bladder and re-scanned (yellow contour).* **(Right)** *Axial CT shows dose colorwash in the same patient. Green: Full bladder GTV; yellow: Emptied bladder GTV; red: Bladder PTV; cyan: Nodal CTV; light yellow: Nodal PTV (0.5 cm).*

TCC (T2a N0 M0)

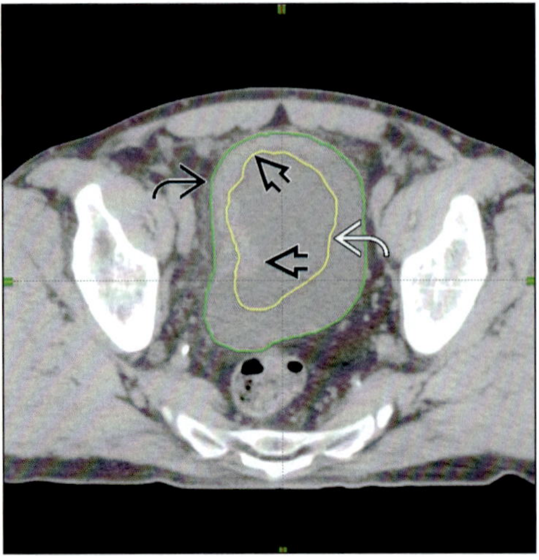

TCC (T2a N0 M0)

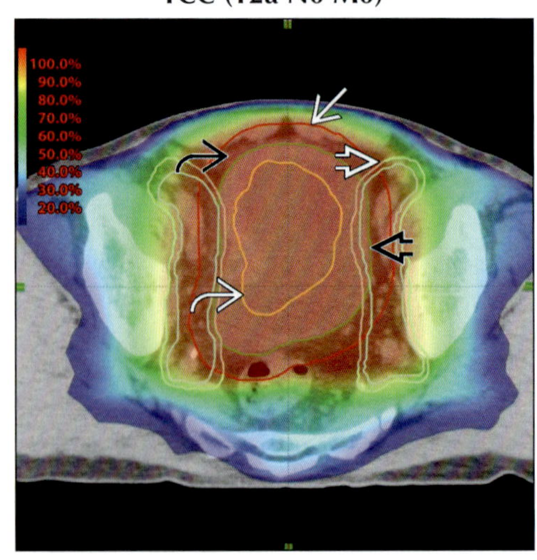

(Left) *Sagittal view in the same patient demonstrates variable bladder filling. Simulation with full bladder (green) and empty bladder contours are superimposed. Variable bladder filling is frequently noted with daily CT, and interfraction filling is reported between 19% and 108%.* **(Right)** *Sagittal CT shows dose colorwash in the same patient. He was treated by creating ITV full/empty bladder and 1 cm margin to PTV, which was verified daily with CT on rails.*

TCC (T2a N0 M0)

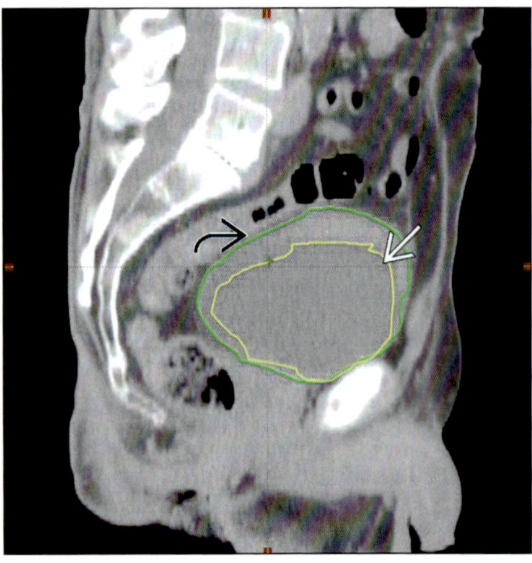

TCC (T2a N0 M0)

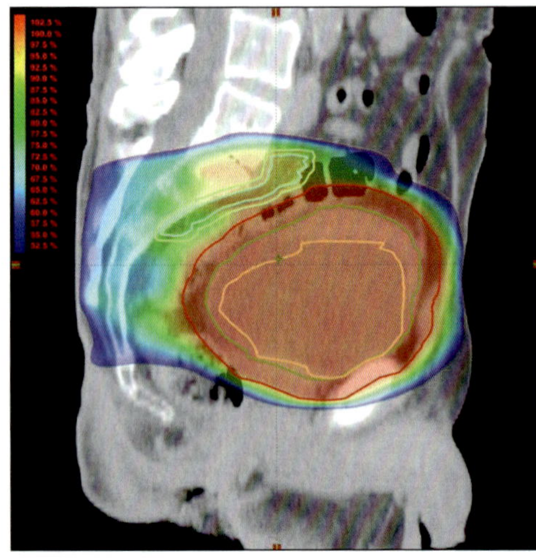

(Left) *Graphic shows IMRT DVH in the same patient with the simultaneous integrated boost technique. The pelvic nodal PTV was prescribed to 5,248 cGy in 32 fractions, with the bladder PTV receiving 6,400 cGy in 32 fractions. Shown are the rectum in dark green, nodal PTV in light green, and the bladder PTV in red.* **(Right)** *Coronal colorwash in the same patient shows dose distribution achieved.*

TCC (T2a N0 M0)

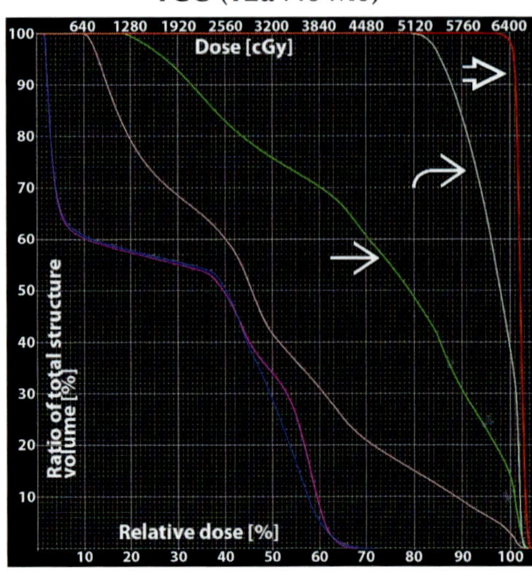

TCC (T2a N0 M0)

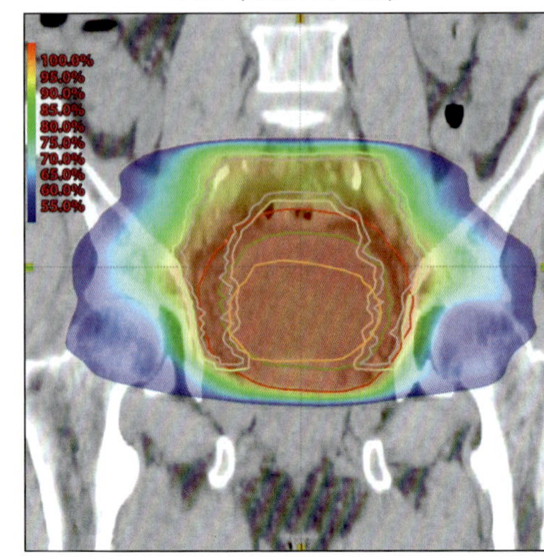

TCC (T2a N1 M0)

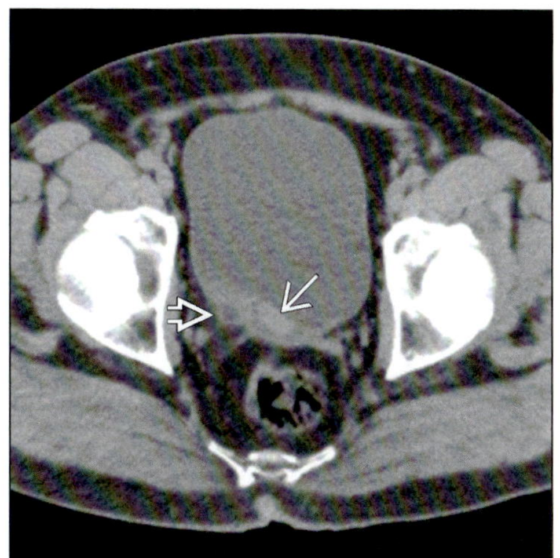

TCC (T2a N1 M0)

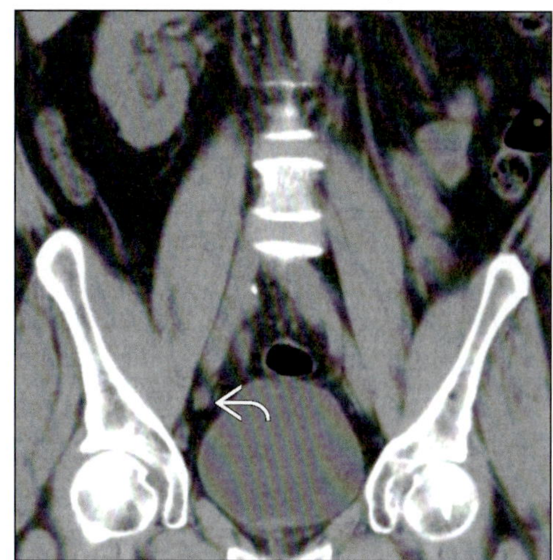

(Left) *Axial CT of a patient who presented with hematuria shows a mass and bladder wall thickening of the posterior-lateral bladder. Note the dilated ureter at the right UVJ.* ***(Right)*** *Coronal CT in the same patient shows an enlarged obturator lymph node called positive. The patient underwent maximal TURBT followed by neoadjuvant chemotherapy prior to planned surgery. The patient changed his mind before surgery and elected definitive chemoRT.*

TCC (T2a N1 M0)

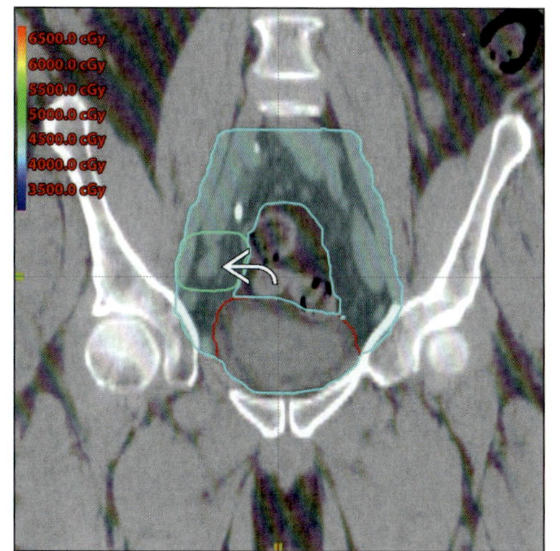

TCC (T2a N1 M0)

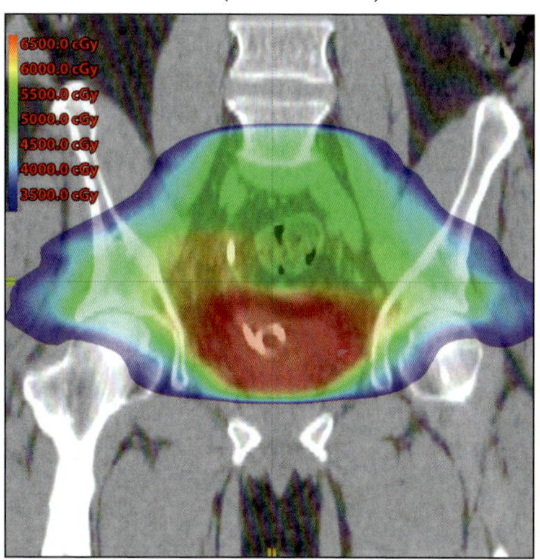

(Left) *Nodal field design in the same patient shows the solitary positive node. Prescription to the pelvic nodal field was to 50.4 Gy. The positive node was boosted to 59.4 Gy, and the entire bladder received 63 Gy.* ***(Right)*** *Dose colorwash in the same patient shows the dose gradients achieved to boost the node and primary.*

TCC (T2a N1 M0)

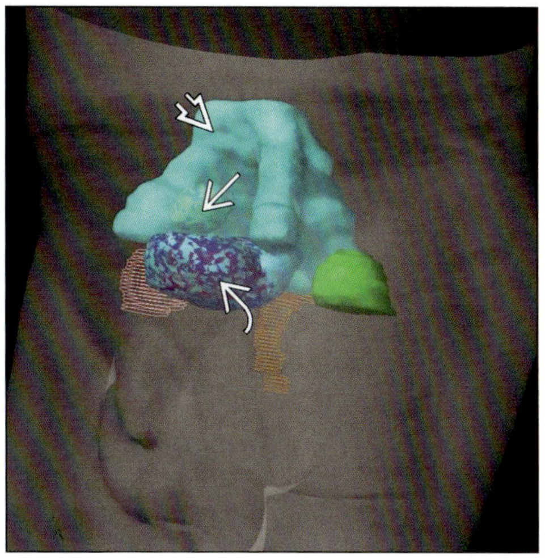

TCC (T2a N1 M0)

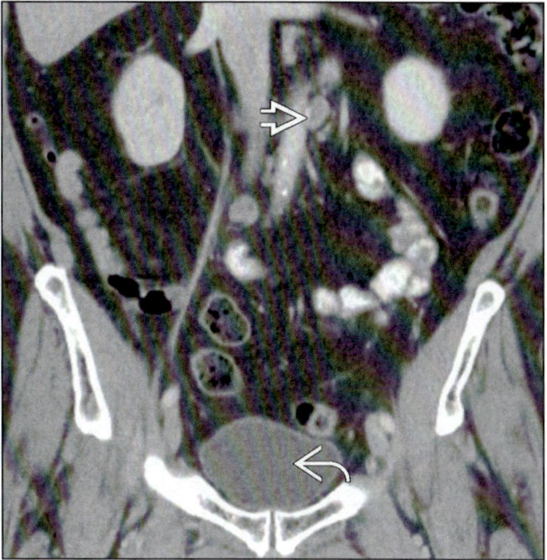

(Left) *Graphic shows various PTVs in the same patient. The nodal PTV went to 50.4 Gy, the positive node was boosted to 59.4 Gy, and the entirety of the bladder went to 63 Gy.* ***(Right)*** *Follow-up scan in the same patient 2 years later shows a normal-appearing bladder. He reported normal urinary and bowel function. The patient remained locally controlled. Unfortunately, he developed a nonregional nodal failure in the paraaortic region.*

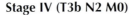

*(**Left**) Axial T2WI MR in a 72-year-old man who presented with painless hematuria shows posterior urinary bladder wall thickening ⇨ with loss of the low signal bladder wall indicating muscle invasion. (**Right**) Axial T1WI C+ FS MR obtained at a higher level in the same patient shows diffuse enhancing wall thickening ➡ involving the dome of the urinary bladder with circumferential thickening of the distal left ureter ➡ due to tumor invasion.*

Stage IV (T3b N2 M0)

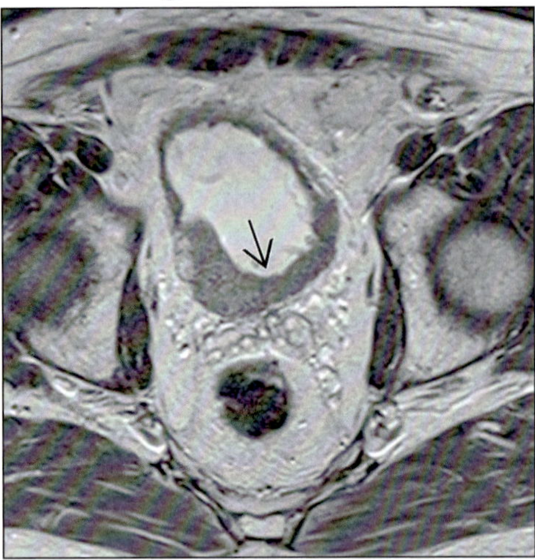

Stage IV (T3b N2 M0)

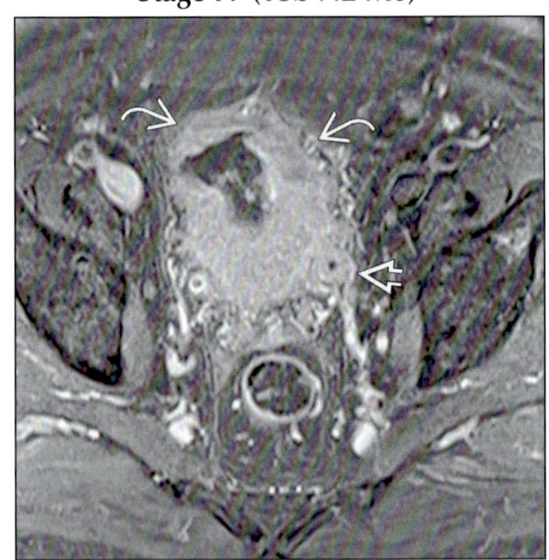

*(**Left**) Axial T2WI MR in the same patient shows 2 enlarged left external iliac lymph nodes ➡. The presence of multiple lymph node metastases within the true pelvis constitutes N2 disease. (**Right**) Axial CECT in the same patient shows contrast material ➡ within the urinary bladder outlining the large necrotic bladder mass ⇨. Note involvement of the ureteric orifice and mild ureteric dilatation ➡. There is a single obturator lymph node ➡, which constitutes N1 disease (stage IV).*

Stage IV (T3b N2 M0)

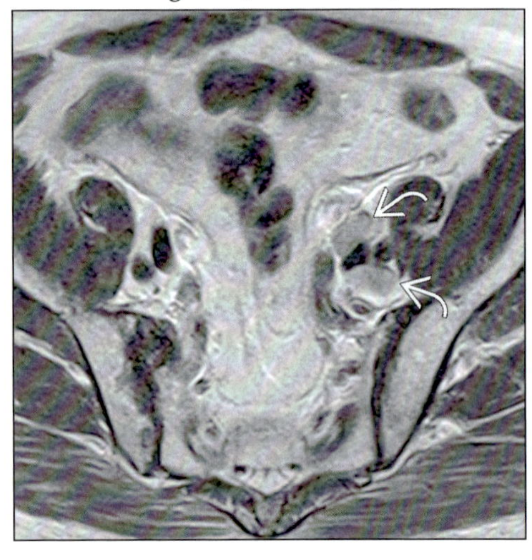

Stage IV (T2b N1 M0)

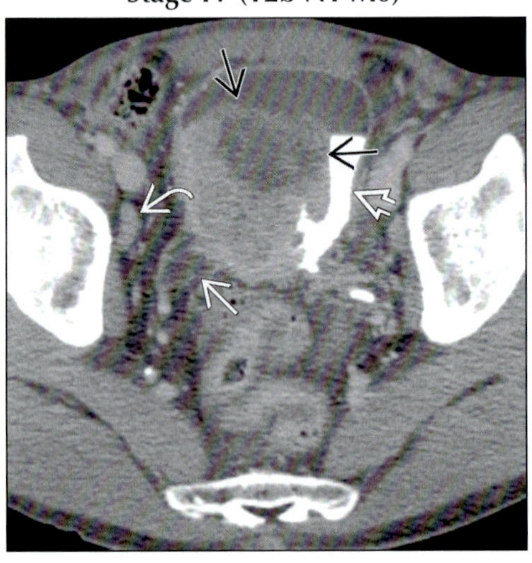

*(**Left**) Sagittal T2WI MR shows marked circumferential thickening of the wall of the urinary bladder ➡, as well as invasion of the rectus muscles anteriorly ➡. (**Right**) Axial CECT in the same patient shows a large dumbbell-shaped polypoid mass that has a large intraluminal component ➡ and a large extraluminal component ⇨. The extraluminal component invades into the anterior abdominal wall ➡.*

Stage IV (T4b N0 M0)

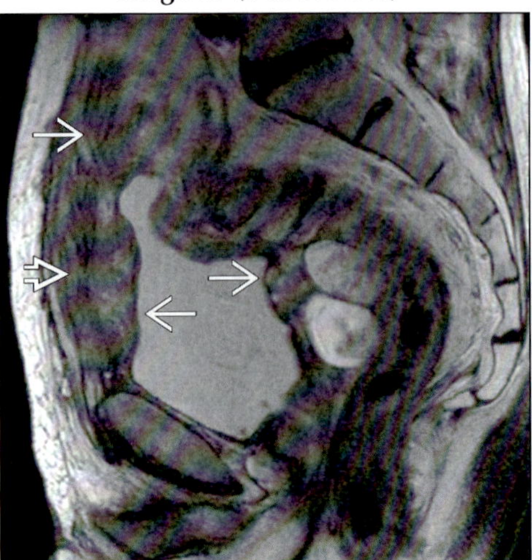

Stage IV (T4b N0 M0)

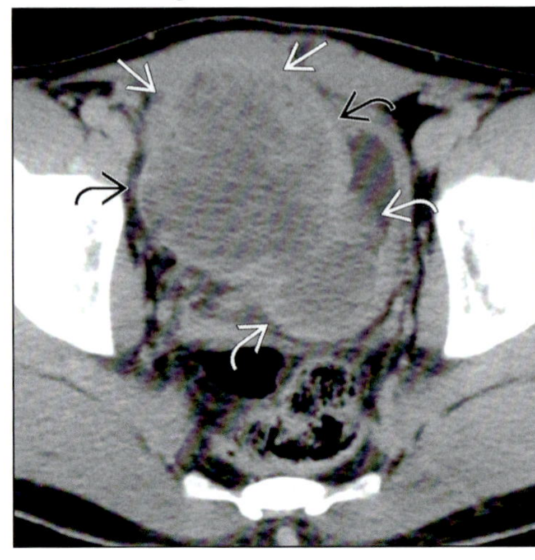

Gross Residual (pT4 N0 M0)

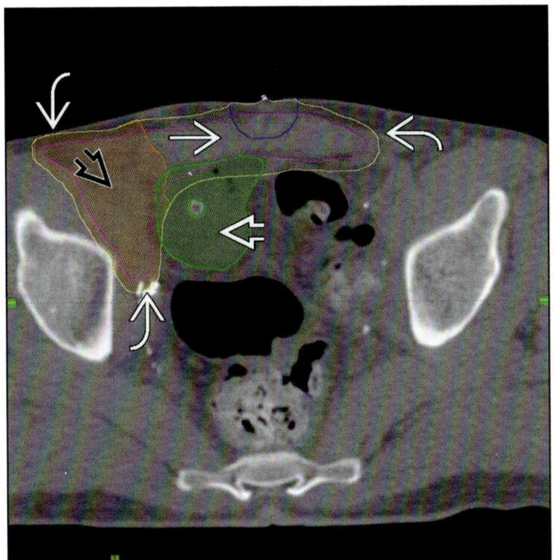

Gross Residual (pT4 N0 M0)

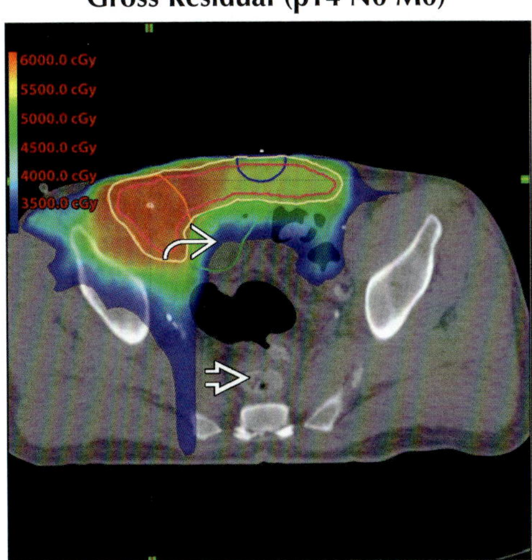

(Left) This 39-year-old man presented with hematuria with invasion of rectus abdominal muscles and underwent cystoprostatectomy and rectus resection. Green: Neobladder ➔; orange: Gross residual PTV ➔; pink: Rectus CTV ➔; yellow: PTV 50.4 Gy ➔. (Right) Axial CT shows dose wash in the same patient treated with IMRT. Avoidance structures were neobladder ➔, rectum ➔, and small bowel. He received combined cisplatin with radiation.

Gross Residual (pT4 N0 M0)

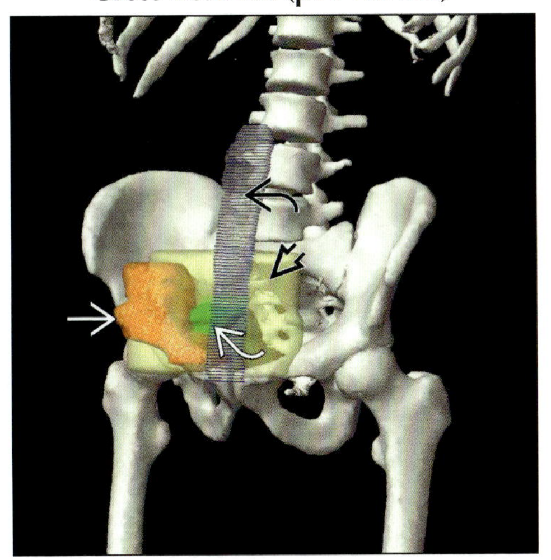

Gross Residual (pT4 N0 M0)

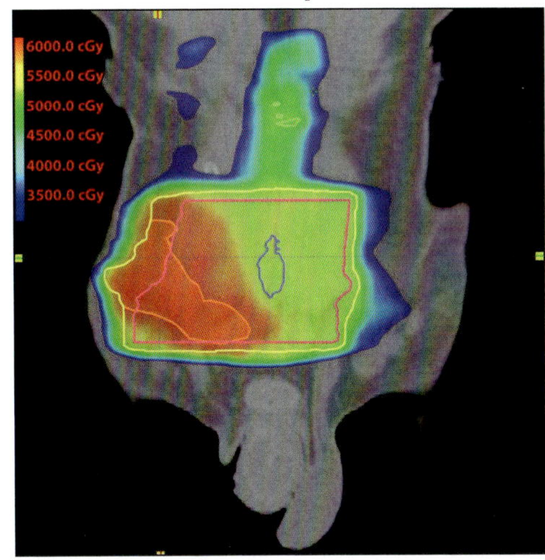

(Left) Model view is shown in the same patient. The entirety of the surgical scar was considered at risk and taken to 50.4 Gy ➔. The gross residual PTV taken to 59.4 Gy is in orange ➔; rectus abdominus PTV was taken to 50.4 Gy in yellow ➔; and neobladder is shown in green ➔. The patient remains free of disease 4 years after completion. (Right) Coronal CT shows dose colorwash in the same patient with IMRT dose gradients.

Gross Residual (pT4 N0 M0)

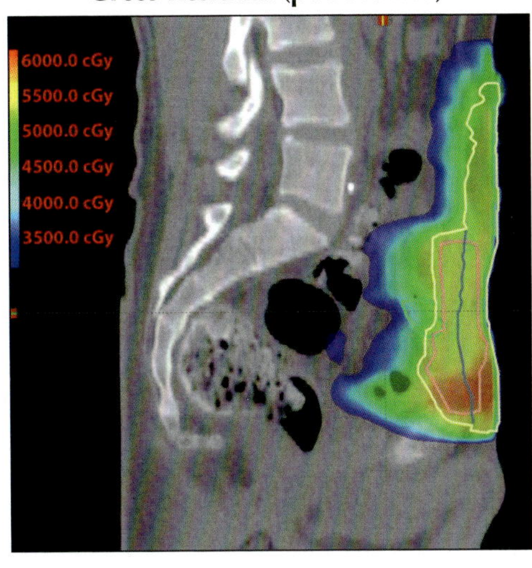

Gross Residual (pT4 N0 M0)

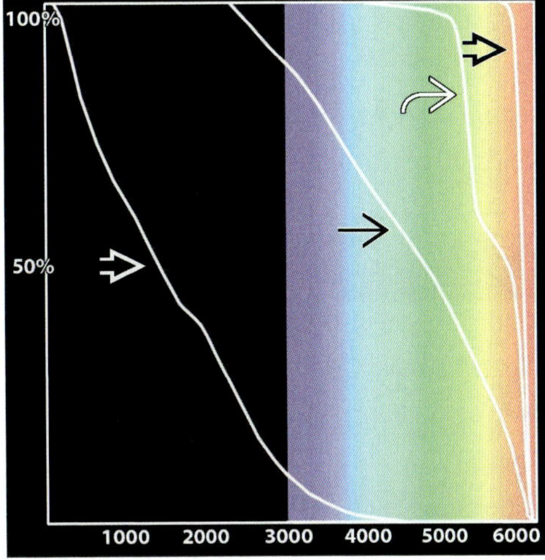

(Left) Sagittal CT shows dose colorwash in the same patient. The dosimetric goal with the normal tissues was to spare the neobladder, small bowel, and rectum to the greatest extent possible. A 7-field IMRT plan was utilized. (Right) Dose volume histogram in the same patient shows small bowel and rectum ➔, neobladder ➔, 50.4 Gy PTV ➔, and 59.4 Gy PTV ➔. The patient reported no bowel toxicity at 4-year follow-up and normal function of his neobladder.

PROSTATE

(T) Primary Tumor

Adapted from 7th edition AJCC Staging Forms.

TNM	*Definitions*
Clinical	
TX	Primary tumor cannot be assessed
T0	No evidence of primary tumor
T1	Clinically inapparent tumor neither palpable nor visible by imaging
T1a	Tumor incidental histologic finding in ≤ 5% of tissue resected
T1b	Tumor incidental histologic finding in > 5% of tissue resected
T1c	Tumor identified by needle biopsy (e.g., because of elevated PSA)
T2	Tumor confined within prostate[1]
T2a	Tumor involves ≤ 1/2 of 1 lobe
T2b	Tumor involves > 1/2 of 1 lobe but not both lobes
T2c	Tumor involves both lobes
T3	Tumor extends through the prostate capsule[2]
T3a	Extracapsular extension (unilateral or bilateral)
T3b	Tumor invades seminal vesicle(s)
T4	Tumor is fixed or invades adjacent structures other than seminal vesicles, such as external sphincter, rectum, bladder, levator muscles, &/or pelvic wall
Pathologic[3]	
pT2	Organ confined
pT2a	Unilateral, ≤ 1/2 of 1 side
pT2b	Unilateral, involving > 1/2 of 1 side but not both sides
pT2c	Bilateral disease
pT3	Extraprostatic extension
pT3a	Extraprostatic extension or microscopic invasion of bladder neck[4]
pT3b	Seminal vesicle invasion
pT4	Invasion of rectum, levator muscles, &/or pelvic wall

(N) Regional Lymph Nodes

Clinical	
NX	Regional lymph nodes were not assessed
N0	No regional lymph node metastasis
N1	Metastasis in regional lymph node(s)
Pathologic	
pNX	Regional nodes not sampled
pN0	No positive regional nodes
pN1	Metastases in regional node(s)

(M) Distant Metastasis

M0	No distant metastasis
M1	Distant metastasis
M1a	Nonregional lymph node(s)
M1b	Bone(s)
M1c	Other site(s) with or without bone disease[5]

[1]*Tumor found in 1 or both lobes by needle biopsy, but not palpable or reliably visible by imaging, is classified as T1c.*
[2]*Invasion into the prostatic apex or into (but not beyond) the prostatic capsule is classified not as T3 but as T2.*
[3]*No pathologic T1 classification.*

[4]Positive surgical margin should be indicated by an R1 descriptor (residual microscopic disease). [5]When > 1 site of metastasis is present, the most advanced category is used. pM1c is most advanced.

(G) Histologic Grade

Adapted from 7th edition AJCC Staging Forms.

TNM	*Definitions*
GX	Gleason score cannot be processed
Gleason ≤ 6	Well differentiated (slight anaplasia)
Gleason 7	Moderately differentiated (moderate anaplasia)
Gleason 8-10	Poorly differentiated/undifferentiated (marked anaplasia)

AJCC Stages/Prognostic Groups

Adapted from 7th edition AJCC Staging Forms.

Stage	*T*	*N*	*M*	*PSA*	*Gleason*
I	T1a-c	N0	M0	PSA < 10	Gleason ≤ 6
	T2a	N0	M0	PSA < 10	Gleason ≤ 6
	T1-2a	N0	M0	PSA X	Gleason X
IIA	T1a-c	N0	M0	PSA < 20	Gleason 7
	T1a-c	N0	M0	10 ≤ PSA < 20	Gleason ≤ 6
	T2a	N0	M0	PSA < 20	Gleason ≤ 7
	T2b	N0	M0	PSA < 20	Gleason ≤ 7
	T2b	N0	M0	PSA X	Gleason X
IIB	T2c	N0	M0	Any PSA	Any Gleason
	T1-2	N0	M0	PSA ≥ 20	Any Gleason
	T1-2	N0	M0	Any PSA	Gleason ≥ 8
III	T3a-b	N0	M0	Any PSA	Any Gleason
IV	T4	N0	M0	Any PSA	Any Gleason
	Any T	N1	M0	Any PSA	Any Gleason
	Any T	Any N	M1	Any PSA	Any Gleason

When either PSA or Gleason is not available, grouping should be determined by T stage &/or either PSA or Gleason as available.

Risk Groups

Risk	*NCCN*	*FCCC*	*MSKCC*
Low	PSA < 10 ng/mL	PSA ≤10 ng/mL	PSA < 10 ng/mL
	Gleason score 2-6	Gleason score 2-6	Gleason score 2-6
	T1a-T2a	T1a-T2c	T1a-T2c
Intermediate	Any of the following	Any of the following	1 of the following
	PSA 10-20 ng/mL	PSA > 10 ≤ 20 ng/mL	PSA > 10 ng/mL
	Gleason score 7	Gleason score 7	Gleason score 7-10
	T2b-T2c		T3-T4
High	Any of the following	Any of the following	2 or more of the following
	PSA > 20 ng/mL	PSA > 20 ng/mL	PSA > 10 ng/mL
	Gleason score 8-10	Gleason score 8-10	Gleason score 7-10
	T3a-T4	T3a-T4	T3a-T4

National Comprehensive Cancer Network (NCCN), Fox Chase Cancer Center (FCCC), Memorial Sloan-Kettering Cancer Center (MSKCC).

Diagram of Gleason Patterns

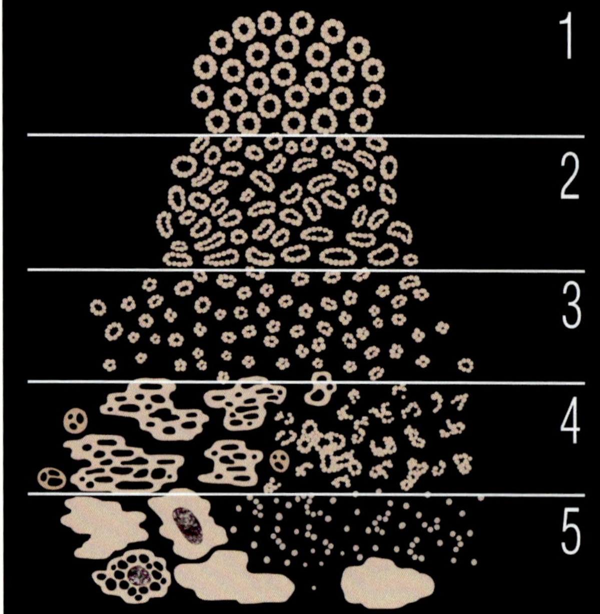

Schematic diagram shows modified Gleason grading system for prostate cancer. Gleason score is powerful prognostic variable in predicting prostate cancer behavior. This grading system is based on glandular architectural patterns divided into 5 histologic categories or grades with decreasing differentiation. (Courtesy R. E. Jimenez, MD.)

Gleason Pattern 3

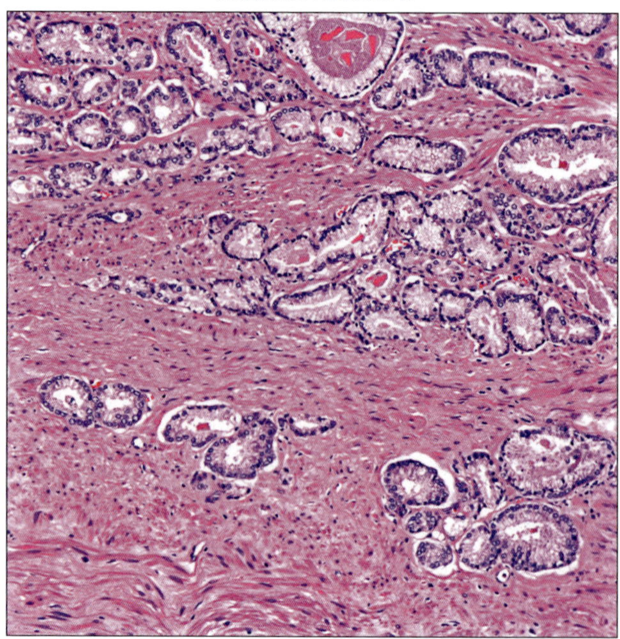

Gleason pattern 3 prostate cancer shows discrete, well-formed glands. These glands are smaller than glands in Gleason patterns 1 or 2 and show an infiltrative pattern of growth. Gleason grade 3 is the most common pattern in the Gleason grading scheme. (Courtesy R. E. Jimenez, MD.)

Gleason Pattern 4

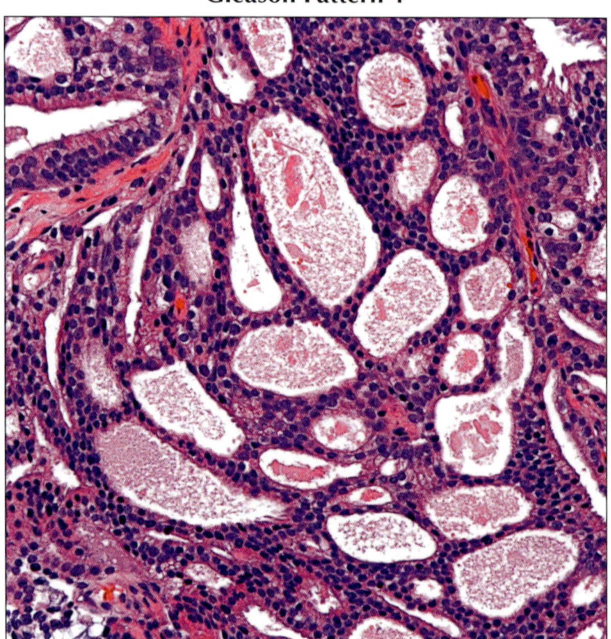

This Gleason pattern 4 cribriform pattern shows a large gland with an irregular outline containing multiple lumina separated by cellular bridges. The presence of necrosis or solid growth in a cribriform gland (not seen here) would warrant designation as Gleason pattern 5. (Courtesy R. E. Jimenez, MD.)

Gleason Pattern 5

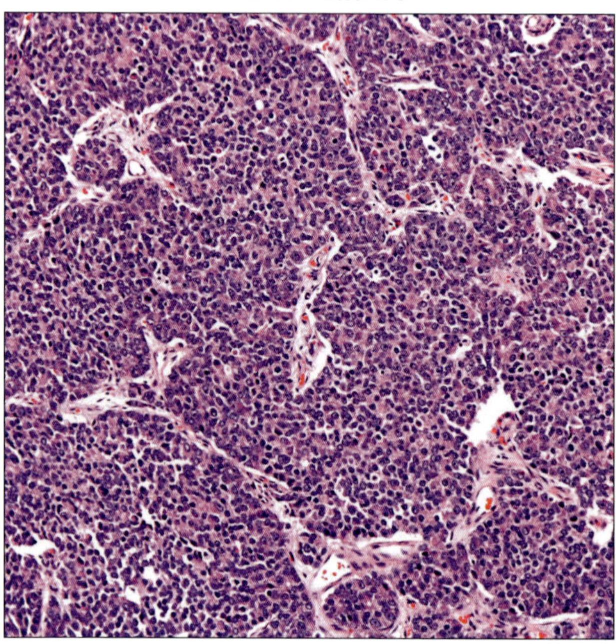

Gleason pattern 5 prostate cancer solid architecture shows diffuse sheet-like growth without lumina. This pattern may be difficult to distinguish from urothelial carcinoma involving the prostate. Use of p63 &/or HMCK (34βE12) immunostains are helpful in making this distinction. (Courtesy R. E. Jimenez, MD.)

Ductal Adenocarcinoma

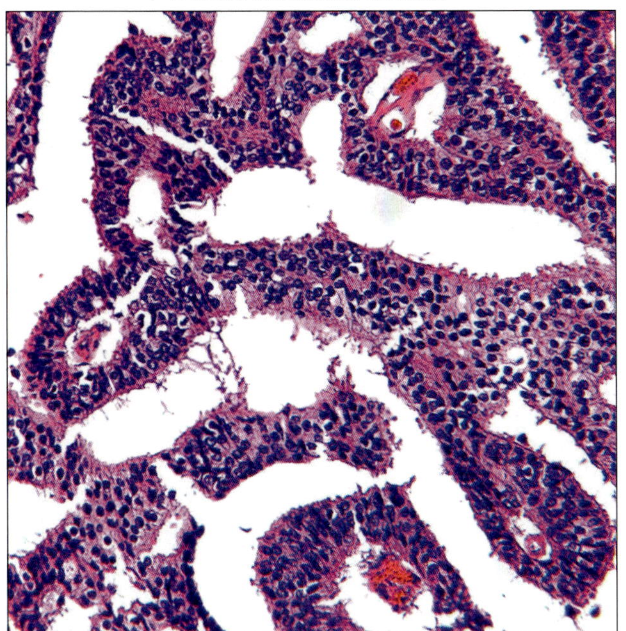

Ductal adenocarcinoma, papillary pattern, shows distinctive papillary architecture with fibrovascular core lined by pseudostratified tall columnar cells. (Courtesy G. P. Paneer, MD.)

Small Cell Carcinoma

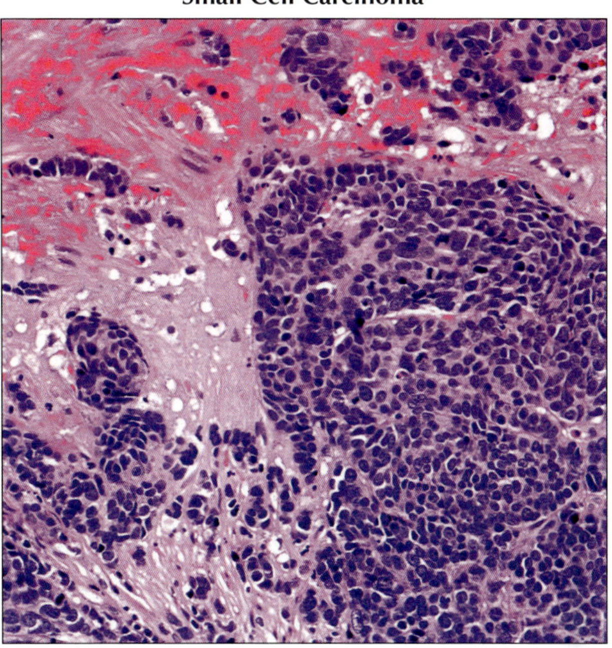

Small cell carcinoma shows diffuse patternless growth and abundant single cell necrosis. Tumor cells are relatively large or intermediate in size with nuclei containing occasional prominent nucleoli. (Courtesy R. E. Jimenez, MD.)

Neuroendocrine Carcinoma

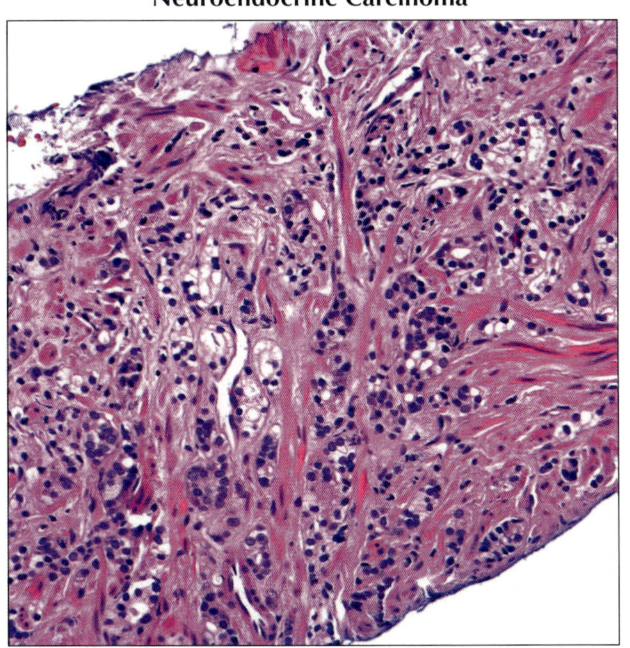

Neuroendocrine carcinoma differentiation in conventional adenocarcinoma shows infiltrative and poorly formed glands of adenocarcinoma, some containing cells with relatively less cytoplasm. (Courtesy R. E. Jimenez, MD.)

Large Cell Neuroendocrine Carcinoma

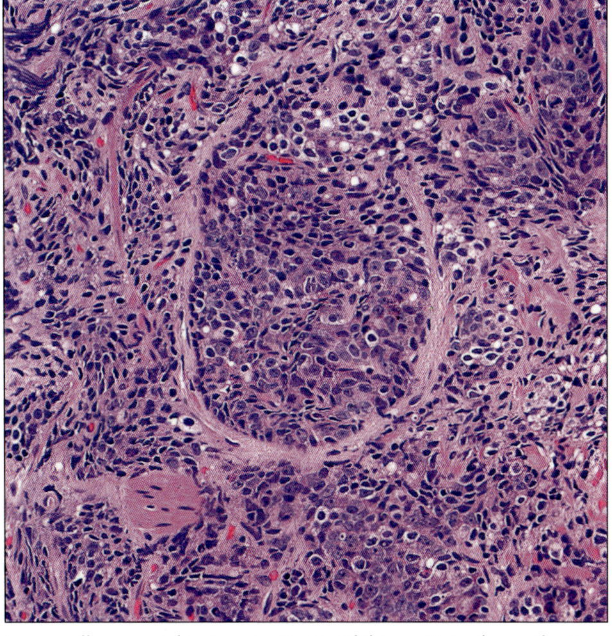

Large cell neuroendocrine carcinoma of the prostate shows sheets of neuroendocrine tumor cells with relatively large nuclei and prominent nucleoli. The tumor cells are less uniform than small cell carcinoma, and some show relatively more cytoplasm. As with small cell carcinoma, an acinar adenocarcinoma component may be present. (Courtesy R. E. Jimenez, MD.)

T2a

Axial graphic demonstrates a localized focus of peripheral zone tumor that involves < 1/2 of 1 lobe of the prostate. This is consistent with T2a disease. T1 disease is neither clinically apparent nor visible on imaging.

T2b

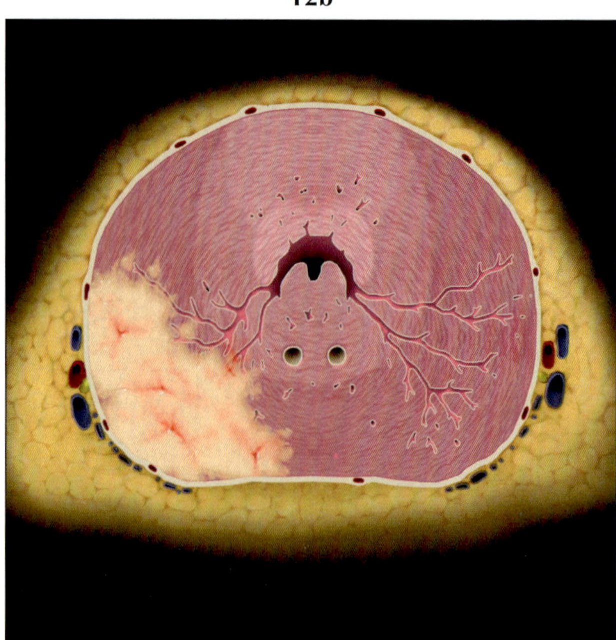

Axial graphic demonstrates a larger focus of peripheral zone tumor that involves > 1/2 of 1 lobe of the prostate but does not cross the midline. The prostatic capsule is intact, and the neurovascular bundle is unaffected by tumor. This is consistent with T2b disease.

T2c

Axial graphic demonstrates a larger focus of peripheral zone tumor that involves > 1/2 of 1 lobe of the prostate and crosses the midline. An additional focus of tumor is present on the contralateral side of the gland. Both of these findings fulfill the criteria for T2c disease.

T3a

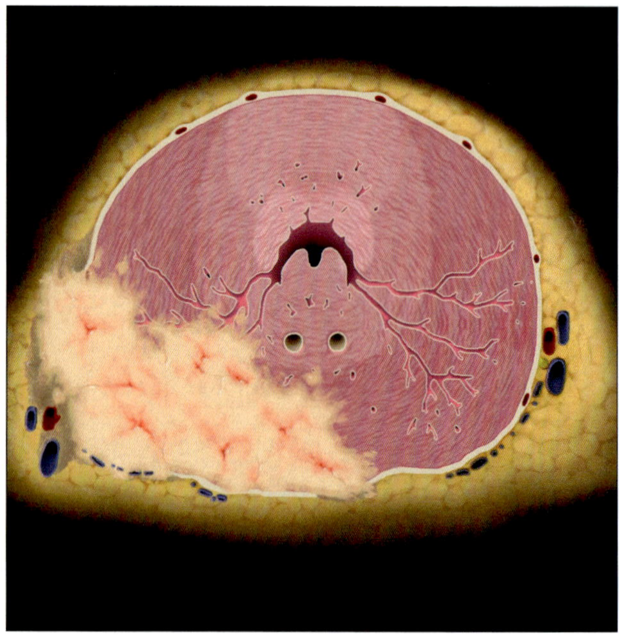

Axial graphic demonstrates a larger focus of peripheral zone tumor with focal bulging of the prostatic contour posteriorly. Additionally, in the posterolateral margin, the capsule is invaded, and tumor spills into the surrounding periprostatic fat and surrounds the neurovascular bundle. This is consistent with T3a disease.

N1

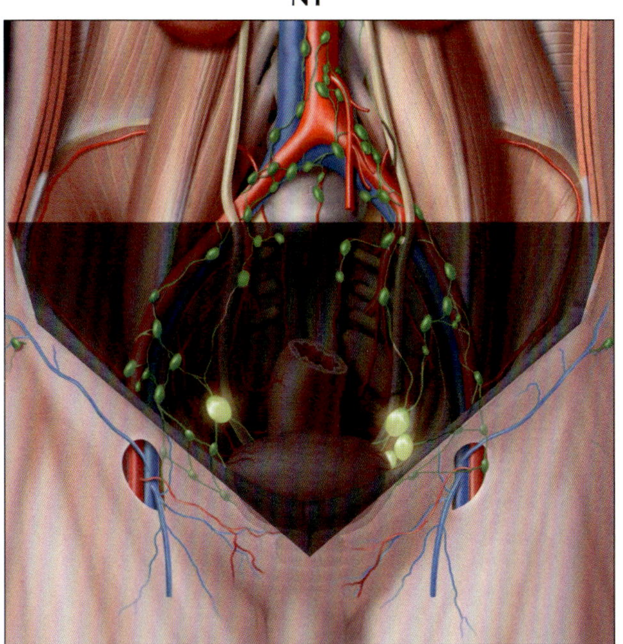

Coronal graphic shows regional lymph nodes shaded in black. Enlarged bilateral internal iliac nodes are present, indicating N1 disease. N1 disease is considered stage IV, regardless of the T stage.

M1a

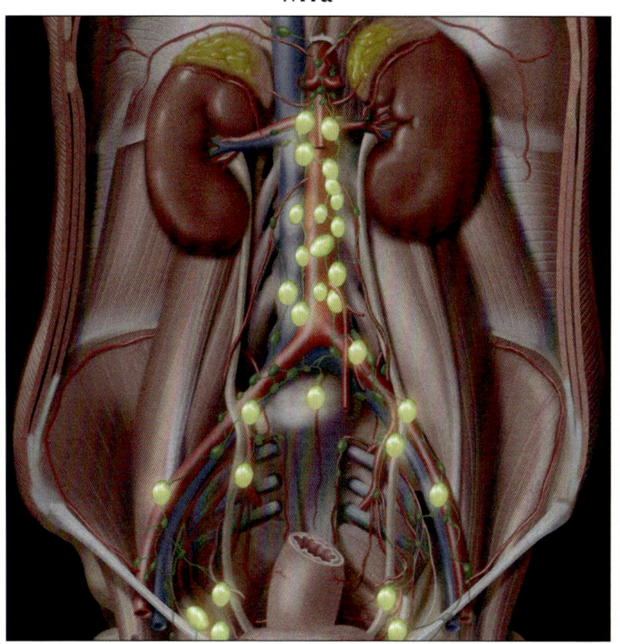

Coronal graphic shows enlarged regional lymph nodes in the pelvis and enlarged nonregional nodes in the common iliac and paraaortic lymph node stations. The presence of nonregional lymph node metastases upgrades disease to M1a.

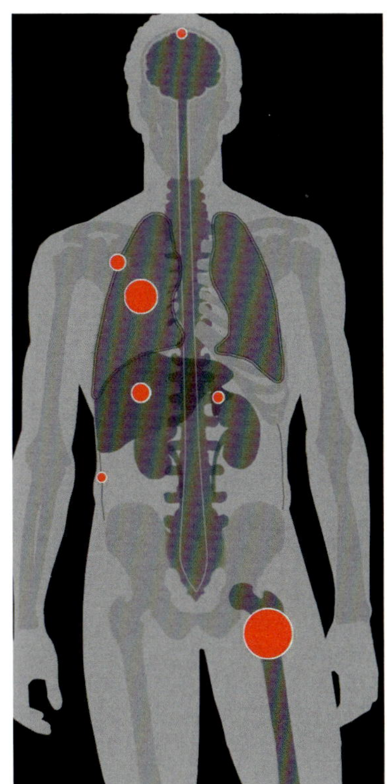

INITIAL SITE OF RECURRENCE

Bone	90%
Lung	46%
Liver	25%
Pleura	21%
Adrenal Gland	13%
Peritoneum	7%
Meninges	6%

Bubendorf L et al: Metastatic patterns of prostate cancer: An autopsy study of 1,589 patients. Hum Pathol. 31(5):578-83, 2000.

PROSTATE

OVERVIEW

General Comments

- Most common noncutaneous cancer in American men
- 1 in 6 men will develop prostate cancer in their lifetime
  - 80% of prostate cancer cases are detected while cancer is localized to prostate gland
  - Screening detects early stage disease well
    - Prostate-specific antigen (PSA) and digital rectal exam (DRE) common screening tests
    - Stage migration has occurred because of widespread PSA screening
      - Overall prevalence of patients with low-risk disease almost 2x greater now than in late 1980s

Classification

- 95% of tumors are adenocarcinoma
- Neuroendocrine and ductal carcinomas rarely occur

NATURAL HISTORY

General Features

- Comments
  - Natural history of prostate cancer varies widely
    - Various risk factors are used to estimate risk of disease progression
      - PSA level (major factor)
      - Gleason score (major factor)
      - T stage (major factor)
      - Percentage of biopsy tissue or cores with cancer (minor factor)
      - Proportion of Gleason pattern 4 or 5 (minor factor)
      - Primary Gleason pattern (i.e., 4+3 versus 3+4) (minor factor)
      - PSA velocity or doubling time (minor factor)
    - Risk grouping is accomplished using established major risk factors
      - Risk may be further stratified using emerging, minor risk factors
  - Untreated prostate cancer can lead to myriad of symptoms, including but not limited to
    - Obstructive &/or irritative urinary symptoms
    - Hematuria or hematospermia
    - Rectal pain or bleeding
    - Painful bone metastasis
    - Neurological pain or weakness from compressive bone or soft-tissue metastasis
    - Lower extremity swelling and edema from pelvic adenopathy

Etiology

- Race
  - United States: African-American males have 60% higher incidence rate compared with white males
  - More common in Western world & rare in Asians (age-adjusted incidence rate 2-10/100,000 men)
  - Difficult to determine specific risk related to race because of socioeconomic confounders
    - Access to health care
    - Income
    - Education
    - Insurance status
- Family history
  - Relative risk (RR) if affected brothers = 3.4 (95% CI: 3.0-3.8)
  - RR if affected fathers = 2.2 (95% CI: 1.9-2.5)
  - Affected male with family history of prostate cancer may present at younger age (6-7 years) than male without such history
- Age
  - < 44 years: Incidence approaches 0
  - 45-54 years: Incidence 8.6%
  - 55-64 years: Incidence 28.0%
  - 65-74 years: Incidence 36.1%
  - 75-84 years: Incidence 22.0%
  - Median age at diagnosis: 69 years
- Diet
  - High-fat diet may increase risk
  - Soy-rich diet may be protective
- Hormonal influence
  - Low testosterone reduces risk
  - 5-α-reductase inhibition reduces risk

Epidemiology & Cancer Incidence

- Number of cases in USA per year
  - 240,890 cases (1st leading cause in men)
  - 33,720 deaths (2nd leading cause in men)

Genetics

- Hereditary prostate cancer accounts for approximately 10% of all prostate cancer cases
  - Unique genetics in early-onset disease (age < 55 years old)
    - Rare autosomal dominant prostate cancer susceptibility genes may account for almost 1/2 of early-onset disease
  - Possible genetic hypotheses include X-linked or recessive inheritance
  - Hereditary prostate cancer 1 (*HPC1*) gene found on chromosome 1q24-25

Gross Pathology & Surgical Features

- Peripheral zone accounts for ~ 80-85% of disease
- Transition zone accounts for ~ 10-15% of disease
  - Site of origin of BPH
- Central zone accounts for ~ 5-10% of disease

Microscopic Pathology

- H&E
  - Gleason score
    - Assignment of histologic grade to predominant (primary) and lesser (secondary) pattern of tumor
    - 2 Gleason grade numbers are summed for a Gleason score
    - Universally accepted and recognized by WHO and AJCC as grading system of choice for prostate cancer
  - Gleason pattern 1
    - Well-differentiated glandular pattern
    - Uniform epithelium, oval nuclei
    - Pale cytoplasm & rare mitotic figures
  - Gleason pattern 2
    - Well-differentiated glandular pattern
    - More intervening stroma between glands
  - Gleason pattern 3
    - Moderately differentiated glandular pattern
    - Distinctly infiltrative margins
  - Gleason pattern 4

- Poorly differentiated glandular pattern
- Irregular masses of neoplastic glands
- Gleason pattern 5
  - Poorly differentiated/anaplastic glandular pattern
  - Only occasional gland formation
  - Sheets of tumor cells, mitoses, cellular atypia
- Histopathologic grading can be complex
  - Morphologic heterogeneity
  - Multifocality
- Special stains
  - Not required routinely
    - May be helpful in specific indications, including
      - Distinguishing prostate cancer from benign mimics and post-treatment changes
      - Distinguishing prostate cancer from nonprostatic malignancies that secondarily involve prostate
  - Broad categories of special stains include
    - Prostate carcinoma-associated marker
    - Antibody stains
    - Epithelial lineage
    - Prostate lineage-specific marker

Routes of Spread

- Local spread
  - Extension through prostatic capsule
  - Seminal vesicle invasion
  - Bladder invasion
  - Rectal invasion
- Lymphatic extension
  - Regional lymph nodes (N1 disease) include nodes of true pelvis; those nodes below bifurcation of common iliac arteries
    - Pelvic nodes NOS
      - 2nd most common site of nodal mets at autopsy
    - Iliac nodes (internal, external, or NOS)
    - Obturator nodes
    - Sacral nodes
    - Hypogastric nodes
  - Distant lymph nodes (M1a disease) are those outside true pelvis
    - Paraaortic nodal disease #1 most common site of nodal mets overall at autopsy
      - May be result of direct nodal seeding from vertebral venous plexus in addition to lymphatic spread
      - Found more frequently when spinal mets are present than when spinal mets are absent
    - Common iliac nodes
    - Mediastinal
      - 3rd most common site of nodal mets
    - Deep and superficial inguinal nodes
      - 4th most common site of nodal mets
- Hematogenous spread
  - Backward venous spread most common source for osteoblastic metastases
    - Prostatic and vesicle venous plexus directly to vertebral (Batson) venous plexus
      - Lumbar spine mets 3x more common than cervical spine mets
      - This pathway may represent early pattern of hematogenous spread
  - Caval route may be later route of dissemination
    - Prostatic venous plexus to iliac veins
    - Inferior vena cava to lungs
    - Lung metastases followed by dissemination to pleura, liver, adrenal glands, etc.
      - Rarely, hematogenous disease will bypass lungs

IMAGING

Staging

- Radionuclide bone scan (Tc-99m whole body bone scan)
  - Most widely used for detecting bone metastases
  - Indication for use dependent on clinical scenario with specific calculated risk of metastatic disease
    - Highly indicated (ACR appropriateness score = 9)
      - T1-2 & GS > 7 & PSA ≥ 20 or ≥ 50% positive core biopsy
      - Clinical T3, seminal vesicle, or bladder neck invasion
    - Indicated (ACR appropriateness score = 8)
      - T1-2 & GS ≤ 6 & PSA > 20 or ≥ 50% positive core biopsy
      - T1-2 & GS 8-10 & PSA < 20 and < 50% positive core biopsy
    - Consider (ACR appropriateness score = 7)
      - T1-2 & GS = 7 & PSA < 20 & < 50% biopsy cores positive
      - PSA in higher part of range or rapid rise in PSA
    - Consider (ACR appropriateness score = 6)
      - T1-2 and GS ≤ 6 and PSA 10-20 and ≥ 50% positive core biopsy
    - Consider for patients with symptomatic bone pain
  - Radiograph, CT, or MR may be used to confirm abnormality seen on bone scan
- CT
  - Most indicated (ACR appropriateness score max = 7)
    - T3-4 or PSA > 20 ng/mL or ≥ 50% positive core biopsy
  - Not accurate in detection of intraprostatic features
  - Otherwise, of limited value for T and N staging
    - Both false-positive and false-negative nodal diagnoses common
    - Poor sensitivity for detecting extracapsular extension (ECE) and seminal vesicle invasion (SVI)
- MR
  - Most indicated (ACR appropriateness score max = 7)
    - T1-2 & GS > 7 & PSA ≥ 20 or ≥ 50% positive core biopsy
    - Clinical T3
  - Accuracy of MR in detection of ECE ranges between 60% and 90%
  - T2WI: Mainly used for local ECE and SVI
    - Best diagnostic clue: Nodular area of ↓ signal in normally high signal peripheral zone
    - Signs of ECE
      - Obliteration of rectoprostatic angle
      - Encroachment of low signal area on neurovascular bundle (NVB)
      - Bulging prostatic outline
      - > 10 mm of low signal area contacting capsule margin suggests capsular invasion but may not be indicative of ECE
    - SVI: Low signal intensity extending into seminal vesicles
    - Urinary bladder or rectal invasion well depicted

PROSTATE

- Osteoblastic bone metastases
  - Low signal intensity on both T1WI & T2WI
  - T1WI: Normal ↑ signal in fatty marrow is replaced by low-intermediate signal intensity
- Functional MR techniques
  - Diffusion-weighted imaging (DWI)
    - Adjunct technique to T2WI with local prostate cancer appearing as areas of high signal on high-b-field DWI
    - Corresponding apparent diffusion coefficient (ADC) is lower than normal tissue in areas of prostate cancer
  - MR spectroscopy
    - Elevated choline peaks or elevated choline + creatine/citrate ratios are malignancy indicators

- FDG PET/CT
  - Little role in primary diagnosis or staging of prostate cancer
  - Difficult to differentiate prostate cancer from BPH and prostatitis
  - Major use is for detection and localization of distant metastases in hormone-refractory prostate carcinoma
- Transrectal ultrasound (TRUS)
  - Poor ability to identify lesions, especially when small
    - Isoechoic to normal peripheral zone (PZ) tissue is not uncommon (30-40%)
  - Poor ability to predict extracapsular tumor extension or seminal vesicle involvement

Restaging

- CT
  - Consider upon biochemical failure (PSA nadir + 2 ng/mL)
- Bone scan
  - Consider upon biochemical failure (PSA nadir + 2 ng/mL)
- MR
  - Local recurrence may manifest as areas of enhancing soft tissue isointense to muscle on T1WI and hyperintense on T2WI
    - Spectroscopy may identify hypermetabolic areas to direct biopsy
  - May also be useful for detecting bony metastases when NM bone scan is equivocal

Screening

- American Cancer Society 2012 guidelines
  - Prior to initiating prostate cancer screening, relative risks and benefits of screening and prostate cancer treatment should be discussed with patient
  - For average-risk male with normal life expectancy (> 10-year overall survival), begin screening with PSA at age 50
  - For high-risk male, begin screening with PSA at age 45
    - African-American males
    - Males with 1st-degree relative diagnosed with prostate cancer < age 65
  - For even higher-risk males, begin screening with PSA at age 40
    - Males with several 1st- and 2nd-degree relatives with prostate carcinoma
- DRE
  - May be helpful for detection of abnormality
- PSA
  - Challenges with false negatives and false positives
    - > 25% of biopsy-proven prostate carcinomas occur in patients with "normal" PSA
    - 70-80% of patients with "elevated" PSA do not have prostate carcinoma
      - May be elevated in BPH
  - Upper limit of PSA levels at which to initiate more definitive testing for prostate cancer has not been established
- No imaging modality yet established as effective for screening

CLINICAL PRESENTATION & WORK-UP

Presentation

- Most asymptomatic at presentation
- Usually detected by screening PSA &/or DRE
  - Controversy exists in regard to benefit of disease detection compared to risk of treatment
- If other significant comorbidities, patient may succumb to death from competing diseases before metastatic prostate cancer

Prognosis

- Prognostic factors
  - PSA
    - Absolute level (major factor)
    - Velocity or doubling time (minor factor)
  - Tumor size
    - T stage (major factor)
    - Percentage of positive biopsy cores or tissue (minor factor)
  - Gleason score
    - Gleason sum (major factor)
    - Primary Gleason pattern (e.g., 4+3 vs. 3+4) (minor factor)
    - Percentage of Gleason pattern 4 or 5 (minor factor)
- 5-year freedom from biochemical failure
  - Low risk: 95%
  - Intermediate risk: 75%
  - High risk: 50%

Work-Up

- Clinical
  - Urinary function
    - American Urologic Association Prostate Symptom Score (AMAPSS)
    - International Prostate Symptom Score (IPSS)
    - Prior urethral surgeries (e.g., transurethral resection of prostate)
  - Erectile function
    - Sexual Health Inventory for Men (SHIM)
  - Gastrointestinal function
    - Number and frequency of bowel movements
    - Symptoms or preexisting conditions (e.g., inflammatory bowel disease)
    - Prior rectal surgeries
  - Comorbidities
    - Anesthetic risk for brachytherapy (BT)
    - Cardiovascular risk for ADT
  - Physical exam

- Particular attention to DRE for clinical T staging
  - Superficial and deep palpation is indicated
  - Firmness or hardness is consistent with cancer
  - Cysts are typically small, smooth, mobile, and can be present after biopsy
  - Obliteration of median raphe suggests bilateral disease
  - Obliteration of lateral sulci suggests ECE
  - Gritty or otherwise irregular texture suggests ECE
  - Rectal mass may require further evaluation
- Radiographic
  - Risk adapted
    - Intermediate or low risk
      - Consider CT and bone scan in selected cases
      - Consider prostate MR to exclude ECE if suspicious on DRE
    - High risk
      - CT abdomen/pelvis and bone scan
      - Baseline bone density measurement by dual energy x-ray absorptiometry for men receiving ADT
- Laboratory
  - Serum PSA and testosterone
  - Baseline fasting blood glucose for men receiving ADT
  - Baseline fasting lipid profile for men receiving ADT

TREATMENT

Major Treatment Alternatives

- Surgery
  - Open prostatectomy
    - Retropubic
    - Perineal
    - Suprapubic transvesicle
  - Laparoscopic or robotic
- External beam RT
  - 3-dimensional conformal RT
  - Intensity-modulated RT with image guidance
- ADT
  - Orchiectomy
  - Anti-androgen
  - Leuteinizing hormone-releasing hormone agonist
- Brachytherapy
  - Permanent BT
    - Low dose rate
  - Temporary BT
    - High dose rate
  - May deliver alone or in combination with external beam RT &/or ADT
- Active surveillance
  - Delays curative treatment until it is warranted based on indicators of disease progression
- Watchful waiting
  - Forgoes curative treatment and initiates intervention only when symptoms arise

Treatment by Risk Category

- Low risk
  - External beam RT
  - Brachytherapy
  - Radical prostatectomy
  - Active surveillance
- Intermediate risk
  - External beam RT
  - External beam RT and BT
  - External beam RT and ADT
  - BT alone
  - Radical prostatectomy
- High risk
  - External beam RT and ADT
  - Combination of external beam RT and BT and ADT
  - Prostatectomy is discouraged
- Post-prostatectomy
  - External beam RT
    - Indications for adjuvant radiation: Positive surgical margin or pT3-4
    - Indications for salvage radiation: Recurrent PSA
  - External beam RT and ADT
    - Consider if salvage (e.g., PSA > 2 ng/mL)
- Other indications
  - Lymph node positive
    - External beam RT and ADT if 10-year life expectancy
  - Palliation of hematuria
    - Usually associated with initial management with ADT alone
      - External beam RT
  - Local recurrence following external beam RT
    - ADT
    - Brachytherapy
    - Cryosurgery
    - Prostatectomy
  - Painful bone metastasis
    - Short course external beam RT
      - 30 Gy in 10 fractions
      - 8 Gy in 1 fraction (non-vertebral)
    - Radiopharmaceuticals
      - Strontium-89
      - Samarium-153

External Beam RT Simulation

- Supine and immobilized
- Comfortably full bladder
- Empty rectum
- CT
- MR

External Beam RT Treatment Planning Scheme

- Intact prostate
  - PTV1 = prostate + proximal seminal vesicles + 8 mm, except posteriorly where 5 mm is used
    - Include any areas suspicious for ECE if T3a
  - PTV2 = distal seminal vesicles + 8 mm, except posteriorly where 5 mm is used
    - Consider including distal seminal vesicles in PTV1 if T3b
  - PTV3 = CTV3 + 5 mm, less if necessary to meet rectal dose constraints
    - Distal common iliac, presacral lymph nodes (S[1]-S[3]), external iliac, internal iliac, and obturator regions included
    - CTV3 = vessels (artery and vein) + 7 mm
    - Bowel, bladder, bone, and muscle should be excluded
- Postoperative
  - PTV1 = prostate bed + 8 mm, except posteriorly where 5 mm is used

PROSTATE

External Beam RT Prescription Doses

- Low risk
  - PTV1: 78 Gy in 2 Gy fractions
- Intermediate risk
  - PTV1: 80 Gy in 2 Gy fractions
- High risk
  - PTV1: 80 Gy in 2 Gy fractions
  - PTV2/PTV3: 56 Gy in 1.4 Gy fractions
- Adjuvant
  - PTV1: 64 Gy in 2 Gy fractions
- Salvage
  - PTV1: 68 Gy in 2 Gy fractions

Other Standard Doses

- Alternative external beam RT (1.8-2 Gy per fraction)
  - Definitive: 76-80 Gy (PTV1), 40-50 Gy (PTV2/PTV3)
  - Postoperative: 64-72 Gy
- Interstitial BT
  - Low dose rate
    - 125-iodine: 140-160 Gy
    - 103-palladium: 110-125 Gy
- Combination external beam RT + BT
  - Low-dose-rate BT
    - 125-iodine: 108-110 Gy
    - 103-palladium: 90-100 Gy
  - High-dose-rate BT
    - 192-iridium: 9.5-10.5 Gy x 2 fractions, 5.5-7.5 Gy x 3 fractions, or 4.0-6.0 Gy x 4 fractions
  - External beam
    - 40-50 Gy (prostate/seminal vesicles)
- ADT
  - Intermediate risk: 4-6 months
  - High risk: 24-36 months

Organs at Risk Parameters

- Normal tissue dose constraints for intensity-modulated RT
  - Rectum (wall and contents from sigmoid flexure to bottom of ischial tuberosities): V60 Gy < 17%, V40 Gy < 35%
    - 90% isodose line extends < 50% of the rectal axial circumference
    - 50% isodose line extends less than the full rectal axial circumference
  - Bladder (wall and contents): V60 Gy < 25%, V40 Gy < 50%
  - Femoral heads (to greater trochanter): V50 Gy < 10% (each)
  - Bowel (potential space): < 150 mL at 40 Gy, otherwise as low as possible

Common Techniques

- Image-guided RT
  - Intact prostate
    - Fiducial markers
      - Electronic portal imaging alignment
      - CT alignment
    - Electromagnetic transponders
    - Cone beam CT alone
      - May be used when fiducial placement is not possible
    - Ultrasound
  - Postoperative
    - CT ± fiducials
    - Electromagnetic transponders

Landmark Trials

- Definitive RT dose escalation: ↑ failure-free survival (FFS) with ↑ dose
  - MD Anderson: 70 vs. 78 Gy (Kuban, 2007)
  - PROG/ACR: 70.2 vs. 79.2 Gy (Zietman, 2010)
  - MRC: 64 vs. 74 Gy (Dearnaley, 2007)
  - Netherlands: 68 vs. 78 Gy (Peeters, 2006)
- Combination RT and ADT vs. RT alone: ↑ FFS with ADT in all trials, and ↑ OS in some
  - RTOG 85-31 (Pilepich, 2005)
  - RTOG 86-10 (Roach, 2008)
  - EORTC (Bolla, 2002)
  - TROG (Denham, 2011)
  - Dana Farber (D'Amico, 2004)
  - RTOG 94-08 (Jones, 2011)
- Combination RT and long-term vs. short-term ADT: ↑ FFS with ADT, and ↑ OS in Bolla trial
  - RTOG 92-02 (Horwitz, 2003)
  - EORTC (Bolla, 2009)
  - Quebec (Laverdiere, 2004)
- Postoperative RT vs. observation: ↑ FFS with ADT in all trials, and ↑ OS in SWOG trial
  - SWOG (Thompson, 2009)
  - EORTC (Bolla, 2005)
  - ARO (Wiegel, 2009)
- Combination RT and ADT vs. ADT alone: ↑ OS in both trials
  - Scandinavia/Swedish (Widmark, 2009)
  - NCIC/MRC (Warde, 2011)

RECOMMENDED FOLLOW-UP

Clinical

- RT alone: DRE annually
- RT and ADT: DRE every 6 months until stabilization of PSA with recovered testosterone, then annually
- Monitor AUA SS, IPSS, and SHIM

Radiographic

- Routine imaging not indicated
- Osteoporosis screening
  - Repeat bone density measurement by dual-energy x-ray absorptiometry after 1 year of ADT, then repeat every 2 years or as clinically indicated

Laboratory

- RT alone: PSA every 6 months; testosterone optional and helpful for evaluation of erectile dysfunction
- RT and ADT: PSA/testosterone every 6 months until stabilization of PSA with recovered testosterone, then annually
- Diabetes and pre-diabetes screening
  - Annual fasting plasma glucose
- Hyperlipidemia screening
  - Fasting lipoproteins

Management for Men Receiving ADT

- Prevention of weight gain
- Reduction in cardiovascular risk factors
  - Smoking cessation
- Regular weight-bearing exercise
- Calcium and vitamin D supplementation
  - 1,200-1,500 mg daily calcium

SELECTED REFERENCES

1. Davis BJ et al: American Brachytherapy Society consensus guidelines for transrectal ultrasound-guided permanent prostate brachytherapy. Brachytherapy. 11(1):6-19, 2012
2. Yamada Y et al: American Brachytherapy Society consensus guidelines for high-dose-rate prostate brachytherapy. Brachytherapy. 11(1):20-32, 2012
3. Denham JW et al: Short-term neoadjuvant androgen deprivation and radiotherapy for locally advanced prostate cancer: 10-year data from the TROG 96.01 randomised trial. Lancet Oncol. 12(5):451-9, 2011
4. Grossmann M et al: Androgen deprivation therapy in men with prostate cancer: how should the side effects be monitored and treated? Clin Endocrinol (Oxf). 74(3):289-93, 2011
5. Jones CU et al: Radiotherapy and short-term androgen deprivation for localized prostate cancer. N Engl J Med. 365(2):107-18, 2011
6. Warde P et al: 3/MRC UK PR07 investigators. Combined androgen deprivation therapy and radiation therapy for locally advanced prostate cancer: a randomised, phase 3 trial. Lancet. 378(9809):2104-11, 2011
7. American Joint Committee on Cancer: AJCC Cancer Staging Manual. 7th ed. New York: Springer. 457-68, 2010
8. Michalski JM et al: Development of RTOG consensus guidelines for the definition of the clinical target volume for postoperative conformal radiation therapy for prostate cancer. Int J Radiat Oncol Biol Phys. 76(2):361-8, 2010
9. Zietman AL et al: Randomized trial comparing conventional-dose with high-dose conformal radiation therapy in early-stage adenocarcinoma of the prostate: long-term results from proton radiation oncology group/ american college of radiology 95-09. J Clin Oncol. 28(7):1106-11, 2010
10. Bolla M et al: Duration of androgen suppression in the treatment of prostate cancer. N Engl J Med. 360(24):2516-27, 2009
11. Lawton CA et al: RTOG GU Radiation oncology specialists reach consensus on pelvic lymph node volumes for high-risk prostate cancer. Int J Radiat Oncol Biol Phys. 74(2):383-7, 2009
12. Thompson IM et al: Adjuvant radiotherapy for pathological T3N0M0 prostate cancer significantly reduces risk of metastases and improves survival: long-term followup of a randomized clinical trial. J Urol. 181(3):956-62, 2009
13. Widmark A et al: Endocrine treatment, with or without radiotherapy, in locally advanced prostate cancer (SPCG-7/ SFUO-3): an open randomised phase III trial. Lancet. 2009 Jan 24;373(9660):301-8. Erratum in: Lancet. 373(9670):1174, 2009
14. Wiegel T et al: Phase III postoperative adjuvant radiotherapy after radical prostatectomy compared with radical prostatectomy alone in pT3 prostate cancer with postoperative undetectable prostate-specific antigen: ARO 96-02/AUO AP 09/95. J Clin Oncol. 27(18):2924-30, 2009
15. Horwitz EM et al: Ten-year follow-up of radiation therapy oncology group protocol 92-02: a phase III trial of the duration of elective androgen deprivation in locally advanced prostate cancer. J Clin Oncol. 26(15):2497-504, 2008
16. Kuban DA et al: Long-term results of the M. D. Anderson randomized dose-escalation trial for prostate cancer. Int J Radiat Oncol Biol Phys. 70(1):67-74, 2008
17. Roach M 3rd et al: Short-term neoadjuvant androgen deprivation therapy and external-beam radiotherapy for locally advanced prostate cancer: long-term results of RTOG 8610. J Clin Oncol. 26(4):585-91, 2008
18. Dearnaley DP et al: Escalated-dose versus standard-dose conformal radiotherapy in prostate cancer: first results from the MRC RT01 randomised controlled trial. Lancet Oncol. 8(6):475-87, 2007
19. Peeters ST et al: Dose-response in radiotherapy for localized prostate cancer: results of the Dutch multicenter randomized phase III trial comparing 68 Gy of radiotherapy with 78 Gy. J Clin Oncol. 24(13):1990-6, 2006
20. Bolla M et al: Postoperative radiotherapy after radical prostatectomy: a randomised controlled trial (EORTC trial 22911). Lancet. 366(9485):572-8, 2005
21. Pilepich MV et al: Androgen suppression adjuvant to definitive radiotherapy in prostate carcinoma--long-term results of phase III RTOG 85-31. Int J Radiat Oncol Biol Phys. 61(5):1285-90, 2005
22. D'Amico AV et al: 6-month androgen suppression plus radiation therapy vs radiation therapy alone for patients with clinically localized prostate cancer: a randomized controlled trial. JAMA. 292(7):821-7, 2004
23. Laverdière J et al: The efficacy and sequencing of a short course of androgen suppression on freedom from biochemical failure when administered with radiation therapy for T2-T3 prostate cancer. J Urol. 171(3):1137-40, 2004
24. Bolla M et al: Long-term results with immediate androgen suppression and external irradiation in patients with locally advanced prostate cancer (an EORTC study): a phase III randomised trial. Lancet. 360(9327):103-6, 2002

(Left) *Grayscale transrectal ultrasound (TRUS) shows an ill-defined, hypoechoic, heterogeneous area* ➔ *in the right peripheral zone. Tumor appears confined to the limits of prostatic capsule. However, TRUS is not sensitive enough to be used to exclude ECE or SVI.* **(Right)** *In same patient, the transducer is rotated to bring nodule to left side of image. Power Doppler ultrasound shows neovascularization* ⤻ *around the mass. Guided biopsy confirmed prostatic carcinoma.*

T2

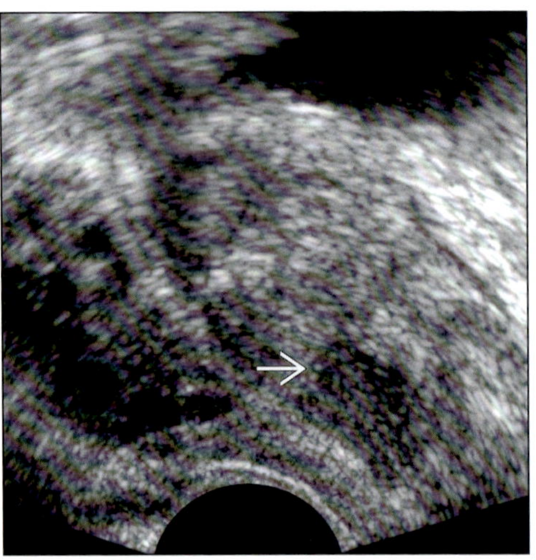

T2

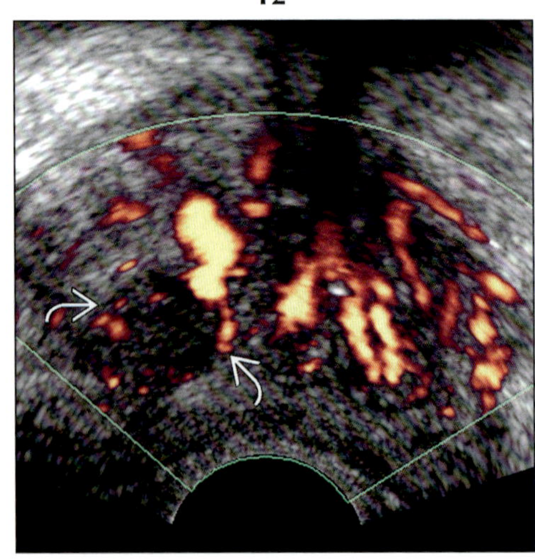

(Left) *Axial T2WI MR without ER coil at 3.0T demonstrates a 9 mm focus of low T2 SI in the right peripheral zone* ➔*, with an intact sharply demarcated T2 dark fibrous band overlying the abnormal focus, suggesting an intact capsule. The normal heterogeneously low T2 SI of the central gland is well demonstrated* ⇩. **(Right)** *Sagittal T2WI MR in the same patient shows the tumor focus* ➔*. Normal high T2 SI is present in the right seminal vesicle* ⤻.

Stage I (pT2a N0 M0, PSA 6, Gleason 6)

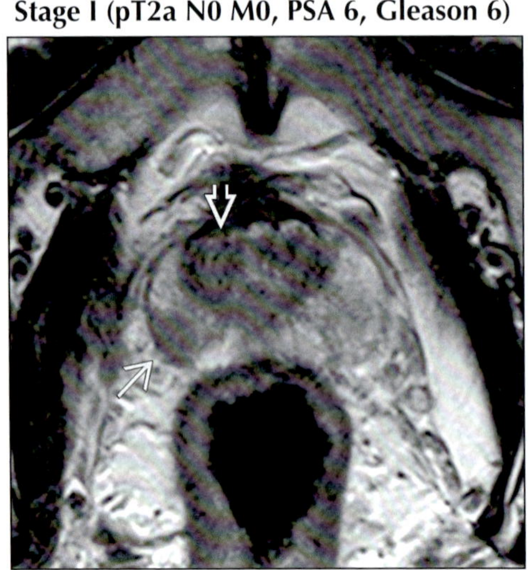

Stage I (pT2a N0 M0, PSA 6, Gleason 6)

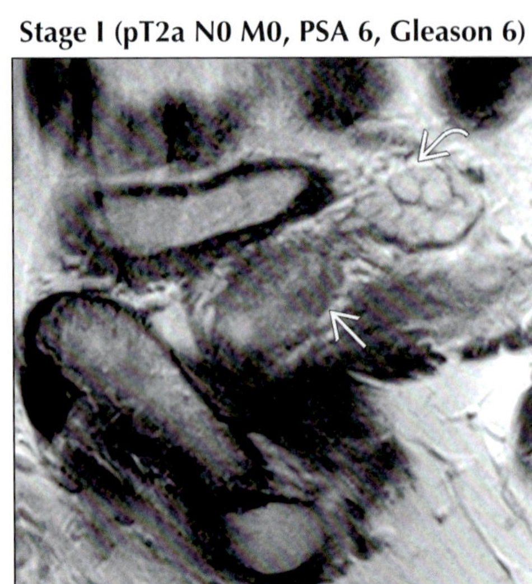

(Left) *Axial T2WI MR without ER coil at 3.0T demonstrates low T2 SI in the right peripheral zone (PZ) mid gland spanning from 7 o'clock to 10:30* ➔*. This area spans more than 1/2 of the left lobe, with normal heterogeneously high T2 SI in the right PZ. An intact neurovascular bundle* ⤻ *is present.* **(Right)** *Coronal T2WI MR from the same patient demonstrates the PZ asymmetry, with abnormal low T2 SI in the right PZ* ➔ *and normal high T2 SI in the left PZ* ⤻.

Stage IIA (T2b N0 M0)

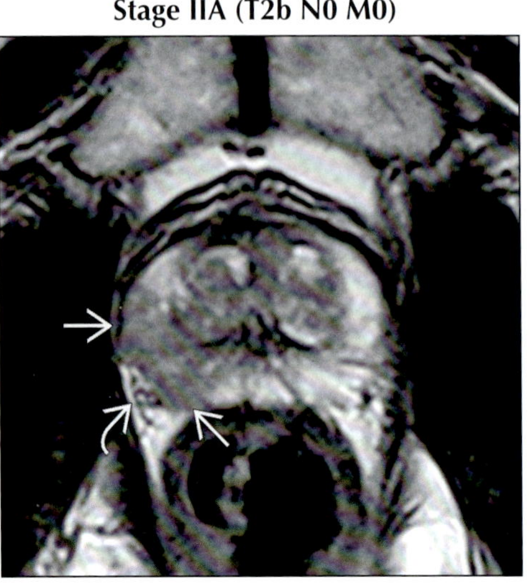

Stage IIA (T2b N0 M0)

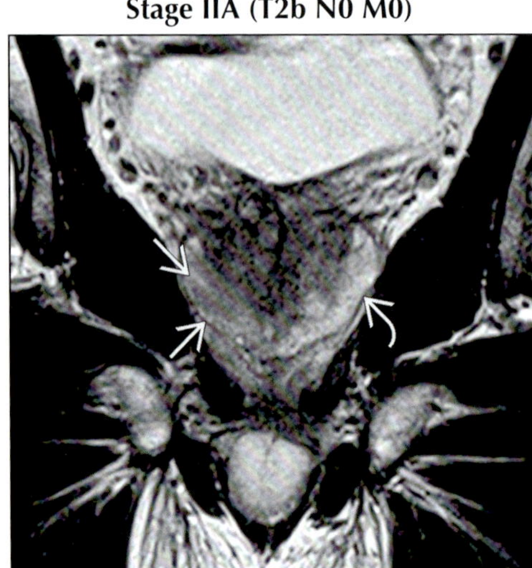

Stage IIB (T2c N0 M0)

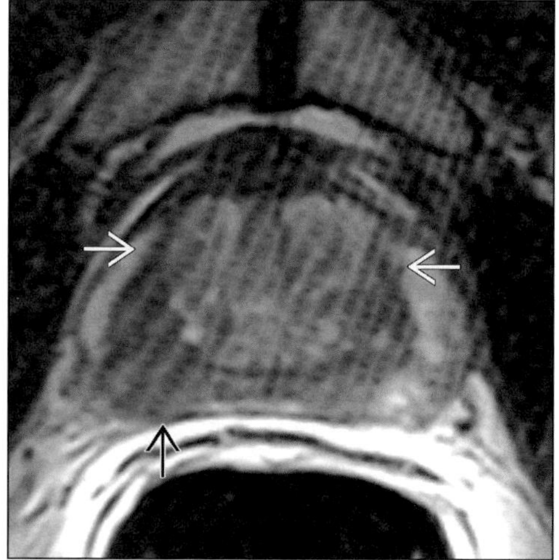

Stage IIB (T2c N0 M0)

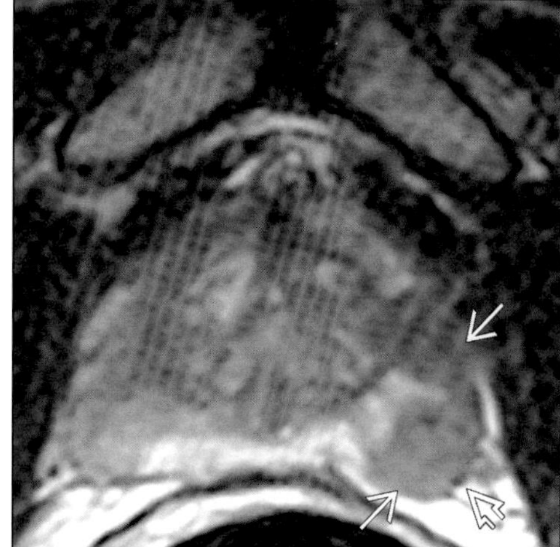

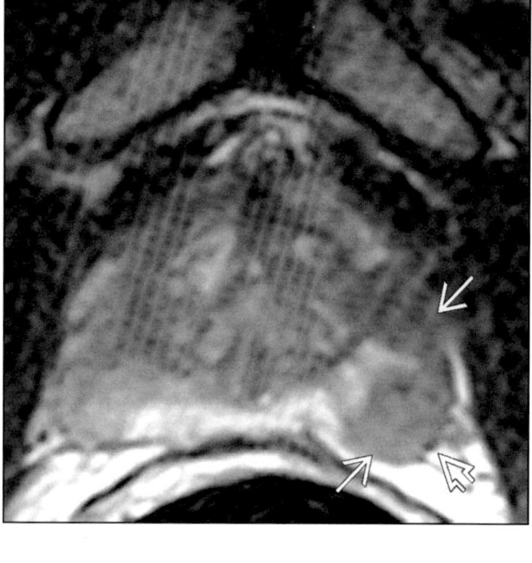

(Left) *Axial T2WI MR with ER coil at the prostate base shows a continuous band of low PZ T2 SI from 1 o'clock to 11 o'clock →. The band abuts both the prostate CZ and the T2 dark fibrous capsule →.* *The capsular margin appears intact.* ***(Right)*** *At the mid gland level in the same patient, a more focal nodule of disease is present on the left → with a bulging rectoprostatic angle →. This is concerning for extracapsular extension. Right-sided low SI tumor is also seen at this level.*

Stage III (pT3a N0 M0, PSA 6, Gleason 7)

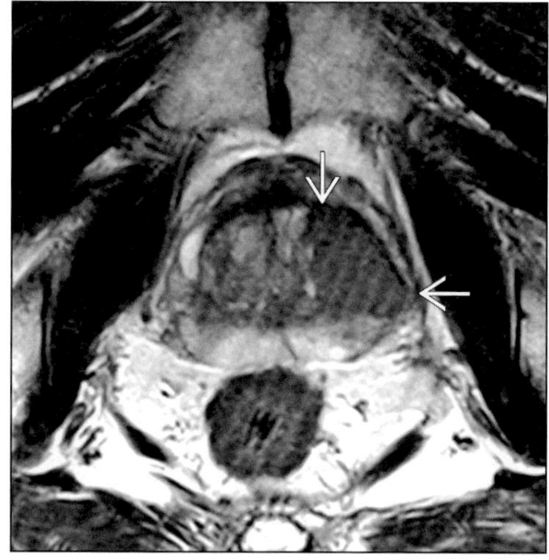

Stage III (pT3a N0 M0, PSA 6, Gleason 7)

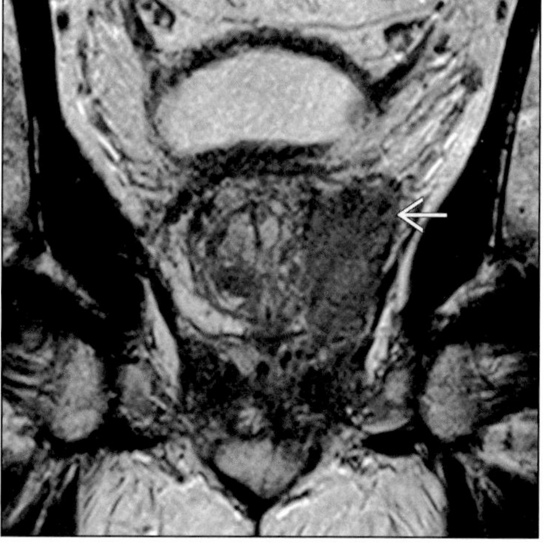

(Left) *Axial T2WI MR without ER coil demonstrates large, homogeneously low T2 SI tumor in the left gland from 2 o'clock to 4 o'clock →. The mass involves the CZ and extends beyond the prostatic capsule. Because the bulk of the tumor is in the anterior portion of the gland, the neurovascular bundle may be spared.* ***(Right)*** *Coronal T2WI MR shows the focal bulge at the lateral base well →. This is consistent with extracapsular extension, which was confirmed at resection.*

Stage III (pT3a N0 M0, PSA 6, Gleason 7)

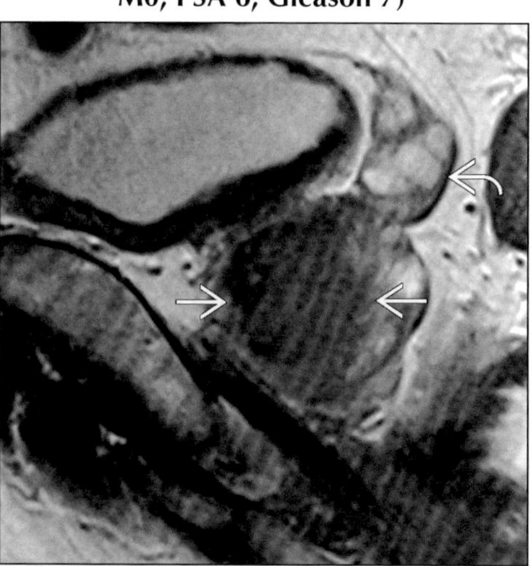

Stage III (pT3a N0 M0, PSA 6, Gleason 7)

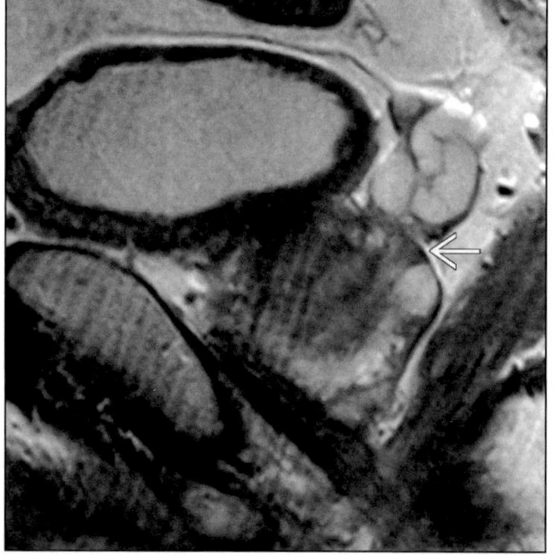

(Left) *Sagittal T2WI MR in the same patient shows the focal low T2 SI area corresponding to tumor on the left →. No definite low SI is present in the seminal vesicle →. The bulk of the tumor is anterior in the prostate, decreasing the likelihood of direct seminal vesicle invasion.* ***(Right)*** *Sagittal T2WI MR on the right in the same patient shows the heterogeneously high PZ T2 SI. A focus of low T2 SI near the prostate base → is concerning for an additional site of disease.*

Stage III (T3a N0 M0)

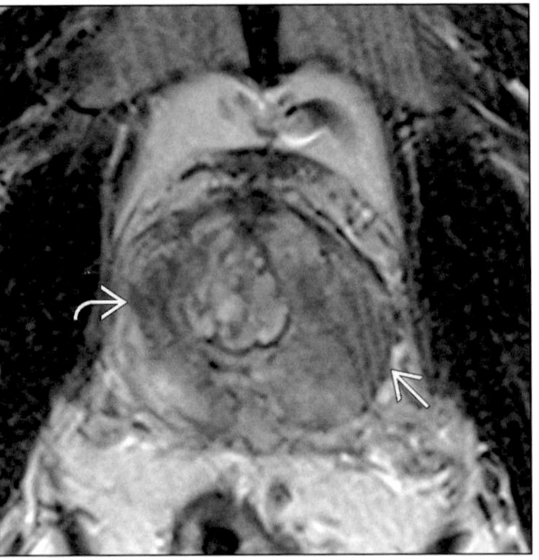

Stage III (T3a N0 M0)

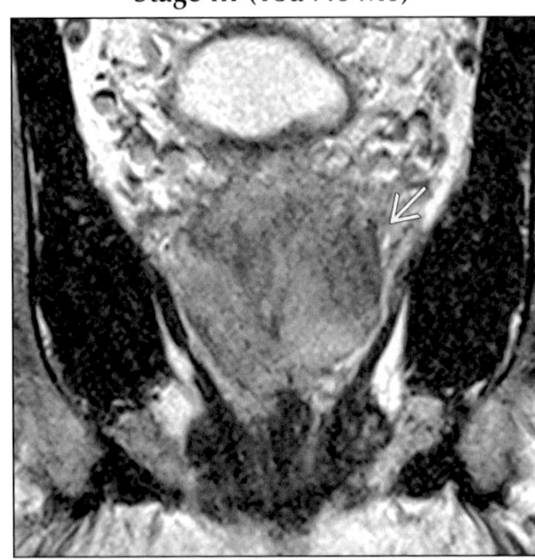

(Left) *Axial T2WI MR shows diffuse low T2 SI throughout the PZ on the left →, with a rim of abnormal signal in the right TZ ↪. The capsule appears intact, but the low T2 SI area in the PZ contacts > 10 mm of the prostate margin.* ***(Right)*** *Coronal T2WI MR in the same patient shows the left-sided low T2 SI nodule with focal bulging and irregularity at the lateral base →. This is evidence of unilateral extracapsular extension. Seminal vesicles were uninvolved.*

Stage III (T3b N0 M0)

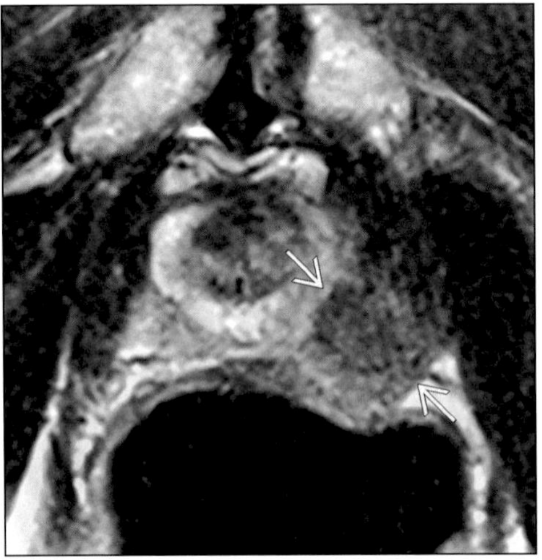

Stage III (T3b N0 M0)

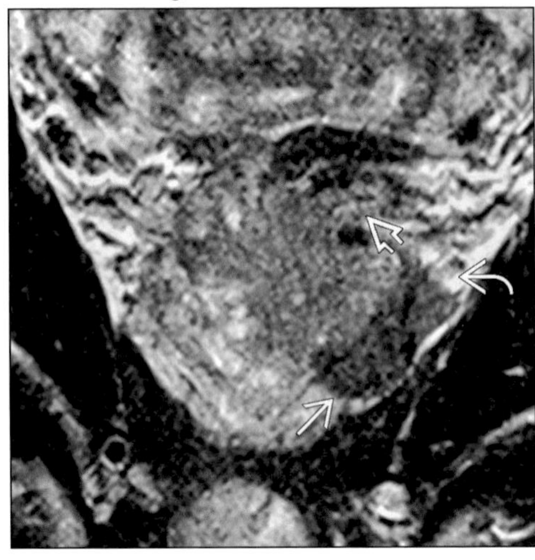

(Left) *Axial T2WI MR shows a focal bulging low T2 SI mass → in the left PZ. This is palpable on DRE as a firm nodule.* ***(Right)*** *Coronal T2WI MR in the same patient shows the focal area of very low T2 SI tumor → extending from the left mid gland to the left base. Extracapsular extension is seen at the base where the tumor extends beyond the capsular margin ↪. Seminal vesicle invasion is present with heterogeneously low T2 SI extending into the SV ⇨.*

Stage III (T3b N0 M0)

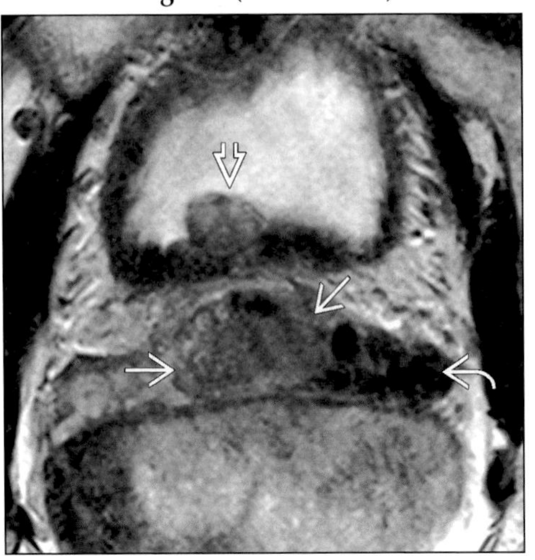

Stage III (T3b N0 M0)

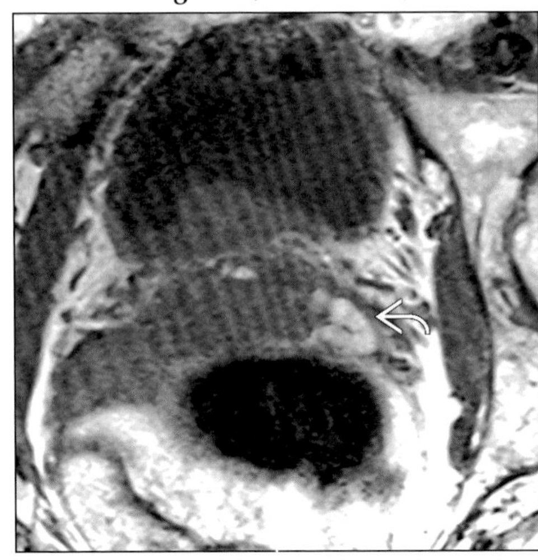

(Left) *Axial T2WI more cranially at the level of the prostate base in the same patient shows the low T2 SI extending into the seminal vesicles → related to the patient's BPH. The tubules of the seminal vesicles on the left demonstrate very dark T2 SI ↪. A prostatic nodule from the patient's BPH protrudes into the bladder base ⇨.* ***(Right)*** *Axial T1WI MR at the same level confirms that the low T2 signal in the seminal vesicles on the left is due to hemorrhage, which is T1 bright ↪.*

Prostate Zonal Anatomy

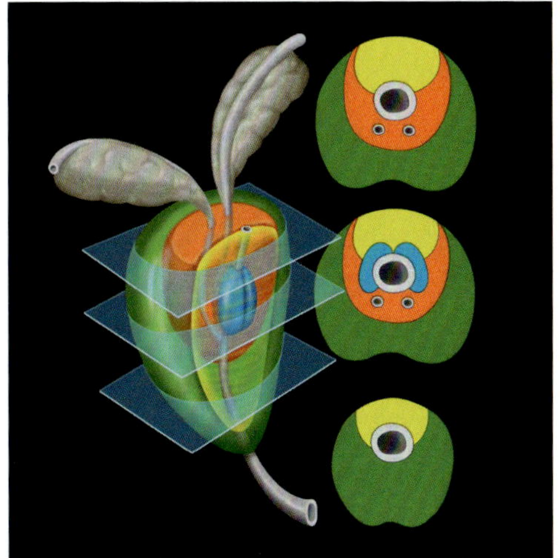

Pelvic Anatomy

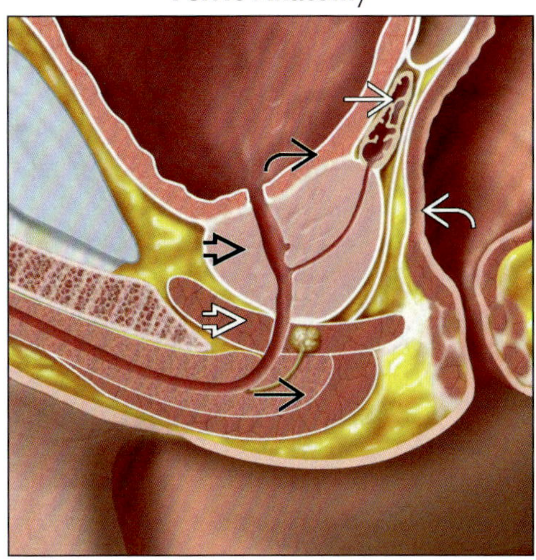

*(**Left**) A schematic of the anatomic zones of the prostate shows the anterior fibromuscular stroma (yellow), central zone (orange), transition zone (blue), and peripheral zone (green). (**Right**) A schematic representation of relevant pelvic anatomy shows the seminal vesicles ➔, bladder wall ↗, rectal wall ↗, prostate ➪, urogenital diaphragm ➔, and penile bulb →.*

Simulation

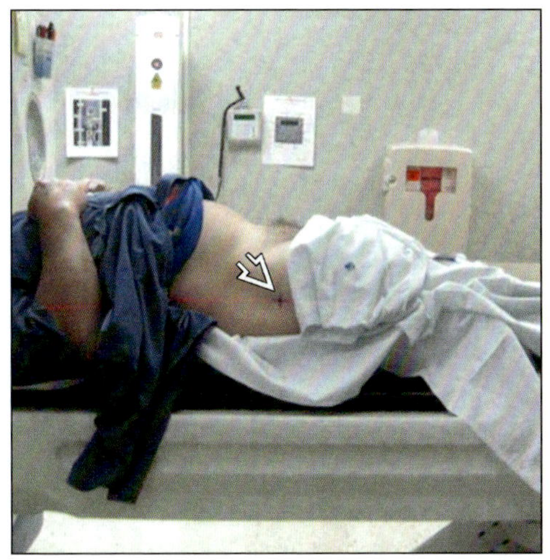

Simulation

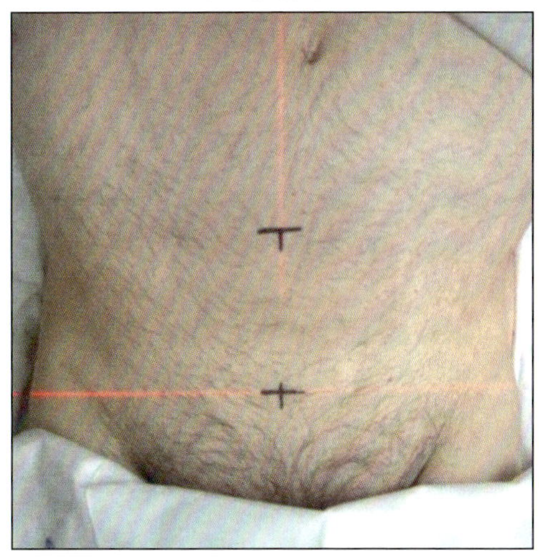

*(**Left**) The patient is simulated in the treatment position lying supine in a customized foam cast. Tattoos triangulate the isocenter and guide patient alignment. Lateral tattoos ➔ gauge axial rotation and straightening of the patient and in-out positioning of the couch. (**Right**) Midline marks and tattoos align the patient in the left-right direction and assist in patient straightening.*

Prostate Contours: Series 1 CT

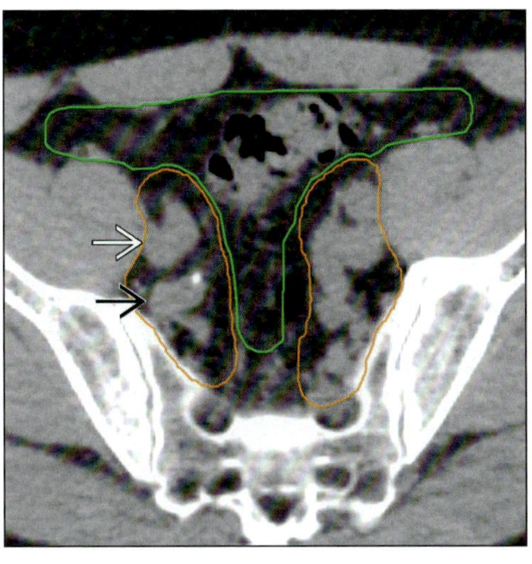

Prostate Contours: Series 1 MR

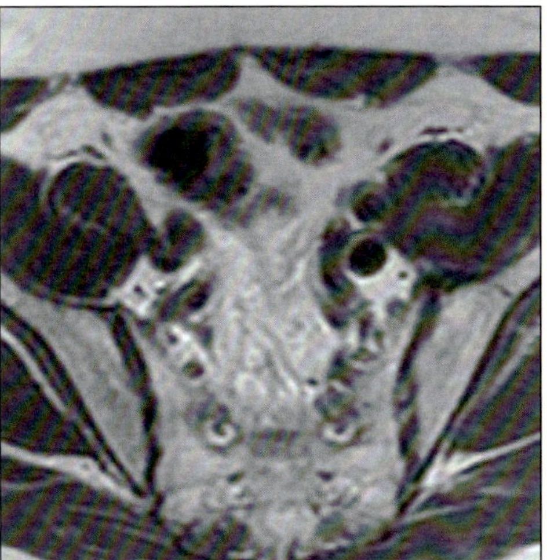

*(**Left**) Pelvic nodal contours (PTV3, orange) above the femoral heads include the external ➔ and internal iliac → vessels with a 7 mm margin. Bowel, bone, and muscle are excluded. The potential space in which the bowel may exist (green) is contoured as an avoidance structure. (**Right**) At this level, MR provides little additional value for the visualization of the pelvic lymph node regions compared to CT.*

PROSTATE

(**Left**) *The potential space containing bowel between 2 lymph node contours (PTV3, orange) can be contoured as a 2nd, separate avoidance structure to achieve greater dose conformality in this region by imposing distinct dose limits to this bowel substructure.* (**Right**) *Bladder and bowel filling can differ between CT and MR. Care should be taken to ensure that all contouring is performed consistently and aligned properly with fiducial markers used for image guidance.*

Prostate Contours: Series 2 CT

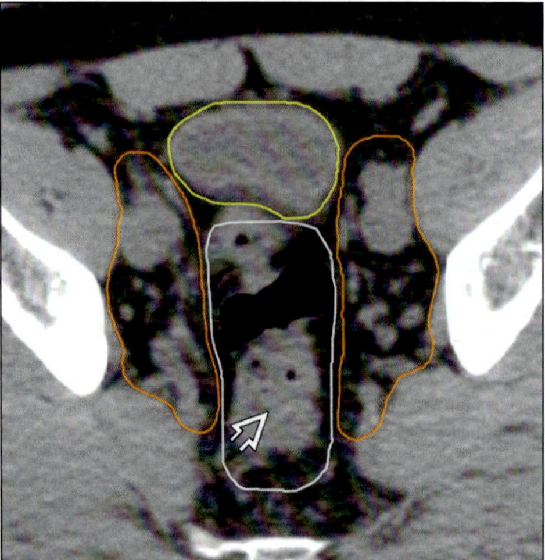

Prostate Contours: Series 2 MR

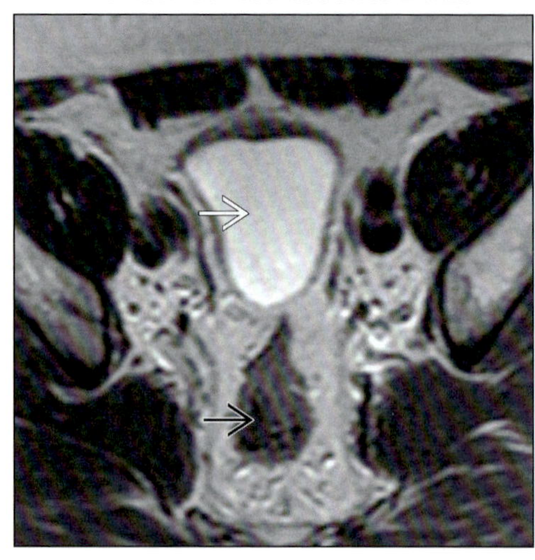

(**Left**) *Below the level of the femoral heads, the lymph node volumes (orange, PTV3) flank the distal seminal vesicles (blue, PTV2) and include the hypogastric and obturator regions. Note the exclusion of the the external iliac vessels at this level.* (**Right**) *The seminal vesicles are distinguished from the high signal intensity of the perirectal fat T2WI.*

Prostate Contours: Series 3 CT

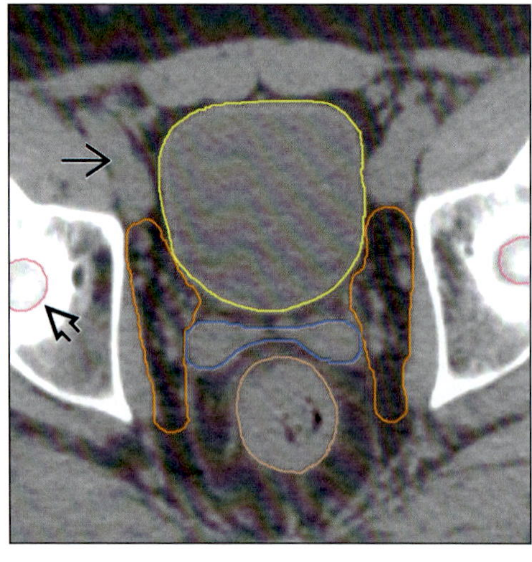

Prostate Contours: Series 3 MR

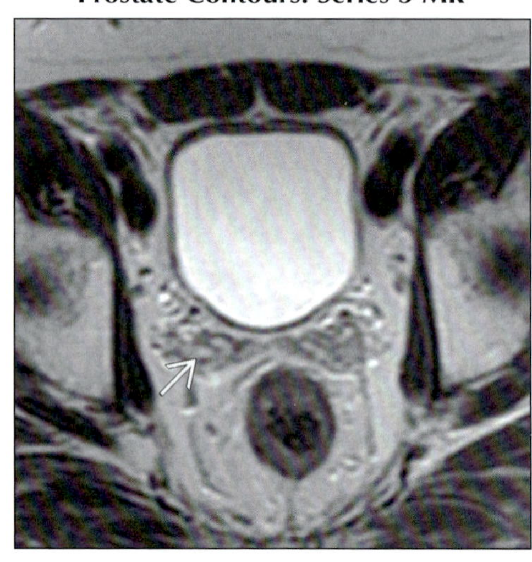

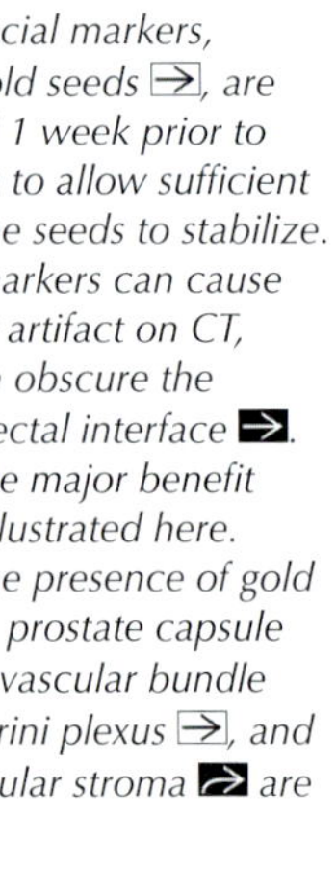

(**Left**) *Fiducial markers, such as gold seeds, are implanted 1 week prior to simulation to allow sufficient time for the seeds to stabilize. Fiducial markers can cause significant artifact on CT, which can obscure the prostate-rectal interface.* (**Right**) *The major benefit of MR is illustrated here. Despite the presence of gold seeds, the prostate capsule, neurovascular bundle, Santorini plexus, and fibromuscular stroma are all seen.*

Prostate Contours: Series 4 CT

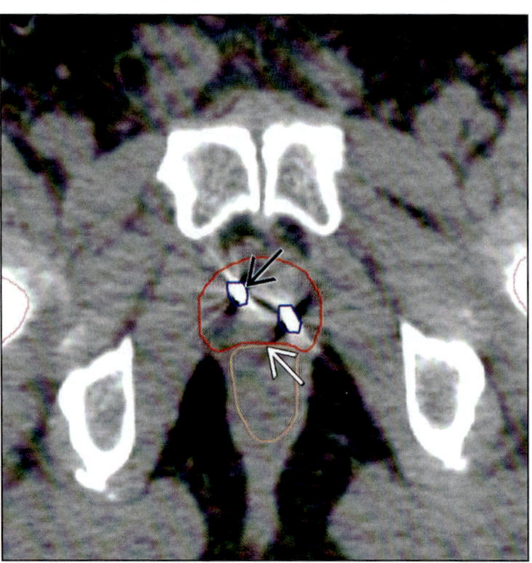

Prostate Contours: Series 4 MR

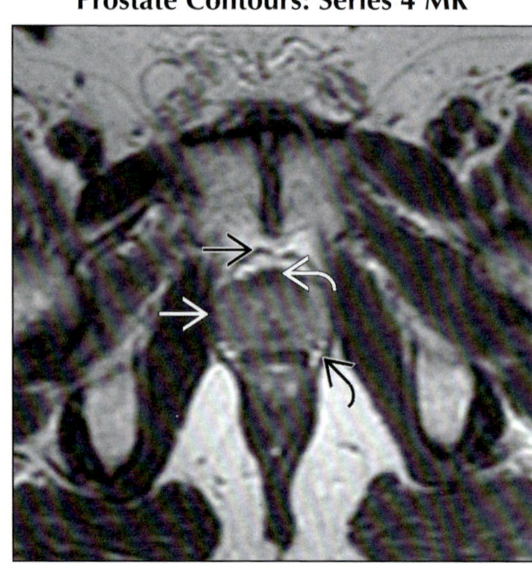

Prostate Contours: Series 5 CT

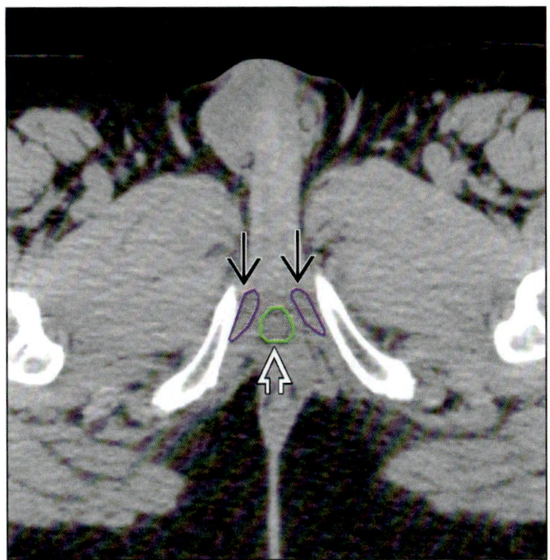

Prostate Contours: Series 5 MR

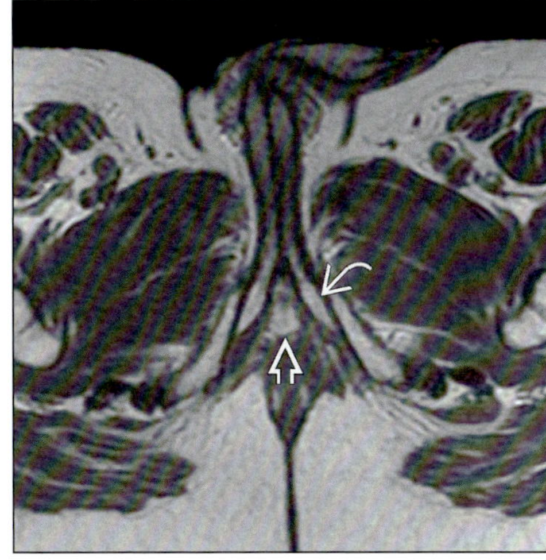

*(**Left**) The penile bulb (green) is defined as the bulbous, proximal portion of the corpora spongiosum and typically measures 1-2 cm in length. The corporal bodies (purple) are defined as the divergent, proximal portions of the corpora cavernosa, typically measuring 2-3 cm in length before their departure from the ischial tuberosities. (**Right**) The erectile tissue is best seen as high signal intensity on T2WI. Note the penile bulb and corporal bodies .*

Intact Prostate, Intensity Modulated RT Treatment Plan

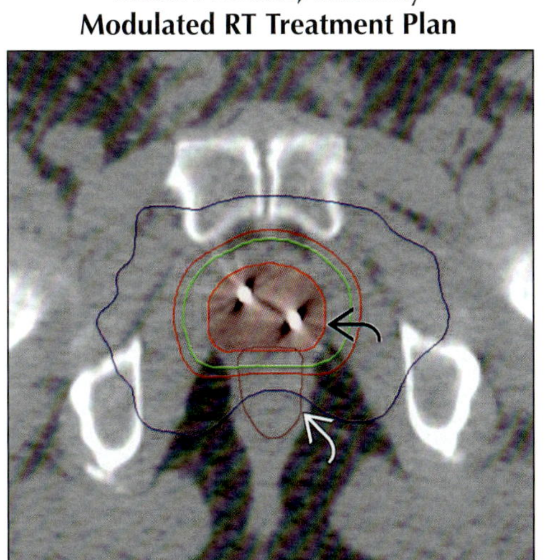

Intact Prostate, Intensity Modulated RT Treatment Plan

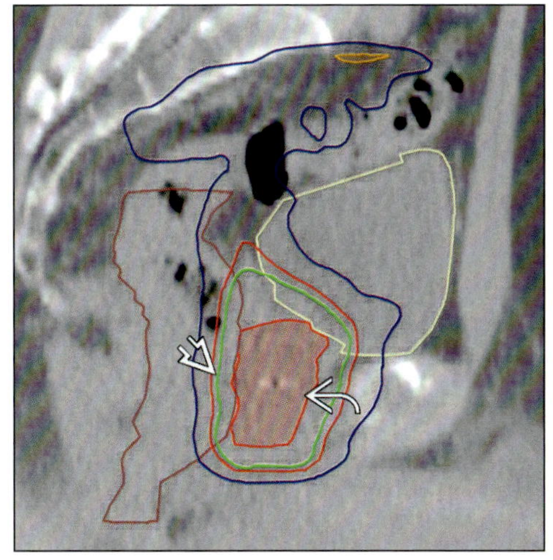

*(**Left**) Axial CT shows arc-based intensity-modulated RT. The 90% isodose line (red) should encompass no more than 1/2 of the rectal width , and the 50% isodose line (blue) should encompass less than full rectal width. The 100% isodose line (green) should be 3-8 mm posterior to the prostate CTV . (**Right**) Sagittal reconstruction confirms conformality of the high dose posteriorly along the prostate CTV to maximize rectal sparing.*

IMRT Treatment Plan

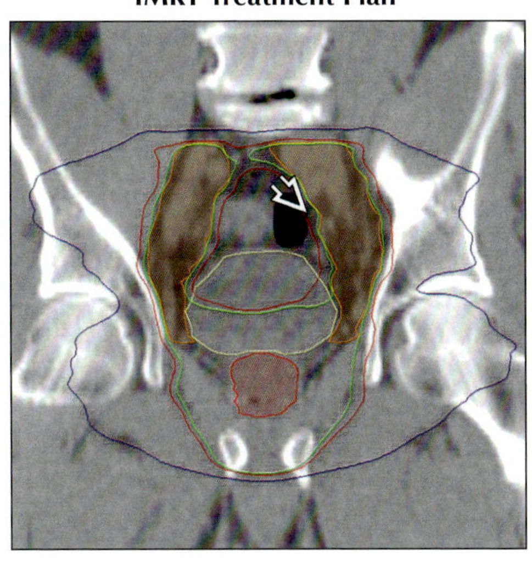

IMRT Treatment Plan

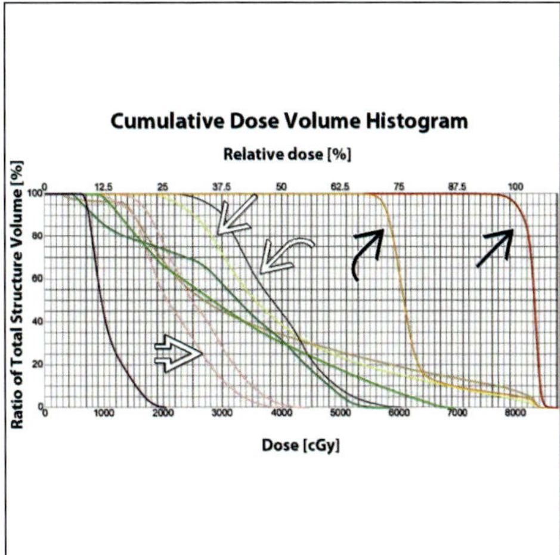

*(**Left**) Conformality of the 100% (green) and 90% (red) isodose lines medially along the nodal volumes (orange) minimizes doses to bowel and bladder. (**Right**) A representative dose-volume histogram for prostate IMRT demonstrates coverage of the prostate/proximal seminal vesicles (PTV1) and distal seminal vesicles/pelvic lymph nodes (PTV2/PTV3) . Organs at risk include the bladder , rectum , and femoral heads .*

(Left) *This is an example of a treatment plan of arc-based intensity-modulated RT. The prostate (CTV) is expanded 5 mm posteriorly and 8 mm in all other directions to create the PTV. The dose is prescribed such that 95% of the PTV receives the prescription dose.* **(Right)** *Differences in bladder and rectal filling on a day-to-day basis may vary the position of the PTV. Image guidance prior to treatment allows the therapist to reposition the patient.*

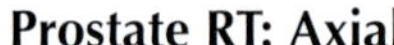

Prostate RT: Axial

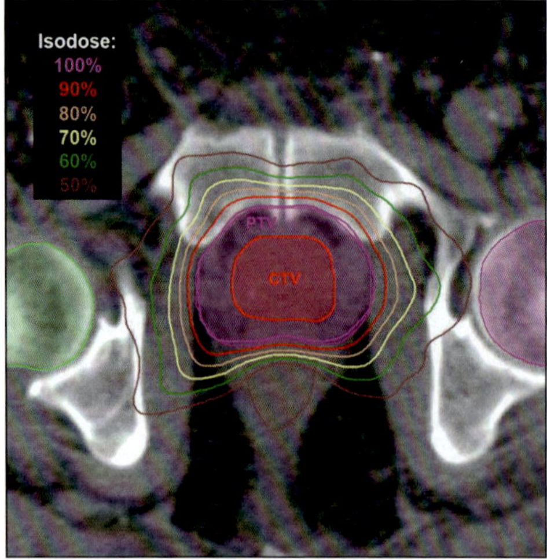

Prostate RT: Sagittal

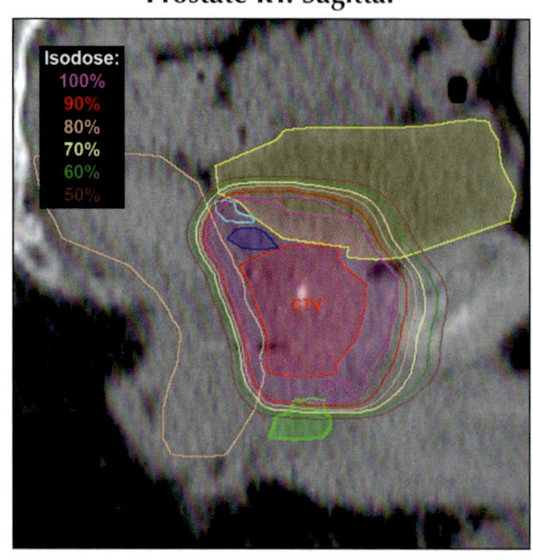

(Left) *Overlaying the DRR (orange) with setup orthogonal images (blue) enables daily prostate location. The contours ➔ are aligned with the gold seeds to determine the required shifts in patient positioning.* **(Right)** *A daily cone beam CT may be generated with the patient in treatment position. This is aligned to the treatment planning DRR to account for interfractional motion of the prostate or prostate bed.*

Image Guidance, Electronic Portal Imaging

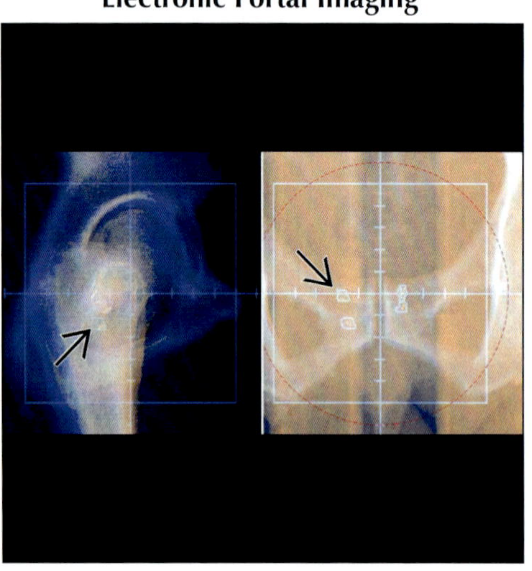

Image Guidance, Cone Beam CT

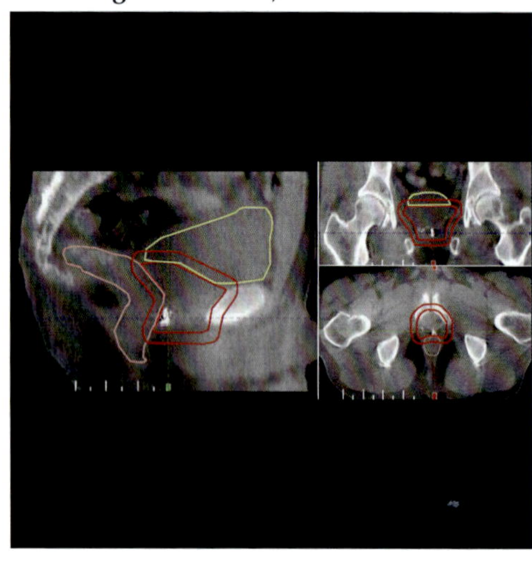

(Left) *Implantation of 3 electromagnetic beacons allows real-time tracking of intrafractional prostate motion in the lateral, longitudinal, and vertical directions. A motion threshold can be used to interrupt treatment for repositioning.* **(Right)** *Motion beyond a threshold ➔ (3 mm here) interrupts treatment for repositioning.*

Electromagnetic Transponders, Daily Log

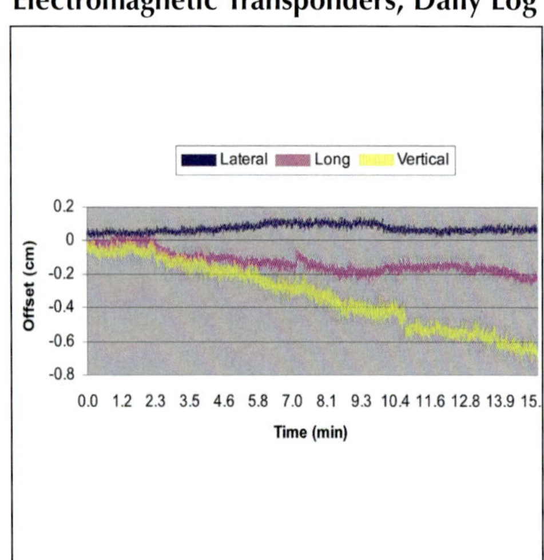

Image Guidance, Electromagnetic Beacons

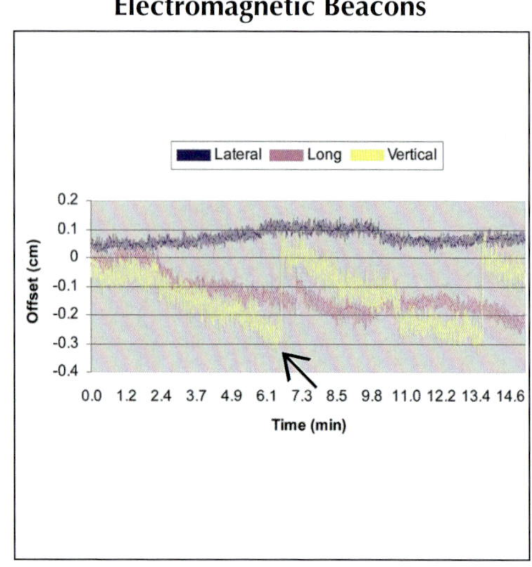

Stage IV (T3b N1 M0)

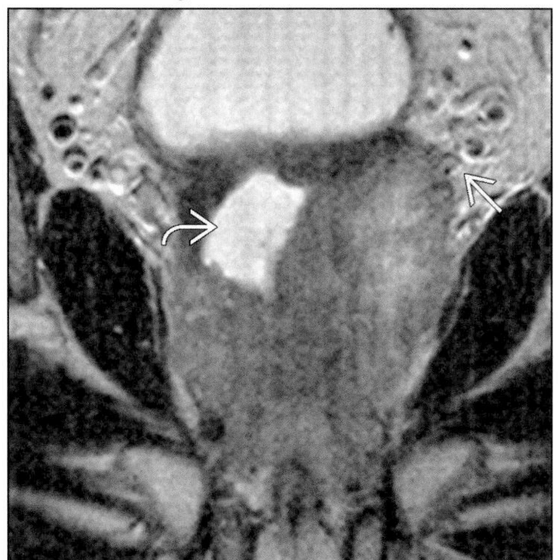

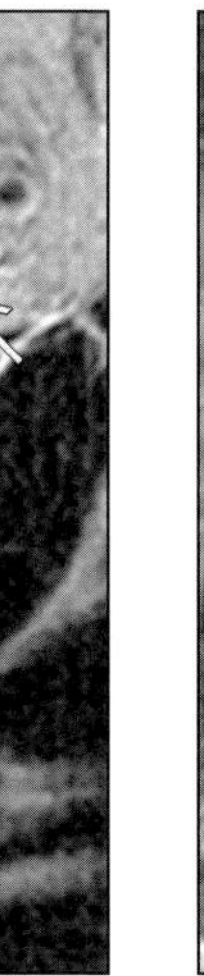

Stage IV (T3b N1 M0)

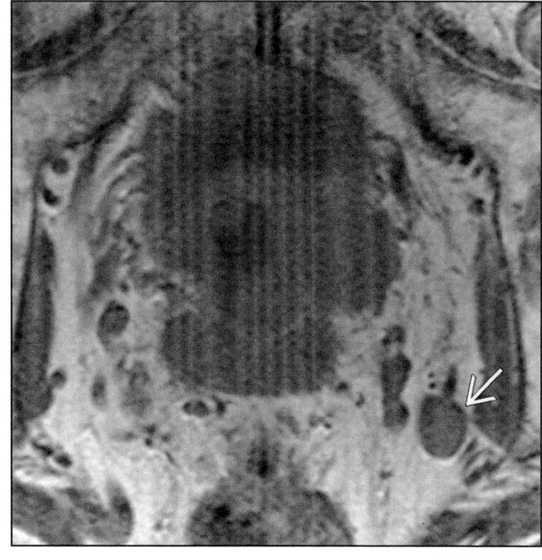

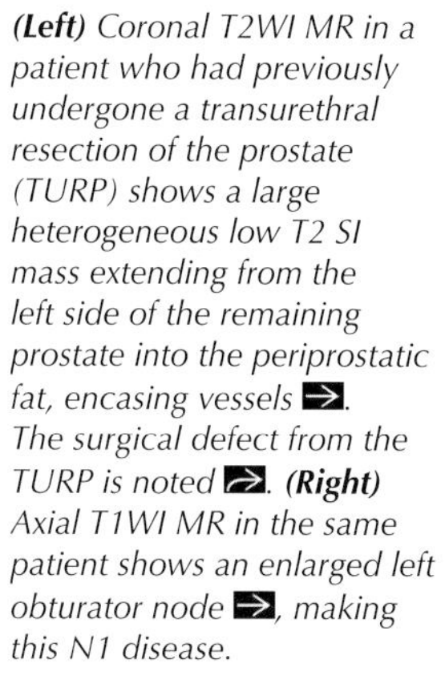

(Left) *Coronal T2WI MR in a patient who had previously undergone a transurethral resection of the prostate (TURP) shows a large heterogeneous low T2 SI mass extending from the left side of the remaining prostate into the periprostatic fat, encasing vessels →. The surgical defect from the TURP is noted ↪.* ***(Right)*** *Axial T1WI MR in the same patient shows an enlarged left obturator node →, making this N1 disease.*

Stage IV (T3b N1 M0, PSA 22, Gleason 9)

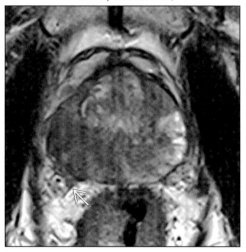

Stage IV (T3b N1 M0, PSA 22, Gleason 9)

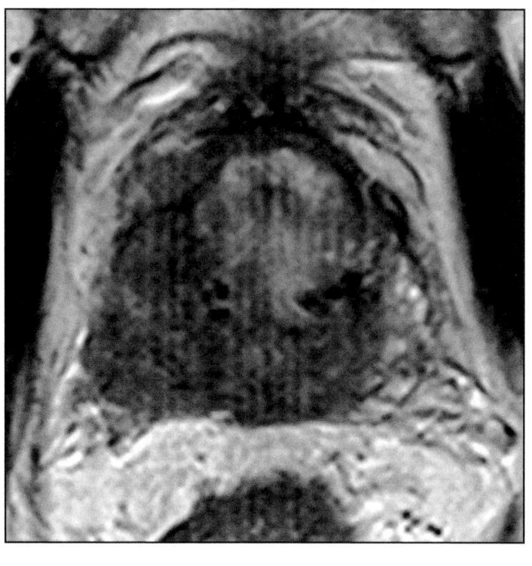

(Left) *Axial T2WI MR at mid gland level shows diffuse low T2 SI throughout the PZ. The margin between PZ and CZ is obscured. The asymmetric bulge on the right, with low T2 SI infiltrating into the region of the neurovascular bundle →, is consistent with ECE and neurovascular bundle involvement.* ***(Right)*** *Axial T2WI MR shows mass-like confluent low T2 SI involving nearly the entire base of the prostate, with definite angularity at right prostatic angle, evidence of ECE.*

Stage IV (T3b N1 M0, PSA 22, Gleason 9)

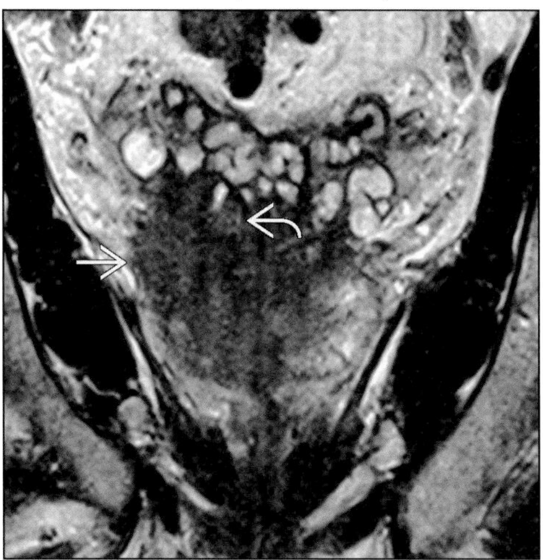

Stage IV (T3b N1 M0, PSA 22, Gleason 9)

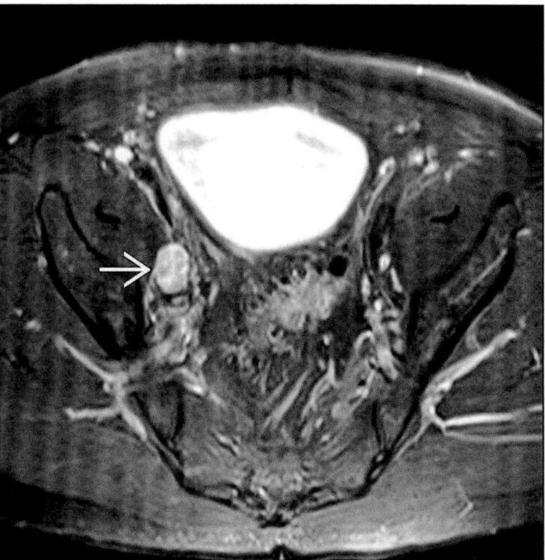

(Left) *Coronal T2WI MR in the same patient shows the abnormal low T2 SI infiltrating from the left side of prostate → into the left seminal vesicles, consistent with seminal vesicle invasion ↪.* ***(Right)*** *Axial T2WI FS MR in the same patient shows an abnormally enlarged right external iliac node →. The metastasis to a regional lymph node is N1 disease. Surgery is not indicated for this stage of disease.*

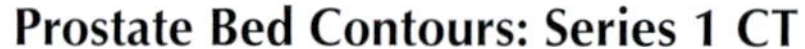

Prostate Bed Contours: Series 1 CT

Prostate Bed Contours: Series 1 MR

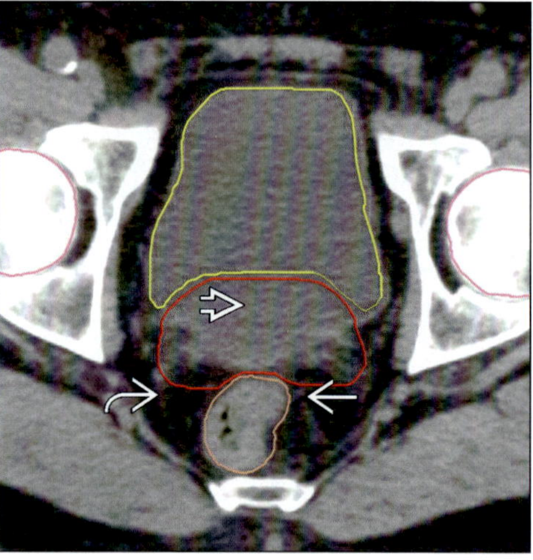

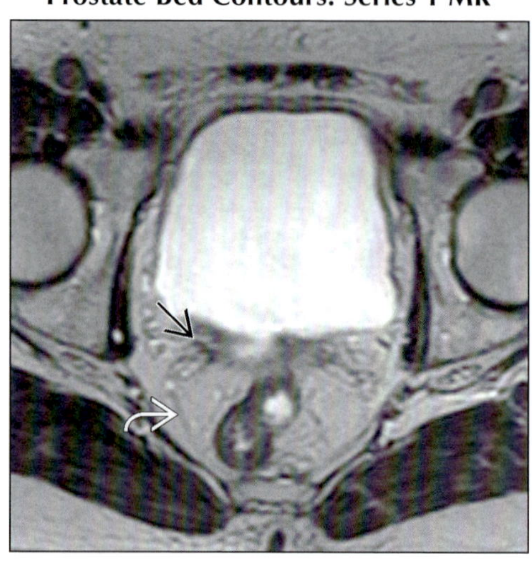

(Left) *The prostate bed (contoured in red) extends posteriorly to the mesorectal fascia ➡ and includes 2-3 cm of the posterior bladder ➡. The sacrorectogenitopubic fascia ➡ marks the lateral border.* ***(Right)*** *The cut end of the vas deferens ➡ marks the superior border of the prostate bed and is best visualized using MR. This typically lies 3-4 cm above the symphysis pubis. The sacrorectogenitopubic fascia ➡ is easily seen on MR.*

Prostate Bed Contours: Series 2 CT

Prostate Bed Contours: Series 2 MR

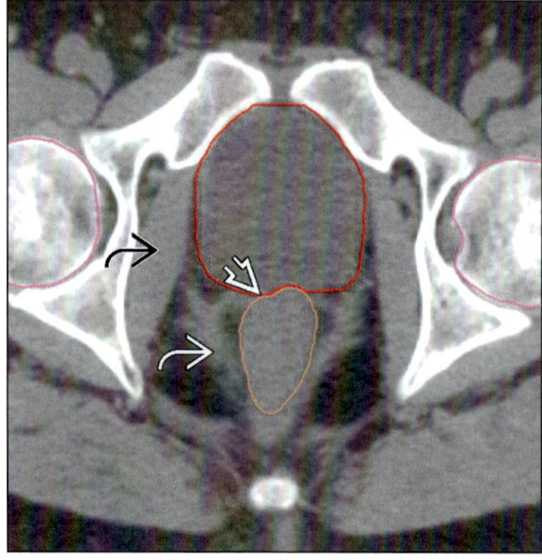

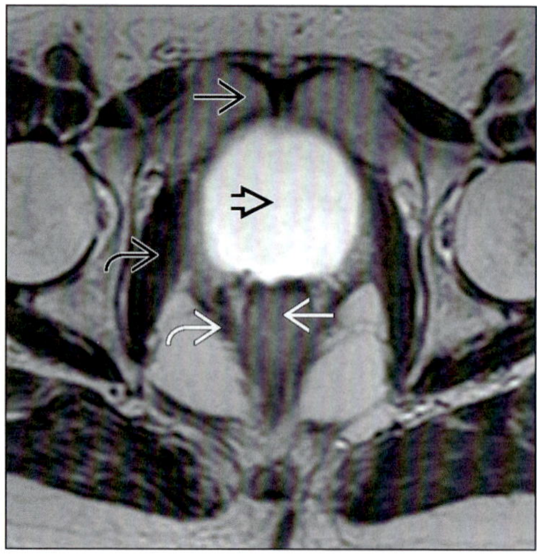

(Left) *Below the level of the symphysis pubis, the prostate bed (contoured in red) extends anteriorly to the posterior pubic rami. Posteriorly, it curves around the anterior rectal wall ➡. The obturator internus ➡ and levator ani muscles ➡ mark the lateral borders at this level.* ***(Right)*** *Obturator internus ➡, levator ani ➡, pubis ➡, rectum ➡, and bladder ➡ are identified.*

Prostate Bed Contours: Sagittal CT

Prostate Bed Contours: Sagittal MR

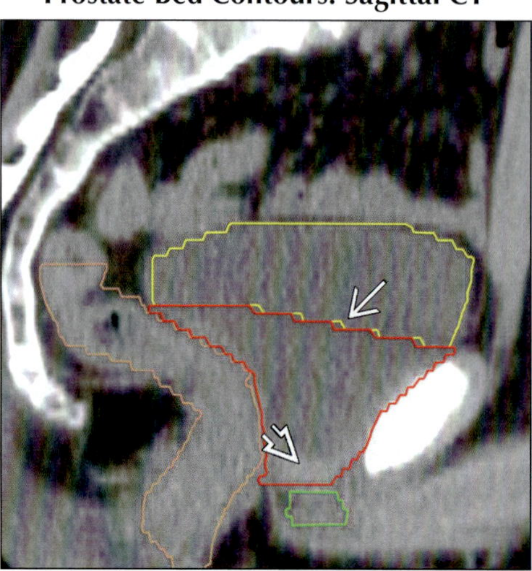

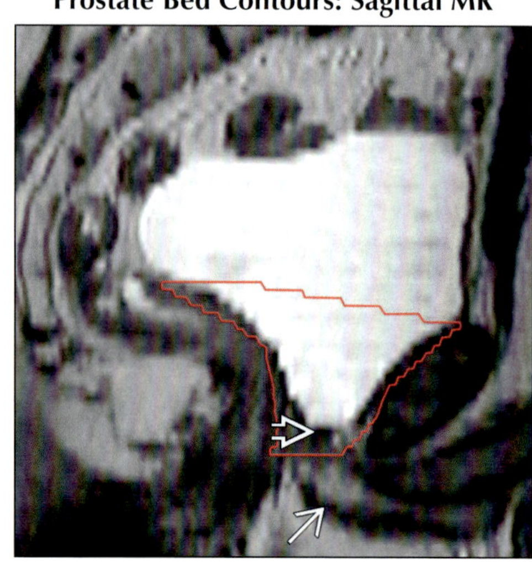

(Left) *The inferior border of the prostate bed volume (red) includes the vesicourethral anastomosis ➡ and extends to the superior aspect of the penile bulb (green). Note that the prostate bed volume gradually tapers posteriorly and superiorly from the superior aspect of the pubis ➡.* ***(Right)*** *MR simulation provides improved visualization of the vesicourethral anastomosis ➡. The penile bulb ➡ is seen as high signal intensity on T2WI.*

Stage IV (TX N1 M1a)

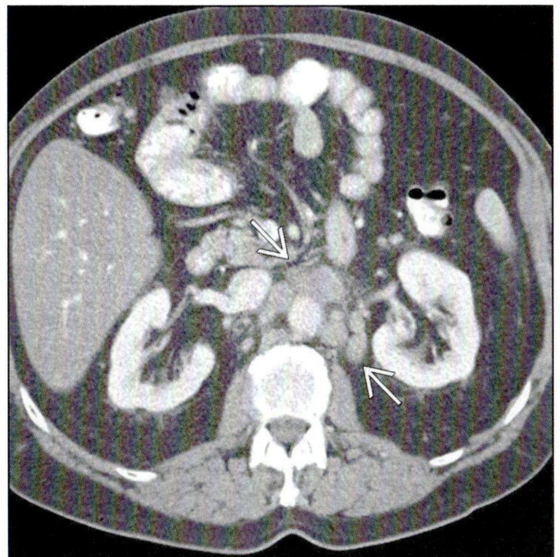

Stage IV (TX N1 M1a)

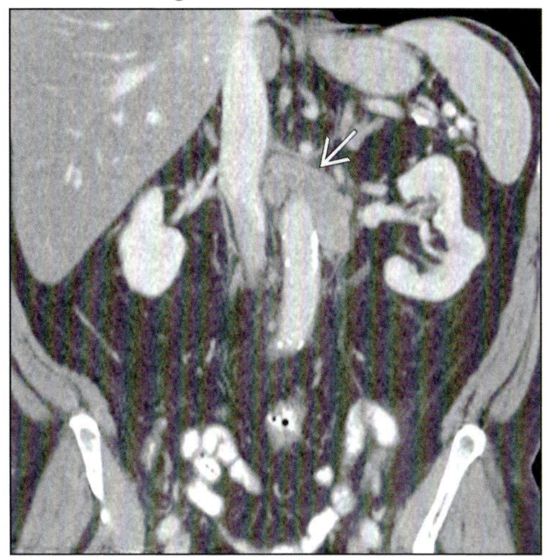

***(Left)** Axial CECT at the level of the right renal vein demonstrates significant paraaortic lymphadenopathy ➡. **(Right)** Coronal CECT in the same patient demonstrates the confluent adenopathy ➡ crossing anterior to the aorta and between the aorta and IVC. Metastases to the paraaortic lymph nodes are the most common sites of nonregional lymphatic spread of disease. These upstage the patient to M1a whereas pelvic regional adenopathy is N1 disease.*

Stage IV (TX N1 M1a)

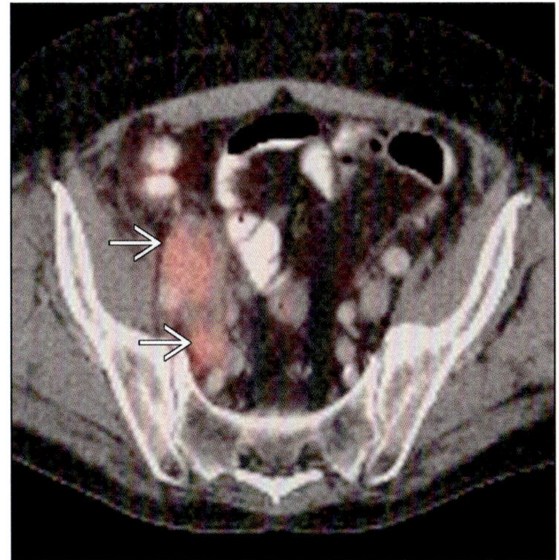

Stage IV (TX N1 M1a)

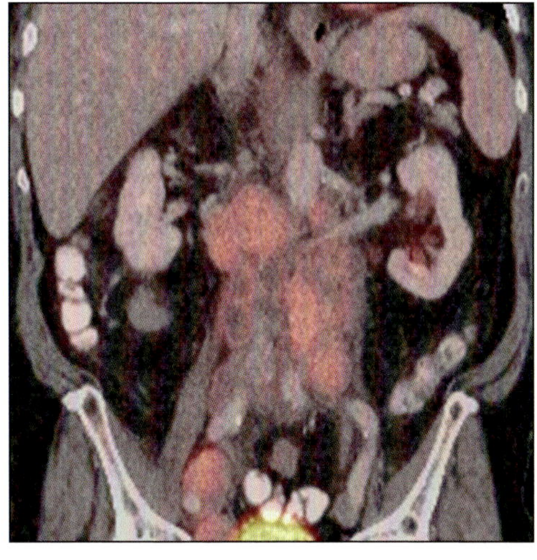

***(Left)** Axial fused PET/CT in the same patient shows the internal and external iliac adenopathy on the right ➡. This regional adenopathy is considered N1 disease. **(Right)** Coronal fused PET/CT in the same patient shows the extensive regional and distant lymphadenopathy. No bone lesions were identified on the PET.*

Stage IV (TX NX M1c)

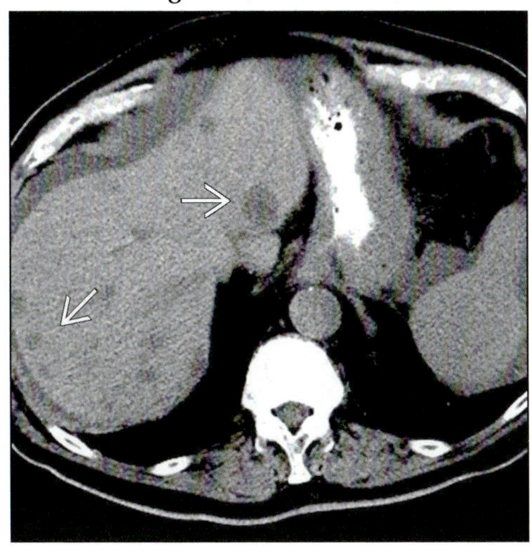

Stage IV (TX NX M1c)

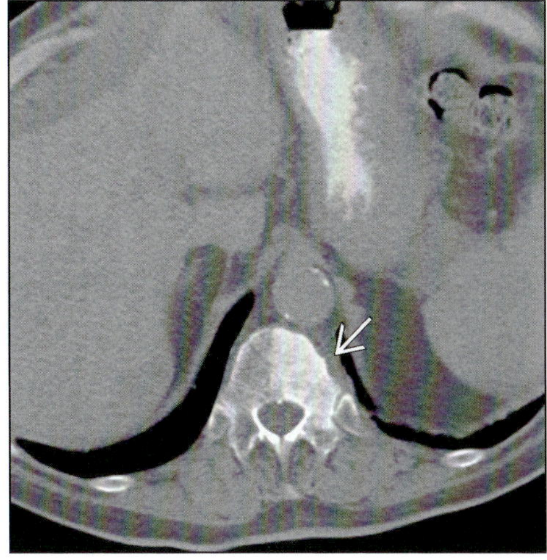

***(Left)** Axial NECT in a patient with a history of prostate cancer (treated > 10 years prior) was performed after liver function test results were found to be abnormal and shows multiple hypoattenuating hepatic lesions ➡. On percutaneous CT-guided biopsy, these were proven to be metastases from prostate cancer. **(Right)** Axial NECT shows that, in addition to the hepatic lesions, a sclerotic bone lesion in the T10 vertebral body ➡ is identified.*

(Left) Frontal chest radiograph demonstrates diffuse pulmonary nodularity in an elderly man with known prostate cancer. (Right) Accompanying lateral radiograph demonstrates the innumerable pulmonary nodules. Additionally, there is the suggestion of sclerosis of the T4 vertebral body ➔. This appearance has been termed an "ivory vertebral body" and is due to near-complete osteoblastic replacement of the vertebra.

Stage IV (TX NX M1c)

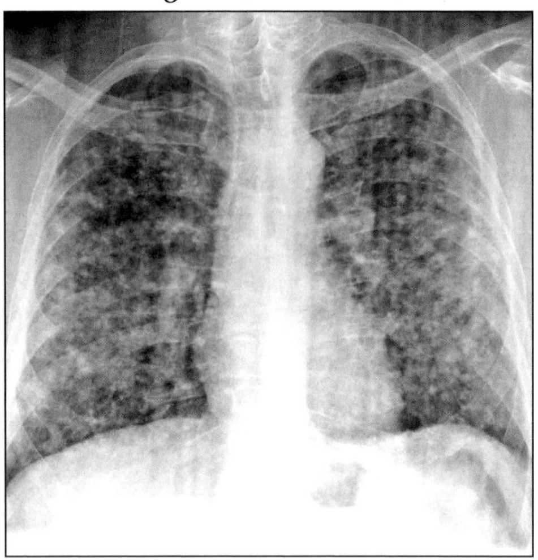

Stage IV (TX NX M1c)

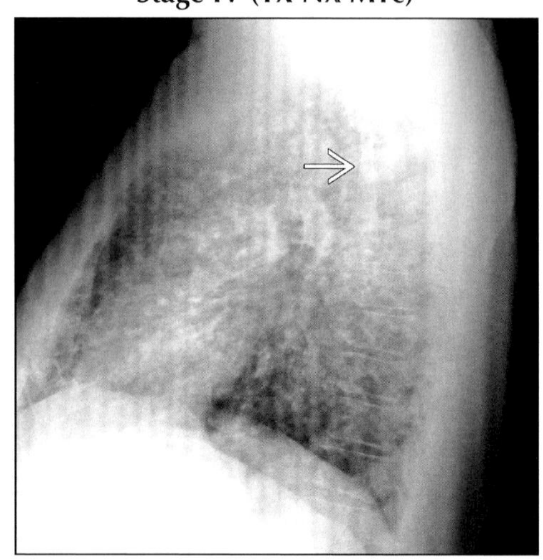

(Left) Axial NECT, lung window (top), in the same patient demonstrates the innumerable pulmonary nodules ➔. Bone window image (bottom) reveals a sclerotic lesion posteriorly in the right 6th rib ➔. (Right) Whole body bone scan in the same patient shows increased uptake in multiple vertebral bodies, including T4, as well as the right 6th rib, the right scapula, and the left pubis. These foci correspond to the sclerotic bone metastases seen on prior imaging.

Stage IV (TX NX M1c)

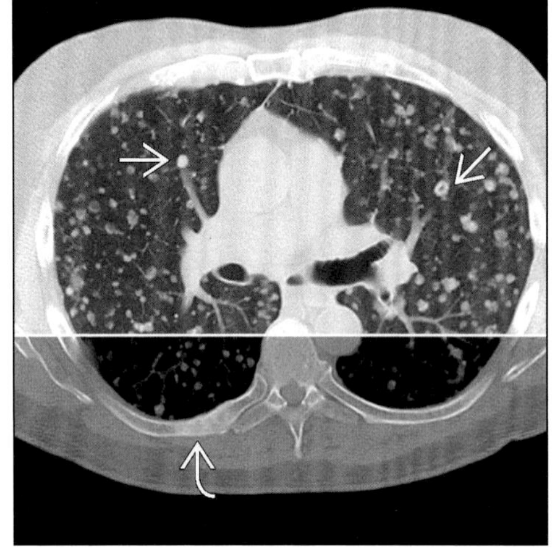

Stage IV (TX NX M1c)

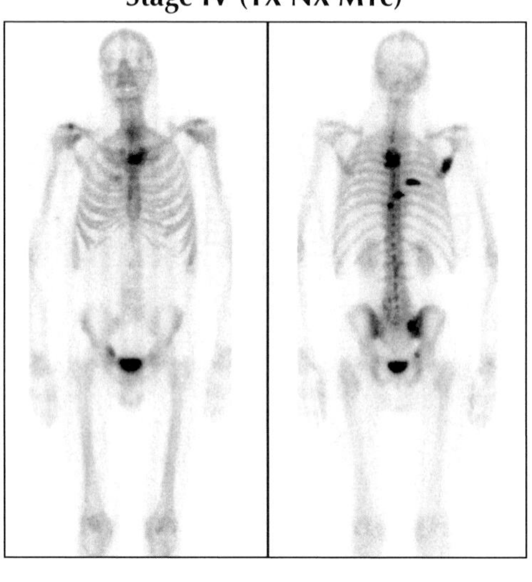

(Left) Coronal In-111 capromab (ProstaScint) SPECT image shows right proximal iliac focal uptake ➔ at the site of a 1.3 cm nodal metastasis. The patient had previously undergone a radical prostatectomy and had a rising PSA, with a PSA doubling time of approximately 6 months. (Right) Axial In-111 capromab (ProstaScint) image from the same patient again shows the node ➔. Normal marrow uptake ➔ is also noted in the iliac bones and vertebral bodies.

Local Recurrence

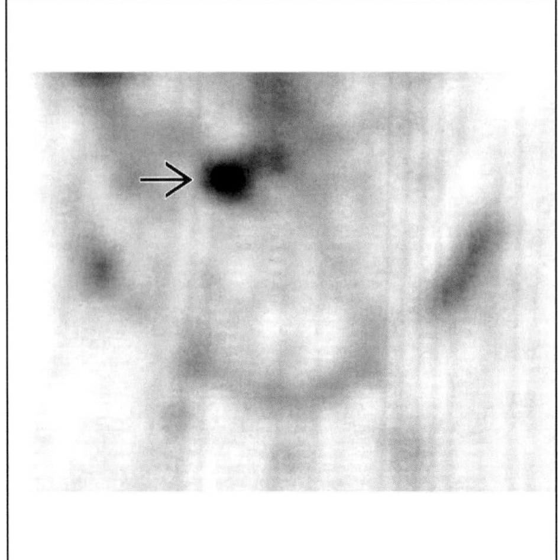

Local Recurrence

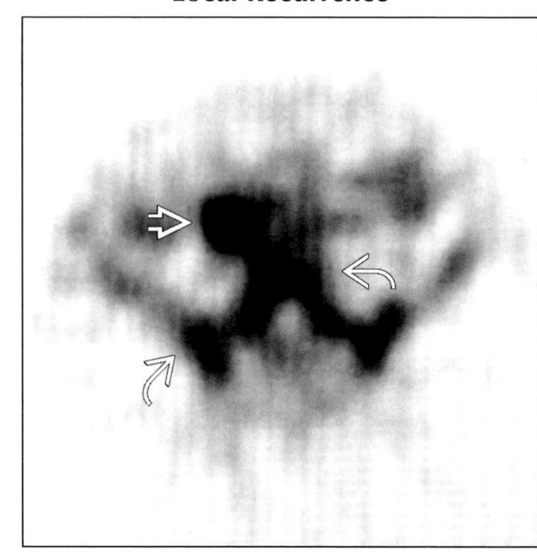

Stage IV (T4 N0 M1b)

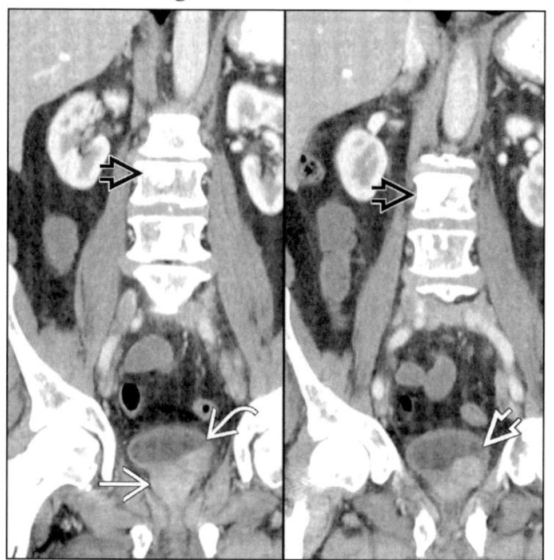

Stage IV (T4 N0 M1b)

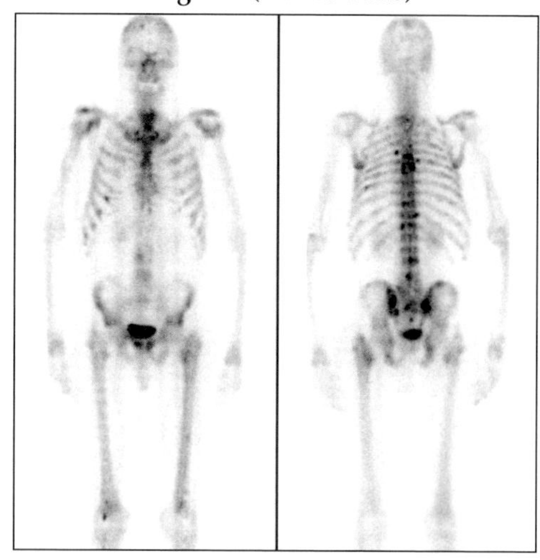

*(**Left**) Coronal CECT images demonstrate a mass extending from the prostate into the bladder base. The right image shows the intraluminal bladder component well. Sclerotic lesions are seen in the lumbar spine. (**Right**) Whole body bone scan in the same patient shows diffuse increased uptake in the spine and bony pelvis, as well as foci of increased uptake in many ribs. With little renal or soft tissue activity, this study approaches a "superscan."*

Stage IV (T2b N0 M1b, PSA 16.5, Gleason 7)

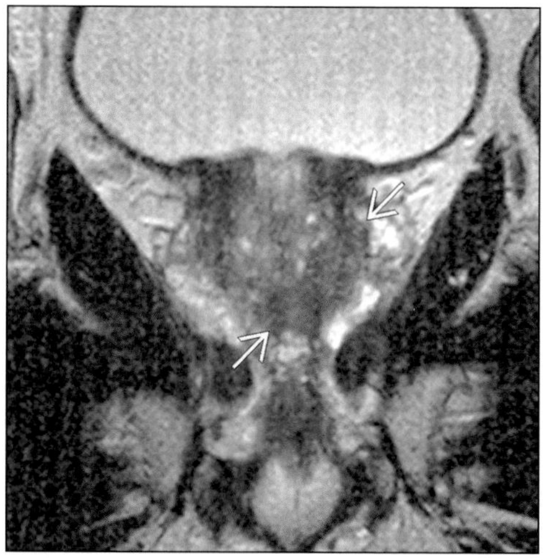

Stage IV (T2b N0 M1b, PSA 16.5, Gleason 7)

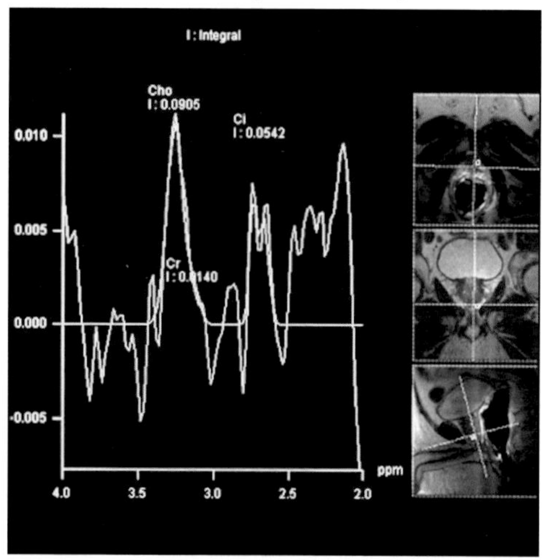

*(**Left**) Coronal T2WI MR shows a band of low T2 SI extending from the apex to base on the left. (Courtesy S. Eberhardt, MD.) (**Right**) Single voxel MR spectroscopy was performed in the same patient by placing a voxel over the area of tumor. This demonstrates a metabolic spectra of elevated choline + creatine/citrate. This spectra is consistent with malignancy. (Courtesy S. Eberhardt, MD.)*

Stage IV (T2b N0 M1b, PSA 16.5, Gleason 7)

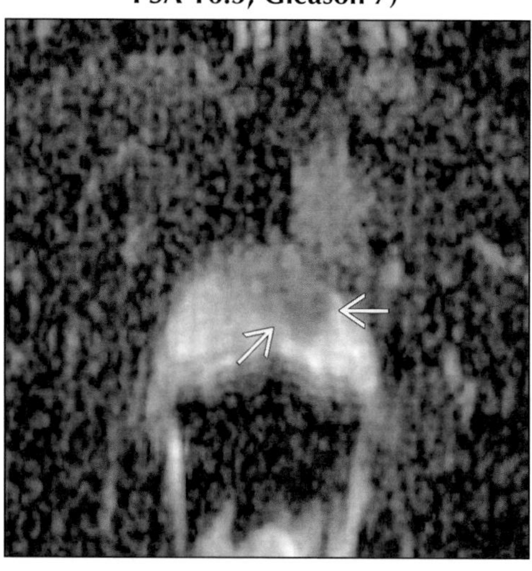

Stage IV (T2b N0 M1b, PSA 16.5, Gleason 7)

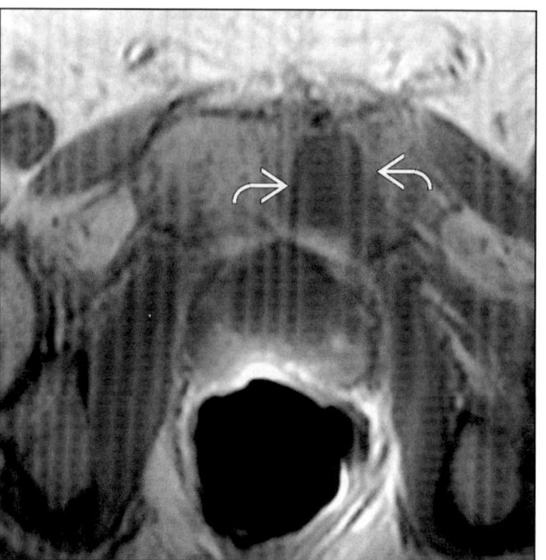

*(**Left**) Axial ADC map from diffusion-weighted imaging in the same patient shows restricted diffusion corresponding to the area of decreased T2 SI. (Courtesy S. Eberhardt, MD.) (**Right**) Coned down axial T1WI MR from the same patient demonstrates a focus of low T1 SI in the left pubis. This is consistent with an osteoblastic bony metastasis. (Courtesy S. Eberhardt, MD.)*

Brachytherapy: Transrectal Ultrasound

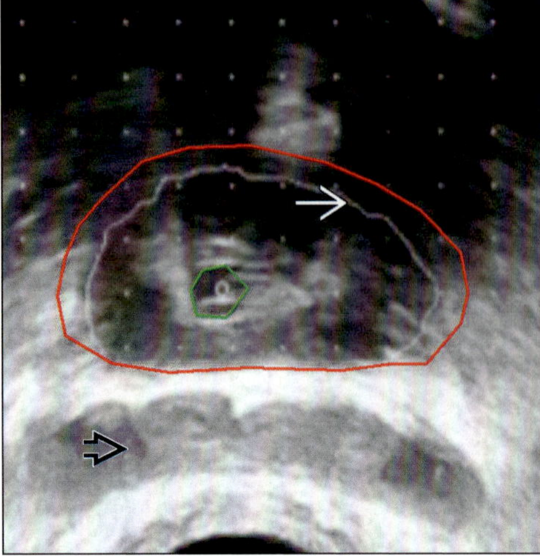

Brachytherapy: Transrectal Ultrasound

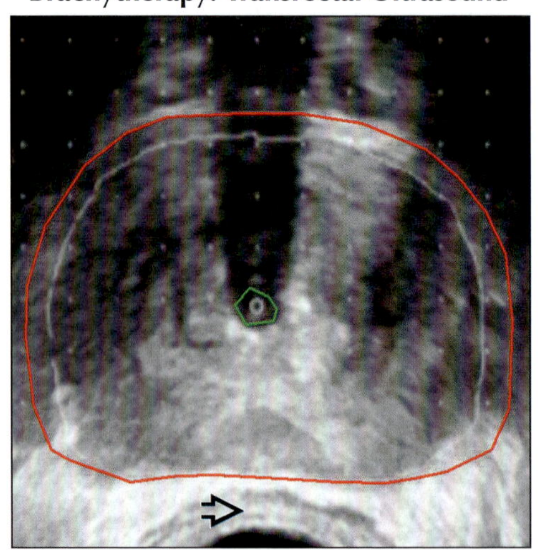

(Left) *During intraoperative planning, the prostate circumference is contoured ➡ on the transrectal ultrasound and captured to the planning system to contour the CTV (red) and urethra (green). Note that the seminal vesicles ⇨ are excluded.* ***(Right)*** *The CTV (red) is created with a 5 mm margin on the prostate. This margin is 0 mm posteriorly to spare the anterior rectal wall ⇨.*

Brachytherapy: Transrectal Ultrasound

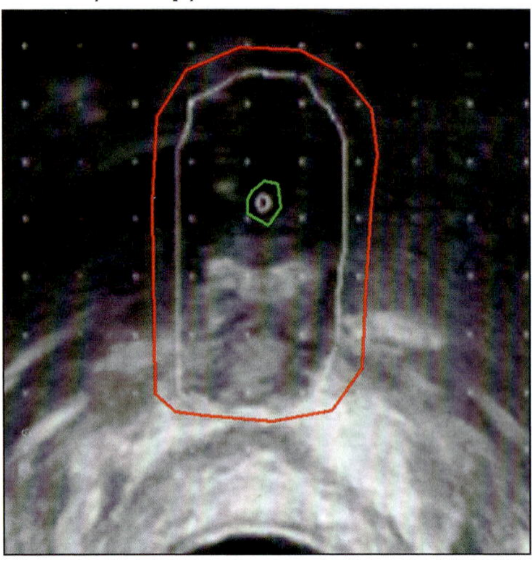

Brachytherapy: Intraoperative Portable Fluroscopy

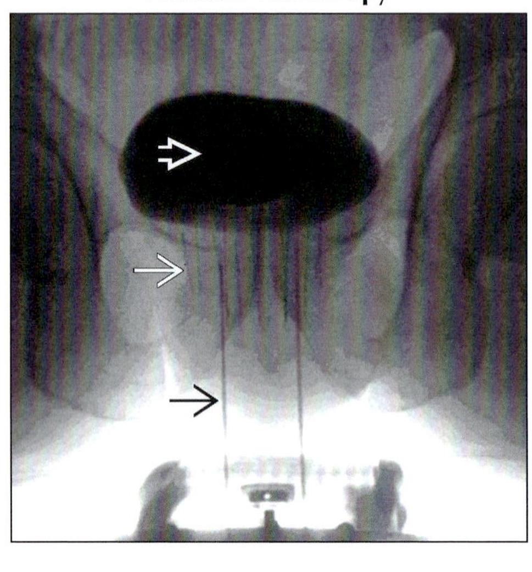

(Left) *A "cap" is contoured on the axial slice 5 mm below the prostate apex to ensure adequate coverage.* ***(Right)*** *X-ray confirms accurate positioning of the low dose rate brachytherapy seeds. Note the strands of seeds throughout the prostate ➡. Contrast is used in the bladder ⇨. Also seen are stabilization needles → that limit prostate motion during the procedure.*

Brachytherapy: 3D Dosimetry Reconstruction

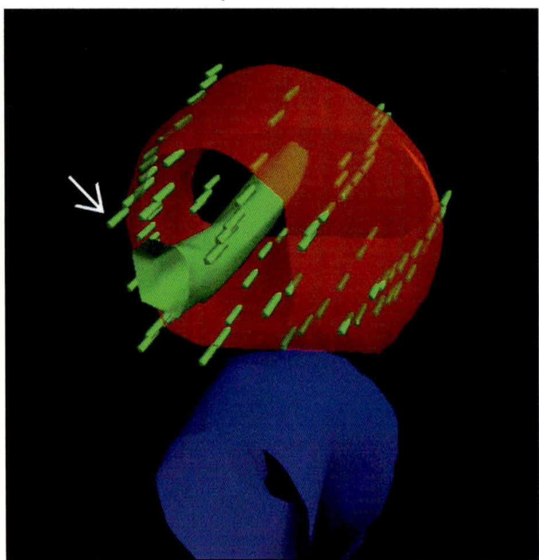

Brachytherapy: Day 0 Dosimetry, CT

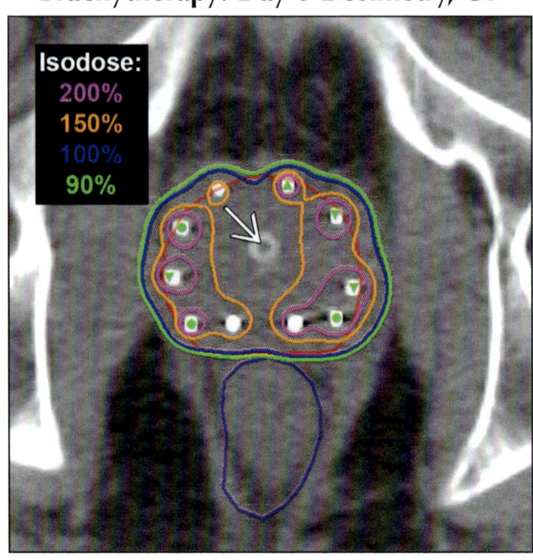

(Left) *Even distribution of seeds ➡ ensures adequate and homogeneous coverage of the prostate (red). Peripheral loading spares dose centrally to the urethra (green).* ***(Right)*** *Peripheral loading avoids high dose to the urethra ➡.*

Local Prostate Recurrence: Endorectal MR

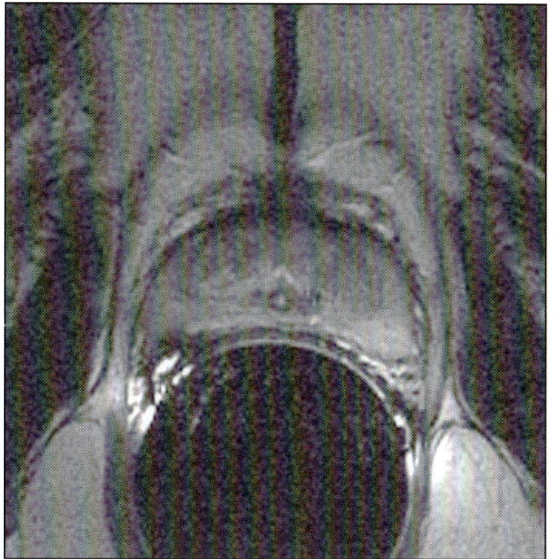

Local Prostate Recurrence: Day 0 Dosimetry, CT

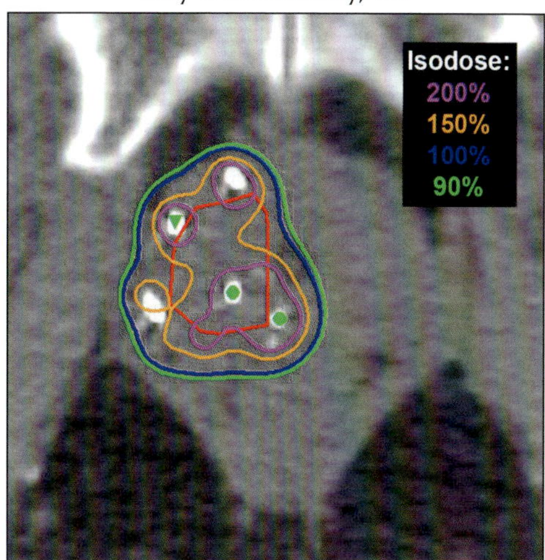

(Left) *Local recurrence is seen 3 years following IMRT. Prostate is small (15 mL) and fibrotic. There is currently no imaging standard for detecting local recurrence although MR spectroscopy or dynamic contrast enhancement may direct biopsies to suspicious areas.* ***(Right)*** *TRUS-guided biopsy shows Gleason 3+3 in right base, mid, and apex that were sites of bulky disease (T2b and > 50% core length involvement). LDR partial prostate implant was used to re-treat right lobe.*

Radiation Proctopathy

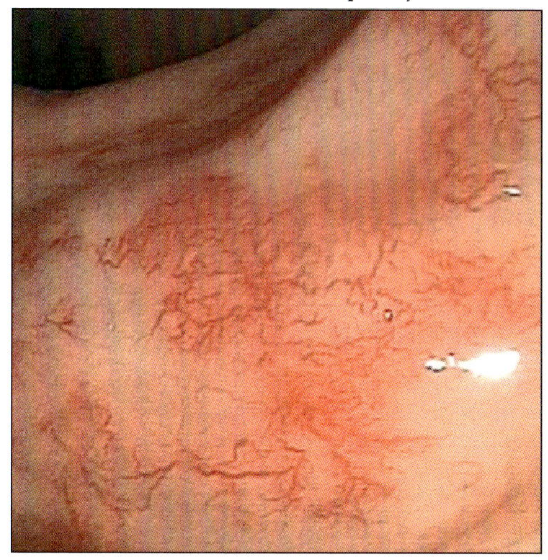

Radiation Proctopathy

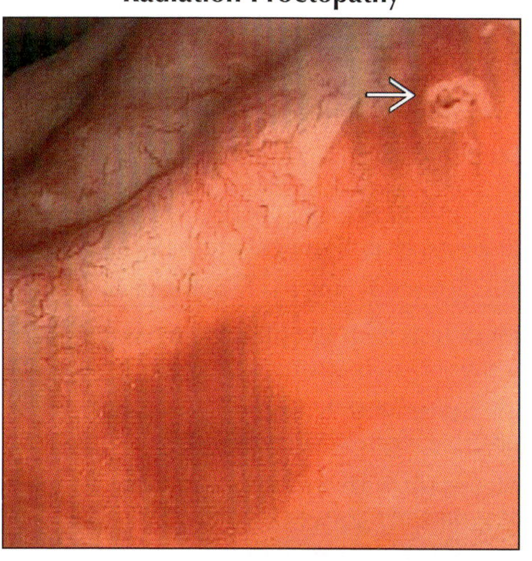

(Left) *Endoscopy shows characteristic telangiectasias of the anterior rectal wall. Painless rectal bleeding occurs in 10-15% of patients and is often self-limited. (Courtesy J. L. Tokar, MD.)* ***(Right)*** *Steroid suppositories can be used to heal bleeding ulcers ➔. Photocoagulation may also be used. Hyperbaric oxygen therapy with pentoxifylline and vitamin E is used for refractory cases. Surgery is rarely necessary. (Courtesy J. L. Tokar, MD.)*

Radiation Cystopathy

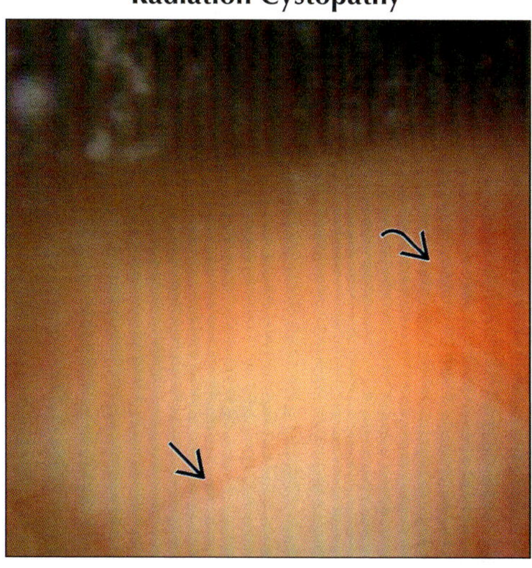

Radiation Cystopathy

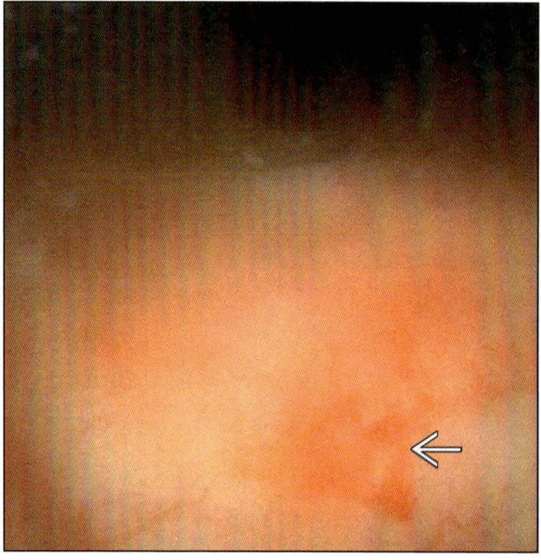

(Left) *Late effects of prostate radiation in the bladder include neovascularization with telangiectasias ➔ and erythema ➔ of the urethral mucosa. This occurs at the trigone, as shown here. (Courtesy R. E. Greenberg, MD, FACS.)* ***(Right)*** *This cystoscopic image demonstrates plumes of blood ➔ arising from the bladder mucosa, indicating hemorrhagic cystopathy. (Courtesy R. E. Greenberg, MD, FACS.)*

TESTIS

(T) Primary Tumor

Adapted from 7th edition AJCC Staging Forms.

TNM	*Definitions*
pTX	Primary tumor cannot be assessed (if no radical orchiectomy has been performed, TX is used)
pT0	No evidence of primary tumor (e.g., histologic scar in testis)
pTis	Intratubular germ cell neoplasia (carcinoma in situ)
pT1	Tumor limited to testis and epididymis without vascular/lymphatic invasion; tumor may invade into tunica albuginea but not tunica vaginalis
pT2	Tumor limited to testis and epididymis with vascular/lymphatic invasion, or tumor extending through tunica albuginea with involvement of tunica vaginalis
pT3	Tumor invades spermatic cord with or without vascular/lymphatic invasion
pT4	Tumor invades the scrotum with or without vascular/lymphatic invasion

(N) Regional Lymph Nodes

Clinical	
NX	Regional lymph nodes cannot be assessed
N0	No regional lymph node metastasis
N1	Metastasis with lymph node mass ≤ 2 cm in greatest dimension; or multiple lymph nodes, none > 2 cm in greatest dimension
N2	Metastasis with lymph node mass > 2 cm but ≤ 5 cm in greatest dimension; or multiple lymph nodes, any one mass > 2 cm but ≤ 5 cm in greatest dimension
N3	Metastasis with a lymph node mass > 5 cm in greatest dimension
Pathological	
pNX	Regional lymph nodes cannot be assessed
pN0	No regional lymph node metastasis
pN1	Metastasis with lymph node mass ≤ 2 cm in greatest dimension and ≤ 5 nodes positive, none > 2 cm in greatest dimension
pN2	Metastasis with lymph node mass > 2 cm but ≤ 5 cm in greatest dimension; or > 5 nodes positive, none > 5 cm; or evidence of extranodal extension of tumor
pN3	Metastasis with lymph node mass > 5 cm in greatest dimension

(M) Distant Metastasis

M0	No distant metastasis
M1	Distant metastasis
M1a	No regional nodal or pulmonary metastasis
M1b	Distant metastasis other than to nonregional lymph nodes and lungs

Except for pTis and pT4, extent of primary tumor is classified by radical orchiectomy. For this reason, a pathologic stage is usually assigned. TX may be used for other categories in the absence of radical orchiectomy.

Serum Tumor Markers (S)

TNM	*Definitions*
SX	Tumor marker studies not available or not performed
S0	Tumor marker study levels within normal limits
S1	LDH < 1.5x normal **and** β-hCG < 5,000 IU/L **and** AFP < 1,000 ng/mL
S2	LDH 1.5-10x normal **or** β-hCG 5,000-50,000 IU/L **or** AFP 1,000-10,000 ng/mL
S3	LDH > 10x normal **or** β-hCG > 50,000 IU/L **or** AFP > 10,000 ng/mL

Serum tumor markers are used as part of tumor stage grouping in testicular cancer. Lactate dehydrogenase (LDH), human chorionic gonadotropin (hCG), α-fetoprotein (AFP).

AJCC Stages/Prognostic Groups

Adapted from 7th edition AJCC Staging Forms.

Stage	*T*	*N*	*M*	*S (Serum Tumor Markers)*
0	pTis	N0	M0	S0
I	pT1-4	N0	M0	SX
IA	pT1	N0	M0	S0
IB	pT2	N0	M0	S0
	pT3	N0	M0	S0
	pT4	N0	M0	S0
IS	Any pT/TX	N0	M0	S1-3 (measured post orchiectomy)
II	Any pT/TX	N1-3	M0	SX
IIA	Any pT/TX	N1	M0	S0
	Any pT/TX	N1	M0	S1
IIB	Any pT/TX	N2	M0	S0
	Any pT/TX	N2	M0	S1
IIC	Any pT/TX	N3	M0	S0
	Any pT/TX	N3	M0	S1
III	Any pT/TX	Any N	M1	SX
IIIA	Any pT/TX	Any N	M1a	S0
	Any pT/TX	Any N	M1a	S1
IIIB	Any pT/TX	N1-3	M0	S2
	Any pT/TX	Any N	M1a	S2
IIIC	Any pT/TX	N1-3	M0	S3
	Any pT/TX	Any N	M1a	S3
	Any pT/TX	Any N	M1b	Any S

T1

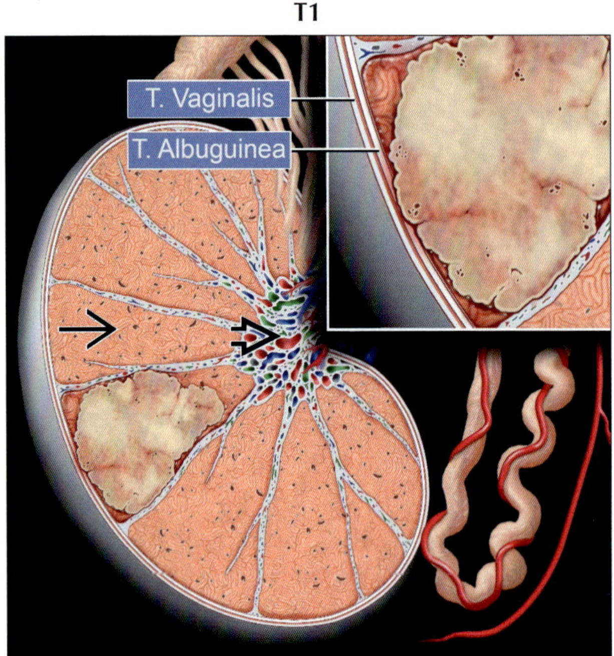

Graphic illustrates tumor limited to the testis and epididymis without vascular/lymphatic invasion. The tumor may invade the tunica albuginea but not the tunica vaginalis (as seen in the inset). Both are classified as T1 disease. Seminiferous tubule ➔ and rete testis ➲ are shown.

T2

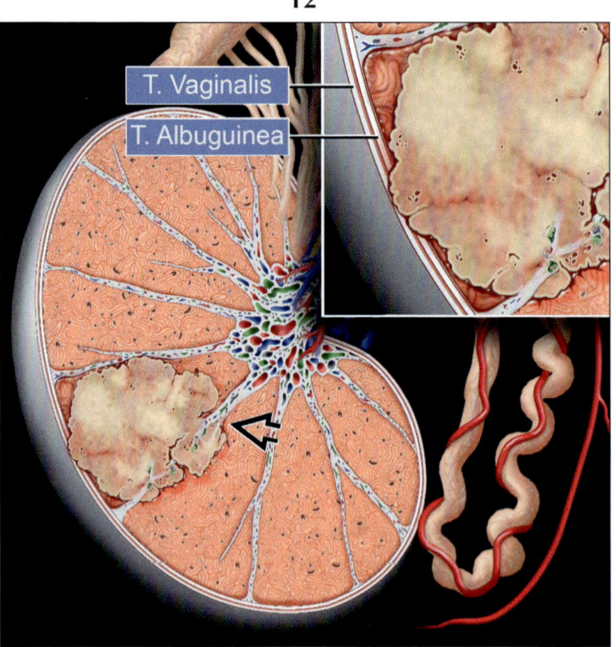

Graphic illustrates tumor limited to the testis and epididymis with vascular/lymphatic invasion ➲. Tumor extending through the tunica albuginea and involving the tunica vaginalis (as seen in the inset) is classified as T2 disease.

T3

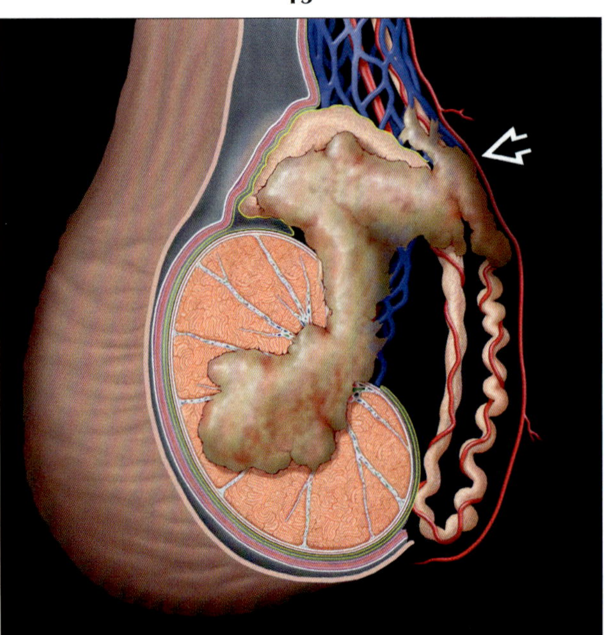

Graphic illustrates tumor invading the spermatic cord ➲ (with or without vascular/lymphatic invasion), compatible with T3 disease.

T4

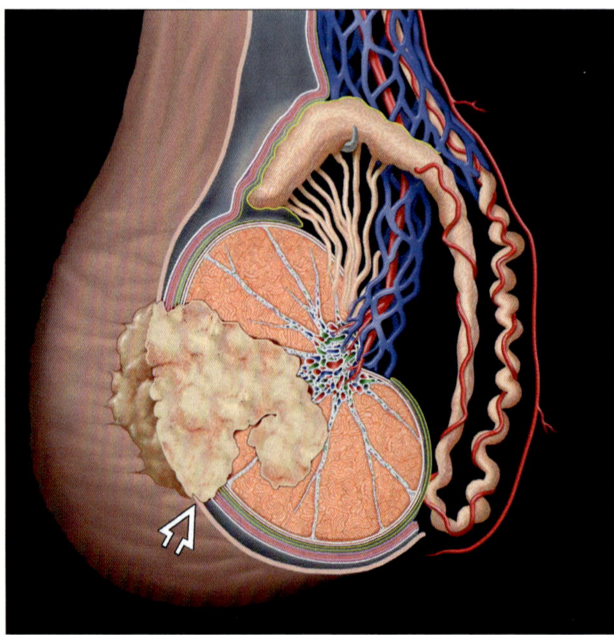

Graphic illustrates tumor invading the scrotum ➲ (with or without vascular/lymphatic invasion), which is considered T4 disease.

N Staging

Prior scrotal or inguinal surgery.

Right testicular nodal spread initially involves nodes around the IVC, including retroperitoneal, aortocaval, and paracaval nodes (dotted white line). If there has been disruption of lymphatics from prior scrotal or inguinal surgery or tumor invasion of the scrotum, then spread is to the inguinal nodes →.

N Staging

After Scrotal or Inguinal surgery.

Left testicular lesion spread typically involves retroperitoneal area bounded by renal vein, aorta, ureter, and IVC as indicated by white dotted line. If lymphatics are disrupted by prior scrotal or inguinal surgery or if tumor invades scrotum, primary spread can be via inguinal lymph nodes →. Size of nodes determines N stage: < 2 cm = N1; 2-5 cm = N2; > 5 cm = N3.

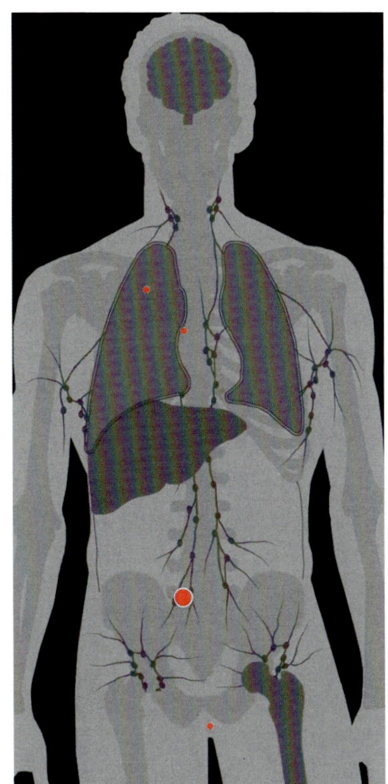

INITIAL SITE OF RECURRENCE	
Abdominopelvic	16%
Groin	0.3%
Lungs	0.1%
Mediastinum	0.1%
Neck/Supraclavicular Fossa	0%
Other	0.3%

Data from 1,558 patients and 263 recurrences following surveillance for stage I seminoma. The vast majority of recurrences occurred in the abdomen or pelvis, although the exact location was not always noted. Known abdominal recurrence occurred in 10% and pelvic in 1%. The remaining abdominopelvic recurrences were not otherwise specified. Martin JM et al: Evidenced-based guidelines for following stage I seminoma. Cancer. 109(11):2248-56, 2007.

TESTIS

OVERVIEW

General Comments

- Testicular cancer is rare and highly curable
  - Most common cancer in men between ages of 15 and 35 years but can occur at any age
    - 2nd peak at age 60 years
  - Lifetime risk of testicular cancer is ~ 1 in 268 (or 0.4%)
- Vast majority (95%) of testicular cancers are germ cell tumors
  - Germ cell tumors may be seminomas or nonseminomas
    - Seminomas are exquisitely sensitive to radiotherapy (RT), and low doses are highly effective in sterilizing microscopic disease and eradicating gross disease
    - RT has no role in the treatment of nonseminoma, with exception of palliation or treatment of brain metastasis

Classification

- Germ cell tumors (95%)
  - Seminoma (40%)
    - Classic (85%)
    - Anaplastic (10%)
    - Spermatocytic (5%)
  - Nonseminoma (60%)
    - Embryonal carcinoma
    - Teratoma
    - Choriocarcinoma
    - Yolk sac tumor
- Sex cord and stromal tumors (5%)
  - Leydig cell tumor
  - Sertoli cell tumor
  - Granulosa cell tumor
  - Fibroma-thecoma

NATURAL HISTORY

General Features

- Comments
  - Seminoma is commonly localized with predictable pattern of spread to regional (retroperitoneal) lymph nodes followed by mediastinum and left supraclavicular fossae
    - Approximately 85% of seminoma is confined to testicle
  - Lifetime risk of metachronous contralateral testicular cancer is 2%, 5x risk of unaffected population
- Location
  - Right testicle is more commonly affected

Etiology

- Risk factors
  - Cryptorchidism
    - 10-15% of seminomas have history of cryptorchidism
    - Intraabdominal or high inguinal have higher risk
    - May present as painful groin mass or abdominal mass
    - Higher metastatic rate
    - Higher incidence of pelvic nodal disease
  - Prior testicular cancer
  - Genetic factors
    - Down syndrome
    - Klinefelter syndrome (47XXY)
    - Increased copies of isochrome 12p
    - Family history
      - 3% of testicular cancers are familial, and vast majority are sporadic
  - Chemical exposures
    - Diethylstilbestrol in utero
    - Agent Orange
    - Solvents to clean jets
  - Race/ethnicity
    - Caucasian men 5x more likely to develop testicular cancer than black men
  - Carcinoma in situ
    - Precursor lesion for most testicular germ cell tumors that originate in utero
  - Infection
    - Some studies suggest that HIV may increase risk of testicular cancer

Epidemiology & Cancer Incidence

- Number of cases in USA per year
  - Lifetime risk of developing testicular cancer is 1 in 270
    - Estimated 8,590 new cases in USA in 2012
  - Lifetime risk of dying of testicular cancer is 1 in 5,000
    - Estimated 360 deaths in USA in 2012
  - Increasing prevalence; > 100% increase in reported cases since 1938
    - Annual percentage change ↑ 2.3% between 1975 and 1989, ↑ 0.8% between 1989 and 2005
- Age of onset
  - Nonseminomas occur at younger age (25-30 years) compared to seminomas (35-39 years)

Gross Pathology & Surgical Features

- Anatomy
  - Testis is composed of wedge-like compartments that contain seminiferous tubules
    - Seminiferous tubules contain spermatogonia and Sertoli cells
  - Seminiferous tubules unite to form rete testis
  - Rete testis joins to form epididymis, which becomes vas deferens then spermatic cord
- Coverings of testis: Tunica albuginea, tunica vaginalis, dartos muscle, external spermatic fascia, cremasteric muscle, internal spermatic fascia, skin

Microscopic Pathology

- H&E
  - Seminoma
    - Uniform cellular morphology resembling primitive germ cells
    - Classic (70-85%)
      - Sheets of large cells with clean cytoplasm
      - Lymphocytic infiltration
    - Anaplastic (10-30%)
      - Worse prognosis than classic
    - Spermatocytic (2-12%)
      - May grow large without spread
      - Intratumor calcification
      - No lymphocytic infiltration
  - Embryonal cell carcinoma

- Papillary tumor with primitive anaplastic epithelial cells resembling early embryonic cells
  - Teratoma
    - Variable appearance with possible ciliated epithelial-lined cysts, densely staining bone and cartilage, and mucin-producing glandular structures
  - Choriocarcinoma
    - Pale-staining cytotrophoblasts surrounded by syncytiotrophoblasts
- Special stains
  - Yolk sac tumor
    - Anti-α-fetoprotein stain positive with brownish deposits within tumor cells

Routes of Spread

- Local spread
  - Through tunica albuginea with involvement of scrotal skin is rare and late finding
- Lymphatic extension
  - Most germ cell tumors spread primarily via lymphatics rather than hematogenously
  - Lymphatic involvement occurs in predictable step-wise fashion
    - Right testis → right-sided retroperitoneal lymph nodes around inferior vena cava (IVC)
      - Most commonly at level of L2
      - Typically ordered spread to interaortocaval region; paracaval, preaortic, and right common iliac and paraaortic lymph nodes
    - Left testis → left retroperitoneal lymph nodes in area bounded by renal vein, aorta, ureter, and inferior mesenteric artery
      - Most commonly at level of L1-L3
      - Typically ordered spread to preaortic and paraaortic regions, then interaortocaval and left common iliac nodes
    - May be spread from right to left, but not from left to right
  - Pelvic adenopathy is uncommon in absence of bulky retroperitoneal disease causing retrograde spread
  - Inguinal lymph node metastases from testicular tumors are reported in 2% of cases, primarily to ipsilateral inguinal nodes
    - Pattern is seen in 2 groups of patients
      - Lymphatic disruption from prior scrotal or inguinal surgery
      - Tumor-contaminated scrotum from biopsy or transscrotal orchiectomy
    - Inguinal nodes are then considered nonregional (M1 disease) unless lymphatic disruption has occurred
  - Nodal disease superior to level of renal hila occurs via direct spread
    - With seminoma, left supraclavicular adenopathy may occur via thoracic duct into posterior mediastinum
- Hematogenous spread
  - Occurs late, except in case of choriocarcinoma
  - Lung is most common location (89%); other sites include liver (73%), brain (31%), bone (30%), kidney (30%), and adrenal (29%)

IMAGING

Detection

- Ultrasound
  - Primary imaging modality for evaluation of testicular lesions
  - Nearly 100% sensitivity for identification of scrotal masses; can almost always differentiate intratesticular from extratesticular mass
  - Ultrasound cannot reliably differentiate tumor subtypes, and orchiectomy is required for detailed pathologic evaluation of tumor
  - Most testicular tumors are hypoechoic to surrounding normal parenchyma
    - Some tumors can be heterogeneous with cystic areas and calcifications
    - Larger tumors tend to be more vascular
  - Ultrasound appearance of different histologic types
    - Seminoma
      - Most commonly uniformly hypoechoic; if larger, can be heterogeneous and may have lobulated nodules
      - May be multifocal &/or bilateral (1-3%), almost always metachronous
    - Embryonal cell carcinoma
      - More heterogeneous and ill defined than seminoma; can hemorrhage and have cystic areas of necrosis
    - Teratoma
      - Complex heterogeneous lesions often with multiple cystic areas and multiple echogenic foci made up of cartilage, calcification, and fibrosis
    - Yolk sac tumor
      - Rarely in pure form in adults, although comprises 80% of childhood tumors, most before age 2
      - Pure forms in childhood have nonspecific imaging findings, sometimes testicular enlargement without focal mass
    - Choriocarcinoma
      - Small echogenic mass, can hemorrhage and have areas of necrosis or calcification
      - Often present with widely metastatic disease
    - Mixed germ cell tumor
      - Imaging variable depending on tumor components
    - Leydig cell tumor
      - Variable sonographic appearance without distinguishing features from germ cell tumors
    - Sertoli cell tumor
      - Often multiple bilateral masses with large calcifications
- Computed tomography (CT)
  - Insensitive for undiagnosed testicular lesion
    - Difficult to distinguish intratesticular from extratesticular lesions
  - Retroperitoneal mass discovered on CT in setting of unknown primary in appropriate patient population warrants further investigation with testicular ultrasound
    - Ultrasound may find primary testicular carcinoma, including possibility of "burned-out" germ cell tumor

- Fluorodeoxyglucose positron emission tomography (FDG PET)
  - Not typically used for initial testicular evaluation
  - FDG PET sensitivity/specificity for seminoma is 100%/80%, respectively
  - SUV > 3 used as cut-off for suspicion of malignancy in primary testicular tumor

Staging

- T staging
  - Primary tumor staging includes evaluation for invasion of testicular vasculature/lymphatics, invasion of tunica albuginea/vaginalis, spermatic cord, and scrotum
    - After identification of intratesticular mass, radical orchiectomy with detailed pathologic evaluation is used for staging
      - In addition to determining extent of tumor invasion, tumor subtype is reported with percentage of each subtype present
- N staging
  - Adenopathy (nodes > 8 mm in short axis) in typical locations concerning for metastatic disease
  - Location of nodal metastases
    - Right testis → right-sided nodes around IVC (most commonly lower retroperitoneal, aortocaval, or paracaval)
    - Left testis → left paraaortic nodes in area bounded by renal vein, aorta, ureter, and inferior mesenteric artery
  - Size of lymph nodes determine nodal staging
    - N1: Single or multiple nodes ≤ 2 cm in short axis
    - N2: Single or multiple nodes > 2 cm but ≤ 5 cm in short axis
    - N3: Single or multiple nodes > 5 cm in short axis
- M staging
  - Nonregional nodes or pulmonary metastasis defines M1a disease
    - Including inguinal nodes if patient did not have scrotal or inguinal surgery, nor tumor invading scrotum
  - Other distant metastasis defines M1b disease
    - Most commonly liver, brain, bone, kidney, or adrenal glands
- Alternate staging
  - Modified Royal Marsden
    - Stage I: Tumor confined to testis
    - Stage II: Infradiaphragmatic adenopathy
      - IIA: Adenopathy < 2 cm
      - IIB: Adenopathy > 2 but < 5 cm
      - IIC: Adenopathy > 5 but < 10 cm
      - IID: Adenopathy > 10 cm
    - Stage III: Supradiaphragmatic adenopathy
    - Stage IV: Parenchymal metastasis
- Magnetic resonance (MR)
  - Offers no advantage over CT in evaluating adenopathy as MR has same limitations in distinguishing reactive from malignant nodes
- FDG PET
  - Offers no statistical advantage for initial staging of testicular germ cell tumors over CT as it is poor at detecting subcentimeter disease

CLINICAL PRESENTATION & WORK-UP

Presentation

- Majority of patients present with painless unilateral testicular mass
- Approximately 15-45% of patients have pain and a mass, which can delay diagnosis
  - Misdiagnosis often attributed to epididymitis, orchitis, or hydrocele
- Diffuse testicular enlargement and evidence of metastatic disease can be seen in approximately 10% of patients

Prognosis

- Seminoma
  - Good prognosis
    - Normal AFP, any hCG, any LDH
    - No nonpulmonary visceral metastases
    - Any primary site
    - 5-year PFS is 82%, 5-year survival is 86%
  - Intermediate prognosis
    - Nonpulmonary visceral metastases present
    - 5-year PFS is 67%, 5-year survival is 72%
  - Poor prognosis: No seminomas are considered poor prognosis

Work-Up

- Clinical
  - Comprehensive history and physical exam
    - Pertinent history includes particular attention to risk factors, prior surgeries, and fertility
    - Physical exam should pay particular attention to palpation of scrotum, groin, abdomen, and left supraclavicular fossa
- Radiographic
  - Abdominal/pelvic CT
    - Evaluation for adenopathy, including retroperitoneal, inguinal, and pelvic
      - Low-attenuating, poorly enhancing lymph nodes in typical retroperitoneal locations, even when small, are concerning for metastatic disease
      - Size criterion of 8 mm in short axis in typical retroperitoneal locations has high specificity but low sensitivity
    - Evaluation of visceral organs, including liver, bones, kidneys, and adrenal glands
      - Presence of horseshoe kidney may preclude use of radiotherapy
  - Chest x-ray
  - Chest CT
    - Indicated if abdominal/pelvic CT is abnormal or abnormal chest x-ray
- Laboratory
  - α-fetoprotein (AFP)
    - Elevated AFP is generally inconsistent with diagnosis of pure seminoma unless liver dysfunction or hepatitis
    - Half-life: 4-7 days
  - β-human chorionic gonadotropin (β-hCG)
    - May be elevated in 10-30% of seminoma
    - May be elevated if marijuana use
    - May be elevated if hypogonadism

    - e.g., Klinefelter syndrome, cryptorchidism, mumps orchitis, hemochromatosis, testicular trauma
  - Half-life: 1-2 days
- Serum lactate dehydrogenase (LDH)
  - Elevated in 50% of germ cell tumors
  - Low sensitivity and specificity

TREATMENT

Treatment Options by Stage

- Seminoma
- Stage I
  - Radical inguinal orchiectomy (RIO) followed by surveillance
    - Surveillance is preferred
    - Relapse: 13-19%; cause-specific survival: 99-100%
    - Surveillance consists of evaluations with history and physical exam, serum markers, chest x-ray, and CT scan
      - History and physical exam, serum markers, chest x-ray, and CT scan every 3-4 months for years 1 & 2, every 6-12 months for years 3 & 4, then annually
      - Abdominal/pelvic CT every 3-4 months for years 1 & 2, every 6-12 months for years 3 & 4, then annually for years 4 & 5
      - Chest x-ray if clinically indicated
  - RIO followed by adjuvant RT
    - Relapse: 3-5%; cause-specific survival: 99-100%
    - RT consisting of 20 Gy in 10 fractions to retroperitoneal lymph nodes (i.e., paraaortic field) is preferred
      - 20 Gy in 10 fractions has been shown to be not inferior to 30 Gy in 10 fractions in Medical Research Council (MRC) trial TE18/European Organisation for the Research and Treatment of Cancer (EORTC) 30942
      - Paraaortic radiotherapy has been shown to be equally effective to paraaortic and ipsilateral hemipelvis radiotherapy in MRC trial TE10
  - RIO followed by adjuvant chemotherapy
    - Chemotherapy may include 1-2 cycles of carboplatin chemotherapy (AUC x 7)
- Stage II
  - Stage IIA/B
    - RIO followed by RT to retroperitoneal and ipsilateral iliac lymph nodes
    - Consider primary etoposide and cisplatin (4 cycles) or bleomycin, etoposide, platinum (3 cycles) chemotherapy in selected IIB patients with lymph nodes > 3 cm
  - Stage IIC
    - RIO followed by combination chemotherapy (with cisplatin-based regime)
- Stage III
  - RIO with multidrug chemotherapy regime
    - Some advocate resection of residual masses > 3 cm or empiric radiation
    - Viable alternative is serial serum markers and CT exam

Organs at Risk Parameters

- 10 cGy: Temporary azoospermia
- 15-60 cGy: Temporary sterility
- 200 cGy: Azoospermia for several years
- 600-800 cGy: Permanent azoospermia

Surveillance vs. Radiotherapy vs. Chemotherapy

- Radiotherapy
  - Adjuvant radiotherapy is highly effective treatment due to inherent radiosensitivity of seminoma
  - RT is associated with adverse late effect
    - Increases relative risk (RR) of secondary malignancy, including (but not limited to) pancreatic (RR: 3.8), colon (RR: 1.9), and gastric (RR: 4.1) cancers
    - Increases risk of cardiac disease after 15 years (standardized mortality ratio = 1.85) not associated with prophylactic mediastinal radiotherapy, radiotherapy dose, age, or stage
  - Despite these concerns, majority (~ 60%) of radiation oncologists recommend adjuvant RT in recent survey of 491 randomly selected American radiation oncologists
  - Surveillance, epidemiology, and end results (SEER) data from 1990-2004 suggests, however, that this proportion may be declining
  - RT is ideally suited to young soldiers who may not have access to routine imaging or laboratory studies required for surveillance of postchemotherapy monitoring
- Chemotherapy
  - Single cycle carboplatin has been shown to be not inferior to adjuvant radiotherapy in MRC TE19/ EORTC 30982 study; 3-year RFS 95.9% with RT and 94.8% for carbo
  - Fewer contralateral testis tumors develop with carbo compared with RT
  - Two cycles of carboplatin were studied prospectively in 2nd Spanish Germ Cell Cancer Cooperative Group study
  - Appropriateness of carboplatin has been questioned for several reasons
    - Risk of relapse has not been shown to be superior to RT
    - Majority of recurrences (~ 75%) occur in the retroperitoneum with carboplatin, requiring radiographic surveillance and salvage radiotherapy
    - Follow-up is short and risk of late toxicity, such as myocardial infarction, hypertension, and hypercholesterolemia, is not fully understood
    - Carboplatin is known to be inferior to cisplatin in disseminated germ cell tumors
- Surveillance
  - Preferred method for almost all seminoma patients because ~ 85% do not require adjuvant treatment, and risks of toxicity associated with overtreatment
  - Reliable and validated risk-adapted strategy that identifies patients at high risk for recurrent seminoma has not been established
  - Recurrence can be successfully salvaged with either radiotherapy or chemotherapy with rates nearing 99%
  - Unfortunately, surveillance does not entirely eliminate risk associated with radiation because radiographic studies are used to screen for recurrence

- Salvage therapy for relapsed stage I seminoma may include more intensive treatment with large-field radiotherapy or full-dose, cisplatin-based chemotherapy, and late toxicity is a concern
- There are concerns that quality of surveillance may be poor, however, and some studies suggest that 30% of all patients receive no imaging or laboratory work in 1st year of surveillance

Radiotherapy Simulation

- CT simulation supine, immobilized in cast with arms at sides
- Identify retroperitoneal vasculature and kidneys
- Scrotal shields should be used (reduces dose by ~ 2-3x)

Radiotherapy Treatment Planning

- General considerations
  - RT should begin within 7 weeks of surgery
  - Patients should receive treatment 5 days a week
  - Antiemetic prophylaxis significantly reduces nausea
- **Stage I**
- Parallel opposed AP/PA technique
  - Conventional RT (bony anatomy based)
    - Superior border: Bottom of T11
    - Inferior border: Bottom of L5
    - Lateral border: From renal hilum to renal hilum (~ 10 cm wide) encompassing transverse process of L3
    - Custom blocking may be used to spare kidneys
    - Radiotherapy dose is prescribed to midplane
  - 3D conformal radiotherapy (volumetric based)
    - CTV = aorta with 1.9 cm margin and inferior vena cava with 1.2 cm margin to include paraaortic, paracaval, interaortocaval, and preaortic lymph node regions
      - Superior and inferior borders are identical to conventional technique (bottom of T11 to bottom of L5)
    - PTV = CTV plus 0.5 cm uniformly
  - Dose
    - 20 Gy in 10 fractions
    - RT dose may be prescribed to mid-plane (7 mm to block edge) or 95% of PTV
- Special considerations
  - Ipsilateral pelvic surgery (e.g., previous inguinal herniorrhaphy)
    - RT to ipsilateral iliac and inguinal lymph node regions is indicated
    - Scar from any prior inguinal surgery (herniorrhaphy) is included
  - Scrotal violation (e.g., transscrotal orchiectomy, transscrotal exploration, biopsy, aspiration, or orchiopexy)
    - Lymphatic drainage of scrotum is different than testis and drains to ipsilateral inguinal region
    - Ipsilateral hemiscrotum and hemipelvis radiotherapy including inguinal region is indicated
- **Stage IIA/B**
- Parallel opposed AP/PA technique
  - **Initial fields**
  - Conventional radiotherapy, modified "dog-leg"
    - Superior border: Bottom of T11
    - Inferior border: Bottom of acetabulum
    - Medial border: Line from tip of contralateral transverse process of L5 to medial border of ipsilateral obturator foramen
    - Lateral border: Line from tip of ipsilateral transverse process of L5 to lateral border of superolateral border of ipsilateral acetabulum
  - 3D conformal radiotherapy
    - GTV = nodal mass
    - CTV = GTV + aorta with 1.9 cm margin and inferior vena cava with 1.2 cm margin to include paraaortic, paracaval, interaortocaval, preaortic, and common and internal iliac lymph node regions
      - Superior and inferior borders are identical to conventional technique (bottom of T11 to top of ipsilateral acetabulum)
    - PTV = CTV plus 0.5 cm uniformly
    - Radiotherapy dose may be prescribed to mid-plane (7 mm to block edge) or 95% of PTV
  - Dose
    - Stages IIA/B: 20 Gy in 10 fractions
      - 25.5 Gy in 15 fractions is an alternative
  - **Cone down field (boost)**
  - Conventional or 3D conformal technique
    - GTV = nodal mass on CT plus 2 cm to block edge
  - Dose
    - Stage IIA: 10 Gy (30 Gy total)
    - Stage IIB: 16 Gy (36 Gy total)

Landmark Trials

- MRC TE18/EORTC 30942
  - 20 Gy in 10 fractions has been shown to be not inferior to 30 Gy in 10 fractions
- MRC trial TE10
  - Paraaortic RT has been shown to be equally effective to paraaortic and ipsilateral hemipelvis RT
- MRC TE19/EORTC 30982
  - Single cycle carboplatin was not inferior to adjuvant RT in terms of recurrence, but regional recurrences in retroperitoneum were higher with carboplatin

RECOMMENDED FOLLOW-UP

Clinical

- In recent years, routine imaging studies that screen for recurrence have been shown to have minor contribution to detection of recurrent disease
  - As a consequence, several guidelines, including National Comprehensive Cancer Network (NCCN), advise fewer imaging studies
- Seminoma stage IA or IB using subdiaphragmatic radiotherapy
  - History and physical exam, AFP, β-hCG, and LDH
    - Every 4 months for years 1 & 2, then annually for years 3-10
  - Abdominal/pelvic CT
    - Annually for 3 years (if paraaortic RT alone is used)
  - Chest x-ray
    - If clinically indicated
- Seminoma stage IIA or IIB status post radiation therapy
  - Abdominal CT at month 4 of year 1
  - Chest x-ray every 3-4 months for years 1 & 2, every 6-12 months for year 3, then annually for years 4 & 5
  - FDG PET/CT used for restaging and evaluation of response to therapy

- Tumor marker elevation in absence of CT findings should prompt FDG PET evaluation for salvage surgery
- FDG PET is best predictor of viable seminoma in residual masses after chemotherapy, may be useful in NSGCT
- Masses with residual malignancy may remain negative on PET for up to 14 days after chemotherapy, "stunned" tumor
- Difficult to differentiate mature teratoma vs. scar, as both have low FDG uptake
- In multirelapse seminoma patients, FDG PET has been shown to change treatment in 57% of cases

SELECTED REFERENCES

1. Arvold ND et al: Barriers to the implementation of surveillance for stage I testicular seminoma. Int J Radiat Oncol Biol Phys. 84(2):383-9, 2012
2. National Comprehensive Cancer Network (NCCN): Clinical Practice Guidelines in Oncology: testicular cancer. www.nccn.org, v.1.2012, 2012
3. Wilder RB et al: Radiotherapy treatment planning for testicular seminoma. Int J Radiat Oncol Biol Phys. 83(4):e445-52, 2012
4. Mead GM et al: Randomized trials in 2466 patients with stage I seminoma: patterns of relapse and follow-up. J Natl Cancer Inst. 103(3):241-9, 2011
5. Oliver RT et al: Randomized trial of carboplatin versus radiotherapy for stage I seminoma: mature results on relapse and contralateral testis cancer rates in MRC TE19/EORTC 30982 study (ISRCTN27163214). J Clin Oncol. 29(8):957-62, 2011
6. American Joint Committee on Cancer: AJCC Cancer Staging Manual. 7th ed. New York: Springer. 469-78, 2010
7. Yu HY et al: Quality of surveillance for stage I testis cancer in the community. J Clin Oncol. 27(26):4327-32, 2009
8. Jones WG et al: Randomized trial of 30 versus 20 Gy in the adjuvant treatment of stage I testicular seminoma: a report on Medical Research Council Trial TE18, European Organisation for the Research and Treatment of Cancer Trial 30942 (ISRCTN18525328). J Clin Oncol. 23(6):1200-8, 2005
9. Travis LB et al: Second cancers among 40,576 testicular cancer patients: focus on long-term survivors. J Natl Cancer Inst. 97(18):1354-65, 2005
10. Classen J et al: Para-aortic irradiation for stage I testicular seminoma: results of a prospective study in 675 patients. A trial of the German testicular cancer study group (GTCSG). Br J Cancer. 90(12):2305-11, 2004
11. Zagars GK et al: Mortality after cure of testicular seminoma. J Clin Oncol. 22(4):640-7, 2004
12. Chung PW et al: Appropriate radiation volume for stage IIA/B testicular seminoma. Int J Radiat Oncol Biol Phys. 56(3):746-8, 2003
13. Classen J et al: Radiotherapy for stages IIA/B testicular seminoma: final report of a prospective multicenter clinical trial. J Clin Oncol. 21(6):1101-6, 2003
14. Fosså SD et al: Optimal planning target volume for stage I testicular seminoma: A Medical Research Council randomized trial. Medical Research Council Testicular Tumor Working Group. J Clin Oncol. 17(4):1146, 1999

TESTIS

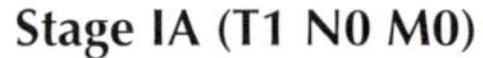

(Left) Longitudinal grayscale ultrasound shows a circumscribed, homogeneous, hypoechoic right testicular mass ➡ in a patient with bilateral testicular microlithiasis ➡. Mass proved to be seminoma at orchiectomy. (Right) Gross pathology in sagittal plane from the same patient demonstrates the testicular mass ➡, which was pure seminoma. The tunica vaginalis is intact ↗, which corresponds to imaging findings.

Stage IA (T1 N0 M0)

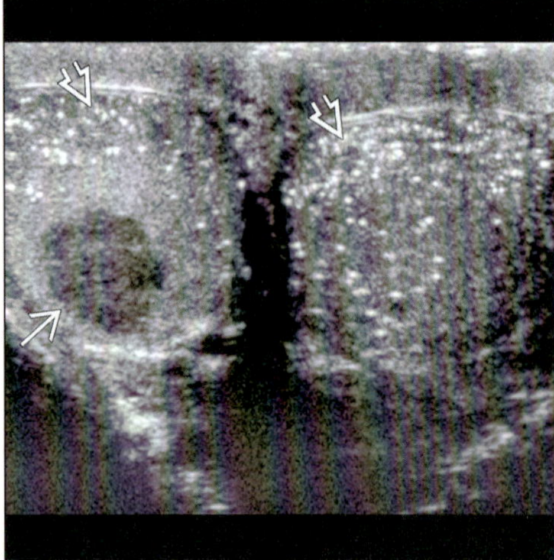

Stage IA (T1 N0 M0)

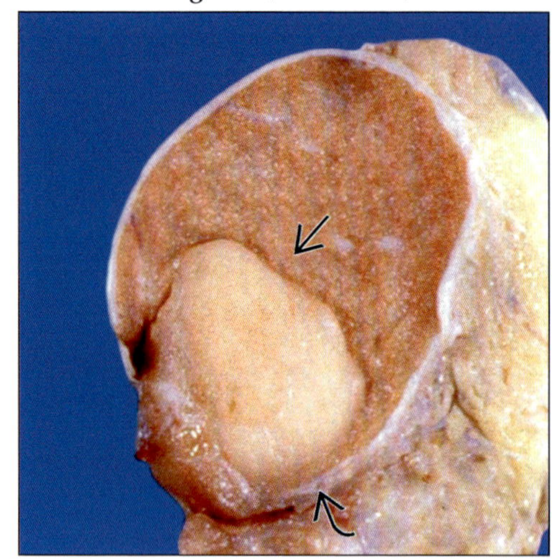

(Left) Gross pathology shows the large mass ➡ replacing the majority of testicular tissue, as well as invasion through the tunica vaginalis ➡. (Right) The field borders laterally are from renal hilum to renal hilum, approximately 10 cm wide, extending superior from the bottom of T11 to the bottom of L5.

Stage IB (T2 N0 M0)

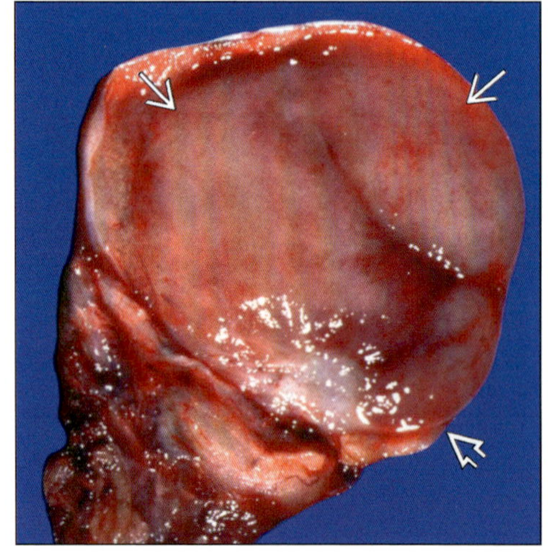

Stage I Conventional Paraaortic Field

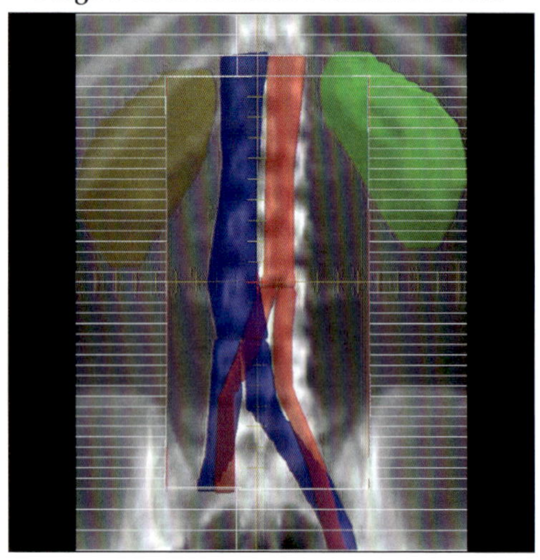

(Left) The CTV includes the aorta with a 1.9 cm margin and the inferior vena cava with a 1.2 cm margin. The PTV includes the CTV with a 0.5 cm margin. A 0.7 cm margin is used for the field edge. A parallel-opposed AP/PA field arrangement is used. (Right) Delayed contrast-enhanced CT images demonstrate a horseshoe kidney ↗ overlying the retroperitoneum. A horseshoe kidney is a contraindication to radiotherapy.

Stage I Conformal Paraaortic Field

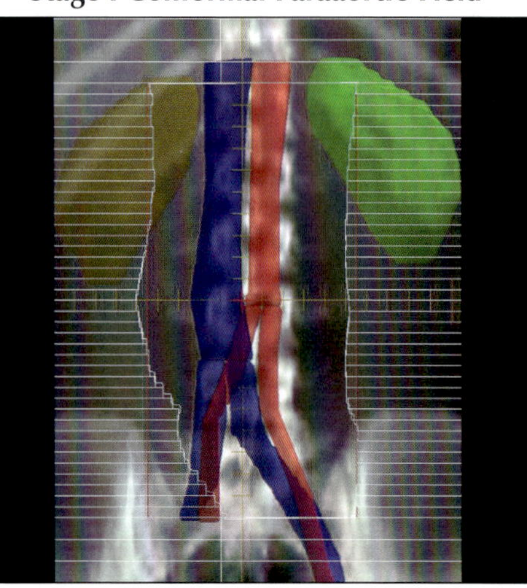

Horseshoe Kidney

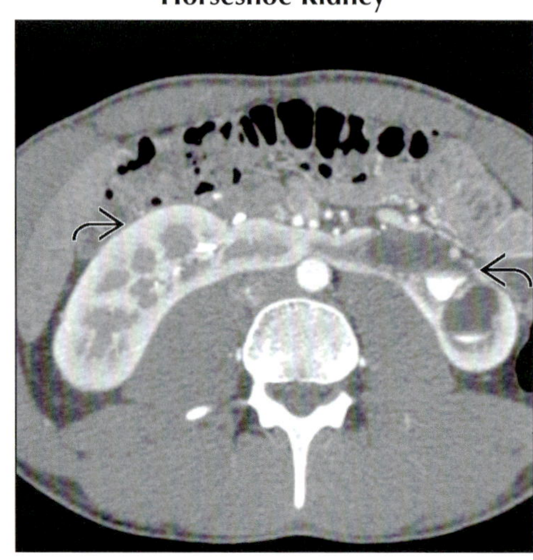

Stage IIA (T1 N1 M0)

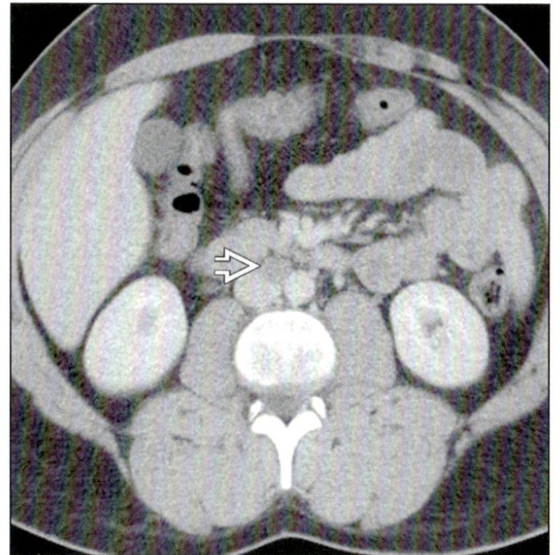

Stage IIB (T2 N2 M0)

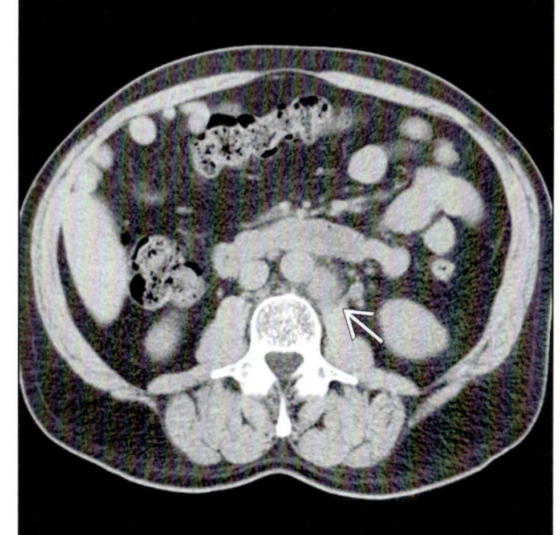

(Left) *Contrast-enhanced CT shows 1.9 cm interaortocaval adenopathy ➩. Regional nodal metastases ≤ 2 cm represents N1 disease.* ***(Right)*** *Axial non-contrast-enhanced CT in a patient with left side seminoma otherwise confined to the testicle shows left paraaortic lymph node ➔. The left testicular lymphatics most commonly follow the testicular artery and vein and attach adjacent to the left renal vessels.*

Stage IIB (T2 N2 M0)

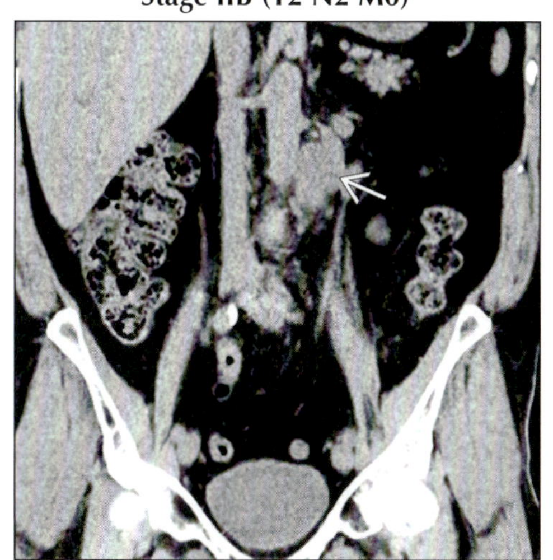

Stage IIA/B, Conventional Dog-Leg AP Field

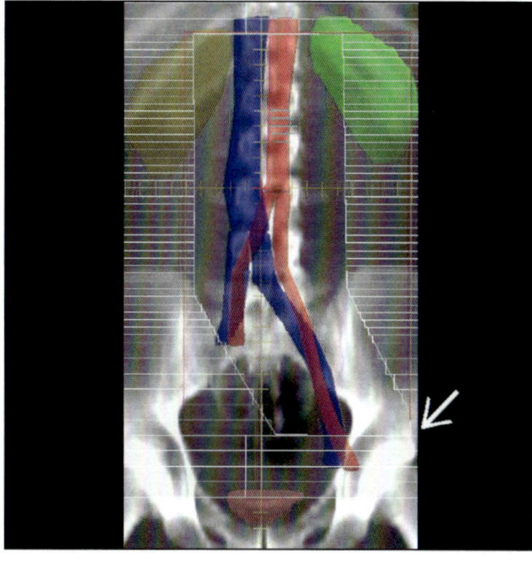

(Left) *Coronal NECT in the same patient shows a 4 cm nodal mass ➔, making this IIB disease. It is also important to consider tumor dimensions because size has implications for treatment (in the case of IIA/B vs. IIIC) and RT dose (in the case of IIA vs. IIB).* ***(Right)*** *In stage II, the paraaortic field is expanded to include the ipsilateral hemipelvis. The lateral border is the lateral aspect of the acetabulum ➔. The inferior border is the roof of the acetabulum.*

Stage IIA/B, Conformal Dog-Leg Field

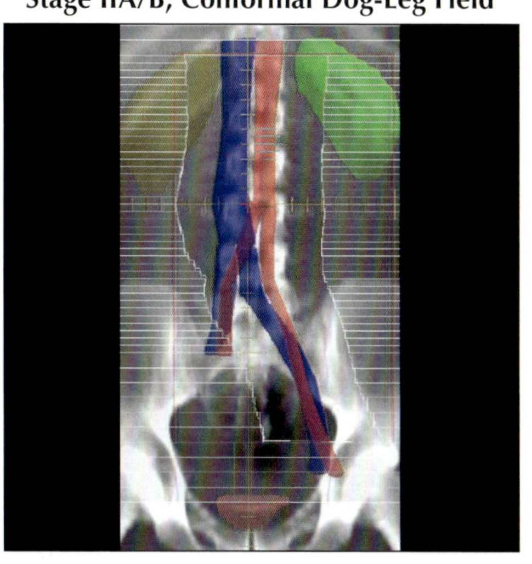

Stage IIA/B, Boost Field to Gross Adenopathy

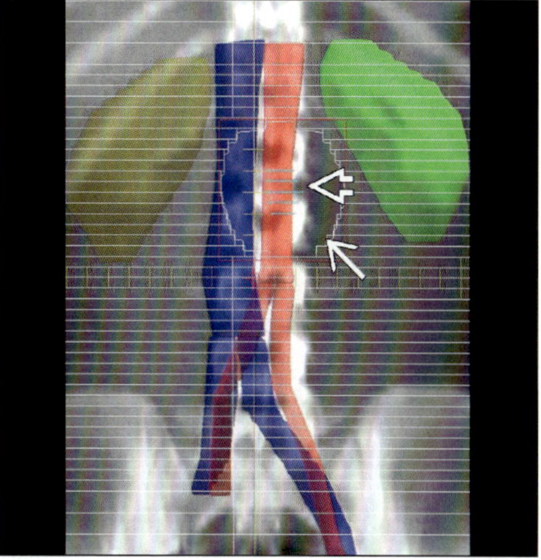

(Left) *The same expansion technique used for stage I is adapted for stage II to include the left internal iliac artery and vein. The inferior border of the field is the roof of the acetabulum.* ***(Right)*** *The field is composed of the gross tumor volume (blue) ➩ with a 2 cm margin ➔ treated with parallel opposed AP/PA field arrangement.*

(Left) Photo shows a Harter holder used to support the scrotum with bolus material ➲. A lucite divider ➲ is used to position the contralateral testicle outside the treatment field. The scrotal scar ➲ is identified to ensure placement in the treatment field. *(Right)* The scrotal scar ➲ and lucite divider → are used to ensure visualization during setup. Verifying an accurate setup clinically is imperative.

Stage I/II: Scrotal Violation

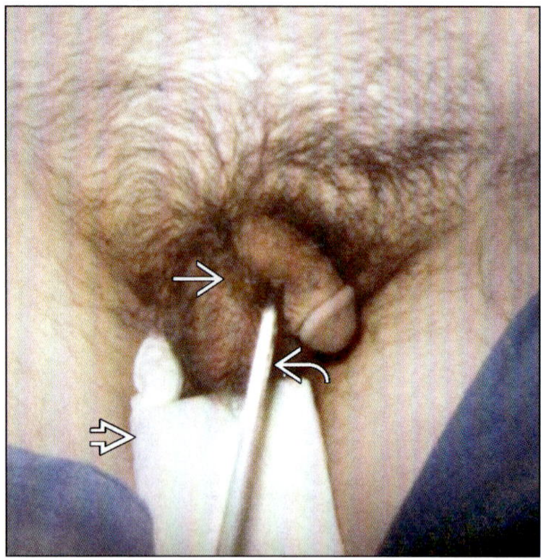

Stage I/II: Scrotal Violation

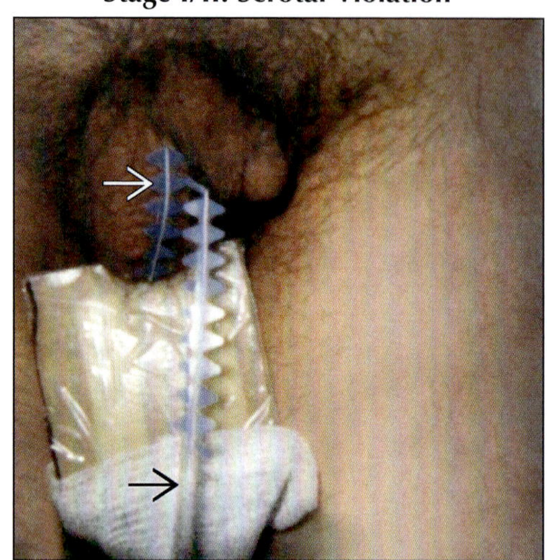

(Left) Bolus material ➲ is also placed over the testicle to ensure full dose to the scrotal skin. In this case, wet gauze measuring 1 cm is used. *(Right)* The Harter holder is fully visualized.

Stage I/II: Scrotal Violation

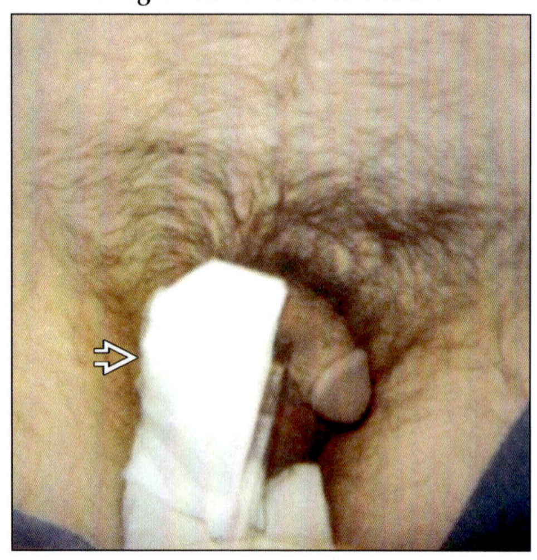

Stage I/II: Scrotal Violation

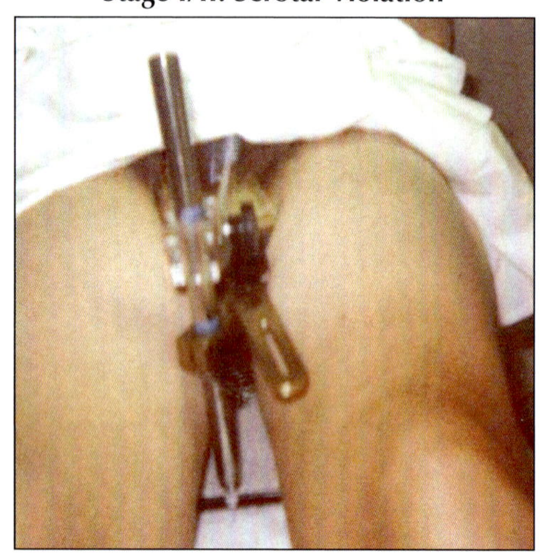

(Left) The hemipelvis field is used to treat the iliac and inguinal regions as well as the hemi-scrotum. Dose is prescribed 3 cm anterior to midplane with an AP/PA technique. The field is matched to a typical paraaortic AP/PA field. The lucite divider can be seen at the field edge ➲. *(Right)* Axial CECT shows the left kidney lying deep in the pelvis ➲, which is a contraindication for pelvic radiotherapy.

Stage I/II: Scrotal Violation

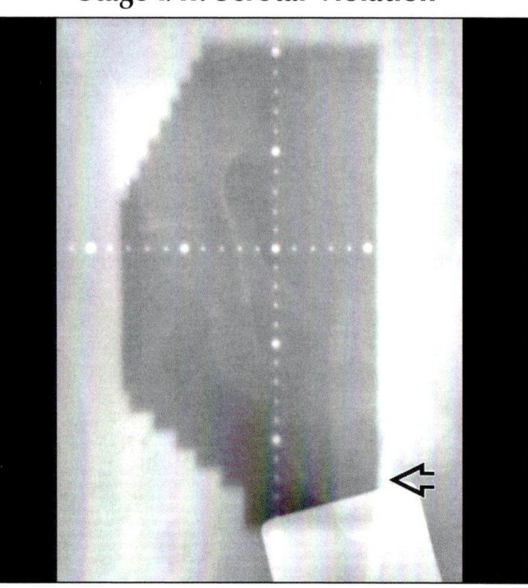

Pelvic Kidney

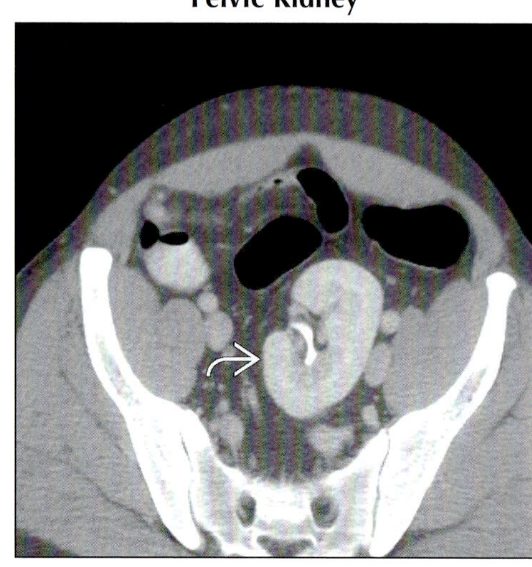

Stage IIC (T1 N3 M0)

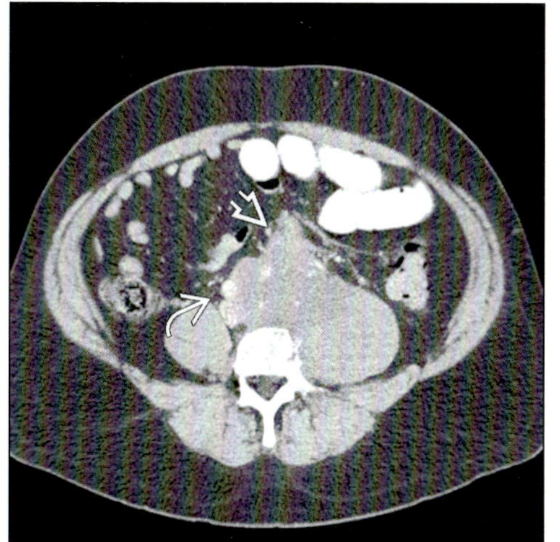

Stage III (T2 N1 M1a)

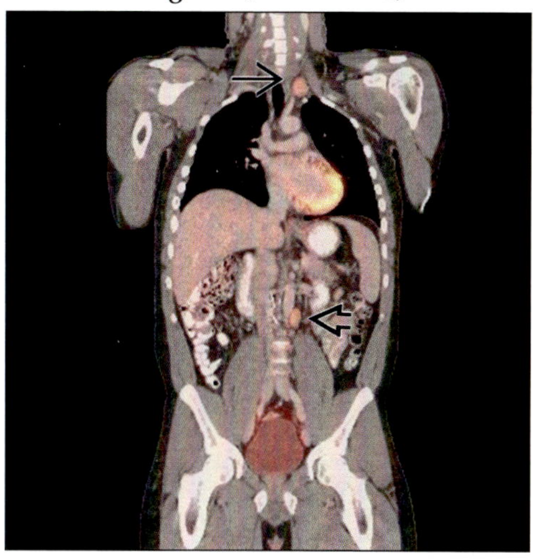

(Left) *Axial CECT shows retroperitoneal mass (> 5 cm)* ➡ *with displacement of infrarenal abdominal aorta* ➡*. Isochromosome 12p can be used to establish diagnosis because nearly all patients with germ cell tumors have increased copies of i(12p). Chemo is the preferred first-line treatment for patients with stage IIC disease.* ***(Right)*** *Coronal PET/CT shows avid left paraaortic* ➡ *and left Virchow lymphadenopathy* ➡*. Left orchiectomy found seminoma with lymphatic invasion.*

Stage IIIC (T1 N3 M1b)

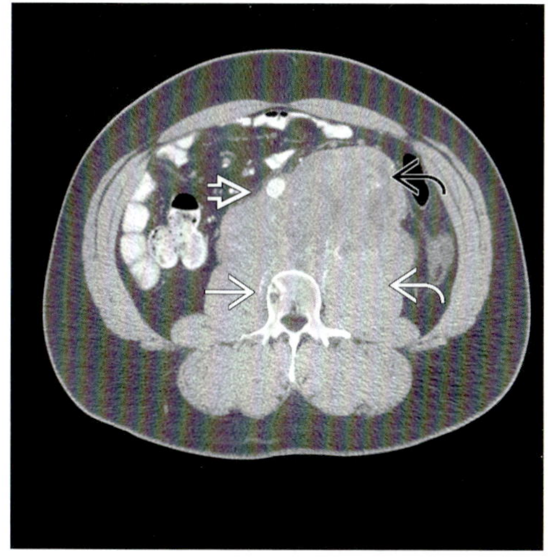

Stage IIIC (T2 N3 M1b)

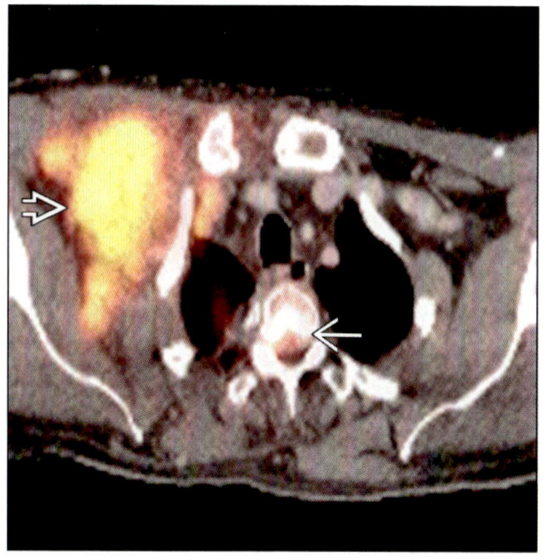

(Left) *Axial contrast-enhanced CT demonstrates a large, heterogeneous retroperitoneal mass* ➡ *displacing the aorta* ➡ *and invading the left psoas muscle* ➡*. Lytic lesion is seen in L3 vertebral body* ➡*.* ***(Right)*** *Axial fused PET/CT demonstrates FDG-avid supraclavicular adenopathy* ➡ *and an FDG-avid vertebral body lesion* ➡ *in a patient with testicular seminoma. The supraclavicular fossa and groin are sites where recurrence is also palpable.*

Lung Metastasis

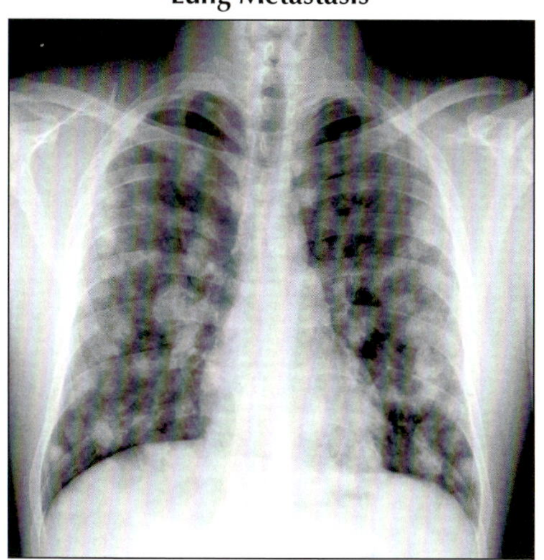

Brain Metastasis

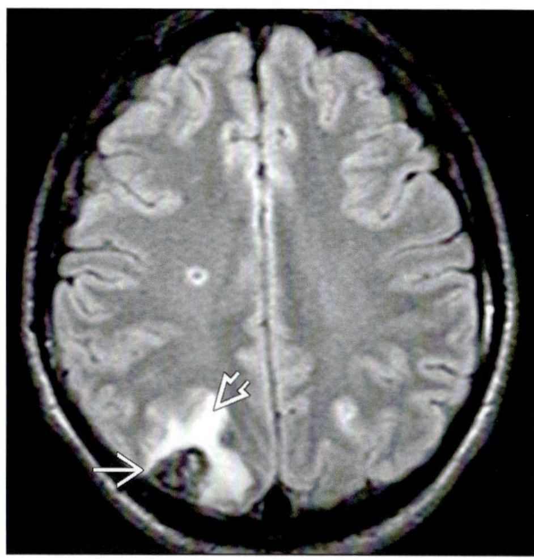

(Left) *Chest x-ray in the same patient shows multiple pulmonary metastatic lesions.* ***(Right)*** *Axial FLAIR MR shows intraaxial metastatic lesion in the right posterior parietal lobe* ➡ *with surrounding vasogenic edema* ➡*. Late recurrences in parenchyma or meninges can occur as the brain is a sanctuary site for seminoma.*

PENIS

(T) Primary Tumor

Adapted from 7th edition AJCC Staging Forms.

TNM	*Definitions*
TX	Primary tumor cannot be assessed
T0	No evidence of primary tumor
Tis	Carcinoma in situ
Ta	Noninvasive verrucous carcinoma
T1a	Tumor invades subepithelial connective tissue without lymphovascular invasion and is not poorly differentiated
T1b	Tumor invades subepithelial connective tissue with lymphovascular invasion or is poorly differentiated
T2	Tumor invades corpus spongiosum or cavernosum
T3	Tumor invades urethra
T4	Tumor invades other adjacent structures

(N) Regional Lymph Nodes

Clinical Staging	
NX	Regional lymph nodes cannot be assessed
N0	No palpable or visibly enlarged inguinal lymph nodes
N1	Palpable mobile unilateral inguinal lymph node
N2	Palpable mobile multiple or bilateral inguinal lymph nodes
N3	Palpable fixed inguinal nodal mass or pelvic lymphadenopathy unilateral or bilateral
Pathologic Staging	
NX	Regional lymph nodes cannot be assessed
N0	No regional lymph node metastasis
N1	Metastasis in a single inguinal lymph node
N2	Metastasis in multiple or bilateral inguinal lymph nodes
N3	Extranodal extension of lymph node metastasis or pelvic lymph node(s) unilateral or bilateral

(M) Distant Metastasis

M0	No distant metastasis
M1	Distant metastasis

AJCC Stages/Prognostic Groups

Adapted from 7th edition AJCC Staging Forms.

Stage	*T*	*N*	*M*
0	Tis	N0	M0
	Ta	N0	M0
I	T1a	N0	M0
II	T1b	N0	M0
	T2	N0	M0
	T3	N0	M0
IIIa	T1-3	N1	M0
IIIb	T1-3	N2	M0
IV	T4	Any N	M0
	Any T	N3	M0
	Any T	Any N	M1

T1/T2

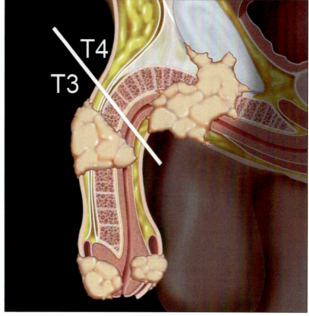

Graphic indicates that T1 tumors invade subepithelial connective tissue. T1a is not poorly differentiated and does not have lymphovascular invasion whereas T1b has 1 or both of those features. T2 invades corpus cavernosum ➔ or spongiosum ➔.

T3/T4

Graphic demonstrates that T3 invades urethra and T4 invades other structures.

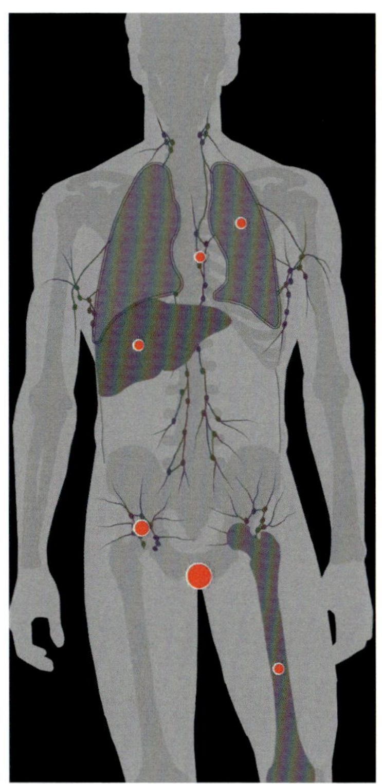

INITIAL SITE OF RECURRENCE

Penis	20%
Regional Nodes	11%
Lung	2%
Distant Nodes	1%
Bone	1%
Liver	1%

de Crevoisier R et al: Long-term results of brachytherapy for carcinoma of the penis confined to the glans (N- or NX). Int J Radiat Oncol Biol Phys. 74(4):1150-6, 2009.

PENIS

OVERVIEW

General Comments

- Penile cancer is a rare entity
- No consensus on care standards (i.e., surgery, chemo, and RT)
- Diagnosis and initial counseling of penile cancer patients is usually performed by urologic surgeons or dermatologists
- Uncommon for any stage penile cancer patient to be referred for consultation by radiation oncology &/or medical oncology
- Psychosexual and urologic complications from radical penectomy can be profound
- Penile preservation techniques and the use of RT instead of surgery for organ preservation should be considered
- Multidisciplinary care team in the treatment of these rare malignancies is important

NATURAL HISTORY

General Features

- Comments
  - Rare in Western countries, but 10-20% of male malignancies in Africa, Asia, and South America
  - Prognosis depends on tumor thickness, lymphovascular space invasion (LVSI), histology, and nodal spread

Etiology

- Risk factors
  - Intact foreskin
    - Mechanism possibly due to poor hygiene
  - Phimosis
  - HPV 16 and 18
    - Viral DNA present in ~ 45% of tumors
  - Bowenoid papulosis
  - Erythroplasia of Queyrat
  - Lichen sclerosis
  - Genital condylomas in adulthood
    - Increases risk 3-8x
- Protective factors
  - Circumcision in infancy
    - 3x risk reduction

Epidemiology & Cancer Incidence

- Number of cases in USA per year
  - 1,570 new cases and 310 deaths annually
  - Fewer than 1 case per 100,000 persons in Western countries
- Age of onset
  - Most common in 6th decade
  - Increases with age

Genetics

- Common translocations
  - *p53* positivity associated with increased risk of adenopathy

Gross Pathology & Surgical Features

- Superficial tumors are often managed with organ-preserving surgery
- T2-T4 tumors require amputative surgical approaches
  - Profound psychological consequences have been reported, including high suicide rate
- Patients with nodal metastases are rarely cured by surgery alone
- Definitive or adjunctive radiotherapy can be used in all stages of disease

Microscopic Pathology

- H&E
  - Most common histologic subtype is squamous cell carcinoma (95%)
    - Squamous cell, not otherwise specified (NOS)
    - Verrucous
    - Papillary squamous
    - Warty squamous
    - Basaloid carcinoma
  - Less common histologies include melanoma, lymphoma, Kaposi sarcoma, and basal cell carcinoma
  - Well-differentiated tumors: 30% node-positive rate
  - Moderate to poorly differentiated: ~ 80% node positive
- Special stains
  - Ki-67 expression showed no correlation with cause-specific or overall survival
  - p16 (INK4A) staining can be used as surrogate marker for HPV infection
    - Lack of p16 (INK4a) expression has been correlated with worse prognosis

Routes of Spread

- Local spread
  - Contiguous skin, corpus spongiosum, corpus cavernosum, urethra, prostate
- Lymphatic extension
  - Penile skin: Bilateral superficial inguinal nodes
  - Glans penis: Bilateral inguinal or iliac nodes
  - Corpora spongiosum or cavernosum: Bilateral deep inguinal and iliac nodes
- Metastatic sites
  - Lung, liver, and bone are most common

IMAGING

Detection

- Common radiologic presentations
  - MR
    - Best for extent of local invasion due to superior soft tissue resolution
    - Can also assess nodes
    - Physical exam has been documented to be superior to MR for T staging of primary lesion
  - Ultrasound
    - Good to assess extent of local invasion
  - CT
    - Primarily used to assess lymphadenopathy and metastatic spread
  - PET/CT
    - Emerging modality, good for assessing nodal and metastatic spread
    - Concern for false-positive adenopathy due to common presentation of reactive inguinal lymph nodes
    - 80.9% sensitivity
    - 92.4% specificity

CLINICAL PRESENTATION & WORK-UP

Presentation

- Presents as visible or painful lesion on penis
- Often difficult to discriminate from genital warts

Prognosis

- Depends on local extent of disease, histologic grade, LVSI, and adenopathy
- 5-year overall survival
  - Stage I: ~ 70-100%
  - Stage II: ~ 65-100%
  - Stage III: ~ 60-90%
  - Stage IV: 50-70%
- Complications
  - Skin necrosis
    - Brachytherapy: 0-23%
    - External beam radiation therapy (EBRT): 1-3%
  - Meatal stenosis/stricture
    - Brachytherapy: 9-45%
    - EBRT: 7-14%
  - Sexual dysfunction in the only prospective study
    - 88% of patients had unchanged erectile function
    - 87% reported unchanged coitus frequency
    - 87% reported unchanged coital satisfaction with accelerated EBRT
  - Suicidal ideation
    - In a series of 29 patients who underwent penectomy, 2 attempted suicide (1 successfully)

Work-Up

- Clinical
  - Careful inspection and palpation of the penis, scrotum, and inguinal nodes are required
  - Imaging to assess lymphadenopathy is required
  - MR is superior technique for delineation of depth of invasion in penis
  - PET/CT can be considered for evaluation of metastatic disease
  - Sentinel node lymphoscintigraphy and biopsy should be considered
    - 22% positive node identification rate in otherwise N0 patients
    - 78% of the time, positive sentinel node is only involved node
    - 8% of procedures result in surgical complications
    - 16% false-negative rate

TREATMENT

Major Treatment Alternatives

- Surgery is most commonly performed treatment
- Brachytherapy and EBRT (± chemotherapy) are alternatives
  - Radiotherapy can achieve durable local control of primary tumor
  - Conventionally fractionated EBRT local control rates are ~ 65%
  - Brachytherapy local control rates are ~ 85%
  - One prospective radiotherapy study at Tata Memorial Hospital
    - 23 stage I/II patients
    - Accelerated regimen of 54-55 Gy in 16-18 fractions of EBRT
    - Local control rate of 92% in stage I patients
  - Salvage penectomy can be used in cases of local failure with local control in ~ 95% range
  - Chemotherapy can be used in adjuvant, neoadjuvant, therapeutic, and palliative setting
    - Adjuvant chemotherapy recommended for N2 disease by European Association of Urology
      - Vincristine/bleomycin/methotrexate combination yielded an 82% 5-year survival vs. 37% in surgery alone in a retrospective study
    - Neoadjuvant regimens with reported response rates
      - Vincristine/bleomycin/methotrexate
      - Cisplatinum/bleomycin/methotrexate
      - Cisplatinum/5-FU
      - Cisplatinum/irinotecan
      - Paclitaxel/cisplatinum/5-FU
    - Concurrent with radiation
      - Cisplatinum weekly or every 3 weeks
      - 5-FU and mitomycin C
      - Cetuximab may be consideration for squamous histologies
    - Palliative
      - All of the above adjuvant regimens
      - Docetaxel and cetuximab

Treatment Options by Stage

- Carcinoma in situ (CIS): Circumcision, local excision, Moh surgery, topical 5-FU, topical imiquimod
  - Brachytherapy, monotherapy, or EBRT can be considered if CIS is extensive and surgery would be disfiguring
- T1-T2, node negative: Due to the rarity of this cancer, no standards of care exist
  - Surgical management
    - Penile-preserving surgery
      - Moh microsurgery
      - Glansectomy
      - Modified partial penectomy
    - Total penectomy
  - Radiation therapy
    - EBRT ± elective nodal radiation ± chemotherapy
    - Brachytherapy ± elective nodal radiation ± chemotherapy
  - Special considerations
    - Lymph node metastases are common and management of the nodes is evolving
      - For surgically managed patients, prophylactic nodal dissection is recommended for T2 or greater lesions, those with LVSI, and all high-grade lesions
      - Sentinel lymph node evaluation should be strongly considered for all patients
  - T3-T4
    - Radical penectomy and bilateral nodal dissection
    - Definitive chemoradiotherapy (CRT) for nonsurgical candidates
  - Any stage, node positive
    - Same surgical &/or RT options as above for primary tumor
    - Pelvic dissection for ≥ 2 pathologically positive inguinal nodes, ECE, or clinically positive nodes is most common practice

- Reports of good control with definitive CRT instead of surgical management of nodes is emerging
- Most extrapolate management of nodes from the vulvar and anal cancer treatment

Standard Doses

- EBRT: Common doses are 60-65 Gy with the pelvis receiving 40-50 Gy
- Brachytherapy: 60 Gy typical with (low dose rate) LDR at 50-65 cGy/hour or pulsed-dose rate
- When combining radiation with chemotherapy, consider anal cancer dose guidelines for primary and nodal basins

Organs at Risk Parameters

- Urethral dose with brachytherapy should receive < 50 Gy
- QUANTEC guidelines for pelvic normal tissue tolerances can be used

Common Techniques

- External beam
  - Early stage lesions of distal penis
    - Mold has to be fashioned to achieve good dose buildup around penile surface
      - Accomplished with wax, perspex, or stacked bolus
  - Locally advanced lesions
    - Tape penis to abdominal wall, use 1 cm bolus "diaper" over penis and inguinals
    - Excellent results with intensity-modulated radiation therapy (IMRT) to primary and nodes with platinum-containing regimens are emerging based on anal cancer experience
- Brachytherapy: Interstitial implants or plesiobrachytherapy molds with embedded sources are most common
  - For lesions of the glans only
  - Contraindicated for lesions > 4 cm or lesions continuous with shaft
  - 2-3 parallel planes of interstitial needles can be held between lucite templates
  - 6 needles are typical, spaced 12-18 mm apart
  - Margin of 10 mm past GTV is recommended

Landmark Trials

- Due to its rarity, no landmark trials have been performed

RECOMMENDED FOLLOW-UP

Clinical

- Clinical evaluation of penis and inguinal nodes every 3-4 months for 1-2 years, then every 6 months until year 5

Radiographic

- No standard of care exists
- Repeat chest, abdomen, and pelvis CT is recommended at 1st follow-up to evaluate regional progression

SELECTED REFERENCES

1. Hakenberg OW et al: Chemotherapy in penile cancer. Ther Adv Urol. 4(3):133-8, 2012
2. Sadeghi R et al: Accuracy of 18F-FDG PET/CT for diagnosing inguinal lymph node involvement in penile squamous cell carcinoma: systematic review and meta-analysis of the literature. Clin Nucl Med. 37(5):436-41, 2012
3. Crook J et al: Penile brachytherapy: technical aspects and postimplant issues. Brachytherapy. 9(2):151-8, 2010
4. Crook J: Radiation therapy for cancer of the penis. Urol Clin North Am. 37(3):435-43, 2010
5. Kroon BK et al: Dynamic sentinel node biopsy in penile carcinoma: evaluation of 10 years experience. Eur Urol. 47(5):601-6; discussion 606, 2005
6. Sarin R et al: Treatment results and prognostic factors in 101 men treated for squamous carcinoma of the penis. Int J Radiat Oncol Biol Phys. 38(4):713-22, 1997

Verrucous Carcinoma

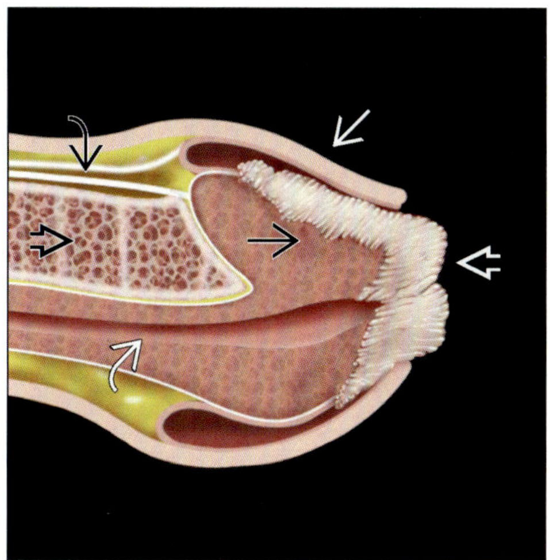

Tis N0 M0

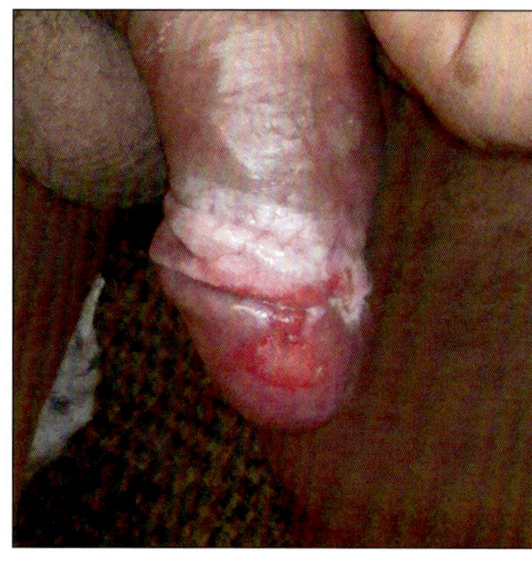

(Left) *Graphic of a verrucous carcinoma highlights the papillary, spiky surface and well-demarcated base. Note the carcinoma ➨, corpus spongiosum →, foreskin ➨, albuginea ↗, corpus cavernosum ⇨, and urethra ➚.* ***(Right)*** *Photo shows the penis of a 31-year-old man with Bowen disease extending from the glans penis onto the corona. Due to the extensive nature of the superficial lesion, conservative surgery was deemed too morbid. Patient failed imiquimod.*

Tis N0 M0

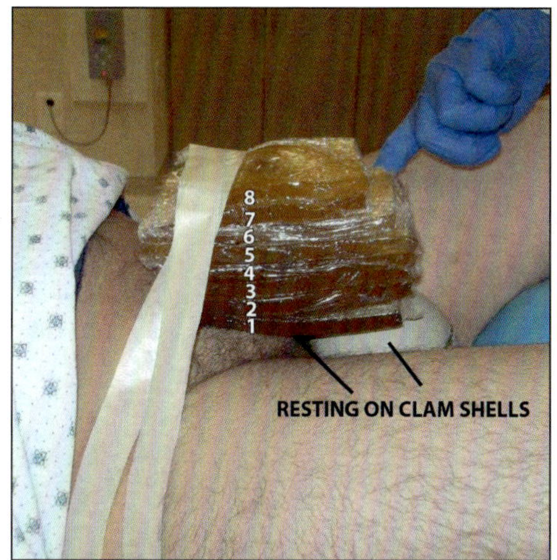

Tis N0 M0

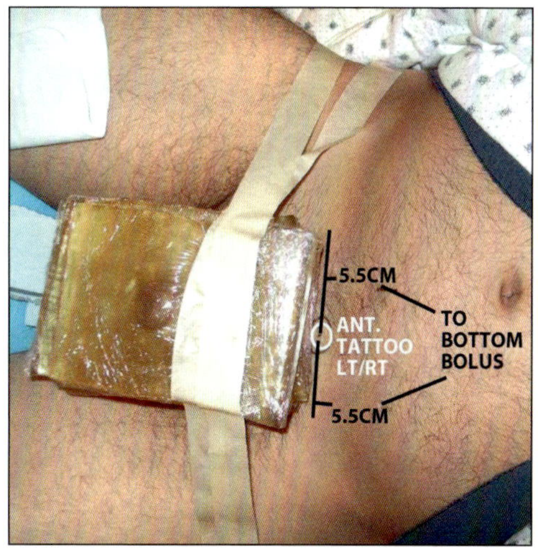

(Left) *Photo shows stacked bolus technique in the same patient. Holes, the diameter of the penis, are cut in the middle of layers of 1 cm bolus and stacked onto the penis. Note "clamshell" shield to protect testis.* ***(Right)*** *Top view of stacked bolus is seen in the same patient. Note detailed setup instructions to guide daily therapy. Swelling can occur during therapy, and the central hole in the bolus may need to be widened to accommodate the swelling.*

Tis N0 M0

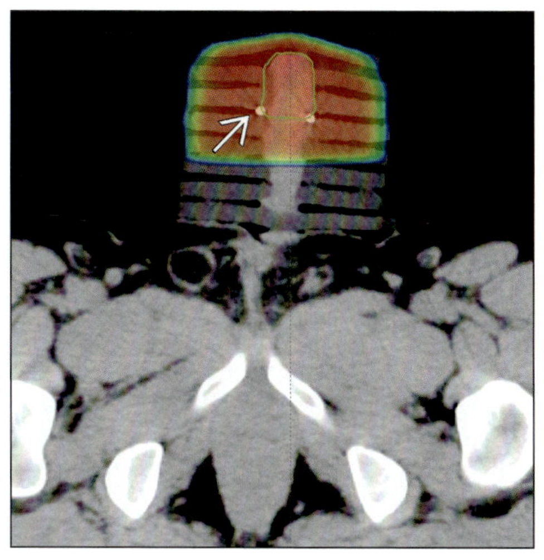

Tis N0 M0

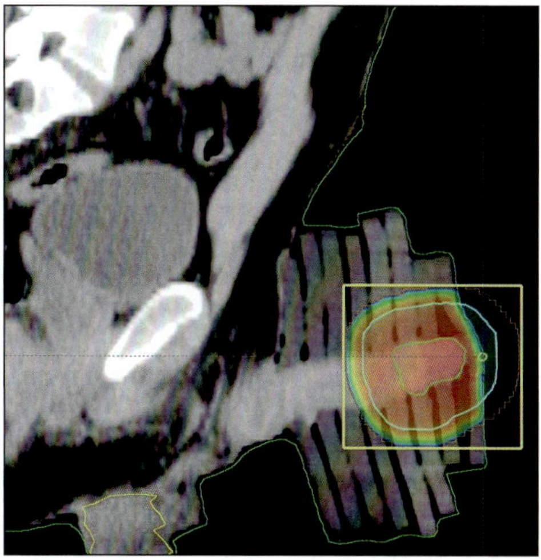

(Left) *Axial view in the same patient shows fiducial markers ➨ placed at the bolus level, marking the most proximal extent of the GTV. 60 Gy was prescribed with a 2 cm proximal margin. Note the dose homogeneity; however, air gaps may be a dosimetric concern.* ***(Right)*** *Sagittal view in the same patient shows that he was treated with daily kV cone-beam image guidance. A measurement from distal tip of the penis to fiducial on bolus was consistent to ensure coverage.*

PENIS

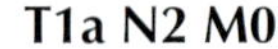

T1a N2 M0

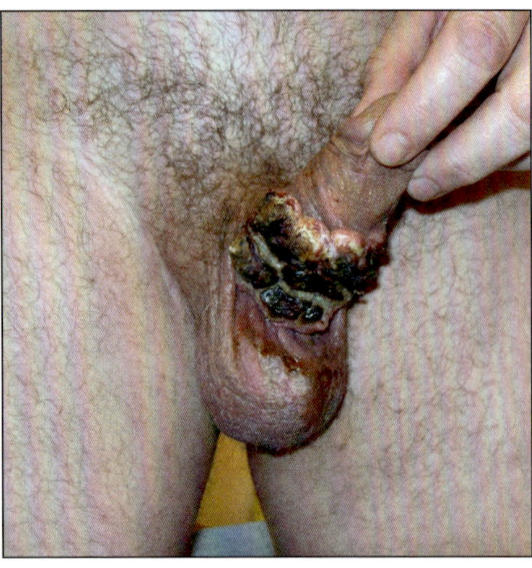

T1a N2 M0

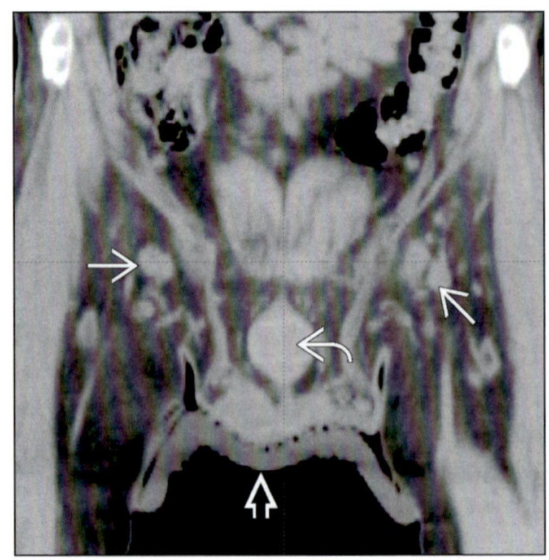

(Left) *Large exophytic squamous cell carcinoma is seen at the base of the penis extending onto the scrotum in a 49-year-old man. Lesion had a foul odor and was causing pain.* ***(Right)*** *Coronal planning CT image in same patient shows bilateral superficial and deep inguinal adenopathy. A 1 cm bolus is used to enhance dose buildup near skin surface. The proximal corpora of the patient appear normal at this cross section.*

T1a N2 M0

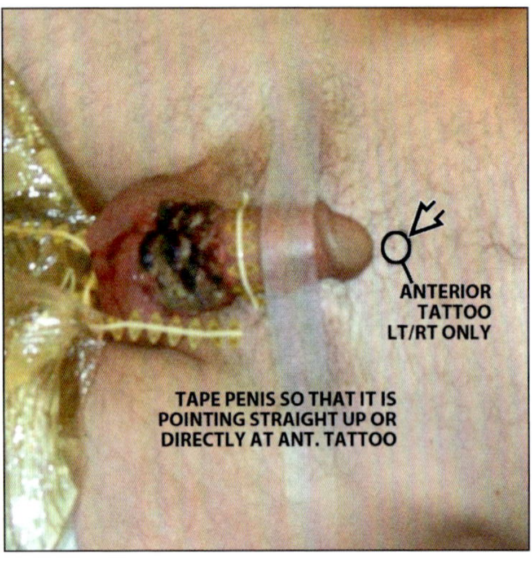

ANTERIOR
TATTOO
LT/RT ONLY
TAPE PENIS SO THAT IT IS
POINTING STRAIGHT UP OR
DIRECTLY AT ANT. TATTOO

T1a N2 M0

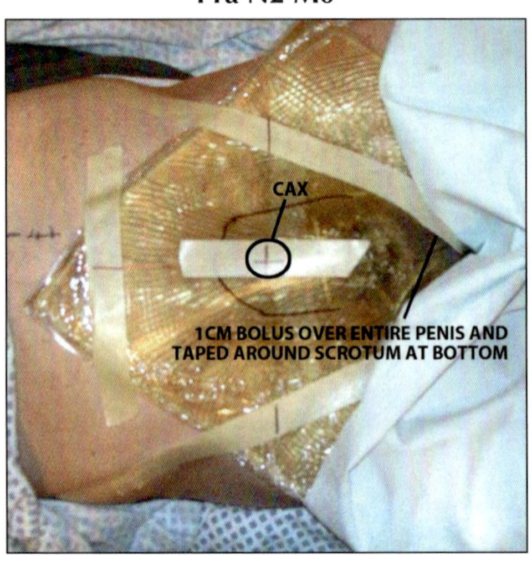

CAX
1CM BOLUS OVER ENTIRE PENIS AND
TAPED AROUND SCROTUM AT BOTTOM

(Left) *Photo in the same patient uses clear instructions to aid in reproducible setup of the penis. Note the use of wire to demarcate lesional borders. Tattoo on midline serves as an important landmark.* ***(Right)*** *Photo in the same patient shows completed setup. Note that a pyramid-shaped 1 cm bolus is used in this so-called "diaper" technique to achieve superficial dose buildup on the primary and inguinal regions.*

T1a N2 M0

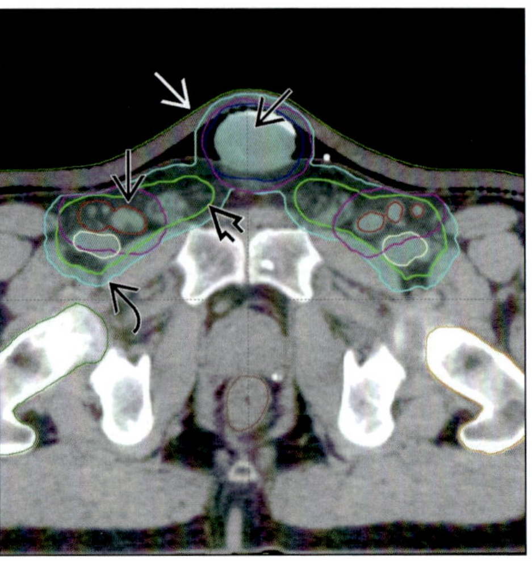

T1a N2 M0

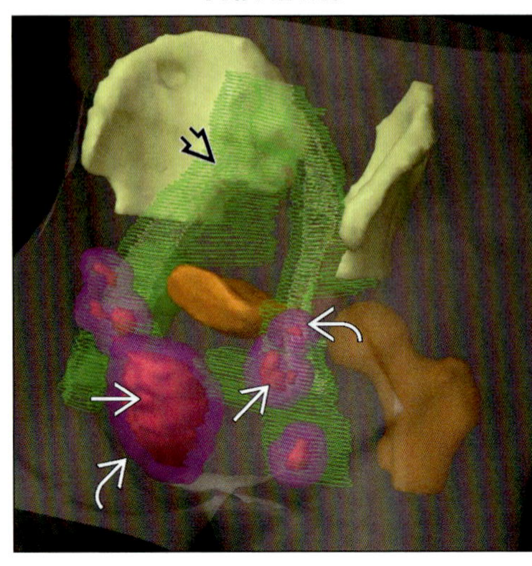

(Left) *Planning axial CT in the same patient demonstrates inguinal nodal contours: GTV, CTV, PTV, and 1 cm bolus "diaper".* ***(Right)*** *DRR in the same patient shows GTV, the boost PTV receiving 55.8 Gy, and the lower risk nodal CTV receiving 45 Gy. He elected definitive organ preserving combined CRT in order to prevent penectomy and inguinal dissection.*

T1a N2 M0

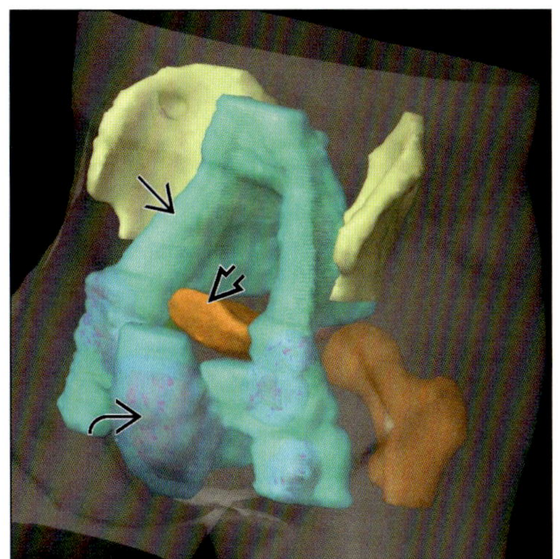

T1a N2 M0

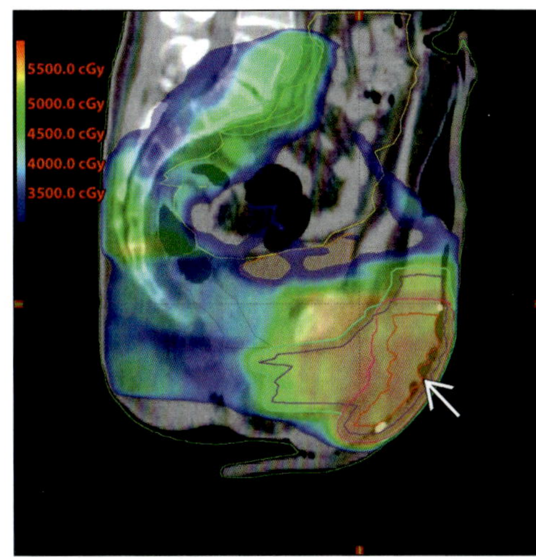

(Left) *DRR in the same patient shows the overall PTV design. Cyan contour → of at-risk nodal groups (superficial and deep inguinal and iliac) receive 45 Gy and maroon contours ↗ with gross disease receive 55.8 Gy. Bladder ➩ is also shown.* ***(Right)*** *Sagittal view of IMRT plan in the same patient shows relative sparing of bowel and bladder. The stippled appearance ➔ of the penile skin is the primary tumor under the bolus "diaper."*

T1a N2 M0

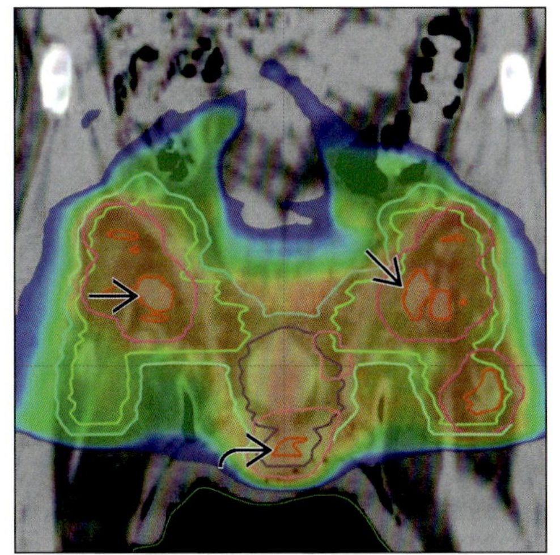

T1a N2 M0

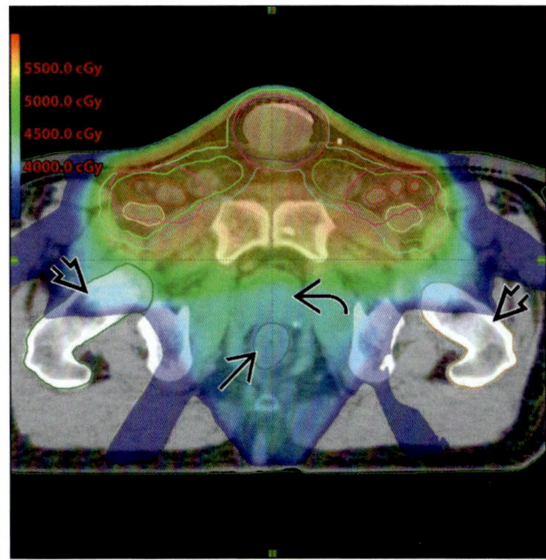

(Left) *Coronal view in the same patient shows IMRT dose distribution and dose painting of the grossly involved inguinal lymph nodes → and primary ↗ region.* ***(Right)*** *Axial view in the same patient shows excellent dose buildup with bolus "diaper" at the inguinal and skin surfaces. Note the relative sparing of the femoral necks ➩, prostate ↗, and rectum →. The patient was highly motivated to preserve his urinary and sexual function.*

T1a N2 M0

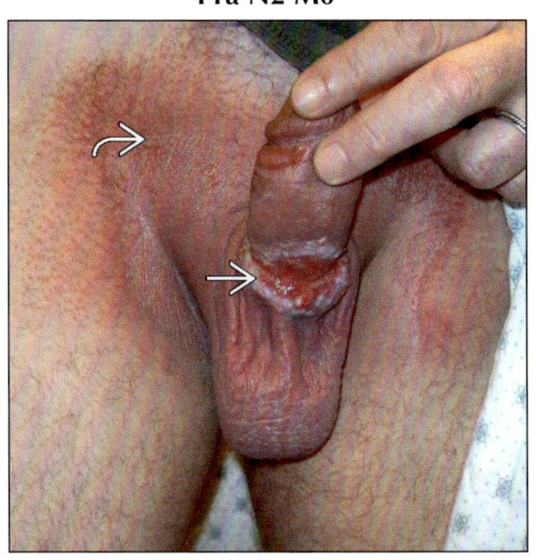

T1a N2 M0

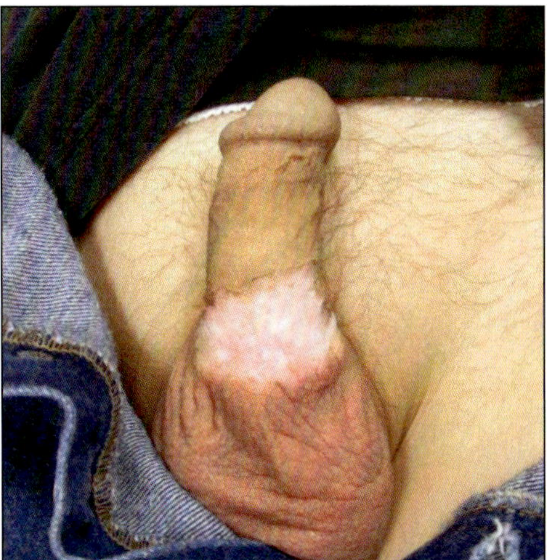

(Left) *Photo shows the same patient on his final treatment day after achieving 55.8 Gy to the primary lesion and inguinals. Brisk erythema is shown on the skin ↗. The tumor has completely regressed and left a crater →.* ***(Right)*** *Same patient 9 months after completing definitive CRT reports being pain free with excellent urologic and sexual function. Note the good cosmetic result with well-healed skin. At 2-year follow-up, he remained NED.*

URETHRA

(T) Primary Tumor

Adapted from 7th edition AJCC Staging Forms.

TNM	*Definitions*
TX	Primary tumor cannot be assessed
T0	No evidence of primary tumor
Ta	Noninvasive papillary, polypoid, or verrucous carcinoma
Tis	Carcinoma in situ
T1	Tumor invades subepithelial connective tissue
T2	Tumor invades any of the following: Corpus spongiosum, prostate, periurethral muscle
T3	Tumor invades any of the following: Corpus cavernosum, beyond prostatic capsule, anterior vagina, bladder neck
T4	Tumor invades other adjacent organs
Urothelial (Transitional Cell) Carcinoma of the Prostate	
Tis pu	Carcinoma in situ, involvement of prostatic urethra
Tis pd	Carcinoma in situ, involvement of prostatic ducts
T1	Tumor invades urethral subepithelial connective tissue
T2	Tumor invades any of the following: Prostatic stroma, corpus spongiosum, periurethral muscle
T3	Tumor invades any of the following: Corpus cavernosum, beyond prostatic capsule, bladder neck (extraprostatic extension)
T4	Tumor invades other adjacent organs (e.g., invasion of bladder)

(N) Regional Lymph Nodes

NX	Regional lymph nodes cannot be assessed
N0	No regional lymph node metastasis
N1	Metastasis in a single lymph node ≤ 2 cm in greatest dimension
N2	Metastasis in a single node > 2 cm in greatest dimension or in multiple nodes

(M) Distant Metastasis

M0	No distant metastasis
M1	Distant metastasis

(G) Histologic Grade

World Health Organization/International Society of Urologic Pathology (WHO/ISUP) Grading System	
LG	Low grade
HG	High grade
General Histologic Grading System	
GX	Grade cannot be assessed
G1	Well differentiated
G2	Moderately differentiated
G3	Poorly differentiated
G4	Undifferentiated

AJCC Stages/Prognostic Groups

Adapted from 7th edition AJCC Staging Forms.

Stage	*T*	*N*	*M*
0a	Ta	N0	M0
0is	Tis	N0	M0
	Tis pu	N0	M0
	Tis pd	N0	M0
I	T1	N0	M0
II	T2	N0	M0
III	T1	N1	M0
	T2	N1	M0
	T3	N0	M0
	T3	N1	M0
IV	T4	N0	M0
	T4	N1	M0
	Any T	N2	M0
	Any T	Any N	M1

Incidence of Primary Urethral Carcinoma

Histologic Subtype	*Incidence in Males*	*Incidence in Females*
Transitional cell carcinoma	70.2%	33.9%
Squamous cell carcinoma	18.4%	31.1%
Adenocarcinoma	11.4%	35.0%

Data from Swartz MA et al: Incidence of primary urethral carcinoma in the United States. Urology. 68(6):1164-8, 2006. Data were calculated from the U.S. SEER database, 1973-2002.

Observed and Overall 1- and 5-Year Survival Rates

Stage	*1-Year Survival*	*5-Year Survival*
0a	97%	79%
0is	93%	62%
I	90%	59%
II	82%	51%
III	79%	28%
IV	59%	22%

Data from American Joint Committee on Cancer: AJCC Cancer Staging Manual. 7th ed. New York: Springer, 2010.

T1 and T2: Female

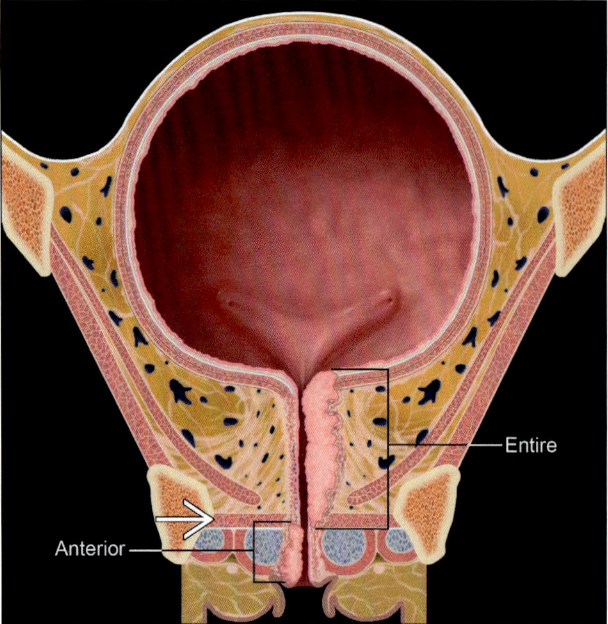

Coronal illustration through the bladder demonstrates primary urethral cancer. The distribution of disease is divided into anterior and entire urethra. Anterior urethral cancer is limited to the distal 1/3 of the urethra, external to the urogenital diaphragm ➡. Entire urethral cancer is usually high grade and locally advanced.

T3 and T4: Female

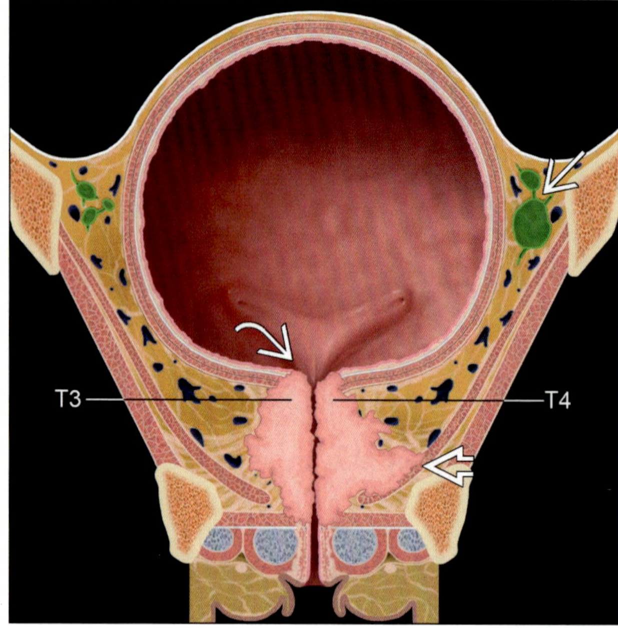

Coronal illustration through the bladder shows T3 disease on the left. This extends into the periurethral soft tissues and may involve the bladder neck ➡. T4 disease, shown on the right, involves the entire urethra and periurethral muscles ➡. N1 disease is illustrated by the enlarged regional lymph node ➡, which measures < 2 cm.

Tis and T1: Male

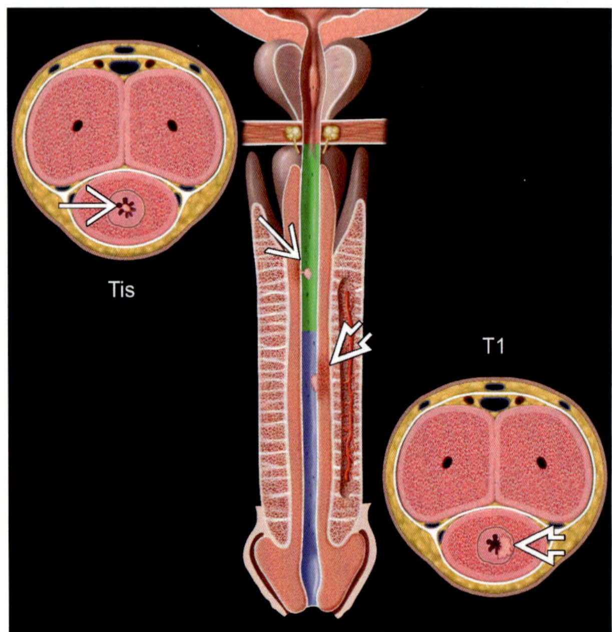

Primary urethral cancer in a male is divided into anterior (penile urethra in blue) and posterior (bulbomembranous urethra in green) distributions. On the left, Tis disease ➡ is papillary and localized, without submucosal invasion. On the right, T1 disease ➡ extends into the submucosal layer.

T2 and T3: Male

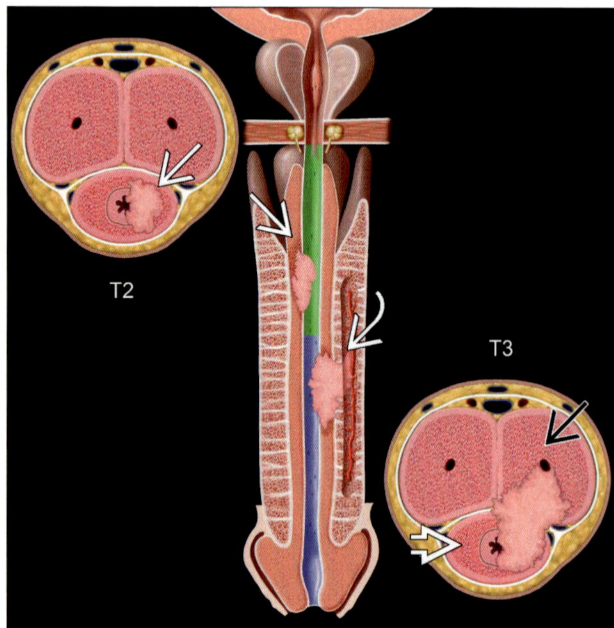

On the left, T2 disease extends into the corpus spongiosum ➡. On the right, T3 disease ➡ extends beyond the corpus spongiosum ➡ into the corpus cavernosum ➡. If prostatic urethra is involved, the etiology is more often prostatic or bladder cancer extending into prostatic urethra.

N1

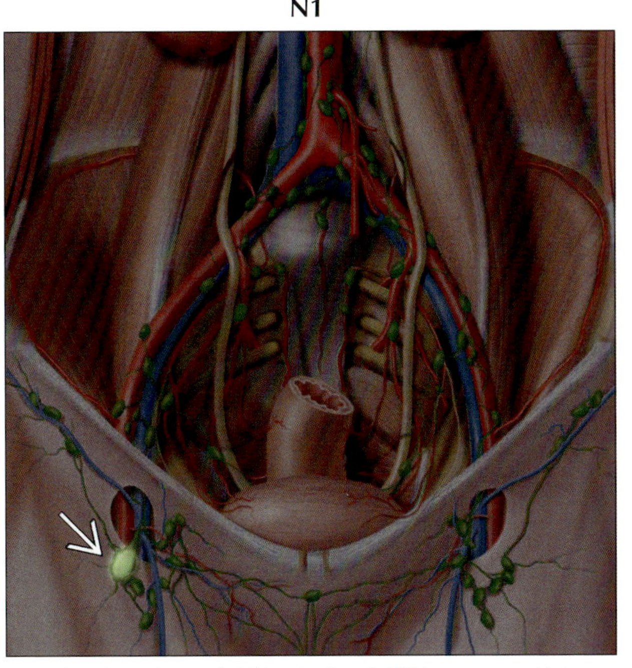

A single enlarged superficial inguinal node ➔ is present, which measures ≤ 2 cm. The presence of N1 disease upgrades disease severity to stage III.

N2

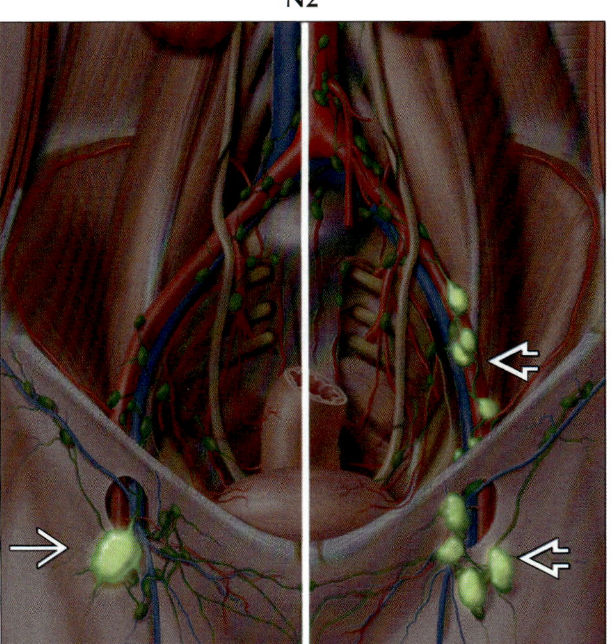

On the left, a single enlarged superficial inguinal node ➔ measures > 2 cm. On the right, multiple nodes and multiple nodal stations are involved ⇨. These are both examples of N2 disease. The presence of N2 disease upgrades disease severity to stage IV.

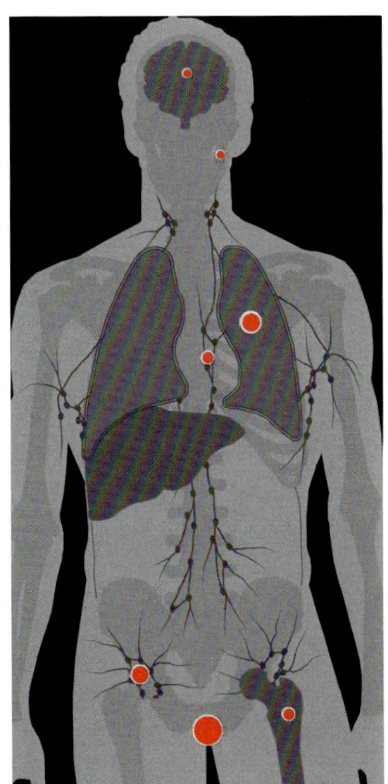

INITIAL SITE OF RECURRENCE

Local	43%
Lung	20%
Inguinal Lymph Nodes	11%
Bone	6%
Brain	2%
Parotid	2%

Data from a report of 46 male cases. Dalbagni G et al: Male urethral carcinoma: analysis of treatment outcome. Urology. 53(6):1126-32, 1999. In a report on 44 female cases, the local, distant, and local and distant recurrence rates were 18%, 9%, and 34%, respectively. Grigsby PW: Carcinoma of the urethra in women. Int J Radiat Oncol Biol Phys. 41(3):535-41, 1998.

URETHRA

OVERVIEW

Classification

- Women: Location is **anterior** or **entire** urethra
  - Anterior tumors exclusively in distal 1/3 of urethra
    - 46% of urethral tumors
    - Squamous cell carcinoma (SCCa) most common
  - Entire urethral tumors usually high grade and locally advanced
- Men: Location is **posterior** or **anterior** urethra
  - Posterior: Prostatic urethra (10%), bulbomembranous urethra (60%)
  - Anterior: Penile urethra (30%)

NATURAL HISTORY

General Features

- Comments
  - Prognosis depends on location, depth of invasion, size, histology, and nodal spread
    - Adenocarcinoma (AC) is an adverse prognostic

Etiology

- Urethral stricture
  - Present in 1/2 of patients with primary urethral carcinoma
- History of sexually transmitted diseases: 1/4 of patients
  - ~ 60% of female patients are HPV(+) (most commonly HPV 16)
- History of bladder cancer
- Chronic urinary tract infections
- Age > 60 years

Epidemiology & Cancer Incidence

- Uncommon; < 1% of all urothelial malignancies
  - Associated with poor outcomes
- Age-adjusted incidence rate: 4.3 cases per 1,000,000 in men and 1.5 cases per 1,000,000 in women
- Usually occurs after 50 years of age
- 2x as common in African-Americans

Microscopic Pathology

- H&E
  - Most common: Transitional cell carcinoma (TCC) 55%, SCCa 22%, and AC 16%
    - In males
      - TCC most common in prostatic urethra
      - SCCa more common in bulbomembranous and penile urethra
      - Undifferentiated subtype associated with bulbomembranous urethra
      - AC from glands of Littré or Cowper
    - In females
      - AC > TCC > SCCa
      - Clear cell AC most common subtype in urethral diverticulum
      - Uncommon tumors include undifferentiated, sarcoma, melanoma, and metastases

Routes of Spread

- Local spread
  - Women: Bladder neck, vagina, vulva
  - Men: Via vascular spaces of corpus spongiosum and periurethral tissues
    - Anterior tumors spread to skin surface
    - Posterior/bulbomembranous tumors spread to perineum
- Lymphatic metastases to regional nodes
  - Anterior urethral cancer nodal distribution
    - Superficial and deep inguinal nodes
    - Occasionally external iliac nodes
  - Posterior urethral cancer nodal distribution
    - Pelvic nodes
  - Palpable inguinal nodes occur in 20%
    - Usually indicative of metastatic disease
  - Female cancer often spreads systemically without regional nodal disease
- Hematogenous spread uncommon, except in
  - TCC of prostatic urethra
  - Advanced local disease

IMAGING

Detection

- **Primary evaluation: Examination under anesthesia**
  - Cystoscopy
  - Bimanual examination
    - External genitalia, urethra, rectum, perineum
    - Flexible sigmoidoscopy if rectal involvement suspected
  - Transurethral or needle biopsy
- **Retrograde cystourethrography**
  - Standard imaging technique for morphologic and functional urethral evaluation
  - Tumor may be incidental finding during evaluation of stricture disease
    - Infiltrating lesions associated with tight stenoses
    - Often difficult or impossible to opacify urethral lumen above lesion
- **Voiding cystourethrogram**
  - Urethral strictures or filling defects
- **MR**
  - Best for depicting local extent of disease
- **Ultrasound**
  - Transperineal, transvaginal, or transrectal
    - Endourethral US with catheter-based transducer
  - Hypo- to isoechoic
  - Irregularly marginated urethral mass

Staging

- **CECT**
  - Limited utility for local disease
    - Difficult to differentiate urethra from vagina/ bladder base
    - May appear as homogeneously or heterogeneously enhancing mass
  - Local soft tissue extension
  - Pelvic lymph node involvement
  - Extension into adjacent bony structures
- **MR**
  - T1WI
    - Low signal intensity mass, difficult to differentiate from urethra
  - T2WI
    - Urethral wall: Signal intensity similar to muscle
    - Urethral cancer
      - Relatively high signal intensity mass disrupting female urethral "target-like" zonal anatomy

- High signal intensity mass invading corpora cavernosa
- T1WI C+
  - Variable enhancement

CLINICAL PRESENTATION & WORK-UP

Presentation

- Urethral bleeding, serosanguineous discharge
- Palpable urethral mass
- Obstructive voiding symptoms
- Urethral fistula, periurethral abscess
- Perineal pain

Prognosis

- Female
  - Anterior urethral cancer
    - Better prognosis
  - Entire urethral cancer
    - Prospects for cure low unless lesions small
      - If < 2 cm, 5-year survival (60%)
      - If > 4 cm, 5-year survival (13%)
- Male
  - Anterior urethral cancer
    - High potential for cure with superficial disease
  - Posterior urethral cancer
    - Low prospects for cure; high local recurrence rates
    - 5-year survival from 15-20%

TREATMENT

Major Treatment Alternatives

- Surgical treatment
  - Options depend on location and extent of disease
  - In men, no demonstrated benefit from prophylactic inguinal lymph node dissection
- Radiation therapy
  - Definitive, adjuvant, neoadjuvant, or chemoradiation therapy (CRT), depending on stage
- Chemotherapy: In clinical trials for metastatic urethral cancer
  - Urethral TCC may respond similarly as bladder TCC

Treatment Options by Stage

- Female: Anterior urethral cancer
  - Stages 0/Tis, Ta: Open excision or electroresection and fulguration or laser vaporization-coagulation, or RT in select cases
  - Stages T1 and T2: EBRT or interstitial radiation or combination or surgical resection of distal 1/3 of urethra
  - T3/recurrent lesions
    - Definitive RT, consider intensity-modulated radiation therapy (IMRT), and consider concurrent chemotherapy
    - Anterior exenteration and urinary diversion ± preoperative radiation and urinary diversion
  - Palpable inguinal nodes: Frozen section tumor confirmation, then ipsilateral node dissection
- Female: Entire urethral cancer
  - Definitive RT, consider IMRT, and consider concurrent chemo (generally EBRT and interstitial implant preferred)
  - Preoperative RT, anterior exenteration and urinary diversion with bilateral pelvic node dissection ± inguinal node dissection
- Male: Anterior urethral cancer
  - Stages 0/Tis, Ta: Open excision or electroresection and fulguration or laser vaporization-coagulation or RT in select cases
  - T1, T2, T3
    - Partial penectomy, negative margins to 2 cm proximal to tumor
    - Penectomy refused
      - Radiation
  - Palpable inguinal nodes: Frozen section tumor confirmation, then ipsilateral node dissection
- Male: Posterior urethral cancer
  - Definitive RT, consider IMRT, and consider concurrent chemo
  - Preoperative RT, cystoprostatectomy, urinary diversion, and penectomy with bilateral pelvic node dissection ± inguinal node dissection

Standard Doses

- 60-66 Gy in definitive cases to gross disease
- 50 Gy to resected nodes
- 50-60 Gy for close margins

Organs at Risk Parameters

- Rectum D2cc < 70 Gy
- Bladder D2cc < 85 Gy

Common Techniques

- 3D conformal or IMRT
- Interstitial boost is well suited for female urethra

RECOMMENDED FOLLOW-UP

Clinical

- Exam every 3-6 months for 1st 2-3 years, q. 6 months for years 4-5, then annually thereafter

Radiographic

- Case and stage dependent

SELECTED REFERENCES

1. American Joint Committee on Cancer: AJCC Cancer Staging Manual. 7th ed. New York: Springer. 507-13, 2010
2. Gillitzer R et al: Single-institution experience with primary tumours of the male urethra. BJU Int. 101(8):964-8, 2008
3. Liedberg F et al: Prospective study of transitional cell carcinoma in the prostatic urethra and prostate in the cystoprostatectomy specimen. Incidence, characteristics and preoperative detection. Scand J Urol Nephrol. 41(4):290-6, 2007
4. Swartz MA et al: Incidence of primary urethral carcinoma in the United States. Urology. 68(6):1164-8, 2006
5. Kawashima A et al: Imaging of urethral disease: a pictorial review. Radiographics. 24 Suppl 1:S195-216, 2004

*(**Left**) Coronal PET/CT demonstrates minimally increased activity in the urethra, corresponding to known site of disease. No discrete lesion was identified on imaging, nor were additional sites of disease identified. (**Right**) Sagittal T2WI FS MR in a male patient demonstrates a low T2 SI expansile ureteral mass in the bulbous portion of the urethra. It involves the corpus spongiosum, but the corpus cavernosum is spared. (Courtesy M. Lockhart, MD, MPH.)*

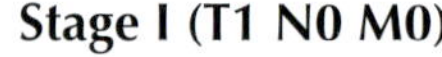

Stage I (T1 N0 M0)

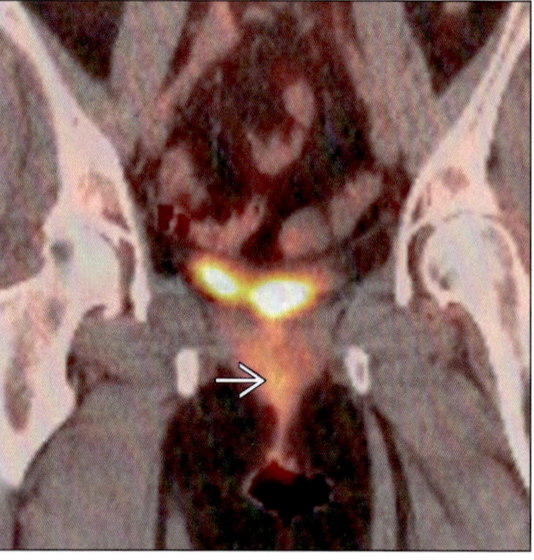

Stage II (T2 N0 M0)

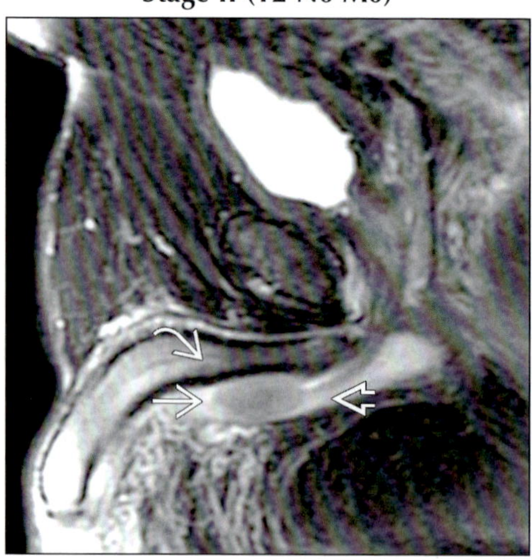

*(**Left**) DRR shows CTV, PTV, and bladder in an elderly male with a poor performance status and multiple unresected, noninvasive, high-grade transitional cell papillomas (Ta). He was not a surgical candidate but was treated for local control (30 Gy/10 fractions) and had a good response. (**Right**) Photo of the same patient uses clear instructions to aid in reproducible setup of the penile and membranous urethra.*

Stage 0a (Ta N0 M0)

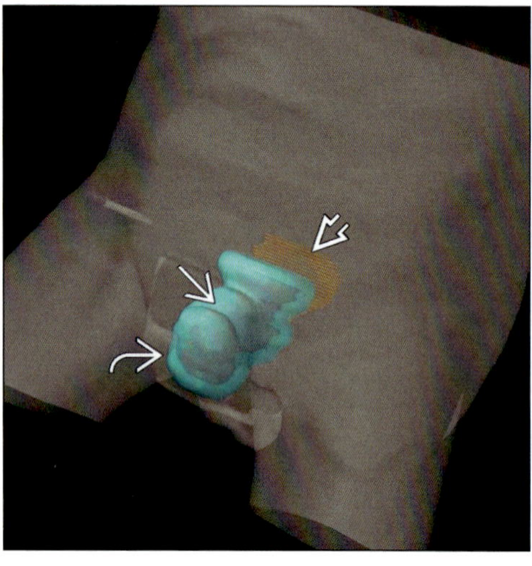

Stage 0a (Ta N0 M0)

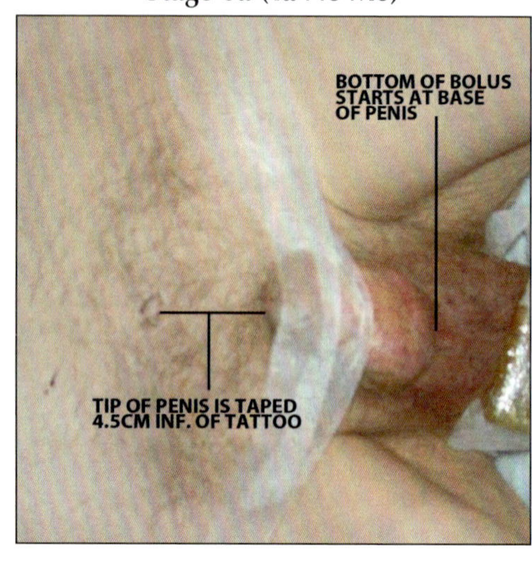
BOTTOM OF BOLUS STARTS AT BASE OF PENIS
TIP OF PENIS IS TAPED 4.5CM INF. OF TATTOO

*(**Left**) Axial CT shows CTV in orange and PTV in blue. Note the presences of bolus to allow full dose buildup. He was treated with a 3-field technique: Anterior, right anterior oblique (RAO), and left posterior oblique (LPO). Red, blue, and yellow indicate the 100%, 90%, and 50% isodose lines, respectively. (**Right**) Sagittal CT in the same patient shows the CTV coming up to the base of the bladder to ensure complete coverage.*

Stage 0a (Ta N0 M0)

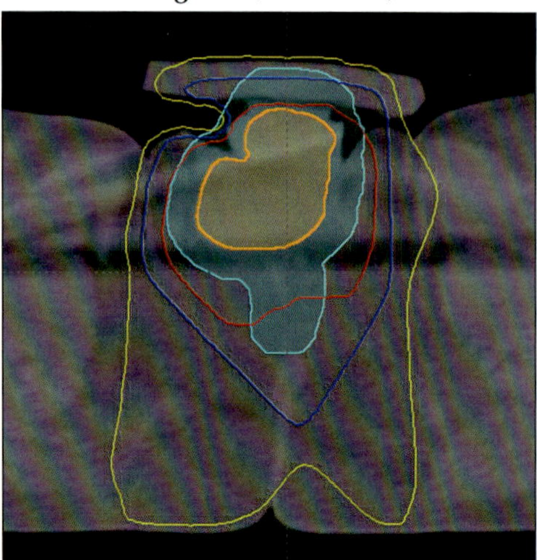

Stage 0a (Ta N0 M0)

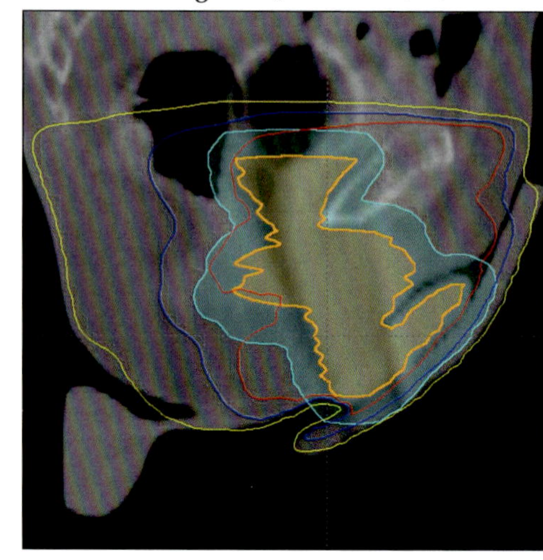

Stage III (T3 N0 M0)

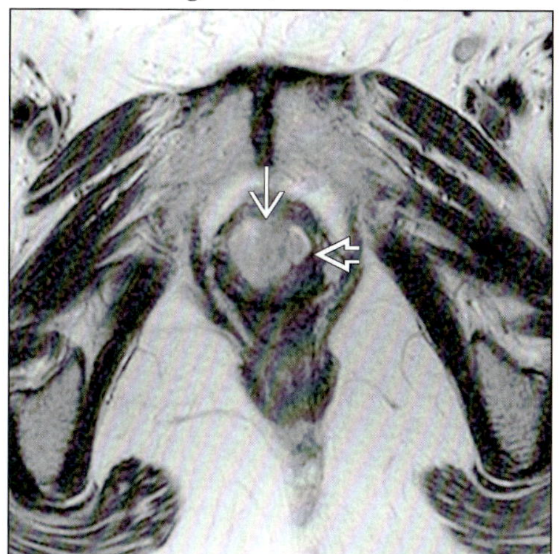

Stage III (T3 N0 M0)

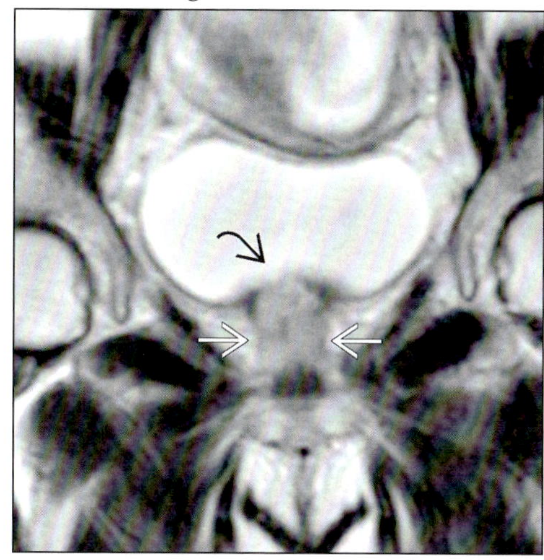

(Left) *On axial T2WI MR, an intermediate signal intensity urethral mass ➡ expands the urethra. The low T2 SI urethral muscular wall ➡ remains intact.* ***(Right)*** *Coronal image shows that the entire urethra is expanded by the mass ➡. Superior extension of the mass into the bladder neck ➡ upstages this to T3 disease.*

Stage IV (T2 N1 M0)

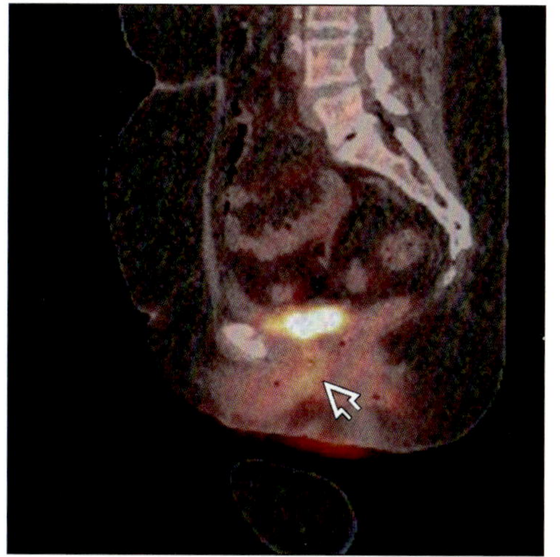

Stage IV (T2 N1 M0)

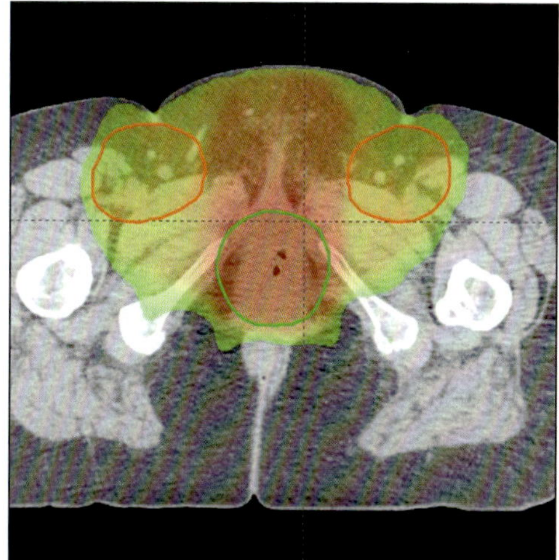

(Left) *Sagittal fused PET/CT shows postoperative activity at the urethra ➡. It is unclear if residual tumor remains. Pathologically, the tumor was completely resected with a 1 mm margin. PET/CT showed lymphadenopathy in a single left external lymph node.* ***(Right)*** *Axial CT in same patient shows a 7-field IMRT plan. The primary was treated to 55 Gy in 30 fractions whereas the inguinal and iliac nodes received 37.5 Gy and 45 Gy, respectively, in 25 fractions.*

Stage IV (T2 N1 M0)

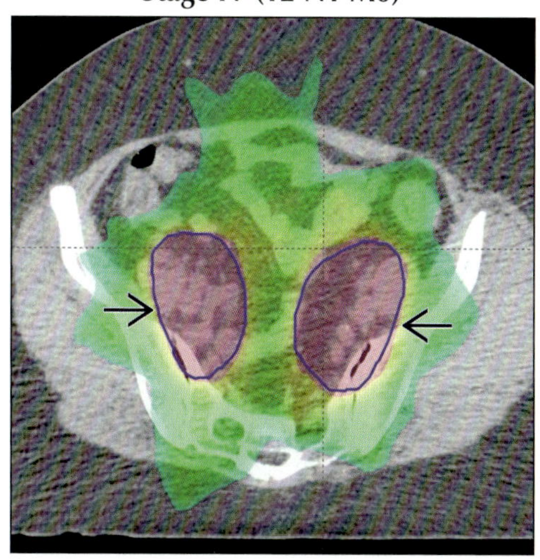

Stage IV (T2 N1 M0)

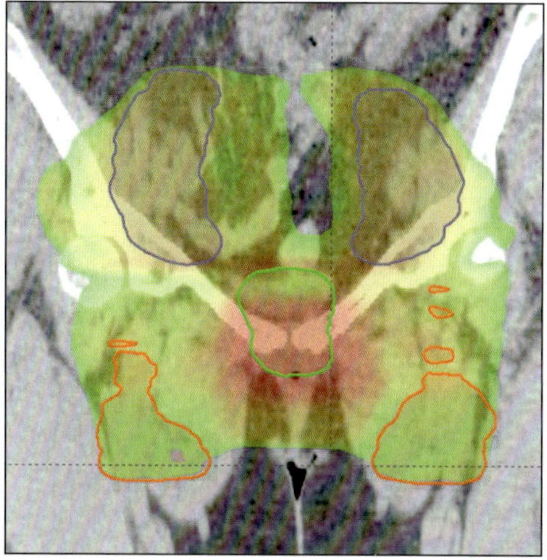

(Left) *IMRT in the same patient demonstrates high conformality to the iliac lymph nodes ➡ while sparing dose to small bowel. The yellow and green show 90% and 50% of the dose, respectively.* ***(Right)*** *Coronal CT in the same patient shows coverage of iliac, inguinal, and primary PTVs. Patient remains disease free 4 years later.*

Stage IV (T2 N0 M1)

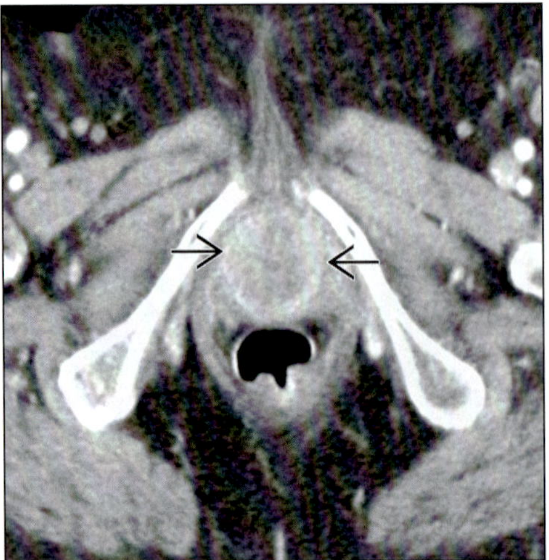

Stage IV (T2 N0 M1)

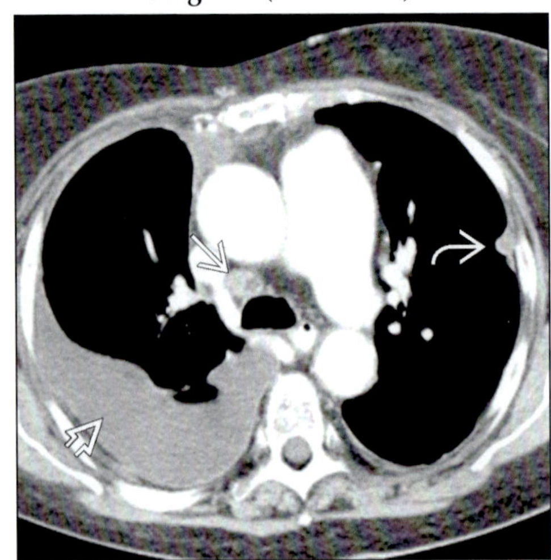

(Left) *Axial CECT shows a heterogeneously enhancing urethral mass ➔; however, the integrity of periurethral tissue planes cannot be determined. Indeed, CT is of limited utility in assessing urethral T stage.* ***(Right)*** *Thoracic CECT in the same patient demonstrates an enlarged enhancing precarinal node ➔, a left pleural nodule ➔, and a right pleural effusion ➔. The extensive thoracic metastatic disease is best demonstrated on CT.*

Stage II (T2 N0 M0)

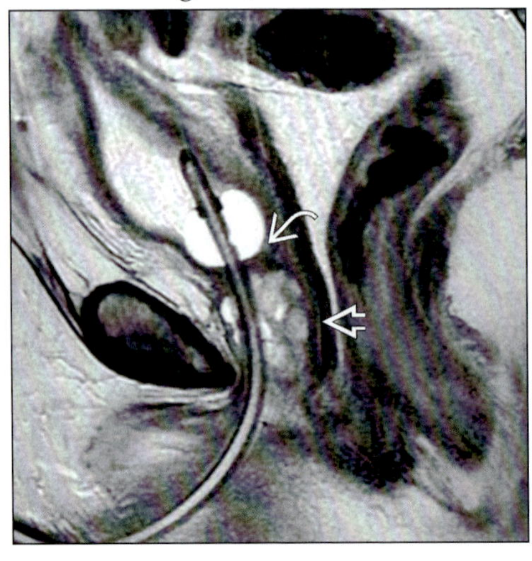

Periurethral Recurrence

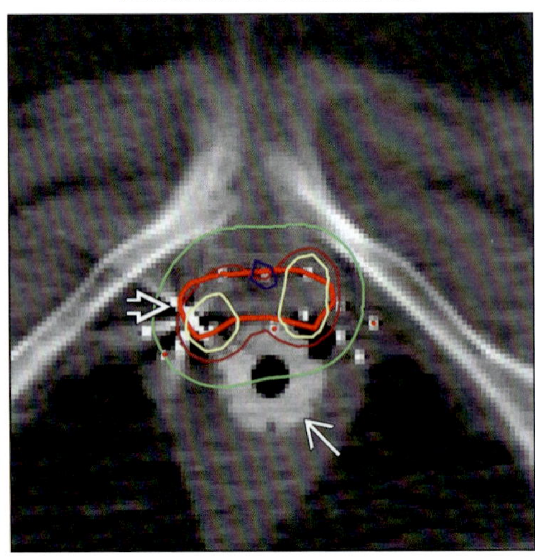

(Left) *Sagittal image in the same patient shows the mass's confinement to the urethral tissues with sparing of the bladder base ➔ and anterior vagina ➔.* ***(Right)*** *Axial CT shows an HDR interstitial implant for a periurethral recurrence from endometrial cancer. Dark red line is CTV, while thin yellow, red, and green lines indicate 150%, 100%, and 50% isodose lines, respectively. Vaginal obturator ➔ and marker seed ➔ are evident. Note rapid dose fall-off with brachytherapy.*

Postoperative Appearance

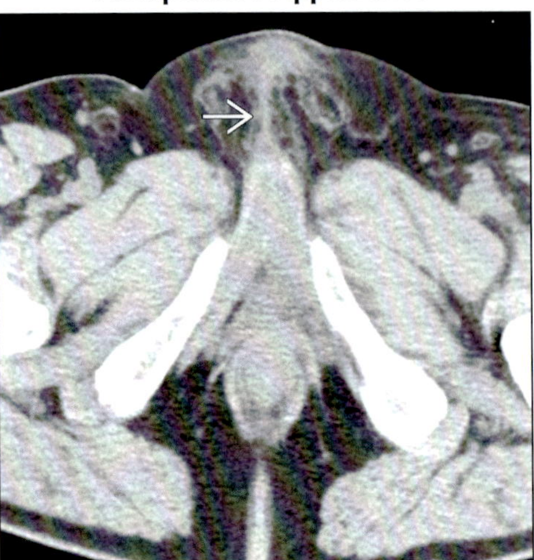

Postoperative Recurrence

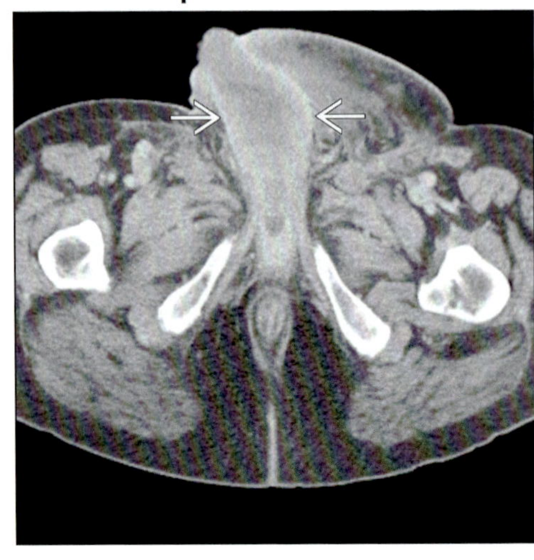

(Left) *Axial CECT shows the postoperative appearance of a partial penectomy ➔ for anterior stage II disease. At this time, no local recurrence is present. Long-term survival has been reported in subjects who undergo this therapy.* ***(Right)*** *Axial NECT in a different patient demonstrates a local recurrence ➔ after partial penectomy. Recurrence developed along the bulbomembranous urethra.*

Stage IV (T4 N0 M0)

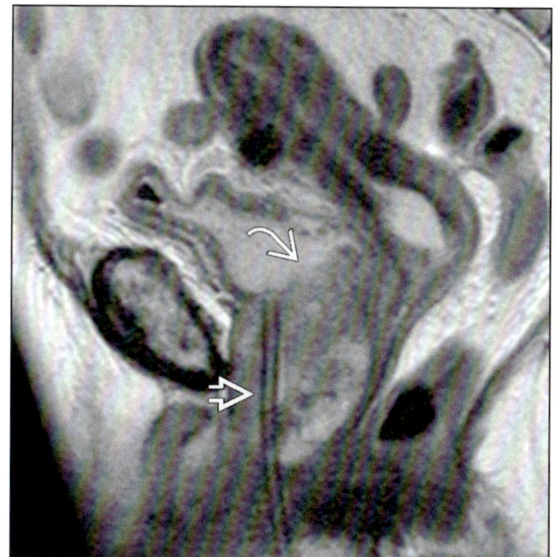

Stage IV (T4 N0 M0)

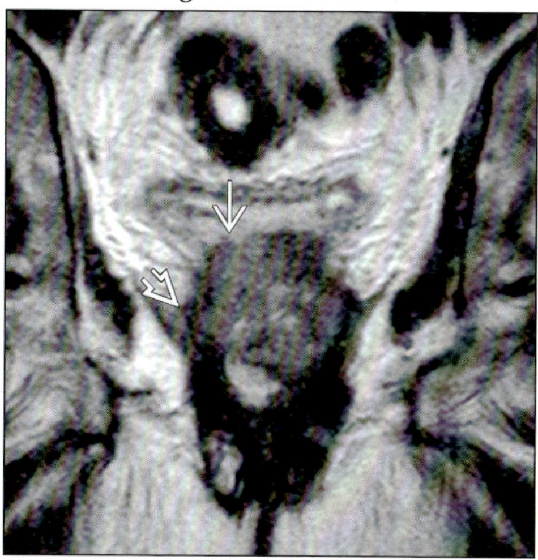

(Left) *Sagittal T2WI MR in the same patient better demonstrates the heterogeneous low T2 SI mass involving the entire urethra and extending cranially to invade the bladder base ➡. A Foley catheter ➡ is present.* ***(Right)*** *Coronal T2WI MR in the same patient demonstrates infiltration beyond the periurethral tissue into the adjacent levator ani muscle complex on the right ➡. Additionally, the mass is seen invading the bladder base ➡.*

Metastatic Disease

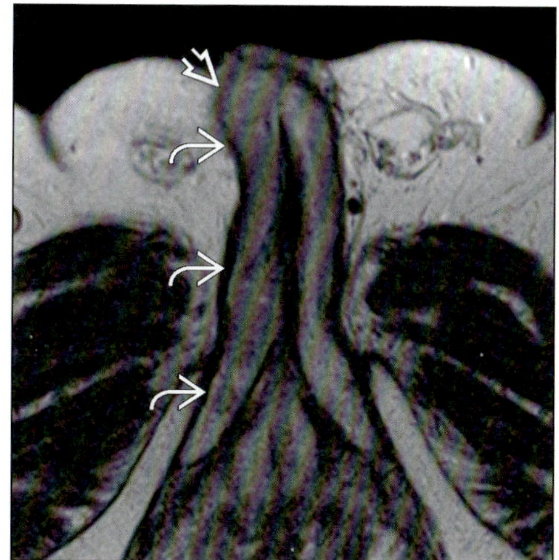

Metastatic Disease

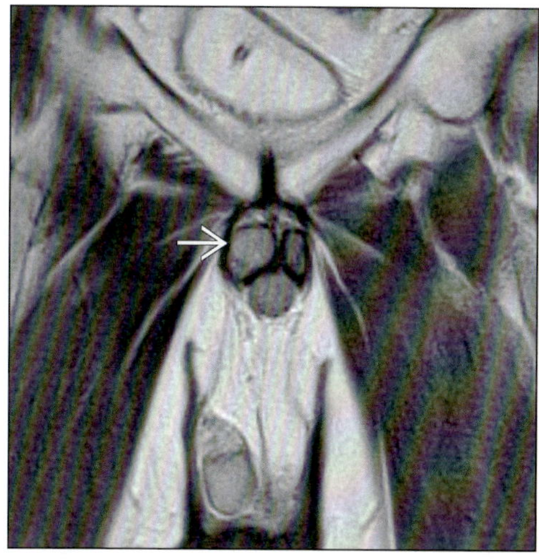

(Left) *Axial T2 MR shows extensive involvement of the right corpus cavernosum ➡ in a 78-year-old man. The urethra was mostly spared. This was biopsy-proven prostate cancer extending down the penile shaft and involving the skin ➡.* ***(Right)*** *Coronal T2WI MR shows expansion of the right corpus cavernosum ➡ compared to the left.*

Metastatic Disease

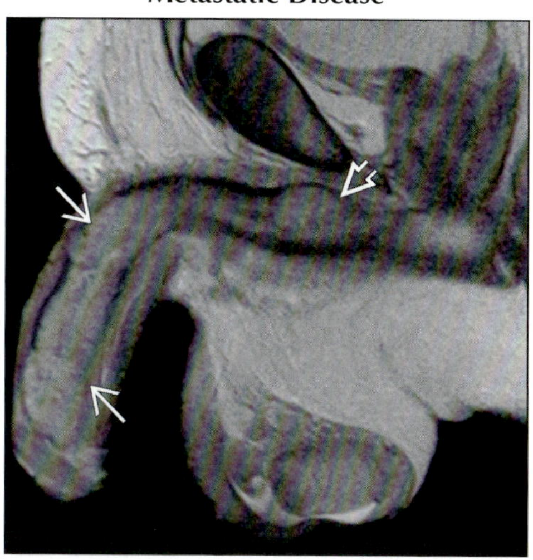

Metastatic Disease

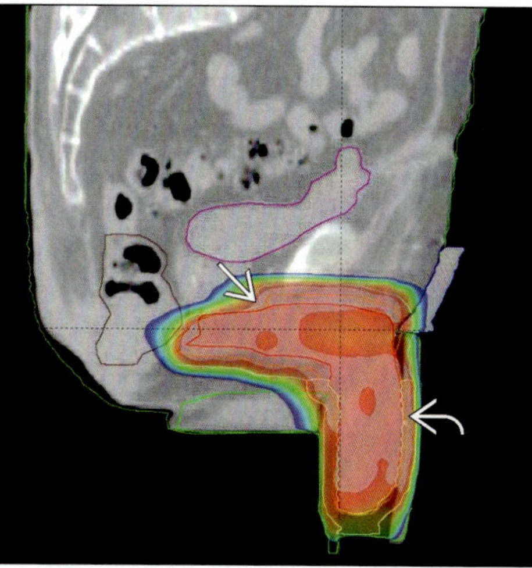

(Left) *Sagittal T2WI MR shows disease involving the proximal ➡ and distal ➡ aspect of the corpus cavernosum.* ***(Right)*** *Sagittal CT shows 7-field IMRT treatment colorwash. The CTV ➡ and PTV ➡ are shown. The presence of bolus is essential in this case to allow full skin dose. The patient had a brisk skin reaction acutely, and also a good palliative response 1 year later.*

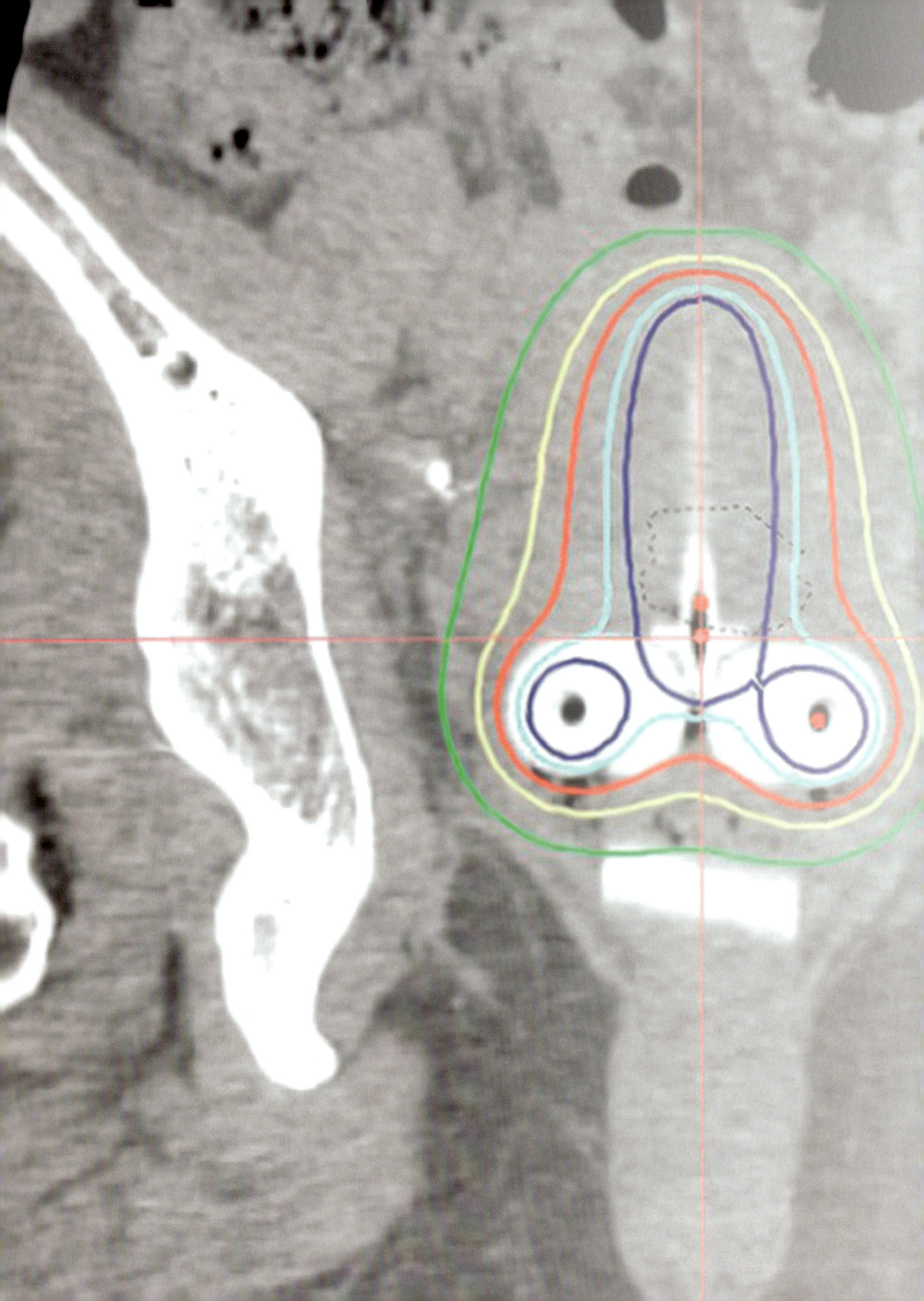

SECTION 7
Gynecology

CERVIX

(T) Primary Tumor

Adapted from 7th edition AJCC Staging Forms.

TNM	*FIGO*	*Definitions*
TX		Primary tumor cannot be assessed
T0		No evidence of primary tumor
Tis[1]		Carcinoma in situ (preinvasive carcinoma)
T1	I	Cervical carcinoma confined to uterus (extension to corpus should be disregarded)
T1a[2]	IA	Invasive carcinoma diagnosed only by microscopy; stromal invasion with a maximum depth of 5.0 mm measured from the base of the epithelium and a horizontal spread of ≤ 7.0 mm; vascular space involvement, venous or lymphatic, does not affect classification
T1a1	IA1	Measured stromal invasion ≤ 3.0 mm in depth and ≤ 7.0 mm in horizontal spread
T1a2	IA2	Measured stromal invasion > 3.0 mm and ≤ 5.0 mm with a horizontal spread ≤ 7.0 mm
T1b	IB	Clinically visible lesion confined to the cervix or microscopic lesions > T1a/IA2
T1b1	IB1	Clinically visible lesion ≤ 4.0 cm in greatest dimension
T1b2	IB2	Clinically visible lesion > 4.0 cm in greatest dimension
T2	II	Cervical carcinoma invades beyond uterus but not to pelvic wall or to lower 1/3 of vagina
T2a	IIA	Tumor without parametrial invasion
T2a1	IIA1	Clinically visible lesion ≤ 4.0 cm in greatest dimension
T2a2	IIA2	Clinically visible lesion > 4.0 cm in greatest dimension
T2b	IIB	Tumor with parametrial invasion
T3	III	Tumor extends to pelvic wall &/or involves lower 1/3 of vagina &/or causes hydronephrosis or nonfunctioning kidney
T3a	IIIA	Tumor involves lower 1/3 of vagina, no extension to pelvic wall
T3b	IIIB	Tumor extends to pelvic wall &/or causes hydronephrosis or nonfunctioning kidney
T4	IVA	Tumor invades mucosa of bladder or rectum &/or extends beyond true pelvis (bullous edema is not sufficient to classify a tumor as T4)

(N) Regional Lymph Nodes

NX		Regional lymph nodes cannot be assessed
N0		No regional lymph node metastasis
N1	IIIB	Regional lymph node metastasis

(M) Distant Metastasis

M0		No distant metastasis
M1	IVB	Distant metastasis (including peritoneal spread, involvement of supraclavicular, mediastinal, or paraaortic lymph nodes, lung, liver, or bone)

[1]*FIGO no longer includes stage 0 (Tis).*

[2]*All macroscopically visible lesions, even with superficial invasion, are T1b/IB.*

AJCC Stages/Prognostic Groups

Adapted from 7th edition AJCC Staging Forms.

Stage	*T*	*N*	*M*
0	Tis	N0	M0
I	T1	N0	M0
IA	T1a	N0	M0
IA1	T1a1	N0	M0
IA2	T1a2	N0	M0
IB	T1b	N0	M0
IB1	T1b1	N0	M0
IB2	T1b2	N0	M0
II	T2	N0	M0
IIA	T2a	N0	M0
IIA1	T2a1	N0	M0
IIA2	T2a2	N0	M0
IIB	T2b	N0	M0
III	T3	N0	M0
IIIA	T3a	N0	M0
IIIB	T3b	Any N	M0
	T1-3	N1	M0
IVA	T4	Any N	M0
IVB	Any T	Any N	M1

Tis

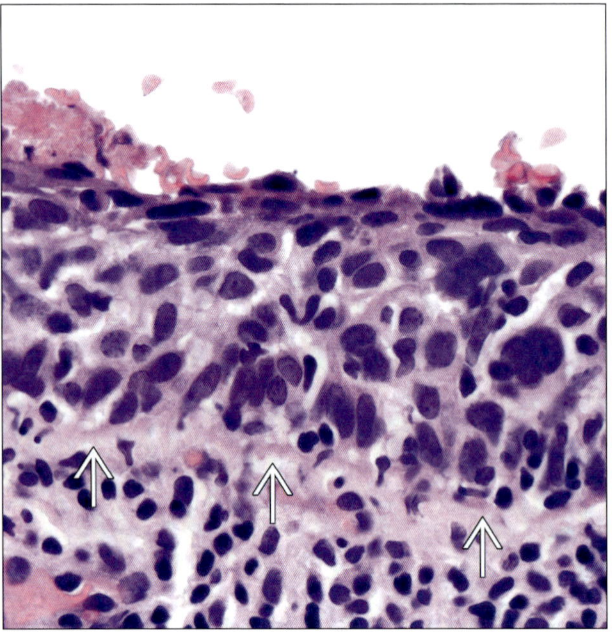

H&E stain shows a high-grade squamous intraepithelial lesion. Cells have hyperchromatic nuclei, lack maturation, lack normal organization, and show indistinct cell membranes. Neoplastic cells are limited by the intact eosinophilic basement membrane ➡, leading to the term "preinvasive carcinoma."

Methods for Microscopic Measurement of Depth of Invasion

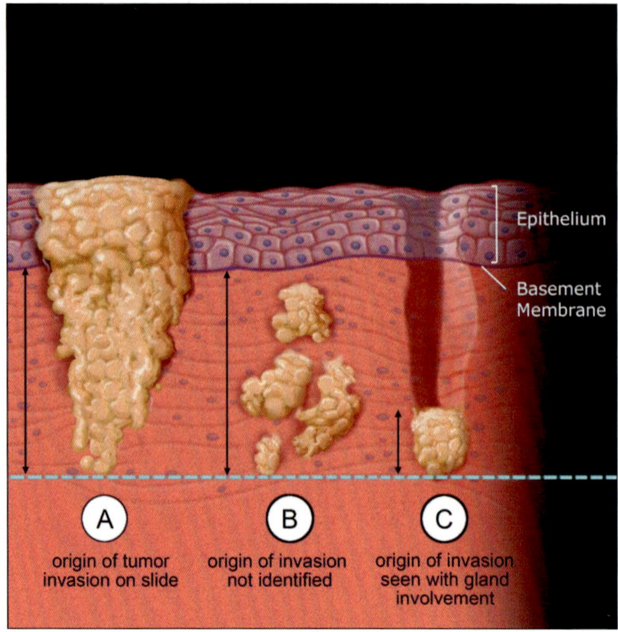

A: Depth of invasion is measured from origin of invasion/basement membrane to the last cell of invasion focus. B: Invasion is measured from basement membrane to the last cell of invasion focus. C: In case no visible basement membrane, invasion is measured from site of origin to the last cell of invasion focus.

IA1

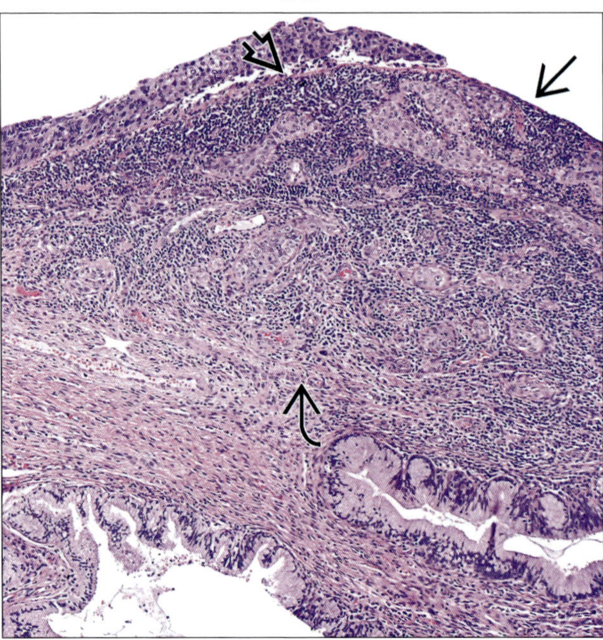

Low-power H&E of cervix shows loss of squamous epithelium on the right ➡ with underlying moderately differentiated carcinoma characterized by irregular nests of squamous cells invading the stroma. Nests ➡ extend to 1.5 mm from the basement membrane ➡. Since depth of invasion is < 3.0 mm, it is an IA1 lesion.

IB1

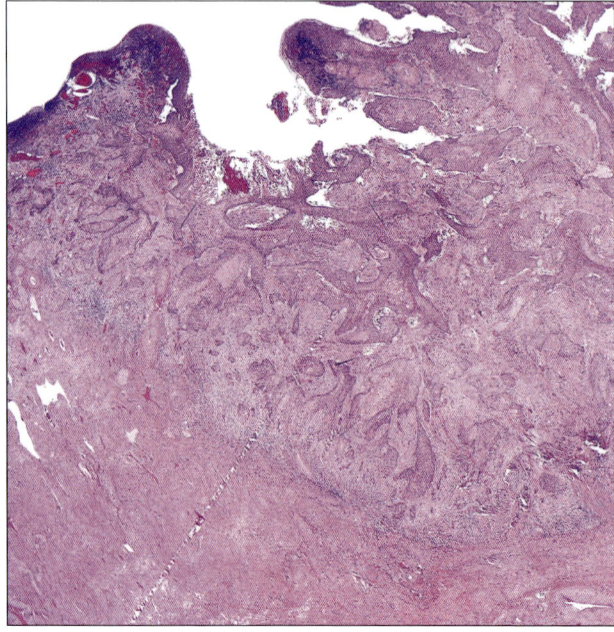

H&E stain shows invasive squamous cell carcinoma with a microscopic depth of invasion of 6 mm. Clinically, this lesion was visible, which also makes it stage IB1. The tumor was confined to the cervix and < 4 cm in greatest dimension.

IA1

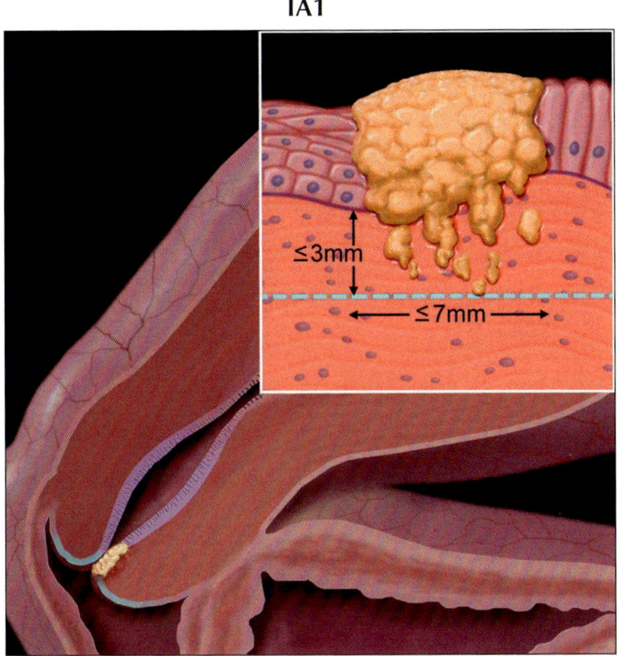

Stage IA1 cervical carcinoma is defined as microscopic tumor with stromal invasion of ≤ 3 mm in depth and ≤ 7 mm in horizontal spread. Stage IA2 is invasion > 3 mm and ≤ 5 mm in depth and ≤ 7 mm in horizontal spread.

IB1

Stage IB1 cervical carcinoma is a microscopic tumor with stromal invasion > 5 mm in depth (inset A) or > 7 mm in horizontal spread (inset B), or a clinical visible lesion confined to the cervix ≤ 4 cm in size.

IB2

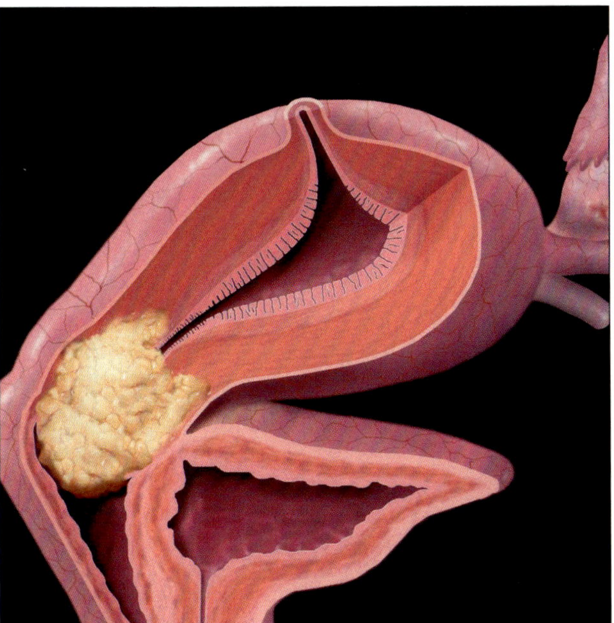

Stage IB2 cervical carcinoma is a clinically visible lesion > 4 cm in size confined to the cervix. Tumor may be exophytic extending into the vaginal vault (barrel-shaped lesion); however, there is no invasion of adjacent structures.

IIA1 and IIA2

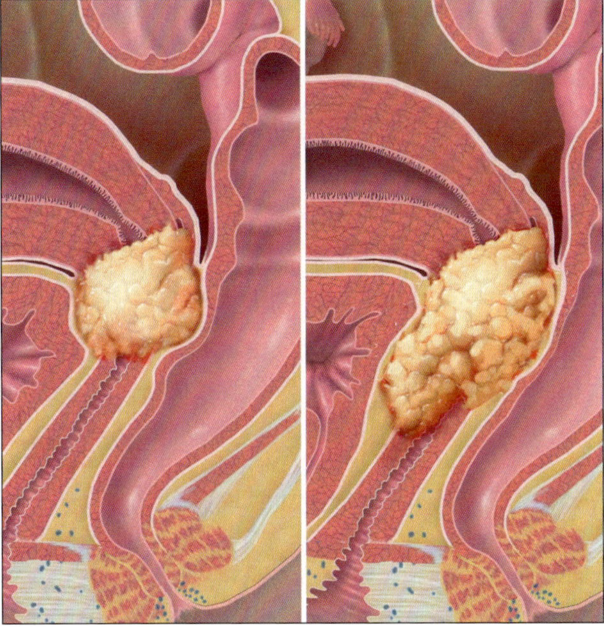

Stages IIA1 and IIA2 tumors extend beyond the cervix to invade the upper 2/3 of the vagina. Graphics are sagittal views of the pelvis showing tumor invading the upper vagina. Left graphic depicts stage IIA1 with tumor ≤ 4 cm in size. Right graphic depicts stage with IIA2 tumor > 4 cm in size.

CERVIX

IIB

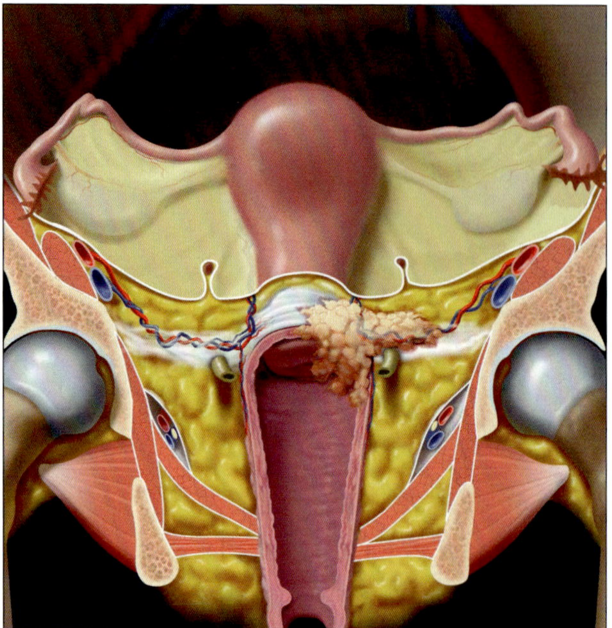

Stage IIB tumor extends beyond the cervix to invade the parametrium. Graphic is a view in the coronal plane depicting tumor invading the parametrium including fat, uterine ligaments, and paracervical vessels. There is encasement of the ureter; however, no hydronephrosis is present.

IIIA

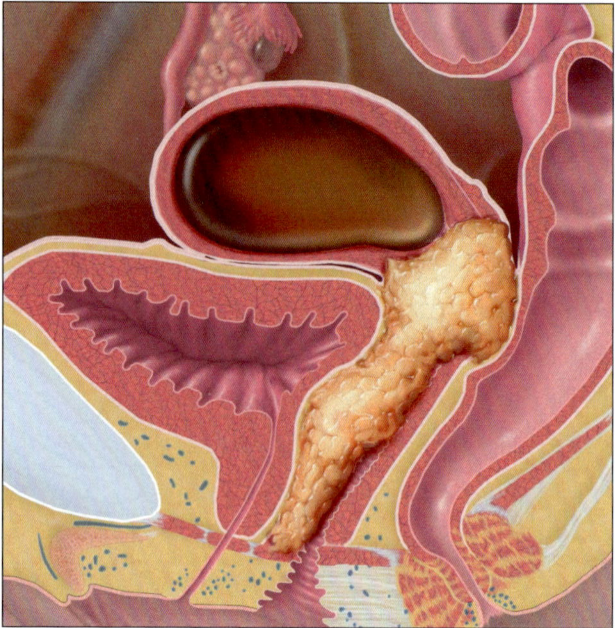

Stage IIIA tumor is an uncommon presentation and invades the lower 1/3 of the vagina. Graphic is a sagittal view of the pelvis showing tumor invading the lower vagina.

IIIB

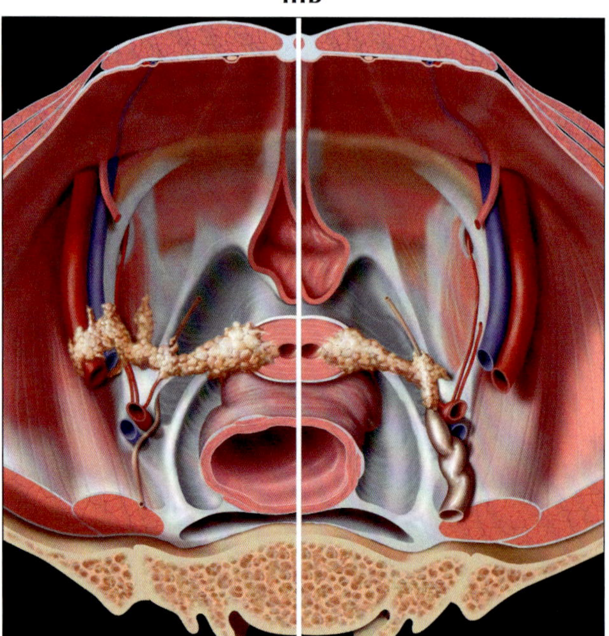

Stage IIIB tumor extends to the pelvic sidewall or causes hydronephrosis. Graphics are looking into the pelvis from above. Left graphic depicts tumor extending to the pelvic sidewall to encase the iliac vessels and invade the musculature. Right graphic depicts tumor invading the ureter, resulting in hydronephrosis.

IIIB

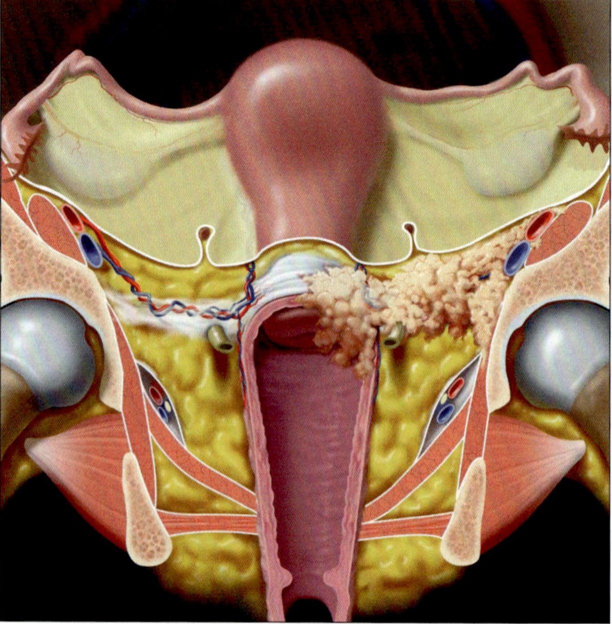

Stage IIIB tumor extends to the pelvic sidewall or causes hydronephrosis. Graphic is a view in the coronal plane showing tumor extending to the pelvic sidewall to encase the external iliac vessels and invade the musculature. Tumor invades the ureter, causing hydronephrosis (not shown).

IVA

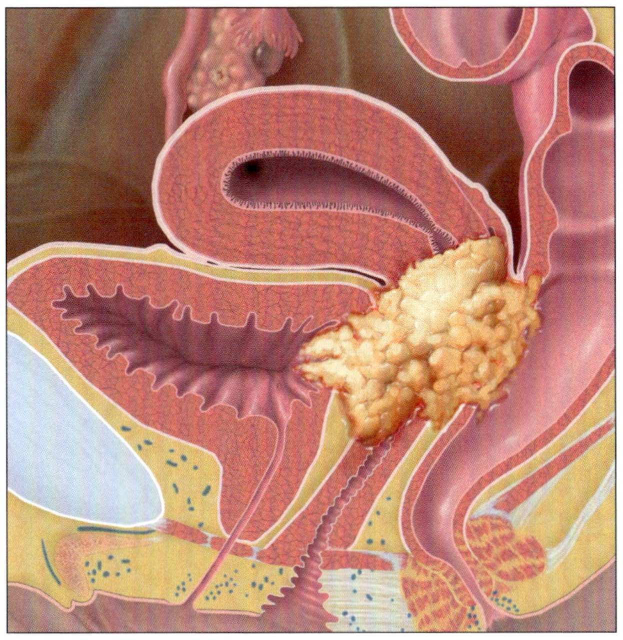

Stage IVA tumor invades the urinary bladder or rectal mucosa. Graphic is a sagittal view of the pelvis showing tumor invading the urinary bladder mucosa anteriorly and the rectal mucosa posteriorly.

N1

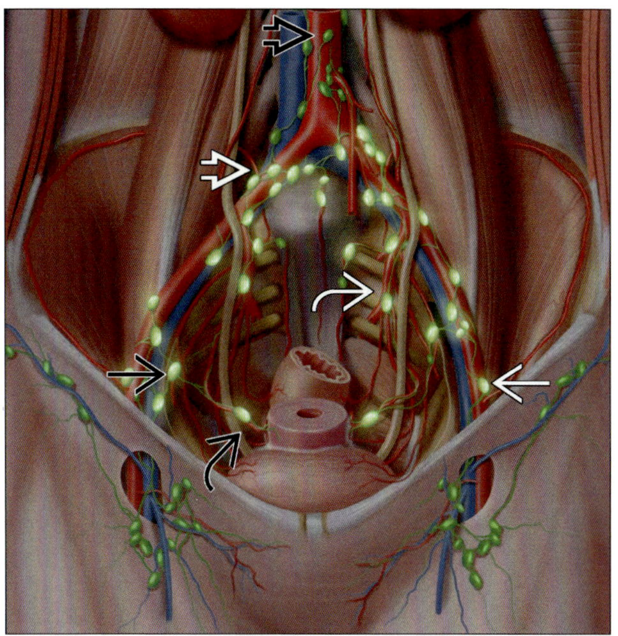

Frontal view of the female pelvis and low abdomen depicts lymph node chains. Regional lymph nodes in cervical carcinoma are highlighted and include parametrial, obturator, internal iliac, external iliac, common iliac, and presacral lymph nodes. Paraaortic lymph nodes are considered distant spread, yet some patients are curable with paraaortic disease.

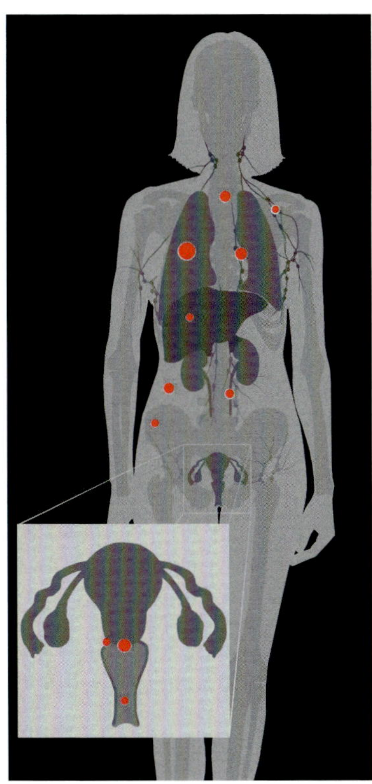

INITIAL SITE OF RECURRENCE	
Lung	21%
Paraaortic Lymph Nodes	11%
Cervix	9%
Abdominal Cavity	8%
Ureter	7%
Supraclavicular Nodes	7%
Spine	7%
Liver	4%
Parametria	3%
Pelvic Wall	3%
Vagina	2%

Pelvic recurrence data obtained from 160 recurrences in 526 patients (Van Nagell et al: Cancer 44(6):2354-61, 1979). Distant recurrence data obtained from 322 mets observed in 1,211 patients (Fagundes et al: IJROBP 24:197-204, 1992).

CERVIX

OVERVIEW

General Comments

- 2nd most common cause of cancer and 3rd most common cause of cancer death in women worldwide
- 80-85% are squamous cell carcinoma

Classification

- Histopathologic types
  - Squamous cell carcinoma in situ
  - Squamous cell carcinoma
    - Invasive
    - Keratinizing
    - Nonkeratinizing
    - Verrucous
  - Adenocarcinoma in situ
  - Invasive adenocarcinoma
  - Endometrioid adenocarcinoma
  - Clear cell adenocarcinoma
  - Adenosquamous carcinoma
  - Adenoid cystic carcinoma
  - Adenoid basal cell carcinoma
  - Small cell carcinoma
  - Neuroendocrine
  - Undifferentiated carcinoma

NATURAL HISTORY

General Features

- Comments
  - Cervical cancer originates at squamocolumnar junction (SCJ)
    - SCJ is originally located in ectocervix (intravaginal)
    - SCJ moves to endocervix with advancing age
    - Cancer arises in transformation zone between old and new SCJ
  - Migration of SCJ accounts for age-related change in tumor growth pattern
    - Young women: Exophytic growth
    - Older women: More commonly endophytic growth
  - Adenocarcinoma and small cell cervical cancer
    - Aggressive histologic subtypes with less favorable survival rates
  - Adenoma malignum
    - Subtype of adenocarcinoma (3%)
    - Arises from columnar epithelium of endocervical canal
    - Composed of well-differentiated endocervical glands
    - History of copious watery discharge
    - Prognosis is poor
      - Early peritoneal metastases
      - Poor response to chemoradiation therapy
    - Associated with Peutz-Jeghers syndrome
  - Clear cell adenocarcinoma
    - Rare histologic subtype of adenocarcinoma
    - Associated with in utero diethylstilbestrol (DES) exposure

Etiology

- Risk factors
  - High-risk strains of human papilloma virus (HPV); 15 high-risk serotypes; 70% of cases are due to HPV 16 or 18
  - 27% of women in USA ages 14-59 years are positive for at least 1 strain of HPV
  - 15.2% are positive for 1 or more high-risk strains
  - Sexual activity at early age
  - Multiple sexual partners
  - Sexually transmitted disease
  - Multiparity
  - Low socioeconomic status
  - Cigarette smoking
  - Immunosuppression/HIV infection
  - Long-term use of oral contraceptives
  - In utero DES exposure
    - Clear cell adenocarcinoma
  - Women with advanced HIV/AIDS have poor prognosis, often rapidly progressive cancer
- Protective factors
  - Barrier contraception

Epidemiology & Cancer Incidence

- Number of cases in USA per year
  - 2nd most common cancer worldwide
  - 12,170 estimated new cases in 2012 and 4,220 estimated deaths
  - Very high incidence in Central and South America, sub-Saharan Africa, and southeast Asia
- 3rd most common gynecologic malignancy following endometrial and ovarian cancer
- Decreased incidence since introduction and widespread use of Papanicolaou smear

Associated Diseases, Abnormalities

- Peutz-Jeghers patients (multiple polyps due to *STK* gene mutation) have a higher incidence

Gross Pathology & Surgical Features

- Gross appearance
  - Poorly circumscribed granular or eroded appearance
  - Nodular, ulcerated lesion or exophytic mass
  - Diffuse enlargement and hardening of cervix
    - Endophytic infiltrative lesion in cervical canal
  - Barrel-shaped cervix
    - Diffusely enlarged, bulky, and > 6 cm
    - Most common with adenocarcinoma

Microscopic Pathology

- H&E
  - Large cell keratinizing squamous cell carcinoma
    - Sheets & nests of malignant squamous cells invade stroma
    - Abundant cytoplasm
    - Large pleomorphic nuclei & inconspicuous nucleoli
    - Keratin pearls & intercellular bridges
    - Occasional mitotic figures
    - Infiltrative growth pattern
  - Large cell nonkeratinizing squamous cell carcinoma
    - Large cells of similar size and shape
    - Moderate cytoplasm
    - May have individual cell keratinization
    - Keratin pearls are absent
    - Prominent nucleoli
    - Mitotic figures are common
    - Invasive edge is smooth

- Histologic grade
  - Degree of differentiation of tumor cells
  - Based on amount of keratin, degree of nuclear atypia, mitotic activity
  - Correlates with frequency of pelvic nodal metastasis
  - Grade 1: Well differentiated
    - Abundant intercellular bridging
    - Cytoplasmic keratinization
    - Keratin pearls
    - Cells are uniform with minimal nuclear pleomorphism
    - Mitotic rate is < 2 mitotic figures per high-power field
  - Grade 2: Moderately differentiated
    - Individual cell keratinization
    - Moderate nuclear pleomorphism
    - Mitotic rate is ≤ 4 mitotic figures per high-power field
  - Grade 3: Poorly differentiated
    - Minimal evidence of squamous differentiation
    - Cells are immature with marked nuclear pleomorphism and scant cytoplasm
    - Mitotic rate is > 4 mitotic figures per high-power field

Routes of Spread

- Local spread
  - Most common mode of spread
  - Caudally to invade
    - Vagina
  - Anteriorly to invade
    - Vesicouterine ligament
    - Urinary bladder
  - Laterally to invade
    - Cardinal ligaments
    - Parametria
      - Fat, vessels, ureters, lymphatics
    - Pelvic sidewall in advanced disease
      - Iliac vessels, pelvic musculature, ilium
  - Posteriorly to invade
    - Uterosacral ligaments
    - Rectum
- Lymphatic extension
  - Significant prognostic indicator
  - ↑ incidence with advancing stage of disease
  - Correlates with ↓ disease-free survival
  - ↑ incidence of recurrence and ~ 50% decrease in survival at each stage with lymph node invasion
  - Lymphatic drainage of cervix
    - Parametrial → obturator → internal/external iliac → common iliac → paraaortic → left supraclavicular fossa
      - Contiguous nodal involvement is common
  - 3 pathways of lymphatic drainage of cervix
    - Lateral route
      - Parallels external iliac vessels
      - Tumor drains 1st to medial external iliac chain, then to middle and lateral chains
      - Deep inguinal lymph nodes drain via lateral route from low vaginal extension
    - Hypogastric route
      - Parallels internal iliac vessels
      - Lymph nodes along internal iliac branches drain to junctional lymph nodes
      - Junctional lymph nodes lie between internal and external iliac vessels
    - Presacral route
      - Along uterosacral ligament
      - Uterosacral ligament → lymphatic plexus anterior to sacrum
  - All 3 routes of lymphatic drainage of cervix drain to common iliac chains
  - Common iliac chains drain to paraaortic lymph nodes
  - Depth of invasion of cervix and adjacent structures and tumor size affect nodal involvement
    - Parametrial and pelvic sidewall invasion
      - Drainage by external iliac lymph nodes
    - Invasion of lower 1/3 of vagina
      - Inguinal lymph node metastases
    - Rectal wall invasion
      - Drainage by inferior mesenteric lymph nodes
- **Peritoneal seeding**
  - Peritoneal metastasis varies from 5-27% in autopsy series
  - Mesenteric or omental metastases are uncommon
  - "Sister Joseph" nodule: 25% due to gyn malignancies, and uncommonly from cervix cancer
    - Umbilical metastasis
    - Direct extension of tumor from anterior peritoneal surface
- Hematogenous spread
  - Liver is most common abdominal organ with metastases
  - Adrenal gland is 2nd most common metastatic site in abdomen
  - Pulmonary metastases are relatively common in autopsy series (33-38%)
    - May be present for significant period of time; however, may remain asymptomatic
    - 1/3 will have mediastinal or hilar adenopathy
    - Lymphangitic carcinomatosis occurs in < 5%

IMAGING

Detection

- **Ultrasound**
  - Inadequate for diagnosis, staging, and surveillance for recurrence
  - Technically limited by body habitus, low signal-to-noise ratio, and lack of tissue characterization
  - Very helpful for uterine tandem placement
  - Transrectal US can identify parametrial invasion
- **CT**
  - Accuracy for staging is 32-80% in various studies
  - Mean sensitivity for parametrial invasion is 64% from literature
  - Mean specificity for parametrial invasion is 81% from literature
  - CT can demonstrate
    - Pelvic sidewall extension
    - Ureteral obstruction
    - Advanced bladder and rectal invasion
    - Adenopathy
    - Extrapelvic spread of disease

- May see distension of uterine cavity with fluid/blood if tumor obstructs endocervical canal
- CT can guide lymph node biopsy and radiation planning
- CT has moderate-high sensitivity and specificity for detection of recurrent tumor
  - Soft tissue mass with variable degrees of necrosis
  - Cystic mass with minimal soft tissue
- Limitations of CT
  - Limited visualization of primary tumor
    - Hypodense or isodense to normal cervical stroma
    - Tumor detection and depth of invasion difficult
  - Limited detection of parametrial invasion
    - Only 30-58% accuracy
    - Parametrial inflammation can mimic parametrial tumor infiltration
    - Paracervical ligaments and vessels may be mistaken for soft tissue strands

- **MR**
  - Ideal for local cervical cancer imaging
    - Superior soft tissue contrast
    - Multiplanar capability
  - Superior to other imaging modalities with regard to tumor characteristics that determine prognosis
    - Tumor size
    - Parametrial invasion
    - Vaginal wall invasion
    - Pelvic sidewall extension
  - Accuracy for stage is 75-96% in various studies, superior to CT
  - Sensitivity for parametrial invasion is 40-57% according to literature
  - Specificity for parametrial invasion is 77-80% according to literature
  - Accuracy of MR is 94% in selecting operative candidates
    - Compared with 76% for CT
  - Including MR in pre-treatment work-up significantly decreases number of procedures and invasive studies
  - Typical MR findings of cervical cancer
    - T2 hyperintense mass disrupting normal hypointense cervical stroma
    - Endophytic: Arises from endocervical canal
    - Exophytic: Arises from ectocervix and extends into vaginal vault
  - MR technique
    - T2WI best for visualization of tumor and local invasion
      - FSE, small field of view (FOV), high resolution
    - Coronal oblique T2WI: Long & short (donut view; perpendicular to the axis of the uterus) axis of cervix
      - Evaluation of depth of cervical stromal invasion
      - Evaluation of parametrial invasion
    - Sagittal T2WI
      - Depth of cervical stromal invasion
      - Visualization of invasion of vagina and urinary bladder
      - Helpful to distend vagina with gel
    - Axial T2WI
      - Parametrial invasion
      - Pelvic sidewall invasion
      - Rectal invasion
    - T2WI with fat saturation
      - Helpful if prominent paracervical venous plexus
    - IV contrast reportedly not helpful for depth of stromal invasion or parametrial involvement
      - Loss of soft tissue contrast due to enhancement of normal cervical stroma and variable tumor enhancement
      - May result in overestimation of tumor size
    - IV contrast is useful in advanced disease to evaluate
      - Rectal, urinary bladder, pelvic sidewall invasion
      - Pelvic fistulas
      - Recurrent/residual disease post radiation or surgery
  - Characteristic features of adenoma malignum
    - Multicystic mass extending from superficial to deep cervical wall
    - Mass may be nodular or annular
    - Mass invades deep into cervical stroma
    - Cystic components are hyperintense on T2WI with intervening low signal septations
    - Solid enhancing components help differentiate adenoma malignum from benign entities
  - Limitations of MR
    - Differentiating tumor recurrence from early radiation change and infection
    - May overestimate parametrial invasion with large tumors
      - Due to surrounding stromal edema from tumor compression or inflammation

- **PET/CT**
  - Excellent for detection of lymphadenopathy and distant metastatic disease
    - Sensitivity is 79-91% and specificity is 95-100% for lymph node detection
    - 100% sensitivity and 94% specificity for distant metastatic disease
    - False positive can be exacerbated by inflammatory states
  - PET is superior to MR and CT for depiction of adenopathy
    - Metabolic changes may precede morphologic changes
    - Moderate to marked increase in FDG uptake relative to normal structures
  - Limitations
    - Lower spatial resolution compared to CT and MR
    - Cannot differentiate malignant from reactive adenopathy
    - Cannot differentiate malignant, infectious, or inflammatory processes
  - Poor anatomic resolution of PET is overcome by fusion with CT

Staging

- **General comments**
  - Important to avoid upstaging at time of surgery
    - Significant increase in morbidity when surgery and radiotherapy are combined
  - International Federation of Gynecology and Obstetrics (FIGO)
    - Clinical staging of cervical cancer
    - Preferred staging system in order to provide uniformity
    - Results of imaging technologies (CT, MR, PET) should **not** be used to determine clinical stage

- Not universally available
- Can be used for prognostic information and treatment planning
- CT is acceptable for evaluating hydronephrosis
  - Surgical and pathologic findings should not change clinical stage
    - Can be used in TNM staging
  - Clinical stage must not be changed for subsequent findings once treatment started
  - If there is doubt regarding stage, the lesser stage should be used
- FIGO staging system is based on
  - Clinical examination (under anesthesia)
  - Chest x-ray
  - Intravenous pyelogram
  - Barium enema
  - Cystoscopy and proctoscopy
  - Aforementioned radiologic and endoscopic studies are often not used in clinical practice
- MR is more accurate for staging compared to clinical FIGO staging
  - Particularly in patients with ≥ stage IIA disease
- MR functional imaging
  - Diffusion-weighted imaging (DWI) measures diffusion of water
  - Apparent diffusion coefficient (ADC) is a quantitative parameter that reflects complexity of biologic diffusion
  - Dynamic contrast-enhanced (DCE) MR measures perfusion in tissue; correlation exists between DCE MR and prognosis
- PET functional imaging
  - FDG evaluates glucose utilization
  - Cu-ATSM measures hypoxia
  - Fluorothymidine detects cellular proliferation
  - Labeled water measures diffusion

- **Stage IA**
  - Microinvasive disease
  - Traditionally not visible on MR
  - Some reports describe area of enhancement in arterial phase on dynamic post-contrast imaging
- **Stage IB**
  - Clinically visible (> 5 mm); however, tumor remains confined to cervix
  - Hyperintense mass disrupting low signal cervical stroma on T2WI
  - Partial stromal invasion
    - Preservation of outer rim of normal low signal cervical stroma on T2WI
    - Parametrial invasion can reliably be excluded if rim of normal stroma is ≥ 3 mm
  - Full thickness stromal invasion
    - No outer rim of normal cervical stroma
    - Parametrial tissue is symmetric and normal in signal intensity
    - Preservation of sharp, distinct parametrial fat planes
    - Excluding parametrial invasion is more difficult with full-thickness invasion
    - If vaginal fornices are not invaded, tumor is likely confined to cervix
  - Exophytic cervical mass can fill and expand vaginal fornices
    - If low signal vaginal wall is preserved (no invasion), this remains stage IB tumor
- **Stage IIA**
  - Invasion of upper 2/3 of vagina
  - Disruption of normal low-signal vaginal wall by hyperintense cervical mass on T2WI
- **Stage IIB**
  - Invasion of parametrial tissues
    - Vessels, fat, and lymphatics between leaves of broad ligament
  - Probability of parametrial invasion is 28% for tumors > 2 cm
  - Specific signs of parametrial invasion
    - Frank extension of mass into parametrial tissues
    - Encasement of parametrial vessels
    - Encasement of ureter (no hydronephrosis)
    - Nodular thickening of uterine ligaments
  - Early parametrial invasion may manifest as
    - Full thickness cervical stromal invasion by tumor with irregularity of outer cervical contour
    - Stranding (> 3-4 mm in thickness) and nodularity of parametrial fat
    - These findings are nonspecific and can be secondary to parametrial inflammation
  - Coronal oblique and sagittal T2WI are best for identifying parametrial involvement
  - T2WI with fat saturation may be helpful in women with prominent paracervical venous plexus
- **Stage IIIA**
  - Invasion of lower 1/3 of vagina
  - Disruption of normal low signal vaginal wall by hyperintense cervical mass on T2WI
  - Best evaluated in axial and sagittal planes
- **Stage IIIB**
  - Hydronephrosis or pelvic sidewall invasion
    - Pelvic sidewall invasion manifests as
      - Tumor extension to within 3 mm of pelvic musculature
      - Invasion of obturator internus and piriformis muscles: Diffuse enlargement or mass
      - Encasement of iliac vessels by tumor
    - Ureteral invasion as manifested by hydronephrosis can be identified with US, CT, or MR
    - Enlarge FOV on coronal fluid-sensitive sequence to evaluate entire urinary tract
  - Radiographically + lymph nodes (cannot be used for clinical staging)
    - Lymph node metastases are detected equally well with CT and MR
    - CT and MR are slightly better than lymphangiography
    - Anatomic imaging uses lymph node size and shape to predict presence of pathology
      - Spherical shape
      - Size > 1 cm in short axis: 75-88% accuracy
    - IV contrast aids in detection of lymph nodes
      - Lymph nodes avidly enhance
      - ↑ conspicuity in hypodense pelvic fat on CT or low signal pelvic fat on T1WI C+ FS MR
    - Central necrosis is highly predictive of metastasis
      - Lack of central enhancement
    - Metabolic imaging with PET utilizes presence of increased glucose metabolism to predict pathology

- Relative increased FDG uptake compared to other lymph nodes is considered positive
    - Detection of micrometastases remains a challenge for both anatomic and metabolic imaging
    - Reactive adenopathy can be difficult to differentiate from malignant adenopathy
- **Stage IVA**
  - Invasion of urinary bladder or rectal mucosa
  - Disruption of normal low signal urinary bladder or rectal wall by high signal tumor on T2WI
  - Eccentric nodular wall thickening
  - Protrusion of tumor into lumen
  - Fistula formation: Tumor to urinary bladder or rectum
    - Enhancing tract on post-contrast sequences
    - Intraluminal air in urinary bladder
  - Bullous edema sign
    - High signal thickening of urinary bladder wall on T2WI
    - Reactive inflammation, not tumor invasion
    - Not stage IVA if occurring in isolation
  - Bladder and rectal mucosal involvement must be confirmed by biopsy and histology
- **Stage IVB**
  - Distant metastatic disease including extrapelvic lymph nodes
  - Metastatic disease is most commonly seen with recurrence or advanced disease
    - 10% have metastatic disease at time of diagnosis
  - Factors influencing incidence of distant metastasis
    - Clinical stage at diagnosis and tumor size
    - Endometrial extension as shown at pre-treatment dilation and curettage
    - Pelvic tumor control with treatment
  - Incidence of distant metastases increases with increasing stage of disease
    - Stage IA (3%) → stage IVA (75%)
  - Most common organs
    - Liver, lungs, abdominal cavity, and GI tract
  - Most common lymph nodes
    - Paraaortic, supraclavicular, and inguinal
  - Most common bones
    - Thoracic and lumbar spine
    - Destructive lesions
    - Usually by contiguous extension from paraaortic lymph node mass
    - Pelvis, ribs, and extremities less frequently involved
  - Liver is most common abdominal organ with metastases
    - Solid mass with variable enhancement on CECT or MR
    - Increased FDG activity compared with background liver on PET/CT
  - Peritoneal carcinomatosis
    - Implants scalloping liver contour
    - Irregular and nodular peritoneal thickening
    - Mass or infiltrative soft tissue in mesentery or omentum
    - Soft tissue masses on serosal surface of bowel
    - Ascites is often present, though nonspecific
  - Pleural involvement
    - Pleural thickening and nodularity
    - Hydrothorax (often seen with ascites)
    - More common with adenocarcinoma
  - Pericardial metastasis is rare
    - Nodular pericardial thickening
    - Pericardial effusion
    - Spread via paraaortic lymph nodes
  - Rare metastatic sites
    - Skin, brain, meninges, heart, and breast
    - Usually occur in recurrent cervical cancer

Restaging

- Recurrence must be preceded by a complete clinical response to distinguish from persistent disease
- Risk factors for recurrence include
  - Histologic grade
  - Tumor size
  - Depth of stromal invasion
  - Lymph node status at presentation
- Most common sites of local recurrence
  - Cervix
  - Vaginal cuff
  - Parametrial tissues
  - Pelvic sidewall
- Local recurrence in pelvis
  - Central
    - At remaining cervix or vaginal cuff
    - Can extend anteriorly to ureter or bladder
    - Posteriorly to invade rectum
      - ± rectovaginal fistula
    - Laterally to pelvic sidewall or lymph nodes
  - Pelvic sidewall
    - Invasion precludes treatment with pelvic exenteration
- CT
  - Overall high sensitivity and specificity in detection of recurrent tumor
  - Limited ability to differentiate early radiation change/fibrosis from recurrence
  - Readily available
  - Short scan time eliminates bowel motion artifact
- MR
  - Contrast-enhanced MR: Accuracy of 82% for distinguishing recurrence from fibrosis
  - Can assess extent of vaginal and pelvic floor involvement
  - Disadvantages include cost and long scan time
- PET/CT
  - Able to differentiate metabolically active tumor from therapy-related fibrosis
  - Whole-body evaluation for distant metastases
  - Poor spatial resolution precludes evaluation of local tumor invasion of adjacent structures

CLINICAL PRESENTATION & WORK-UP

Presentation

- Average age of presentation is 50 years
- Most common symptoms are vaginal bleeding and discharge
- Precursor is cervical intraepithelial neoplasia (CIN)
  - CIN 1: Minor dysplasia
  - CIN 2: Moderate dysplasia
  - CIN 3: Severe dysplasia

- 40% progress to invasive cancer if not treated
- Average time to progression is 10-15 years

Prognosis

- Major factors influencing prognosis
  - Histologic type and grade
  - Stage
  - Tumor volume
  - Depth of stromal invasion
  - Adjacent tissue extension
  - Lymphatic spread
  - Vascular invasion

Work-Up

- Clinical
  - Complete H&P including detailed gynecologic history, biopsy, and detailed pelvic examination with EUA if needed
- Radiographic
  - PET/CT preferred for evaluation of lymph nodes and distant metastases
  - MR preferred for soft tissue delineation and surgical or RT planning
  - Chest x-ray
  - Cystoscopy and proctoscopy optional
- Laboratory
  - Complete blood count (particular attention to hemoglobin); liver function tests and creatinine

TREATMENT

Major Treatment Alternatives

- Surgical resection
  - Trachelectomy
    - Maintains fertility
    - Depends on tumor size and relationship of tumor to internal os
  - Wertheim-Meigs operation (radical hysterectomy)
    - Total abdominal hysterectomy
    - Resection of upper 1/3 of vagina
    - Excision of parametrial and uterosacral ligaments
    - Pelvic and paraaortic lymph node dissection
- Radiation therapy
  - External beam pelvic radiation and intracavitary brachytherapy for stages IB2-IVA
  - Intracavitary brachytherapy is integral part of advanced cervix cancer treatment
  - For patients with positive nodes, parametria, or margins after hysterectomy chemoradiotherapy improves overall survival (OS)
  - After hysterectomy, if 2 of these are present (large tumor size, LVSI, or deep stromal invasion) then RT improves disease-free survival
  - Can extend radiation field to include paraaortic lymph nodes
    - Long-term disease control if low volume (< 2 cm) nodal disease below L3
    - Cure rate about 25% with paraaortic involvement
- Chemotherapy
  - Survival advantage in stage IB2-IVA disease when concurrent with radiation therapy
  - 40 mg/m2 cisplatin weekly is most common
  - Risk of death is decreased by 30-50%
  - Palliative in patients with recurrence or stage IVB
    - Cisplatin is the most active single agent

Major Treatment Roadblocks/ Contraindications

- Frequent in low socioeconomic groups with limited access to health care
- Large tumor size or parametrial infiltration may obviate en bloc resection
- RT should be delivered in facilities with expertise, in < 8 weeks, and with brachytherapy if possible

Treatment Options by Stage

- IA1-IB1 often treated with hysterectomy, or trachelectomy for fertility preservation
  - RT may be used if surgery is not an option
  - Advantage of surgery is ovarian preservation
- 1B1-select IIA may be treated with chemoradiation therapy (CRT) or surgery
- IB2-IVA CRT is preferred
- IVB chemotherapy
- Postop RT or CRT if Sedlis or Peters criteria apply

Dose Response

- Squamous cell cancers are responsive
- Adenocarcinomas may respond slower and less completely
- With a combination of external beam radiation therapy (EBRT) and brachytherapy, cervix receives a very high dose

Standard Doses

- After hysterectomy, 45-50 Gy is preferred
- Gross nodes boosted to 60-70 Gy depending on adjacent normal structures
- Sidewall 60 Gy if large IIIB or parametria + after EBRT
- For advanced cases, pelvis and nodes are treated to 45 Gy and then brachytherapy
- Cumulative dose 85 Gy to point A for LDR; for HDR, 30 Gy in 5 fractions is common after 45 Gy to pelvis
- Point A &/or CTV 80-84 EQD2 (Gy)

Organs at Risk Parameters

- Limit rectum and sigmoid D2 mL < 75 Gy, and D2 mL for bladder to < 90 Gy
- ICRU 38 points for bladder < 75 Gy and rectum < 70-75 Gy

Common Techniques

- 3D CRT is standard for IB2-IVA
- IMRT should be reserved for centers with expertise due to tumor regression and organ motion
- IMRT or 3D may be used after hysterectomy
  - Limit dose to small bowel
- Image-guided brachytherapy (IGBT) provides an accurate dose to tumor and sparing of organs at risk (OAR)
  - High-risk CTV (HR CTV) for IGBT includes cervix, gross tumor, and palpable abnormalities at time of brachytherapy
  - Dose to point A should be recorded
- Interstitial brachytherapy is a good option for recurrent disease or stage IIIA
- SBRT has been reported to be useful for some nodal and central recurrences

Landmark Trials

- GOG 92: ↑ PFS, but not OS for patients with 2 of 3 (large tumor size, deep stromal invasion, and LVSI) after radical hysterectomy
- GOG 109: 10% ↑ in OS with 5-FU and cisplatin + RT after radical hysterectomy in patients with + parametria, margins, or nodes
- Landoni: No difference in OS between RT and surgery in stages I and II
- RTOG 9001: 26% ↑ in OS with 5-FU and cisplatin and pelvic RT vs. extended field RT at 7 years
- GOG 120: 19% ↑ in OS with cisplatin and RT vs. hydroxyurea and RT at 10 years

RECOMMENDED FOLLOW-UP

Clinical

- Pelvic examination with Pap smear every 3 months for 1st 2 years, then 2x yearly through year 5, then annually
- Vaginal dilator after RT

Radiographic

- PET/CT 1x at 3 months, then additional imaging as needed

SELECTED REFERENCES

1. Mayr NA et al: Characterizing tumor heterogeneity with functional imaging and quantifying high-risk tumor volume for early prediction of treatment outcome: cervical cancer as a model. Int J Radiat Oncol Biol Phys. 83(3):972-9, 2012
2. Siegel R et al: Cancer statistics, 2012. CA Cancer J Clin. 62(1):10-29, 2012
3. Pötter R et al: Clinical outcome of protocol based image (MRI) guided adaptive brachytherapy combined with 3D conformal radiotherapy with or without chemotherapy in patients with locally advanced cervical cancer. Radiother Oncol. 100(1):116-23, 2011
4. American Joint Committee on Cancer: AJCC Cancer Staging Manual. 7th ed. New York: Springer. 395-402, 2010
5. Kidd EA et al: Lymph node staging by positron emission tomography in cervical cancer: relationship to prognosis. J Clin Oncol. 28(12):2108-13, 2010
6. National Institutes of Health. Cervical cancer treatment. www.cancer.gov/cancertopics/pdq/treatment/cervical/HealthProfessional. Accessed October 23, 2009
7. Rezvani M et al: Imaging of cervical pathology. Clin Obstet Gynecol. 52(1):94-111, 2009
8. Akin O et al: Imaging of uterine cancer. Radiol Clin North Am. 45(1):167-82, 2007
9. Loft A et al: The diagnostic value of PET/CT scanning in patients with cervical cancer: a prospective study. Gynecol Oncol. 106(1):29-34, 2007
10. Sala E et al: MRI of malignant neoplasms of the uterine corpus and cervix. AJR Am J Roentgenol. 188(6):1577-87, 2007
11. Amit A et al: The role of hybrid PET/CT in the evaluation of patients with cervical cancer. Gynecol Oncol. 100(1):65-9, 2006
12. Haie-Meder C et al: Recommendations from Gynaecological (GYN) GEC-ESTRO Working Group (I): concepts and terms in 3D image based 3D treatment planning in cervix cancer brachytherapy with emphasis on MRI assessment of GTV and CTV. Radiother Oncol. 74(3):235-45, 2005
13. Eifel PJ et al: Pelvic irradiation with concurrent chemotherapy versus pelvic and para-aortic irradiation for high-risk cervical cancer: an update of radiation therapy oncology group trial (RTOG) 90-01. J Clin Oncol. 22(5):872-80, 2004
14. Unger JB et al: Detection of recurrent cervical cancer by whole-body FDG PET scan in asymptomatic and symptomatic women. Gynecol Oncol. 94(1):212-6, 2004
15. Jeong YY et al: Uterine cervical carcinoma after therapy: CT and MR imaging findings. Radiographics. 23(4):969-81; discussion 981, 2003
16. Kaur H et al: Diagnosis, staging, and surveillance of cervical carcinoma. AJR Am J Roentgenol. 180(6):1621-31, 2003
17. Metser U et al: MR imaging findings and patterns of spread in secondary tumor involvement of the uterine body and cervix. AJR Am J Roentgenol. 180(3):765-9, 2003
18. Okamoto Y et al: MR imaging of the uterine cervix: imaging-pathologic correlation. Radiographics. 23(2):425-45; quiz 534-5, 2003
19. Scheidler J et al: Imaging of cancer of the cervix. Radiol Clin North Am. 40(3):577-90, vii, 2002
20. Pannu HK et al: CT evaluation of cervical cancer: spectrum of disease. Radiographics. 21(5):1155-68, 2001
21. Nicolet V et al: MR imaging of cervical carcinoma: a practical staging approach. Radiographics. 20(6):1539-49, 2000
22. Peters WA 3rd et al: Concurrent chemotherapy and pelvic radiation therapy compared with pelvic radiation therapy alone as adjuvant therapy after radical surgery in high-risk early-stage cancer of the cervix. J Clin Oncol. 18(8):1606-13, 2000
23. Yang WT et al: Comparison of dynamic helical CT and dynamic MR imaging in the evaluation of pelvic lymph nodes in cervical carcinoma. AJR Am J Roentgenol. 175(3):759-66, 2000
24. Fulcher AS et al: Recurrent cervical carcinoma: typical and atypical manifestations. Radiographics. 19 Spec No:S103-16; quiz S264-5, 1999
25. Rose PG et al: Concurrent cisplatin-based radiotherapy and chemotherapy for locally advanced cervical cancer. N Engl J Med. 340(15):1144-53, 1999
26. Sedlis A et al: A randomized trial of pelvic radiation therapy versus no further therapy in selected patients with stage IB carcinoma of the cervix after radical hysterectomy and pelvic lymphadenectomy: A Gynecologic Oncology Group Study. Gynecol Oncol. 73(2):177-83, 1999
27. Landoni F et al: Randomised study of radical surgery versus radiotherapy for stage Ib-IIa cervical cancer. Lancet. 350(9077):535-40, 1997
28. Yamashita Y et al: Adenoma malignum: MR appearances mimicking nabothian cysts. AJR Am J Roentgenol. 162(3):649-50, 1994
29. Hricak H et al: Invasive cervical carcinoma: comparison of MR imaging and surgical findings. Radiology. 166(3):623-31, 1988
30. LaPolla JP et al: The influence of surgical staging on the evaluation and treatment of patients with cervical carcinoma. Gynecol Oncol. 24(2):194-206, 1986
31. Van Nagell JR Jr et al: The staging of cervical cancer: inevitable discrepancies between clinical staging and pathologic findinges. Am J Obstet Gynecol. 110(7):973-8, 1971

Stage IB1 (T1b1 N0 M0)

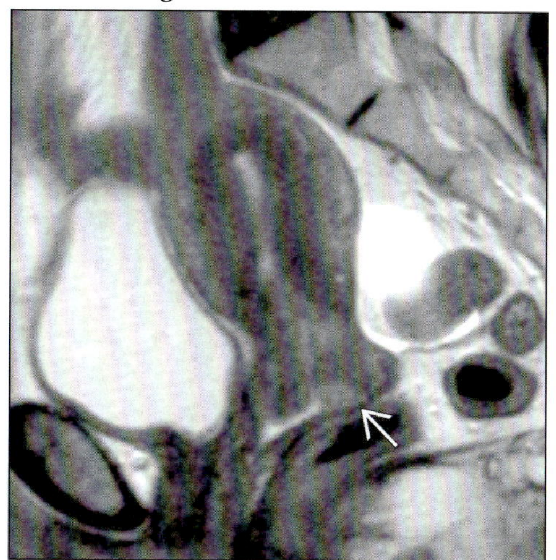

Stage IB1 (T1b1 N0 M0)

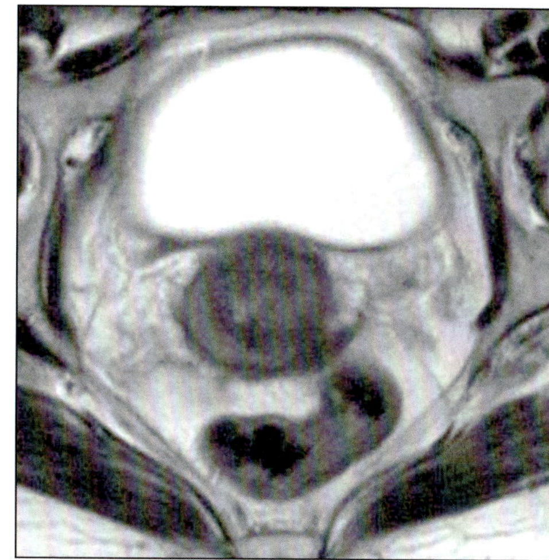

(Left) *Sagittal T2WI FSE MR shows a small hyperintense cervical mass ➔ at the expected location of the squamo-columnar junction in the ectocervix.* ***(Right)*** *Coronal oblique (short axis) T2WI FSE MR in the same patient shows the small hyperintense cervical mass.*

Stage IB1 (T1b1 N0 M0)

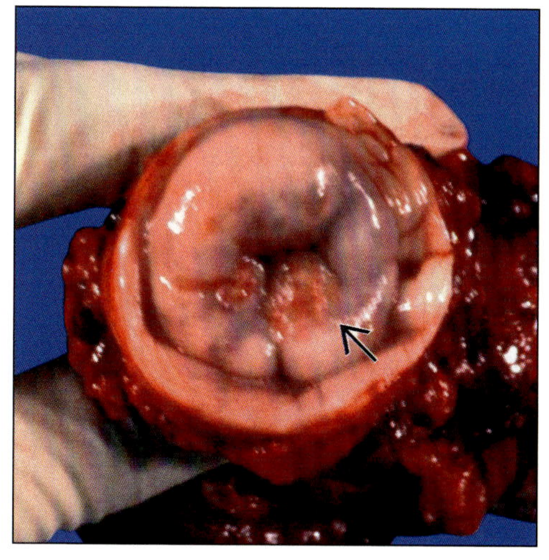

Stage IB1 (T1b1 N0 M0)

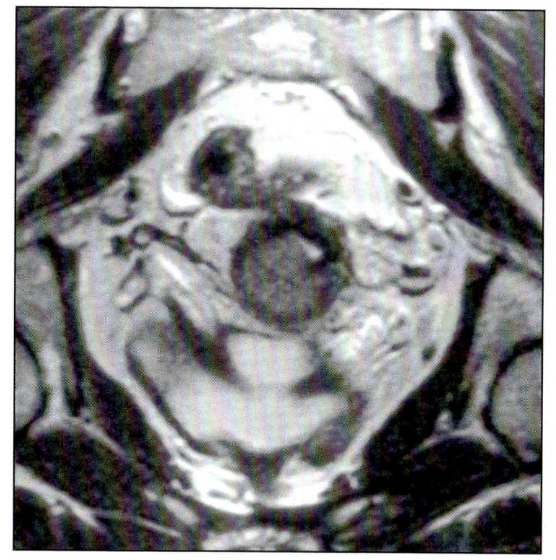

(Left) *Gross surgical specimen from the same patient shows the small exophytic mass ➔ at the external os of the cervix arising from the expected location of the squamo-columnar junction.* ***(Right)*** *T2WI FSE MR shows a hyperintense cervical mass with preservation of a rim of normal low signal cervical stroma.*

Adenoma Malignum

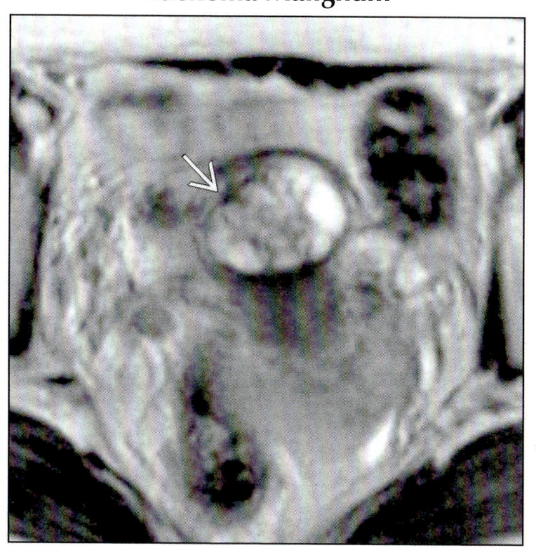

Adenoma Malignum

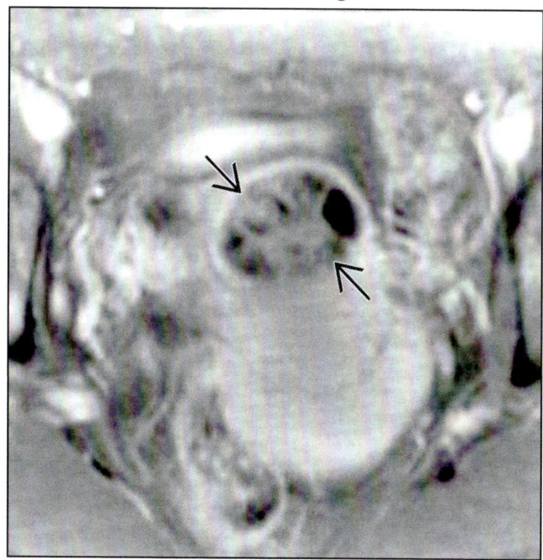

(Left) *T2WI FSE MR shows a multicystic cervical mass ➔ penetrating deep into the cervical stroma.* ***(Right)*** *T1WI C+ FS MR in the same patient shows solid enhancing nodules ➔ in the multicystic cervical mass.*

CERVIX

External Beam Planning

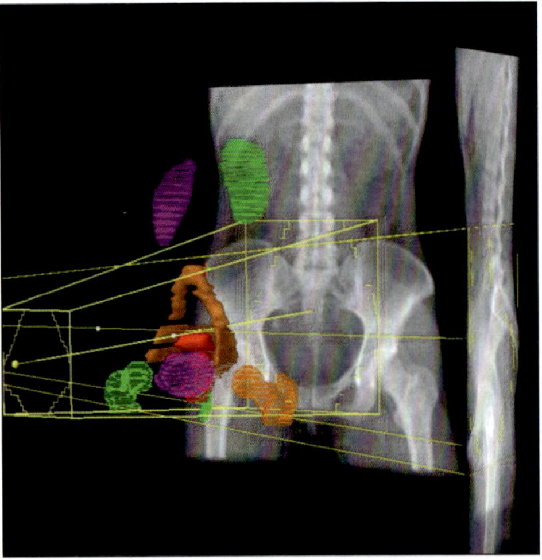

External Beam Planning

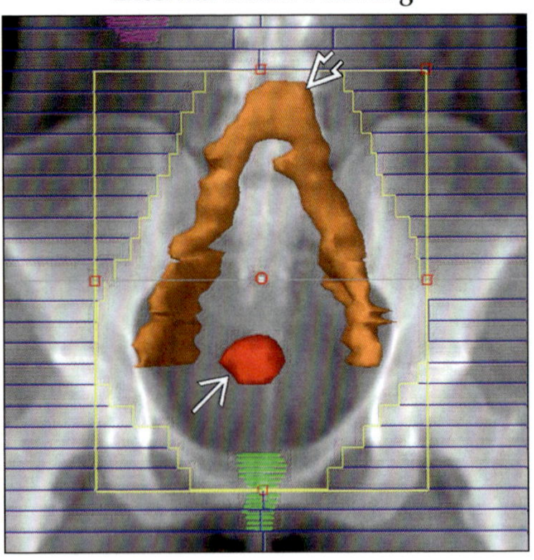

(Left) *Digital reconstructed radiograph allows DVH analysis for CTV and OARs. Care needs to be taken to cover nodal drainage patterns in cervix cancer and not miss typical routes of tumor spread (e.g., uterosacral ligament involvement in stages IIB-IVA cases).* ***(Right)*** *In carcinoma of the cervix, the common iliac chain should be covered. The aortic bifurcation is often above the L4/5 interspace. In this case, it is at the mid L4 level ➔. The GTV is outlined in red ➔ and the nodal CTV is shown in orange.*

External Beam Planning

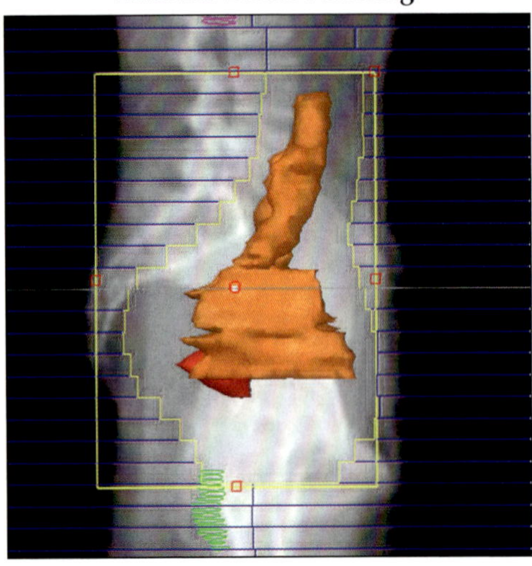

IMRT vs. 3D DVH

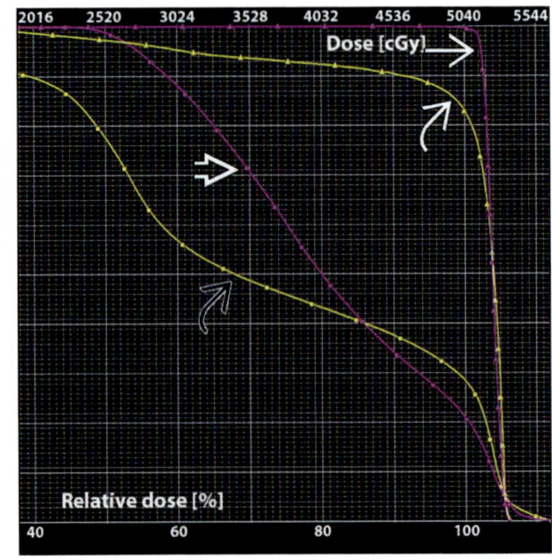

(Left) *In this stage IB1, the entire sacrum is not covered, and as much anus (green) was excluded as safety permitted. In advanced cases, it is prudent to cover the sacral hollow to fully encompass the uterosacral ligaments.* ***(Right)*** *DVH comparison of IMRT (9 fields) vs. 3D (4 fields) in postoperative cervix cancer case shows reduction in dose to bladder and rectum. IMRT OARs for bladder ➔ and rectum ➔ and 3D OARs for bladder ➔ and rectum ➔ are shown.*

Brachytherapy

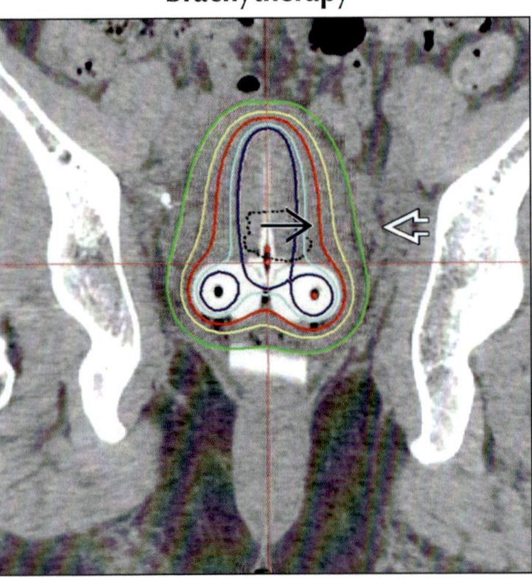

Brachytherapy

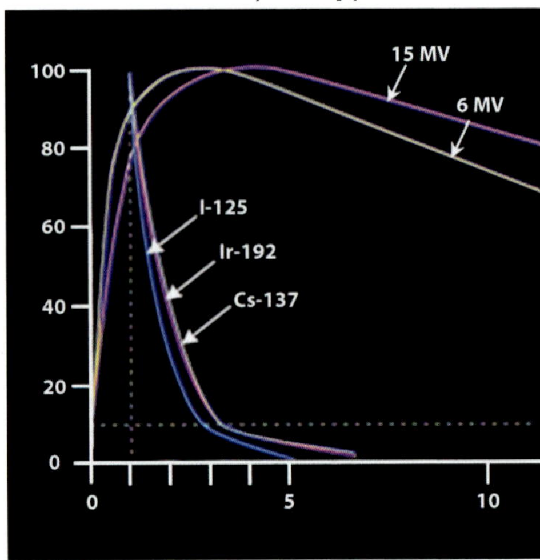

(Left) *This is a pear-shaped isodose surface from coronal CT. 200% (dark blue), 150% (light blue), 100% (red), 75% (yellow), and 50% (green) isodose lines are shown. Point A ➔ is defined as 2 cm above the vaginal fornix and 2 cm lateral from the tandem, and point B is an additional 3 cm lateral ➔.* ***(Right)*** *Brachytherapy is well suited for gynecologic applications. The more rapid dose fall-off for brachytherapy isotopes compared with common photon beams limits dose to OARs.*

Image-Guided Brachytherapy

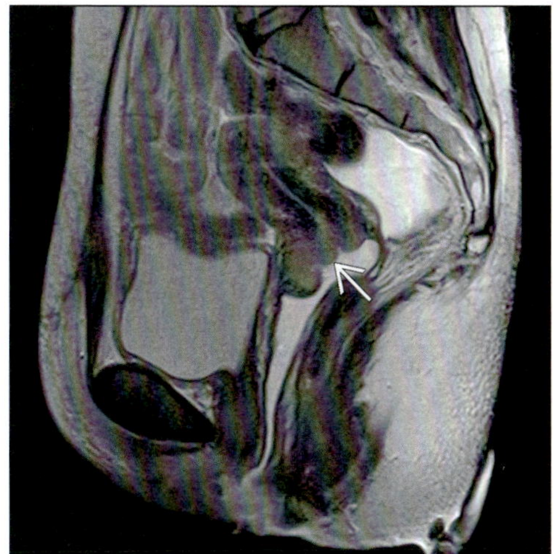

Image-Guided Brachytherapy

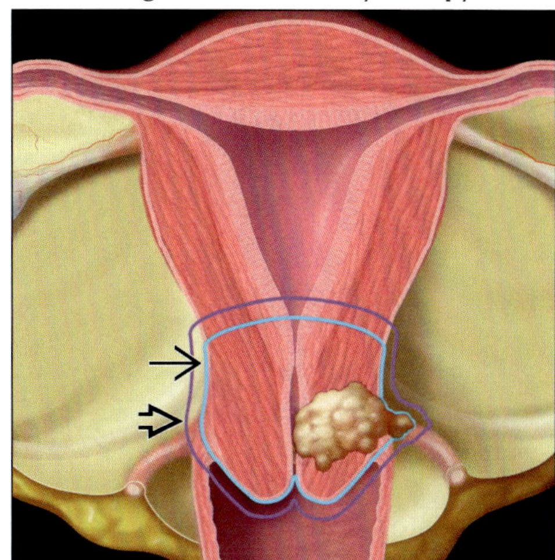

(Left) Sagittal T2WI shows a 3.5 cm lesion confined to the cervix; hence stage IB1. Cervix tumor is hyperintense and well delineated →. Surgilube is placed in the vagina to distend the fornices and provide contrast. *(Right)* The high-risk (HR) CTV → is shown in blue and includes gross disease, cervix, and palpable abnormalities at brachytherapy. The intermediate risk CTV → is shown in purple and is the HR CTV + 5-15 mm.

Image-Guided Brachytherapy

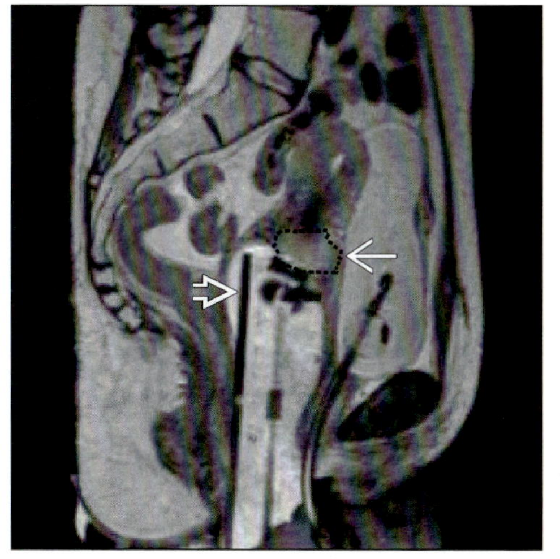

Image-Guided Brachytherapy

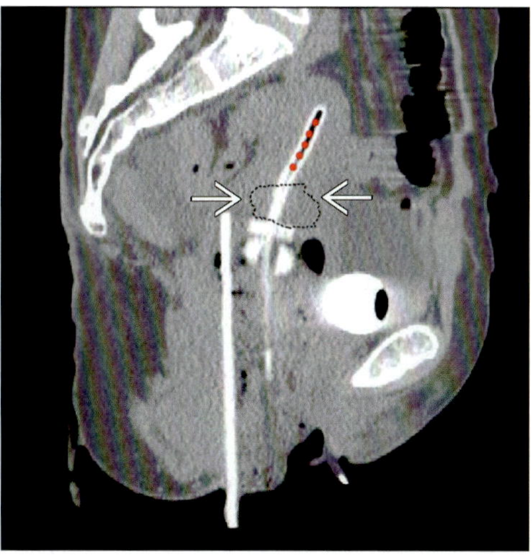

(Left) Sagittal T2WI in the same patient on 1st implant shows a good response to CRT. The HR CTV → is marked with the dotted line and includes gross disease, cervix, and palpable abnormalities at brachytherapy. In this case, a rectal blade → was used. *(Right)* Sagittal simulation CT was performed for the 1st implant in the same patient. CT is not able to delineate the cervix well in this case. MR/CT fusion was performed to display the HR CTV →.

Image-Guided Brachytherapy

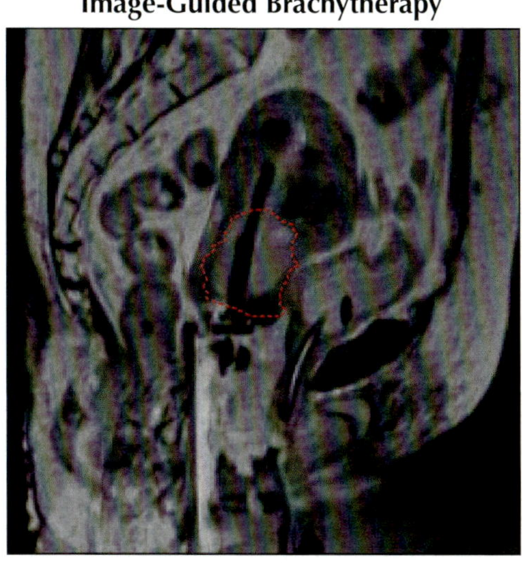

Image-Guided Brachytherapy

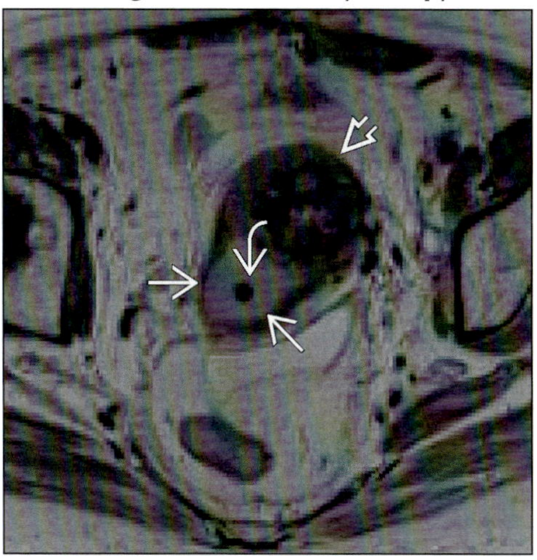

(Left) Sagittal MR T2WI shows a moderate response after 4 weeks of CRT. The HR CTV is shown within the dotted red line. When contouring the HR CTV, it is important to check accuracy in different imaging planes. *(Right)* MR T2WI axial plane is shown in the same patient. MR-compatible uterine tandem → and ovoid is used. An eccentric fibroid is present →. The hyperintense cervical tumor → is easily identified in this case.

Image-Guided Brachytherapy

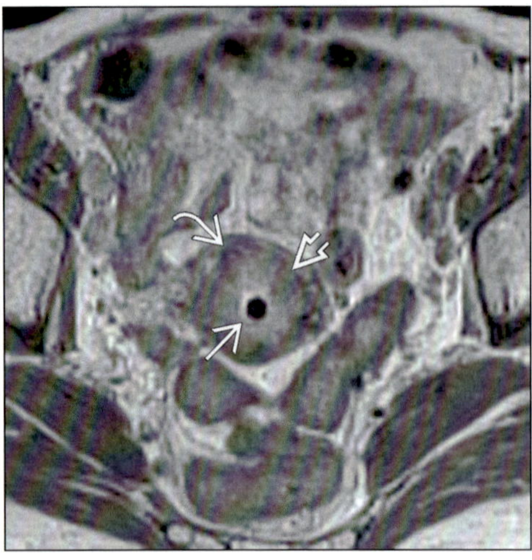

Image-Guided Brachytherapy

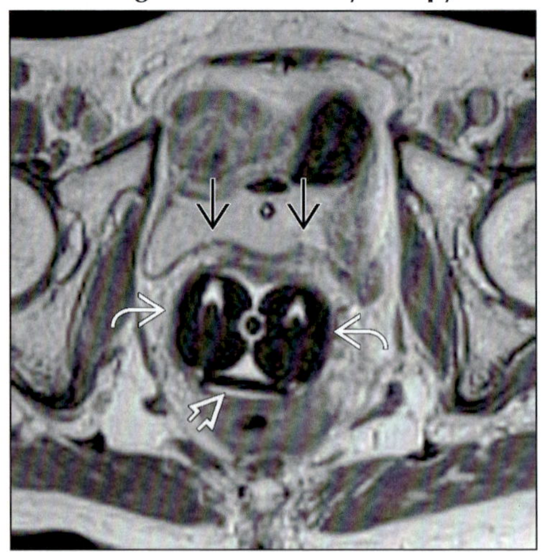

*(**Left**) Axial T2WI MR reveals the uterine tandem located centrally in the endocervical canal and surrounded by mildly hyperintense tumor. The transition to hypointense normal cervix shows examples of gray zones that should be included in the HR CTV. (**Right**) Axial T2WI MR image in the same patient shows ovoids appropriately positioned in the upper vagina. Note rectal blade pushing rectum posteriorly, and the vaginal ovoids are pushing anteriorly into bladder.*

Image-Guided Brachytherapy Inverse Planning vs. Standard Planning

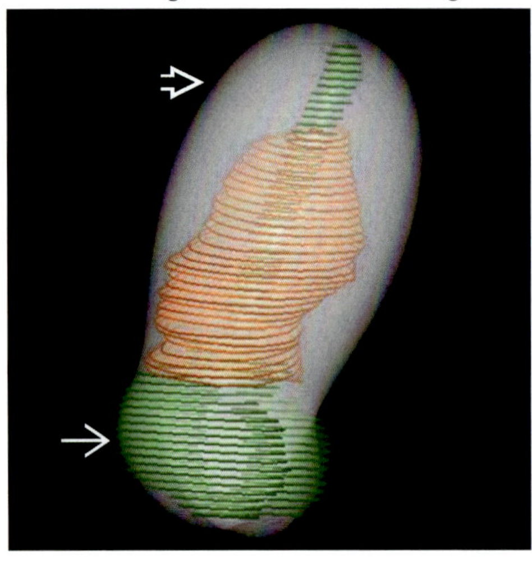

Image-Guided Brachytherapy Inverse Planning vs. Standard Planning

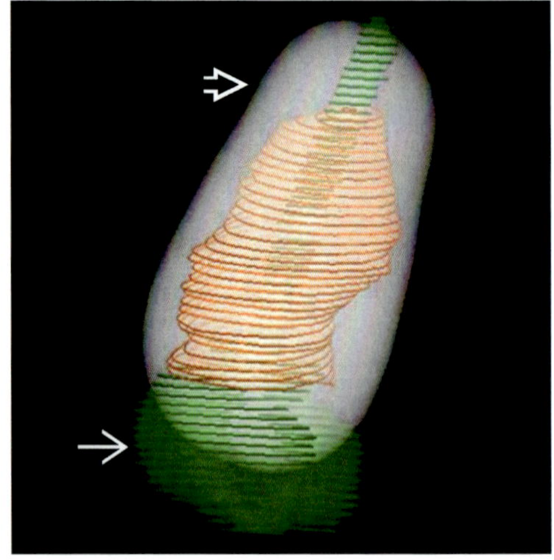

*(**Left**) DRR wire diagram shows HR CTV in orange and uterine tandem and ovoid in green. Dose envelope is 100% isodose surface. Standard point A classic pear-shaped plan was made. Note generous coverage cephalad at uterine fundus and caudad by the ovoids. (**Right**) Dose was prescribed to the HR CTV by inverse planning. Note the dose is more conformal. There is less coverage of the cephalad extent of the uterus and of the vagina distally, resulting in less dose to OAR.*

Image-Guided Brachytherapy Inverse Planning vs. Standard Planning

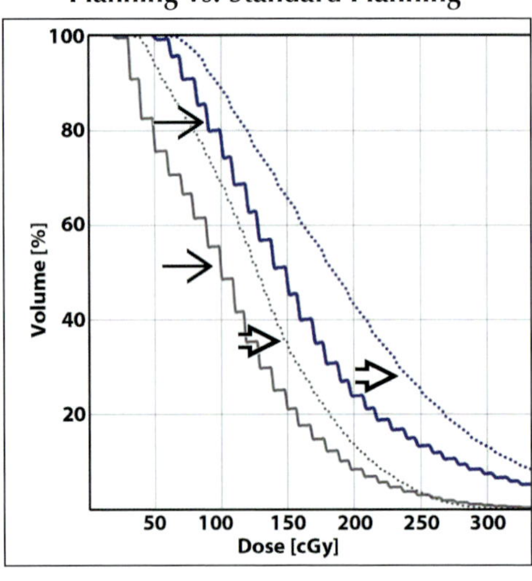

Functional Imaging (PET)

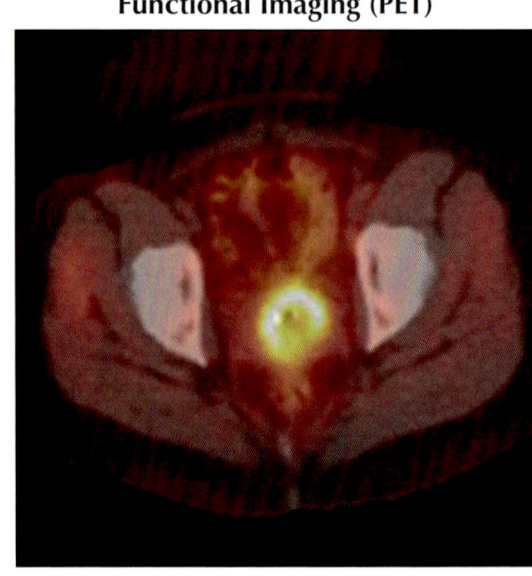

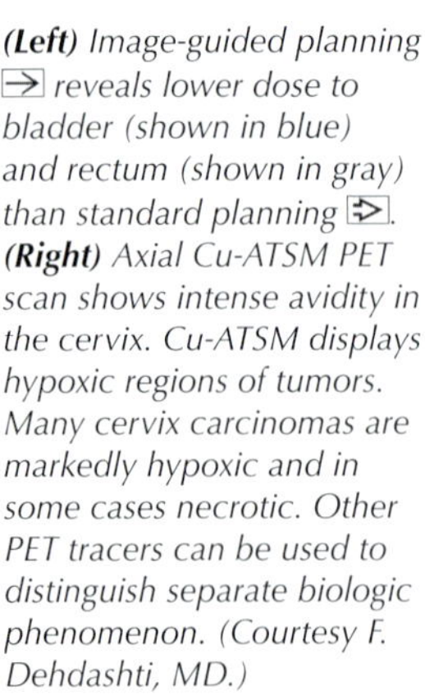

*(**Left**) Image-guided planning reveals lower dose to bladder (shown in blue) and rectum (shown in gray) than standard planning. (**Right**) Axial Cu-ATSM PET scan shows intense avidity in the cervix. Cu-ATSM displays hypoxic regions of tumors. Many cervix carcinomas are markedly hypoxic and in some cases necrotic. Other PET tracers can be used to distinguish separate biologic phenomenon. (Courtesy F. Dehdashti, MD.)*

Functional Imaging

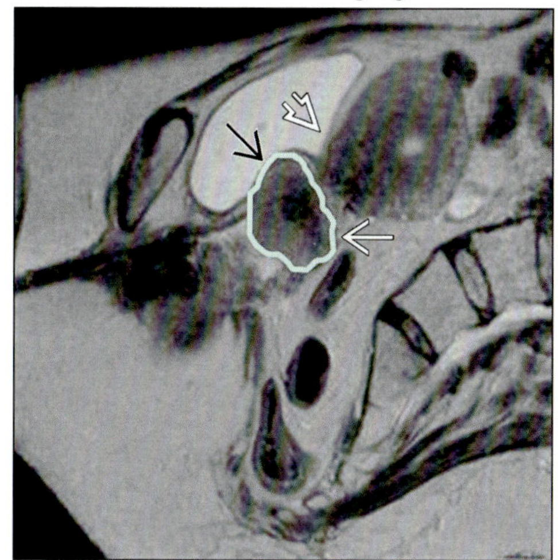

Functional Imaging (DWI MR)

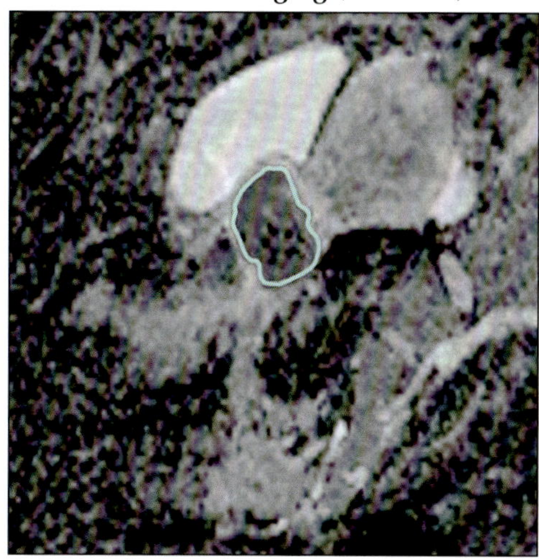

(Left) *T2WI shows tumor pushing toward bladder ➔ and rectum ➔. Note sharp transition at cervicouterine isthmus ➔. (Courtesy J. Schwarz, MD, PhD; P. Grigsby, MD.)* ***(Right)*** *Image shows low signal intensity of tumor, indicating restricted diffusion (increased cellularity and abnormal architecture). DWI measures diffusion of water. Apparent diffusion coefficient is quantitative and reflects complexity of diffusion in biologic tissues. (Courtesy J. Schwarz, MD, PhD, P. Grigsby, MD.)*

Functional Imaging

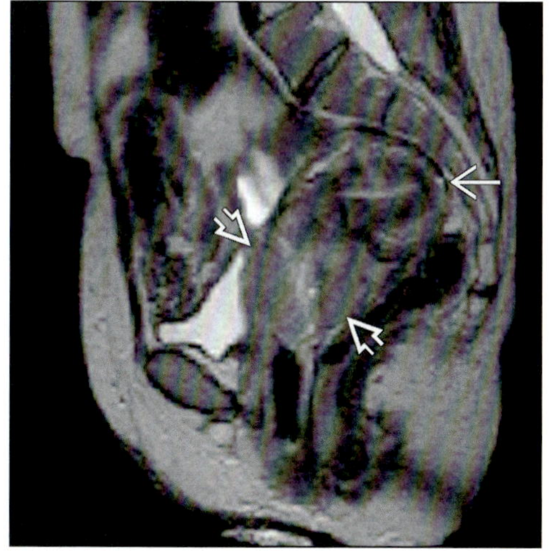

Functional Imaging (DCE MR)

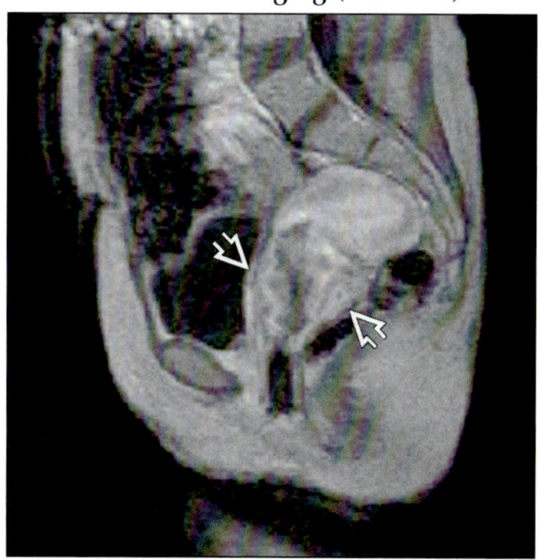

(Left) *Sagittal T2WI shows a large cervical mass ➔ with retroflexed uterus ➔. Note the uterus abuts the sacrum. (Courtesy N. Mayr, MD.)* ***(Right)*** *DCE MR in same patient shows mass ➔ displaying heterogeneous enhancement with contrast. DCE MR measures perfusion and has been found to be an early response indicator of survival. (Courtesy N. Mayr, MD.)*

Stage IB2 (T1b2 N0 M0)

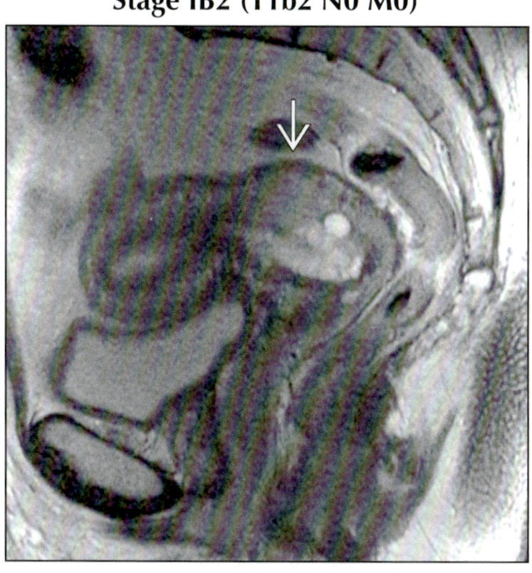

Stage IB2 (T1b2 N0 M0)

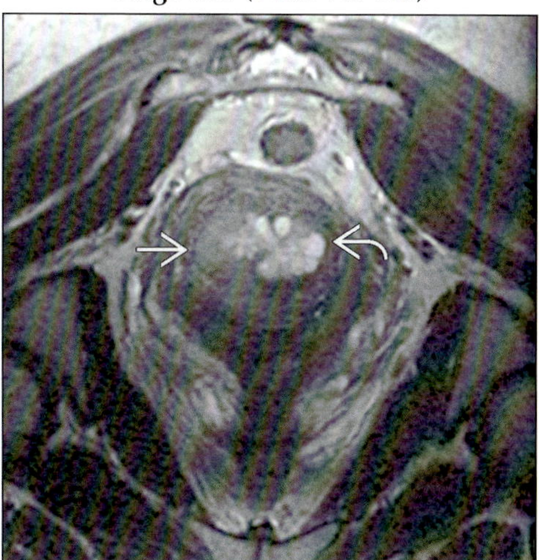

(Left) *Sagittal T2WI FSE MR shows partial thickness invasion of the posterior cervix with preservation of a rim of normal low signal stroma ➔.* ***(Right)*** *Coronal oblique (short axis) T2WI FSE MR in the same patient shows a hyperintense cervical mass ➔ obliterating the normal low signal stroma. Contrast the superficial location of nabothian cysts ➔ with the deep invasion of tumor.*

CERVIX

Stage IB2 (T1b2 N1 M0)

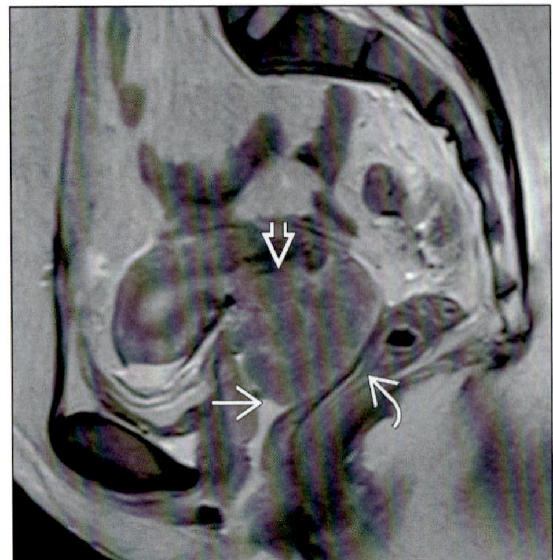

Stage IB2 (T1b2 N1 M0)

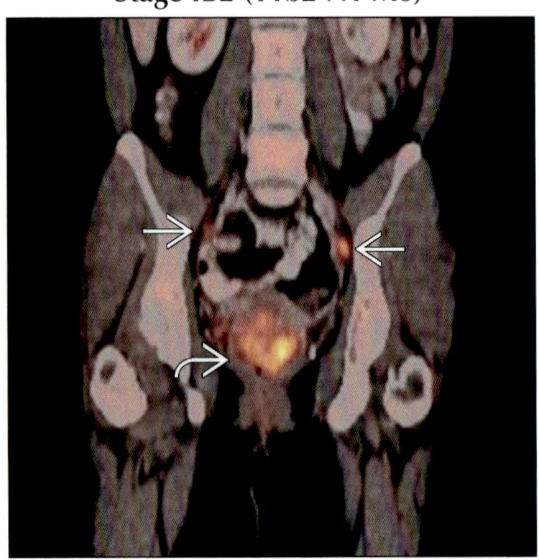

(Left) Sagittal T2WI shows a large cervical mass ⇨ compressing the rectum ⇨ and protruding down the vaginal canal ⇨. Patient presented with bleeding and sensation of prolapse. *(Right)* Coronal PET/CT in the same patient shows bilateral common iliac adenopathy ⇨ and an FDG-avid cervical tumor ⇨.

Stage IB2 (T1b2 N1 M0)

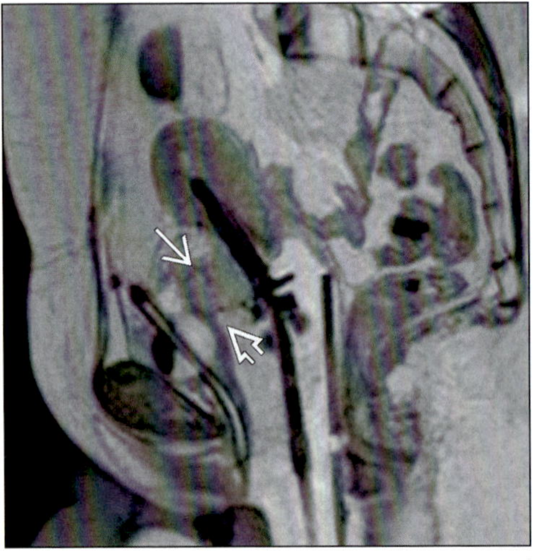

Tumor Regression

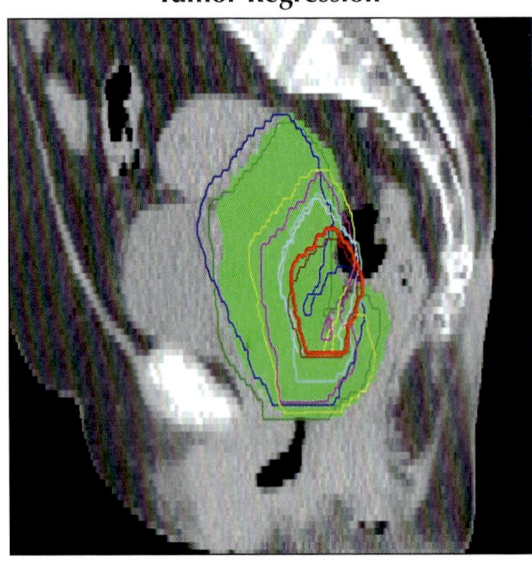

(Left) Sagittal T2WI shows dramatic tumor regression ⇨ in the same patient after CRT at 1st implant. A residual nodule was present only on the anterior cervix. Due to obliteration of the fornices, little packing was able to be placed between the cervix and the bladder ⇨. *(Right)* Weekly sagittal CT reveals successive tumor regression during EBRT. The red outline is the final size of the cervix prior to brachytherapy. (Courtesy A. Jhingran, MD.)

Tumor Regression and Mobility

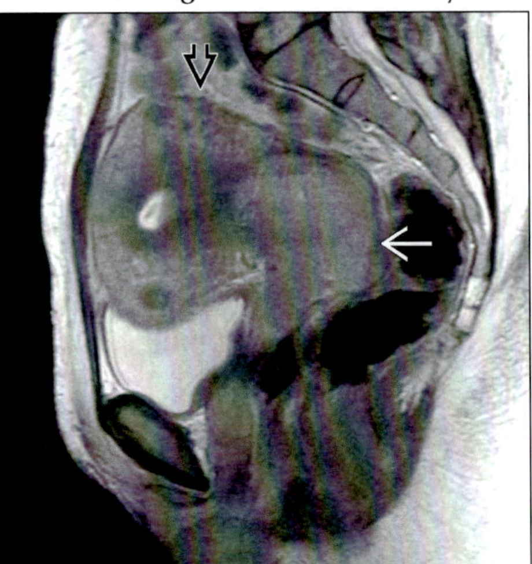

Tumor Regression and Mobility

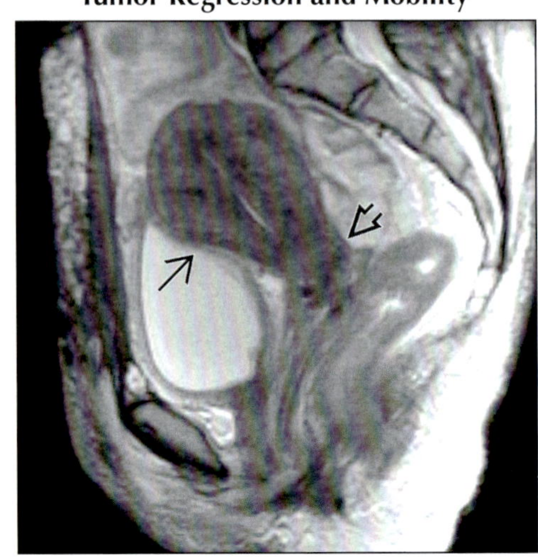

(Left) Sagittal T2WI shows anteverted uterus ⇨ and large cervical tumor ⇨. (Courtesy A. Jhingran, MD.) *(Right)* Sagittal T2WI in the same patient after EBRT and chemotherapy shows cervical tumor ⇨ regression and the bladder ⇨ pushing the uterus cephalad. (Courtesy A. Jhingran, MD.)

Stage IIA1 (T2a1 N0 M0)

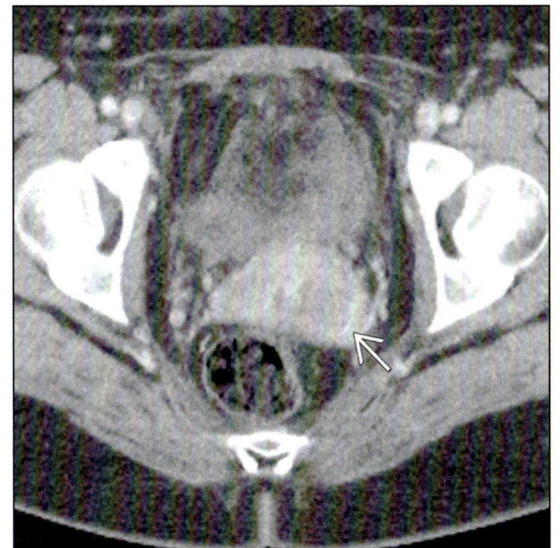

Stage IIA1 (T2a1 N0 M0)

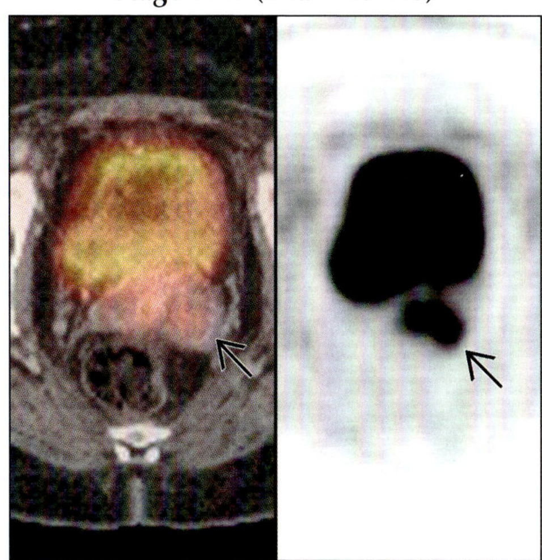

(Left) *Axial CECT shows a hypoenhancing mass ➔ in the cervix. The mass is difficult to see due to poor soft tissue contrast, which is typical of cervical cancer on CT.* ***(Right)*** *Axial fused PET/CT and PET in the same patient clearly demonstrate a hypermetabolic cervical mass ➔. No adenopathy or metastatic disease was found.*

Stage IIA1 (T2a1 N0 M0)

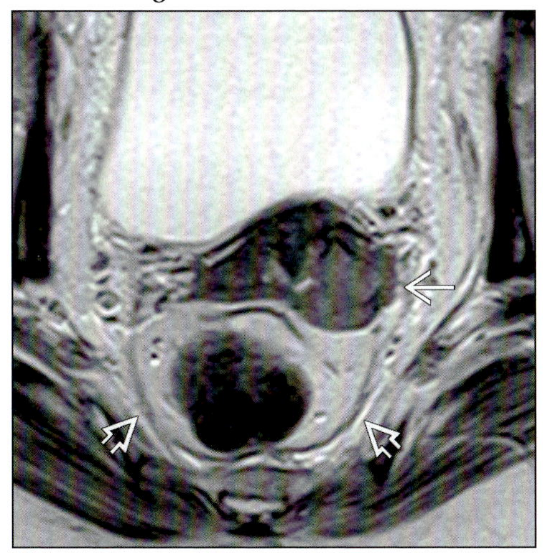

Stage IIA1 (T2a1 N0 M0)

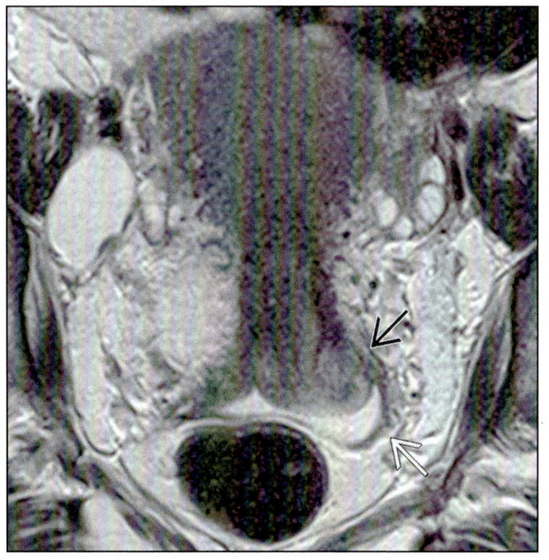

(Left) *Coronal oblique T2WI MR in the same patient shows a hyperintense, partially exophytic cervical mass ➔. Thin, smooth uterosacral ligaments ➔ and normal parametrial fat indicate absence of parametrial invasion.* ***(Right)*** *Coronal oblique T2WI MR in the same patient shows a hyperintense, partially exophytic cervical mass focally invading the upper vagina ➔. Note preservation of the normal low signal ➔ in the remainder of the vaginal wall.*

Stage IIA1 (T2a1 N0 M0)

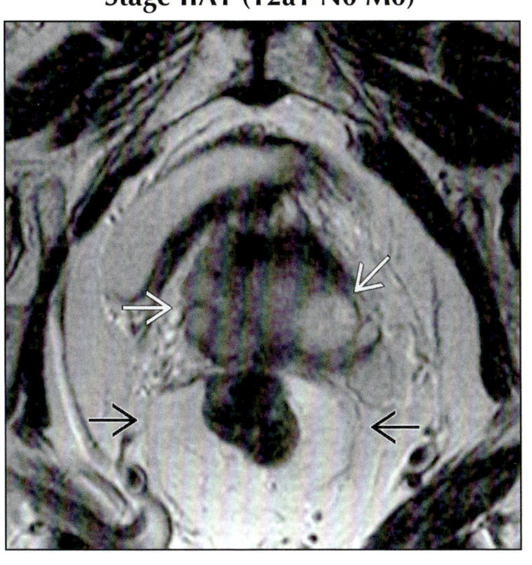

Stage IIA2 (T2a2 N0 M0)

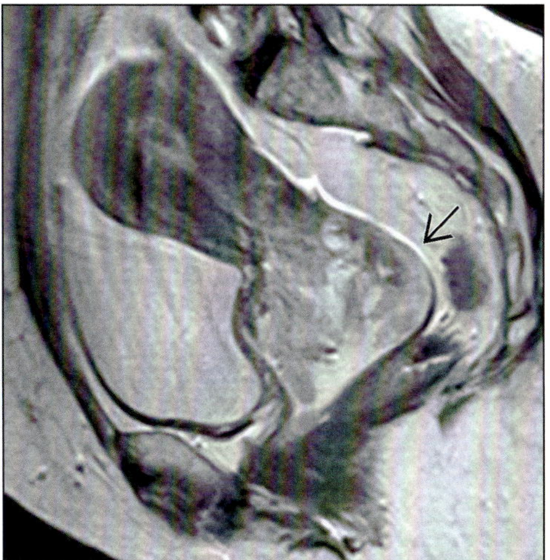

(Left) *Coronal oblique T2WI FSE MR shows a hyperintense cervical mass ➔. The parametrium-tumor interface is sharp with preservation of fat planes suggesting no invasion. Note normal thin uterosacral ligaments ➔.* ***(Right)*** *Sagittal T2WI FSE MR shows a large exophytic cervical mass expanding the vaginal fornices with disruption of the normal low signal vaginal wall ➔. The external contour of the tumor is smooth and parametrial fat is preserved.*

CERVIX

(Left) *Sagittal T2WI FSE MR shows a hyperintense cervical mass ➔ invading the upper anterior wall of the vagina. Note distention of the uterine cavity due to obstruction by the cervical mass.* ***(Right)*** *Gross surgical specimen (hysterectomy) from the same patient shows the large exophytic cervical mass.*

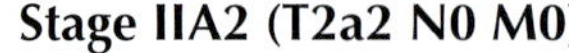

Stage IIA2 (T2a2 N0 M0)

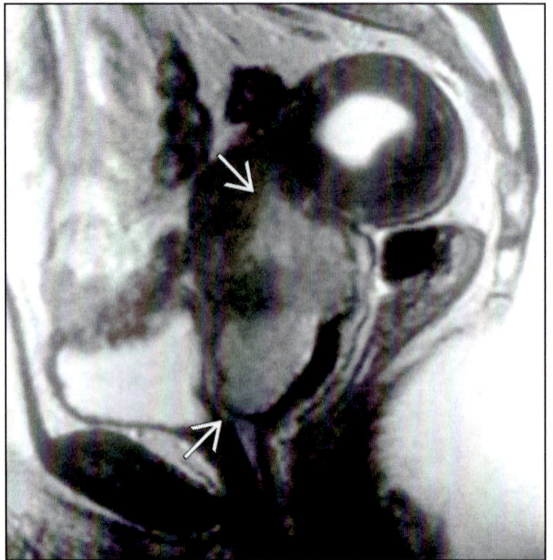

Stage IIA2 (T2a2 N0 M0)

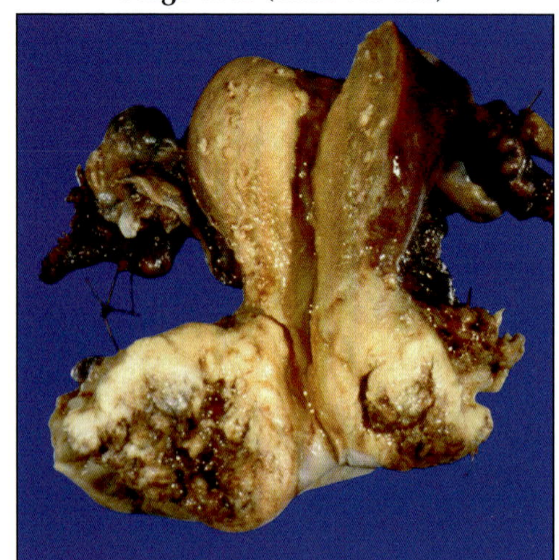

(Left) *Coronal oblique T2WI FSE MR shows a hyperintense mass ➔ obliterating the cervix and invading the parametrial tissues →.* ***(Right)*** *Axial CECT shows a cervical mass with full thickness cervical stromal invasion and extension into the uterus. The cervical contour is ill defined, and the paracervical fat is increased in density. These nonspecific findings can be due to parametrial inflammation or tumor invasion.*

Stage IIB (T2b N0 M0)

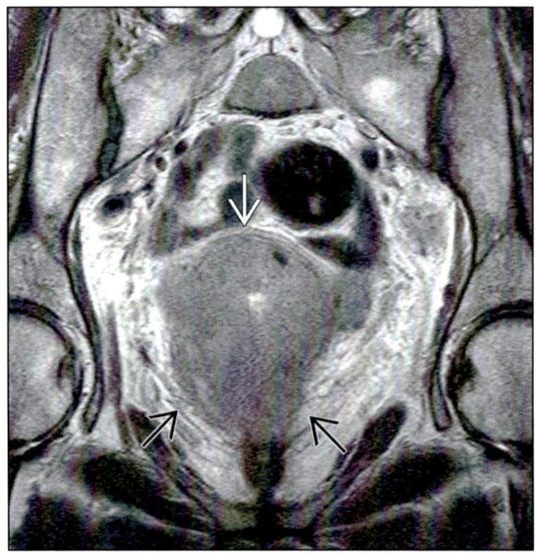

Stage IIB (T2b N0 M0)

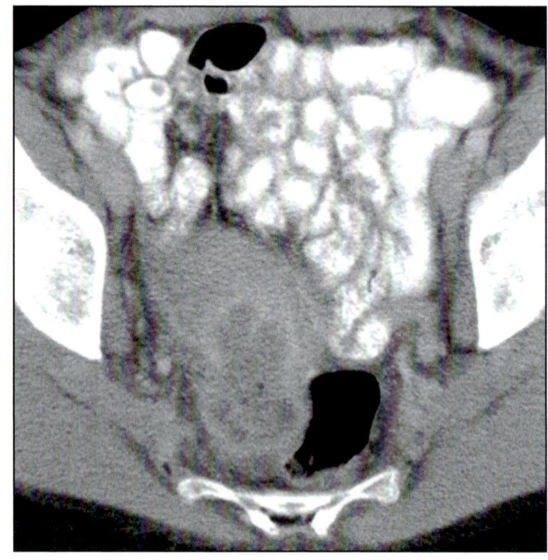

(Left) *Coronal oblique T2WI FSE MR (long axis) shows an exophytic cervical mass expanding the left vaginal fornix. There is full thickness invasion on the left with tumor extension into the parametrium ⇨.* ***(Right)*** *Coronal oblique T2WI FSE MR (donut view) in the same patient shows the cervical mass disrupting the normal stroma and expanding the endocervical canal. Note the contrast between the normal hypointense cervical stroma ➔ and the hyperintense mass ⇨.*

Stage IIB (T2b N0 M0)

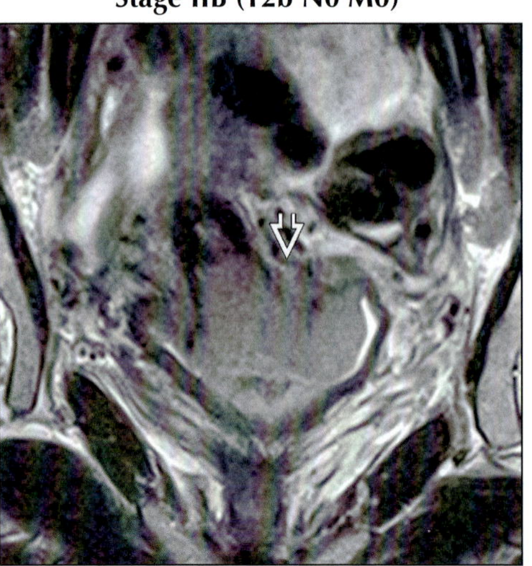

Stage IIB (T2b N0 M0)

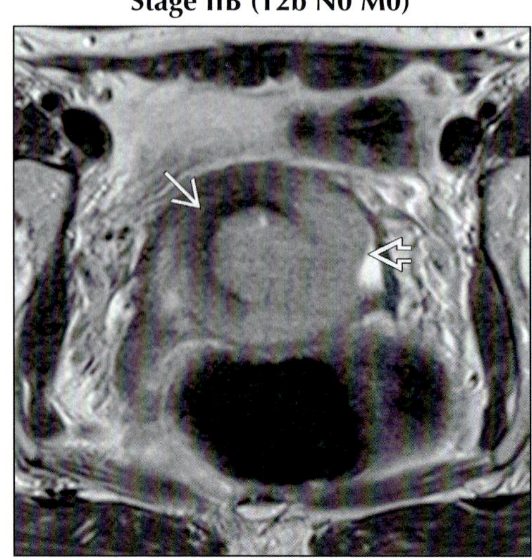

Stage IIIA (T3a N1 M0)

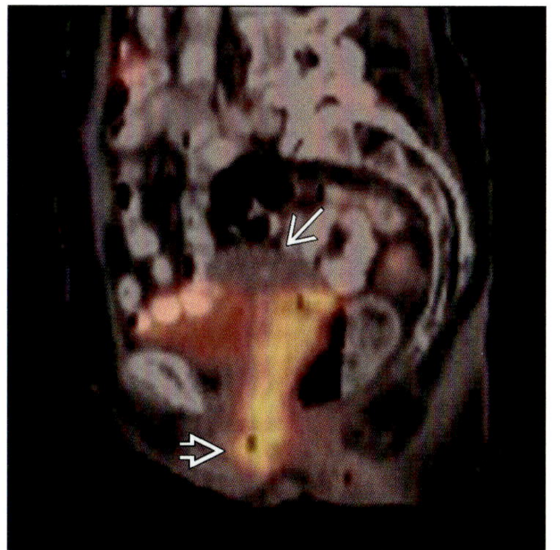

Stage IIIA (T3a N1 M0)

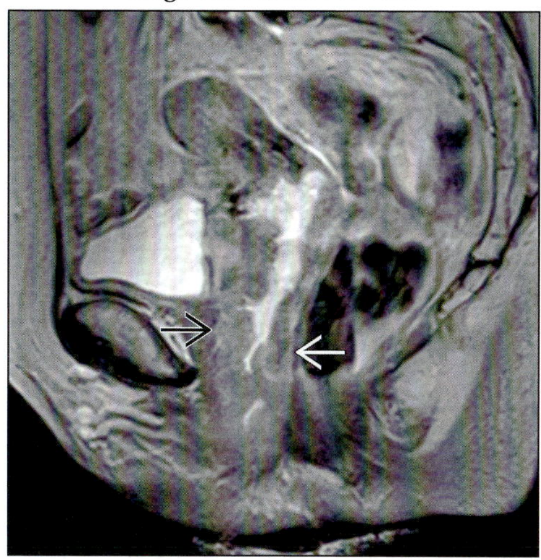

*(**Left**) Sagittal PET/CT shows avid tumor extending to the introitus ➲ in this octogenarian. Note the small, nonavid uterus ➡. (**Right**) Sagittal T2WI MR in the same patient shows markedly irregular and thickened vaginal contours anteriorly → and posteriorly ➡. Surgilube is present in the vagina.*

Stage IIIA (T3a N1 M0)

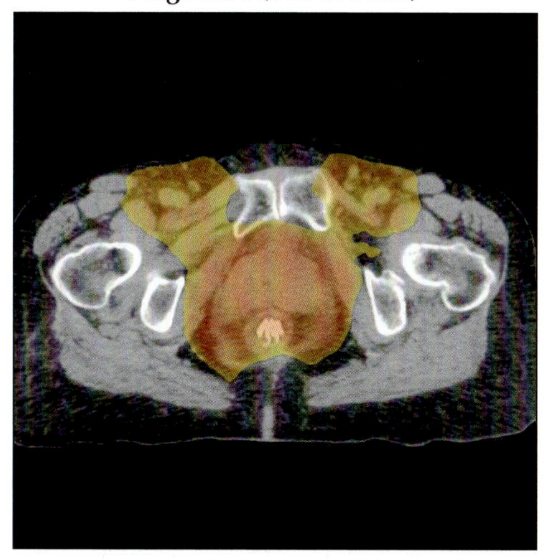

Stage IIIA (T3a N1 M0)

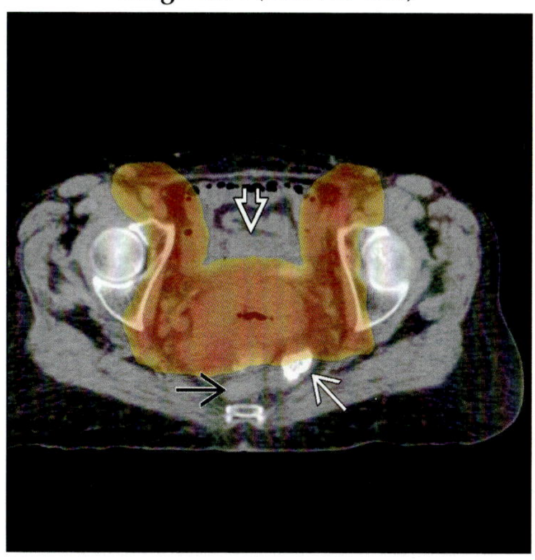

*(**Left**) Due to tumor extension to the lower 1/3 of the vagina and introitus in the same patient, it is necessary to treat the inguinal lymph nodes. Shown in orange is the 90% isodose surface in this IMRT treatment. (**Right**) In the same patient at the level of the femoral heads, IMRT permits relative sparing of the bladder ➲, rectum →, and sigmoid colon ➡. Shown in orange is the 90% isodose surface.*

Stage IIIA (T3a N1 M0)

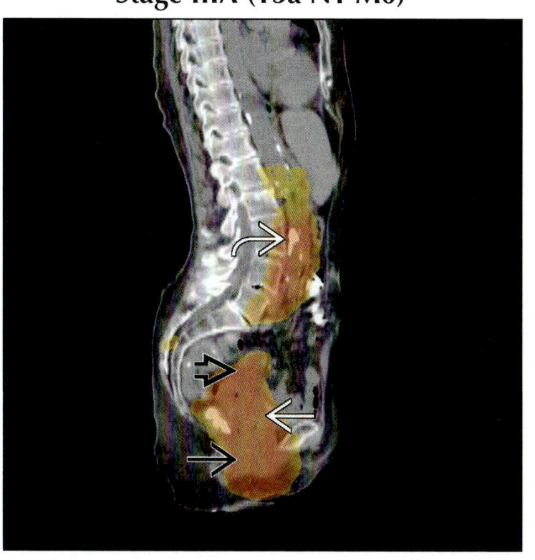

Stage IIIA (T3a N1 M0)

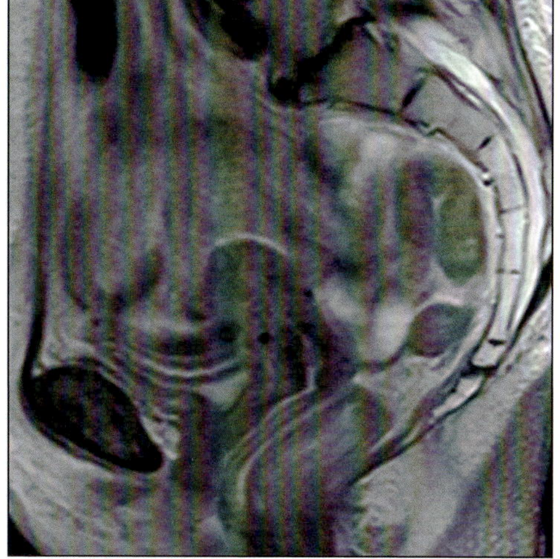

*(**Left**) Sagittal CT in the same patient shows the 90% isodose surface in this IMRT treatment. The vagina →, cervix ➡, and uterus ➲ are covered as well as the paraaortic chain. Note the extensive calcifications ➡ seen in the aorta. (**Right**) After 50.4 Gy external beam, the same patient had a complete clinical and radiographic response demonstrating the chemoradiosensitivity of squamous cell carcinomas.*

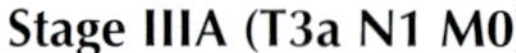

Stage IIIA (T3a N1 M0)

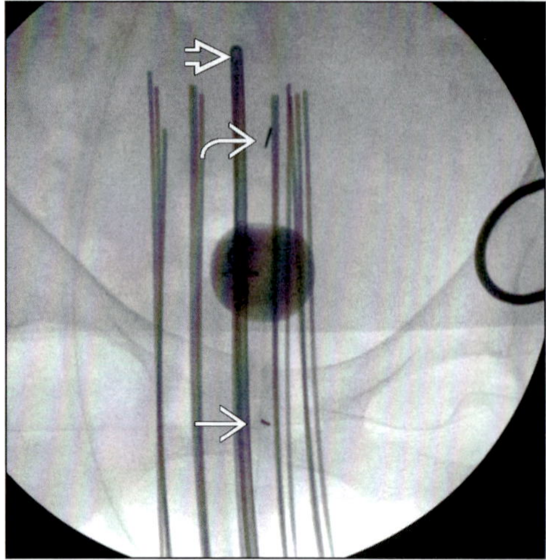

Stage IIIA (T3a N1 M0)

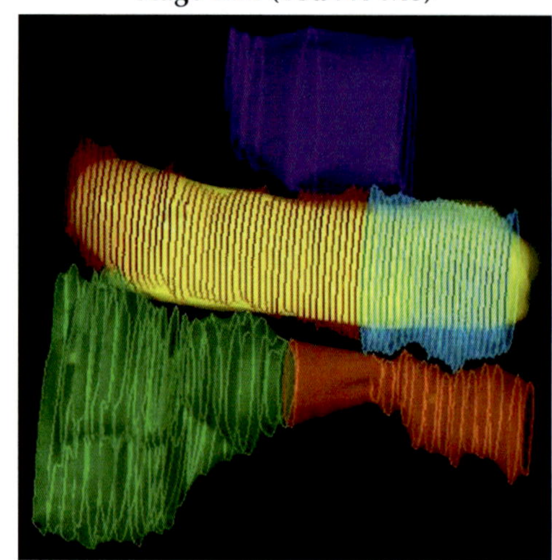

(Left) *In the same patient, intraoperative x-ray is used for interstitial needle placement. The presence of a uterine tandem is very important for good dosimetry. Fiducials mark the cephalad and caudal extent of tumor.* ***(Right)*** *DRR shows wire diagrams of bladder (purple), rectum (brown), and sigmoid colon (green). Yellow shows the 100% isodose surface. In this case, the lower vagina (blue) was intentionally prescribed a lower dose than the upper vagina (red).*

Stage IIIA (T3a N1 M0)

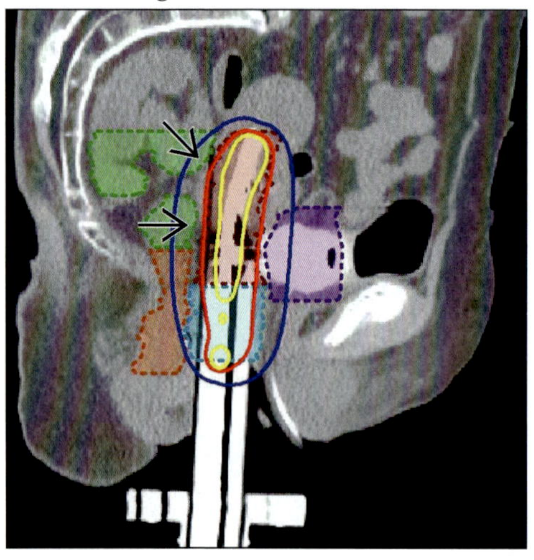

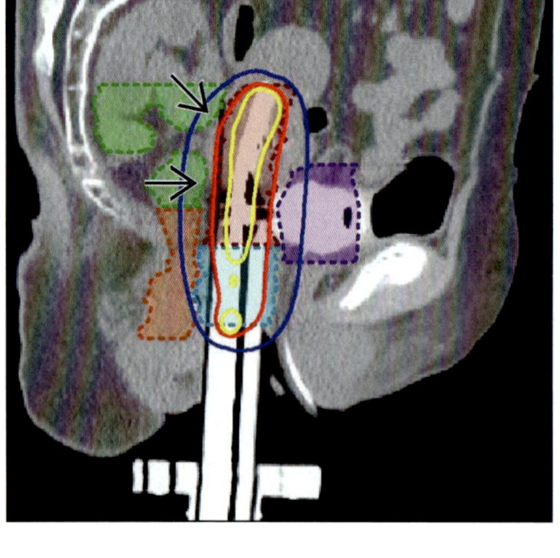

Stage IIIA (T3a N1 M0)

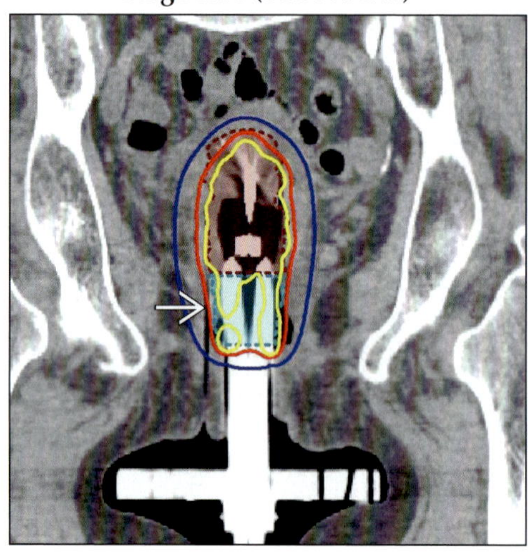

(Left) *Sagittal CT in the same patient reveals organs at risk, including bladder (purple), rectum (brown), and sigmoid colon (green). Note the proximity of parts of the sigmoid colon to the high dose region.* ***(Right)*** *Coronal CT in the same patient shows lower vagina (light blue) was given a lower dose due to the ↓ radiation tolerance of the distal vagina. Note the 100% isodose constriction seen in red. Also shown is the 150% isodose line in yellow and the 50% isodose line in blue.*

Stage IIIA (T3a N1 M0) Brachytherapy DVH

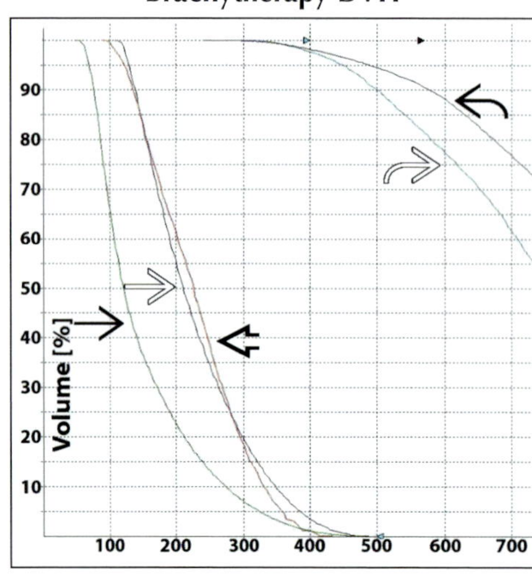

Extended Field Technique

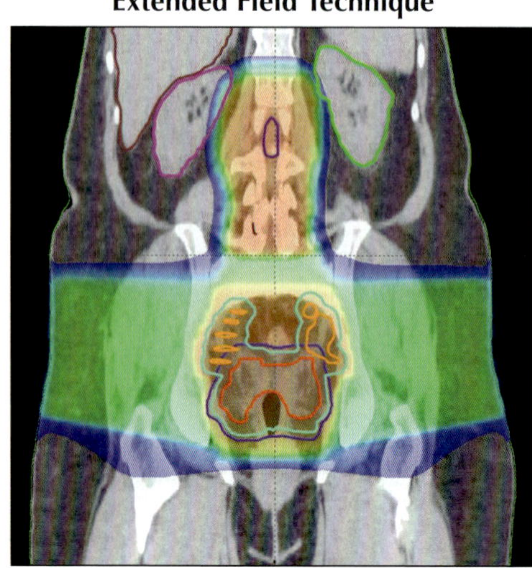

(Left) *As seen in the same patient, a principle advantage of brachytherapy is the dose separation of OARs from the CTV. In this case, the upper and lower vagina were contoured separately so they could receive different doses. OARs shown include sigmoid colon, bladder, and rectum.* ***(Right)*** *A common method to treat an extended field encompassing the paraaortic lymph nodes is AP/PA to the paraaortics and 4 field to the pelvis.*

Stage IIIB with Bullous Edema Sign

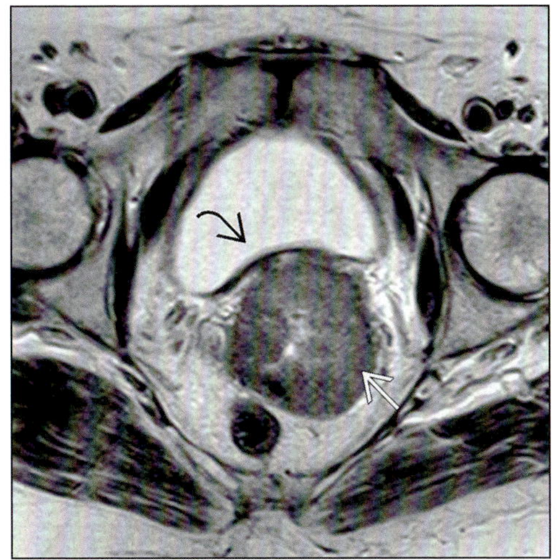

Stage IIIB with Bullous Edema Sign

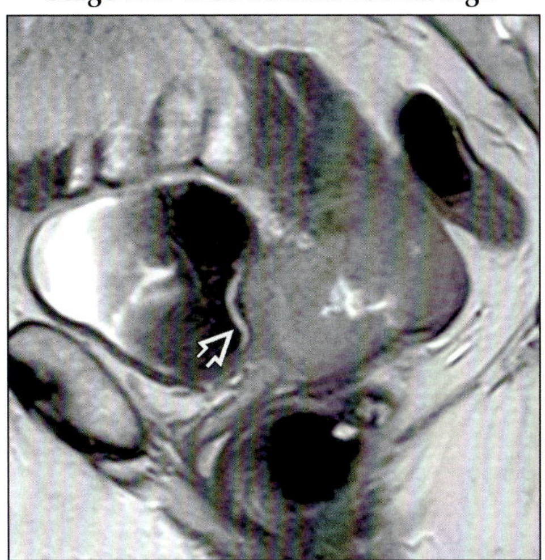

(Left) *Axial T2WI FSE MR shows hyperintense cervical mass ➡ invading the vesicouterine ligament. There is reactive T2 hyperintense thickening of the urinary bladder mucosa ↪, however no disruption of the low signal wall is present to suggest invasion. Left hydronephrosis was seen (not shown).* ***(Right)*** *Sagittal T2WI MR after intravenous contrast better demonstrates the reactive urinary bladder wall edema ➡, which is outlined by dense, low-signal gadolinium.*

Stage IIIB (T3b N0 M0)

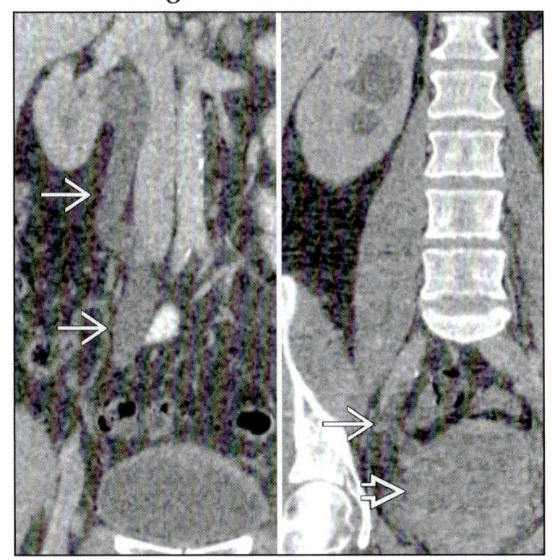

Stage IIIB (T3b N0 M0)

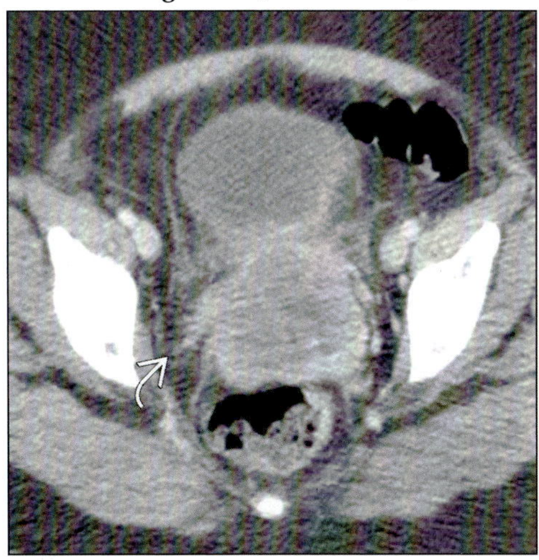

(Left) *Coronal CECT shows right hydronephrosis ➡ to the level of the cervical mass ➡, consistent with right ureteral invasion.* ***(Right)*** *Axial CECT in the same patient shows a heterogeneous cervical mass with frank extension into the paracervical fat on the right ↪. There is abrupt termination of the ureteral dilation in the previous figure at this level, making this a FIGO stage IIIB tumor.*

Stage IIIB (T3b N1 M0)

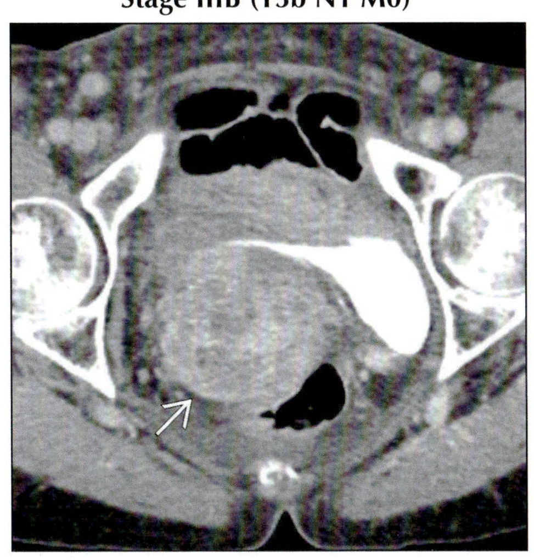

Stage IIIB (T3b N1 M0)

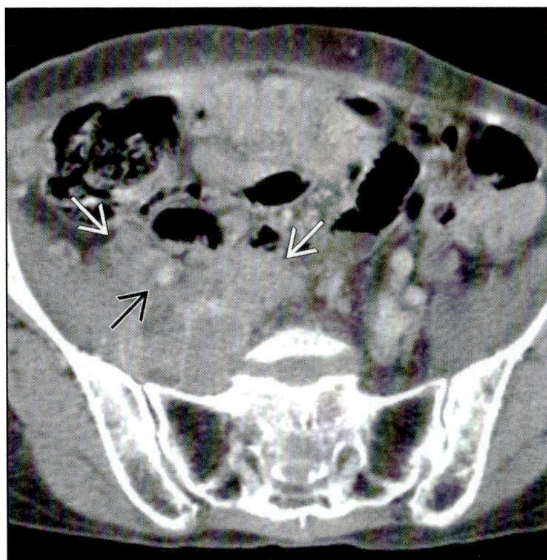

(Left) *Axial CECT shows a heterogeneous cervical mass ➡ placing mass effect on the urinary bladder and rectum without definite mucosal invasion.* ***(Right)*** *Axial CECT in the same patient shows extension of the cervical mass ➡ to encase the right external iliac artery ➡, consistent with pelvic sidewall invasion.*

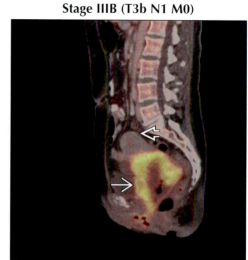

(**Left**) *Coronal CECT shows massive cervical tumor, bilateral hydronephrosis, and right common iliac adenopathy →.* (**Right**) *Sagittal PET/CT in same patient shows massive tumor adjacent to urinary bladder → and sparing the uterine fundus →. This young patient developed a vesicovaginal fistula during CRT.*

Stage IIIB (T3b N1 M0)

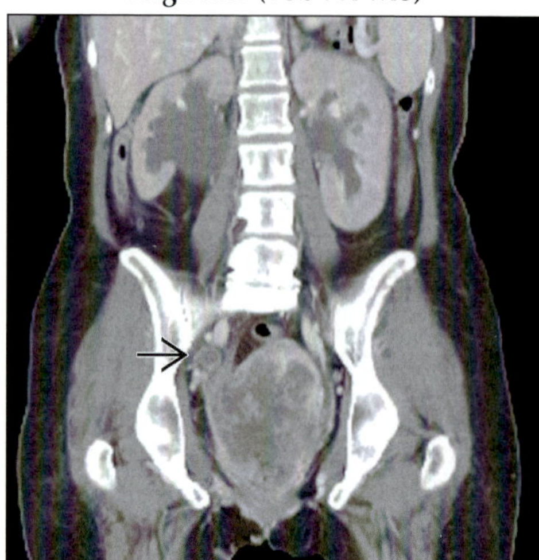

Stage IIIB (T3b N1 M0)

(**Left**) *Axial PET/CT in same patient shows bilateral iliac adenopathy →.* (**Right**) *AP radiograph depicts same patient. Due to the bilateral hydronephrosis, ureteral stents were placed. Anterograde contrast is shown filling the left ureter → during US-guided percutaneous placement.*

Stage IIIB (T3b N1 M0)

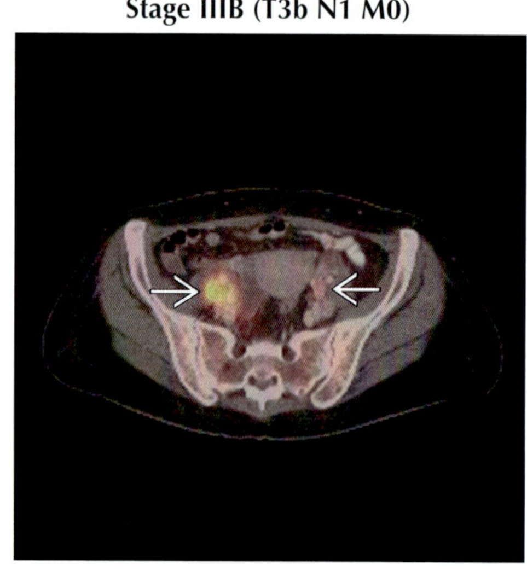

Stage IIIB (T3b N1 M0)

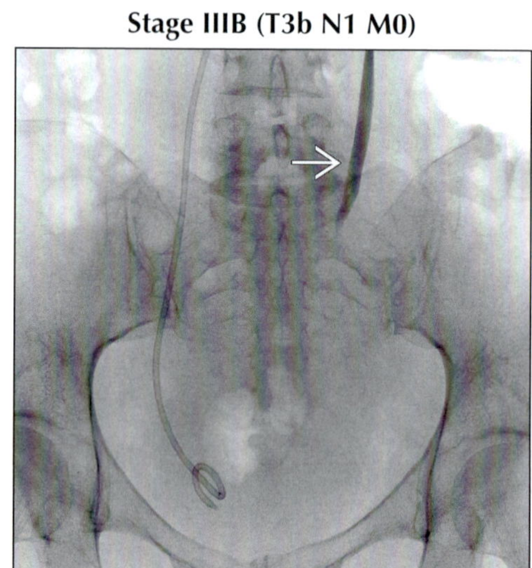

(**Left**) *Sagittal PET/CT 3 months after completion of CRT in same patient shows suspicious FDG at the cervix →. The vesicovaginal fistula spontaneously closed 2 years after treatment, and at 4 years out the patient remains free of disease.* (**Right**) *Sagittal CECT shows large cervical mass → compressing rectum → with a hematogenous metastasis to the pubis →.*

Stage IIIB (T3b N1 M0)

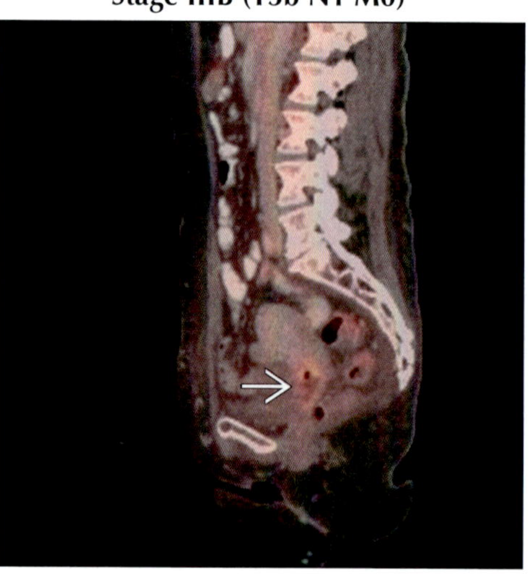

Stage IVB (T4a N1 M1)

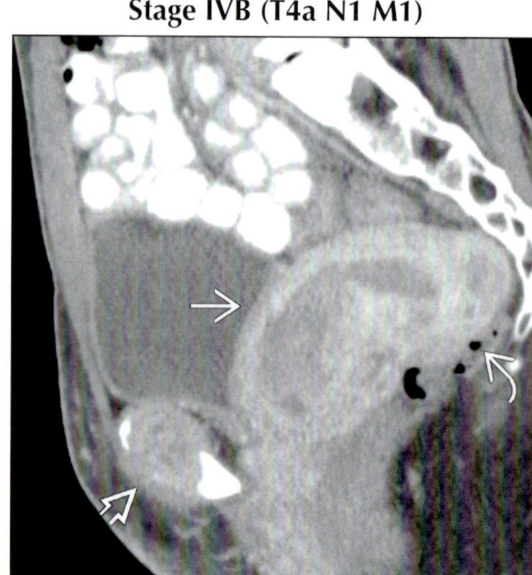

Stage IVB (T2b N1 M1)

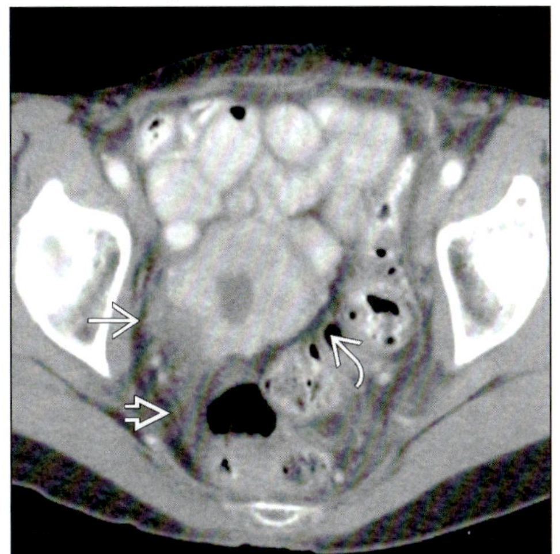

Stage IVB (T2b N1 M1)

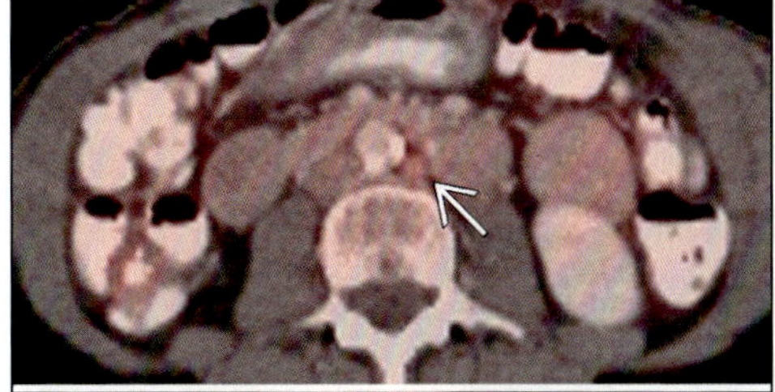

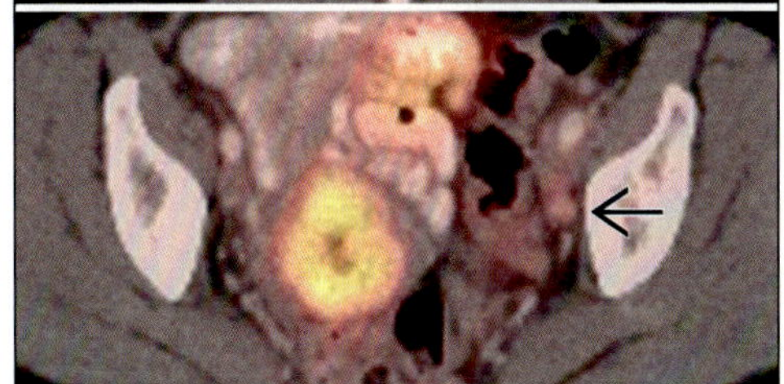

(Left) *Axial CECT shows a cervical mass. Irregularity of the right tumor-fat interface, increased density of the parametrial fat, and thickening of the right uterosacral ligament are consistent with parametrial invasion. The left parametrial fat is preserved.* **(Right)** *Axial PET/CT in the same patient shows the hypermetabolic cervical mass. Small left obturator and paraaortic nodes are not enlarged but hypermetabolic, upstaging this patient.*

Stage IVB (T1b2 N1 M1)

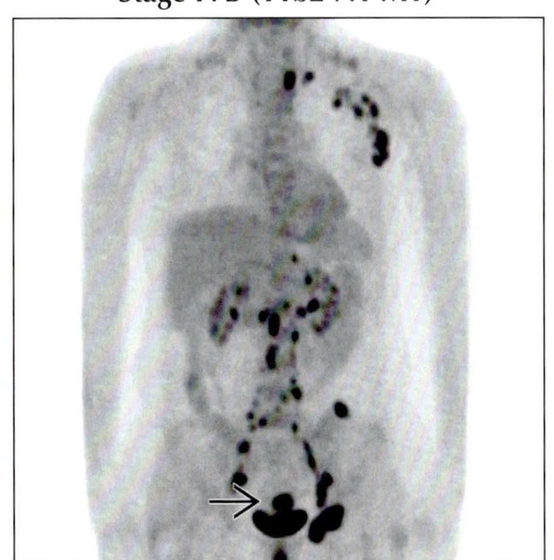

Stage IVB (T2b N0 M1)

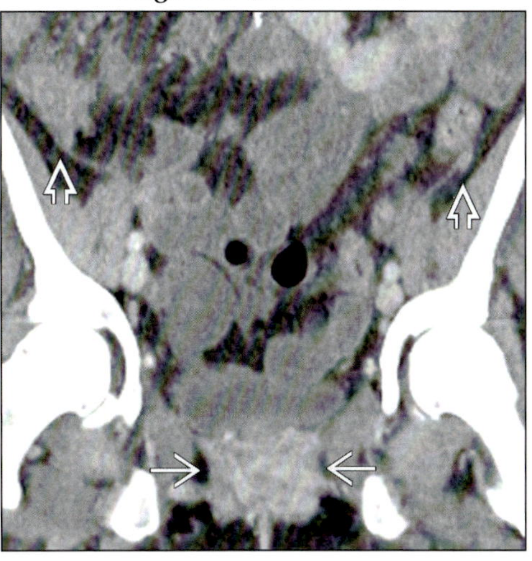

(Left) *Whole-body PET image shows overall disease burden in a patient with metastatic cervical cancer. Note the FDG-avid primary tumor, as well as metastases in the inguinal, iliac, periaortic, supraclavicular, and axillary lymph nodes.* **(Right)** *Coronal CECT shows an enhancing urethral mass in a patient with metastatic cervical cancer. Also note peritoneal carcinomatosis. Numerous pulmonary nodules, although present, are not shown.*

Stage IVB (T2a N1 M1)

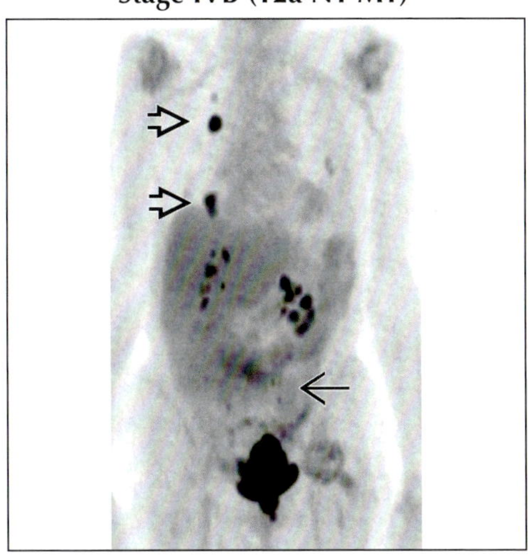

Stage IVB (T2a2 N0 M1)

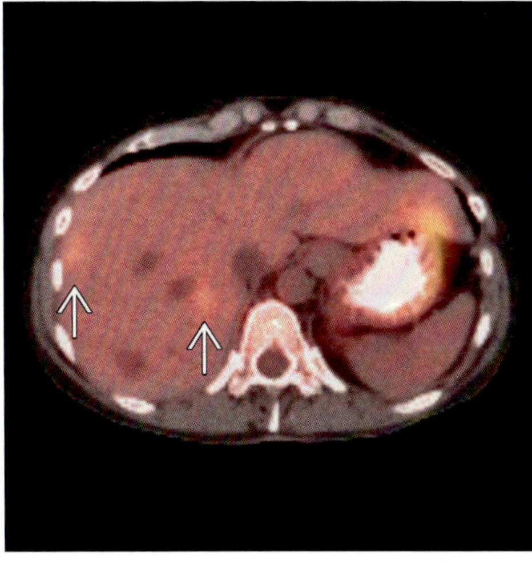

(Left) *Whole-body PET image shows FDG-avid, subcentimeter common iliac lymph nodes and lung nodules. The findings changed the treatment from curative to palliative.* **(Right)** *Axial fused PET/CT shows 2 focal areas of increased FDG activity in the liver, compatible with hepatic metastatic disease.*

CERVIX

*(**Left**) Axial CECT shows replacement of the cervix by a mass that invades anteriorly into the urinary bladder lumen. Note nodular thickening of the left uterosacral ligament. (**Right**) Axial CECT in the same patient after administration of rectal contrast better shows eccentric wall thickening of the left rectum and luminal irregularity indicative of mucosal invasion with clear loss in intervening fat plane.*

Stage IVA (T4 N0 M0)

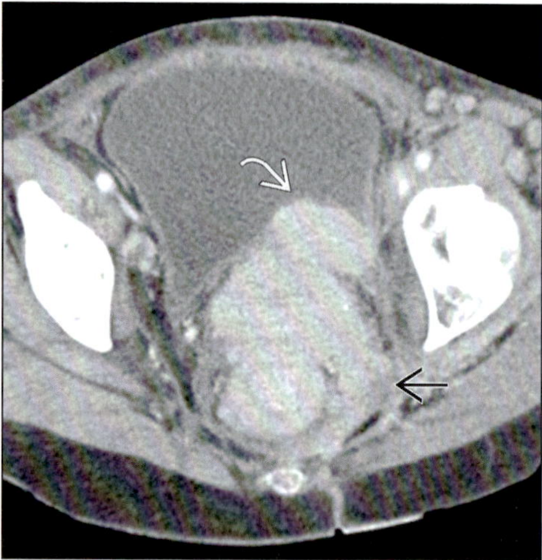

Stage IVA (T4 N0 M0)

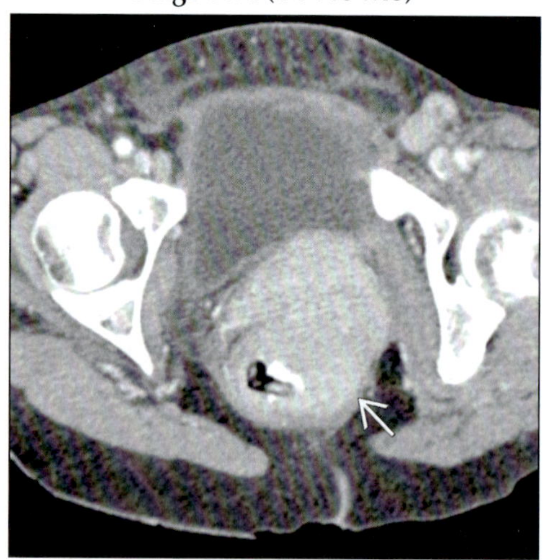

*(**Left**) Coronal PET shows metastatic clear cell carcinoma arising in the posterior aspect of the cervix and extensive pelvic, paraaortic, and biopsy-proven supraclavicular adenopathy. Due to metastatic disease, she was treated 1st with cisplatin-based chemotherapy. (**Right**) Coronal T2WI MR in the same patient shows mass effect into the bowel and rectal invasion, which was demonstrated on colonoscopy.*

Stage IVB (T4 N1 M1)

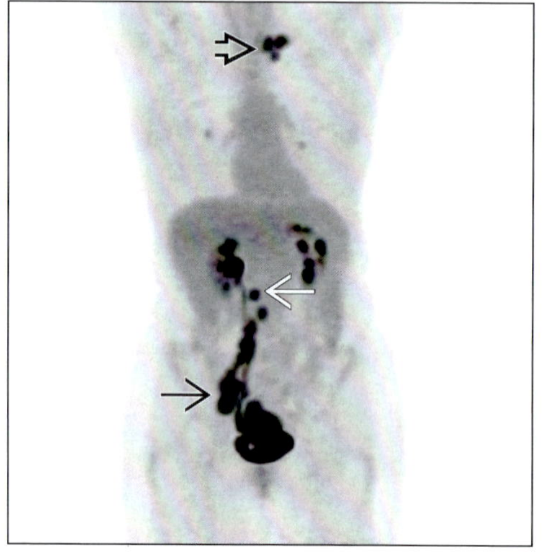

Stage IVB (T4 N1 M1)

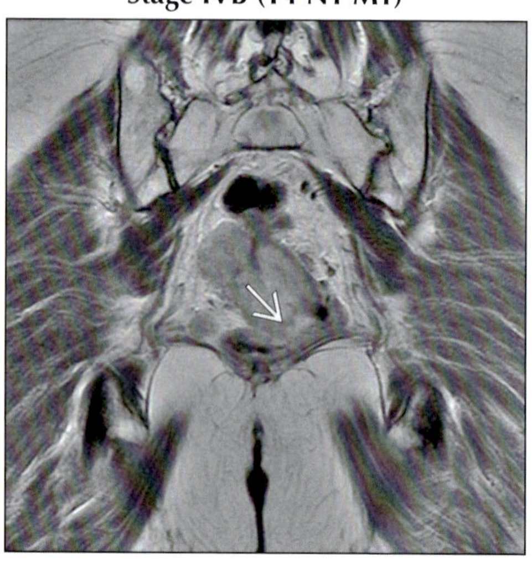

*(**Left**) In the same patient, sagittal T2WI MR shows a large heterogeneous cervical mass. (**Right**) In the same patient after cisplatin-based chemotherapy, sagittal PET/CT revealed a near-complete PET response to the cervical mass and the paraaortic disease. During chemotherapy, the supraclavicular node increased in size, and the patient was subsequently treated with external beam.*

Stage IVB (T4 N1 M1)

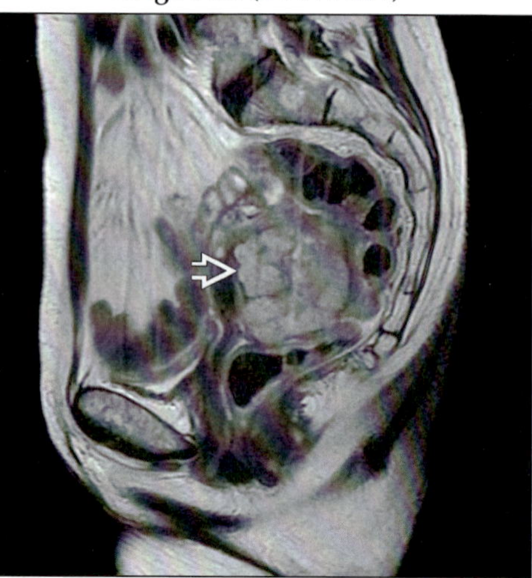

Stage IVB (T4 N1 M1)

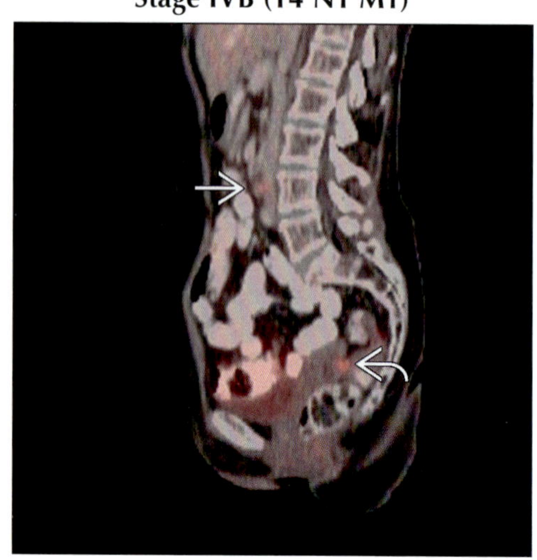

Cystic Pelvic Sidewall Recurrence

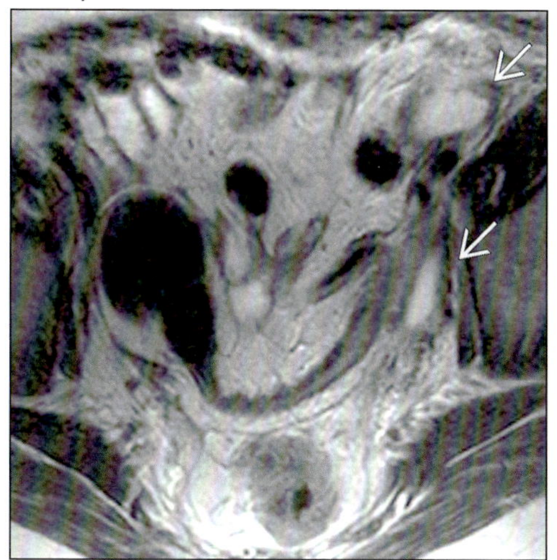

Central Recurrence

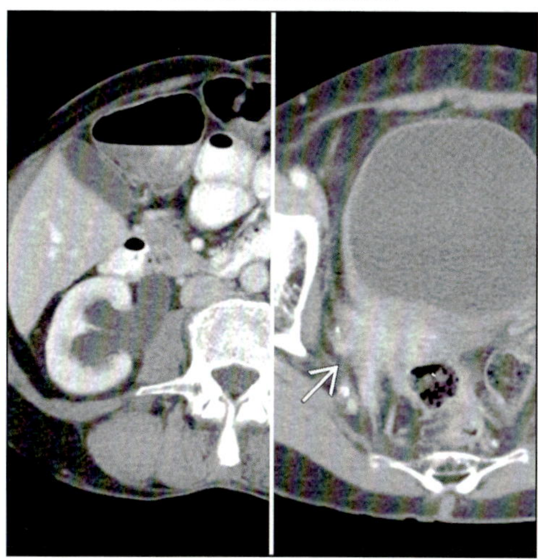

(Left) *Axial T2WI FSE MR shows 2 cystic masses ➡ at the left pelvic sidewall in this patient with cervical cancer status post remote hysterectomy.* ***(Right)*** *Axial CECT shows right hydronephrosis with obstruction of the ureter by an irregular enhancing mass at the right vaginal cuff. The mass ➡ extends into the parametrial tissues, up to the obturator internus muscle, to the thickened urinary bladder and rectum with loss of intervening fat planes.*

Recurrence

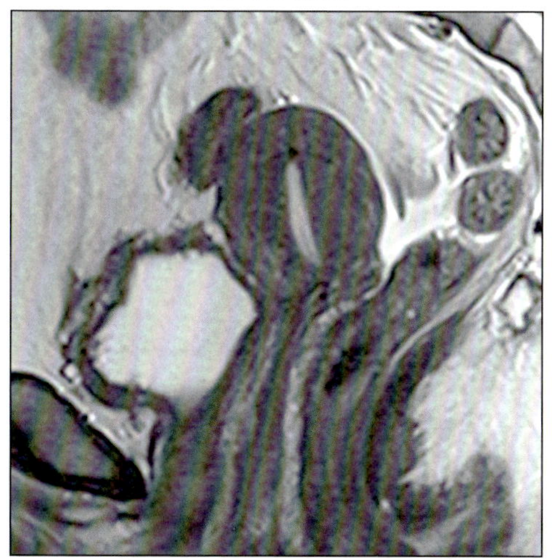

Recurrence

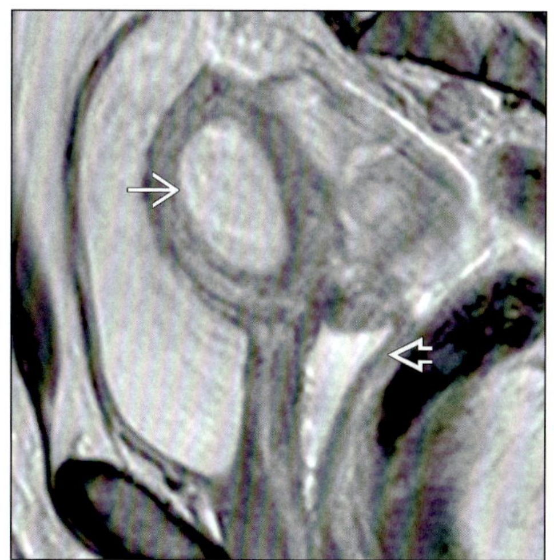

(Left) *Sagittal T2WI FSE MR in a patient with cervical cancer shows the normal post-trachelectomy appearance with absence of the cervix.* ***(Right)*** *Sagittal T2WI FSE MR in the same patient 1 year later demonstrates distension of the uterine cavity ➡ with fluid, concerning for tumor recurrence and obstruction. Note distension of the vagina ➡ with Surgilube.*

Recurrence

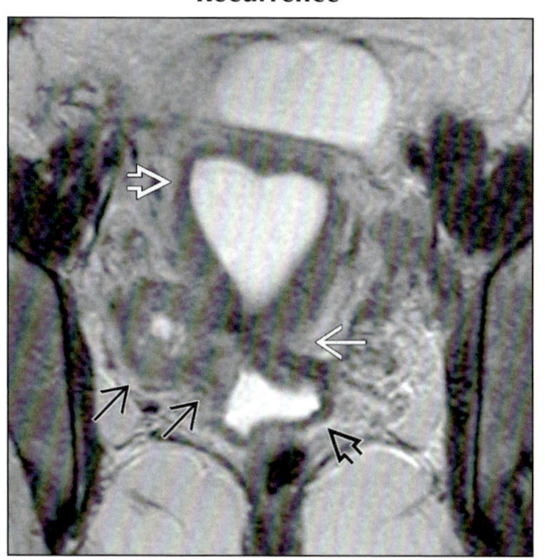

Recurrence

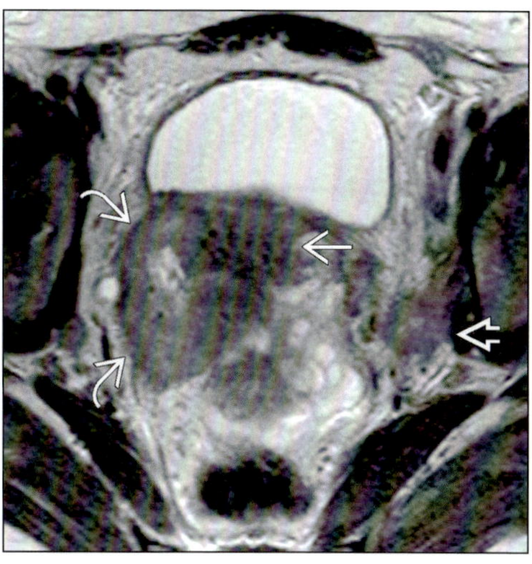

(Left) *Coronal oblique T2WI FSE MR in the same patient shows the uterine cavity distended ➡ with fluid and stenosis ➡ with an associated T2 hyperintense exophytic mass ➡ at the level of the trachelectomy. Note the utility of distending the vagina ➡ with Surgilube.* ***(Right)*** *Coronal oblique (donut) T2WI FSE MR in the same patient at the level of the stenosis ➡ shows the exophytic recurrent tumor ➡ and pelvic adenopathy ➡.*

UTERUS

(T) Primary Tumor for Uterine Carcinomas

Adapted from 7th edition AJCC Staging Forms.

TNM	*FIGO*	*Definitions*
TX		Primary tumor cannot be assessed
T0		No evidence of primary tumor
Tis[1]		Carcinoma in situ (preinvasive carcinoma)
T1	I	Tumor confined to corpus uteri
T1a	IA	Tumor limited to endometrium or invades < 1/2 of the myometrium
T1b	IB	Tumor invades ≥ 1/2 of the myometrium
T2	II	Tumor invades stromal connective tissue of cervix but does not extend beyond uterus[2]
T3a	IIIA	Tumor invades serosa &/or adnexa (direct extension or metastasis)
T3b	IIIB	Vaginal involvement (direct extension or metastasis) or parametrial involvement
T4	IVA	Tumor invades bladder mucosa &/or bowel mucosa (bullous edema is not sufficient to classify a tumor as T4)

[1]*FIGO no longer includes stage 0 (Tis).*

[2]*Endocervical glandular involvement only should be considered as stage I and not as stage II.*

(N) Regional Lymph Nodes for Uterine Carcinomas

Adapted from 7th edition AJCC Staging Forms.

TNM	*FIGO*	*Definitions*
NX		Regional lymph nodes cannot be assessed
N0		No regional lymph node metastasis
N1	IIIC1	Regional lymph node metastasis to pelvic lymph nodes
N2	IIIC2	Regional lymph node metastasis to paraaortic lymph nodes ± positive pelvic lymph nodes

(M) Distant Metastasis for Uterine Carcinomas

Adapted from 7th edition AJCC Staging Forms.

TNM	*FIGO*	*Definitions*
M0		No distant metastasis
M1	IVB	Distant metastasis (includes metastasis to inguinal lymph nodes intraperitoneal disease, or lung, liver, or bone; excludes metastasis to paraaortic lymph nodes, vagina, pelvic serosa, or adnexa)

AJCC Stages/Prognostic Groups for Uterine Carcinomas*

Adapted from 7th edition AJCC Staging Forms.

Stage	*T*	*N*	*M*
0	Tis	N0	M0
I	T1	N0	M0
IA	T1a	N0	M0
IB	T1b	N0	M0
II	T2	N0	M0
III	T3	N0	M0
IIIA	T3a	N0	M0
IIIB	T3b	N0	M0
IIIC1	T1-T3	N1	M0
IIIC2	T1-T3	N2	M0
IVA	T4	Any N	M0
IVB	Any T	Any N	M1

**Carcinosarcomas should be staged as carcinoma.*

(T) Primary Tumor for Leiomyosarcoma and Endometrial Stromal Sarcoma[1]

Adapted from 7th edition AJCC Staging Forms.

TNM	*FIGO*	*Definitions*
TX		Primary tumor cannot be assessed
T0		No evidence of primary tumor
T1	I	Tumor limited to the uterus
T1a	IA	Tumor ≤ 5 cm in greatest dimensions
T1b	IB	Tumor > 5 cm
T2	II	Tumor extends beyond the uterus, within the pelvis
T2a	IIA	Tumor involves adnexa
T2b	IIB	Tumor involves other pelvic tissues
T3	III[2]	Tumor infiltrates abdominal tissues
T3a	IIIA	1 site
T3b	IIB	> 1 site
T4	IVA	Tumor invades bladder or rectum

[1]*Simultaneous tumors of the uterine corpus and ovary/pelvis in association with ovarian/pelvic endometriosis should be classified as independent primary tumors.*

[2]*In this stage, lesions must infiltrate abdominal tissues and not just protrude into the abdominal cavity.*

(N) Regional Lymph Nodes for Leiomyosarcoma and Endometrial Stromal Sarcoma

Adapted from 7th edition AJCC Staging Forms.

TNM	*FIGO*	*Definitions*
NX		Regional lymph nodes cannot be assessed
N0		No regional lymph node metastasis
N1	IIIC	Regional lymph node metastasis

UTERUS

(M) Distant Metastasis for Leiomyosarcoma and Endometrial Stromal Sarcoma

Adapted from 7th edition AJCC Staging Forms.

TNM	*FIGO*	*Definitions*
M0		No distant metastasis
M1	IVB	Distant metastasis (excluding adnexa, pelvic and abdominal tissues)

(T) Primary Tumor for Adenosarcoma[1]

Adapted from 7th edition AJCC Staging Forms.

TNM	*FIGO*	*Descriptions*
TX		Primary tumor cannot be assessed
T0		No evidence of primary tumor
T1	I	Tumor limited to the uterus
T1a	IA	Tumor limited to the endometrium/endocervix
T1b	IB	Tumor invades to < 1/2 of the myometrium
T1c	IC	Tumor invades ≥ 1/2 of the myometrium
T2	II	Tumor extends beyond the uterus, within the pelvis
T2a	IIA	Tumor involves adnexa
T2b	IIB	Tumor involves other pelvic tissues
T3	III[2]	Tumor involves abdominal tissues
T3a	IIIA	1 site
T3b	IIIB	> 1 site
T4	IVA	Tumor invades bladder or rectum

[1]*Simultaneous tumors of the uterine corpus and ovary/pelvis in association with ovarian/pelvic endometriosis should be classified as independent primary tumors.*

[2]*In this stage, lesions must infiltrate abdominal tissues and not just protrude into the abdominal cavity.*

(N) Regional Lymph Nodes for Adenosarcoma

Adapted from 7th edition AJCC Staging Forms.

TNM	*FIGO*	*Descriptions*
NX		Regional lymph nodes cannot be assessed
N0		No regional lymph node metastasis
N1	IIIC	Regional lymph node metastasis

(M) Distant Metastasis for Adenosarcoma

Adapted from 7th edition AJCC Staging Forms.

TNM	*FIGO*	*Definitions*
M0		No distant metastasis
M1	IVB	Distant metastasis (excluding adnexa, pelvic and abdominal tissues)

AJCC Stages/Prognostic Groups for Uterine Sarcomas

Adapted from 7th edition AJCC Staging Forms.

Stage	*T*	*N*	*M*
I	T1	N0	M0
IA[1]	T1a	N0	M0
IB[1]	T1b	N0	M0
IC[2]	T1c	N0	M0
II	T2	N0	M0
IIIA	T3a	N0	M0
IIIB	T3b	N0	M0
IIIC	T1, T2, T3	N1	M0
IVA	T4	Any N	M0
IVB	Any T	Any N	M1

[1]*Stage IA and IB differ from those applied for leiomyosarcoma and endometrial stromal sarcoma.*

[2]*Stage IC does not apply for leiomyosarcoma and endometrial stromal sarcoma.*

Stage IA-IB (T1a-T1b N0 M0)

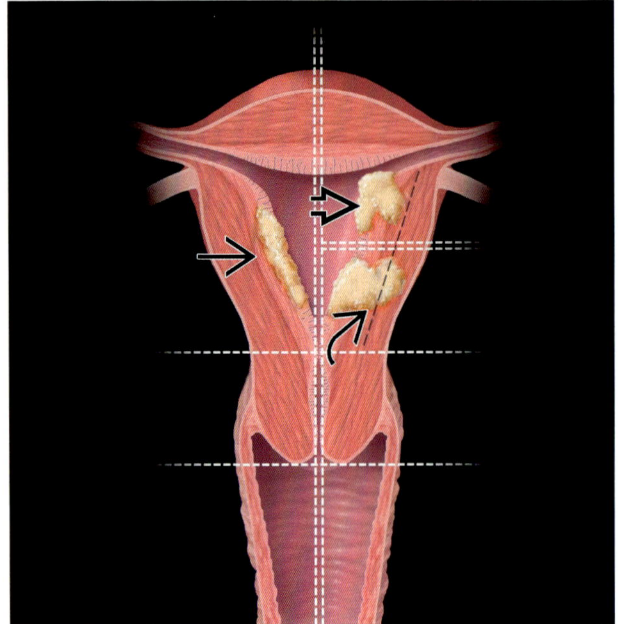

Coronal graphic shows T1 tumors, those confined to corpus uteri. T1a tumors are limited to the endometrium or involve < 1/2 of the myometrium. T1b tumors invade 1/2 or more of the myometrium indicated by the tumor traversing the dotted horizontal line, marking the halfway plane of the myometrium.

Stage II (T2 N0 M0)

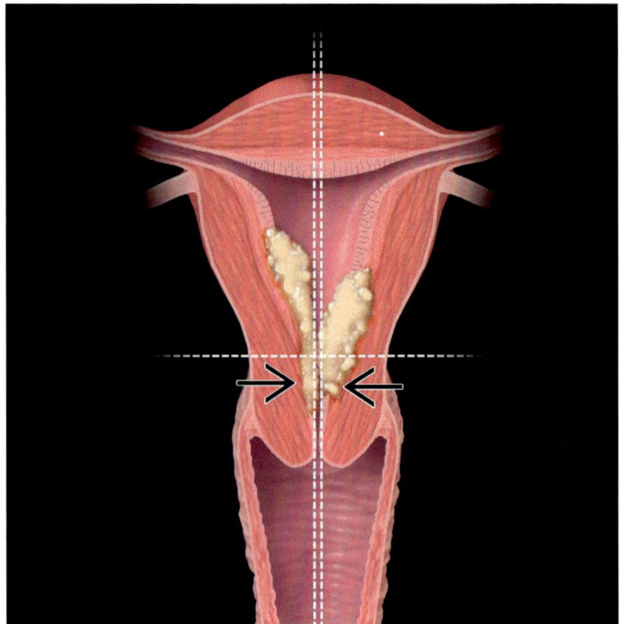

Coronal graphic shows a typical T2 tumor, which invades the cervix but does not extend beyond the uterus. Endocervical glandular involvement only should be considered stage I and not stage II.

Stage IIIA-B (T3a-T3b N0 M0)

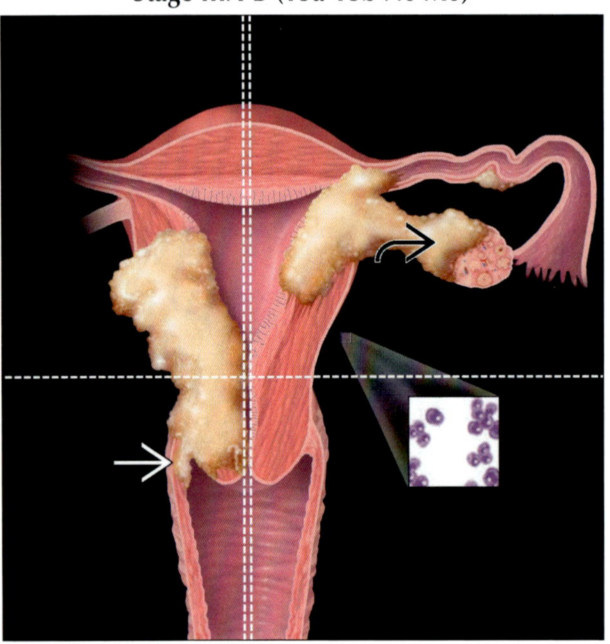

Coronal graphic shows stage III disease, both T3a, which is a tumor involving the serosa &/or adnexa, and T3b, which is a tumor that involves the vagina by direct extension or metastases or parametrial involvement.

Stage IVA (T4 N0 M0)

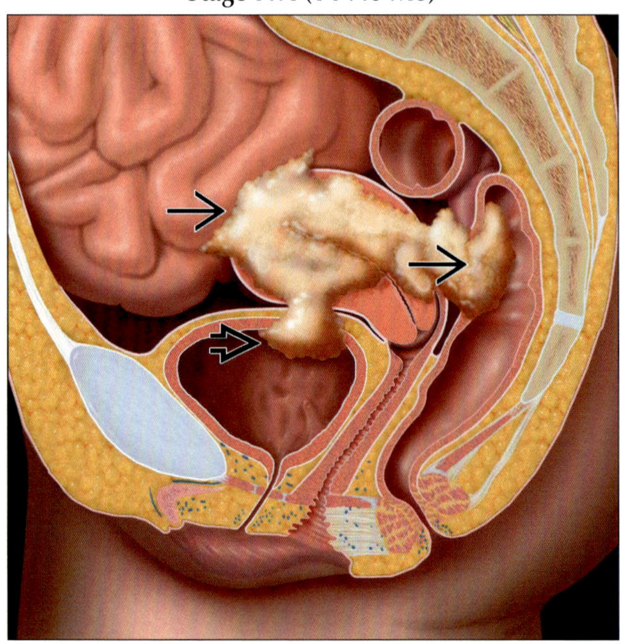

Sagittal graphic shows stage IVA disease with a tumor that invades the bladder mucosa &/or bowel mucosa. However, bullous edema is not sufficient to classify a tumor as T4. Stage IVB is defined as distant metastasis, including metastasis to inguinal lymph nodes, peritoneum, lung, liver, or bone.

Stages IIIC1 and IIIC2

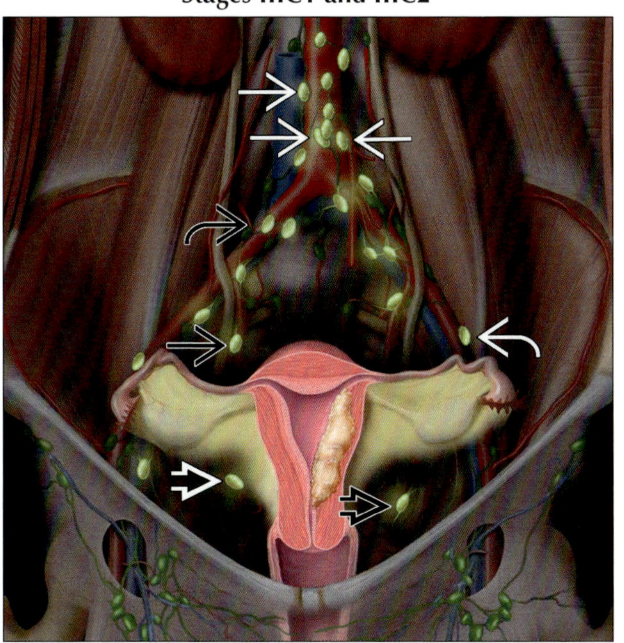

Coronal graphic shows an example of stage IIIC1 (pelvic adenopathy, N1) and stage IIIC2 (paraaortic lymph nodes ➔ ± positive pelvic lymph nodes, N2). Within the pelvis are parametrial ➔, obturator ➔, internal iliac ➔, external iliac ➔, and common iliac lymph nodes ➔.

Endometrioid Adenocarcinoma

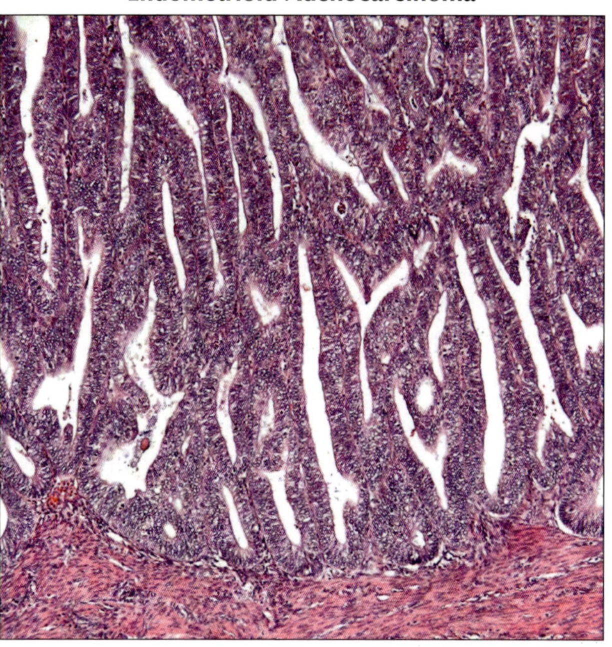

Endometrial adenocarcinoma, endometrioid type is characterized by back-to-back glands with no intervening stroma. The term "endometrioid" reflects the similarity of the tumor to normal endometrium. (Courtesy M. Nucci, MD.)

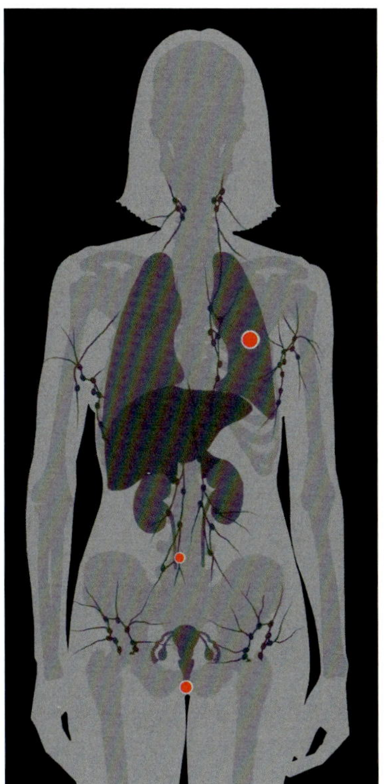

INITIAL SITE OF RECURRENCE

Distant	12%
Vagina	7%
Pelvis	5%

Data represent 75 failures in 364 patients, of which 238 received RT in the pre-CT era. Stage distribution: 84%, 11%, 4%, and 1% for stages I, II, III, and IV, respectively. Salazar OM et al: IJROBP. 2:1101-1107, 1977.

UTERUS

OVERVIEW

General Comments

- Corpus uteri carcinoma is the most common gynecologic cancer in USA
  - Also the most common gynecologic cancer in many other developed countries
- 95% of uterine malignancies are carcinomas
- Endometrial cancer can be divided into 2 types
  - **Type I**
    - Includes endometrioid histology
    - Makes up to 70-80% of new diagnoses in USA
    - Association with chronic estrogen exposure
    - Premalignant disease, such as endometrial hyperplasia, often precedes cancer
    - More commonly estrogen and progesterone receptor positive
  - **Type II**
    - Nonendometrioid histology
    - Includes papillary serous and clear cell carcinomas
    - Aggressive clinical course
    - No association with estrogen exposure has been identified
    - Not associated with readily observable premalignant disease

Classification

- **Primary malignant tumors (WHO classification)**
  - **Endometrial carcinoma**
    - Endometrioid adenocarcinoma
    - Mucinous adenocarcinoma
    - Serous adenocarcinoma
    - Clear cell adenocarcinoma
    - Mixed cell adenocarcinoma
    - Squamous cell carcinoma
    - Transitional cell carcinoma
    - Small cell carcinoma
  - **Mesenchymal tumors**
    - Endometrial stromal and related tumors
      - Endometrial stromal sarcoma, low grade
      - Endometrial stromal nodule
      - Undifferentiated endometrial sarcoma
    - Smooth muscle tumors
      - Leiomyosarcoma (epithelioid and myxoid variants)
      - Smooth muscle tumor of uncertain malignant potential
      - Leiomyoma, not otherwise specified
    - Miscellaneous mesenchymal tumors
  - **Mixed epithelial and mesenchymal tumors**
    - Carcinosarcoma
    - Adenosarcoma
    - Carcinofibroma
    - Adenofibroma
    - Adenomyoma
  - **Gestational trophoblastic disease**
    - Trophoblastic neoplasms
      - Choriocarcinoma
      - Placental site trophoblastic tumor
      - Epithelioid trophoblastic tumor
    - Molar pregnancies
      - Hydatiform mole
    - Nonneoplastic
      - Nonmolar trophoblastic lesions
  - **Miscellaneous tumors**
    - Sex cord-like tumors
    - Neuroectodermal tumors
    - Melanotic paraganglioma
    - Tumors of germ cell type
    - Others
  - **Lymphoid and hematopoietic tumors**
    - Malignant lymphoma
    - Leukemia

NATURAL HISTORY

General Features

- Comments
  - Endometrioid adenocarcinoma
    - Represents 75-80% of endometrial cancers

Epidemiology & Cancer Incidence

- Age of onset
  - Most common in 6th and 7th decades of life
- Estimated 2012 statistics in USA for endometrial cancer
  - 47,130 new cases: 4th highest incidence for women after breast, lung, and colorectal cancer
  - 8,010 deaths: 8th highest death rate
  - Chance of endometrial cancer is 1 in 38 from birth to death
- Represents 6% of all cancers in women
- **Risk factors**
  - Estrogen hormone replacement therapy
    - Increases risk 2-10x
  - Obesity
    - Increases risk 2-20x
  - Polycystic ovarian syndrome (PCOS)
    - Increases risk 3x
  - Chronic anovulation and infertility
    - Increases risk 3x
  - Tamoxifen
    - Increases risk 2-3x
  - Nulliparity
    - Increases risk 2-3x
  - Early menarche
    - Increases risk 2-3x
  - Late menopause
    - Increases risk 2-3x
  - Hypertension
    - Increases risk 2-3x
  - Diabetes
    - Increases risk 2-3x
  - Pelvic RT
  - History of polyps and other benign uterine growths
  - Sedentary lifestyle
- Demographics
  - **Ethnicity**
    - Common in eastern Europe and USA
    - Uncommon in Asia

Genetics

- Lynch syndrome (hereditary nonpolyposis colorectal cancer)
  - Autosomal dominant disease due to mutations in mismatch repair genes: *MLH1*, *MSH2*, *MSH6*, and *PMS2*
    - 2-7% of all colorectal cancers

- Associated with ↑ risk of colorectal, endometrial, ovarian, stomach, hepatobiliary, upper urinary, brain, and skin cancers
- Endometrial cancer
  - 2-5% of all endometrial cancers due to Lynch syndrome
  - Lifetime risk is 40-60%, which is likely > risk of colorectal cancer
  - Annual screening after age 30

- **Type I endometrial cancers**
  - Microsatellite instability
  - *KRAS* mutations
  - *PTEN* mutations
  - DNA mismatch repair defects
  - Mutations in *p53*
    - Less frequent
    - Late occurrence in development (differing from type II cancers)
- **Type II endometrial cancers**
  - Mutations in *p53*
    - Common mutation
  - Nondiploid karyotype
  - Her-2/neu (c-erB-2) overexpression

Associated Diseases, Abnormalities

- Endometrial hyperplasia
  - Atypical hyperplasia 40% chance of progressing to carcinoma

Microscopic Pathology

- H&E
  - Histological patterns can be broadly divided into type I and type II endometrial cancers
    - Endometrioid histology
    - Nonendometrioid histology
  - Histopathologic types
    - Endometrioid carcinomas
      - Most common endometrial cancer (75-80% of cases)
      - Most are well differentiated
      - Back-to-back glandular proliferation of endometrium lacking intervening stroma
    - Villoglandular adenocarcinoma
      - Many villous fronds
      - Delicate central fibrovascular cores of villi and simpler branching pattern differentiates it from papillary serous carcinoma
    - Adenocarcinoma with benign squamous elements, squamous metaplasia, or squamous differentiation (adenoacanthoma)
    - Adenosquamous carcinoma (mixed adenocarcinoma and squamous cell carcinoma)
    - Mucinous adenocarcinoma
    - Serous adenocarcinoma (papillary serous)
      - Bizarre nuclei
      - Scant cytoplasm
      - Nuclear stratification
      - Marked nuclear atypia
      - Complex papillary architecture
      - Psammoma bodies (seen in 30% of cases)
      - Aggressive nature
      - Often presents late
    - Clear cell carcinoma
      - Possible patterns include tubulocystic, papillary, or solid
      - Psammoma bodies may be present but not as commonly as in papillary serous tumors
      - Clear cell appearance due to glycogen
      - Myometrial invasion is common (80% of carcinomas)
      - Aggressive nature
      - Often presents late
    - Squamous cell carcinoma
    - Undifferentiated carcinoma
    - Malignant mixed mesodermal tumors
- Special stains
  - Most tumors are CEA(-) and vimentin(+)
  - Grades 1 and 2 cancers
    - 84% ER(+) and 83% PR(+)

Routes of Spread

- Local spread
  - Most common
- Lymphatic extension
  - Common nodes include
    - Pelvic (N1)
    - Paraaortic (N2)
    - Inguinal nodes (less common)
- Hematogenous spread
  - Lungs
  - Liver
  - Bone
  - Skin
  - Brain (uncommon)
- **Peritoneal spread**
  - Intraperitoneal implants
  - Common in papillary serous carcinoma

IMAGING

Detection

- **Key diagnostic clues**
  - Endometrial mass resulting in uterine cavity expansion
  - Localized tumors
    - Polypoid masses superficially attached to endometrium
  - Diffuse tumors
    - Extensive endometrial invasion
- **Location**
  - Uterine cavity abnormalities
  - Invasion into myometrium, cervix, or adjacent structures may be seen in some patients
- **Morphology**
  - Polypoid masses or diffuse thickening of endometrium
- **General T-staging imaging characteristics**
  - **Ultrasound**
    - Variable appearance
      - Typically nonspecific
    - Thickened endometrial complex
      - Hyperechoic with well-defined borders
    - Areas of decreased echogenicity can be seen within thickened endometrial complex
    - Mass-like lesion may be heterogeneous or homogeneous
    - Subendometrial halo intact
    - Margins irregular or ill defined

- Extension of normal echogenicity into inner myometrium
- Disruption of subendometrial halo may be focal or diffuse
- 3D ultrasound
  - May offer superior endometrial cancer volume measurement as compared to thickness measurement in detecting endometrial cancer
- Transvaginal ultrasound (TVUS) findings
  - Subendometrial halo disruption is suggestive of myometrial invasion
  - Uterine cancer appears as a polypoid mass or diffuse thickening in endometrial cavity
  - Evaluation of cervix, parametrium, and lymph nodes is limited in TVUS

- **CT**
  - **NECT**
    - Difficult to differentiate between cancer and normal uterine tissue
  - **CECT**
    - Diffuse thickening or a discrete mass may be visualized in uterine cavity
    - Compared to myometrium, uterine carcinoma is relatively low attenuation
    - Myometrial invasion is indicated by irregular tumor-myometrial border
    - Local staging limited due to lack of accurate demonstration of deep myometrial invasion and cervical involvement
- **MR**
  - Assessing depth of myometrial invasion
    - Sensitivity: 69-94%
    - Specificity: 64-100%
  - **T2WI**
    - Heterogeneous intermediate signal intensity compared to hyperintense endometrium
      - Deep myometrial invasion can be excluded if junctional zone is intact
      - If junctional zone not well seen, as in postmenopausal women, then irregular endometrium/myometrium border is suggestive of myometrial invasion
    - Pitfalls of T2WI
      - Thinning of myometrium in postmenopausal women
      - Tumor extension into cornua
      - Myometrial compression from a polypoid tumor
      - Poor tumor-myometrial contrast
      - Leiomyomas/adenomyosis
  - **T1WI**
    - Tumor is isointense to normal hypodense endometrium and myometrium
  - **T1WI C+**
    - Endometrial cancer less avidly enhancing relative to myometrium and cervix
      - Max contrast between tumor and myometrium is at 50-120 seconds
      - Most important phase in dynamic imaging for assessment of depth of invasion
    - Endometrial tumor enhances earlier than normal endometrium
    - Dynamic post-contrast images
      - Highly valuable in visualizing myometrial and cervical invasion
      - Valuable in differentiating endometrial cancer from fluid or blood in uterine cavity
      - Useful in detection of lymph nodes
  - **DWI**
    - Increased water restriction in malignancies relative to myometrium due to greater cellularity of tumors
    - May improve accuracy of MR for depth of myometrial invasion
    - Decreased apparent diffusion coefficient (ADC) values
      - Corresponds to high signal intensity on DWI images
- **PET**
  - F18 FDG PET valuable in detection of adenopathy, metastases, and surveillance for recurrences
  - Not helpful for evaluating primary tumor or for assessing myometrial or cervical involvement
  - Sensitivity 63% and specificity of 95% for detection of malignant adenopathy, improves with nodal size
- **Recommendations**
  - Best imaging tool
    - TVUS can be used in initial evaluation, particularly in cases of abnormal bleeding
      - Most common modality for detection
      - Endometrial sampling should be performed in presentation of postmenopausal bleeding with an endometrial complex > 5 mm in size
    - CT, MR, and PET/CT useful in detecting adenopathy or distant disease
    - MR best for tumor-related detail for image-guided brachytherapy
  - Protocol advice
    - MR imaging protocol should include
      - T1WI: Axial, large field of view, including entire pelvis
      - T2WI: Axial, sagittal, and coronal small field of view
      - T1WI C+: Dynamic and sagittal

Staging

- T staging
  - **Ultrasound**
    - Greatest accuracy in early stage disease with small tumors
    - Overstaging can be seen in large, polypoid lesions
    - Early stages
      - Pulsed Doppler: Benign and malignant thickening of endometrium show significant overlap in resistive index and pulsatility
      - Color Doppler: Mild to moderate vascularity with multiple feeding vessels
  - **CECT**
    - Early stages
      - Focal/diffuse thickening of the endometrium
      - Tumor mass hypodense to myometrium
      - Mass located centrally
      - Lack of zonal anatomy results in decreased accuracy (65-75%)
  - **MR**
    - Most accurate imaging modality in local staging
    - Zonal anatomy loss in postmenopausal women: Potential problem in staging and decreases MR accuracy
    - Early stages

- T1WI: Hypointense to isointense relative to endometrium or myometrium and detects hematometra
- T2WI: Hypointense or isointense relative to endometrium (100%) and isointense or hyperintense relative to outer myometrium (70%)

- N staging
  - Criteria in defining lymph nodes as pathologic
    - Oval nodes ≥ 1 cm in short axis
    - Round nodes ≥ 0.8 cm in diameter
  - Enhancement of nodes or node signal is not predictive of metastatic lymphadenopathy
  - CT and MR show equal accuracy in assessing involvement of pelvic and paraaortic lymph nodes
  - Nodal metastases may skip
    - Metastasizes to paraaortic lymph nodes through the ovarian lymphatics without pelvic lymphadenopathy
  - **CT**
    - CECT detects adenopathy
    - CT, MR, and PET are chosen modalities in detecting adenopathy
      - 60-90% accuracy
  - **MR**
    - **T1WI**
      - Detects adenopathy
    - **T2WI**
      - Detects pelvic &/or paraaortic adenopathy
    - Increased sensitivity for nodal metastases with MR enhanced by ultrasmall superparamagnetic iron oxide (USPIO)
  - **PET**
    - Increased sensitivity for nodal metastases with F18 FDG PET
    - Insensitive for small nodal metastases < 6-7 mm
    - High positive predictive value when nodes 7-15 mm demonstrate increased activity
- M staging
  - **CT**
    - Most common modality for serial evaluation of patients with uterine malignancies
    - **CECT**
      - Frequently used modality in assessing distant metastases
  - **MR**
    - More often used as problem-solving tool for indeterminate lesions seen on US or CT
  - **PET/CT**
    - PET/CT valuable in detecting lesions in organs as well as nodes
    - Some uterine malignancies are not FDG avid or less FDG avid (leiomyosarcoma)
    - Metastatic lesions may also have variable FDG activity compared to that of primary tumor

Restaging

- **CT**
  - Most frequently used modality for restaging patients
  - Helpful for differentiating scar vs. residual/recurrent tumor
  - More sensitive than PET for detecting early carcinomatosis or peritoneal spread
- **MR**
  - Used for problem solving or indeterminate lesions on other modalities
- **PET/CT**
  - Can be helpful for detecting occult disease
  - Pitfalls
    - Inability to detect early carcinomatosis and occasionally non-FDG-avid lesions on PET
    - Need to look at CT images even if performed at low dose to look for peritoneal involvement

CLINICAL PRESENTATION & WORK-UP

Presentation

- Abnormal vaginal bleeding
  - 75-90% of patients present with postmenopausal bleeding
  - May also present with leukorrhea
- Other signs and symptoms resulting from metastatic disease in more advanced cancers may occur
  - Dysuria
  - Constipation
  - Pain

Prognosis

- Typically diagnosed earlier, as majority of women seek evaluation following vaginal bleeding, which is seen in most cases
- Majority of patients diagnosed with surgical stage I disease (70-75% of cases)
- **Prognostic factors**
  - Histologic grade of tumor
  - Depth of myometrial invasion
  - Stage of disease
  - Lymph node involvement
- **5-year overall survival (OS) rates for endometrial cancer in > 21,000 cases**
  - Stage IA: 88.4%
  - Stage IB: 75.1%
  - Stage II: 68.9%
  - Stage IIIA: 58.1%
  - Stage IIIB: 49.9%
  - Stage IIIC: 46.6%
  - Stage IVA: 16.8%
  - Stage IVB: 15.2%

Work-Up

- Clinical
  - H&P with focus on gynecologic issues
  - Endometrial biopsy
  - Consider genetic counseling in women < 50 years old and with a strong family history
- Radiographic
  - Chest x-ray is standard
  - Pre- and postoperative assessment is clinician dependent
- Laboratory
  - Complete blood count
  - Consider renal function tests, liver function tests, and chemistries

TREATMENT

Major Treatment Alternatives

- Multimodality treatment plan based on disease stage
  - Surgery
    - Total hysterectomy (TH) and bilateral salpingo-oophorectomy (BSO)
    - Nodal assessment is part of FIGO staging; however, 2 randomized trials showed no survival benefit for pelvic node evaluation
  - Brachytherapy or external beam radiation therapy (EBRT) or both depending on stage
  - Chemotherapy depending on stage
  - Hormonal treatments depending on stage
    - Commonly include progestational agents

Major Treatment Roadblocks/ Contraindications

- Comorbid conditions and advanced age

Treatment Options by Stage

- **Stage I**
  - TH and BSO
  - Pelvic and paraaortic lymph nodes should be evaluated in grade 3 lesions or stage IB, otherwise up to the discretion of surgeon
  - Brachytherapy and EBRT depending on pathologic findings
- **Stage II**
  - TH, BSO, and pelvic and paraaortic node evaluation
    - May be combined with intracavity and EBRT given preoperatively for large clinical stage II
  - Postoperatively: EBRT + brachytherapy ± chemotherapy
- **Stage III**
  - Postoperative management is controversial: Chemoradiation, chemotherapy, or radiation alone
    - Hormonal therapy is an option
- **Stage IV**
  - Treatment plan guided by sites of metastatic lesions and resulting symptoms
  - Radiation used for stage IVA or for palliation ± chemotherapy ± hormonal therapy

Standard Doses

- 45-50 Gy in adjuvant setting is standard
- 55-65 Gy for gross nodal disease
- 7 Gy x 3 at 5 mm is often used in vaginal brachytherapy

Common Techniques

- 4 field or intensity-modulated radiation therapy (IMRT)

Landmark Trials

- Aalders: Local recurrence 1.9% with EBRT vs. 6.9% without; no difference in OS
- PORTEC1: Local regional recurrence (LRR) 6% with EBRT vs. 15% without; no difference in OS
- PORTEC2: LRR 5.1% with vaginal brachytherapy vs. 2.1% with EBRT; no difference in OS
- GOG 99: Recurrence 3% with EBRT vs. 12% without; high intermediate-risk cohort recurrence 6% with RT vs. 26% without
- ASTEC: LRR 3.2% with EBRT vs. 6.1% without; no difference in OS; > 50% of patients in each arm had vaginal brachytherapy
- ASTEC and Benedetti-Panici showed no survival benefit for pelvic lymphadenectomy
- Japanese and Italian trials: RT vs. CAP chemo; no difference in OS
- GOG 122: 5-year stage-adjusted survival 55% with chemotherapy vs. 42% with whole-abdominal radiation
- NSGO/EORTC (Hogberg): Chemotherapy improved progression-free survival (PFS), but not OS after surgery and RT vs. no adjuvant chemo

RECOMMENDED FOLLOW-UP

Clinical

- Pelvic exam every 3-4 months for 2 years, then every 6 months or annually

Radiographic

- Consider annual chest x-ray and vaginal cytology; abdominal imaging dependent on stage and clinical scenario

Laboratory

- CA125 optional

SELECTED REFERENCES

1. Beddy P et al: FIGO staging system for endometrial cancer: added benefits of MR imaging. Radiographics. 32(1):241-54, 2012
2. Creutzberg CL et al: Fifteen-year radiotherapy outcomes of the randomized PORTEC-1 trial for endometrial carcinoma. Int J Radiat Oncol Biol Phys. 81(4):e631-8, 2011
3. Hogberg T et al: Sequential adjuvant chemotherapy and radiotherapy in endometrial cancer--results from two randomised studies. Eur J Cancer. 46(13):2422-31, 2010
4. ASTEC/EN.5 study group et al: Adjuvant external beam radiotherapy in the treatment of endometrial cancer (MRC ASTEC and NCIC CTG EN.5 randomised trials): pooled trial results, systematic review, and meta-analysis. Lancet. 373(9658):137-46, 2009
5. Grigsby PW: Role of PET in gynecologic malignancy. Curr Opin Oncol. 21(5):420-4, 2009
6. Benedetti Panici P et al: Systematic pelvic lymphadenectomy vs. no lymphadenectomy in early-stage endometrial carcinoma: randomized clinical trial. J Natl Cancer Inst. 100(23):1707-16, 2008
7. Susumu N et al: Randomized phase III trial of pelvic radiotherapy versus cisplatin-based combined chemotherapy in patients with intermediate- and high-risk endometrial cancer: a Japanese Gynecologic Oncology Group study. Gynecol Oncol. 108(1):226-33, 2008
8. Maggi R et al: Adjuvant chemotherapy vs radiotherapy in high-risk endometrial carcinoma: results of a randomised trial. Br J Cancer. 95(3):266-71, 2006

Surgical Staging

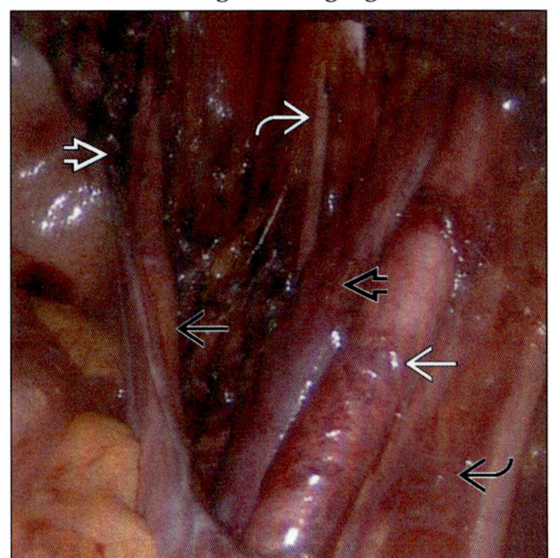

Stage IA

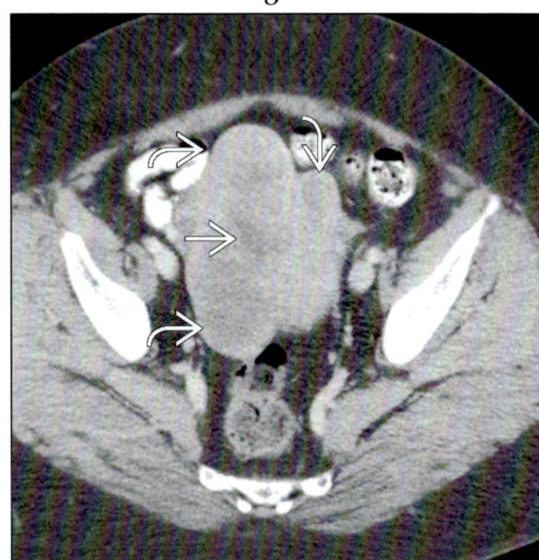

(Left) *Laparoscopic view into pelvis shows vessels are devoid of lymph nodes. Clip → is placed on anterior branch of internal iliac artery, which is overlying ureter →. Psoas muscle →, external iliac artery →, vein →, and obturator nerve → are demonstrated. (Courtesy M. Dodson, MD.)* ***(Right)*** *Axial CECT shows enlarged uterus with multiple leiomyomas → and slightly prominent endometrium →. Pathology revealed 2 cm mass that did not involve myometrium, compatible with stage IA.*

Stage IA

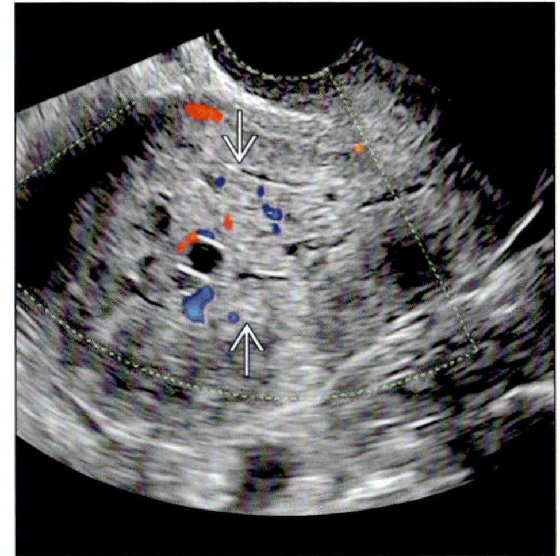

Stage IA

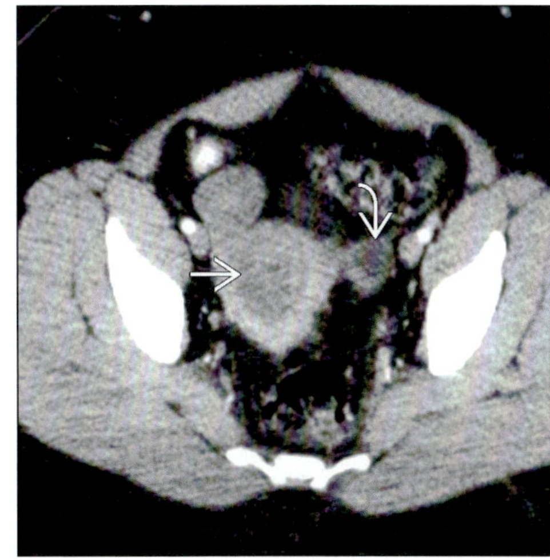

(Left) *Color Doppler ultrasound shows areas of increased color (blood flow) to the thickened endometrium →. Pathology revealed endometrial carcinoma that had developed within a polyp in this patient that had been on tamoxifen. Disease limited to the endometrium is stage IA.* ***(Right)*** *Axial CECT shows nonspecific endometrial enlargement → and a left ovarian cyst → in this patient with recently diagnosed stage IA endometrial carcinoma.*

Stage I Medically Inoperable

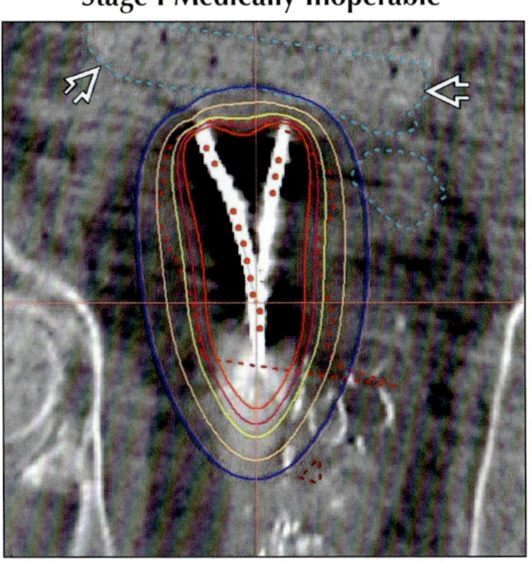

Stage I Medically Inoperable

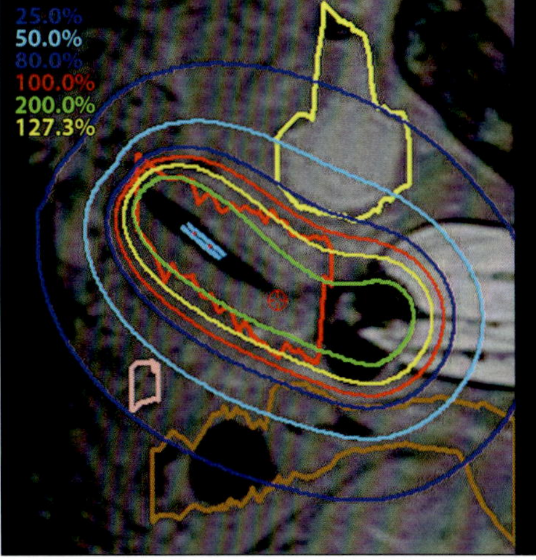

(Left) *Coronal CT shows dual tandem inserted into cornu of uterus to aid in optimal dose coverage. Orange, yellow, and blue lines represent the 600, 400, and 200 cGy lines, respectively. Sigmoid → is just cephalad to the uterus. (Courtesy L. Lee, MD.)* ***(Right)*** *Sagittal MR shows tandem and ovoids. Low-grade tumors that are not deeply invasive are ideal cases for brachytherapy alone without external beam. MR is superior for soft tissue delineation. (Courtesy A. Viswanathan, MD, MPH.)*

Stage IB

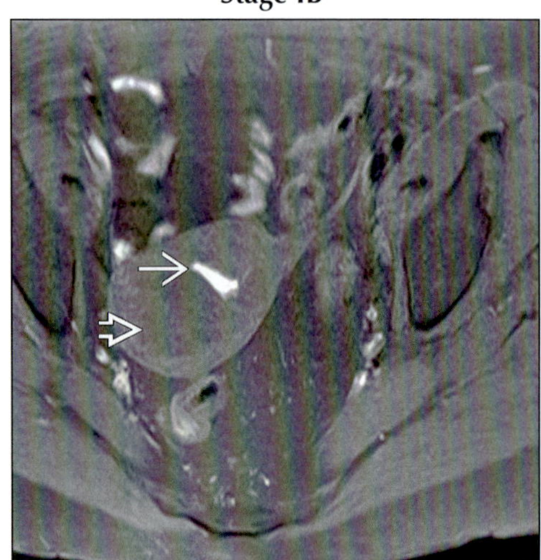

Stage IB

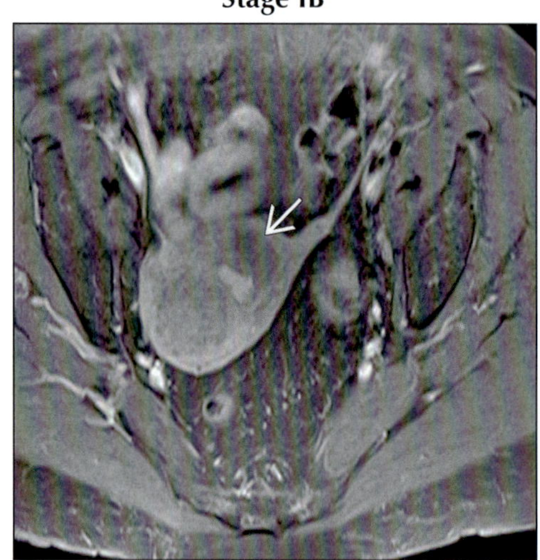

*(**Left**) Axial T1WI MR before contrast is given shows high signal ➡ likely due to recent biopsy. T2WI MR showed a large fibroid ➡ in the right aspect of the uterus. (**Right**) Axial T1WI MR post contrast reveals a hypoenhancing mass ➡ penetrating > 1/2 of myometrium. This is in contrast to the brightly enhancing normal myometrium.*

Stage IB

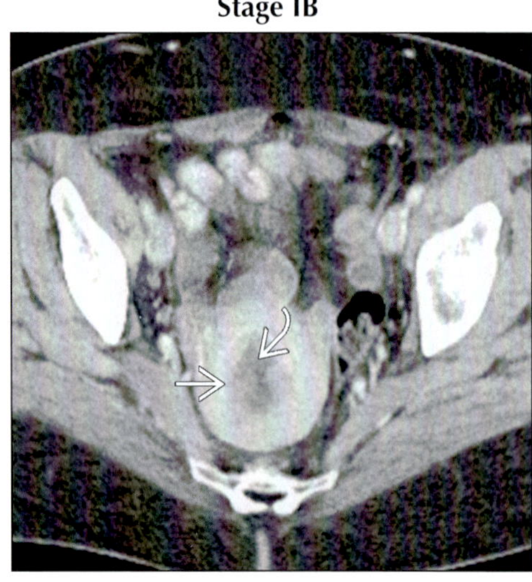

Stage IB

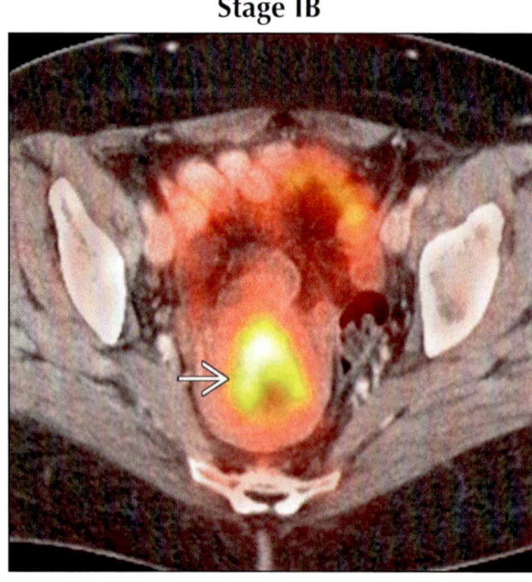

*(**Left**) Axial CECT shows irregularly thickened endometrium ➡ with some fluid/debris in the endometrial canal ➡ in this patient with postmenopausal bleeding. (**Right**) Axial PET/CT in the same patient shows intense FDG ➡ activity in the thickened endometrium compatible with recently diagnosed endometrial carcinoma. FDG activity in the endometrium in a postmenopausal woman should be further evaluated to exclude carcinoma.*

Stage IB

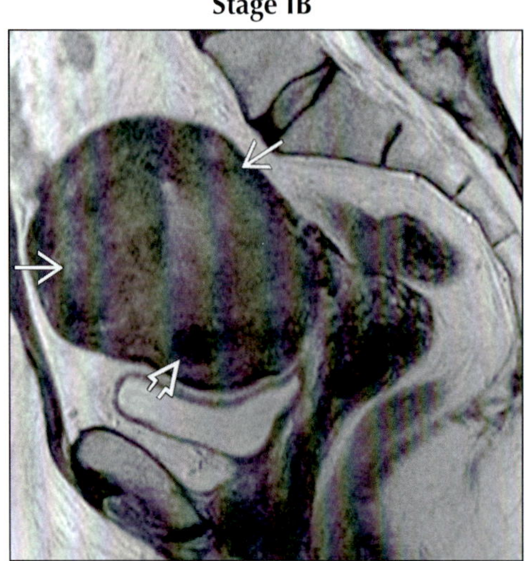

Stage IB

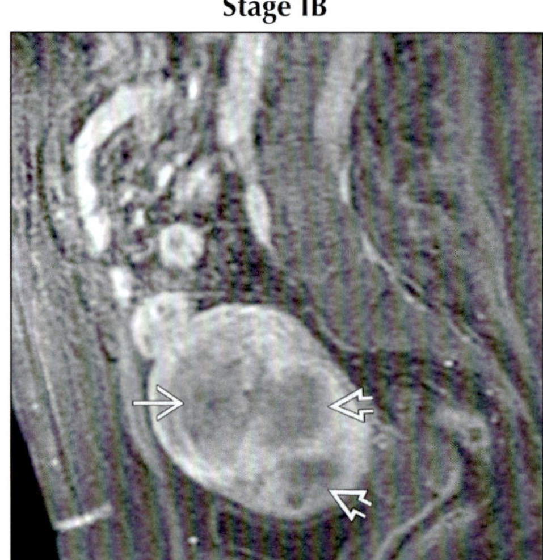

*(**Left**) Sagittal T1WI C+ MR shows a tumor ➡ in a bulky uterus with multiple leiomyomas ➡ with an indistinct junctional zone, raising the suspicion of myometrial invasion. (**Right**) Sagittal T2WI FS MR in the same patient shows the higher signal mass ➡ in a bulky uterus with a better view of the multiple low signal intensity leiomyomas ➡.*

Stage IB

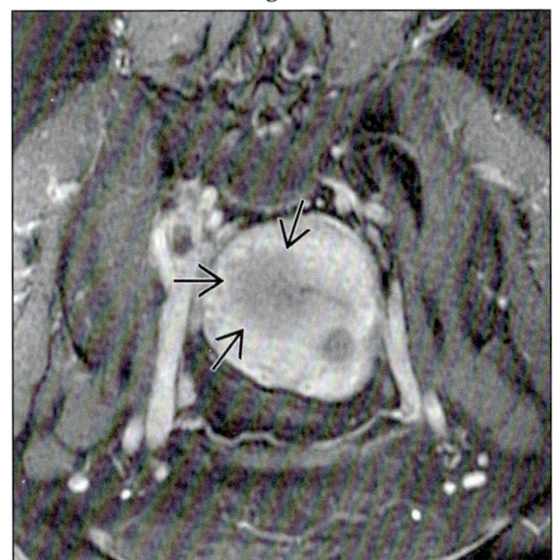

Stage IB

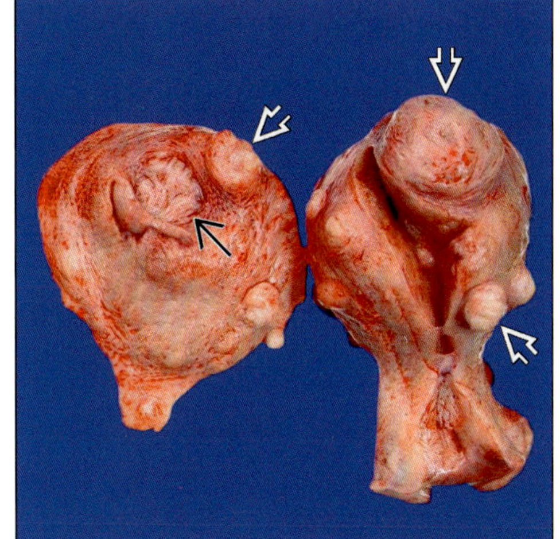

(Left) *Coronal T1WI C+ FS MR post gadolinium administration in the same patient shows that the tumor* ➙ *involves > 50% of the myometrium, making this a T1b lesion or stage IB.* ***(Right)*** *Cut gross hysterectomy specimen from the same patient shows the presence of stage IB endometrial cancer* ➙*. Also note multiple leiomyomata* ➙*.*

Brachytherapy in Early Endometrial Cancer

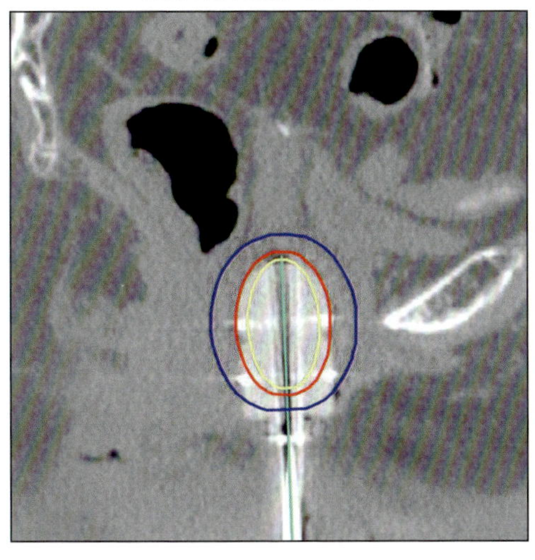

Brachytherapy in Early Endometrial Cancer

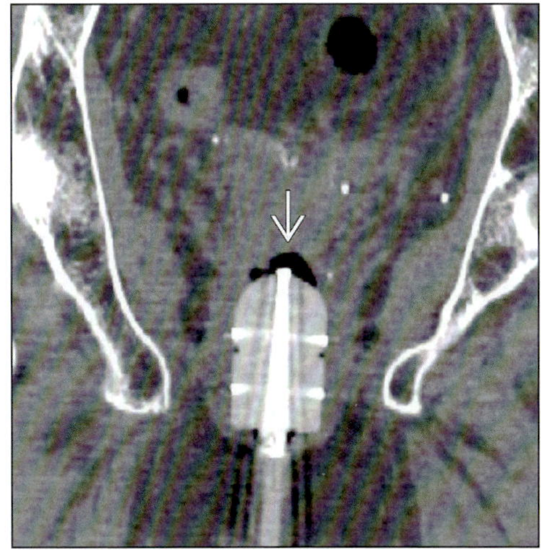

(Left) *In this patient with a T1b grade 2 lesion penetrating 60% through the myometrium with no LVSI, a 3 cm length of the vagina was treated. The blue, red, and yellow lines represent the 50%, 100%, and 150% isodose surfaces, respectively.* ***(Right)*** *Coronal CT shows an air gap* ➙ *present at the cephalad aspect of the cylinder. Care should be taken to minimize air gaps to prevent poor dosimetry. The vaginal mucosa needs to be in approximation to the cylinder.*

Brachytherapy in Early Endometrial Cancer

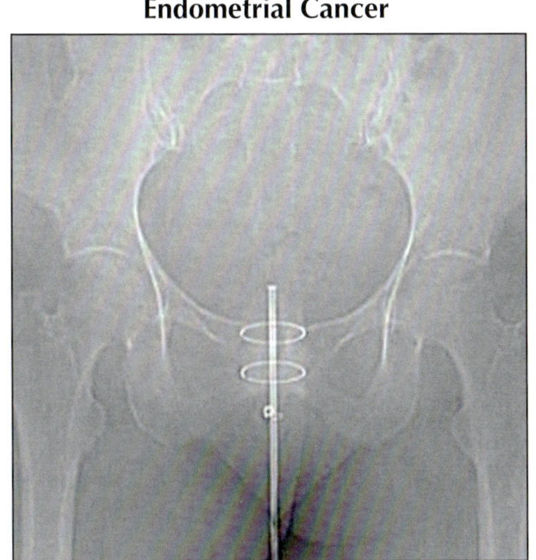

Brachytherapy in Early Endometrial Cancer

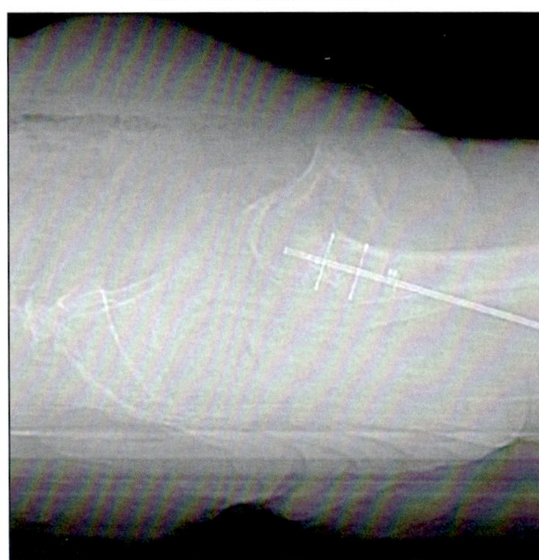

(Left) *To achieve maximal dose at the vaginal mucosa and spare organs at risk (OAR) as much as possible, the largest diameter cylinder should be used. The length of vagina treated is a clinical decision. The cylinder should be centered, secured, and without air gaps present.* ***(Right)*** *Lateral scout view shows the cylinder is not in the same plane as the patient. This positioning is incorrect and can lead to overdosing OAR such as the bladder.*

UTERUS

(Left) Sagittal T1WI MR shows an endometrial mass ➔ with extension into the endocervical canal. The low signal intensity junctional zone is disrupted anteriorly, compatible with > 50% myometrial extension. Pathology showed invasion of cervical stromal tissue. (Right) Axial PET/CT shows intense FDG activity ➔ correlating with the bulky endometrial mass. Although not routinely used to evaluate the primary mass, PET/CT can be used for initial treatment decision making.

Stage II

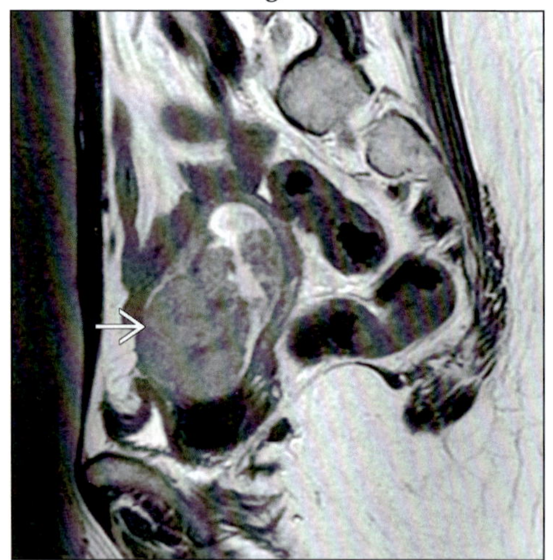

Stage II

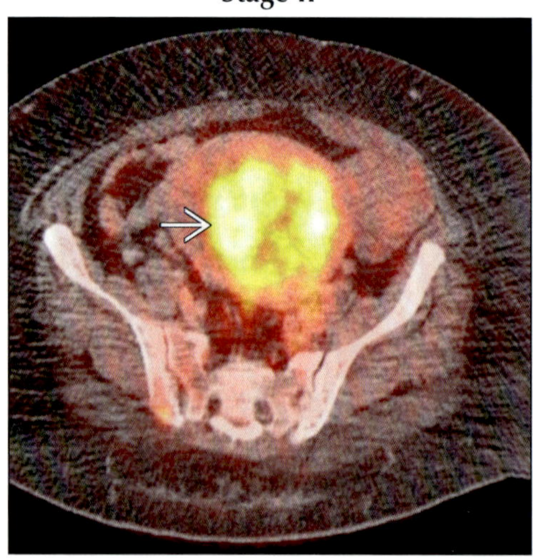

(Left) Axial NECT shows vaginal CTV with a generous margin around vagina ➔ to account for motion. Obturator internus ➔ and levator ani ➔ muscles are seen. A clip is present in the perirectal space, along with free fluid ➔. (Right) Axial NECT shows nodal CTV encompassing the internal ➔ and external iliac ➔ vessels. If the vessels are contoured often a 7 mm expansion is used for the CTV. Bowel, muscle, and bone should be excluded from the CTV.

Vaginal CTV

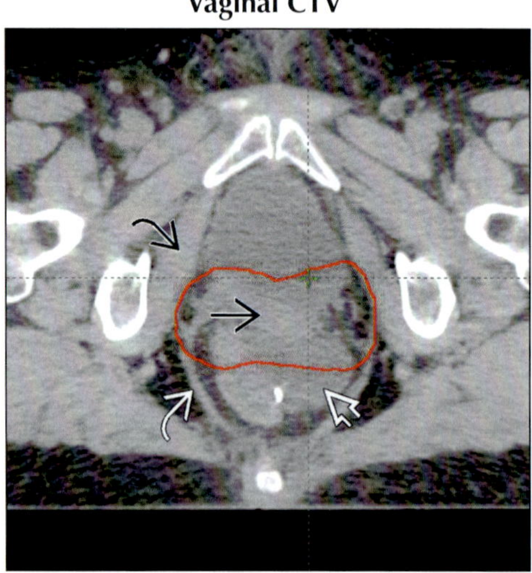

Nodal CTV

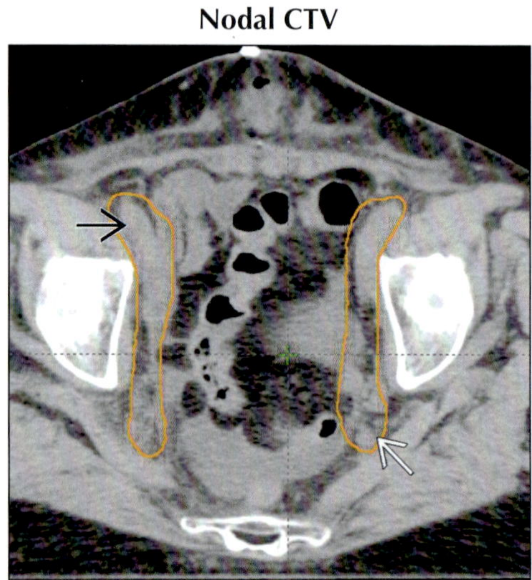

(Left) A belly board device can be very helpful in displacing small bowel out of the pelvis for a prone patient. The prone position is not as stable as supine and hence, for IMRT, the supine position may be preferred. (Right) In this 3-field treatment, the small bowel is excluded from the pelvis. The full bladder ➔ is also aiding in displacing the small bowel.

EBRT Dosimetry

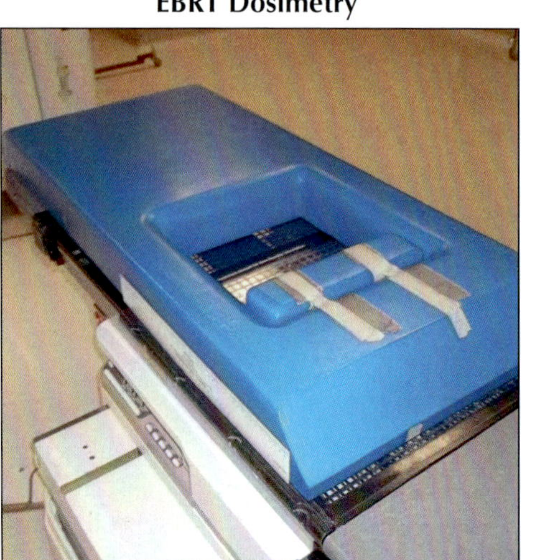

EBRT Dosimetry

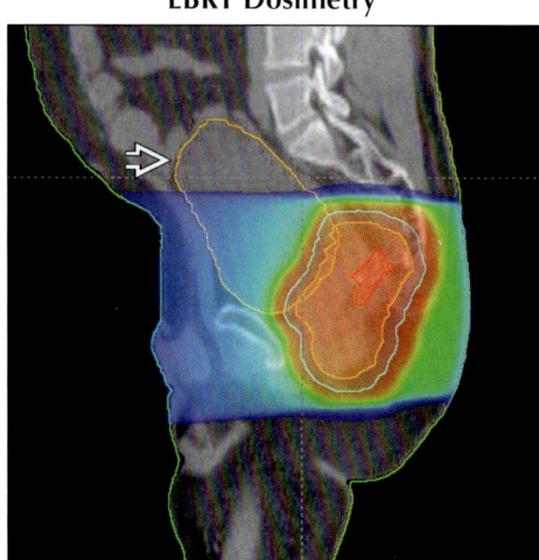

EBRT Dosimetry: 4 Field

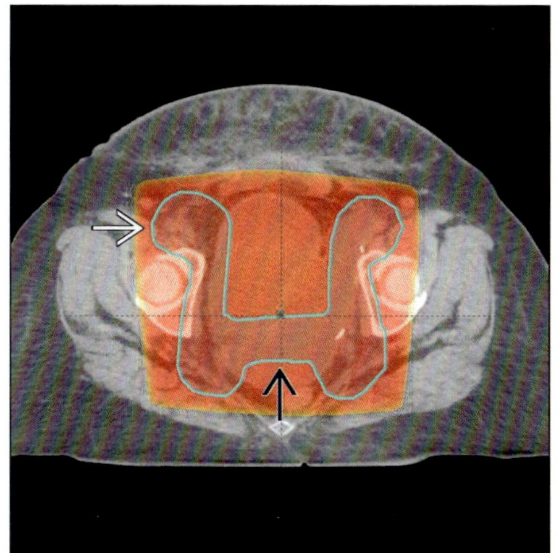

EBRT Dosimetry: IMRT

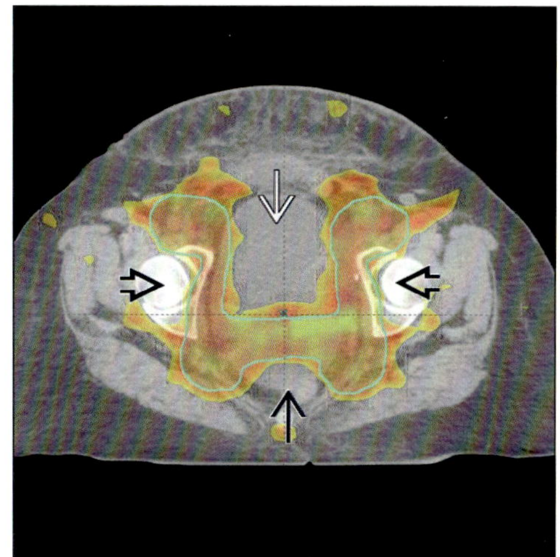

*(**Left**) Planning CT shows the nodal ➡ and vaginal PTVs ⇨ are merged. The colorwash is the 90% isodose surface. (**Right**) An example of IMRT dosimetry for the same case is shown at the level of the femoral heads. The colorwash is the 90% isodose surface. There is relative sparing of high-dose regions to the bladder ➡, rectum ⇨, and femoral heads ⇨.*

EBRT Dosimetry: 4 Field

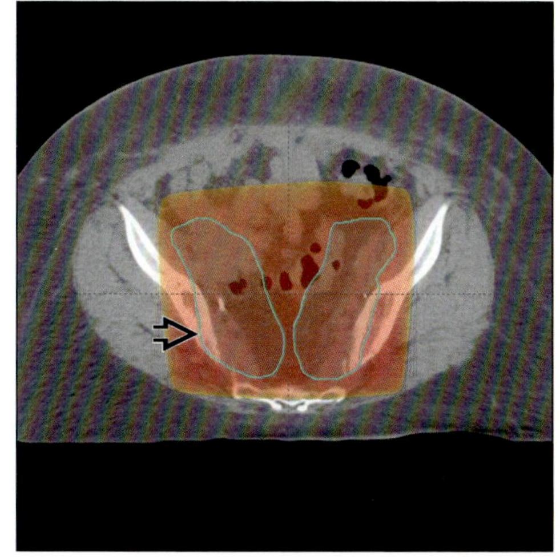

EBRT Dosimetry: IMRT

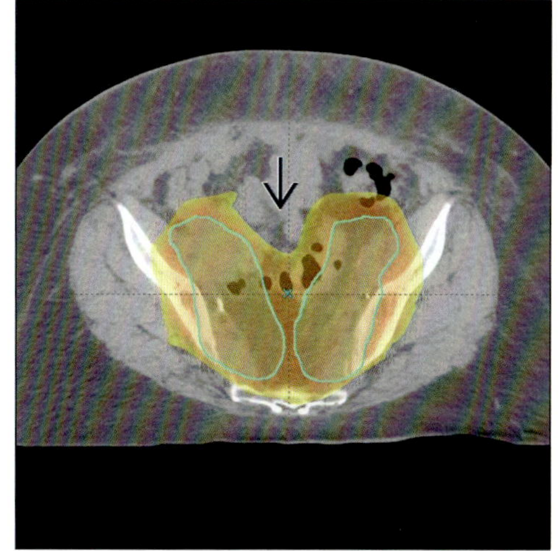

*(**Left**) This is an example of 4-field dosimetry for endometrial cancer at the level of the sciatic notch. The nodal PTV is shown ⇨. The colorwash is the 90% isodose surface. (**Right**) IMRT dosimetry is shown for the same patient at the level of the sciatic notch. The nodal PTV is shown. The colorwash is the 90% isodose surface. There is relative sparing of high-dose regions to the small bowel ⇨.*

EBRT Dosimetry

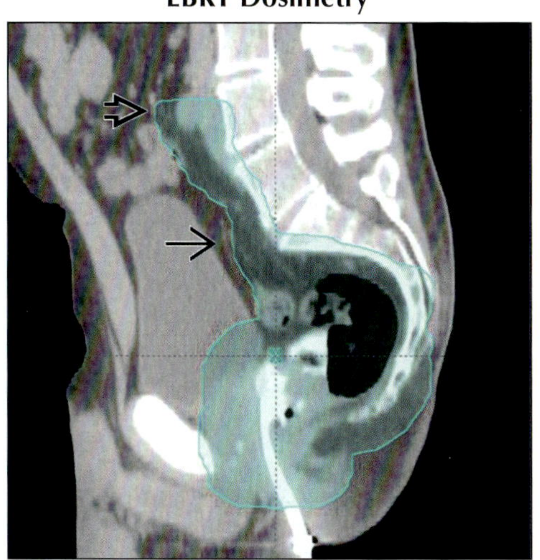

EBRT Dosimetry

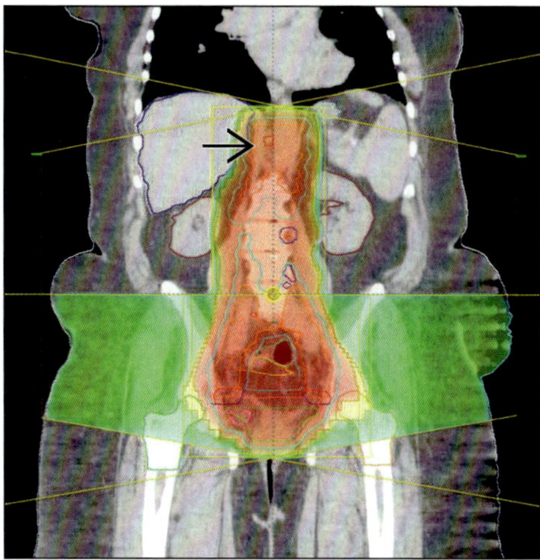

*(**Left**) A small pelvic field ⇨ commonly ends at the sacral promontory or L5/S1 junction, whereas a large pelvic field covering the bifurcation ⇨ increases the size dramatically, as in this case. (**Right**) A common technique utilized to cover an extended field is a split beam: 4 field to the pelvis and AP/PA to the paraaortic lymph nodes ⇨. This technique avoids appreciable dose to the kidneys. A high-energy beam should be used to limit dose to the spinal cord.*

Stage IIIA

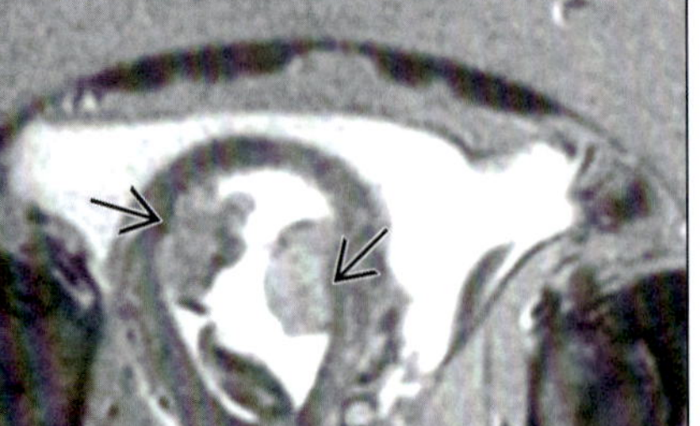

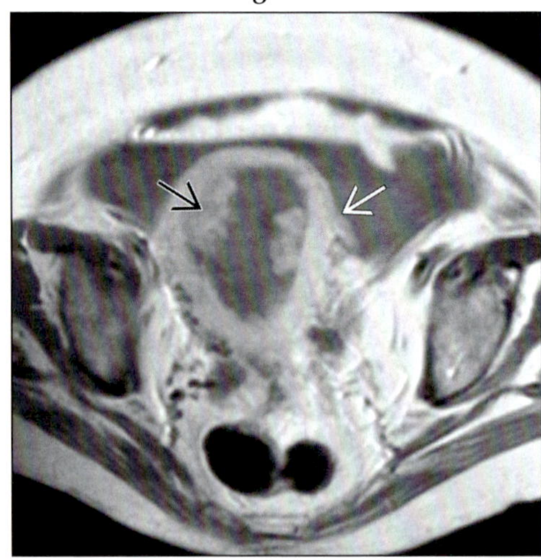

__(Left)__ Axial T2WI MR shows the uterus markedly distended with fluid and enhancing polypoid tumor masses →. No deep invasion of the myometrium is seen here. __(Right)__ Axial T1WI C+ MR in the same patient shows the polypoid masses → and irregular enhancing outer uterine wall →, suggesting serosal extension which was evident on pathology, making this stage IIIA.

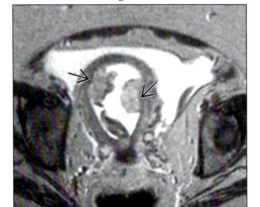

Stage IIIB

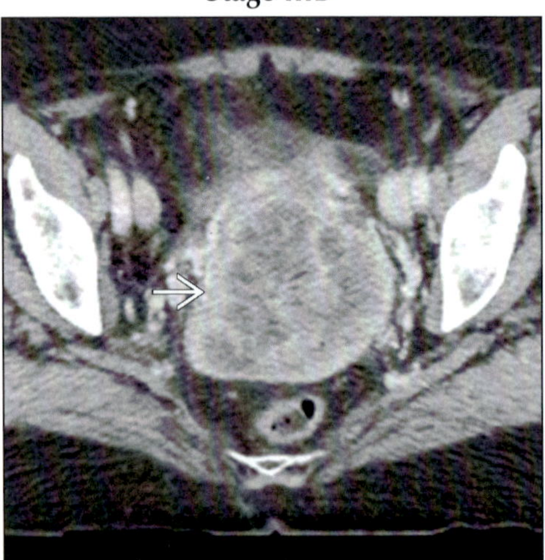

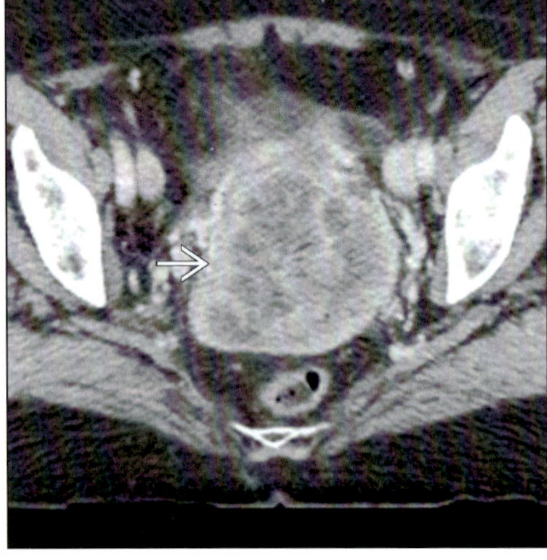

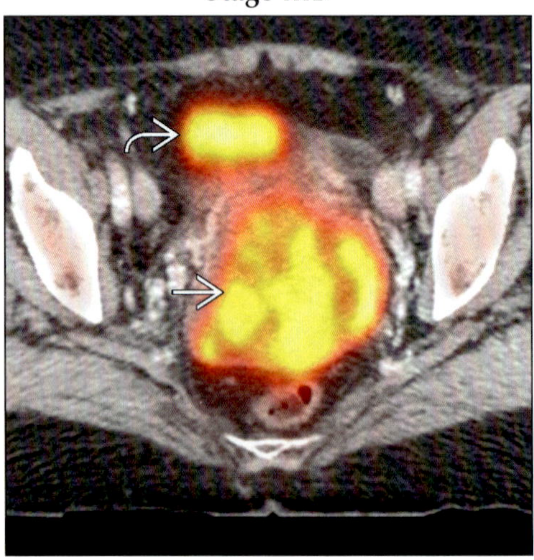

__(Left)__ Axial CECT shows a large heterogeneously enhancing mass → with an enlarged uterus in this patient with recently diagnosed endometrial carcinoma. __(Right)__ Axial PET/CT in the same patient shows diffuse intense FDG activity in the large endometrial mass → occupying the whole uterus. Involvement of the vagina makes this a T3b lesion. FDG activity anteriorly ↷ is normal excretory FDG in the bladder.

Stage IIIC1

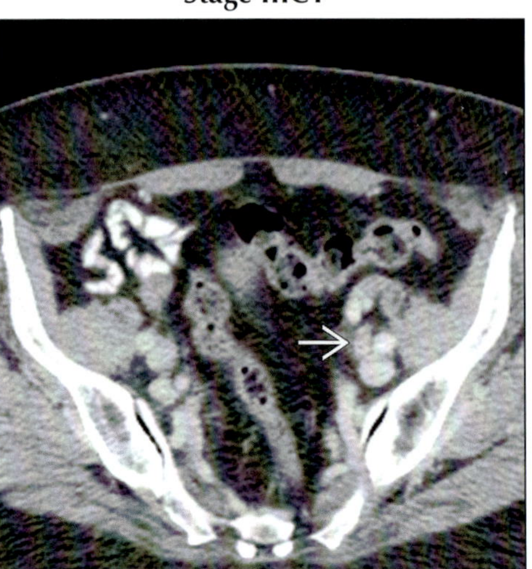

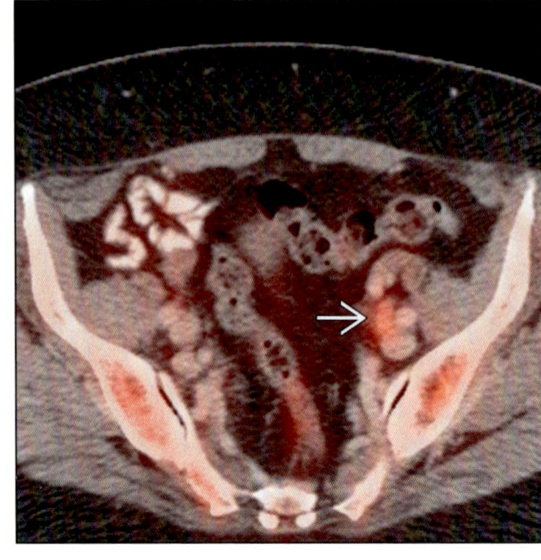

__(Left)__ In this patient with a newly diagnosed endometrial carcinoma, axial CECT shows a subtle, borderline, enlarged but nonspecific left external iliac node → without any additional specific features to suggest malignancy. __(Right)__ Axial PET/CT in the same patient shows mild FDG activity within the lymph node →. Pathologic staging is required for correct stage assignment. Paraaortic node involvement is stage IIIC2.

Stage IVA

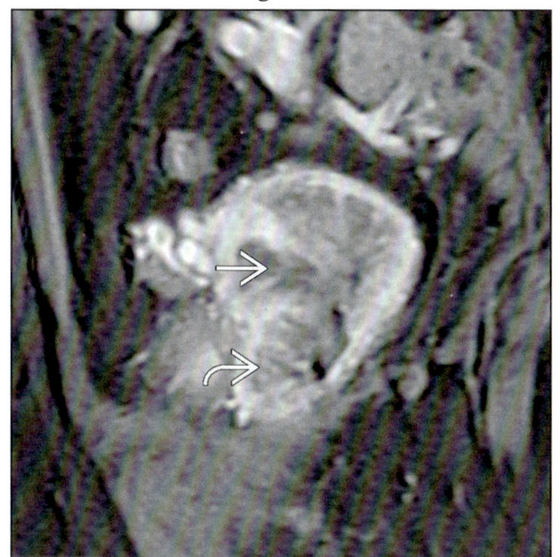

Stage IVA

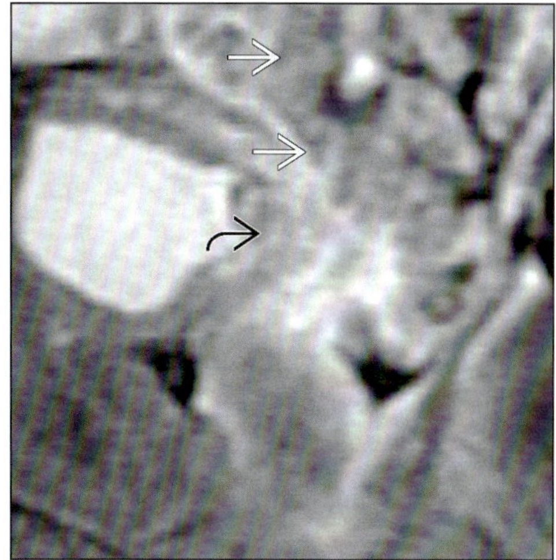

(Left) *Sagittal T1WI C+ FS MR shows a large mass → involving the majority of the endometrium, extending into the endocervix →, and involving more than 50% of the myometrium.* ***(Right)*** *Sagittal T1 C+ FS MR (smaller field of view in the same patient) shows the primary mass → with obvious abnormal enhancement of the posterior wall of the bladder →, compatible with a T4 lesion or stage IVA.*

Stage IVB

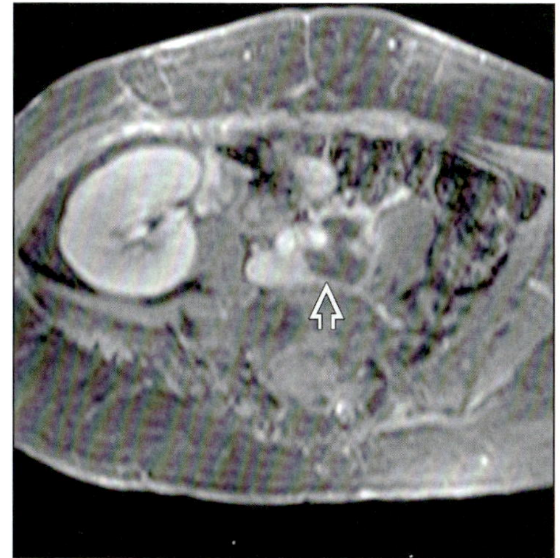

Stage IVB

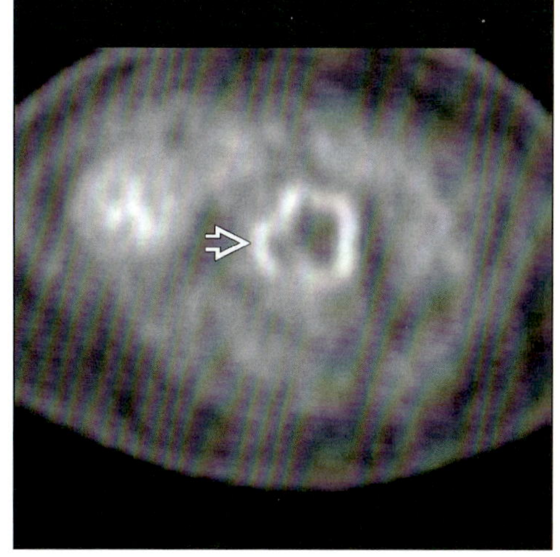

(Left) *Axial T1WI C+ FS MR shows a cystic mass → surrounding the proximal common iliac vessels. The mass shows abnormally enhancing wall with central necrosis, compatible with metastatic disease.* ***(Right)*** *FDG PET scan in the same patient shows abnormal rim-like intense FDG activity → correlating with the mass surrounding the proximal common iliac vessels. Note the center of the cystic mass is not avid.*

Stage IVB

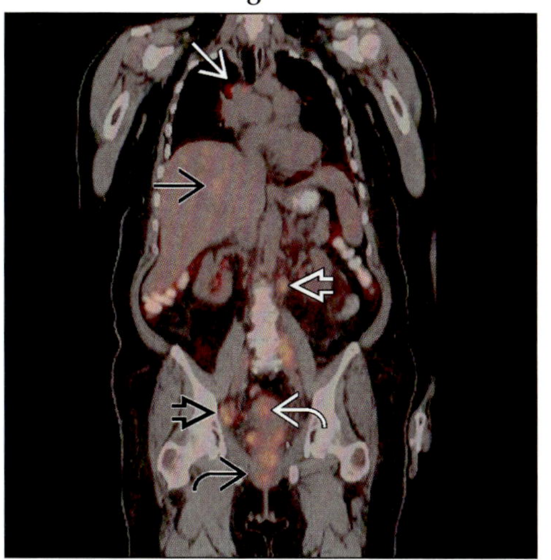

Stage IVB

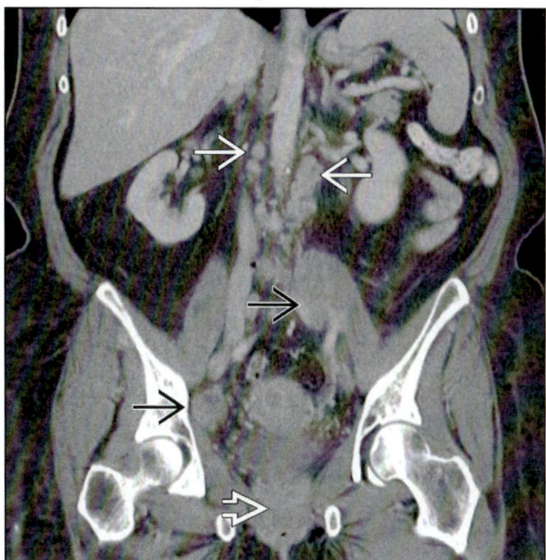

(Left) *Coronal PET/CT is depicted in a patient with pelvic pain and vaginal bleeding. Pelvic exam revealed a tumor extending down the anterior vagina to the introitus. Biopsy showed grade 3 adenocarcinoma. PET/CT shows avidity in hilar nodes →, liver →, paraaortic → and pelvic nodes →, uterus →, and vagina →.* ***(Right)*** *Coronal CECT shows bulky pelvic → and paraaortic → lymphadenopathy, and a vaginal mass → extending to the introitus.*

*(**Left**) Axial fused PET/CT in same patient shows bilateral inguinal lymph nodes → and avid vaginal mass →. Despite avidity in the rectum ↷, colonoscopy was negative. (**Right**) Axial CECT in the same patient shows enlarged heterogeneous right inguinal lymph node →. The irregular vaginal mass → is readily identified.*

Stage IVB

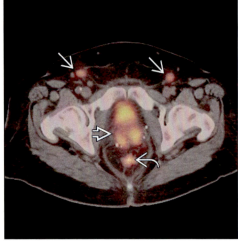

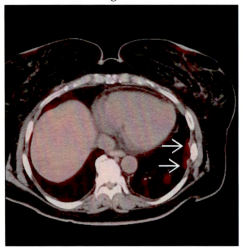

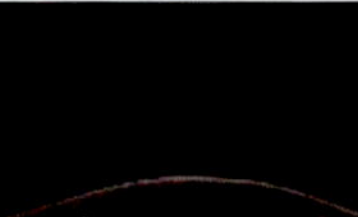

Stage IVB

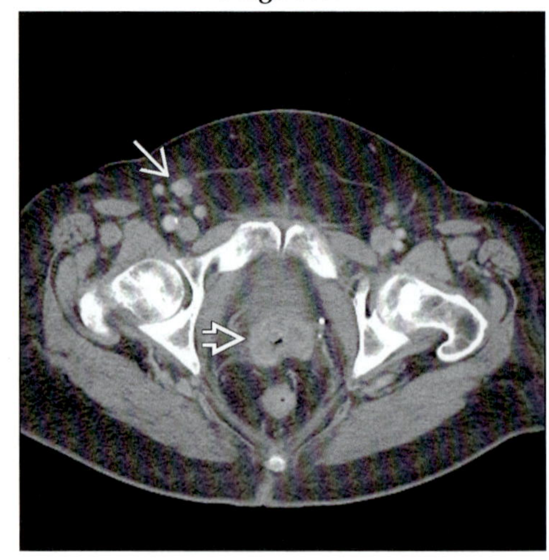

*(**Left**) Axial fused PET/CT in the same patient shows avid pleural masses →. Small avid lung masses were identified as well (not shown). (**Right**) Due to pain, patient was treated with palliative RT to 37.5 Gy in 15 fractions to the pelvis and paraaortic lymph nodes. Follow-up CT 8 weeks later demonstrates reduction in vaginal mass →, pelvic → and paraaortic lymphadenopathy, and explosion of disease in liver → and spleen ↷.*

Stage IVB

Stage IVB

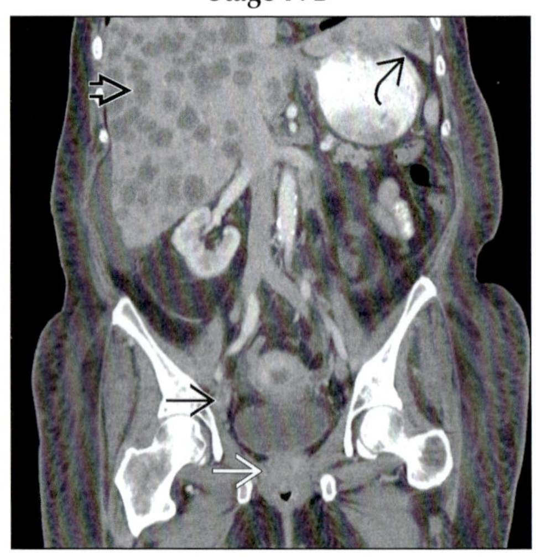

*(**Left**) This patient was treated with hysterectomy and subsequently developed a large right-sided pelvic recurrence. She was treated with 4-field EBRT to 40 Gy and then an IMRT boost for 26 Gy. Boost plan is shown. Tumor was too large to consider brachytherapy. (**Right**) Axial colorwash diagram in the same patient shows blue, green, yellow, and orange representing the 20%, 60%, 80%, and 100% isodose surfaces, respectively. The CTV → is depicted.*

Sidewall Recurrence

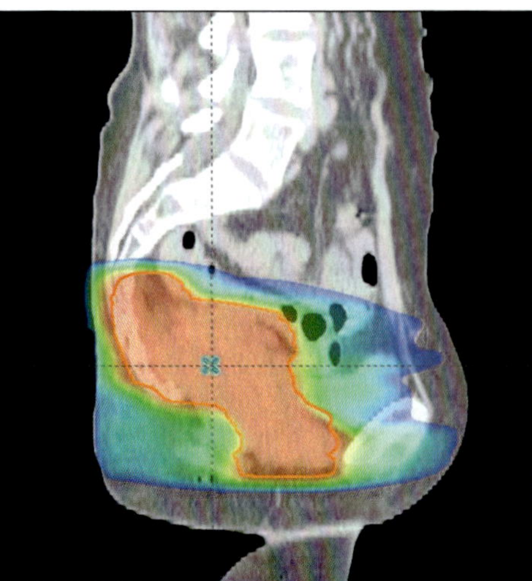

Sidewall Recurrence

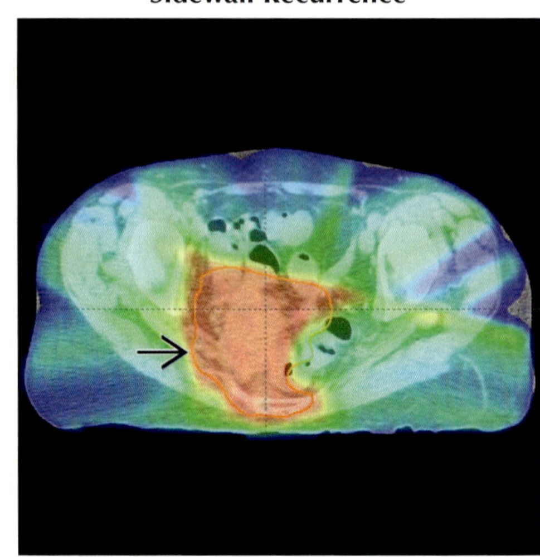

Sidewall Recurrence

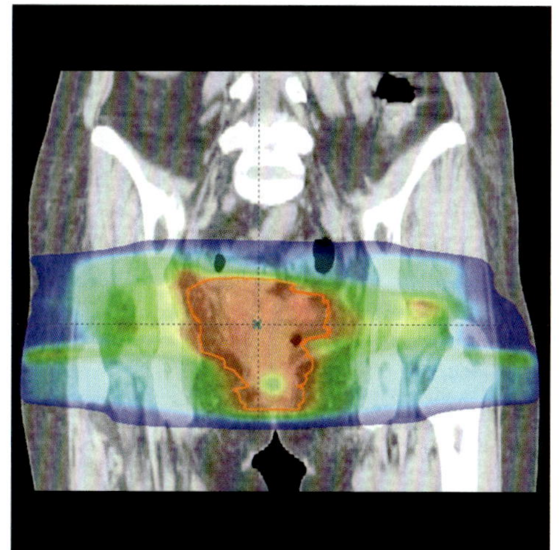

Cuff and Nodal Recurrence

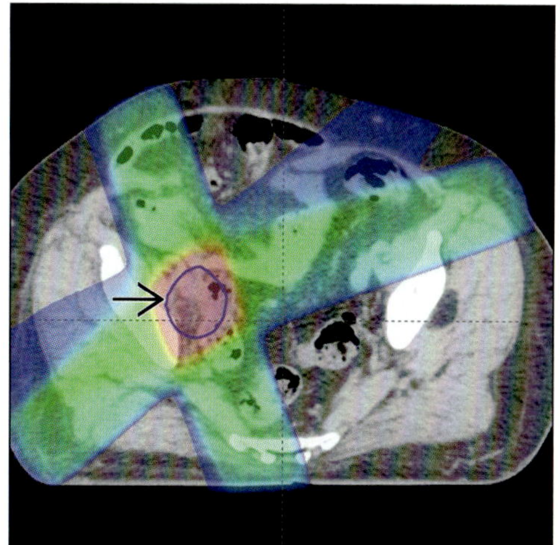

*(**Left**) Axial isodose colorwash diagram depicts boost plan. Same patient remains without recurrence at 5 years. (**Right**) Patient was treated with hysterectomy and developed recurrence at the vaginal cuff and external and common iliac lymph nodes. She was treated by a 4-field plan, 45 Gy to the pelvis followed by a 9 Gy 4-field oblique plan, which is shown. The nodal PTV is shown ⇒. Beam orientation was chosen to reduce dose to bowel.*

Cuff and Nodal Recurrence

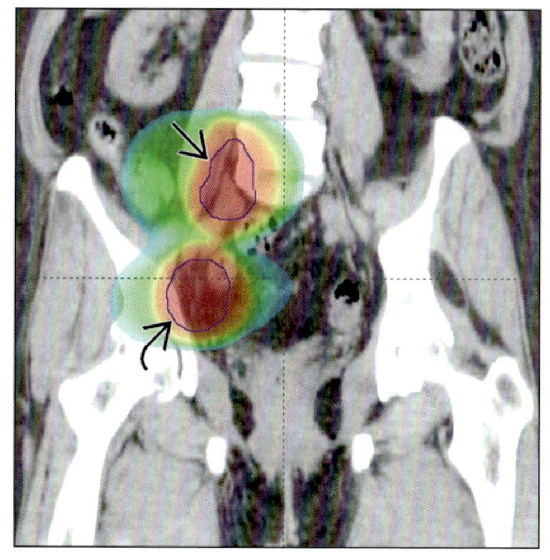

Cuff and Nodal Recurrence

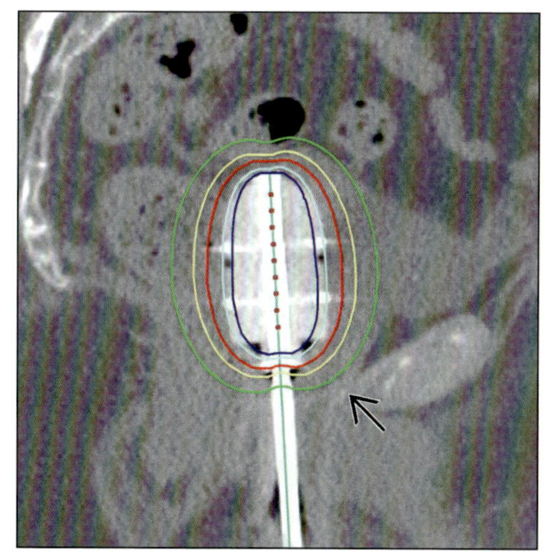

*(**Left**) Coronal CT in the same patient shows good conformality to the common iliac ⇒ and external iliac nodal ⇒ PTVs. Blue, green, yellow, and orange colorwash represent the 20%, 60%, 80%, and 100% isodose surfaces, respectively. (**Right**) In the same patient at brachytherapy, there was < 5 mm of disease at the cuff. 7 Gy was prescribed at 5 mm from the surface and given 3 times. The entire vaginal length was treated in this recurrent case down to the base of the pubis ⇒.*

Perineal Recurrence

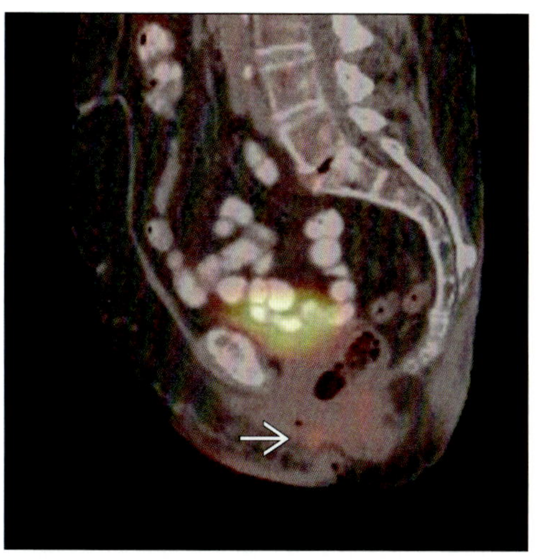

Perineal Recurrence

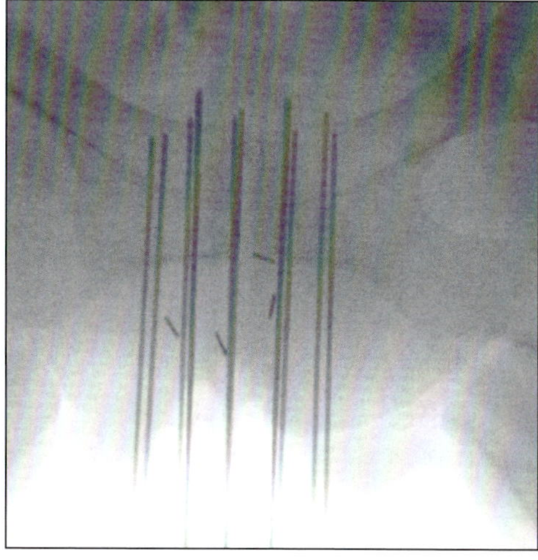

*(**Left**) Patient presented with a 12 mm perineal mass ➡ adjacent to the anus as shown by sagittal PET/CT 1 year after external beam and brachytherapy for a IB, grade 3 lesion. (**Right**) Intraoperative fluoroscopic image in the same patient shows good coverage by interstitial needles that were placed via a perineal template. Marker seeds were placed to bracket the lesion.*

(Left) In the same patient, the 100% isodose line (thin red line ➔) covers the PTV well (dark red line). The green line is the 50% isodose line. *(Right)* Coronal planning CT is shown in a 53-year-old patient who developed a suburethral recurrence. Two years previous, she underwent a hysterectomy for a grade 1 lesion confined to the endometrial lining. Separate photon fields were used to supplement the dose to the groins ➔.

Perineal Recurrence

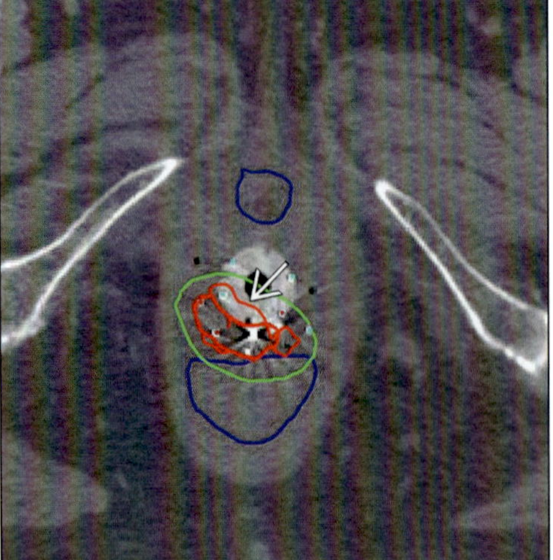

Suburethral Recurrence

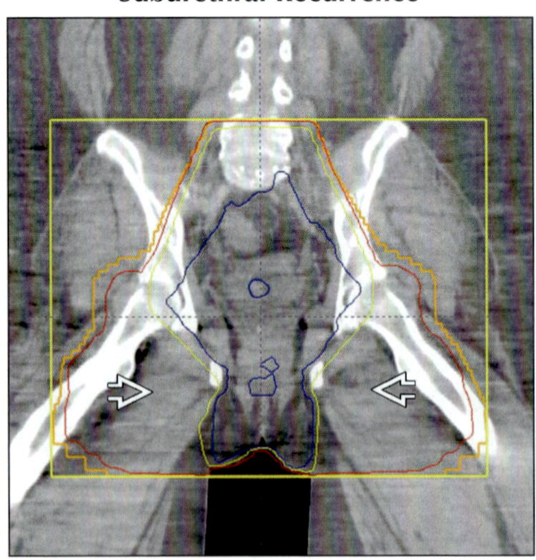

(Left) Axial CT in the same patient shows the 100%, 90%, and 60% isodose lines in blue, yellow, and red, respectively. Due to the patient's large size, the supplemental anterior groin fields were treated with 15 MV photons. *(Right)* Interstitial implant boost in the same patient shows the PTV in dark red. The 100%, 75%, and 50% isodose lines are shown in red, yellow, and green, respectively. Most of the urethra ➔ is receiving < 50% of the dose. Patient remains free of disease.

Suburethral Recurrence

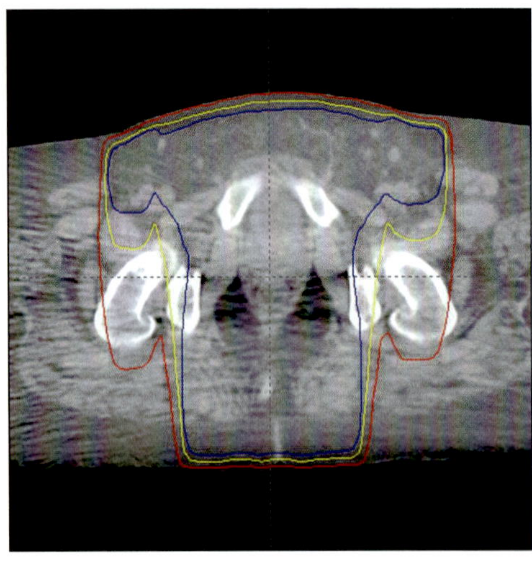

Suburethral Recurrence

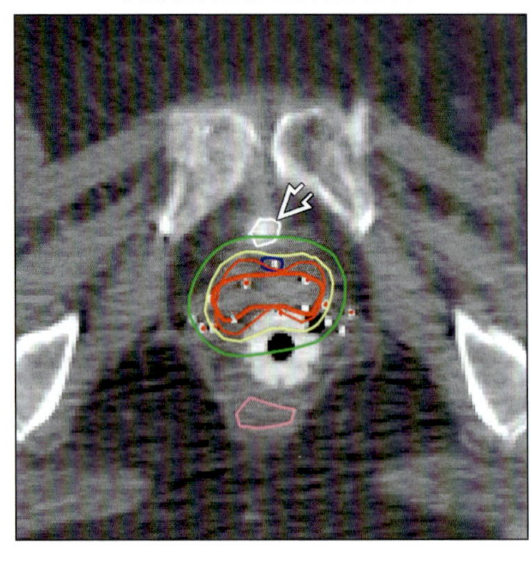

(Left) Patient underwent hysterectomy and had no EBRT. Sagittal T2WI MR shows hematogenous metastasis to S1 ➔. Cortical bone destruction and a protruding soft tissue mass ➔ are readily apparent. *(Right)* In the same patient, axial T1 FSE + contrast shows hyperintense mass ➔ eroding 1/2 of the S1 vertebral body. The tumor mass is pushing the iliac vessels anteriorly ➔.

Isolated Sacral Recurrence

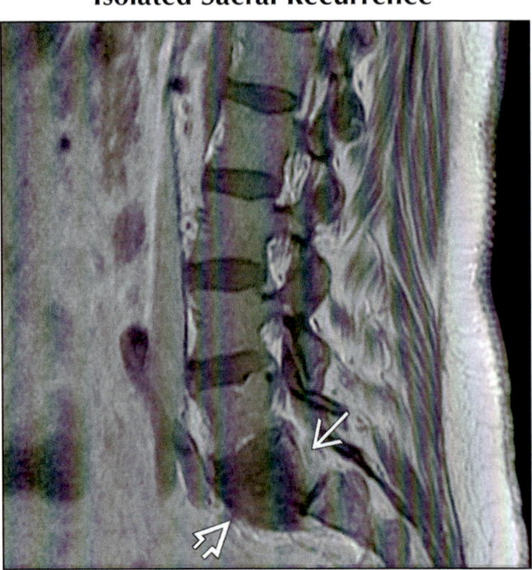

Isolated Sacral Recurrence

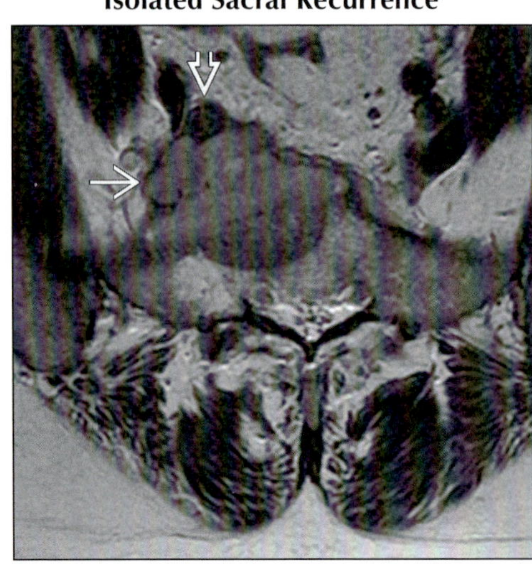

Isolated Sacral Recurrence

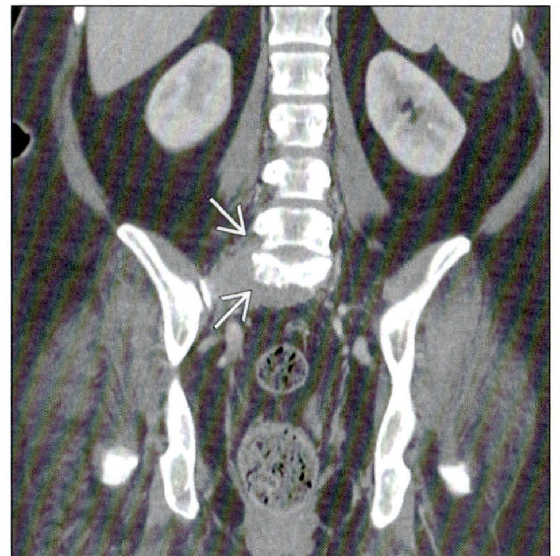

Isolated Sacral Recurrence

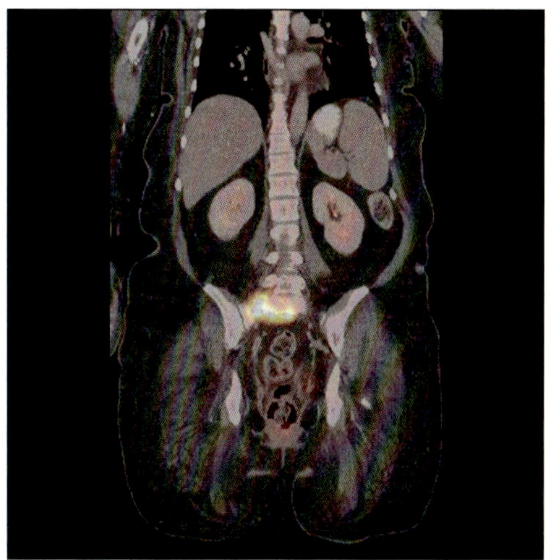

*(**Left**) Coronal CECT in the same patient reveals extensive soft tissue component of the mass. Tumor is encroaching on the intervertebral foramina ➡ surrounding S1 on the right. (**Right**) FDG PET/CT in the same patient shows markedly avid solitary mass. Patient underwent aggressive RT.*

Late Effect of EBRT

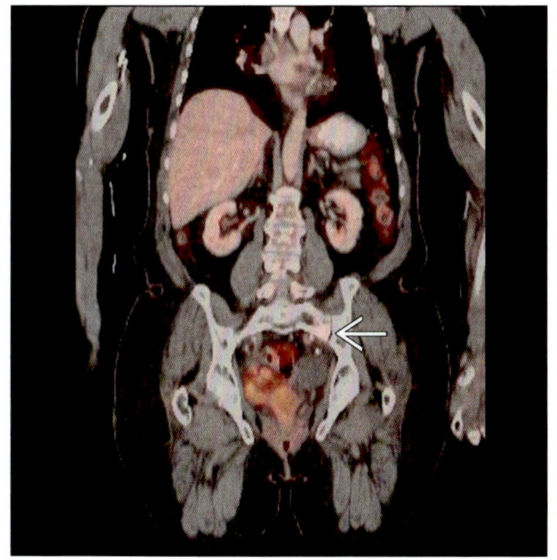

Leiomyosarcoma, Stage IB (T1b N0 M0)

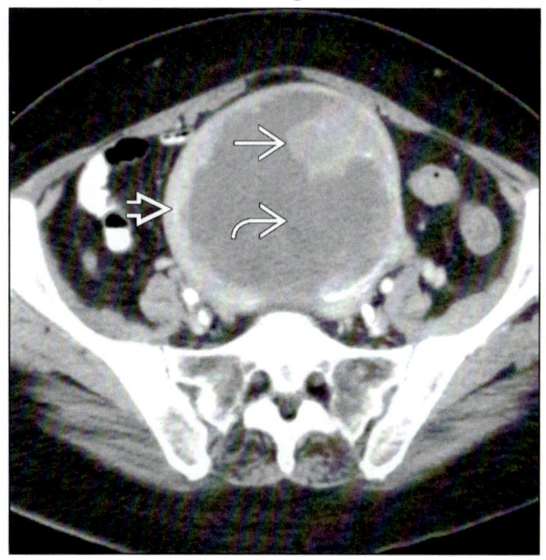

*(**Left**) Coronal PET/CT is shown in a patient with back pain 2 years after EBRT. PET/CT demonstrated an SUV of 3.9 and an area of sclerosis ➡ that was suspicious for a sacral insufficiency fracture. MR can be used if need be to render a diagnosis. (**Right**) Axial CECT in a patient with newly diagnosed uterine leiomyosarcoma measuring > 5 cm shows uterine wall thickening ➡, areas of polypoid abnormal enhancing soft tissue ➡, and extensive central necrosis ➡.*

Leiomyosarcoma, Stage IB (T1b N0 M0)

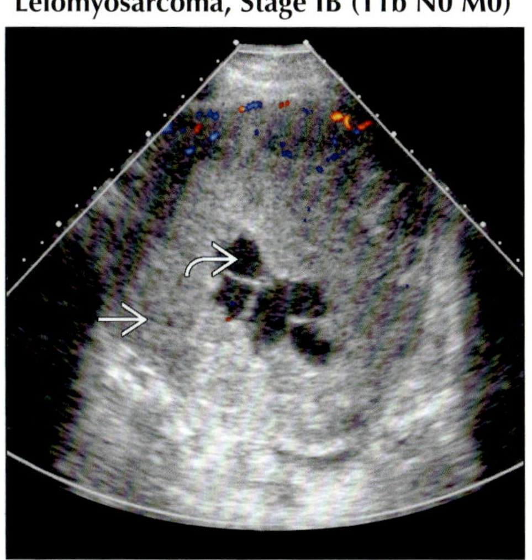

Leiomyosarcoma, Stage IB (T1b N0 M0)

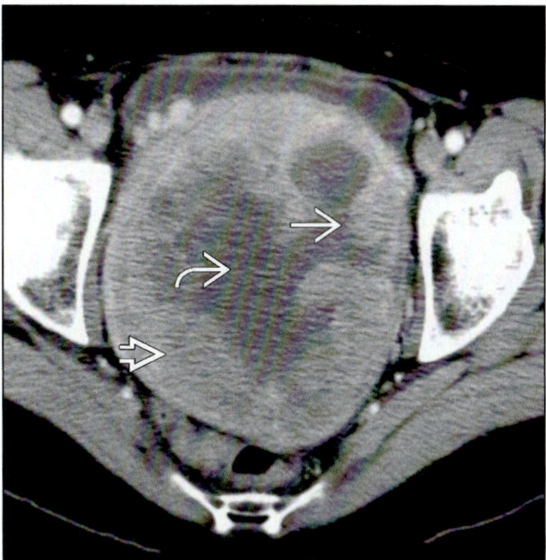

*(**Left**) Transverse color Doppler ultrasound shows a heterogeneous mass ➡ with central hypoechogenic areas of necrosis ➡ in a patient with abdominopelvic pain. (**Right**) Axial CECT in the same patient shows irregular uterine wall thickening ➡, areas of polypoid abnormal enhancing soft tissue ➡, and extensive central necrosis ➡, all findings frequently seen with sarcomas. Surgery revealed uterine leiomyosarcoma.*

*(**Left**) Axial CECT shows a cystic → and solid recurrence ↗ of leiomyosarcoma 1 year after complete resection for uterine-confined disease in a 46-year-old woman. Initially, she received chemo and no RT. Upon recurrence, she was treated with additional chemotherapy with planned resection and possible IORT. (**Right**) Axial CECT in same patient shows gross total resection. Due to adherence to left sidewall, 18 Gy IORT to the surface was delivered with a HAM applicator.*

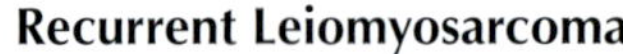

Recurrent Leiomyosarcoma

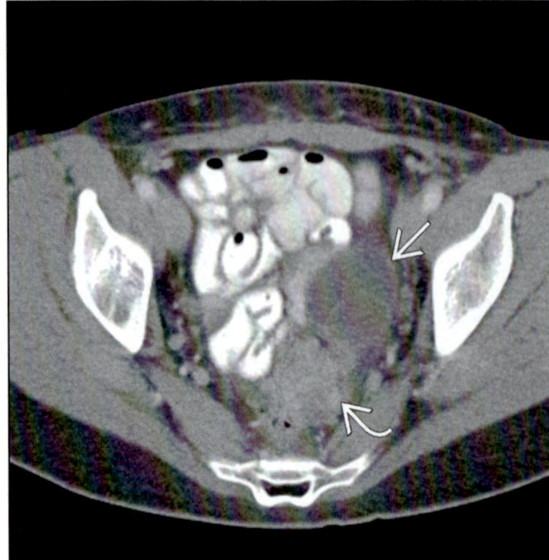

Recurrent Leiomyosarcoma

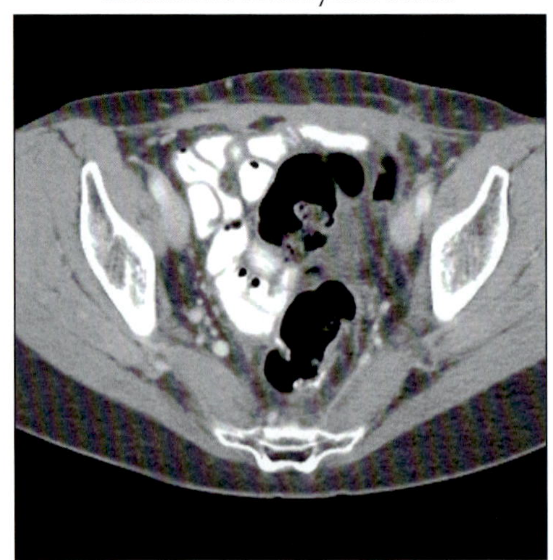

*(**Left**) Axial CT shows the nodal and parametrial/vaginal CTVs and PTV in blue. After IORT, same patient was treated with a 4-field approach to cover the peritoneal surfaces to a dose of 40 Gy in 20 fractions. The 100%, 70%, and 50% isodose lines are shown. (**Right**) Sagittal CT in the same patient shows a likely metastatic focus ↗ in the ileum. The field was expanded to cover this site.*

Recurrent Leiomyosarcoma

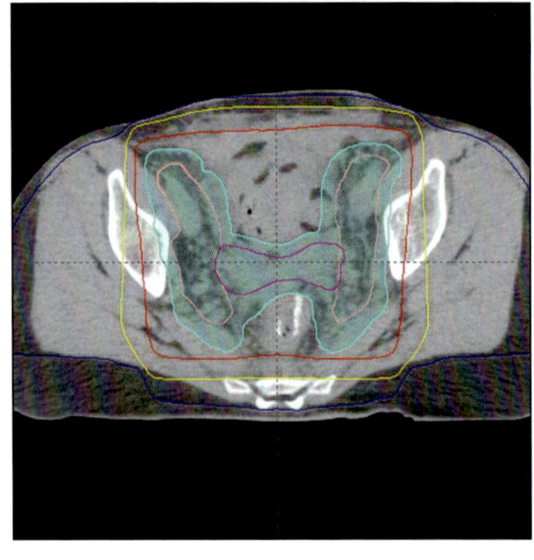

Recurrent Leiomyosarcoma

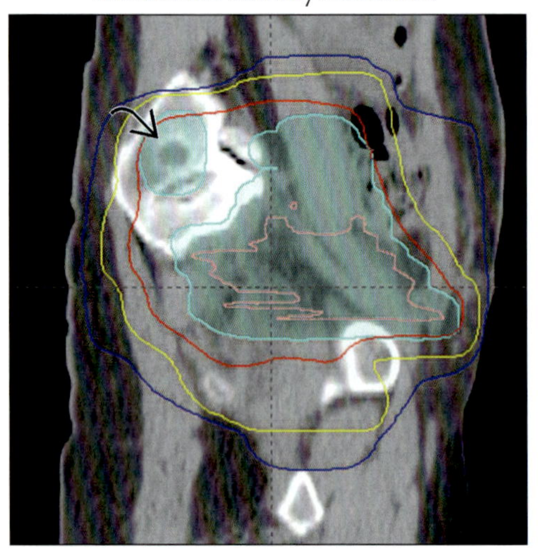

*(**Left**) The same patient was free of disease for 14 months until this coronal CECT showed extensive ascites and solid areas of omental ↗ and peritoneal nodules →. (**Right**) The same patient underwent paracentesis and salvage chemotherapy. This patient has had a partial response with residual disease in the pelvis →.*

Recurrent Leiomyosarcoma

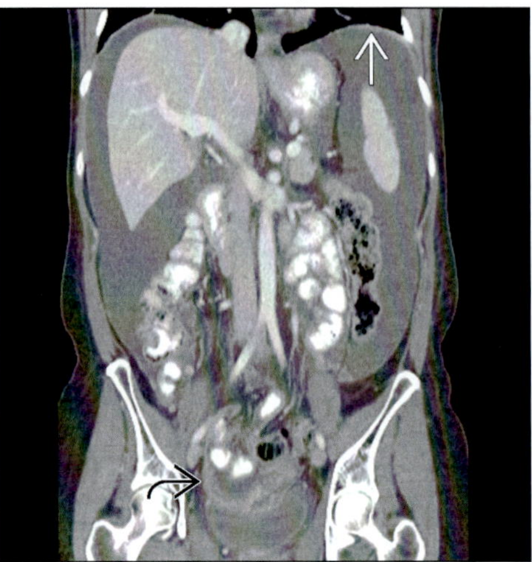

Recurrent Leiomyosarcoma

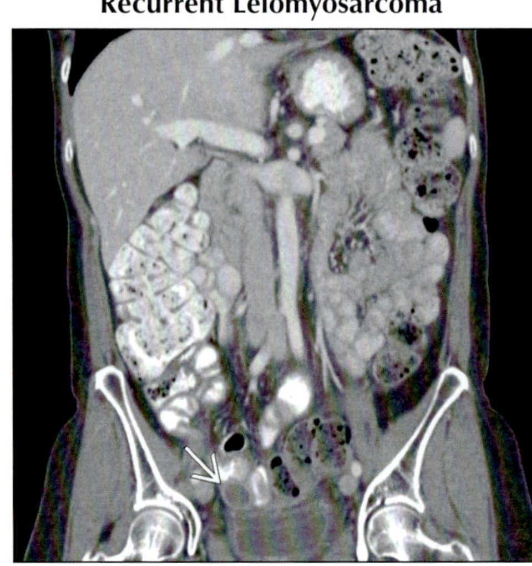

Recurrent Uterine Sarcoma

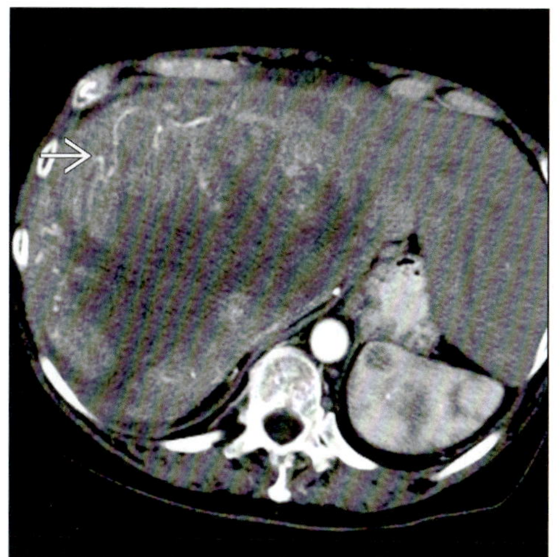

Recurrent Uterine Sarcoma

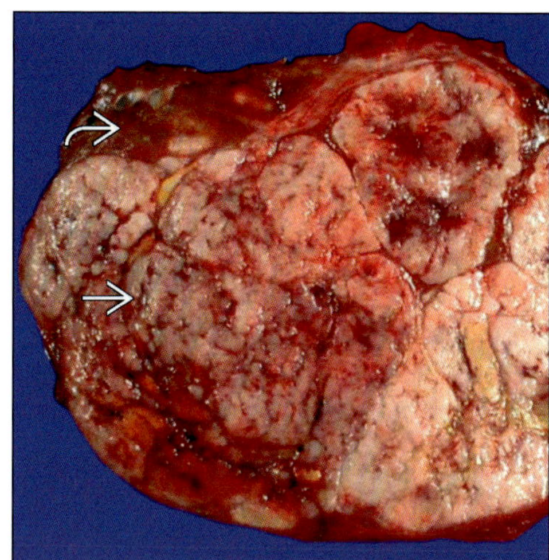

(Left) *Axial CECT during the hepatic arterial phase shows extensive vascularity ➡ within this recurrent uterine leiomyosarcoma of the liver. Sarcomas often outgrow their blood supply and become necrotic centrally.* ***(Right)*** *Gross pathology specimen in the same patient shows the large resected hepatic lesion ➡ against the minimal amount of normal hepatic tissue seen along the right upper border ➡.*

Recurrent Uterine Sarcoma

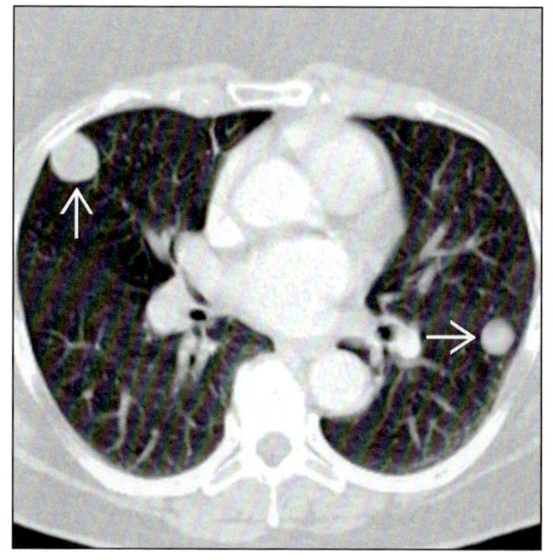

Recurrent Uterine Sarcoma

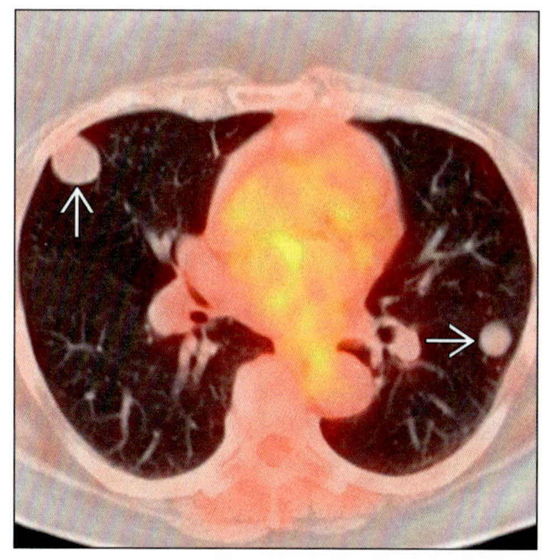

(Left) *Axial CECT shows bilateral well-circumscribed large lesions ➡ in a patient with a history of uterine leiomyosarcoma, very worrisome for metastatic disease.* ***(Right)*** *Axial fused PET/CT from the same patient shows no increased FDG activity in the lesions ➡ above background lung. Subsequent CT-guided biopsy revealed metastatic uterine leiomyosarcoma.*

Recurrent Uterine Sarcoma

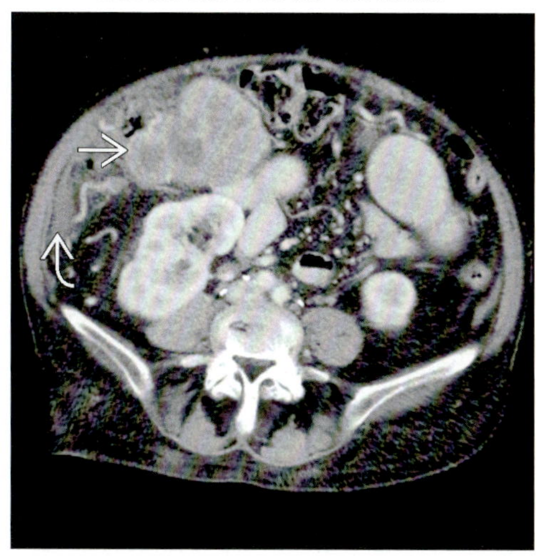

Recurrent Uterine Sarcoma

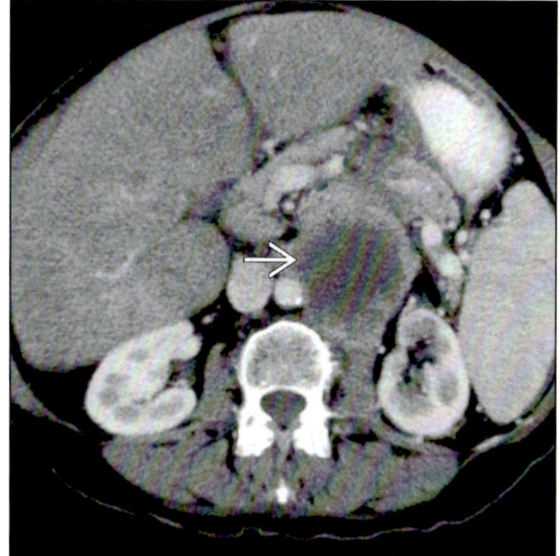

(Left) *Axial CECT shows recurrent tumor ➡ within the small bowel mesentery in this patient with a history of uterine leiomyosarcoma. Also note early nodular carcinomatosis ➡ along the right side of the omentum.* ***(Right)*** *Axial CECT shows a large necrotic left paraaortic mass ➡ in this patient with a history of uterine leiomyosarcoma, compatible with recurrence.*

OVARY AND FALLOPIAN TUBE

(T) Primary Tumor

Adapted from 7th edition AJCC Staging Forms.

TNM	*FIGO*	*Definitions*
TX		Primary tumor cannot be assessed
T0		No evidence of primary tumor
T1	I	Tumor limited to ovaries (1 or both)
T1a	IA	Tumor limited to 1 ovary; capsule intact, no tumor on ovarian surface; no malignant cells in ascites or peritoneal washing
T1b	IB	Tumor limited to both ovaries; capsules intact, no tumor on ovarian surface; no malignant cells in ascites or peritoneal washings
T1c	IC	Tumor limited to 1 or both ovaries with any of the following: Capsule ruptured, tumor on ovarian surface, malignant cells in ascites or peritoneal washings
T2	II	Tumor involves 1 or both ovaries with pelvic extension
T2a	IIA	Extension &/or implants on uterus &/or tube(s); no malignant cells in ascites or peritoneal washings
T2b	IIB	Extension to &/or implants on other pelvic tissues; no malignant cells in ascites or peritoneal washings
T2c	IIC	Pelvic extension &/or implants with malignant cells in ascites or peritoneal washings
T3	III	Tumor involves 1 or both ovaries with peritoneal metastasis outside pelvis
T3a	IIIA	Microscopic peritoneal metastasis beyond pelvis (no macroscopic tumor)
T3b	IIIB	Macroscopic peritoneal metastasis beyond pelvis ≤ 2 cm in greatest dimension
T3c	IIIC	Peritoneal metastasis beyond pelvis > 2 cm in greatest dimension &/or regional lymph node metastasis

(N) Regional Lymph Nodes

NX		Regional lymph nodes cannot be assessed
N0		No regional lymph node metastasis
N1	IIIC	Regional lymph node metastasis

(M) Distant Metastasis

M0		No distant metastasis
M1	IV	Distant metastasis (excludes peritoneal metastasis)

AJCC Stages/Prognostic Groups

Adapted from 7th edition AJCC Staging Forms.

Stage	*T*	*N*	*M*
I	T1	N0	M0
IA	T1a	N0	M0
IB	T1b	N0	M0
IC	T1c	N0	M0
II	T2	N0	M0
IIA	T2a	N0	M0
IIB	T2b	N0	M0
IIC	T2c	N0	M0
III	T3	N0	M0
IIIA	T3a	N0	M0
IIIB	T3b	N0	M0
IIIC	T3c	N0	M0
	Any T	N1	M0
IV	Any T	Any N	M1

T1a

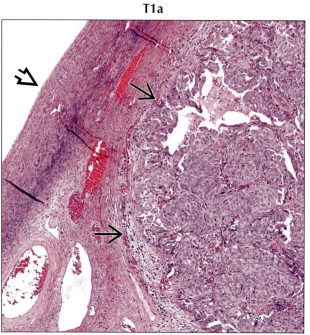

Low-power magnification of H&E shows ovarian carcinoma that is limited to 1 ovary with intact capsule (T1a). Sheets of tumor cells → are seen with intact capsule ⇨.

T1a

High-power magnification shows sheets of serous carcinoma cells → and an intact capsule ⇨ overlying ovarian stroma.

T1c

Low-power magnification shows ovarian tumor extending through the capsule to the ovarian surface (T1c). The H&E stain shows ovarian tumor ⇨ extending to the ovarian surface →. Note normal ovarian tissue on the right side of the photomicrograph.

T1c

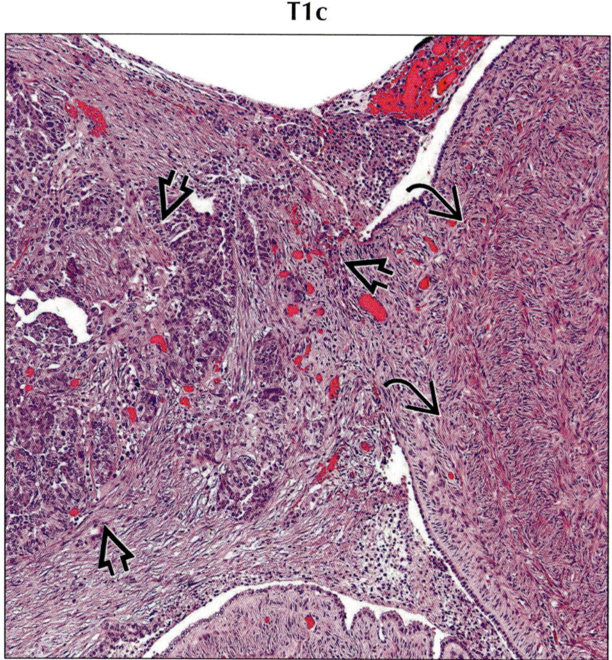

Higher magnification shows a close-up of the cords and nests of tumor cells ⇨ and ovarian plump spindle stromal cells ↷.

T2a

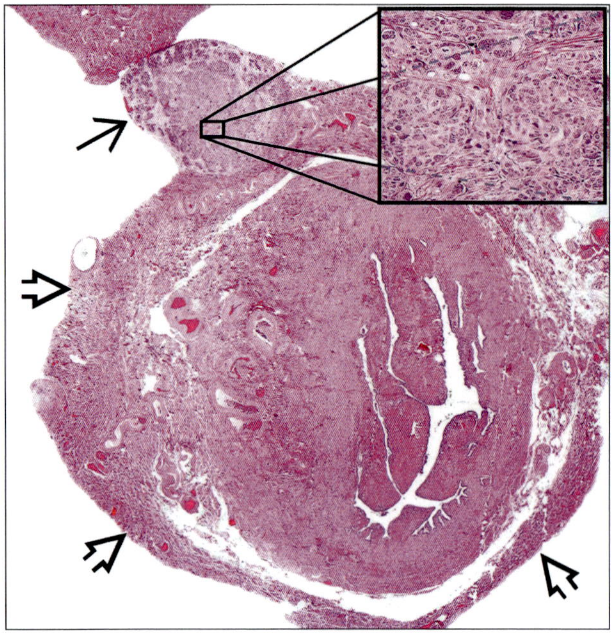

Low-power magnification of H&E stain shows a cross section of a fallopian tube ⇨ with ovarian tumor nodule → implanted on the serosal aspect. The inset shows a high-magnification view of the neoplastic malignant cells of the nodule.

T2b

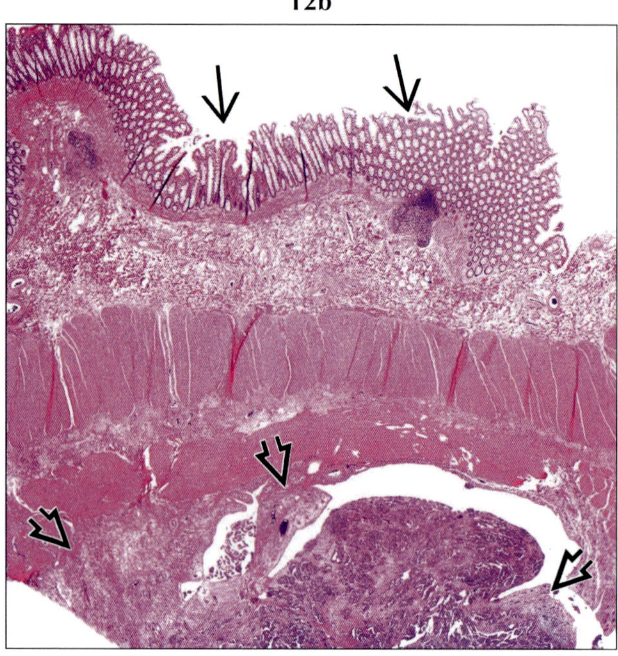

Low-power magnification of H&E stain shows an implanted ovarian nodule to the serosal surface of the rectosigmoid colon (T2b). The mucosal side of the rectosigmoid is highlighted →, as well as the tumor nodule ⇨.

T3

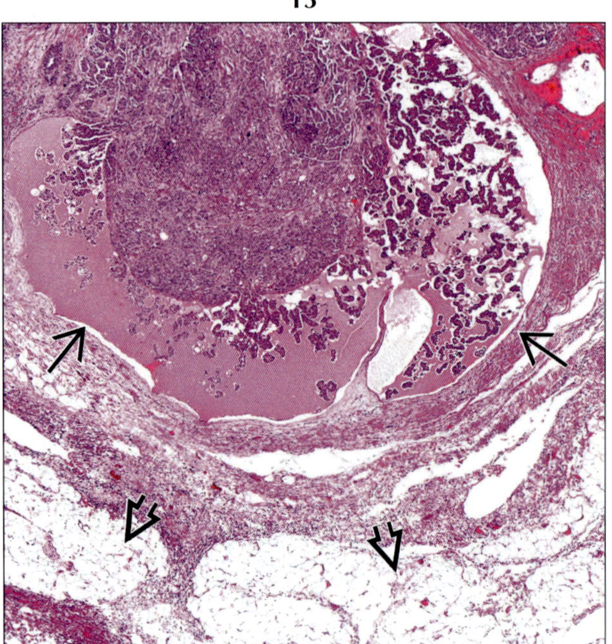

H&E section shows peritoneal metastasis of ovarian papillary serous carcinoma outside the pelvis (T3). The nodule in the upper part of the slide → represents the metastatic tumor and is implanted in the fibrofatty tissue ⇨ of the peritoneum (lower aspect of the slide).

T3c

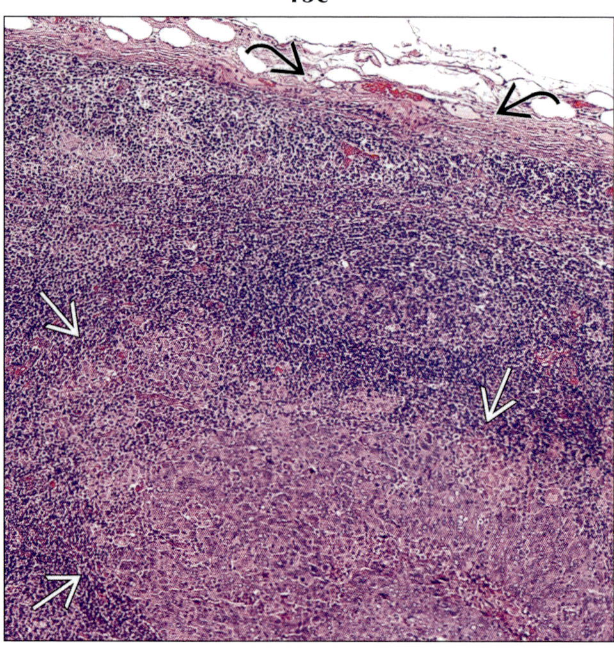

Low-power magnification of H&E stain shows a metastatic ovarian carcinoma to a regional lymph node (T3c). The lymph node capsule is highlighted ↷; tumor nest ➡ is present within the lymph node.

T1a (FIGO IA)

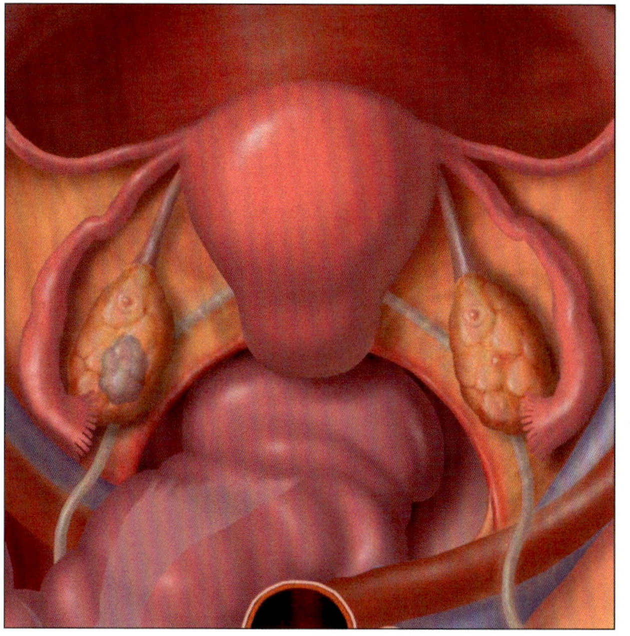

T1a tumors are limited to 1 ovary with an intact capsule, no tumor on the ovarian surface, and no malignant cells in ascites or peritoneal washings.

T1b (FIGO IB)

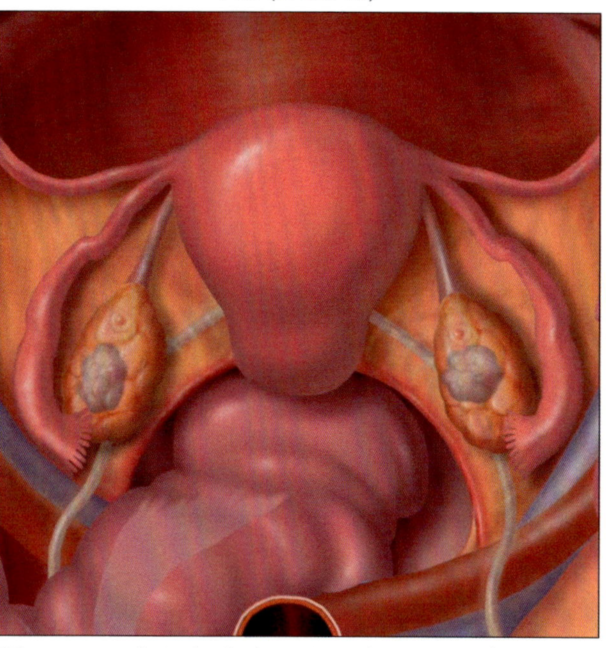

T1b tumors are limited to both ovaries with intact capsules, no tumor on the ovarian surface, and no malignant cells in ascites or peritoneal washings.

T1c (FIGO IC)

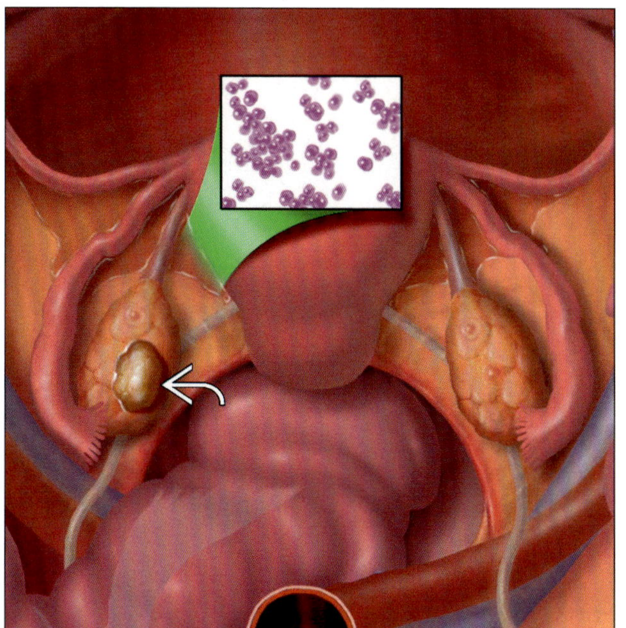

T1c tumors are limited to 1 or both ovaries with capsule rupture, tumor on the ovarian surface ➔, or malignant cells in ascites or peritoneal washings.

T2a (FIGO IIA)

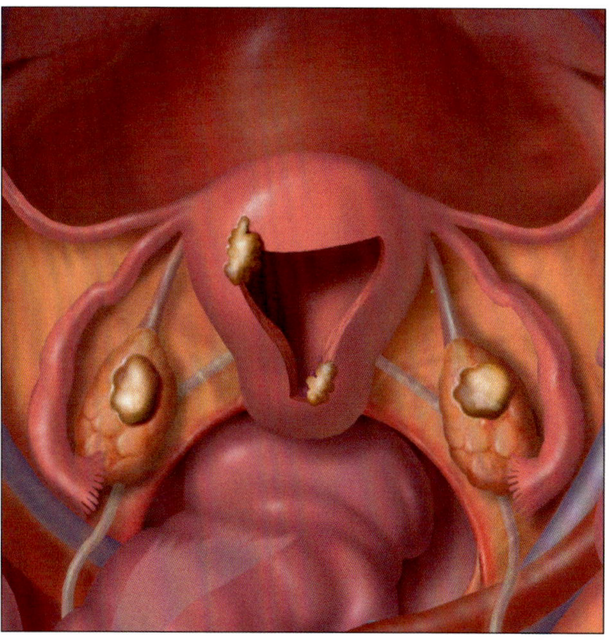

T2a tumors involve 1 or both ovaries with pelvic extension to the uterus or fallopian tube. No malignant cells are found in ascites or peritoneal washings.

OVARY AND FALLOPIAN TUBE

T2b (FIGO IIB)

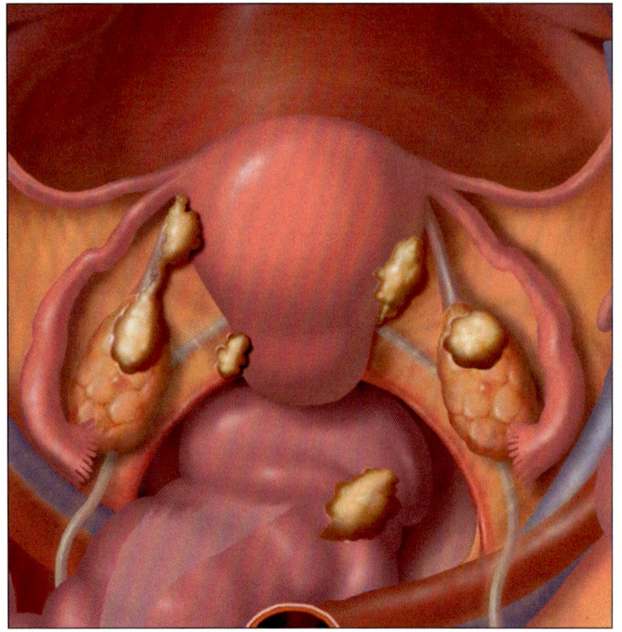

T2b tumors involve 1 or both ovaries with pelvic extension &/or implants to other pelvic organs. No malignant cells in ascites or peritoneal washings are found.

T2c (FIGO IIC)

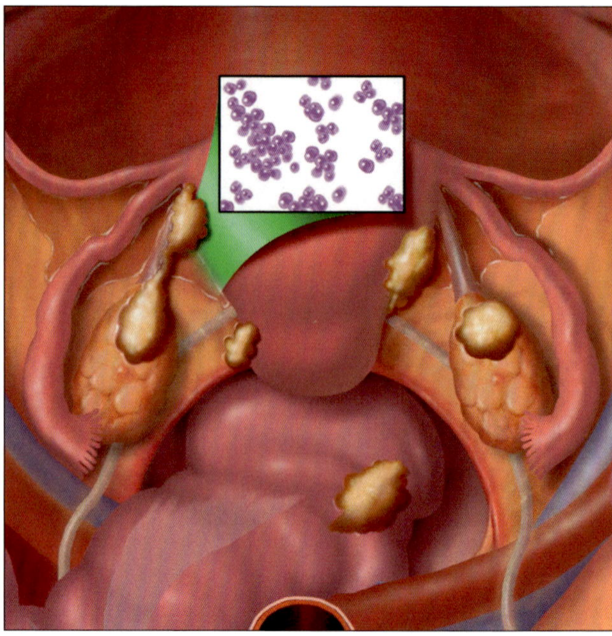

T2c tumors involve 1 or both ovaries with pelvic extension &/or implants, with malignant cells in ascites or peritoneal washings.

T3a (FIGO IIIA)

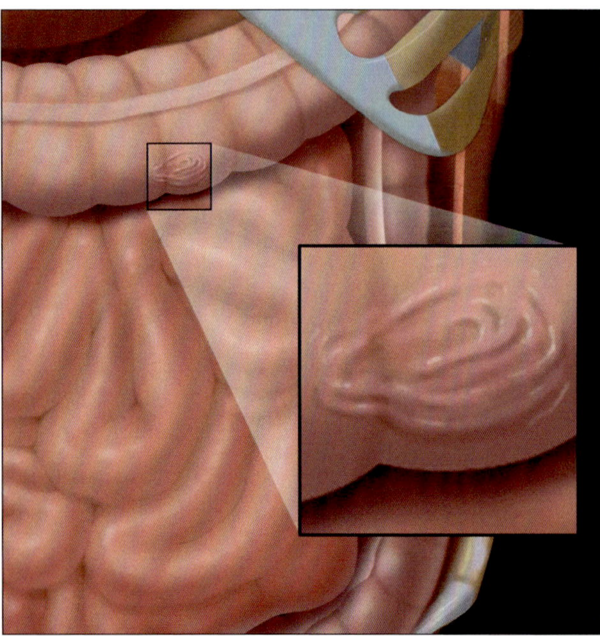

T3a tumors involve microscopic peritoneal metastases beyond the pelvis. This cannot be visualized by imaging; rather, it is found through peritoneal biopsy at staging laparotomy.

T3b (FIGO IIIB)

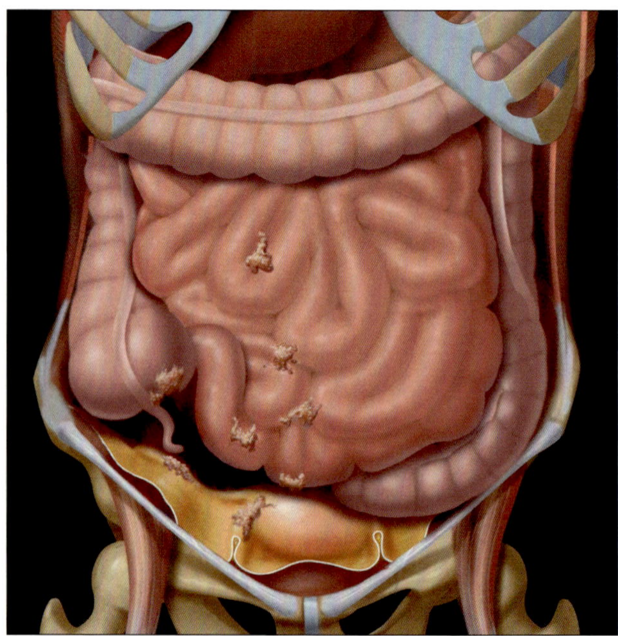

T3b tumors feature macroscopic peritoneal metastases beyond the pelvis that are ≤ 2 cm in greatest dimension.

T3c (FIGO IIIC)

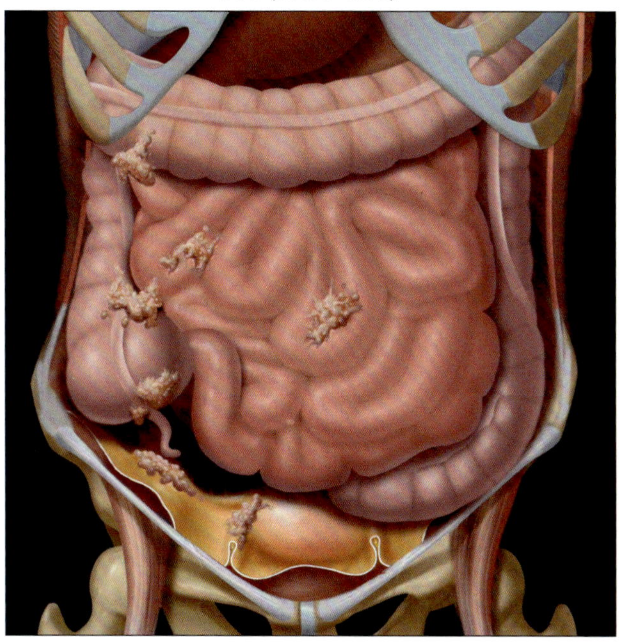

T3c tumors involve macroscopic peritoneal metastases beyond the pelvis (> 2 cm in greatest dimension) &/or regional nodal metastases.

Nodal Drainage of Ovary

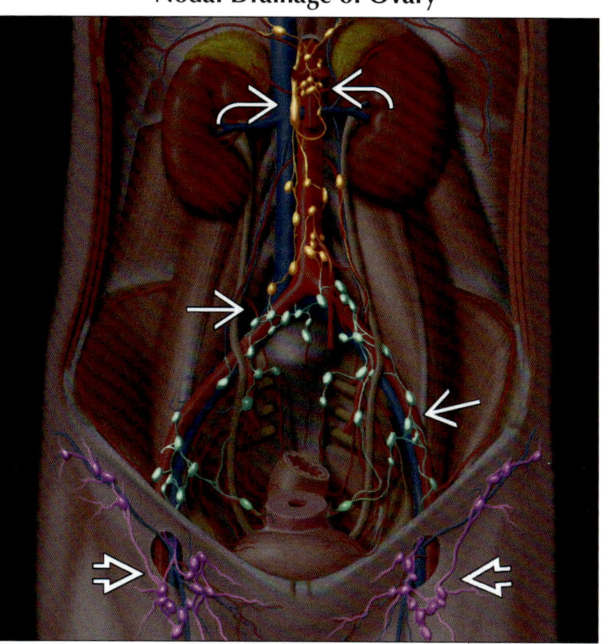

The main ovarian lymphatics follow the ovarian veins to the paraaortic lymph nodes. Lymphatic spread may also occur through the broad ligament to the pelvic lymph nodes and along the round ligament to the inguinal lymph nodes.

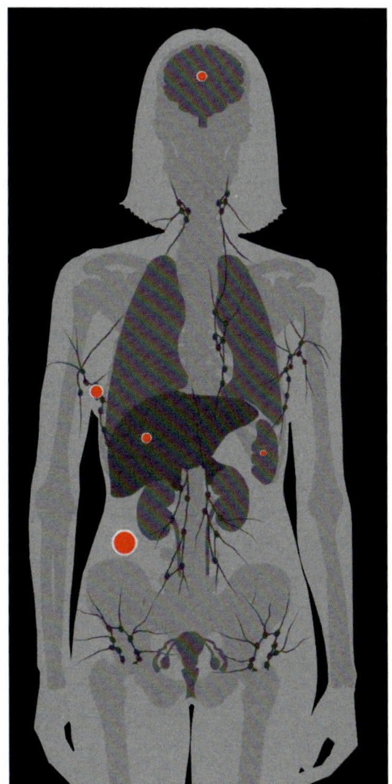

INITIAL SITE OF RECURRENCE

Site	%
Abdominal Carcinomatosis	37%
Multiple Nodules	16%
Lymph Nodes	7%
Single Nodule	6%
Liver	3%
Brain	2%
Spleen	1%

Data from 270 stage III/IV patients, most of whom received chemotherapy. The recurrence rate was 18% for 58 stage I/II patients. The anatomic sites listed refer to discrete lesions and are included in single and multiple nodules. Ferrandina G et al: Impact of patterns of recurrence on clinical outcomes of ovarian cancer patients. Clinical Considerations. Eur J Cancer: 42:2296-2302, 2006.

OVARY AND FALLOPIAN TUBE

OVERVIEW

General Comments

- Primary peritoneal carcinoma (unusual tumor of similar histiogenic origin) included in 7th edition of AJCC staging manual

Classification

- Primary ovarian carcinomas are differentiated by cell origin
  - Epithelial ovarian tumors (EOT): 90% of ovarian carcinomas
    - Serous cystadenocarcinoma (60%)
    - Endometrioid carcinoma (10%)
    - Clear cell carcinoma (10%)
    - Carcinosarcoma (10%)
    - Mixed (5%)
    - Mucinous cystadenocarcinoma (3%)
      - Less common than initially thought
      - Many are actually metastatic from GI primary
    - Undifferentiated carcinoma (1%)
    - Brenner tumor (< 1%)
  - Nonepithelial ovarian tumors: 10% of ovarian carcinomas
    - Germ cell tumors
      - Dysgerminoma
      - Embryonal carcinoma
      - Immature teratoma
      - Polyembryoma
      - Choriocarcinoma
      - Mixed tumors
    - Tumor of sex cord or stroma
      - Malignant granulosa cell tumor
- Nonepithelial primary ovarian cancers may be staged using TNM classification system

NATURAL HISTORY

Etiology

- Factors known to increase risk of developing ovarian cancer include
  - Family history (strongest known risk factor)
    - ~ 10% of cases are thought to have hereditary basis
    - Women who have had breast cancer or who have family history of breast or ovarian cancer are at increased risk
  - Nulliparity, early menarche, and late menopause
  - Estrogen use alone as postmenopausal hormone therapy
  - Obesity may be associated with increased risk
- Pregnancy and long-term use of oral contraceptives reduce risk of developing ovarian cancer

Epidemiology & Cancer Incidence

- Approximately 3% of all cancers among women
- 2nd most common gynecological malignancy after endometrial carcinoma
- Leading cause of death from gynecological cancers and 9th leading cause of cancer death in women
- Number of cases in USA per year
  - Estimated 22,280 new cases in USA in 2012
  - Estimated 15,500 deaths in USA in 2012

Genetics

- Lifetime risk of ovarian cancer: 15-30% in women carrying genes responsible for most hereditary ovarian cancers (*BRCA1*, *BRCA2*)
- Hereditary nonpolyposis colon cancer (Lynch syndrome) has also been associated with endometrial and ovarian cancers

Gross Pathology & Surgical Features

- General features
  - 2/3 of cases involve both ovaries
  - Range from microscopic to about 20 cm in diameter
  - Typically multilocular and cystic, with intracystic, soft, friable papillae
    - Cysts contain serous, turbid, or bloody fluid
  - External surfaces may be smooth or bosselated and may display grossly exophytic papillary tumor on surface (at least T1c)
  - Solid areas and intracystic nodules are more common in carcinomas than in cystadenomas
  - Hemorrhage and necrosis are often present
- Endometrioid carcinoma arising in endometrioma
  - Gross findings of endometriotic cyst containing chocolate-colored fluid
  - 1 or more solid mural nodules reflecting foci of malignant transformation

Microscopic Pathology

- Major histologic types
  - **Serous cystadenocarcinoma**
    - Most common type of ovarian cancer
      - Accounts for > 50%
    - Complex papillary and solid patterns with marked nuclear atypia; qualify as high-grade carcinomas
    - Characteristic pattern is lace-like or labyrinthine pattern
      - May be focal but often diffuse
      - Characterized by extensive bridging and coalescence of papillae resulting in solid sheets of tumor cells with interspersed slit-like spaces
    - Serous carcinomas that display extensive solid areas are usually composed of uniform sheets of cells with high-grade nuclear atypia
      - Usually there are focal areas with papillary architecture that permit diagnosis of serous carcinoma as opposed to undifferentiated carcinoma
    - Psammoma bodies are present in 25% of cases
  - **Endometrioid carcinoma**
    - Well-differentiated endometrioid adenocarcinoma accounts for most cases
    - Confluent or cribriform proliferation of glands lined by tall stratified columnar epithelium with sharp luminal margins
    - Villoglandular growth pattern also occurs
    - Squamous differentiation is present in 50% of cases
  - **Mucinous adenocarcinoma**
    - Stromal invasion measuring > 5 mm
    - Stromal invasion in primary ovarian mucinous neoplasms is characterized by 3 different patterns
      - Confluent glandular growth with crowded glands without intervening stroma

- Clusters of single cells with abundant eosinophilic cytoplasm surrounded by clear spaces
      - Glands of varying sizes infiltrating stroma in haphazard pattern
    - Cytoplasm is scant and eosinophilic with irregular borders and occasional mucin droplets
  - **Brenner tumor**
    - Rounded nests of transitional or squamous cell-like epithelium and glandular structures of cylindrical cells within abundant fibrous nonepithelial tissue
    - Microscopically resembles urothelial transitional cell carcinoma
  - **Clear cell adenocarcinoma**
    - Ovarian epithelial tumor in which most cells have clear cytoplasm
    - High association with pelvic endometriosis

Routes of Spread

- Understanding pattern of spread is crucial for adequate radiological and surgical staging
- **Local spread**
  - Direct extension to surrounding pelvic structures
    - Commonly: Fallopian tubes, uterus, and contralateral adnexa
    - Less commonly: Rectum, bladder, and pelvic sidewall
  - Uterine involvement
    - Independent primary tumors of low histologic grade, usually of endometrioid type, with involvement limited to endometrium and ovary
      - Favorable prognosis; often no additional treatment
    - Tumors metastasizing from uterus to ovary or from ovary to uterus
      - Worse prognosis; adjuvant therapy is generally indicated
    - Distinction between primary vs. secondary involvement relies on histological examination
      - Genetic studies may help in some cases
- **Peritoneal seeding**
  - Most common mode of tumor spread
  - Malignant cells are distributed by gravity into cul-de-sac or follow normal routes of peritoneal fluid circulation
    - Preferential flow and seeding along right paracolic gutter, liver capsule, and right hemidiaphragm
  - Peritoneal fluid normally drains through rich lymphatic capillary network of diaphragm to supradiaphragmatic lymph nodes
    - Occlusion of these lymphatics by tumor cells blocks absorption of peritoneal fluid
    - Contributes to accumulation of malignant ascites
  - Most common sites of peritoneal metastases
    - Cul-de-sac
    - Greater omentum
    - Paracolic gutters
    - Small and large bowel surface
    - Liver surface
    - Subphrenic spaces
  - Other potential sites of metastases
    - Porta hepatis
    - Fissure for ligamentum teres
    - Lesser sac
    - Gastrosplenic and gastrohepatic ligaments
    - Splenic hilum
  - Primary peritoneal carcinoma
    - Unusual tumor of similar histiogenic origin
    - Primary tumor of peritoneum that diffusely involves peritoneal surface but spares or only superficially involves ovaries
    - Generally diagnosed in state of peritoneal carcinomatosis
    - Poor prognosis
    - Biopsy important to differentiate primary peritoneal carcinoma from peritoneal carcinomatosis (due to other cancers, mesothelioma, lymphomatosis, or tuberculous peritonitis)
  - Pseudomyxoma peritonei
    - Growing body of immunohistochemical and molecular studies suggest that majority are secondary to appendiceal tumors in both men and women
    - Those that are ovarian in origin probably originated from mucinous tumors arising in teratomas
- **Lymphatic spread**
  - 3 primary pathways for lymphatic drainage
    - Main lymphatics follow ovarian veins → paraaortic and aortocaval lymph nodes at level of renal veins
    - Through broad ligament → pelvic lymph nodes, including external iliac, hypogastric, and obturator nodes
    - Along round ligament → inguinal lymph nodes
- **Hematogenous spread**
  - Least common mode of spread
  - Usually not present at initial diagnosis but can be found at restaging
    - In up to 50% of patients at autopsy

IMAGING

Detection

- Primary goal of radiologic assessment is differentiation of malignant from benign tumors
- CA 125 is a glycoprotein that is assessed by monoclonal antibody CA 125
  - ↑ CA 125 serum level ≥ 30 U/mL indicates presence of malignancy
  - False-positive results
    - Conditions affecting peritoneal surface, such as endometriosis
  - False-negative results
    - Early-stage invasive disease and borderline ovarian tumors
- **General imaging findings suggestive of malignancy**
  - Most predictive imaging findings for malignancy are
    - Solid mass, especially when necrosis is present
    - Presence of nonfat nodular components in cystic lesion
  - Other findings suggestive of malignancy
    - Irregular, thick wall or septa (> 3 mm)
    - Vascularity in solid mass or papillary projections
      - Doppler demonstration of blood flow
      - Enhancement on CT and MR
  - Ancillary findings that are strong indicators of malignancy

- Ascites
- Peritoneal metastases
- Lymphadenopathy
- Pelvic organ or sidewall invasion
- **Special tumor features** may be present and can suggest specific type
  - Calcification in cystic or partially cystic tumor
    - Serous epithelial tumor
  - Associated endometrial hyperplasia or carcinoma
    - Endometrioid epithelial tumor (20-30% of patients)
  - Variable density (echogenicity) within loculi of multilocular tumor
    - Mucinous epithelial tumor
  - Pseudomyxoma peritonei virtually never occurs in association with primary ovarian mucinous tumors
- **Ultrasound (US)**
  - Low cost and wide availability
  - Modality of choice to evaluate suspected or palpable adnexal mass
    - Adnexal masses are found on US in about 10% of premenopausal women
    - US seems to be similar with CT and MR in differentiation of malignant from benign ovarian tumors
      - Pattern recognition on US correctly classified 93% of lesions as benign or malignant (in experienced hands)
  - Transvaginal ultrasound (TVU) and transabdominal ultrasound (TAU) should be used together
    - TVU allows best evaluation of pelvic masses but limited field of view
    - TAU is better for large mass or if ovaries are displaced by enlarged leiomyomatous uterus
  - Ovarian volumes
    - Premenopausal women: Up to 20 mL
    - Postmenopausal women: Up to 8-10 mL
    - Ovarian volumes progressively decrease with age and years post menopause
    - Enlarged ovary for age, or ovary > 2x volume of other ovary, may be early indication of ovarian neoplasm
  - Spectral Doppler findings suggestive of malignancy
    - Low-resistance waveforms due to tumor neovascularity and arteriovenous shunting
    - Resistance index < 0.4 and pulsatility index < 1
    - Considerable overlap with benign physiological lesions
    - More suspicious in postmenopausal women, in whom benign lesions are less frequent
    - Color Doppler flow imaging alone is significantly inferior to combined US techniques, morphologic assessment alone, and contrast-enhanced US in diagnosis of ovarian cancer
  - Hemorrhagic cysts may appear similar to neoplasm
    - Repeat scanning 4-6 weeks following initial detection of indeterminate ovarian mass
  - Mixed results reported for use of US ± CA 125 in screening for ovarian cancer
    - Routine US screening of asymptomatic women → ↑ false-positive results → unnecessary laparoscopy or laparotomy
    - Positive predictive value for invasive cancer is 3.7% for abnormal CA 125, 1% for abnormal TVU, and 23.5% if both tests are abnormal
- **CT**
  - Increased number of incidental ovarian lesions discovered due to widespread use of CT
  - Recent advances in CT technology and availability of multidetector CT (MDCT) allow better detection and improved characterization of adnexal masses
  - MDCT: Sensitivity (90%), specificity (89%), positive predictive value (78%), negative predictive value (95%), and overall accuracy in diagnosing malignancy (89%)
- **MR**
  - Used mainly as problem-solving tool in setting of sonographically indeterminate or complex adnexal mass
  - Can provide tissue characterization based on signal properties
    - MR is superior to US and CT in differentiation of benign from malignant masses
  - Adequate evaluation of adnexal masses on MR imaging requires
    - T1WI and T2WI to delineate pelvic anatomy and tumor
    - Fat-saturated T1WI to distinguish between fat and hemorrhage
    - Gadolinium-enhanced T1WI to improve detection of solid components
  - Dynamic contrast-enhanced MR imaging has been used to analyze perfusion of solid components contained in ovarian tumors
    - Can differentiate among benign, borderline, and malignant tumors
    - Different parameters have been used
      - Include enhancement amplitude (EA), time of half rising (Tmax), and maximal slope (MS)
    - Invasive tumors tend to show early intense and persistent enhancement
- **FDG PET/CT**
  - May detect unexpected ovarian cancers during staging of other tumors
  - Low specificity since benign lesions, such as corpus luteum cyst in premenopausal women, can increase ovarian uptake
    - Increased ovarian FDG uptake in postmenopausal women, in whom benign lesions are less likely, is usually associated with malignancy
  - May detect ovarian carcinoma in so-called normal-sized ovary carcinoma syndrome (NOCS)
    - NOCS occurs when diffuse metastatic malignant disease with normal-sized ovaries is noted, but no origin is assigned by preoperative or intraoperative evaluation
  - May be useful in identifying recurrent disease, especially whether isolated or diffuse, to decide which further therapy is best for the patient including surgery, chemo, or RT

Staging

- Staging is surgical, based on FIGO system
  - Requires staging laparotomy
    - Total abdominal hysterectomy
    - Bilateral salpingo-oophorectomy
    - Omentectomy

  - Retroperitoneal lymph node sampling
  - Peritoneal and diaphragmatic biopsies
  - Cytological evaluation of peritoneal washings
- Preoperative imaging staging of ovarian carcinoma
  - CT is primary imaging modality for preoperative staging of ovarian cancer
  - MR is at least as accurate as CT
    - Used when CT is contraindicated
      - e.g., in patients with poor renal function or allergy to iodinated contrast
    - 3.0T MR can achieve staging of ovarian cancer accuracy comparable to surgical staging
    - Adding DWI to routine MR improves sensitivity and specificity for depicting peritoneal metastases
      - Sensitivity and specificity of 90% and 95.5%, respectively
      - Peritoneal tumor shows restricted diffusion on DWI and ascites of low signal intensity, increasing tumor conspicuity
  - FDG PET/CT
    - FDG PET is limited in resolution and not optimal for detecting lesions < 0.5 cm in size
  - CT and pelvic MR have replaced barium enema and IVP
- Goals of preoperative imaging
  - Detection of metastatic lesions
    - Prevent understaging
    - Allow adequate intraoperative sampling of suspected lesions
  - Recognition of extensive, unresectable disease
- Factors generally indicating inoperable disease include
  - Invasion of pelvic sidewall, rectum, sigmoid colon, or bladder
  - Bulky peritoneal disease in
    - Porta hepatis
    - Intersegmental fissure of liver
    - Lesser sac
    - Gastrosplenic ligament
    - Gastrohepatic ligament
    - Subphrenic space
    - Small bowel mesentery
    - Supracolic omentum
    - Presacral space
  - Suprarenal and splenic adenopathy
  - Hepatic and splenic (parenchymal), pleural, or pulmonary metastases
- Preoperative CT and MR imaging are highly accurate in
  - Detection of inoperable tumor
  - Prediction of suboptimal debulking
- **Malignant ascites**
  - Ascites can result from increased production by tumor, peritoneal metastases, or decreased absorption
    - Diaphragmatic lymphatic blockage, indicating stage III disease
  - Any peritoneal fluid in postmenopausal women and more than small amount of fluid in premenopausal women is abnormal
  - Presence of ascites: Positive predictive value (75%) for presence of peritoneal metastases
- **Peritoneal disease**
  - Microscopic peritoneal disease is undetectable with imaging
  - Small peritoneal implants ≤ 2 cm are difficult to detect with imaging
  - Omentum is most common site of peritoneal spread of tumor
    - Early omental disease
      - Subtle, fine, reticular nodularity
    - Advanced omental disease
      - Mass-like omental thickening (omental cakes)
  - Common sites of involvement should be carefully evaluated, including subphrenic space, mesentery, and paracolic gutters
  - Presence of ascites or calcifications of peritoneal nodules make implants more conspicuous and easy to detect
  - Pseudomyxoma peritonei
    - Accumulation of mucinous ascites → hepatic, splenic, and mesenteric scalloping
    - When found, should raise possibility of primary appendiceal neoplasm with ovarian metastases rather than primary mucinous ovarian neoplasm
- **Local extension**
  - Local tumor extension involving surrounding pelvic organs is suggested by
    - Distortion or irregular interface between tumor and myometrium
    - Obscuration of tissue planes with either urinary bladder or colon
    - < 3 mm between tumor and pelvic sidewall
    - Displacement or encasement of iliac vessels
  - Local extension is easier to identify with MR than with either CT or US
    - Superior soft tissue contrast
- **Nodal disease**
  - Frequency of nodal metastases in M1 patients: 65%
  - Major limitation of CT and MR: Dependence on size of lymph node to determine nodal involvement
    - Enlarged lymph node is likely to be involved
    - Not possible to exclude metastatic disease in normal-sized node
  - Using short axis size threshold of ≥ 1 cm to define abnormal lymph nodes
    - Sensitivity of preoperative CT (50%), MR (83%)
    - Specificity of preoperative CT (92%), MR (95%)
  - Cardiophrenic nodes are detected in approximately 15% of patients with advanced disease
    - Often indicates poor prognosis; usually considered stage IV disease
    - Enlargement is defined as short axis diameter > 5 mm
  - Functional evaluation of lymph nodes
    - DWI MR is accurate in distinguishing malignant from benign pelvic lymph nodes
    - FDG PET
      - Detect metastases in normal-sized lymph nodes
      - Verify malignant tissue in enlarged nodes
- **Small bowel involvement**
  - Commonly occurs and is frequent cause of morbidity
    - Either due to serosal implants or frank wall invasion
- **Liver involvement**
  - Important to distinguish implants on liver capsule (stage III) from true parenchymal metastases (stage IV)

- Capsular implants are considered resectable, whereas parenchymal metastases generally are not
- Capsular masses are usually smooth, well defined; have elliptic or biconvex appearance and sharp interface with liver parenchyma
- Parenchymal metastases are less defined and surrounded by liver parenchyma
- Capsular metastases may invade liver parenchyma
  - Fuzzy interface between mass and liver parenchyma

- **Pleural effusion**
  - Most common finding in stage IV disease
  - Presence of effusion is not sufficient for designation of stage IV disease
    - Cytologic evaluation is required
  - Pleural masses, nodularity, or thickening makes likelihood of pleural metastases extremely high

Restaging

- Imaging recommendations
  - Patients treated for ovarian cancer are followed up with serial measurements of CA 125 and either CT scan or MR imaging of abdomen and pelvis
    - Serial serum CA 125 levels are accurate measure of disease burden for most women
  - PET/CT demonstrates greater accuracy and less interobserver variability than CT alone
  - Chest CT should not be performed routinely
    - Used if ↑ tumor markers and no sites of recurrence are detected on abdominal and pelvic CT
  - MR is more sensitive than PET/CT for detecting local pelvic recurrence and peritoneal lesions in recurrent ovarian carcinoma

CLINICAL PRESENTATION & WORK-UP

Presentation

- Symptoms are usually nonspecific
- Common symptoms
  - Abdominal pressure, fullness, swelling, or bloating
  - Urinary urgency
  - Pelvic discomfort or pain
  - Women who experience such symptoms daily for more than a few weeks should seek medical evaluation
- Other signs and symptoms
  - Persistent indigestion, gas, or nausea
  - Unexplained changes in bowel habits, including diarrhea or constipation
  - Changes in bladder habits, including urinary frequency
  - Loss of appetite, unexplained weight loss or gain, increased abdominal girth
  - Dyspareunia
  - Low back pain
  - Abnormal vaginal bleeding is rare symptom of ovarian cancer

Prognosis

- Prognosis of ovarian cancer is generally poor, mainly due to late detection
  - Percentage of tumor stage at diagnosis
    - Stage I: 34%
    - Stage II: 8%
    - Stage III: 43%
    - Stage IV: 11%
- Staging is most important prognostic factor
  - 5-year survival rate depends on tumor stage
    - Stage IA: 87.6%
    - Stage IB: 84.5%
    - Stage IC: 81.7%
    - Stage IIA: 69.3%
    - Stage IIB: 70.2%
    - Stage IIC: 64.1%
    - Stage IIIA: 52.2%
    - Stage IIIB: 45.3%
    - Stage IIIC: 32.1%
    - Stage IV: 15.3%
  - Other prognostic factors include volume of residual disease, tumor grade, histologic subtype, age, and malignant ascites
  - Preoperative CA 125 usually reflects volume of disease and is not an independent prognostic factor; however, postoperative CA 125 does have prognostic value

TREATMENT

Treatment Options by Stage

- Stage I
  - Total abdominal hysterectomy + bilateral salpingo-oophorectomy + omentectomy
  - Undersurface of diaphragm should be visualized and biopsied; pelvic and abdominal peritoneal biopsies and pelvic and paraaortic lymph node biopsies are required
  - Peritoneal washings should be obtained routinely
  - Unilateral salpingo-oophorectomy
    - Alternative for selected patients who desire childbearing and have grade 1 tumors on histologic examination
    - May be associated with ↑ risk of recurrence
  - No further treatment if low-grade cancer; possible combination chemotherapy if high-grade cancer
    - 2 randomized trials show that platinum-based adjuvant chemotherapy improves overall survival and recurrence-free survival in high-risk, early-stage ovarian carcinoma
- Stage II
  - Total abdominal hysterectomy + bilateral salpingo-oophorectomy + debulking of as much tumor as possible + sampling of lymph nodes and other suspected tissues
  - Following surgery, combination chemotherapy ± radiation therapy
- Stage III
  - Same as stage II
  - Possible follow-up surgery to remove any remaining tumor
  - Neoadjuvant chemotherapy
- Stage IV
  - Debulking surgery to remove as much tumor as possible, followed by combination chemotherapy
  - Neoadjuvant chemotherapy
- Radiation therapy

- Identification of active chemotherapy has limited the use of RT
  - ↑ evidence that RT benefits a subset of patients
- Dominant route of dissemination is throughout the abdominal cavity; hence, traditionally, RT has consisted of whole-abdominal/pelvic radiation
  - Several studies have shown that whole-abdominal/pelvic RT is superior to single-agent alkylating chemo
  - 5 trials have shown curative potential of abdominopelvic RT, but rates are determined by stage at presentation and volume of residual disease after surgery
    - 32-62% of patients with residual disease < 2 cm were cured with abdominopelvic RT
    - In stage II disease, cure rates were higher in patients whose pelvises were treated to higher doses
    - For patients with residual disease in excess of 2 cm, probability of cure ranged from 0-14%
  - Dembo et al defined classification for patients with low residual disease into 3 risk groups with recommended adjuvant therapy, and this was verified by other groups
  - Some studies have shown advantage of use of consolidation whole-abdominal/pelvic RT after chemo with lower doses
  - Studies that compared whole-abdominal/pelvic RT to chemo are flawed
    - Toxicity is much less with chemo and therefore preferred
  - Side effects of abdominal/pelvic RT is main reason for limiting use
    - GI side effects (both acute and chronic are the major side effects): One study reported 14% late GI toxicity
    - Myelosuppression in one study showed that 10% of patients could not complete their treatment
    - Other late side effects include basal pneumonitis or fibrosis
  - Recent studies have shown the limitation to chemo, especially in clear cell carcinoma, and local RT is being explored in setting of recurrent disease

Standard Doses

- Whole abdominal/pelvic RT consists of treatment to the entire peritoneal cavity and pelvis
  - Dose to abdomen/pelvis is 22-30 Gy at 1-1.2 Gy per day with limits to kidney to 18-20 Gy
  - Pelvis is boosted to 45-50 Gy
  - Single fields have less toxicity than moving strips

Organs at Risk Parameters

- Liver: Mean < 30 Gy
- Kidney (bilateral): Mean < 15-18 Gy
- Small bowel: V45 < 195 mL

Common Techniques

- AP/PA ± laterals for pelvic boost

RECOMMENDED FOLLOW-UP

Clinical

- Laboratory blood work and physical exams are recommended every 3 months for 1st year, every 4 months for next year, and then every 6 months until 5 years out

Radiographic

- No routine imaging is recommended unless patient is symptomatic or has elevated CA 125 or other indications for imaging

Laboratory

- CA 125 is usually recommended, but sensitivity is unclear

SELECTED REFERENCES

1. Hoskins PJ et al: Low-stage ovarian clear cell carcinoma: population-based outcomes in British Columbia, Canada, with evidence for a survival benefit as a result of irradiation. J Clin Oncol. 30(14):1656-62, 2012
2. Hauspy J et al: Role of adjuvant radiotherapy in granulosa cell tumors of the ovary. Int J Radiat Oncol Biol Phys. 79(3):770-4, 2011
3. Lee M et al: Comparison of the efficacy and toxicity between radiotherapy and chemotherapy in nodal and isolated nonnodal recurrence of ovarian cancer. Int J Gynecol Cancer. 21(6):1032-9, 2011
4. American Joint Committee on Cancer: AJCC Cancer Staging Manual. 7th ed. New York: Springer. 419-28, 2010
5. Nagai Y et al: Postoperative whole abdominal radiotherapy in clear cell adenocarcinoma of the ovary. Gynecol Oncol. 107(3):469-73, 2007
6. Chen M et al: Differentiation between malignant and benign ovarian tumors by magnetic resonance imaging. Chin Med Sci J. 21(4):270-5, 2006
7. Woodward PJ et al: From the archives of the AFIP: radiologic staging of ovarian carcinoma with pathologic correlation. Radiographics. 24(1):225-46, 2004
8. Seidman JD et al: Pathology of ovarian carcinoma. Hematol Oncol Clin North Am. 17(4):909-25, vii, 2003
9. Trimbos JB et al: European Organisation for Research and Treatment of Cancer-Adjuvant ChemoTherapy in Ovarian Neoplasm. Impact of adjuvant chemotherapy and surgical staging in early-stage ovarian carcinoma: European Organisation for Research and Treatment of Cancer-Adjuvant ChemoTherapy in Ovarian Neoplasm trial. J Natl Cancer Inst. 95(2):113-25, 2003
10. Coakley FV: Staging ovarian cancer: role of imaging. Radiol Clin North Am. 40(3):609-36, 2002
11. Hruby G et al: WART revisited: the treatment of epithelial ovarian cancer by whole abdominal radiotherapy. Australas Radiol. 41(3):276-80, 1997
12. Carey MS et al: Testing the validity of a prognostic classification in patients with surgically optimal ovarian carcinoma: a 15-year review. Int J Gynecol Cancer. 3(1):24-35, 1993
13. Martinez A et al: Postoperative radiation therapy for epithelial ovarian cancer: the curative role based on a 24-year experience. J Clin Oncol. 3(7):901-11, 1985

Stage IA (T1a N0 M0)

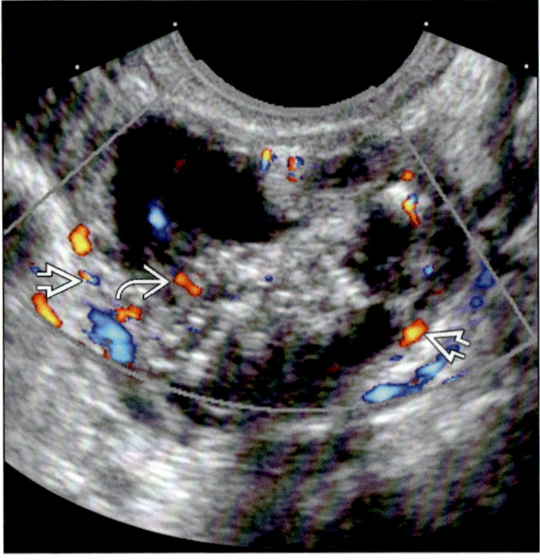

Stage IA (T1a N0 M0)

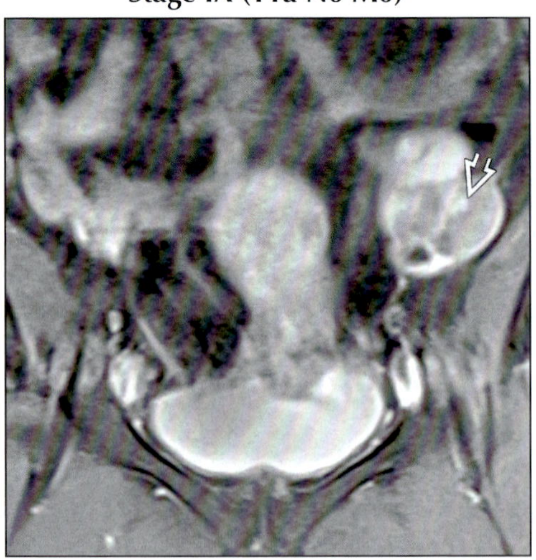

(Left) *Longitudinal color Doppler ultrasound shows a mixed solid-cystic left ovarian mass with a large solid component. There is blood flow within both the solid component ➔ and the wall ➔. The other ovary was normal; there is no ascites.* ***(Right)*** *Coronal T1 C+ FS MR shows enhancement of the intracystic papillary lesion ➔, which proved to be clear cell. Clear cell and endometrioid adenocarcinoma are the 2 histologic types that develop within endometriomas.*

Stage IB (T1b N0 M0)

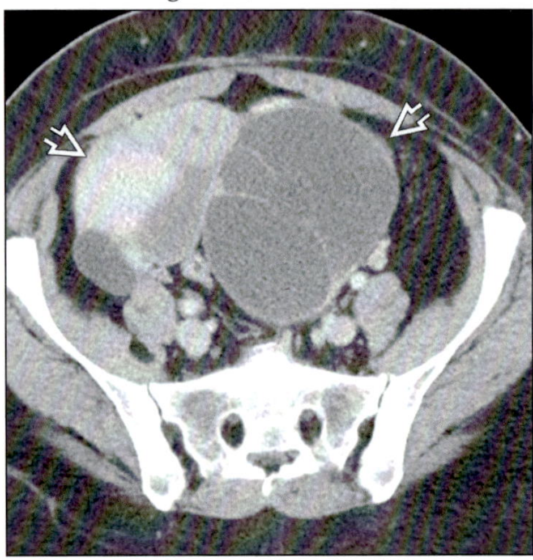

Stage IC (T1c N0 M0)

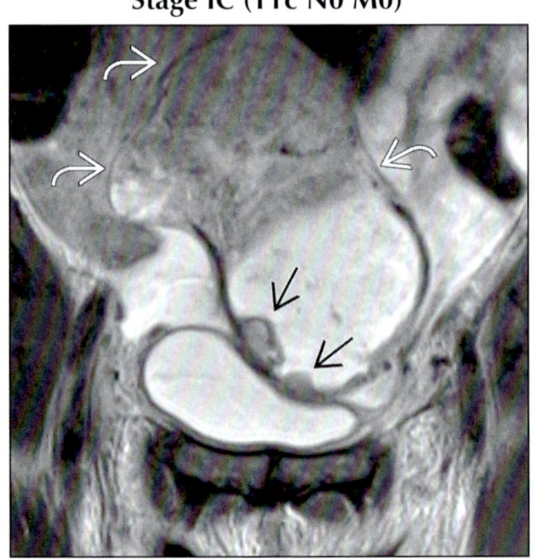

(Left) *Axial CECT shows bilateral ovarian masses ➔. The presence of multiple loculi of different attenuation in an ovarian mass is a feature of mucinous tumors.* ***(Right)*** *Coronal T2WI MR shows a mixed solid-cystic ovarian mass ➔ with mural nodules ➔. At surgery, malignant cells were found in the ascitic fluid. The size of an ovarian mass does not affect staging as long as the tumor is limited to the ovary and there is no capsular rupture.*

Stage IIB (T2b N0 M0)

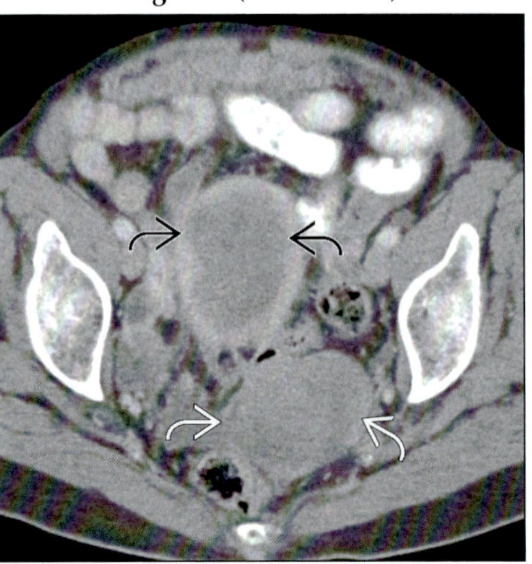

Stage IIIC (T3c N0 M0)

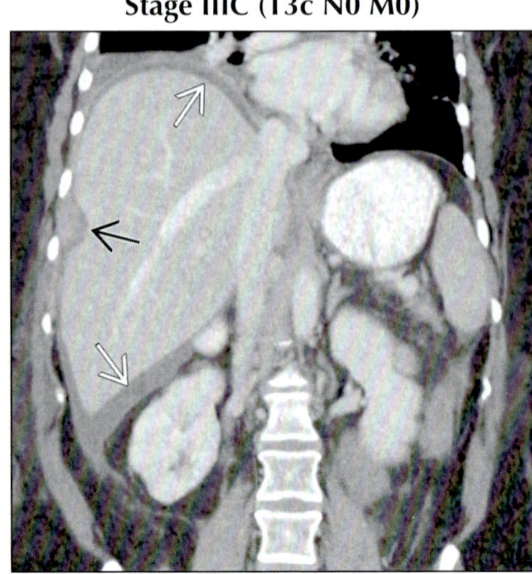

(Left) *Axial CECT shows a heterogeneous left ovarian mass ➔ and another heterogeneous mass ➔ that fills the uterine cavity. Histology revealed a primary ovarian tumor with metastasis to the uterus.* ***(Right)*** *Coronal reformat CECT in the same patient shows a perihepatic peritoneal implant ➔ with no parenchymal invasion. Perihepatic ascites is also seen ➔. Coronal reformat better delineates capsular implants and confirms the peritoneal.*

Stage IIIC (T3c N0 M0)

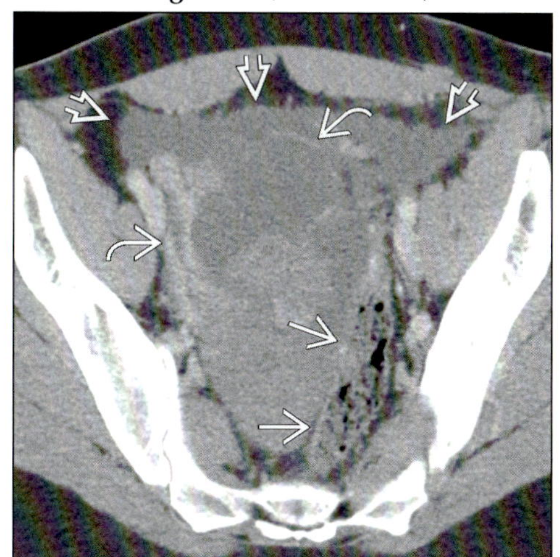

Stage IIIC (T3c N0 M0)

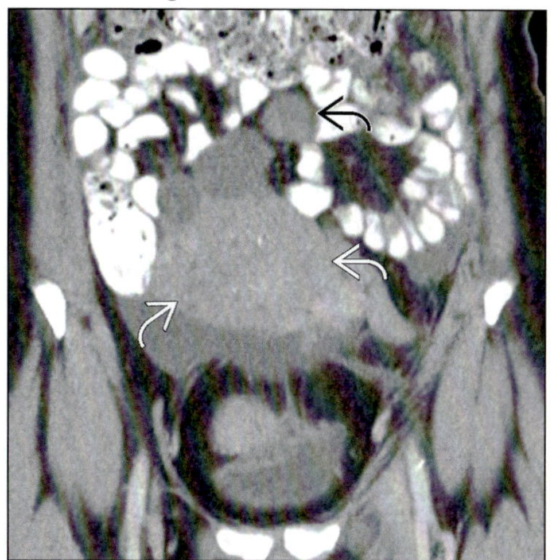

*(**Left**) Axial CECT in a 37-year-old woman who presented with abdominal distension and was found to have pelvic masses on vaginal exam shows a mixed solid and cystic right ovarian mass ➔. Ascites is present ➔. The mass displaces the colon ➔ without obvious invasion. (**Right**) Coronal CECT in the same patient shows the left ovarian mass ➔ with a separate peritoneal metastatic lesion ➔.*

Stage IIIC (T1a N1 M0)

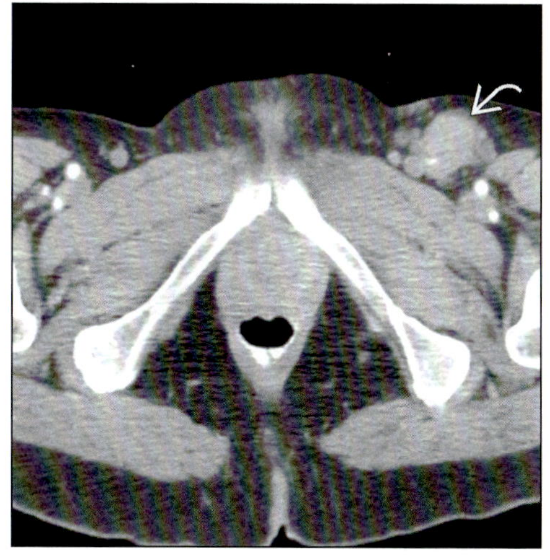

Stage IIIC (T2b N1 M0)

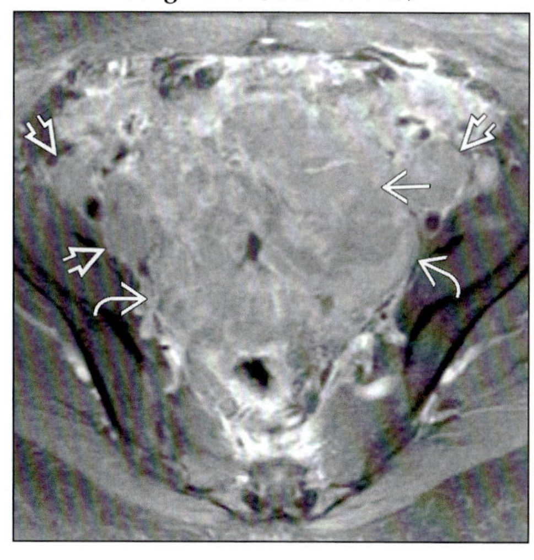

*(**Left**) Axial CECT shows an enlarged left inguinal lymph node ➔. Metastases to inguinal nodes result from tumor spread through lymphatics along the round ligament. (**Right**) Axial T1WI C+ FS MR shows a large mass occupying almost the entire pelvis. There is an irregular interface between the tumor and the uterus ➔ due to uterine invasion. The tumor comes within 3 mm of the pelvic sidewall ➔. Bilateral external iliac nodes are also seen ➔.*

Stage IIIC (T2b N1 M0)

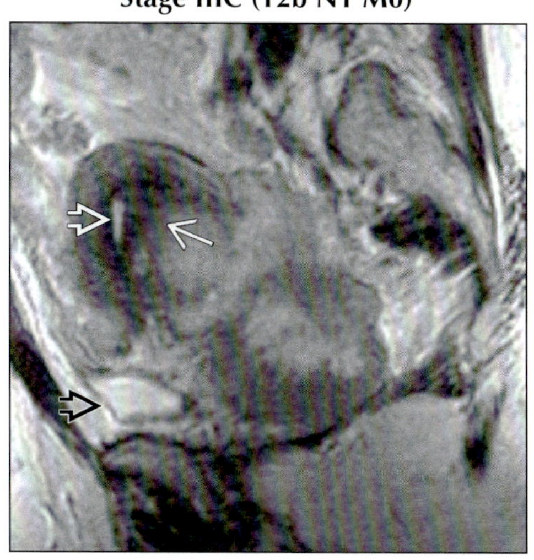

Stage IIIC (T2b N1 M0)

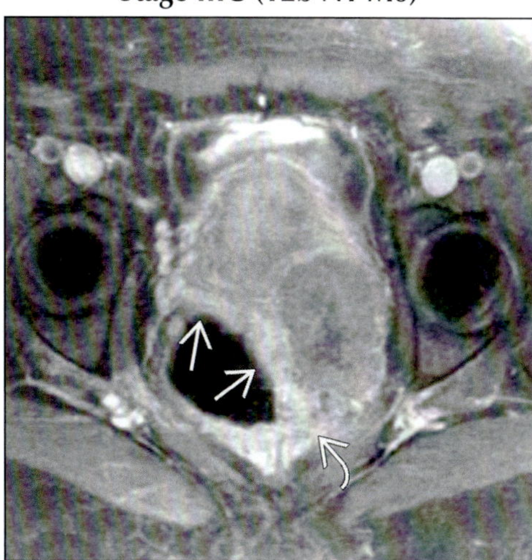

*(**Left**) Sagittal T2WI MR in the same patient shows invasion of the posterior wall of the uterus ➔ sparing the endometrium ➔. The urinary bladder ➔ is not involved. (**Right**) Axial T1WI C+ FS MR in the same patient shows enhancing tumor ➔ invading and wrapping around the rectum to involve the uterosacral ligament ➔.*

Stage IIIC (T3b N1 M0)

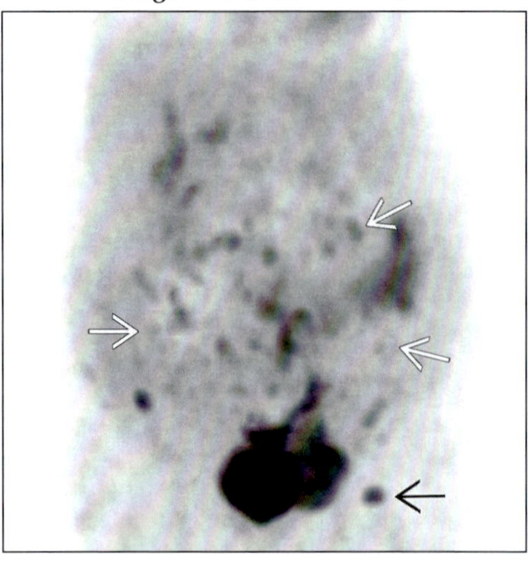

Stage IV (T3c N0 M1)

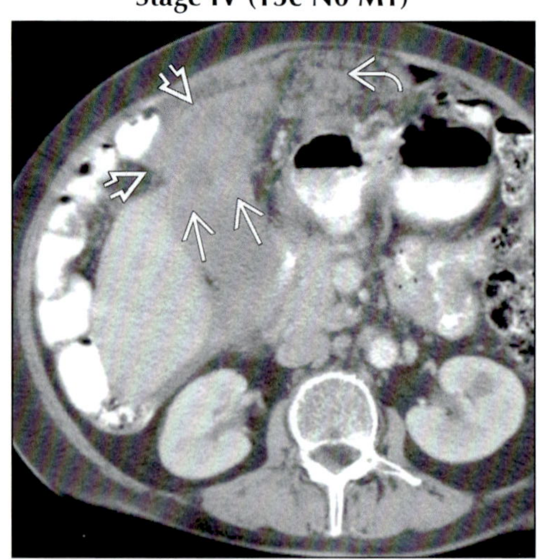

(Left) *Coronal PET shows extensive peritoneal metastatic disease ➔. Peritoneal lesions are < 2 cm in greatest dimension. The left inguinal node ➔ shows increased metabolic activity.* ***(Right)*** *Axial CECT shows omental metastases ➔ with a large omental mass ➔ invading the fundus of the gallbladder ➔. Large peritoneal metastases (> 2 cm) within the abdomen constitute T3c disease, and invasion of the gallbladder constitutes M1 disease.*

Stage IV (T3c N1 M1)

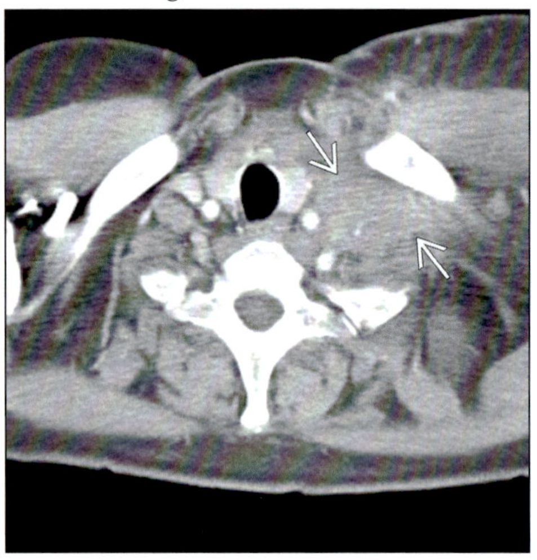

Recurrent Clear Cell Carcinoma

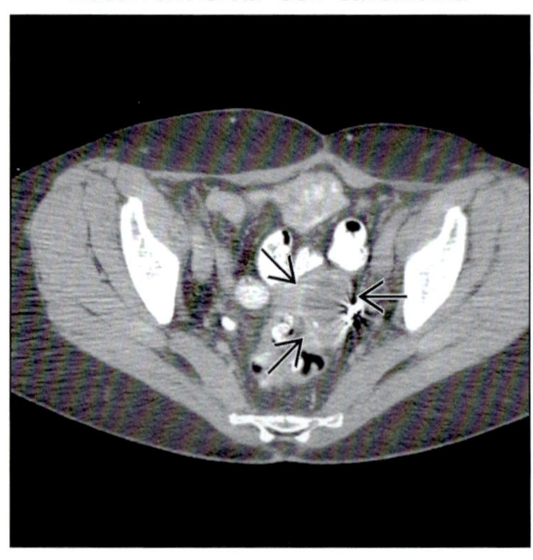

(Left) *Axial CECT in a patient with advanced local disease shows an enlarged left supraclavicular lymph node ➔. Metastatic disease to supraclavicular nodes constitutes M1 disease.* ***(Right)*** *Axial CECT in a patient with recurrent clear cell carcinoma of the ovary ➔ in 2006 shows the recurrent mass in the left ovary surrounded by surgical clips. Disease extends cephalad as well. Patient was diagnosed in 2004, treated with surgery and multiple courses of chemotherapy.*

Recurrent Clear Cell Carcinoma

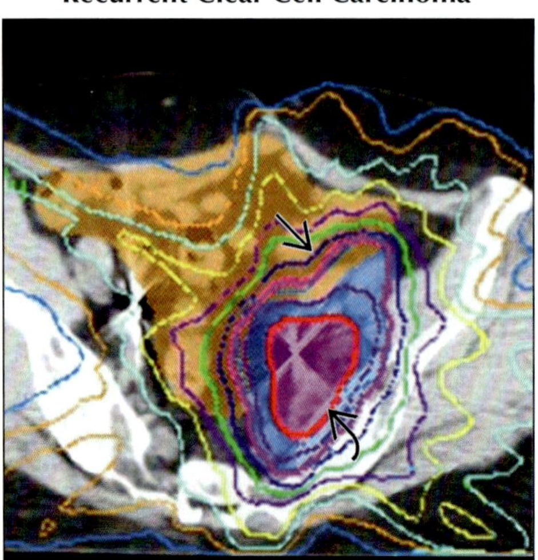

Recurrent Clear Cell Carcinoma

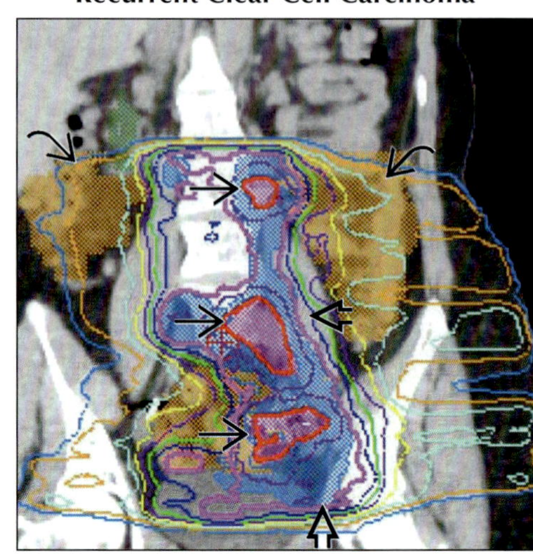

(Left) *Axial view of the IMRT plan in the same patient ➔ shows a red line, which is the 63 Gy line that covers the entire mass. The 50 Gy line ➔ covers the entire ipsilateral nodal chain.* ***(Right)*** *Coronal image of the same patient shows the 3 areas of gross disease, all receiving 63 Gy ➔ and microscopic disease receiving 50 Gy ➔ to the ipsilateral nodal chain. IMRT spares normal tissues such as the bowel (in light brown ➔).*

Recurrent Clear Cell Carcinoma

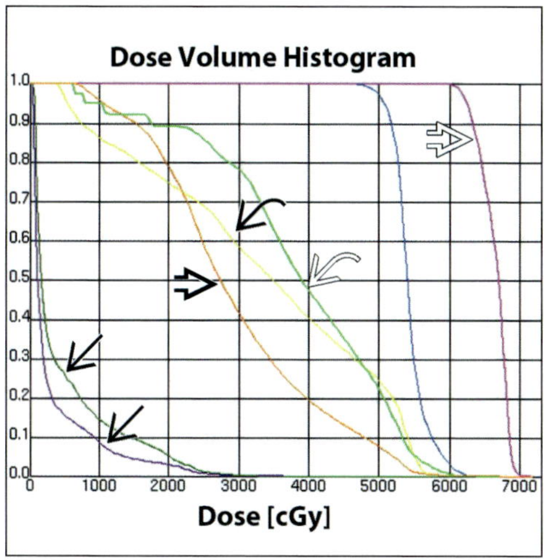

Recurrent Clear Cell Carcinoma

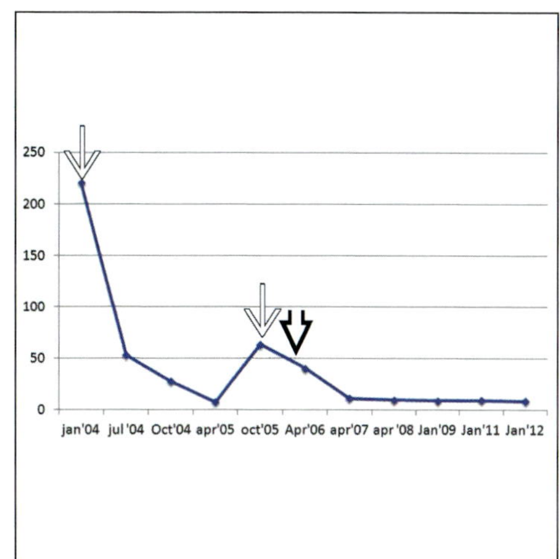

(Left) *DVH in same patient shows dose to the kidneys, which are spared, and dose to the tumor, which is 63 Gy. It also shows relative sparing of the small bowel, bladder, and rectum with these IMRT doses.* ***(Right)*** *Graph shows CA 125 of same patient. The time space between the 2 white arrows represents the time the patient was on continuous chemotherapy. Black arrow shows when RT was given. The patient received no further therapy and is NED 6 years out.*

Granulosa Cell Carcinoma of Ovary

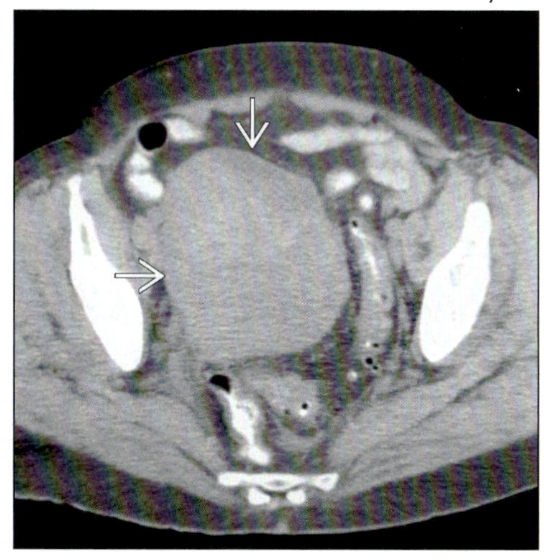

Granulosa Cell Carcinoma of Ovary

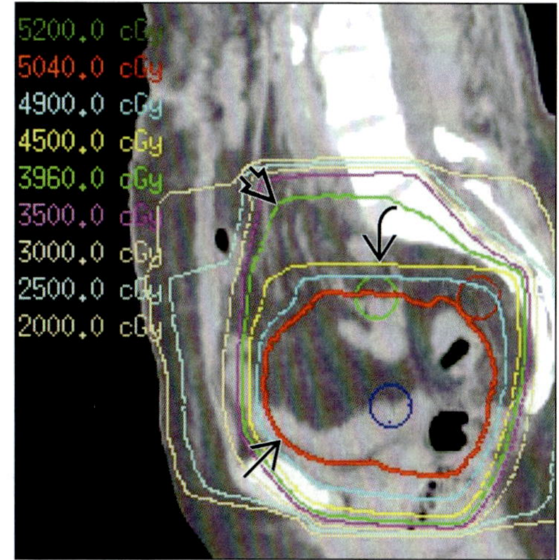

(Left) *Axial CECT shows a large solid mass arising in the right ovary. Pathology showed a 9.7 cm granulosa tumor adherent to right pelvic sidewall musculature, bladder, and vagina, and was completely removed (stage IIB).* ***(Right)*** *Sagittal view in the same patient shows the 50.40 Gy line, 45 Gy line, and 39.6 Gy line. This is a good representation of a 3D conformal plan, which shows how the entire pelvis in the field receives full dose.*

Granulosa Cell Carcinoma of Ovary

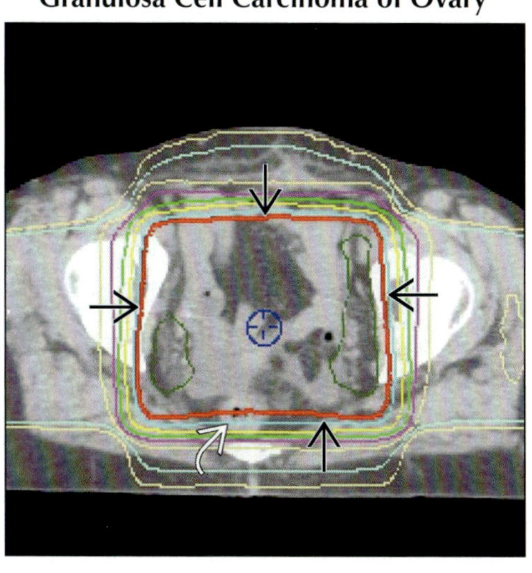

Granulosa Cell Carcinoma of Ovary

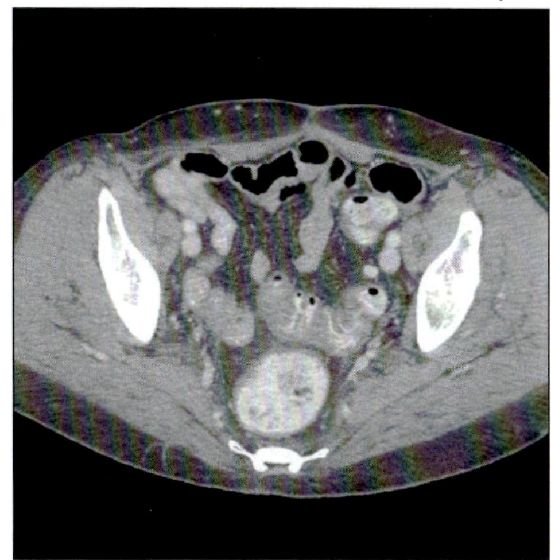

(Left) *Axial plane in the same patient shows a typical 4-field postoperative RT plan to the pelvis. The 50.4 Gy line is seen in red. At this level, the rectum is bisected by the prescription dose.* ***(Right)*** *Follow-up axial CECT showed no sign of recurrent disease. Patient is 6 years out from surgery and RT with no recurrent disease and no side effects.*

*(**Left**) Axial PET/CT from 2012 shows recurrent masses in the vaginal cuff ➔ and in the presacral region ↪. Biopsy was positive for low-grade serous carcinoma. Patient was initially diagnosed in 2006, treated with neoadjuvant chemotherapy, surgery, and more chemotherapy. The carcinoma recurred in 2009, and the patient was treated with stem cell transplant. (**Right**) Axial CT in the same patient shows the vaginal mass ➔ and the presacral mass ↪.*

Recurrent Low-Grade Serous Carcinoma

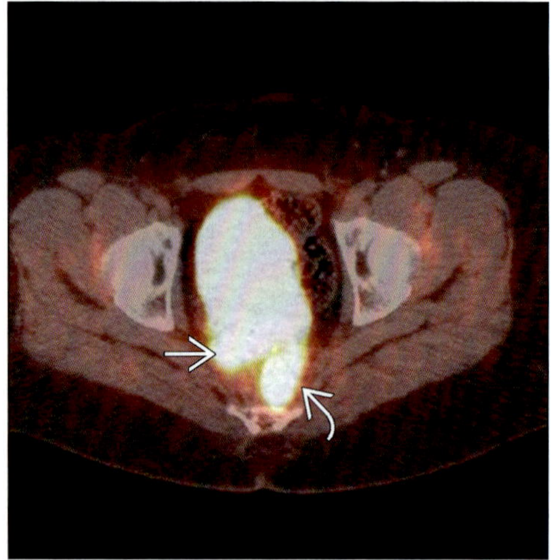

Recurrent Low-Grade Serous Carcinoma

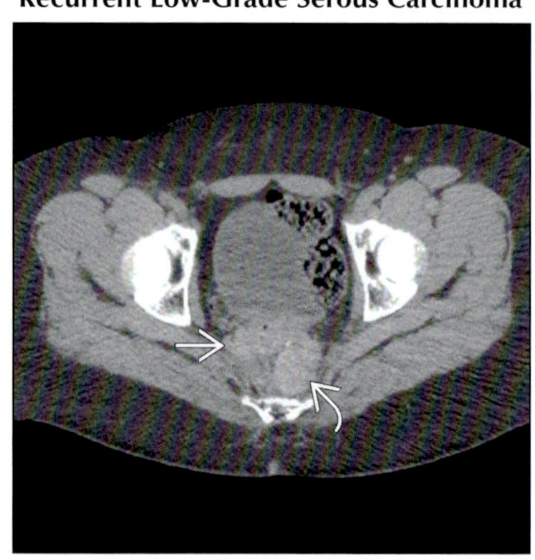

*(**Left**) Axial CT scan in the same patient (more cephalad) shows the full extent of the sacral recurrence ↪. No other sites of disease were noted. (**Right**) This image compares a proton plan ➔ and IMRT plan ⇨ in the same patient. The major difference is the amount of low-dose radiation that is given to the rest of the body by the IMRT plan.*

Recurrent Low-Grade Serous Carcinoma

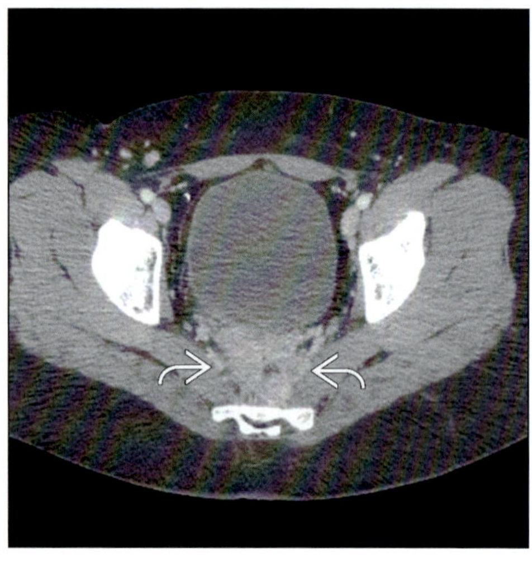

Recurrent Low-Grade Serous Carcinoma

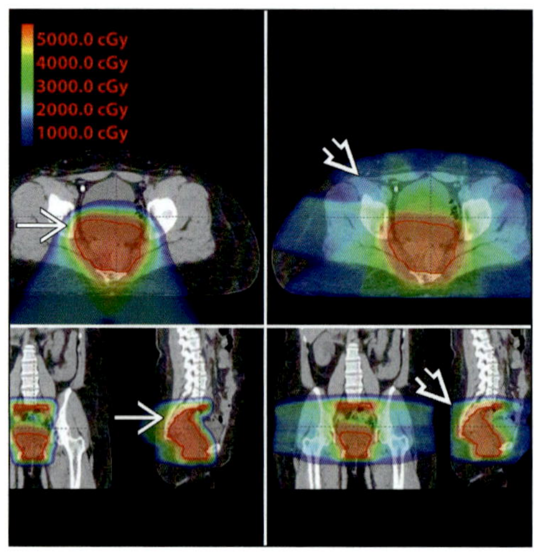

*(**Left**) Image shows the comparison of the DVH between the proton and IMRT plan. Protons gave less dose to both rectum (green lines) → and bladder (pink lines) ➔ than the IMRT plan to rectum ↪ and bladder ↪. (**Right**) Due to insurance reasons, patient was treated with IMRT as shown in this axial CT. The light blue represents the 50.4 Gy line ↪, and the dark blue represents the 56 Gy line →. Additionally, a 10 Gy focal boost was performed (total dose: 66 Gy).*

Recurrent Low-Grade Serous Carcinoma

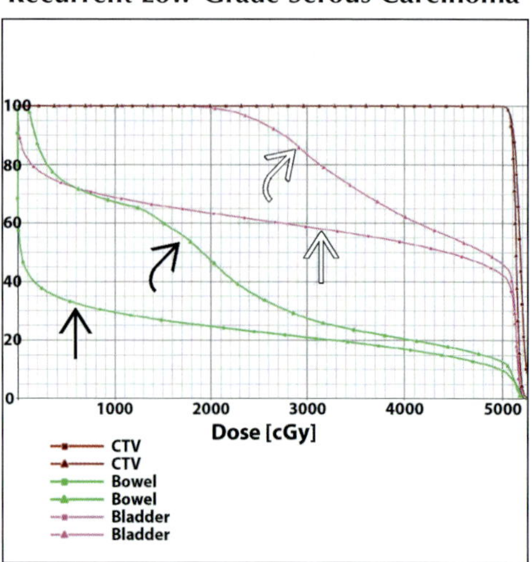

Recurrent Low-Grade Serous Carcinoma

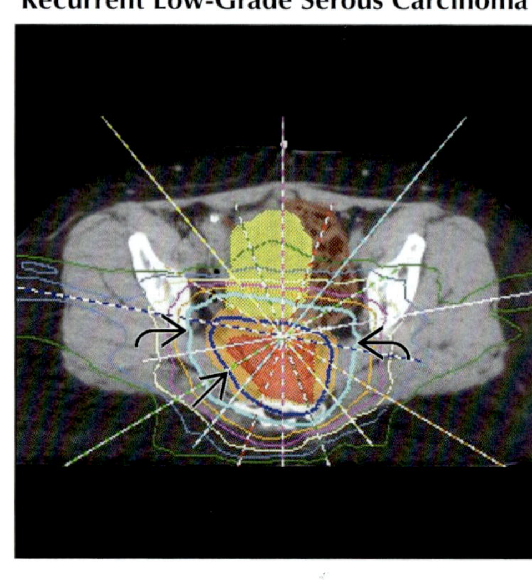

Recurrent Undifferentiated Carcinoma

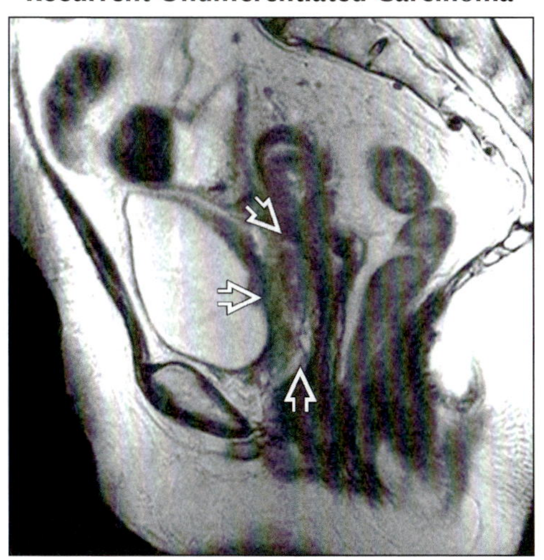

Recurrent Undifferentiated Carcinoma

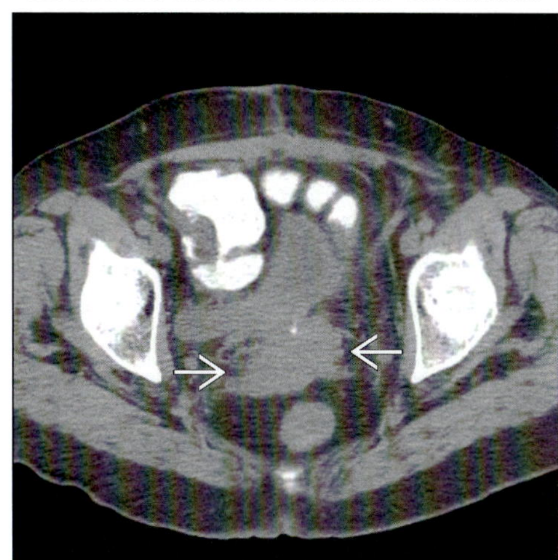

(Left) *This patient was diagnosed with ovarian cancer in 2002 & treated with surgery & chemotherapy. The patient received no further therapy, & this sagittal T2WI MR was done in 2005 due to symptoms. MR shows an area anterior to the vagina that was thought to be an abscess or thickening, & the patient was observed.* ***(Right)*** *Axial CECT scan from the same patient in 2005 shows retrovesical mass (positive biopsy) extending to apex of vagina with no other sites of disease.*

Recurrent Undifferentiated Carcinoma

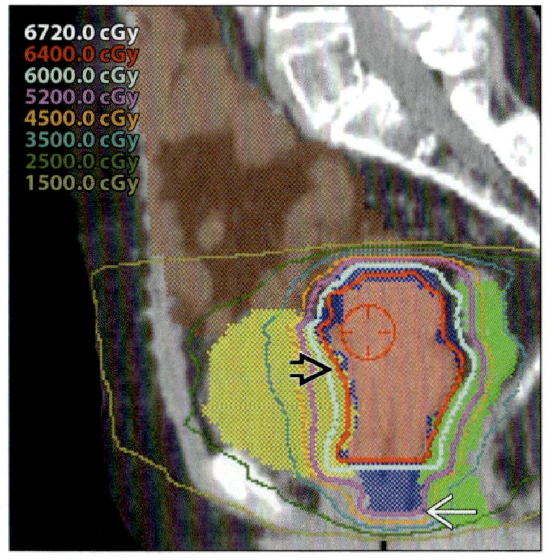

Recurrent Undifferentiated Carcinoma

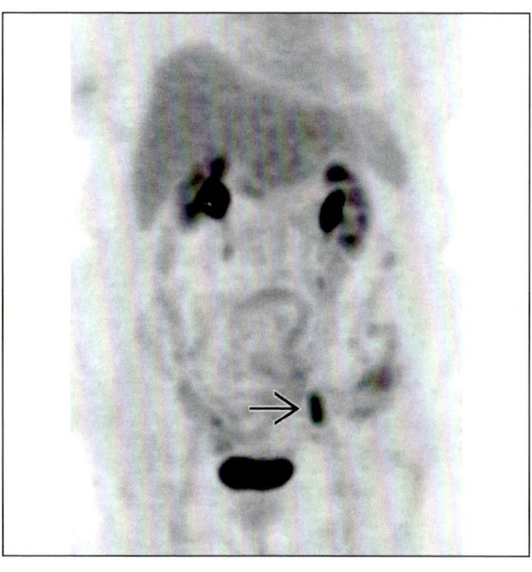

(Left) *IMRT plan (sagittal view) of the same patient shows that just the vaginal mass (covered by 64 Gy) was treated due to the time from initial treatment to relapse. 52 Gy covered microscopic disease in vagina.* ***(Right)*** *Coronal PET image in the same patient shows the left external node as the only site of recurrent disease 1.5 years out from RT to the vaginal mass with no other treatment. Biopsy was positive for recurrent cancer.*

Recurrent Undifferentiated Carcinoma

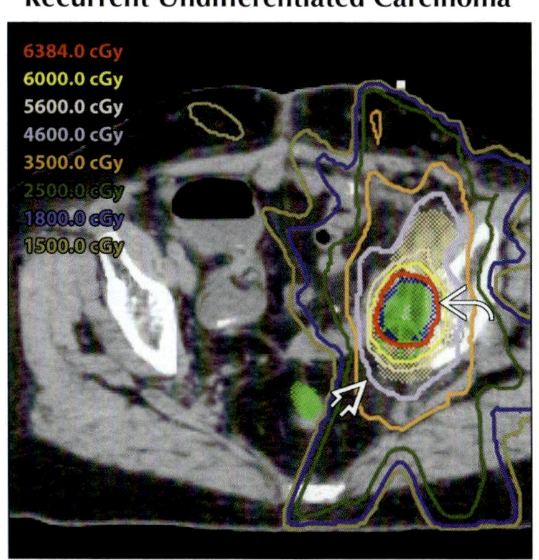

Recurrent Undifferentiated Carcinoma

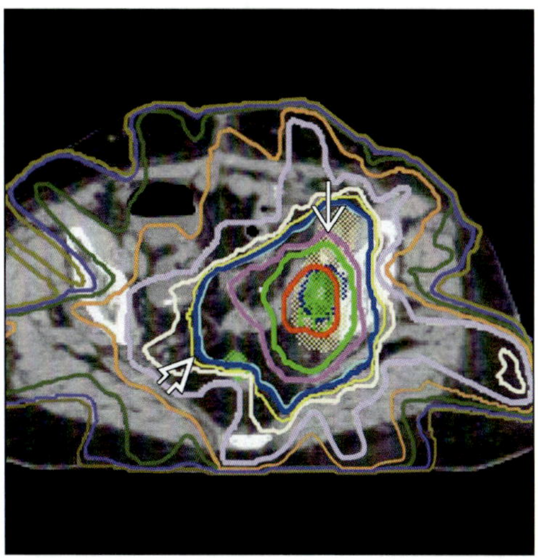

(Left) *Axial CT of IMRT on the same patient shows treatment only to the recurrent node. This was mostly above the previous treatment to the vaginal mass. The 63.8 Gy line covering the node is shown. The 45 Gy line covered the ipsilateral nodes . Most of the normal tissues were spared.* ***(Right)*** *Axial CT shows composite plan from both old and new treatments in the same patient. The 80 Gy line is in pink and the 63.8 Gy line is in dark blue .*

Recurrent Undifferentiated Carcinoma

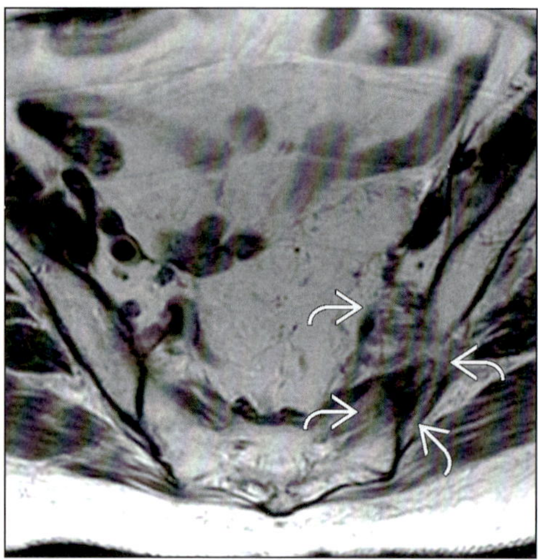

Recurrent Undifferentiated Carcinoma

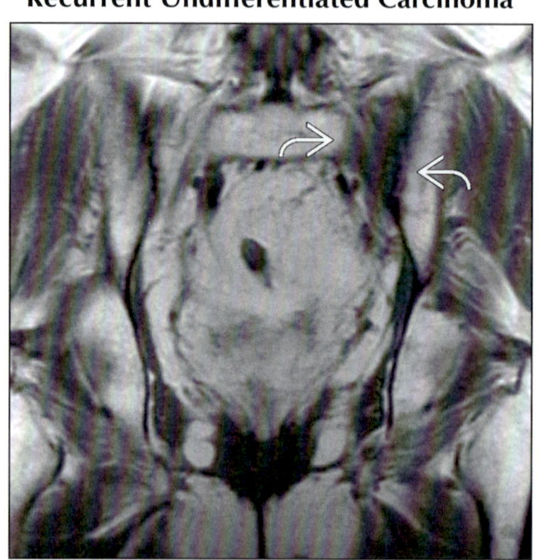

(Left) *In 2008, the same patient presented with pain in the left side, and this axial T1WI MR shows ischemic changes and stress fracture at the left sacroiliac joint. This is the same area that probably received about 80 Gy total. There were no sites of recurrent disease.* ***(Right)*** *Coronal T1WI MR shows the same patient at the same time point. The area of fracture remains evident. She was treated with risedronate and rest.*

Recurrent Undifferentiated Carcinoma

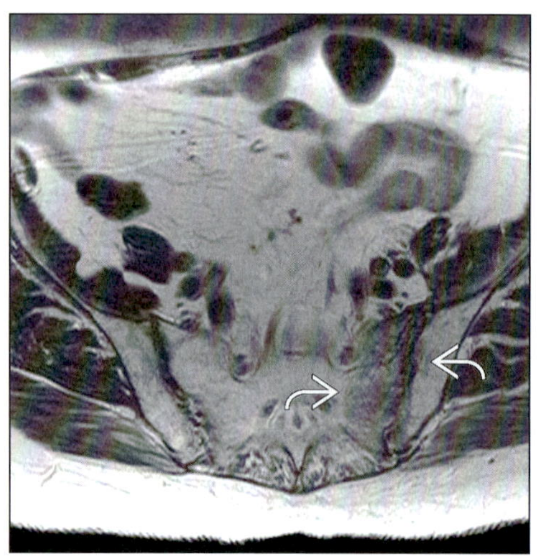

Recurrent Anaplastic Carcinoma

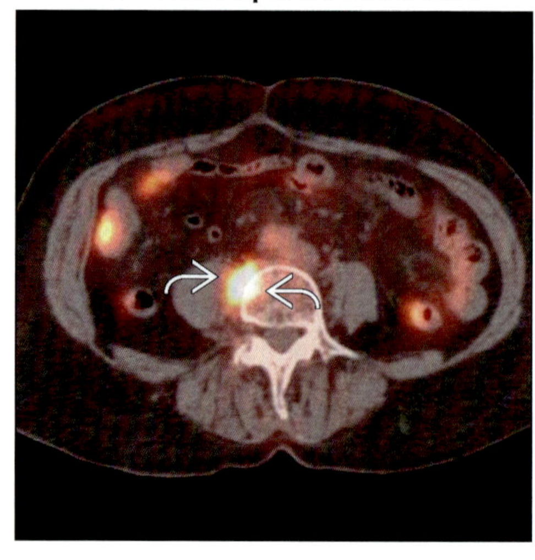

(Left) *Axial T1WI MR in same patient from 2010 shows healing fracture. The patient's symptoms had completely resolved. Patient remained NED from her ovarian cancer; however, she died of head and neck cancer in 2012.* ***(Right)*** *Fused PET/CT done in 2007 shows an avid right perivertebral soft tissue mass. Patient was diagnosed in 1991 and treated with surgery/chemo. The cancer recurred in the left supraclav in 2005 and was treated with chemo and maintenance letrozole.*

Recurrent Anaplastic Carcinoma

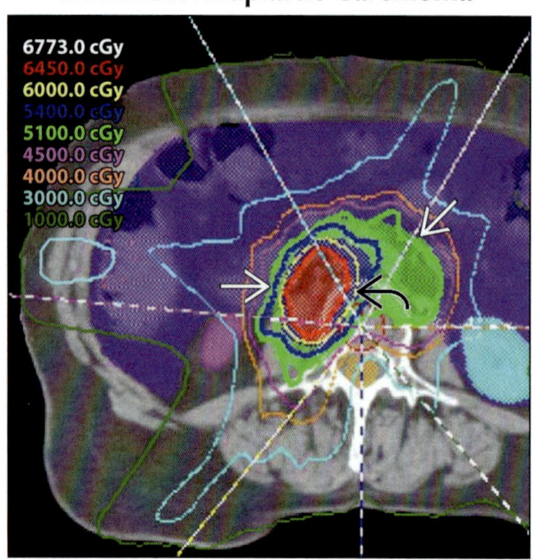

Recurrent Anaplastic Carcinoma

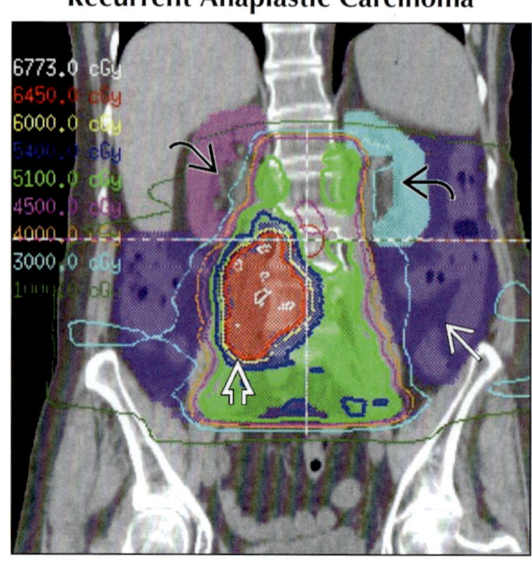

(Left) *Mass was biopsied, proving positive for anaplastic carcinoma. Since this was the only site of disease, the same patient was treated with IMRT to the mass and remaining paraaortic nodes. This is an axial image of the IMRT plan. The GTV was treated to 64.5 Gy, and microscopic nodal disease to 51 Gy (green line).* ***(Right)*** *Coronal image of plan shows good sparing of normal tissues, including kidneys and bowel. The GTV boost is shown.*

Recurrent Anaplastic Carcinoma

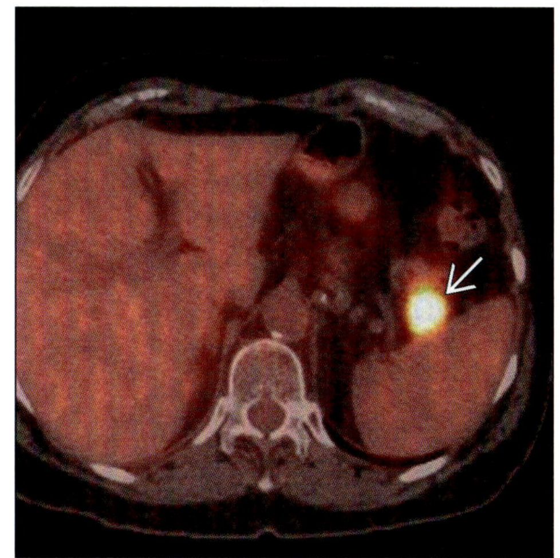

Recurrent Anaplastic Carcinoma

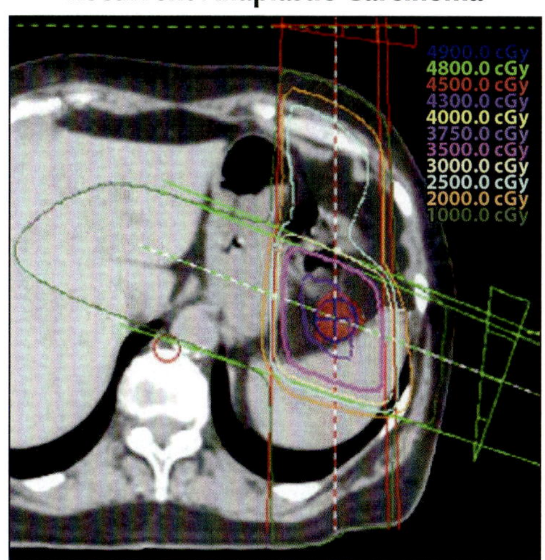

(Left) *Same patient was disease free until this axial PET/CT showed a parasplenic mass with no other sites of disease in 2009.* ***(Right)*** *Since the same patient was not tolerating chemotherapy, she was treated with palliative RT to the parasplenic mass using 3D conformal plan as seen on axial CT. She was treated to 35 Gy in 14 fractions.*

Recurrent Anaplastic Carcinoma

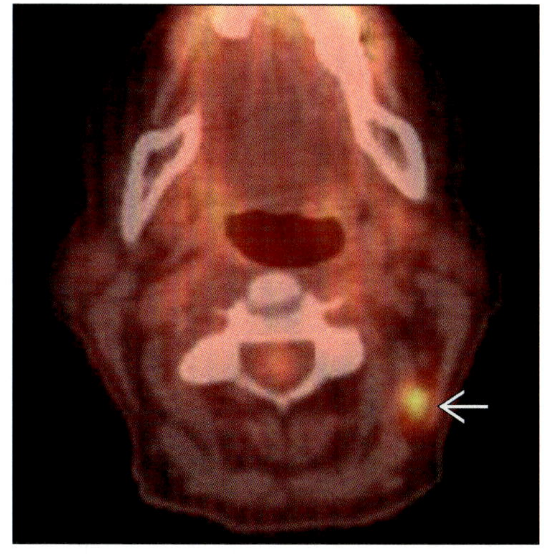

Recurrent Anaplastic Carcinoma

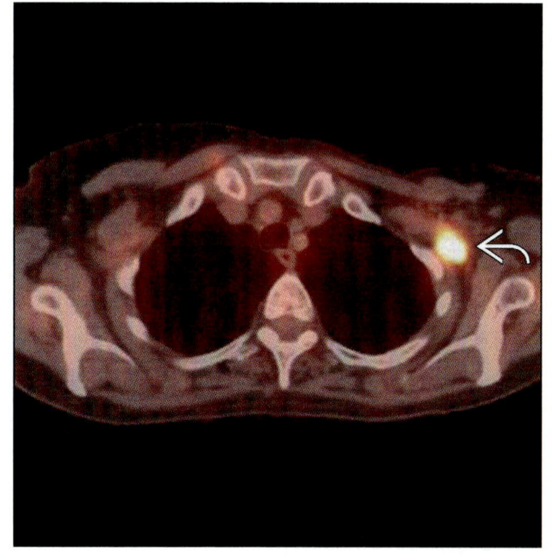

(Left) *Patient did well until 2010 when she had a left axillary node positive for adenocarcinoma. She was treated on a phase I protocol. Restaging in 2011 included this fused PET/CT that showed this left posterior neck node .* ***(Right)*** *Axial PET/CT from 2011 in the same patient also showed this axillary node , as well as an internal mammary node. Patient was treated with Doxil and etoposide for 9 months.*

Recurrent Anaplastic Carcinoma

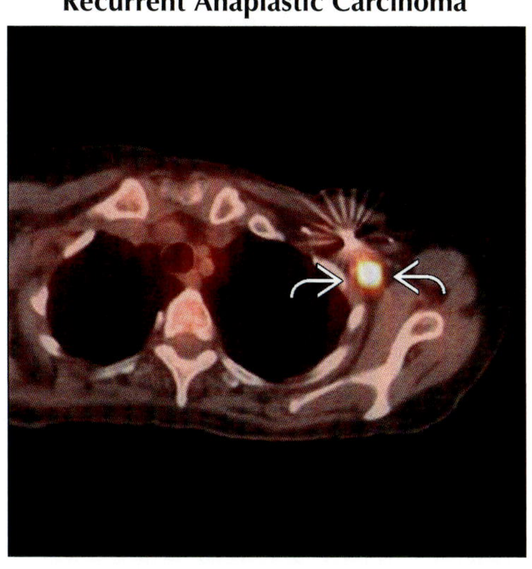

Recurrent Anaplastic Carcinoma

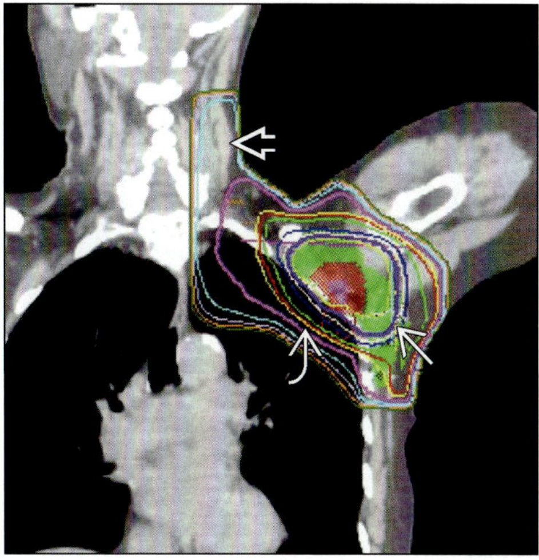

(Left) *Axial PET/CT from later in 2011 reimaging showed only this left axillary node ; the other nodes including the high neck nodes as well as the internal mammary nodes all had resolved. No other sites of disease were noted.* ***(Right)*** *Coronal representation shows 3D plan treating the axillary node as well as the high neck nodes. The axillary node got a boost to 62 Gy , the axilla was taken to 50 Gy , and the entire neck to 40 Gy .*

(Left) Follow-up axial PET/CT in the same patient 3 months later shows inflammation but no residual disease. *(Right)* This patient was initially diagnosed in 2005 and treated with surgery and no further therapy. In 2008, she had a recurrence, shown in this axial CECT. It shows a mass anterior to the bladder ➡. Patient underwent a 2nd surgery with pathology positive for recurrent disease. No other sites were noted, and it was the same site as the previous scar.

Recurrent Anaplastic Carcinoma

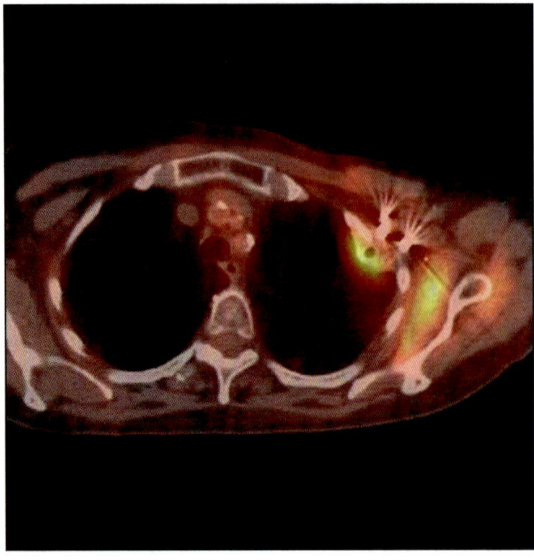

Recurrent Granulosa Cell Carcinoma

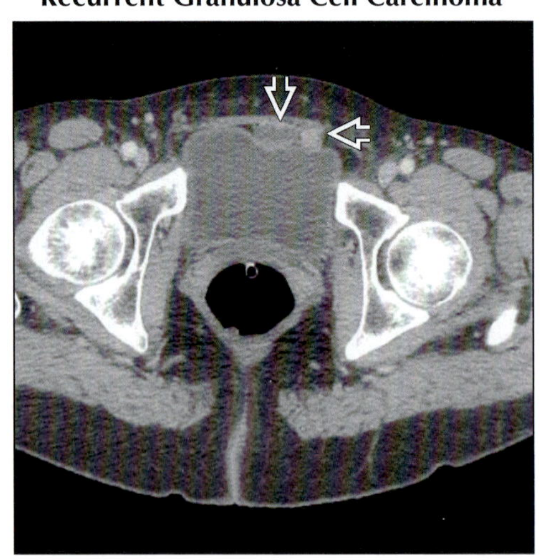

(Left) DRR in the same patient shows photon field of the postoperative RT field purposely drawn to include the previous scar ➡. *(Right)* Skin rendering in the same patient shows the electron field. Patient was treated with combination of electrons and photon to spare the normal tissues underneath, including bowel and bladder. A photon contribution is often added to decrease the skin dose &/ or increase the coverage at depth.

Recurrent Granulosa Cell Carcinoma

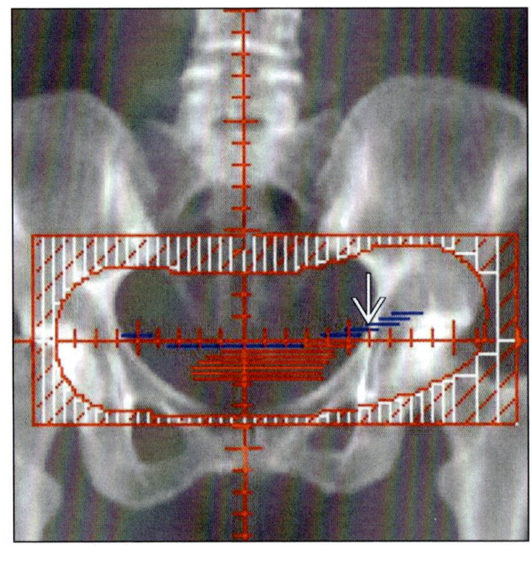

Recurrent Granulosa Cell Carcinoma

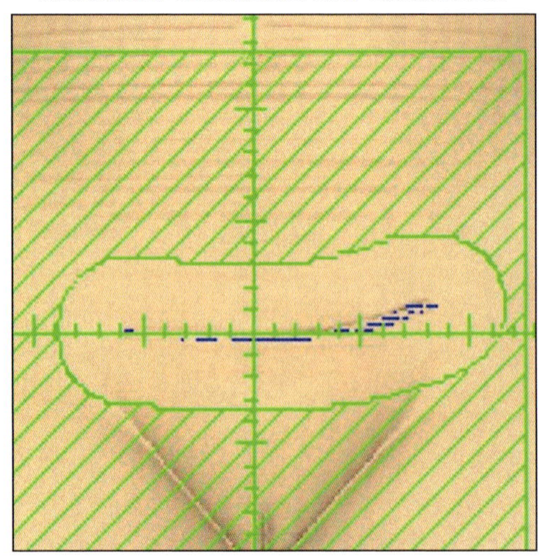

(Left) Sagittal image of the plan in the same patient shows how the combination of photons and electrons spared the normal tissue, especially the bladder in yellow. Red line represents the 50.5 Gy line, and the pink line is the 30 Gy line ➡. The target is shown ➡. *(Right)* Axial view of the same plan shows how the postoperative bed in red is covered by the 50 Gy line (red line) ➡. 20 Gy is depicted by the light blue line ➡.

Recurrent Granulosa Cell Carcinoma

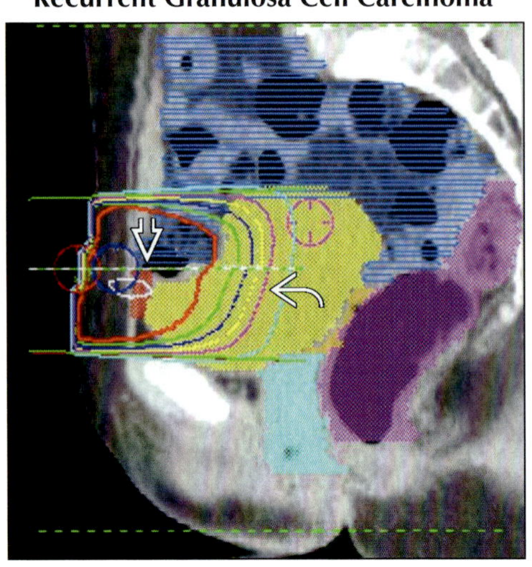

Recurrent Granulosa Cell Carcinoma

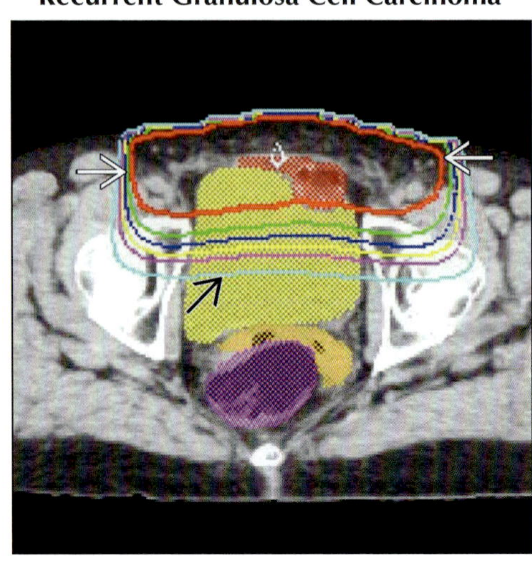

Recurrent Granulosa Cell Carcinoma

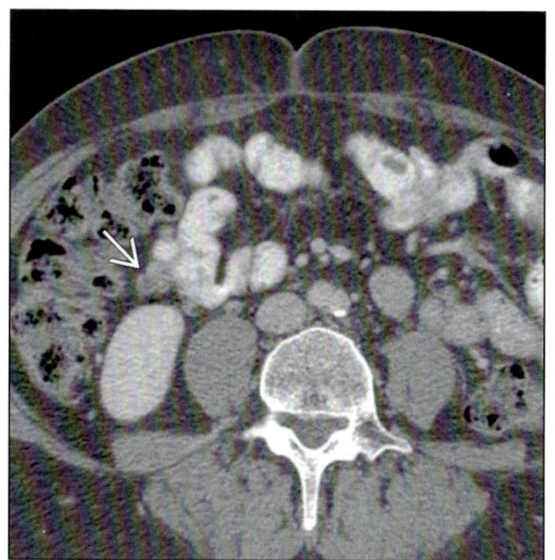

Recurrent Granulosa Cell Carcinoma

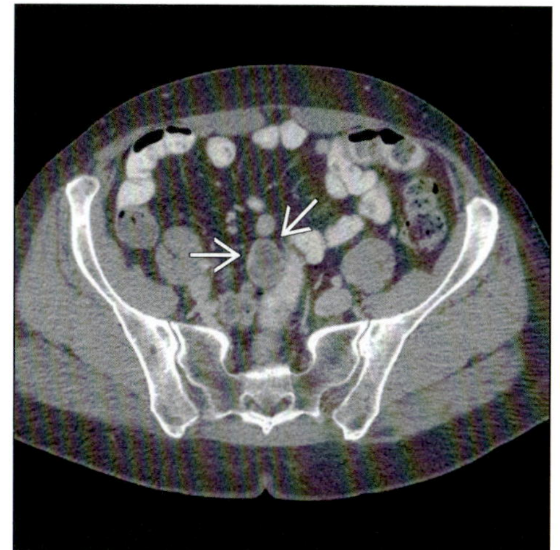

(Left) *Axial CT from 2011 shows recurrence in the same patient. She was noted to have several nodules, including the one visible in this image ➔.* ***(Right)*** *Axial CT image (more inferior) in same patient on same date shows another nodule ➔. She was treated with surgical resection of 7 nodules in 2011, followed by 6 courses of chemotherapy. Six months later, she had no evidence of disease.*

Recurrent Ovarian Carcinoma to Adrenal

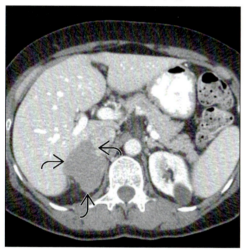

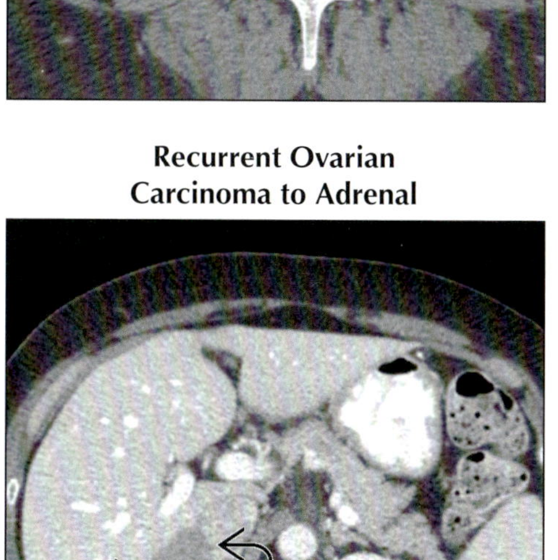

Recurrent Ovarian Carcinoma to Adrenal

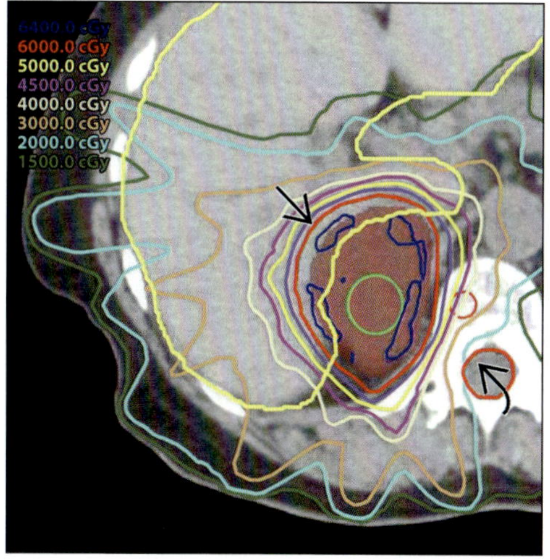

(Left) *Axial CECT shows a 5.6 cm x 5.0 cm right adrenal mass ↷. Patient was originally diagnosed in 2001 and treated with surgery/chemo. The cancer recurred in right adrenal in 2010 and was again treated with surgery/chemo. This scan from 2012 shows an isolated 2nd recurrence in the same area.* ***(Right)*** *The same patient was treated with SBRT 60 Gy (red line) ➔ in 10 fractions. IMRT minimizes dose to OARs including the cord ↷, liver, bowel, and kidneys.*

Recurrent Ovarian Carcinoma to Adrenal

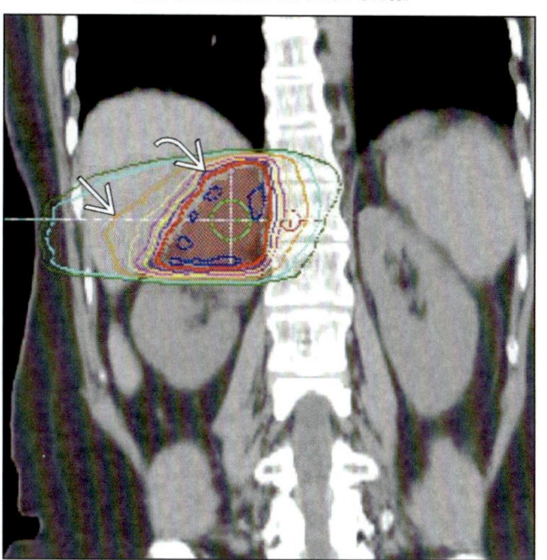

Recurrent Ovarian Carcinoma to Adrenal

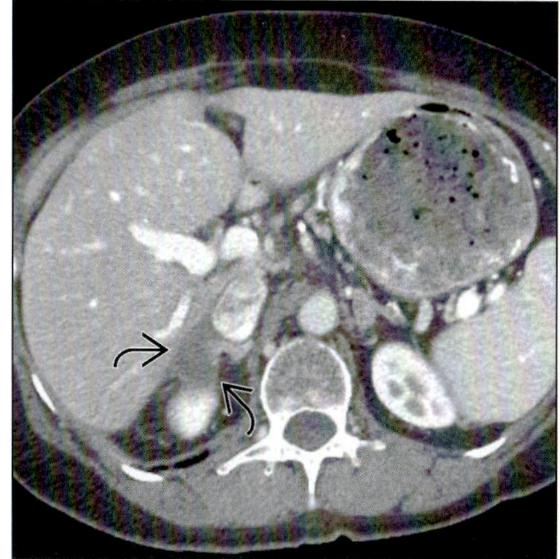

(Left) *Coronal image in the same patient demonstrates the conformal coverage of the PTV (red volume) by the prescription dose (60 Gy) ↷. Daily image-guided CT scans were used to ensure accuracy. The 30 Gy line is shown in orange ➔.* ***(Right)*** *Axial CECT 3 months after completion of RT in the same patient shows the reduction in the size of the adrenal mass ↷. There were no other sites of disease.*

VAGINA

(T) Primary Tumor

Adapted from 7th edition AJCC Staging Forms.

TNM	*FIGO*	*Definitions*
TX		Primary tumor cannot be assessed
T0		No evidence of primary tumor
Tis[1]		Carcinoma in situ (preinvasive carcinoma)
T1	I	Tumor confined to vagina
T2	II	Tumor invades paravaginal tissues but not to pelvic wall
T3	III	Tumor extends to pelvic wall[2]
T4	IVA	Tumor invades mucosa of bladder or rectum &/or extends beyond true pelvis (bullous edema is not sufficient evidence to classify a tumor as T4)

(N) Regional Lymph Nodes

NX		Regional lymph nodes cannot be assessed
N0		No regional lymph node metastasis
N1	III	Pelvic or inguinal lymph node metastasis

(M) Distant Metastasis

M0		No distant metastasis
M1	IVB	Distant metastasis

[1]*FIGO no longer includes stage 0 (Tis).*

[2]*Pelvic wall is defined as muscle, fascia, neurovascular structures, or skeletal portions of the bony pelvis. On rectal examination, there is no cancer-free space between the tumor and pelvic wall.*

AJCC Stages/Prognostic Groups

Adapted from 7th edition AJCC Staging Forms.

Stage	*T*	*N*	*M*
0	Tis	N0	M0
I	T1	N0	M0
II	T2	N0	M0
III	T1-T3	N1	M0
	T3	N0	M0
IVA	T4	Any N	M0
IVB	Any T	Any N	M1

Tis

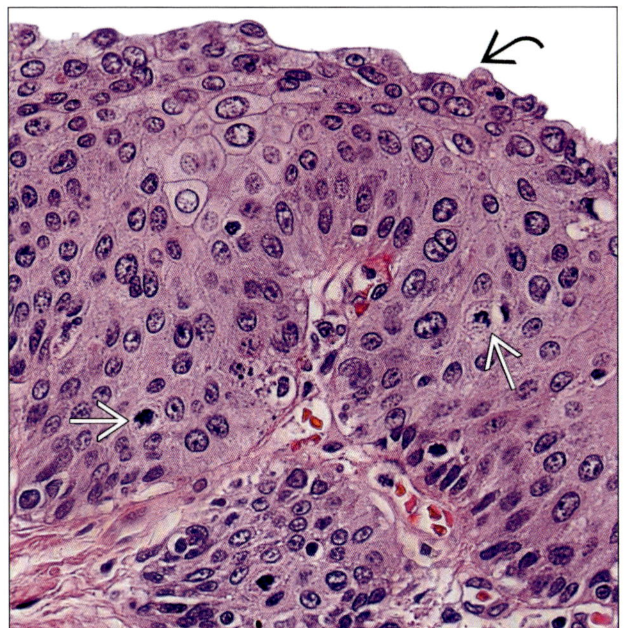

H&E stain shows dysplastic cells with enlarged and pleomorphic nuclei and high nuclear:cytoplasmic ratio involving the full thickness of the mucosa. Numerous dysplastic cells extend all the way to the surface. Mitotic figures are evident.

T1: Invasive Squamous Cell Carcinoma

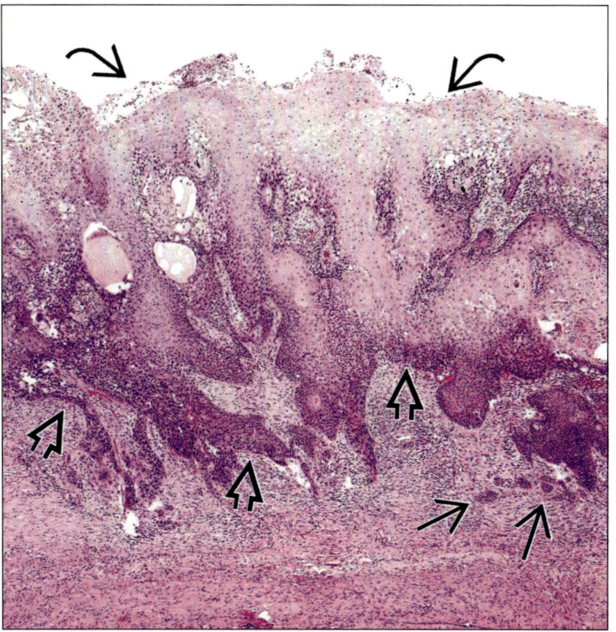

Low-power magnification of H&E stain shows nonstratified squamous epithelium of vaginal mucosa with invasive squamous cell carcinoma. Both the mucosal surface and irregular basement membrane are highlighted. Few nests are noted deeper in the submucosa.

T1: Invasive Squamous Cell Carcinoma

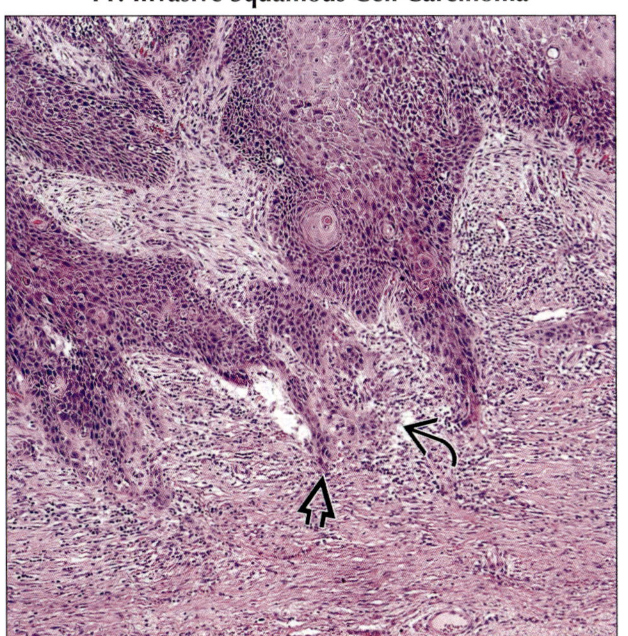

Higher magnification of the lower aspect of the mucosa shows irregular basement membrane with projections of cords and nests of cells, indicating an invasive component to the submucosa.

T3

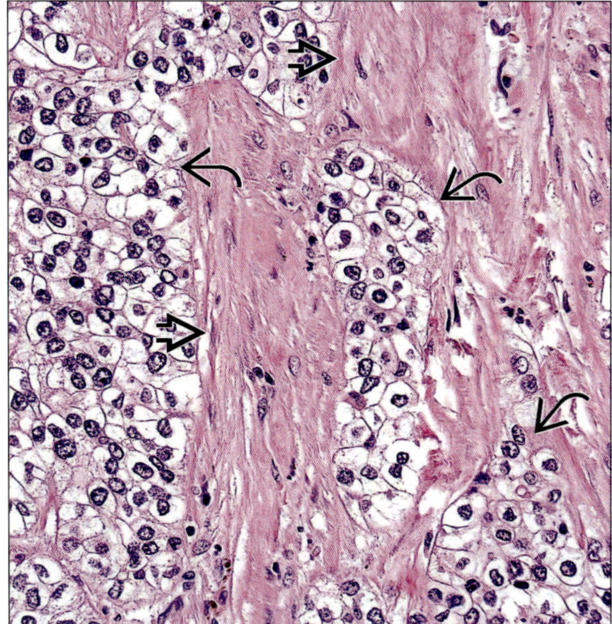

Tumor extends to the pelvic wall (T3). H&E stain from pelvic wall nodule shows vaginal squamous carcinoma. Note the nests and sheets of neoplastic squamous cells invading into the fibroconnective tissue and fascia of the pelvic wall.

VAGINA

T1

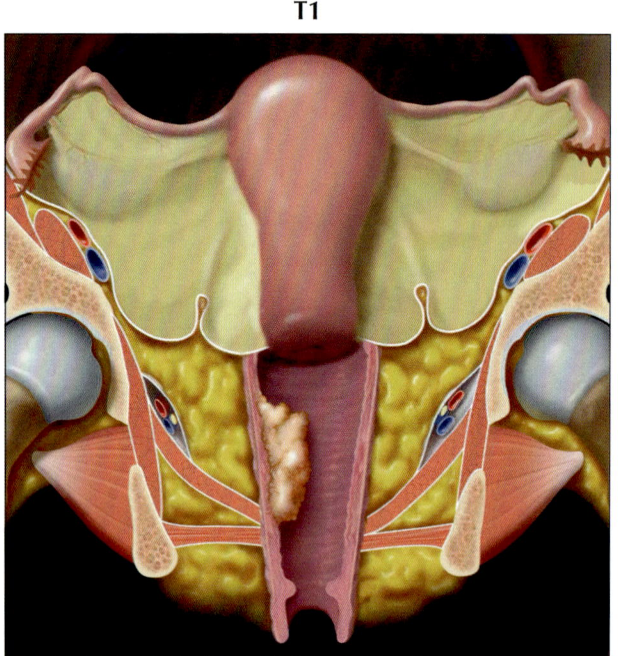

Graphic illustrates T1 tumor. Tumor is confined to the vagina without invasion of the paravaginal tissues.

T2

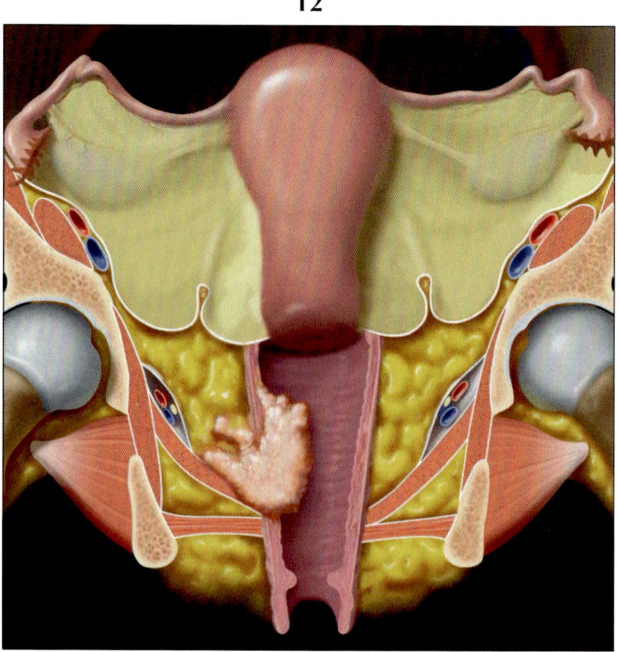

Graphic illustrates T2 tumor. Tumor invades paravaginal tissues but does not reach to the pelvic wall.

T3

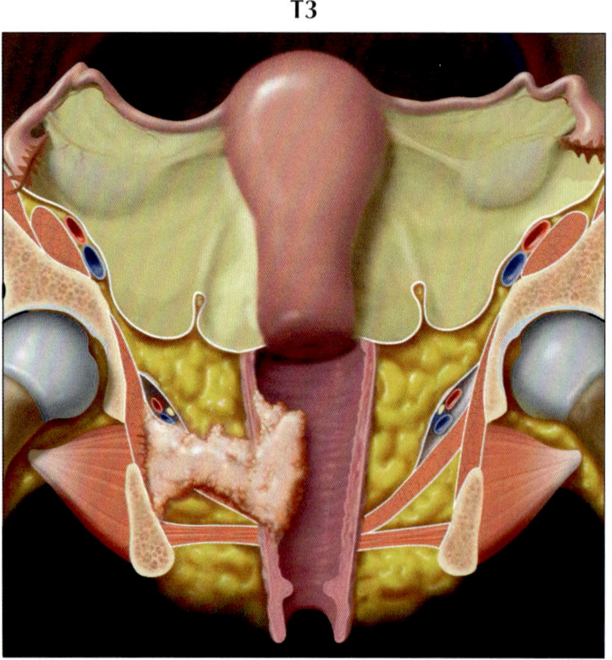

Graphic illustrates T3 tumor. Tumor invades paravaginal tissues and extends to the pelvic wall. Pelvic wall is defined as muscle, fascia, neurovascular structures, or bony pelvis.

T4

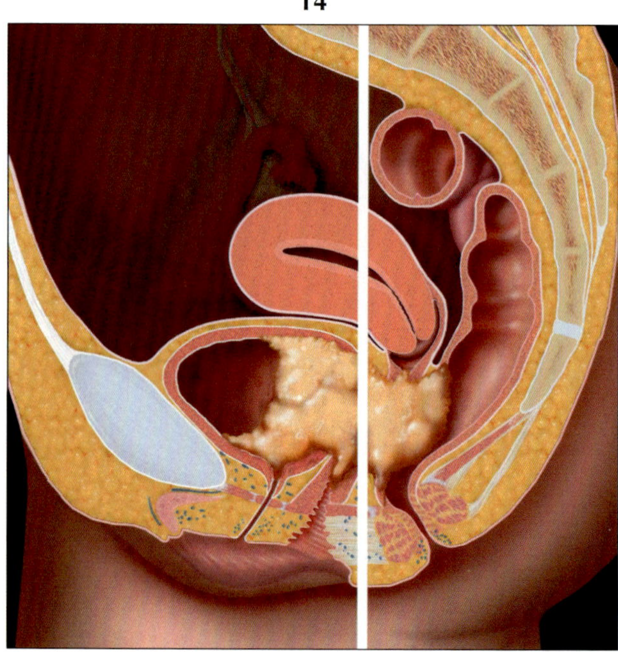

Graphic illustrates T4 tumor. Tumor invades mucosa of bladder (to the left of the divider) or rectum (to the right of the divider) &/or extends beyond the true pelvis.

Nodal Drainage of the Vagina

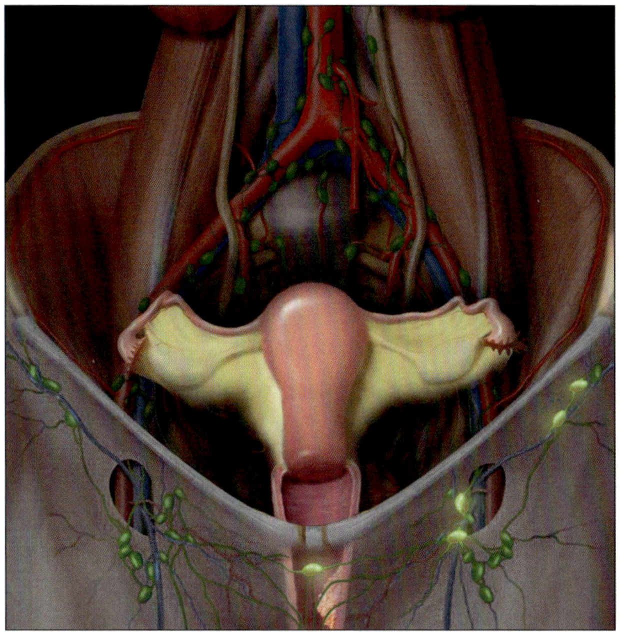

Graphic illustrates nodal drainage of tumors arising in the lower 1/3 of the vagina. Those tumors spread to inguinal and femoral lymph nodes.

Nodal Drainage of the Vagina

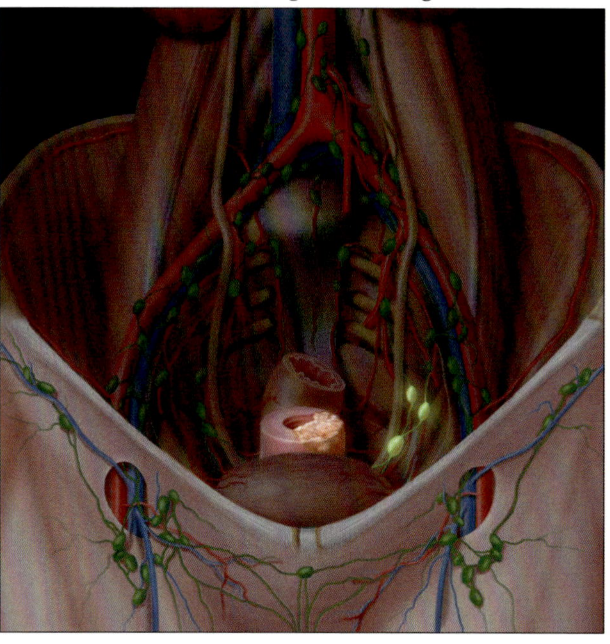

Graphic illustrates nodal drainage of tumors arising in the upper 2/3 of the vagina. Those tumors spread to pelvic lymph nodes, including obturator and internal and external iliac nodes.

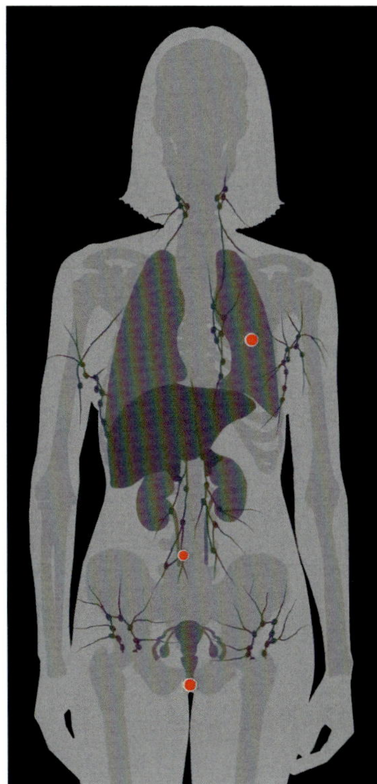

INITIAL SITE OF RECURRENCE	
Distant	9%
Vagina	7%
Pelvis	6%
Vagina and Pelvis	3%
Pelvis and Distant	3%
Vagina and Distant	2%

Data represent 147 patients that underwent definitive RT at MDACC. Stage distribution was 26%, 50%, 20%, and 4% for stages I, II, III, and IVA, respectively. Frank et al IJROBP 62(1):138-147, 2005.

VAGINA

OVERVIEW

General Comments

- Vaginal involvement with malignant disease occurs more commonly from metastatic spread
  - Most commonly due to adjacent cancers from female urogenital tract
- Vaginal carcinoma should be diagnosed only if other gynecologic malignancies have been excluded
  - Tumor involving cervix, including external os, should always be assigned to carcinoma of cervix
  - Tumor involving vulva and extending to vagina should always be assigned to carcinoma of vulva
  - Different clinical approaches in treatment of cervical and vulvar carcinoma

Classification

- Histology
  - Squamous cell carcinoma
    - Approximately 85-90% of cases
  - Adenocarcinoma
    - Approximately 10% of cases
    - Clear cell carcinoma associated with exposure to diethylstilbestrol (DES) in utero
  - Adenosquamous carcinoma
    - Approximately 1-2% of cases
  - Melanoma
  - Sarcoma including sarcoma botryoides (rhabdomyosarcoma variant)
  - Germ cell tumors (very rare)

NATURAL HISTORY

Etiology

- Risk factors
  - Squamous cell carcinoma
    - Squamous carcinoma of vagina is associated with human papilloma virus (HPV)
      - HPV viral particles can be identified in approximately 60% of invasive squamous cancers of vagina
      - Up to 30% of patients have history of intraepithelial or invasive carcinoma of cervix or vulva
  - Adenocarcinoma
    - Thought to arise from
      - Areas of vaginal adenosis
      - Foci of endometriosis
      - Wolffian rest remnants
      - Periurethral glands
    - Clear cell carcinoma
      - 2/3 have history of in utero exposure to DES
      - Develop in up to 2% of women exposed in utero to DES
      - Associated with congenital T-shaped uterus

Epidemiology & Cancer Incidence

- Uncommon tumor comprising 1-2% of gynecologic malignancies
  - 5th in frequency behind carcinoma of ovary, uterus, cervix, and vulva
- Number of cases in USA per year
  - 2,680 estimated new cases in USA in 2012
    - Highest incidence among African-American women (1.24 per 100,000 person-years)
  - 840 estimated deaths in USA in 2012
- Age of onset
  - Age of presentation depends on histologic type
    - Squamous cell carcinoma
      - Predominantly in postmenopausal women
      - Mean age ± standard deviation at diagnosis was 65.7 ± 14.3 years
    - Adenocarcinoma
      - Typically occurs in younger women ages 14-21 years (peak age: 19 years)
      - Majority are clear cell histology

Associated Diseases, Abnormalities

- Vaginal carcinoma frequently found in association with vaginal intraepithelial neoplasia

Gross Pathology & Surgical Features

- Most common patterns of presentation of vaginal squamous cell carcinoma are
  - Ulcerating lesion (50%)
  - Fungating mass (30%)
  - Annular constricting mass (20%)
- Tumor location in vagina depends on tumor histologic type
  - Squamous cell carcinoma
    - Occurs mainly in upper 1/3 on posterior wall
  - Adenocarcinoma
    - Occurs mainly in upper 1/3 on anterior wall

Microscopic Pathology

- Squamous cell carcinoma
  - Tumor composed of malignant squamous cells
  - Tumors can be graded as
    - Well differentiated
    - Moderately differentiated
    - Poorly differentiated
    - Undifferentiated
  - Squamous cell carcinoma can be
    - Keratinizing
    - Nonkeratinizing
  - Subtypes of squamous cell carcinoma include
    - Verrucous
    - Warty
    - Spindle
- Adenocarcinoma
  - Clear cell adenocarcinoma
    - Tumor cells have clear or eosinophilic cytoplasm
    - Type of vaginal adenocarcinoma related to DES exposure
    - May be seen next to areas of adenosis in older women
  - Endometrioid adenocarcinoma
    - Closely resemble morphology of uterine endometrial carcinoma
    - May be seen in association with adenosis or endometriosis
  - Mucinous adenocarcinoma
    - Rare in vagina
    - Can be of endocervical or enteric (contain goblet cells) types
  - Mesonephric adenocarcinoma

VAGINA

Routes of Spread

- Local spread
  - Tumor spreads locally into paravaginal soft tissues and eventually to pelvic sidewall, mucosa of bladder, or rectum
- Lymphatic extension
  - Early spread to regional lymph nodes
    - 1/3 of patients have pelvic or groin lymph node involvement at diagnosis
  - Nodal spread usually depends on site of primary tumor
    - Expected nodal disease
      - Upper and middle 1/3 → pelvic obturator nodes, internal and external iliac nodes, common iliac and paraaortic nodes
      - Lower 1/3 → inguinal and femoral nodes
      - Disease progression or tumor involving whole length of vagina may → inguinal and iliac nodes
  - Lymphatic drainage does not always follow expected lymphatic channels predicted anatomically based on tumor location
- Hematogenous spread
  - Most common sites of distant metastases are lung, liver, and bone

IMAGING

Detection

- CT
  - Detection of vaginal carcinoma is difficult with CT
    - In one study, CT detected vaginal carcinoma in only 43% of patients
  - Tumors are only seen if large enough to alter vaginal contour
- MR
  - Location and extent best assessed with high-resolution T2-weighted imaging (T2WI)
  - Improved detection of vaginal pathology by intravaginal instillation of ultrasound gel
  - Appearance on MR imaging correlates with macroscopic patterns of disease
    - Ill-defined, irregular, diffuse mass (ulcerating pattern of disease)
    - Well-defined lobulated mass (fungating pattern of disease)
    - Circumferential thickening (annular constricting pattern of disease)
  - T1WI
    - Isointense to muscle
    - May be difficult to see unless large enough to alter vaginal contour
  - T2WI
    - Mass of homogeneous intermediate signal intensity distinct from low signal intensity of vaginal wall
    - Hyperintense to muscles, lower than that of fat
    - Presence of high signal intensity foci likely due to tumoral necrosis should raise possibility of
      - Poorly differentiated squamous cell carcinoma
      - Adenosquamous carcinoma
      - Mucinous adenocarcinoma
- FDG PET
  - In one study, FDG PET identified abnormal vaginal uptake in 100% of patients with primary vaginal carcinoma

Staging

- T staging
  - MR
    - Valuable in demonstrating
      - Tumor location
      - Parametrial extension
      - Pelvic sidewall involvement
      - Local extension to bladder or urethra and rectum
      - Regional lymph node involvement
    - T1
      - Tumor limited to vaginal mucosa
      - Appears as mass or plaque of tissue of intermediate signal intensity on T2WI, expanding and filling vagina
      - Preservation of low signal intensity of outer vaginal muscularis layer
    - T2
      - Extension into paravaginal tissue
      - Paravaginal fat is of abnormal low signal intensity on T1WI
      - Loss of low signal intensity of vaginal muscularis layer
    - T3
      - Tumor extends to pelvic sidewall (defined as muscle, fascia, neurovascular structures, or skeletal portions of bony pelvis)
      - Best seen on axial and coronal T2WI
      - Intermediate signal intensity tumor extends to and infiltrates low signal intensity muscles of pelvic sidewall and floor
    - T4
      - Invasion of bladder or rectal mucosa
      - Spreads beyond pelvis and may involve peritoneum and small or large bowel loops
      - Best evaluated on T2WI
      - Invasion through low signal intensity of bladder or rectal wall
      - Loss of fat planes between vagina and bladder or rectum
      - Presence of bullous edema is not sufficient evidence to classify a tumor as T4
  - CT
    - Except in advanced disease, CT is not helpful for local staging
      - Poor soft tissue characterization
- N staging
  - CT and MR can be equally useful in evaluating regional lymph nodes
  - PET/CT is superior to CT in identification of nodal metastases
  - Lymphoscintigraphy can be helpful in detection of nodal metastases
    - Nodal metastases do not always follow predicted patterns
    - May result in change of radiation field
- M staging
  - CT or PET/CT are modalities of choice for evaluation of distant metastases
  - Lung metastatic nodules from squamous cell carcinoma frequently cavitate

Restaging

- CT or PET/CT is useful for detection of recurrent or metastatic tumor

CLINICAL PRESENTATION & WORK-UP

Presentation

- Patients usually present with following symptoms
  - Painless vaginal bleeding (65-80%)
  - Abnormal discharge (30%)
  - Urinary symptoms (20%)
  - Pelvic pain (15-30%)
  - Feeling of vaginal mass (10%)
  - Asymptomatic (10-27%)

Prognosis

- 5-year survival depends on stage
  - Stage 0: 85%
  - Stage I: 61%
  - Stage II: 48%
  - Stage III: 34%
  - Stage IVA: 22%
  - Stage IVB: 11%
- Exophytic tumors are associated with significantly better prognosis than infiltrative ones
  - Possibly because exophytic tumors tend to grow more superficially whereas ulcerative lesions are more likely to invade adjacent pelvic structures

Work-Up

- Clinical
  - Complete H&P with a detailed gynecologic history and complete pelvic exam
  - Other tumors need to be excluded
  - Exam under anesthesia if needed with fiducial placement
- Radiographic
  - MR is preferable for evaluation of local extent along with clinical exam
  - PET/CT or CT is preferred for evaluation of adenopathy and distant metastases
- Laboratory
  - Complete blood count with attention to hemoglobin
  - Chemistries including creatinine and liver function tests

TREATMENT

Major Treatment Alternatives

- Discrete T1 lesions may be amenable to resection
- Radiotherapy is primary modality of most lesions (T1-T4)
- Addition of concurrent chemotherapy is uncertain, may be preferred in physiologically young patients

Major Treatment Roadblocks/ Contraindications

- Many patients are elderly and may have comorbid conditions

Treatment Options by Stage

- Squamous cell carcinoma in situ
  - Wide local excision ± skin grafting
  - Partial or total vaginectomy with skin grafting for multifocal or extensive disease
  - Intravaginal chemotherapy with 5% fluorouracil cream
  - Laser therapy
  - Intracavitary radiation therapy delivering 60-70 Gy to mucosa
    - Entire vaginal mucosa should be treated due to potential field effect
- Stage I squamous cell carcinoma
  - Superficial lesions < 0.5 cm thick
    - Intracavitary radiation therapy
    - External beam radiation therapy (EBRT) for bulky lesions + brachytherapy
    - For lesions of lower 1/3 of vagina, elective radiation therapy to low pelvis ± inguinal lymph nodes
    - Wide local excision or total vaginectomy with vaginal reconstruction, especially in lesions of upper vagina
    - In cases with close or positive surgical margins, adjuvant radiation therapy should be considered
  - Lesions > 0.5 cm thick
    - Select cases: Radical vaginectomy + pelvic lymphadenectomy ± construction of neovagina
      - Adjuvant RT in cases with close or positive surgical margins, or positive nodes
    - Most cases should be treated with EBRT and brachytherapy
      - Interstitial brachytherapy is preferred for lesions with > 5 mm residual thickness after EBRT
      - Inguinal lymph nodes should be treated for lesions involving lower 1/3 of vagina
    - Elective radiation therapy to pelvic ± inguinal lymph nodes
- Stage II squamous cell carcinoma or adenocarcinoma
  - Combination of brachytherapy and EBRT
    - Concurrent chemotherapy could be considered
  - For lesions of lower 1/3 of vagina, elective radiation therapy to inguinal lymph nodes
  - Radical vaginectomy or pelvic exenteration ± radiation therapy
- Stages III and IVA squamous cell carcinoma or adenocarcinoma
  - Combination of EBRT and brachytherapy
    - Interstitial brachytherapy is preferred for lesions with > 5 mm residual thickness after EBRT
  - Elective RT to inguinal lymph nodes if lower 1/3 of vagina is involved
  - Consider concurrent chemotherapy
  - Definitive EBRT should be performed if entire lesion is not able to be implanted (IMRT may be advantageous)
- Stage IVB squamous cell carcinoma or adenocarcinoma
  - Radiation (for palliation of symptoms) ± chemotherapy

Dose Response

- Several studies have noted importance of dose in local control

Standard Doses

- For Tis lesions: 60-70 Gy intracavitary
- 45-50 Gy EBRT for stages I-IVA to low pelvis ± inguinal lymph nodes
- Cumulative 80 Gy to upper vaginal lesions
- Cumulative 70 Gy to lower vaginal lesions
  - Distal vagina has lower RT tolerance
- Definitive EBRT 65-75 Gy

Organs at Risk Parameters

- In absence of well-defined data, use criteria for cervix cancer
- Keep rectum and sigmoid colon D2 mL < 75 Gy and D2 mL bladder < 90 Gy

Common Techniques

- EBRT
  - 4 field
  - Broad anterior photon field, narrower posterior photon field and electrons to inguinal nodes
  - IMRT: Be sure to account for vaginal motion due to bladder and rectal filling
  - Brachytherapy
    - Fiducials should be placed prior to EBRT
    - Intracavitary if < 5 mm thick
    - Interstitial if > 5 mm thick

RECOMMENDED FOLLOW-UP

Clinical

- Pelvic examination every 3 months for 2 years, then 2-3x annually until year 5, then annually
- Vaginal cytology should be considered

Radiographic

- Per clinical discretion

Laboratory

- Per clinical discretion

SELECTED REFERENCES

1. Beriwal S et al: American Brachytherapy Society consensus guidelines for interstitial brachytherapy for vaginal cancer. Brachytherapy. 11(1):68-75, 2012
2. Siegel R et al: Cancer statistics, 2012. CA Cancer J Clin. 62(1):10-29, 2012
3. Ghia AJ et al: Primary vaginal cancer and chemoradiotherapy: a patterns-of-care analysis. Int J Gynecol Cancer. 21(2):378-84, 2011
4. American Joint Committee on Cancer: AJCC Cancer Staging Manual. 7th ed. New York: Springer. 387-93, 2010
5. Shah CA et al: Factors affecting risk of mortality in women with vaginal cancer. Obstet Gynecol. 113(5):1038-45, 2009
6. Griffin N et al: Magnetic resonance imaging of vaginal and vulval pathology. Eur Radiol. 18(6):1269-80, 2008
7. Parikh JH et al: MR imaging features of vaginal malignancies. Radiographics. 28(1):49-63; quiz 322, 2008
8. Taylor MB et al: Magnetic resonance imaging of primary vaginal carcinoma. Clin Radiol. 62(6):549-55, 2007
9. Frank SJ et al: Definitive radiation therapy for squamous cell carcinoma of the vagina. Int J Radiat Oncol Biol Phys. 62(1):138-47, 2005
10. Lamoreaux WT et al: FDG-PET evaluation of vaginal carcinoma. Int J Radiat Oncol Biol Phys. 62(3):733-7, 2005
11. Mock U et al: High-dose-rate (HDR) brachytherapy with or without external beam radiotherapy in the treatment of primary vaginal carcinoma: long-term results and side effects. Int J Radiat Oncol Biol Phys. 56(4):950-7, 2003
12. Kucera H et al: Radiotherapy alone for invasive vaginal cancer: outcome with intracavitary high dose rate brachytherapy versus conventional low dose rate brachytherapy. Acta Obstet Gynecol Scand. 80(4):355-60, 2001
13. Yeh AM et al: Patterns of failure in squamous cell carcinoma of the vagina treated with definitive radiotherapy alone: what is the appropriate treatment volume? Int J Cancer. 96 Suppl:109-16, 2001
14. Perez CA et al: Irradiation in carcinoma of the vulva: factors affecting outcome. Int J Radiat Oncol Biol Phys. 42(2):335-44, 1998
15. Urbański K et al: Primary invasive vaginal carcinoma treated with radiotherapy: analysis of prognostic factors. Gynecol Oncol. 60(1):16-21, 1996
16. Corn BW et al: Improved treatment planning for the Syed-Neblett template using endorectal-coil magnetic resonance and intraoperative (laparotomy/laparoscopy) guidance: a new integrated technique for hysterectomized women with vaginal tumors. Gynecol Oncol. 56(2):255-61, 1995
17. Kucera H et al: Radiation management of primary carcinoma of the vagina: clinical and histopathological variables associated with survival. Gynecol Oncol. 40(1):12-6, 1991

VAGINA

Stage I (T1 N0 M0)

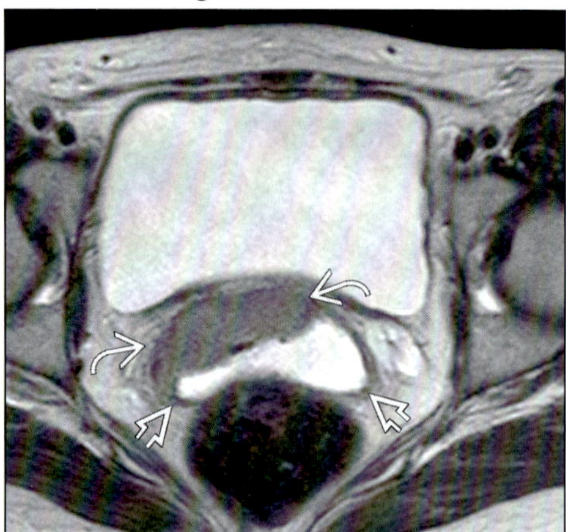

Stage I (T1 N0 M0)

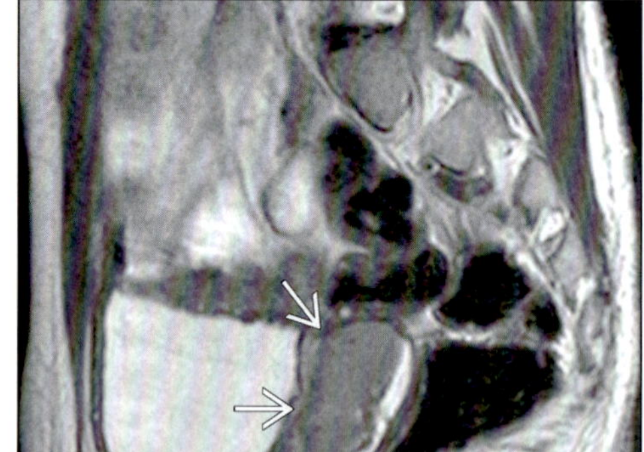

*(**Left**) Axial T2WI MR in a 52-year-old woman who had a hysterectomy at the age of 40 due to uterine leiomyomas shows an intermediate signal tumor involving the right anterior aspect of the gel-filled vagina. Tumor is limited by the vaginal wall with no invasion of the paravaginal tissues. (**Right**) Sagittal T2WI MR in the same patient shows the tumor involving the upper and middle 1/3 of the vagina.*

Stage I (T1 N0 M0)

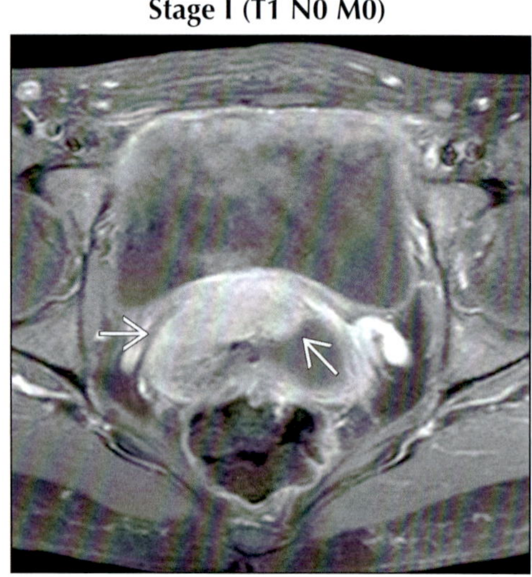

Stage I (T1 N0 M0)

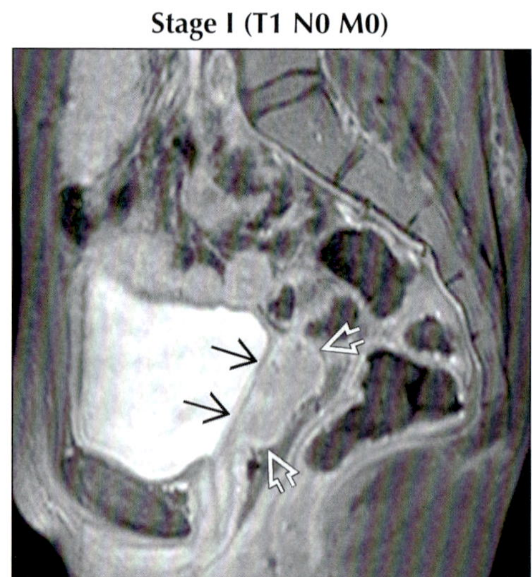

*(**Left**) Axial T1WI C+ FS MR in the same patient shows enhancement of the vaginal tumor with no enhancing nodules extending into the paravaginal fat. (**Right**) Sagittal T1WI C+ FS MR in the same patient shows enhancing tumor with clear plane between the vaginal tumor and the contrast-filled urinary bladder.*

Stage I (T1 N0 M0)

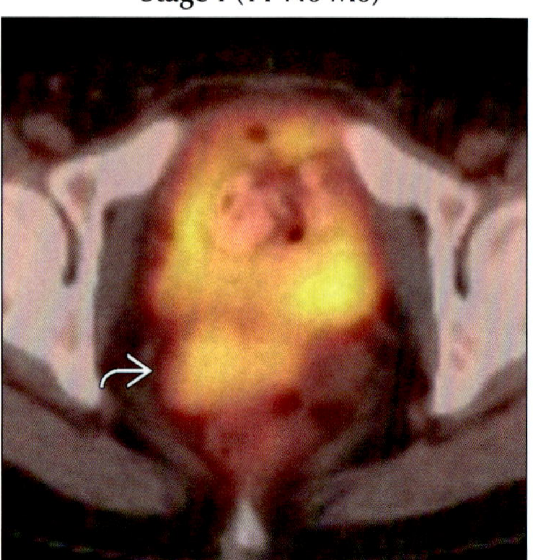

Stage I (T1 N0 M0)

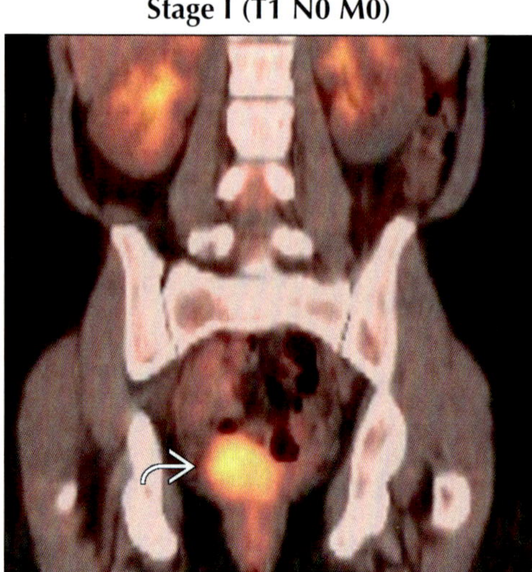

*(**Left**) Axial PET/CT in the same patient shows increased metabolic activity within the vaginal mass. (**Right**) Coronal PET/CT in the same patient shows increased metabolic activity within the vaginal mass. No other metastatic lesions were detected. Tumor limited to the vagina without paravaginal involvement constitutes T1 disease.*

Stage II (T2 N0 M0)

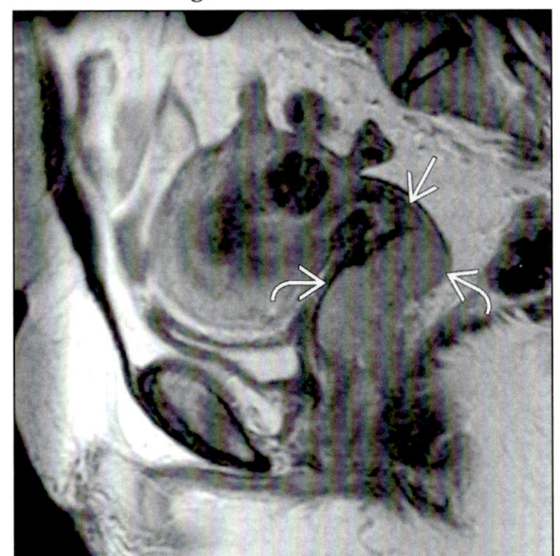

Stage II (T2 N0 M0)

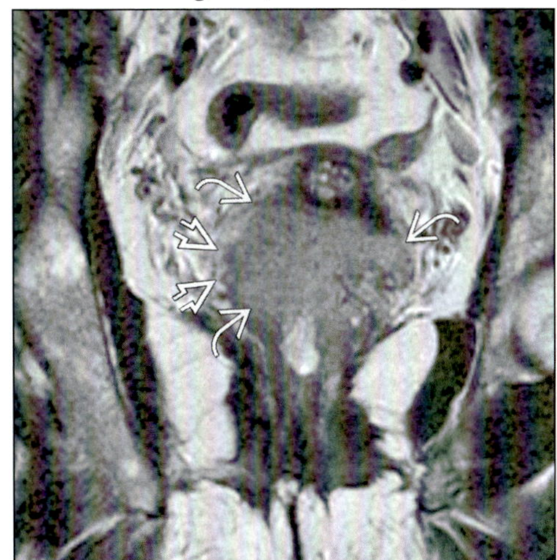

(Left) *Sagittal T2WI MR shows a large polypoid mass* ➔ *expanding the vaginal lumen. The cervix* ➔ *is not involved.* ***(Right)*** *Coronal T2WI MR in the same patient shows a vaginal mass* ➔ *with irregular nodular interface* ➔ *with the paravaginal tissues due to paravaginal fat invasion. Paravaginal fat invasion without extension to pelvic wall represents T2 disease.*

Stage II (T2 N0 M0)

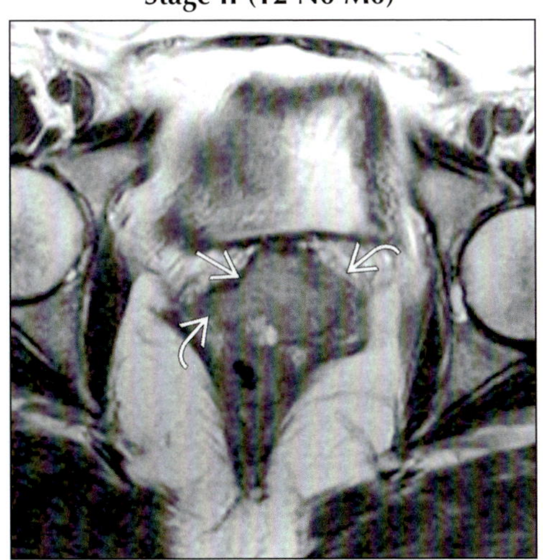

Stage II (T2 N0 M0)

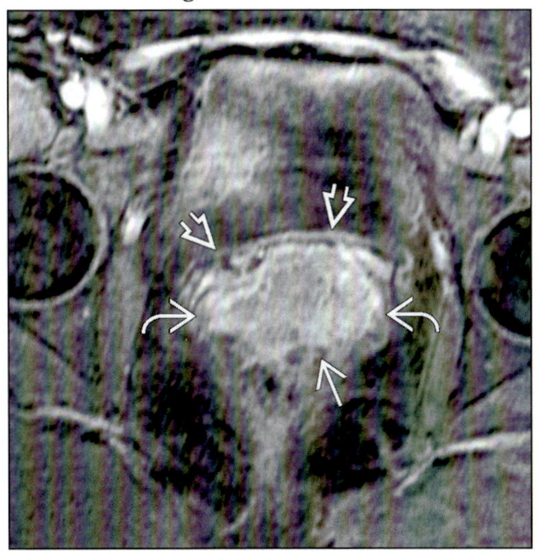

(Left) *Axial T2WI MR in the same patient shows a tumor* ➔ *filling the vagina, with paravaginal invasion* ➔ *disrupting the low signal intensity vaginal wall.* ***(Right)*** *Axial T1WI C+ MR in the same patient shows an enhancing vaginal mass* ➔ *with bilateral extension into the paravaginal fat* ➔*. Note the clear interface* ➔ *anteriorly between the vagina and the posterior wall of the urinary bladder.*

Stage III (T3 N0 M0)

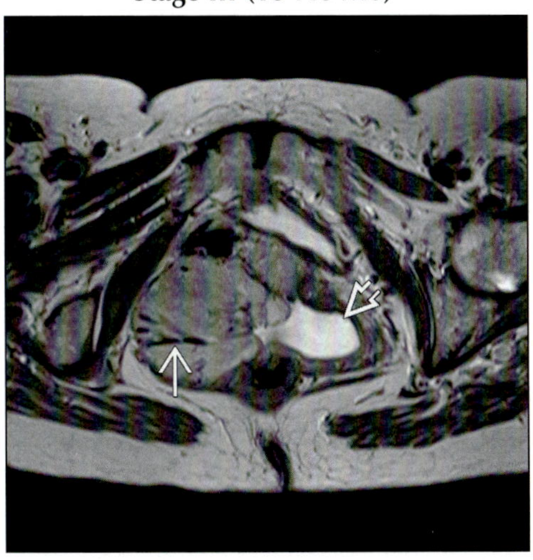

Stage III (T3 N0 M0)

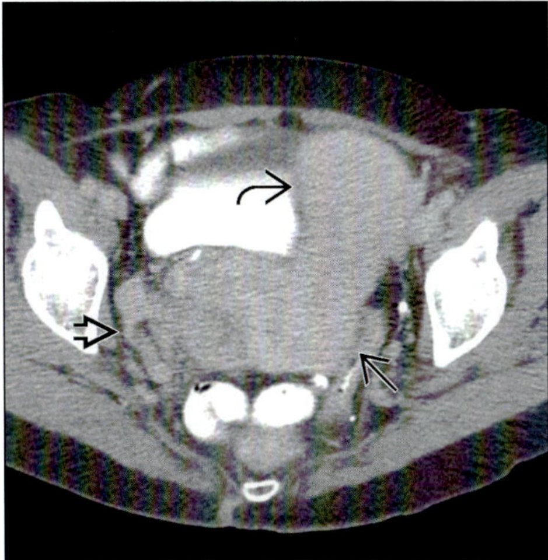

(Left) *Axial T2WI shows right-sided vaginal lesion abutting sidewall. Flow voids* ➔ *are seen in this vascular carcinosarcoma of the midvagina. Surgilube in the vagina* ➔ *is displaced to the left.* ***(Right)*** *Axial CECT shows vaginal lesion pushing cervix* ➔ *and uterus* ➔ *to the left. The parametria* ➔ *is infiltrated on the right.*

(Left) Sagittal T2WI shows a 7 cm hyperintense mass ➨ displacing the bladder anteriorly ➨ and the rectum posteriorly ➨. *(Right)* T2WI oblique donut view reveals flow voids ➨ in the vascular mass. The cervix ➨ is displaced to the left.

Stage III (T3 N0 M0)

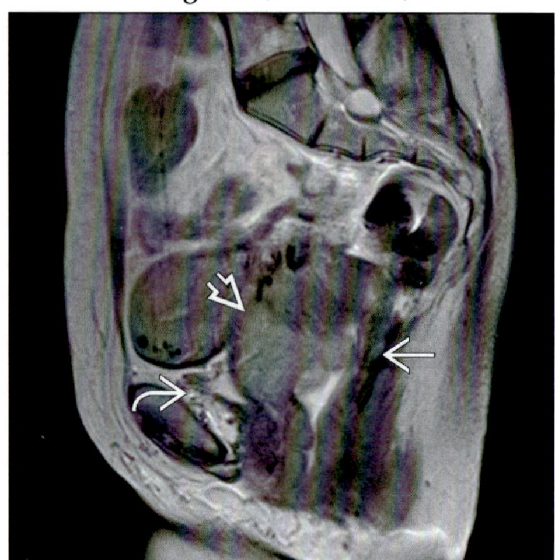

Stage III (T3 N0 M0)

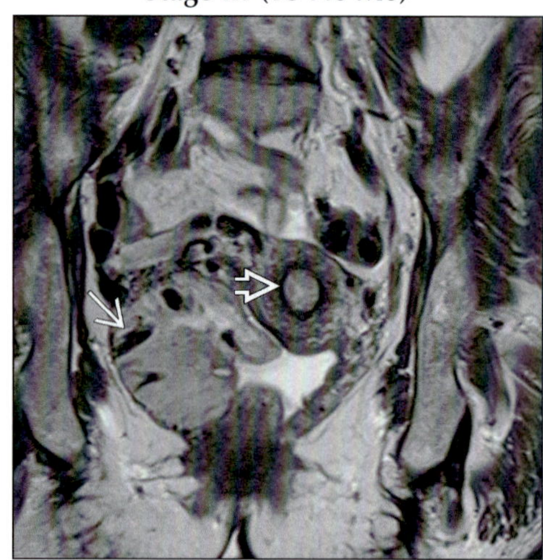

(Left) 3D planning for vaginal cancer shows the high-dose coverage of the primary ➨ and inguinal lymph nodes ➨, due in part to unequal weighting of the beams. *(Right)* Mid and low vaginal lesions should have the inguinal nodes covered. The CTV ➨ and the PTV ➨ are shown. The 100% isodose surface is shown by the colorwash. The introitus is covered in this case due to the low vaginal extent of tumor.

EBRT Planning: 3D

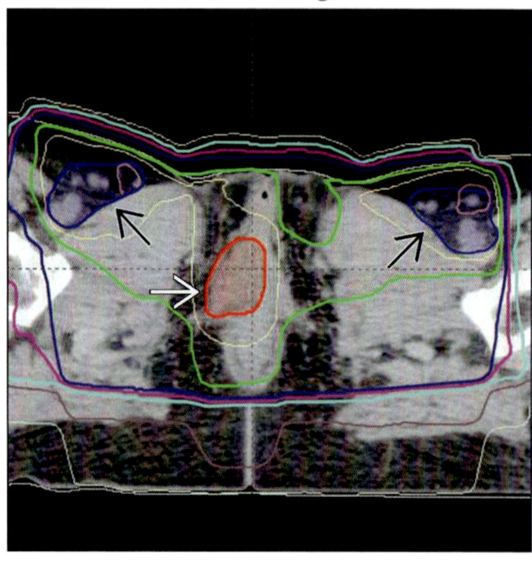

EBRT Planning: IMRT

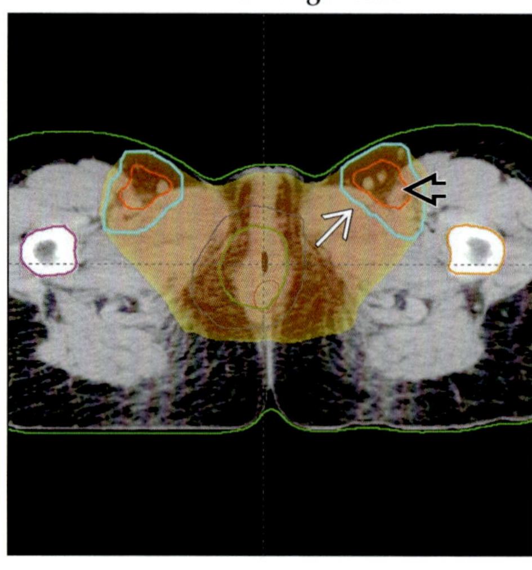

(Left) After a complete response to 45-50 Gy with < 5 mm of residual disease, a cylinder can be used. If there is multifocality, or if the tumor is large, the entire vagina should be treated. The blue, red, and yellow lines represent the 50%, 100%, and 150% isodose lines, respectively. A common prescription is 7 Gy x 3 at 5 mm. *(Right)* Coronal CT shows the entire vagina being treated to the level of the introitus ➨.

Cylinder Dosimetry

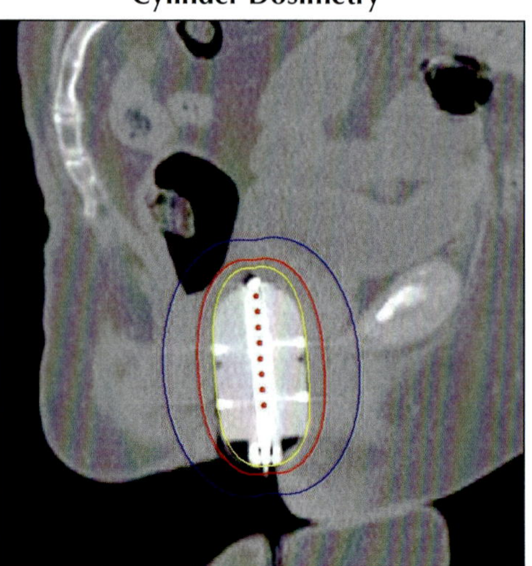

Cylinder Dosimetry

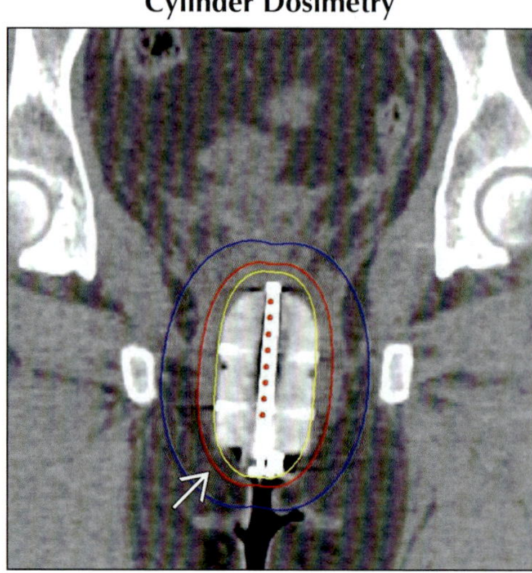

Stage IVA (T4 N1 M0)

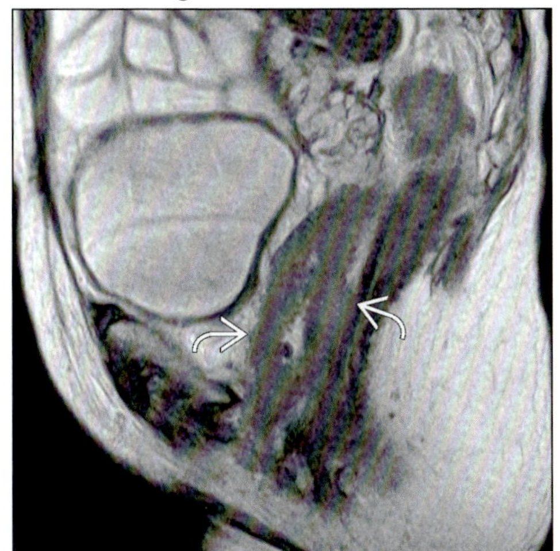

Stage IVA (T4 N1 M0)

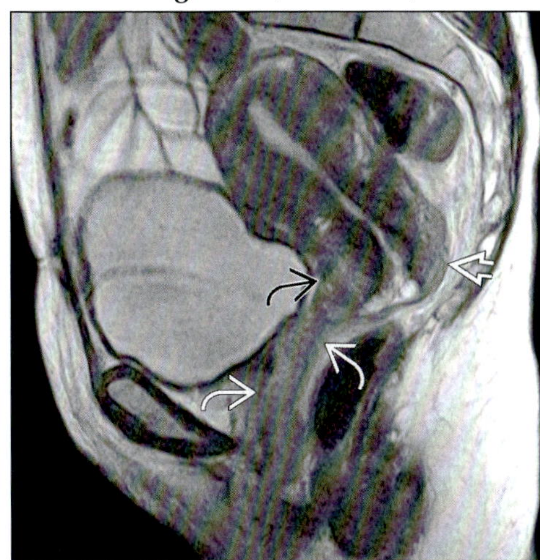

(Left) *Sagittal T2WI MR to the right of the midline in a 45-year-old woman, who presented with vaginal bleeding and discharge, shows circumferential thickening of the vaginal wall involving almost the entire length of the vagina.* ***(Right)*** *Sagittal T2WI MR in the same patient close to the midline shows thickening of the vaginal wall. The cervix is normal. Tumor extends into the anterior vaginal fornix.*

Stage IVA (T4 N1 M0)

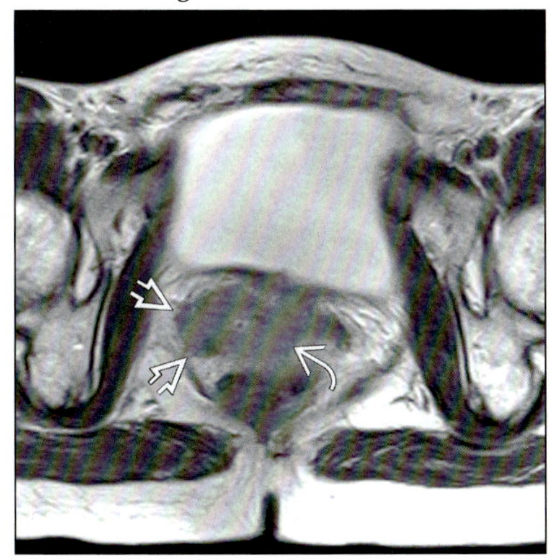

Stage IVA (T4 N1 M0)

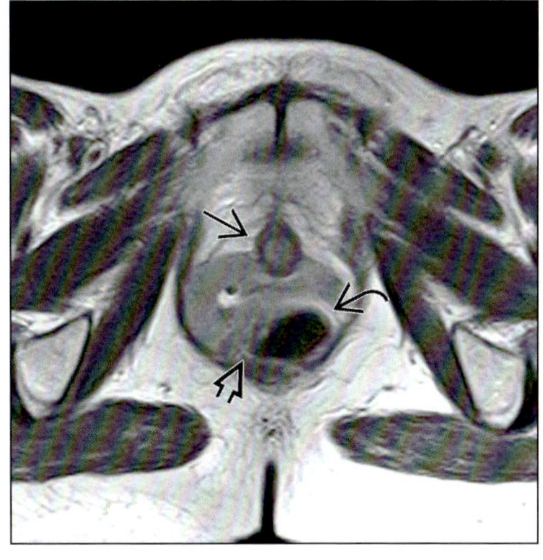

(Left) *Axial T2WI MR in the same patient shows thickening of the vaginal wall with extension into the right paravaginal fat.* ***(Right)*** *Axial T2WI MR in the same patient shows tumor extension to involve the right side of the rectum. Compare this to the clear fat plane between the vagina and anterior aspect of the rectum. The low signal intensity around the urethra is preserved with no evidence of tumor invasion.*

Stage IVA (T4 N1 M0)

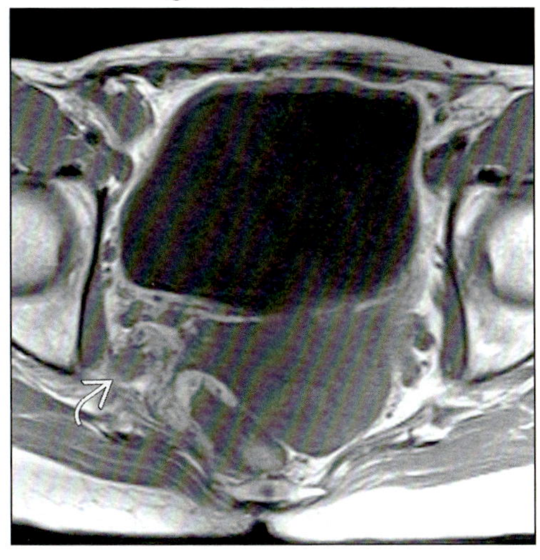

Stage IVA (T4 N1 M0)

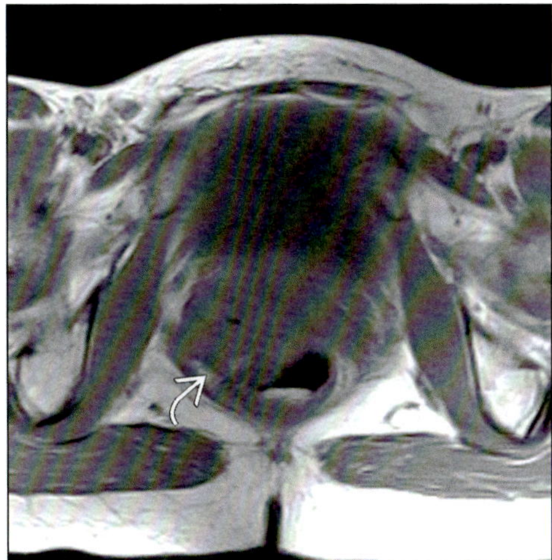

(Left) *Axial T1WI MR in the same patient shows a rounded and irregular right pelvic lymph node.* ***(Right)*** *Axial T1WI MR in the same patient shows tumor extending into the paravaginal fat. MR imaging should include imaging without fat suppression to allow visualization of intermediate signal intensity or nodular tumor extension into paravaginal fat.*

*(**Left**) Sagittal CT of an anterior vaginal lesion demonstrates excellent conformality of the 100% isodose line in yellow to the CTV shown in the red dotted line. Rapid dose fall-off limits dose to rectum and bladder. (**Right**) Axial T2WI MR shows a left-sided vaginal lesion. T2WI MRV is depicted in the dotted red line. The blue, yellow, and black lines represent the 50%, 100%, and 200% isodose lines, respectively. MR-guided brachytherapy allows superior tumor visualization.*

Interstitial Dosimetry

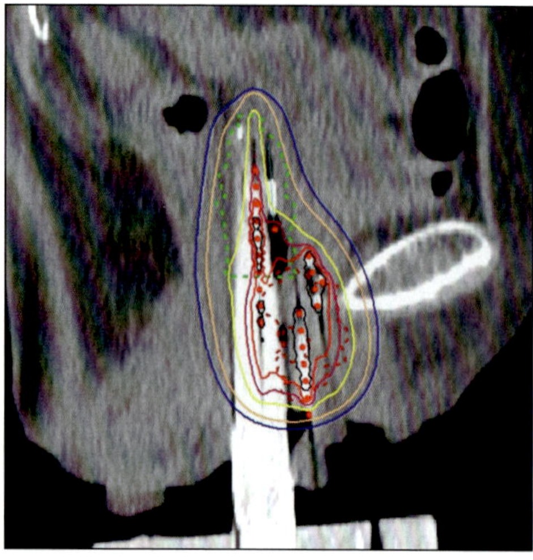

Interstitial Dosimetry

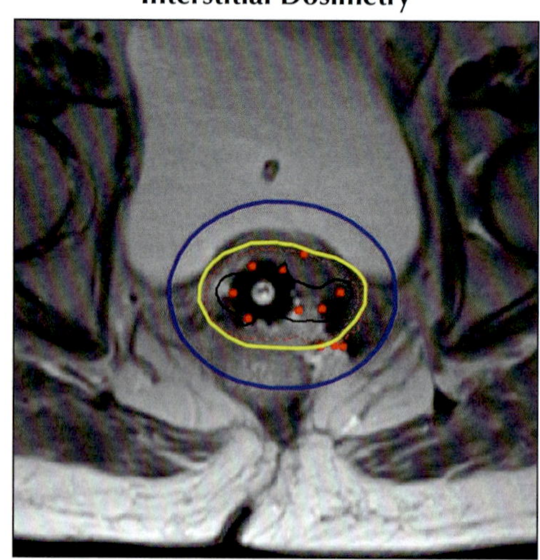

*(**Left**) Sagittal T2WI shows rectum, bladder, and sigmoid colon contoured in brown, yellow, and blue, respectively. The 100% isodose surface corresponds well to the CTV in dotted orange and red. (**Right**) Coronal T2WI MR in the same patient in plane with the vaginal obturator shows the isodose lines conforming to the larger extent of the tumor mass at the vaginal cuff ➔. High dose rate (HDR) brachytherapy allows precise dosimetry by alteration of dwell positions and times.*

Interstitial Dosimetry

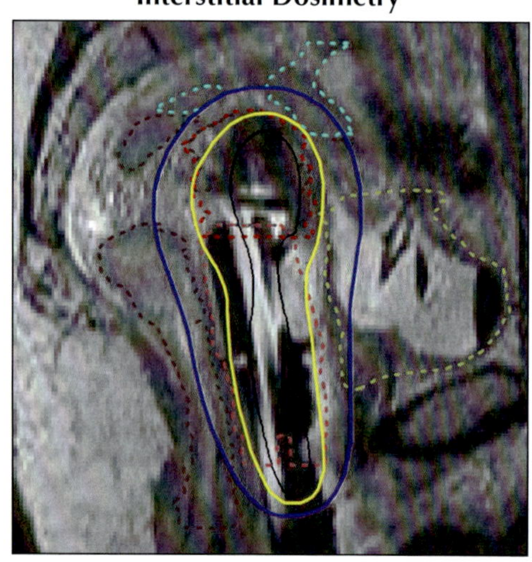

Interstitial Dosimetry

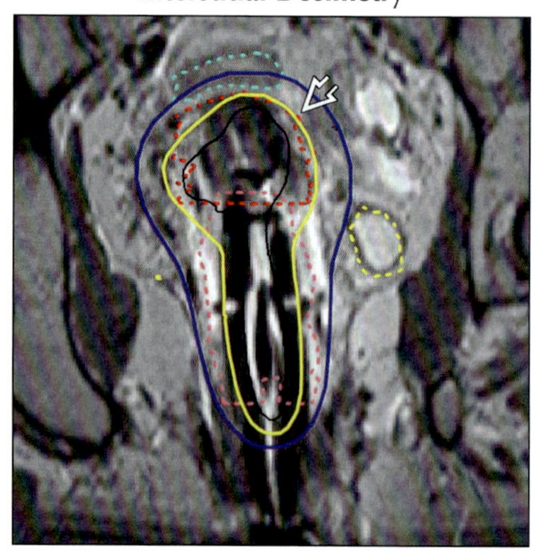

*(**Left**) Axial T2WI MR in a 65-year-old woman who presented with vaginal bleeding shows a vaginal mass ➔ of intermediate signal intensity that extends through the paravaginal fat to involve the pelvic sidewall ➔ and rectum ➔. (**Right**) Axial T1WI C+ FS MR in the same patient shows intense enhancement of the vaginal mass ➔ with enhancing soft tissue extending to involve the pelvic sidewall ➔ and rectum ➔.*

Stage IVA (T4 N0 M0)

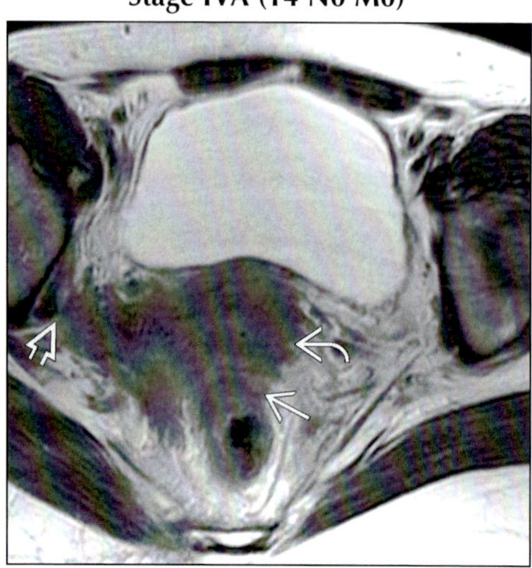

Stage IVA (T4 N0 M0)

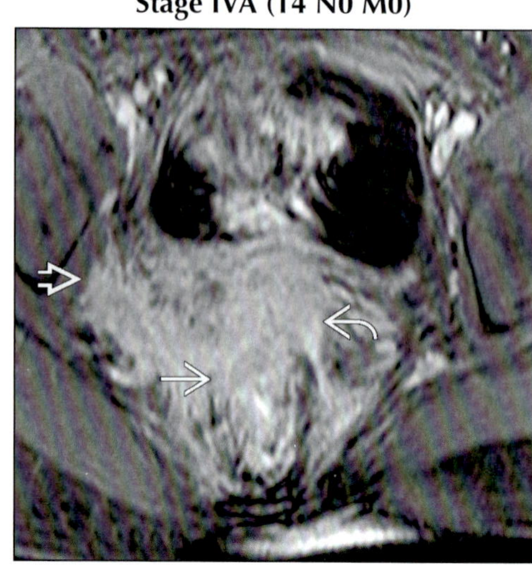

Stage IVA (T4 N0 M0)

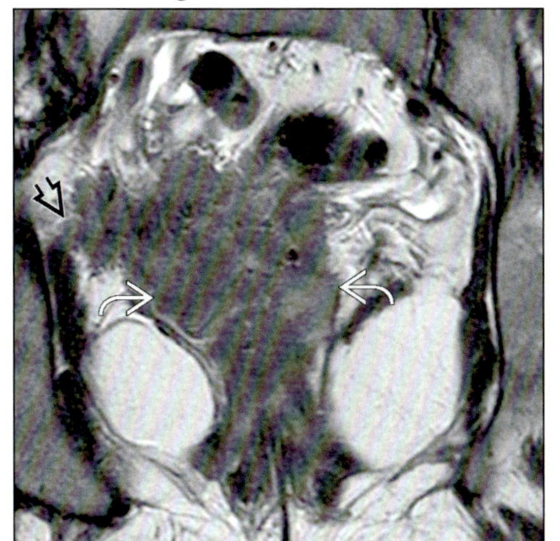

Stage IVA (T4 N0 M0)

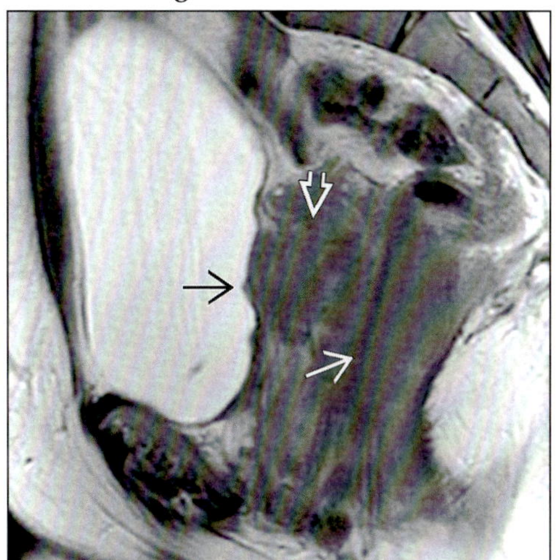

(Left) Coronal T2WI MR in the same patient shows the vaginal mass ➡ with lateral extension to the pelvic sidewall ➡. (Right) Sagittal T2WI MR in the same patient shows a vaginal mass ➡ with anterior extension to involve the posterior wall of the urinary bladder ➡ and posterior extension to involve the rectum ➡.

Metastatic Vaginal Carcinoma

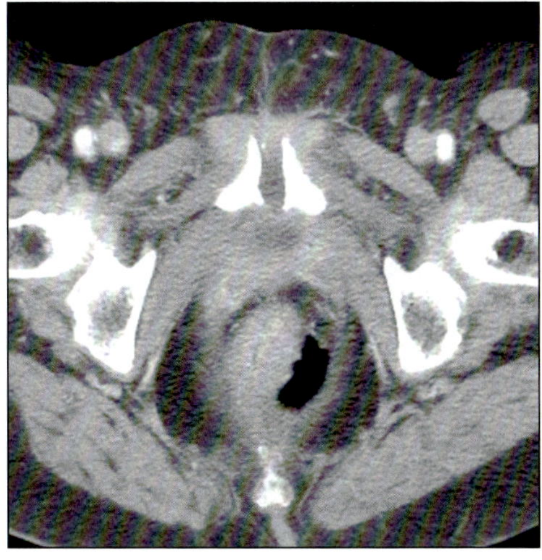

Metastatic Vaginal Carcinoma

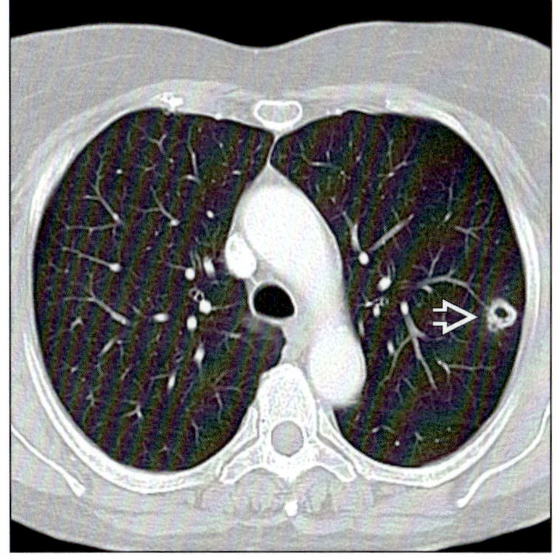

(Left) Axial CECT in a 79-year-old woman who underwent radical vaginectomy for stage II vaginal squamous carcinoma shows no evidence of local recurrence. (Right) Axial CECT lung window in the same patient shows a cavitary lung lesion ➡. Metastases from squamous carcinoma frequently cavitate. CT can be useful for follow-up in patients for detection of local recurrence or metastatic disease.

Locally Recurrent Vaginal Carcinoma

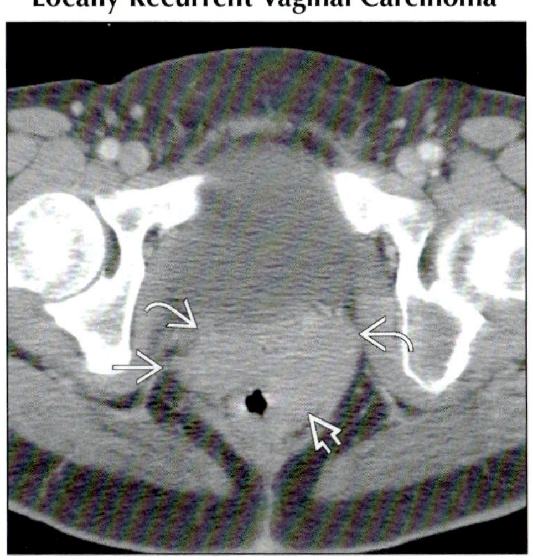

Locally Recurrent Vaginal Carcinoma

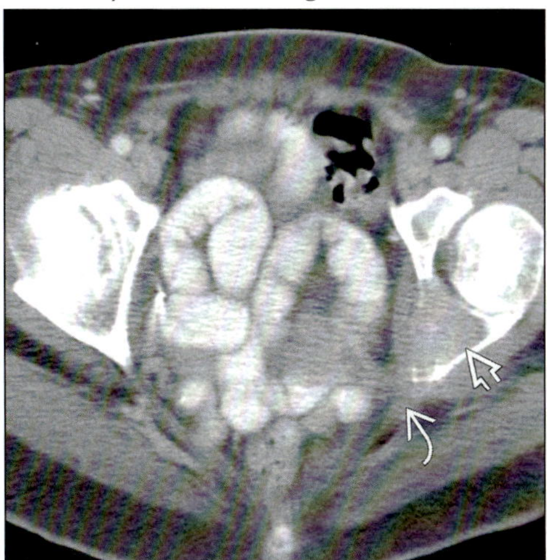

(Left) Axial CECT in a 75-year-old woman who presented with stage III vaginal carcinoma and underwent radiation treatment shows a vaginal mass ➡ with extension to the paravaginal tissue ➡ and to the rectum ➡. (Right) Axial CECT in the same patient also shows extension to the pelvic muscles ➡ and left ischium ➡.

Locally Recurrent Vaginal Carcinoma

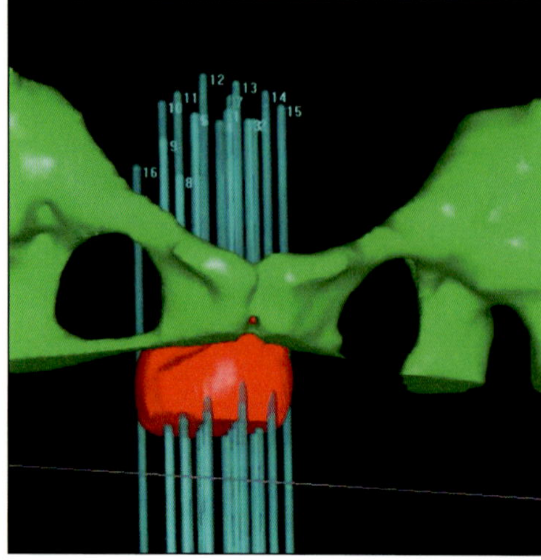

Locally Recurrent Vaginal Carcinoma

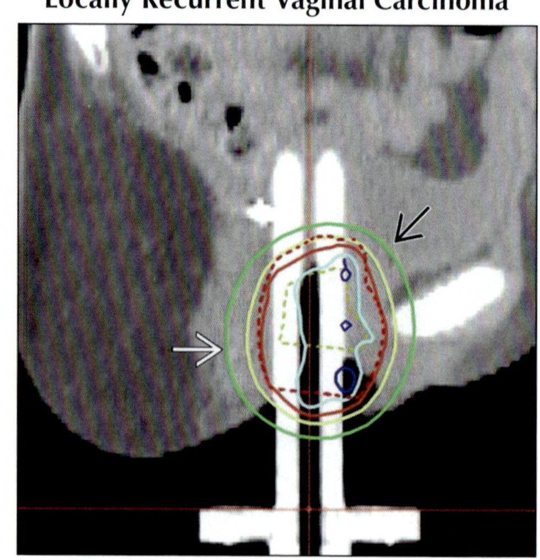

(Left) *Preplan determines needle placement. The CTV is shown in red.* ***(Right)*** *Sagittal CT shows nice conformality to the CTV shown in the dotted red line. The solid red line is the 100% isodose line and green is the 50% line. Note the sparing of dose to bladder → and anus →.*

Locally Recurrent Vaginal Carcinoma

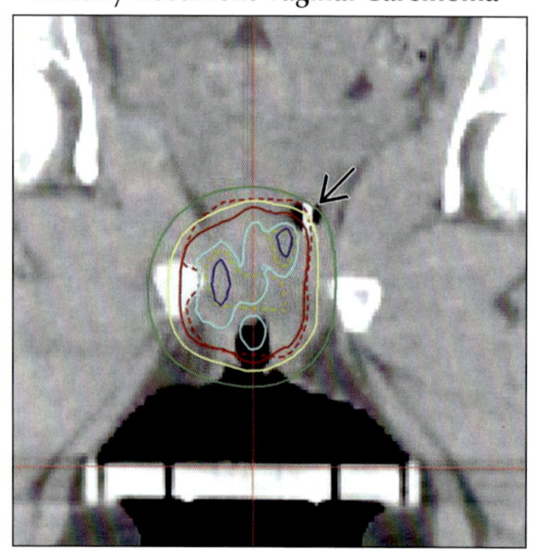

Locally Recurrent Vaginal Carcinoma

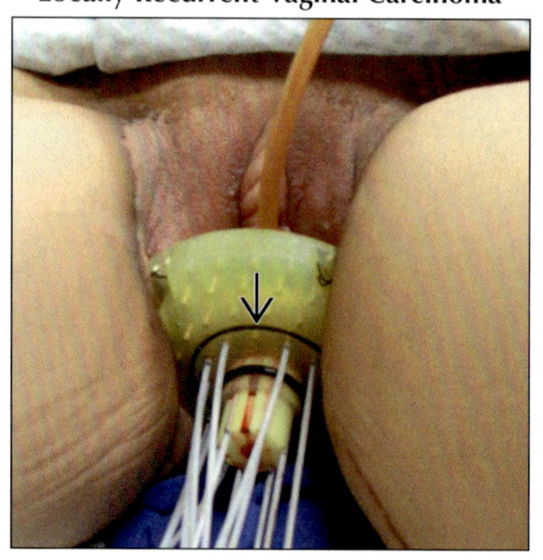

(Left) *Coronal CT shows the solid red 100% isodose line conforming well to the CTV. A clip → is placed to mark the cephalad extent of the tumor.* ***(Right)*** *Perineal template at time of treatment with HDR: Note absence of anterior needle → to avoid trauma to the urethra. Fluoroscopy was used to guide needle depth.*

Locally Recurrent Vaginal Carcinoma

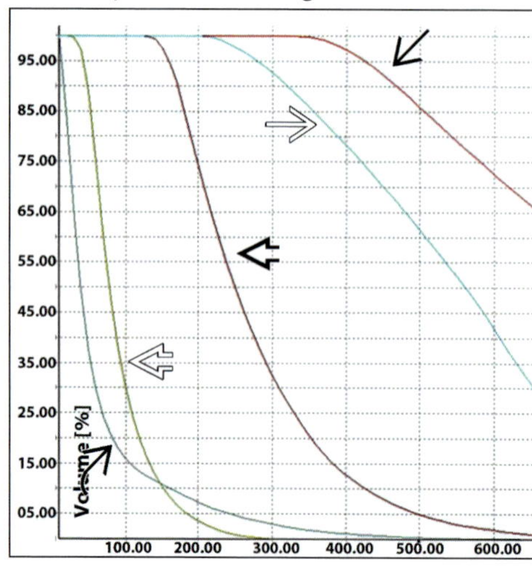

Locally Recurrent Vaginal Carcinoma

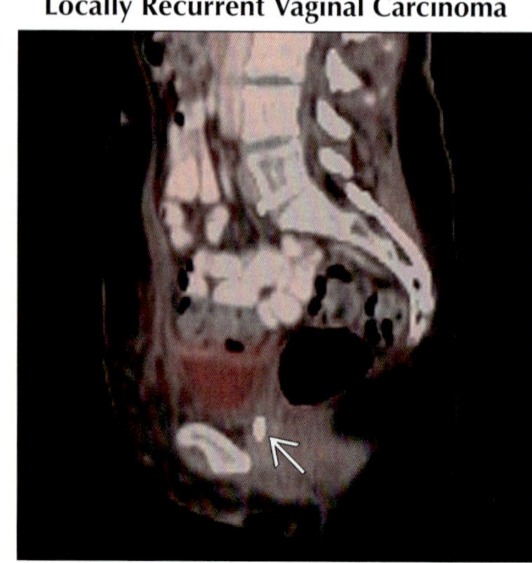

(Left) *DVH shows favorable coverage of the CTV → and sparing of urethra →, anus →, bladder →, and rectum →. Brachytherapy avoids high dose to OARs due to rapid dose fall-off.* ***(Right)*** *Axial PET/CT 6 months after treatment shows no avidity and no mass. Pelvic exam demonstrated a clinical complete response. Clip → is present in paravaginal tissues from brachytherapy.*

Locally Recurrent Vaginal Carcinoma

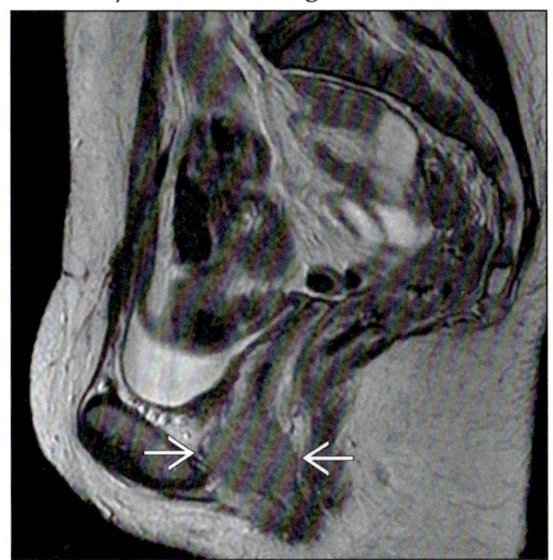

Locally Recurrent Vaginal Carcinoma

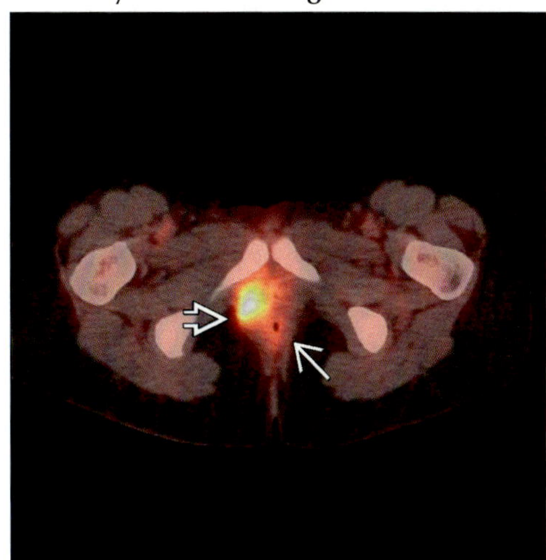

(Left) *Sagittal T2WI MR shows a 4.5 cm squamous cell carcinoma ➡ at the introitus.* ***(Right)*** *Axial PET/CT in the same patient shows a discrete lesion ⇨ in the low vagina, just superior to the anus ➡. Inguinal lymph nodes were not clinically involved.*

Locally Recurrent Vaginal Carcinoma

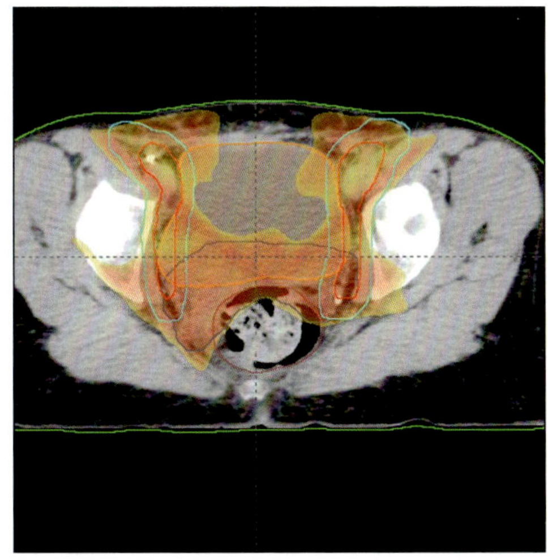

Locally Recurrent Vaginal Carcinoma

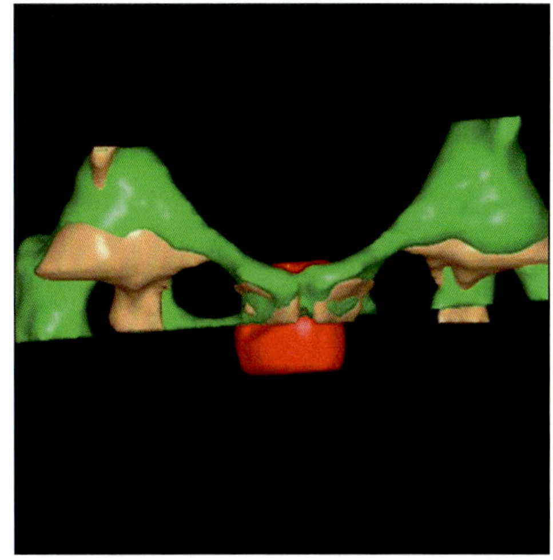

(Left) *In this isolated recurrence, the pelvis and inguinal lymph nodes were treated to 45 Gy with IMRT. The 90% isodose surface is shown in colorwash. Nodal CTV and PTVs are displayed.* ***(Right)*** *MR-CT fusion was performed for image-guided brachytherapy. Note alignment of the pelvic bones. The CTV is shown in red.*

Locally Recurrent Vaginal Carcinoma

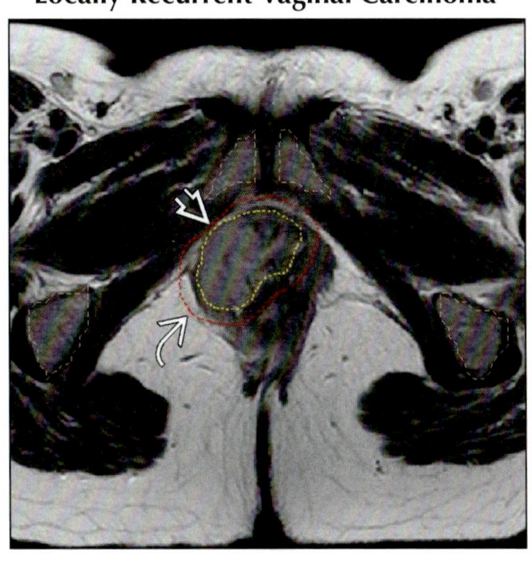

Locally Recurrent Vaginal Carcinoma

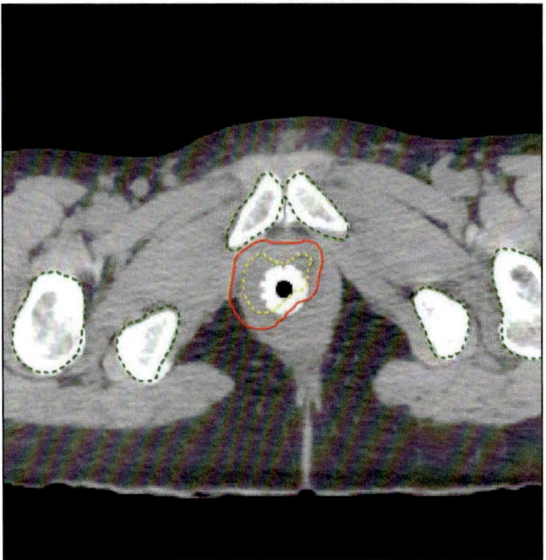

(Left) *Axial T2WI MR shows the GTV nicely (dotted yellow line) ⇨. A margin is added to encompass microscopic tumor spread for the CTV (dotted red line) ↪ for brachytherapy preplanning.* ***(Right)*** *Axial CT at simulation with vaginal obturator in place: CT does not permit the soft tissue resolution of the mass that was nicely seen by MR. The CTV is shown in red.*

VULVA

(T) Primary Tumor

Adapted from 7th edition AJCC Staging Forms.

TNM	*FIGO*	*Definitions*
TX		Primary tumor cannot be assessed
T0		No evidence of primary tumor
Tis[1]		Carcinoma in situ (preinvasive carcinoma)
T1a	IA	Lesions ≤ 2 cm in size, confined to the vulva or perineum and with stromal invasion[2] ≤ 1.0 mm
T1b	IB	Lesions > 2 cm in size **or** any size with stromal invasion > 1.0 mm, confined to the vulva or perineum
T2[3]	II/III	Tumor of any size with extension to adjacent perineal structures (lower/distal 1/3 urethra, lower/distal 1/3 vagina, anal involvement)
T3[4]	IVA	Tumor of any size with extension to any of the following: Upper/proximal 2/3 of urethra, upper/proximal 2/3 vagina, bladder mucosa, rectal mucosa, or fixed to pelvic bone

(N) Regional Lymph Nodes

NX		Regional lymph nodes cannot be assessed
N0		No regional lymph node metastasis
N1		1 or 2 regional lymph nodes with the following features
N1a	IIIA	1 or 2 lymph node metastases each < 5 mm
N1b	IIIA	1 lymph node metastasis ≥ 5 mm
N2	IIIB	Regional lymph node metastasis with the following features
N2a	IIIB	≥ 3 lymph node metastases each < 5 mm
N2b	IIIB	≥ 2 lymph node metastases ≥ 5 mm
N2c	IIIC	Lymph node metastasis with extracapsular spread
N3	IVA	Fixed or ulcerated regional lymph node metastasis

(M) Distant Metastasis

M0		No distant metastasis
M1	IVB	Distant metastasis (including pelvic lymph node metastasis)

[1]*FIGO no longer includes stage 0 (Tis).* [2]*The depth of invasion is defined as the measurement of the tumor from the epithelial-stromal junction of the adjacent most superficial dermal papilla to the deepest point of invasion.* [3]*FIGO uses the classification T2/T3. This is defined as T2 in TNM.* [4]*FIGO uses the classification T4. This is defined as T3 in TNM.*

AJCC Stages/Prognostic Groups

Adapted from 7th edition AJCC Staging Forms.

Stage	*T*	*N*	*M*
0	Tis	N0	M0
I	T1	N0	M0
IA	T1a	N0	M0
IB	T1b	N0	M0
II	T2	N0	M0
IIIA	T1, T2	N1a, N1b	M0
IIIB	T1, T2	N2a, N2b	M0
IIIC	T1, T2	N2c	M0
IVA	T1, T2	N3	M0
	T3	Any N	M0
IVB	Any T	Any N	M1

Tis

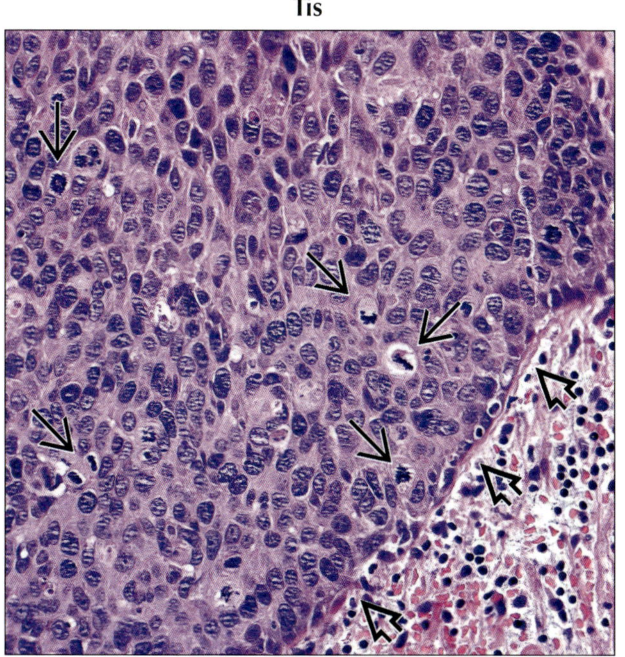

High magnification shows crowded, pleomorphic, and dysplastic cells that lack maturation. The nuclei are hyperchromatic with many mitotic figures →. Note that the basement membrane ⇨ is intact with no invasive component.

T1

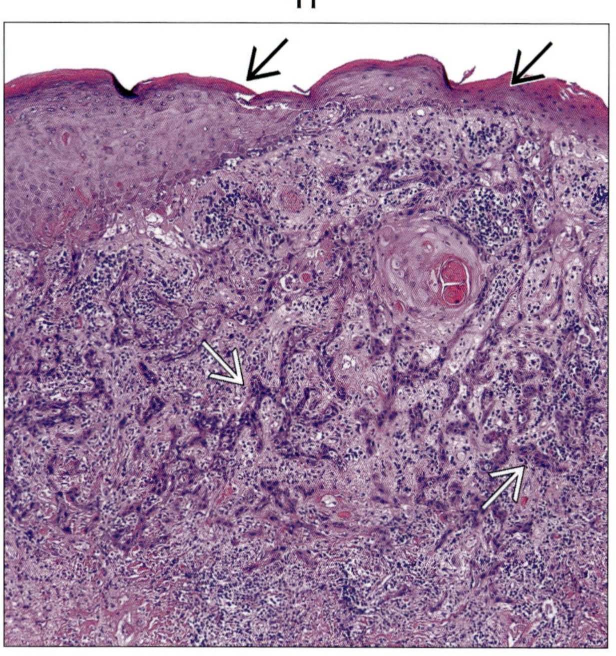

Vulvar biopsy specimen shows overlying stratified squamous epithelium → with an invasive squamous cell carcinoma. High magnification shows nonkeratinized cords ➡ and nests of malignant cells in a desmoplastic stroma.

T1

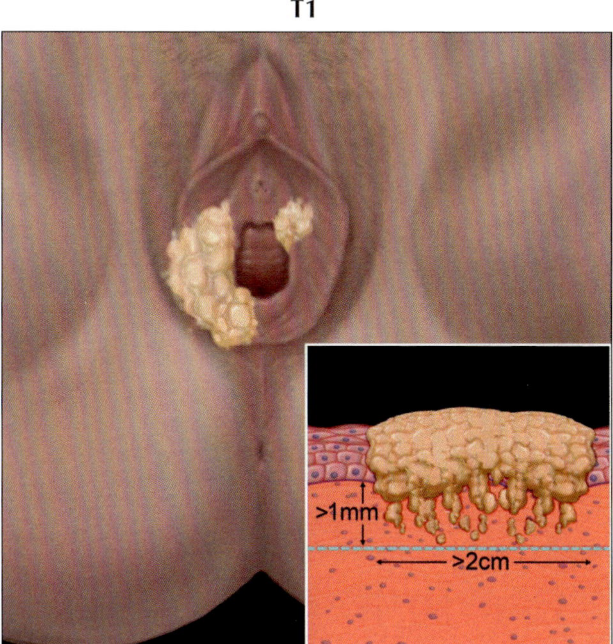

This picture shows a multifocal tumor confined to the vulva > 2 cm in greatest dimension. T1 tumors are confined to the vulva or perineum. T1a lesions are ≤ 2 cm with stromal invasion ≤ 1 mm, and T1b lesions are > 2 cm or with > 1 mm of stromal invasion.

T2

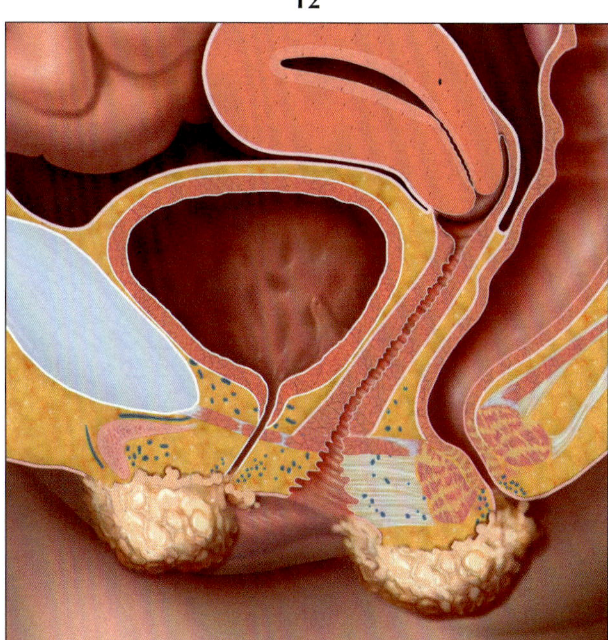

Sagittal view of the pelvis depicts vulvar tumor invading the lower urethra, lower vagina, and anus. Invasion of the distal 1/3 of adjacent perineal structures characterizes tumor stage T2.

T3

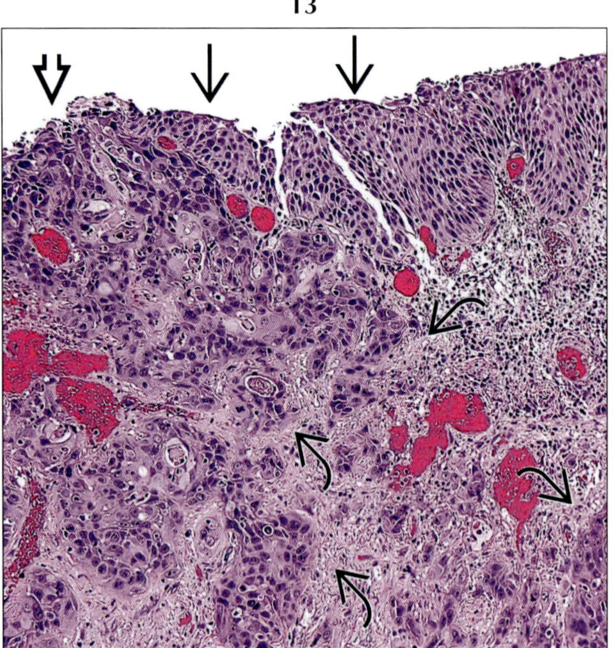

H&E stain of a biopsy specimen from the urinary bladder shows bladder mucosa with transitional epithelium ➡. Invasive vulvar carcinoma involves the wall of the bladder ↷ and extends to involve the bladder mucosa in the left upper corner ⇨.

T3

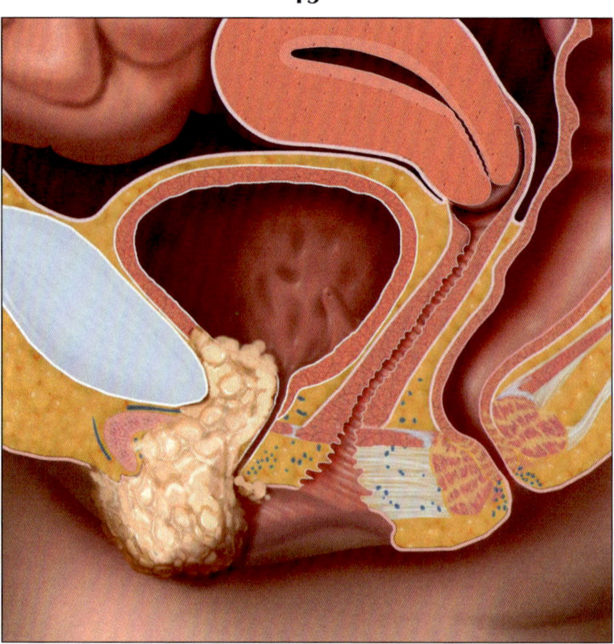

Sagittal view of the pelvis depicts vulvar tumor extending to the upper urethra, urinary bladder, and pubic bone. Invasion of the proximal urethra and bladder mucosa constitutes tumor stage T3, as does tumor fixed to the pelvic bone and rectum (not shown).

N1a and N1b

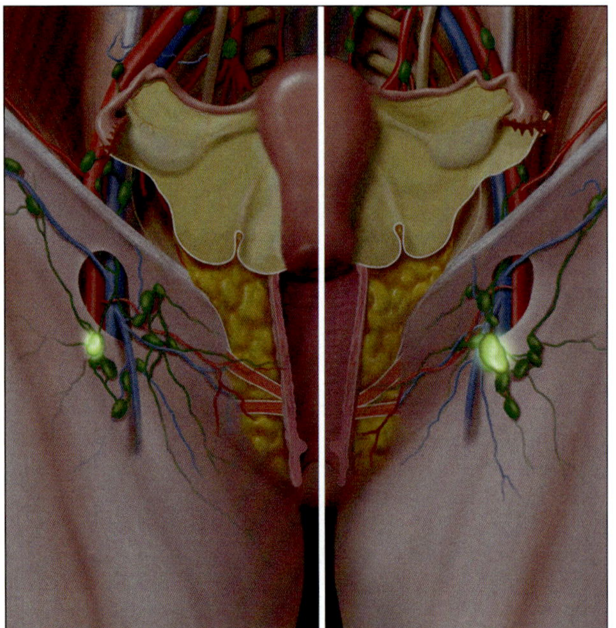

Graphic shows the inguinofemoral lymph node basin. The image on the left depicts 1 lymph node metastasis ≤ 5 mm. Only 1 or 2 regional lymph nodes with metastases < 5 mm can be involved for nodal stage N1a. The image on the right depicts 1 lymph node metastasis ≥ 5 mm, which constitutes stage N1b.

N2a and N2b

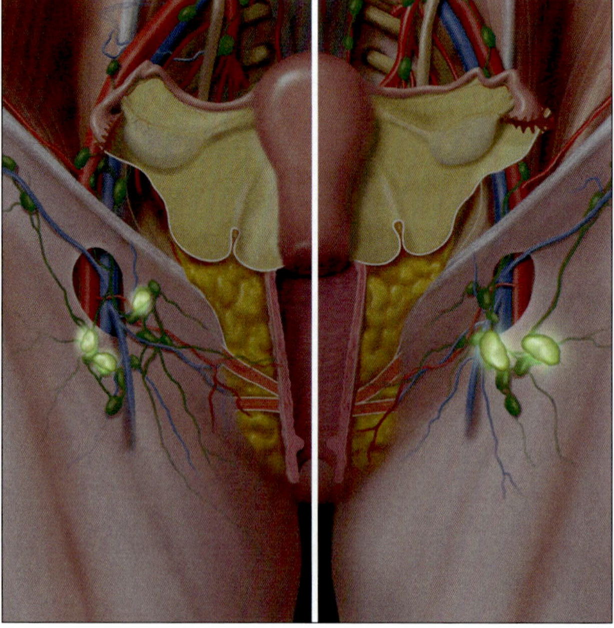

The image on the left depicts 3 lymph node metastases, each < 5 mm. For nodal stage N2a, 3 or more regional lymph nodes with metastases < 5 mm can be involved. The image on the right depicts 2 lymph node metastases ≥ 5 mm. For nodal stage N2b, 2 or more lymph nodes with metastases ≥ 5 mm can be involved.

N2c

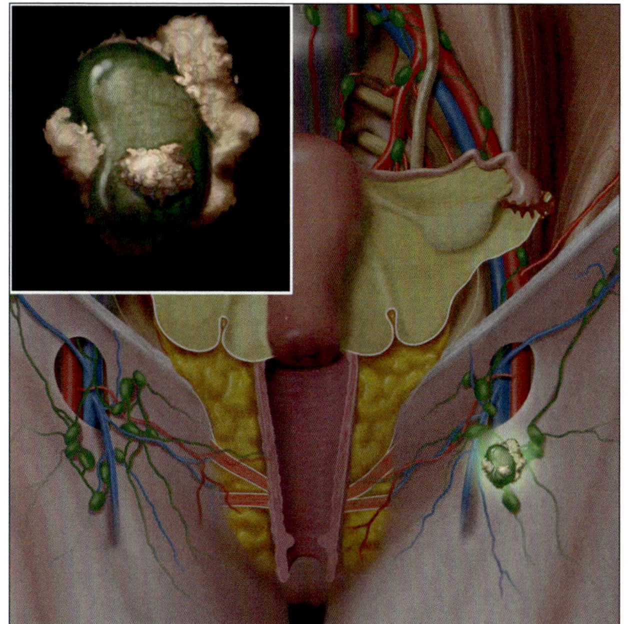

This graphic shows the inguinofemoral lymph node basin with a magnified lymph node metastasis inset. A regional lymph node metastasis with extracapsular spread of tumor constitutes nodal stage N2c.

N3

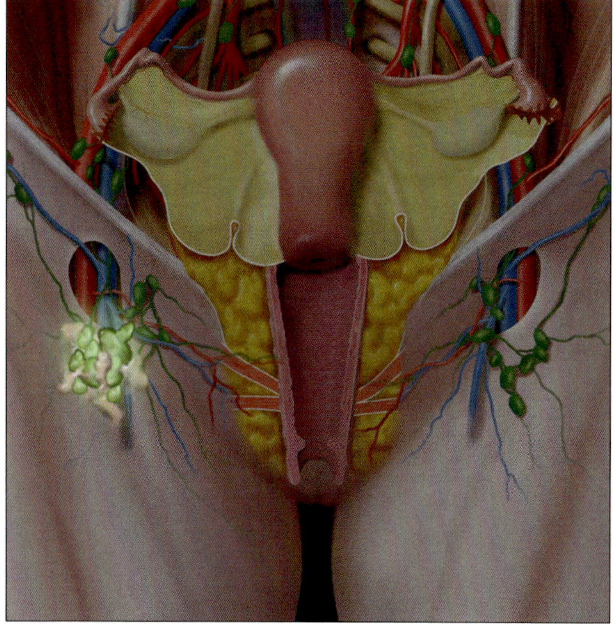

Graphic of the inguinofemoral lymph node basin depicts regional lymph node metastases with the nodal mass fixed to surrounding tissues. Fixation or ulceration of adjacent tissues constitutes nodal stage N3.

INITIAL SITE OF RECURRENCE

Groin	14%
Distant	12%
Local (Vulva)	8%
Pelvis	4%
Vulva and Distant	4%

Data represent 111 node-positive patients treated on GOG 37 (Homesley trial). Kunos C et al: Obstetrics and Gynecology, 114(3):537-546, 2009.

VULVA

OVERVIEW

General Comments

- 4th most common gynecologic malignancy in the developed world
- 4% of female genital tract malignancies
- 90% are squamous cell carcinoma (SCCa)

Classification

- Histopathologic types
  - Squamous cell carcinoma
  - Verrucous carcinoma
  - Paget disease of vulva
  - Adenocarcinoma, not otherwise specified (NOS)
  - Basal cell carcinoma, NOS
  - Bartholin gland carcinoma
- Mucosal malignant melanoma is not included in this classification and staging

NATURAL HISTORY

Etiology

- Risk factors
  - Cigarette smoking
  - Vulvar dystrophy
  - Vulvar intraepithelial neoplasia (VIN) or cervical intraepithelial neoplasia (CIN)
  - Human papilloma virus (HPV) infection
  - Immunodeficiency syndromes
  - History of cervical cancer
  - Northern European ancestry

Epidemiology & Cancer Incidence

- 4,490 new cases in USA and 950 deaths estimated for 2012
- Rate of invasive cancer has been stable for 2 decades
- Incidence of VIN (in situ) has doubled

Genetics

- S-phase fraction (proliferation index) ↑ in tumors from patients with lymphatic spread
- HPV-encoded oncoproteins E6 and E7
  - Can bind tumor suppressor gene products (p53 protein and retinoblastoma protein), causing loss of growth suppression
- Epidermal growth factor receptor positivity
  - ↑ nodal metastases and ↓ patient survival
- HER2/neu positivity: ↑ risk of nodal metastases

Associated Diseases, Abnormalities

- Synchronous 2nd malignancy in up to 22%, most commonly cervical neoplasia
- HPV
  - Responsible for 60% of vulvar cancers
  - HPV 16, 18, and 33 are most common
  - HPV-related cancer found in younger women
    - Increasing incidence of HPV-related VIN in young women
    - Tend to present with earlier stage disease and may be multifocal
  - Risk factors associated with HPV infection
    - Early age at 1st intercourse
    - Multiple sexual partners
    - HIV infection
    - Cigarette smoking
- Vulvar dystrophies
  - Includes lichen sclerosus and squamous cell hyperplasia
  - Cancer occurs in older women
  - Not associated with HPV and tends to be unifocal

Gross Pathology & Surgical Features

- Location
  - 50% in labia majora
  - 15-20% in labia minora
  - 10-15% in clitoris
  - Infrequently in other sites
  - 10% of lesions are too extensive to determine site of origin
- 5% of cases are multifocal
- Verrucous cancer is typically exophytic, may be large, infiltrates locally

Microscopic Pathology

- H&E
  - Squamous cell carcinoma is most common
  - Usually well differentiated
  - If high grade, may have areas of glandular differentiation
  - Clitoral tumors may be more anaplastic
  - VIN and keratosis may occur at margins

Routes of Spread

- Local spread
  - Influenced by histology
    - Well differentiated: Superficial spread with minimal invasion
    - Anaplastic: More likely to be deeply invasive
  - Posteriorly to anus and rectum
  - Anteriorly to urethra, rarely to urinary bladder and pubic bone
  - Cephalad to vagina
  - Usually slowly infiltrates local tissues, followed by lymph node spread
- Lymphatic extension
  - Typical lymphatic drainage
    - Superficial inguinal → deep femoral → external iliac lymph nodes
    - Superficial inguinal lymph nodes
      - Subcutaneous along medial inguinal ligament
      - Along saphenous vein, near saphenofemoral junction
    - Deep femoral lymph nodes
      - Along femoral artery and vein, within femoral sheath
      - Can be involved without superficial inguinal adenopathy
    - External iliac lymph nodes
      - Cloquet node: Most caudal lymph node in this chain, at entrance of femoral canal
      - Cloquet node signals likelihood of pelvic node metastases
  - Drainage based on tumor location
    - Lateral lesions spread to ipsilateral lymph nodes
    - Central lesions may spread to ipsilateral, contralateral, or both lymph nodes
      - Lesions within 1 cm of vulvar midline
      - Anterior lesions (area immediately posterior to clitoris)

- Posterior lesions drain mainly to superficial inguinal lymph nodes
  - Likelihood of lymphatic spread increases with each millimeter of depth
    - ≤ 1 mm: 0%
    - 1.1-2 mm: 5.4%
    - > 5 mm: 32%
  - Other patterns of lymphatic spread
    - Bilateral groin metastasis
      - Drainage from midline structures: Perineum and clitoris
    - Direct spread to pelvic nodes
      - Rarely occurs with central cancers
      - Direct drainage via internal pudendal chain to internal iliac nodes
    - Subcutaneous and dermal lymphatics
      - Obstruction of typical lymphatic drainage
      - Involves vulva, mons pubis, upper thighs, lower abdomen
    - Obturator or internal iliac nodes
      - Involved if invasion of vagina or bladder
  - Risk factors for lymph node metastases
    - Clinical node status
    - Age
    - Grade
    - Stage, size, and depth of stromal invasion
    - Lymphovascular space invasion (LVSI)
- Hematogenous spread
  - Distant metastases are rare and usually fatal, occur late and rarely without nodal metastases

IMAGING

Detection

- **CT**
  - Small superficial tumors
    - Often not seen
    - May appear as irregularity of vulvar surface
  - Large exophytic tumors
    - Enhancing solid mass
    - Surface irregularity may indicate ulceration
- **MR**
  - Tumor characteristics
    - Hypointense on T1WI
    - Intermediate to high signal on T2WI
  - IV contrast not helpful for tumor detection
  - Limited visualization of small tumors & plaque-like lesions

Staging

- Surgically staged malignancy
- **Primary tumor**
  - Borders: Mons pubis anteriorly, genitocrural folds laterally, and perineum posteriorly
  - Imaging of limited utility in early stage (small superficial) tumors
  - Exam under anesthesia may be needed
- **Lymphatic metastases**
  - Regional lymph nodes → femoral & inguinal
  - Likelihood of lymphatic spread is very low if ≤ 1 mm stromal invasion
    - Lymph node dissection (LND) is optional for stage IA disease
  - Unilateral lesions with ≥ 3 mm stromal invasion have ≥ 2.8% rate of bilateral groin metastases
  - Traditionally nodal staging has been surgical
    - Inguinal-femoral lymphadenectomy has morbidity
      - Lower extremity lymphedema (up to 69% of cases)
      - Wound breakdown or infection
      - Lymphocysts
      - Psychosexual consequences
  - Unilateral dissection performed if < 1% risk of contralateral metastasis
    - Unifocal tumor < 2 cm
    - Lateral lesion (> 1 cm from vulvar midline)
    - No palpable adenopathy in either groin
    - No lymph node metastases at time of unilateral LND
  - Bilateral dissection performed if
    - Tumor > 2 cm or
    - Central lesion (< 1 cm from vulvar midline) or
    - Metastasis found at unilateral LND
  - Clinical palpation is unreliable
    - Sensitivity is 57%, specificity is 62%
    - Allows evaluation of only superficial lymph nodes
    - Limited by body habitus, small lymph node size, scar tissue, and reactive nodal tissue
  - Ultrasound
    - Helpful for evaluation of groin adenopathy
      - Sensitivity is 86%, specificity is 96%
    - Characteristics of malignant lymph nodes
      - Round shape, irregular contour
      - Short axis diameter > 8 mm
      - Long axis/short axis ratio < 2
      - Loss of echogenic fatty hilum
      - ↑ thickness & ↓ echogenicity of cortex
      - Peripheral vascularity, high resistance flow
    - Advantages
      - Can evaluate superficial and deep lymph nodes
      - Can guide surgery or cytology
    - Limitations
      - Operator dependent
      - May be difficult to reproduce findings
      - False-positives due to reactive lymph nodes
      - Morphologically normal lymph nodes may harbor micrometastases
  - Ultrasound-guided fine needle aspiration (FNA) cytology
    - Most reliable: Combines morphology & cytology
      - Sensitivity is 93%, specificity is 100%
    - More sensitive than cytology alone (sensitivity of 75% due to sampling error)
    - Limitations
      - Operator dependent
      - Micrometastases
  - CT
    - Inferior to US and guided FNA in detecting malignant adenopathy
  - MR
    - Sensitivity is inconsistent among studies
      - 40-50% in 1 study, but 86% and 89% in others
      - Significant overlap in size of benign and malignant lymph nodes
    - High specificity: 97-100%
    - Malignant lymph node characteristics
      - Short axis diameter > 8 mm

- Irregular or round shape
- ↑ SI on STIR or heterogeneous SI on T2WI
- Advantages
  - Not operator dependent, reproducible
  - Multiplanar imaging allows assessment of size, shape, and signal intensity
- Future directions: MR lymphography
  - Ultrasmall iron particles accumulate in normal lymph nodes
  - ↓ SI in normal lymph nodes on T2WI post contrast
  - Metastatic lymph nodes are replaced by tumor cells → do not accumulate iron oxide → no change in SI post contrast
  - May improve sensitivity of MR
  - May be able to detect micrometastases
- PET
  - Poor sensitivity for metastatic lymph nodes
    - Sensitivity is 67%, specificity is 95%
  - Limitations
    - False-positives (acute or chronic inflammation, post-radiotherapy reactions)
    - Micrometastases
- Lymphoscintigraphy & sentinel node biopsy (SNB)
  - In one multi-institutional study of 276 patients, groin recurrence rate was 3.0% in those with negative sentinel lymph node (SLN)
  - Highly accurate in predicting nodal metastases
  - Learning curve for successful application
  - Absence of tracer uptake may indicate lymph node completely replaced by tumor

- **Distant metastases**
  - Any site beyond regional lymph nodes, including pelvic nodes
    - Lung, liver, extragenital skin, bone, intraabdominal sites, heart, central nervous system
    - Pelvic nodes are M1; however, some patients with pelvic adenopathy are cured with radical chemoradiation therapy (CRT)
  - Rare in most common types of vulvar cancer
  - Can be seen with melanoma and rare sarcomas

Restaging

- Recurrence
  - Poor prognosis, usually fatal if recurrence is in the groin
  - Predictors of recurrence
    - Size of lesion
    - Close margins at resection
      - Need > 8 mm tumor-free margin
    - Metastases in ≥ 2 groin nodes, and size of nodal metastases
  - 80% of recurrence occurs within 2 years of primary treatment
  - Location
    - Vulva/groin
    - Skin bridge
      - Between vulvar & groin incisions
    - Pelvic lymph nodes
    - Distant sites
      - Rare except with melanoma or sarcoma

CLINICAL PRESENTATION & WORK-UP

Presentation

- Elderly women, mean age of 65 at diagnosis
  - Data suggest age at diagnosis is trending down
    - May be related to ↑ in VIN in young women
- Signs and symptoms
  - Asymptomatic
  - Vulvar plaque, ulcer, or mass
  - Pruritus
  - Bleeding or discharge
  - Dysuria
  - Enlarged groin lymph node

Prognosis

- Lymph nodes are most important prognostic indicator
  - 90% survival if negative groin nodes
  - 50-60% survival if positive groin nodes
  - Poor prognostic indicators
    - Bilateral malignant nodes
    - Unilateral malignant adenopathy involving multiple nodes
    - Tumor penetration of lymph node capsule
    - Increasing size of metastatic focus in node
- Primary tumor characteristics are important in prognosis
  - Tumor size
    - Recently thought to be less important in predicting survival (independent of other factors)
  - Depth of tumor invasion
    - Measured from epithelial-stromal junction of adjacent most superficial dermal papilla to deepest point of invasion
    - Infiltrative growth pattern
  - LVSI
    - Documented at histologic evaluation
    - Correlates with incidence of nodal metastases
  - High grade
  - Margins < 8 mm
  - Midline and periclitoral lesions

Work-Up

- Clinical
  - Complete H&P with detailed gynecologic history
  - Biopsy of primary ± biopsy of suspicious lymph nodes
- Radiographic
  - Consider PET/CT to evaluate nodal and distant spread in larger lesions and for RT planning
  - Consider MR to evaluate extent of invasion in larger lesions and for RT planning
  - CT of chest/abdomen/pelvis
- Laboratory
  - Complete blood count

TREATMENT

Major Treatment Alternatives

- Surgery
  - Radical vulvectomy
    - Removal of vulva to level of deep thigh fascia
    - Removal of periosteum of pubis

- Removal of inferior fascia of urogenital diaphragm
  - Simple vulvectomy spares clitoris
  - Partial vulvectomy: Most conservative
  - Inguinofemoral lymphadenectomy
    - En bloc resection with vulvectomy
    - Morbidity reduced with separate groin incisions
- Radiation therapy (RT)
  - Primary radiation therapy or CRT
    - Patient unable to tolerate surgery or declines surgery, or surgery extremely morbid
  - Adjuvant radiation therapy
    - Surgical margin < 8 mm, LVSI, > 5 mm thickness
    - Radiation therapy to groin if node positive (some debate about a single positive node)

Treatment Options by Stage

- Early stage disease
  - Microinvasive disease (< 1 mm invasion)
    - Wide excision (5-10 mm)
  - Lateralized tumor confined to vulva < 2 cm, invasion < 5 mm, clinically node negative
    - Radical local excision/partial vulvectomy
    - Unilateral lymphadenectomy
  - Tumor confined to vulva & perineum > 2 cm
    - Modified radical vulvectomy
    - Bilateral inguinofemoral LND
    - Adjuvant local radiation therapy if surgical margin < 8 mm (reexcision usually considered 1st), extensive LVSI, or positive lymph nodes
  - If patient is unable to tolerate surgery, treat with radiation
- Advanced stage disease
  - Radical vulvectomy + en bloc inguinofemoral LND
    - Depending on tumor extent, may require removal of involved structures or pelvic exenteration
    - RT or CRT: Margins narrow (< 8 mm), extensive LVSI
    - RT to groin if positive lymph nodes (± ipsilateral deep pelvic lymph nodes, ± contralateral groin) → improves survival per GOG 37
  - If patient is unable to tolerate surgery, radiation therapy ± chemotherapy
  - Neoadjuvant CRT or RT → surgery
- Survival predominantly determined by lymph node metastases
  - Unilateral lymphadenopathy, 70% 5-year survival
  - ≥ 3 unilateral lymph nodes involved, 30% 5-year survival
- Recurrent disease
  - Local recurrence without regional LND
    - Radical excision: 5-year survival is 56%
  - Local recurrence > 2 years after treatment
    - Excision & radiation: 5-year survival > 50%

Standard Doses

- 50 Gy to resected lymph nodes
- 60-66 Gy to gross nodal disease and primary
- 50-60 Gy for close margins

Common Techniques

- Intensity-modulated radiation therapy (IMRT)
- Broad anterior photons, narrow posterior photons, and supplemental electrons to groins ± primary tumor
- 4 field or 2 field

Landmark Trials

- Homesley: After vulvectomy and groin dissection, RT ↑ OS by 14% compared to pelvic lymphadenectomy
  - Clinically suspicious and fixed ulcerated groin nodes and ≥ 2 groin nodes were poor prognostic factors

RECOMMENDED FOLLOW-UP

Clinical

- Pelvic exam every 3-4 months for 1st 2 years, then 2x yearly until year 5, then annually
- Vaginal dilator should be offered to decrease vaginal stenosis

Radiographic

- Consider PET/CT, MR, or CT for large lesions (T3/T4) or node-positive cases at 3 months

SELECTED REFERENCES

1. American Joint Committee on Cancer: AJCC Cancer Staging Manual. 7th ed. New York: Springer. 379-86, 2010
2. McMahon CJ et al: Lymphatic metastases from pelvic tumors: anatomic classification, characterization, and staging. Radiology. 254(1):31-46, 2010
3. Oonk MH et al: The role of sentinel node biopsy in gynecological cancer: a review. Curr Opin Oncol. 21(5):425-32, 2009
4. Van der Zee AG et al: Sentinel node dissection is safe in the treatment of early-stage vulvar cancer. J Clin Oncol. 26(6):884-9, 2008
5. Land R et al: Routine computerized tomography scanning, groin ultrasound with or without fine needle aspiration cytology in the surgical management of primary squamous cell carcinoma of the vulva. Int J Gynecol Cancer. 16(1):312-7, 2006
6. Oonk MH et al: Prediction of lymph node metastases in vulvar cancer: a review. Int J Gynecol Cancer. 16(3):963-71, 2006
7. Singh K et al: Accuracy of magnetic resonance imaging of inguinofemoral lymph nodes in vulval cancer. Int J Gynecol Cancer. 16(3):1179-83, 2006
8. Hall TB et al: The role of ultrasound-guided cytology of groin lymph nodes in the management of squamous cell carcinoma of the vulva: 5-year experience in 44 patients. Clin Radiol. 58(5):367-71, 2003
9. Sohaib SA et al: Imaging in vulval cancer. Best Pract Res Clin Obstet Gynaecol. 17(4):543-56, 2003
10. Sohaib SA et al: MR imaging of carcinoma of the vulva. AJR Am J Roentgenol. 178(2):373-7, 2002
11. Heaps JM et al: Surgical-pathologic variables predictive of local recurrence in squamous cell carcinoma of the vulva. Gynecol Oncol. 38(3):309-14, 1990
12. Homesley HD et al: Radiation therapy versus pelvic node resection for carcinoma of the vulva with positive groin nodes. Obstet Gynecol. 68(6):733-40, 1986

*(**Left**) Coronal PET/CT shows minimal soft tissue and increased FDG uptake in the left vulva →. No enlarged or FDG-avid lymph nodes were seen. On physical examination, this tumor was estimated to be 1 x 1 cm; however, on pathologic examination the largest diameter was 2.1 cm, making it a T1b tumor. (**Right**) Coronal T2WI MR shows an intermediate signal mass → arising from the labia majora and extending up to invade the lower urethra.*

Stage IB (T1b N0 M0)

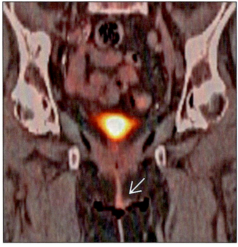

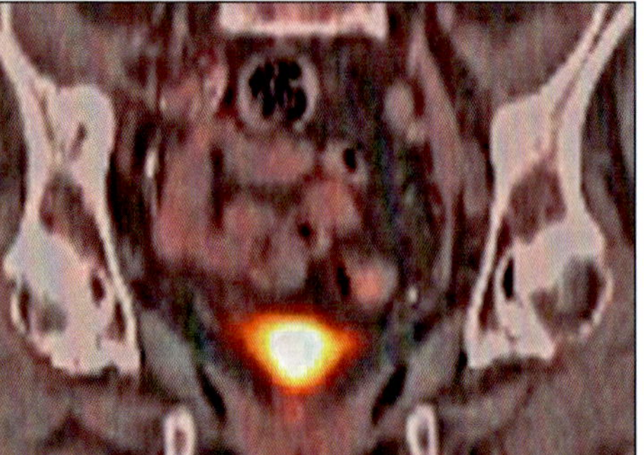

Stage II (T2 N0 M0)

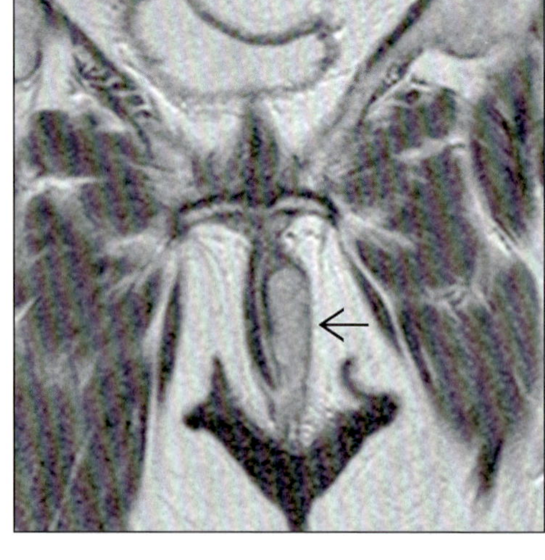

*(**Left**) Axial T1WI C+ FS MR in the same patient shows avid enhancement of the vulvar mass. No regional or pelvic adenopathy was seen on this exam. (**Right**) Axial and coronal CECT images show a right inguinal lymph node → with central hypodensity. The fatty hilum is obliterated and the node is replaced by soft tissue centrally. The metastatic focus is > 5 mm; however, there is no extracapsular spread of tumor.*

Stage II (T2 N0 M0)

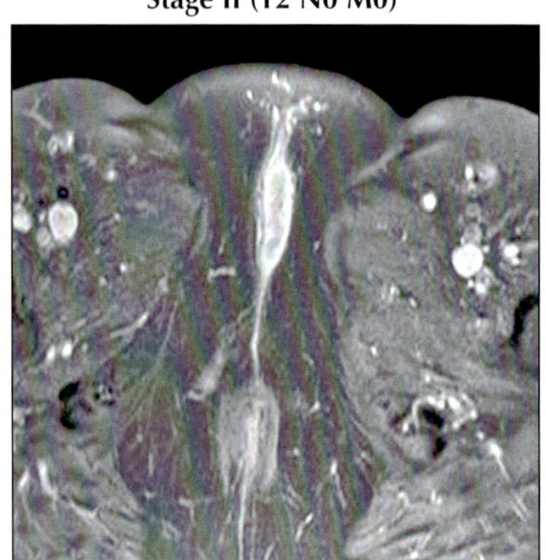

Stage IIIA (T1b N1b M0)

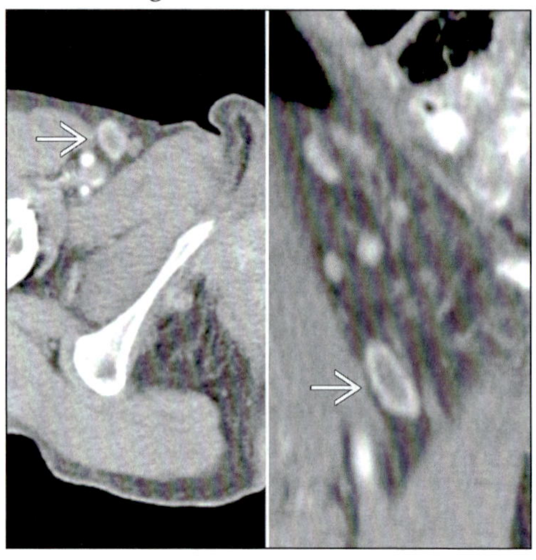

*(**Left**) Photo shows infiltrative right labial lesion with involvement of the anus; hence, T2. A satellite lesion → is shown demonstrating multifocality. (**Right**) A much more advanced, ulcerative lesion displays subcutaneous and dermal lymphatic infiltration and a satellite lesion →.*

T2

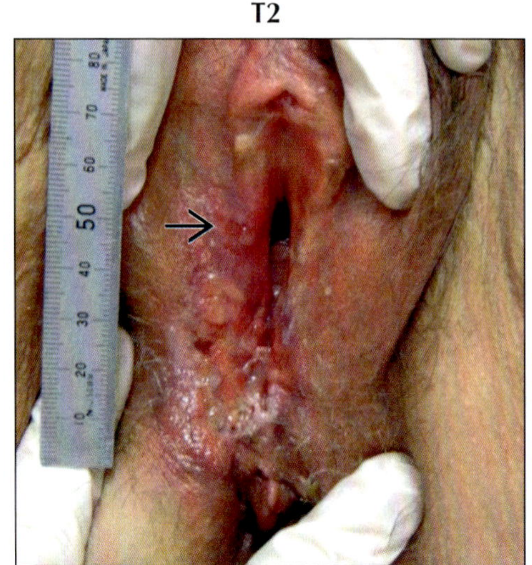

T2

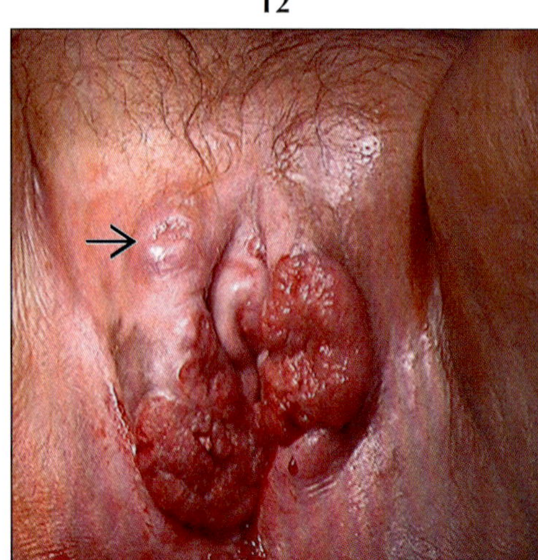

Stage IIIB (T2 N2b M0)

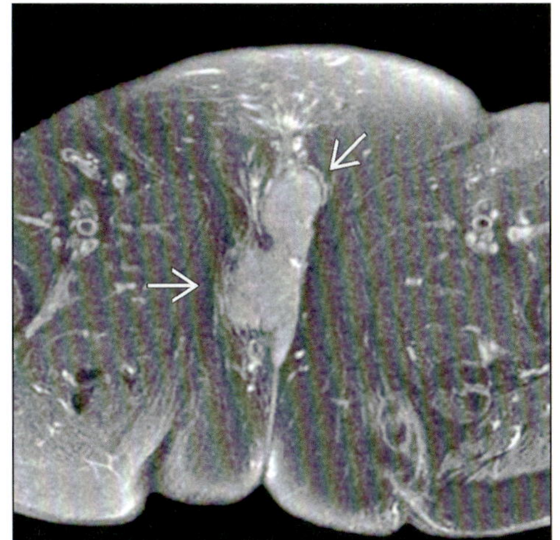

Stage IIIB (T2 N2b M0)

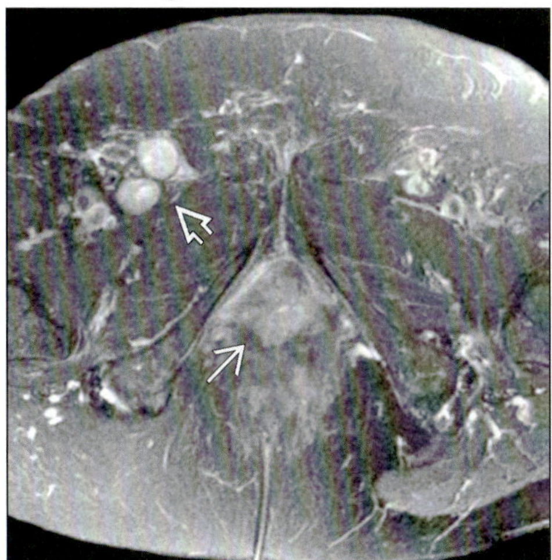

(Left) *Axial T1WI C+ FS MR shows an enhancing vulvar mass ➡.* ***(Right)*** *Axial T1WI C+ FS MR in the same patient shows cephalad extension of the vulvar mass ➡ to invade the distal urethra. In addition, there are 2 enlarged, round, enhancing right inguinal lymph nodes ➡ with loss of the fatty hila, corresponding to nodal stage N2b.*

EBRT

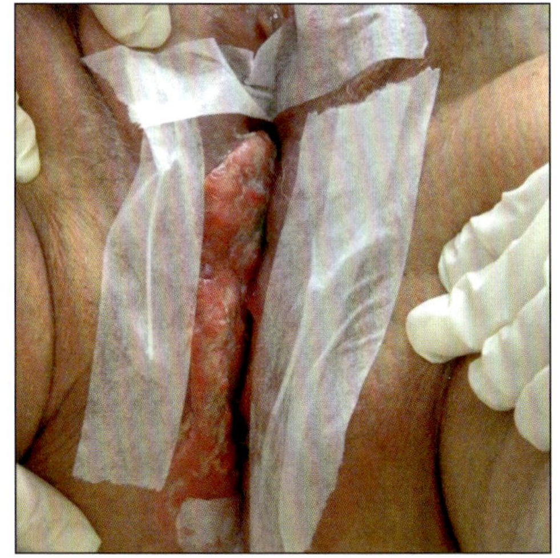

EBRT

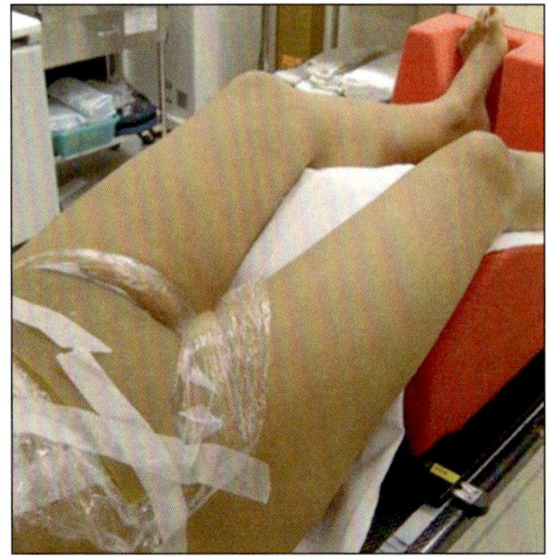

(Left) *Wires used at the time of simulation can be invaluable for planning. Additionally, wires can be used to mark scars, lymph nodes, and normal structures such as the anus.* ***(Right)*** *Effective treatment requires rigid and reproducible immobilization (note foot rests and knee sponges). Bolus is essential to fully dose inguinal lymph nodes and the primary. In most cases, in vivo dosimetry should be used.*

EBRT

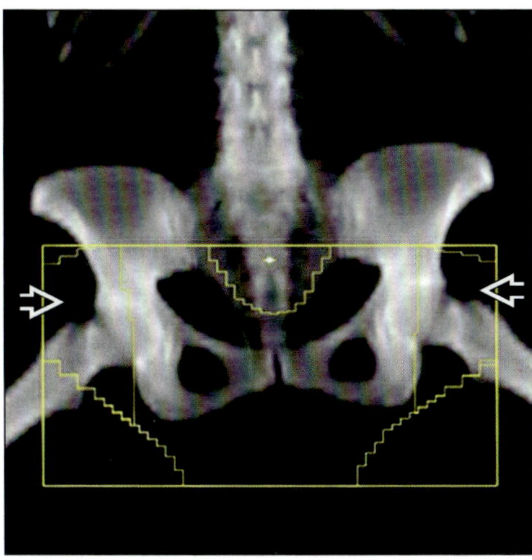

EBRT

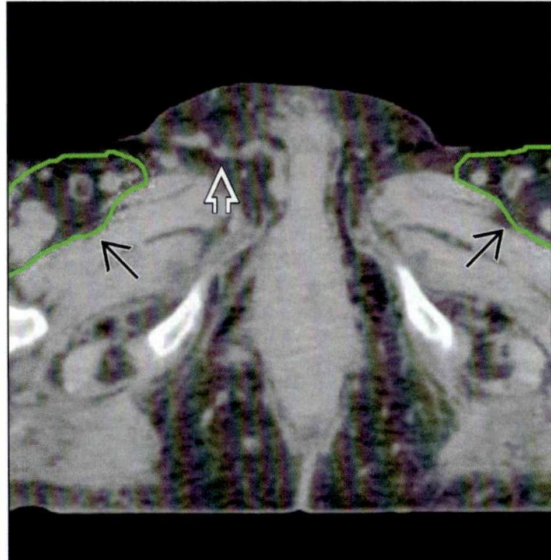

(Left) *A common technique is a broad anterior photon field, narrow posterior photon field, and supplemental electron fields ➡ to the inguinal nodes. Note the frog-leg position to reduce skin overlap in the inguinal region and between the upper thighs.* ***(Right)*** *Axial CT shows a large vessel ➡ communicating to the inguinal lymph nodes from the primary. This highlights the importance of including the skin bridge between the 2 structures. The nodal CTV ➡ is depicted.*

EBRT

IMRT DVH

*(**Left**) An en face electron beam is often an ideal boost technique, or it can be used in small primary lesions that are node negative. Bolus is essential in these cases. (**Right**) This is a DVH of an advanced lesion treated to a final boost dose of 60 Gy with IMRT. The median doses to the rectum, left and right femoral heads, bladder, bone marrow, and bowel were 20 Gy, 25 Gy, 20 Gy, 28 Gy, 21 Gy, and 23 Gy, respectively.*

Nodal Boost With IMRT

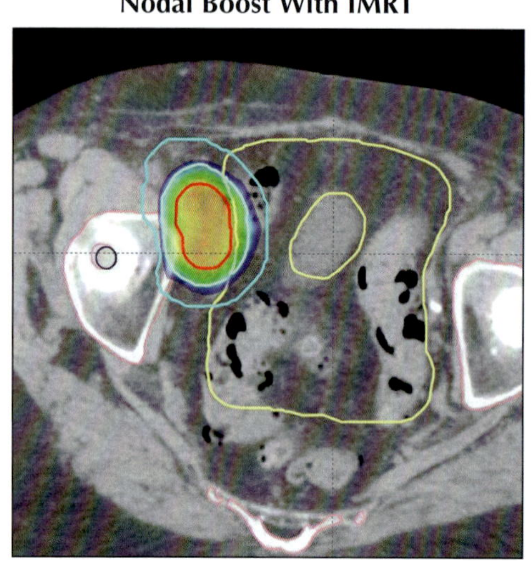

Nodal Boost With IMRT

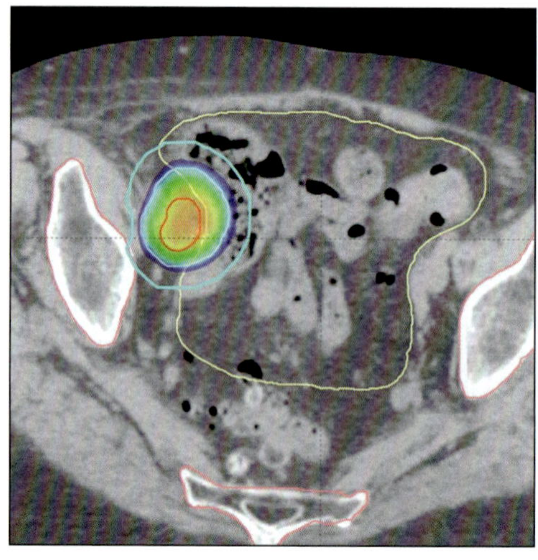

*(**Left**) Axial CT shows a boost plan for a nearly 4 cm node. Orange, green, and blue represent 63 Gy, 61 Gy, and 57 Gy, respectively. (**Right**) Axial CT in the same patient shows marked regression of the right pelvic lymph node, necessitating a replan after the initial fields. Orange, green, and blue represent 63 Gy, 61 Gy, and 57 Gy, respectively.*

EBRT

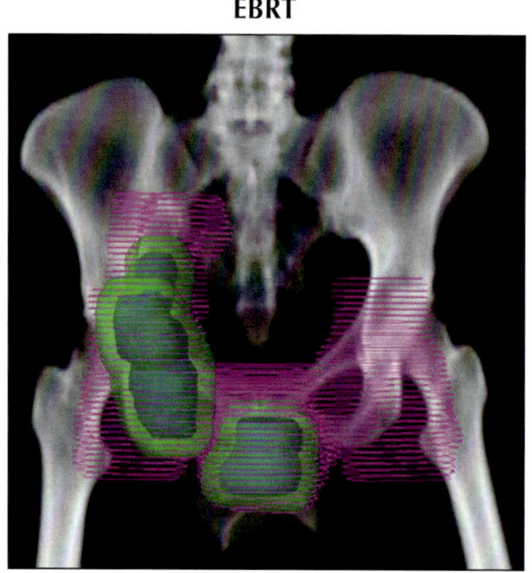

EBRT

*(**Left**) The pink shows the 50 Gy PTV (primary, and inguinal and pelvic nodes). Light green shows the 54 Gy PTV boost, and dark green shows the final cone-down boost to 60-64 Gy (GTV + 7 mm). (**Right**) DRR shows wire diagram of PTV. Coverage of the Iliac lymph nodes ➔ is shown.*

IMRT

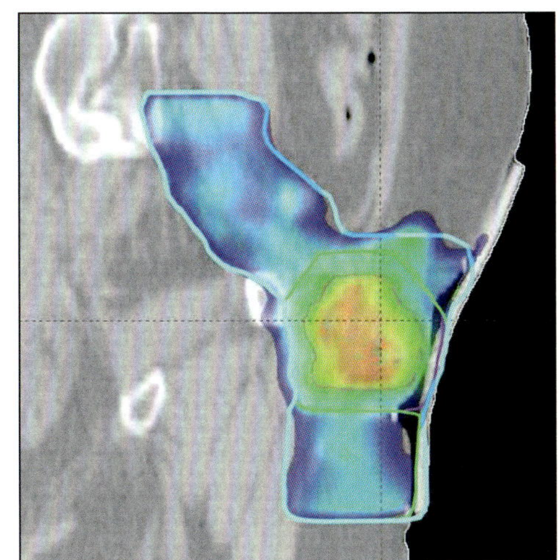

IMRT

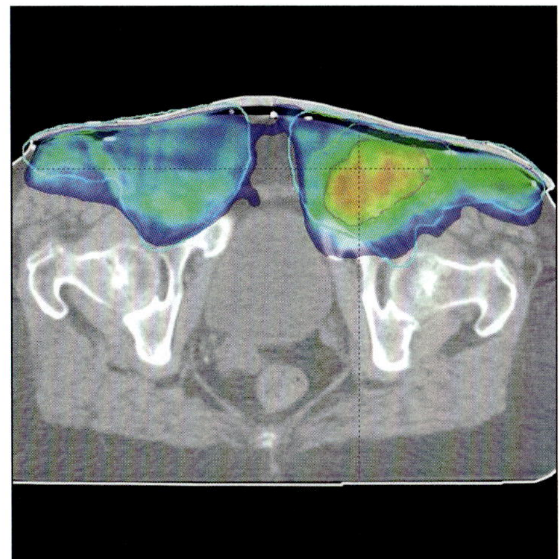

(Left) *Sagittal CT shows IMRT plan and coverage for the 3 PTVs. Orange, green, and blue represent 63 Gy, 56 Gy, and 48 Gy, respectively.* ***(Right)*** *Axial CT in the same patient shows IMRT plan and coverage for the 3 PTVs. Orange, green, and blue represent 63 Gy, 56 Gy, and 48 Gy, respectively. Significant sparing of OARs is achieved with IMRT.*

Stage IVA (T1b N3 M0)

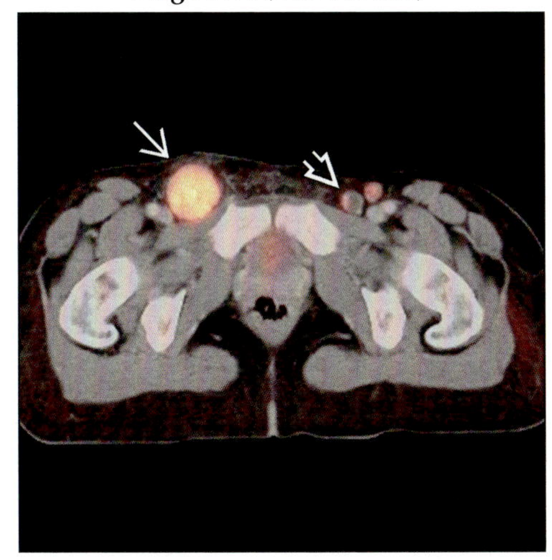

Stage IVA (T1b N3 M0)

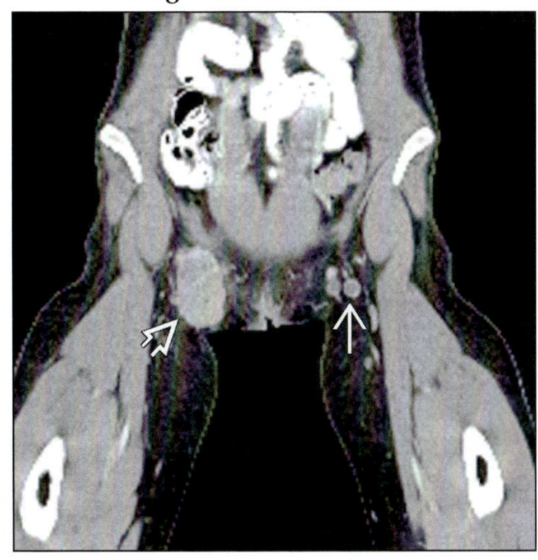

(Left) *Axial PET/CT shows bulky right adenopathy ➔. On the left, FDG avidity ➔ is restricted to the periphery of the lymph node, which is frequently observed pathologically. This young patient underwent ovarian transposition to preserve ovarian function.* ***(Right)*** *Coronal CECT in the same patient shows hypodense central necrosis in the left inguinal lymph node ➔ and bulky right-sided adenopathy ➔.*

Stage IVA (T1b N3 M0)

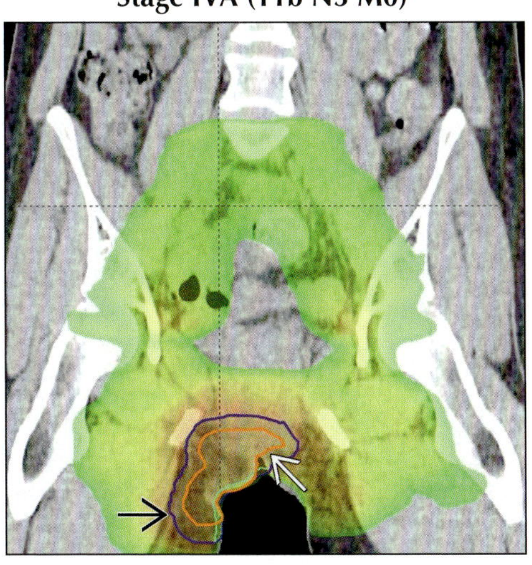

Stage IVA (T1b N3 M0)

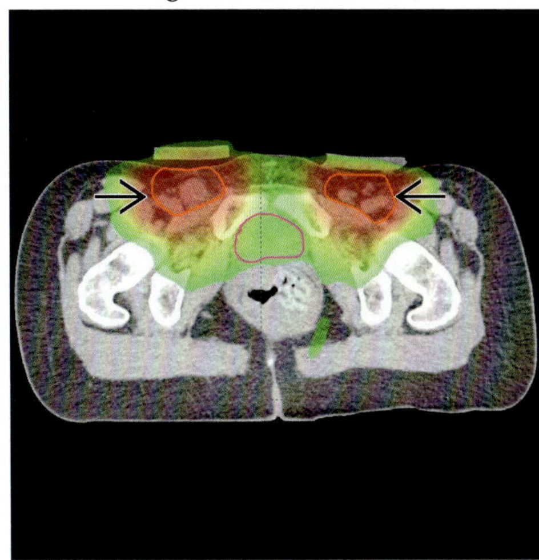

(Left) *In the same patient, coronal IMRT colorwash demonstrates primary and nodal coverage. The primary was treated to 59.4 Gy, and the uninvolved lymph nodes 45 Gy. The CTV ➔ and PTV ➔ are shown for the primary.* ***(Right)*** *In the same patient, axial IMRT colorwash demonstrates nodal coverage (green = 40 Gy, red = 64 Gy). The inguinal CTVs ➔ are shown and were treated to 64.8 Gy. Follow-up PET/CT and clinical exam demonstrated a complete response.*

*(**Left**) Picture of the perineum shows a large mass centered in the right labia majora with extensive surface ulceration and necrosis. (**Right**) Image of the pelvis from whole-body PET shows the large hypermetabolic vulvar mass ➔ and right inguinal lymph node ➔. There was no distant metastatic disease, including no pelvic lymphadenopathy.*

Stage IIIC (T2 N2c M0)

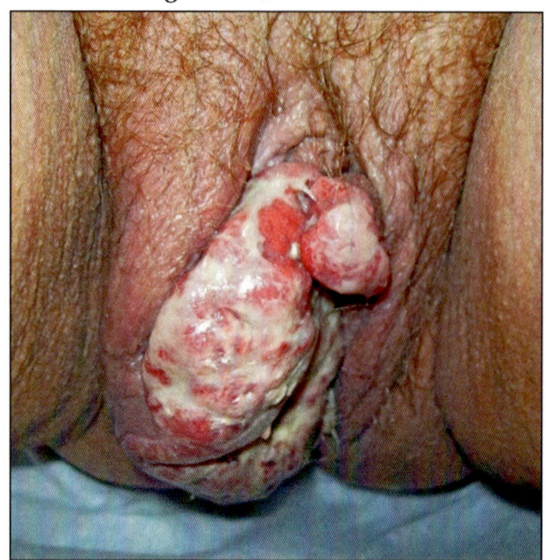

Stage IIIC (T2 N2c M0)

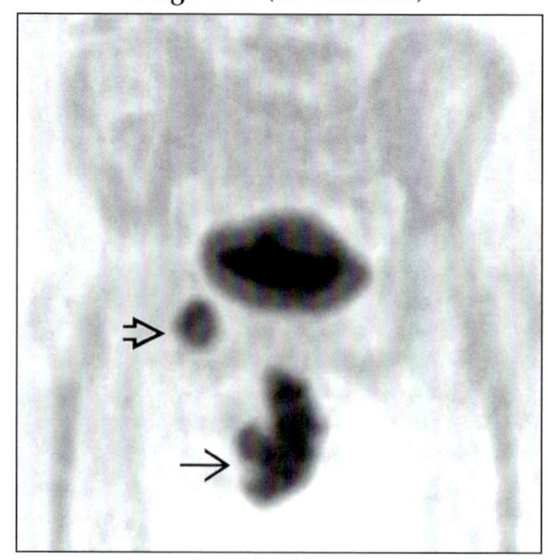

*(**Left**) Axial T1WI C+ FS MR through the vulvar mass ➔ shows dermal thickening and enhancement of the right labia majora ➔, consistent with dermal invasion. (**Right**) Axial T1WI C+ FS MR in the same patient shows multiple, hyperenhancing right inguinal lymph nodes. The largest ➔ has irregular, ill-defined margins, suggestive of extracapsular spread.*

Stage IIIC (T2 N2c M0)

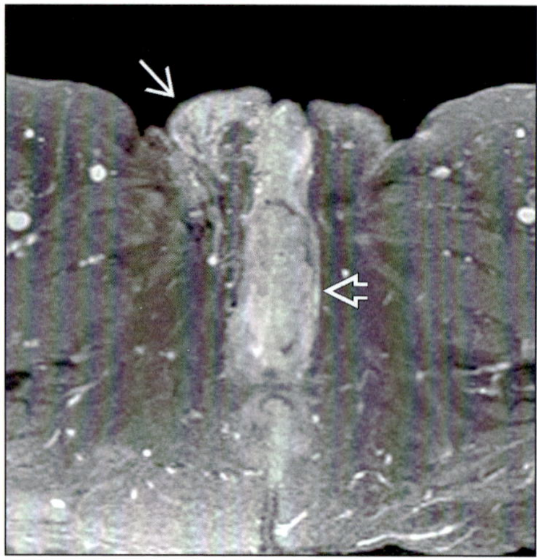

Stage IIIC (T2 N2c M0)

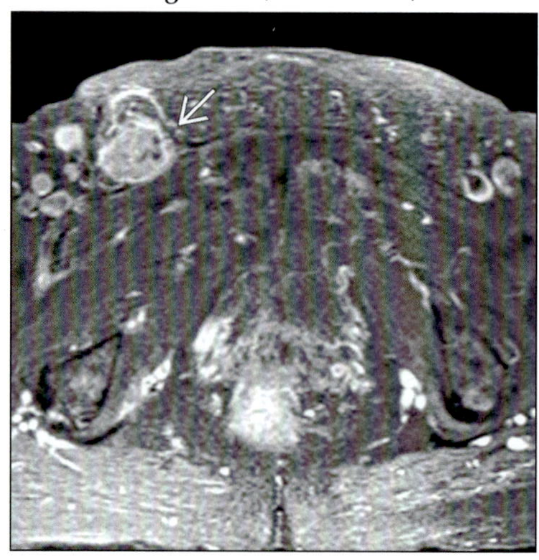

*(**Left**) Axial CECT shows an enhancing vulvar mass ➔ with a large exophytic component. The right labia majora ➔ is partially visualized with skin thickening and enhancement, concerning for dermal invasion. (**Right**) Axial CECT in the same patient shows a large right inguinal lymph node ➔ with foci of central necrosis. The lymph node margins are irregular and ill defined, suggestive of extracapsular spread.*

Stage IIIC (T2 N2c M0)

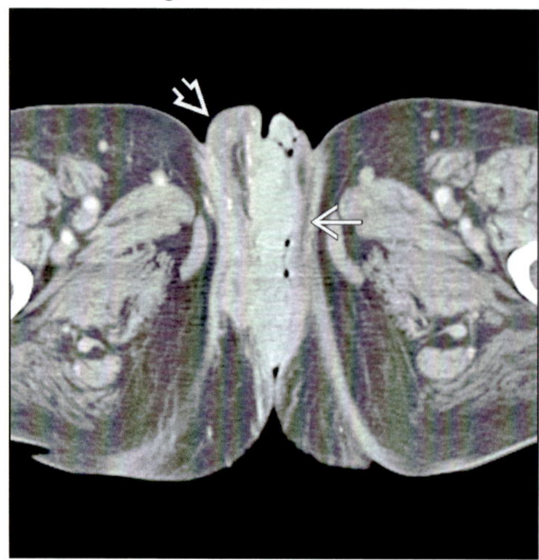

Stage IIIC (T2 N2c M0)

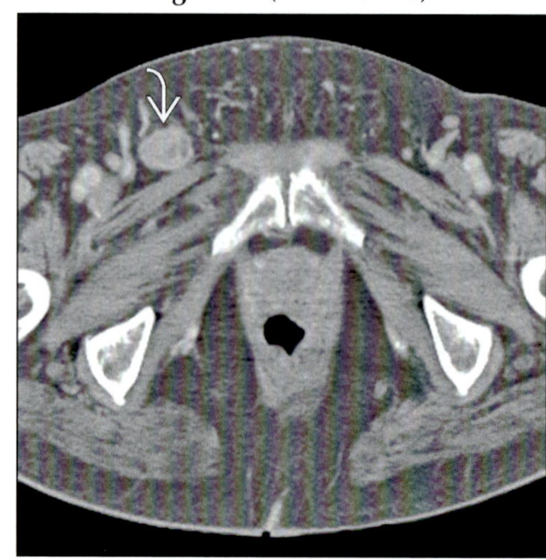

Stage IIIC (T2 N2c M0)

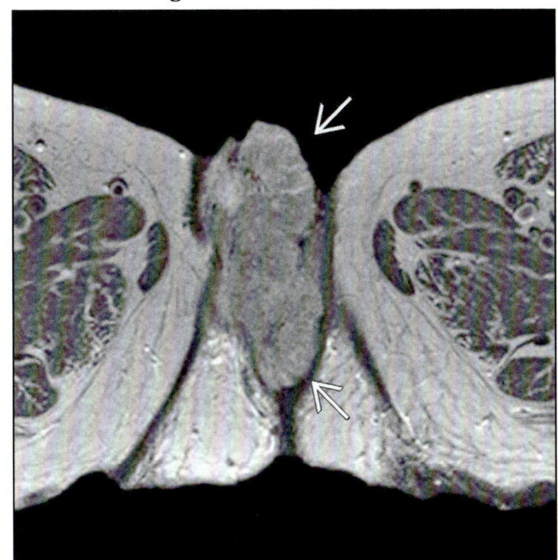

Stage IIIC (T2 N2c M0)

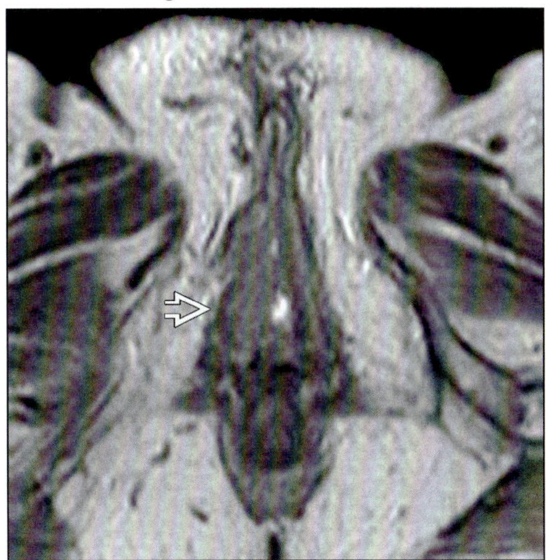

(Left) *Axial T2WI FSE MR in the same patient shows a large, exophytic, intermediate signal vulvar mass ➡.* ***(Right)*** *Axial T2WI FSE MR in the same patient obtained more cephalad to the previous image shows the intermediate signal mass invading the right lower vaginal wall ➡ and the right crus of the clitoris, as well as obliterating the lower urethra.*

Stage IIIC (T2 N2c M0)

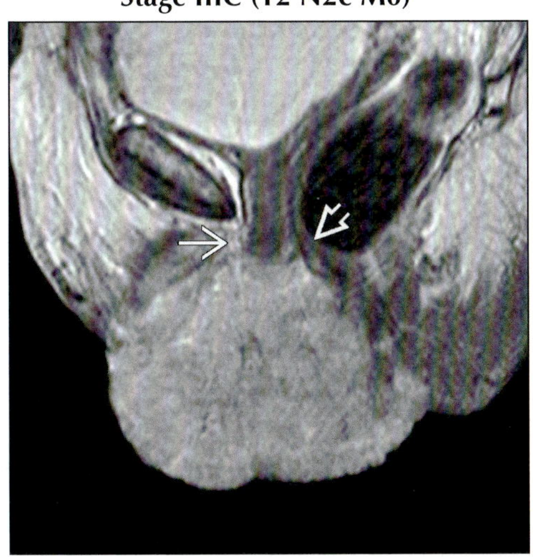

Stage IIIC (T2 N2c M0)

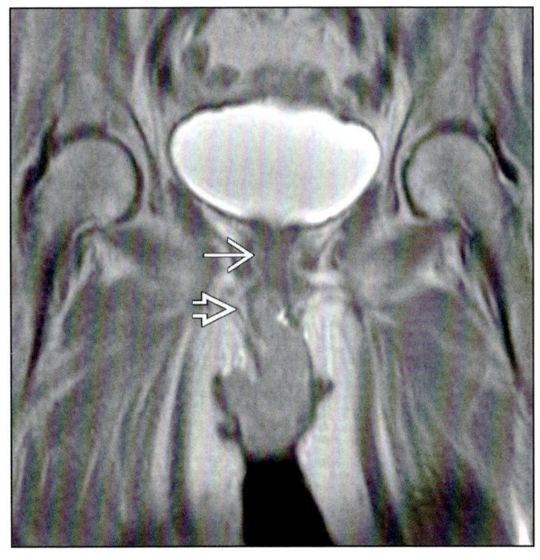

(Left) *Sagittal T2WI FSE MR in the same patient shows the large exophytic vulvar mass. Note extension to the lower urethra ➡ and vagina ➡.* ***(Right)*** *Coronal T2WI MR in the same patient shows the vulvar mass invading the lower urethra ➡. Note the normal, low signal upper urethra ➡.*

Stage IIIC (T2 N2c M0)

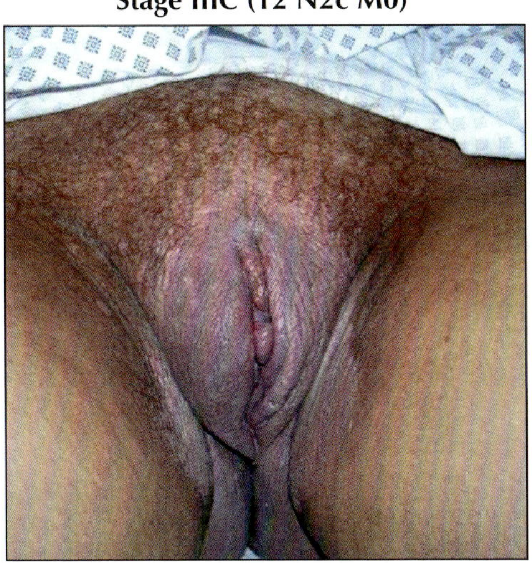

Stage IIIC (T2 N2c M0)

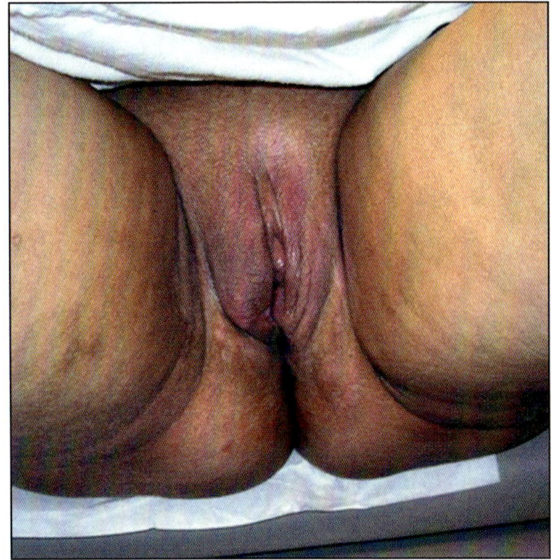

(Left) *Photo shows same patient with brisk erythema of the inguinal folds and perineal regions with a near-complete response at 48.6 Gy EBRT with sensitizing cisplatin.* ***(Right)*** *Photo shows same patient at 3 months with a complete response. The cumulative dose was 64 Gy. PET scan confirmed a complete metabolic response.*

(Left) Coronal fused PET/CT in a 57 year old shows a 10 cm vulvar SCCa replacing the entire ipsilateral labia, and invading into introitus/ distal vagina, distal urethra, and clitoris. Lymph nodes were not palpable, but PET/ CT revealed bilateral inguinal (N2b) and right external iliac LN involvement (M1). Patients with pelvic lymph nodes should still be treated definitively. ***(Right)*** Coronal T2WI MR in the same patient reveals the long but not deeply invasive lesion ➔.

Stage IVB (T2 N2b M1)

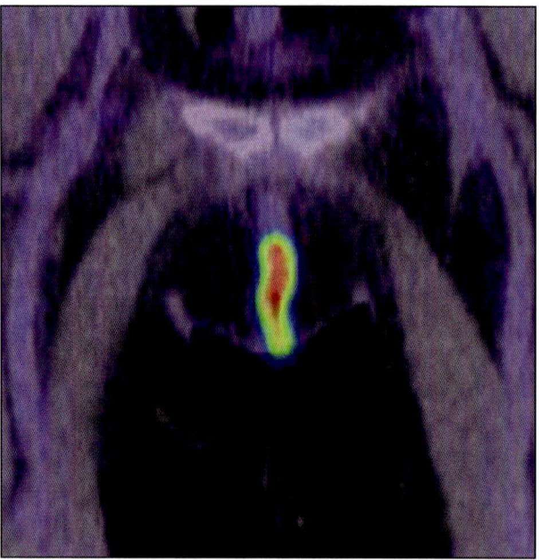

Stage IVB (T2 N2b M1)

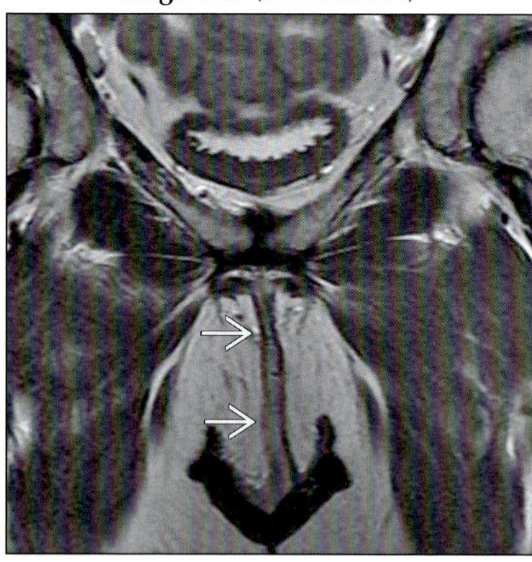

(Left) Sagittal fused PET/ CT shows FDG-avid mass occupying the entire right labia ➔. ***(Right)*** Sagittal CT demonstrates the extensive mass at midline ➔. Patient was treated with 60 Gy IMRT with concurrent cisplatin to primary lesion and involved nodes, and 50.4 Gy to uninvolved pelvic lymph nodes.

Stage IVB (T2 N2b M1)

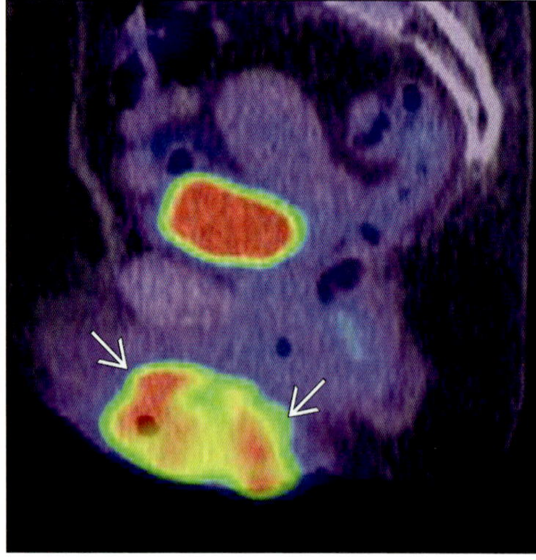

Stage IVB (T2 N2b M1)

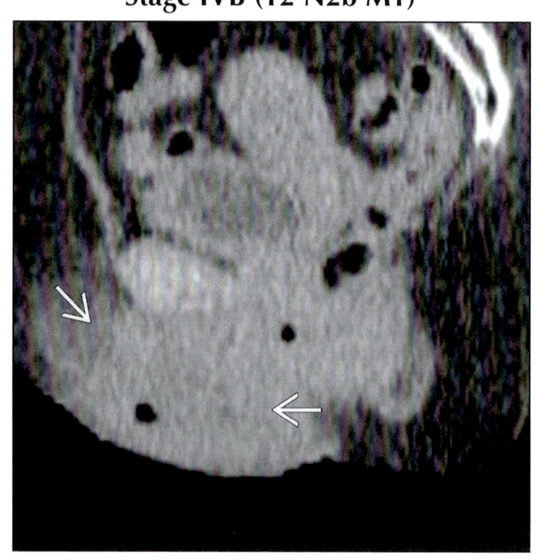

(Left) Sagittal fused PET/CT 1 year later shows a complete response. After CRT, the lesion reduced in size from 10 cm to 2 cm. At 4 months post RT, the patient had a wide local excision. The residual lesion was 15 mm with clear margins. ***(Right)*** Sagittal CT confirms the complete response. Patient remains free of disease at 18 months after completion.

Stage IVB (T2 N2b M1)

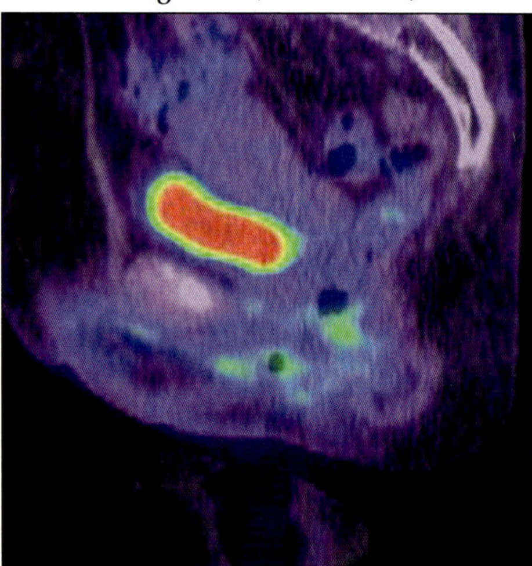

Stage IVB (T2 N2b M1)

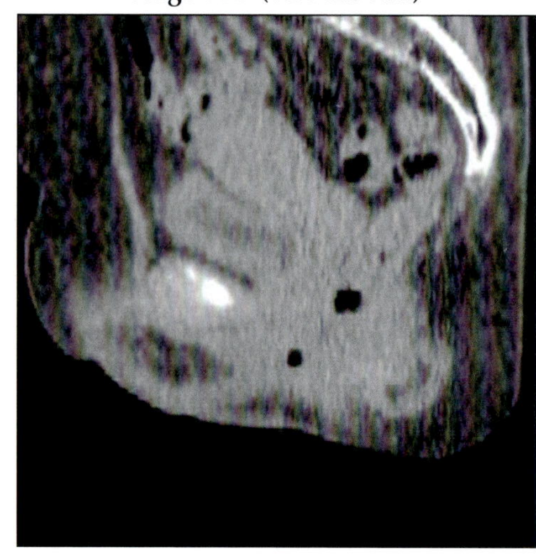

Stage IVA (T3 N0 M0)

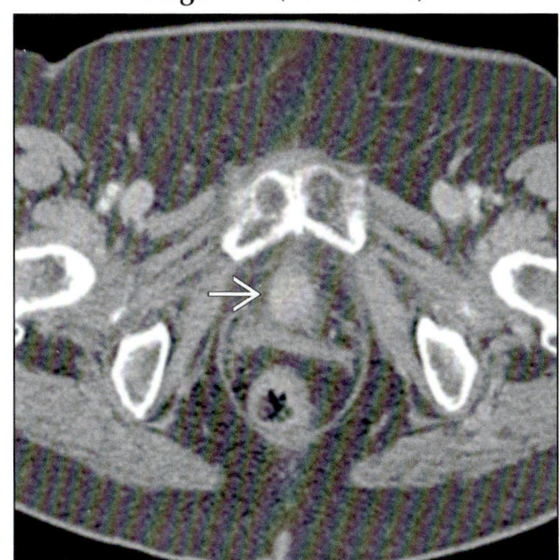

Stage IVA (T3 N0 M0)

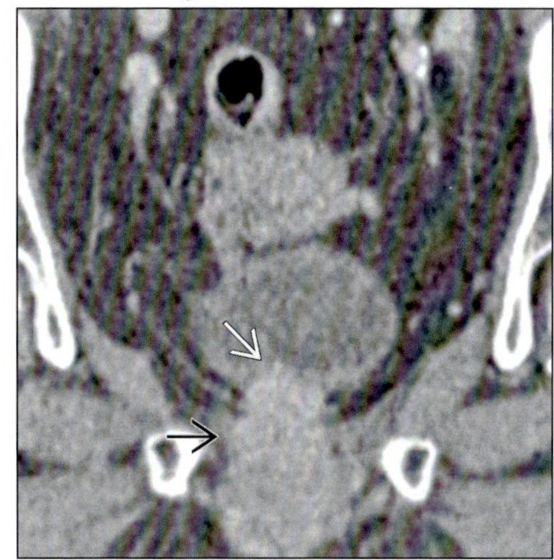

(Left) *Axial CECT shows an enhancing, ill-defined tumor encasing the urethra ➔.* ***(Right)*** *Coronal CECT in the same patient shows an enhancing, ill-defined mass encasing the urethra ➔ and invading the base of the urinary bladder ➔.*

Recurrence

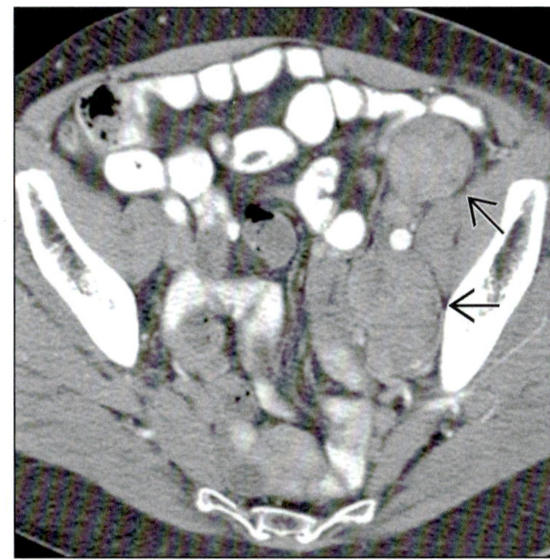

Recurrence

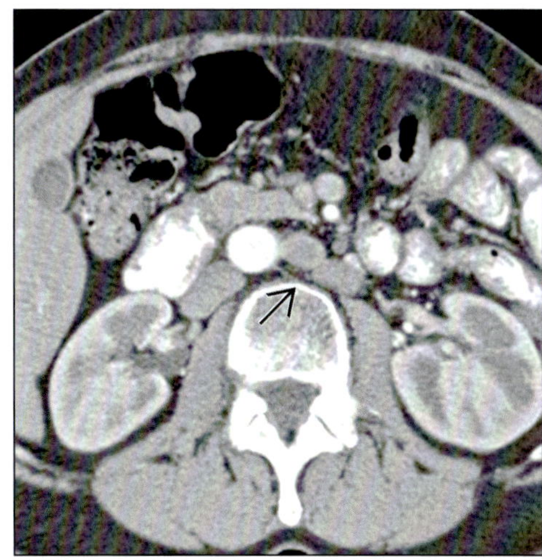

(Left) *Axial CECT in a patient with a history of vulvar cancer status post left vulvectomy shows bulky left external iliac adenopathy ➔.* ***(Right)*** *Axial CECT in the same patient shows necrotic left paraaortic adenopathy ➔. The prognosis is poor and usually fatal.*

Telangiectasias

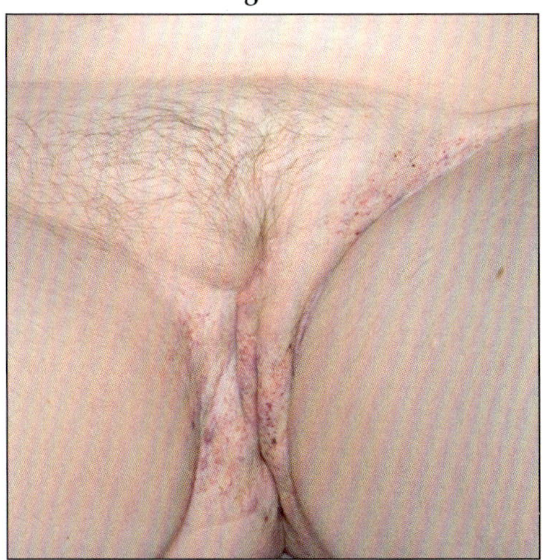

Telangiectasias

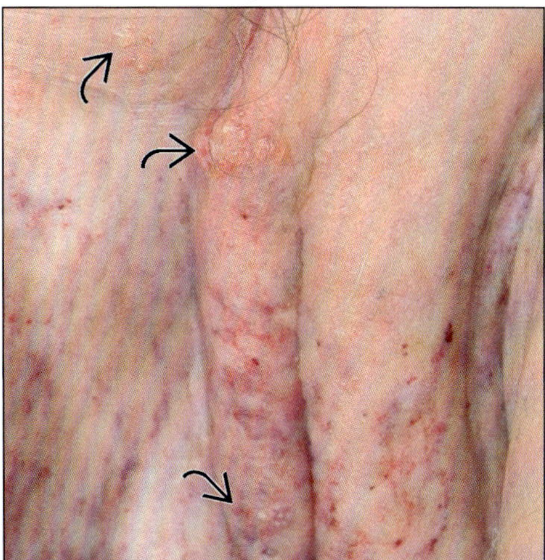

(Left) *Photo depicts telangiectasias that have developed 14 years after surgery and RT to the vulva and left groin. Alopecia, induration, and fragile-appearing skin are evident on the perineum and left groin.* ***(Right)*** *Close-up photo reveals lymphangioma circumscripta ➔: Fluid-filled vesicles secondary to longstanding lymphedema.*

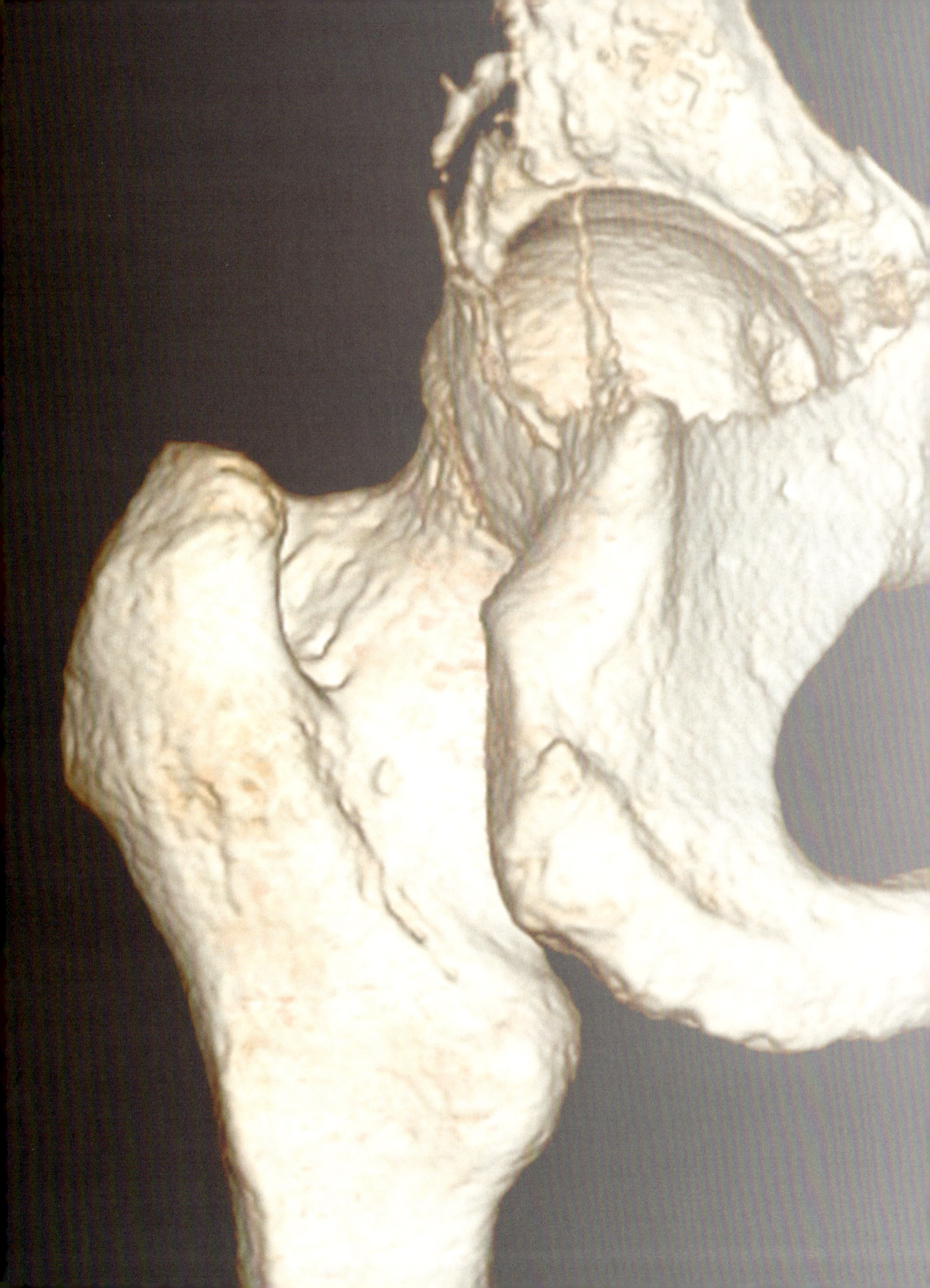

SECTION 8
Mesenchymal Tumors

SARCOMA

(T) Primary Tumor

Adapted from 7th edition AJCC Staging Forms.

TNM	*Definitions*
TX	Primary tumor cannot be assessed
T0	No evidence of primary tumor
T1	Tumor ≤ 5 cm in greatest dimension
T1a	Superficial tumor ≤ 5 cm in greatest dimension
T1b	Deep tumor ≤ 5 cm in greatest dimension
T2	Tumor > 5 cm in greatest dimension
T2a	Superficial tumor > 5 cm in greatest dimension
T2b	Deep tumor > 5 cm in greatest dimension

(N) Regional Lymph Nodes

NX	Regional lymph nodes cannot be assessed
N0	No regional lymph node metastasis
N1	Regional lymph node metastasis

(M) Distant Metastasis

M0	No distant metastasis
M1	Distant metastasis

(G) Histologic Grade

GX	Grade cannot be assessed
G1	Grade 1 (FNCLCC score 2-3)
G2	Grade 2 (FNCLCC score 4-5)
G3	Grade 3 (FNCLCC score 6-8)

Fédération Nationale des Centres de Lutte Contre le Cancer (FNCLCC) is the histologic grading method preferred by AJCC.

Additional descriptors that can be utilized include residual tumor (R) and combined lymphovascular invasion (LVI). Residual tumor is coded as cannot be assessed = RX, is not present = R0, is microscopically present = R1, or is macroscopically present = R2. LVI is described as not present/not identified, present/identified, not applicable, or unknown/indeterminate.

AJCC Stages/Prognostic Groups

Adapted from 7th edition AJCC Staging Forms.

Stage	*T*	*N*	*M*	*G*
IA	T1a, T1b	N0	M0	G1, GX
IB	T2a, T2b	N0	M0	G1, GX
IIA	T1a, T1b	N0	M0	G2, G3
IIB	T2a, T2b	N0	M0	G2
III	T2a, T2b	N0	M0	G3
	Any T	N1	M0	Any G
IV	Any T	Any N	M1	Any G

The American Joint Committee on Cancer (AJCC) staging system is commonly utilized, as well as the Surgical Staging System of the Musculoskeletal Tumor Society. Please see the chapter text for further description of the Surgical Staging System.

T1a

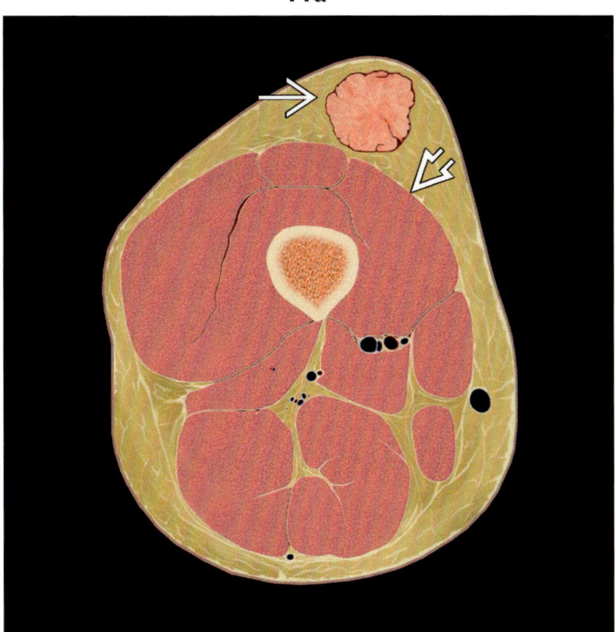

Axial graphic shows a T1a ➡ soft tissue sarcoma. These tumors must be ≤ 5 cm in greatest dimension. The "a" designation refers to the tumor being located superficial to, and not involving, the superficial fascia ⇨.

T1b

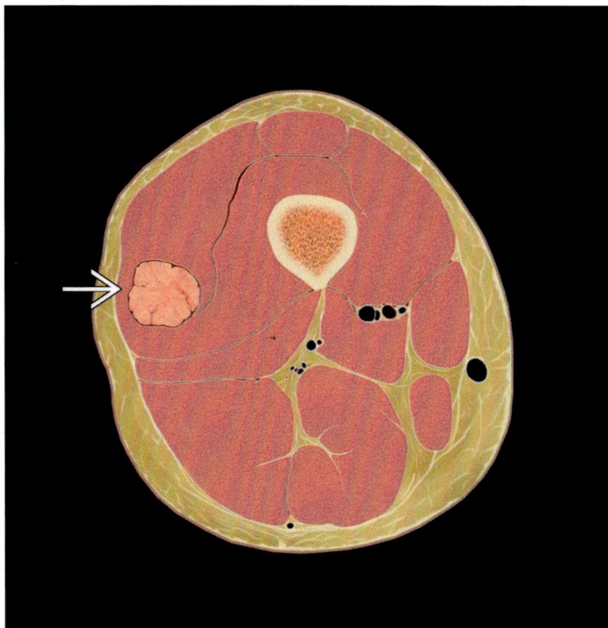

Axial graphic shows a T1b ➡ soft tissue sarcoma. These lesions must be ≤ 5 cm in diameter. The "b" designation refers to a deep lesion. Any involvement of the superficial fascia or a location exclusively deep to the fascia is defined as a deep tumor.

T2a

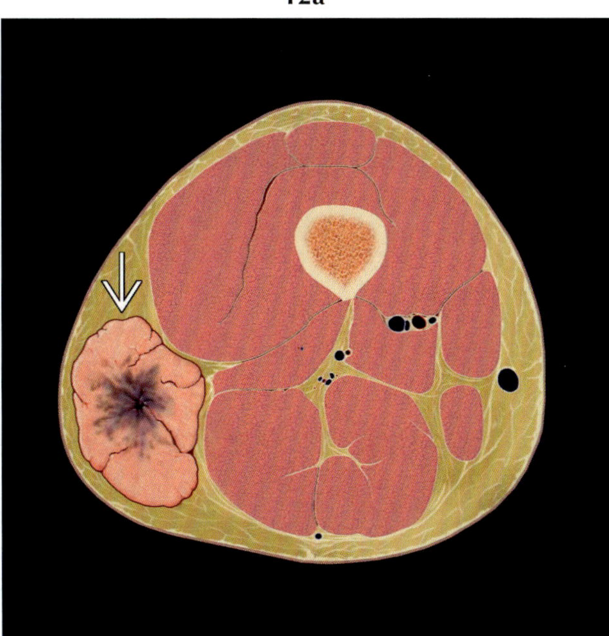

Axial graphic shows a T2a ➡ soft tissue sarcoma. These tumors are > 5 cm in greatest dimension. The "a" designation indicates that the mass is located superficial to the superficial fascia, without any fascial involvement.

T2b

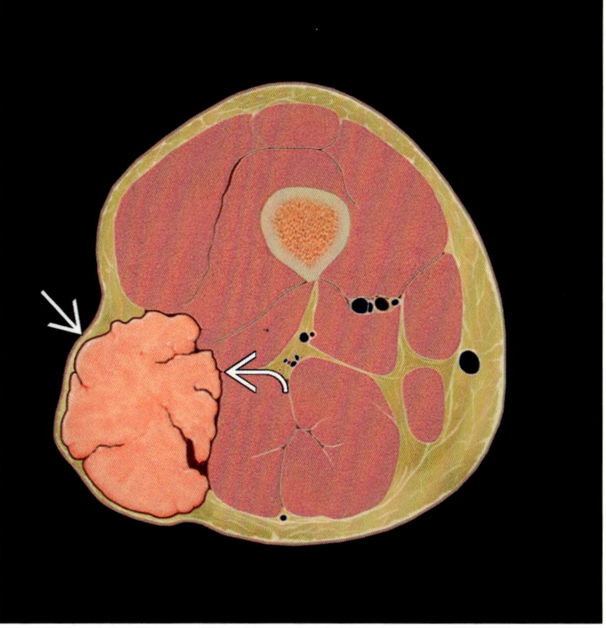

Axial graphic shows a T2b ➡ soft tissue sarcoma. This tumor measures > 5 cm. Although it is located superficial to the superficial fascia ↩, the nonvisualization of an intact fat plane between the tumor and fascia makes it suspicious for fascial involvement, which would cause this to be designated a deep lesion.

T2b

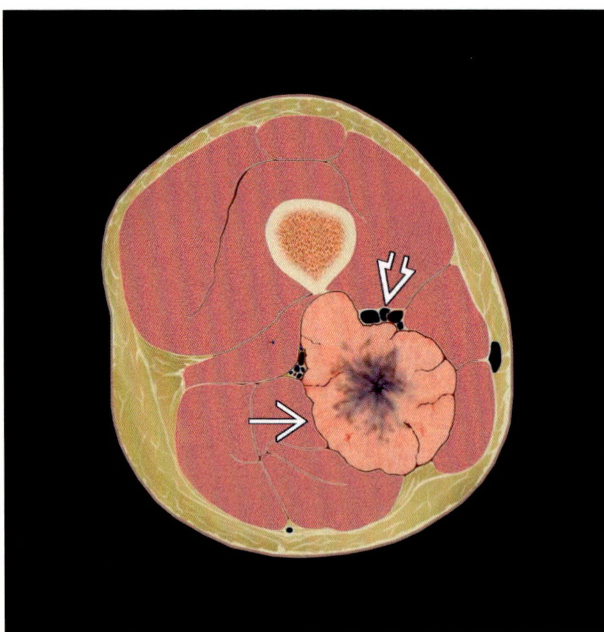

Axial graphic shows another type of T2b ➔ soft tissue sarcoma. This tumor is > 5 cm and is located deep to the superficial fascia. Note that this tumor abuts adjacent to neurovascular structures ⇨. Neurovascular involvement was included in earlier staging systems but is not included in the current staging system.

Stage I

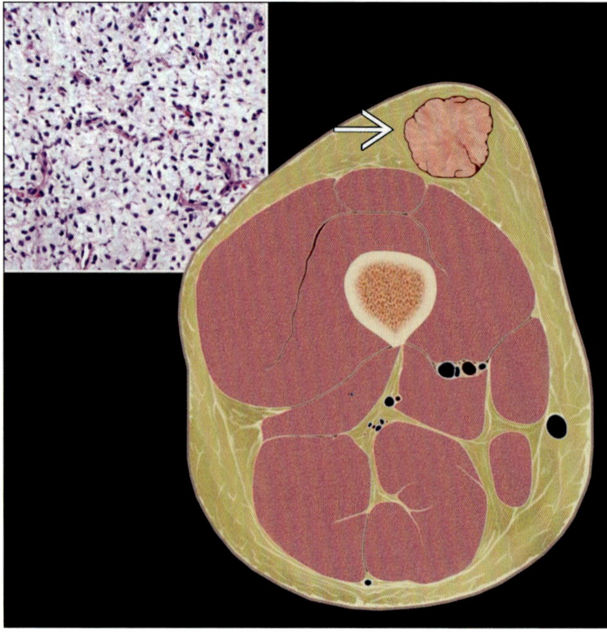

Axial graphic of a stage I soft tissue sarcoma illustrates a T1a mass ➔. The key characteristic of a stage I soft tissue sarcoma is that the lesion is low grade. The inset shows an example of low-grade pathology. Stage I tumors can be any size and may be located either superficial or deep to the fascia.

Stage II

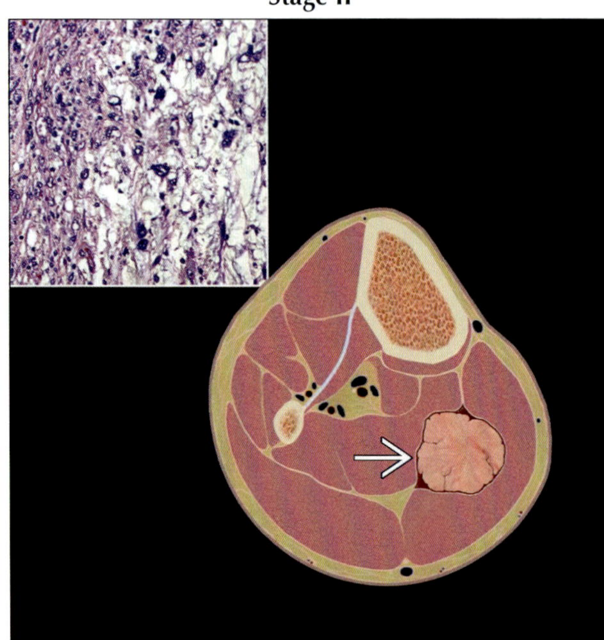

Axial graphic shows a stage II soft tissue sarcoma. These lesions are all G2 or G3 tumors. The inset shows an example of high-grade pathology. If the mass is ≤ 5 cm in size, it may be either G2 or G3 and may be located superficial (T1a) or deep (T1b ➔) to the fascia. However, if the mass is > 5 cm, then it must be T2.

Stage III

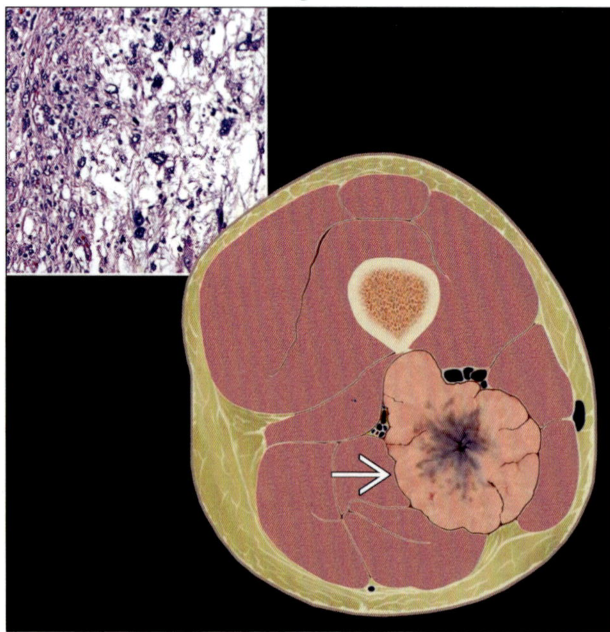

Axial graphic shows a stage III soft tissue sarcoma. These tumors measure > 5 cm, may be superficial (T2a) or deep (T2b ➔) to the superficial fascia, and are high-grade (G3) tumors. The inset shows an example of high-grade pathology. Nodal metastases, with any lesion size, location, or grade, also confer stage III disease.

Stage III

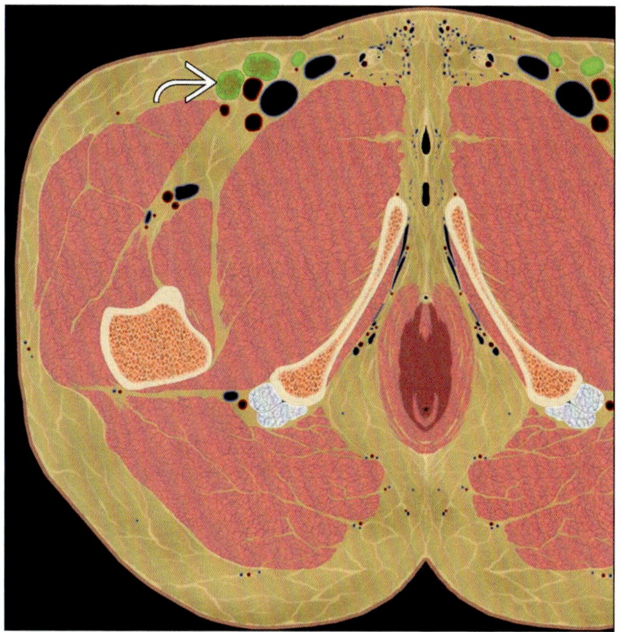

Axial graphic through the low pelvis shows inguinal adenopathy. The presence of lymph nodes involved with the tumor makes this stage III disease. The primary tumor can be any size, located at any depth, and have any histologic grade. The previous staging system designated nodal metastases as stage IV disease.

Stage IV

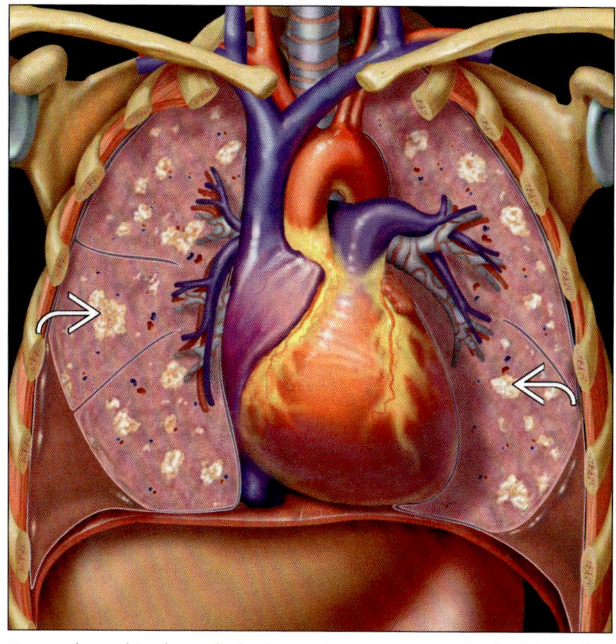

Coronal graphic through the lungs demonstrates multiple bilateral pulmonary metastases. The presence of distant metastases makes this stage IV disease. Stage IV primary tumors can be any size, have any depth, and have any histologic grade.

INITIAL SITE OF RECURRENCE

Lung	> 75%
Other	Varies based on tumor type

Sites of soft tissue sarcoma metastatic disease are highly dependent on the tumor type. Overall, the majority of metastases involve the lung. There is a relatively low incidence of lymph node metastasis, although some sarcoma subtypes are more prone to lymph node metastases. These include rhabdomyosarcoma, angiosarcoma, clear cell sarcoma, synovial sarcoma, and epithelioid sarcoma. Myxoid liposarcoma has a tendency to metastasize to other soft tissue sites. Retroperitoneal sarcomas have an increased incidence of metastasis to the liver. Surveillance for metastatic disease should be tailored to the patient's tumor type.

SARCOMA

OVERVIEW

General Comments

- Soft tissue sarcoma (STS) represents ~ 1% of malignancies
  - Derived from mesenchymal tissue
    - Often have cytogenetic abnormalities
- Associated with high mortality rate if high grade and large size
  - 5-year survival 50-60%
  - Prognostic factors include tumor grade, tumor size, and depth of invasion
- Lymph node metastasis rare
  - Except with select histologic subtypes including clear cell sarcoma, epithelioid cell sarcoma, synovial cell sarcoma, angiosarcoma, rhabdomyosarcoma
- ~ 25 major categories of malignant and borderline STS, ~ 60 types when all subcategories are considered, and > 300 synonyms for these 60 types
  - Classified by histogenesis (tumor type)
  - Most common in adults are liposarcoma, malignant fibrous histiocytoma, leiomyosarcoma, synovial sarcoma, rhabdomyosarcoma, unclassified STS

Classification

- American Joint Committee on Cancer (AJCC) Staging System, 7th edition
  - Unified classification with International Union Against Cancer (UICC) in 1987
  - Based on tumor histologic grade (3-grade system), primary tumor size & depth, and presence of nodal disease and distant metastases
  - Does not take into account anatomic site or whether tumor extends outside compartment of origin
  - Extraskeletal osteosarcoma, extraskeletal Ewing sarcoma, angiosarcoma, dermatofibrosarcoma protuberans, and extraskeletal chondrosarcoma are included in this staging system
  - Not applicable to rhabdomyosarcoma, Kaposi sarcoma, desmoid tumor, mesothelioma, infantile fibrosarcoma, inflammatory myofibroblastic tumor, and gastrointestinal stromal tumor
  - Also not applicable to sarcomas arising from dura mater, brain, parenchymal organs, or hollow viscera
- Surgical Staging System, Musculoskeletal Tumor Society (a.k.a. Enneking staging system)
  - Commonly used by orthopedic oncologic surgeons
  - Emphasizes whether tumor is confined to compartment of origin
  - Useful information for surgical planning
  - Has not been proven as predictor of survival
  - Current Enneking staging has 3 grades
  - Does take into account tumor size (≥ 5 cm), tumor location (superficial or deep to fascia), or nodal status
  - Does not apply to rhabdomyosarcoma or tumors of marrow/reticuloendothelial origin
- Staging of rhabdomyosarcoma
  - Most used staging system for rhabdomyosarcoma
  - Separates patients into 4 clinical groups based on
    - Complete resection vs. varying degrees of partial resection
    - Extent of tumor beyond muscle or organ of origin
    - Nodal involvement
    - Distant metastases
  - Risk groups are based on histology, stage, and group

NATURAL HISTORY

General Features

- Comments
  - Can occur anywhere in body
  - Locally invasive in direction of least resistance; initially tends to be radial, but fascial plans direct growth longitudinally
    - Present substantive local problem
  - Characterized by a pseudocapsule
    - Not a true capsule or anatomic boundary but admixture of neovascular cells, tumor cells, and edema
  - Generally respect fascial planes
  - Metastases are often seen in lungs (majority), retroperitoneal lymph nodes, and liver (typically from retroperitoneal sarcoma)
  - Most sarcomas do not spread to lymph nodes
- Location
  - 60% of STS located in extremities or torso (45% for lower extremity and 15% for upper extremity)
    - Thigh most commonly involved
  - 30% in retroperitoneum and trunk (15% retroperitoneal and 15% trunk, respectively)
  - 10% in head and neck

Etiology

- Etiology generally unknown
- Environmental exposures can increase risk
  - External beam radiotherapy, typically 10-15 years post exposure
  - Herbicides & pesticides
  - Thorotrast
  - Arsenic
- Viral infection & immunodeficiency
  - Human herpes virus 8 → Kaposi sarcoma
  - Epstein-Barr virus → smooth muscle tumors
  - Chronic lymphedema → angiosarcoma (postulated due to regional acquired immunodeficiency)
- Uncertain association with scar tissue, fractures, surgical implants, trauma
  - Trauma generally thought to draw attention to the area, not true causative agent

Epidemiology & Cancer Incidence

- Number of cases in USA per year
  - ~ 11,000-12,000
  - Annual incidence: 30 per 1,000,000 population
- Sex predilection
  - Slight male predominance
- Age of onset
  - Occurs in all ages, with 80% in patients > 40 years old

Genetics

- Molecular markers & cytogenetic alterations are used for tissue diagnosis but not for staging
- Numerous cytogenetic changes are associated with different tumor types
  - Changes range from simple to complex
- Surgical specimens, core biopsy, or fine-needle aspiration (FNA) samples can be used for cytogenetic studies

- DNA probe sets are commercially available for some tumor types
- High risk of STS
  - Li-Fraumeni syndrome (*TP53* mutation)
  - Autosomal dominant retinoblastoma (*RB1* mutation)
- Common translocations
  - t(X;18)(p11;q11) seen in synovial sarcoma; t(12;16)(q13; p11) seen in myxoid liposarcoma
  - t(2;13)(q35;q14) seen in alveolar rhabdomyosarcoma

Associated Diseases, Abnormalities

- Neurofibromatosis type 1 = ↑ malignant peripheral nerve sheath disease

Gross Pathology & Surgical Features

- May have deceptively encapsulated appearance
  - Can lead to incomplete resection & markedly worsened prognosis
- Tissue from potential sarcomas should have special handling
  - Fresh tissue sent for cytogenetics
  - Snap-frozen tissue for molecular analysis
  - Snap-frozen sample for tissue banking
  - Special fixative for electron microscopy
- Clear & accurate orientation of specimen necessary for margin identification

Microscopic Pathology

- H&E
  - Complex, extensive classification scheme
    - Some tumors have uncertain differentiation
  - Exact classification may not always be possible
  - Consultation with centers having subspecialty expertise is recommended
    - Can be significant interinstitutional discrepancy with diagnosis due to inexperience diagnosing these lesions
  - Histologic grading based on differentiation, mitotic activity, and necrosis
    - 3-grade system recommended for use over 2- and 4-grade systems
    - Fédération Nationale des Centres de Lutte Contre le Cancer (FNCLCC) is preferred grading method for AJCC staging system
- Special stains
  - Immunohistochemistry profiles help identify lines of differentiation
    - MDM2 often expressed in liposarcoma and others
    - Wild-type p53 expression in many types of STS

Routes of Spread

- Local spread
  - Locally invasive growth, often in direction of least resistance; typically radial initially, but fascial planes direct growth longitudinally
- Hematogenous spread
  - Most common metastatic site is lung
- Metastatic sites
  - Lung, liver
- Most common site of metastatic spread is dependent on tumor type
  - Extremity sarcoma = lung
  - Retroperitoneal sarcoma = liver
- Overall, regional involvement of lymph nodes is uncommon
  - Slightly common in rhabdomyosarcoma, angiosarcoma, synovial sarcoma, epithelioid sarcoma, & clear cell sarcoma
- Myxoid liposarcoma has predisposition to metastasize to other soft tissue sites (retroperitoneal lymph nodes and liver)
- Iatrogenic spread of tumor to adjacent tissue compartments by poorly planned biopsy or subtotal resection

IMAGING

Detection

- Common radiologic presentations
  - MR is highly recommended to stage primary STS, and CT scans are commonly used to look for metastasis regionally and distantly
- MR
  - T1 contrast fat-suppression and T2 fat-suppression sequences are helpful in most cases
  - Most have nonspecific, heterogeneous signal intensity on T1WI & fluid-sensitive sequences
    - Some tissue signal types can help suggest specific sarcoma type
      - Adipocytic sarcomas: Low signal on fat-suppressed sequences ± high signal foci on T1WI
      - Fibroblastic sarcomas: Intermediate to low signal foci on T1WI & T2WI sequences
      - Fibrohistiocytic sarcomas: Marked heterogeneity
  - Most helpful modality for assessing primary tumor
    - Delineates size & relationship to adjacent critical structures
  - Gadolinium enhancement should be utilized to establish local extent of tumor
    - Peritumoral edema (no enhancement) defined by T2 images can be difficult to differentiate from tumor (enhancement) if gadolinium not utilized
    - For tumors with high T1WI signal, consider subtraction postprocessing of pre- and post-gadolinium fat-suppressed T1WI
- Radiography
  - Limited usefulness for soft tissue tumor detection
  - Evaluate for calcification & ossification
  - Assess involvement of adjacent bone
- CT
  - Evaluate primary tumor if MR cannot be performed
  - Can establish gross extent of tumor
    - Involvement of &/or relationship to neurovascular structures, fascial planes
  - May suggest tumor type
    - Presence of fat or large blood vessels
  - Percutaneous biopsy guidance
    - Best demonstrates compartmental anatomy
    - Enhancing regions best for biopsy (avoid necrotic regions)
    - Prebiopsy consultation with oncologic surgeon essential to plan biopsy approach
    - Biopsy trajectory must correspond to planned surgical approach or may necessitate more extensive surgery than would have been necessary
- FDG PET/CT

- Promising technology but not currently standard for diagnosis or staging since not all types of STS are FDG avid
- May be helpful to establish extent of disease, especially unsuspected metastases
- Can identify most metabolically active portion of mass for biopsy
- Heterogeneity of tracer uptake within mass has been suggested to indicate worse prognosis

- Ultrasound
  - May exclude benign causes for soft tissues masses
  - Often used judiciously to guide biopsies so as not to contaminate other tissue compartments

Staging

- Nuances of staging
  - Tumor grade also contributes to overall stage
  - If surgery happens after neoadjuvant radiation, stage as "p"
- Tumor size
  - Size can be measured either radiologically or clinically
    - Deep STS are best measured utilizing MR
    - Gadolinium enhancement on MR differentiates tumor from reactive edema; suspicious peritumoral edema may contain microscopic tumor
- Regional lymph nodes
  - MR, CT, and PET/CT are all excellent modalities to evaluate nodal status
    - Nodes in inguinal region can normally measure up to 3 cm in long axis dimension
    - Nodes that are > 1 cm in short axis dimension with obliteration of fatty hilum are typically considered suspicious
    - PET/CT demonstrates increased tracer uptake in malignant nodes
  - Nodal involvement is uncommon & should initiate further work-up for distant metastases
  - Formerly, nodal involvement had the same prognostic implications as distant metastasis but now downgraded to AJCC stage III disease
    - Lymph node involvement in sclerosing epithelioid sarcoma is less clinically significant than with other sarcomas
  - Surgical staging system does not include nodal status
- Distant metastasis
  - Chest CT to be performed for all sarcoma cases
  - Abdominopelvic CT additionally performed if sarcoma has retroperitoneal location or certain histology subtypes such as myxoid liposarcoma of extremity
  - FDG PET might be helpful for certain types of STS, but not all kinds of STS are FDG-avid lesions
- Histologic grade
  - One of the most important prognostic factors
- Additional descriptors
  - Special case descriptors use lower case letters
    - Multiple primary tumors in single site = (m); added parenthetically after T in TNM classification (e.g., T[m]NM)
    - Pathologic staging = p; prefix to TNM (e.g., pTNM)
    - Clinical staging = c; prefix to TNM (e.g., cTNM)
    - Classified during or after multimodality therapy = y; prefix to TNM (e.g., ycTNM)
    - Staged recurrence after disease-free interval = r; prefix to TNM (e.g., rTNM)
    - Staged at autopsy = a; prefix to TNM (e.g., aTNM)

Restaging

- Before definitive excision but after preoperative chemotherapy &/or radiotherapy
  - MR of primary tumor site and closest regional lymph nodes if possible
    - Use change in gadolinium enhancement to assess response to treatment
    - Mild enhancement post therapy may be seen with either residual viable tumor **or** entirely necrotic tumor with enhancement of neovascularization
  - CT scans of chest without contrast can be used for restaging in many types of STS mainly for pulmonary metastasis
- After definitive surgical excision
  - MR of operative bed & regional area to establish baseline appearance
  - Gadolinium enhancement for MR is useful
    - Enhancement in disrupted tissues of operative bed is normal: Do not overcall postoperative changes as tumor
      - Suspicious enhancement patterns include mass-like, nodular, or enlarging findings
    - Consider subtraction postprocessing of pre- and post-contrast-enhancement images for detection of subtle lesions
    - Recommend short-term interval follow-up for equivocal findings, usually 3 months
- Asymptomatic interval follow-up
  - Complicated management process based on several variables
    - Success of tumor excision: Wide margins vs. incomplete or marginal excision
    - Risk of metastasis based on tumor type, e.g., synovial sarcoma, dedifferentiated liposarcoma, angiosarcoma, rhabdomyosarcoma, angiosarcoma, unclassified high-grade STS
    - Risk of metastasis based on size: Progressive risk with sizes > 5 cm
    - Tumor histologic grade
    - Pattern of practice; individual vs. multidisciplinary effort
  - High-risk patient
    - MR of primary tumor area + chest CT q. 3 months for 1st 2 years
    - MR of primary tumor area + chest CT q. 6 months for next 3 years
    - MR of primary tumor area + chest CT annually thereafter
  - Low-risk patient
    - MR of primary tumor area + chest CT q. 6 months for 1st 2 years
    - MR of primary tumor area + chest CT annually thereafter
  - Recurrence is not common after 10 years
- After recurrence
  - MR (contrast-enhanced CT if MR contraindicated) of primary tumor area
  - Chest CT
  - Tissue biopsy or surgical resection to definitively document recurrence prior to treatment

CLINICAL PRESENTATION & WORK-UP

Presentation

- Most commonly presents as painless, extremity mass
  - May have history of trauma to area, thus relatively common to be initially misdiagnosed as hematoma
  - Neurovascular compression = pain &/or edema
- Paraneoplastic symptoms are rare
- Location influences size at presentation
  - Retroperitoneal > proximal extremity > distal extremity
- Superficial soft tissue masses > 5 cm have 10% chance of being sarcoma

Prognosis

- Survival is most directly related to risk of metastatic disease; 5-year survival rates below for extremity STS
  - Stage I: 90%
  - Stage II: 80%
  - Stage III: 56%
  - Stage IV: 10-20%
- Risk of metastasis increases with high grade and ↑ tumor size

Work-Up

- Clinical
  - History and physical examination
- Radiographic
  - Both CT and MR are widely used to assess primary
    - Contrast-enhanced CT is used if MR is contraindicated
  - Role of PET/CT not clear
  - CT of chest is commonly used to look for pulmonary metastasis
    - CT of abdomen/pelvis is often used if it is for retroperitoneal sarcoma or myxoid liposarcoma and other histologies
- Laboratory
  - Core biopsy is primary diagnostic tool

TREATMENT

Major Treatment Alternatives

- Surgery: Referral to tertiary care center where multidisciplinary sarcoma clinic is available
  - Wide resection: Negative margins (R0 resection) necessary, not "shelling out"
    - Preoperative radiation therapy (RT) followed by wide resection is commonly recommended for majority of STS
    - Wide resection is recommended in the following circumstances
      - Sarcoma histology is not established after initial biopsy/biopsies
      - Small sarcoma (typically < 3 cm superficial): Postoperative RT might not be required if negative margin
      - Low-grade sarcoma and adjuvant postoperative RT is not anticipated after resection
      - Prolonged wound-healing problem is highly anticipated
  - Compartmental resection: Seldom used anymore
  - Limb amputation: Seldom used anymore
- RT: Referral to tertiary or quaternary center where multidisciplinary sarcoma clinic is available
  - Decreases local recurrence rate to < 10% in patients after margin-negative resection
  - Given for close or positive margins or large high-grade sarcoma
  - External beam radiotherapy (EBRT): Either preop or postop, &/or in combination with brachytherapy or intraoperative RT
    - Intensity-modulated radiation therapy (IMRT) or 3D chemoradiation therapy (CRT) is recommended to spare normal tissue including a longitudinal strip of tissue from high-dose RT
    - Local control and survival are similar, but toxicity profiles are different with preoperative vs. postoperative radiotherapy, based on results from phase III NCIC SR2 trial
    - Preop EBRT
      - Often recommended because of decrease in chronic radiation morbidities, radiation dose, and target volume
      - May also decrease tumor seeding during surgery and, occasionally, tumor mass, which may facilitate complete resection
      - Wide resection typically occurs in 4-8 weeks after preoperative EBRT
    - Postop EBRT
      - Commonly given 4-6 weeks after resection and wound healing are complete
      - Potential advantages include complete histology examination after resection and reduced opportunity for wound complication
  - Brachytherapy (low dose rate [LDR], high dose rate [HDR], or intraoperative radiation therapy [IORT]) can be given as boost combined with EBRT to high-risk margin predicted for recurrence
  - Adjuvant brachytherapy (LDR or HDR) can be given after sarcoma resection
  - Brachytherapy (LDR or HDR) can also be given after resection in patients whose tumor site was previously irradiated
  - For certain pediatric sarcomas such as rhabdomyosarcoma, RT can be used as alternative to surgery for local control if surgery would result in significant functional problems
- Chemotherapy
  - Adriamycin-ifosfamide-based chemotherapy considered first-line regiment
  - Commonly for patients with nodal or distant metastatic disease
  - Controversial for patients with localized STS
    - Adjuvant chemotherapy provided a small survival benefit (local recurrence-free survival of 6% vs. overall recurrence-free survival of 10%) on meta-analysis
    - Certain types of adult STS might be sensitive to both chemotherapy and RT
      - Rhabdomyosarcoma, synovial sarcoma, myxoliposarcoma (round cell liposarcoma), and angiosarcoma
      - Still debated whether to treat other types of adult high-grade STS including MFH, dedifferentiated liposarcoma, &/or unclassified STS

- Neoadjuvant chemotherapy alone prior to resection is investigational since results of previous EORTC study failed to show survival benefit
  - Neoadjuvant chemotherapy prior to or concurrent with RT is preferred in some institutions
  - May be easy to monitor and alter or terminate therapy in patients who do not appear to be deriving any benefit
- Retroperitoneal sarcoma: Majority with tumors > 10 cm in size die from local complications related to uncontrolled primary
  - Surgery
    - Complete resection is a mainstay in treatment of retroperitoneal sarcoma
      - Unresectable retroperitoneal sarcoma: Extremely poor outcome
    - Local recurrence rate of 30-80% if surgical resection alone
    - Positive margin and high grade associated with poor survival
  - Radiotherapy of retroperitoneal sarcoma
    - Radiation treatment: Either EBRT alone or in combination with intraoperative brachytherapy
      - Preoperative RT is highly recommended to avoid high-dose RT to adjacent normal tissue structures such as small bowels, kidneys, stomach, etc., that would fill tumor bed
      - IMRT highly recommended to maximize normal tissue sparing during radiotherapy
      - IORT can be used to boost high-risk margin either pre- or post EBRT; alternatively, IMRT with simultaneously integrated boost can be used to boost high-risk margin only
    - Chemotherapy for retroperitoneal sarcoma: Role of neoadjuvant or adjuvant chemotherapy unclear
      - Switch to preoperative RT if sarcoma does not respond
      - Patients might not be able to tolerate adjuvant chemotherapy after aggressive margin-negative resection (kidney resection &/or bowel resection)
  - STS of head and neck and other sites
    - Surgery: Same principles in treatment of extremity STS apply
      - Wide resection alone recommended for small low-grade STS
      - Wide resection combined with RT recommended for intermediate- to high-grade or close-to-positive margin

Major Treatment Roadblocks/ Contraindications

- Tissue contamination or violation from biopsy (typically nonlongitudinal for extremity sarcoma)
- Nononcological planned resection with microscopically positive margins
  - Often leaves residual tumor behind
  - Reexcision of operative bed followed by radiation is standard care
    - Options would be preoperative RT followed by surgical resection
- Large retroperitoneal sarcoma that are not resectable
- Treatment complications associated with radiation treatment
  - Increased risk of secondary malignancy for all primary tumor locations, especially in young patients
  - Head & neck → cataracts, dry mouth, dental abnormalities, growth & intellectual delay (children)
  - Abdominal & retroperitoneal → GI toxicities including bowel obstruction, perforation, fistula, and renal insufficiency
  - Extremity → osteonecrosis, osteochondromas, osteitis, and bony fracture
  - Major acute wound complications more associated with preoperative RT (35%) than postoperative RT (17%)
    - Major acute wound complications often seen in lower extremity and rarely seen in upper extremity
    - Major acute wound complications defined in phase III randomized trial (SR2) as follows
      - Secondary operations required for wound treatment
      - Readmission to hospital for wound care
      - Invasive procedure required for wound care (drainage of hematoma, seroma, or infected wound)
      - Deep wound packing required for any wound measuring at least 2 cm in length
      - Prolonged dressing changes
      - Failure of epithelialization of skin graft by 4 weeks after resection
  - Radiation-related morbidities include subcutaneous fibrosis, edema, and joint stiffness associated more with postop RT than preop RT
    - Directly related to field size and radiation dose
  - Second primary cancer
    - May be related to genetic abnormality and high radiation dose

Treatment Options by Stage

- Therapy chosen has significant variation based on individual tumor characteristics & treatment facility
- Stage T1-2 N0 M0 G1 STS in any site
  - Margin-negative wide resection is required
  - Postop RT may be recommended if positive margin
- Stage T1a N0 M0 G2-3 STS of extremity and body wall
  - Margin-negative wide resection is required
  - Postoperative radiation recommended if positive or close margin
  - For initial nononcological resection with close/ positive margin, re-resection combined with RT (either before or after) is often recommended
    - Preoperative RT followed by wide resection is preferred
- Stage T1b N0 M0 G2-3 STS of extremity and body wall
  - Wide resection
  - Radiation (either preop or postop) often recommended if high grade &/or involvement in neurovascular bundle
- Stage T2a N0 M0 G1 of soft tissue sarcoma of extremity and trunk
  - Wide resection
  - Preop RT recommended if margin-negative resection is not anticipated to be achieved and postop RT is expected
  - Postop RT recommended after resection with positive margin
- Stage T2 N0 M0 G2-3 of STS of extremity and trunk

- Combination of RT and wide resection is often recommended regardless of margin status
    - Preop radiation recommended unless prolonged wound complication is highly anticipated
    - Postop radiation recommended if wide resection is already completed
  - Chemotherapy may be considered for certain histology subtypes such high-grade myxoid liposarcoma, synovial sarcoma, dedifferentiated liposarcoma, etc.
    - Neoadjuvant chemotherapy recommended if chemotherapy is indicated
- Localized retroperitoneal sarcoma
  - Preop IMRT is highly recommended, followed by surgery
  - Postop RT should be avoided if possible; after resection, it may be prudent to observe and treat when it recurs
  - Role of chemotherapy remains unclear; important to closely monitor tumor response and not to miss window opportunity for resection if neoadjuvant chemotherapy given
- Stage IV STS with limited metastasis
  - Better outcomes with slow-growing sarcoma
  - Definitive treatment (surgery combined with radiation) of primary STS is often recommended
    - Chemotherapy may be recommended prior to or after resection of primary STS
  - Resection or other ablative treatment is recommended to treat limited metastasis
    - Cryosurgery or SBRT or radiofrequency ablation considered if the limited metastasis is not surgically or medically resectable
- Stage IV with disseminated involvement
  - Palliative surgery, chemotherapy, or RT
  - Radiofrequency ablation, cryoablation, or embolization for local control or pain relief
  - Supportive care
- Unresectable localized soft tissue sarcoma at any site (surgically &/or medically)
  - Definitive RT is alternative option even though local control rate with RT is inferior to surgery combined with RT
  - Chemotherapy might be considered to maximize tumor response &/or to sensitize definitive RT
    - Neoadjuvant &/or concurrent chemotherapy is often recommended

Dose Response

- RECIST criteria using MR (preferred) or CECT is often used to measure tumor response, but often inadequate in STS
  - Choi criteria incorporates not only size, but change in attenuation
    - Choi criteria remains investigational in STS

Standard Doses

- Preop EBRT for STS of extremity and trunk: Typically, a dose of 50 Gy in 25 fx is prescribed
- RT simulation: Treatment position should be individualized
  - Upper extremity, typically arm above head in either prone or supine position
    - Biopsy site should be marked and included in field
  - Lower extremity: Typically, affected leg is straight and unaffected leg is in frog-leg position for maximal separation
  - Either CT-MR simulation or pretreatment MR of primary tumor site in same position for radiotherapy CT planning is highly recommended to add target volume definition
    - Axial T1 MR with gad contrast and T2 with fat suppression are recommended
  - Based on results of NCIC phase III SR2 trial, typical margins for 2D RT are 5 cm margin superior and inferior, and 2 cm margin radial to the gross tumor
  - GTV and CTV for 3D CRT or IMRT are recommended below for preop RT by RTOG sarcoma radiation oncologists
- Additional boost to positive margin is generally recommended
  - Tumor bed should be marked with radiopaque seeds or clips to define postop boost volume
    - Postop boost can be given either IORT or brachytherapy (HDR or LDR) or EBRT
    - IORT: 10-12.5 Gy for microscopic, 15-17.5 Gy for macroscopic, 20 Gy for large residual or unresectable disease often prescribed at 90% isodose line
      - Limiting toxicity is peripheral neuropathy associated with > 15 Gy
    - Interstitial brachytherapy: LDR 16 Gy in < 100 cGy per hour or HDR 3.4 Gy x 4 fx starting at day 5 postoperatively
      - Often prescribed at 1 cm from isotope source or to > 90% planning target volume using intensity modulation (HDR)
    - EBRT 16 Gy in 8 fx given after complete wound healing
- Target volume definition for preop RT used in RTOG 0630 phase II of IGRT sarcoma trial for primary extremity sarcoma
  - Definition of CTV for grades 2-3 sarcoma (> 8 cm): CTV includes gross tumor and clinical microscopic margins
    - Typically CTV = GTV + 3 cm margins in longitudinal directions covering suspicious edema
    - Suspicious edema defined by T2 MR
    - Radial margin from lesion should be 1.5 cm including any portion of tumor not confined by intact fascial barrier, bone, or skin surface
  - Definition of CTV for low-grade or other small G2-3: CTV includes GTV and clinical microscopic margins; CTV = GTV + 2 cm margins in longitudinal directions covering suspicious edema
    - Radial margin from lesion should be 1 cm including any portion of tumor not confined by intact fascial barrier, bone, or skin surface
    - Suspicious edema defined by T2 MR
  - PTV margin is 5 mm when daily IGRT used
- Postoperative EBRT for STS of extremity and trunk
  - Total dose of 60-66 Gy in 1.8-2.0 Gy per fx, with successive field decrease; median dose of 63 Gy in 35 fx for margin-negative resection
    - Dose of 45-50 Gy given if IORT or brachytherapy (LDR or HDR) planned as mentioned above
  - GTV reconstructed using preoperative images (MR preferred)

- CTV1: Add 1.5 cm radial margins and 4 cm longitudinal margins to GTV
  - CTV1 should be inside the skin and longer than the scar
- PTV1 margin is generated through autoexpansion of CTV1, but PTV margins vary by institutional protocols, including use of IGRT
- Bolus 5 mm thick is often placed over incision site and drainage site only
- Dose of 45-50 Gy in 1.8-to-2 Gy per fx is typically prescribed to PTV1

- Definitive RT for unresectable localized STS at any site (surgically &/or medically)
  - > 70 Gy in 35 fx or equivalent may be required to optimize local control
- Pediatric sarcomas often have reduced dose regimen

Organs at Risk Parameters

- Every effort should be made to avoid treating full circumference of extremity
- If tumor is close to the following structures
  - Typically < 50% volume of anus and vulva should receive 3,000 cGy
  - ≤ 50% of a longitudinal strip of skin and subcutaneous tissue of an extremity should receive 2,000 cGy
  - ≤ 50% of normal weight-bearing bone within radiation field should receive 50 Gy, except when
    - Tumor invades bone
    - There is circumferential involvement of tumor > 1/4 of bone
    - Bone will be later resected

Common Techniques

- CT-based 3D conformal radiation or IMRT
- MR simulation or fusion of MR and treatment planning CT in same treatment position

Landmark Trials

- Amputation vs. limb-sparing surgery with radiation
  - No survival benefit for amputation
- Surgery alone vs. surgery and brachytherapy
  - Local control ↑ for high-grade lesions only
- Preop RT vs. postop RT
  - No difference in local control or survival

RECOMMENDED FOLLOW-UP

Clinical

- H&P every 3-6 months for 2-3 years, then every 6 months for years 4 and 5, then annually
- Evaluation for rehabilitation with physical and occupational therapy until maximal function achieved

Radiographic

- Postoperative baseline exam

Laboratory

- Specific biomarkers in blood and urine are unknown for sarcoma

SELECTED REFERENCES

1. Haas RL et al: Radiotherapy for management of extremity soft tissue sarcomas: why, when, and where? Int J Radiat Oncol Biol Phys. 84(3):572-80, 2012
2. Wang D et al: Phase II trial of neoadjuvant/adjuvant imatinib mesylate for advanced primary and metastatic/ recurrent operable gastrointestinal stromal tumors: long-term follow-up results of Radiation Therapy Oncology Group 0132. Ann Surg Oncol. 19(4):1074-80, 2012
3. Wang D et al: RTOG sarcoma radiation oncologists reach consensus on gross tumor volume and clinical target volume on computed tomographic images for preoperative radiotherapy of primary soft tissue sarcoma of extremity in Radiation Therapy Oncology Group studies. Int J Radiat Oncol Biol Phys. 81(4):e525-8, 2011
4. Wang D et al: Variation in the gross tumor volume and clinical target volume for preoperative radiotherapy of primary large high-grade soft tissue sarcoma of the extremity among RTOG sarcoma radiation oncologists. Int J Radiat Oncol Biol Phys. 81(5):e775-80, 2011
5. American Joint Committee on Cancer: AJCC Cancer Staging Manual. 7th ed. New York: Springer. 291-6, 2010
6. Garner HW et al: Benign and malignant soft-tissue tumors: posttreatment MR imaging. Radiographics. 29(1):119-34, 2009
7. Moore LF et al: Radiation-induced pseudotumor following therapy for soft tissue sarcoma. Skeletal Radiol. 38(6):579-84, 2009
8. Navarro OM et al: Pediatric soft-tissue tumors and pseudo-tumors: MR imaging features with pathologic correlation: part 1. Imaging approach, pseudotumors, vascular lesions, and adipocytic tumors. Radiographics. 29(3):887-906, 2009
9. NCCN Soft Tissue Sarcoma Clinical Practice Guidelines in Oncology (Version 1.2009). © 2009 National Comprehensive Cancer Network, Inc. Available at: www.nccn.org/professionals/physician_gls/ f_guidelines.asp. Accessed June 29, 2009
10. Shapeero LG et al: Post-treatment complications of soft tissue tumours. Eur J Radiol. 69(2):209-21, 2009
11. Eary JF et al: Spatial heterogeneity in sarcoma 18F-FDG uptake as a predictor of patient outcome. J Nucl Med. 49(12):1973-9, 2008
12. Hueman MT et al: Management of extremity soft tissue sarcomas. Surg Clin North Am. 88(3):539-57, vi, 2008
13. Hueman MT et al: Management of retroperitoneal sarcomas. Surg Clin North Am. 88(3):583-97, vii, 2008
14. Kaushal A et al: The role of radiation therapy in the management of sarcomas. Surg Clin North Am. 88(3):629-46, viii, 2008
15. Loeb DM et al: Pediatric soft tissue sarcomas. Surg Clin North Am. 88(3):615-27, vii, 2008
16. Park K et al: The role of radiology in paediatric soft tissue sarcomas. Cancer Imaging. 8:102-15, 2008
17. Toner GC et al: PET for sarcomas other than gastrointestinal stromal tumors. Oncologist. 13 Suppl 2:22-6, 2008
18. van de Luijtgaarden AC et al: Promises and challenges of positron emission tomography for assessment of sarcoma in daily clinical practice. Cancer Imaging. 8 Suppl A:S61-8, 2008
19. Peterson JJ: F-18 FDG-PET for detection of osseous metastatic disease and staging, restaging, and monitoring response to therapy of musculoskeletal tumors. Semin Musculoskelet Radiol. 11(3):246-60, 2007
20. Rubin BP et al: Pathology of soft tissue sarcoma. J Natl Compr Canc Netw. 5(4):411-8, 2007
21. Skubitz KM et al: Sarcoma. Mayo Clin Proc. 82(11):1409-32, 2007
22. Tzeng CW et al: Soft tissue sarcoma: preoperative and postoperative imaging for staging. Surg Oncol Clin N Am. 16(2):389-402, 2007

Clinical Target Volume

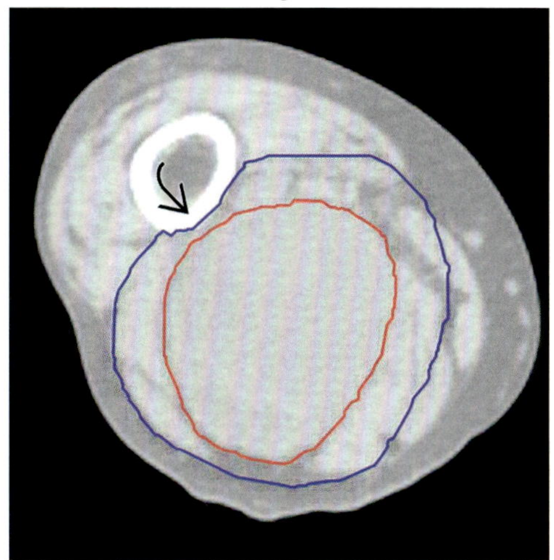

T2b N0 M0 G3

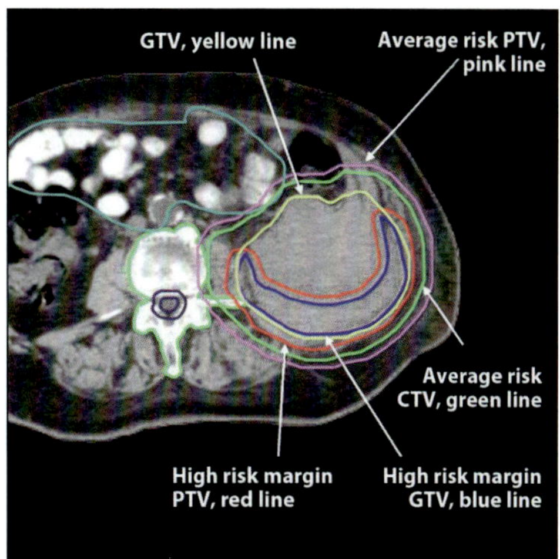

(Left) *Axial CT shows representative GTV and CTV of large, high-grade sarcoma for preoperative RT. Note that CTV is curved ➲ at the edge of anatomic boundaries such as bone and fascia.* ***(Right)*** *Axial CT shows large, high-grade retroperitoneal sarcoma. Arrows point to representative risk target volume (primary GTV, average risk CTV and PTV, high-risk margin GTV, CTV, and PTV) for preop IMRT with boost to the high-risk margin predicted for recurrence.*

Stage IA (T1a N0 M0 G1)

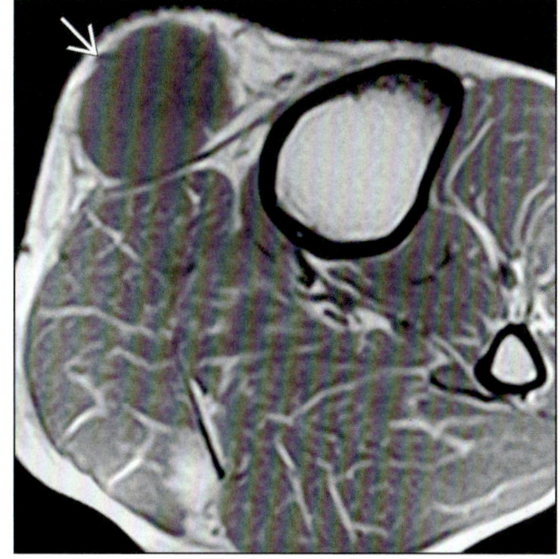

Stage IA (T1a N0 M0 G1)

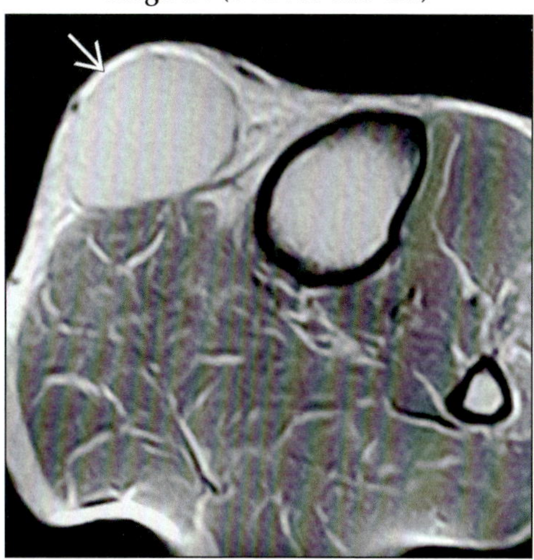

(Left) *Axial T1WI MR shows an intermediate-grade myxoid liposarcoma ➡. The mass is well defined and located in the subcutaneous fat in the proximal medial calf.* ***(Right)*** *Axial T2WI MR in the same patient shows the myxoid liposarcoma ➡ to have homogeneous high signal. The lesion has no identifiable fat signal intensity, which is not uncommon for myxoid liposarcomas. Without contrast, this lesion would be difficult to differentiate from a benign cystic lesion.*

T2b

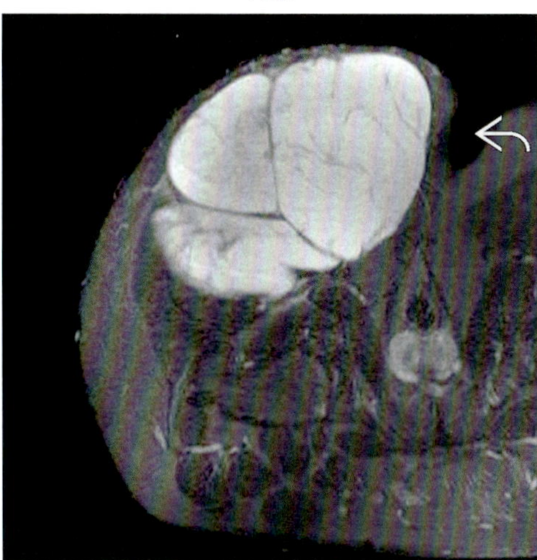

T2b

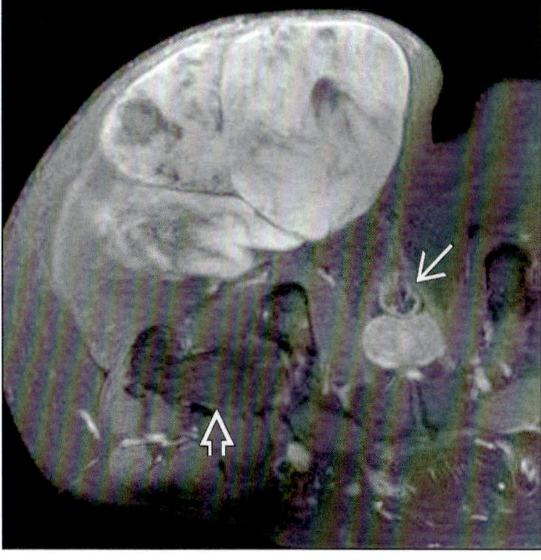

(Left) *T2WI FS MR shows a large, high-grade myxoid liposarcoma in a 42-year-old man. MR simulation was performed for preop IMRT. Note the roll of cloth towel ➲ that was used to separate the buttocks.* ***(Right)*** *T1WI C+ FS MR shows a myxoid liposarcoma of right buttock in the same patient. Preoperative IMRT was given to avoid high dose to right femur head/neck ➡. In addition, preoperative RT dose to anus and rectum ➡ would be less than postoperative RT dose.*

SARCOMA

(**Left**) *T1WI C+ FS MR shows a high-grade epithelioid sarcoma ➡ involving the right thigh in a 34-year-old woman. MR simulation was performed for preop IMRT (50 Gy in 25 fx).* (**Right**) *T2WI FS MR in the same patient shows a large, high-grade epithelioid sarcoma involving the right thigh. Note the peritumoral edema ➡. It is crucial to contour the suspicious peritumoral edema into the CTV for preoperative RT since it might harbor microscopic disease.*

T2b N0 M0 G3

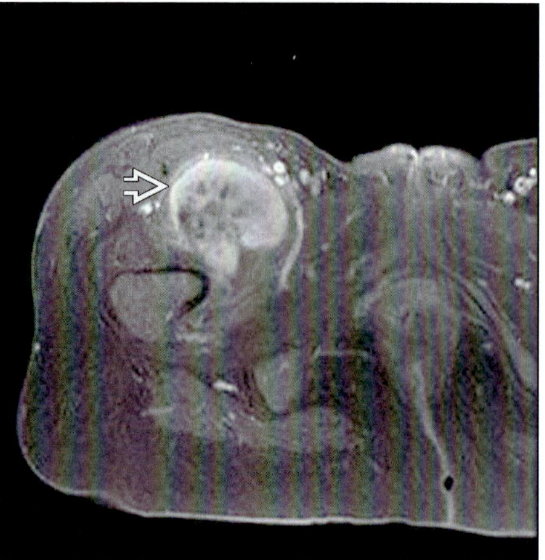

T2b N0 M0 G3

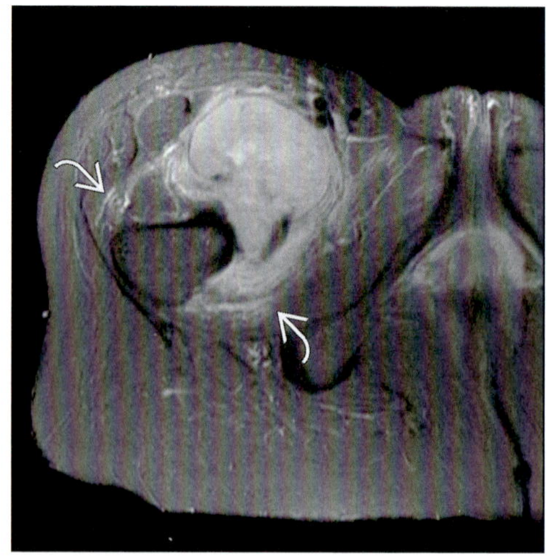

(**Left**) *Coronal T2WI FS MR in the same patient shows a large, high-grade epithelioid sarcoma of the right thigh. Note the cephalad extent of disease ➡ and the extent of peritumoral edema caudally ➡.* (**Right**) *Sagittal T1WI FS MR of the same patient shows a large, high-grade epithelioid sarcoma ➡ of the right thigh in the sagittal plane.*

T2b N0 M0 G3

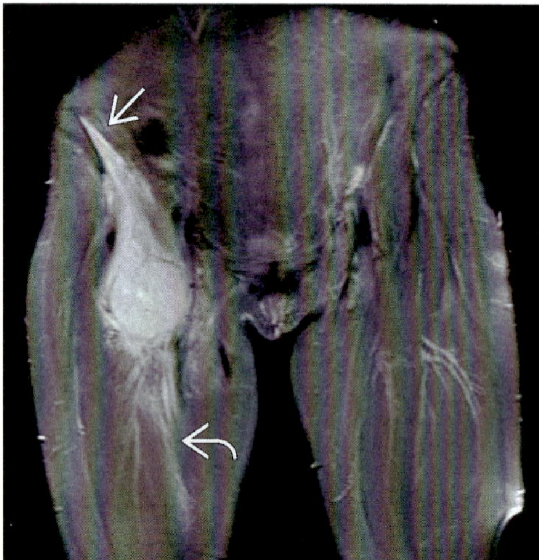

T2b N0 M0 G3

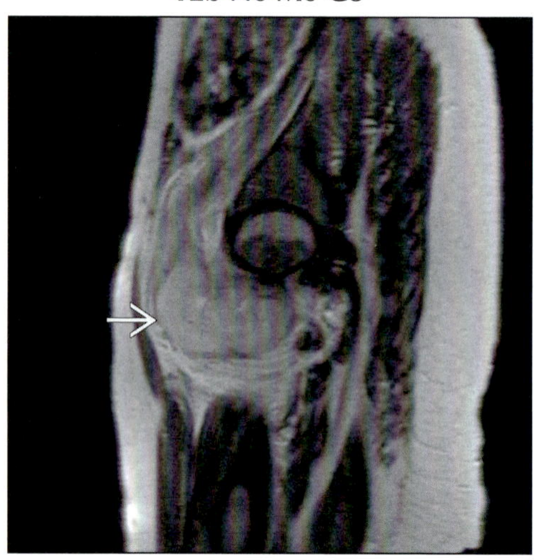

(**Left**) *Axial T1WI C+ FS MR shows a large, high-grade unclassified sarcoma ➡ involving right gluteal/perineal region in a 39-year-old man. MR simulation was performed for preop IMRT.* (**Right**) *Axial T2WI FS MR shows a sarcoma involving the gluteal/perineal region in the same patient. There is a limited amount of edema ➡. Genitals should be immobilized during treatment. The patient was advised to have sperm banking prior to treatment.*

T2b

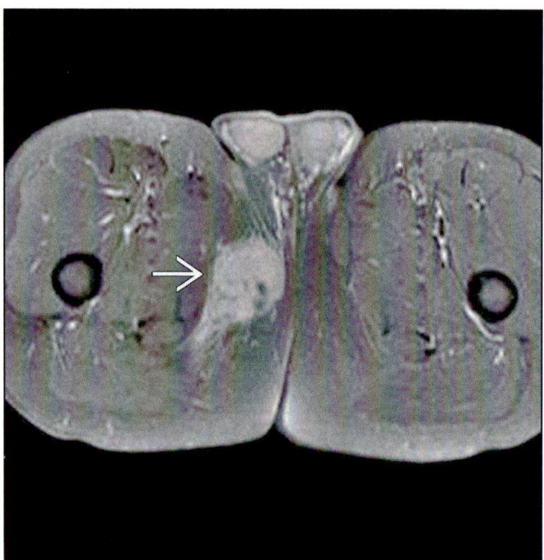

T2b

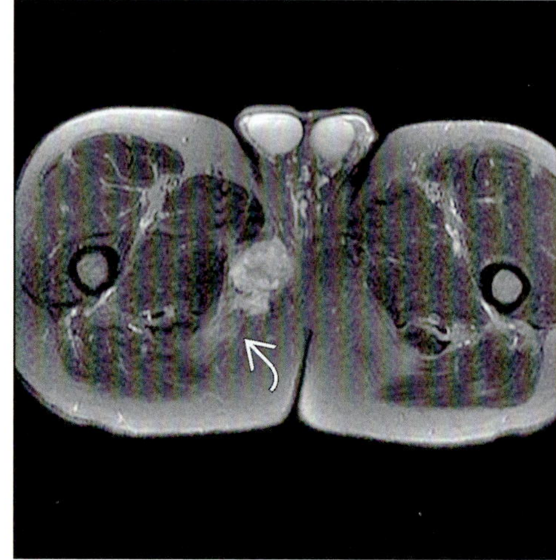

T2b Fibrosarcoma

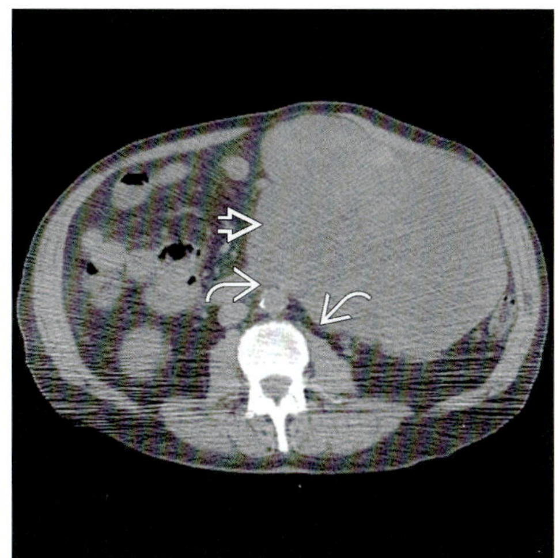

T2b Fibrosarcoma

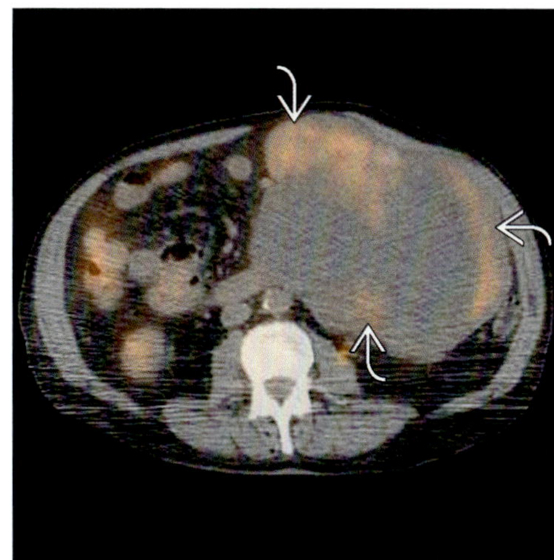

*(**Left**) Axial CT component of PET shows a large, high-grade retroperitoneal fibrosarcoma ➡ in a 73-year-old man. There is high-risk margin ➡ predicted for recurrence after resection. Preoperative IMRT with a dose of 45 Gy/57.5 Gy was prescribed to the primary tumor PTV/high-risk margin PTV using SIB technique. (**Right**) Axial fused PET/CT shows a large, high-grade retroperitoneal fibrosarcoma in the same patient. There is peripheral FDG uptake only ➡.*

T2b Fibrosarcoma

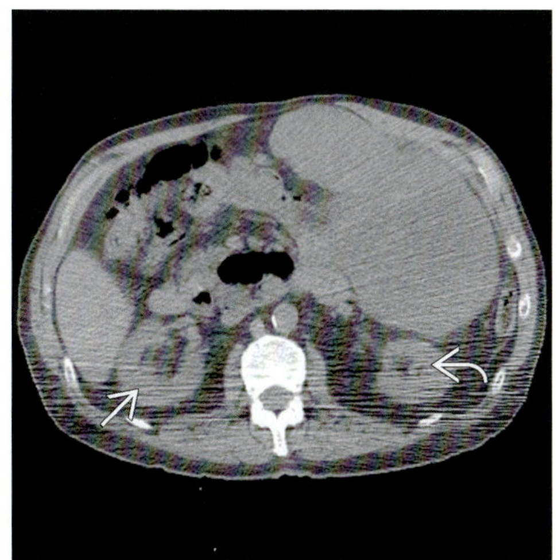

T2b Fibrosarcoma

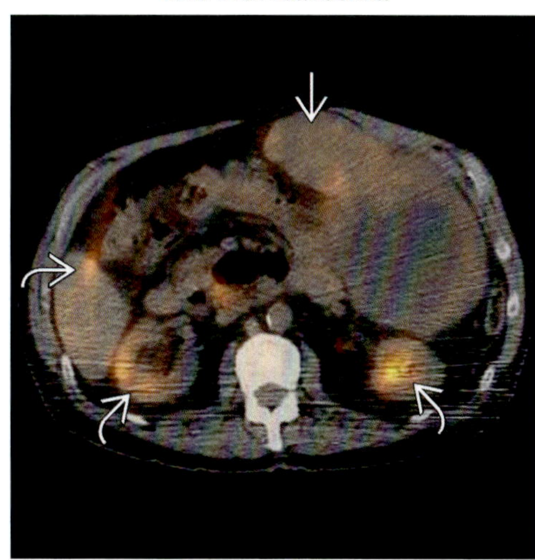

*(**Left**) Axial CT component of PET/CT shows a large, retroperitoneal fibrosarcoma in the same patient. The left kidney ➡ is very close to the sarcoma and is less protected. Renogram or contrast CT should be used to assess right renal function ➡. CT with oral small bowel contrast was used for RT planning. (**Right**) Axial fused PET/CT shows a retroperitoneal fibrosarcoma ➡ in the same patient. There is nonspecific uptake in the kidneys and liver ➡.*

T2b Leiomyosarcoma

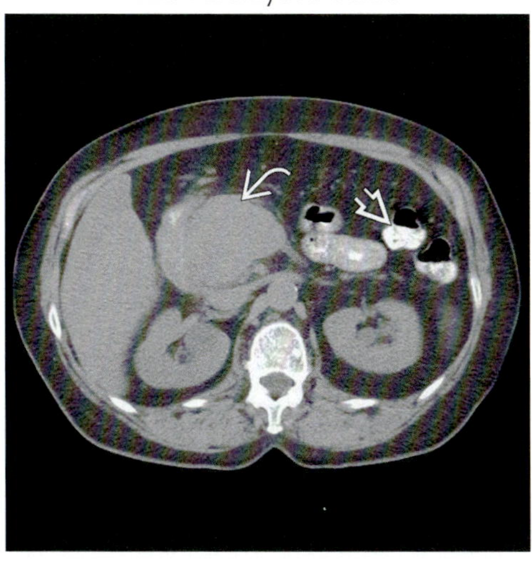

T2b Leiomyosarcoma

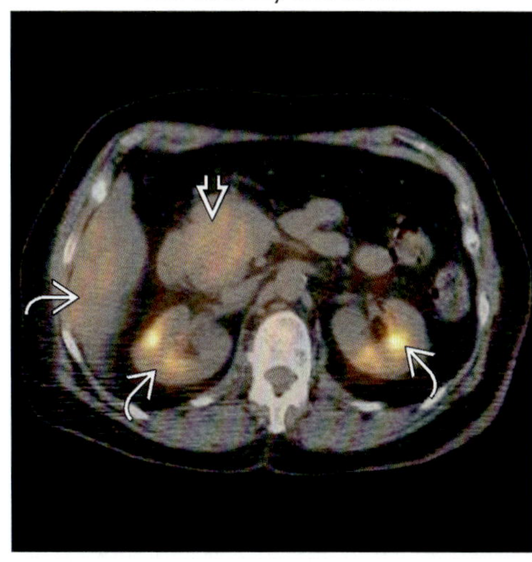

*(**Left**) Axial CT shows a large, high-grade leiomyosarcoma ➡ in a 50-year-old woman. Preoperative IMRT was prescribed. CT contrast or renogram should be performed to assess the right renal function. Normal structures including small bowel, liver, kidneys, and cord should be contoured and protected in IMRT. Note the small bowel contrast ➡. (**Right**) Axial fused PET/CT in the same patient shows the FDG avid sarcoma ➡. Note the nonspecific uptake ➡.*

T2b Myxoid Liposarcoma

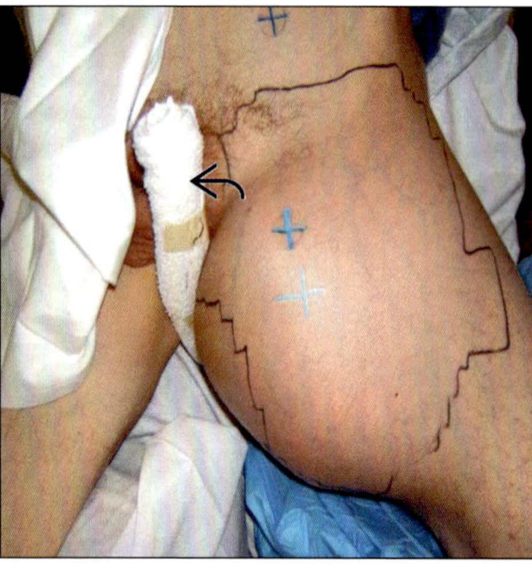

T2b Myxoid Liposarcoma

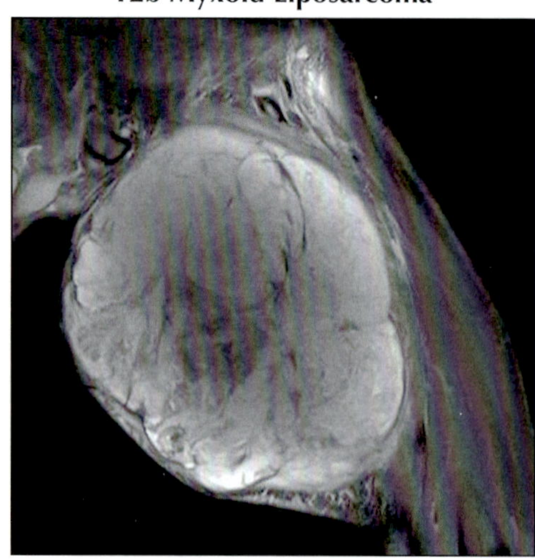

(Left) *Photo shows a large, high-grade myxoid liposarcoma involving the left upper thigh in a 55-year-old man with limited liver metastasis. A roll of cloth towel ➔ was placed in the left inguinal region to displace the scrotum and penis in the treatment position for preoperative RT planning.* ***(Right)*** *Coronal MR in the same patient shows the somewhat heterogeneous, large liposarcoma.*

T2b Myxoid Liposarcoma

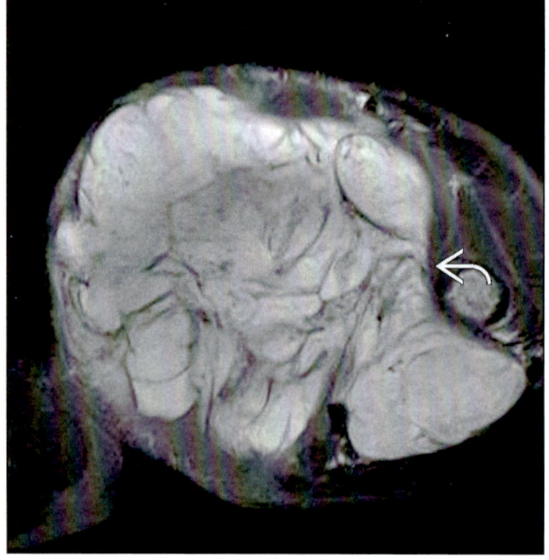

T2b Myxoid Liposarcoma

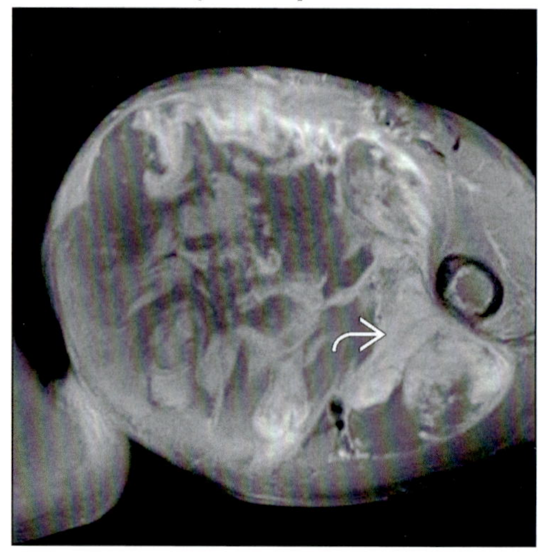

(Left) *Axial T2WI FS MR shows the massive, high-grade liposarcoma ➔ involving most of the left upper thigh in the same patient.* ***(Right)*** *Axial T1WI C+ FS MR shows the large, high-grade liposarcoma with marked areas of heterogeneous enhancement ➔ of the left upper thigh in the same patient.*

T2b Myxoid Liposarcoma

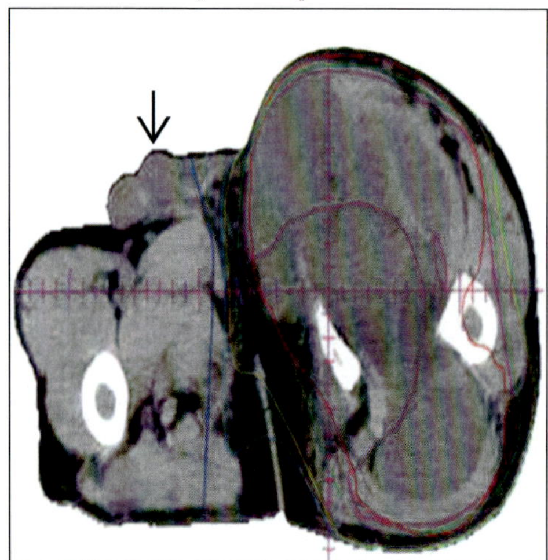

T2b Myxoid Liposarcoma

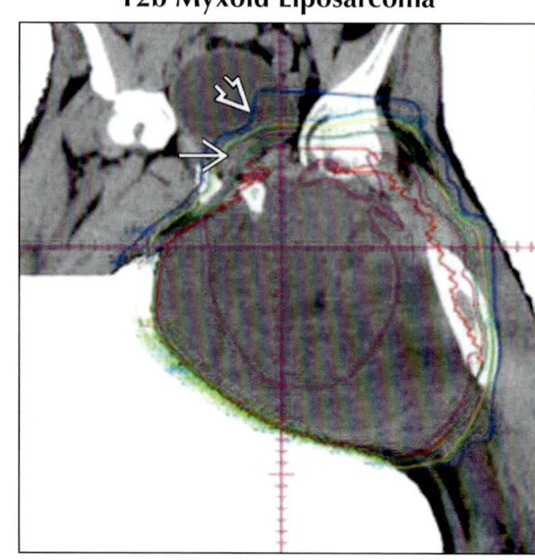

(Left) *Axial CT (RT planning) shows dose distribution of a large liposarcoma in the same patient. Immobilizing the genitals ➔ to the contralateral side aids in reducing the dose.* ***(Right)*** *Coronal CT (RT planning CT) shows the dose distribution in a large liposarcoma in the same patient. An advantage of preoperative RT is that less normal tissue is treated. The proximity of the tumor necessitates treating a fraction of the prostate ➔ and bladder ➔.*

T2b Epithelioid Sarcoma

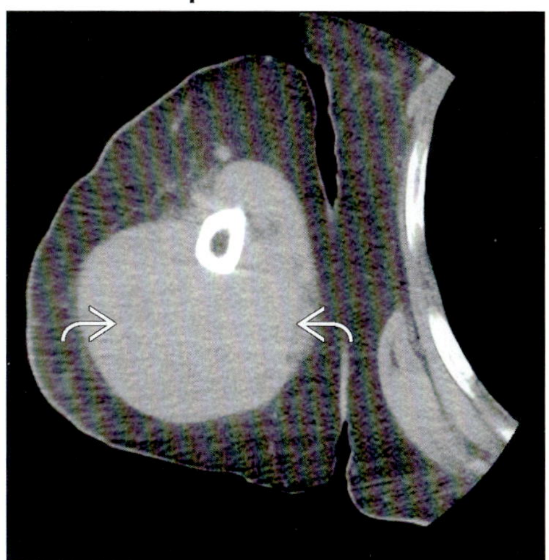

T2b Epithelioid Sarcoma

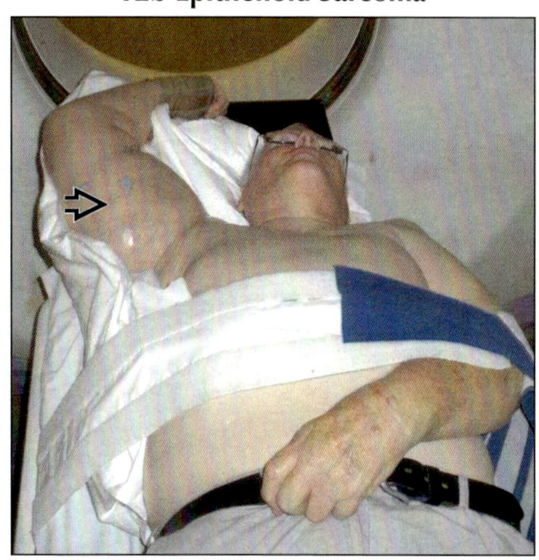

(Left) *Axial diagnostic CT with contrast shows a large, high-grade epithelioid sarcoma involving the right triceps muscle (upper arm) in a 74-year-old man. MR was not performed due to pacemaker. Sarcoma* ➔ *extends the entire width of arm in this arm-down position.* ***(Right)*** *AP treatment simulation for preop RT planning shows a large, epithelioid sarcoma* ⇨ *involving the right upper arm in the same patient. Arm elevated above the head can maximize beam positions.*

T2b Epithelioid Sarcoma

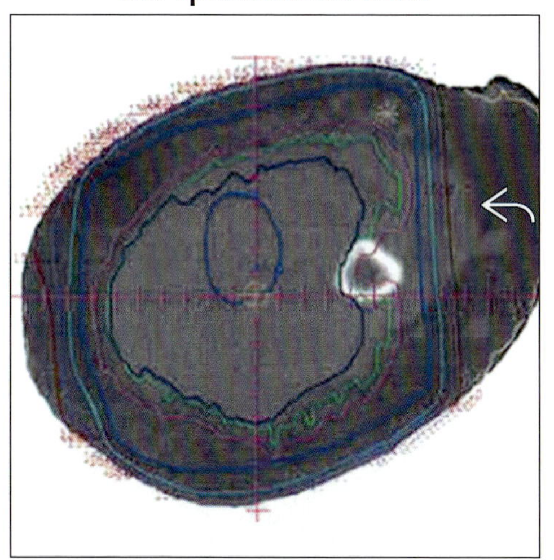

T2b Epithelioid Sarcoma

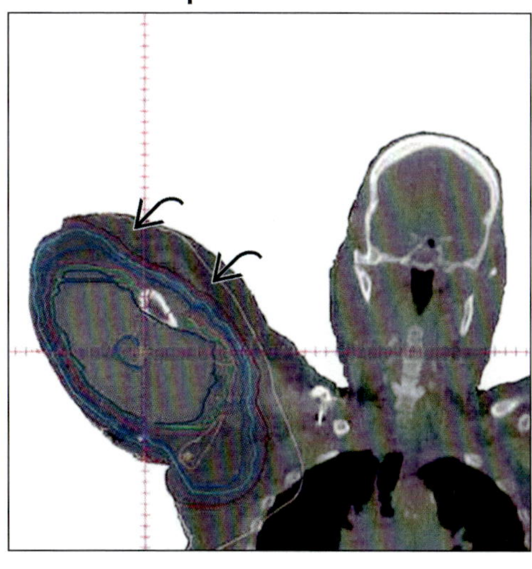

(Left) *Axial CT for RT planning shows a large sarcoma of right upper arm in the treatment position with dose distribution. There is a strip of normal tissue* ➔ *that was spared from RT secondary to the elevated arm treatment position.* ***(Right)*** *Axial CT for RT planning shows a large sarcoma involving the right upper arm in the same patient. There is a strip of normal tissue* ➔ *that was spared from RT in the elevated arm treatment position.*

T1b Leiomyosarcoma

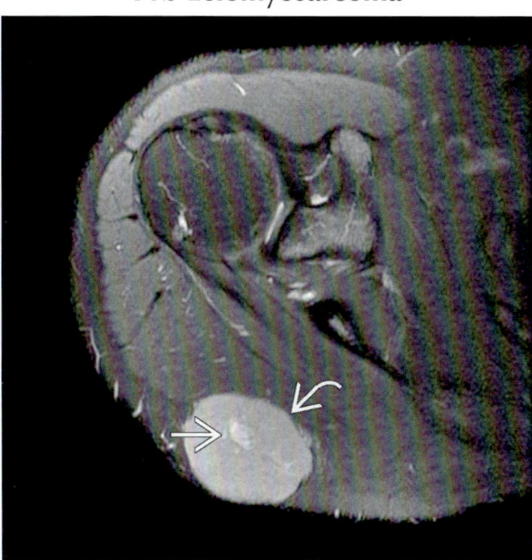

T1b Leiomyosarcoma

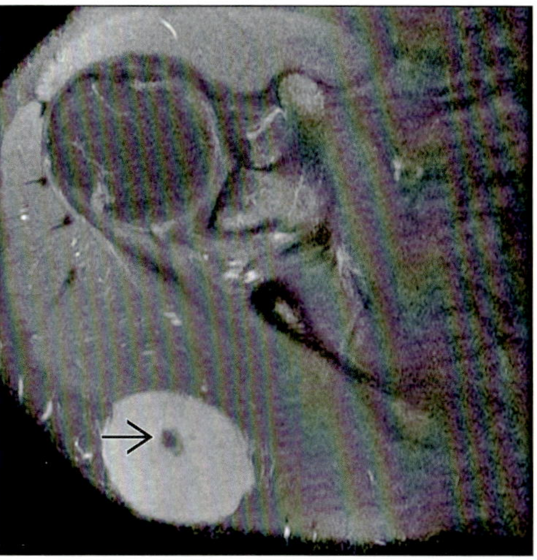

(Left) *T2WI FS MR shows a small (3.8 cm in maximal dimension) but high-grade leiomyosarcoma with central necrosis* ➔ *involving the subcutaneous fat of the right shoulder in a 25-year-old woman. The sarcoma displaced the deltoid muscle and fascia* ➔ *and contacted the skin in the right posterior shoulder.* ***(Right)*** *Axial T1WI C+ FS MR shows a small sarcoma involving subcutaneous fat in the same patient. Note central necrosis* ➔*.*

T2b Spindle Cell Sarcoma

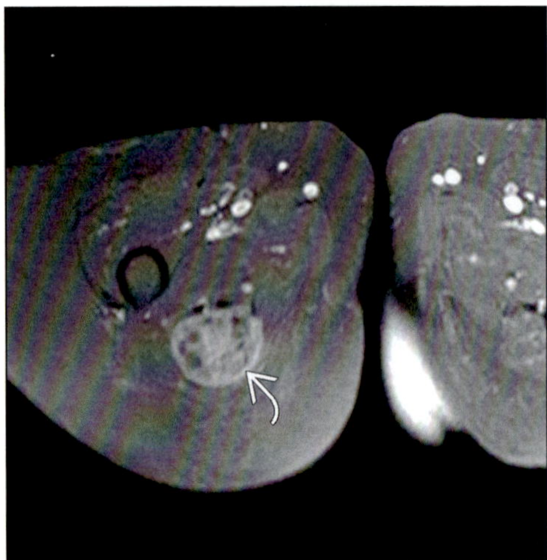

T2b Spindle Cell Sarcoma

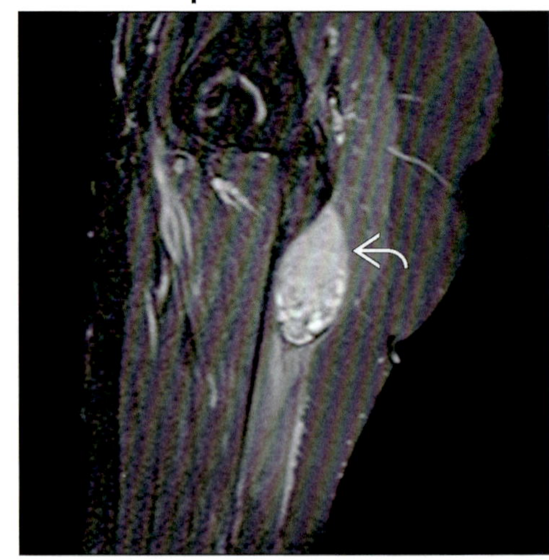

(Left) *Axial T1WI C+ FS MR shows a high-grade unclassified spindle cell sarcoma ➔ of the right thigh in a 50-year-old woman who has a history of pelvic radiotherapy for endometrial carcinoma 5 years prior.* ***(Right)*** *Sagittal T2WI FS MR in the same patient shows the spindle cell sarcoma ➔, which is sharply demarcated from surrounding muscle.*

T2b Spindle Cell Sarcoma

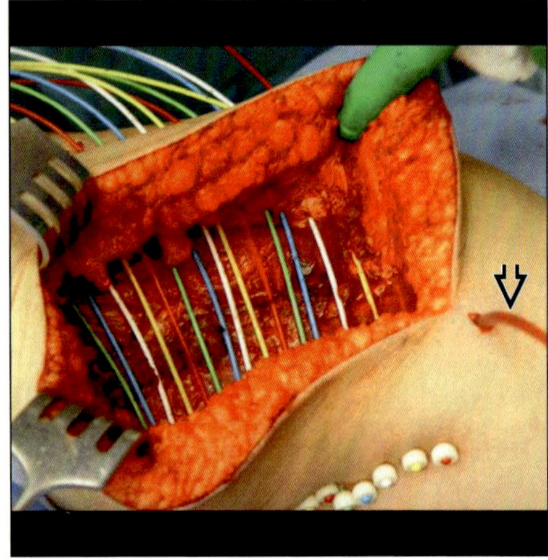

T2b Spindle Cell Sarcoma

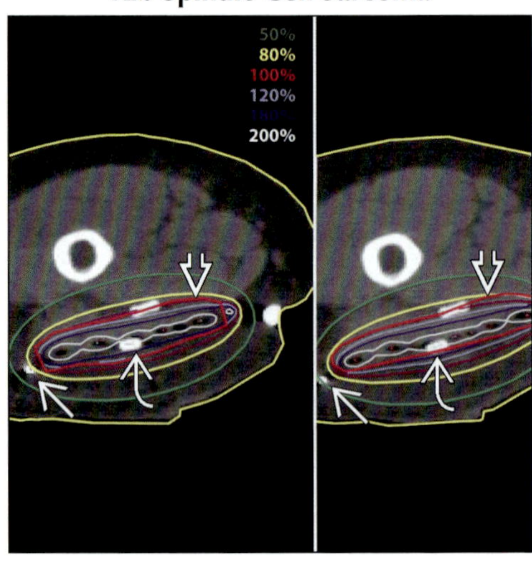

(Left) *Fourteen catheters were placed in the same patient for adjuvant HDR brachytherapy after resection. The catheters were obliquely placed in approximately 1 cm intervals after resection. Note the drainage tube ⇨ placement.* ***(Right)*** *Axial CT for HDR brachytherapy shows dose distribution (34 Gy in 10 fx, b.i.d. > 6-hour intervals) prescribed to 90% PTV ➔ defined by gold seeds ➔ placed at the edge of tumor bed. Note the drainage tube ➔ placed under the catheters.*

Stage IA (T1b N0 M0 G1)

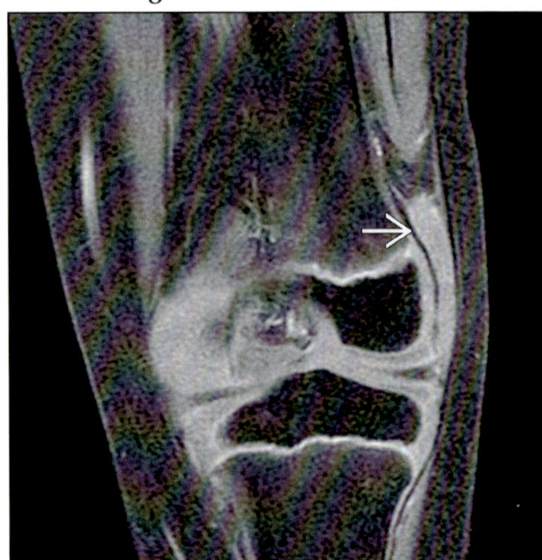

Stage IA (T1b N0 M0 G1)

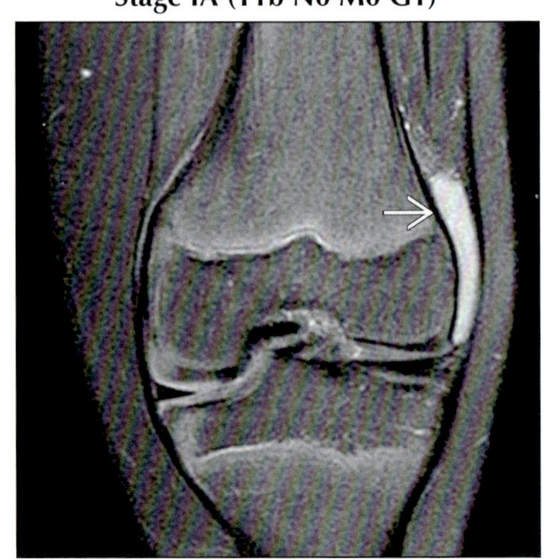

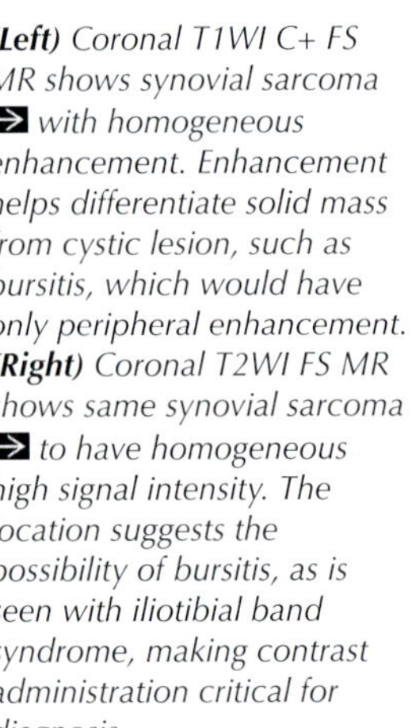

(Left) *Coronal T1WI C+ FS MR shows synovial sarcoma ➔ with homogeneous enhancement. Enhancement helps differentiate solid mass from cystic lesion, such as bursitis, which would have only peripheral enhancement.* ***(Right)*** *Coronal T2WI FS MR shows same synovial sarcoma ➔ to have homogeneous high signal intensity. The location suggests the possibility of bursitis, as is seen with iliotibial band syndrome, making contrast administration critical for diagnosis.*

T2b Pleomorphic Sarcoma

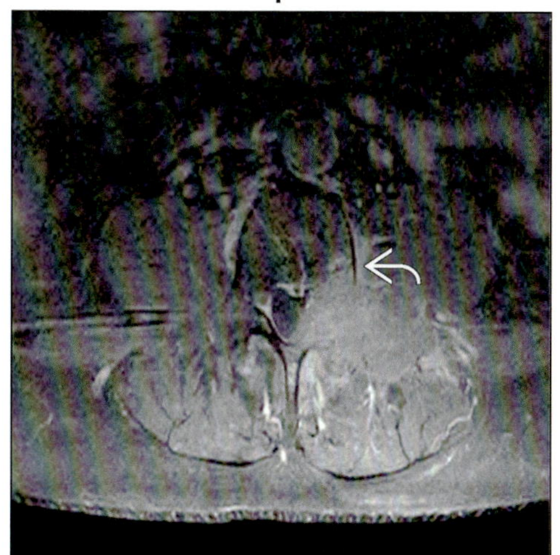

T2b Pleomorphic Sarcoma

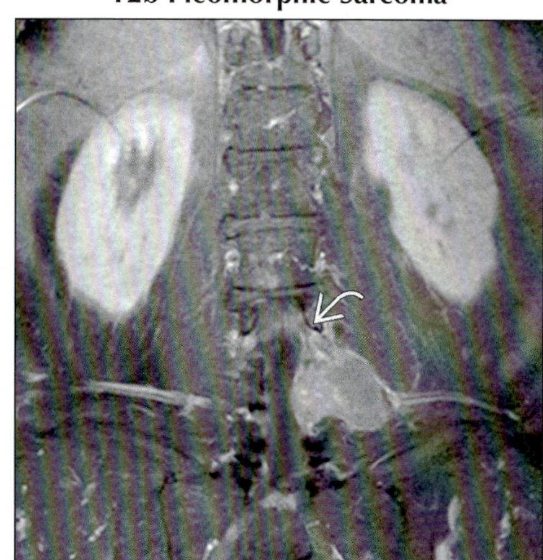

*(**Left**) Axial T1WI C+ MR shows a pleomorphic sarcoma involving the left psoas muscle at T4 with bony invasion ➦ in a 74-year-old patient. Definitive CRT was prescribed. Neoadjuvant chemotherapy (3 cycles) was given prior to RT. After 4 years, the patient remains alive without disease. (**Right**) Coronal T2WI FS MR shows the sarcoma involving the left psoas muscle in the same patient. Bone invasion ➦ is evident.*

T2b

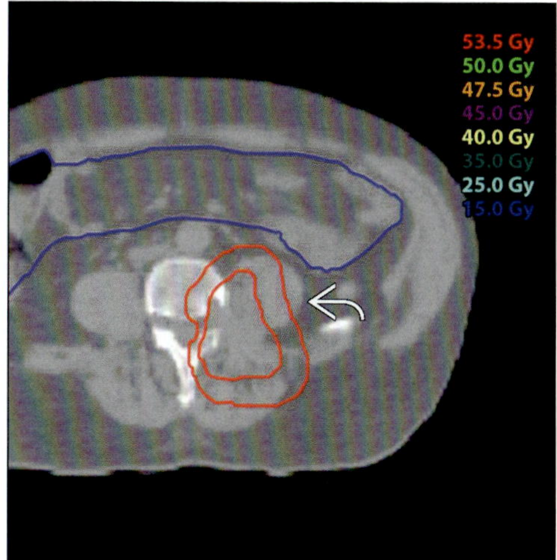

T2b

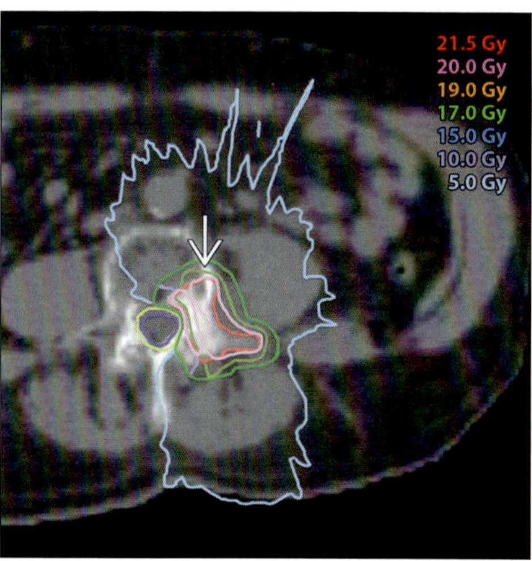

*(**Left**) Axial CT from the fused PET/CT was used for initial RT planning in the same patient. PET/CT shows significant tumor reduction after chemotherapy. Tomotherapy with a dose of 50 Gy ➦ in 25 fx was prescribed. This was followed by an SBRT boost with 20 Gy in 5 fx to the residual tumor after the initial tomotherapy. (**Right**) Axial CT shows the SBRT boost plan in the same patient. The 20 Gy isodose line and residual tumor ➔ are depicted.*

T2b Chondrosarcoma

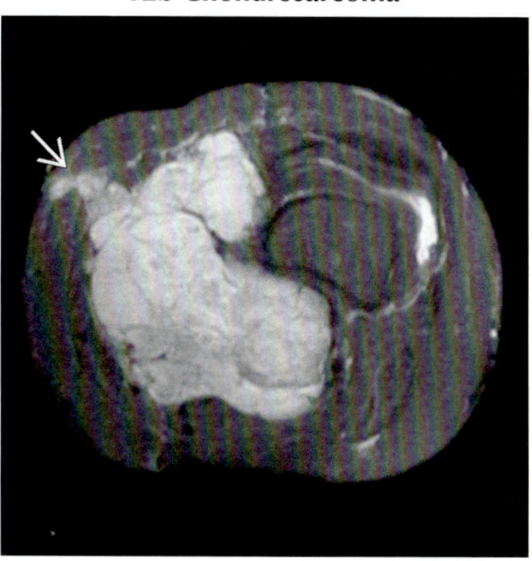

T2b Chondrosarcoma

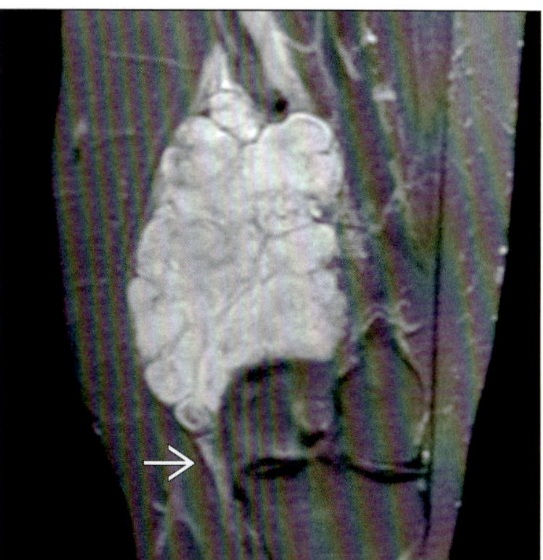

*(**Left**) Axial T2WI FS MR shows a large intermediate-grade extraskeletal chondrosarcoma involving left distal thigh in a 53 year old. Tumor ➔ can be seen tracking along the core needle biopsy site. (**Right**) Sagittal T2WI FS MR shows extraskeletal chondrosarcoma involving left distal thigh in same patient. Note peritumoral edema ➔. Preop RT was recommended to minimize knee joint toxicity with understanding of high risk for wound-healing problem.*

ISCL/EORTC Revision to the Classification of Mycosis fungoides and Sézary Syndrome

From Olsen E et al: Revisions to the staging and classification of mycosis fungoides and Sézary syndrome: A proposal of the International Society for Cutaneous Lymphomas (ISCL) and the cutaneous lymphoma task force of the European Organization of Research and Treatment of Cancer (EORTC). Blood. 110(6):1713-22, 2007.

TNM	*Definitions*
Skin	
T1	Limited patches[1], papules, &/or plaques[2] covering < 10% of the skin surface; may further stratify into T1a (patch only) vs. T1b (plaque ± patch)
T2	Patches, papules, or plaques covering ≥ 10% of the skin surface; may further stratify into T2a (patch only) vs. T2b (plaque ± patch)
T3	1 or more tumors[3] (≥ 1 cm diameter)
T4	Confluence of erythema covering ≥ 80% of body surface area

[1]*"Patch" indicates any size skin lesion without significant elevation or induration. Presence/absence of hypo/hyperpigmentation, scale, crusting, &/or poikiloderma should be noted.*

[2]*"Plaque" indicates any skin lesion that is elevated or indurated. Presence or absence of scale, crusting, &/or poikiloderma should be noted. Histologic features such as folliculotropism or large cell transformation (> 25% large cells), CD30(+) or CD30(-), and clinical features such as ulceration are important to document.*

[3]*For skin, "tumor" indicates at least one 1 cm diameter solid or nodular lesion with evidence of depth &/or vertical growth. Note total number of lesions, total volume of lesions, largest size lesion, and region of body involved. Also note if histologic evidence of large cell transformation has occurred. Phenotyping for CD30 is encouraged.*

ISCL/EORTC Revision to the Classification of Mycosis fungoides and Sézary Syndrome (continued)

From Olsen E et al: Revisions to the staging and classification of mycosis fungoides and Sézary syndrome: A proposal of the International Society for Cutaneous Lymphomas (ISCL) and the cutaneous lymphoma task force of the European Organization of Research and Treatment of Cancer (EORTC). Blood. 110(6):1713-22, 2007.

TNM	*Definitions*
Node	
N0	No clinically abnormal peripheral lymph nodes[4]; biopsy not required
N1	Clinically abnormal peripheral lymph nodes; histopathology Dutch grade 1 or NCI LN0-2
N1a	Clone negative[5]
N1b	Clone positive[5]
N2	Clinically abnormal peripheral lymph nodes; histopathology Dutch grade 2 or NCI LN3
N2a	Clone negative[5]
N2b	Clone positive[5]
N3	Clinically abnormal peripheral lymph nodes; histopathology Dutch grades 3-4 or NCI LN4; clone positive or negative
NX	Clinically abnormal peripheral lymph nodes; no histologic confirmation
Viscera	
M0	No visceral organ involvement
M1	Visceral involvement (must have pathology confirmation[6], and organ involved should be specified)
Peripheral Blood Involvement	
B0	Absence of significant blood involvement: ≤ 5% of peripheral blood lymphocytes are atypical (Sézary) cells[7]
B0a	Clone negative[5]
B0b	Clone positive[5]
B1	Low blood tumor burden: > 5% of peripheral blood lymphocytes are atypical (Sézary) cells but does not meet the criteria of B2
B1a	Clone negative[5]
B1b	Clone positive[5]
B2	High blood tumor burden: ≥ 1,000/μL Sézary cells[7] with positive clone[5]

[4]For node, "abnormal peripheral lymph node(s)" indicates any palpable peripheral node that on physical examination is firm, irregular, clustered, fixed, or ≥ 1.5 cm in diameter. Node groups palpated include cervical, supraclavicular, epitrochlear, axillary, and inguinal. Central nodes, which are not generally amenable to pathologic assessment, are not currently considered in the nodal classification unless used to establish N3 histopathologically.

[5]A T-cell clone is defined by PCR or Southern blot analysis of the T-cell receptor (TCR) gene.

[6]For viscera, spleen and liver may be diagnosed by imaging criteria.

[7]For blood, Sézary cells are defined as lymphocytes with hyperconvoluted cerebriform nuclei. If Sézary cells are not able to be used to determine tumor burden for B2, then 1 of the the following modified ISCL criteria along with a positive clonal rearrangement of the TCR may be used instead: 1) Expanded CD4(+) or CD3(+) cells with CD4/CD8 ratio ≥ 10; 2) expanded CD4(+) cells with abnormal immunophenotype including loss of CD7 or CD26.

ISCL/EORTC Revision to the Staging of Mycosis fungoides and Sézary Syndrome

From Olsen E et al: Revisions to the staging and classification of mycosis fungoides and Sézary syndrome: A proposal of the International Society for Cutaneous Lymphomas (ISCL) and the cutaneous lymphoma task force of the European Organization of Research and Treatment of Cancer (EORTC). Blood. 110(6):1713-22, 2007.

Stage	*T*	*N*	*M*	*Peripheral Blood Involvement*
IA	T1	N0	M0	B0, B1
IB	T2	N0	M0	B0, B1
IIA	T1, T2	N1, N2	M0	B0, B1
IIB	T3	N0-2	M0	B0, B1
III	T4	N0-2	M0	B0, B1
IIIA	T4	N0-2	M0	B0
IIIB	T4	N0-2	M0	B1
IVA1	T1-4	N0-2	M0	B2
IVA2	T1-4	N3	M0	B0-2
IVB	T1-4	N0-3	M1	B0-2

Histopathologic Staging of Lymph Nodes in Mycosis fungoides and Sézary Syndrome

From Olsen E et al: Revisions to the staging and classification of mycosis fungoides and Sézary syndrome: A proposal of the International Society for Cutaneous Lymphomas (ISCL) and the cutaneous lymphoma task force of the European Organization of Research and Treatment of Cancer (EORTC). Blood. 110(6):1713-22, 2007.

Updated ISCL/EORTC Classification	*Dutch System*	*NCI-VA Classification*
N1	Grade 1: Dermatopathic lymphadenopathy (DL)	LN0: No atypical lymphocytes
		LN1: Occasional and isolated atypical lymphocytes (not arranged in clusters)
		LN2: Many atypical lymphocytes or in 3-6 cell clusters
N2	Grade 2: DL; early involvement by MF (presence of cerebriform nuclei > 7.5 µm)	LN3: Aggregates of atypical lymphocytes; nodal architecture preserved
N3	Grade 3: Partial effacement of LN architecture; many atypical cerebriform mononuclear cells (CMCs)	LN4: Partial/complete effacement of nodal architecture by atypical lymphocytes or frankly neoplastic cells
	Grade 4: Complete effacement	

St. Jude Staging System

From Murphy SB et al: Non-Hodgkin's lymphomas of childhood: An analysis of the histology, staging, and response to treatment of 338 cases at a single institution. J Clin Oncol. 7(2):186-93, 1989.

Stage	*Definitions*
I	A single tumor (extranodal) or single anatomic area (nodal), with the exclusion of mediastinum or abdomen
II	A single tumor (extranodal) with regional node involvement
	≥ 2 nodal areas on the same side of the diaphragm
	2 single (extranodal) tumors with or without regional node involvement on the same side of the diaphragm
	A primary gastrointestinal tract tumor, usually in the ileocecal area, with or without involvement of associated mesenteric nodes only[1]
III	2 single tumors (extranodal) on opposite sides of the diaphragm
	≥ 2 nodal areas above and below the diaphragm
	All primary intrathoracic tumors (mediastinal, pleural, thymic)
	All extensive primary intraabdominal disease[1]
	All paraspinal or epidural tumors, regardless of other tumor site(s)
IV	Any of the above with initial central nervous system &/or bone marrow involvement[2]

[1]*A distinction is made between apparently localized gastrointestinal tract lymphoma and more extensive intraabdominal disease because of their quite different patterns of survival after appropriate therapy. Stage II disease typically is limited to 1 segment of the gut ± the associated mesenteric nodes only and the primary tumor can be completely removed grossly by segmental excision. Stage III disease typically exhibits spread to paraaortic and retroperitoneal areas by implants and plaques in mesentery or peritoneum, or by direct infiltration of structures adjacent to the primary tumor. Ascites may be present, and complete resection of all gross tumor is not possible.*

[2]*If the marrow involvement is present initially, the number of abnormal cells must be ≤ 25% in an otherwise normal marrow aspirate with a normal peripheral blood picture.*

LYMPHOMA

Diffuse Large B-Cell Lymphoma (DLBCL)

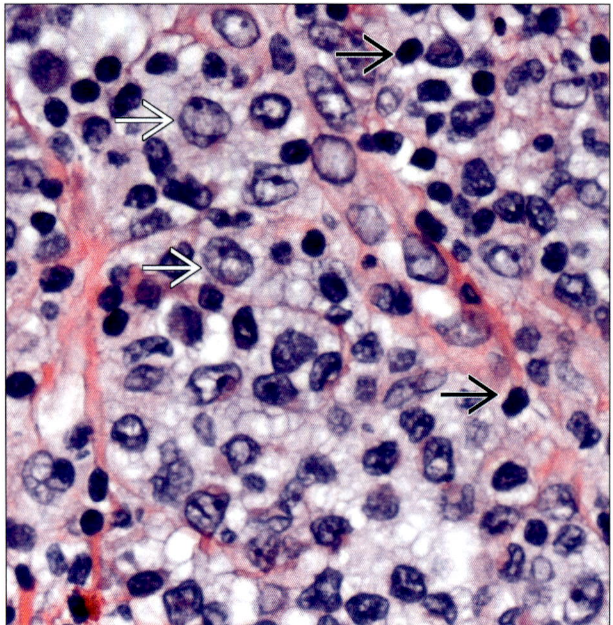

Typical centroblasts ➡ are large, noncleaved with vesicular chromatin, and have membrane-bound nucleoli. Reactive small lymphocytes are also present ➡. DLBCL are CD20(+), CD3(-), CD5(-), and CD45(+). (Courtesy F. Vega, MD, PhD.)

Follicular Lymphoma (FL), Grade 3

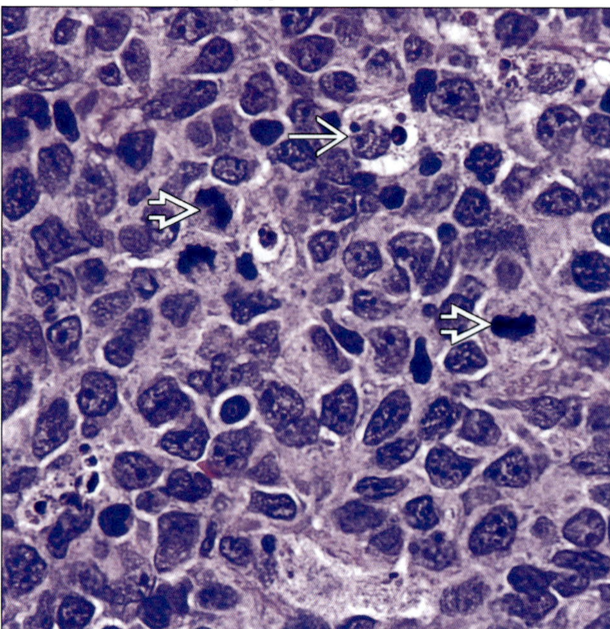

The architecture is replaced by neoplastic follicles composed of numerous centroblasts. In this neoplastic follicle, mitotic figures ➡ and tingible body macrophages ➡ are seen. No small centrocytes are noted. FL are CD20(+), CD3(-), CD10(+), and CD5(-). (Courtesy C. C. Yin, MD, PhD.)

Marginal Zone B-Cell Lymphoma

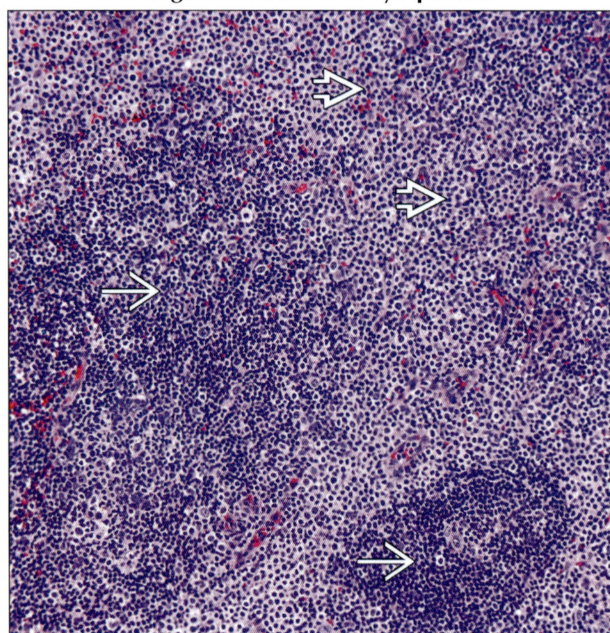

Neoplastic monocytoid (pale) cells expand interfollicular areas ➡. Two residual germinal centers are present ➡; one is nearly replaced by the neoplasm while the other shows marked follicular colonization by the neoplastic cells. Marginal zone lymphomas are CD20(+), CD3(-), CD10(-), CD5(-), and CD23(-). (Courtesy P. Lin, MD.)

Small Lymphocytic Lymphoma

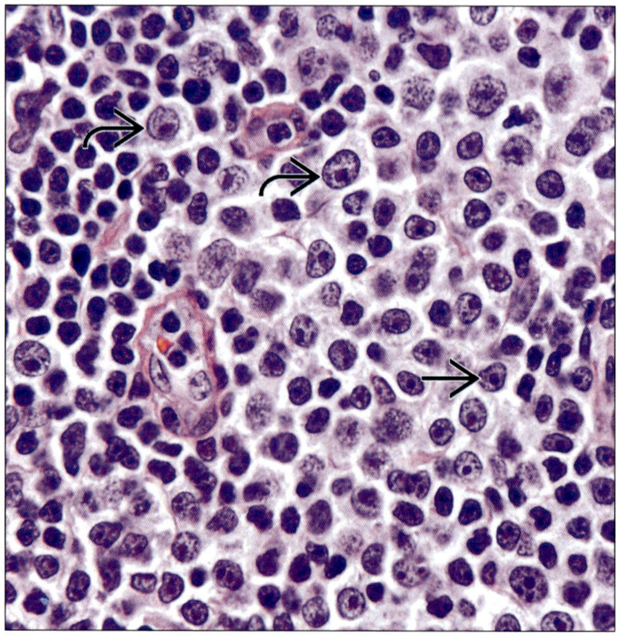

This entity is histologically the same as chronic lymphocytic leukemia. The lymph node proliferation center is composed of small lymphocytes, prolymphocytes ➡, and paraimmunoblasts ↗. (Courtesy C. E. Bueso-Ramos, MD.)

Mycosis Fungoides

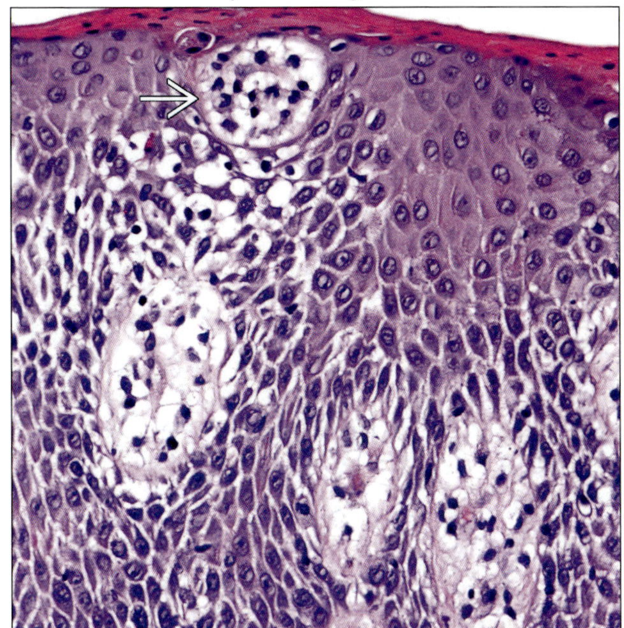

The plaque stage of mycosis fungoides (MF) shows the presence of a Pautrier microabscess ➔ containing small atypical tumor cells. MF shows an elevated CD4/CD8 ratio, +/- clonal T cell gene receptor rearrangement, and frequent depletion of CD2, CD3, CD5, and CD7 positive cells. (Courtesy S. A. Wang, MD.)

Nodular Sclerosing Hodgkin Lymphoma

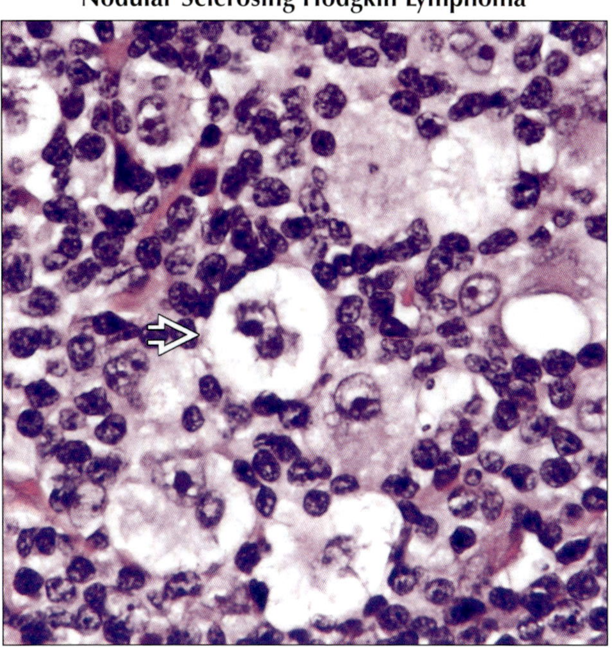

High-power view shows Reed-Sternberg (RS) cells with retraction artifact of cytoplasm as an empty or lacunar space. Hence, these cells are known as lacunar cells. An example of an "owl's eye" cell ➔ is shown. Hodgkin lymphoma is CD15(+) and CD30(+). (Courtesy C. C. Yin, MD, PhD.)

Lymphocyte Deplete Hogkin Lymphoma

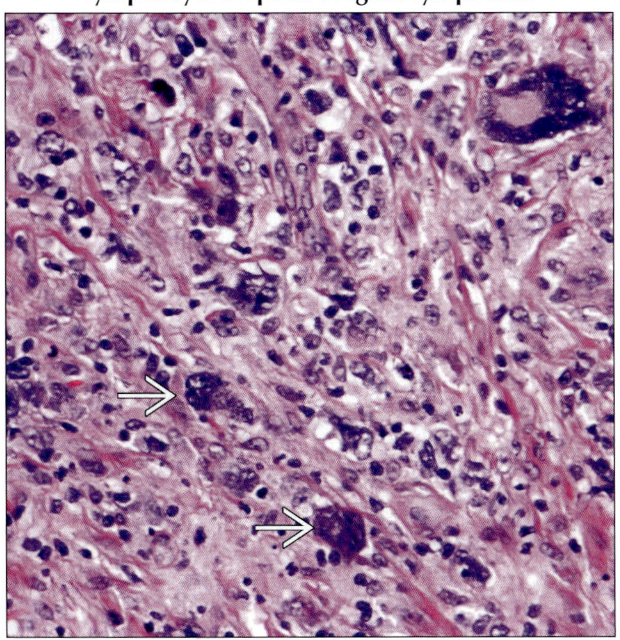

Reed-Sternberg cells ➔ are numerous and pleomorphic, and small lymphocytes are depleted. (Courtesy C. C. Yin, MD, PhD.)

Nodular Lymphocyte Predominant Hodgkin Lymphoma (NLPHL)

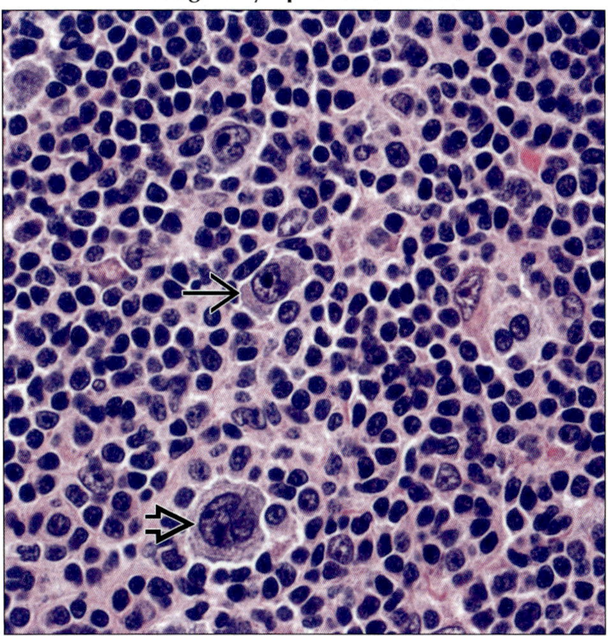

This H&E of NLPHL shows various morphologic appearances of LP cells, including "popcorn" cells ➔ and one with a prominent nucleolus ➔, similar to the RS cells of classic Hodgkin lymphoma.

LYMPHOMA

Stage I

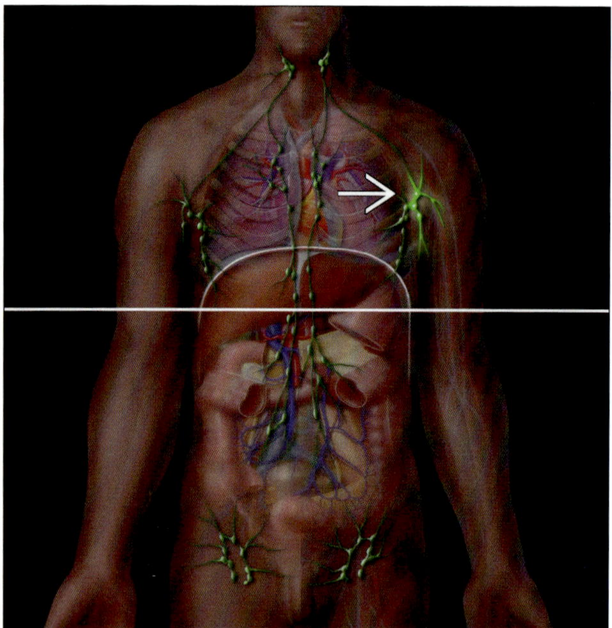

Graphic shows multiple malignant left axillary lymph nodes (LNs) ➔. Stage I is defined as involvement of a single lymphatic site (i.e., nodal region, Waldeyer ring, thymus, or spleen) (I) or localized involvement of a single extralymphatic organ or site in the absence of any lymph node involvement (IE).

Stage II

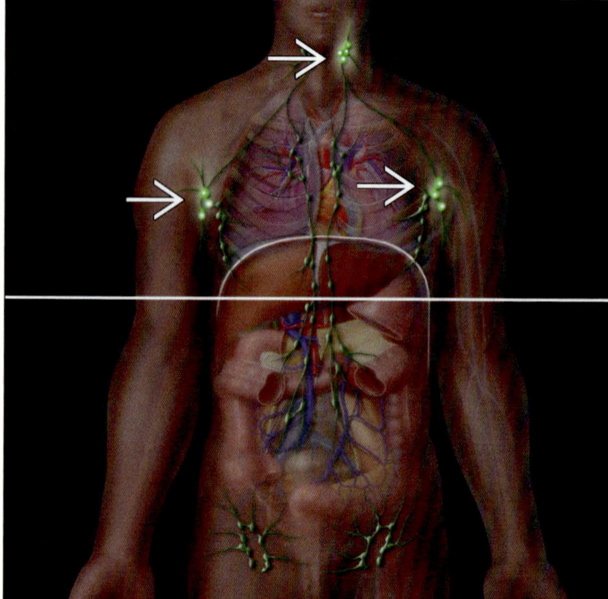

Graphic shows nodal disease ➔ above the diaphragm. Stage II is confined to one side of the diaphragm; it may involve 2 or more LN groups or localized involvement of a single extralymphatic organ or site in association with regional LN involvement with or without involvement of other LN regions (IIE).

Stage III

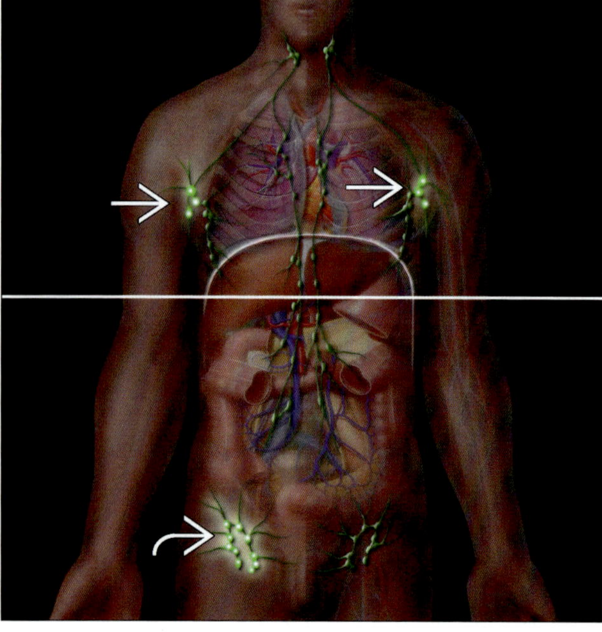

Graphic shows multiple LN groups above ➔ and below ➔ the diaphragm. Stage III is defined as involvement of the LN regions on both sides of the diaphragm, which may also be accompanied by extralymphatic extension in association with adjacent LN involvement (IIIE) or by involvement of the spleen (IIIS) or both.

Stage IV

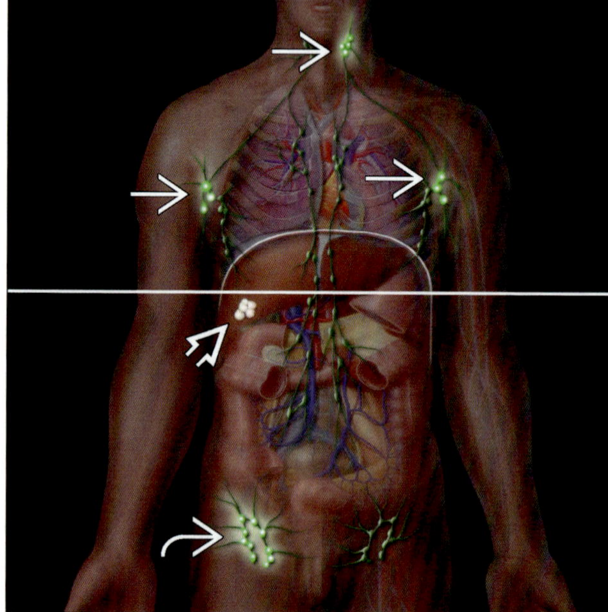

Graphic shows liver involvement ➔ and multiple LN groups above ➔ and below ➔ the diaphragm. Stage IV is diffuse involvement of 1 or more extralymphatic organs, ± associated LN involvement, or isolated extralymphatic organ involvement in the absence of adjacent regional LN involvement, but with distant disease.

Stage IV

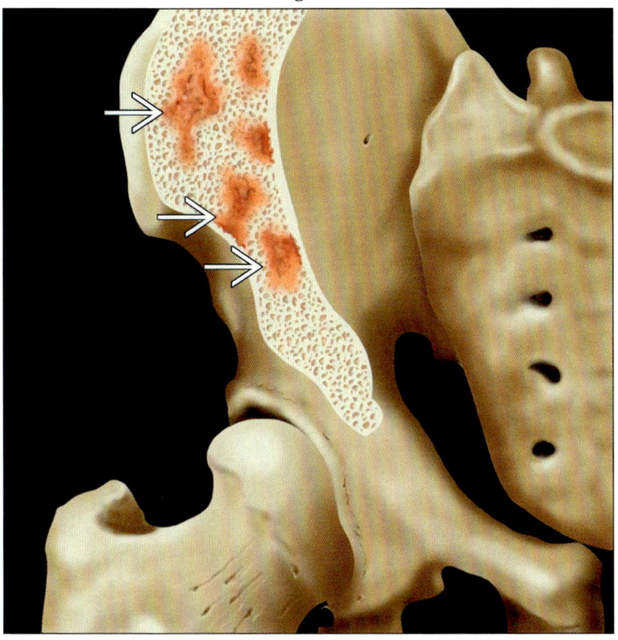

Coronal graphic shows multiple infiltrative lesions within the right hemipelvis, compatible with lymphoma. Osseous involvement with lymphoma is considered stage IV disease.

Stage IV

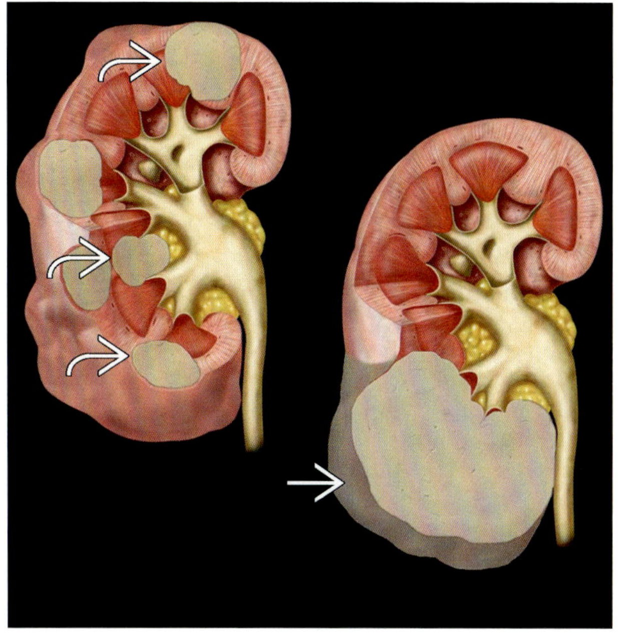

Coronal graphic shows 2 patterns of renal involvement with lymphoma, which may present in a multifocal pattern or as a single, large, often infiltrating mass. Diffuse involvement of an extralymphatic organ is considered stage IV disease.

INITIAL SITE OF RECURRENCE

Distant	20%
Untreated Lymph Nodes	19%
Local Failure (in Field)	10%

Patterns of failure after RT for aggressive lymphomas treated primarily with radiation alone. Cox JD et al: Cancer 29:1043-51, 1972; Kun LE et al: Radiology 141:791-4, 1981.

LYMPHOMA

OVERVIEW

General Comments

- Lymphoma: Neoplastic disease of lymphocytes with heterogeneous characteristics
  - Clonal expansion of lymphocytes
    - B cells
    - T cells
    - NK cells
- Non-Hodgkin lymphoma (NHL) represents 85% of all malignant lymphomas
- NHL, compared to Hodgkin lymphoma, is more likely to disseminate extranodally

Classification

- Lymphoma broadly divided into 2 groups
  - Hodgkin lymphoma (HL)
  - NHL
- **Primary malignant tumors (WHO classification)**
  - **B-cell neoplasms**
    - Peripheral (mature) B-cell neoplasms
      - Chronic lymphocytic leukemia (CLL)/small lymphocytic lymphoma (SLL)
      - B-cell prolymphocytic leukemia
      - Lymphoplasmacytic lymphoma
      - Splenic marginal zone lymphoma
      - Hairy cell leukemia
      - Plasmacytoma/multiple myeloma including solitary plasmacytoma of bone and extraosseous plasmacytoma
      - Extranodal marginal zone B-cell lymphoma, also called mucosa-associated lymphoid tissue (MALT) lymphoma (MALToma)
      - Nodal marginal zone B-cell lymphoma
      - Follicular lymphoma, grades 1-3
      - Mantle cell lymphoma
      - Diffuse large B-cell lymphoma (DLBCL)
      - Mediastinal (thymic) large cell lymphoma
      - Intravascular large B-cell lymphoma
      - Primary effusion lymphoma
      - Burkitt lymphoma/leukemia
  - **Immunodeficiency-associated lymphoproliferative disorders**
    - Associated with a primary disorder, HIV, methotrexate
    - Post transplant
    - Primary CNS lymphoma most often but not exclusively associated with AIDS
  - **T-cell and NK-cell neoplasms**
    - Precursor T-cell lymphoblastic leukemia/ lymphoma
    - Peripheral (mature) T-cell neoplasms
      - T-cell prolymphocytic leukemia
      - T-cell large granular lymphocytic leukemia
      - Aggressive NK-cell leukemia
      - Adult T-cell leukemia/lymphoma
      - Extranodal NK-/T-cell lymphoma, nasal type
      - Enteropathy-type T-cell lymphoma
      - Hepatosplenic T-cell lymphoma
      - Blastic NK lymphoma
      - Subcutaneous panniculitis-like T-cell lymphoma
      - Mycosis fungoides/Sézary syndrome
      - Primary cutaneous anaplastic large cell lymphoma
      - Peripheral T-cell lymphoma, not otherwise specified (NOS)
      - Angioimmunoblastic T-cell lymphoma
      - Anaplastic large cell lymphoma
  - **Hodgkin lymphoma, NOS**
    - Nodular lymphocyte-predominant Hodgkin disease (NLPHD) (5%)
    - Classical Hodgkin lymphoma (95%)
      - Nodular sclerosis (only type more common in women than men)
      - Lymphocyte rich
      - Lymphocyte depleted
      - Mixed cellularity

NATURAL HISTORY

General Features

- Comments
  - NHL
    - Diverse neoplasms with differing prognoses
      - B-cell lymphomas (90%)
      - T-cell lymphomas (10%)
    - More often involving extranodal sites than HL
  - Hodgkin lymphoma
    - Reed-Sternberg (RS) cells comprise minority of the tumor mass
    - Contiguous nodal involvement in central sites is most common
- Location
  - B-cell lymphomas arise from the lymph node follicles
  - T-cell lymphomas arise in the paratrabecular region of lymph nodes

Etiology

- Risk factors
  - Immunodeficiency states
  - Epstein-Barr virus (EBV) is associated with African Burkitt lymphoma and some AIDS-associated lymphomas
  - Human T-lymphotropic virus type 1 (HTLV-1) associated with aggressive T-cell leukemia/lymphoma
  - *H. pylori* associated with gastric MALTomas
  - *Chlamydia psittaci* associated with orbital MALTomas

Epidemiology & Cancer Incidence

- Number of cases in USA per year
  - NHL
    - 70,130 estimated new cases of NHL with 18,940 deaths in 2012
    - 7th highest incident cancer in men and women
    - 9th cause of cancer death in men and 7th cause of cancer death in women
    - Probability of NHL from birth to death
      - Males: 1 in 43
      - Females: 1 in 51
- Sex predilection
  - Males > females
- Age of onset
  - NHL median age 67; HL has bimodal peak at 30 and 70 years of age

Genetics

- Common translocations

- t(14;18), t(11;14), and some t(8;14) probably occur in primitive B cells in the marrow
- Immunoglobulin gene rearrangements occur in B-cell neoplasms
- T-cell receptor gene rearrangements occur in T-cell neoplasms
- DLBCL
  - *BCL6* mutations, t(14;18), and others
- Follicular lymphomas
  - t(14;18) causes dysregulation of *BCL2* and blocks apoptosis
- Mantle cell lymphoma
  - *BCL1* mutations, t(11;14)
- Lymphoplasmacytic lymphoma
  - *PAX5*/IgH mutations, t(9;14)
- Marginal zone lymphoma
  - *AP12*/*MLT* mutations, t(11;18)
- Burkitt lymphoma
  - *c-MYC* translocations, t(8;n)
- Anaplastic large cell lymphoma
  - *NPM*/*ALK* mutations, t(2;5)

Associated Diseases, Abnormalities

- NHL: 8% of patients have an autoimmune disease
- HL: 9% of patients have or develop an autoimmune disease
  - Most common are Sjögren syndrome, thyroiditis, polymyositis, scleroderma, and glomerulonephritis
  - Paraneoplastic neurologic manifestations in HL include subacute cerebellar degeneration, limbic encephalitis, subacute necrotic myelopathy, and subacute motor neuropathy

Gross Pathology & Surgical Features

- Heterogeneous gross pathologies vary among subtypes of NHL
- Hepatosplenomegaly depending on histology

Microscopic Pathology

- H&E
  - Histological findings are heterogeneous in NHL, with morphology varying among subtypes
  - Both low- and high-power views are important to assess nodal architecture
- Special stains
  - Immunohistochemistry is essential: B- &/or T-cell markers may be expressed depending on subtype
  - Flow cytometry often valuable
  - Cytogenetics often valuable
  - Molecular studies growing in importance

Routes of Spread

- Local spread
  - Large mediastinal masses may invade chest wall, pericardium, or other thoracic structures
- Lymphatic extension
  - NHL typically spreads to noncontiguous lymph nodes, leading to widely disseminated pattern of nodal involvement
    - Stages III and IV more common than stages I and II
    - NHL commonly spreads to extranodal sites
  - Hodgkin lymphoma typically spreads to contiguous lymph nodes, leading to pattern of nodal spread within same region
    - Stages I and II more common than stages III and IV
    - Rarely spreads to extranodal sites
- Metastatic sites
  - Common sites include
    - Spleen
    - Liver
    - Bone
    - Kidney

IMAGING

Detection

- **General**
  - Choice of modality often depends on specific factors, such as anatomic location
    - Often palpable abnormality, such as lymphadenopathy, may be initially evaluated with CT
  - Lymphoma is frequently a systemic disease; patients are routinely evaluated with CT or PET/CT
    - Initial evaluation most often includes axial coverage from skull base through pelvis
- **Ultrasound**
  - Useful modality in initial evaluation of NHL for directing/guiding interventional diagnostic procedures
  - Evaluation of anatomic sites located superficially (i.e., neck, breast, axilla, extremities)
  - Will often see multiple, bilateral, nonnecrotic enlarged nodes
    - Despite large lymph node size, cystic necrosis is uncommon
  - Can also be used in assessment of spleen and kidneys
    - Right kidney may be imaged better than left kidney
- **Radiograph**
  - Fairly limited in overall assessment with some exceptions, such as pulmonary NHL
  - Cavitating lesions may mimic tuberculosis
  - Because radiographic features are nonspecific, can be confused for variety of other processes, particularly infectious etiologies
- **Mammography**
  - Can detect primary or metastatic NHL of breast
    - Primary lymphoma of breast is uncommon
  - Breast involvement appears as solitary mass without calcification
    - May also present with multiple masses, which makes differentiation of primary disease from metastatic disease impossible
    - Margins may be distinct or indistinct
- **CT**
  - NECT
    - Cannot distinguish etiology of enlarged lymph nodes on NECT and CECT
    - Can detect diffusely enlarged spleen but may miss focal lesions without contrast enhancement
  - CECT
    - Optimal modality for detection in addition to FDG PET (PET/CT)
    - Will more accurately depict lesions that may be missed on NECT, particularly when there is organ involvement
    - Typically, portal venous phase of imaging is sufficient

- Primary modality for overall evaluation of lymphoma
- Primary head and neck extranodal lymphoma
  - NHL imaging findings may be identical to squamous cell carcinoma of pharyngeal mucosal space
    - Can arise from tonsils, mandible, hard palate, nasopharynx, parotid glands, nasal cavity, paranasal sinuses, pharynx, larynx, thyroid gland, and ocular adnexa
    - Most common sites of occurrence in pharyngeal mucosal space: Faucial (palatine) tonsil > nasopharyngeal adenoids > lingual tonsil (i.e., Waldeyer ring)
  - Accounts for up to 20% of all NHL cases
- Thoracic lymphoma
  - CT and radiographs are primary modalities for evaluation of chest involvement
  - Radiologically, appearance of intrathoracic involvement in NHL may be similar to that of HL
  - Unlike HL, NHL is relatively evenly distributed in all mediastinal compartments, and posterior mediastinal lymphadenopathy is relatively common
  - CT can be used to evaluate for possible superior vena cava syndrome
- CT is also used to evaluate abdomen, pelvis, genitourinary tract, and gastrointestinal tract

- **MR**
  - Indicated for CNS imaging
  - Otherwise used as problem-solving tool
- **PET/CT**
  - Can be used for initial diagnosis or detection of lymphoma
    - For example, in patients with retroperitoneal adenopathy not easily accessible by percutaneous means
    - PET may be falsely negative for some cell types such as MALT, mantle cell lymphoma, and small lymphocytic lymphoma
  - Optimally performed with contrast-enhanced CT as part of exam
  - Increasingly important as an early response indicator to therapy
- **Nuclear medicine**
  - In general, PET/CT has replaced gallium-67 (Ga-67) for evaluating patients with lymphoma
  - Ga-67 sensitivity
    - Higher for more common histologic subtypes of low-grade NHL than for rare types
    - About equivalent for HL and high-grade NHL
- **Image-guided FNA**
  - Often CT- or ultrasound (US)-guided
    - With sufficient sample, sensitivity and specificity > 90-95% may be achieved
    - In certain diagnostic settings, core biopsy or open resection may be preferred to evaluate nodal architecture
  - Residual masses
    - Open procedures may be preferred over percutaneous procedure
      - Fibrotic tissue increases likelihood of false negatives

Staging

- **Nodal disease**
  - **Ultrasound**
    - Not often used for primary staging
    - Abnormal architecture in clinically suspected lymphadenopathy can establish presence of metastasis
    - US can be used to direct tissue sampling
  - **CT**
    - CECT used in detection of mediastinal nodes
      - NECT also capable of detection, but contrast facilitates measurement
      - Slice thickness between 5 and 10 mm generally sufficient to visualize chest nodes
      - Slight to moderate uniform enhancement following IV contrast, marked enhancement unusual (low attenuation in 20% of cases)
    - Calcification in affected lymph nodes prior to treatment is rarely seen
    - Lymphomatous masses more often encase and displace mediastinal structures than invade or constrict them
    - Retroperitoneal
      - Mantle of soft tissue adenopathy surrounding aorta and inferior vena cava
      - Nodes may displace aorta from spine (unusual for nodal mets not due to lymphoma)
      - Enlarged nodes (> 1.5 cm in short axis) involving bilateral retroperitoneal nodal chains
      - 25% of newly diagnosed HL patients have positive paraaortic nodes at presentation, compared to 50% with NHL
    - Abdominal
      - Involvement of peripancreatic nodes from NHL results in large peripancreatic mass (pancreatic lymphoma)
      - Involvement of mesenteric nodes more common with NHL (> 50%) than HL (< 5%)
      - Lymphoma (HL & NHL) arises in periportal areas due to high content of lymphatic tissue
  - **MR**
    - T1WI: Lymph nodes exhibit homogeneous low signal intensity (SI), similar to muscle
    - T2WI: Homogeneous high SI or areas of low SI (fibrotic tissue) and high SI (cystic degeneration or necrosis)
    - Usually mild enhancement post Gd-DTPA
- **Metastatic disease**
  - **General**
    - 30% of systemic lymphoma patients have skeletal involvement
      - Lytic, permeative bone destruction ± soft tissue mass
      - Vertebral involvement often spreads over multiple levels
      - May cross disc spaces
    - Epidural extension from adjacent vertebral/ paraspinous disease common
      - Best imaging tool: MR C+ fat-saturated T1WI
      - Epidural spread: Enhancing epidural mass ± vertebral involvement
      - Leptomeningitic spread: Smooth/nodular pial enhancement

- Intramedullary spread: Poorly defined enhancing mass
  - Peritoneum, mesentery, peritoneal ligaments
    - Omental caking, soft tissue implants on peritoneal surface are best diagnostic clues
  - Breast: Consider in differential of breast masses lacking typical features of breast carcinoma (e.g., spiculation and microcalcifications)
- **Ultrasound**
  - NHL of thyroid: Rapidly enlarging, solid, noncalcified thyroid mass in elderly woman with history of Hashimoto thyroiditis
    - Primary thyroid NHL is defined as extranodal, extralymphatic lymphoma that arises from thyroid gland
- **CT**
  - Most common manifestation is lymphadenopathy that may involve nodes above &/or below diaphragm
  - Infiltrative involvement of liver, spleen, and bone marrow may not be accurately detected with CT
    - Organomegaly is poor predictor of tumor involvement
    - ~ 30% of patients with splenic enlargement do not have malignant involvement
    - Sensitivity: 15-37% for infiltrative splenic disease and 19-33% for infiltrative liver disease
  - Liver metastases present as lobulated low-density masses
  - Ascites, nodular thickening/enhancement of peritoneum, hypovascular omental masses on CECT
- **MR**
  - Potentially superior to CT in evaluating
    - Small adrenal masses
    - Hepatic tumors
    - Renal tumors
    - Pelvic organs
    - Vertebral lesions, particularly when vertebral collapse has occurred
    - Superior vena cava syndrome and other venous obstructions when iodinated contrast is contraindicated
    - Thoracic wall invasion
- **PET/CT**
  - Baseline PET/CT should be considered for all newly diagnosed NHL and HL patients
    - Contrast enhancement for CT portion is preferable or separate CECT
  - High-grade NHL: Multiple enlarged lymph nodes or nodal groups with intense FDG activity ± splenic/other organ involvement
    - Splenic involvement better assessed with PET/CT than with CT alone
  - Low-grade NHL: Enlarged lymph nodes, extranodal mass with low to intense FDG uptake
    - Considerable heterogeneity may be seen between lesions of same histologic subtype
    - Overlap between tumor grades is not uncommon
  - Marked FDG uptake may represent high-grade transformation in patients with low-grade lymphomas
  - Infiltrative osseous involvement may show diffuse uptake greater than that of liver
    - PET can be used to direct bone marrow biopsy to most metabolically active sites
  - Upstaging of extranodal disease observed mostly in stages I and II disease
  - Chronic/small cell lymphocytic lymphoma (CLL/SLL): PET of limited use in staging secondary to ↓ FDG uptake (sensitivity [58%])
    - SUV > 3.5 suggests Richter transformation of CLL/SLL → DLBCL (sensitivity [91%], specificity [80%], PPV [53%], NPV [97%])
  - Marginal zone lymphoma (MZL): FDG PET staging sensitivity (71%) (lower for extranodal)
    - Most common sites of involvement on PET/CT are stomach, lung, orbit, and parotid gland
  - MALT lymphoma: Typically no or low FDG uptake; SUV > 3.5 suggests plasmacytic differentiation
  - Cutaneous T-cell lymphoma (CTCL): FDG PET useful in staging
    - CTCL: Intense nodal sites suspicious for large cell transformation
  - Follicular lymphoma (FL): FDG PET useful in staging all grades (sensitivity [94%], specificity [100%])
    - Wide overlap between FDG uptake by lower (SUV 2.3-13) and higher grade (SUV 3.2-43) FL
    - Emergence of sites of ↑ FDG uptake (SUV > 10): Transformation to higher grade (specificity [81%])
  - Brown fat is common pitfall
    - Young adults who have been exposed to cold environment may demonstrate brown fat uptake on PET
    - Often manifests as symmetric high uptake in suboccipital, cervical, supraclavicular, mediastinal, and paraspinal areas
  - As many as 100% of patients with positive PET scan after chemotherapy have early relapse, while in > 80% of patients with negative PET, long-term remission occurs
- **Nuclear medicine**
  - PET and Ga-67 for HL
    - Should be performed prior to treatment for initial staging, as 1 dose of chemotherapy may decrease uptake/sensitivity
    - Focal uptake more specific than diffuse uptake
    - Abnormally increased uptake in spleen or liver

Restaging

- **General**
  - **Ultrasound**
    - Limited utility for restaging
  - **CT**
    - Conventional imaging modalities, such as CT and MR, can demonstrate only a decrease in lesion size, and findings are poor predictors of clinical outcome after treatment for lymphoma
      - On long-term follow-up, < 50% of patients with positive CT findings have disease relapse or other evidence of residual tumor
    - Patients with infiltrative marrow involvement have no bone destruction and are usually asymptomatic; their lesions may be difficult to detect on CT
      - To be detected on CT, osseous involvement must be focal and associated with bone destruction

- Isolated chest wall lesions without direct extension can occur, especially in cases of recurrence
  - **MR**
    - Superior for imaging of CNS
    - Otherwise used as problem-solving tool
  - **PET/CT**
    - Excellent for predicting prognosis in aggressive NHL and HL after therapy
      - Usefulness of follow-up scan hinges on existence of pretherapy scan indicating FDG-avid disease
    - Can be positive months before histological confirmation of asymptomatic relapse
      - Especially for DLBCL patients
    - Absence of metabolic activity on FDG PET following treatment has high predictive value for disease-free survival (DFS)
    - Persistent metabolic activity on FDG PET following treatment has moderate predictive value for recurrence
    - G-CSF and recombinant erythropoietin can result in diffusely increased FDG uptake in bone marrow and spleen, limiting sensitivity
      - Uptake due to growth factors usually returns to baseline by 1 month post therapy
    - Chemotherapy can cause marrow hyperplasia and also generalized FDG uptake
    - FDG PET demonstrates poor sensitivity for predicting likelihood of response/progression in patients with indolent lymphoma
    - Allow for treatment of residual/progressive disease before it spreads further
    - HL: Residual masses after treatment may not represent active disease; PET aids in differentiating
    - In patients with lymphoma, 30-64% have residual mass after completion of therapy
      - FDG accumulates in viable tumor but not in fibrotic or necrotic tissue
    - High FDG uptake is associated with high proliferation rate
      - Higher SUV of diffuse large B-cell lesion → worse prognosis
- **Nuclear medicine**
  - Ga-67 scintigraphy
    - Ga-67-citrate less sensitive and specific than FDG PET for aggressive lymphoma
    - Useful in differentiating residual mediastinal disease from post-treatment fibrosis
    - Can be used to monitor responses to treatment
    - Sensitivity of 85% for high-grade NHL
    - Sensitivity is poor for low-grade NHL
    - Sarcoid anterior mediastinal lymphadenopathy may also show uptake

CLINICAL PRESENTATION & WORK-UP

Presentation

- Non-Hodgkin and Hodgkin lymphoma most commonly present with peripheral lymphadenopathy (> 2/3 of cases)
  - Rapid, progressive enlargement of nodes is associated with aggressive NHL
  - Waxing and waning of nodes is associated with indolent lymphomas
    - Nodes may completely disappear and reappear
- Low-grade lymphoma
  - Peripheral adenopathy (most common presentation)
    - Painless
    - Slowly progressive
  - Enlarged lymph nodes spontaneously regress
    - May clinically be confused with infectious etiology
  - Bone marrow involvement
    - Cytopenia
  - Physical exam findings
    - Peripheral adenopathy
    - Splenomegaly
      - Seen in 40% of patients
      - Uncommon for spleen to be sole site of involvement at presentation
    - Hepatomegaly
  - Uncommon presentations
    - Primary extranodal involvement
    - B symptoms
      - Fever: Unexplained temperature > 38° C
      - Drenching night sweats
      - Unexplained weight loss > 10% of baseline in past 6 months
    - Fatigue
    - Weakness
    - Pruritus
    - Alcohol intolerance
- Intermediate- and high-grade lymphomas
  - Presentation often varies
  - Adenopathy
    - Bulky retroperitoneal lymphadenopathy may result in secondary obstructive hydronephrosis
  - Extranodal involvement
    - Seen in > 1/3 of patients
    - Common locations of extranodal involvement include
      - GI tract
      - Skin
      - Bone marrow
      - Sinuses
      - GU tract
      - Thyroid
      - CNS
      - Lung
      - Liver
  - B symptoms are more common than in low-grade lymphomas (30-40%)
  - Lymphoblastic lymphoma typically presents with
    - Large mass in abdomen
    - Bowel obstruction symptoms
  - Physical exam findings
    - Lymphadenopathy that grows rapidly and is bulky in nature
    - Splenomegaly
    - Hepatomegaly
    - Large mass in abdomen (usually seen in Burkitt lymphoma)
    - Testicular mass
    - Skin lesions
      - Associated with cutaneous T-cell lymphoma (mycosis fungoides), anaplastic large cell lymphoma, angioimmunoblastic lymphoma

Prognosis

- NHL can be categorized into 2 prognostic groups
  - Indolent lymphomas
  - Aggressive lymphomas
  - This division is important in therapeutic decision making as well
- Risk factors in International Prognostic Index (IPI)
  - Age ≥ 60 years
  - Ann Arbor stages III or IV
  - Elevated LDH
  - Eastern Cooperative Oncology Group (ECOG) performance status ≥ 2
    - Grade 0: Fully active, able to carry on all pre-disease performance without restriction
    - Grade 1: Restricted in physically strenuous activity but ambulatory and able to carry out work of a light or sedentary nature, e.g., light housework, office work
    - Grade 2: Ambulatory and capable of all self-care but unable to carry out any work activities
      - Up and about for > 50% of waking hours
    - Grade 3: Capable of only limited self-care, confined to bed or chair for > 50% of waking hours
    - Grade 4: Completely disabled, cannot carry on any self-care, totally confined to bed or chair
    - Grade 5: Dead
  - > 1 extranodal site
- 5-year overall survival (OS) and relapse-free status
  - 0-1 IPI risk factors: 75%
  - 2-3 IPI risk factors: 50%
  - 4-5 IPI risk factors: 25%

Work-Up

- Clinical
  - H&P with attention to B symptoms, alcohol intolerance, pruritus, fatigue, performance status
  - Bone marrow biopsy for HL stages IB-IV
  - PFTs depending on regimen
  - Evaluation of ejection fraction for doxorubicin-containing regimens
  - Fertility counseling, smoking cessation
    - Semen cryopreservation; or IVF, ovarian tissue, or oocyte cryopreservation
  - Pneumococcal, H-flu, meningococcal vaccines in select histologies, particularly if spleen is being irradiated
  - Hepatitis panel in many NHL diagnoses
- Radiographic
  - PET/CT preferred in most cases, CECT in others
  - Consider chest x-ray for HL, and head and neck CECT in select cases
- Laboratory
  - CBC, ESR, LDH, LFT, albumin, chemistries, pregnancy test, HIV test if risk factors
  - Excisional or core biopsy
  - Other labs depending on specific diagnosis

TREATMENT

Major Treatment Alternatives

- NHL
  - Radiation therapy
    - Organ involvement: Include whole organ (i.e., whole stomach in gastric MALT or total unilateral parotid)
    - Bone treated with margin, whole bone not necessary
      - MR may be useful in many bone cases
    - Involved field is most appropriate; regional or extended fields not usually recommended
    - Often follows chemotherapy (e.g., DLBCL)
      - In post-chemo setting, treat post-chemo volume in transverse diameter for mediastinum, abdomen, and pelvis
    - Margins influenced by the quality of imaging and clinical information
  - Chemotherapy
    - Most common modality
      - Disseminated lymphomas often cured
    - Many regimens depending on diagnosis
  - Immunotherapy
    - Monoclonal antibodies, such as rituximab and Campath-1H
    - Interferon therapy (not widely used in United States but more common in Europe)

Major Treatment Roadblocks/ Contraindications

- NHL
  - Cardiotoxicity with anthracyclines
  - Therapy-induced malignancies (e.g., AML from etoposide)
  - Immunosuppression
  - Anemia, thrombocytopenia, and neutropenia
  - Radiation-induced secondary malignancies not seen overall in NHL patients
    - Present in young patients only

Treatment Options by Stage

- NHL
  - RT
    - Used solely in early stage (I/II) low-grade NHL
    - Consolidation in aggressive histologies post chemo
    - Effective for palliation
  - Chemotherapy
    - Used with curative intent in most settings
    - Low-grade lymphomas (follicular) stage III/IV
      - Chemo frequently held until symptoms appear
    - High-dose chemotherapy and stem cell rescue used often in relapsed setting
- HL
  - RT
    - Consolidation post chemo except in limited stage NLPHD
    - RT can be used alone in rare cases where morbidity or age precludes chemotherapy
  - Chemotherapy
    - Initial therapy most often
    - Regimens include ABVD, Stanford V, BEACOPP, and others

Dose Response

- Local control 58% at 20 Gy, 74% at 25 Gy, 93% at 30 Gy, and 97% for 31-40 Gy for RT alone in HL

Standard Doses

- NHL

- Follicular NHL: 24-30 Gy
- MALT NHL: Stomach 30 Gy, other organs 24-30 Gy
- Early stage mantle NHL: 30 Gy
- Consolidation for DLBCL
  - CR to chemo: 30-36 Gy
  - PR to chemo: 40-50 Gy
- Palliation for advanced-stage low-grade NHL 2 x 2 Gy
- HL
  - Nonbulky stage I/II
    - ABVD: 20-30 Gy
    - Stanford V: 30 Gy
  - Bulky sites (all stages)
    - ABVD: 30-36 Gy
    - Stanford V: 36 Gy
  - RT alone for NLPHD
    - Involved regions: 30-36 Gy
    - Uninvolved regions: 25-30 Gy

Common Techniques

- AP/PA is often a good method to treat midline structures
- Shrinking field techniques should be used to limit lung and cardiac dose

Landmark Trials

- Aggressive NHL
  - SWOG 8736: CHOP x 8 vs. CHOP x 3 + RT (40 Gy + 10 Gy boost); ↑ OS with CHOP + RT and ↓ cardiac morbidity
  - ECOG: CHOP x 8 vs. CHOP x 8 + RT (CR randomized to ± 30 Gy, PR given 40 Gy), ↑ DFS, no difference in OS
  - GELA LN93-4: CHOP x 4 vs. CHOP x 4 + RT (40 Gy); no difference in OS
  - GELA LN93-1: CHOP x 3 + RT vs. ACVBP; OS ↑ with ACVBP, complicated regimen, not widely adopted
  - GELA LNH03-2B: ACVBP-R vs. CHOP-R; ↑ OS and ↑ PFS with ACVBP-R, ↑ in adverse events with ACVBP-R arm
  - Mexico (residual): ± RT for residual disease (< 5 cm) after CHOP, ↑ OS with RT
  - Mexico (Waldeyer): Stage I NHL of Waldeyer ring: Randomized to chemo, CRT, or RT, ↑ OS with RT
  - Mexico (stage IV): ± RT for patients with stage IV, ↑ OS with RT
- HL
  - HD4: EFRT 40 Gy vs. EFRT 30 Gy; 30 Gy adequate for uninvolved sites
  - SWOG S9133: Subtotal lymphoid irradiation (STLI) vs. STLI + doxo, vinblastine, CRT superior to STLI
  - EORTCH8: Favorable disease, chemo x 3 + IFRT best; unfavorable disease, chemo x 4 + IFRT best
  - German HD7: RT vs. ABVD x 2 + RT, CRT better
  - HD10: Favorable disease, ABVD x 2 or 4 and IFRT 20 Gy or 30 Gy (2 x 2); ABVD x 2 and 20 Gy is the new standard

RECOMMENDED FOLLOW-UP

Clinical

- H&P every 3 months for years 1-2, then 3-6 months for years 2-5, then annually for > 5 years
- HL after 5 years
  - Pneumococcal revaccination after 5 years
  - Meningococcal and H-flu vaccines in select cases
  - Annual influenza vaccine in high-risk cases (e.g., thoracic RT, bleomycin)

Radiographic

- Chest imaging (x-ray or CT) every 6-12 months for years 1-5, consider abdominal/pelvic CT for years 1-3
- PET/CT: Beware of false positives; clinical decisions should not be made on PET findings alone
- In HL for late-effect monitoring
  - Mammograms and MR 8 years post treatment or at age 40, whichever comes first
  - Consider chest CT in patients at risk for lung cancer (e.g., thoracic RT or smoking history)

Laboratory

- CBC, ESR, TSH if high thoracic or neck RT
- HL after 5 years
  - Lipid panel

SELECTED REFERENCES

1. Bakst R et al: Radiation therapy for chloroma (granulocytic sarcoma). Int J Radiat Oncol Biol Phys. 82(5):1816-22, 2012
2. Hoppe RT et al: Hodgkin lymphoma. J Natl Compr Canc Netw. 9(9):1020-58, 2011
3. Récher C et al: Intensified chemotherapy with ACVBP plus rituximab versus standard CHOP plus rituximab for the treatment of diffuse large B-cell lymphoma (LNH03-2B): an open-label randomised phase 3 trial. Lancet. 378(9806):1858-67, 2011
4. Zelenetz AD et al: Non-Hodgkin's lymphomas. J Natl Compr Canc Netw. 9(5):484-560, 2011
5. American Joint Committee on Cancer: AJCC Cancer Staging Manual. 7th ed. New York: Springer. 599-615, 2010
6. Engert A et al: Reduced treatment intensity in patients with early-stage Hodgkin's lymphoma. N Engl J Med. 363(7):640-52, 2010
7. Aiken AH et al: Imaging Hodgkin and non-Hodgkin lymphoma in the head and neck. Radiol Clin North Am. 46(2):363-78, ix-x, 2008
8. Allen-Auerbach M et al: The impact of fluorodeoxyglucose-positron emission tomography in primary staging and patient management in lymphoma patients. Radiol Clin North Am. 46(2):199-211, vii, 2008
9. Anis M et al: Imaging of abdominal lymphoma. Radiol Clin North Am. 46(2):265-85, viii-ix, 2008
10. Bae YA et al: Cross-sectional evaluation of thoracic lymphoma. Radiol Clin North Am. 46(2):253-64, viii, 2008
11. Iagaru A et al: Perspectives of molecular imaging and radioimmunotherapy in lymphoma. Radiol Clin North Am. 46(2):243-52, viii, 2008
12. Kwee TC et al: Imaging in staging of malignant lymphoma: a systematic review. Blood. 111(2):504-16, 2008
13. Lee WK et al: Abdominal manifestations of extranodal lymphoma: spectrum of imaging findings. AJR Am J Roentgenol. 191(1):198-206, 2008
14. Matasar MJ et al: Overview of lymphoma diagnosis and management. Radiol Clin North Am. 46(2):175-98, vii, 2008
15. Bar-Shalom R: Normal and abnormal patterns of 18F-fluorodeoxyglucose PET/CT in lymphoma. Radiol Clin North Am. 45(4):677-88, vi-vii, 2007
16. Bonnet C et al: CHOP alone compared with CHOP plus radiotherapy for localized aggressive lymphoma in elderly patients: a study by the Groupe d'Etude des Lymphomes de l'Adulte. J Clin Oncol. 25(7):787-92, 2007
17. Engert A et al: Two cycles of doxorubicin, bleomycin, vinblastine, and dacarbazine plus extended-field radiotherapy is superior to radiotherapy alone in early

favorable Hodgkin's lymphoma: final results of the GHSG HD7 trial. J Clin Oncol. 25(23):3495-502, 2007
18. Even-Sapir E et al: Fluorine-18 fluorodeoxyglucose PET/CT patterns of extranodal involvement in patients with Non-Hodgkin lymphoma and Hodgkin's disease. Radiol Clin North Am. 45(4):697-709, vii, 2007
19. Fermé C et al: Chemotherapy plus involved-field radiation in early-stage Hodgkin's disease. N Engl J Med. 357(19):1916-27, 2007
20. Margolis DJ et al: Molecular imaging techniques in body imaging. Radiology. 245(2):333-56, 2007
21. Podoloff DA et al: PET and PET/CT in management of the lymphomas. Radiol Clin North Am. 45(4):689-96, vii, 2007
22. Seam P et al: The role of FDG-PET scans in patients with lymphoma. Blood. 110(10):3507-16, 2007
23. Avilés A et al: Residual disease after chemotherapy in aggressive malignant lymphoma: the role of radiotherapy. Med Oncol. 22(4):383-7, 2005
24. Isasi CR et al: A metaanalysis of 18F-2-deoxy-2-fluoro-D-glucose positron emission tomography in the staging and restaging of patients with lymphoma. Cancer. 104(5):1066-74, 2005
25. Reyes F et al: ACVBP versus CHOP plus radiotherapy for localized aggressive lymphoma. N Engl J Med. 352(12):1197-205, 2005
26. Avilés A et al: Adjuvant radiotherapy in stage IV diffuse large cell lymphoma improves outcome. Leuk Lymphoma. 45(7):1385-9, 2004
27. Horning SJ et al: Chemotherapy with or without radiotherapy in limited-stage diffuse aggressive non-Hodgkin's lymphoma: Eastern Cooperative Oncology Group study 1484. J Clin Oncol. 22(15):3032-8, 2004
28. Kumar R et al: Utility of fluorodeoxyglucose-PET imaging in the management of patients with Hodgkin's and non-Hodgkin's lymphomas. Radiol Clin North Am. 42(6):1083-100, 2004
29. Israel O et al: Clinical pretreatment risk factors and Ga-67 scintigraphy early during treatment for prediction of outcome of patients with aggressive non-Hodgkin lymphoma. Cancer. 94(4):873-8, 2002
30. Kostakoglu L et al: Comparison of fluorine-18 fluorodeoxyglucose positron emission tomography and Ga-67 scintigraphy in evaluation of lymphoma. Cancer. 94(4):879-88, 2002
31. Buchmann I et al: 2-(fluorine-18)fluoro-2-deoxy-D-glucose positron emission tomography in the detection and staging of malignant lymphoma. A bicenter trial. Cancer. 91(5):889-99, 2001
32. Dühmke E et al: Low-dose radiation is sufficient for the noninvolved extended-field treatment in favorable early-stage Hodgkin's disease: long-term results of a randomized trial of radiotherapy alone. J Clin Oncol. 19(11):2905-14, 2001
33. Press OW et al: Phase III randomized intergroup trial of subtotal lymphoid irradiation versus doxorubicin, vinblastine, and subtotal lymphoid irradiation for stage IA to IIA Hodgkin's disease. J Clin Oncol. 19(22):4238-44, 2001
34. Miller TP et al: Chemotherapy alone compared with chemotherapy plus radiotherapy for localized intermediate- and high-grade non-Hodgkin's lymphoma. N Engl J Med. 339(1):21-6, 1998
35. Avilés A et al: Treatment of non-Hodgkin's lymphoma of Waldeyer's ring: radiotherapy versus chemotherapy versus combined therapy. Eur J Cancer B Oral Oncol. 32B(1):19-23, 1996

(**Left**) *Graphic shows lymph node regions. The white regions (neck, infraclavicular, axillary, hilar, epitrochlear, iliac, and inguinal/femoral) are paired structures. It is helpful to indicate the number of involved regions with a subscript when staging.* (**Right**) *Coronal graphic depicts an involved field treatment border in yellow → and an involved node treatment in light blue ↷. With more intensive systemic treatment, involved node treatment may be a reasonable option.*

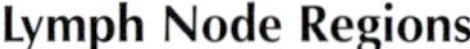

Lymph Node Regions

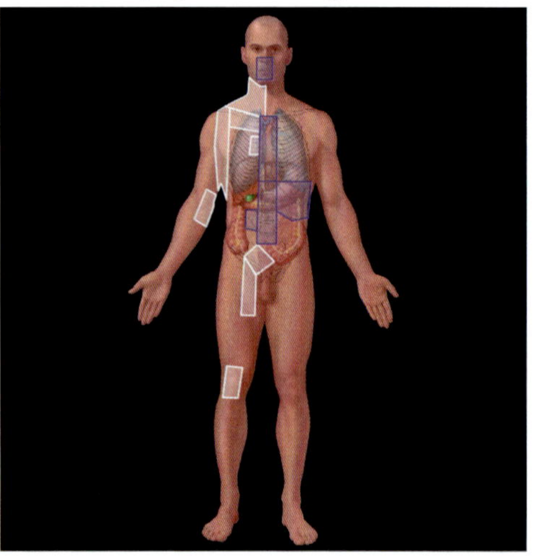

Involved Field vs. Involved Node

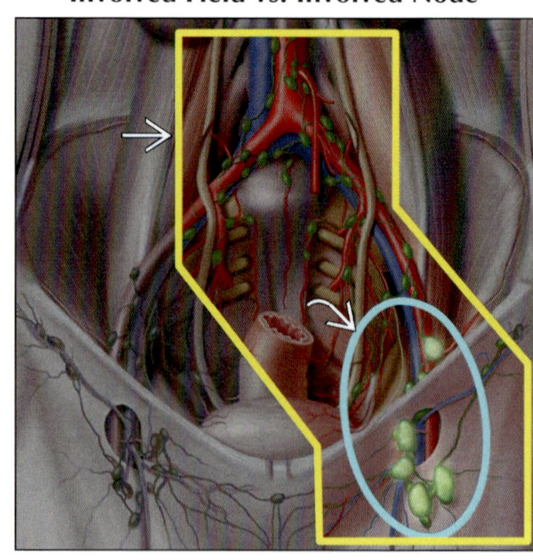

(**Left**) *Sagittal PET/CT shows FDG avidity involving the paraaortic region ⇨. Lymphadenopathy was incidentally observed on CT.* (**Right**) *FNA CT-guided biopsy in the same patient of a retroperitoneal lymph node ⇨ showed that atypical lymphocytes and malignancy could not be excluded. Open biopsy was performed, and pathology showed lymphocyte-predominant (LP) Hodgkin lymphoma. Early stage LP Hodgkin lymphoma is well treated with localized RT.*

Stage IA LP Hodgkin Lymphoma

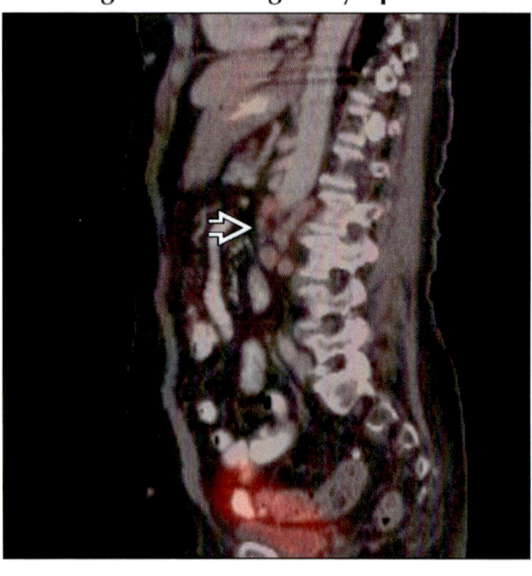

Stage IA LP Hodgkin Lymphoma

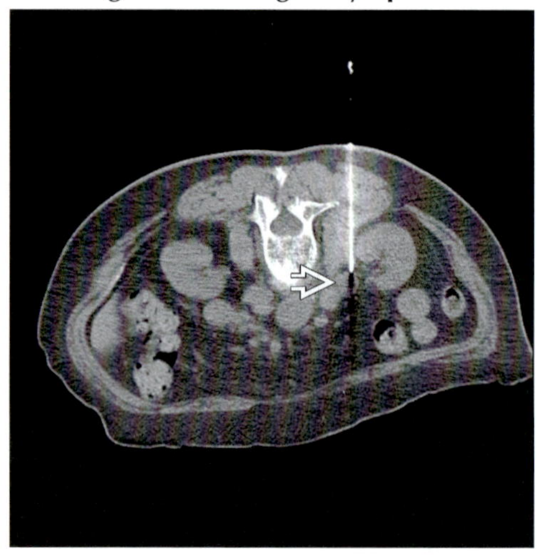

(**Left**) *Axial CT in the same patient shows colorwash diagram of 4-field treatment. Beam angles were chosen to minimize kidney dose. Red, green, and blue are covered by the 30 Gy, 20 Gy, and 10 Gy isodose surface, respectively. Patient was treated to 30.6 Gy in 17 fractions.* (**Right**) *Coronal CT in the same patient shows colorwash with outlined CTV →. Follow-up PET/CT was normal. LP HL can relapse late and hence patients should receive prolonged follow-up care.*

Stage IA LP Hodgkin Lymphoma

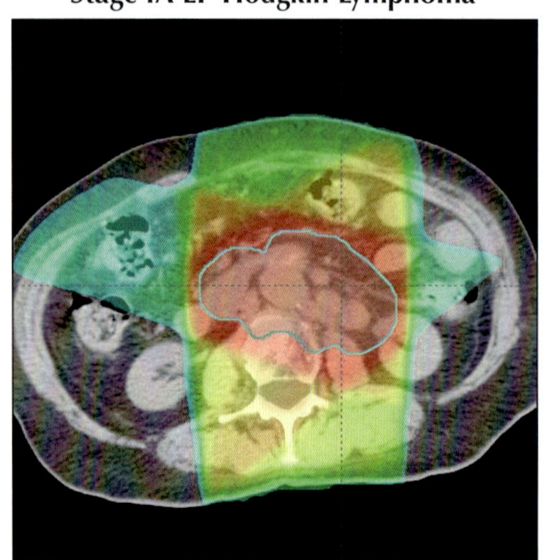

Stage IA LP Hodgkin Lymphoma

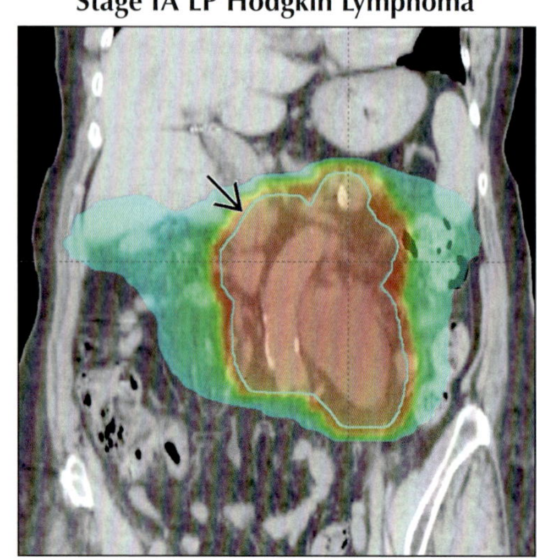

Stage IE

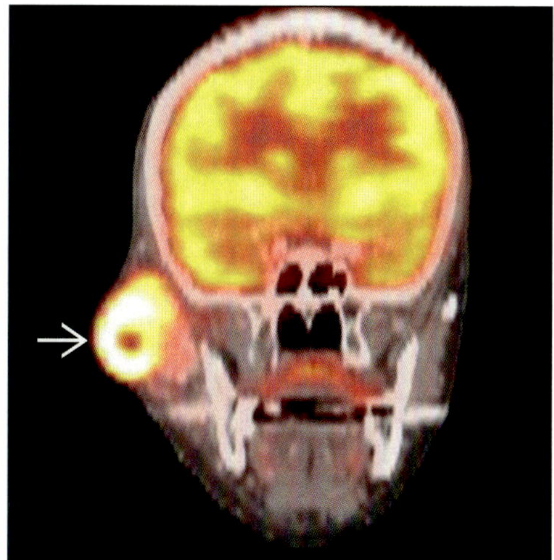

Stage IA DLBCL

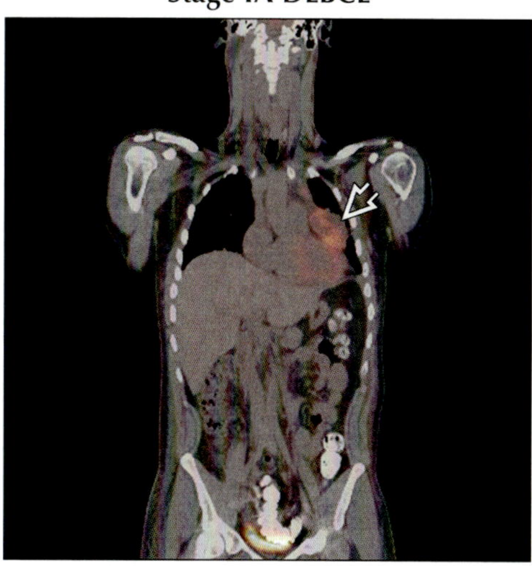

(Left) *Coronal fused PET/CT shows intense FDG activity ➡ in the right parotid mass, compatible with a high-grade lymphoma. CT revealed that the parotid mass had a necrotic center.* ***(Right)*** *Fused PET/CT in a young man with anterior mediastinal lymphoma shows heterogeneous uptake in the mass ➡. Chamberlain procedure showed diffuse large B-cell lymphoma (DLBCL). He was treated with R-CHOP x 3 and had a complete response by PET criteria prior to RT.*

Stage IA DLBCL

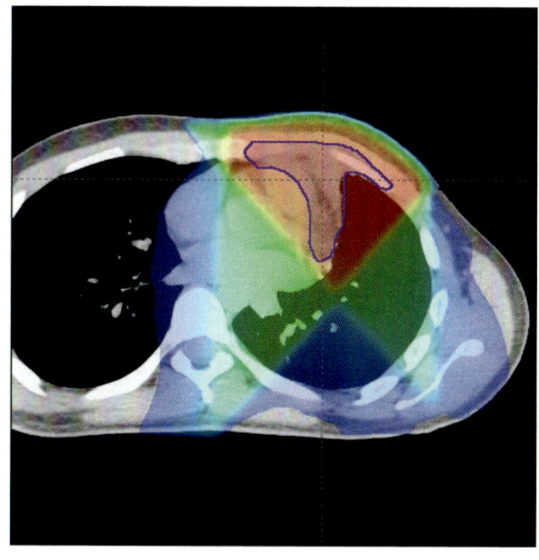

Stage IA DLBCL

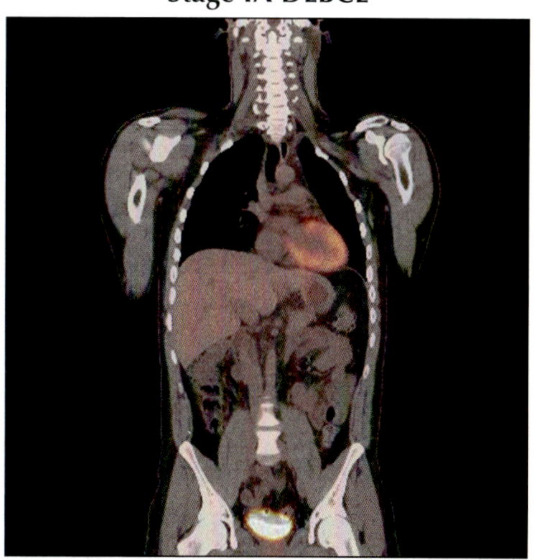

(Left) *It is customary to treat AP/PA; however, axial CT in same patient shows that a wedge pair was used in this case due to the anterior location of the lymphadenopathy and to decrease dose to heart and lung. The red, green, and blue represent the 36 Gy, 22 Gy, and 6 Gy lines, respectively.* ***(Right)*** *Follow-up coronal PET/CT in the same patient shows that he remains free of disease after chemotherapy and 36 Gy in 20 fractions.*

Cutaneous B-Cell Lymphoma

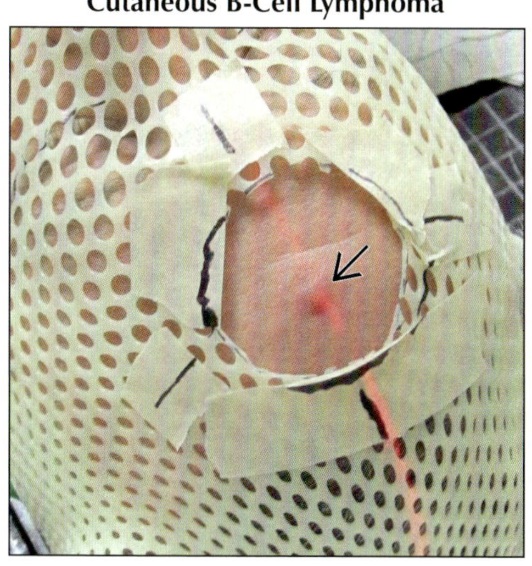

Stage IA Mycosis Fungoides

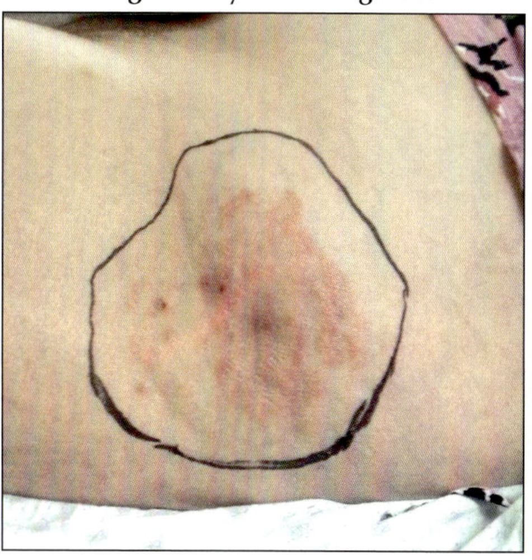

(Left) *Violaceous solitary cutaneous B-cell lymphoma ➡ is shown at simulation. A generous margin is used since these have a tendency to recur locally.* ***(Right)*** *This isolated erythematous plaque was shown to be mycosis fungoides (MF) on biopsy. The raised and scaly mass is typical of MF lesions. A generous 2 cm margin was used. Bolus is essential in treating these cases.*

LYMPHOMA

Stage IA DLBCL

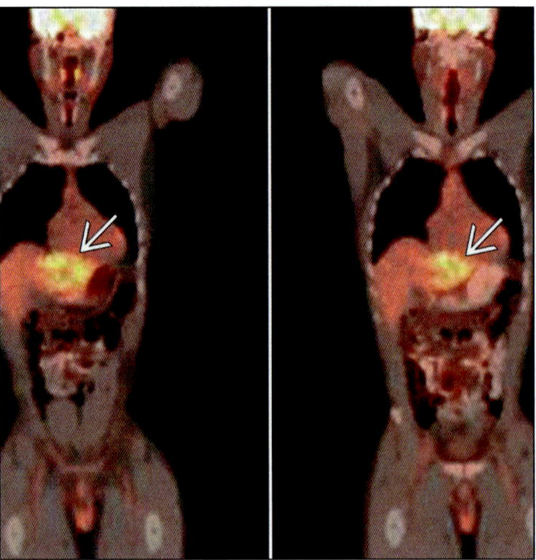

Stage IA DLBCL

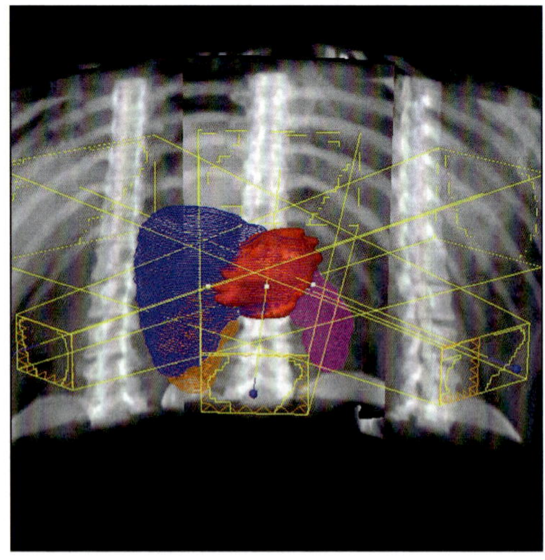

(Left) *Coronal PET/CT reveals marked avidity of the left hepatic lobe ➔. Biopsy showed diffuse large B-cell lymphoma. The patient was treated with R-CHOP and had a complete response.* ***(Right)*** *In the same patient, a 3-field technique was used, all from the anterior direction. The right hepatic lobe is shown in blue, and the PTV (left hepatic lobe) is shown in red. The kidneys are shown in orange and pink.*

Stage IA DLBCL

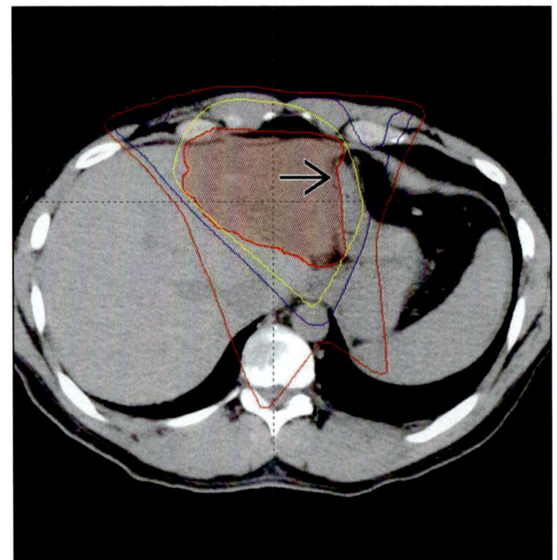

Stage IA DLBCL

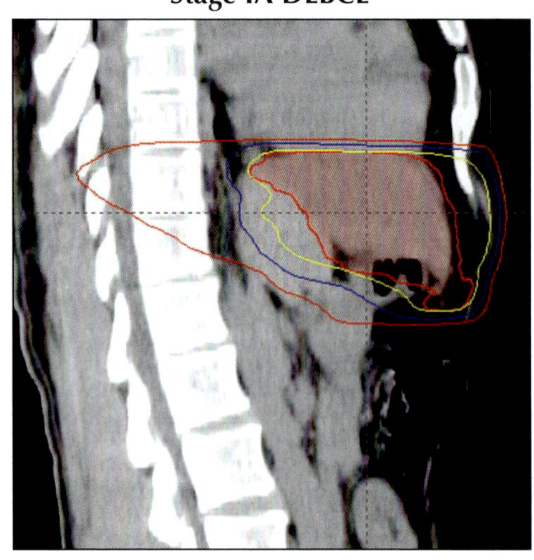

(Left) *Axial CT in the same patient shows the PTV in red ➔. The yellow, blue, and red lines indicate the 95%, 70%, and 40% isodose lines, respectively.* ***(Right)*** *Sagittal CT in the same patient shows reduced dose to posterior structures with this 3-field approach for this anterior hepatic NHL.*

Stage IS

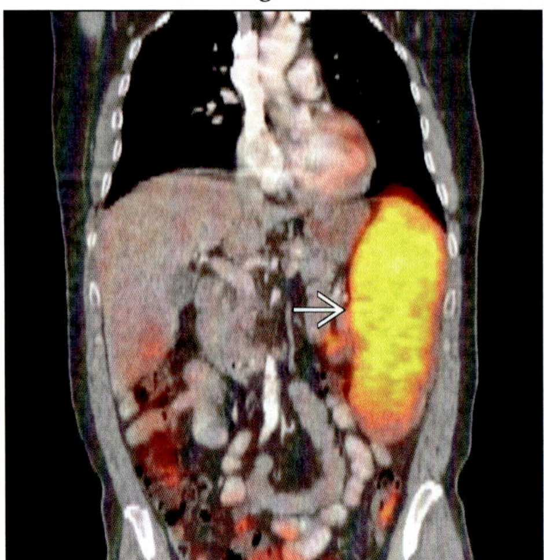

Stage IS

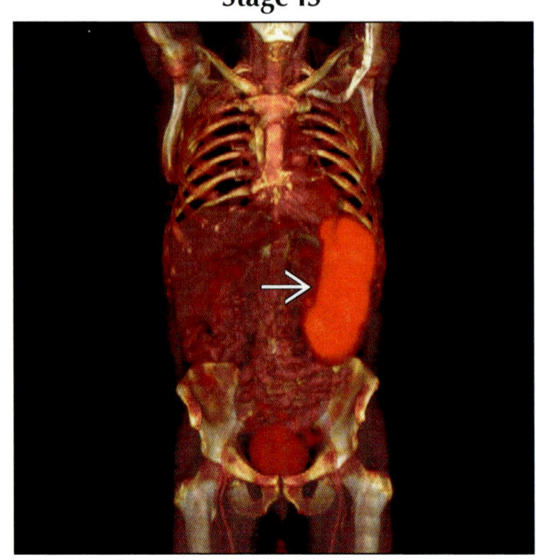

(Left) *Coronal fused PET/CT in the same patient shows marked craniocaudal enlargement of the spleen ➔. Although rare, non-Hodgkin lymphoma with only splenic involvement is considered stage IS.* ***(Right)*** *Coronal fused PET/CT volumetric reconstruction in the same patient shows relative hypermetabolism in the spleen ➔ compared to the remaining structures, a finding suggestive of a high-grade lymphoma.*

Stage I

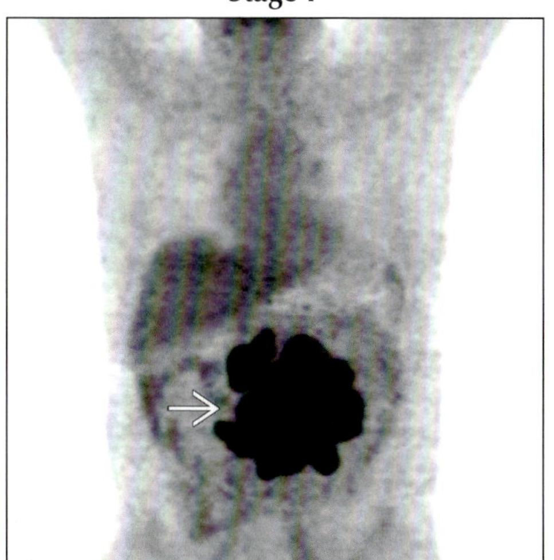

Stage I

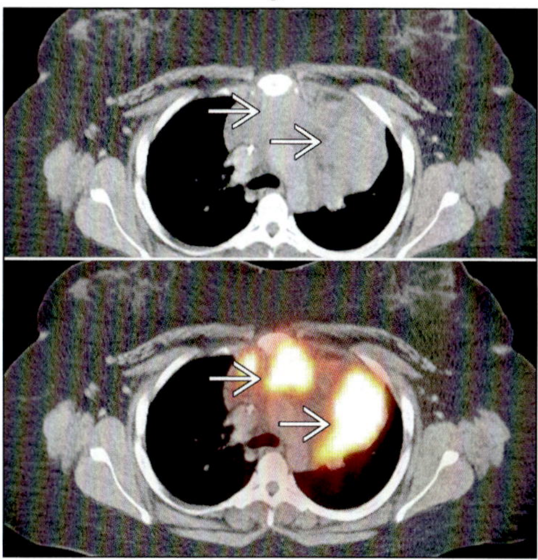

(Left) *Coronal PET shows an example of stage I lymphoma with a large cluster of hypermetabolic mesenteric lymph nodes ➔ but no other lymph node regions involved and no disease above the diaphragm.* ***(Right)*** *Axial CECT and fused PET/CT show a hypermetabolic soft tissue mass ➔ in the anterior mediastinum, compatible with stage I non-Hodgkin lymphoma. Involvement of a single lymph node region or lymphatic structure, such as the thymus, is considered stage I.*

Stage II

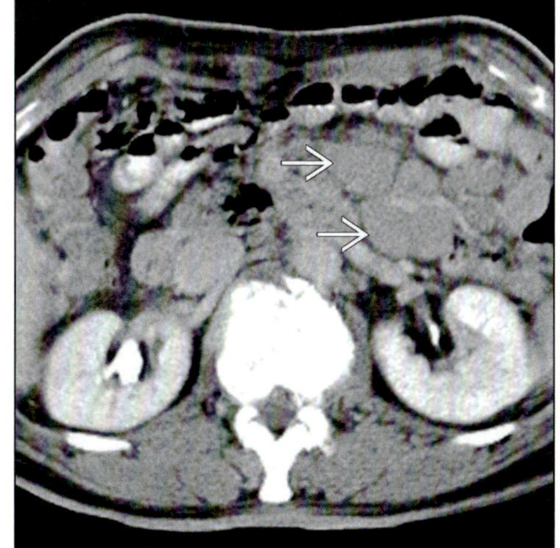

Stage II

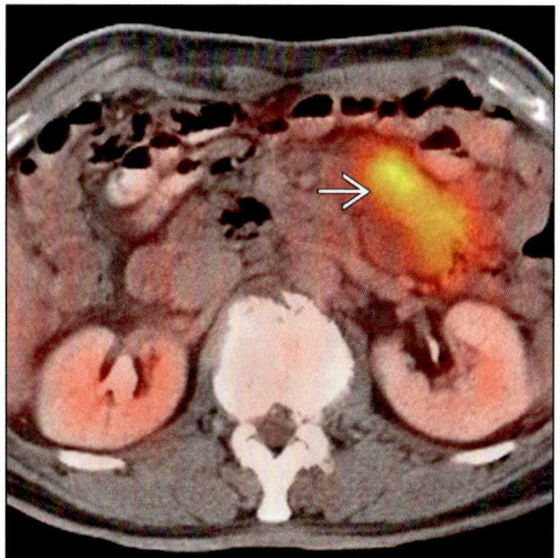

(Left) *Axial CECT shows extensive bulky mesenteric adenopathy ➔ in this patient with newly diagnosed non-Hodgkin lymphoma. The patient had additional areas of adenopathy beneath the diaphragm, compatible with stage II disease.* ***(Right)*** *Axial fused PET/CT in the same patient shows intense FDG activity ➔ corresponding to the mesenteric adenopathy and compatible with a high-grade lymphoma.*

Stage II, Post Treatment

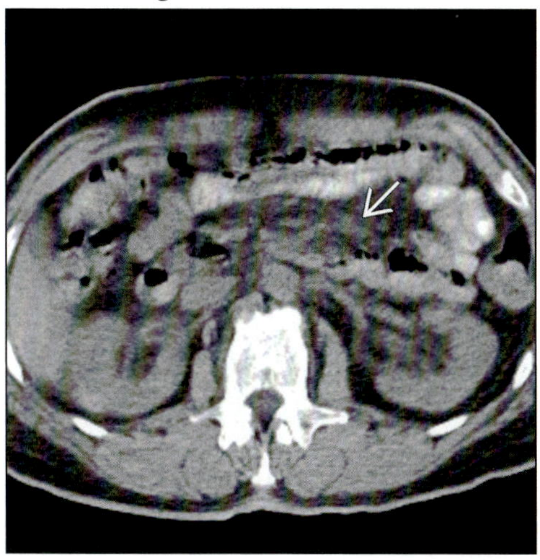

Stage II, Post Treatment

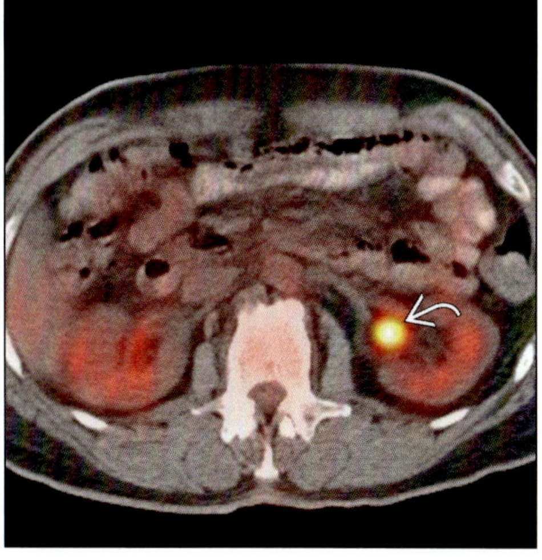

(Left) *Axial NECT in the same patient following chemotherapy shows a marked response to therapy with almost complete resolution ➔ of the abnormal lymph nodes seen in the small bowel mesentery.* ***(Right)*** *Axial fused PET/CT in the same patient shows no residual metabolic activity, compatible with a complete metabolic response. Normal FDG excretion ➔ should not be confused with pathologic uptake. PET/CT is increasingly being used to assess early response to chemotherapy.*

LYMPHOMA

Stage II

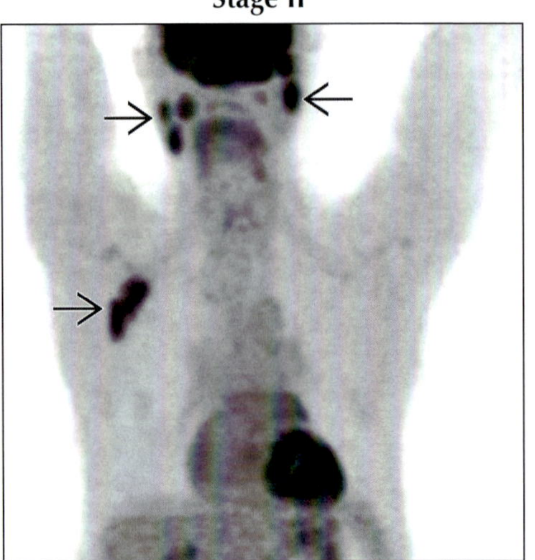

Stage II

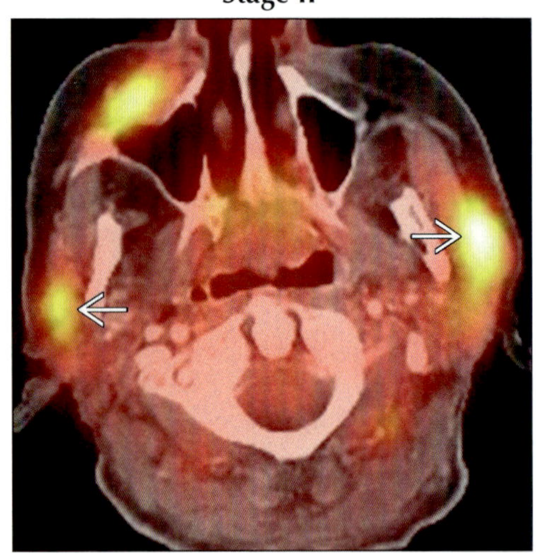

(Left) *Coronal PET shows bilateral cervical hypermetabolic adenopathy ➔ as well as abnormal nodes in the right axillary region, compatible with stage II non-Hodgkin lymphoma.* ***(Right)*** *Axial fused PET/CT demonstrates areas of hypermetabolism ➔ corresponding to enlarged nodes on the CT portion of the exam (not shown) and compatible with the patient's history of newly diagnosed follicular lymphoma.*

Stage IIE

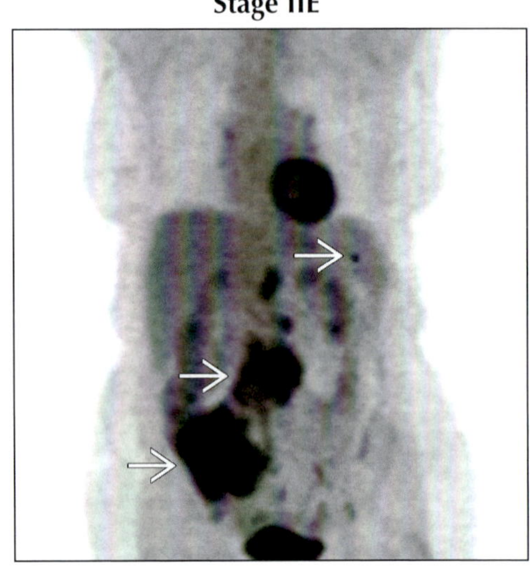

Stage IIE

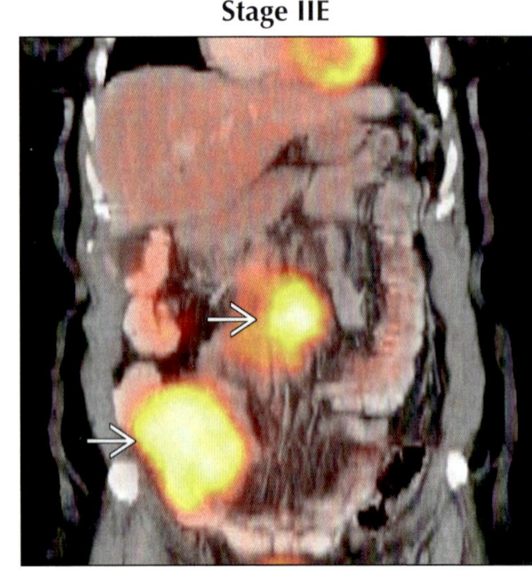

(Left) *Coronal PET shows multiple abnormal areas of increased metabolism ➔ in this patient with newly diagnosed non-Hodgkin lymphoma. Note that there are no abnormal areas of increased FDG activity above the diaphragm.* ***(Right)*** *Coronal fused PET/CT in the same patient shows the areas of increased metabolic activity ➔ relative to the underlying anatomy, with probable bowel involvement.*

Stage IIE

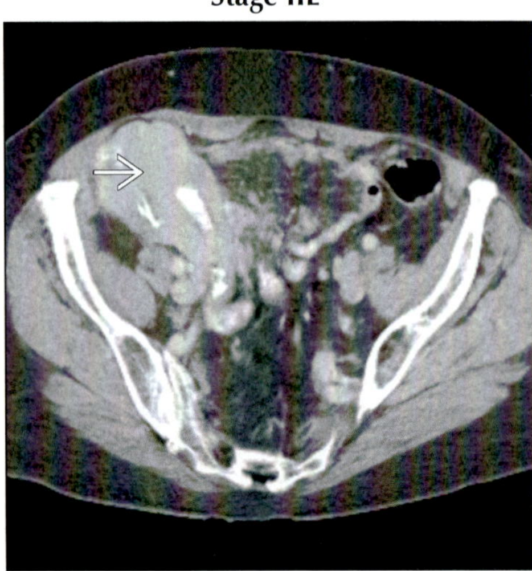

Stage IIE

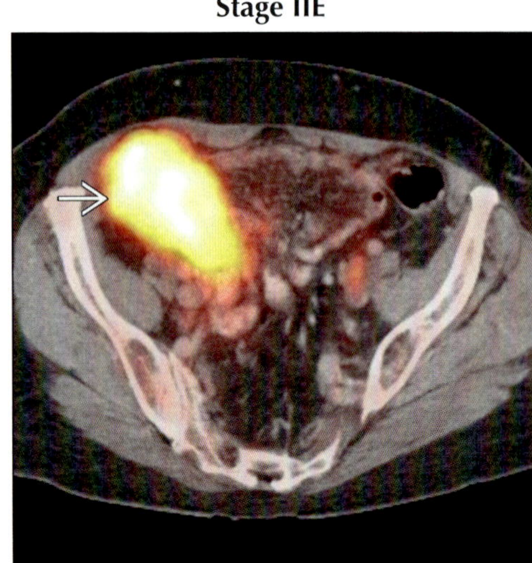

(Left) *Axial CECT in the same patient shows diffuse small bowel wall thickening ➔, compatible with involvement with lymphoma. Involvement of an extralymphatic structure with additional lymph node groups is compatible with stage IIE.* ***(Right)*** *Axial fused PET/CT in the same patient shows marked increased metabolic activity ➔ within the thickened small bowel loops, compatible with a high-grade lymphoma.*

Stage IIBX Hodgkin Lymphoma

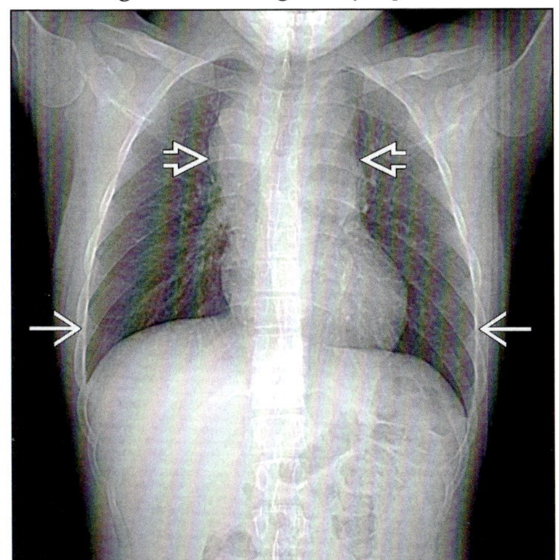

Stage IIBX Hodgkin Lymphoma

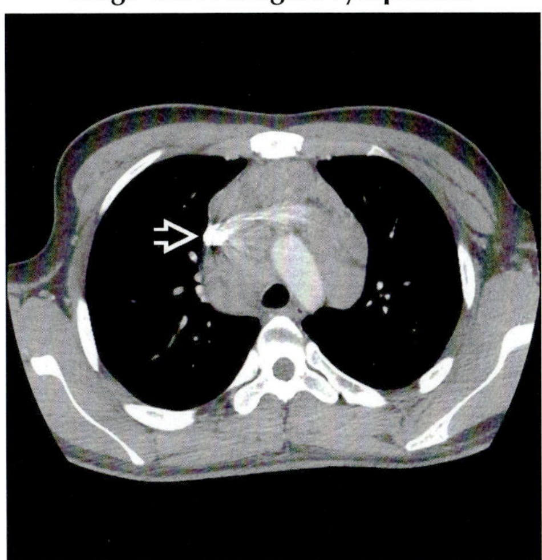

(Left) PA chest x-ray shows bulky bilateral mediastinal adenopathy that was > 1/3 of the thoracic diameter and > 10 cm. Patient had night sweats and thus was diagnosed with stage IIBX nodular sclerosing (NS) Hodgkin lymphoma. (Right) Axial CECT reveals the bilateral adenopathy in the same patient and also shows a widely patent superior vena cava (SVC) in this case.

Stage IIBX Hodgkin Lymphoma

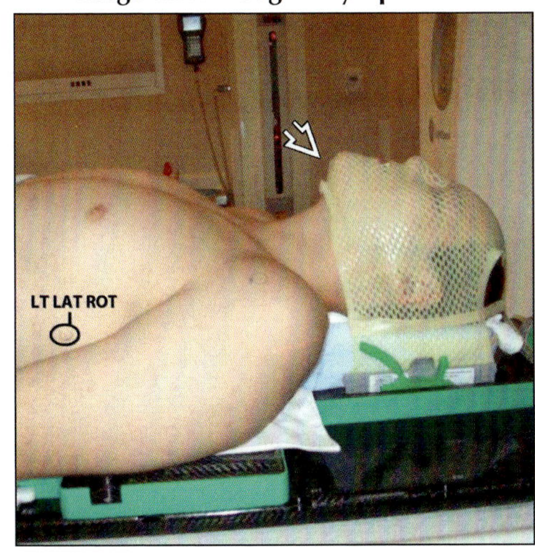

Stage IIBX Hodgkin Lymphoma

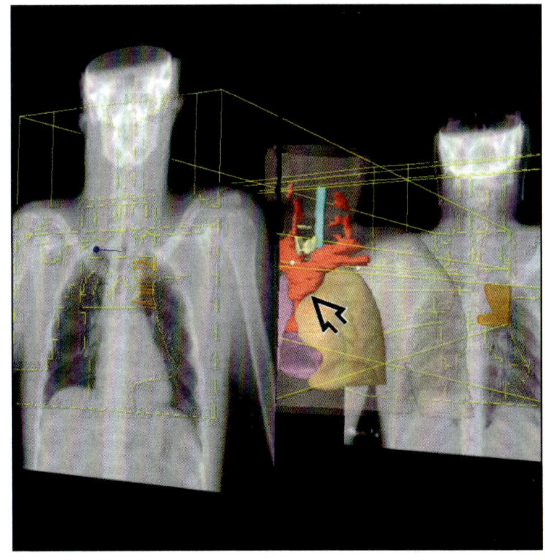

(Left) Photograph shows immobilization of the same patient treated for a modified mantle. Patient had a PR after ABVD chemotherapy. Great attention must be paid to correct positioning of the chin to reduce dose to the oral cavity and to the occiput in mid to high neck presentations. (Right) DRR in same patient demonstrates the large degree of divergence in large modified mantle fields. The red volume reveals the CTV.

Stage IIBX Hodgkin Lymphoma

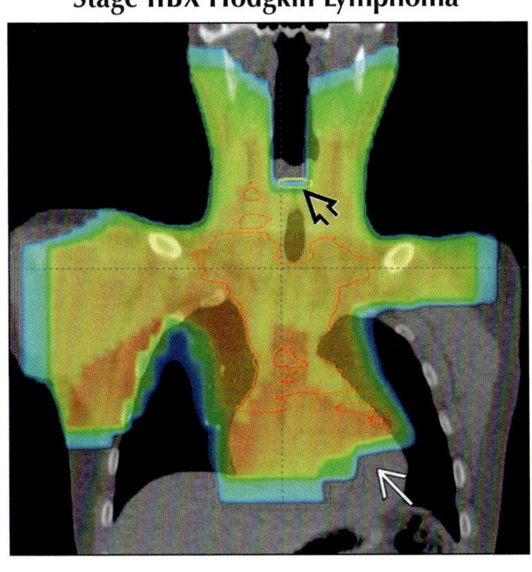

Stage IIBX Hodgkin Lymphoma

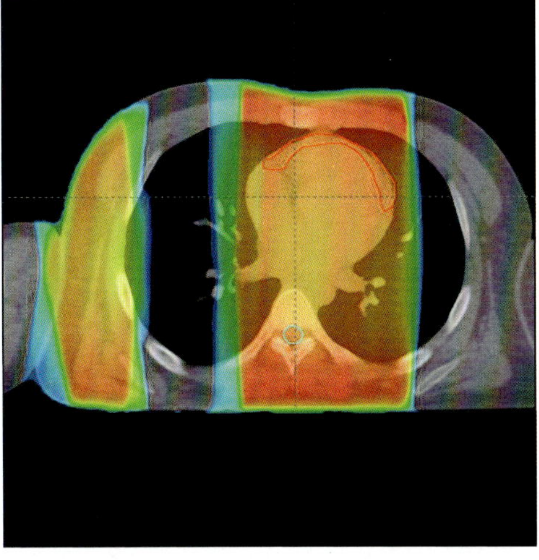

(Left) Coronal CT in the same patient shows the larynx contoured in yellow. Great care should be taken to avoid OARs if possible. The heart was excluded as much as possible. (Right) Planning CT in the same patient shows axial view of dosimetry. Red, green, and blue represent the 30 Gy, 20 Gy, and 10 Gy isodose surfaces, respectively. Patient was treated with 30.6 Gy in 17 fractions and remains free of disease.

LYMPHOMA

(**Left**) *PET MIP view shows level II ➡ and level V ➡ neck adenopathy in a patient with Sjögren syndrome. Patient presented with a unilateral palpable mass over the parotid. Biopsy showed MALT lymphoma.* (**Right**) *Axial fused PET/CT in same patient shows FDG avidity in the parotids ➡ bilaterally with an SUV of > 6 and bilateral adenopathy ➡. Due to bilaterality and concerns of xerostomia, the patient opted to be treated with rituximab and has had a clinical complete response.*

Stage IIAE MALT Lymphoma

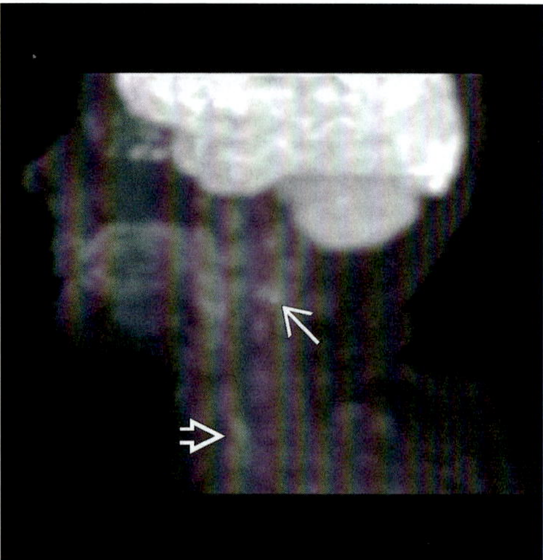

Stage IIAE MALT Lymphoma

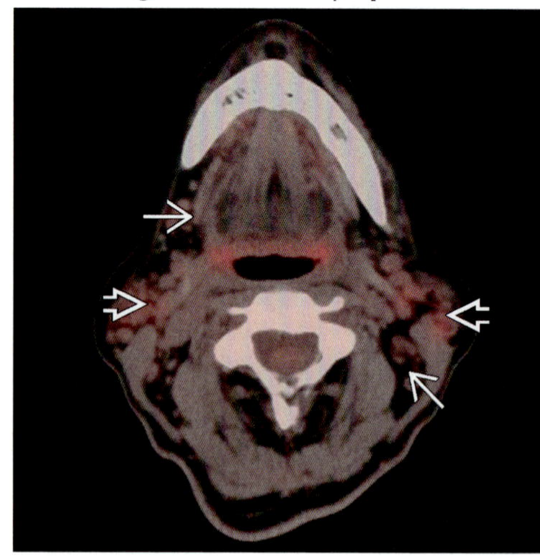

(**Left**) *Sagittal CT shows PTV outlined ➡ in a patient with a late relapse after being disease free for 6 years from a diagnosis of concurrent NHL and HL. He initially was treated with chemotherapy alone. He developed night sweats, and biopsy revealed LP Hodgkin lymphoma.* (**Right**) *The same patient was treated with a 7F IMRT plan. The small bowel is shaded in purple. The red, green, and blue show the 100%, 60%, and 20% isodose surfaces, respectively.*

Relapsed Stage IIB LP HL

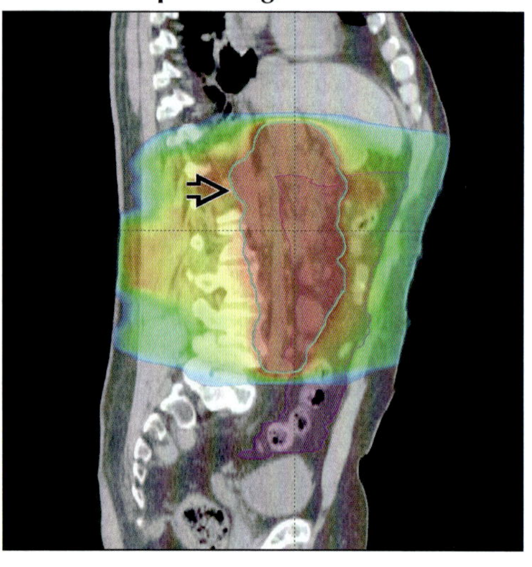

Relapsed Stage IIB LP HL

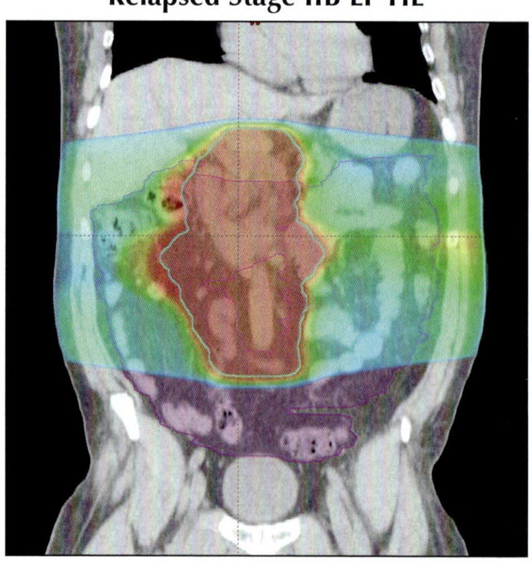

(**Left**) *Axial view in the same patient shows a 7F IMRT treatment. Patient had a complete response with localized RT and remains free of disease.* (**Right**) *In the same patient, DVH shows that IMRT was used to reduce dose to OAR. Significant dose reduction was achieved to small bowel with the IMRT plan ➡ vs. 3D ➡, and for the kidneys with the IMRT plan ➡ vs. 3D ➡.*

Relapsed Stage IIB LP HL

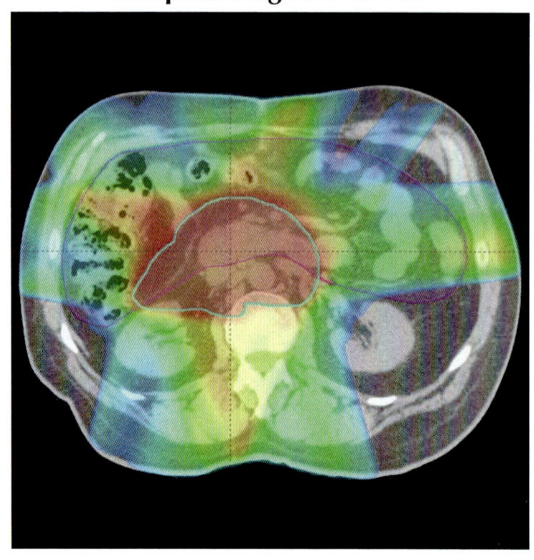

Relapsed Stage IIB LP HL

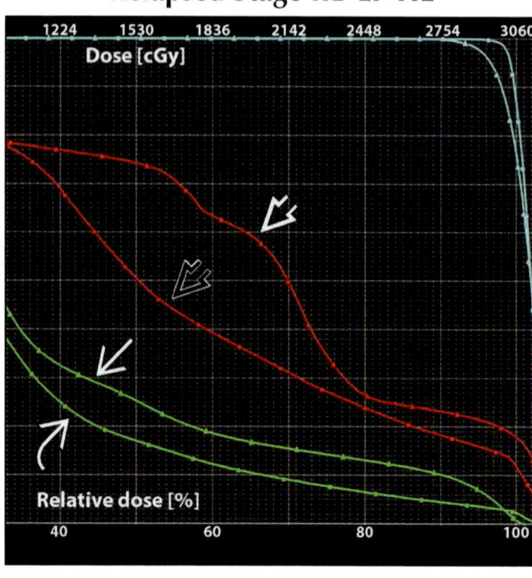

Stage IIA NS Hodgkin Lymphoma

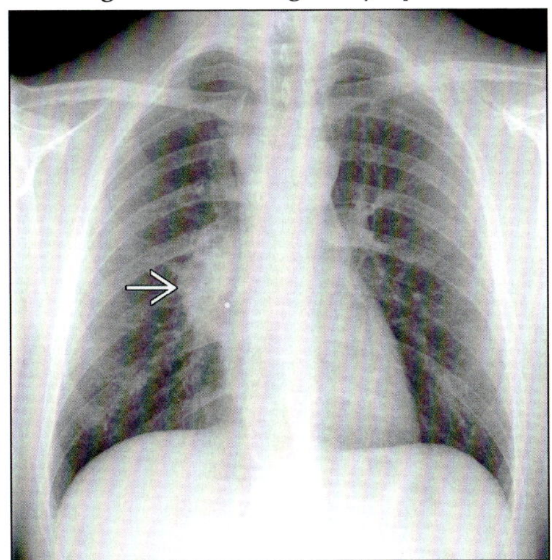

Stage IIA NS Hodgkin Lymphoma

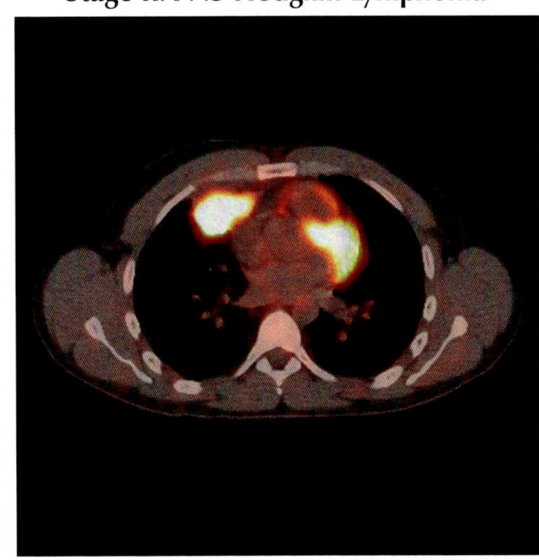

(Left) *PA chest x-ray shows 6 cm discrete right mediastinal adenopathy ➔ in a young patient who presented with chest pain.* ***(Right)*** *Fused PET/CT in the same patient shows avid mass with an SUV of 17. Patient also had supraclavicular disease and hence was stage II.*

Stage IIA NS Hodgkin Lymphoma

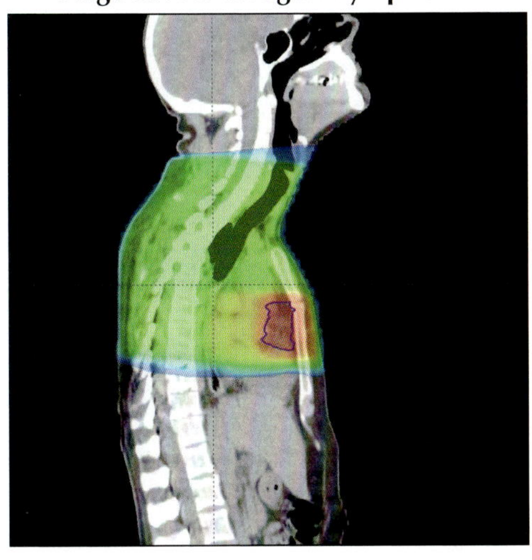

Stage IIB NS Hodgkin Lymphoma

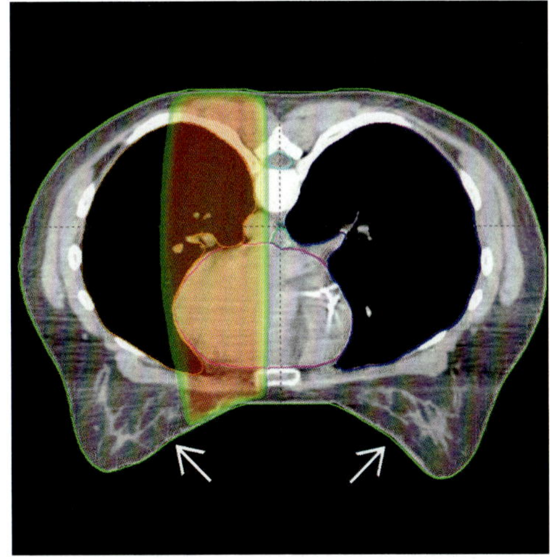

(Left) *The same patient was treated to 25.2 Gy followed by a boost to 36 Gy to areas of PR after chemo. The red, yellow, and blue represent the 36 Gy, 25 Gy, and 10 Gy isodose surfaces, respectively. The extended head position prevents dose to the oral cavity.* ***(Right)*** *CT shows prone positioning for this young woman with HL. Secondary breast cancers are markedly elevated in young females. A specialized breast board with wedges was used to displace the breasts ➔ laterally out of field.*

Stage IIB NS Hodgkin Lymphoma

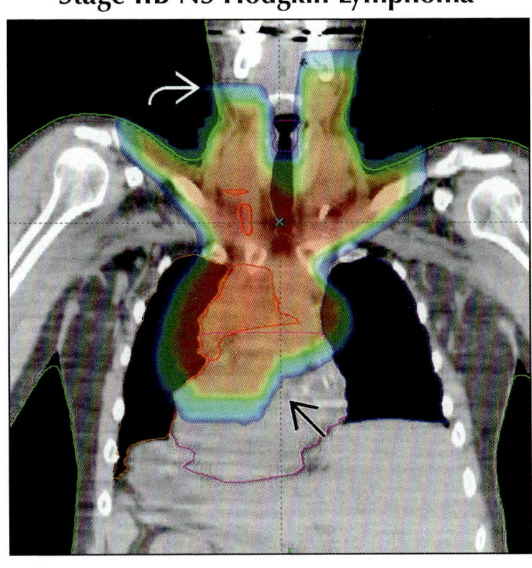

Stage IIB NS Hodgkin Lymphoma

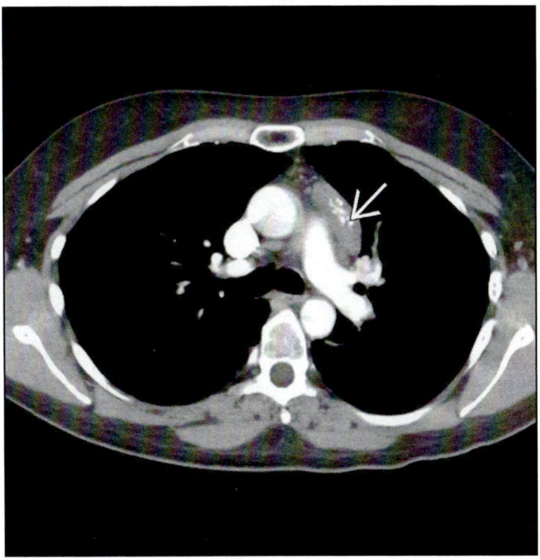

(Left) *Coronal CT in the same patient shows shaping to avoid as much heart ➔ as possible and to reduce coverage of the left neck ➔ due to the less cephalad adenopathy compared to the right.* ***(Right)*** *Follow-up CECT of the same patient shows stable mass with marked calcifications in the left mediastinum ➔. PET/CT showed no FDG uptake. These findings are common and should be followed.*

LYMPHOMA

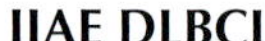

(Left) Coronal CT shows a large nasal mass ➔ that has eroded the nasal septum. Bilateral neck adenopathy was present. Patient had a CR to R-CHOP x 3. **(Right)** Axial CT in the same patient shows sparing of the eyes, chiasm, and brainstem with IMRT (36 Gy in 20 fractions). The PTV is shown in light blue, and the red, yellow, and blue lines represent the 95%, 80%, and 50% isodose lines, respectively. The patient remains locally controlled 7 years later.

IIAE DLBCL

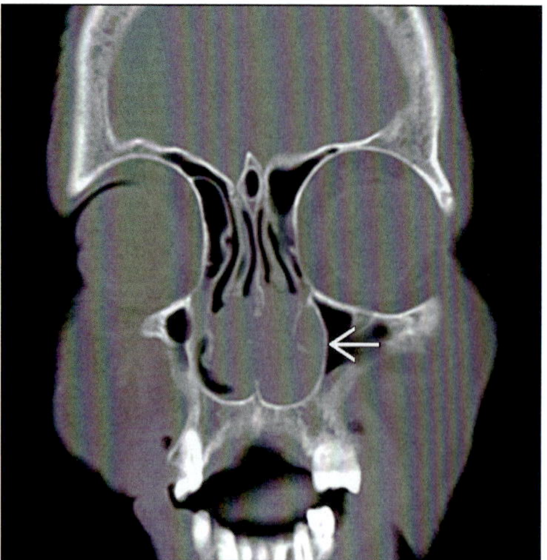

Stage IIAE DLBCL

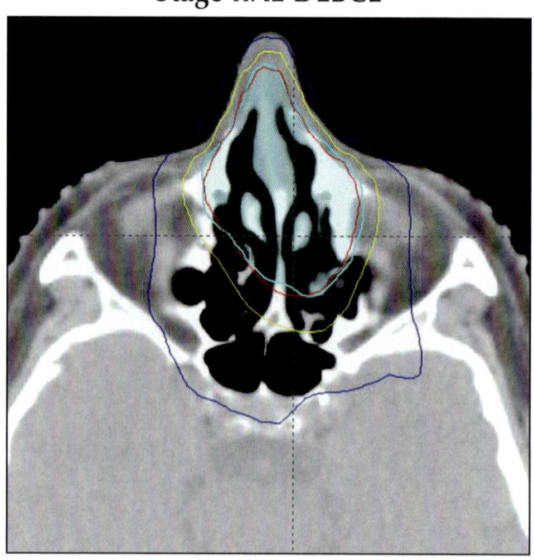

(Left) Young patient presented with pneumonia and 80 lb weight loss. Coronal fused PET/CT shows heterogeneous avidity with an SUV of 22. **(Right)** Biopsy in the same patient showed a gray zone lymphoma. These are biphenotypic, and this tumor had areas of classic HL and DLBCL. The patient was treated with R-CHOP-14 x 6 and had a CR by PET. A 4D scan was used to reduce the margins, and IMRT was used. Blue line shows the integrated target volume (ITV) from the 4D scan.

Gray Zone Lymphoma, Stage IIBX

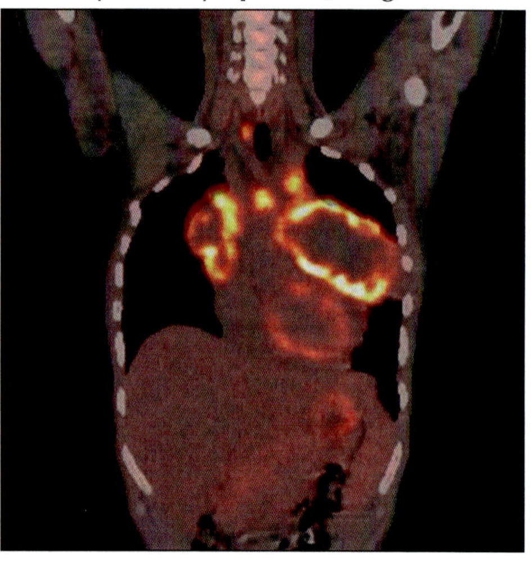

Gray Zone Lymphoma, Stage IIBX

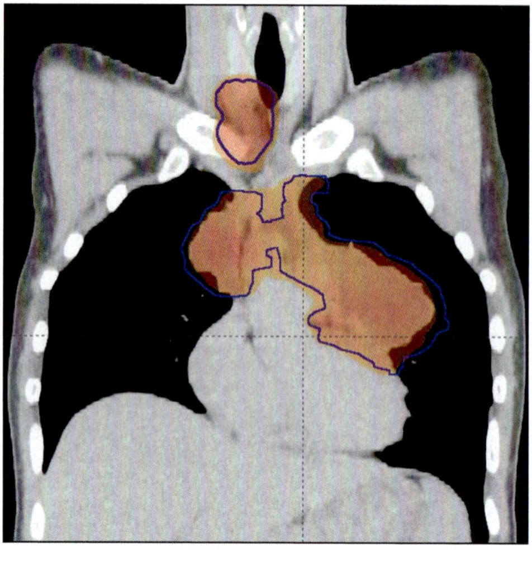

(Left) The red shaded region in the same patient is the 36 Gy line. IMRT permits conformal treatment of this irregularly shaped mass. **(Right)** In the same patient, a post-chemotherapy mass ⇨ can be seen. This is common with large tumors and needs to be adequately covered.

Gray Zone Lymphoma, Stage IIBX

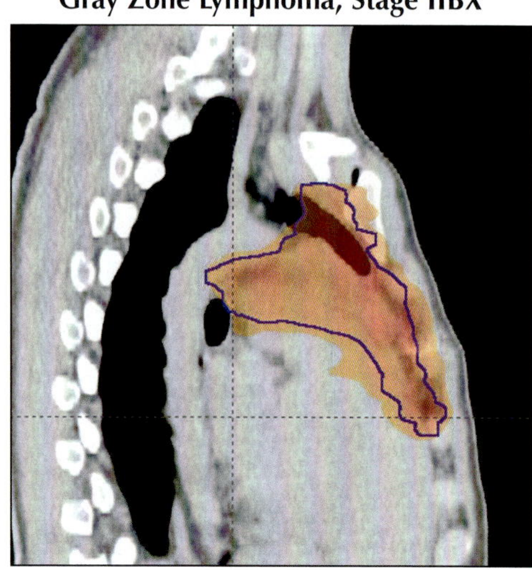

Gray Zone Lymphoma, Stage IIBX

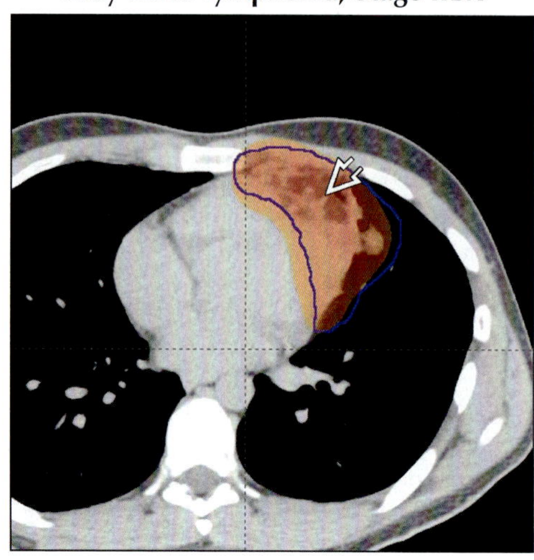

Stage III

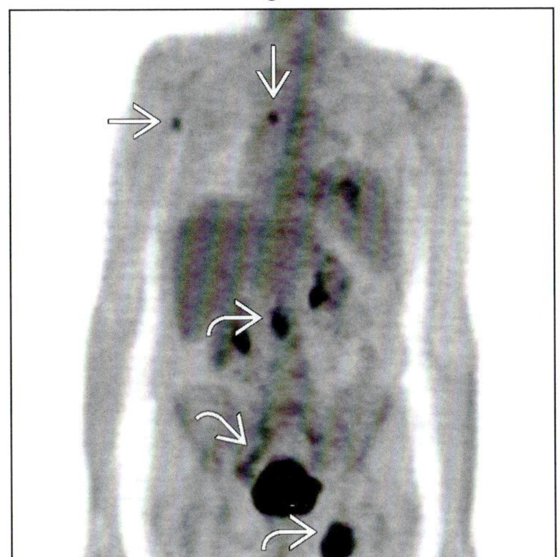

Stage III

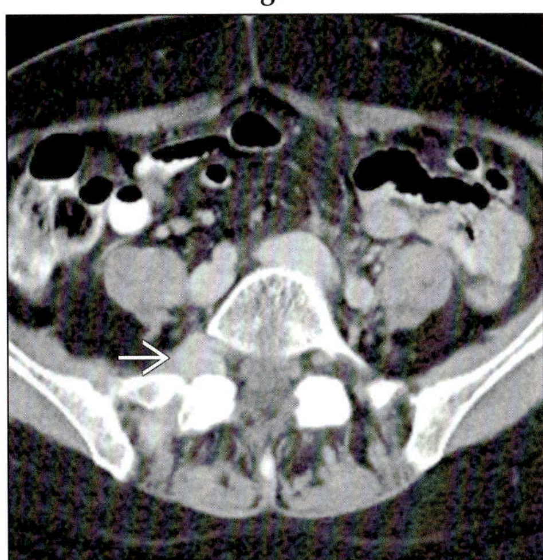

(Left) *Coronal PET shows areas of hypermetabolism in the right retroperitoneal and left inguinal regions ➩ in this patient with recently diagnosed non-Hodgkin lymphoma after a biopsy of the left inguinal mass. However, 2 small foci above the diaphragm ➡ make this stage III.* ***(Right)*** *Axial CECT in the same patient shows an enhancing mass ➡ adjacent to the right hemisacrum encroaching on the neuroforamen on the right.*

Stage III

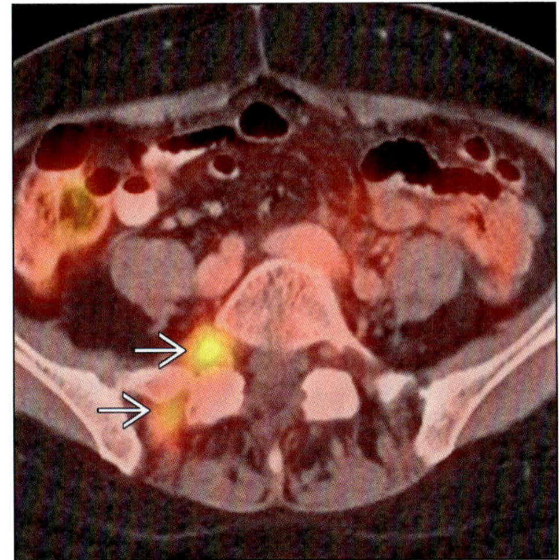

Stage IIIS

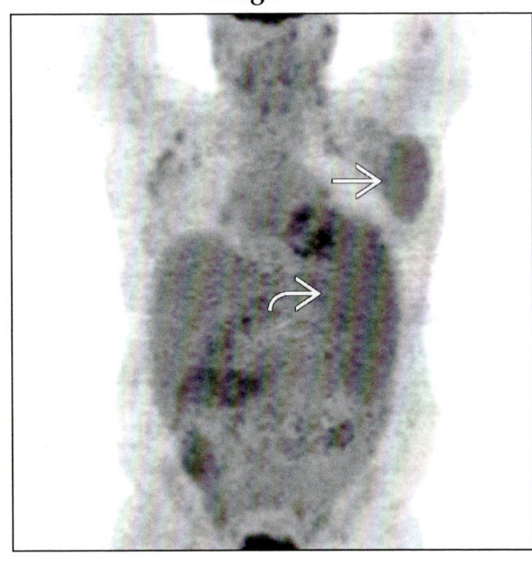

(Left) *Axial fused PET/CT in the same patient shows areas of increased metabolic activity ➡ corresponding to the abnormal soft tissue seen on CT and compatible with malignancy.* ***(Right)*** *Coronal PET in this patient with suspected lymphoma shows an enlarged spleen ➩ with metabolic activity that is slightly above that of normal liver. In addition, there is mildly increased FDG activity corresponding to bilateral axillary adenopathy ➡, the left much larger than the right.*

Stage IIIS

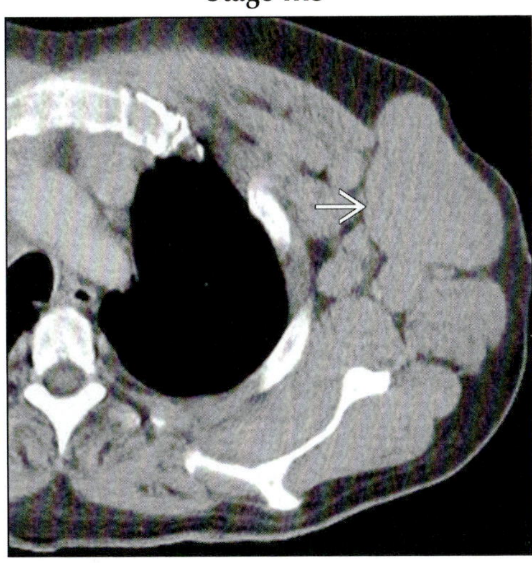

Stage IIIS

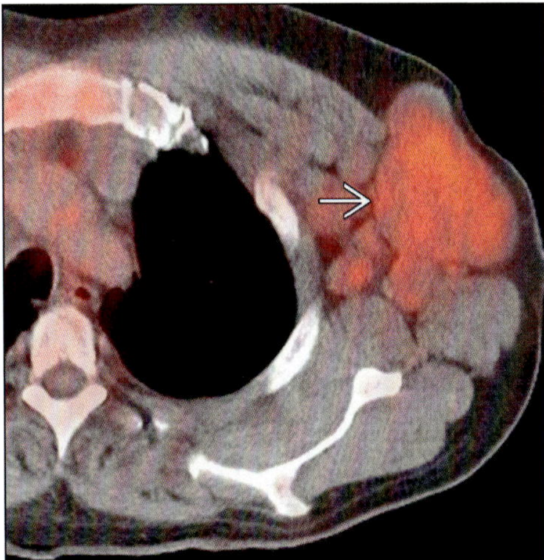

(Left) *Axial NECT in the same patient shows large, bulky left axillary adenopathy ➡ worrisome for malignancy.* ***(Right)*** *Axial fused PET/CT in the same patient shows only mildly increased metabolic activity ➡ within the adenopathy. Low-grade increased metabolic activity in the areas of involvement is a fairly typical finding in patients with chronic lymphocytic leukemia. Subsequent biopsy confirmed the diagnosis.*

(Left) *Axial CECT shows no discrete abnormality despite good portal venous phase contrast enhancement.* **(Right)** *Axial PET/CT in the same patient shows focal intense FDG activity ➔ in the posterior aspect of the spleen, compatible with lymphoma. An added benefit of PET/CT is detecting lesions that may not be seen on CT. Note physiologic gastric FDG activity ➔. Disease above the diaphragm (not shown) with splenic involvement makes this stage IIIS.*

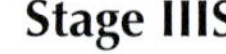

Stage IIIS

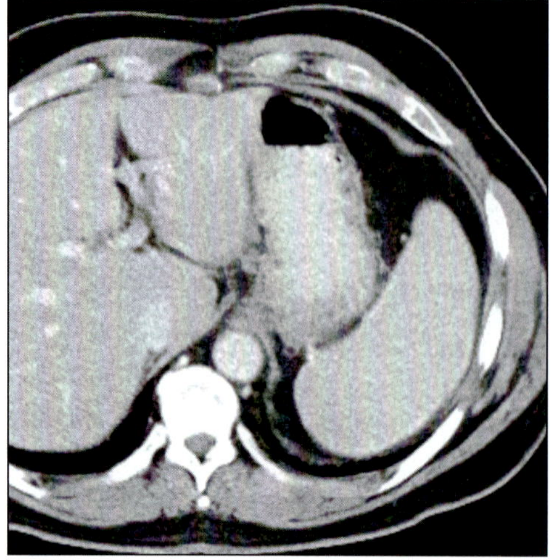

Stage IIIS

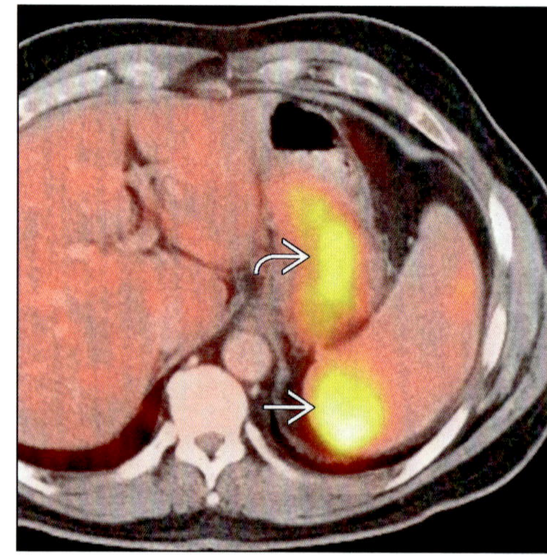

(Left) *Patient required multiple biopsies before a diagnosis of Hodgkin lymphoma could be made. PET/CT reveals extensive mediastinal disease ➔, bilateral supraclavicular disease ➔, and left axillary disease ➔. Patient had minimal disease below the diaphragm (not shown); hence, she was stage IIIBX.* **(Right)** *CECT in the same patient shows marked collateral flow due to obstruction of the vena cava.*

IIIBX Hodgkin Lymphoma

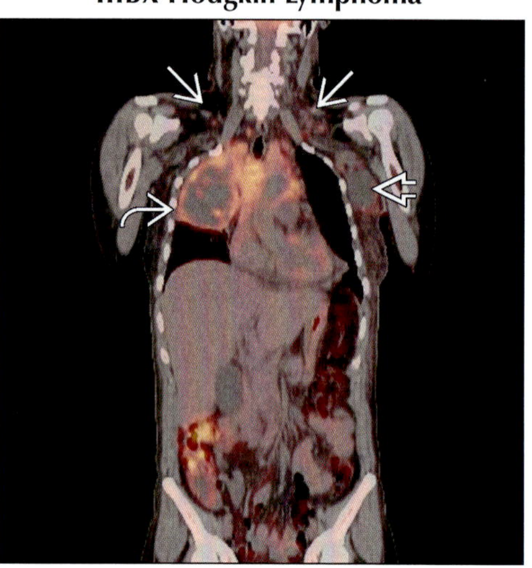

IIIBX Hodgkin Lymphoma

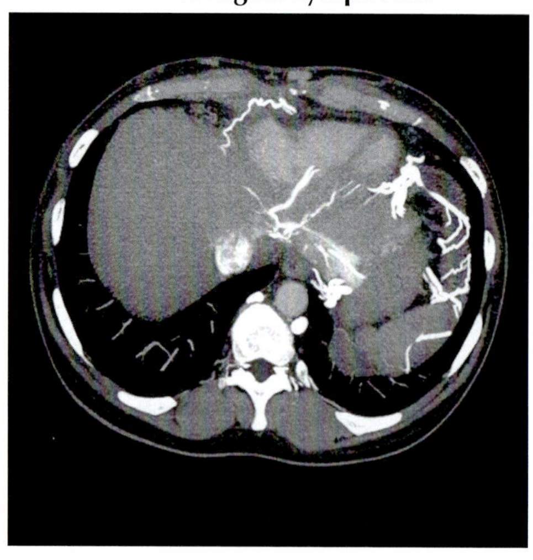

(Left) *Setup is challenging in modified mantle patients. A large mask should be employed that will immobilize the upper thorax. Fields should be drawn on to aid in reproducibility.* **(Right)** *Axial CT in the same patient shows the PTV. She had a CR by PET after chemotherapy. The neck, mediastinum, and axilla were treated to 21.6 Gy, the mediastinum and neck to 28.8 Gy, and the mediastinal mass to 36 Gy.*

IIIBX Hodgkin Lymphoma

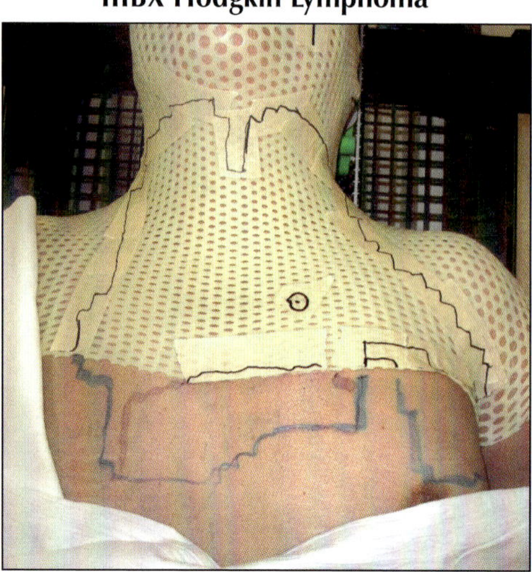

IIBX Hodgkin Lymphoma

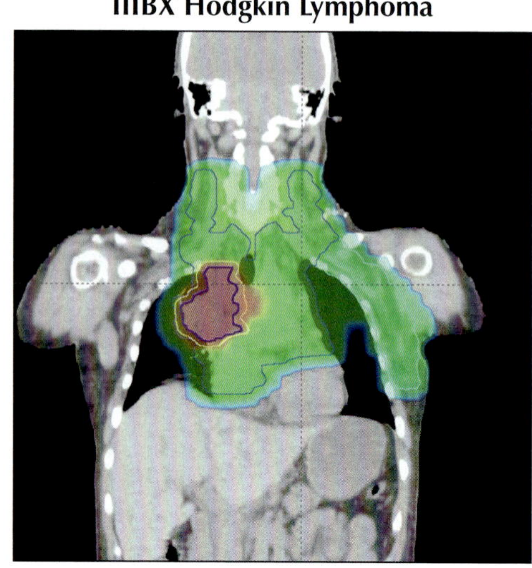

Stage IV

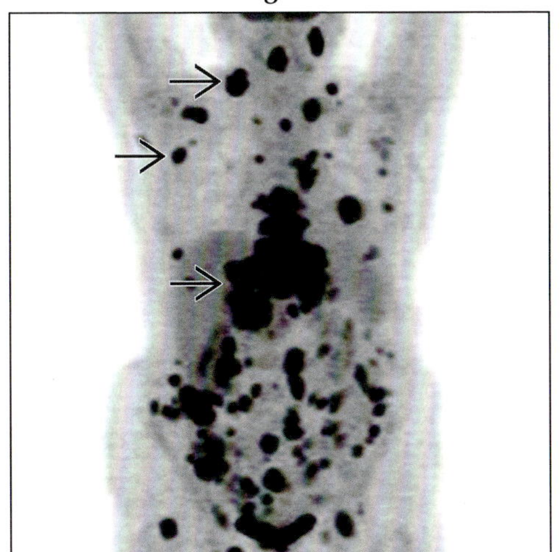

Stage IV, Post Treatment

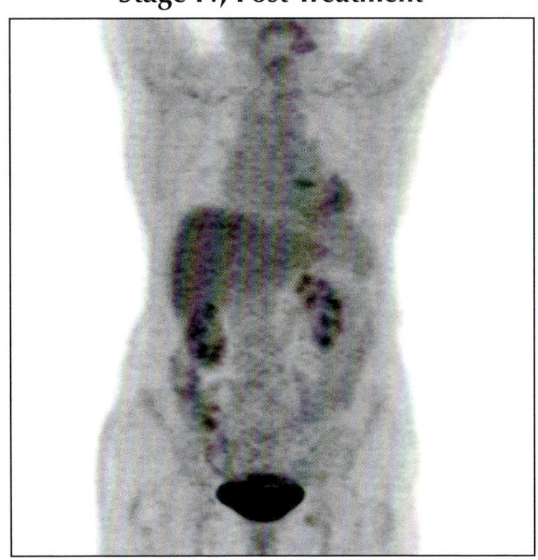

(Left) *Coronal PET shows extensive involvement with multiple lesions ➔ that are intensely FDG avid throughout the soft tissue and osseous structures. Diffuse osseous involvement makes this stage IV.* ***(Right)*** *Coronal PET in the same patient after 2 cycles of chemotherapy shows a complete metabolic response. FDG PET can be used to help assess early response to chemotherapy in patients with high-grade non-Hodgkin and Hodgkin lymphoma.*

Stage IV

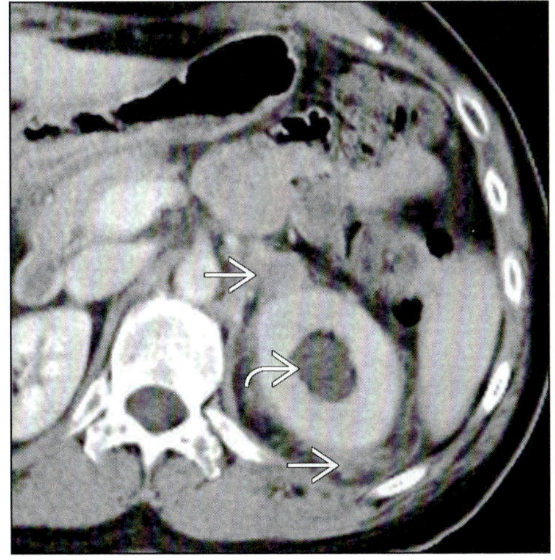

Stage IV

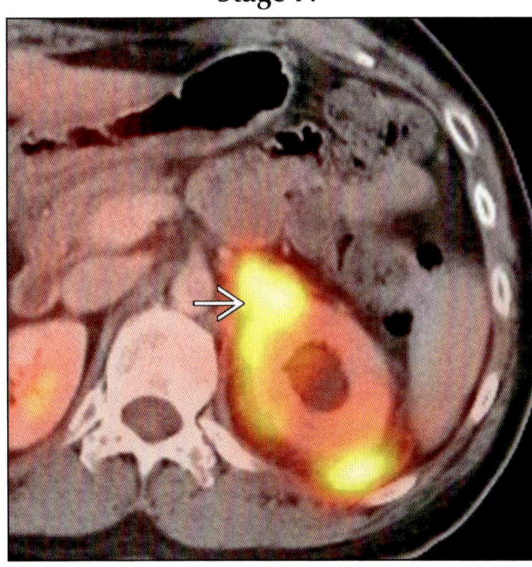

(Left) *Axial CECT in a patient with newly diagnosed lymphoma shows multiple nodular and infiltrative soft tissue lesions ➔ in the left perirenal space. Also note hydronephrosis ➔.* ***(Right)*** *Axial fused PET/CT in the same patient shows intense FDG activity ➔ surrounding the left kidney corresponding to the left perirenal lesions and compatible with malignancy.*

Stage IV

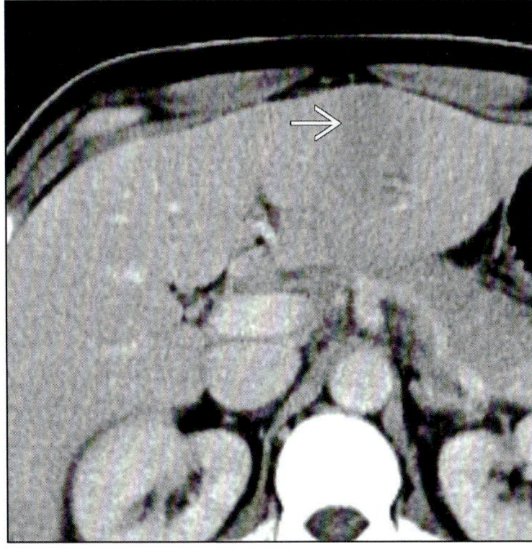

Stage IV

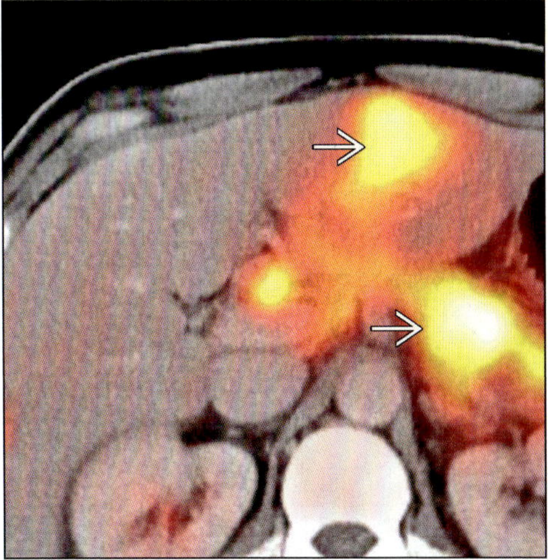

(Left) *Axial CECT in the same patient shows no definite abnormality although there is a suggestion of a geographic area ➔ of low attenuation in the left hepatic lobe.* ***(Right)*** *Axial fused PET/CT in the same patient shows multiple areas of hypermetabolism ➔ in the liver, pancreas, and periportal area, compatible with involvement with lymphoma. Involvement of the kidneys and the liver makes this stage IV disease.*

LYMPHOMA

(**Left**) *Axial CECT in a patient with recently diagnosed diffuse large B-cell lymphoma shows a nonspecific subcutaneous lesion ➡ in the region of the left shoulder.* (**Right**) *Axial fused PET/CT in the same patient shows intense FDG activity corresponding to the subcutaneous lesion ➡ and compatible with high-grade lymphoma.*

Stage IV

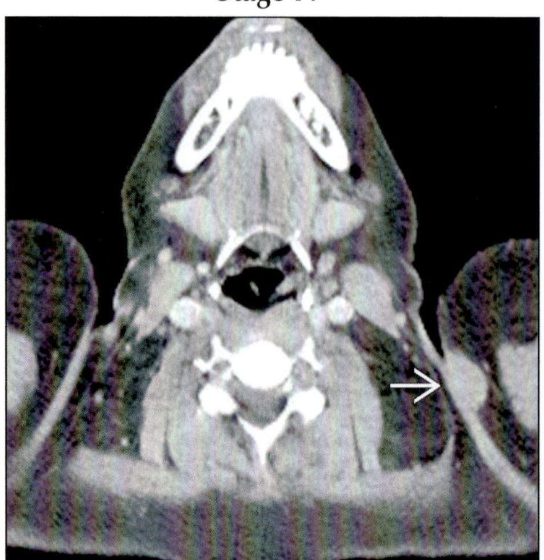

Stage IV

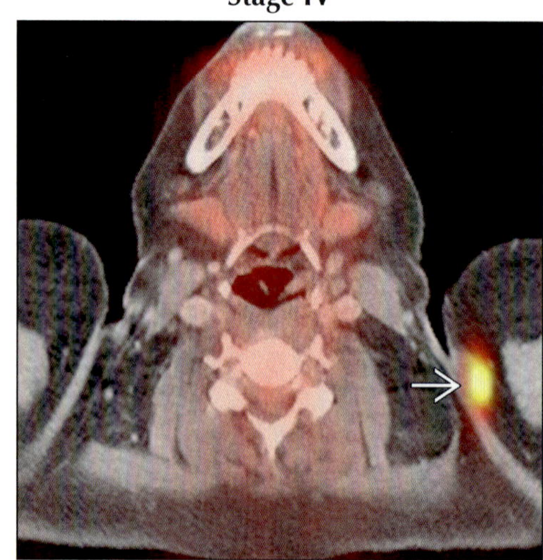

(**Left**) *Axial CECT in the same patient shows nonspecific nodularity ➡ within the breasts, possibly representing normal breast tissue.* (**Right**) *Axial fused PET/CT in the same patient shows intense FDG activity ➡ within the breasts, compatible with lymphoma. Typical physiologic FDG activity within the breasts is usually minimal unless the patient is lactating.*

Stage IV

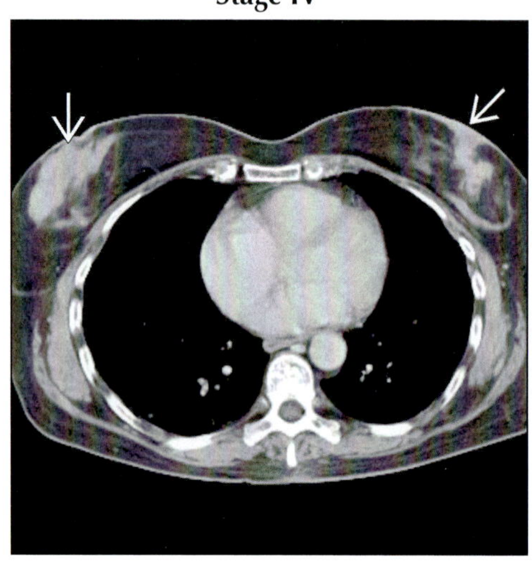

Stage IV

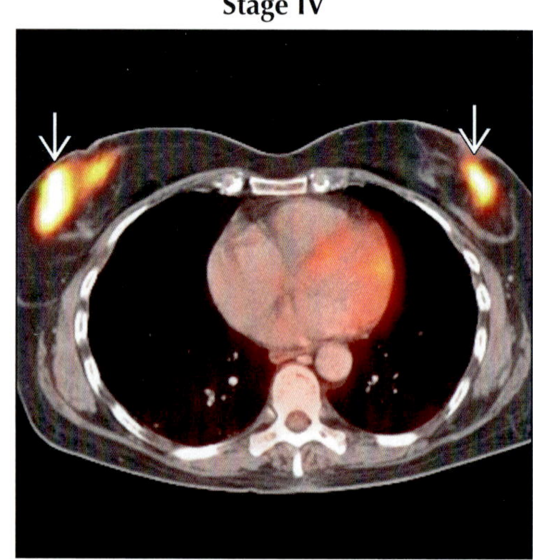

(**Left**) *Axial fused PET/CT in the same patient shows intense metabolic activity within bilobar hepatic lesions ➡, compatible with malignancy.* (**Right**) *Axial simulation CT is fused to T1 post-gadolinium MR obtained 2 years after treatment. Fibrosis ➡ is depicted in left atrial wall. This stage IVAEX DLBCL patient was treated with R-CHOP and involved field RT. The red, blue, and yellow lines show the 95%, 50%, and 30% isodose lines, respectively. (Courtesy A. Harrison, MD.)*

Stage IV

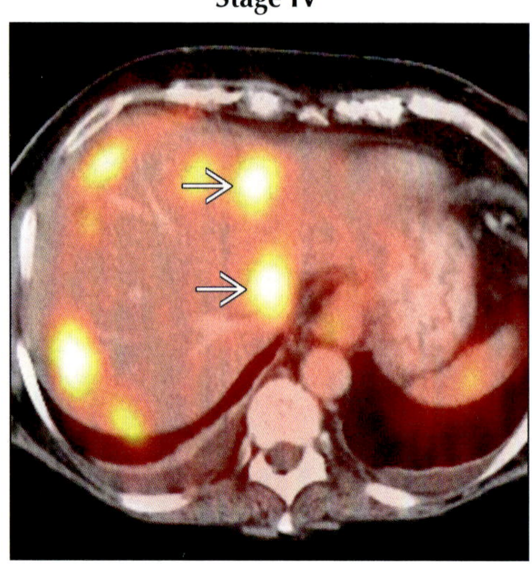

Late Effects

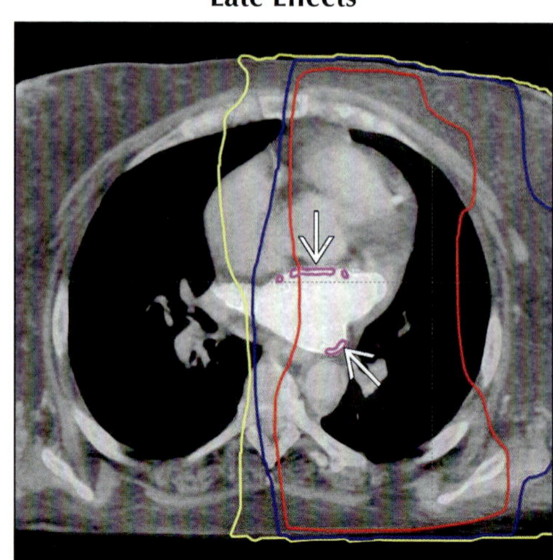

Stage IVBEX DLBCL

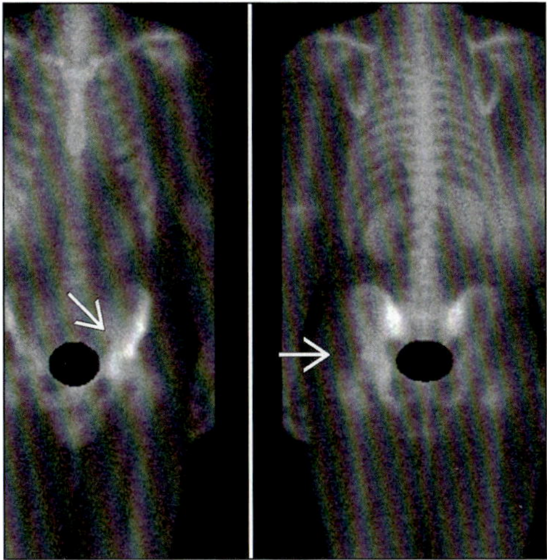

Stage IVBEX DLBCL

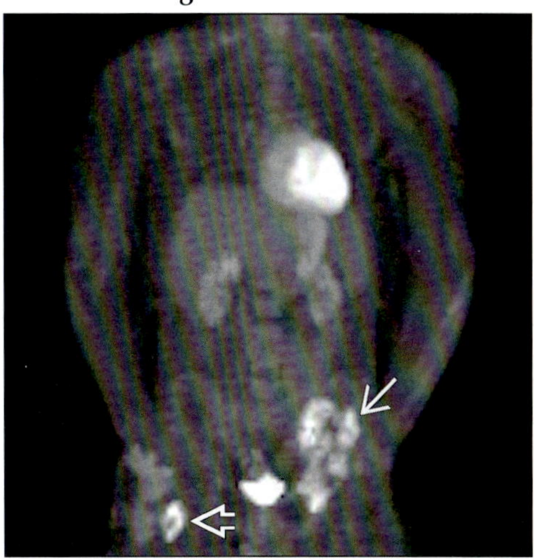

(Left) *Bone scan in a young man with hip pain shows increased uptake in left ileum ➡.* ***(Right)*** *PET image in same patient shows extensive left hip mass ➡ as well as right femoral ⇨ lesion. Biopsy revealed DLBCL.*

Stage IVBEX DLBCL

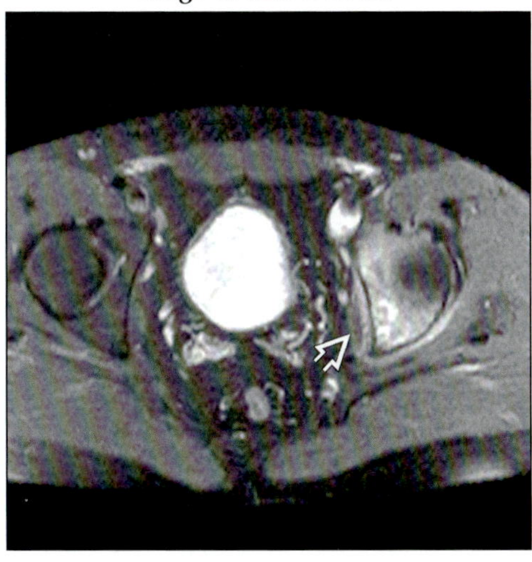

Stage IVBEX DLBCL

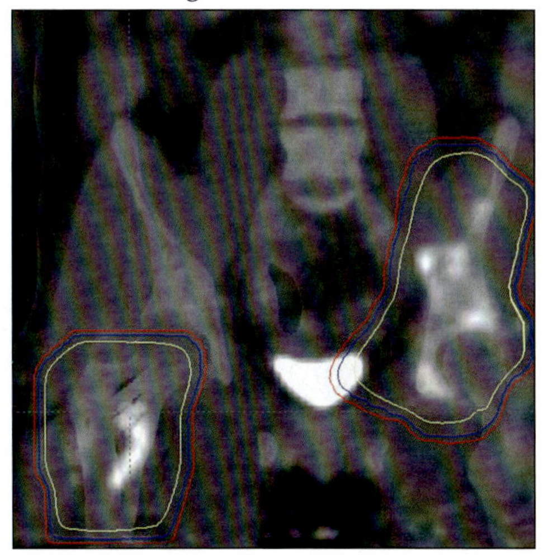

(Left) *Axial fat-saturated MR in the same patient shows extensive replacement of the left acetabulum ⇨. Disease extended into the ischium and significantly up the iliac wing.* ***(Right)*** *Coronal simulation CT in the same patient is fused to PET/CT for treatment planning. After R-CHOP-14 x 6, patient underwent RT. A shield was used to limit dose to the testicles. The yellow, blue, and red lines indicate the 95%, 80%, and 50% isodose surfaces, respectively.*

Stage IVBEX DLBCL

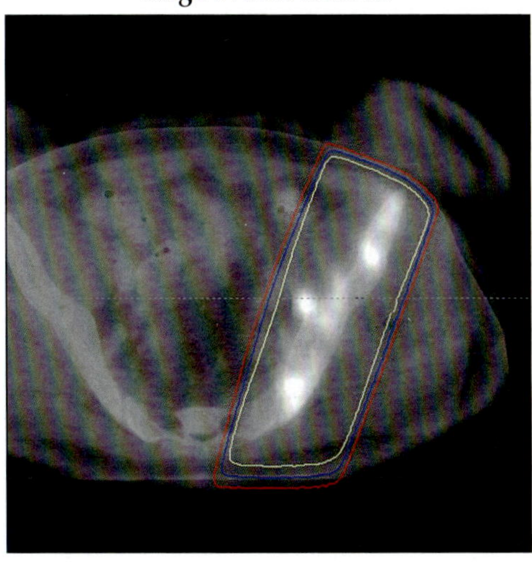

Relapsed Lymphoma

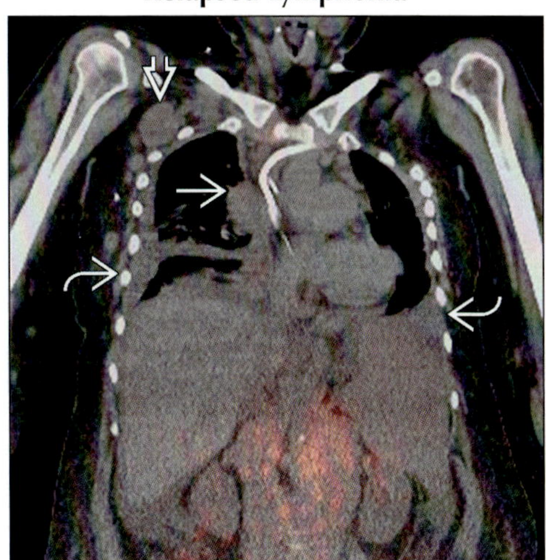

(Left) *The patient's left hip lesion was treated with opposed obliques to limit dose to the bowel. The patient was treated to 34 Gy in 17 fractions and remains in complete remission.* ***(Right)*** *Coronal fused PET/CT in a different patient shows extensive abdominal disease, mediastinal ➡ and axillary adenopathy ⇨, and bilateral pleural effusions ➡.*

(**Left**) *Photo shows advanced mycosis fungoides (MF) with lesions of varying severity. Scaly plaque lesions are evident over the anterior axillary fold* → *and infraclavicular region* ⇨. *The ulcerated lesions* ⇨ *can easily become infected in these immunocompromised patients. MF lesions often respond well to low doses of RT.* (**Right**) *Photo shows MF lesion with a 2 cm margin around the lesion for palliative electron beam. A small area of ulceration* ➡ *is seen.*

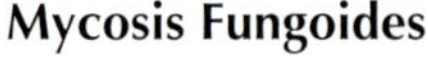

Mycosis Fungoides

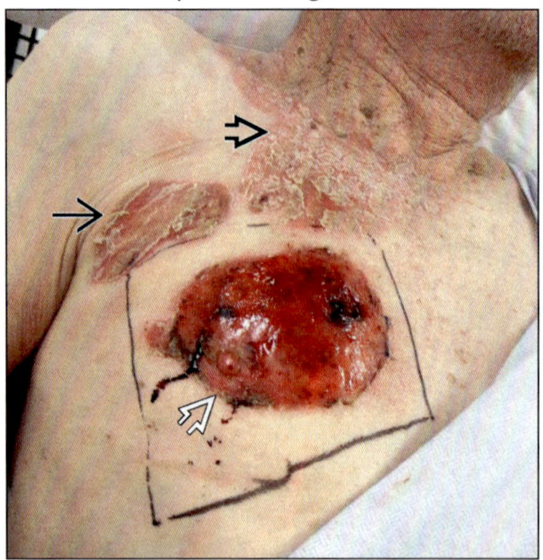

Mycosis Fungoides

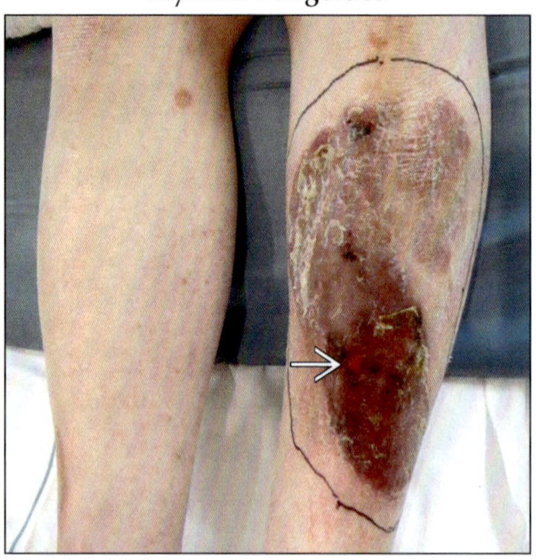

(**Left**) *Patient was diagnosed 1 year previously and treated with R-CVP chemotherapy. At relapse, axial CECT scan shows marked gastric wall thickening* ➡. (**Right**) *Coronal CECT in the same patient shows gastric thickening* ➡ *and right retroperitoneal adenopathy* ⇨.

Relapsed Stage IV MALT NHL

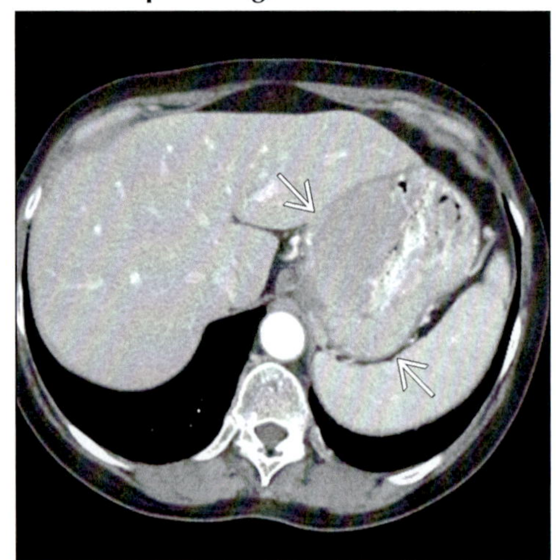

Relapsed Stage IV MALT NHL

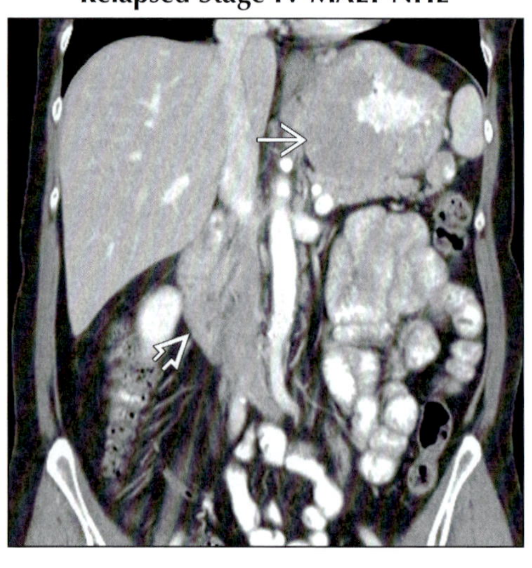

(**Left**) *Axial simulation CT shows the block edge in blue and the yellow and red represent the 97% and 90% isodose lines, respectively. A 4-field approach was used: 27 Gy in 15 fractions.* (**Right**) *Follow-up CECT shows a CR. Patient remains free of disease 2 years later.*

Relapsed Stage IV MALT NHL

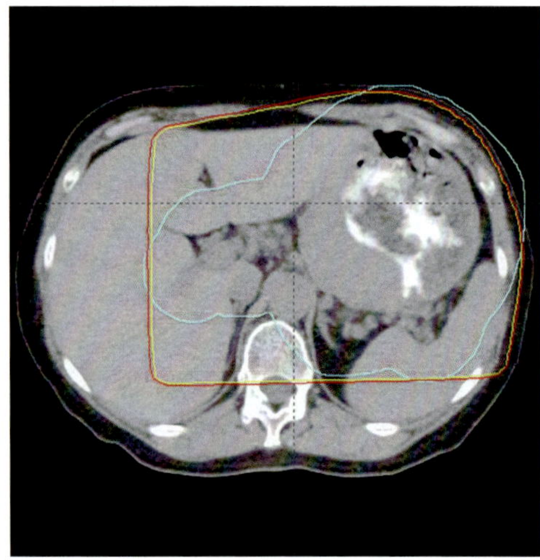

Relapsed Stage IV MALT NHL

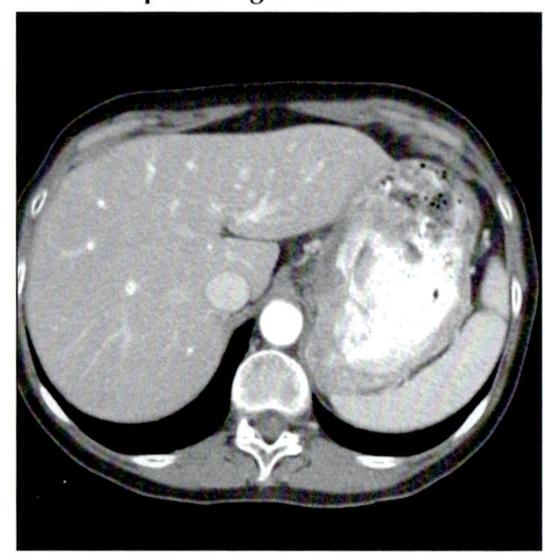

Relapsed Lymphoma

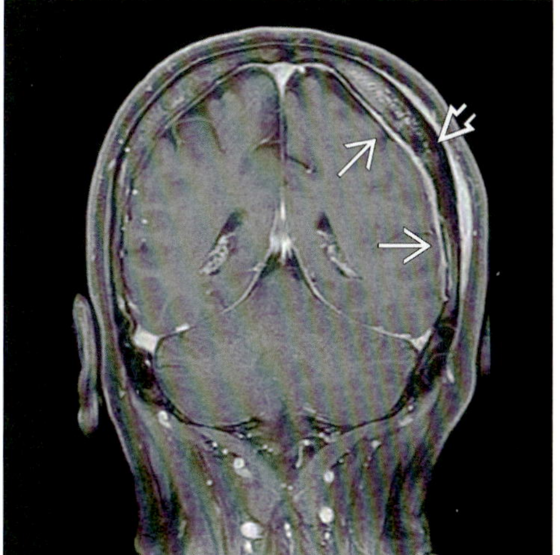

Relapsed Lymphoma

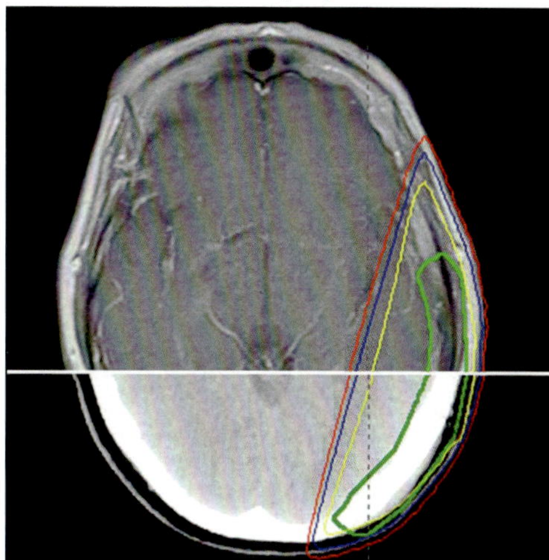

(Left) *Coronal post-contrast MR shows dural thickening ➔ without leptomeningeal disease. There is replacement of the normal fatty marrow ➙ in the left parietal bone.* ***(Right)*** *Fused MR (anteriorly) to CT (posteriorly) allows precise targeting and sparing of brain parenchyma. The same patient with recurrent lymphoma and headaches was treated with 10 Gy in 5 fractions, had progression 1 year later, and was retreated with good results.*

Chloroma

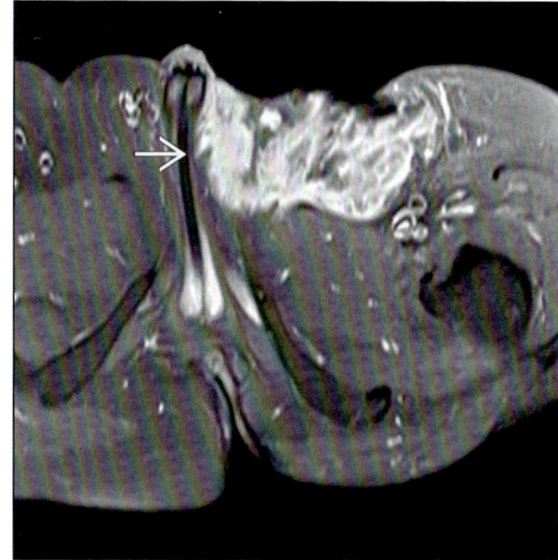

Chloroma

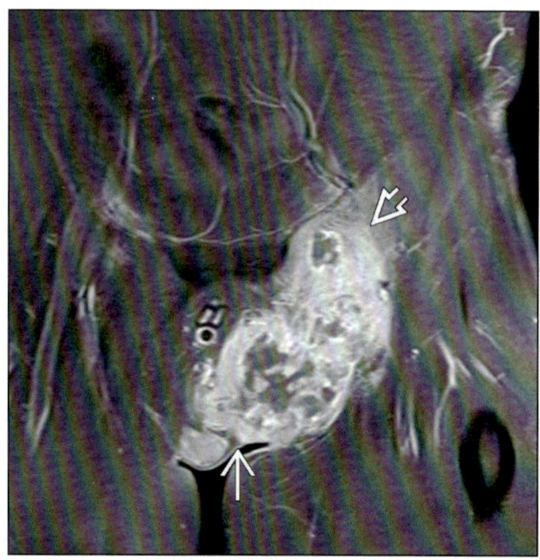

(Left) *Axial T1WI post-contrast FS MR shows brightly enhancing mass invading the penis ➔ in a young man with a history of Fournier gangrene and AML M5. After high-dose chemotherapy and stem cell rescue, he presented with an enlarging mass in the left groin.* ***(Right)*** *Coronal T1WI post-contrast FS MR in the same patient shows scrotal invasion ➔ and ipsilateral pelvic adenopathy ➙.*

Chloroma

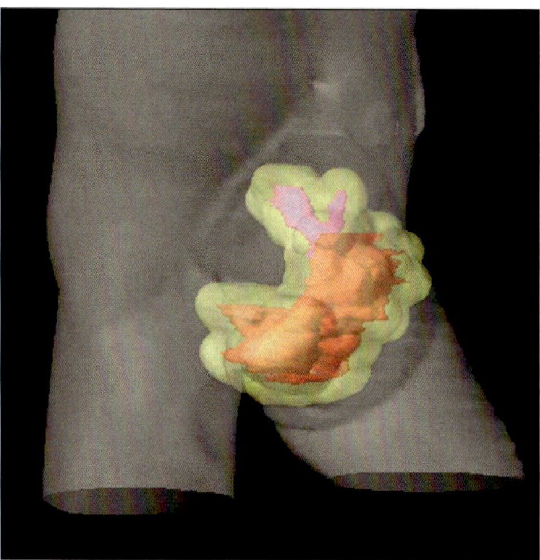

Chloroma

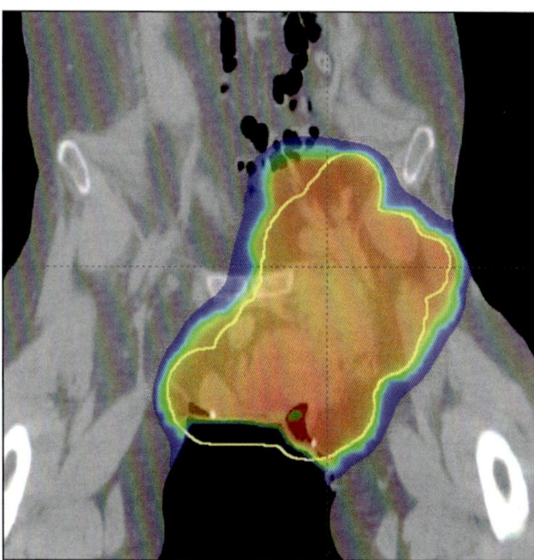

(Left) *DRR in the same patient shows the primary GTV in orange, nodal GTV in pink, and PTV in yellow. Chloromas can invade along fascial planes.* ***(Right)*** *Coronal CT in the same patient shows the PTV in yellow, and the orange, green, and blue represent 98%, 60%, and 15% isodose surfaces, respectively. Patient was treated to 24 Gy in 12 fractions.*

MULTIPLE MYELOMA

Durie and Salmon PLUS Staging System

Classification	*Bone Marrow*	*Laboratory Parameters*	*Imaging Parameters*[1]
Monoclonal gammopathy of undetermined significance (MGUS): Not included in staging	< 10% plasma cells		No intra- or extramedullary disease
Smoldering multiple myeloma (SMM): Stage IA[2]	≥ 10% plasma cells	All of the following: Hemoglobin > 10 g/dL; sCa++ ≤12 mg/dL; low M-component production; IgG < 5.0 g/dL; IgA < 3.0 g/dL; urine M-protein < 4g/24h	Limited disease (definition evolving)
Multiple myeloma (MM): Stages IB-III	≥ 10% plasma cells &/or plasmacytoma + end organ damage[3]	Variable by stage	Variable by stage
Stage IB[2]		Same as stage IA	< 5 focal lesions[4]; mild diffuse disease[5] on T1 MR
Stage IIA/B[2]		Neither stage I nor stage III	5-20 focal lesions[4]; moderate diffuse disease[5] on T1 MR
Stage IIIA/B[2]		1 or more of the following: Hemoglobin < 8.5 g/dL; sCa++ > 12 mg/dL; IgG > 7.0 g/dL; IgA > 5.0 g/dL; urine M-protein > 12g/24h	> 20 focal lesions[4]; severe diffuse disease[5] on T1 MR

[1]*The imaging appearance of bone marrow is variable. Patients with stage III myeloma by clinical criteria can have a normal MR appearance of bone marrow, which is associated with a more favorable prognosis.*

[2]*A: Serum creatinine < 2.0 mg/dL & no extramedullary disease; B: Serum creatinine > 2.0 mg/dL &/or extramedullary disease.*

[3]*End organ damage includes calcium elevation, renal insufficiency, anemia, or bone abnormalities.*

[4]*Focal lesions ≥ 5 mm.*

[5]*Degree of diffuse disease is evaluated on T1 images. Mild = micronodular or "salt and pepper" pattern of infiltration; moderate = diffuse lower T1 signal than normal marrow but with contrast between vertebral bone marrow and disc; severe = low T1 signal throughout the vertebral bone marrow with signal less than that of the adjacent disc.*

International Staging System

Stage	*Criteria*
I	Serum β2-microglobulin < 3.5 mg/L
	Serum albumin ≥ 3.5 g/dL
II	Not stage I or III
III	Serum β2-microglobulin ≥ 5.5 mg/L

The International Staging System is useful in imaging facilities without advanced imaging with MR or PET and as a measure of survival. Median survival for stage I: 62 months; stage II: 44 months; stage III: 29 months.

Stage I (Durie and Salmon PLUS)

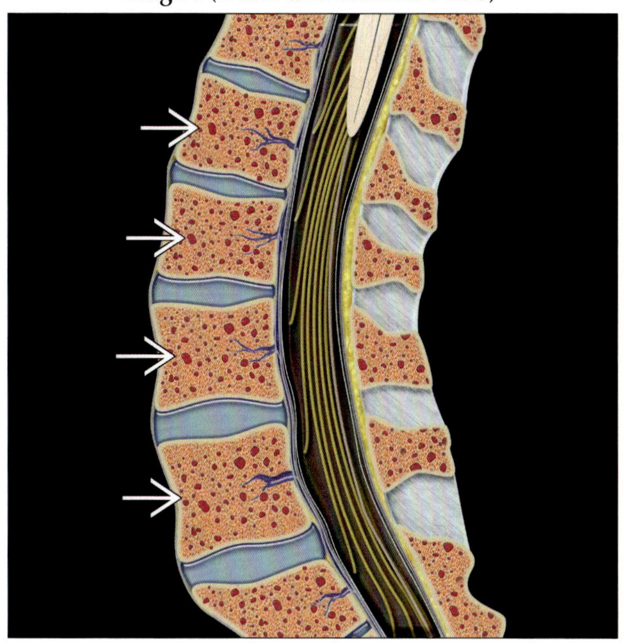

This sagittal graphic depicts micronodular foci ➔ of plasma cells within the axial bone marrow of the lumbar spine. Normal bone marrow by imaging is also associated with stage I disease.

Stage II/III (Durie and Salmon PLUS)

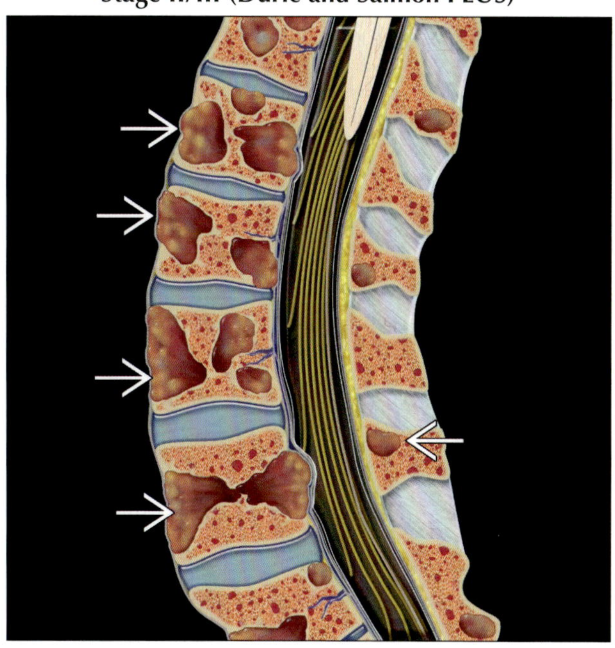

This sagittal graphic demonstrates multifocal disease ➔ within the lumbar spine, which is associated with more advanced (stage II/III) disease. Moderate diffuse infiltration or 5-20 focal lesions is stage II disease whereas > 20 focal lesions or severe diffuse disease is stage III disease.

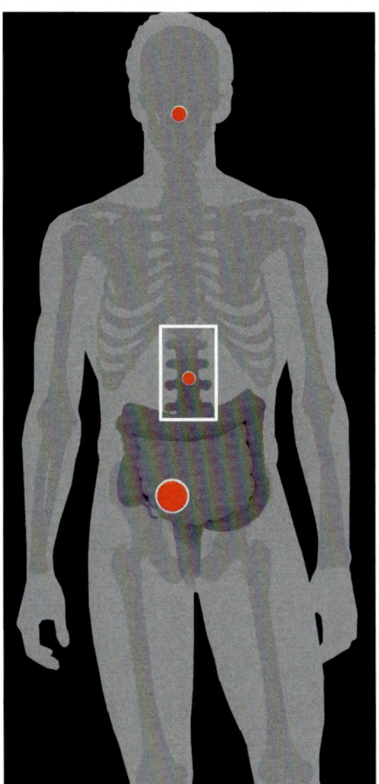

INITIAL SITE OF RECURRENCE

Conversion to Multiple Myeloma	46-56%
Development of Sequential Solitary Plasmacytomas	10-25%
Local Failure After RT	4-12%

Data represent 7 studies of solitary plasmacytoma of bone. Corresponding data for extramedullary plasmacytoma from 5 studies show conversion to MM in 8-36% of cases, local failure after RT in 4-17%, and development of sequential solitary plasmacytomas of 5-10%. Wasserman TH: Myeloma and Plasmacytoma. In Principles and Practices of Radiation Oncology. 3rd ed. Philadelphia: Lippincott-Raven, 1998.

MULTIPLE MYELOMA

OVERVIEW

General Comments

- Heterogeneous plasma cell (PC) disorder
- Characterized by bone marrow (BM) infiltration
- Diagnosed by combination of blood tests, BM biopsy and aspirate, urine protein studies, and x-rays
- Chemotherapy improves survival but is not curative unless an allogeneic transplant is performed

Classification

- Based on increasing malignant potential
  - Monoclonal gammopathy (MG) of undetermined significance (MGUS)
    - Progression risk → multiple myeloma (MM) = 1% per year
    - < 3 g/dL serum M-protein & < 10% BM PCs
    - When progression occurs, it usually leads to MM or Waldenström macroglobulinemia
    - Potentially can also progress to
      - Primary amyloidosis
      - Chronic lymphocytic leukemia
      - Lymphoma
    - MG of borderline significance (MGBS)
      - Subclassification (not universally used)
      - Higher risk of progression to MM than MGUS
      - Difference = ↑ PC number in BM (10-30% for MGBS vs. < 10% for MGUS)
  - Smoldering multiple myeloma (SMM)
    - ≥ 3g/dL serum M-protein & ≥10% BM PCs
    - No end organ damage (EOD) (asymptomatic)
    - Higher risk of progression to MM
  - Multiple myeloma
    - Symptomatic: EOD present
    - EOD includes any of the following (CRAB)
      - **C**alcium elevation
      - **R**enal insufficiency
      - **A**nemia
      - **B**one abnormalities (lytic or osteopenic)
    - Nonsecretory
      - No elevated M-protein in urine or blood
      - Disease best followed by PET/CT
    - POEMS syndrome
      - **P**olyneuropathy, **o**rganomegaly, **e**ndocrinopathy, **m**-protein, **s**kin changes
      - Sclerotic bone lesions
    - PC leukemia is characterized by > 20% circulating PCs at any time

NATURAL HISTORY

General Features

- Comments
  - Disorder with abnormal proliferation of BM PCs
  - Aggressiveness varies 2° to genetic alterations in PCs
  - Plasmacytoma generally refers to solitary lesion
  - Receptor activator of nuclear factor-κB ligand (RANKL) activates osteoclasts → bone resorption → hypercalcemia
- Location
  - Bone marrow
  - Extramedullary plasmacytomas most commonly occur in upper respiratory tract

Etiology

- Unknown
- Exposure to herbicides, insecticides, benzene, and ionizing radiation may contribute

Epidemiology & Cancer Incidence

- Number of cases in USA per year
  - 21,700 estimated new cases in 2012 with 10,710 deaths
- Sex predilection
  - M > F
- Most common primary bone malignancy
- 10% of all hematologic malignancies
- 2x ↑ incidence for African-Americans

Genetics

- Common translocations
  - Chromosomal abnormalities of 14 and 13 seen (~ 50% of cases each)
- Rarely hereditary
- Multiple PC genetic subclassifications
  - Poor prognostic factors
    - Del chromosome (chr) 13 → retinoblastoma-1 (RB1) mutation
    - ↑ PC proliferation index
    - Del chr 17p13 → inactivation of *p53* tumor suppressor gene
    - t(4;14) → upregulation of fibroblast growth factor (FGF) receptor 3
    - t(14;16) → upregulation of MAF transcription factor
  - Neutral/favorable prognostic factors
    - Absence of poor prognostic factors, plus 1 of the following
      - t(11;14) → upregulation of cyclin D1
      - t(6;14) → upregulation of cyclin D3
      - Hyperdiploidy

Associated Diseases, Abnormalities

- Myelofibrosis
- Fanconi syndrome type II (renal tubular acidosis)

Gross Pathology & Surgical Features

- Focal or widespread BM infiltration by genetically altered PCs
- Focal extramedullary disease is termed plasmacytoma

Microscopic Pathology

- H&E
  - % of BM PCs important for classification of MM
  - BM analysis: May be subject to sampling error
    - Aspirate can underestimate or overestimate number of PCs
    - BM biopsy more accurate
- Special stains
  - Wright-Giemsa considered superior
  - CD138 immunohistochemistry most accurate
  - Typically positive for CD56, CD38, and CD138 and negative for CD19 and CD45

Routes of Spread

- Primarily intramedullary spread
- Extramedullary spread, especially in advanced disease
- Plasmacytoma of bone progresses to MM in 50-60% of cases

- Extramedullary plasmacytomas progress to MM in ~ 15% of cases
  - Useful in imaging facilities without MR or PET
  - Useful as measure of survival

IMAGING

Detection

- Solitary plasmacytoma
  - Detected via biopsy of solitary lesion
  - MR or FDG PET/CT used to exclude systemic disease
- Radiographic skeletal survey (RSS)
  - 20% of patients with normal axial MR showed extremity lesions by RSS
  - More sensitive than bone scan in 38%
  - Lytic lesions (< 5, 5-20, > 20) or osteopenia
    - Number of lytic lesions is important for staging
  - If RSS without lytic lesions
    - Whole-body MR vs. MR spine/pelvis
    - If no MR, FDG PET/CT preferred over CT alone
- Bone scan
  - Insensitive for MM; of limited usefulness
- CT
  - More sensitive than RSS for detecting lytic lesions
  - Number of lytic lesions ≥ 5 mm important for staging
- MR
  - 52% of normal RSS demonstrate lesions by MR
  - Whole-body MR most sensitive
  - T2 FS and STIR sequences most sensitive
  - T1 post gadolinium does not add to detection
  - Number of lesions ≥ 5 mm important for staging
  - Patterns of bone marrow disease visualized by MR
    - Normal (all patients with MGUS and early MM or MM associated with better prognosis)
    - Micronodular (a.k.a. variegated, "salt and pepper")
    - Focal lesions
    - Diffuse
      - Mild = micronodular or "salt and pepper"
      - Moderate = lower T1 signal than normal BM but with contrast between vertebral BM and disc
      - Severe = low T1 signal throughout vertebral BM with signal ≤ adjacent disc
    - May have combinations of the above 3
  - Normal and micronodular BM patterns: Associated with stage I disease
  - Active lesions → fluid-sensitive signal intensity ↑
- FDG-PET
  - Assesses metabolic activity, evaluates extramedullary disease, & identifies nonmyeloma lesions
  - More readily detects disease in extramedullary sites, ribs, and scapulae than MR
  - Number of lytic lesions ≥ 5 mm important for staging
  - Especially valuable for evaluating disease burden in nonsecretory multiple myeloma
  - Active lesions have ↑ activity above background
  - Absence of FDG uptake seen in all patients with MGUS and early stage MM or disease associated with better prognosis

Staging

- Durie and Salmon PLUS staging system
  - Incorporates advanced imaging with MR and PET
- International staging system (ISS)

CLINICAL PRESENTATION & WORK-UP

Presentation

- Symptomatic
  - Bone pain or constitutional symptoms
- Laboratory findings
  - Elevated β2-microglobulin
  - Serum and urine M-protein (except nonsecretory)
  - Calcium elevation
  - Renal insufficiency
  - Anemia

Prognosis

- Due to heterogeneity, survival varies among patients
- Median survival in patients treated with melphalan and steroids ~ 2.5 years
- Median survival with modern treatment ~ 8.5 years

Work-Up

- Clinical
  - H&P
  - Bone marrow biopsy and aspirate, cytogenetics
- Radiographic
  - Skeletal survey and whole-body MR or PET/CT if available
  - Some cases may require CT (avoid contrast)
  - Bone densitometry if bisphosphonates are used or in certain circumstances
- Laboratory
  - CBC, calcium, albumin, creatinine, LDH
  - B2-microglobulin
  - Serum protein electrophoresis (SPEP) and serum immunofixation electrophoresis (SIFE)
  - Urine protein electrophoresis (UPEP) and urine immunofixation electrophoresis (UIFE)
  - Some cases may require serum viscosity analysis and HLA typing

TREATMENT

Major Treatment Alternatives

- Chemotherapy (chemo)
  - Typically proteosome inhibitor (Bortezomib) + steroids ± antiangiogenic (i.e., thalidomide or lenalidomide)
  - If transplant is not an option, then melphalan and prednisone may be good option
- ↑ dose chemo with auto transplantation → ↑ survival
  - Autologous transplantation performed in patients < 65 years old and those older who can tolerate intensive treatment
  - 1 study showed superiority of chemopreparative regimen compared to 8 Gy TBI + melphalan
- Allogeneic transplantation (rare)
  - Potentially curative; however, mortality rate of 5-10%
  - Minitransplants: 1 trial showed ↑ overall survival (OS) with 2 Gy TBI + fludarabine for patients with HLA identical sibling, but also ↑ nonrelapse death

MULTIPLE MYELOMA

- Bisphosphonates recommended for all patients receiving active treatment
- Solitary plasmacytoma of bone
  - Local control: 88-96% in 7 studies and conversion to MM 46-56%
  - Multiple sequential solitary plasmacytomas may develop in 10-25%
- Extramedullary plasmacytoma
  - Local control: 83-96% in 5 studies and conversion to MM 8-36%
  - Solitary plasmacytomas of bone may develop in 5-10%
- Focal palliative treatment
  - RT for epidural disease if chemo does not cause rapid decompression
    - Limited fields should be used to spare bone marrow
  - Kypho-/vertebroplasty for symptomatic compression

Major Treatment Roadblocks/ Contraindications

- Age and functional status

Treatment Options by Stage

- Solitary plasmacytoma (stage IA): Radiation
- Stage IB-III: Systemic therapy

Dose Response

- In 1 study, palliation was observed in 98% when > 10 Gy was used

Standard Doses

- ≥ 45 Gy for both solitary plasmacytoma and extramedullary plasmacytoma
  - Treat GTV + 2-3 cm margin
  - For extramedullary plasmacytoma, consider including primary draining lymphatics
- For cord compression, 1 study showed 30 Gy in 10 fractions was more durable than short course

RECOMMENDED FOLLOW-UP

Clinical

- Bone marrow biopsy and aspirate

Radiographic

- Annual skeletal survey
- MR or PET/CT as indicated

Laboratory

- CBC, calcium, albumin, creatinine, LDH
- β2-microglobulin
- Quantitative immunoglobulins

SELECTED REFERENCES

1. Anderson KC et al: Multiple myeloma. J Natl Compr Canc Netw. 9(10):1146-83, 2011
2. Björkstrand B et al: Tandem autologous/reduced-intensity conditioning allogeneic stem-cell transplantation versus autologous transplantation in myeloma: long-term follow-up. J Clin Oncol. 29(22):3016-22, 2011
3. Hanrahan CJ et al: Current concepts in the evaluation of multiple myeloma with MR imaging and FDG PET/CT. Radiographics. 30(1):127-42, 2010
4. Dimopoulos M et al: International myeloma working group consensus statement and guidelines regarding the current role of imaging techniques in the diagnosis and monitoring of multiple myeloma. Leukemia. 23(9):1545-56, 2009
5. Shortt CP et al: Whole-Body MRI versus PET in assessment of multiple myeloma disease activity. AJR Am J Roentgenol. 192(4):980-6, 2009
6. Baur-Melnyk A et al: Whole-body MRI versus whole-body MDCT for staging of multiple myeloma. AJR Am J Roentgenol. 190(4):1097-104, 2008
7. Kyle RA et al: Multiple myeloma. Blood. 111(6):2962-72, 2008
8. Avet-Loiseau H et al: Genetic abnormalities and survival in multiple myeloma: the experience of the Intergroupe Francophone du Myélome. Blood. 109(8):3489-95, 2007
9. Breyer RJ 3rd et al: Comparison of imaging with FDG PET/CT with other imaging modalities in myeloma. Skeletal Radiol. 35(9):632-40, 2006
10. Durie BG: The role of anatomic and functional staging in myeloma: description of Durie/Salmon plus staging system. Eur J Cancer. 42(11):1539-43, 2006
11. Greipp PR et al: International staging system for multiple myeloma. J Clin Oncol. 23(15):3412-20, 2005
12. Angtuaco EJ et al: Multiple myeloma: clinical review and diagnostic imaging. Radiology. 231(1):11-23, 2004
13. Moreau P et al: Comparison of 200 mg/m(2) melphalan and 8 Gy total body irradiation plus 140 mg/m(2) melphalan as conditioning regimens for peripheral blood stem cell transplantation in patients with newly diagnosed multiple myeloma: final analysis of the Intergroupe Francophone du Myélome 9502 randomized trial. Blood. 99(3):731-5, 2002
14. Leigh BR et al: Radiation therapy for the palliation of multiple myeloma. Int J Radiat Oncol Biol Phys. 25(5):801-4, 1993
15. Frassica DA et al: Solitary plasmacytoma of bone: Mayo Clinic experience. Int J Radiat Oncol Biol Phys. 16(1):43-8, 1989

Stage I

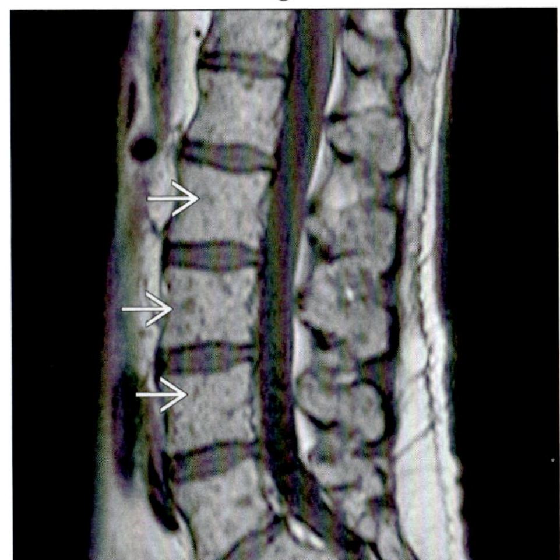

Stage II

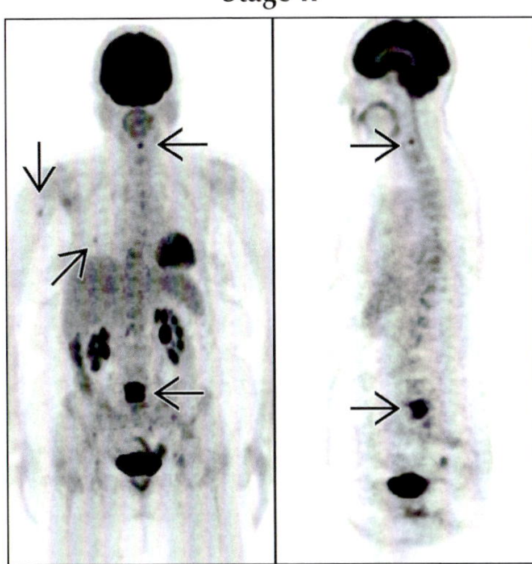

(Left) *Sagittal T1WI MR through the lumbar spine demonstrates replacement of the normal fatty bone marrow with micronodular foci ➔ of low T1 signal, consistent with myeloma infiltration.* ***(Right)*** *MIP (left) and sagittal (right) FDG-PET images in a patient with stage II disease demonstrate focal areas of increased FDG uptake → in L4, right humerus, C5, and a posterior right rib with low background marrow activity (SUV < 2.5).*

Stage III

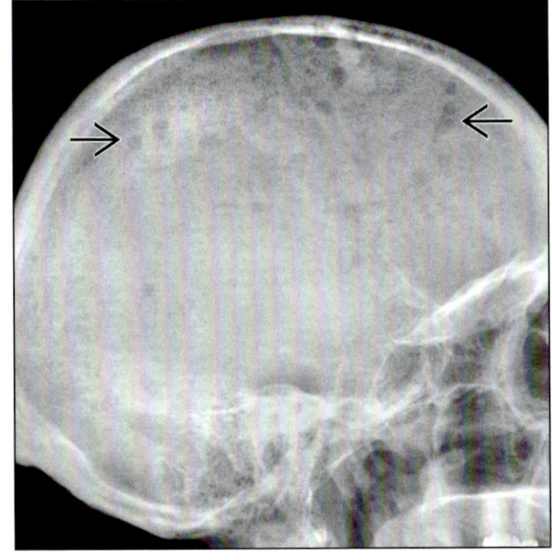

Stage IIIB

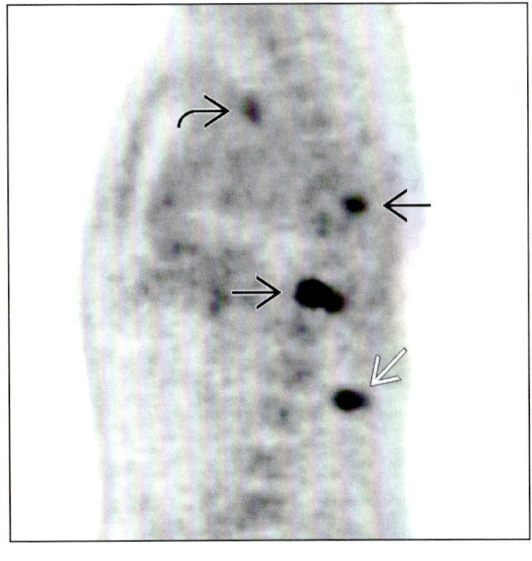

(Left) *Sagittal radiograph through the skull demonstrates numerous subcentimeter lytic foci →. More than 20 lytic foci indicate stage III disease.* ***(Right)*** *Sagittal FDG-PET demonstrates focal areas of increased uptake in vertebrae → and spinous process ➔ marrow. Uptake within mediastinal lymph node ↷ is suggestive of extramedullary uptake that elevates the patient's disease to substage B.*

Stage IIIB

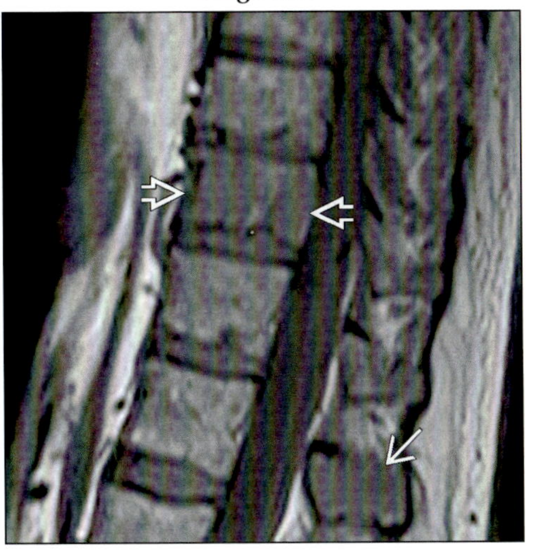

Stage IIIB

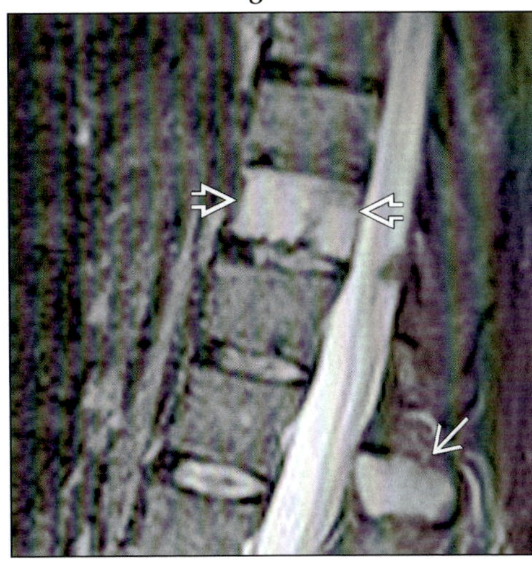

(Left) *Sagittal T1WI MR in the same patient through the thoracolumbar spine demonstrates replacement of normal fatty marrow with low T1 signal foci of myeloma infiltration involving the vertebral body ➔ and the spinous process marrow ➔.* ***(Right)*** *Sagittal STIR MR from the same patient demonstrates increased STIR signal involving the vertebra ➔ and the spinous process ➔. MR and PET readily identified disease in the spinous process, which was not identified on x-ray.*

MULTIPLE MYELOMA

(Left) A young adult presented with incontinence and an inability to ambulate. Sagittal CT shows destruction of the posterior aspect of T10. A significant mass can be seen filling the spinal canal ➡. (Right) Axial CT in the same patient shows the severe bony destruction, including the posterior elements ↪ and the large soft tissue mass ➡.

Plasmacytoma of Bone

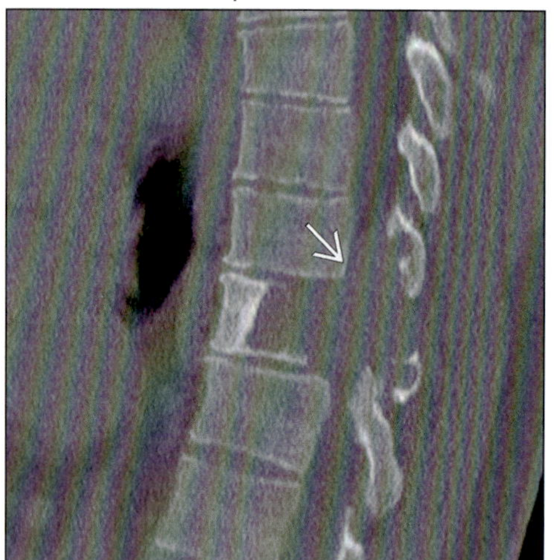

Plasmacytoma of Bone

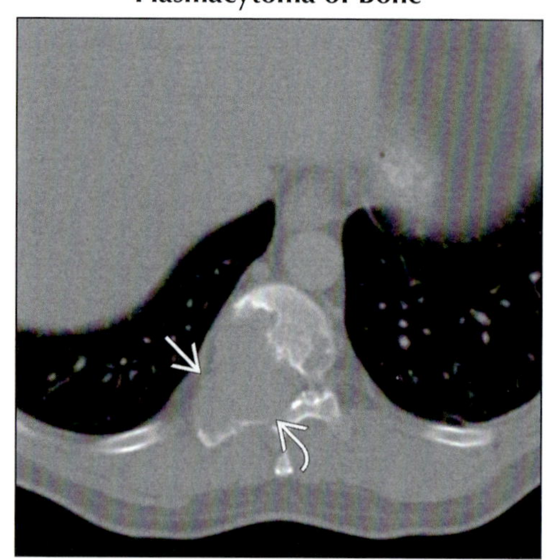

(Left) 3D DRR of T10 vertebral body in the same patient shows large lytic region ➡. These reconstructions can aid surgical reconstruction. (Right) Lateral x-ray in the same patient demonstrates posterior fixation to promote long-term stability.

Plasmacytoma of Bone

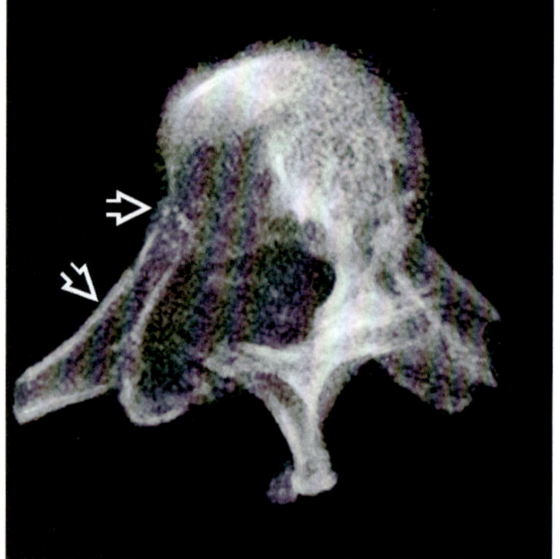

Plasmacytoma of Bone

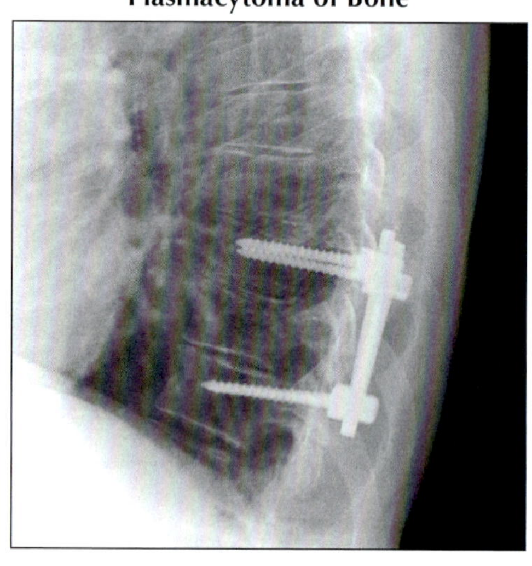

(Left) Axial CT in the same patient shows the red, yellow, and blue isodose lines representing 105%, 96%, and 90%, respectively. An anterior beam was used to supplement dose to the anterior aspect of the vertebral body. Patient had a full neurologic recovery after 40 Gy in 20 fractions. (Right) TBI is one preparatory regimen for multiple myeloma. Partial transmission lung blocks are shown ➡. Chemo preparatory regimens have shown less morbidity than TBI regimens.

Plasmacytoma of Bone

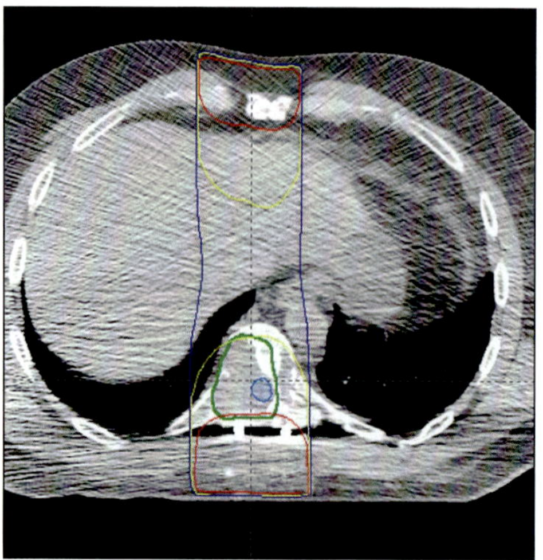

Total Body Irradiation

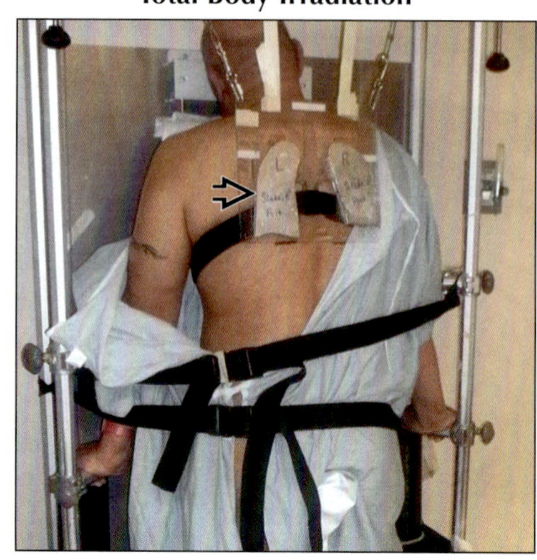

Skull Base Plasmacytoma

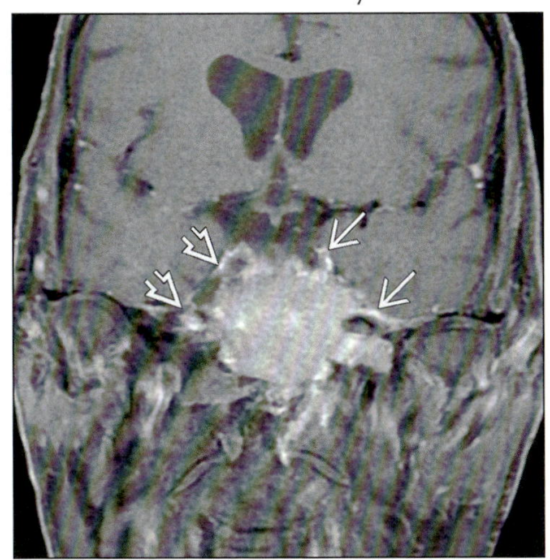

Skull Base Plasmacytoma

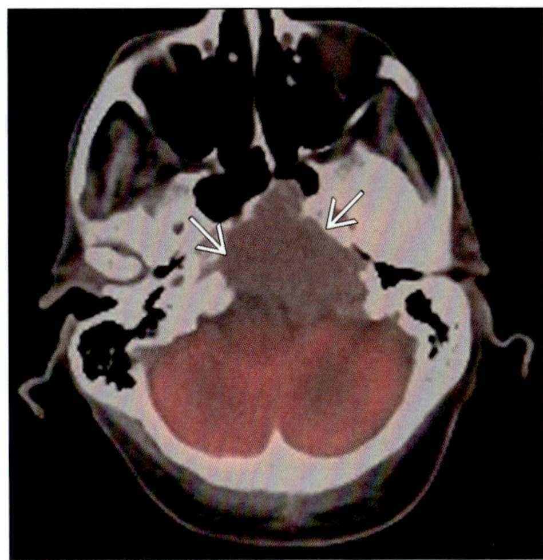

*(**Left**) Coronal T1WI post-contrast MR shows a brightly enhancing mass occupying the sphenoid and temporal bone. The tumor encased the carotid on the left ➡ and abutted the carotid on the right ➡. (**Right**) Axial fused PET/CT in the same patient shows the mass ➡ is not FDG avid. Normal avidity is seen in the cerebellum. Bone scan also showed no increased uptake, which is common for myeloma. Bone destruction is readily apparent on CT.*

Skull Base Plasmacytoma

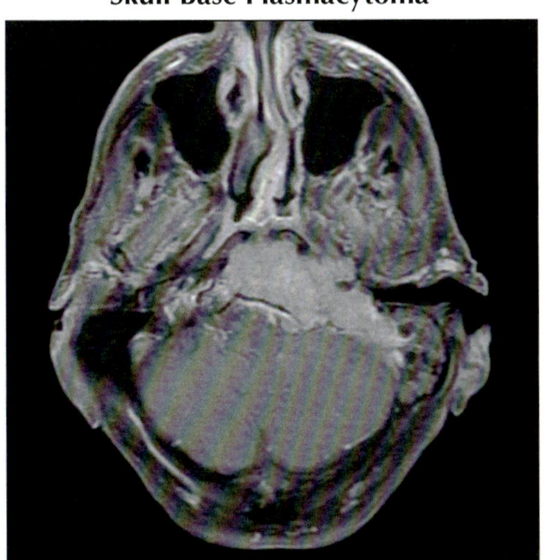

Skull Base Plasmacytoma

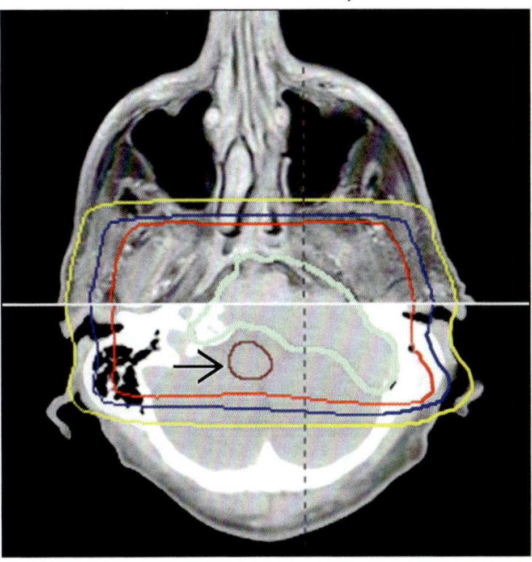

*(**Left**) Axial T1WI post-contrast MR in the same patient shows extensive enhancement in the temporal bone. (**Right**) Fused MR T1WI post FS anteriorly to NECT posteriorly in the same patient shows the GTV in light green. The red, blue, and yellow show the 100%, 90%, and 50% isodose surfaces, respectively. 44 Gy was delivered in 22 fractions with a good neurologic response. Brain stem ➡ is contoured in brown. MR/CT fusion permits much greater precision for the GTV.*

Extramedullary Plasmacytoma of the Trachea

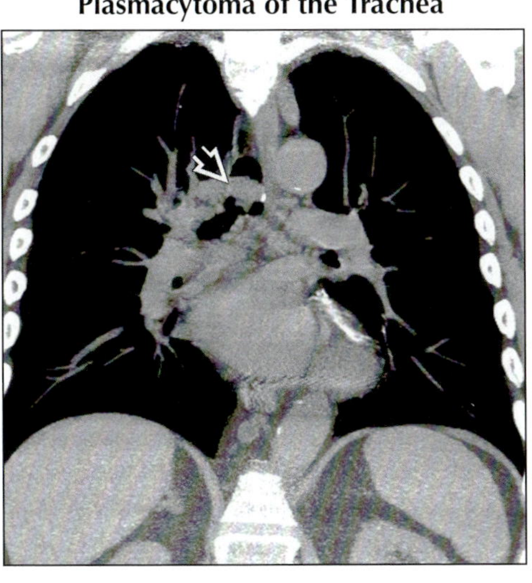

Extramedullary Plasmacytoma of the Trachea

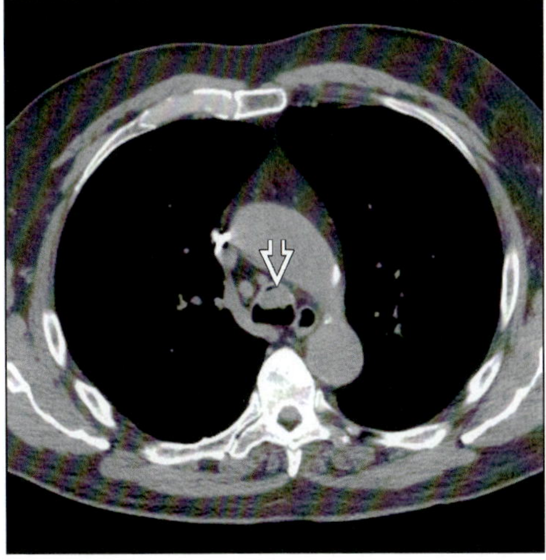

*(**Left**) Coronal CECT shows tracheal mass ➡ just superior to the carina. Extramedullary plasmacytomas can occur in various locations; however, the upper respiratory tract is most common. (**Right**) Axial CECT in the same patient reveals mass on the axial aspect of the trachea ➡.*

(Left) *Sagittal CECT in the same patient shows tracheal lesion* ➔ *filling ~ 50% of the lumen of the trachea.* **(Right)** *After endobronchial resection in the same patient, sagittal NECT demonstrates the preresection location of the mass in green. Red, yellow, and blue represent the 100%, 90%, and 50% isodose lines, respectively. Patient was treated to 20 Gy in 10 fractions after complete resection. Myeloma can be well palliated with low doses.*

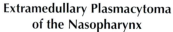

Extramedullary Plasmacytoma of the Trachea

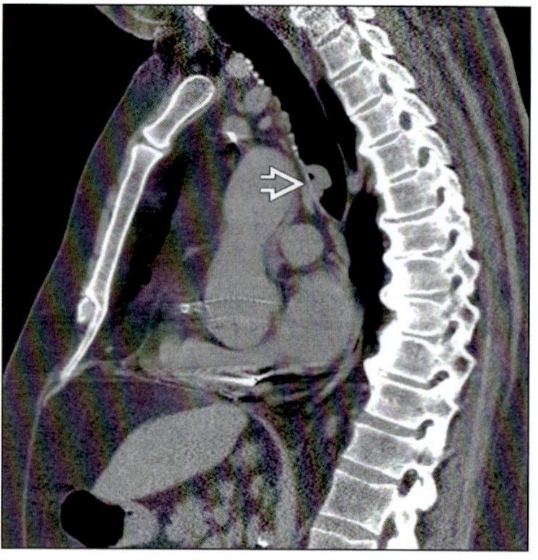

Extramedullary Plasmacytoma of the Trachea

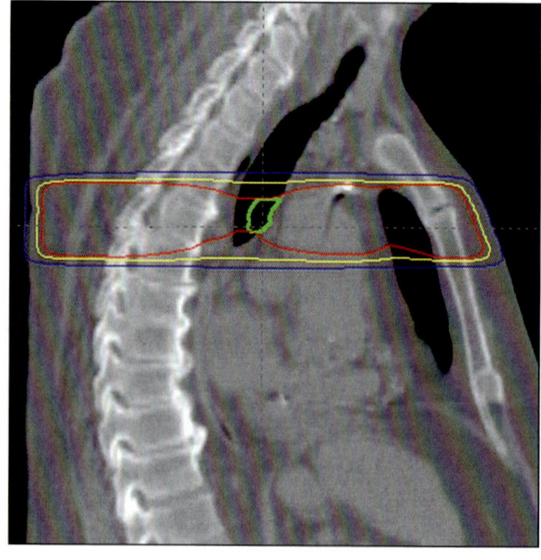

(Left) *Coronal T1WI post-contrast MR shows 9 mm by 9 mm mass* ➔ *adjacent to the torus tubarius in the right nasopharynx.* **(Right)** *Axial T1WI post-contrast MR in the same patient shows 9 mm by 9 mm mass* ➔ *brightly enhancing.*

Extramedullary Plasmacytoma of the Nasopharynx

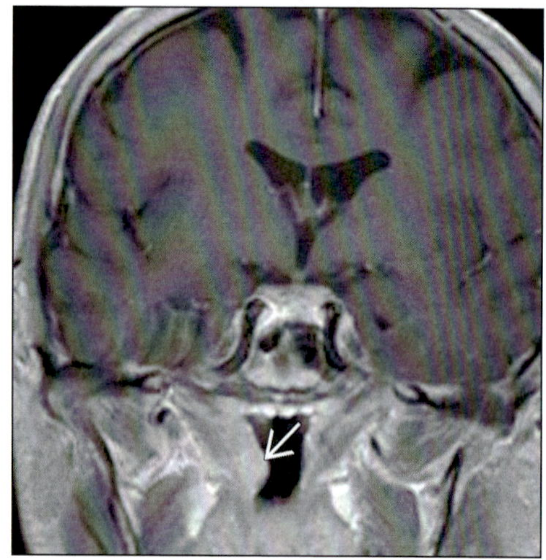

Extramedullary Plasmacytoma of the Nasopharynx

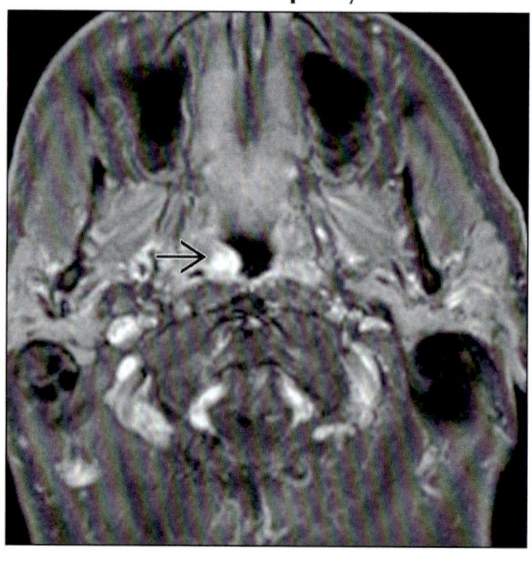

(Left) *Sagittal T1WI post-contrast MR in the same patient was fused to CT. The PTV is shown in yellow. The thin pink, green, and purple lines represent the 95%, 80%, and 20% isodose lines, respectively.* **(Right)** *Coronal T1WI post-contrast MR in the same patient shows sharp dose fall-off with this 7F IMRT plan. Note the sparing of the right parotid* ➔*. The advantage of IMRT here is the reduction of high-dose regions to OARs. 45 Gy was delivered in 25 fractions.*

Extramedullary Plasmacytoma of the Nasopharynx

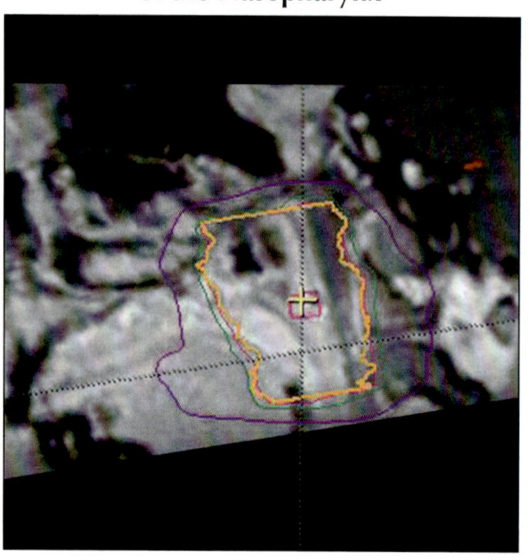

Extramedullary Plasmacytoma of the Nasopharynx

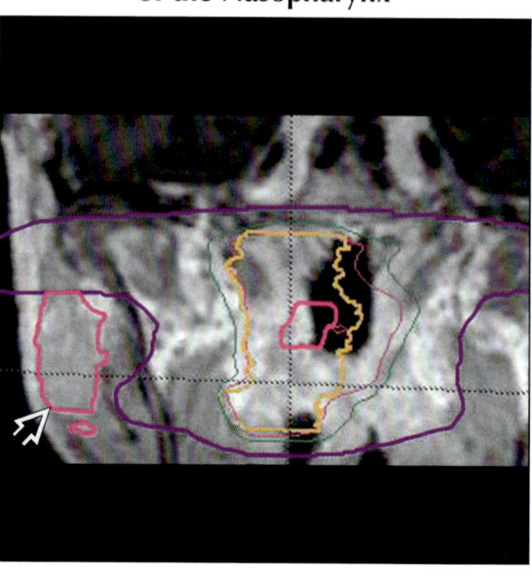

Plasmacytoma of Bone

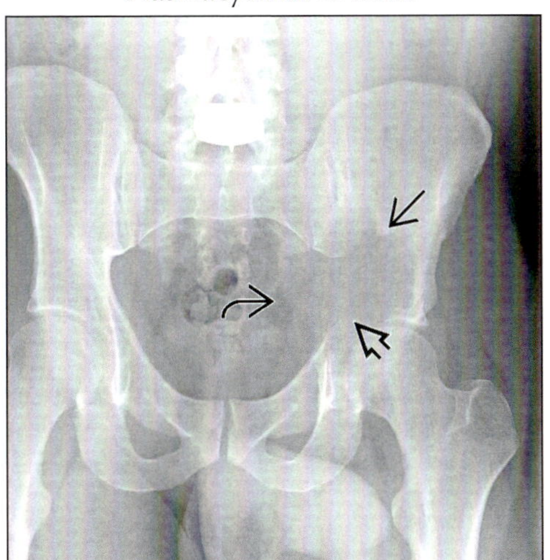

Plasmacytoma of Bone

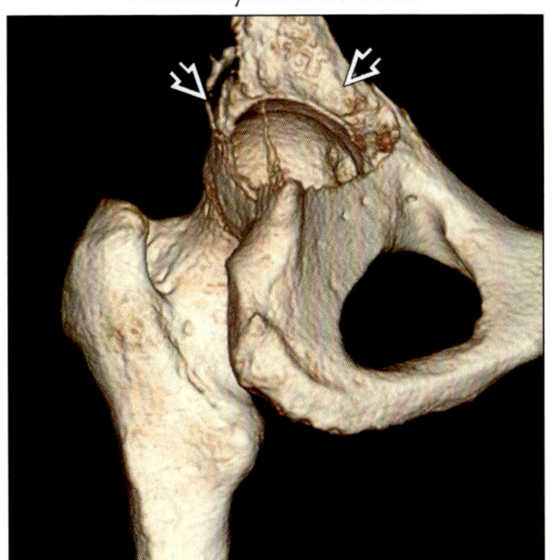

*(**Left**) Anterior x-ray shows a large lytic mass ➔ in the left ileum with destruction of the acetabulum ➢. A soft tissue component ↗ can be seen encroaching into the pelvis. (**Right**) DRR shows destruction of the acetabulum in the same patient. These model reconstructions can aid the surgeons in reconstruction of the bony defect ➢.*

Plasmacytoma of Bone

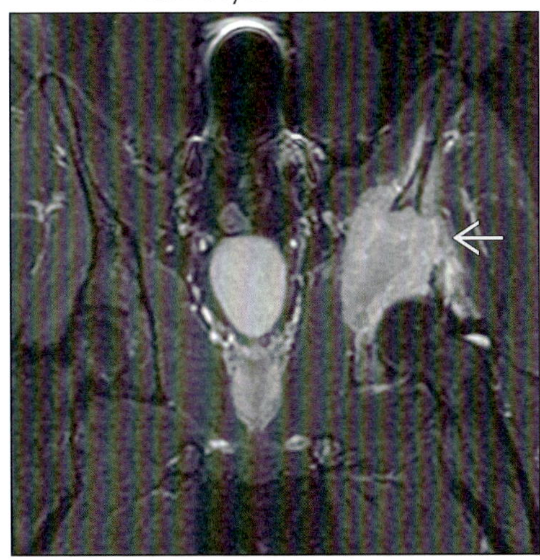

Plasmacytoma of Bone

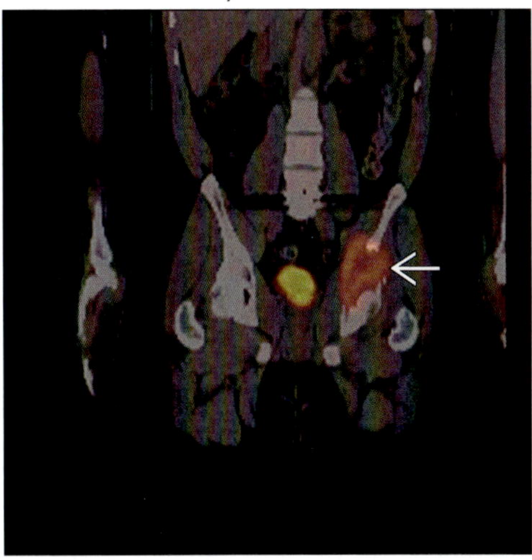

*(**Left**) Coronal STIR MR in the same patient shows the brightly enhancing tumor ➔. Whole-body MR failed to reveal other lesions; hence, a plasmacytoma was diagnosed. (**Right**) Coronal fused PET/CT in the same patient shows that, in this case, the mass ➔ is FDG avid. The CT confirms the lytic destruction of bone by the plasmacytoma.*

Plasmacytoma of Bone

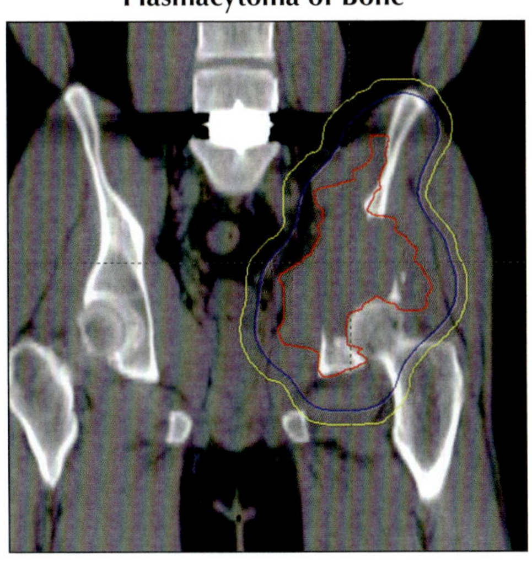

Plasmacytoma of Bone

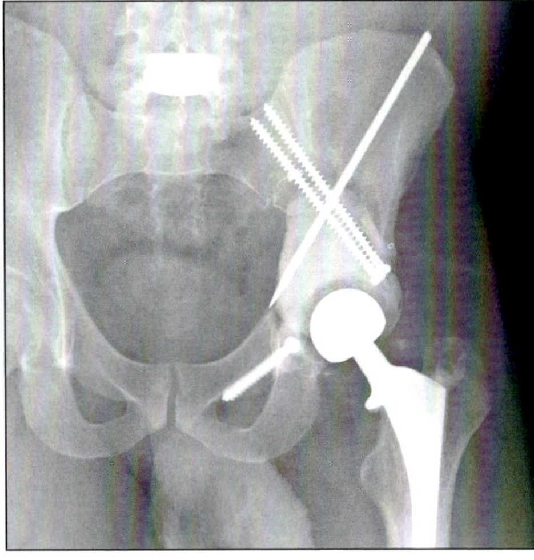

*(**Left**) Coronal NECT in the same patient shows the GTV in red. The blue and yellow lines indicate the 95% and 75% lines, respectively. The patient was treated with opposed obliques to 44 Gy in 22 fractions. (**Right**) Post RT, the same patient underwent fixation to promote stability and prevent fracture.*

MELANOMA

(T) Primary Tumor

Adapted from 7th edition AJCC Staging Forms.

TNM	*Definitions*
TX	Primary tumor cannot be assessed (e.g., curettaged or severely regressed melanoma)
T0	No evidence of primary tumor
Tis	Melanoma in situ
T1	Melanomas ≤ 1.0 mm in thickness
T1a	Melanomas ≤ 1.0 mm in thickness without ulceration and mitosis < 1/mm²
T1b	Melanomas ≤ 1.0 mm in thickness with ulceration or mitoses ≥ 1/mm²
T2	Melanomas 1.01-2.0 mm
T2a	Melanomas 1.01-2.0 mm without ulceration
T2b	Melanomas 1.01-2.0 mm with ulceration
T3	Melanomas 2.01-4.0 mm
T3a	Melanomas 2.01-4.0 mm without ulceration
T3b	Melanomas 2.01-4.0 mm with ulceration
T4	Melanomas > 4.0 mm
T4a	Melanomas > 4.0 mm without ulceration
T4b	Melanomas > 4.0 mm with ulceration

(N) Regional Lymph Nodes

NX	Patients in whom regional nodes cannot be assessed (e.g., previously removed for another reason)
N0	No regional metastases detected
N1	1 metastatic node
N1a	1 metastatic node and micrometastasis[1]
N1b	1 metastatic node and macrometastasis[2]
N2	2-3 metastatic nodes
N2a	2-3 metastatic nodes and micrometastasis[1]
N2b	2-3 metastatic nodes and macrometastasis[2]
N2c	2-3 metastatic nodes and in-transit met(s)/satellite(s) **without** metastatic nodes
N3	≥ 4 metastatic nodes, or matted nodes, or in-transit met(s)/satellite(s) **with** metastatic node(s)

(M) Distant Metastasis

M0	No detectable evidence of distant metastases
M1a	Metastases to skin, subcutaneous tissues, or distant lymph nodes
M1b	Metastases to lung
M1c	Metastases to all other visceral sites or distant metastases to any site associated with elevated serum LDH

[1]*Micrometastases are diagnosed after sentinel lymph node biopsy and completion lymphadenectomy (if performed).*
[2]*Macrometastases are defined as clinically detectable nodal metastases confirmed by therapeutic lymphadenectomy or when nodal metastasis exhibits gross extracapsular extension.*

Clinical and Pathologic AJCC Stages/ Prognostic Groups

Adapted from 7th edition AJCC Staging Forms.

Clinical Stage[1]	*Clinical T*	*Clinical N*	*Clinical M*	*Pathologic Stage*[2]	*Pathologic T*	*Pathologic N*	*Pathologic M*
0	Tis	N0	M0	0	Tis	N0	M0
IA	T1a	N0	M0	IA	T1a	N0	M0
IB	T1b	N0	M0	IB	T1b	N0	M0
	T2a	N0	M0		T2a	N0	M0
IIA	T2b	N0	M0	IIA	T2b	N0	M0
	T3a	N0	M0		T3a	N0	M0
IIB	T3b	N0	M0	IIB	T3b	N0	M0
	T4a	N0	M0		T4a	N0	M0
IIC	T4b	N0	M0	IIC	T4b	N0	M0
III	Any T	≥ N1	M0	IIIA	T(1-4)a	N1a	M0
					T(1-4)a	N2a	M0
				IIIB	T(1-4)b	N1a	M0
					T(1-4)b	N2a	M0
					T(1-4)a	N1b	M0
					T(1-4)a	N2b	M0
					T(1-4)a	N2c	M0
				IIIC	T(1-4)b	N1b	M0
					T(1-4)b	N2b	M0
					T(1-4)b	N2c	M0
					Any T	N3	M0
IV	Any T	Any N	M1	IV	Any T	Any N	M1

[1]*Clinical staging includes microstaging of the primary melanoma and clinical/radiologic evaluation for metastases. By convention, it should be used after complete excision of the primary melanoma with clinical assessment for regional and distant metastases.*

[2]*Pathologic staging includes microstaging of the primary melanoma and pathologic information about the regional lymph nodes after partial or complete lymphadenectomy. Pathologic stage 0 or stage IA patients are the exception; they do not require pathologic evaluation of their lymph nodes.*

MELANOMA

Clark Level II

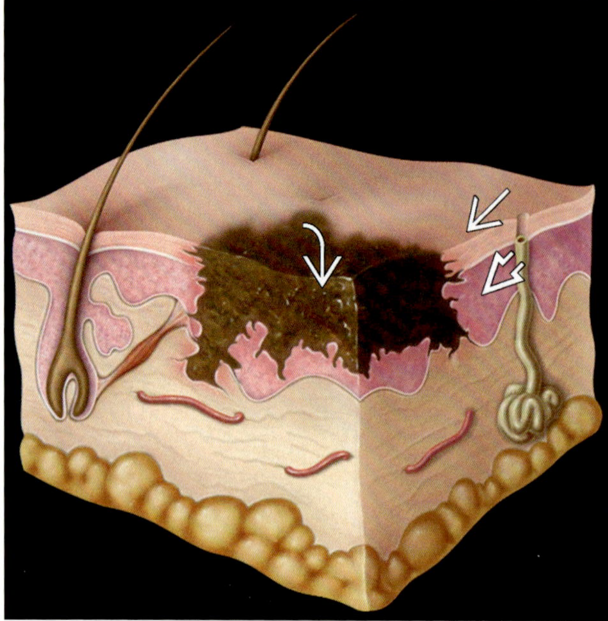

Graphic shows a Clark level II melanoma ➡ with invasion through the epidermis ➡ into papillary dermis ➡. Though widely used for < 40 years, Clark levels are not as reproducible among pathologists nor reflect prognosis as accurately as tumor thickness. Clark levels have thus been dropped from 7th edition AJCC staging.

Clark Level III

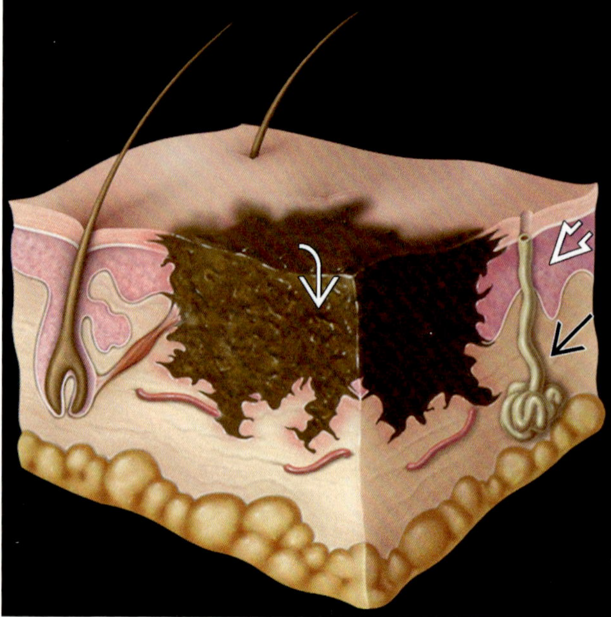

Graphic shows a Clark level III melanoma ➡ with invasion to the junction of the papillary dermis ➡ and the reticular dermis ➡.

Clark Level IV

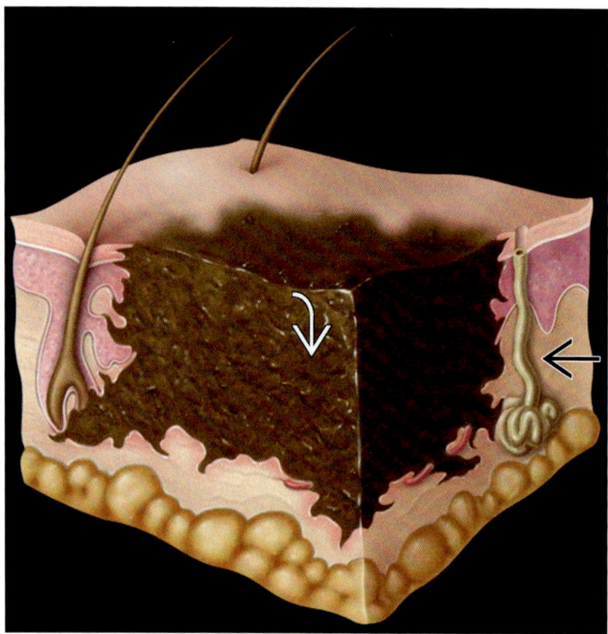

Graphic shows a Clark level IV melanoma ➡ with invasion into the reticular dermis ➡.

Clark Level V

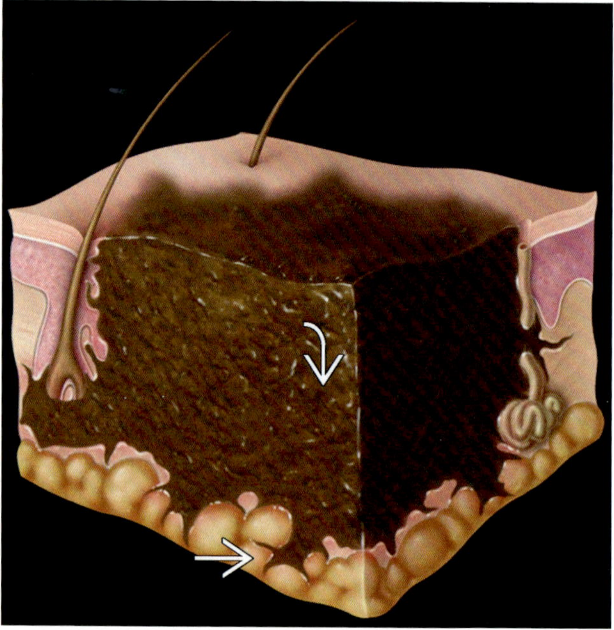

Graphic shows a Clark level V melanoma ➡ with invasion into the subcutaneous fat ➡.

T1a

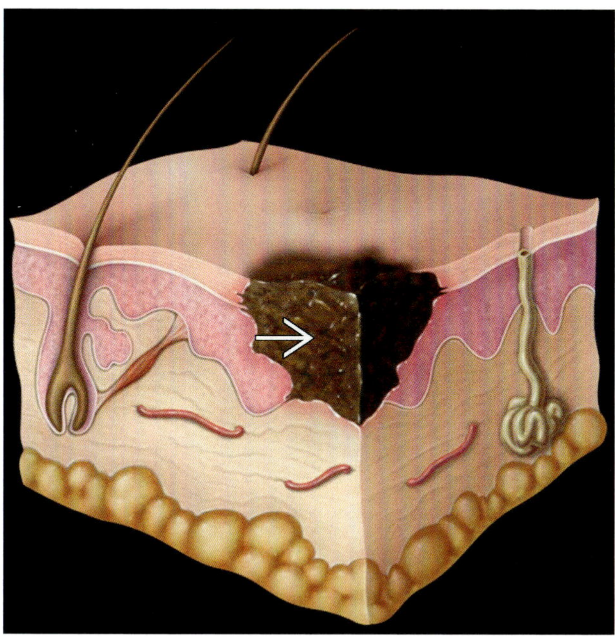

Graphic shows a T1a lesion ➡, which is ≤ 1 mm in thickness, with absence of ulceration and mitotic rate < 1/mm². By definition, T1 melanoma lesions are ≤ 1 mm in thickness.

T1b

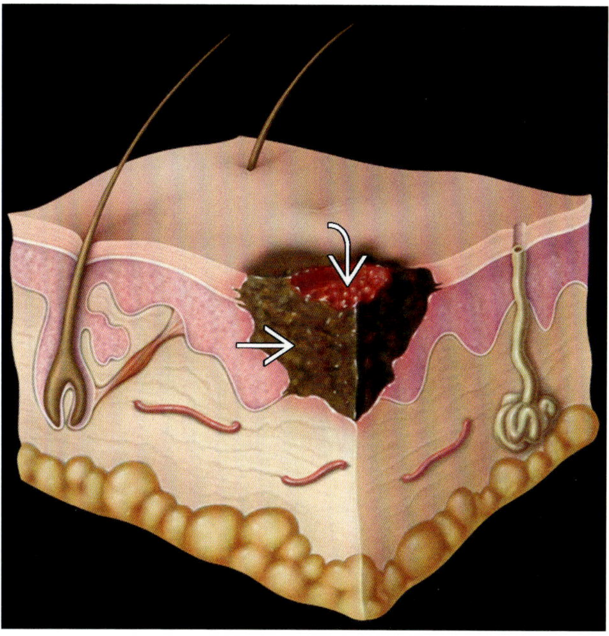

Graphic illustrates a T1b lesion, which is defined as a melanoma ➡ ≤ 1 mm in thickness with a mitotic rate > 1 mitosis/mm², or ulceration ➦.

T2a

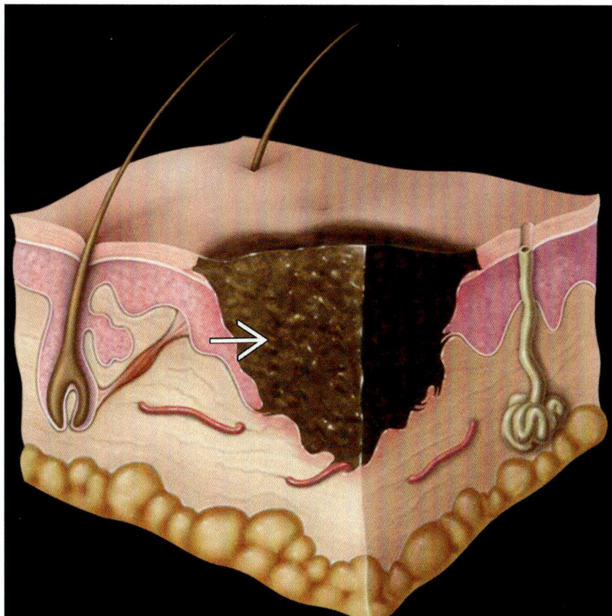

Graphic shows a T2a melanoma ➡. It is thicker than 1 mm but ≤ 2 mm and lacks ulceration.

T2b

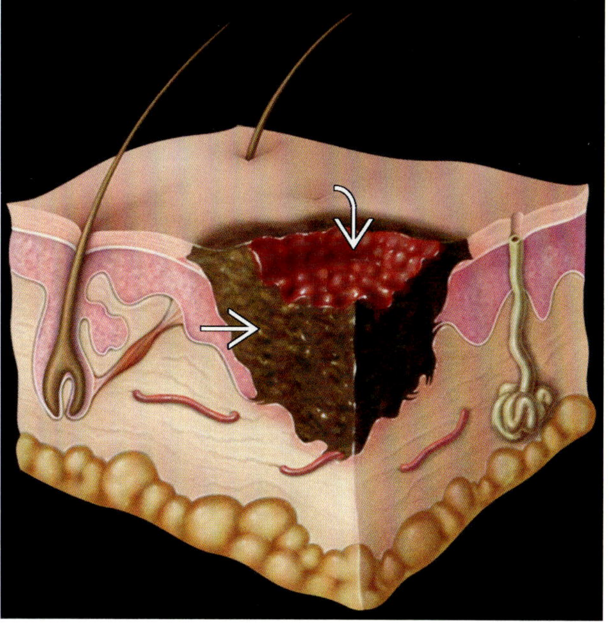

Graphic shows a T2b lesion ➡, which is > 1 mm but ≤ 2 mm in thickness with ulceration ➦.

MELANOMA

T3a

Graphic shows a T3a melanoma, which is > 2 mm but ≤ 4 mm in thickness without ulceration.

T3b

Graphic shows a T3b lesion. Its thickness (> 2 mm but ≤ 4 mm) makes it T3, and the ulceration subclassifies it as T3b.

T4a

Graphic shows a T4a lesion, which is > 4 mm in thickness without ulceration.

T4b

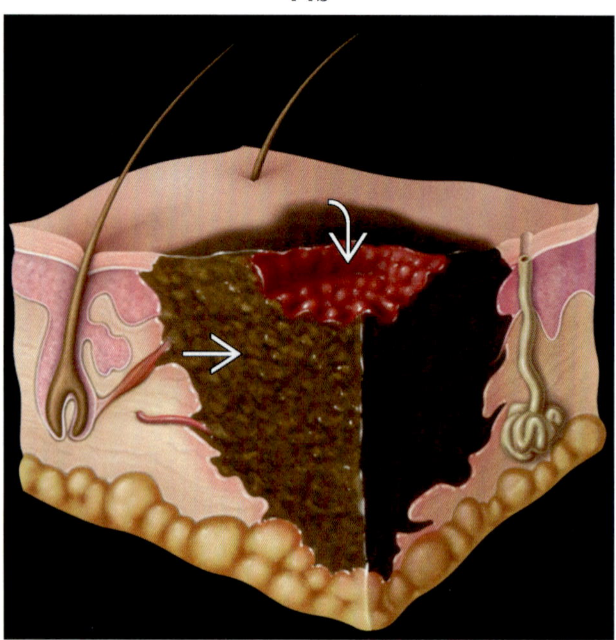

Graphic shows a T4b melanoma, which is thicker than 4 mm with ulceration.

N1, N2, and N3

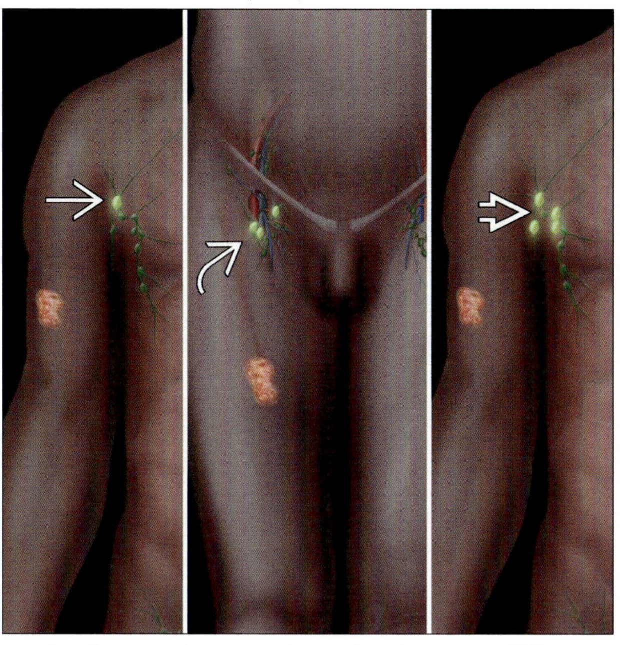

Graphic shows N1 disease, single lymph node metastasis ; N2 disease, 2-3 metastatic nodes ; and N3 disease, 4 or more metastatic nodes , matted nodes, or in-transit metastases/ satellite(s) with metastatic nodes. Both N1 and N2 can be subdivided into a (micrometastasis) and b (macrometastasis).

M1a and M1b

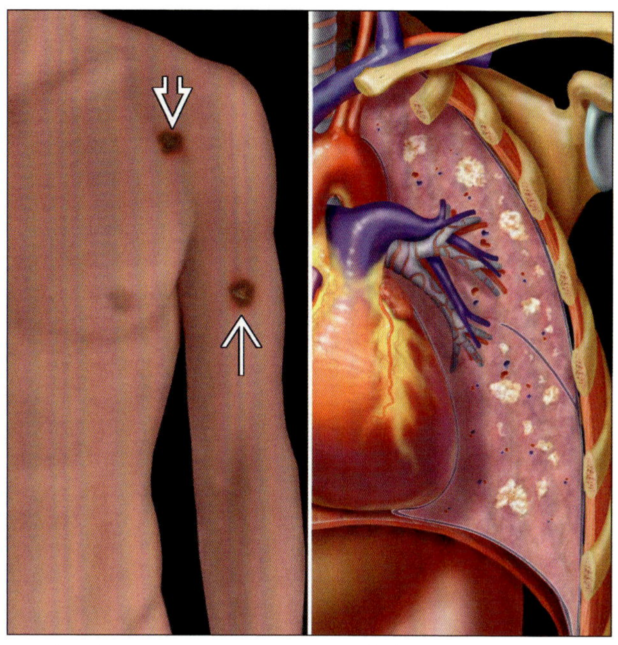

Graphic shows a primary site on the arm with metastasis to the subcutaneous tissues and skin of the shoulder (M1a). Distant lymph nodes would also be M1a. Lung metastases (right) are M1b. Metastases to all other visceral sites or distant metastases to any site associated with an elevated serum LDH are considered M1c.

INITIAL SITE OF RECURRENCE

Distant Only	30%
Lymph Node Field Only	21%
Distant + Any Locoregional Site	12%
Local or In Transit	3%
Lymph Node Field + Local or In Transit	2%

Data represent results of 126 patients randomized to observation after resection of palpable lymphadenopathy from TROG/ANZMTG trial. In the adjuvant RT group, lymph node field only relapsed to 7%, but 40% failed distantly alone (Burmeister et al, 2012). Most common sites for distant disease in decreasing order include lung, brain, distant skin & subcutaneous tissue, liver, nonregional lymph nodes, & bone (Agrawal et al, 2009).

MELANOMA

OVERVIEW

General Comments

- Malignant tumor of pigment-producing melanocytes usually located in skin
- Relative to other skin malignancies, melanoma is characterized by aggressive nature
  - Represents small fraction of total skin cancers (4%)
  - Responsible for majority of deaths from skin cancer (74%)
- Incidence of melanoma has been steadily increasing

Classification

- Melanocytic tumors (WHO classification)
  - Malignant melanoma
    - Superficial spreading melanoma
    - Nodular melanoma
    - Lentigo maligna
    - Acral lentiginous melanoma
    - Desmoplastic melanoma
    - Melanoma arising from blue nevus
    - Melanoma arising in giant congenital nevus
    - Melanoma of childhood
    - Nevoid melanoma
    - Persistent melanoma
- Major melanoma subtypes (organized by histological characteristics)
  - Superficial spreading melanoma
  - Nodular melanoma
  - Lentigo maligna melanoma
  - Acral lentiginous melanoma
  - Desmoplastic melanoma

NATURAL HISTORY

General Features

- Comments
  - Heterogeneous cancer with varying gross pathological and histological characteristics
- Location
  - Can occur anywhere on skin

Etiology

- Risk factors
  - UV radiation (e.g., sun & tanning beds)
  - Genetic susceptibilities
- Protective factors
  - Screening skin for concerning lesions
  - Protection from UV radiation
    - Sunscreen with zinc oxide &/or titanium dioxide

Epidemiology & Cancer Incidence

- Number of cases in USA per year
  - Estimated 2012 statistics for USA
    - 76,250 new cases of melanoma
    - 9,180 deaths from melanoma
      - Survival rates are improving over time
- Sex predilection
  - 1.4:1 male predominance
- Age of onset
  - Wide age range at diagnosis
  - 18% of all patients diagnosed before age 45
  - Median age of onset is 61 years
- Risk factors
  - Intense or prolonged sun exposure
    - Increased risk in areas near equator or with sunny climates
  - Fair-skinned phenotype
  - History of
    - Large number of nevi
    - Dysplastic nevi
    - Congenital nevi
  - History of blistering sunburns as child or adolescent
- Genetic diseases with highly increased risk
  - Xeroderma pigmentosum
  - Familial atypical mole melanoma syndrome

Genetics

- High-risk mutations can lead to uninhibited progression of cell cycle resulting in tumorigenesis
  - Implicated genes include
    - *CDKN2A* (a.k.a. *MTS1*, *p16INK4a*, and *CDKN2*)
    - *CDK4*
- Moderate- to low-risk mutations include
  - *BRCA2*
  - Retinoblastoma
  - Melanocortin-1 receptor genes
  - 1p22 gene locus

Associated Diseases, Abnormalities

- Hereditary melanomas are linked with increased risk of pancreatic cancer and brain tumors

Gross Pathology & Surgical Features

- Characterized by varying morphological appearance
- ABCDE criteria
  - Asymmetry
  - Border irregularities
  - Color variegation (varying colors in specified region)
  - Diameter > 6 mm
  - Evolution (changes in lesion over time)
- Macular areas correspond to radial growth phase
- Raised areas correspond to vertical growth phase

Microscopic Pathology

- Melanoma exhibits wide degree of histological diversity
- Main histologic subtypes
  - **Superficial spreading melanoma**
    - Frequency: ~ 70% of all melanomas
    - Location: Trunk in men and women & legs in women
    - Age: Median onset in 4th-6th decades
    - Appearance: Commonly exhibits ABCDE warning criteria
    - Histology
      - Dominant cells seen in radial and vertical growth phases are epithelioid cells
      - Epidermis may range from normal to hyperplastic
      - Diffuse pagetoid pattern is seen
  - **Nodular melanoma**
    - Frequency: ~ 15-30% of all melanomas
    - Location: Legs and trunk in men and women
    - Age: Median onset in 6th decade
    - Appearance: Often lacks ABCDE warning criteria
      - May be clinically amelanotic
      - Commonly involves elevation, ulceration with bleeding, or both
    - Histology
      - Lack of radial growth phase

- Dominant cells in vertical growth phase are epithelioid cells
- **Lentigo maligna melanoma**
  - Frequency: ~ 4-15% of all melanomas
  - Location: Head, neck, and arms in areas of chronically sun-damaged skin
  - Age: Median onset in 7th decade
  - Appearance: Development of elevated blue-black nodules within in situ lesion, which often appears dark brown to black
  - Histology
    - Often involves a junctional confluent proliferation of melanocytes and extension along adnexal structures
    - In radial growth phase, lentiginous pattern is seen and atrophy is present in epidermis
    - Spindle and epithelioid cells are commonly seen in radial and vertical growth phases
    - Desmoplasia and neurotropism are common
- **Acral lentiginous melanoma**
  - Frequency: ~ 2-3% of all melanomas
    - 9-72% of melanomas in dark-skinned individuals (i.e., African-Americans, Asians, & Hispanics)
    - Only ~ 2% of melanomas in non-Hispanic whites
  - Location: Palms, soles, beneath nail plate (subungual)
  - Age: Median onset in 7th decade
  - Appearance: Darkly pigmented areas on skin or longitudinal brown, tan, or black streak on a nail bed
  - Histology
    - In radial growth phase, lentiginous pattern is seen and epidermis is hyperplastic
    - Spindle and epithelioid cells are commonly seen in radial and vertical growth phases
    - Desmoplasia and neurotropism are common
- **Desmoplastic melanoma**
  - Frequency: < 5% of all melanomas
  - Location: Sun-exposed areas of head & neck
  - Age: Median onset in 7th decade
  - Appearance: Macular area of pigmentation, or firm, amelanotic nodule or scar
  - Histology: Frequently exhibits deep invasion and perineural involvement
- Stains
  - Immunohistochemistry can offer further diagnostic value in addition to H&E stain
  - Commonly used monoclonal antibodies that bind to melanoma antigens include
    - S100
    - Melan-A/MART-1
    - HMB-45

Routes of Spread

- Local spread
  - Some melanomas exhibit in situ growth phase (radial growth) before potential dermal invasion (vertical growth)
    - e.g., superficial spreading, lentigo maligna, and acral lentiginous melanoma
  - Nodular melanoma exhibits vertical growth phase from onset
    - Accounts for its aggressiveness
  - Desmoplastic melanoma has a propensity for deep invasion with lower risk for nodal and metastatic spread
- Lymphatic extension
  - Most common sites of spread are regional lymph nodes
    - Autopsy series showed nodal metastases in nearly 3/4 of patients
  - Satellite metastases: Grossly visible cutaneous &/ or subcutaneous metastases occurring ≤ 2 cm of primary
  - Microsatellites: Microscopic and discontinuous &/ or subcutaneous metastases found on pathologic examination adjacent to primary
  - In transit: Clinically evident cutaneous &/or subcutaneous metastases identified > 2 cm from primary
- Hematogenous spread
  - Lung, brain, distant skin & subcutaneous tissue, liver, nonregional nodes, bone

IMAGING

Disease Evaluation

- Primary
  - Imaging not generally used for detection or assessment of primary because lesion is almost always cutaneous
  - For rare noncutaneous melanomas, consider contrast-enhanced CT of chest, abdomen, and pelvis, PET/CT, or MR
- Nodes
  - **Tc-99m sulfur colloid sentinel lymph node mapping**
    - Directs surgeon to appropriate lymph node basin for sentinel lymph node biopsy
    - Tracer is injected subcutaneously around site of primary lesion hours before wide local excision
    - Recommended if Breslow depth > 1 mm or 0.76-1 mm in presence of ulceration &/or ≥ 1 mitoses/ mm^2
  - **Ultrasound**
    - Abnormal lymph nodes can have abnormal shape, thickened cortex, and loss of fatty hilum
    - Intraoperative ultrasound can also be performed
  - **CT**
    - Not sensitive for small nodal metastases
      - Relatively high level of false positives
    - Metastatic lymph nodes appear round with loss of fatty hilum on CT
    - Other features suggestive of malignancy include necrosis or abnormal enhancement
  - **PET/CT**
    - In a clinically negative axilla, FDG PET is not generally sensitive for detection of regional lymph node metastases
      - However, small nodes with increased FDG activity do generally represent metastases
- Metastases
  - **CT**
    - Thoracic CECT is main modality in imaging pulmonary metastases

MELANOMA

- Often > 5 pulmonary metastases seen in metastatic melanoma to lung
- Abdominopelvic CT scan
  - Used in evaluation of metastatic disease to GI tract
  - Most liver metastases are of lower attenuation than normal parenchyma
- **MR**
  - Greater sensitivity than CT for CNS metastases
    - Typical appearance involves multiple areas of T1 hypointensity and heterogeneous T2 hyperintensity
    - Due to melanin content of tumor, metastases may also appear T1 hyperintense and T2 hypointense
    - Brain parenchymal lesions show ring, homogeneous, or nodular staging
    - Lepto-/pachymeningeal enhancement can be seen
    - Metastases often hemorrhage with characteristic appearance
    - Hemorrhage also seen in tumors such as renal cell carcinoma, anaplastic lung carcinoma, thyroid carcinoma, choriocarcinoma, and hypernephroma
  - More accurate in detection of metastases to liver and bone (e.g., spine) than CT
    - Hepatic metastases ≤ 1 cm have bright signal on T1WI
  - Detection of bone metastases, especially to spine
- **PET/CT**
  - Valuable in assessment of possibly resectable stage IV disease
  - Detection of metastases in advanced disease
    - More sensitive with either equal or better specificity than CT or MR
  - Sensitivity greatest in metastases with diameter > 1 cm
    - ≥ 90% sensitivity
    - PET/CT is possibly superior for bone metastasis, as it has higher sensitivity for osteolytic lesions than Tc-99m MDP bone scanning
- **Echocardiography**
  - Assesses for cardiac metastases and associated pericardial effusion

Recommendations for Staging

- Stages I and II
  - Imaging work-up not required unless there are clinical findings or symptoms suspicious for metastases
- Stage IIIA
  - Consider CT, PET/CT, &/or MR (including brain) for baseline imaging &/or to evaluate specific symptoms
- Stages IIIB-C
  - Recommend CT, PET/CT, &/or MR (including brain) for baseline imaging &/or to evaluate specific symptoms
- Stage IV
  - Encourage CT, PET/CT, &/or MR (including brain) for baseline imaging &/or to evaluate specific symptoms

Restaging

- **General**
  - Consider CT, PET/CT, &/or MR to evaluate response to treatment for unresectable or metastatic patients
  - Elevated laboratory markers or clinical evidence of recurrence should prompt reimaging
    - e.g., increased serum lactate dehydrogenase (LDH)
- **PET/CT**
  - FDG PET detects recurrent disease with sensitivity 74% and specificity 86%
    - Baseline study helpful for assessing response to therapy
    - Inclusion of upper and lower extremities improves sensitivity
  - Cytokine therapy promotes symmetric hypermetabolism in normal lymph tissue (tonsils, nodes) for several months
  - Recent skin biopsy site may show FDG uptake
  - Non-attenuation-corrected images best for evaluating skin recurrence

CLINICAL PRESENTATION & WORK-UP

Presentation

- Appearance of melanoma upon visual examination of skin surface (ABCDE criteria)
- Less common symptoms in pigmented lesion that may indicate melanoma
  - Bleeding
  - Itching
  - Ulceration
  - Pain

Prognosis

- Melanoma often begins as new or changing mole on skin
  - May grow at cutaneous level before potentially spreading through various routes
- Melanoma diagnosed at early stage has relatively better outlook for curative treatment
  - After metastases, median survival of 6-9 months
- 2 most important prognostic factors
  - Tumor thickness
  - Presence of ulceration
- 5-year survival rates in pathologically staged patients
  - Nonulcerated melanoma (Ta)
    - IA: 95%
    - IB: 89%
    - IIA: 79%
    - IIB: 67%
    - IIIA: 67%
    - IIIB: 54%
    - IIIC: 28%
  - Ulcerated melanoma (Tb)
    - IB: 91%
    - IIA: 77%
    - IIB: 63%
    - IIC: 45%
    - IIIB: 52%
    - IIIC: 24%

Work-Up

- Clinical
  - H&P, with emphasis on skin and nodal basins

- Laboratory
  - LDH recommended in stage IV patients

TREATMENT

Major Treatment Alternatives

- Surgical excision of primary site
  - Size of margins determined by thickness of tumor
- Surgical removal of metastatic sites
- Adjuvant therapy
  - Common immunotherapies include interferon, interleukin-2, and biochemotherapy
- Radiation and chemotherapy may be used for advanced metastatic sites

Major Treatment Roadblocks/ Contraindications

- Potentially severe toxicity from interactions between radiation and systemic agents need to be considered
  - e.g., interferon-α2b concurrent with radiation therapy may cause significant toxicity
- Melanoma has potential to metastasize to every organ
  - Level of metastases is often underestimated

Treatment Options by Stage

- Stage 0
  - Surgical excision with margin of ~ 0.5 cm
  - Consider RT for lentigo maligna patients with positive margins or if surgery potentially very morbid
- Stage I
  - If thickness < 1 mm, excision with margin of 1 cm
  - If thickness 1-2 mm, margin of 1-2 cm
  - Margin > 2 cm is not necessary for stage I melanoma
  - Consider sentinel lymph node biopsy for thickness 0.76-1.0 mm if other high-risk features present
- Stage II
  - If thickness 1-2 mm, margin of 1-2 cm
  - If thickness > 2 mm, margin of 2 cm
  - For positive sentinel node biopsy, lymph node dissection should be performed
  - Adjuvant systemic therapy may be warranted for more serious cases, including
    - Melanoma thickness > 4 mm
- Stage III
  - Similar treatment guidelines to stage II with respect to surgical excision margins at primary site
  - Lymph node dissection is often performed in stage III tumors
  - Adjuvant systemic therapy may also provide benefit
  - Adjuvant radiation to macroscopically involved nodal bed may improve regional control
- Stage IV
  - Treatment alternatives for metastatic sites include
    - Systemic therapy
      - Ipilimumab
      - Vemurafenib for *BRAF* V600E mutated tumors
      - Imatinib for C-kit mutated tumors
      - Immunotherapy
    - Surgical removal
    - Radiation

Dose Response

- Melanoma responds to a variety of dose schedules
  - When radiating gross disease in palliative setting, clinical complete response (CR) rates range from 17-69%, with 49-97% receiving either partial response (PR) or CR
- Early in vitro studies of melanoma cell lines depicted wide initial shoulders on survival curves
  - This caused a misconception that melanoma is radioresistant and thus requires large dose per fraction
- Phase III studies have shown no difference in outcomes for various fractionation schedules

Organs at Risk Parameters

- Dependent on dose & fractionation
- 60 Gy in 30 fractions
  - Spinal cord < 45 Gy, brachial plexus < 60 Gy, larynx mean dose ≤ 20 Gy
- 50 Gy in 20 fractions
  - Brain & spinal cord < 40 Gy, brachial plexus < 45 Gy, larynx < 45 Gy, mandible < 45 Gy
- 30-36 Gy in 5-6 fractions (2 fractions/week)
  - Brain & spinal cord < 24 Gy, brachial plexus < 30 Gy, small bowel < 24 Gy

Common Techniques

- Technique highly dependent on treatment intent & target location
  - May involve photons, electrons, or combination of both
  - Clinical setup may be adequate for some cutaneous targets
  - CT simulation recommended if depth of target is in question
  - IMRT may provide benefit in organs at risk (OAR) sparing (e.g., head & neck location)

Landmark Trials

- TROG 02.01/ANZMTG 01.02 (Burmeister BH, 2012)
  - Phase III trial of 250 patients with palpable nodal disease S/P lymphadenectomy & with LDH < 1.5x normal
  - Randomized to observation vs. adjuvant nodal basin radiation
  - Inclusion criteria: Pathology showing ≥ 1 parotid, ≥ 2 cervical or axillary, or ≥ 3 ilio-inguinal nodes, maximum node diameter ≥ 3 cm in neck or ≥ 4 cm in groin or axilla, or nodal extracapsular extension
  - RT decreased risk of nodal relapse (HR 0.56) but no difference in relapse-free survival (RFS) or overall survival (OS)
- RTOG 83-05 (Sause WT, 1991)
  - Phase III trial of 167 patients with melanoma lesions measurable clinically or radiographically
  - Randomized to 50 Gy in 20 daily fractions of 2.5 Gy vs. 32 Gy in 4 weekly fractions of 8 Gy
  - No difference in outcome, with CR rates at 23% vs. 24% and PR rates at 34% vs. 35%
- Chapman PB, 2011
  - Phase III trial of 675 patients with metastatic melanoma with the *BRAF* V600E mutation
  - Randomized to vemurafenib or dacarbazine
  - Vemurafenib resulted in superior OS, progression-free survival (PFS), and response rates
- Flaherty KT, 2012

- Phase III trial of 322 patients with metastatic disease and *BRAF* mutation
- Randomized to receive MEK inhibitor or chemotherapy
- MEK inhibitor resulted in improved PFS & OS

- SWOG S0008 (Flaherty LE, 2012)
  - Phase III trial of 432 patients, stage IIIA (≥ N2a) through stage IIIC
  - Randomized to high-dose interferon vs. biochemotherapy (dacarbazine, cisplatin, vinblastine, IL-2, and interferon)
  - Biochemotherapy improved median RFS to 4.0 vs. 1.9 years; no difference in OS
- Hodi FS, 2010
  - Phase III trial of 676 patients with unresectable stage III or IV disease
  - Randomized to receive ipilimumab alone (monoclonal antibody that blocks CTCLA-4 to promote antitumor immunity), gp100 alone (cancer vaccine), or ipilimumab plus gp100
  - Superior median (10 months vs. 6.4 months) and 2-year OS (24% vs. 14%) for ipilimumab vs. gp100 alone

RECOMMENDED FOLLOW-UP

Clinical

- IA-IIA
  - H&P (with emphasis on nodes & skin) every 3-12 months for 5 years, then as indicated
- IIB-IV
  - H&P (with emphasis on nodes & skin) every 3-6 months for 2 years, then every 3-12 months for 3 years, then as indicated

Radiographic

- IA-IIA
  - Routine imaging not recommended
- IIB-IV
  - Consider CT &/or PET/CT scans every 3-12 months & annual MR brain to screen for recurrent/metastatic disease; after 5 years, routine imaging is not recommended

SELECTED REFERENCES

1. Burmeister BH et al: Adjuvant radiotherapy versus observation alone for patients at risk of lymph-node field relapse after therapeutic lymphadenectomy for melanoma: a randomised trial. Lancet Oncol. 13(6):589-97, 2012
2. Flaherty KT et al: Improved survival with MEK inhibition in BRAF-mutated melanoma. N Engl J Med. 367(2):107-14, 2012
3. Flaherty LE et al: Phase III trial of high-dose interferon alpha-2b versus cisplatin, vinblastine, DTIC plus IL-2 and interferon in patients with high-risk melanoma (SWOG S0008): An intergroup study of CALGB, COG, ECOG, and SWOG. J Clin Oncol. 30 (suppl; abstr 8504), 2012
4. Chapman PB et al: Improved survival with vemurafenib in melanoma with BRAF V600E mutation. N Engl J Med. 364(26):2507-16, 2011
5. American Joint Committee on Cancer: AJCC Cancer Staging Manual. 7th ed. New York: Springer. 325-44, 2010
6. Hodi FS et al: Improved survival with ipilimumab in patients with metastatic melanoma. N Engl J Med. 2010 Aug 19;363(8):711-23. Epub 2010 Jun 5. Erratum in: N Engl J Med. 363(13):1290, 2010
7. Agrawal S et al: The benefits of adjuvant radiation therapy after therapeutic lymphadenectomy for clinically advanced, high-risk, lymph node-metastatic melanoma. Cancer. 115(24):5836-44, 2009
8. Beadle BM et al: Radiation therapy field extent for adjuvant treatment of axillary metastases from malignant melanoma. Int J Radiat Oncol Biol Phys. 73(5):1376-82, 2009
9. Krug B et al: Role of PET in the initial staging of cutaneous malignant melanoma: systematic review. Radiology. 249(3):836-44, 2008
10. Scarsbrook AF et al: Pearls and pitfalls of radionuclide imaging of the lymphatic system. Part 1: sentinel node lymphoscintigraphy in malignant melanoma. Br J Radiol. 80(950):132-9, 2007
11. Kumar R et al: Fluorodeoxyglucose-PET in the management of malignant melanoma. Radiol Clin North Am. 43(1):23-33, 2005
12. Essner R: Surgical treatment of malignant melanoma. Surg Clin North Am. 83(1):109-56, 2003
13. Mijnhout GS et al: Systematic review of the diagnostic accuracy of (18)F-fluorodeoxyglucose positron emission tomography in melanoma patients. Cancer. 91(8):1530-42, 2001
14. Sause WT et al: Fraction size in external beam radiation therapy in the treatment of melanoma. Int J Radiat Oncol Biol Phys. 20(3):429-32, 1991
15. Harwood AR: Conventional fractionated radiotherapy for 51 patients with lentigo maligna and lentigo maligna melanoma. Int J Radiat Oncol Biol Phys. 9(7):1019-21, 1983

SLN Biopsy

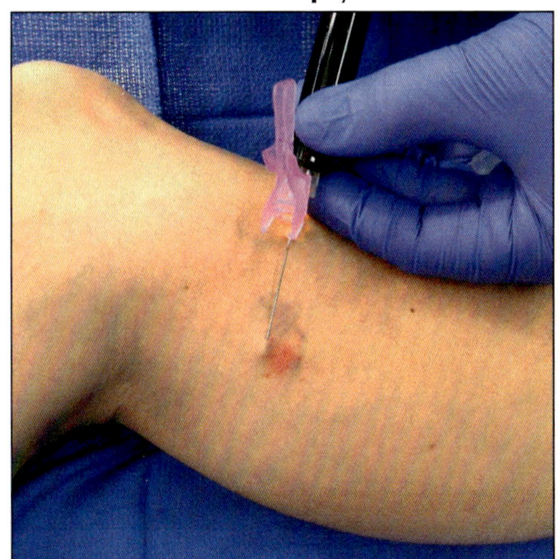

SLN Biopsy

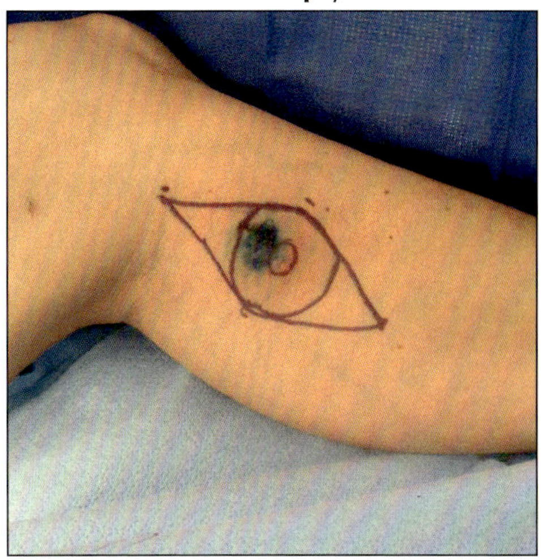

(Left) *Methylene blue is being injected intradermally into the left medial calf for intraoperative lymphatic mapping. Prior shave biopsy showed a T2a melanoma with 2 mitoses/mm². (Courtesy R. H. I. Andtbacka, MD, CM.)* ***(Right)*** *In the same patient, a 1.5 cm radial excision margin is drawn around the initial biopsy site. Fusiform lines are then drawn in the long axis to guide the incision. The site where methylene blue was injected is clearly visible. (Courtesy R. H. I. Andtbacka, MD, CM.)*

SLN Biopsy

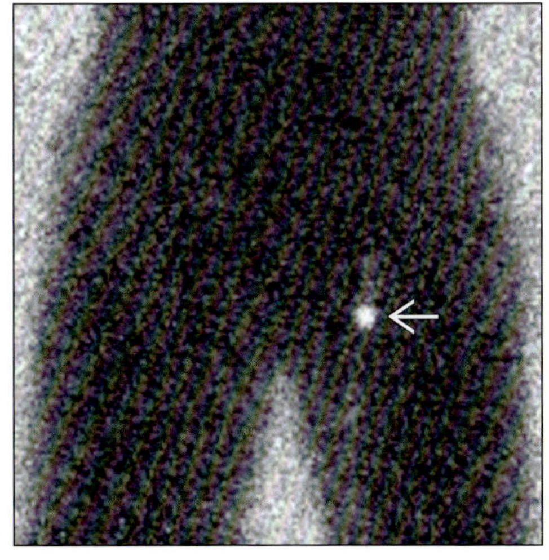

SLN Biopsy

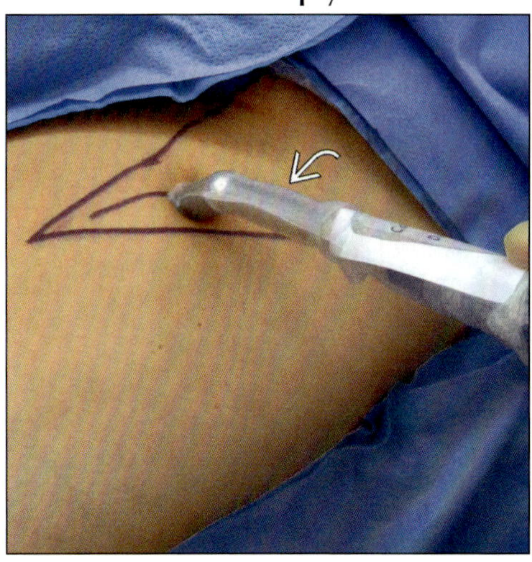

(Left) *Preoperative lymphoscintigraphy with 110 uCi Tc-99m sulfur colloid shows a single radioactive sentinel lymph node (SLN) in the left groin ➔ of the same patient.* ***(Right)*** *A gamma probe ➔ is used to identify the site of the radioactive groin node in the same patient. (Courtesy R. H. I. Andtbacka, MD, CM.)*

SLN Biopsy

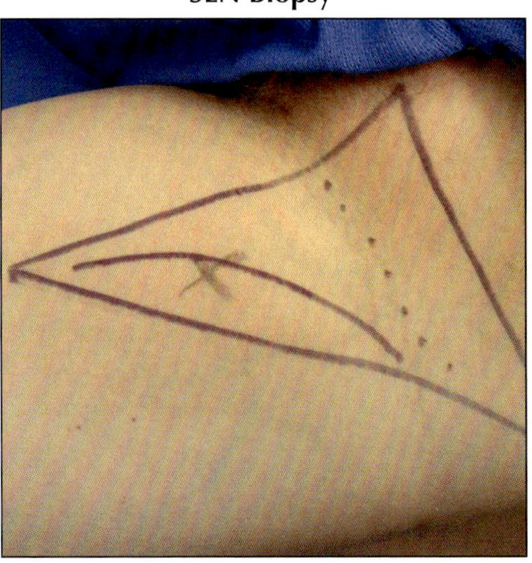

SLN Biopsy

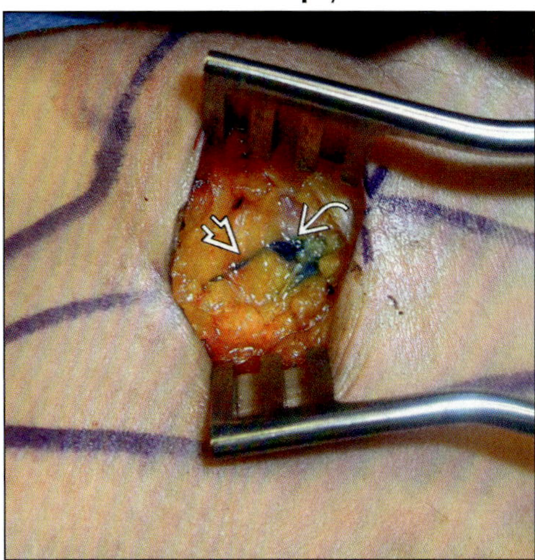

(Left) *The femoral triangle is drawn on the skin of the same patient, with the radioactive node site marked with an X. (Courtesy R. H. I. Andtbacka, MD, CM.)* ***(Right)*** *An incision is made along the curved line crossing the X. Blue lymphatic channels ➔ are found coursing toward a blue and radioactive SLN ➔. (Courtesy R. H. I. Andtbacka, MD, CM.)*

MELANOMA

SLN Biopsy

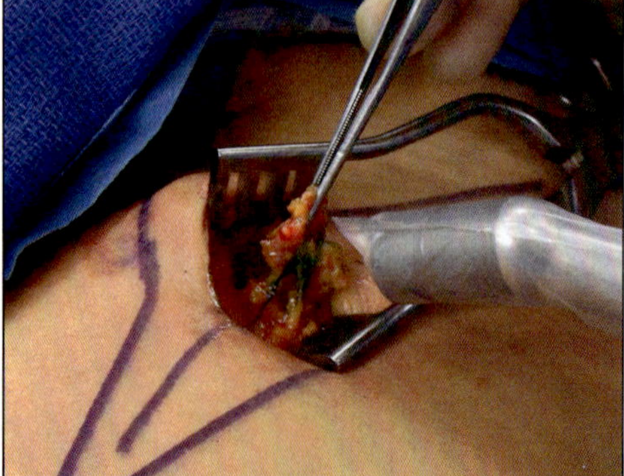

SLN Biopsy

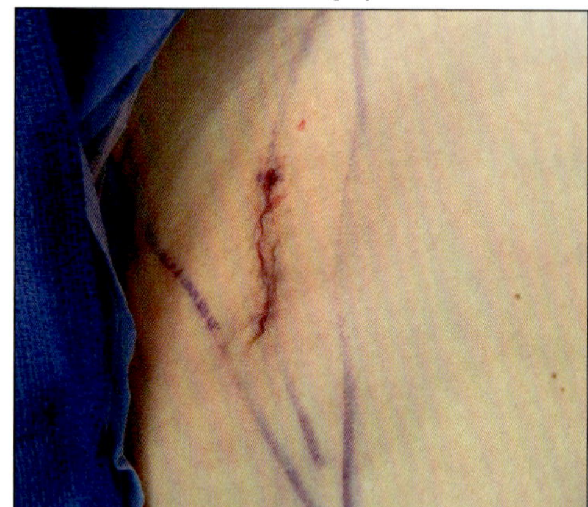

(Left) *A gamma probe is used in the same patient to confirm that the blue node is radioactive. It is 3 mm and not grossly suspicious for metastatic disease. (Courtesy R. H. I. Andtbacka, MD, CM.)* ***(Right)*** *The superficial thigh fascia in the same patient is reapproximated with interrupted sutures, after which the skin is closed with a subcuticular running suture. (Courtesy R. H. I. Andtbacka, MD, CM.)*

Wide Local Excision

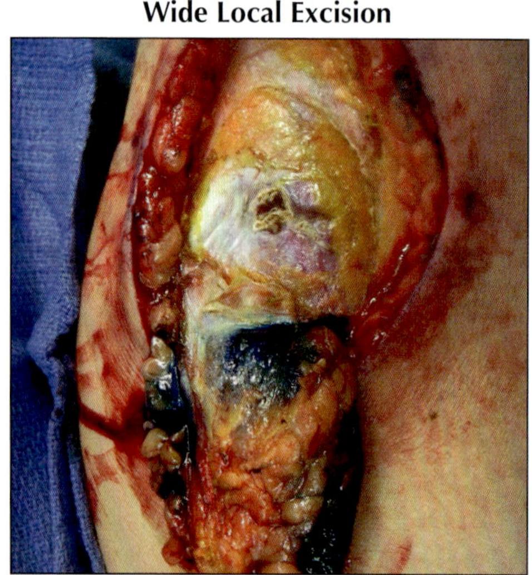

Wide Local Excision

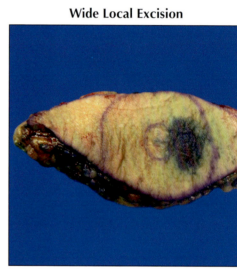

(Left) *Following SLN removal in the same patient, dissection of the primary specimen is taken down through the fascia of the underlying musculature. It is removed along the previously drawn fusiform lines. (Courtesy R. H. I. Andtbacka, MD, CM.)* ***(Right)*** *The operative specimen from the same patient measures 11 x 6 cm and contains the initial biopsy site. (Courtesy R. H. I. Andtbacka, MD, CM.)*

Wide Local Excision

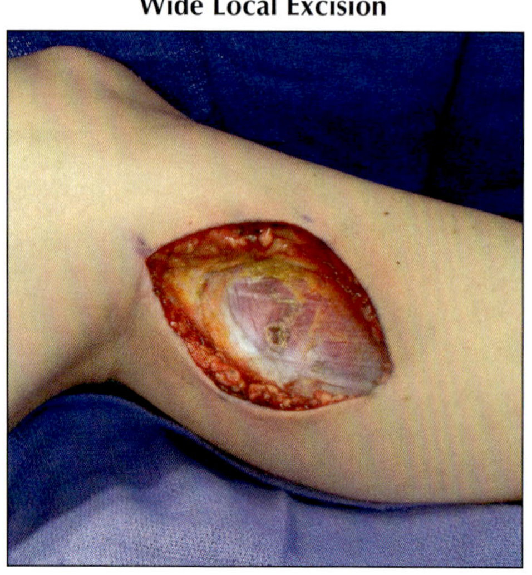

Wide Local Excision

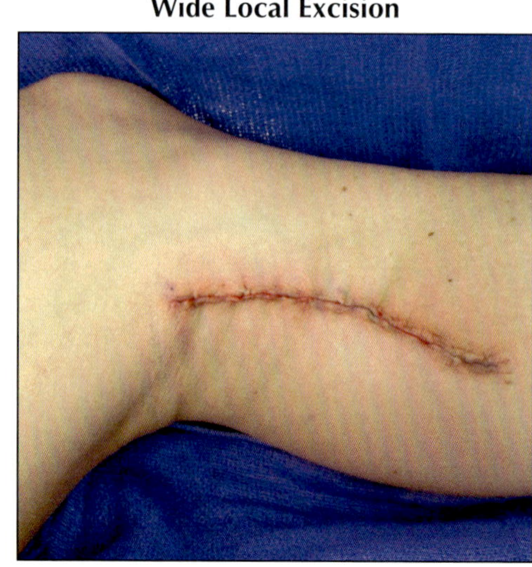

(Left) *Photo shows the wide local excision operative site in the same patient. (Courtesy R. H. I. Andtbacka, MD, CM.)* ***(Right)*** *Fusiform shape of operative site in same patient facilitates closure by decreasing wound tension compared to a circular shape. In this case, prefascial advancement flaps are created 3 cm circumferentially around wound. (Courtesy R. H. I. Andtbacka, MD, CM.)*

Pathologic Stage IIC (T4b N0 M0)

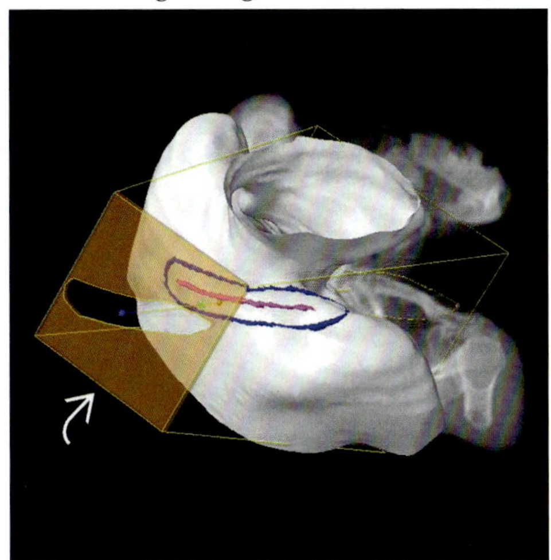

Pathologic Stage IIC (T4b N0 M0)

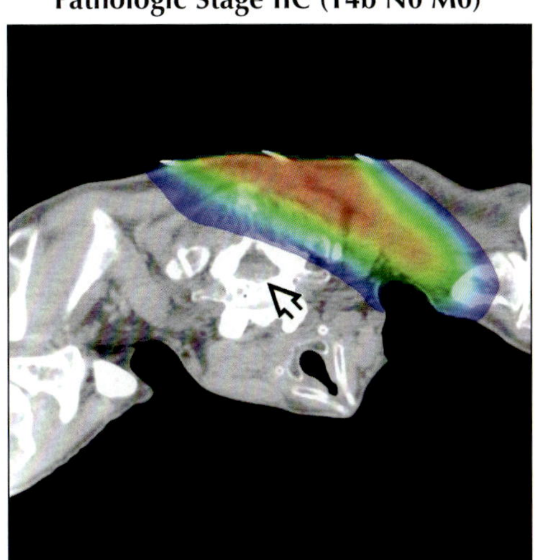

(Left) *Skin rendering was performed on a 90-year-old man found to have a 16 mm deep neurotropic desmoplastic melanoma, Clark Level V, extending to the deep margin. A 2 cm circumferential margin (blue) around scar guided electron block creation ➡.* ***(Right)*** *Axial NECT in the same patient shows dose colorwash using 12 MeV electrons with 1 cm bolus. RT delivery was oriented to avoid the spinal cord ⇨. A dose of 36 Gy given in 6 twice weekly fractions was delivered.*

Stage IIIB (T1b N2c M0)

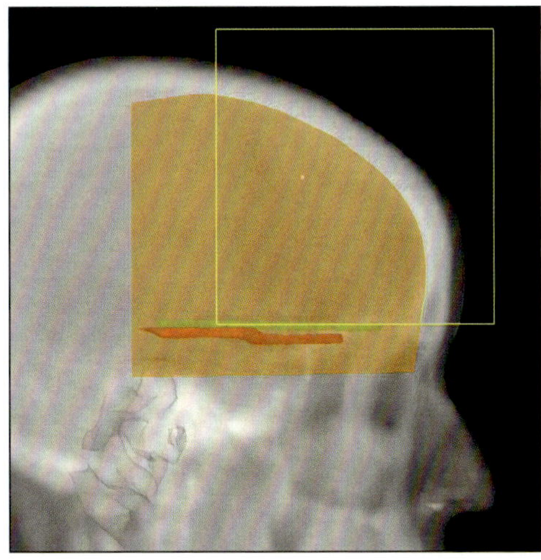

Stage IIIB (T1b N2c M0)

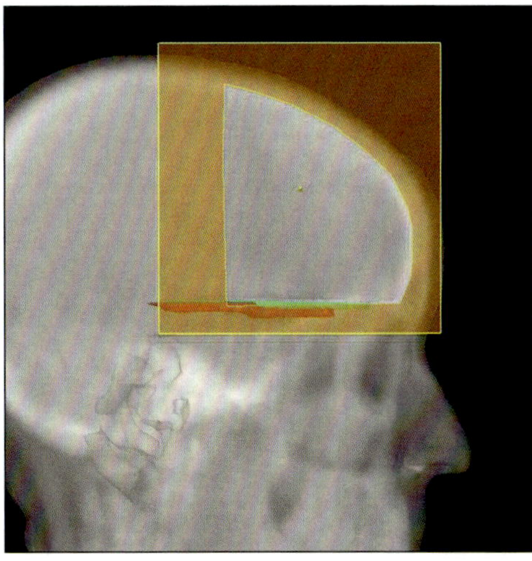

(Left) *Lateral DRR shows a peripheral 6 MV photon field in a 49-year-old woman with positive margins and in-transit metastases. Re-resection was not recommended due to likelihood of further positive margins.* ***(Right)*** *In the same patient, after delineating the photon field borders, the 6 MeV electron field is created, thus completing the "helmet technique." Wires placed on the right (red) and left (green) side of the scalp at the time of simulation delineate the inferior border.*

Stage IIIB (T1b N2c M0)

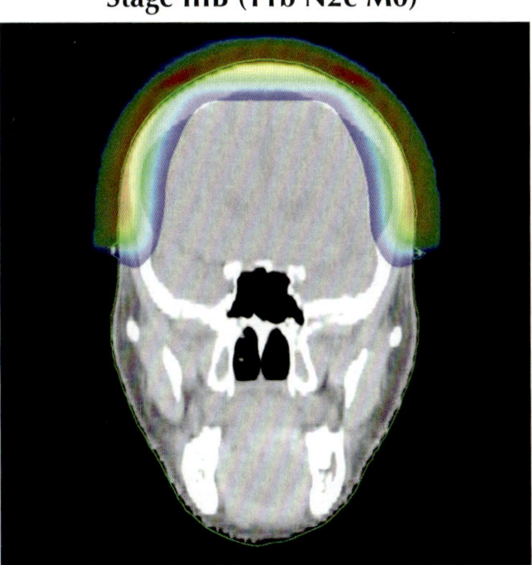

Stage IIIB (T1b N2c M0)

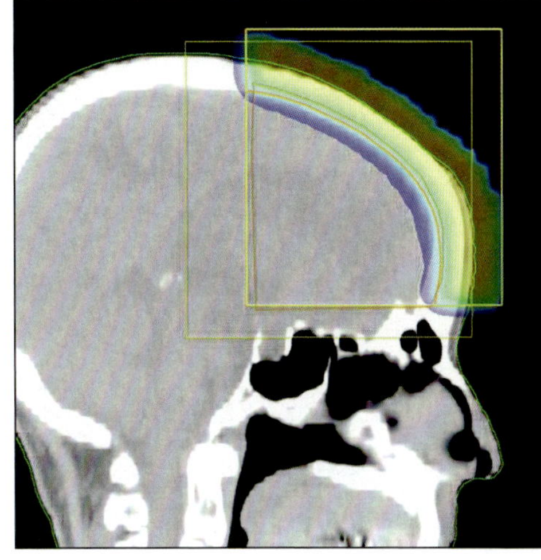

(Left) *Coronal CT dose colorwash in the same patient shows the significant brain sparing this technique allows. The lowest dose shown in blue represents 10% of the prescription dose of 60 Gy, which was given over 30 fractions with 1/2 cm of bolus.* ***(Right)*** *Sagittal CECT in the same patient shows slight overlap of the electron field over the photon field to decrease potential cold spots in the dosimetry.*

*(**Left**) Photo shows visual extent of hyperpigmented lentigo maligna (LM) ➔. Patient refused surgery & imiquimod due to cosmesis concerns. (Courtesy G. M. Bowen, MD.) (**Right**) Wood lamp exam in same patient revealed more extensive disease requiring a larger field ➔. Setup photo shows custom wax-covered block ⇨; 1/2 cm of bolus was placed on skin; 50 Gy in 20 fractions was prescribed. Consider dosimeter placement.*

Stage 0 (Tis N0 M0) Lentigo Maligna

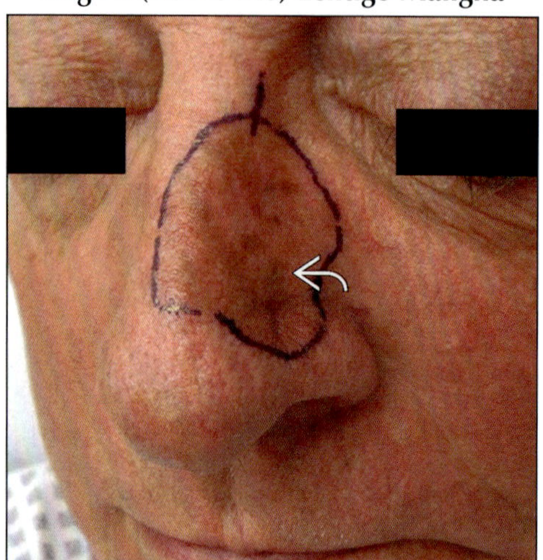

Stage 0 (Tis N0 M0) Lentigo Maligna

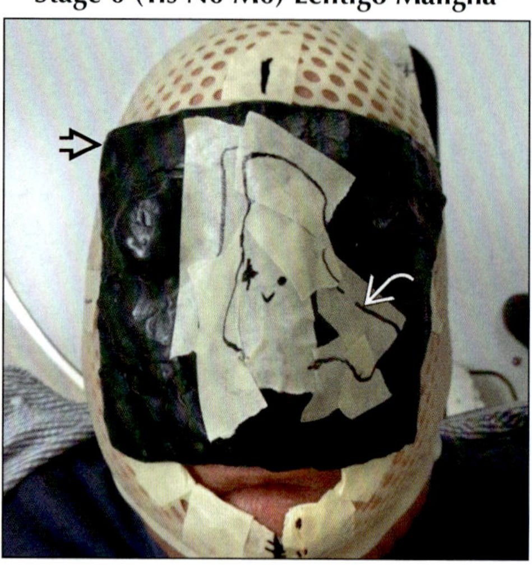

*(**Left**) Photo of the same patient shows persistent hyperpigmentation ➔ 4 months after RT. The black marker ⇨ indicates incisional biopsy location. (Courtesy G. M. Bowen, MD.) (**Right**) In the same patient, pathology showed persistent LM with irregular proliferation of atypical pigmented epithelioid melanocytes in the epidermis ⇨. Pagetoid scatter and extension down epithelial structures of adnexa are present. No invasion was noted. (Courtesy K. Duffy, MD.)*

Stage 0 (Tis N0 M0) Lentigo Maligna

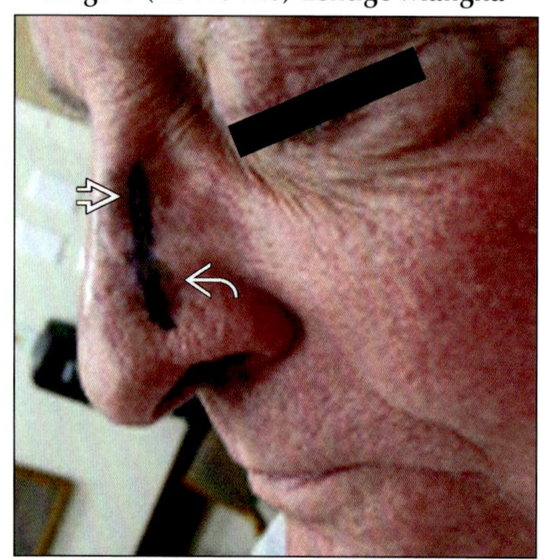

Stage 0 (Tis N0 M0) Lentigo Maligna

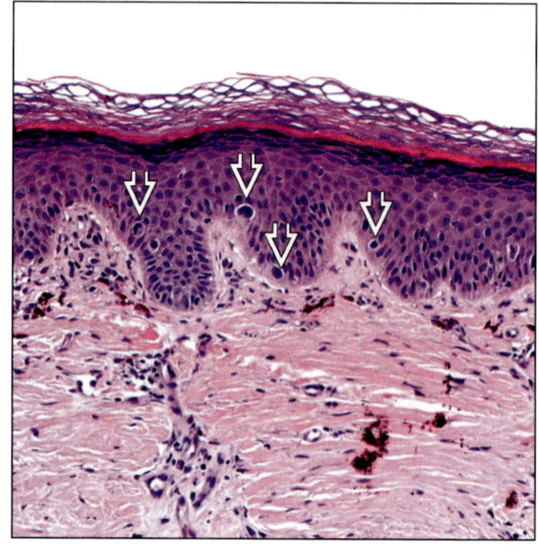

*(**Left**) Because of residual disease in the same patient, imiquimod was used topically for 6 weeks. Photo taken 9 months after initial course of RT and 3.5 months after use of imiquimod shows no residual skin hyperpigmentation. In this case, a good cosmetic outcome was achieved. (Courtesy G. M. Bowen, MD.) (**Right**) Repeat biopsy from the same patient shows only a dermal scar and no residual LM. (Courtesy K. Duffy, MD.)*

Stage 0 (Tis N0 M0) Lentigo Maligna

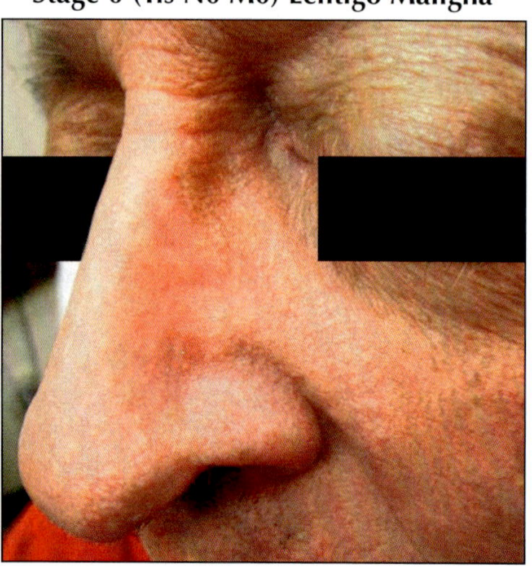

Stage 0 (Tis N0 M0) Lentigo Maligna

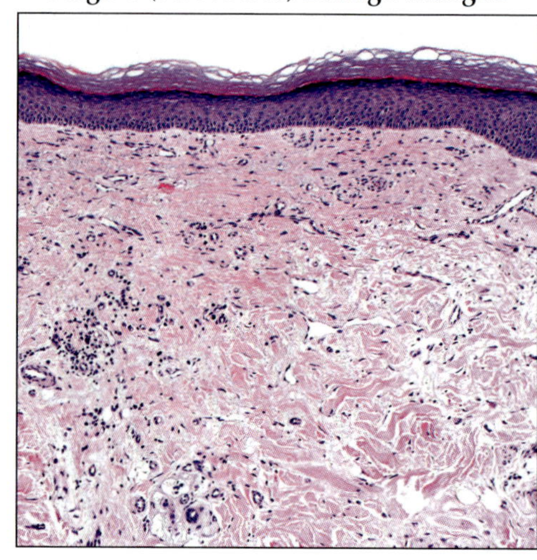

Stage IIB (T4a N0 M0) Lentigo Maligna Melanoma

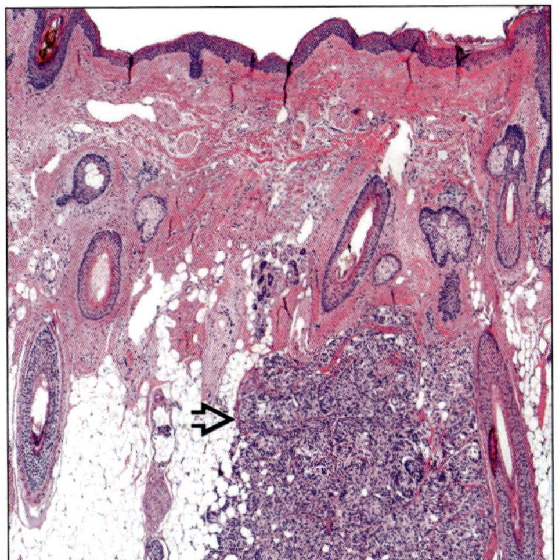

Stage IIB (T4a N0 M0) Lentigo Maligna Melanoma

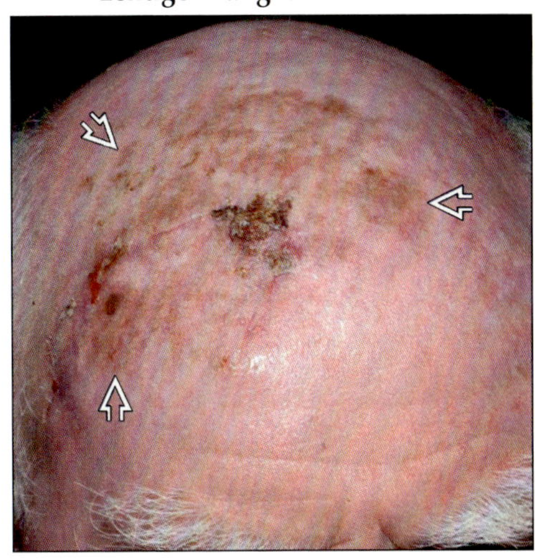

(Left) *Pathology shows lentigo maligna melanoma (LMM) ⇨ invading the deep dermis and subcutaneous tissue. (Courtesy K. Duffy, MD.)* ***(Right)*** *Photo shows an 84-year-old man S/P excision of LMM with a close deep margin and LM at the lateral margins ➡. Adjuvant RT was given to 36 Gy/20 fx with 6 MV tangents followed by 10 Gy/5 fx en face 6 MeV electron boost, both with 1 cm of bolus. (Courtesy G. Fogarty, MD.)*

Stage IIB (T4a N0 M0) Lentigo Maligna Melanoma

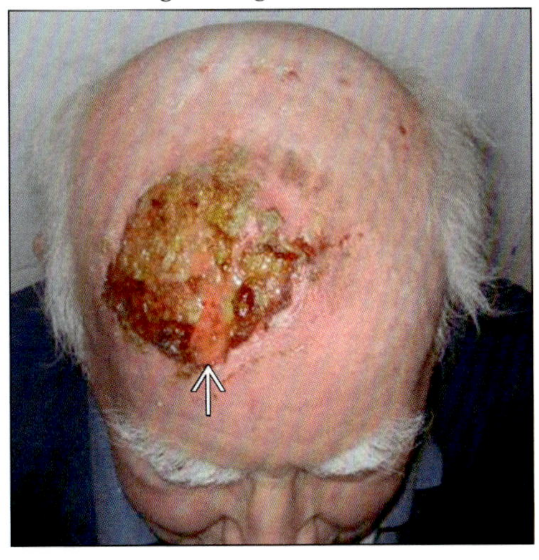

Stage IIB (T4a N0 M0) Lentigo Maligna Melanoma

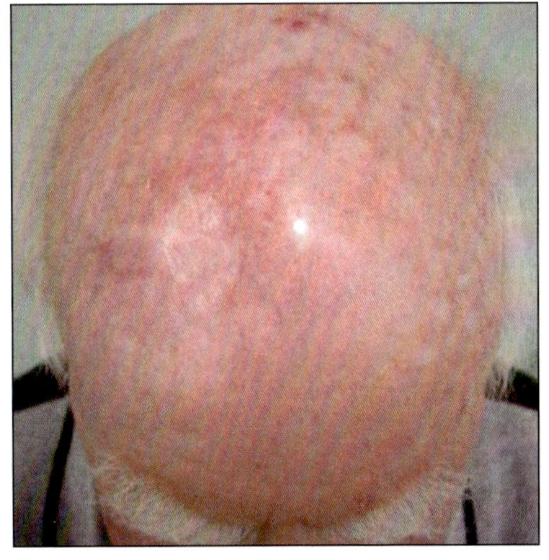

(Left) *Photo of the same patient 1 week after RT shows point of maximum skin reaction. Note moist desquamation ➡, consistent with CTCAE grade 3 dermatitis. TLDs were used to ensure the 90% isodose straddled the skin surface. (Courtesy G. Fogarty, MD.)* ***(Right)*** *Photo of the same patient 6 months after RT shows complete response and excellent cosmesis. (Courtesy G. Fogarty, MD.)*

Open Neck, Adjuvant RT

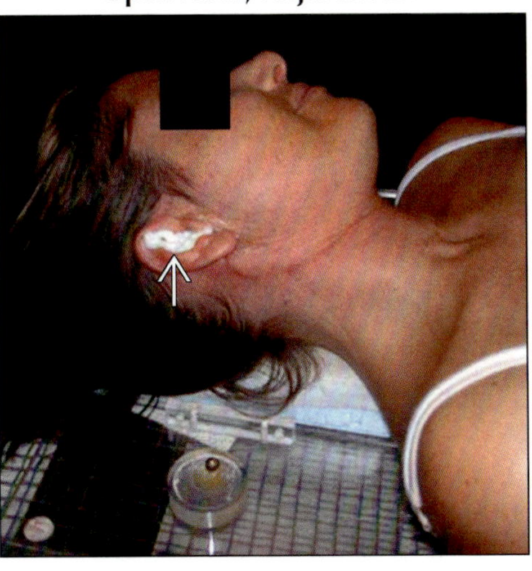

Open Neck, Adjuvant RT

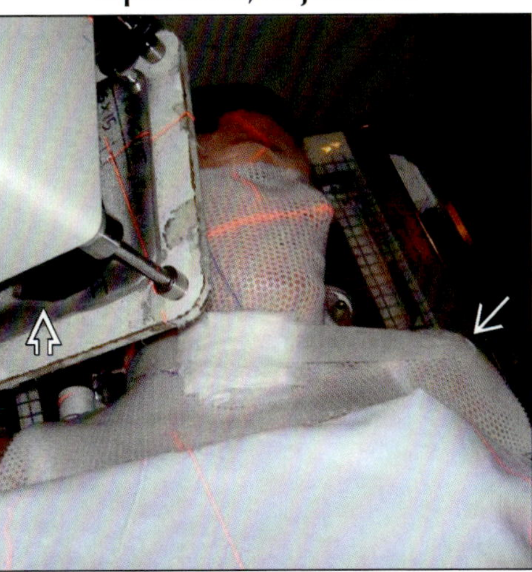

(Left) *Photo shows CT simulation for treatment of levels I-V due to nodal disease. Note wet gauze ➡ in ipsilateral ear canal used as tissue equivalent bolus. (Courtesy B. Burmeister, MD.)* ***(Right)*** *Orfit mask ➡ was applied to same patient for immobilization, head turned to allow for maximum flatness of plane formed by trapezius, sternocleidomastoid, & mandible. Note electron field with block in place ➡ for en face treatment. (Courtesy B. Burmeister, MD.)*

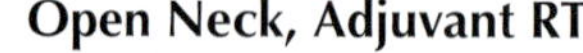

Open Neck, Adjuvant RT

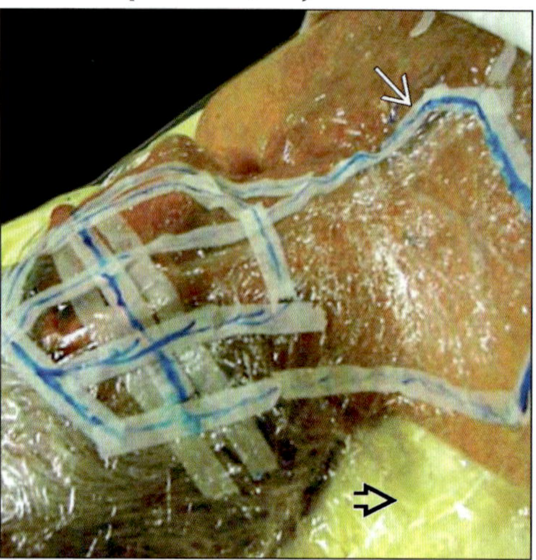

Open Neck, Adjuvant RT

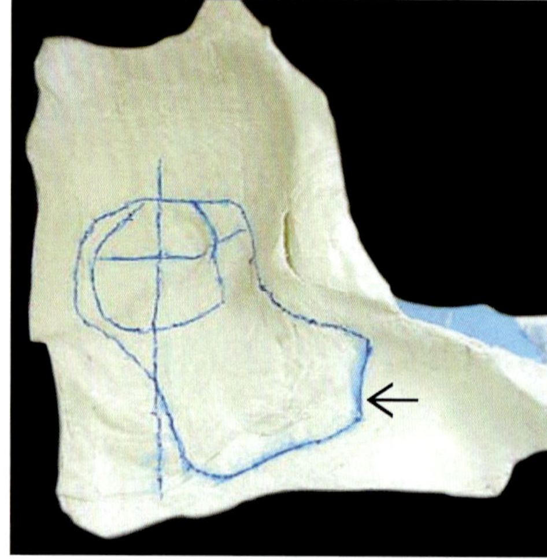

(Left) *Photo shows setup with the same patient kept in position using personalized wax cast* ➲. *Treatment area is delineated by marker, then covered using polyurethane wrap with reference lines superimposed on tape affixed to the wrap* ➡. *(Courtesy G. Fogarty, MD.)* ***(Right)*** *Plaster of Paris is poured over the polyethylene to make a mask for the same patient. Reference lines* ➲ *bleed into underside of mask and are then traced. Mask is then used at setup. (Courtesy G. Fogarty, MD.)*

Open Neck, Adjuvant RT

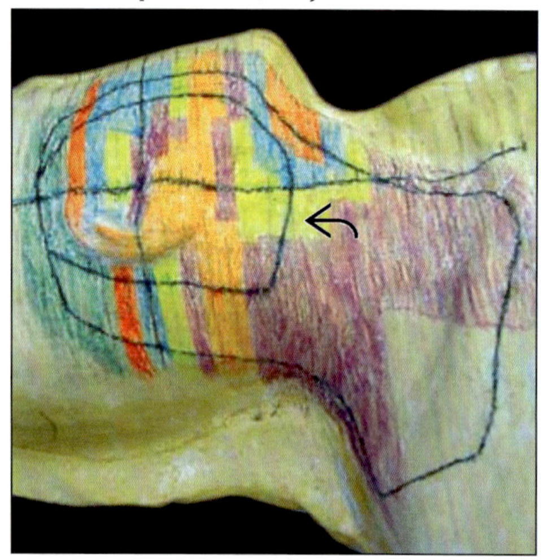

Open Neck, Adjuvant RT

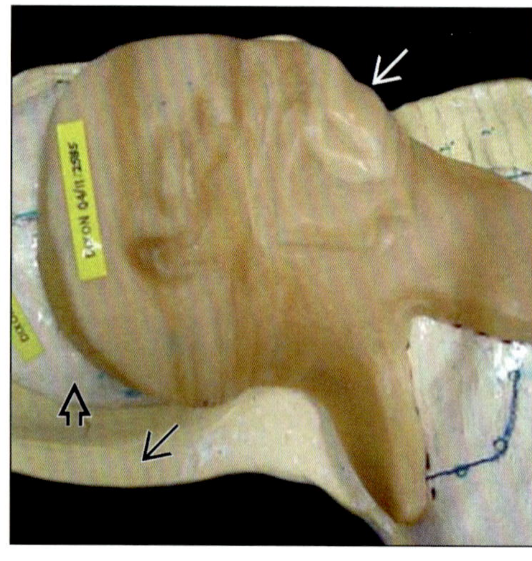

(Left) *After wiring the field borders for the same patient, CT simulation is performed, and volumes are contoured. Next, the plaster mask is color coded to delineate differing depths of the CT target volume. The deepest areas to be treated (e.g., level II nodes* ➲*) will have the thinnest bolus. (Courtesy G. Fogarty, MD.)* ***(Right)*** *For safe storage, the custom wax bolus* ➡ *rests on a sturdy polyethylene mask* ➲ *cast from the original plaster mask* ➲ *for the same patient. (Courtesy G. Fogarty, MD.)*

Open Neck, Adjuvant RT

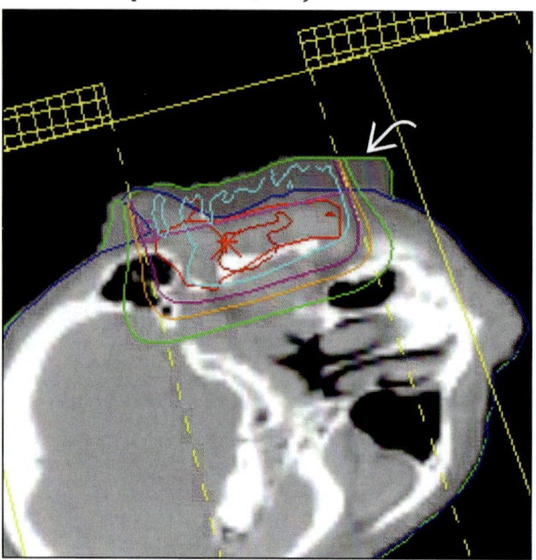

Open Neck, Adjuvant RT

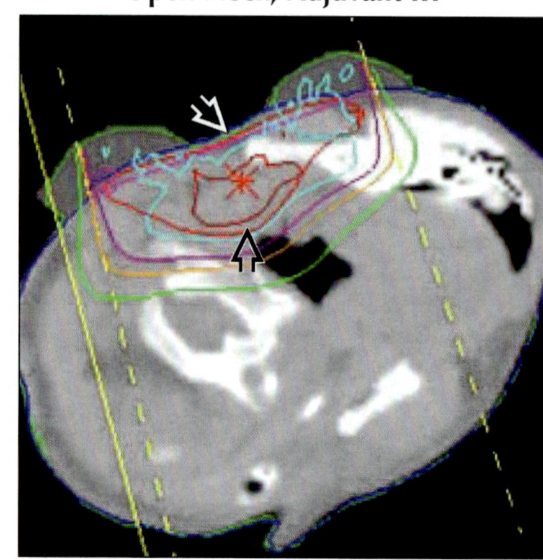

(Left) *Bolus* ➡ *allows adequate build-up of dose to the surface of the target volume in the same patient, while attenuating the dose to deeper uninvolved areas (red = target, blue = 90%, purple = 70%, orange = 50%, green = 20%). (Courtesy B. Burmeister, MD.)* ***(Right)*** *Note absence of bolus* ➡ *in the region of neck nodal level II in the same patient to allow for coverage of the deep portion* ➲ *of the target volume (red). (Courtesy B. Burmeister, MD.)*

Cervical Lymphadenopathy

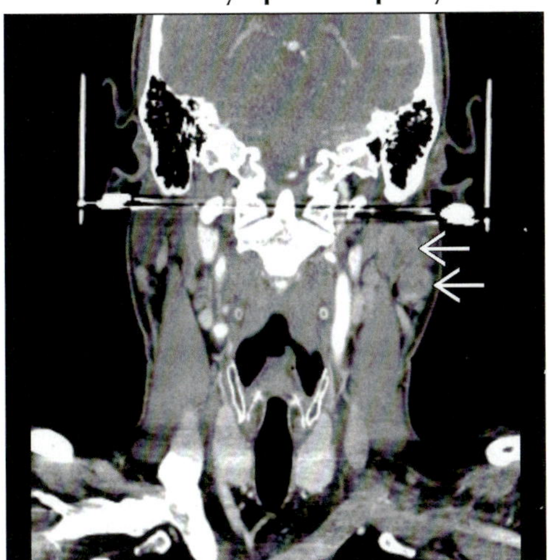

DVH: IMRT vs. 3D Conformal RT

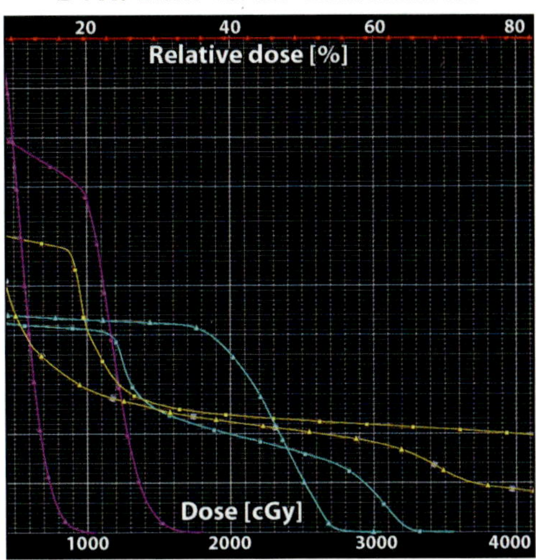

(Left) *Coronal CECT of a 29-year-old man shows intraparotid nodes ➔. He presented with a neck mass, but no primary was identified. Lymphadenectomy showed 3 positive parotid nodes, largest 2.5 cm, and none with extracapsular extension. The other 57 level II-V nodes were uninvolved (stage IIIB).* ***(Right)*** *DVH from the same patient shows no clinically significant difference between the IMRT (triangle) and 3D (square) plans (orange = mandible, cyan = cord, purple = oral cavity).*

IMRT vs. 3D Conformal RT

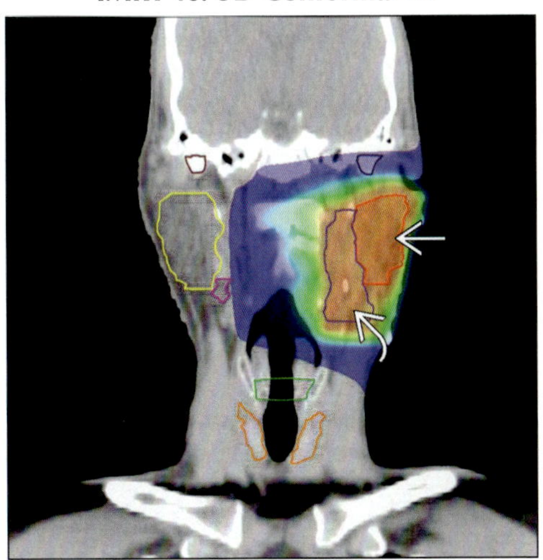

IMRT vs. 3D Conformal RT

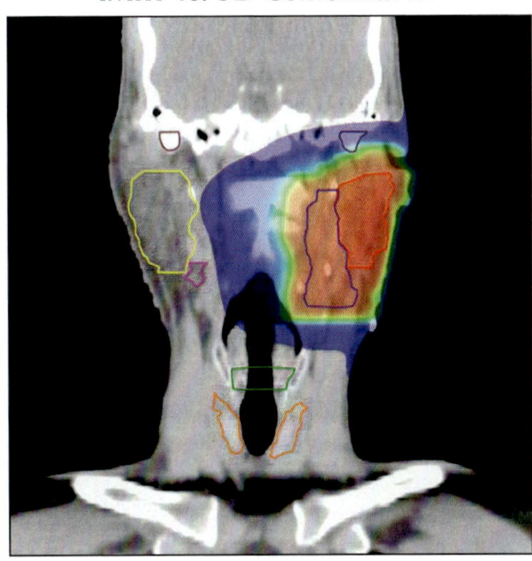

(Left) *Coronal NECT from the same patient shows 3D conformal plan with dose colorwash. Lowest dose level is set to 3% of the prescription dose. Note larynx and thyroid are out of the RT field. (Blue = level II nodal region ➔, red = parotid/operative bed ➔.)* ***(Right)*** *IMRT plan in same patient shows no significant difference from the 3D conformal plan.*

IMRT vs. 3D Conformal RT

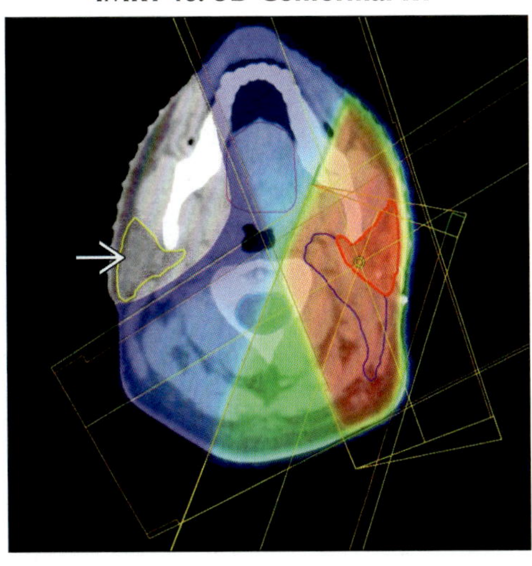

IMRT vs. 3D Conformal RT

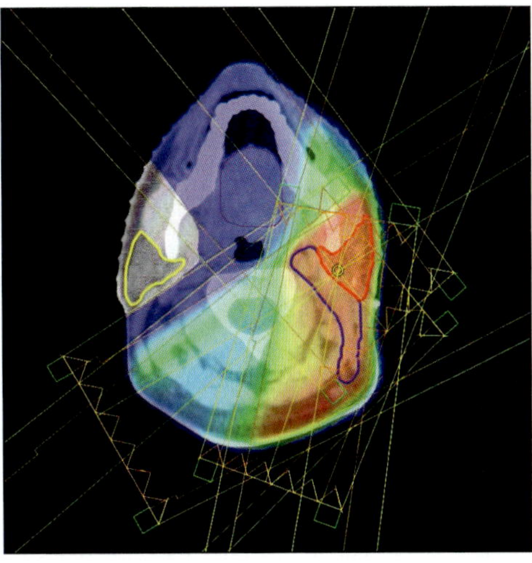

(Left) *3D conformal plan with axial NECT of the same patient shows lowest level of dose colorwash set to 3% of the prescription dose. 50 Gy in 20 fractions was planned to the remaining left parotid, operative bed, and level II node. Note excellent sparing of the parotid ➔.* ***(Right)*** *Corresponding IMRT plan on same axial NECT slice shows very slightly lower dose to the oral cavity. Due to approximate equivalence of the plans, the 3D plan was chosen instead of IMRT.*

Cervical Lymphadenopathy

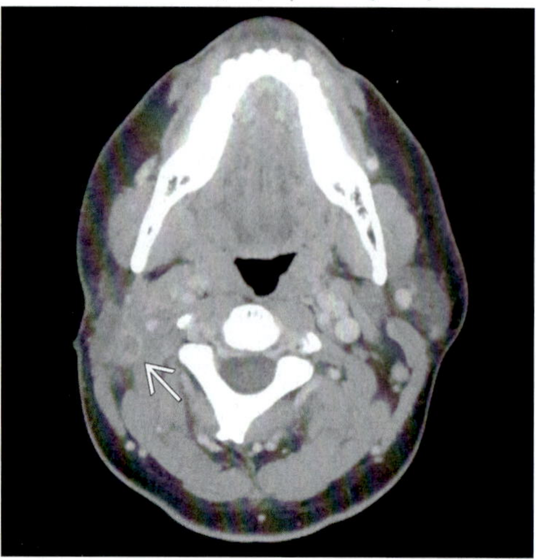

DVH: IMRT vs. 3D Conformal RT

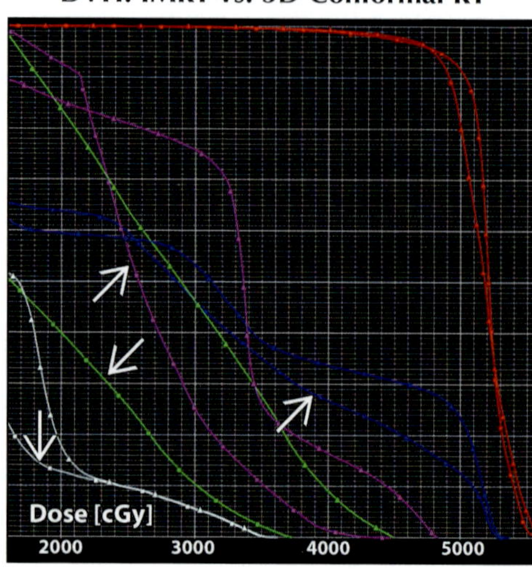

*(**Left**) Axial CECT shows level II nodal involvement ➔ in a 27-year-old man who had a 0.9 mm ulcerated lesion resected 3 years prior. Lymphadenectomy revealed 2 intraparotid and 2 level II nodes involved with disease, none with ECE, with the largest node 2.6 cm. (**Right**) DVH from the same patient shows lower dose to OARs with IMRT (squares ➔) compared to 3D (triangles). Mandible = blue, oral cavity = magenta, right cochlea = green, and spinal cord = blue.*

IMRT vs. 3D Conformal RT

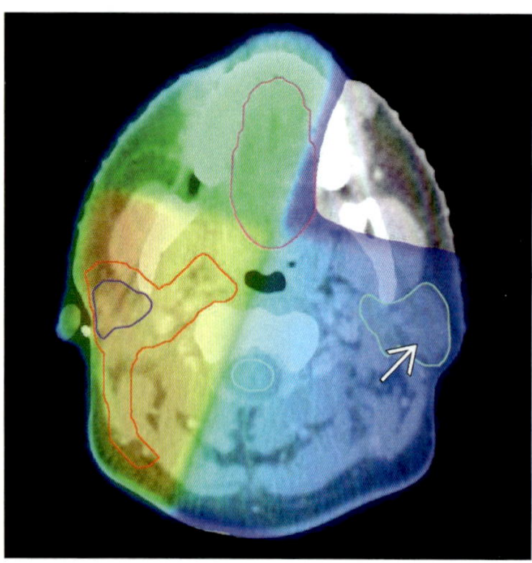

IMRT vs. 3D Conformal RT

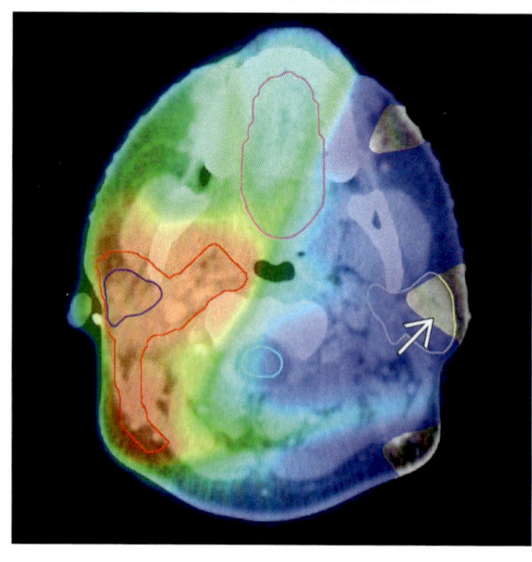

*(**Left**) 3D conformal plan with axial NECT of same patient shows lowest level of dose colorwash set to 10% of the prescription dose. 50 Gy in 20 fractions was planned to the remaining right parotid, operative bed, and levels IB-V nodes. Note the opposite parotid ➔ covered by the dose. (**Right**) IMRT plan is shown on same axial CT slice. Note improved OAR sparing (e.g., oral cavity and left parotid ➔), which led to the choice of IMRT instead of the 3D plan.*

IMRT vs. 3D Conformal RT

IMRT vs. 3D Conformal RT

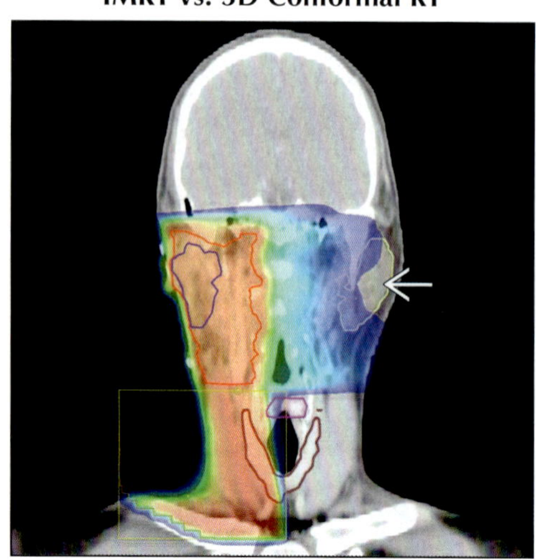

*(**Left**) 3D conformal plan with coronal NECT of the same patient shows inferior extent of target volume. Lowest level of dose colorwash again set to 10% of the prescription dose. (**Right**) IMRT dose wash is shown on coronal NECT, with decreased dose noted to the left parotid ➔. Using an AP field for the low neck decreases the dose to the larynx, thyroid, cervical esophagus, and cord compared to using IMRT for the entire field.*

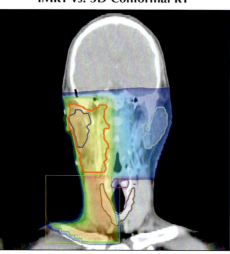

Axillary Lymphadenopathy

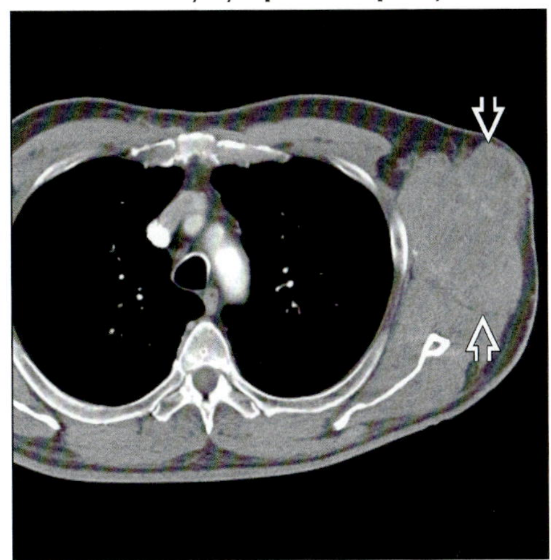

Axillary Lymphadenopathy

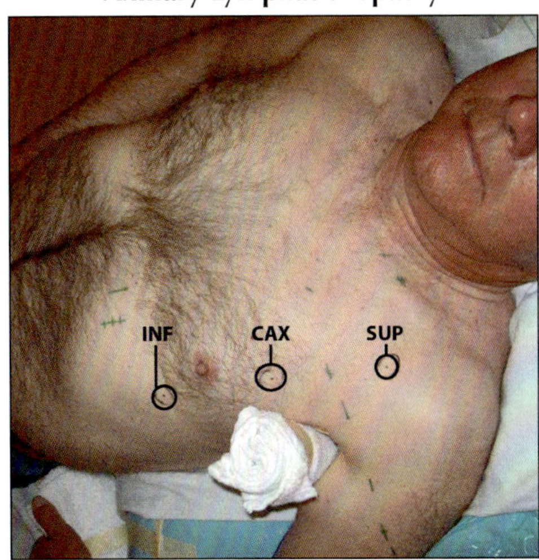

(Left) *Axial CECT shows a 69-year-old man with a history of T3a N0 M0 back melanoma, now with matted axillary lymphadenopathy ➡. Lymphadenectomy revealed 2 of 22 involved nodes, both from level I. Each node had ECE, and the largest was 8 cm.* *(Right)* *Photo shows CT simulation in the same patient, with arm abducted to decrease the axillary skin fold. An α cradle was used for immobilization and a custom towel roll was placed to improve setup reproducibility.*

Axillary EBRT, Standard Field

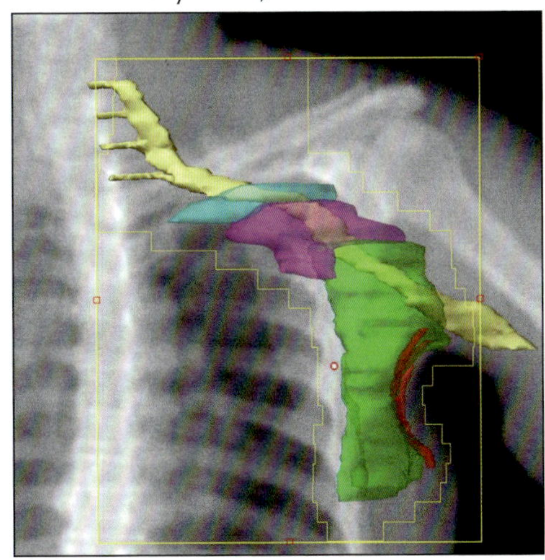

Axillary EBRT, Reduced Field

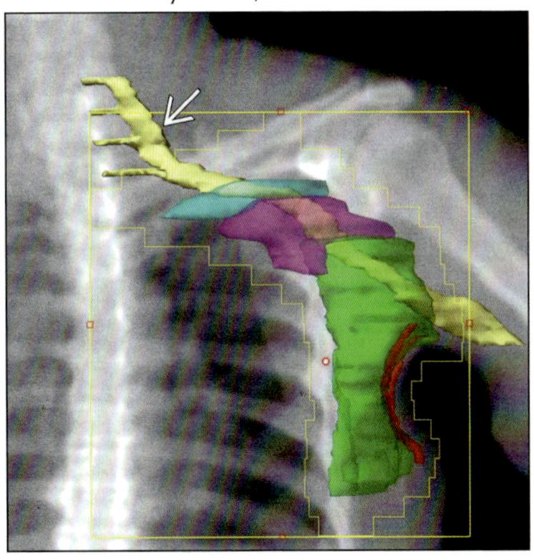

(Left) *AP DRR from the same patient shows field borders including axillary levels I (green), II (magenta), III (cyan), supraclavicular fossa, and surgical scar (red). Note field contains majority of the proximal brachial plexus (yellow). 30 Gy in 5 fractions was prescribed.* *(Right)* *AP DRR from the same patient shows exclusion of the SCV fossa and brachial plexus ➡. Published data shows decreased toxicity without worse disease control.*

Post RT Imaging

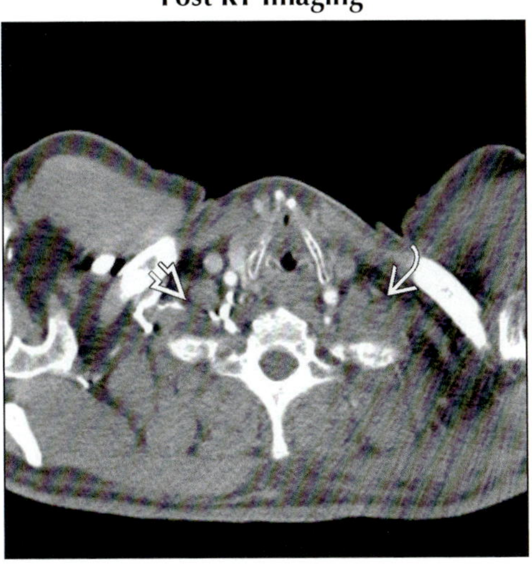

Post RT Imaging

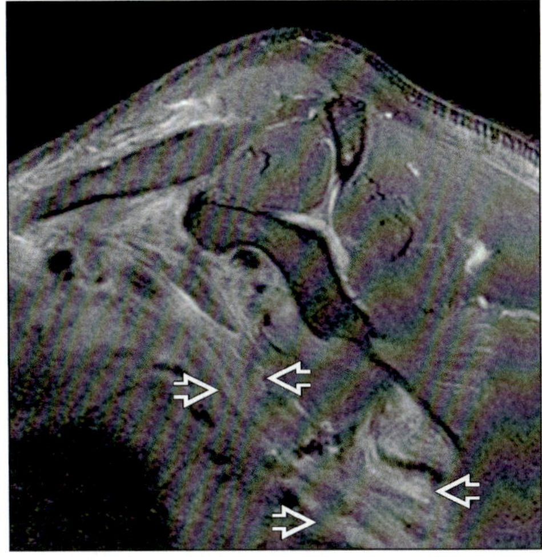

(Left) *Axial CECT from the same patient shows thickening and indistinct fat planes of the left supraclavicular paraspinal soft tissue ➡ compared to the right ➡, due to RT.* *(Right)* *Sagittal T2WI MR 1 year post RT in the same patient shows thickening and indistinct borders of the hyperintense brachial plexus ➡. EMG was consistent with brachial plexopathy. He presented with weakness and pain, which improved significantly from physical therapy and pregabalin.*

(Left) *Axial CECT of a 70-year-old woman who felt a groin mass 5 months after diagnosis of a stage IIB, T3b N0 M0 left heel melanoma shows a 25 mm left inguinal enhancing node ➔ with central areas of necrosis. Lymphadenectomy revealed 9 of 12 involved nodes, with ECE present, and the largest node at 2.3 cm.* **(Right)** *At simulation in the same patient, an α cradle was used for immobilization with the leg abducted to minimize the groin skin fold ➔.*

Groin Lymphadenopathy

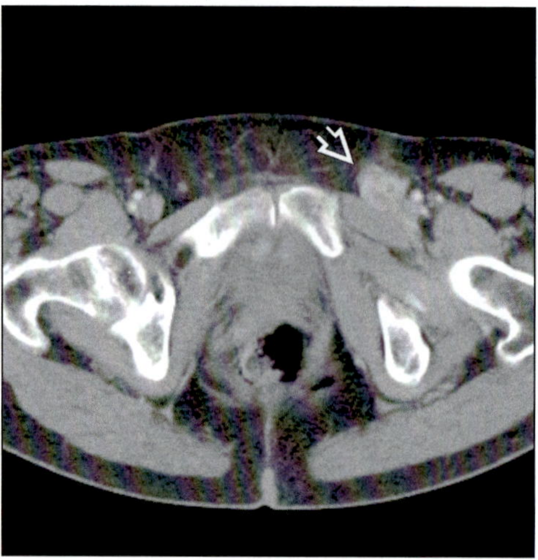

Groin Lymphadenopathy

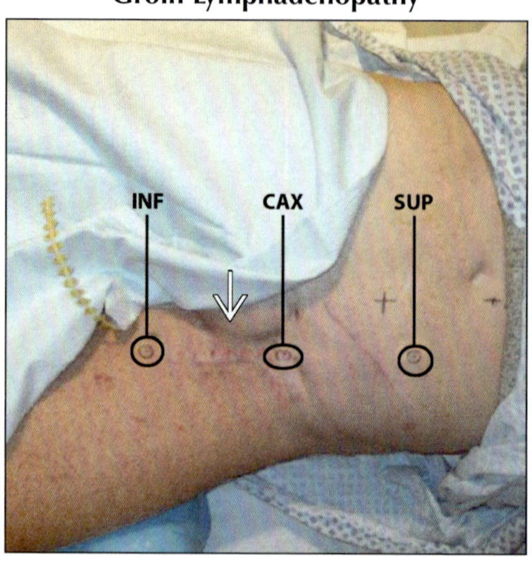

(Left) *AP DRR in the same patient shows the majority of the femoral neck (blue) as well as part of the bladder (yellow), bowel (pink), and vagina/uterus (purple) in the field covering the left inguinal preop GTV (red) and CTV (cyan).* **(Right)** *Axial NECT in the same patient with dose colorwash set to 10% of the prescription dose shows partial inclusion of OARs in the RT field.*

Groin Lymphadenopathy

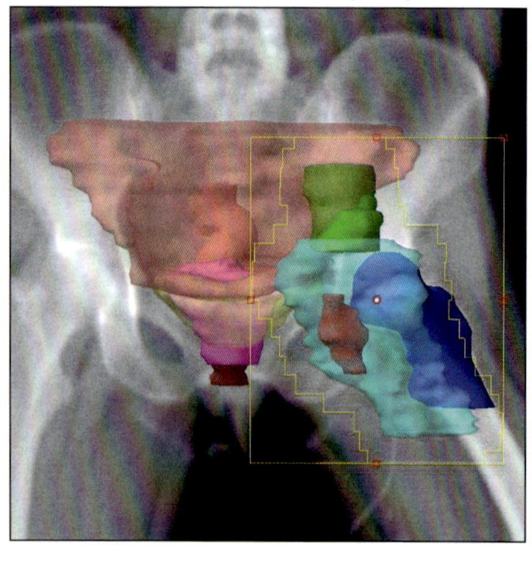

Groin Lymphadenopathy

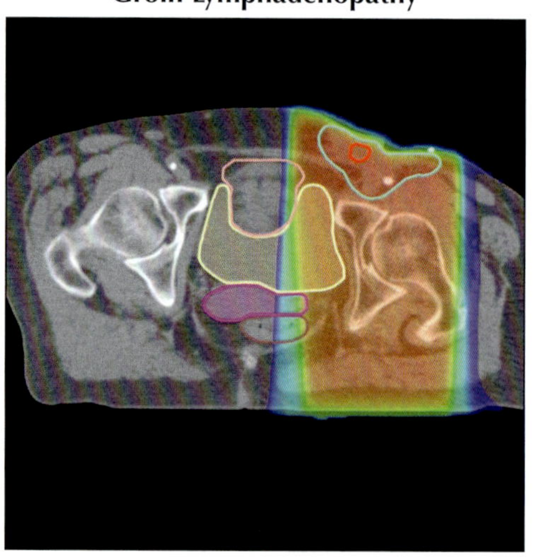

(Left) *Axial NECT with 3-field plan in the same patient shows increased OAR sparing from the high-dose region. However, note the increased volume of small bowel ➔ receiving low-dose RT.* **(Right)** *DVH in the same patient shows higher OAR doses for the AP/PA ➔ vs. the 3-field ➔ plan (PTV = cyan). The only exception is the 3F plan increases the small bowel volume receiving < 20 Gy (not shown).*

Groin Lymphadenopathy

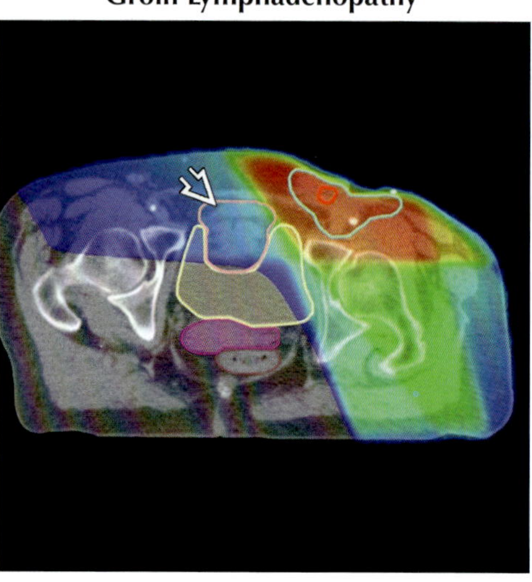

Groin Lymphadenopathy

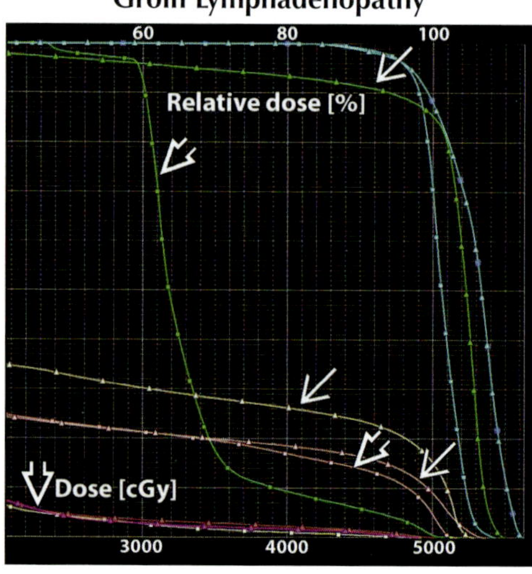

Spine Metastases

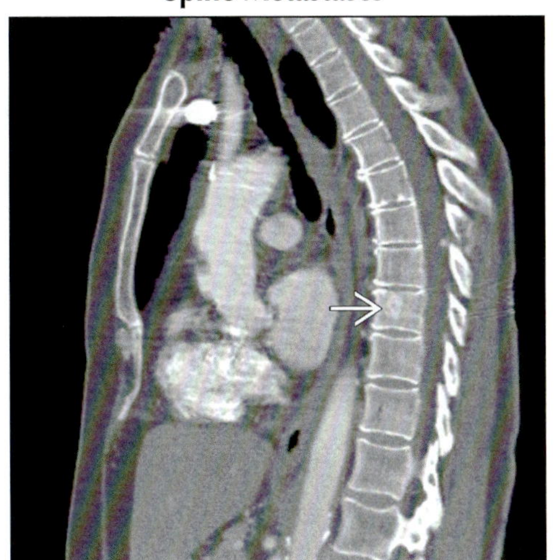

Spine Metastases

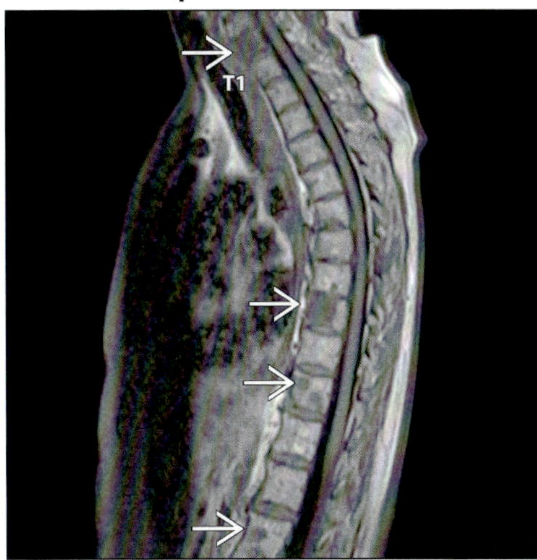

(Left) *CECT in the same patient performed due to report of new back pain following RT shows a new, poorly defined sclerotic lesion in the T9 vertebral body* ➡. ***(Right)*** *Sagittal T1WI MR of the spine in the same patient a few days later shows extensive disease denoted by T1 hypointense lesions* ➡. *MR is more sensitive than CT for evaluation of spinal metastases.*

External Iliac Recurrence

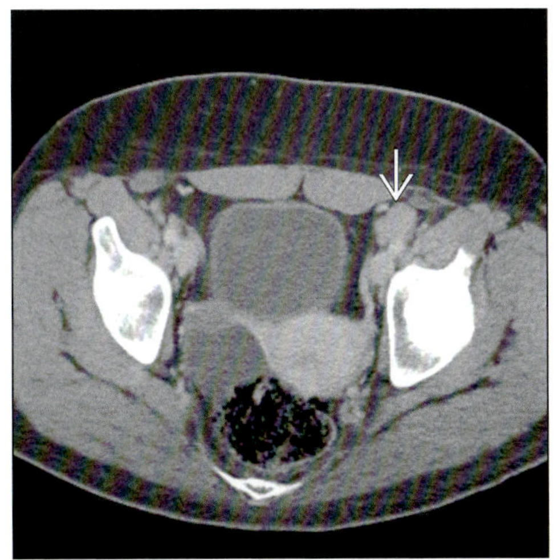

External Iliac Recurrence

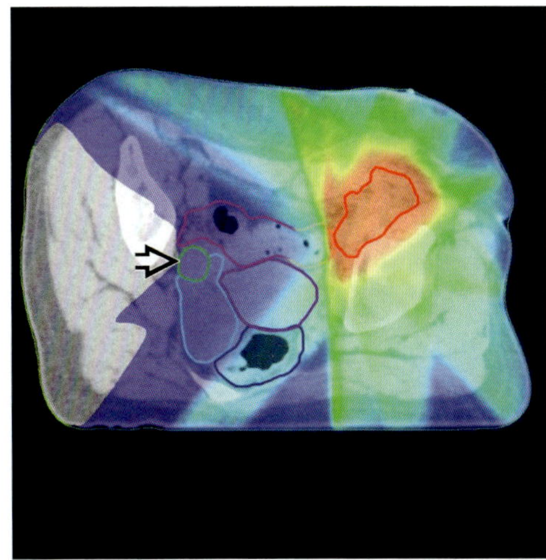

(Left) *CECT in a 33-year-old woman with history of stage IIIB left calf melanoma shows a 2.1 cm left external iliac node* ➡. *At diagnosis, 3 of 11 inguinal nodes were positive for disease.* ***(Right)*** *NECT shows IMRT dose colorwash set at a minimum of 3 Gy. The right ovary* ⇨ *received a median dose of 6 Gy (Dmin 3.2 Gy). The left ovary (not shown) Dmin was 22 Gy. Although IMRT was used to spare bowel, the ovarian dose caused cessation of menses.*

Brain Recurrence

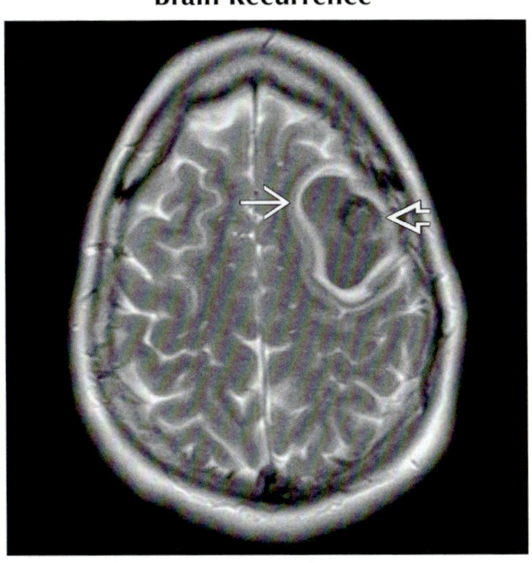

Brain Recurrence

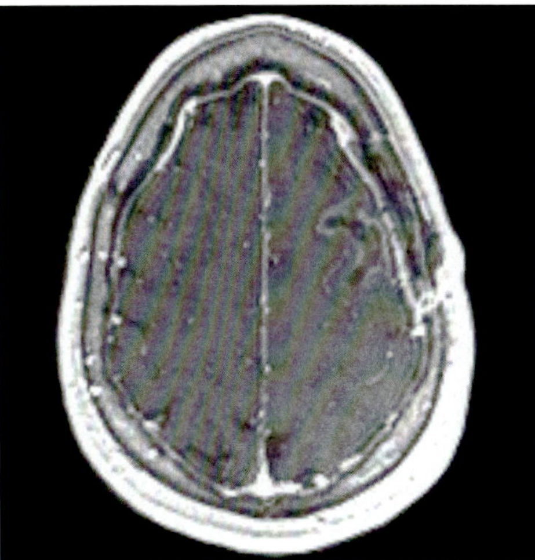

(Left) *In the same patient, seizures occurred 8 months post RT. Axial T2WI MR of the brain reveals a 4 cm hemorrhagic lesion in the left frontal lobe* ➡ *with a solid, hemorrhagic 1.3 cm lesion* ⇨. ***(Right)*** *In the same patient, axial T1WI C+ SPGR MR of the brain 1 month following resection of the mass in preparation for SRS shows marked contracture of the operative bed. 24 Gy in 1 fraction was delivered.*

Head & Neck Recurrence

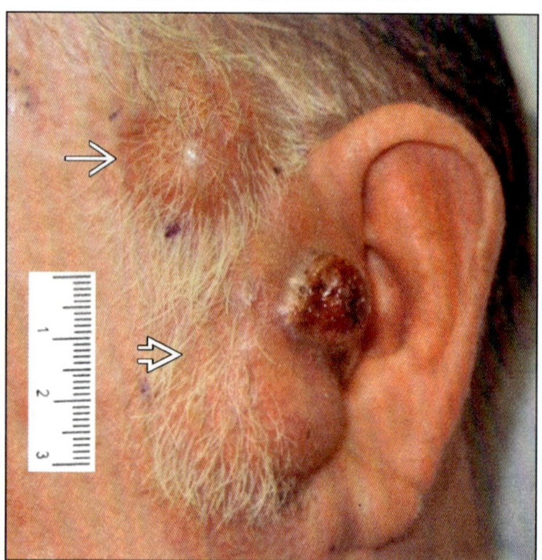

Head & Neck Recurrence

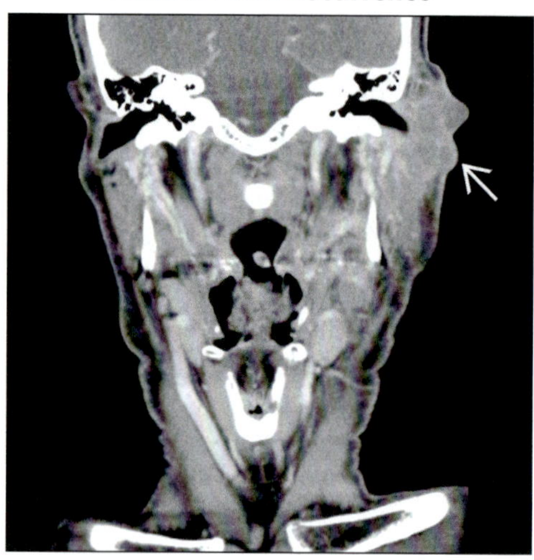

(Left) *Photo shows a 67-year-old man 8 months after resection of a left temple T3b N0 M0 melanoma. Disease recurred in the left preauricular → & parotid ⇨ regions, as well as left cervical levels II-V. Progression occurred despite treatment 2 months prior with a cancer vaccine.* ***(Right)*** *Coronal CECT in the same patient shows nodal conglomerate with peripherally enhancing, centrally low-density masses completely replacing the left parotid parenchyma →.*

Head & Neck Recurrence

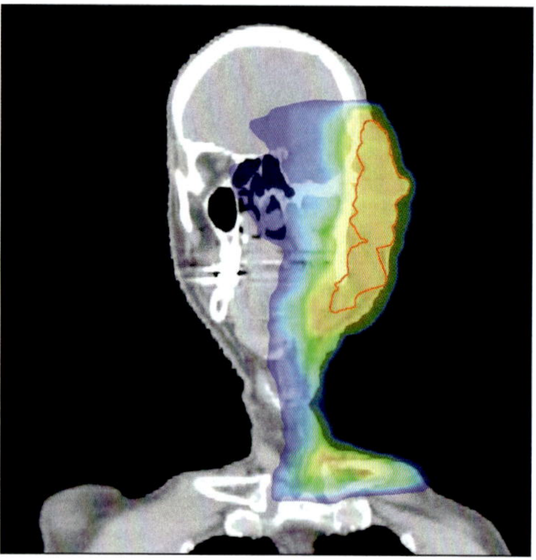

Post Treatment

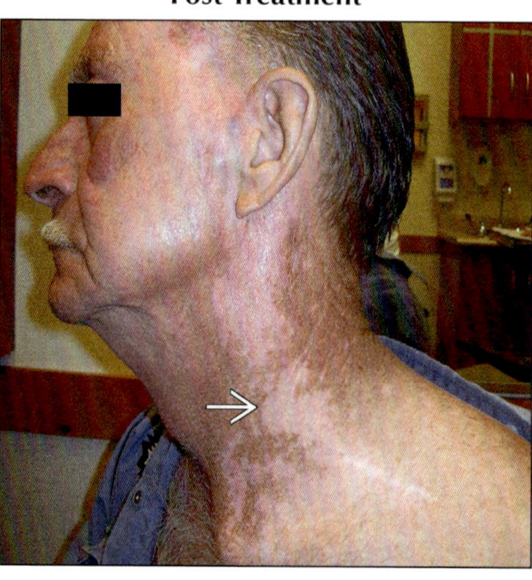

(Left) *Coronal NECT with dose colorwash in the same patient shows ≥ 10% (blue) of the prescription dose. 50 Gy in 20 fractions using a 6-field IMRT plan with 1/2 cm bolus was started 2 weeks after his 1st of 4 ipilimumab infusions, which were given every 3 weeks.* ***(Right)*** *Photo of the same patient 8 months after radiation shows a CR was achieved, with some residual hypopigmentation of the skin →.*

Post Treatment

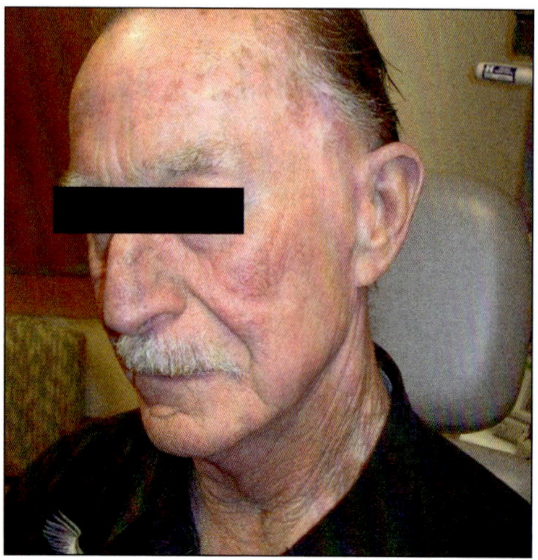

Post Treatment

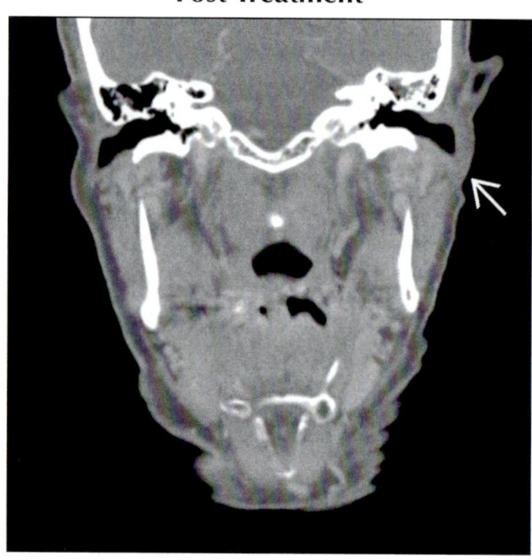

(Left) *Photo of the same patient 14 months after RT and ipilimumab shows excellent cosmetic outcome.* ***(Right)*** *Coronal CECT in the same patient shows his CR is still durable 18 months after treatment, with no evidence of lymphadenopathy in its pre-RT location →.*

Unresectable Stage III (T4b N3 M0)

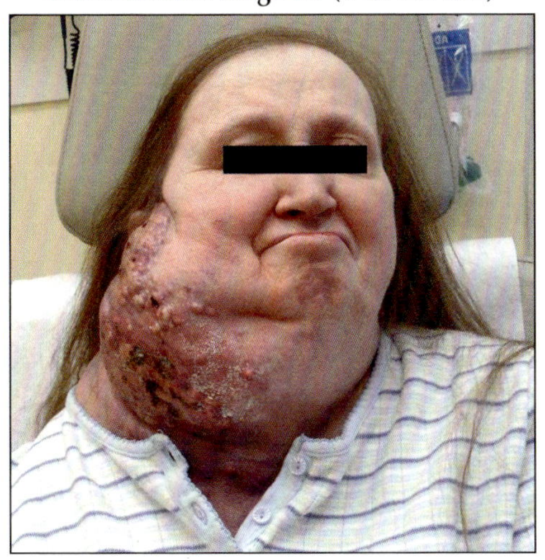

Unresectable Stage III (T4b N3 M0)

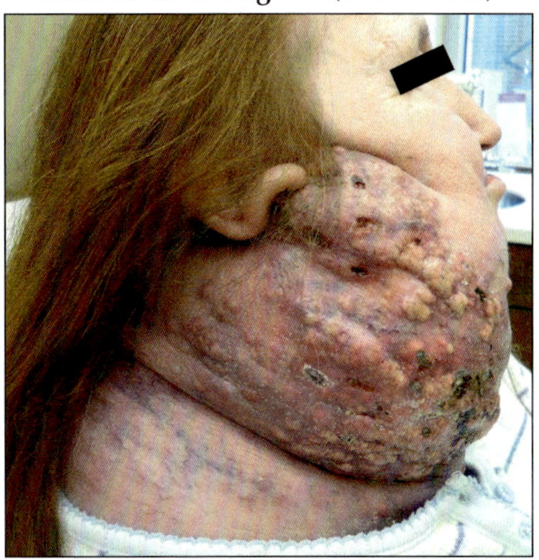

*(**Left**) Photo shows extensive lymphadenopathy in a 65-year-old woman found to have a deeply invasive (> 5 mm) scalp primary. (**Right**) Lateral photo of the same patient shows lymphadenopathy in all levels of the right neck, with tumor infiltration into the subcutaneous tissue. She was found to have the BRAF V600E mutation, but progressed despite a BRAF inhibitor. (Courtesy K. Grossmann, MD, PhD.)*

Unresectable Stage III (T4b N3 M0)

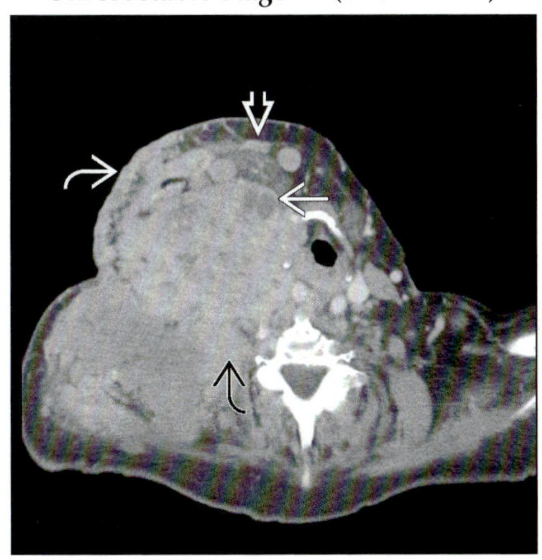

Unresectable Stage III (T4b N3 M0)

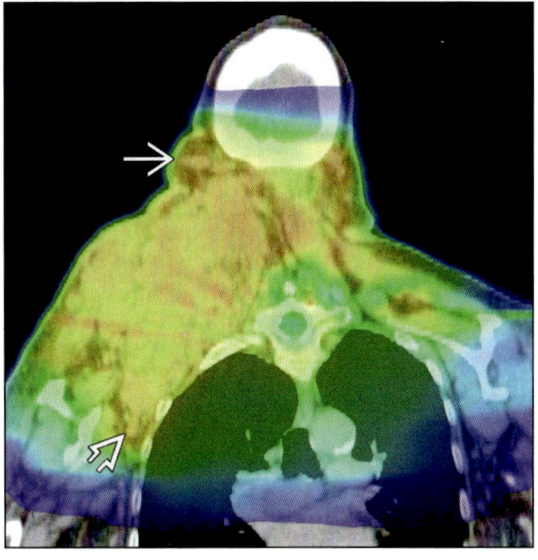

*(**Left**) Axial CECT in the same patient shows tumor infiltration into subcutaneous tissue ➔ and neck musculature (SCM, platysma ➔, paraspinal). There are areas of solid enhancement ➔ with multiple areas of nonenhancement ➔ indicative of cystic changes or necrosis. (**Right**) Coronal NECT with dose colorwash in the same patient shows tumor extension from the right suboccipital region ➔ to the infraclavicular fossa, superior mediastinum, and axilla ➔.*

Unresectable Stage III (T4b N3 M0)

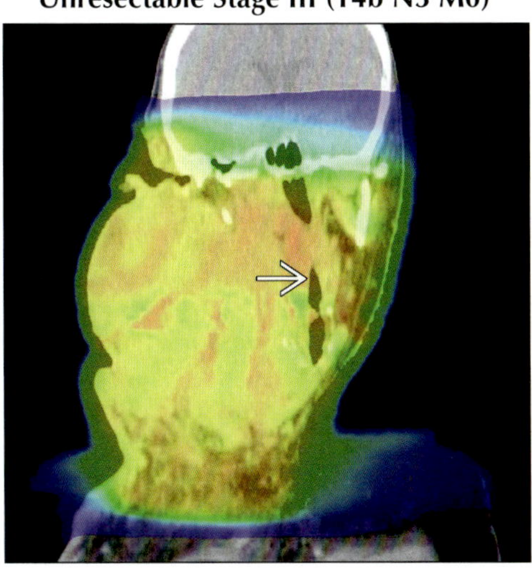

Unresectable Stage III (T4b N3 M0)

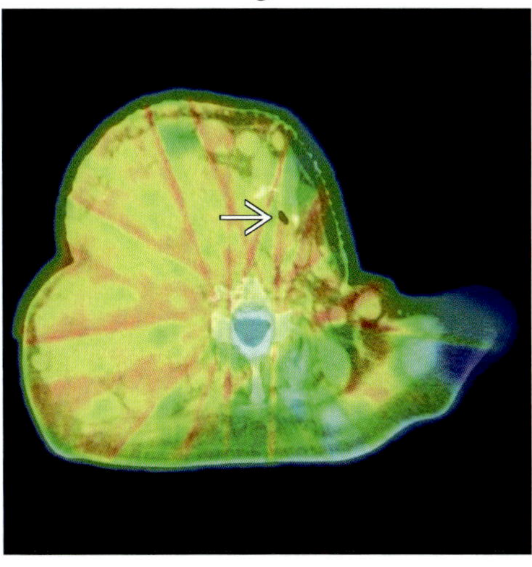

*(**Left**) Coronal NECT shows the same patient with dose colorwash set at 10% (blue) of the prescription dose of 50 Gy/20 fx. The mass is causing leftward displacement of the airway ➔. (**Right**) Axial NECT with dose colorwash in the same patient shows significant leftward displacement of the larynx, with marked narrowing of the airway ➔. Patient refused tracheostomy before proceeding with RT, and died shortly following completion of RT from airway compromise.*

(Left) *Photo shows a 69-year-old man with history of T3b N0 M0 right scalp nodular melanoma with lymphovascular invasion (LVI), with in-transit recurrence noted 9 months later ➔.* **(Right)** *Coronal NECT in same patient shows dose colorwash at 50%, covering right frontotemporal in-transit metastases with a 3 cm margin to block edge. 50 Gy in 20 fractions was delivered using a 6 MeV electron beam with 1/2 cm bolus daily.*

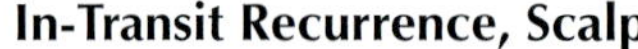

In-Transit Recurrence, Scalp

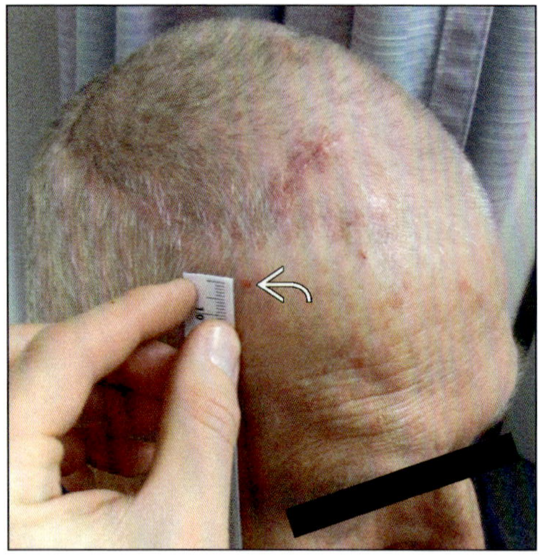

In-Transit Recurrence, Scalp

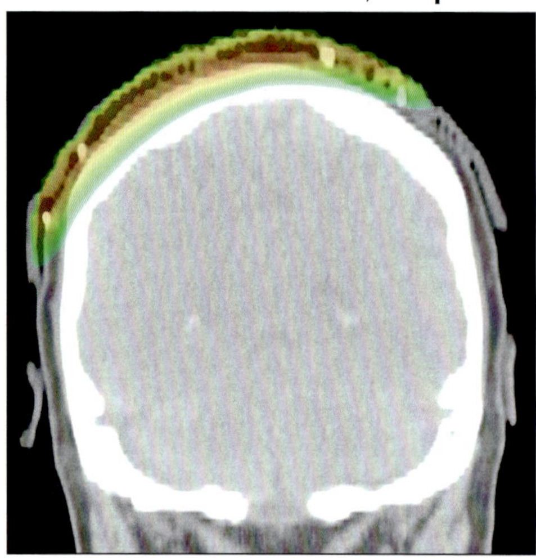

(Left) *Photo of the same patient 8 months after RT shows predominately in-field progression. Due to his request for 1 treatment, he was given a single 15 Gy fx with 1/2 cm bolus over the right temporal ➔ and vertex ➔ areas, which overlapped with his prior field.* **(Right)** *Photo of the same patient shows out-of-field recurrence on the left scalp with a field drawn around the bleeding lesion. 18 Gy in 1 fx was prescribed using 6 MeV electrons with 1/2 cm of bolus.*

In Transit Recurrence, Scalp

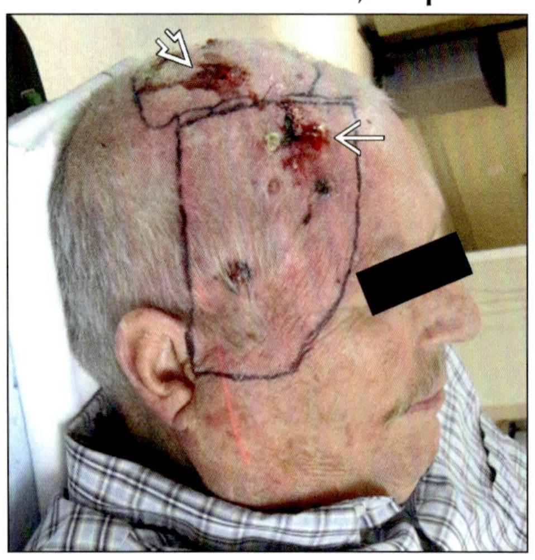

In-Transit Recurrence, Scalp

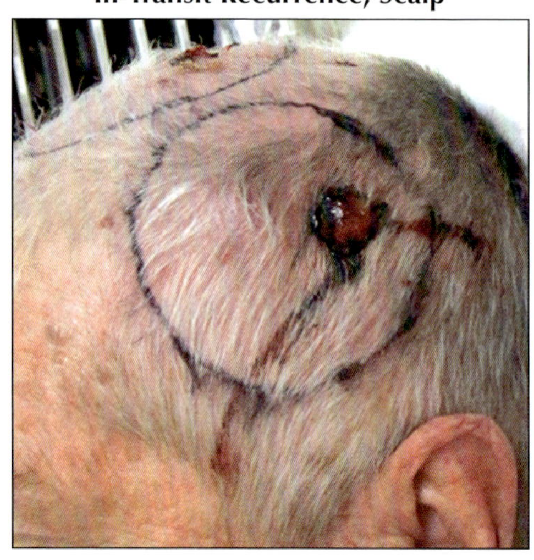

(Left) *Photo shows right lateral scalp of the same patient 3 months after single fx RT course. Note excellent regression of all treated metastases, coincident with cessation of bleeding.* **(Right)** *Photo shows left lateral scalp of the same patient 3 months after single fx RT course, again with impressive regression of the bleeding in-transit metastasis →. Alopecia is noted, which matches prior RT fields ➔.*

In-Transit Recurrence, Scalp

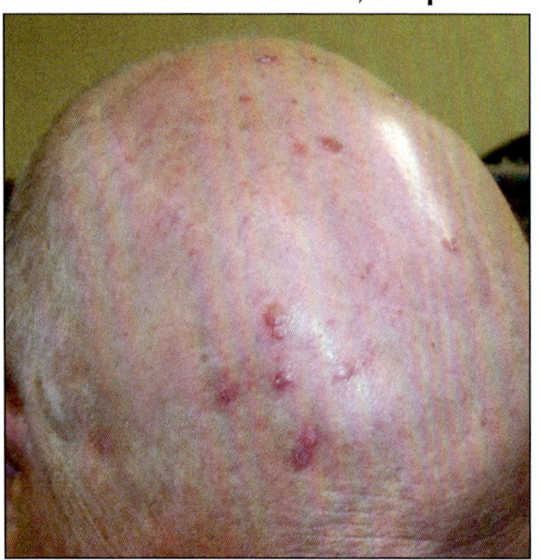

In-Transit Recurrence, Scalp

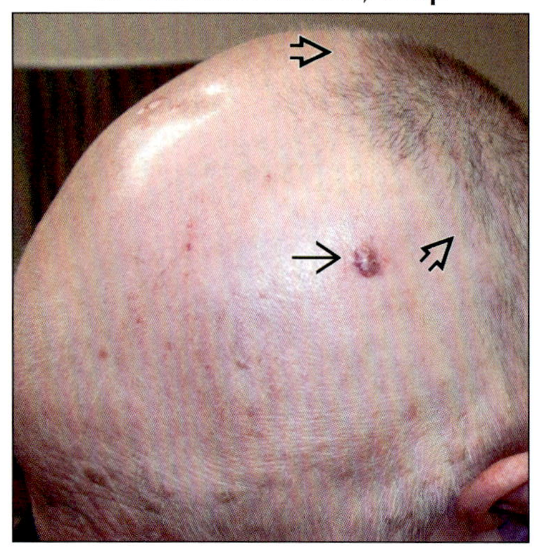

In-Transit Recurrence, Scalp

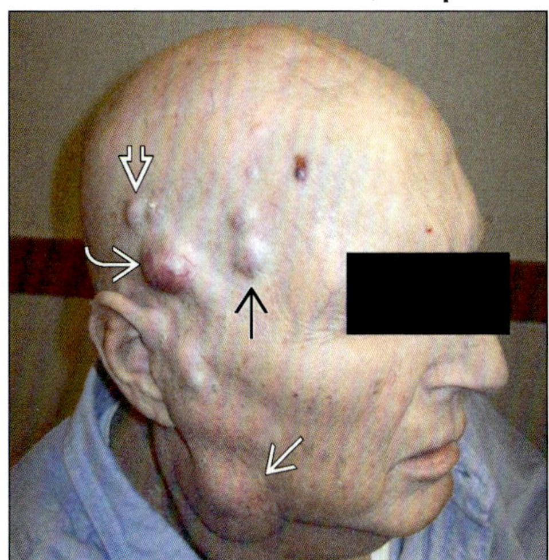

In-Transit Recurrence, Scalp

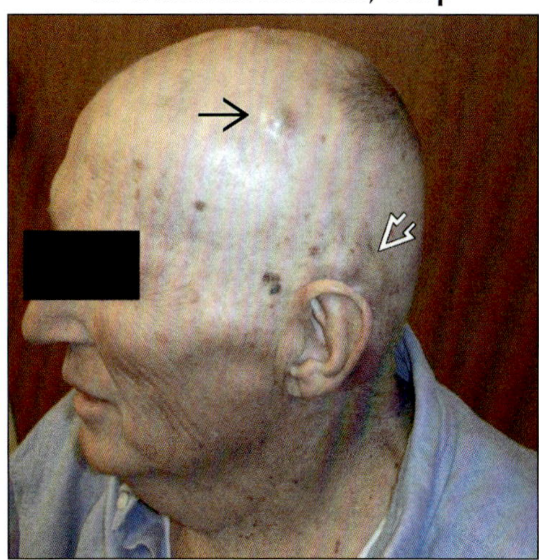

*(**Left**) Photo shows the same patient 10 months after 1st RT course. One month prior, he had completed RT to painful, progressive disease in the neck with significant reduction in his disease ➡. Progression within ⇒, at the margin ➡, and out ➡ of the prior RT fields have occurred. (**Right**) Left lateral photo shows slight progression of scalp lesion treated 10 months prior ⇒, as well as rapid growth of new out-of-field posterior auricular nodes ➡.*

In-Transit Recurrence, Upper Extremity

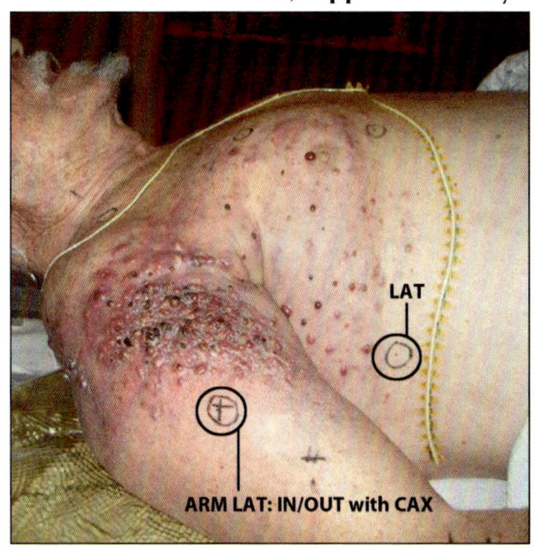

In-Transit Recurrence, Upper Extremity

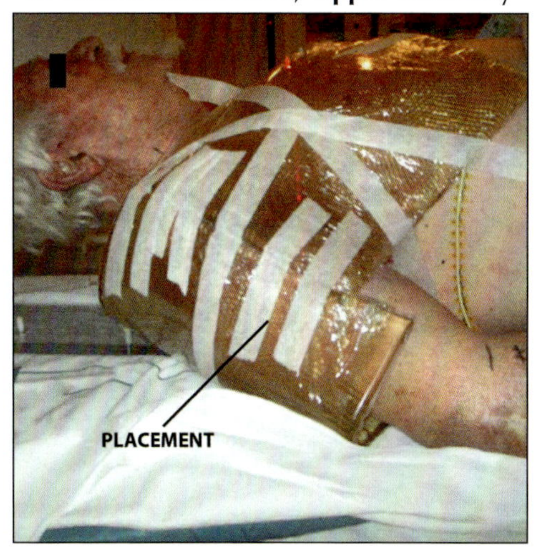

*(**Left**) Photo shows simulation for an 85-year-old man 1 year after diagnosis of a T3a N1a M0 right shoulder melanoma without LVI. Adjuvant therapy was refused, and after an in-transit recurrence he progressed despite BCG injections. Due to 10/10 pain, radiation was considered. (**Right**) At simulation, his right arm was abducted and 1 cm of bolus was wrapped front to back to cover his disease. He later refused treatment, and died shortly after starting hospice.*

In-Transit Recurrence, Lower Extremity

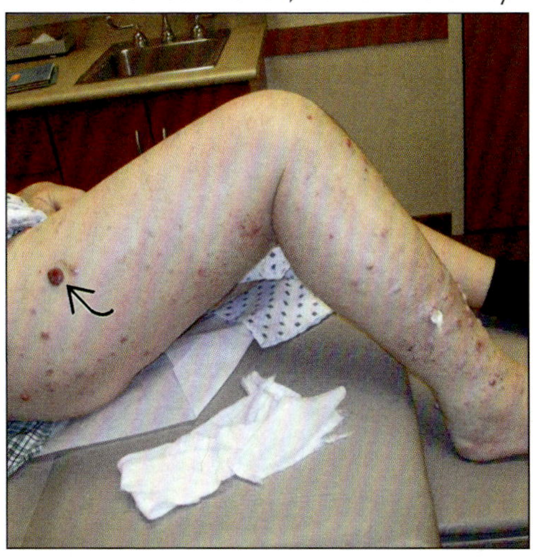

In-Transit Recurrence, Lower Extremity

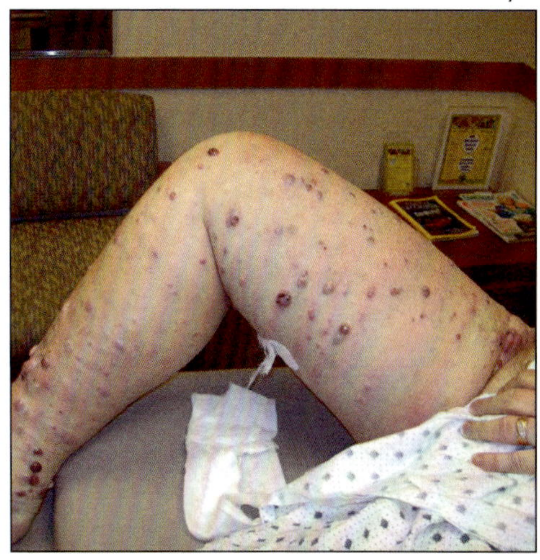

*(**Left**) Photo shows a 51-year-old man with a T3b N2a melanoma of the right great toe diagnosed 1 year previously, with 3/16 positive inguinal nodes but no LVI. 6 months later, he recurred and had a toe amputation, and an in-transit metastasis was resected at the same time. Lateral leg photo 6 months later shows progression of widespread in-transit metastases despite ipilimumab and IL-2. Note exophytic, painful thigh lesion ⇗. (**Right**) Photo shows medial view of leg.*

MELANOMA

(**Left**) Photo of the same patient shows raised, painful in-transit lesions on the medial right ankle. The field marked by black dots ➡ was treated to 28 Gy in 4 fractions, given 2x weekly, using 9 MeV electrons with 1/2 cm of bolus. (**Right**) Photo of the same patient shows painful lesions in the groin. Initially an electron field was planned with the field border shown by black dots. However, the disease was noted to be much deeper at CT simulation.

In-Transit Recurrence, Lower Extremity

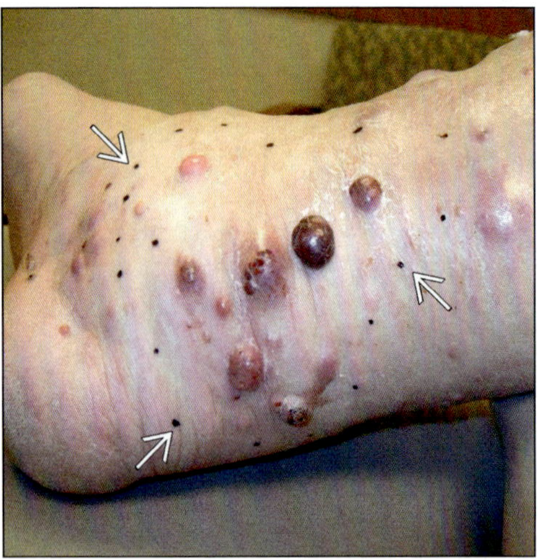

In-Transit Recurrence, Lower Extremity

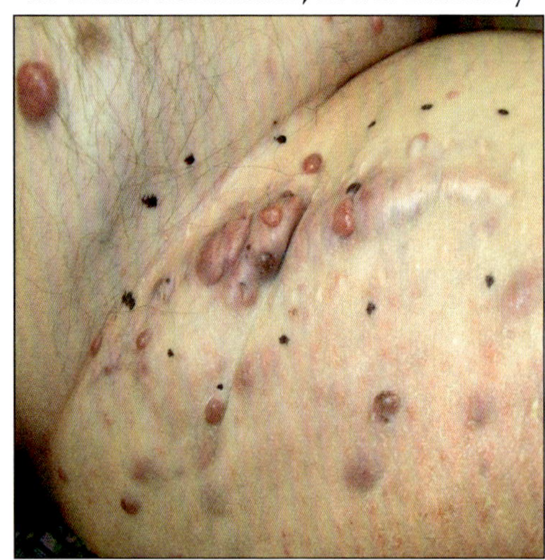

(**Left**) Axial NECT in the same patient shows groin dose colorwash from 10 MV fields arranged AP/PA, with 1 cm of bolus in place ➡. Note the large, exophytic lesion on his lateral thigh ➡, which was treated with electrons, located superficially to lymphatic vessels ➡ engorged from tumor spread. (**Right**) Coronal NECT in the same patient shows engorgement of the lymphatic vasculature ➡ from tumor, as well as nodules ➡ in the right thigh region.

In-Transit Recurrence, Lower Extremity

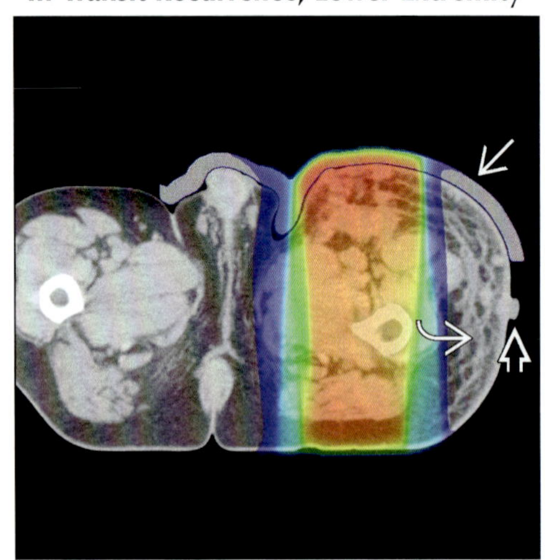

In-Transit Recurrence, Lower Extremity

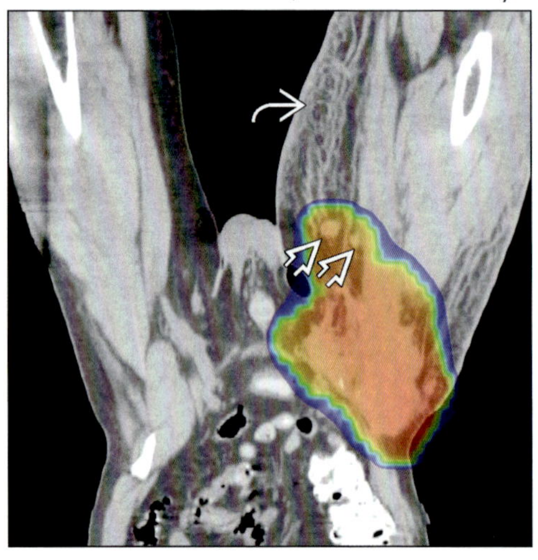

(**Left**) Photo of the same patient 3 months later shows erythema and slight regression of disease over the medial ankle ➡. However, there is an overall progression of disease, with marked asymmetry of the legs noted. (**Right**) Photo taken the same day shows slight regression of disease over his groin ➡ and lateral thigh ➡ with decreased pain and bleeding from the lesions. However, because of an overall progression of disease, hospice was recommended.

In-Transit Recurrence, Lower Extremity

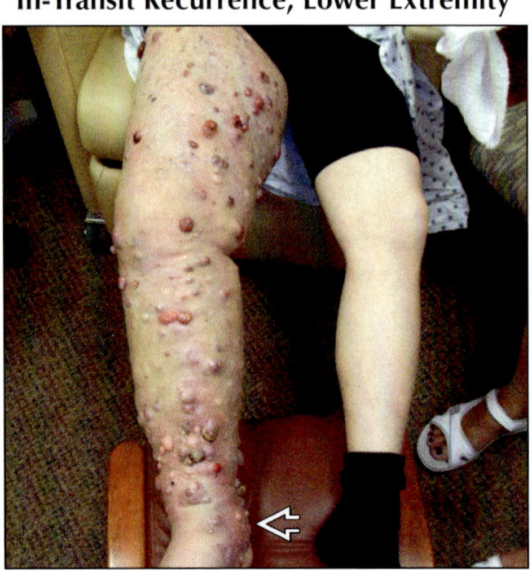

In-Transit Recurrence, Lower Extremity

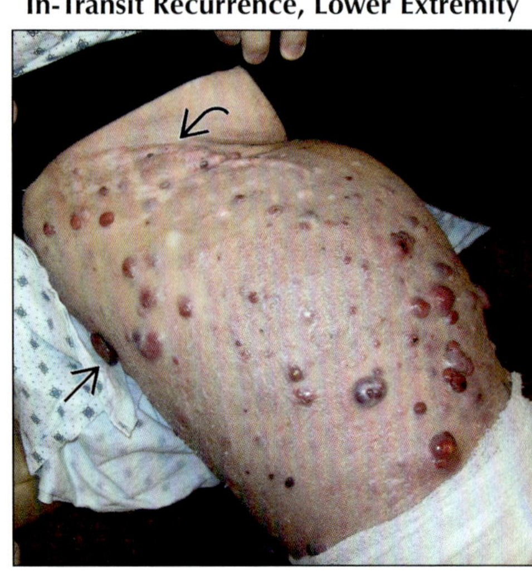

Distant Recurrence

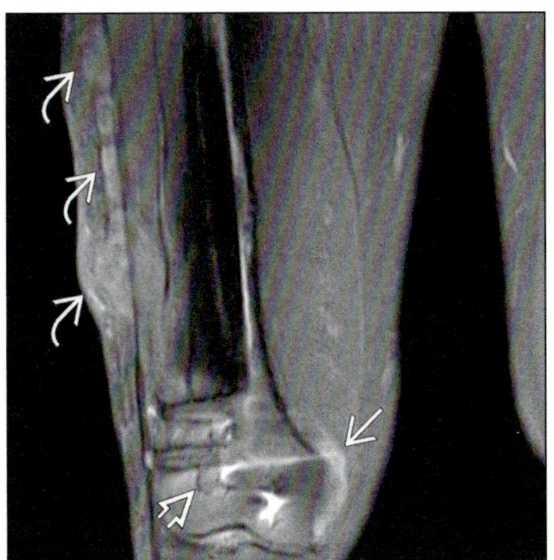

Distant Recurrence

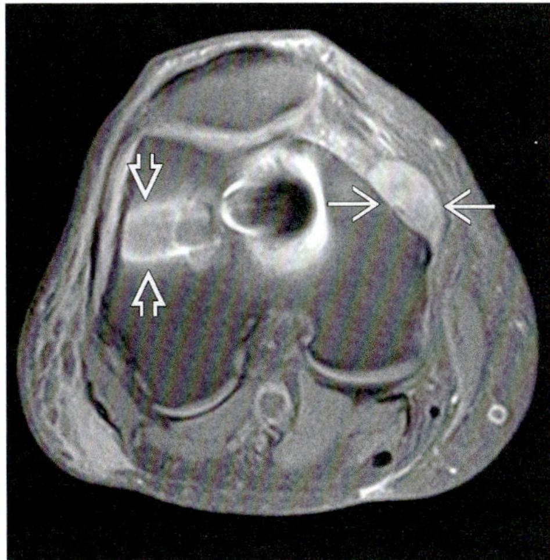

*(**Left**) Coronal T1WI C+ MR of a man with history of stage IIIB preauricular melanoma shows a multilobulated lateral thigh mass infiltrating the subcutaneous fat and dermis ➔. A lytic lesion ➔ is in the distal lateral femoral metaphysis. A mass is noted in the distal vastus medialis ➔. (**Right**) Axial T1WI C+ MR in the same patient shows the femoral ➔ and vastus medialis ➔ metastases. One month after 37.5 Gy/15 fx, his pain dropped from 10 to 1/10 and he no longer needed narcotics.*

Distant Recurrence

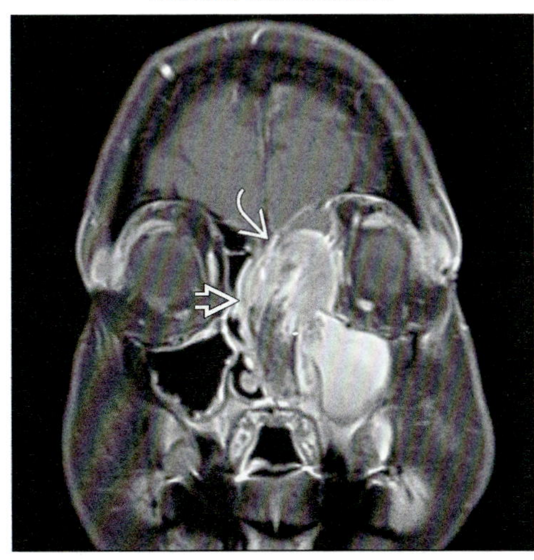

Distant Recurrence

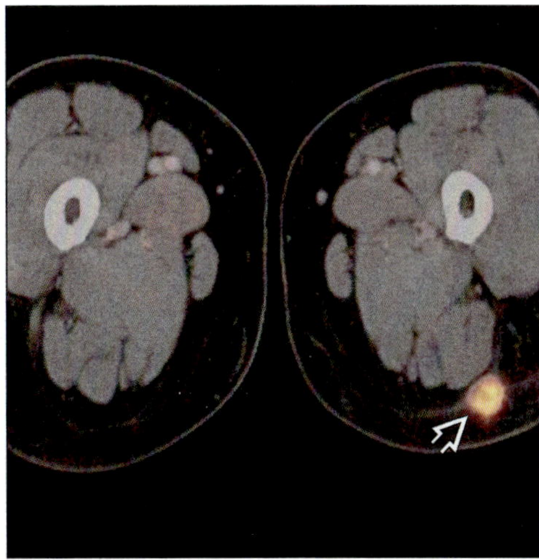

*(**Left**) Because of headaches and left-sided proptosis, MR was obtained in this 62-year-old woman who had a stage IIA right calf melanoma resected 12 years previously. Coronal T1WI C+ SPGR MR shows a hyperintense mass displacing the nasal septum to the right ➔. The lesion eroded the anterior skull base and extended into the anterior cranial fossa ➔. (**Right**) Axial PET/CT in the same patient shows a subcutaneous metastasis ➔ superficial to the hamstring.*

Distant Recurrence

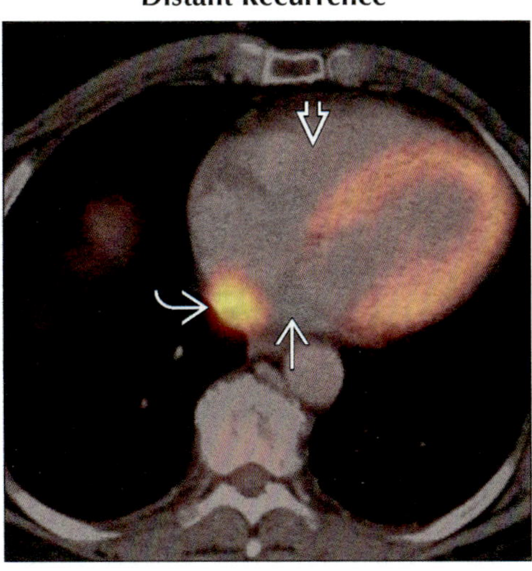

Distant Recurrence

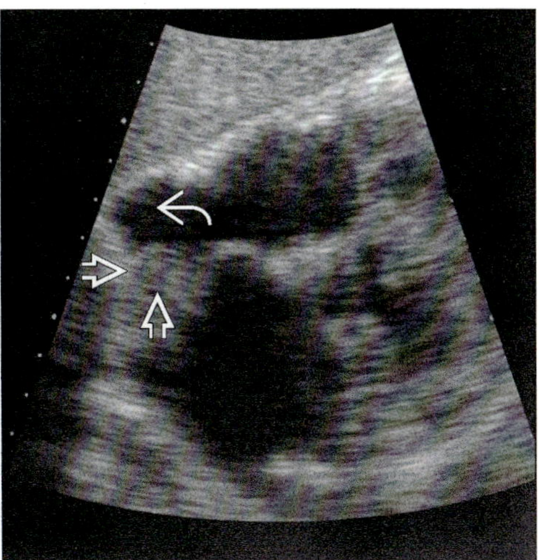

*(**Left**) Axial PET/CT in the same patient shows a 25 mm mass ➔ along the posterior inferior wall of the right atrium. (Right ventricle ➔; left atrium ➔.) (**Right**) Transthoracic echocardiogram in the same patient confirms the mass ➔ in the right atrium ➔. A Holter monitor worn for the next 2 days revealed no significant abnormalities. Following 4 cycles of biochemotherapy, her lesions significantly decreased in size and metabolic activity.*

MELANOMA

(**Left**) *Photo shows a subconjunctival metastasis in a 38-year-old man with a history of stage IIIA, T2b N1a M0, left anterior chest melanoma resected 9 years previously. Following his initial diagnosis, he received 1 year of adjuvant interferon-α. (Courtesy J. Carver, MD.)* (**Right**) *Oblique view of the same patient shows the subconjunctival metastasis. Following a subtotal resection, he receives vemurafenib and remains disease free 1 year later. (Courtesy J. Carver, MD.)*

Distant Recurrence

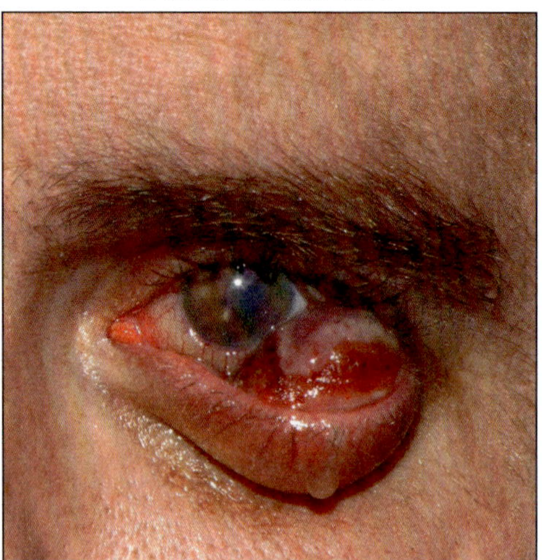

Distant Recurrence

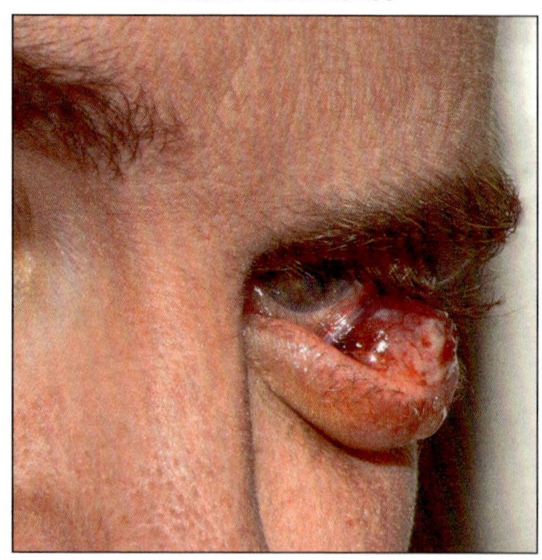

(**Left**) *Axial T1WI C+ FS BLADE MR in a 51-year-old man with history of stage IIIB right forearm melanoma shows an ependymal-based lesion ➔ extending into the left lateral ventricle. He received SRS to this and 3 other lesions.* (**Right**) *Four weeks later, the same patient developed acute right extremity weakness. Axial NECT shows development of intraparenchymal ➔ and intraventricular ➔ hemorrhage. Despite EVD placement and intubation, he died 2 weeks later.*

Distant Recurrence

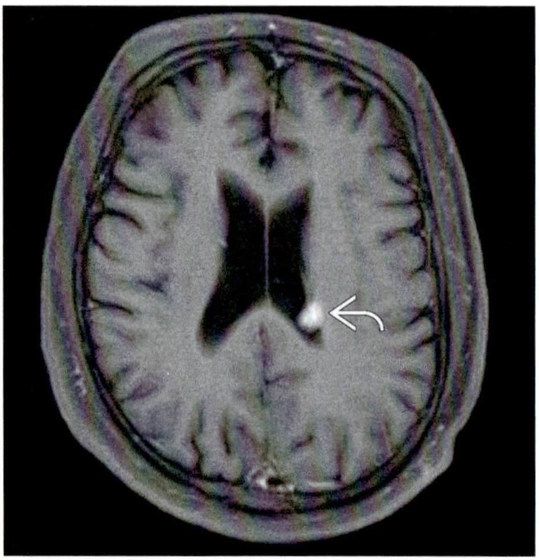

Distant Recurrence

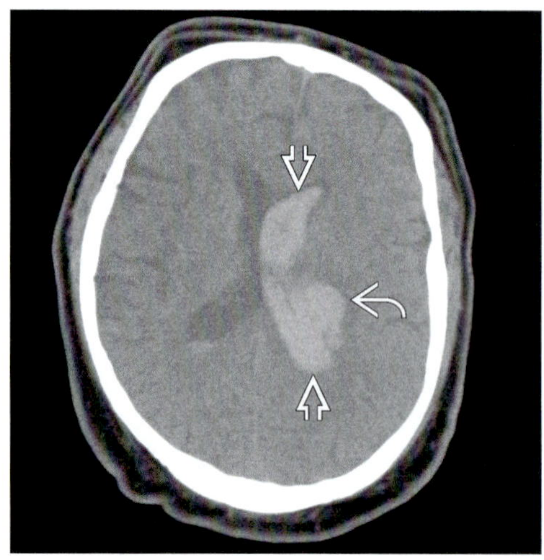

(**Left**) *Axial T1WI C+ MR of the brain in a 33-year-old man who developed diplopia and ataxia shows enhancing leptomeningeal disease around the brainstem ➔ and cerebellum ➔.* (**Right**) *The same patient had saddle anesthesia, back pain, and urinary incontinence. Sagittal T1WI C + FS spine MR shows diffuse leptomeningeal enhancement of the lumbar spinal cord ➔ and lumbosacral nerve roots ➔. He died 3 weeks after 30 Gy/10 fx to the brain & spine.*

Distant Recurrence

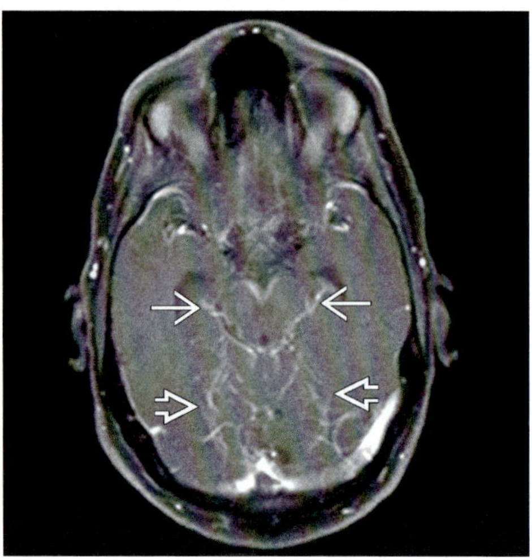

Distant Recurrence

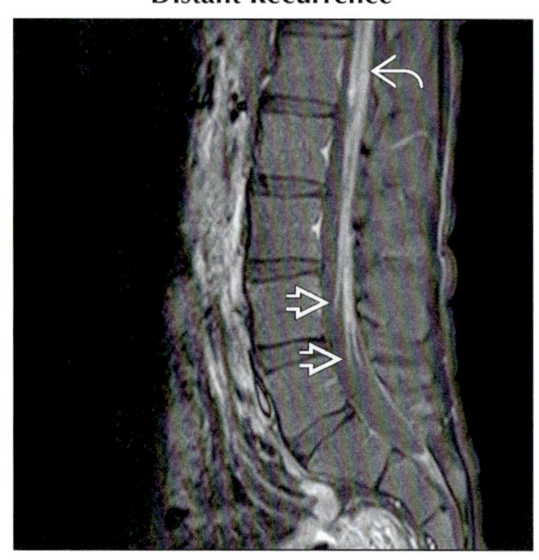

Distant Lung Recurrence

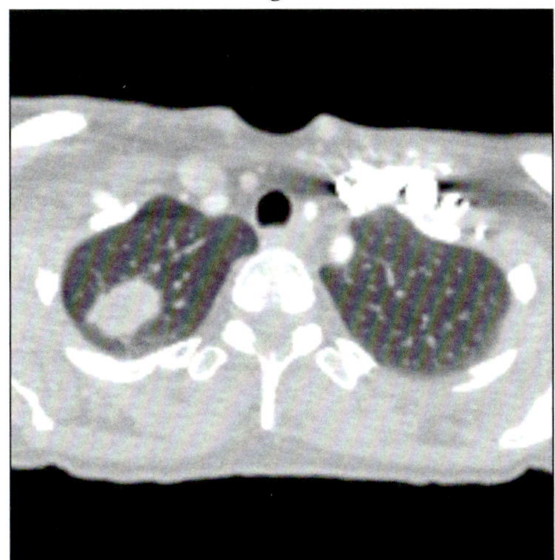

Distant Lung Recurrence

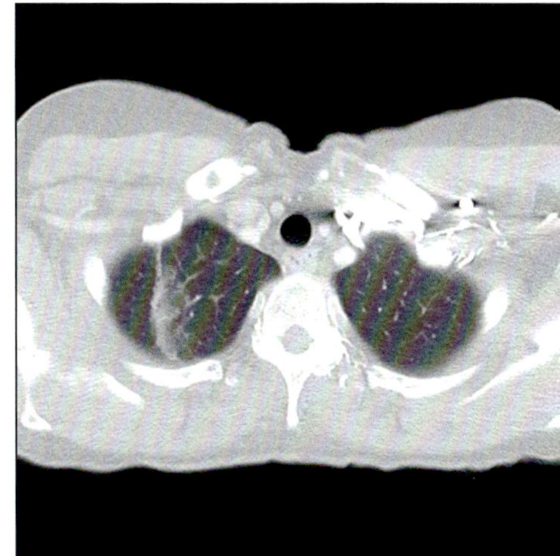

(Left) *For this 48-year-old woman with a history of stage IIIC melanoma of the forearm, surveillance axial CECT revealed a 2.7 cm RUL nodule. The metastasis was treated with SBRT to 50 Gy/5 fractions given QOD.* ***(Right)*** *Axial CECT in the same patient 1 year later shows a non-rounded opacity consistent with parenchymal scarring. Of note, 4 months post RT, subcutaneous nodules and abdominal lymphadenopathy developed, with a CR achieved from a BRAF inhibitor.*

Distant Nodal Recurrence

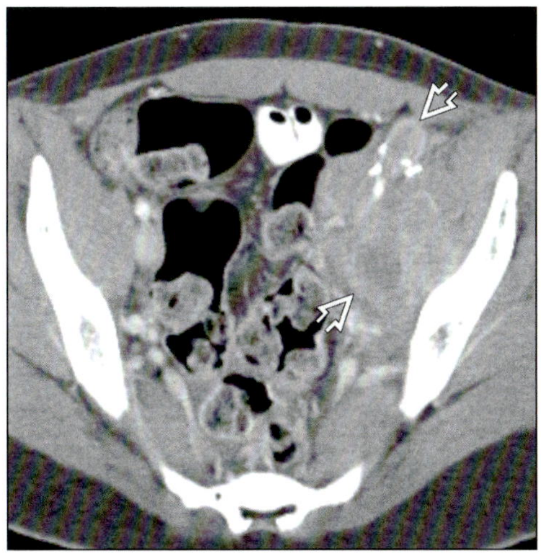

Distant Nodal Recurrence

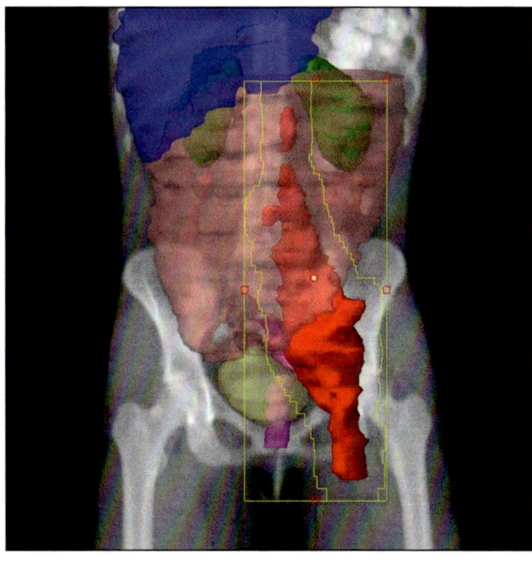

(Left) *Axial CECT shows progressive lymphadenopathy ➲ in a 24-year-old female with T2 N2a M0 melanoma of the left 4th toe diagnosed 7 years ago. This occurred despite repeat nodal dissections, limb perfusion, temozolomide, IL-2, tumor-infiltrating lymphocyte harvest & infusion, & ipilimumab. Disease extended from the paraaortic to inguinal regions, & caused 10/10 pain.* ***(Right)*** *AP DRR in same patient shows RT field, with GTV in red (bowel = pink, vagina = purple).*

Distant Nodal Recurrence

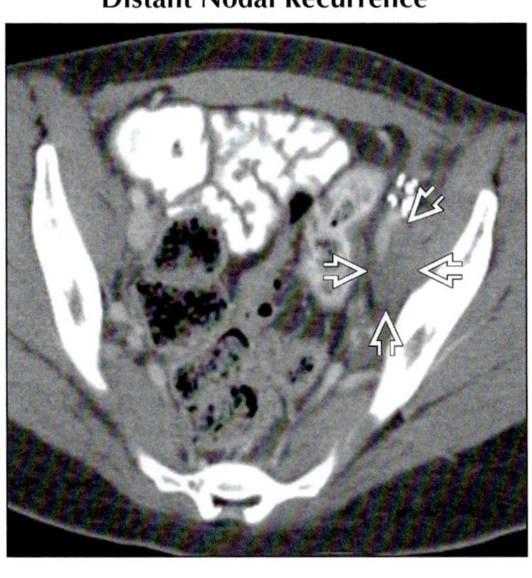

Distant Nodal Recurrence

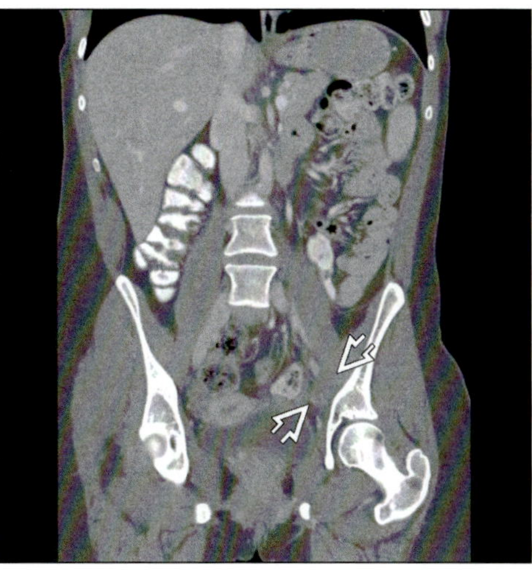

(Left) *The same patient received 37.5 Gy/15 fx concurrent with cisplatin 40 mg/m². During CRT grade 3 nausea and vomiting lasted 1 day but was then well controlled medically. Her pain completely resolved by the end of CRT, and she stopped all narcotics. Next she had biochemotherapy. Axial CECT 8 months post CRT shows reduction of her disease to a single, stable 3 cm external iliac node ➲.* ***(Right)*** *Coronal CECT in the same patient shows minimal residual disease ➲.*

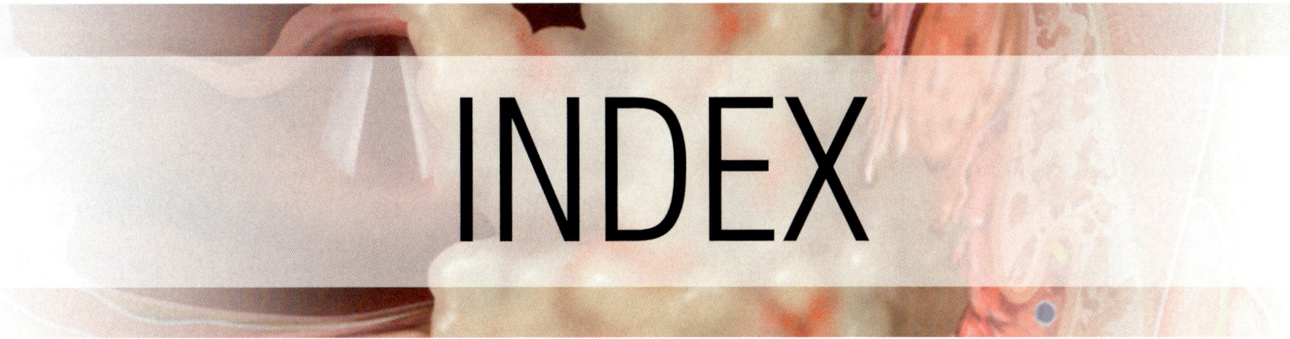

INDEX

Locators refer to Chapter:page number

A

INDEX

INDEX

C

INDEX

INDEX

D

INDEX

INDEX

F

G

INDEX

H

I

J

K

INDEX

L

INDEX

N

INDEX

INDEX

INDEX

P

INDEX

INDEX

R

S

INDEX

T

INDEX

INDEX